CORONARY ARTERY DISEASE AND ITS CONSEQUENCES

Collected Reprints
(1971-2017)

By

WILLIAM C. ROBERTS, MD

and

COLLEAGUES

ISBN: 979-8-88862-143-1
Printed in the United States of America on acid-free paper.

Table of Contents

134.*   **The pathology of acute myocardial infarction** 1
Roberts WC. *Hosp Pract.* 1971;6(12):88-104.

137.   **Coronary arteries in fatal acute myocardial infarction** 13
Roberts WC. *Circulation.* 1972;45(1):215-230.

138.   **Relationship between coronary thrombosis and myocardial infarction** 29
Roberts WC. *Mod Concepts Cardiovasc Dis.* 1972;41(2):7-10.

143.   **The frequency and significance of coronary arterial thrombi and other observations in fatal acute myocardial infarction: a study of 107 necropsy patients** 33
Roberts WC, Buja LM. *Am J Med.* 1972;52(4):425-443.

150.   **Left ventricular papillary muscles. Description of the normal and a survey of conditions causing them to be abnormal** 52
Roberts WC, Cohen LS. *Circulation.* 1972;46(1):138-154.

166.   **Left-to-right shunt at atrial level after rupture of papillary muscle from acute myocardial infarction** 69
Nagel MR, Ronan JA Jr, Roberts WC. *Am Heart J.* 1973;86(1):112-116.

177.   **Does thrombosis play a major role in the development of symptom-producing atherosclerotic plaques?** 74
Roberts WC. *Circulation.* 1973;48(6):1161-1166.

179.   **Coronary thrombosis and fatal myocardial ischemia** 80
Roberts WC. *Circulation.* 1974;49(1):1-3.

183.   **Steroid therapy during acute myocardial infarction. A cause of delayed healing and of ventricular aneurysm** 83
Bulkley BH, Roberts WC. *Am J Med.* 1974;56(2):244-250.

201.   **Coronary thrombosis in myocardial infarction. Report of a workshop on the role of coronary thrombosis in the pathogenesis of acute myocardial infarction** 90
Chandler AB, Chapman I, Erhardt LR, Roberts WC, Schwartz C, Sinapius D, Spain DM, Sherry S, Ness PM, Simon TL. *Am J Cardiol.* 1974;34(7):823-833.

226.   **Myocardial embolus to coronary artery: result of rupture of papillary muscle during acute myocardial infarction** 101
Hammer WJ, Ferrans VJ, Roberts WC. *Chest.* 1975;68(6):843-844.

234.   **Acute myocardial infarction and angiographically normal coronary arteries. An unproven combination** 103
Arnett EN, Roberts WC. *Circulation.* 1976;53(3):395-400.

236.   **Atherosclerotic narrowing of the left main coronary artery. A necropsy analysis of 152 patients with fatal coronary heart disease and varying degrees of left main narrowing** 109
Bulkley BH, Roberts WC. *Circulation.* 1976;53(5):823-828.

244. **Angiographically normal arteries after healing of acute myocardial infarction**.. 115
Arnett EN, Roberts WC. *Practical Cardiology.* 1976;2:13-19.

258. **Site of myocardial infarction. A determinant of the cardiovascular changes induced in the cat by coronary occlusion** 122
Corr PB, Pearle DL, Hinton JR, Roberts WC, Gillis RA. *Circ Res.* 1976;39(6):840-847.

260. **Coronary heart disease: a review of abnormalities observed in the coronary arteries** 130
Roberts WC. *Cardiovasc Med.* 1977;2:29-49.

282. **The coronary arteries in ischemic heart disease: facts and fancies** 145
Roberts WC. *Triangle.* 1977;16(2):77-90.

311. **Fatal coronary heart disease: is the coronary atherosclerosis focal or diffuse?** 159
Roberts WC. *Med Times.* 1978;106(6):30-32.

316. **Coronary embolism: a review of causes, consequences, and diagnostic considerations** 162
Roberts WC. *Cardiovasc Med.* 1978;3:699-710.

326. **Location of myocardial infarcts: a confusion of terms and definitions** 170
Roberts WC, Gardin JM. *Am J Cardiol.* 1978;42(5):868-872.

328. **Right ventricular infarction complicating left ventricular infarction secondary to coronary heart disease. Frequency, location, associated findings and significance from analysis of 236 necropsy patients with acute or healed myocardial infarction** 175
Isner JM, Roberts WC. *Am J Cardiol.* 1978;42(6):885-894.

329. **Location of acute myocardial infarcts** 185
Gardin JM, Roberts WC. *Practical Cardiol.* 1979;5:25-32.

344. **Quantitation of coronary arterial narrowing at necropsy in sudden coronary death: analysis of 31 patients and comparison with 25 control subjects** 192
Roberts WC, Jones AA. *Am J Cardiol.* 1979;44(1):39-45.

348. **Coronary artery narrowing in coronary heart disease: comparison of cineangiographic and necropsy findings** 199
Arnett EN, Isner JM, Redwood DR, Kent KM, Baker WP, Ackerstein H, Roberts WC. *Ann Intern Med.* 1979;91(3):350-356.

350. **Thrombocytosis, coronary thrombosis and acute myocardial infarction** 206
Virmani R, Popovsky MA, Roberts WC. *Am J Med.* 1979;67(3):498-506.

354. **Quantification of coronary arterial narrowing in clinically-isolated unstable angina pectoris. An analysis of 22 necropsy patients** 215
Roberts WC, Virmani R. *Am J Med.* 1979;67(5):792-799.

361. **Structure-function correlations in cardiovascular and pulmonary diseases (CPC). Disappearance of symptomatic coronary heart disease and death from a noncardiac condition** 223
Virmani R, Roberts WC. *Chest.* 1980;77(1):91-93.

363. **Clinical pathologic conference. Left and right ventricular myocardial infarction in idiopathic dilated cardiomyopathy** 226
Isner JM, Virmani R, Itscoitz SB, Roberts WC. *Am Heart J.* 1980;99(2):235-242.

367. **Quantification of coronary arterial narrowing at necropsy in acute transmural myocardial infarction. Analysis and comparison of findings in 27 patients and 22 controls** 234
Roberts WC, Jones AA. *Circulation.* 1980;61(4):786-790.

370. **Left ventricular aneurysm, intraaneurysmal thrombus and systemic embolus in coronary heart disease** 239
Cabin HS, Roberts WC. *Chest.* 1980;77(5):586-590.

375. **Sudden death while running in conditioned runners aged 40 years or over** 244
Waller BF, Roberts WC. *Am J Cardiol.* 1980;45(6):1292-1300.

376. **Quantification of coronary arterial narrowing and of left ventricular myocardial scarring in healed myocardial infarction with chronic, eventually fatal, congestive cardiac failure** 253
Virmani R, Roberts WC. *Am J Med.* 1980;68(6):831-838.

389. **Status of the coronary arteries at necropsy in diabetes mellitus with onset after age 30 years. Analysis of 229 diabetic patients with and without clinical evidence of coronary heart disease and comparison to 183 control subjects** 261
Waller BF, Palumbo PJ, Lie JT, Roberts WC. *Am J Med.* 1980;69(4):498-506.

396. **True left ventricular aneurysm and healed myocardial infarction. Clinical and necropsy observations including quantification of degrees of coronary arterial narrowing** 270
Cabin HS, Roberts WC. *Am J Cardiol.* 1980;46(5):754-763.

398. **Cross-sectional area of the proximal portions of the three major epicardial coronary arteries in 98 necropsy patients with different coronary events. Relationship to heart weight, age and sex** 280
Roberts CS, Roberts WC. *Circulation.* 1980;62(5):953-959.

400. **Amount of narrowing by atherosclerotic plaque in 44 nonbypassed and 52 bypassed major epicardial coronary arteries in 32 necropsy patients who died within 1 month of aortocoronary bypass grafting** 287
Waller BF, Roberts WC. *Am J Cardiol.* 1980;46(6):956-962.

405. **Quantification of amounts of coronary arterial narrowing in patients with types II and IV hyperlipoproteinemia and in those with known normal lipoprotein patterns** 294
Cabin HS, Roberts WC. *Am Heart J.* 1981;101(1):52-58.

415. **Running to death** 301
Waller BF, Csere RS, Baker WP, Roberts WC. *Chest.* 1981;79(3):346-349.

417. **Significance of coronary arterial thrombus in transmural acute myocardial infarction. A study of 54 necropsy patients** 305
Brosius FC III, Roberts WC. *Circulation.* 1981;63(4):810-816.

419.   **Coronary arterial disease in systemic lupus erythematosus: quantification of degrees of narrowing in 22 necropsy patients (21 women) aged 16 to 37 years** 312
Haider YS, Roberts WC. *Am J Med.* 1981;70(4):775-781.

420.   **Transmural myocardial infarction in hypertrophic cardiomyopathy: a cause of conversion from left ventricular asymmetry to symmetry and from normal-sized to dilated left ventricular cavity** 319
Waller BF, Maron BJ, Epstein SE, Roberts WC. *Chest.* 1981;79(4):461-465.

421.   **Non-fatal healed transmural myocardial infarction and fatal non-cardiac disease. Qualification and quantification of coronary arterial narrowing and of left ventricular scarring in 18 necropsy patients** 324
Virmani R, Roberts WC. *Br Heart J.* 1981;45(4):434-441.

423.   **Accuracy of angiographic determination of left main coronary arterial narrowing. Angiographic-histologic correlative analysis in 28 patients** 332
Isner JM, Kishel J, Kent KM, Ronan JA Jr, Ross AM, Roberts WC. *Circulation.* 1981;63(5):1056-1064.

433.   **Fatal cardiac arrest during cardiac catheterization for angina pectoris: analysis of 10 necropsy patients** 341
Cabin HS, Roberts WC. *Am J Cardiol.* 1981;48(1):1-8.

434.   **Survival for 20 years or longer after transmural acute myocardial infarction: analysis of eight well-documented necropsy patients** 349
McManus BM, Roberts WC. *Am Heart J.* 1981;102(2):176-182.

442.   **Comparison of degree and extent of coronary narrowing by atherosclerotic plaque in anterior and posterior transmural acute myocardial infarction** 356
Brosius FC III, Roberts WC. *Circulation.* 1981;64(4):715-722.

443.   **Type III hyperlipoproteinemia: Quantification, distribution, and nature of atherosclerotic coronary arterial narrowing in five necropsy patients** 364
Cabin HS, Schwartz DE, Virmani R, Brewer HB Jr, Roberts WC. *Am Heart J.* 1981;102(5):830-835.

445.   **Sudden death while playing professional football** 370
Roberts WC, Maron BJ. *Am Heart J.* 1981;102(6 Pt 1):1062-1063.

473.   **Coronary narrowing in types II, III, and IV hyperlipoproteinemia and in known normal lipoprotein patterns** 373
Cabin HS, Roberts WC. *Cardiovasc Rev Rep.* 1982;3:699-708.

480.   **Comparison of amount of extent of coronary narrowing by atherosclerotic plaque and of myocardial scarring at necropsy in anterior and posterior healed transmural myocardial infarction** 383
Cabin HS, Roberts WC. *Circulation.* 1982;66(1):93-99.

487.   **Sudden death in Prinzmetal's angina with coronary spasm documented by angiography. Analysis of three necropsy patients** 390
Roberts WC, Curry RC Jr, Isner JM, Waller BF, McManus BM, Mariani-Constantini R, Ross AM. *Am J Cardiol.* 1982;50(1):203-210.

488.   **Relation of healed transmural myocardial infarct size to length of survival after acute myocardial infarction, age at death, and amount and extent of coronary arterial narrowing by atherosclerotic plaques: analysis of 70 necropsy patients** 398
Cabin HS, Roberts WC. *Am Heart J.* 1982;104(2 Pt 1):216-220.

493.   **Relation of serum total cholesterol and triglyceride levels to the amount and extent of coronary arterial narrowing by atherosclerotic plaque in coronary heart disease. Quantitative analysis of 2,037 five mm segments of 160 major epicardial coronary arteries in 40 necropsy patients** 403
Cabin HS, Roberts WC. *Am J Med.* 1982;73(2):227-234.

499.   **Embolus to the left main coronary artery** 411
Waller BF, Dixon DS, Kim RW, Roberts WC. *Am J Cardiol.* 1982;50(3):658-660.

502.   **Quantitative comparison of extent of coronary narrowing and size of healed myocardial infarct in 33 necropsy patients with clinically recognized and in 28 with clinically unrecognized (silent?) previous acute myocardial infarction** 414
Cabin HS, Roberts WC. *Am J Cardiol.* 1982;50(4):677-681.

514.   **Status of the major epicardial coronary arteries 80 to 150 days after percutaneous transluminal coronary angioplasty. Analysis of 3 necropsy patients** 419
Waller BF, McManus BM, Gorfinkel HK, Kishel JC, Schmidt ECH, Kent KM, Roberts WC. *Am J Cardiol.* 1983;51(1):81-84.

516.   **Cardiovascular disease in the very elderly. Analysis of 40 necropsy patients aged 90 years or over** 423
Waller BF, Roberts WC. *Am J Cardiol.* 1983;51(3):403-421.

522.   **Coronary arterial rupture during coronary angioplasty** 442
Saffitz JE, Rose TE, Oaks JB, Roberts WC. *Am J Cardiol.* 1983;51(5):902-904.

535.   **Extravasated erythrocytes, iron, and fibrin in atherosclerotic plaques of coronary arteries in fatal coronary heart disease and their relation to luminal thrombus: frequency and significance in 57 necropsy patients and in 2958 five mm segments of 224 major epicardial coronary arteries** 445
Virmani R, Roberts WC. *Am Heart J.* 1983;105(5):788-797.

552.   **Thrombocytosis and fatal coronary heart disease** 455
Saffitz JE, Phillips ER, Temesy-Armos PN, Roberts WC. *Am J Cardiol.* 1983;52(5):651-652.

561.   **The "blessing" of angina pectoris** 457
Roberts WC. *Am J Cardiol.* 1983;52:1154.

562.   **Fatal cardiac arrest during cardiac catheterization for angina pectoris. A marker of quadruple vessel disease** 458
Warnes CA, Kishel JC, Roberts WC. *Chest.* 1983;84(5):631-632.

572.   **Amounts of coronary arterial narrowing by atherosclerotic plaques in clinically isolated, chronic, pure aortic regurgitation: analysis of 37 necropsy patients older than 30 years** 460
Day PJ, McManus BM, Roberts WC. *Am J Cardiol.* 1984;53(1):173-177.

584.   **When I have an acute myocardial infarction take me to the hospital that has a cardiac catheterization laboratory and open cardiac surgical facilities** 465
Roberts WC. *Am J Cardiol.* 1984;53(9):1410.

593.   **Sudden coronary death: relation of amount and distribution of coronary narrowing at necropsy to previous symptoms of myocardial ischemia, left ventricular scarring and heart weight** 466
Warnes CA, Roberts WC. *Am J Cardiol.* 1984;54(1):65-73.

597.   **The coronary artery surgery study (CASS): Do the results apply to your patient?** 475
Roberts WC, Manning DM. *Am J Cardiol.* 1984;54:440-443.

607.   **Comparison at necropsy by age group of amount and distribution of narrowing by atherosclerotic plaque in 2995 five-mm long segments of 240 major coronary arteries in 60 men aged 31 to 70 years with sudden coronary death** 479
Warnes CA, Roberts WC. *Am Heart J.* 1984;108(3 Pt 1):431-435.

613.   **Sudden coronary death: comparison of patients with to those without coronary thrombus at necropsy** 484
Warnes CA, Roberts WC. *Am J Cardiol.* 1984;54:1206-1211.

614.   **Formation of new coronary arteries within a previously obstructed epicardial coronary artery (intraarterial arteries): a mechanism for occurrence of angiographically normal coronary arteries after healing of acute myocardial infarction** 490
Roberts WC, Virmani R. *Am J Cardiol.* 1984;54(10):1361-1362.

640.   **Occluding clot in the left main coronary artery with survival long enough to develop massive left ventricular wall necrosis** 492
Mas IJ, Barth CW III, Shutlk PK, Sheilh MU, Roberts WC. *Am J Cardiol.* 1985;55:1218-1220.

641.   **Right ventricular infarction with electrocardiographic anterior left ventricular infarction and thrombosis of the left anterior descending coronary artery** 495
Barbour DJ, Saulino PF, Roberts WC. *Am J Cardiol.* 1985;55:1220-1221.

667.   **Severe atherosclerotic coronary artery disease, healed myocardial infarction and chronic congestive heart failure: analysis of 81 patients studied at necropsy** 497
Ross EM, Roberts WC. *Am J Cardiol.* 1986;57:44-50.

668.   **Severe atherosclerotic coronary arterial narrowing and chronic congestive heart failure without myocardial infarction: analysis of 18 patients studied at necropsy** 504
Ross EM, Roberts WC. *Am J Cardiol.* 1986;57:51-56.

669.   **Intussusception of a coronary artery associated with sudden death in a college football player** 510
Roberts WC, Silver MA, Sapala JC. *Am J Cardiol.* 1986;57:179-180.

686.   **Amounts of coronary arterial narrowing by atherosclerotic plaques in clinically isolated mitral valve stenosis: analysis of 76 necropsy patients older than 30 years** 512
Reis RN, Roberts WC. *Am J Cardiol.* 1986;57:1117-1123.

689.   **Relation of size of transmural acute myocardial infarct to mode of death, interval between infarction and death and frequency of coronary arterial thrombus** 519
Saffitz JE, Fredrickson RC, Roberts WC. *Am J Cardiol.* 1986;57:1249-1254.

691.   **Sudden cardiac death: definitions and causes** 525
Roberts WC. *Am J Cardiol.* 1986;57:1410-1413.

699.   **Rupture of a left ventricular papillary muscle during acute myocardial infarction: analysis of 22 necropsy patients** 529
Barbour DJ, Roberts WC. *J Am Coll Cardiol.* 1986;8(3):558-565.

702.   **The senile cardiac calcification syndrome** 537
Roberts WC. *Am J Cardiol.* 1986;58:572-574.

712. **Morphologic findings in sudden coronary death: a comparison of those with and those without previous symptoms of myocardial ischemia** 540
Warnes CA, Roberts WC. *Cardiol Clin.* 1986;4(4):607-615.

736. **Cardiac findings associated with sudden death secondary to atherosclerotic coronary artery disease: comparison of patients with and those without previous angina pectoris and/or healed myocardial infarction** 549
Barbour DJ, Warnes CA, Roberts WC. *Circulation.* 1987;75(3 Pt 2):II9-II11.

748. **Calcification of healed myocardial infarcts** 552
Roberts WC, Kaufman RJ. *Am J Cardiol.* 1987;60:28-32.

753. **Rupture of the ventricular septum or left ventricular free wall from acute myocardial infarction early after coronary artery bypass grafting** 557
Mann JM, Kalan JM, Wallace RB, Roberts WC. *Am J Cardiol.* 1987;60:374-375.

757. **Fatal rupture of both left ventricular free wall and ventricular septum (double rupture) during acute myocardial infarction: analysis of seven patients studied at necropsy** 559
Mann JM, Roberts WC. *Am J Cardiol.* 1987;60:722-724.

761. **Delayed clinical evidence of coronary arterial disruption after presumably successful percutaneous transluminal coronary angioplasty for angina pectoris** 562
Potkin BN, Myler RK, Motamed HE, Mann JM, Hendel JL, Sperling DC, Stertzer S, Roberts WC. *Am J Cardiol.* 1987;60:909-911.

764. **Cardiac morphologic observations after operative closure of acquired ventricular septal defect during acute myocardial infarction: analysis of 16 necropsy patients** 565
Mann JM, Roberts WC. *Am J Cardiol.* 1987;60:981-987.

790. **Aneurysmal coronary artery disease in cerebrotendinous xanthomatosis** 572
Potkin BN, Hoeg JM, Connor WE, Salen G, Quyyumi AA, Brush JE Jr, Roberts WC, Brewer HB Jr. *Am J Cardiol.* 1988;61:1150-1152.

794. **Acquired ventricular septal defect during acute myocardial infarction: analysis of 38 unoperated necropsy patients and comparison with 50 unoperated necropsy patients without rupture** 575
Mann JM, Roberts WC. *Am J Cardiol.* 1988;62:8-19.

813. **Location of an acute myocardial infarct in patients with a healed myocardial infarct: analysis of 129 patients studied at necropsy** 587
Potkin BN, Roberts WC. *Am J Cardiol.* 1988;62:1017-1023.

814. **Frequency of acute and healed myocardial infarcts in fatal cardiac amyloidosis** 594
Barbour DJ, Roberts WC. *Am J Cardiol.* 1988;62:1134-1135.

831. **Morphologic changes in coronary artery seen late after endarterectomy** 596
Kragel AH, McIntosh CM, Roberts WC. *Am J Cardiol.* 1989;63(11):757-759.

833. **Frequency of rupture of the left ventricular free wall or ventricular septum among necropsy cases of fatal acute myocardial infarction since introduction of coronary care units** 599
Reddy SG, Roberts WC. *Am J Cardiol.* 1989;63:906-911.

839. **Qualitative and quantitative comparison of amounts of narrowing by atherosclerotic plaques in the major epicardial coronary arteries at necropsy in sudden coronary death, transmural acute myocardial infarction, transmural healed myocardial infarction and unstable angina pectoris** 605
Roberts WC. *Am J Cardiol.* 1989;64:324-328.

840. **Extensive multifocal myocardial infarcts from cloth emboli after replacement of mitral and aortic valves with cloth-covered, caged-ball prostheses** 610
Dollar AL, Pierre-Louis ML, McIntosh CL, Roberts WC. *Am J Cardiol.* 1989;64:410-412.

858. **Morphometric analysis of the composition of atherosclerotic plaques in the four major epicardial coronary arteries in acute myocardial infarction and in sudden coronary death** 613
Kragel AH, Reddy SG, Wittes JT, Roberts WC. *Circulation.* 1989;80(6):1747-1756.

861. **Mode of death, frequency of healed and acute myocardial infarction, number of major epicardial coronary arteries severely narrowed by atherosclerotic plaque, and heart weight in fatal atherosclerotic coronary artery disease: analysis of 889 patients studied at necropsy** 623
Roberts WC, Potkin BN, Solus DE, Reddy SG. *J Am Coll Cardiol.* 1990;15(1):196-203.

864. **Sudden cardiac death: A diversity of causes with focus on atherosclerotic coronary artery disease** 631
Roberts WC. *Am J Cardiol.* 1990;65:13B-19B.

865. **Quantitative analysis of amounts of coronary arterial narrowing in cocaine addicts** 638
Dressler FA, Malekzadeh S, Roberts WC. *Am J Cardiol.* 1990;65:33-38.

870. **Diffuse extent of coronary atherosclerosis in fatal coronary artery disease** 644
Roberts WC. *Am J Cardiol.* 1990;65:2-6.

873. **Coronary arterial morphology 10 years after endarterectomy** 649
Kragel AH, McIntosh CL, Roberts WC. *Clin Cardiol.* 1990;13(3):224-226.

874. **Cardiac morphologic findings in patients with acute myocardial infarction treated with recombinant tissue plasminogen activator** 652
Gertz SD, Kalan JM, Kragel AH, Roberts WC. Braunwald E; TIMI Investigators. *Am J Cardiol.* 1990; 65:953-961.

875. **Rupture of the left ventricular free wall during acute myocardial infarction without hemopericardium** 661
Roberts WC. *Am J Cardiol.* 1990;65:1033-1034.

879. **Coronary artery imaging with intravascular high-frequency ultrasound** 663
Potkin BN, Bartorelli AL, Gessert JM, Neville RF, Almagor Y, Roberts WC, Leon MB. *Circulation.* 1990; 81(5):1575-1585.

884. **Morphometric analysis of the composition of coronary arterial plaques in isolated unstable angina pectoris with pain at rest** 674
Kragel AH, Reddy SG, Wittes JT, Roberts WC. *Am J Cardiol.* 1990;66:562-567.

887. **Myocarditis or acute myocardial infarction associated with interleukin-2 therapy for cancer** 680
Kragel AH, Travis WD, Steis RG, Rosenberg SA, Roberts WC. *Cancer.* 1990;66(7):1513-1516.

888. **Comparison of coronary and myocardial morphologic findings in patients with and without thrombolytic therapy during fatal first acute myocardial infarction** 684
Gertz SD, Kragel AH, Kalan JM, Braunwald E, Roberts WC; TIMI Investigators. *Am J Cardiol.* 1990; 66:904-909.

893. **Sudden death behind the wheel from natural disease in drivers of four-wheeled motorized vehicles** 690
Antecol DH, Roberts WC. *Am J Cardiol.* 1990;66:1329-1335.

894. **Hemodynamic shear force in rupture of coronary arterial atherosclerotic plaques** 697
Gertz SD, Roberts WC. *Am J Cardiol.* 1990;66:1368-1372.

895. **Ages at death and sex distribution in age decade in fatal coronary artery disease** 702
Roberts WC, Kragel AH, Potkin BN. *Am J Cardiol.* 1990;66:1379-1381.

902. **Composition of atherosclerotic plaques in the coronary arteries in homozygous familial hypercholesterolemia** 705
Kragel AH, Roberts WC. *Am Heart J.* 1991;121(1 Pt 1):210-211.

911. **Composition of atherosclerotic plaques in coronary arteries in women <40 years of age with fatal coronary artery disease and implications for plaque reversibility** 707
Dollar AL, Kragel AH, Fernicola DJ, Waclawiw MA, Roberts WC. *Am J Cardiol.* 1991;67:1223-1227.

912. **Composition of atherosclerotic plaques in the four major epicardial coronary arteries in patients 90 years of age** 712
Gertz SD, Malekzadeh S, Dollar AL, Kragel AH, Roberts WC. *Am J Cardiol.* 1991;67:1228-1233.

928. **Morphologic comparison of frequency and types of acute lesions in the major epicardial coronary arteries in unstable angina pectoris, sudden coronary death and acute myocardial infarction** 718
Kragel AH, Gertz SD, Roberts WC. *J Am Coll Cardiol.* 1991;18(3):801-808.

931. **The heart in fatal unstable angina pectoris** 726
Roberts WC, Kragel AH, Gertz SD, Roberts CS, Kalan JM. *Am J Cardiol.* 1991;68:22B-27B.

952. **Reported frequency of coronary arterial narrowing by angiogram in patients with valvular aortic stenosis** 732
Mautner GC, Roberts WC. *Am J Cardiol.* 1992;70:539-540.

953. **The heart in Tangier disease. Severe coronary atherosclerosis with near absence of high-density lipoprotein cholesterol** 734
Mautner SL, Sanchez JA, Rader DJ, Mautner GC, Ferrans VJ, Fredrickson DS, Brewer HB Jr, Roberts WC. *Am J Clin Pathol.* 1992;98(2):191-198.

958. **Degrees of coronary arterial narrowing at necropsy in men with large fusiform abdominal aortic aneurysm** 742
Mautner GC, Berezowski K, Mautner SL, Roberts WC. *Am J Cardiol.* 1992;70:1143-1146.

959. **Amounts of coronary arterial narrowing by atherosclerotic plaque at necropsy in patients with lower extremity amputation** 746
Mautner GC, Mautner SL, Roberts WC. *Am J Cardiol.* 1992;70:1147-1151.

960. **Composition of atherosclerotic plaques in the epicardial coronary arteries in juvenile (Type I) diabetes mellitus** 751
Mautner GC, Mautner SL, Roberts WC. *Am J Cardiol.* 1992;70:1264-1268.

963. **Scarring of the left ventricular papillary muscles in sickle-cell disease** 756
Berezowski K, Roberts WC. *Am J Cardiol.* 1992;70:1368-1370.

964. **Comparison of composition of atherosclerotic plaques in saphenous veins used as aortocoronary bypass conduits with plaques in native coronary arteries in the same men** 759
Mautner SL, Mautner GC, Hunsberger SA, Roberts WC. *Am J Cardiol.* 1992;70:1380-1387.

969. **Amounts of coronary arterial luminal narrowing and composition of the material causing the narrowing in Buerger's disease** 767
Mautner GC, Mautner SL, Lin F, Roggin GM, Roberts WC. *Am J Cardiol.* 1993;71:486-490.

978. **Comparison in women versus men of composition of atherosclerotic plaques in native coronary arteries and in saphenous veins used as aortocoronary conduits** 772
Mautner SL, Lin F, Mautner GC, Roberts WC. *J Am Coll Cardiol.* 1993;21(6):1312-1318.

980. **Subepicardial myocardial lesions** 779
Shirani J, Roberts WC. *Am Heart J.* 1993;125(5 Pt 1):1346-1352.

1001. **Effects of tissue plasminogen activator therapy on the frequency of acute right ventricular myocardial infarction associated with acute left ventricular infarction** 786
Kalan JM, Gertz SD, Kragel AH, Berger PB, Roberts WC, Ryan TJ. *Int J Cardiol.* 1993;38(2):151-158.

1006. **Out-of-hospital sudden death from left ventricular free wall rupture during acute myocardial infarction as the first and only manifestation of atherosclerotic coronary artery disease** 794
Shirani J, Berezowski K, Roberts WC. *Am J Cardiol.* 1994;73:88-92.

1008. **Status of the major epicardial coronary arteries at necropsy in paraplegia and quadriplegia** 799
Shirani J, Roberts WC. *Am J Cardiol.* 1994;73:207-208.

1020. **Coronary arteries in unstable angina pectoris, acute myocardial infarction, and sudden coronary death** 801
Roberts WC, Kragel AH, Gertz SD, Roberts CS. *Am Heart J.* 1994;127(6):1588-1593.

1021. **Radiation-induced cardiovascular disease including stenosis of coronary ostium, coronary and carotid arteries, and aortic valves** 807
Harvey LAC, DeMaio SJ, Roberts WC. *Proc Bayl Univ Med Cent.* 1994;7(3):33-36.

1025. **Coronary artery calcification: assessment with electron beam CT and histomorphometric correlation** 811
Mautner GC, Mautner SL, Froehlich J, Feuerstein IM, Proschan MA, Roberts WC, Doppman JL. *Radiology.* 1994;192(3):619-623.

1037. **Major cardiac findings at necropsy in 366 American octogenarians** 816
Shirani J, Yousefi, J, Roberts WC. *Am J Cardiol.* 1995;75:151-156.

1038. **Factors involved in the development of symptom-producing atherosclerotic plaques** 822
Roberts WC. *Am J Cardiol.* 1995;75:1B-2B.

1042. **Clinical features and pathogenesis of intracerebral hemorrhage after rt-PA and heparin therapy for acute myocardial infarction: the Thrombolysis in Myocardial Infarction (TIMI) II Pilot and Randomized Clinical Trial combined experience** 824
Sloan MA, Price TR, Petito CK, Randall AMY, Solomon MHS, Terrin ML, Gore J, Collen D, Kleiman N, Feit F, Babb J, Herman M, Roberts WC, Sopko G, Bovill E, Forman S, Knatterud GL; TIMI Investigators. *Neurology.* 1995;45(4):649-658.

1060. **Sudden death in young competitive athletes. Clinical, demographic, and pathological profiles** 834
Maron BJ, Shirani J, Poliac LC, Mathenge R, Roberts WC, Mueller FO. *JAMA* 1996;276:199-204.

1067. **Frequency and characteristics of coronary thrombosis in the epicardial coronary arteries after cardiac transplantation** 840
Arbustini E, Bello BD, Morbini P, Grosso M, Diegoli M, Fasani R, Pilotto A, Bellini O, Pellegrini C, Martinelli L, Campana C, Gavazzi A, Specchia G, Vigano M, Roberts WC. *Am J Cardiol.* 1996;78:795-800.

1083. **Liver transplantation after coronary artery bypass grafting** 846
Pelosi F Jr, Klintmalm GBG, Simon WB, Roberts WC. *Am J Cardiol.* 1997;79:1405-1407.

1106. **Severe mitral regurgitation late after healing of myocardial infarction from calcification of the posteromedial left ventricular papillary muscle** 849
Gottdiener JS, Roberts WC. *Am J Cardiol.* 1998;81:662.

1124. **Comparison of cardiac findings at necropsy in octogenarians, nonagenarians, and centenarians** 850
Roberts WC, Shirani J. *Am J Cardiol.* 1998;82:627-631.

1146. **Operative therapy of coronary arterial aneurysm** 855
Harandi S, Johnston SB, Wood RE, Roberts WC. *Am J Cardiol.* 1999;83:1290-1293.

1174. **Twenty questions on atherosclerosis** 859
Roberts WC. *Proc Bayl Univ Med Cent.* 2000;13(2):139-143.

1182. **Wide open coronary arteries at 103 years of age** 864
Roberts WC. *Am J Geriatr Cardiol.* 2000;9(4):227.

1191. **Comparison of modes of death and cardiac necropsy findings in fatal acute myocardial infarction in men and women >75 years of age** 865
Shirani J, Alaeddini J, Roberts WC. *Am J Cardiol.* 2000;86:1010-1012.

1247. **Thrombotic occlusion of the aortic ostia of saphenous venous grafts early after coronary artery bypass grafting by using the Symmetry aortic connector system** 868
Donsky AS, Schussler JM, Donsky MS, Roberts WC, Hamman BL. *J Thorac Cardiovasc Surg.* 2002; 124(2):397-399.

1284. **Syndrome of protein C deficiency and anterior wall acute myocardial infarction at a young age from a single coronary occlusion with otherwise normal coronary arteries** 871
Peterman MA, Roberts WC. *Am J Cardiol.* 2003;92:768-770.

1291. **Late (>6 years) results of combined coronary artery bypass grafting and mitral valve replacement for severe mitral regurgitation secondary to acute myocardial infarction** 874
Theleman KP, Stephan PJ, Isaacs MG, Hebeler RF Jr, Henry AC III, Roberts WC. *Am J Cardiol.* 2003; 92:1086-1090.

1292.	**Krakatoa—the ultimate heart attack** 879
Roberts WC. *Am J Cardiol.* 2003;92:1140.

1315.	**Acute myocardial infarction at 25 years of age** 880
Falcone MW, Grayburn PA, Roberts WC. *Proc Bayl Univ Med Cent.* 2004;17(3):363-365.

1323.	**Clinical and necropsy findings in patients with calcified myocardial infarcts** 883
Cameron CS, Roberts WC. *Proc Bayl Univ Med Cent.* 2004;17(4):420-424.

1355.	**Angina pectoris, dyspnea, fatigue, and edema after a non-ST-segment-elevation myocardial infarct** 888
Glancy DL, Roberts WC. *Proc Bayl Univ Med Cent.* 2006;19(1):52-53.

1399.	**Quantitative comparison of amounts of cross-sectional area narrowing in coronary endarterectomy specimens in patients having coronary artery bypass grafting to amounts of narrowing in the same artery in patients with fatal coronary artery disease studied at necropsy** 890
Roberts WC, Turnage TA II, Whiddon LL. *Am J Cardiol.* 2007;99:588-592.

1409.	**Fatal cardiac arrest in the hospital during transfer from Gurney to operating table for planned coronary artery bypass grafting and mitral valve repair** 895
Roberts WC, Williams SL, Ko JM, Kuiper JJ. *Am J Geriatr Cardiol.* 2007;16(3):192-196.

1413.	**Comparison of body mass index among patients with versus without angiographic coronary artery disease** 900
Phillips SD, Roberts WC. *Am J Cardiol.* 2007;100:18-22.

1547.	**Natural history, clinical consequences, and morphologic features of coronary arterial aneurysms in adults** 905
Roberts WC. *Am J Cardiol.* 2011;108:814-821.

1638.	**Commonalities of cardiac rupture (left ventricular free wall or ventricular septum or papillary muscle) during acute myocardial infarction secondary to atherosclerotic coronary artery disease** 913
Roberts WC, Burks KH, Ko MJ, Filardo G, Guileyardo JM. *Am J Cardiol.* 2015;115:125-140.

1687.	**Relation of left ventricular free wall rupture and/or aneurysm with acute myocardial infarction in patients with aortic stenosis** 929
Sheilkh IN, Roberts WC. *Proc (Bayl Univ Med Cent).* 2017;30(2):161-162.

1690.	**Coronary arterial aneurysms in previously transplanted (donor) hearts** 931
Kondapalli N, Roberts WC. *Proc (Bayl Univ Med Cent).* 2017; 30(3):303-304.

1701.	**Frequency of coronary endarterectomy in patients undergoing coronary artery bypass grafting at a single tertiary Texas hospital 2010 to 2016 with morphologic studies of the operatively excised specimens** 933
Roberts WC, Berry AE. *Am J Cardiol.* 2017; 120(12):2164-2169.

*Articles are numbered based on WCR's CV.

The Pathology of Acute Myocardial Infarction

WILLIAM C. ROBERTS *National Heart and Lung Institute*

The relationship of coronary thrombosis to myocardial necrosis needs reassessment:
the evidence, from systematic histologic study of the major coronary arteries in
consecutive patients, suggests that thrombi are more likely to be the result of acute
myocardial infarction than the cause. Support for this view comes also from
the fact that thrombi are found much more often when death has not been instantaneous.

Nearly 60 years ago James Herrick recorded several observations in reference to heart disease that were to influence medical thinking for many years to follow. One was that acute obstruction of a major coronary artery, or even of a main trunk, was not necessarily lethal. It has since been amply documented that while "acute coronary occlusion" is often fatal it is not invariably so, as Herrick correctly observed. He drew a further inference from his work that also gained general acceptance: that the usual cause of coronary arterial occlusion is thrombus.

Indeed, after Herrick, the terms "coronary thrombosis" and "coronary occlusion" came into wide usage as synonyms to describe events leading to myocardial necrosis. Among many clinicians and pathologists alike the belief persists to this day that without thrombotic occlusion of a major coronary artery, acute myocardial infarction is unlikely to occur. Moreover, coronary arterial thrombosis is considered a prerequisite for myocardial necrosis.

It is not difficult to see why this assumption has taken so firm a hold. Clinically, acute myocardial infarction is often a dramatic event. A patient apparently well to that point is suddenly in cardiovascular collapse; death may come within minutes and often does. Even with a history of cardiac disease there is likely to be an abrupt change in the patient's status at onset of the fatal attack. The pathologist, pressed for an explanation, looks for some new finding in the coronary arteries to account for the acute clinical event. Given the long association of thrombotic occlusion and infarction, both he and the clinician expect to find a fresh arterial thrombus; if none is there the implication may be that it was somehow missed. A thrombus is found often enough to perpetuate the view that acute myocardial infarction usually results from thrombotic occlusion of a coronary artery.

Careful examination of the facts, however, leads one to question seriously whether there is a causal relationship; rather, the evidence would suggest that arterial thrombi may occur as consequences of acute myocardial infarction and not the other way around.

Reports over the years have indicated a wide range of incidence of coronary arterial thrombi in patients dying of acute myocardial infarction – from as low as 21% in some studies to as high as 100% in others. This discrepancy in itself might argue against a causal role, although other factors, such as differences in techniques of examining coronary arteries, could explain some of it.

Strict definition of terms is a requirement for collecting meaningful incidence data. It must also be taken into account that gross inspection of coronary arteries is not sufficient for assessing their status. Several distinguishing features of thrombi must be confirmed histologically: A true thrombus is adherent at some point along its length (more often distally than proximally) to the luminal surface of the artery; it is composed of platelets or fibrin or both, and usually also of erythrocytes and leukocytes. Actually the composition of a thrombus may differ substantially along its length (usually about 1 cm): Distally it is more likely to consist chiefly of platelets or fibrin or both (white thrombus), whereas proximally it is more often composed chiefly of erythrocytes, with lesser quantities of fibrin, platelets, and leukocytes (red thrombus). Early in their formation, however, thrombi are likely to be composed almost entirely of platelets.

Too often when coronary arteries are sectioned at autopsy, an arterial thrombus is all that is looked for; if something red is spotted it is usually assumed to be a thrombus. But hemorrhage into an old atherosclerotic plaque may closely resemble a thrombus grossly, as may postmortem clot, although close inspection would show

Dr. Roberts is Chief, Section of Pathology, National Heart and Lung Institute; Clinical Associate Professor of Pathology, Georgetown University; and Assistant Professor of Pathology, the Johns Hopkins University.

that the latter is nonadherent and composed chiefly of erythrocytes. Histologic examination must be done, therefore, to distinguish a true thrombus from a postmortem clot or from hemorrhage into an old plaque.

A coronary arterial thrombus may not necessarily totally occlude the vessel containing it; this must be kept in mind in considering whether thrombus formation is likely to be causally related to acute myocardial necrosis. When the terms "occlusion" and "thrombosis" are used interchangeably, as they often are, it is overlooked that the occlusion may be only partial rather than complete and that a coronary artery may be occluded by material other than that which forms a thrombus. In the patients with fatal transmural infarction that we have studied, about 80% of the thrombi found were totally occlusive; the remainder were partially occlusive or nonocclusive mural thrombi. Young thrombi composed purely of platelets are usually small and nonocclusive.

Nonocclusive thrombi probably have little functional significance. Indeed, as will become evident, even occlusive thrombi-under some circumstances may be of little functional significance. Thus, it is not enough to know whether or not a coronary artery contains a thrombus; knowledge of whether it is totally or only partially occlusive and other facts of the situation are required before its significance can be judged.

In clarifying the relationship of thrombosis to myocardial necrosis, it is important to consider the type of infarction present. Reported variations in incidence of arterial thrombi in fatal acute myocardial infarction may largely reflect the patient group studied: Incidence of death differs sharply in transmural infarction involving virtually the entire thickness of the myocardial wall, as compared with incidence in subendocardial infarction, with necrosis limited to the inner half of the myocardial wall. There is a third possibility to take into account as well: Sudden death may result from an arrhythmia before subendocardial or transmural necrosis has a chance to evolve.

It has been recognized for some time that coronary arterial thrombi are rarely present at necropsy in sudden death cases, whether or not there was a prior history of heart disease; coronary thrombosis is also uncommon in patients with subendocardial infarction. Thrombosis has, however, been closely associated with acute transmural infarction; observations implicating thrombosis etiologically in acute myocardial infarction have been based chiefly on cases of the latter type.

In examining major coronary arteries of patients who died of acute myocardial infarction, we were unable to find either gross or histologic evidence of arterial thrombosis in many patients in whom this might have been expected. In search of more information we decided to examine the coronary arteries systematically in consecutive patients who died of extensive myocardial infarction. In each patient at least three sections of left ventricular wall were obtained for histologic study. Before the ventricles were opened the major extramural coronary arteries (left main, left anterior descending, left circumflex, and right) were excised intact. Each major vessel was extended to full length and sectioned transversely in 5 mm segments. A key step in the procedure was decalcification of the vessels — both before and after sectioning — to avoid crushing and distortion of the vessel by cutting. This was essential for accurate measurement of the degree of luminal narrowing by old atherosclerotic plaques. Since we were questioning the importance of arterial thrombus formation in precipitating acute myocardial necrosis it seemed essential to explore other factors that might prove important.

Another important step in the procedure was to imbed the arteries in paraffin at precise right angles so that they could be cut directly across in

Frequency of Coronary Thrombosis in Acute Myocardial Infarction

Author	Year	Number of Patients	Number (%) with Coronary Thrombosis
Herrick	1919	3	3 (100)
Nathanson	1925	113	24 (21)
Davenport	1928	50	30 (60)
Parkinson and Bedford	1928	51	33 (64)
Levine	1929	46	23 (50)
Lisa and Ring	1932	32	13 (41)
Saphir et al.	1935	34	18 (53)
Friedberg and Horn	1939	153	119 (78)
Mallory et al.	1939	100	70 (70)
Blumgart et al.	1940	16	14 (88)
Foord	1948	315	274 (87)
Yater et al.	1948	68	34 (50)
Miller et al.	1951	143	92 (64)
Branwood and Montgomery	1956	61	13 (21)
Spain and Bradess	1960	200	109 (55)
Ehrlich and Shinohara	1964	130	57 (44)
Mitchell and Schwartz	1965	26	21 (81)
Baroldi	1965	449	211 (47)
Meadows	1965	100	30 (30)
Kurland et al.	1965	127	70 (55)
Harland and Holburn	1966	53	48 (91)
Chapman	1968	292	278 (95)
Kagan et al.	1968	176	87 (49)
Spain and Bradess	1970	391	115 (29)
Walston et al.	1970	37	19 (51)
Bouch and Montgomery	1970	100	66 (66)
Page et al.	1971	36	30 (83)
Roberts and Buja (*in press*)	1972	107	42 (39)
Totals		3,409	1,943 (57)

(Specific references for the above list, with annotations by the author, may be requested from HOSPITAL PRACTICE.*)*

segments of uniform size. For identification of arterial thrombi two histologic sections were prepared from each 5 mm segment (one stained by hematoxylin and eosin, and the second by Movat's method). By examining the many sections in each patient, it seemed unlikely that arterial thrombi might be present but remain undetected. Each section was examined by light microscopy and the maximal degree of luminal narrowing was recorded.

If a thrombus was found, its composition was noted (an unstained section of thrombus was treated with phosphotungstic-acid hematoxylin to aid in quantifying the several components). The condition of the coronary artery at the site was carefully observed, in particular whether the lumen there or close by was already narrowed, and to what degree, by old atherosclerotic plaques. The presence of hemorrhage into plaques was recorded as well, since this too has been implicated in precipitating acute infarction.

Of 107 patients investigated in this manner, 74 had acute transmural infarcts, nine had acute infarcts limited to the subendocardium, and 24 patients died suddenly before myocardial necrosis was detectable by histologic examination. (In our studies sudden death was defined as death occurring within six hours following onset of acute symptoms.) It is assumed that necrosis would have developed in these patients also if they had lived longer; perhaps early signs of necrosis prior to death would be more evident with improved techniques for recognizing it.

An association between thrombosis and transmural infarction, although by no means a consistent one, was clearly confirmed, as was the relative absence of arterial thrombi in the other two groups. Specifically, only two of the 24 sudden death cases had coronary thrombi, and none of the nine cases of subendocardial infarction had coronary thrombi. In contrast, thrombi were present in more than half (40 of 74) of the cases of fatal transmural infarction. (As indicated earlier, the thrombi were totally occlusive in most but not all of these cases)

Hemorrhage into atherosclerotic plaques proved fairly common, occurring in 24% of the 107 cases studied.

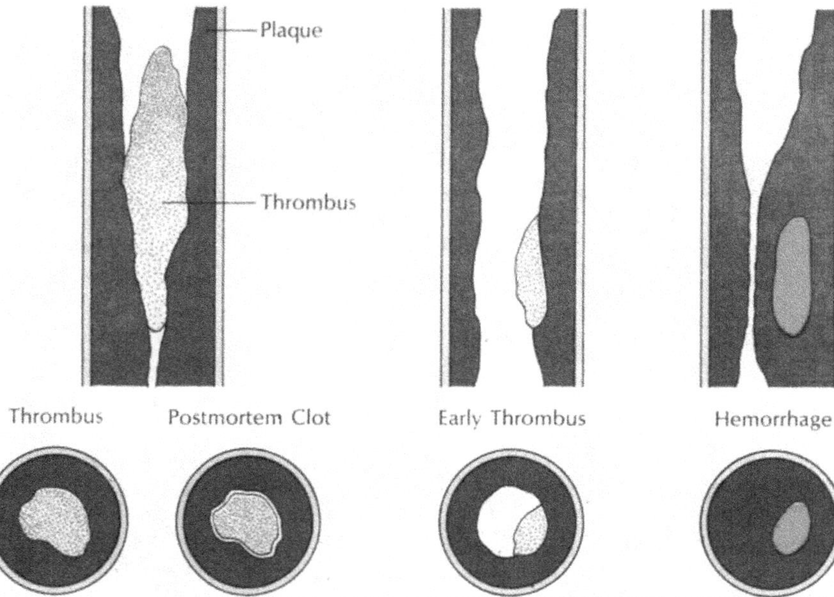

of luminal narrowing by atherosclerotic plaques; platelets, and later platelets and fibrin, are chief thrombus components, whereas a hemorrhage into an old plaque or postmortem clot is composed chiefly of erythrocytes. Thrombus and postmortem clot also differ in the adherence of the former to luminal surface.

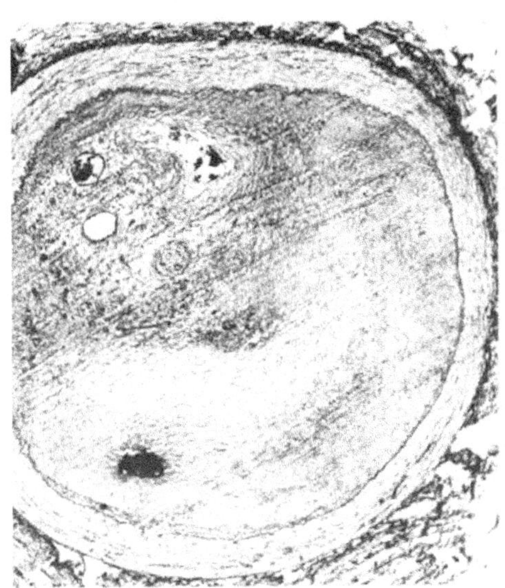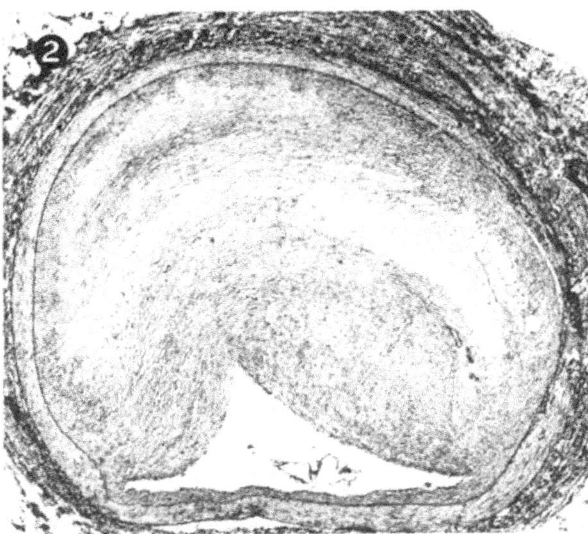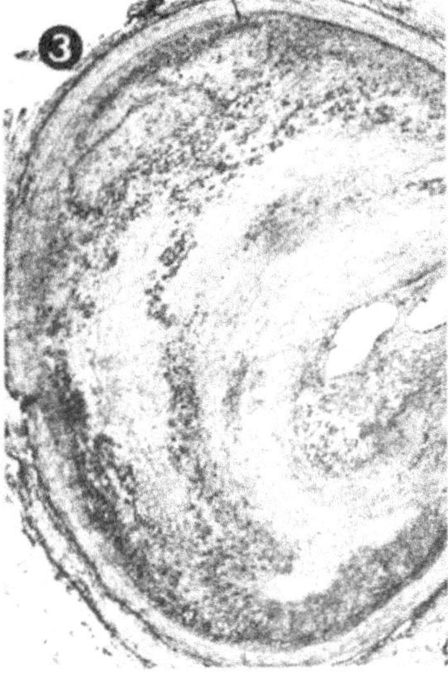

Atherosclerotic plaques accounted for virtually all narrowing of extramural vessels in a 26-year-old female victim of coronary disease; sections of the right (1), the left circumflex (2), and the left anterior descending (3) coronary arteries are shown at the sites of their maximal narrowing. Each of the photomicrographs was taken at the same magnification.

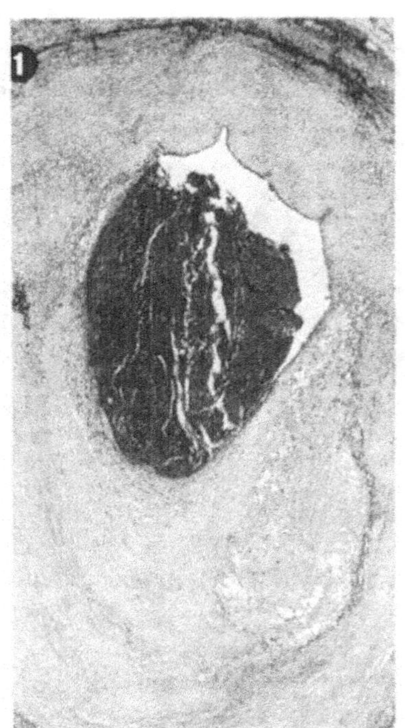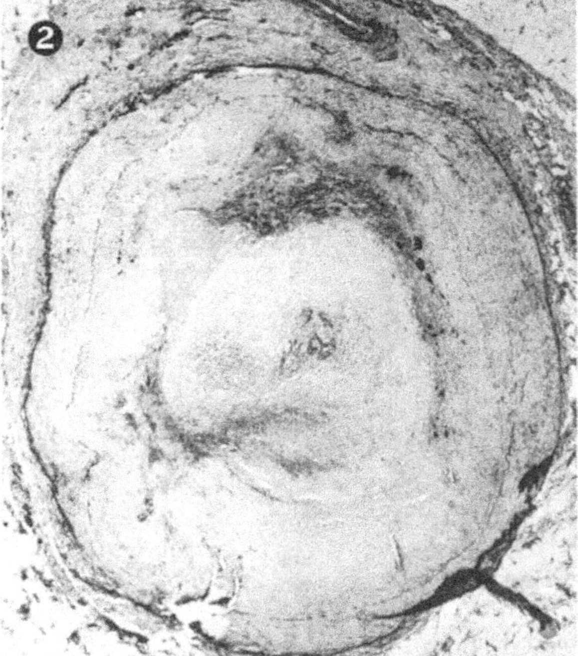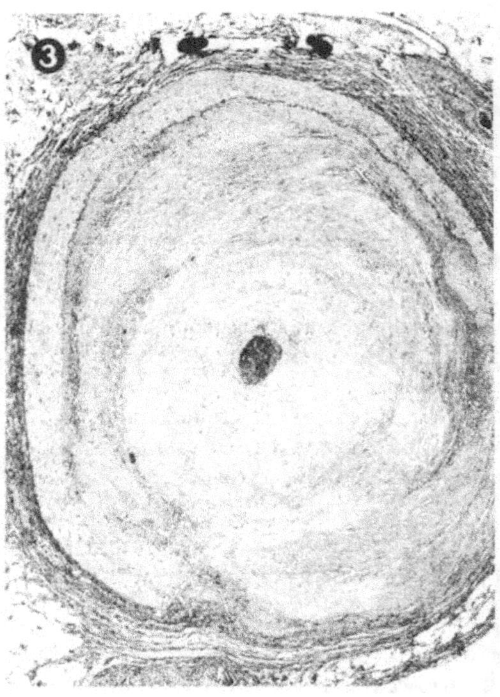

Sectioning of right coronary artery of 52-year-old woman revealed a partially occluding thrombus (1) and a totally occluding atherosclerotic plaque (2) just distal to it. As suggested schematically (right) and shown histologically (3) presence of an arterial thrombus may have little functional significance in acute myocardial infarction if diffuse atherosclerotic plaquing has already narrowed

These seemed to be of little functional significance in terms of initiating infarction. In only one of the 26 patients with hemorrhage into an atherosclerotic plaque was the arterial lumen compromised by the extravasated blood. Such hemorrhages appear to form from either breaks in the fibrous capsule covering a plaque or from rupture of a small vascular channel within a plaque, although either of these mechanisms is difficult to prove in the individual patient. In some patients, hemorrhages into old plaques apparently keep occurring over lengthy periods. In any case, hemorrhage probably has little to do with the onset of acute myocardial infarction.

Our systematic examination of major coronary arteries made clear that "nothing new" appears in these vessels at the time of acute myocardial infarction in most patients stricken. The low incidence of arterial thrombosis in patients dying suddenly of coronary disease, and its presence in only about half of those with myocardial necrosis, strengthened our conviction that a causal relation to myocardial infarction was unlikely. Even in patients in whom fresh thrombi were present it would be difficult to say whether they developed before or after the infarction.

It has been suggested that fresh coronary thrombi present before death may be undetected at necropsy because of postmortem lysis of thrombi due to excessive fibrinolysin production. Several observations tend to discount this hypothesis. If lysis of thrombi did occur, there should be evidence of the fact in the form of blood or blood products in the affected coronary arteries. This is rarely the case. Indeed, necropsies performed within 15 minutes of death from acute myocardial infarction have disclosed no evidence of lysed or partially lysed thrombi. It is also unlikely that postmortem lysis of thrombi would occur so selectively as to liquefy thrombi in patients with subendocardial but not in those with transmural myocardial necrosis. When the same investigators have checked for the appearance of thrombi in two widely separated studies they have tended to find a similar incidence of thrombus formation on both occasions. This would be unlikely if lysis is a factor, since it would occur by chance.

Looked at another way, the absence of arterial thrombi in many patients with acute myocardial infarction may in part explain the lack of clear-cut benefit from anticoagulant therapy. The initial rationale given for use of anticoagulants in patients with coronary artery disease was a presumed causal relationship between thrombosis and infarction and the presumed ability of these drugs to reduce arterial thrombus formation or extension. Yet it has been learned that the incidence of coronary arterial thrombosis in fatal acute myocardial infarction is similar in patients receiving and those not receiving anticoagulant therapy.

On several grounds, then, it is time to consider the alternative hypothesis in reference to coronary arterial thrombosis. Rather than being causally related to acute myocardial infarction, does coronary arterial thrombosis occur as a consequence of advancing myocardial necrosis?

When we analyzed our transmural infarction cases, a provocative finding emerged. Arterial thrombi appeared to develop only in certain patients dying of myocardial necrosis — those who experienced cardiogenic shock and/or congestive heart failure for a time before death. In the patient with uncomplicated acute transmural infarction — whose death was due not to pump failure but to a lethal arrhythmia — arterial thrombi were rarely present at necropsy.

Interestingly, similar findings were obtained in a study by Walston and

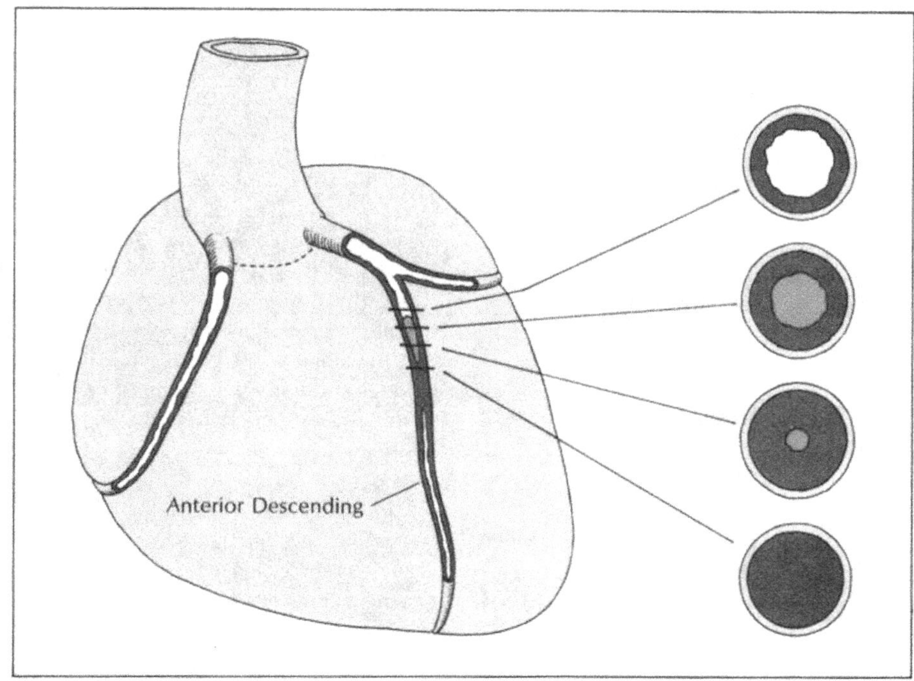

extramural arteries severely. The small thrombus present in the anterior descending artery (3) could have caused only minimal luminal narrowing. Patient was a 59-year-old woman who died six weeks following onset of myocardial infarction.

coworkers on patients who died of acute myocardial infarction. The presence of antemortem arterial thrombi could be linked to the occurrence of the "power failure syndrome" – in essence an inability of the myocardium to maintain a level of cardiac output necessary for adequate organ perfusion. In the 37 cases studied, Walston et al. found arterial thrombi at necropsy in 71% of patients who before death had manifested the power failure syndrome and in only 15% of those who had not.

These findings, and ours along the same line, suggested that a markedly diminished cardiac output and the consequent slowdown in coronary blood flow might be required for arterial thrombus formation in association with acute myocardial infarction (we have since become increasingly convinced that this is the case). Other observations began to shed further light on conditions favoring the appearance of arterial thrombi in association with acute myocardial infarction. For example, thrombi were most often located at sites of luminal narrowing; frequently the degree of narrowing was greater than 75% at the distal attachment. It seemed possible, if still speculative, that thrombus formation at this location might be related to introduction of high-velocity gradients as luminal narrowing increases, since this tends to favor platelet aggregation.

One certainty was that examination of the entire coronary tree yielded an unexpected discovery about the condition of the coronary arteries in patients who died of myocardial infarction. Many believe the process of atherosclerosis underlying coronary heart disease is usually localized, with atherosclerotic plaquing often confined to one major vessel. Our studies showed unequivocally that the entire extramural coronary tree is likely to be affected. The degree of luminal narrowing differed in each particular coronary artery and in each patient studied, but there was some atherosclerotic plaquing on the intimal surface of nearly every millimeter of artery examined, not only within the major extramural arteries themselves

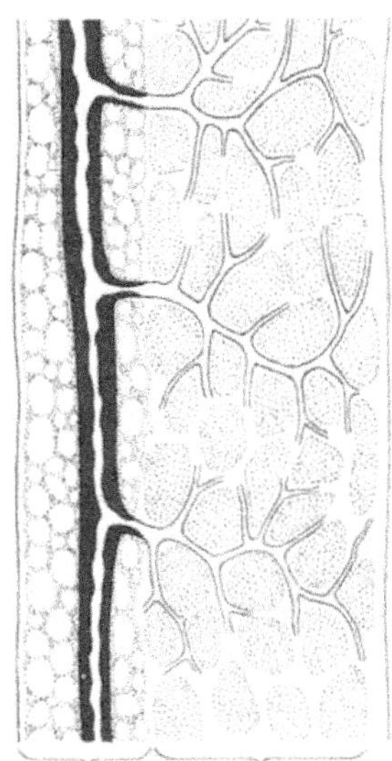

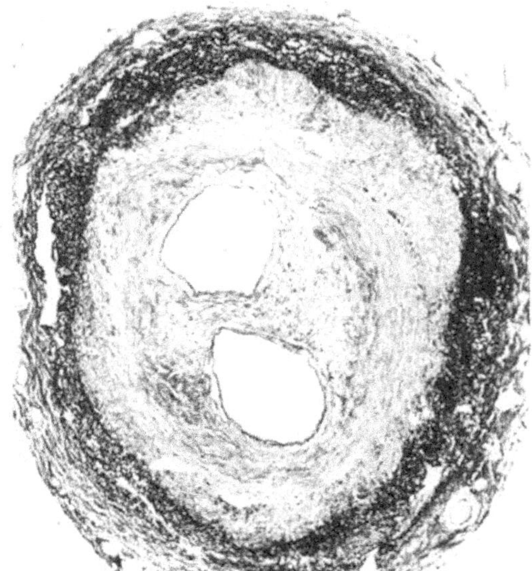

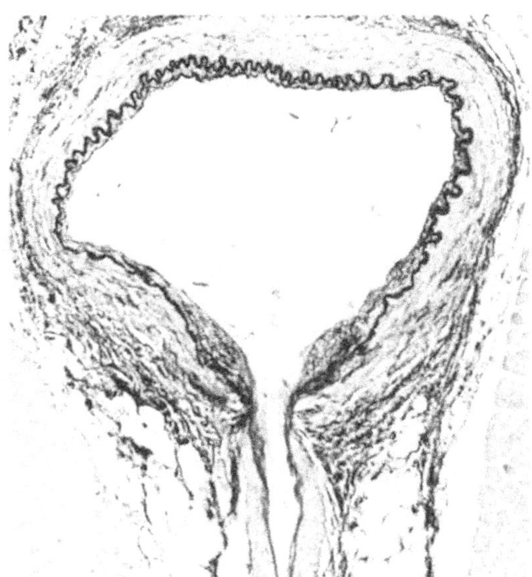

Extensive atherosclerosis usually seen in main extramural arteries and epicardial branches almost never extends into intramural coronary arteries (diagram). For example, in autopsy study of sudden death victim with known severe hypertension, severe luminal narrowing was found in left circumflex and other extramural arteries (above) but intramural arteries were essentially normal (right).

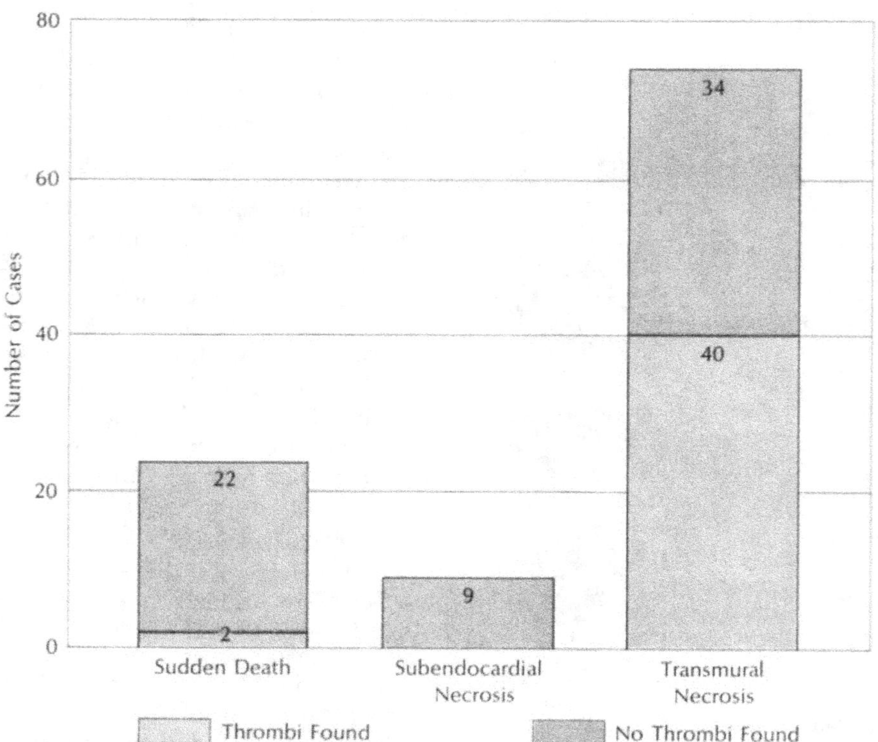

Confirmation of an association between thrombosis and transmural infarction was obtained in the study of 107 patients dying of acute myocardial infarction. Its relative absence in cases of subendocardial infarction or sudden death was also demonstrated.

but in the smaller extramural branches as well. In all, several thousand histologic sections were examined and only four sections were free of old atherosclerotic plaques, excluding three patients with coronary arterial emboli.

We were aware that despite considerable atherosclerosis a coronary artery may still carry sufficient blood to the myocardium; in general, coronary flow is unlikely to be seriously reduced, with the patient in the basal state, until the original lumen is decreased by 75% or more. Thus our interest was in the degree of luminal narrowing produced by atherosclerotic plaquing.

Sites of maximal narrowing showed wide variation, but with examination of a large number of cases definable patterns emerged. For example, the lumen of the left main coronary artery was rarely severely stenosed by atherosclerotic plaques; indeed, this vessel was narrowed by more than 75% in only two of the 107 patients studied. On the other hand, the left anterior descending, left circumflex, and right coronary arteries were often narrowed to that degree and more. The average number of these latter three vessels narrowed by more than 75% was 2.4

per patient in the group with transmural infarction, 2.1 in patients with subendocardial necrosis, and 2.4 in the sudden death patients. Vessel narrowing by 90% or more was frequent.

Significantly, from the point that the affected artery actually enters the myocardial wall of the heart and distally it is likely to appear entirely normal. It seems generally true that conditions involving the extramural coronary arteries do not involve the intramural coronary arteries; likewise, diseases affecting the intramural coronary arteries infrequently affect the extramural coronary arteries. Admittedly, there are dissenting opinions on this point; in our experience, however, this intramural-extramural difference does appear to hold. In the 107 patients studied, none had significant abnormalities of the intramural coronary arteries.

It would appear that the intramural coronary arteries are somehow protected from intimal proliferation and luminal narrowing by the contracting adjacent myocardium. Even in the presence of systemic hypertension the intramural coronary arteries remain normal or virtually normal; perhaps this is because they are not exposed

to systemic systolic pressures, since they are perfused mainly in ventricular diastole. The contracting myocardium may further lower intraluminal pressure in these small vessels. It may seem puzzling that the intramural arteries remain free of significant coronary atherosclerosis, but there is no doubt that they do. A typical finding: Epicardial branches of major extramural arteries showing almost total luminal narrowing by atherosclerotic plaques suddenly were seen to be wide open as they penetrated the myocardium.

It cannot be assumed that any part of the extramural coronary arterial tree is entirely normal, but some sites are more predisposed to severe narrowing than are others. Typically, in our patients, maximal narrowing of the left anterior descending and left circumflex arteries was found to occur within 2 cm of the bifurcation of the left main coronary artery; in the right coronary artery, the proximal and midportions tended to show greater degrees of luminal narrowing by old plaques than did the distal portion, but this was not always the case. It is worth noting that the main function of the right coronary artery is to supply the posterior wall of the left ventricle via its posterior descending branches; it begins perfusing the left ventricle only after traversing the right atrioventricular sulcus for about 12 cm. Thus, significant narrowing of the right coronary artery 11 cm from its aortic ostium may be as important functionally as similar narrowing much closer to its aortic ostium. In contrast, since the left coronary arterial tree begins supplying the left ventricle about 2 cm from its aortic origin, marked narrowing of the left anterior descending artery far downstream may be of little myocardial consequence if significant proximal narrowing is not present. Since arterial thrombi tended to develop at or proximal to a site of severe luminal narrowing, thrombi in the left anterior descending or left circumflex arteries were usually within 2 cm of the bifurcation of the left main. In the right coronary artery, they occurred with about equal frequency in the proximal, middle, and distal portions.

Almost always, if a thrombus was present in fatal acute myocardial infarction, it was located in the coronary

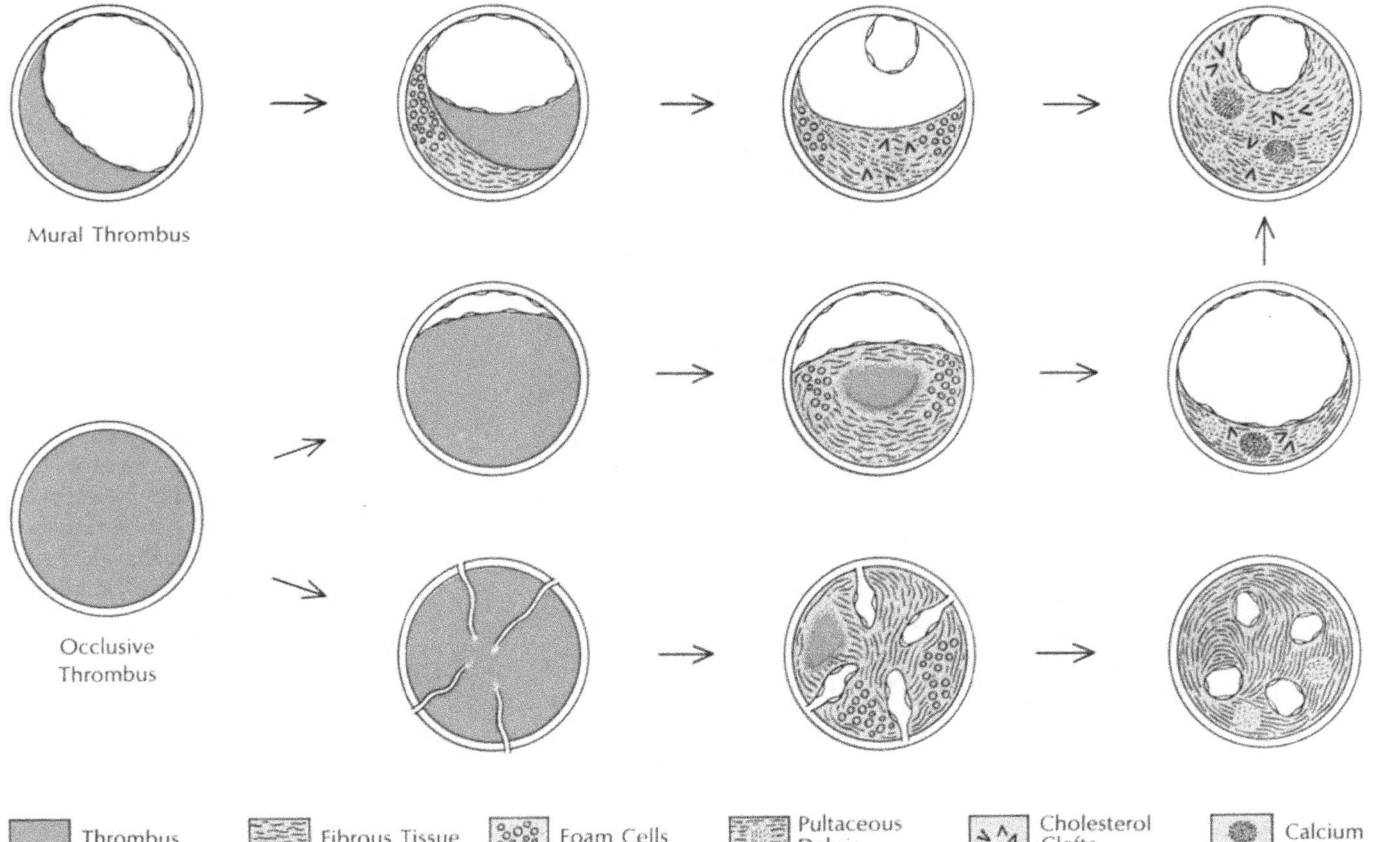

Thesis that both mural and occlusive thrombi may be incorporated into arterial intima as plaques is posed in diagram of postulated sequence of events in formation of both thrombus types. Organization of mural thrombi, beginning with ingrowth of overlying endothelial cells and connective tissue, leads to formation of atherosclerotic-type lesions. An occlusive thrombus may organize similarly; alternatively, capillaries growing into its base may dilate as thrombus retracts, resulting in plaque with recanalized channels.

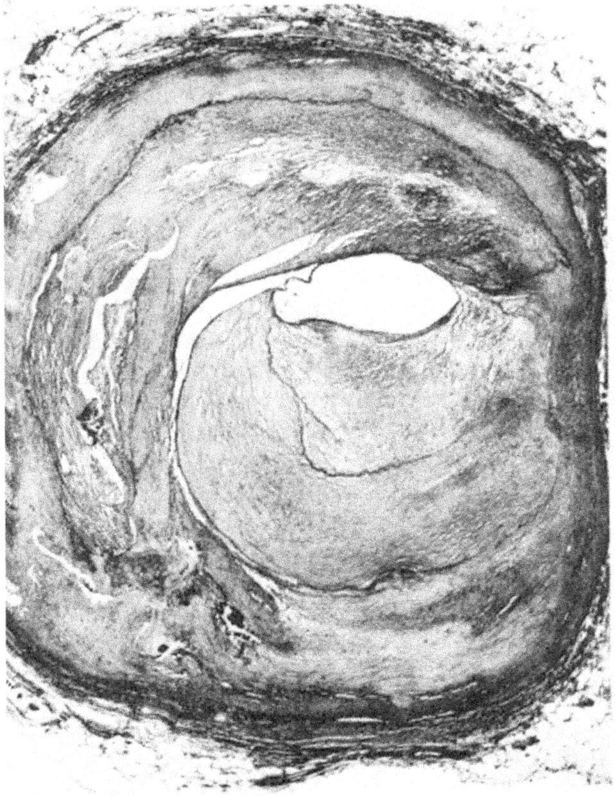

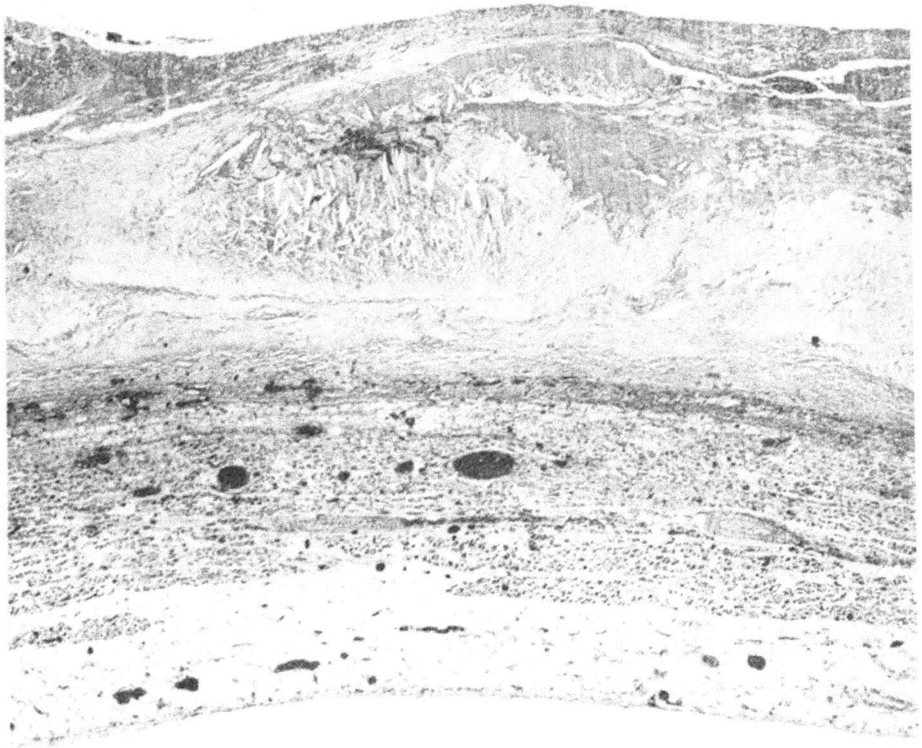

Section of right coronary artery of 65-year-old man (left) shows extensive atherosclerotic plaquing and almost total luminal narrowing. Demarcation lines suggest plaques are of varying ages.

Right: Cholesterol clefts, pultaceous debris, and calcific deposits – key components of arterial atherosclerotic plaques – were all present in left atrial thrombus in patient with mitral stenosis.

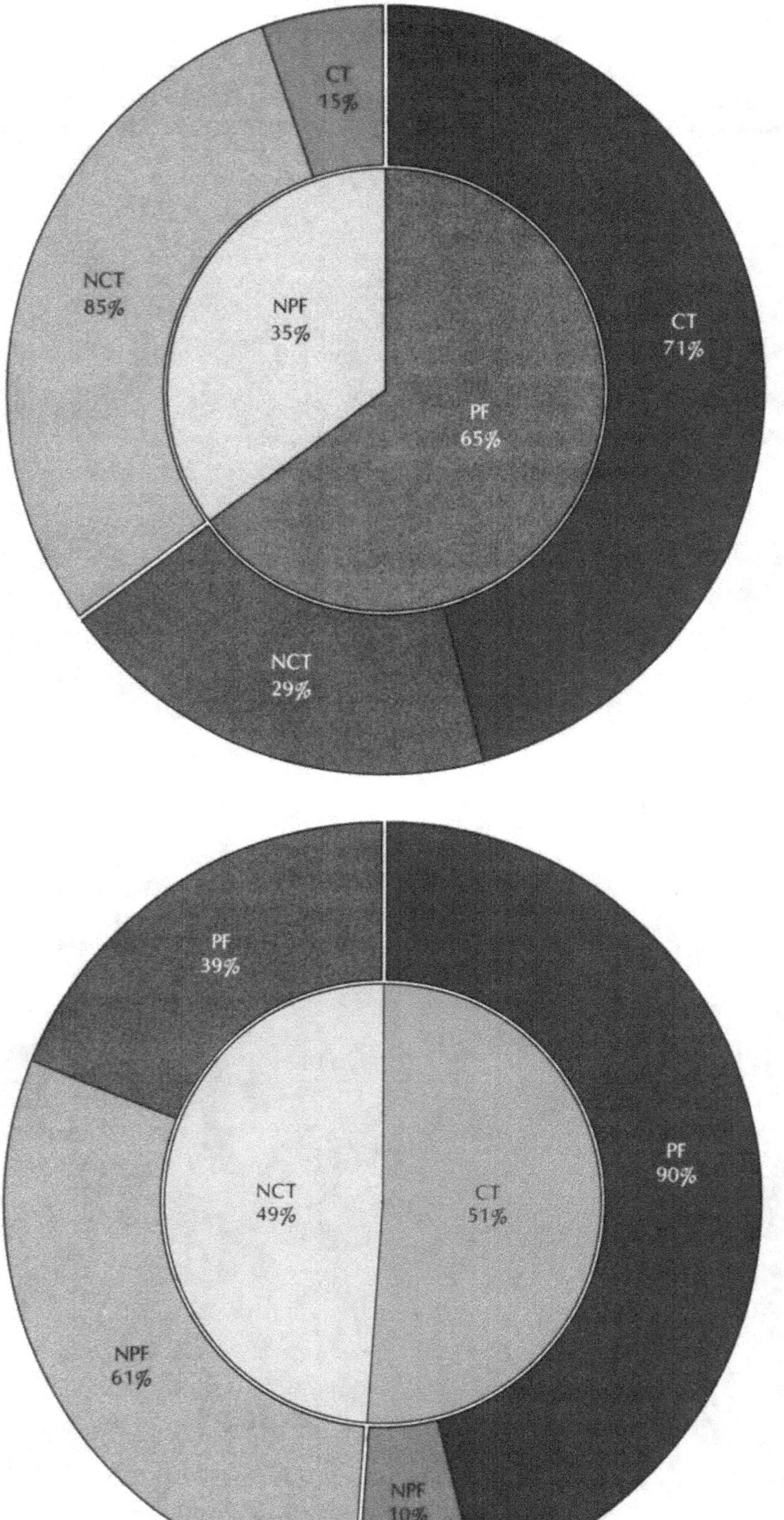

PF = Power Failure
NPF = No Power Failure

CT = Coronary Thrombus
NCT = No Coronary Thrombus

In an analysis by Walston and coworkers, coronary thrombus formation proved clearly related to the occurrence of power failure, as shown in upper diagram; among cases with thrombosis, fully 90% were associated with power failure (lower diagram). Relationship suggests a severely diminished cardiac output may be needed for thrombus formation.

artery that supplied the infarcted area. Thus, in infarction involving the anterior wall of the left ventricle, the anterior descending coronary artery was the site of thrombus formation, while posterior wall infarction was associated with thrombosis of the right coronary artery.

It is noteworthy that in previous studies relating coronary arterial thrombosis to acute myocardial infarction the condition of the artery distal to the thrombus has not been considered. The focus of attention has been on the coronary arterial segment containing the thrombus; a number of investigators have carefully examined this portion of the vessel by serial sectioning techniques. Usually the inquiry has stopped there, implying that finding a fresh arterial thrombus more or less establishes its functional significance.

But if a coronary artery is already severely narrowed distally – and in nearly all the patients we studied in whom thrombi were found the degree of distal luminal narrowing was severe, greater than 75% – the significance of a proximal thrombus must be sharply questioned. That distal narrowing was found in so many of the patients we studied was an important influence moving us to consider thrombus formation more likely the result than the cause of acute infarction. The same inference has been drawn by others from comparisons of the histologic ages of coronary thrombi and of acute myocardial infarcts. Since it is difficult to judge the age of a coronary thrombus histologically, this approach is not reliable.

Nonetheless, several observations, some already alluded to, strongly suggest that fresh coronary thrombi present at death develop only after the myocardial necrotic process is already under way. Not the least of these is the fact that coronary thrombi do not occur in all patients with acute myocardial infarction. The clinical events in fatal cases may hold the explanation. When Spain and Bradess examined the clinical courses in some 400 fatal cases, they found that in general the longer the interval between onset of symptoms and death, the greater the likelihood of coronary arterial thrombus formation. Thus the incidence of thrombi increased from 17% among

(continued on page 101)

patients surviving less than an hour to 36% in patients surviving one to eight hours, and 54% in patients who survived 24 hours or more before death. This finding would indicate that a certain but variable period of survival must elapse after onset of myocardial necrosis in order for an arterial thrombus to form, although it does not identify the factors that influence thrombus formation.

Whether severely decreased coronary flow leads directly to formation of arterial thrombi remains to be established; from the evidence it does seem a possibility worth exploring further. If valid, the slow-flow hypothesis would have to account for occurrence of arterial thrombi at sites of, and proximal to, severe stenosis caused by old atherosclerotic plaques. Sometimes thrombi can be seen covering cracks in plaques and it has been suggested by some that rupture of the innermost layer of plaque may precipitate arterial thrombosis. The evidence given is that rupture occurs particularly in fibrous tissue covering deposits of pultaceous debris; this leads to discharge of necrotic material into the arterial lumen or to bleeding into plaques. The abrupt change in volume of the plaque caused by discharge of plaque material into the lumen or from hemorrhage into the plaque via the rupture causes abnormalities in flow patterns favoring platelet thrombosis, it is further suggested.

However, the postulated relationship between rupture of necrotic plaques and formation of coronary arterial thrombi has yet to be confirmed. Observing cracks in plaques requires serial sectioning techniques, and even when these are done interpretation may be difficult. In our studies, most thrombi formed over plaques with intact surfaces. It should be borne in mind too that rupture of a plaque may sometimes result from cutting an artery and fixing it without prior support of its wall. When Fulton and coworkers injected coronary arteries with a solid supporting medium before sectioning, no plaque ulceration or cracking was observed in the 25 cases of coronary heart disease (14 of acute myocardial infarction) that were studied.

Even with our limited understand-

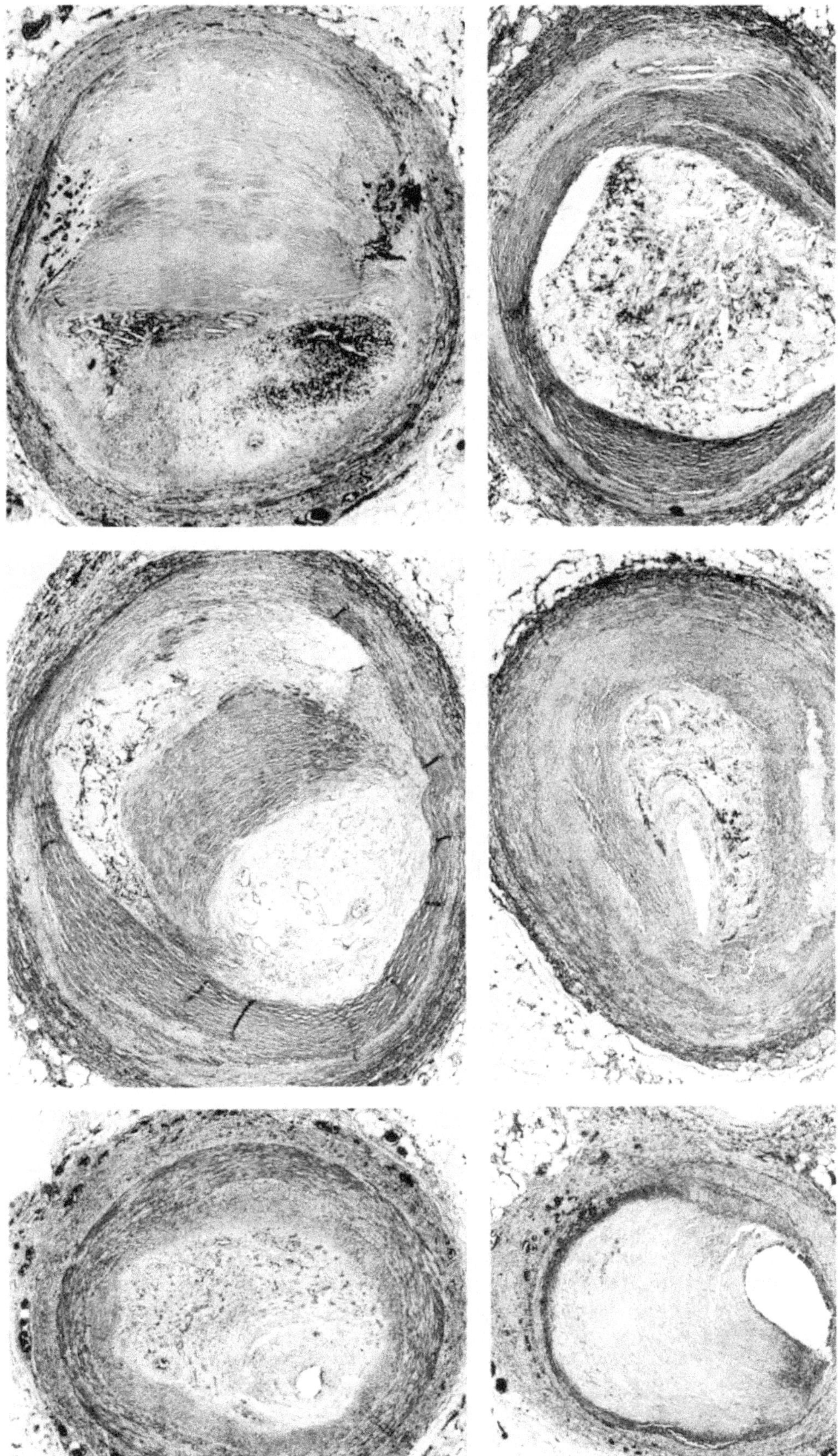

These six sections were taken from a 2 cm segment of the posterior descending artery of a 49-year-old man who died suddenly. A year earlier, this patient had suffered an acute posterior wall infarction. Atherosclerotic plaques apparent in all sections vary greatly in composition. Hemorrhage has occurred into several plaques.

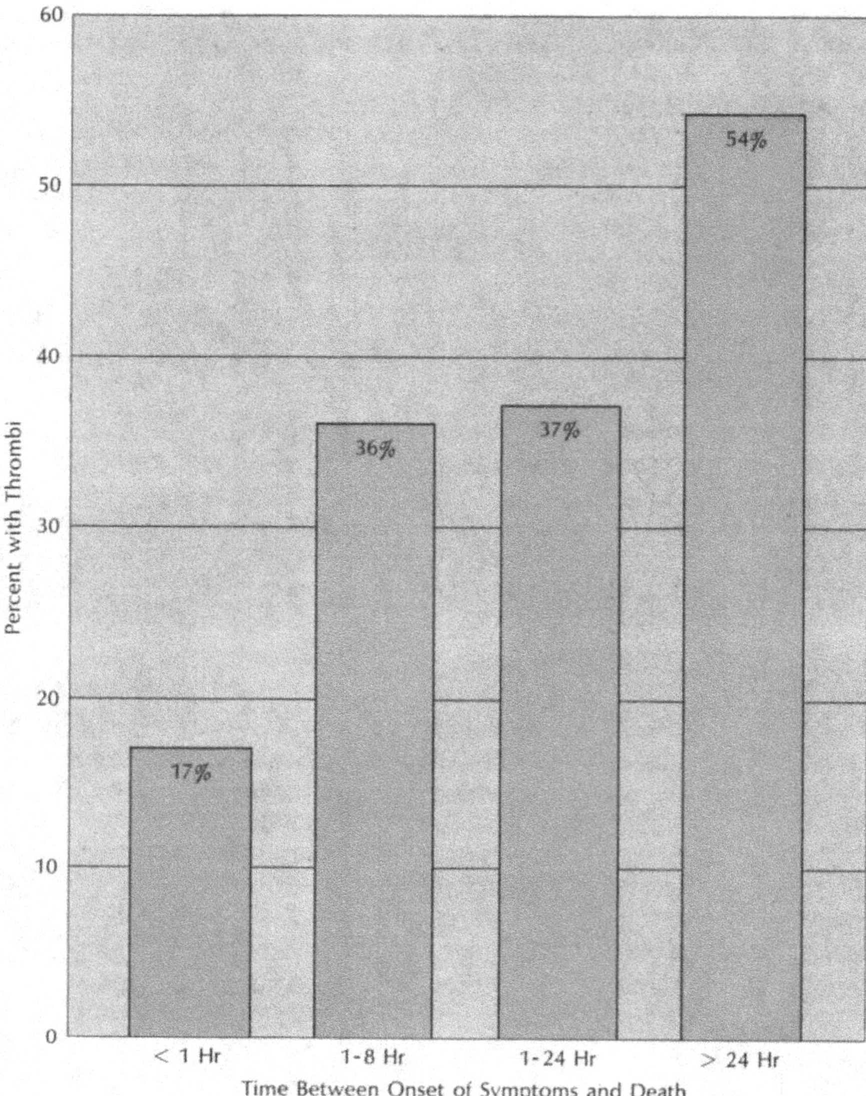

Thrombus formation proved closely related to survival time in close to 400 fatal infarction cases studied by Spain and Bradess; thus incidence of thrombi increased from 17% in patients who survived less than an hour to 54% in those who lived 24 hours or more.

ing of conditions favoring formation of arterial thrombi it is now clear that we must look elsewhere for the events that precipitate myocardial necrosis. But if thrombus formation is not the critical factor, what is? We know that fatal acute myocardial infarction is associated with diffuse coronary artery disease that presumably has been progressing for some time prior to the acute episode. Against this setting, is it possible that even minor disturbances in coronary artery perfusion could shift the balance from adequate to inadequate flow, producing ischemia and necrosis in myocardium? Perhaps one additional pin on the elephant's back, so to speak, is all that is required to tip the scales.

Another question: Is it possible that although thrombosis appears not to be a precipitating cause of acute infarction, it figures in the early development of coronary atherosclerosis? This possibility would return coronary thrombosis very much to the center of the stage, though in a very different role than that of curtain ringer. Despite the apparent paradox, the most logical explanation of atherosclerotic plaquing does seem to be the laying down and organization of mural thrombi.

As is known, atherosclerotic lesions may be primarily fatty (yellow) or fibrous in composition, or may be "complicated" plaques usually composed of cholesterol clefts, pultaceous debris, calcific deposits, and few, if any, foam cells. The atherosclerotic

plaques in coronary arteries in fatal acute myocardial infarction are chiefly of the complicated type. Routinely seen in extramural coronary arteries in the patients we examined, they were never present in intramural coronary arteries. That formation and organization of mural thrombi contribute significantly to development of these complicated atherosclerotic plaques is supported, for one, by the presence of fibrin and platelets, both thrombus constituents, in the plaques. This has been demonstrated by immunofluorescent techniques; fibrin has also been shown both histologically and by electron microscopy. To strengthen the relationship, there is the finding of atherosclerotic-type lesions (containing cholesterol clefts, foam cells, pultaceous debris, and calcific deposits) in organized thrombi, such as those found in the left atrium in mitral stenosis.

The possibility that atherosclerotic plaques may be thrombus derived has been discounted in part because histologic evidence is often obscured. As a thrombus becomes covered by a new endothelium, the underlying endothelium is replaced by connective tissue from the intima and the original line of demarcation disappears.

Recent findings suggest that organization of thrombi occurs by ingrowth of overlying endothelial cells and connective tissue; modified smooth muscle cells capable of synthesizing collagen, elastin, and probably mucopolysaccharides – all present in connective tissue of arterial intima – then invade the bases of attached thrombi. Although small mural thrombi usually organize by an avascular process, larger mural thrombi become vascularized; capillaries from the new overlying endothelium provide a direct blood supply from the lumen and from vasa vasorum penetrating thrombi at their bases. With an increased blood supply, enhanced fibrinolysis may contribute to the resolution of the thrombus as it becomes organized. The capillaries may later atrophy or they may become a source of hemorrhage into plaques.

It appears that both occlusive and nonocclusive (mural) thrombi may be incorporated into the arterial intima as atherosclerotic plaques. However, occlusive thrombi that retract before endothelialization is complete may appear later as mural or nonocclusive plaques.

The source of lipids in atherosclerotic plaques is of course a matter of great interest. Among other findings, the fact that fatty degeneration can occur in any thrombus suggests that thrombus components, such as platelets and erythrocytes, may contribute to lipid accumulation. The erythrocyte component of thrombi contains less lipid than does the platelet component; nonetheless, repeated hemorrhages might lead to accumulation of considerable amounts of lipid, especially cholesterol. Lipoproteins present in both fresh and organizing thrombi also contribute to lipid accumulation in atherosclerotic plaques.

Experimental findings lend support to the view that thrombosis may be important in development of atherosclerosis: When whole blood clots are injected into systemic veins of rabbits, fibrous intimal plaques containing little lipid form in pulmonary arteries; thromboemboli, at first occlusive, organize by retracting into eccentric plaques. Injection of platelet-rich thrombi rather than whole blood clots results in typical atherosclerotic plaque formation, with plaques containing foam cells and calcific deposits.

As our histologic studies have made clear, atherosclerotic plaques are much like fingerprints—no two are completely alike. Indeed, our examination of the coronary arterial tree revealed tremendous variation in the composition of adjacent plaques. Whereas some contained lipid and large quantities of pultaceous debris, others were composed primarily of fibrous tissue. Differences in composition of atherosclerotic plaques may be explained in part on the basis of differences in composition of underlying thrombi.

It is known, for example, that mixed white and red thrombi tend to form plaques that contain some foam cells but fewer than do plaques derived chiefly from platelet-rich or white thrombi. Occlusive platelet thrombi undergoing transformation to fibrofatty plaques usually do not accumulate fibrin, whereas mural platelet thrombi are usually partially or totally replaced by fibrin before undergoing organization; consequently the plaques that form are chiefly fibromuscular.

Enough may have been said con-

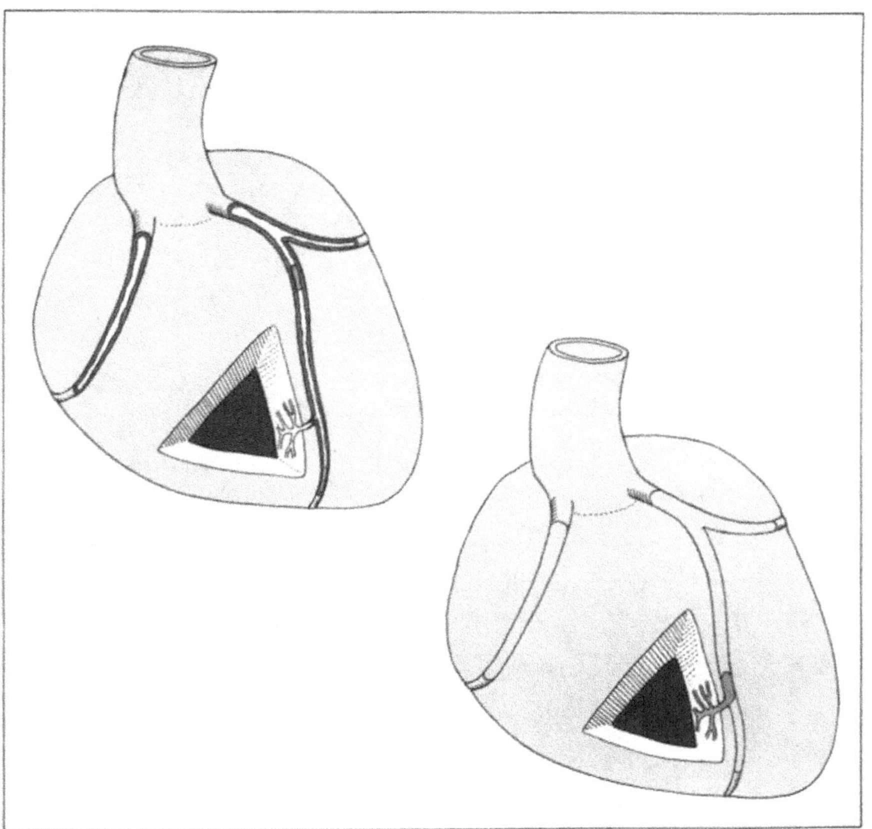

Key differences between coronary arterial thrombosis (left) and embolism (right), as diagrammed above, include the distal occurrence of the latter and its extension into intramural arteries. In addition, the coronary tree is usually devoid of atherosclerotic plaquing.

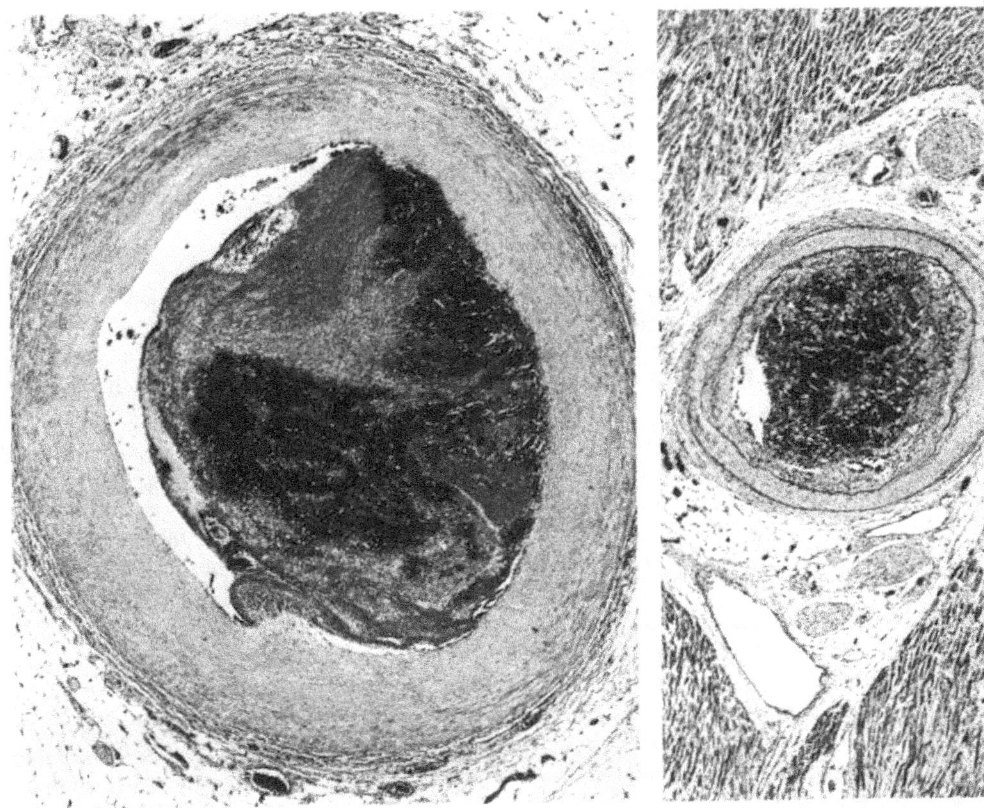

Extension of an arterial embolus to intramural vessels is shown in section of the left anterior descending artery (left) and its intramural branches (right) in man who died of anteroseptal wall infarction. No significant old atherosclerotic plaque is present.

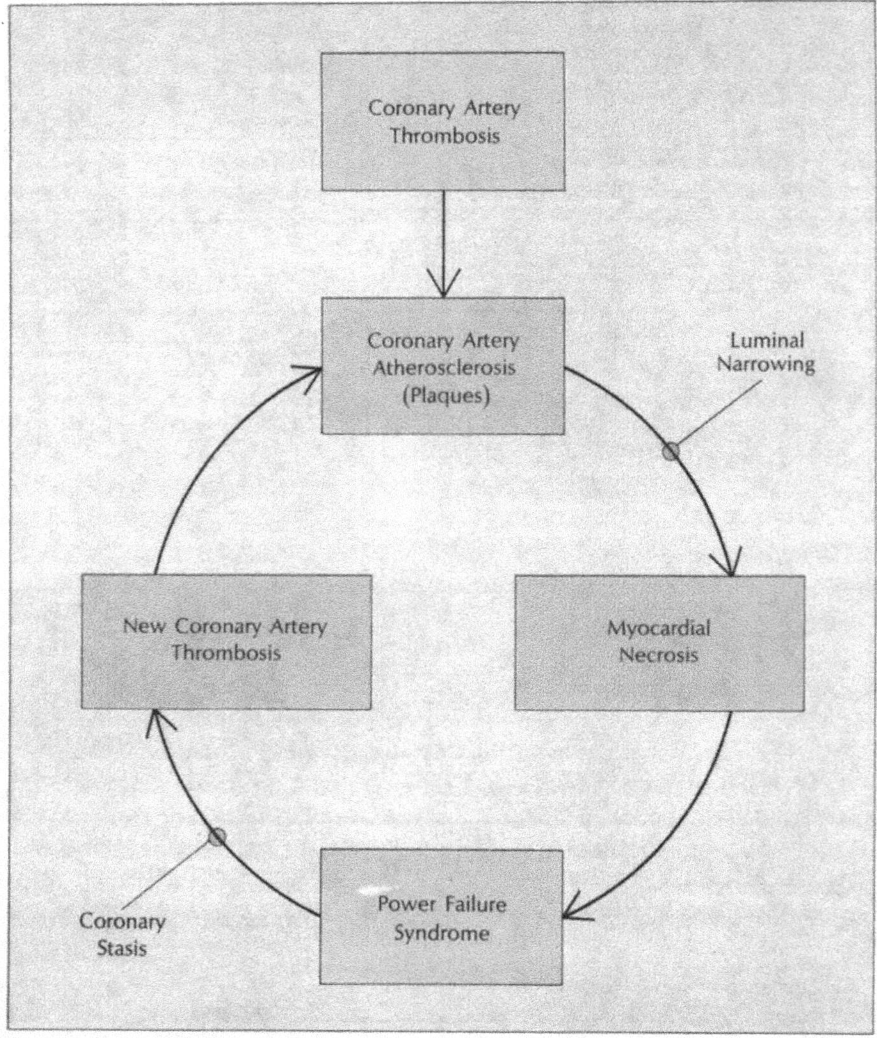

Postulated relationship of coronary artery thrombosis to acute myocardial infarction includes the possibility of a primary role in development of atherosclerosis; in addition, thrombus formation at the time of infarction appears linked to the occurrence of power failure, suggesting that coronary stasis may be required for thrombosis.

cerning a possible relationship of thrombosis to atherogenesis to suggest that it warrants much more investigation. This leaves still unanswered, however, the question of what precipitates acute myocardial infarction. If not arterial thrombosis, then what? Although the answer is unknown, possibly coronary arterial embolism may be involved on rare occasions.

Admittedly, coronary arterial emboli occur far less frequently than arterial thrombi in acute myocardial infarction. (Only three emboli vs 39 arterial thrombi were found in our 107 patients.) Nonetheless, coronary arterial embolism may occur more often than is generally recognized. The presence of a clot in the distal portion of a major extramural coronary artery should suggest embolism and not thrombosis; the latter is more often located proximally in the arterial tree. The two can be more accurately distinguished if the following and other differences are kept in mind: In coronary arterial embolism the clot usually extends into the small epicardial branches of major extramural arteries and into intramural coronary vessels as well. As indicated earlier, in thrombosis the intramural coronary arteries are uninvolved and the small epicardial branches of extramural arteries are less often affected than the major vessels themselves. A key distinction is that in the presence of arterial embolism the extramural coronary tree is relatively free of old atherosclerotic plaques while, as we have seen, quite the opposite is true in cases of arterial thrombosis. Also, patients with arterial emboli are usually relatively young in comparison with those with thrombosis. Predisposing factors such as the presence of arrhythmias, infective endocarditis, and intracardial mural thrombosis should also suggest that an arterial clot is embolic in origin.

Actually, in studies to date concerning acute myocardial infarction the thrust has been essentially descriptive, aimed at recording significant clinical events and anatomic findings associated with acute myocardial ischemia and necrosis. More quantitative anatomic information is needed. It would be useful, for example, to have more accurate data on the composition of arterial thrombi, in hope of explaining why they often differ distally and proximally; why some consist almost entirely of fibrin, others of red cells and a few fibrin strands; why some contain few platelets and others many. Also, quantitative data on the size of myocardial infarcts would be useful. The area of myocardial necrosis weighs how many grams compared with the weight of the non-necrotic or fibrotic left ventricular myocardium? What percent of left ventricular myocardium needs to remain intact for survival? What percent of necrotic myocardium is fatal?

Another question is why cardiogenic shock and congestive failure develop in some cases of acute myocardial infarction and not in others. The answer may relate primarily to the amount of myocardium infarcted: the larger the infarct the greater the likelihood of reduced cardiac output, reduced blood flow, and pump failure. Recently, Page and associates showed that in patients with fatal acute myocardial infarction associated with shock, more than 40% of the left ventricular myocardium was either necrotic or fibrotic, and in patients without shock, less than 35% of the left ventricular wall was destroyed. The likelihood of thrombus formation is known to be increased with increasing infarct size; perhaps the occurrence of arterial thrombosis in patients with acute transmural infarction complicated by shock or congestive heart failure can be explained on this basis.

The major question centers on the relative roles of thrombosis and lipids in development and progression of coronary atherosclerosis. □

Coronary Arteries in Fatal Acute Myocardial Infarction

By William C. Roberts, M.D.

SUMMARY

The coronary arteries are diffusely involved by atherosclerotic plaques in fatal acute myocardial infarction (AMI). The degree of luminal narrowing may vary but plaques are present in practically every millimeter of extramural coronary artery. Usually the lumens of at least two of the three major coronary arteries are narrowed >75% by old plaques in patients who die suddenly (<6 hours) from cardiac disease with or without myocardial necrosis. Coronary thrombi occur in about 10% of patients who die suddenly or in whom necrosis is limited to the left ventricular subendocardium, and in about 50% of patients with transmural myocardial necrosis. Coronary thrombi usually indicate the presence of shock or congestive heart failure or both during the development of myocardial necrosis. The infrequency of coronary thrombi in patients dying suddenly of cardiac disease and in those with transmural necrosis who never have shock or congestive heart failure suggests that the thrombi may be consequences rather than causes of AMI.

Although it may not precipitate AMI, coronary thrombosis may still be the underlying cause of the atherosclerosis. The finding of fibrin deposits in old atherosclerotic plaques and the findings of atherosclerotic-type lesions (cholesterol clefts, foam cells, pultaceous debris, calcific deposits) in organized known thrombi (as in the left atrium in mitral stenosis) suggest a strong relationship between thrombosis and atherosclerosis.

Coronary arterial emboli are not rare; they are located in distal portions of the coronary tree and are present in the small epicardial branches as well as in intramural coronary arteries. In contrast, coronary thrombi are located in proximal portions of major extramural vessels, are infrequent in the small epicardial branches, and are absent in intramural coronary arteries. Coronary atherosclerosis is limited to the extramural coronary arteries and spares the intramural coronary arteries.

Additional Indexing Words:

Atherosclerosis	Coronary thrombosis	Coronary hemorrhages	Shock
Congestive cardiac failure	Coronary embolism	Intramural coronary arteries	

T HIS PAPER focuses attention on the coronary arteries in fatal acute myocardial infarction (AMI) and attempts to present evidence that the following conclusions about this condition are valid: (1) that the extramural coronary arteries are diffusely involved by old atherosclerotic plaques; (2) that thrombi in extramural coronary arteries are infrequent in patients dying suddenly and in those with only subendocardial necrosis; (3) that thrombi, when found in extramural coronary arteries in transmural infarction, generally indicate the presence of pump failure for some time before death; (4) that thrombi in coronary arteries usually are located at, and just proximal to, sites already severely narrowed by old atherosclerotic plaques; (5) that although coronary arterial thrombi do not appear to precipitate AMI, thrombosis, nevertheless, may cause the underlying atherosclerosis; (6) that coronary atherosclerosis does not involve intramural coronary arteries; and (7) that coronary arterial emboli are not rare and that their pathology is usually distinctive.

From the Section of Pathology, National Heart and Lung Institute, National Institutes of Health, Bethesda, Maryland.

Diffuse Nature of Extramural Coronary Arterial Atherosclerosis in Fatal AMI

The extramural coronary arteries are diffusely involved by old atherosclerotic plaques in patients dying of AMI[1] (figs. 1 and 2). The degree of luminal narrowing varies, but some plaques are present on the intimal surface of virtually every millimeter of major artery. The extent of the coronary arterial atherosclerotic process in fatal AMI was dramatically demonstrated to Roberts and Buja by examination of three histologic sections in every 5-mm segment of the entire left main, left anterior descending, left circumflex, and right coronary arteries.[1] Of several thousand histologic sections of coronary arteries examined in 74 patients with transmural necrosis, in nine patients with subendocardial necrosis and in 24 patients who died suddenly (<6 hours after onset of symptoms, but with no myocardial necrosis), only four sections (excluding those in three patients with coronary arterial emboli) were free of old atherosclerotic plaques. A coronary artery, however, may contain a considerable amount of atherosclerosis and yet be capable of transporting substantial quantities of blood to the myocardium. When the degree of coronary narrowing decreases the original lumen by more than 75%, the flow in the vessel is significantly decreased. In the carotid artery, a detectable reduction in flow and pressure does not occur until the degree of luminal narrowing is $>80\%$.[2] Among the 107 necropsy patients studied by Roberts and Buja, the average number of major coronary arteries (three per patient, excluding the left main) narrowed $>75\%$ by old atherosclerotic plaques were: 2.4 in 74 patients with transmural necrosis; 2.1 in nine patients with only subendocardial necrosis; and 2.4 in 24 patients who died suddenly. Similar observations had been made by Saphir and associates,[3] Blumgart et al.[4] and Yater et al.[5] who found "complete occlusions" of usually two major coronary arteries in patients dying with angina pectoris or of AMI. The degree of coronary arterial luminal narrowing by old atherosclerotic plaques is identical in patients with fatal AMI who have coronary thrombi and in those without coronary thrombi.[6]

The sites of maximal narrowing of major extramural coronary arteries are highly variable from patient to patient, but certain patterns emerge when large groups of patients with fatal AMI are examined. The lumen of the left main coronary artery is infrequently narrowed $>75\%$ by old atherosclerotic plaques. In two of the 107 patients studied by Roberts and Buja this vessel was narrowed to this degree. Maximal narrowing of the left anterior descending and left circumflex coronary arteries is usually within 2 cm of the bifurcation of the left main artery. The proximal and midportions of the right coronary artery also appear to be predisposed to greater degrees of luminal narrowing by old plaques than does the distal portion. The main function of the right coronary artery is to supply the posterior wall of left ventricle via its posterior descending branches. Thus, narrowing of the right coronary artery at any site proximal to the origins of the posterior descending branches might have similar functional significance. In other words, the left coronary arterial tree begins supplying the left ventricle with oxygen about 2 cm from its origin from the aorta; the right coronary artery does not begin perfusing the left ventricle until it has traveled in the right atrioventricular sulcus for about 12 cm. Thus, severe narrowing of the right coronary artery 11 cm from its aortic ostium might be as significant a lesion as a similar narrowing 2 cm from its ostium. In contrast, severe narrowing of the left anterior descending coronary artery 11 cm downstream without significant proximal narrowing may have minor myocardial consequences.

Atherosclerotic lesions generally have been classified into three types:[7] (1) yellow (fatty) streaks or dots; (2) fibrous plaques; and (3) complicated plaques. The latter plaques contain calcific deposits, cholesterol clefts, thrombus, or all three, and they may ulcerate (into the arterial lumen) or weaken the vessel wall so that it dilates. The atherosclerotic plaques

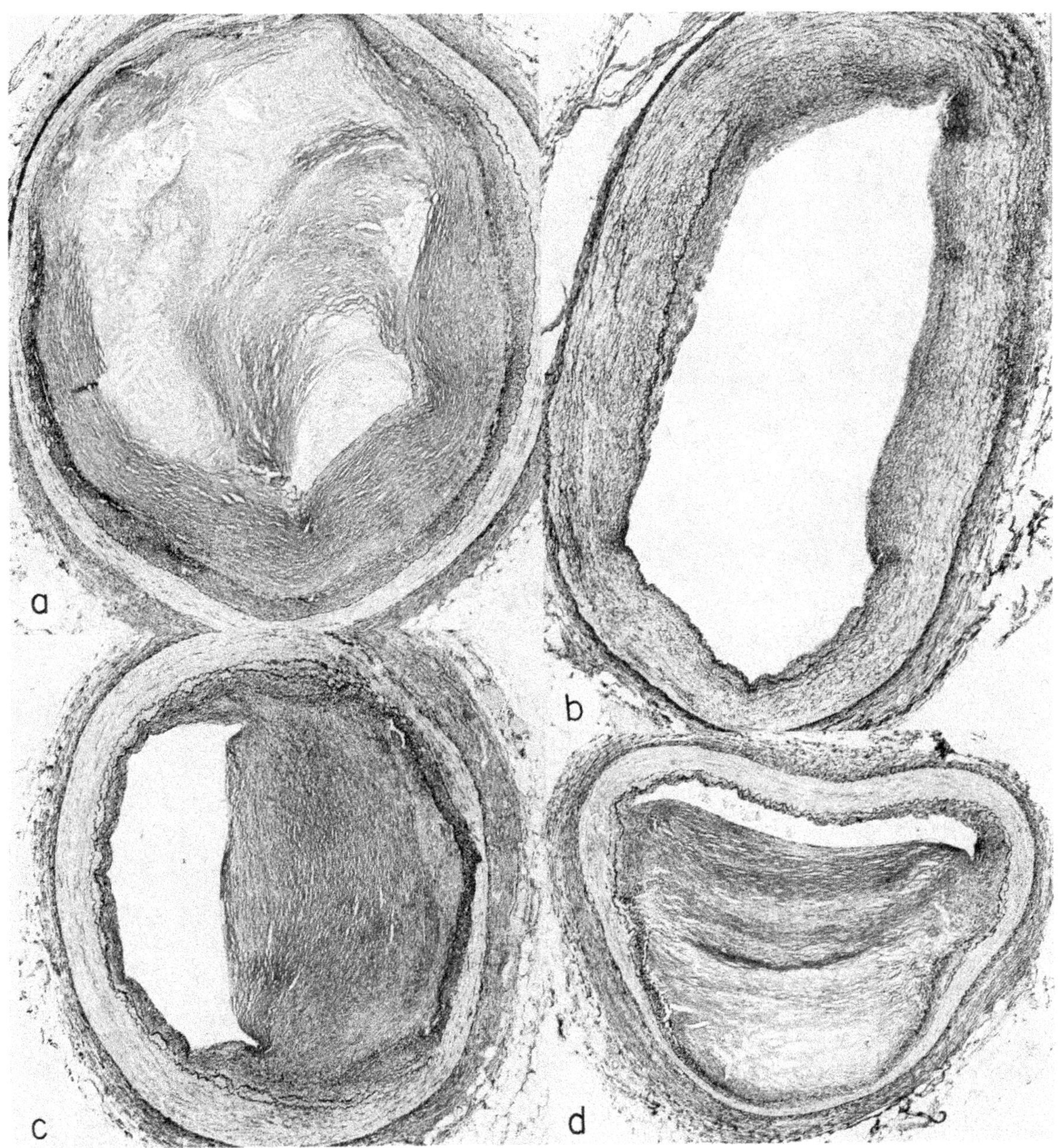

Figure 1

Major extramural coronary arteries at site of maximal narrowing in a 54-year-old woman (SH#A4571) who died suddenly at home. She had had angina pectoris for several years but never a myocardial infarct or congestive cardiac failure. At autopsy, the heart weighed 300 g, and no foci of myocardial necrosis or fibrosis were present. (a) Right coronary artery 3 cm from the aortic ostium. The lumen is >90% obliterated. (b) Left main artery. (c) Left circumflex artery in the first 1 cm. (d) Left anterior descending artery 3 cm from the bifurcation of the left main artery. The luminal narrowing in each vessel is due entirely to old plaques. No thrombi or hemorrhages into plaques were found. (Elastic van Gieson stains, each × 31.)

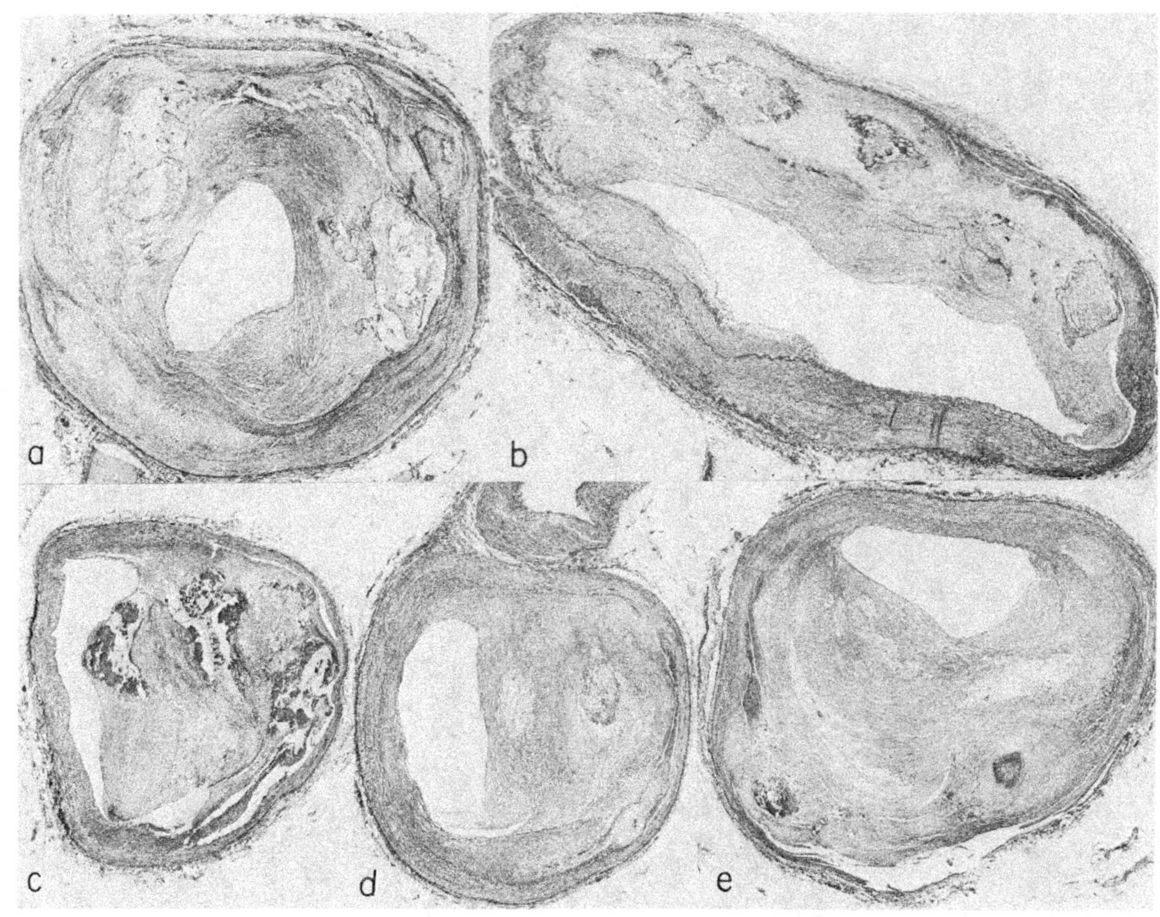

Figure 2

Major coronary arteries at sites of maximal narrowing in a 71-year-old man (SH#A4489) who died suddenly of left ventricular free-wall rupture 9 days after onset of acute myocardial infarction. At no time during his life was congestive cardiac failure or shock noted. At autopsy, the heart weighed 390 g, and no thrombi or hemorrhages were observed in the coronary arteries. (a) Right artery. (b) Left main artery. (c) Left marginal artery. (d) Left circumflex artery. (e) Left anterior descending artery. The major arteries (excluding left main and left marginal) were narrowed >75% by old plaques. (Movat stains, each × 20.)

observed in extramural coronary arteries in fatal AMI are of the complicated type. Significant degrees of coronary arterial luminal narrowing do not result from foam-cell lesions alone, except possibly in patients with type III hyperlipoproteinemia.[8] In most complicated plaques few foam cells are present and the luminal narrowing is caused primarily by fibrous tissue, with or without calcific deposits, and pultaceous debris (presumably the end result of the breakdown of foam cells). Why calcific deposits are absent in coronary arteries of some patients with fatal AMI and extensive in others is unknown. Calcific deposits in these vessels increase with age (>95% of patients in the U.S.A. >80 years of age have coronary arterial calcific deposits[9]), and these deposits are more frequent and extensive in patients with systemic hypertension as compared to normotensive patients.[9] Patients with diabetes mellitus also appear to have larger and more extensive coronary calcific deposits than non-diabetics.

Incidence and Significance of Coronary Arterial Thrombi in Fatal AMI

AMI is generally considered to result from thrombotic occlusion of a major extramural coronary artery. Indeed, *coronary thrombosis* was the name applied originally and used for years to describe AMI both clinically and pathologically. Although many clinicians and pathologists expect to find a thrombus in a coronary artery in fatal AMI, the reported incidence of such thrombosis has varied from 7 to 91%.[1, 3, 10–30] Inclusion of cases of subendocardial infarction and sudden death ("acute cardiovascular collapse in the absence of acute myocardial necrosis")[31] with cases of transmural infarction may be the major cause for the variation in incidence.

Coronary arterial thrombi are infrequent in patients who die suddenly with or without previous histories of cardiac disease and in those with only subendocardial necrosis (limited to the inner one half of the myocardium). Among 24 patients who died suddenly (<6 hours from onset of symptoms) studied by Roberts and Buja[1] two (8%) had a thrombus in a coronary artery; and of nine patients with only subendocardial necrosis, none had coronary arterial thrombus. It contrast, of 74 patients with transmural myocardial necrosis studied in a similar manner by the same authors, 40 (54%) had a thrombus in a coronary artery.

A true thrombus is adherent to the surface of the artery bordering the lumen, and it is composed of platelets or fibrin or both and usually also of erythrocytes and leukocytes. Coronary arterial thrombi are usually about 1 cm in length, and although they are adherent distally they may not be adherent proximally. The composition of a thrombus at varying levels may differ; distally it is likely to consist of platelets or fibrin or both (white thrombus), and more proximally it is likely to be composed of erythrocytes, lesser quantities of fibrin, few platelets, and some leukocytes (red thrombus). Early thrombi may be composed purely of platelets, and they are usually small and nonocclusive.

Thrombi occurring in patients dying of AMI are, except in cases of embolism, superimposed on old atherosclerotic plaques (fig. 3). Usually the artery containing the thrombus is $>50\%$ narrowed already by old atherosclerotic plaques and frequently the degree of luminal narrowing is $>75\%$ at the distal attachment. In nearly all patients with fatal AMI and coronary arterial thrombi the lumen of the artery distal to the thrombus is $>75\%$ narrowed by old plaques. Of 40 patients with coronary arterial thrombi and fatal transmural AMI studied by Roberts and Buja, the artery distal to the thrombus was already $>75\%$ narrowed by old atherosclerotic plaques in 36 (90%). In three of the remaining four patients, embolism rather than in situ thrombosis was the cause. Although many investigators have examined by serial sections the coronary arterial segment containing the thrombus, the status of the artery distal to the thrombus has been poorly studied until recently[1] (fig. 3). In a few patients studied by Roberts and Buja the thrombus occurred in a segment of artery between two sites of extreme narrowing by old plaques. Experimentally, the site of predilection of a thrombus has been within such a segment or at the beginning of the poststenotic luminal expansion.[32]

Why fresh thrombi are located at sites of narrowing is unclear. Several investigators[1, 3, 6, 33–40] have observed thrombi covering cracks in old atherosclerotic plaques, and some[36–38, 40] have considered rupture of the innermost layer of plaques the important precipitating cause of coronary arterial thrombosis. Ruptures occur particularly in fibrous tissue covering deposits of pultaceous debris and lead to discharge of necrotic debris into the arterial lumens or to bleeding into plaques. The break in the plaque exposes collagen to the flowing blood, and this site is said to be a strong stimulus for platelet accumulation.[41] The sudden change in volume of the plaque by discharge of plaque material into the lumen or from hemorrhage into the plaque via the rupture also creates alterations in flow patterns which favor platelet thrombosis.[36] Jørgensen[6] has suggested that the pathogenesis of coronary thrombi associated

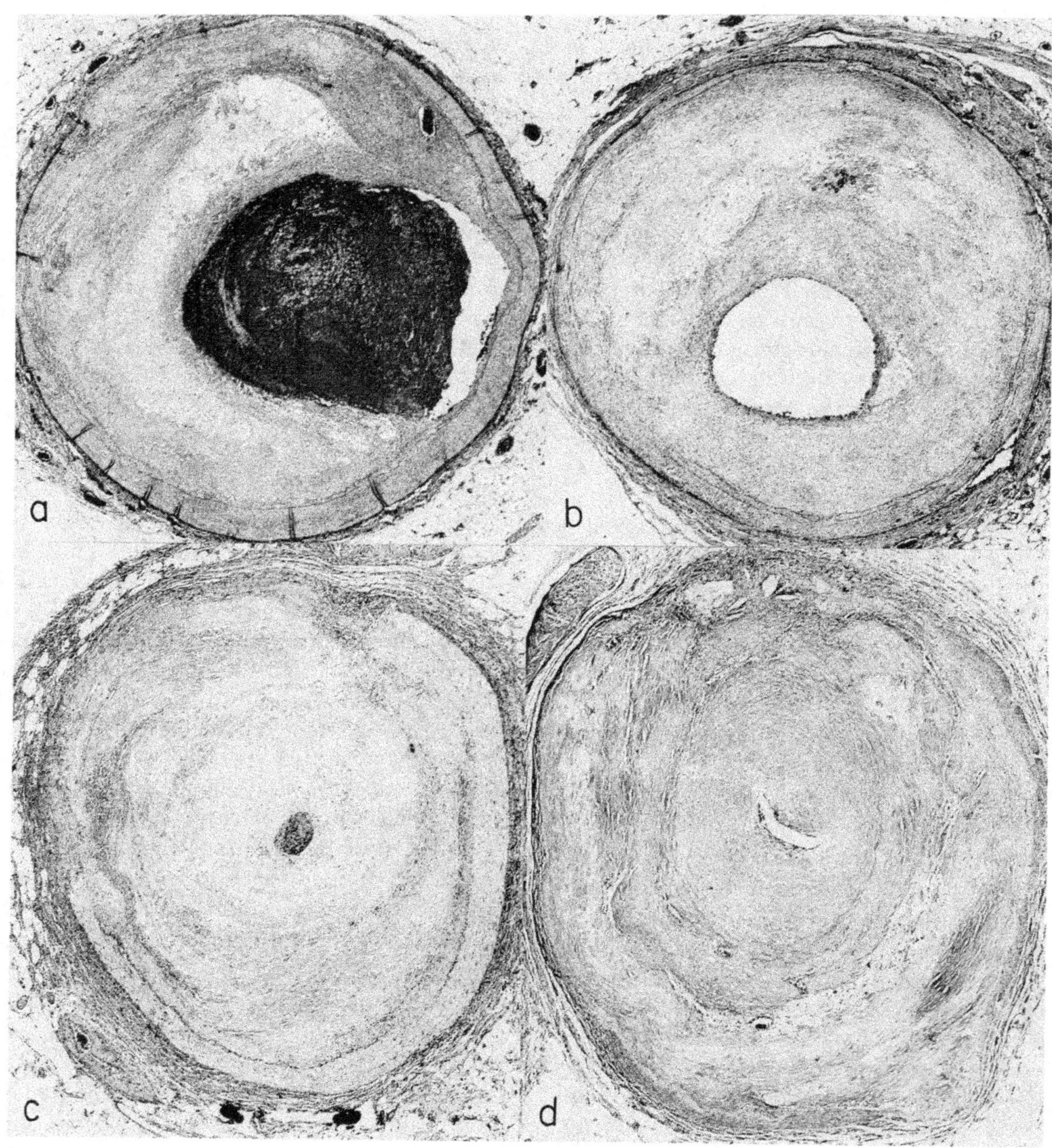

Figure 3

One coronary artery in each of two patients, both of whom had thrombi. (a and b) Left circumflex coronary artery in a 57-year-old woman (A69-131) who died 4 days after onset of acute transmural myocardial infarction. (a) The thrombus is firmly attached to an old plaque. The retraction of the thrombus on one side is an artifact. (b) Distal to the thrombus, the lumen is > 75% narrowed by an old plaque. (Movat stains, each × 21.)

(c and d) Anterior descending coronary artery 6–7 cm from the aortic ostium in a 59-year-old woman (A68-285) who had the onset of acute transmural myocardial infarction 48 hours before death. She had the onset of intermittent chest pain 2 months earlier and systemic hypertension for 10 years. Her final 2 days were characterized by shock, pulmonary edema, and bradycardia. At autopsy, a "massive" anterior-wall infarct, which was aneurysmally dilated, was present. The lumens of all three major coronary arteries were >75% narrowed by old plaques. In addition, a small occluding thrombus was present in the left anterior descend-

with ruptures of necrotic plaques is different from that unassociated with rupture. That coronary arterial thrombi are related to rupture of necrotic plaques, however, is far from proven. Serial sections are usually necessary to observe cracks in plaques, and even by this means interpretation is often difficult. Such cracks were infrequently observed beneath thrombi in the patients studied by Roberts and Buja, and probably most thrombi form over plaques with intact surfaces.[42, 43] Rupture of a plaque may result at times from cutting an artery and fixing it without prior support of its wall by injection. Fulton[43] injected coronary arteries with a solid supporting medium before sectioning, and in few did the intima produce convexity of the lining. In none of his 25 patients who died of coronary heart disease (14 with AMI) was ulceration of a plaque observed. Interpretation of whether a plaque is cracked or, if present, an artifact or real is fraught with too much difficulty, in my opinion, to give this possible mechanism of thrombosis undue weight.

The thrombus in fatal AMI is practically always located in the coronary artery responsible for supplying blood to the myocardium which was made necrotic: i.e., if the infarct involves the anterior wall of the left ventricle, and if a thrombus occurs, it will be located in the anterior descending coronary artery; posterior-wall necrosis is associated with thrombosis of the right coronary artery. When thrombi occur in either the left anterior descending or circumflex coronary arteries, they are usually located within 2 cm of the bifurcation of the left main (or within 4 cm of the left aortic) ostium. The left main artery is virtually never the site of thrombosis. The proximal portion of the right coronary artery, however, does not appear to be a more frequent site of thrombus formation than does the mid- or distal portion. Thrombi are infrequently seen in the small epicardial branches of the major extramural coronary arteries and never occur, other than as platelet aggregates, to my knowledge, in intramural coronary arteries. (See "Coronary Arterial Embolism" below, for comparison.)

Not all coronary arterial thrombi are totally occluding. (The term "occlusion" is not synonymous with "thrombosis" as implied in many reports, since occlusion may be partial as well as complete, and since the vessel may be occluded by material other than that which forms a thrombus.) Partially occluding mural or nonocclusive thrombi were found in seven (18%), and totally occluding (*occlusive*) thrombi in 33 (82%), of 40 patients with thrombi and fatal transmural myocardial necrosis studied by Roberts and Buja. Pure platelet thrombi, as mentioned earlier, are usually small and infrequently totally occlude lumens. Nonocclusive thrombi, since they are small, may have little functional significance. Even totally occluding thrombi when formed in arteries already >90% occluded by old atherosclerotic plaque also may have little functional significance. Thus, it is not enough to know whether or not a coronary artery contains a thrombus. Information regarding the degree of luminal narrowing by an old atherosclerotic plaque at the site of, and distal to, the thrombus, and whether the thrombus is totally or only partially occlusive is required before the significance of a coronary arterial thrombus can be judged.

The role of coronary thrombosis in AMI is unclear. For several decades coronary thrombosis was considered the cause of AMI. Clinically, AMI represents a sudden change for the patient compared to his preinfarction status. This often dramatic clinical event has been equated at autopsy with the finding of a "fresh" thrombus in a coronary artery. However, only about 50% of patients with transmural myocardial necrosis and about 10% of patients with subendocardial necrosis or "sudden cardiovascular collapse without necrosis"

---

ing vessel (c). (Movat stain, × 25.) The percent of narrowing caused by the thrombus is small, however, compared to the percent of narrowing resulting from old atherosclerotic plaques. The lumen distal (d) to the thrombus is already severely narrowed by an old plaque. (Hematoxylin and eosin stain, × 25.)

have a thrombus in a coronary artery at necropsy. Thus, nothing new is found in the coronary arteries in the majority of patients dying of cardiac disease. The lack of finding coronary arterial thrombi in patients dying suddenly of cardiac disease and in only about one half of those with myocardial necrosis has given rise to the concept that coronary arterial thrombi are *consequences* rather than *causes* of AMI. Comparison of histologic ages of coronary arterial thrombi and of acute myocardial infarcts has indicated to some observers[20] that thrombosis follows rather than precedes myocardial necrosis. Judging the age of a coronary thrombus, however, is difficult and probably inaccurate, and therefore this comparison is unreliable.

An examination of the clinical events during the period of myocardial infarction has provided a possible explanation for the occurrence of coronary arterial thrombi in some patients with AMI and their absence in others. Spain and Bradess[16, 28] have shown that the frequency of thrombi increased, up to a point, with increasing intervals between the onset of symptoms of myocardial ischemia and death, rising from 17% of 80 patients surviving < 1 hour, to 36% of 22 patients surviving 1–8 hours, and to 57% of 100 patients surviving > 8 hours. Thus, a certain but variable period of survival after infarction begins is usually necessary for a thrombus to form.

The presence of coronary arterial thrombi in AMI also has been found to correlate with the presence of the power-failure syndrome (a form of cardiogenic shock resulting in "an inability of the myocardium to maintain the level of cardiac output necessary for adequate organ perfusion. There is evidence of under-perfusion of one or more organ systems").[30] Walston and associates[30] in a clinicopathologic study of 37 patients who died of AMI found thrombi in 17 (71%) of 24 patients with and in only two (15%) of 13 patients without the power-failure syndrome. Of their 37 patients, 19 had coronary arterial thrombi, 17 (90%) of whom had the power-failure syndrome; of their 18 patients without coronary arterial thrombi, seven (39%) had had the power-

failure syndrome. Similar correlations between the presence of pump failure (shock or overt congestive cardiac failure or both) were observed by Roberts and Buja.[1] Thus, a severely diminished cardiac output and consequently slowed coronary arterial blood flow is usually required for a thrombus to form in a coronary artery. It has also been observed at necropsy that the larger the area of myocardial necrosis the more likely will a thrombus be present in a coronary artery. Of course, the larger the infarct, the more likely will pump failure occur.

The type of activity of patients at the time of onset of AMI also may reflect slowed blood flow. Master, Dack, and Jaffe[44] interviewed 890 patients with AMI and found that symptoms of myocardial necrosis appeared in 73% of them during sleep, rest, or mild activity (table 1). For myocardial necrosis to begin during inactivity is in direct contrast to angina pectoris, which appears during activity, but is associated with similar degrees of coronary arterial luminal narrowing.[4, 45–47] It would appear that decreased coronary arterial blood flow, i.e., relative stasis, is necessary for a thrombus to form in a coronary artery and that shock, congestive cardiac failure, and inactivity all decrease coronary flow. The slow-flow concept, however, does not explain the occurrence of coronary arterial thrombi at sites of, and proximal to, severe stenoses caused by old atherosclerotic plaques. Luminal narrowing, however, does introduce points

Table 1

Types of Activity at Onset of Acute Myocardial Infarction

	Attacks	
Activity	No.	%*
1. Sleep	198	22
2. Rest (lying or sitting)	277	31
3. Mild activity	180	20
4. Moderate activity (excludes walking)	76	9
5. Walking	141	16
6. Unusual or severe exertion	18	2
	890	100

*The percentages for these six activities are very similar to those occurring in most individual's daily lives.

of high-velocity gradients which appear to favor platelet aggregation.[48] A high shearing stress also may damage erythrocytes,[49] followed by release of adenosine diphosphate[50] and platelet damage.

Several explanations have been offered for the absence of coronary arterial thrombi in patients dying of AMI or of "acute cardiovascular collapse without myocardial necrosis." Postmortem lysis of thrombi as a result of excessive production of fibrinolysins has not been proved or disproved although several observations tend to discount this explanation. In fatal AMI or sudden death the major coronary arteries in patients without definite thrombi are frequently free of blood or blood products. If fresh thrombi had been lysed immediately postmortem, partially liquified blood or a remnant of a thrombus within the lumen would be expected, and this has not been the case. Necropsies performed within 15 min on patients with coronary heart disease dying suddenly have not disclosed evidence of partially lysed thrombi.[28] It is unlikely that postmortem lysis of thrombi could be so selective as to liquefy only those thrombi which allegedly might have been present in patients with subendocardial necrosis and not lyse those thrombi associated with transmural necrosis. It is unlikely that postmortem lysis, an artifact, which in a sense occurs by chance, could account for identical percentages of thrombi being present in separate but similar studies carried out a decade apart by the same investigators.[16, 28]

Inadequate examination of the coronary tree so that thrombi, though actually present, were not observed is highly unlikely. At least three histologic sections of every 5-mm segment of the entire extramural coronary arterial tree were examined in the study of 107 patients with fatal AMI by Roberts and Buja.[1] The chance of missing a thrombus by this technique is unlikely.

The absence of thrombi in coronary arteries of many patients with AMI may explain in part the lack of clear-cut benefits provided to patients with AMI treated with anticoagulants. After the use of these drugs for 20 years,

controversy still continues as to whether or not they are beneficial to patients with AMI. Of factors favoring the use of anticoagulants in patients with AMI, the purported ability of these drugs to inhibit the formation or extension of a thrombus in a coronary artery has been high on the list. This factor, however, had been based on the supposition that AMI is usually caused by coronary thrombosis. The incidence of coronary arterial thrombi in fatal AMI in patients treated with anticoagulants is similar to that in patients not receiving anticoagulants.[6]

Although it may not be the precipitating cause of AMI, thrombosis may still cause the underlying coronary atherosclerosis. Indeed, there is little doubt that organization of thrombi contributes to the development of the complicated atherosclerotic plaque. The presence of fibrin and platelets in atherosclerotic plaques strongly connects atherosclerosis with thrombosis. Each has been found in plaques by immunofluorescent techniques,[51, 52] and fibrin is commonly found in plaques by histologic and electron-microscopic examination. Histologic evidence that a plaque is derived from a thrombus, however, is frequently obscured.[53] As a thrombus is covered by new endothelium, the underlying endothelium is replaced by connective tissue from the intima which obliterates the original line of demarcation (fig. 4). Thrombi appear to organize by ingrowth of overlying endothelial cells and by connective tissue from the intima.[54] Modified smooth-muscle cells,[55-57] which are capable of synthesizing collagen, elastin, and probably mucopolysaccharides[55, 58] and which are present in connective tissue of arterial intima (they also may be derived from endothelium[55]), invade the bases of attached thrombi. Small mural thrombi organize by an avascular process[53, 59] whereas larger thrombi become vascularized.[60] Capillaries extend from the new overlying endothelium to provide a direct blood supply from the lumen and from vasa vasora to penetrate thrombi at their bases.[60, 61] Vascularization is considered the hallmark of an organized thrombus.[60] Capillaries growing into a thrombus have

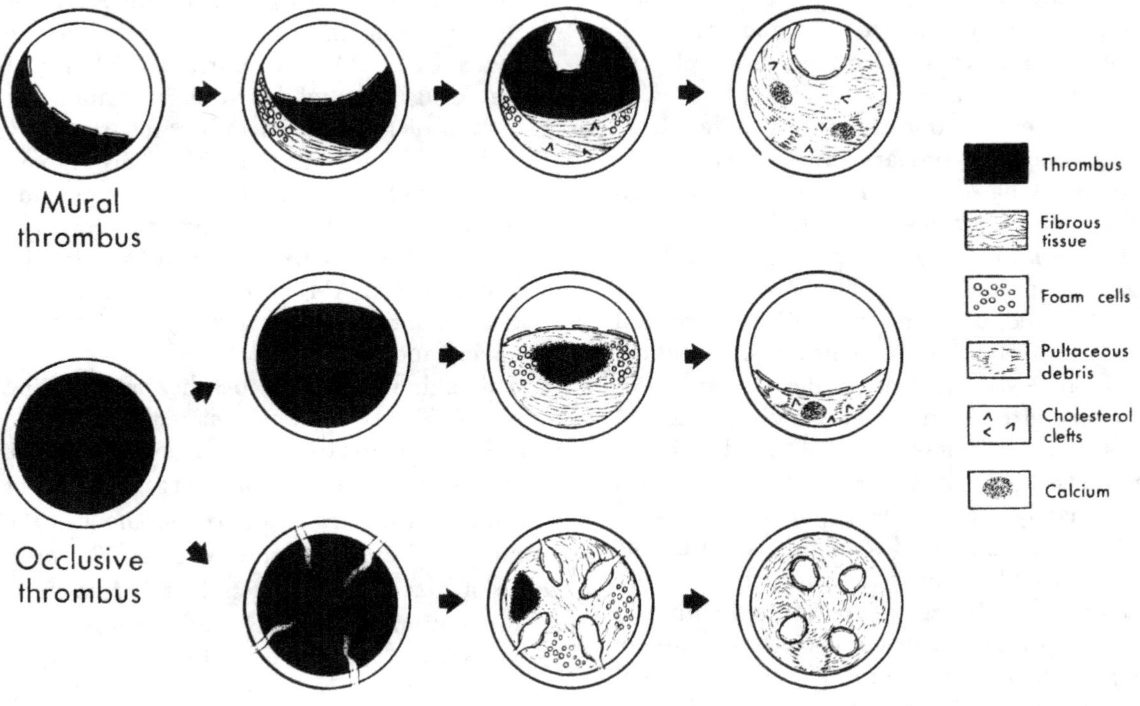

Figure 4

Diagram depicting formation of coronary arterial atherosclerotic plaques from mural and occlusive thrombi. The mural thrombus initially contacts only a portion of the intimal lining. The fibrin-platelet thrombus is covered by endothelial cells, and retraction occurs as it organizes into fibrous tissue. Foam cells appear. Another mural thrombus follows, and the process of organization is repeated. The lines of demarcation between the separate thrombi gradually fade so that at the final stage histologic study makes recognition of previous components of the thrombus difficult.

Organization of an occlusive thrombus may occur in two ways. In one, the thrombus retracts from one intimal surface to form a single channel. As it organizes, the surface of the thrombus exposed to the lumen is covered by endothelial cells. Organization takes place from the overlying newly grown endothelium and from preexisting intima to encase in fibrous tissue the residual thrombus, which may undergo fatty degeneration. Alternatively, organization may occur by capillaries growing into the thrombus at its base. The capillaries may dilate as the thrombus retracts during organization finally leading to the plaque with recanalized channels.

fibrinolytic activity,[62] which contributes to resolution of a thrombus as it organizes. These capillaries, which may later atrophy, can be a source of hemorrhage into plaques. Occlusive thrombi, like mural thrombi, may be incorporated into the intima of arteries as atherosclerotic plaques.[53] Occlusive thrombi may retract before endotheliazation is complete and thereby appear later as mural or nonocclusive plaques (fig. 4).

The source of lipids in atherosclerotic plaques is unclear. Fatty degeneration may occur in any thrombus or hematoma; organization of a left atrial thrombus in mitral stenosis, for example, may result in a structure apparently identical to an atherosclerotic plaque (fig. 5). Platelets, erythrocytes, and plasma all may provide lipids to plaques. When whole blood clots are injected into systemic veins of rabbits, fibrous intimal plaques (containing little lipid) form in pulmonary arteries.[63] Even though the emboli

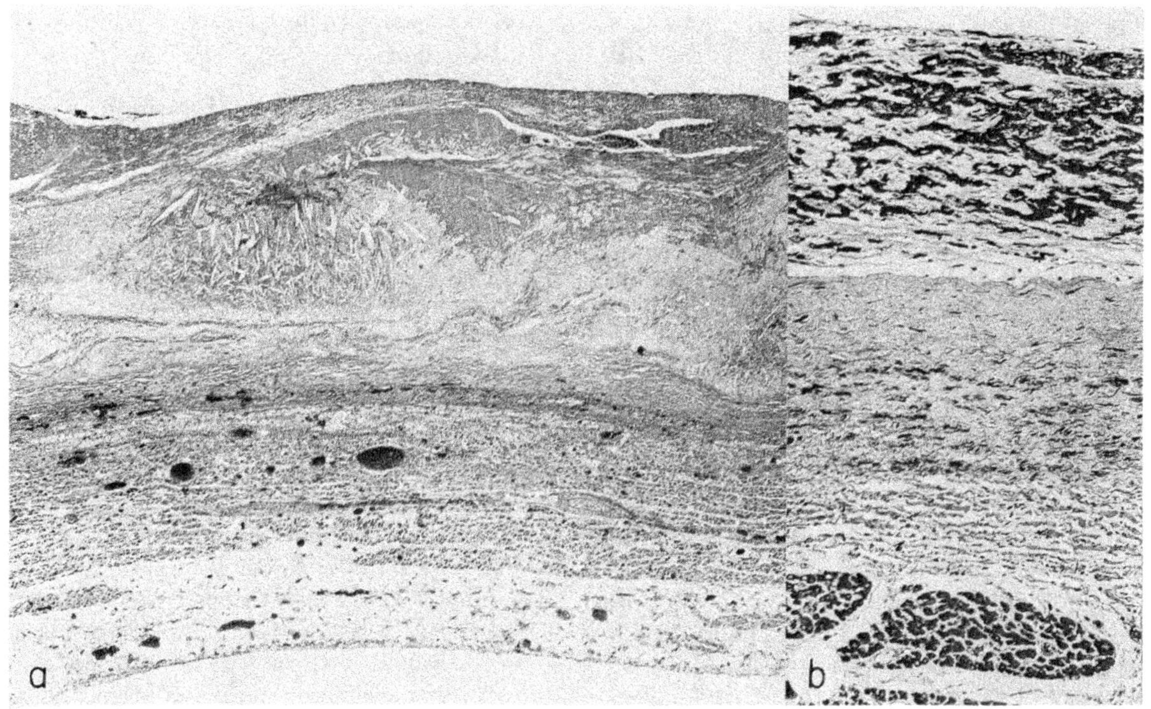

Figure 5

Left atrial thrombi in each of two patients with mitral valvular disease. Organization of these thrombi may result in plaques that may look identical to complicated atherosclerotic plaques. (a) Section of left atrial wall in a 50-year-old woman (A67-210) with a huge thrombus. Organization of portions of the thrombus led to development of numerous cholesterol clefts, pultaceous debris, and calcific deposits, as well as fibrous tissue—components of arterial atherosclerotic plaques. (Hematoxylin and eosin stain, $\times$ 20.)

(b) Section of portion of left atrial wall in a 60-year-old man (A70-280) with severe mitral regurgitation. Mitral valve replacement was performed 50 days before death. Organizing mural thrombus was found in the left atrium at autopsy. The section shows strands of fibrin (dark) interspersed with strands of fibrous tissue (light) on the endocardial surface of the left atrium. This process represents organization of a thrombus—probably 50 days old—and is virtually identical to the fibrin-fibrous tissue lesions that occur in coronary arteries. (Phosphotungstic acid-hematoxylin stain, $\times$ 100.)

are occlusive they organize by retracting into eccentric plaques. The conversion of thromboemboli to plaques is important evidence for the thrombotic origin of atherosclerosis. When platelet-rich thombi rather than whole blood clots are injected, typical fatty atherosclerotic plaques containing many foam cells and foci of calcium develop.[64] Erythrocytes contain less lipid than do platelets, but repeated small hemorrhages may lead to accumulation of large amounts of lipid, especially cholesterol.[65] The plasma supplies lipoproteins, which are found in both recent and organizing thrombi[66] as well as in old plaques.[67]

Atherosclerotic plaques are like fingerprints. No two are alike. In a study of the entire coronary tree of 107 patients with fatal AMI, tremendous variation in the composition of adjacent plaques was noted.[1] Some plaques contained lipid and large quantities of pultaceous debris, whereas others were composed primarily of fibrous tissue. Differences in composition of original thrombi may explain differences in composition of atherosclerotic plaques. Mixed white and red thrombi form plaques that contain some foam cells,[68] but not in the quantity found in plaques derived from platelet-rich or white thrombi.[64] The type of thrombus, whether mural (nonocclusive) or occlusive, also may affect the composition of a plaque. Occlusive platelet thrombi usually do not accumulate fibrin while undergoing transformation to fibrofatty plaques.[64] Mural platelet thrombi, in contrast, appear to be partially or totally replaced by fibrin before undergoing organization, and consequently the plaques that form are mainly fibromuscular.[69–71]

Hemorrhages into Atherosclerotic Plaques

Hemorrhages into old atherosclerotic plaques are common, occurring in 26 (24%) of 107 patients studied by Roberts and Buja,[1] but they probably are of little functional significance. In only one of the 26 patients with hemorrhages into plaques studied by Roberts and Buja did the lumen of the artery appear to have been compromised by the extravasated blood. In contrast to thrombi in coronary arteries in fatal AMI, hemorrhages often occur in coronary arteries unrelated to the area of necrosis, and they may occur in more than one artery or in multiple sites in the same artery. Hemorrhages appear to form from either breaks in the fibrous capsule covering a plaque or from rupture of a small vascular channel within a plaque. Each of these mechanisms is difficult to prove in the individual patient. Possibly small hemorrhages into old plaques occur chronically and have little to do with AMI. It is possible that some hemorrhages into old plaques may be produced artifactually during cutting and processing of coronary arteries for histologic study. A possible detrimental effect of hemorrhages into plaques is the occurrence of superimposed thrombi. This association, however, is not as frequent as once supposed. The two may occur together, presumably when a crack in a plaque is the responsible mechanism. Fulton,[43] Jørgensen et al.,[6] and Roberts and Buja[1] did not find an association between hemorrhages into plaques and coronary thrombosis, probably because the majority of thrombi were observed over plaques that consisted predominantly of fibrous tissue.[43] The incidence of hemorrhages into plaques does not appear to be increased by the use of anticoagulants.[6, 43]

Coronary Arterial Embolism

The occurrence of a clot in the distal portion of a major extramural coronary artery suggests that the cause is embolism rather than thrombosis. This situation occurred in three of 107 patients with fatal AMI studied by Roberts and Buja. Coronary arterial embolism differs from thrombosis in the following manner: (1) the clot is located distally, not proximally, and is usually in the anterior descending coronary artery; (2) the clot extends into intramural coronary arteries and into the epicardial branches of the major extramural vessel (in thrombosis, no clot is found in intramural coronary arteries and uncommonly in the small epicardial branches of major vessels); and (3) the entire extramural coronary arterial tree is relatively free of old atherosclerotic plaques. It is difficult to make the diagnosis of embolism anatomically if the lumens of the coronary arteries are >50% narrowed by old plaque. Also, patients with emboli are usually relatively young and the predisposing circumstances exist for embolism to occur (arrhythmia, infective endocarditis, intracardiac mural thrombosis, etc.).[72–76]

Intramural Coronary Arteries in Fatal AMI

Much has been written about disease of the small coronary arteries. That intramural coronary arteries are narrowed in certain conditions, particularly the neurogenic heart diseases (Friedrich's ataxia, progressive muscular dystrophy, myotonic congenita), is now a well-established fact.[77] In my view, conditions that involve extramural coronary arteries have not been shown also to involve the intramural coronary arteries. There are dissenting views, however, on this point.[78–81] Likewise, conditions that clearly involve intramural coronary arteries tend to spare the extramural coronary arteries. With the exception of the small arteries in the left ventricular papillary muscles, which are subjected to maximal systolic intraventricular pressure over the entire circumference of their surfaces, diseases that affect the intramural coronary arteries do not affect the extramural coronary arteries, and vice versa. Other than insignificant minimal fibrous intimal proliferation in a rare intramural coronary artery, and that usually is in the left ventricular papillary muscles, no abnormality was observed in the intramural coronary arteries in any of the 107 patients with fatal AMI studied by Roberts and Buja. Indeed the intramural vessels in the heart appear to be protected from intimal proliferation and luminal narrowing by the contracting adjacent myocardium. In coronary atherosclerosis, plaques occur routinely in epicardial branches of major extramural arteries, but as soon as these branches penetrate into myocardium the lumen is suddenly wide open again. Even in systemic hypertension, the intramural coronary arteries are not affected as are other small systemic arteries in this condition. The coronary arteries are not exposed to the high systolic pressure because they are perfused mainly in diastole. The contracting ventricular myocardium may further lower the intraluminal pressure in these small vessels. Although patients with diabetes mellitus have been reported to have disease of intramural coronary arteries,[79] this finding has not been observed by this author. Foam cells, cholesterol clefts, and pultaceous debris—components of plaques in extramural coronary arteries—are virtually never found in intramural vessels. Thus, significant involvement of intramural coronary arteries does not occur in patients with significant luminal narrowing of extramural coronary arteries.

References

1. Roberts WC, Buja LM: The frequency and significance of coronary arterial thrombi and other observations in fatal acute myocardial infarction: A study of 107 necropsy patients. Amer J Med. In press

2. Brice JG, Dowsett DJ, Lowe RD: The effect of constriction on carotid bloodflow and pressure gradient. Lancet 1: 84, 1964

3. Saphir O, Priest WS, Hamburger WM, Katz LN: Coronary arteriosclerosis, coronary thrombosis and the resulting myocardial changes. Amer Heart J 10: 567, 1935

4. Blumgart HL, Schlesinger MJ, Davis D: Studies on the relation of the clinical manifestations of angina pectoris, coronary thrombosis, and myocardial infarction to the pathologic findings with particular reference to the significance of the collateral circulation. Amer Heart J 19: 1, 1940

5. Yater WM, Traum AH, Brown WG, Fitzgerald RP, Geisler MA, Wilcox BB: Coronary artery disease in men 18 to 39 years of age: Report of 866 cases, 450 with necropsy examination. Amer Heart J 36: 334, 481, 683, 1948

6. Jørgensen L, Chandler AB, Borchgrevink CF: Acute lesions of coronary arteries in anticoagulant-treated and in untreated patients. Atherosclerosis 13: 21, 1971

7. Classification of atherosclerotic lesions. Report of a Study Group, WHO Techn Rep Ser (no. 143), 1958

8. Roberts WC, Levy RI, Fredrickson DS: Hyperlipoproteinemia: A review of the five types with first report of necropsy findings in type 3. Arch Path (Chicago) 90: 46, 1970

9. Frink RJ, Achor RWP, Brown AL Jr, Kincaid OW, Brandenberg RO: Significance of calcification of the coronary arteries. Amer J Cardiol 26: 241, 1970

10. Barnes AB, Ball RG: The incidence and situation of myocardial infarction in one thousand consecutive postmortem examinations. Amer J Med Sci 183: 215, 1932

11. Lisa JR, Ring A: Myocardial infarction or gross fibrosis: Analysis of 100 necropsies. Arch Intern Med (Chicago) 50: 131, 1932

12. Friedberg CK, Horn H: Acute myocardial infarction not due to coronary artery occlusion. JAMA 112: 1675, 1939

13. Foord AG: Embolism and thrombosis in coronary heart disease. JAMA 138: 1009, 1948

14. Miller RD, Burchell HB, Edwards JE: Myocardial infarction with and without acute coronary occlusion: A pathologic study. Arch Intern Med (Chicago) 88: 597, 1951

15. Branwood AW, Montgomery GL: Observations on the morbid anatomy of coronary artery disease. Scot Med J 1: 367, 1956

16. Spain DM, Bradess VA: Frequency of coronary thrombi as related to duration of survival from onset of acute fatal episodes of myocardial ischemia. Circulation 22: 816, 1960

17. Spain DM, Bradess VA: The relationship of coronary thrombosis to coronary atherosclerosis and ischemic heart disease: A necropsy study covering a period of 25 years. Amer J Med Sci 240: 701, 1960

18. Kurland GS, Weingarten C, Pitt B: The relation between the location of coronary occlusions and the occurrence of shock in acute myocardial infarction. Circulation 31: 646, 1965

19. Meadows R: Coronary thrombosis and myocardial infarction. Med J Australia 2: 409, 1965

20. Ehrlich JC, Shinohara Y: Low incidence of coronary thrombosis in myocardial infarction: A restudy by serial block technique. Arch Path (Chicago) 78: 432, 1964

21. Mitchell JRA, Schwartz CJ: Arterial Disease. Philadelphia, F.A. Davis, 1965

22. Baroldi G: Acute coronary occlusion as a cause of myocardial infarct and sudden coronary heart death. Amer J Cardiol 16: 859, 1965

23. Harland WA, Holburn AM: Coronary thrombosis and myocardial infarction. Lancet 2: 1158, 1966

24. Kagan A, Livsic AM, Sternby N, Vihert AM: Coronary-artery thrombosis and the acute attack of coronary heart-disease. Lancet 2: 1199, 1968

25. Chapman I: Relationships of recent coronary artery occlusion and acute myocardial infarction. J Mt Sinai Hosp 35: 149, 1968

26. Jørgensen L, Hoerem JW, Chandler AB, Borchgrevink CF: The pathology of acute coronary death. Acta Anaesth Scand (suppl) 29: 193, 1968

27. Hackel DB, Estes EH, Walston A, Koff S, Day E: Some problems concerning coronary artery occlusion and acute myocardial infarction. Circulation 40 (suppl IV): IV-31, 1969

28. Spain DM, Bradess VA: Sudden death from coronary heart disease: Survival time, frequency of thrombi, and cigarette smoking. Dis Chest 58: 107, 1970

29. Bouch DC, Montgomery GL: Cardiac lesions in fatal cases of recent myocardial ischemia from a coronary care unit. Brit Heart J 32: 795, 1970

30. Walston A, Hackel DB, Estes EH: Acute coronary occlusion and the "power failure" syndrome. Amer Heart J 79: 613, 1970

31. Edwards JE: What is myocardial infarction? Circulation 40 (suppl IV): IV-5, 1969

32. Jørgensen L: Experimental platelet and coagulation thrombi: A histologic study of arterial and venous thrombi of varying age in untreated and heparinized rabbits. Acta Path Microbial Scand 62: 189, 1964

33. Leary T: Coronary spasm as a possible factor in producing sudden death. Amer Heart J 10: 338, 1934

34. Clark E, Graef I, Chasis H: Thrombosis of the aorta and coronary arteries: With special reference to the fibrinoid lesions. Arch Path (Chicago) 22: 183, 1936

35. Osborn GR: The Incubation Period of Coronary Thrombosis. London, Butterworths, 1963

36. Chapman I: Morphogenesis of occluding coronary artery thrombosis. Arch Path (Chicago) 80: 256, 1965

37. Constantinides P: Plaque fissures in human coronary thrombosis. J Atheroscler Res 6: 1, 1966

38. Friedman M, Van den Bovenkamp GJ: The pathogenesis of a coronary thrombus. Amer J Path 48: 19, 1966

39. Jørgensen L: Thrombosis and the complications of atherosclerosis. In: Atherosclerois, Proceedings of the Second International Symposium, edited by RJ Jones. New York, Springer-Verlag, 1970

40. Friedman M: The coronary thrombus: Its origin and fate. Human Path 2: 81, 1971

41. Hovig T, Jørgensen L, Packham MA, Mustard JF: Platelet adherence to fibrin and collagen. J Lab Clin Med 71: 29, 1968

42. Anitschkow N: Morphodynamik der Koronarsklerose des Herzens. Acta Path Microbiol Scand 49: 426, 1960

43. Fulton WFM: The Coronary Arteries: Arteriography, Microanatomy, and Pathogenesis of Obliterative Coronary Artery Disease. Springfield, Illinois, Charles C Thomas, 1965

44. Master AM, Dack S, Jaffe HL: Activities associated with the onset of acute coronary artery occlusion. Amer Heart J 18: 434, 1939

45. Zoll PM, Wessler S, Blumgart HL: Angina

pectoris, clinical and pathologic correlations. Amer J Med **11**: 331, 1951

46. LENEGRE J, HIMBERT J: Critical study of the relationship between angina pectoris and coronary atherosclerosis. Amer Heart J **58**: 539, 1959

47. ALLISON RB, RODRIGUEZ FL, HIGGINS EA JR, LEDDY JP, ABELMANN WH, ELLIS LB, ROBBINS SL: Clinicopathologic correlations in coronary atherosclerosis: Four hundred thirty patients studied with postmortem coronary angiography. Circulation **27**: 170, 1963

48. DINTENFASS L, ROZENBERG MC: The influence of the velocity gradient on *in vitro* blood coagulation and artificial thrombosis. J Atheroscler Res **5**: 276, 1965

49. NEVARIL CG, LYNCH EC, ALFREY CP JR, HELLUMS JD: Erythrocyte damage and destruction induced by shearing stress. J Lab Clin Med **71**: 784, 1968

50. HARRISON MJG, MITCHELL JRA: The influence of red blood-cells on platelet adhesiveness. Lancet **2**: 1163, 1966

51. WOOLF N, CRAWFORD T: Fatty streaks in aortic intima studied by an immuno-histochemical technique. J Path Bact **80**: 405, 1960

52. WOOLF N, CARSTAIRS KC: Infiltration and thrombosis in atherosclerosis: A study using immunofluorescent techniques. Amer J Path **51**: 373, 1967

53. DUGUID JB: Thrombosis as a factor in the pathogenesis of coronary atherosclerosis. J Path Bact **58**: 207, 1946

54. CRAWFORD T, LEVENE CI: Incorporation of fibrin in the aortic intima. J Path Bact **64**: 523, 1952

55. HAUST DM, MORE RH, MOVAT HZ: The role of smooth muscle cells in the fibrogenesis of arteriosclerosis. Amer J Path **37**: 377, 1960

56. GEER JC, McGILL HC JR, STRONG JP: The fine structure of the human atherosclerotic lesions. Amer J Path **31**: 263, 1961

57. WISSLER RW: The arterial medial cell, smooth muscle or multifunctional mesenchyme? J Atheroscler Res **8**: 201, 1968

58. GETZ GS, VESSELINOVITCH D, WISSLER RW: A dynamic pathology of atherosclerosis. Amer J Med **46**: 657, 1969

59. HAUST MD, MORE RH, MOVAT HH: The

60. GEIRINGER E: Intimal vascularization and atherosclerosis. J Path Bact **63**: 201, 1951

61. MORGAN AD: The Pathogenesis of Coronary Occlusion. Springfield, Illinois, Charles C Thomas, 1956

62. TODD AS: Localization of fibrinolytic activity in tissues. Brit Med Bull **20**: 210, 1964

63. HARRISON CV: Experimental pulmonary atherosclerosis. J Path Bact **60**: 289, 1948

64. HAND RA, CHANDLER AB: Atherosclerotic metamorphosis of autologous pulmonary thromboemboli in the rabbit. Amer J Path **40**: 469, 1962

65. HARTROFT WS: Ceroid-like pigments, hemoceroid and hyaloceroid, in atheromatous lesions of human subjects. Amer J Path **28**: 526, 1952

66. WOOLF N, PILKINGTON TRE, CARSTAIRS KC: The occurrence of lipoproteins in thrombi. J Path Bact **91**: 383, 1966

67. KAO VCY, WISSLER RW: A study of the immunohistochemical localization of serum lipoproteins and other plasma proteins in human atherosclerotic lesions. Exp Molec Path **4**: 457, 1965

68. FILSHIE I, SCOTT GBD: The organization of experimental venous thrombi. J Path Bact **76**: 71, 1958

69. JØRGENSEN L, ROWSELL HC, HOVIG T, MUSTARD JF: Resolution and organization of platelet-rich mural thrombi in carotid arteries of swine. Amer J Path **51**: 681, 1967

70. WOOLF N, BRADLEY JWP, CRAWFORD T, CARSTAIRS KC: Experimental mural thrombi in the pig aorta: The early natural history. Brit J Exp Path **49**: 257, 1968

71. WOOLF N, CASTAIRS KG: The survival time of platelets in experimental mural thrombi. J Path **97**: 595, 1969

72. SAPHIR O: Coronary embolism. Amer Heart J **8**: 312, 1933

73. HAMMAN L: Coronary embolism. Amer J Med **21**: 401, 1941

74. SHRADER EL, BAWELL MB, MORAGUES V: Coronary embolism. Circulation **14**: 1159, 1956

75. WENGER NK, BAUER S: Coronary embolism: Review of the literature and review of fifteen cases. Amer J Med **25**: 549, 1958

76. OAKLEY C, YUSUF R, HOLLMAN A: Coronary embolism and angina in mitral stenosis. Brit Heart J 23: 357, 1961

77. JAMES TN: Etiologic concept concerning the obscure myocardiopathies. Progr Cardiovasc Dis 7: 43, 1964

78. SAPHIR O, OHRINGER L, WONG R: Changes in the intramural coronary branches in coronary arteriosclerosis. Arch Path (Chicago) 62: 159, 1956

79. BLUMENTHAL HT, ALEX M, GOLDENBERG S: A study of lesions of the intramural coronary artery branches in diabetes mellitus. Arch Path (Chicago) 70: 13, 1960

80. DONOMAE I, MATSUMOTO Y, KOKUBU T, KOIDE R, KOBAYASHI R, IKEGAMI H, UEDA E, FUJISAWA T, FUJIMOTO S: Pathological studies of coronary atherosclerosis: Especially of sclerosis of intramuscular coronary arteries. Jap Heart J 3: 423, 1962

81. MORE BM, SOMMERS SC: The status of the myocardial arterioles in angina pectoris. Amer Heart J 64: 323, 1962

Relationship Between Coronary Thrombosis and Myocardial Infarction

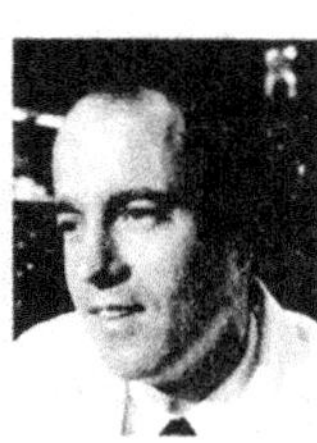

■ **William C. Roberts, M.D.**

Chief, Section of Pathology
National Heart and Lung Institute
National Institutes of Health
Bethesda, Maryland 20014

Although many clinicians and pathologists apparently consider coronary arterial thrombosis to be the cause of fatal acute myocardial infarction (AMI), the reported incidence of such thrombosis has varied from 21% to 91%.[1-21] The major cause for the variation in incidence is probably the inclusion of cases of subendocardial infarction and sudden death ("acute cardiovascular collapse in the absence of myocardial necrosis") with cases of transmural necrosis. In a recent study,[21] coronary arterial thrombi were infrequently found in patients who died suddenly with or without previous histories of cardiac disease, or in patients in whom necrosis was limited to the inner one-half of the left ventricular wall (subendocardium). In this study, a coronary thrombus was found in only 2 (8%) of 24 patients who died suddenly (less than six hours from onset of symptoms), in none of 9 patients with only subendocardial necrosis, but in 40 (54%) of 74 patients with fatal transmural myocardial necrosis.[21]

Although the type of myocardial infarct is probably the most important factor, differing techniques of examining coronary arteries at necropsy and differing definitions of what constitutes a true thrombus also may contribute to the varied reported incidence of coronary thrombosis in fatal AMI. Studies utilizing only gross inspection of these vessels without histological confirmation of the presence or absence of thrombus are inadequate. Postmortem clots, hemorrhage into old atherosclerotic plaques, and even highly vascularized old plaques may be confused grossly with antemortem thrombi. True (antemortem) thrombi are adherent to the luminal surfaces of the arteries, are composed of platelets, or fibrin, or both, and usually also of erythrocytes and leukocytes. Coronary arterial thrombi are always adherent distally, but not always proximally. The composition of a thrombus at varying levels may differ: distally, it is more likely to consist of platelets, or fibrin, or both (white thrombus), whereas proximally it is more likely to be composed of erythrocytes, lesser quantities of fibrin, few platelets, and some leukocytes (red thrombus). Early thrombi may be composed purely of platelets. The postmortem or false thrombus, in contrast, is nonadherent and composed mainly of erythrocytes. Lysis of a thrombus, either before or after death, as a result of excessive production of fibrinolysins has been suggested to explain the varied frequency of coronary thrombi found in patients with fatal AMI, but the available data are against this contention.

Thrombi occurring in patients dying of AMI are, except in cases of embolism, superimposed on old atherosclerotic plaques. Usually the artery containing the thrombus is already more than 50% narrowed by the atherosclerotic plaques, and in about 90% of patients with fatal

AMI and coronary arterial thrombi, the lumen of the artery distal to the thrombus is >75% narrowed by old plaques.[21] Why fresh thrombi are located at, or proximal to, sites of narrowing is unclear. Thrombi may be seen over cracks in old atherosclerotic plaques and intimal rupture of plaques may be an important precipitating cause of coronary arterial thrombosis.[19] Such ruptures, which occur particularly in fibrous tissue covering deposits of pultaceous debris, can lead to discharge of necrotic debris into the arterial lumen or to hemorrhage within the plaque. The break in the plaque exposes its contents to the flowing blood and is said to be a strong stimulus for platelet accumulation. That coronary arterial thrombi are related to rupture of necrotic plaques, however, is not established. Study of serial sections is usually necessary to observe cracks in plaques and even then interpretation is often difficult. At times, rupture of a plaque may result from fixing and cutting an artery without providing prior support of its wall by injection.

The thrombus in fatal AMI is practically always located in the coronary artery that supplies the infarcted myocardium. If the infarct involves the anteroseptal wall of the apical part of the left ventricle, and if a thrombus occurs, it will be located in the anterior descending coronary artery, whereas posterior wall necrosis at the base is associated with thrombosis of the right or left circumflex coronary artery. Thrombi in either the left anterior descending or the left circumflex coronary artery generally are located within 2 cm of the bifurcation of the left main artery (or within 4 cm of the left aortic ostium), although the left main coronary artery itself is rarely the site of thrombosis. In contrast, thrombosis in the proximal portion of the right coronary artery may not be more frequent than thrombosis in its mid or distal portions. Thrombi are infrequently seen in the small epicardial branches of the major extramural coronary arteries and never occur, other than as platelet aggregates, in intramural coronary arteries.

Not all coronary arterial thrombi produce total luminal occlusion. (The term "occlusion" is not synonymous with "thrombosis," since occlusion may be partial as well as complete and since the vessel may be occluded by material other than that which forms a thrombus.) In the patients with fatal transmural myocardial necrosis who had coronary thrombi found at autopsy, the thrombus was partially occluding *(mural)* in about 20% and totally occluding *(occlusive)* in

about 80%.[21] Pure platelet thrombi are usually small and infrequently totally occlude lumens. Before the significance of a coronary arterial thrombus can be judged, it is necessary to know whether the thrombus is totally or only partially occlusive and the degree of luminal narrowing by old atherosclerotic plaques at the site of, and distal to, the thrombus.

The role of coronary thrombosis in AMI is unclear. For several decades, coronary thrombosis was considered the cause of AMI. Clinically, AMI represents a sudden change for the patient compared to his preinfarction status. This often dramatic clinical event has been equated at necropsy with the finding of a "fresh" thrombus in a coronary artery. In our study, however, only 54% of patients with transmural myocardial necrosis and about 10% of patients with subendocardial necrosis or "sudden cardiovascular collapse without myocardial necrosis" had a thrombus in a coronary artery at necropsy.[21] The virtual absence of coronary arterial thrombi in patients dying suddenly of cardiac disease and their presence in only about one-half of those with myocardial necrosis support the concept that coronary arterial thrombi are *consequences* rather than *causes* of AMI.[4, 6, 7, 10] In support of this theory, the age of the myocardial necrosis has sometimes been judged to be older than the age of the coronary thrombus,[7] but judging accurately the age of a thrombus is particularly difficult and thus this comparison may not be reliable.

The examination of clinical events following an AMI has provided a possible explanation for the occurrence of coronary arterial thrombi in some patients with AMI and their absence in others. Spain and Bradess[6, 17] demonstrated that the frequency of finding coronary thrombi rises with increasing intervals between the onset of symptoms of myocardial ischemia and death. In their study in 1960,[6] the frequency rose from 16% in 303 patients surviving less than one hour, to 37% in 65 patients surviving one to 24 hours, and to 54% in 200 patients surviving longer than 24 hours. In their 1970 study of other patients,[17] the frequency rose from 17% in 80 patients surviving less than one hour, to 36% in 22 patients surviving one to eight hours, and to 57% in 100 patients surviving longer than eight hours. Thus, the longer the period of survival after infarction the more likely is a coronary thrombus to be found up to a point.

The presence of coronary arterial thrombi in AMI also has been found to correlate positively with the incidence of the power failure syndrome.[15, 18, 20] Walston and associates,[18] in a clinicopathological study of 37 patients with fatal AMI, found thrombi in 17 (71%) of 24 patients with the power failure syndrome and in only 2 (15%) of 13 patients without this syndrome. Of their 37 patients, 19 had coronary arterial thrombi and 17 (90%) of these had the power failure syndrome; of their 18 patients without coronary arterial thrombi, 7 (39%) had had the power failure syndrome. Thus, a patient with a severely diminished cardiac output is much more likely to have a thrombus at autopsy. In addition, the larger the area of myocardial necrosis, the more likely will a thrombus be present in a coronary artery. Of course, the larger the infarct, the more likely will pump failure occur.[20]

The occurrence of a clot in the distal portion of a major extramural coronary artery suggests that the cause is embolism rather than thrombosis. This situation occurred in 3 of the 107 patients with fatal AMI studied by Roberts and Buja.[21] Coronary arterial embolism differs from thrombosis in several ways: (1) the clot is located distally, not proximally, and is usually in the anterior descending coronary artery; (2) the clot extends into intramural coronary arteries and into the epicardial branches of the major extramural vessel (in thrombosis, no clot is found in intramural coronary arteries and uncommonly in the small epicardial branches of major vessels); and (3) the entire extramural coronary arterial tree is relatively free of old atherosclerotic plaques. Also, patients with emboli are usually relatively young and have certain predisposing conditions (dysrhythmia, infective endocarditis, intracardiac mural thrombosis, etc.).

Although thrombosis may not always be the precipitating cause of AMI, organization of thrombi may still play a major contributing role in the production of the complicated atherosclerotic plaque. Although both fibrin and platelets have been detected occasionally in atherosclerotic plaques by immunofluorescent techniques, histological evidence that a plaque is derived from thrombus is frequently obscure. Differences in composition of atherosclerotic plaques may be related to differences in composition of thrombi contributing to the plaque. Mixed white and red thrombi form plaques that contain some foam cells, but not in the quantity found in plaques derived from platelet-rich or white thrombi. The type of thrombus, whether mural or occlusive, also may affect the composition of a plaque. Occlusive platelet thrombi usually do not accumulate fibrin while undergoing transformation to fibrofatty plaques. Nonocclusive platelet thrombi, in contrast, appear to be partially or totally replaced by fibrin before undergoing organization, and consequently the plaques that form are mainly fibromuscular.

In our study, hemorrhages in old atherosclerotic plaques of coronary arteries were found in about 25% of patients with fatal AMI or fatal sudden cardiovascular collapse.[21] Although they rarely actually cause luminal narrowing, hemorrhages are often observed in plaques with superimposed thrombi. More frequently, however, they are not associated with thrombi and, in AMI, may be seen in coronary arteries unrelated to areas of myocardial necrosis. Indeed, they may occur in more than one artery or in multiple sites in the same artery. Hemorrhages appear to form either from breaks in the fibrous capsule covering a plaque or from rupture of a small vascular channel within a plaque. Small hemorrhages into old plaques may possibly occur chronically and have little to do with AMI. Also, possibly some hemorrhages are produced artifactually during cutting and processing of coronary arteries for histological study. The incidence of hemorrhages into plaques does not appear to be increased by the use of anticoagulants.

Nearly all patients with symptomatic ischemic heart disease have *diffuse* and *severe* coronary arterial atherosclerosis. Roberts and Buja[21] examined several thousand histological sections of coronary arteries in 107 patients with fatal AMI and found only four sections without atherosclerotic plaquing. The degree of luminal narrowing, however, varied, but some plaque formation was present in virtually every millimeter of major coronary artery. In patients with fatal AMI or fatal sudden cardiovascular collapse (sudden death), the lumen of at least one of the three major extramural coronary arteries is nearly always narrowed more than 75% by old atherosclerotic plaques. Among the 107 necropsy patients studied,[21] the average number of major coronary arteries (3 per patient; excludes left main) narrowed by more than 75% by old atherosclerotic plaques was: 2.4 in 74 patients with transmural necrosis; 2.3 in 9 patients with only subendocardial necrosis; and 2.4 in 24 patients who died suddenly. A coronary artery, however, may have considerable atherosclerosis and yet be able to transport considerable quantities of blood. When the degree of coronary narrowing decreases the original lumen by more than 75%, however, the flow in the vessel is significantly decreased.

Much has been written about disease of the small coronary arteries. It is now well established that intramural coronary arteries are narrowed in certain conditions, particularly the neuromyopathic heart diseases (Friedreich's ataxia, progressive muscular dystrophy, myotonic muscular dystrophy). Conditions involving *extramural* coronary arteries, however, have not been shown also to involve the *intramural* coronary arteries with the exception of those in the left ventricular papillary muscles. There are dissenting views, however, on this point. Likewise, conditions that clearly involve intramural coronary arteries tend to spare the extramural coronary arteries. Indeed, the intramural coronary arteries appear to be protected from intimal proliferation and luminal narrowing by the contracting adjacent myocardium. In coronary atherosclerosis, plaques occur routinely in epicardial branches of major extramural arteries, but as soon as these branches penetrate the myocardium, the lumen is suddenly wide open again and plaques are not encountered. Although patients with diabetes mellitus have been reported to have disease of intramural coronary arteries, this finding is debated. Foam cells, cholesterol clefts, and pultaceous debris—components of plaques in extramural coronary arteries—are virtually never found in intramural vessels.

It is difficult to explain the occurrence of an acute myocardial infarction in patients in whom no acute occlusion of a coronary artery is found. Explanations that have been offered include inadequate pathological examination and lysis of an antemortem thrombus or of transient platelet aggregates. In addition, in patients with a critical balance between myocardial oxygen supply and demand, infarction can result from anything that causes an acute decrease in supply (decrease in perfusion pressure, etc.) or an acute increase in oxygen demand (hypertension, tachycardia, etc.).

Conclusions

Among patients with ischemic heart disease, coronary arterial thrombi are infrequent in patients who die suddenly and in those with only subendocardial necrosis. Coronary thrombi are found in just over 50% of patients with fatal transmural myocardial necrosis. Thrombi are more likely to be found in patients who survive longer following the onset of chest pain and in patients who have the power failure syndrome. Coronary thrombi in fatal acute myocardial infarction (AMI) usually are located at, or just proximal to, sites previously severely narrowed by old atherosclerotic plaques. In nearly all patients with fatal AMI, the extramural (epicardial) coronary arteries are diffusely involved by old atherosclerotic plaques, whereas the intramural coronary arteries are characteristically spared.

R E F E R E N C E S

1. **Harrison CV, Wood P:** Hypertensive and ischaemic heart disease: A comparative clinical and pathological study. Brit Heart J 11:205-229, 1949

2. **Miller RD, Burchell HB, Edwards JE:** Myocardial infarction with and without acute coronary occlusion: A pathologic study. Arch Intern Med (Chicago) 88:597-604, 1951

3. **Snow PJD, Morgan Jones A, Daber KS:** Coronary disease: A pathological study. Brit Heart J 17:503-510, 1955

4. **Branwood AW, Montgomery GL:** Observations on the morbid anatomy of coronary artery disease. Scot Med J 1:367-375, 1956

5. **Snow PJD:** Coronary occlusion and myocardial infarction. Amer Heart J 58:645-647, 1959

6. **Spain DM, Bradess VA:** Relationship of coronary thrombosis to coronary atherosclerosis and ischemic heart disease: A necropsy study covering a period of 25 years. Amer J Med Sci 240:701-710, 1960

7. **Ehrlich JC, Shinohara Y:** Low incidence of coronary thrombosis in myocardial infarction: A restudy by serial block technique. Arch Path (Chicago) 78:432-445, 1964

8. **Baroldi G:** Acute coronary occlusion as a cause of myocardial infarct and sudden coronary heart death. Amer J Cardiol 16:859-880, 1965

9. **Kurland GS, Weingarten C, Pitt B:** Relation between the location of coronary occlusions and the occurrence of shock in acute myocardial infarction. Circulation 31:646-650, 1965

10. **Meadows R:** Coronary thrombosis and myocardial infarction. Med J Aust 2:409-411, 1965

11. **Harland WA, Holburn AM:** Coronary thrombosis and myocardial infarction. Lancet 2:1158-1160, 1966

12. **Rona G:** Pathogenesis of human myocardial infarction. Canad Med Ass J 95:1012-1019, 1966

13. **Chapman I:** Relationships of recent coronary artery occlusion and acute myocardial infarction. J Mount Sinai Hosp NY 35:149-154, 1968

14. **Kagan A, Livsic AM, Sternby N, Vihert AM:** Coronary-artery thrombosis and the acute attack of coronary heart-disease. Lancet 2:1199-1202, 1968

15. **Haekel DB, Estes EH, Walston A, Koff S, Day E:** Some problems concerning coronary artery occlusion and acute myocardial infarction. Circulation 39 and 40 (suppl IV): IV-31–IV-35, 1969

16. **Davis NA:** Incidence of thrombosis in myocardial infarction. Aust Ann Med 19 (suppl I): 60-62, 1970

17. **Spain DM, Bradess VA:** Sudden death from coronary heart disease: Survival time, frequency of thrombi, and cigarette smoking. Chest 58:107-110, 1970

18. **Walston A, Haekel DB, Estes EH:** Acute coronary occlusion and the "power failure" syndrome. Amer Heart J 79:613-619, 1970

19. **Friedman M:** Coronary thrombus: Its origin and fate. Hum Path 2:81-128, 1971

20. **Page DL, Caulfield JB, Kastor JA, DeSanctis RW, Sanders CA:** Myocardial changes associated with cardiogenic shock. New Eng J Med 285:133-137, 1971

21. **Roberts WC, Buja LM:** Frequency and significance of coronary arterial thrombi and other observations in fatal acute myocardial infarction: A study of 107 necropsy patients. To be published in Amer J Med

The Frequency and Significance of Coronary Arterial Thrombi and Other Observations in Fatal Acute Myocardial Infarction

A Study of 107 Necropsy Patients

WILLIAM C. ROBERTS, M.D.
L. MAXIMILIAN BUJA, M.D.
Bethesda, Maryland

From the Section of Pathology, National Heart and Lung Institute, National Institutes of Health, Bethesda, Maryland 20014. Requests for reprints should be addressed to Dr. William C. Roberts. Manuscript received August 31, 1971.

Observations made from histologic study of the entire extramural coronary arterial tree are described in 107 patients who died of acute ischemic heart disease: seventy-four had transmural left ventricular myocardial infarction, nine had necrosis limited to the inner one half of the left ventricular myocardium (acute subendocardial infarcts) and twenty-four died suddenly (less than six hours from onset of symptoms of myocardial ischemia) without histologically detectable myocardial necrosis. Old atherosclerotic plaquing was diffuse and extensive in the extramural coronary arteries in 104 of the 107 patients. The lumens of at least two of the three major extramural coronary arteries (right, left anterior descending and left circumflex) were narrowed more than 75 per cent by old atherosclerotic plaques in 101 of the 107 patients.

Coronary arterial thrombi were found in forty (54 per cent) of the seventy-four patients with transmural necrosis, in none of the nine with only subendocardial necrosis and in two (8 per cent) of the twenty-four who died suddenly. In thirty-seven of the forty-two patients with antemortem coronary arterial clots the lumen of the vessel containing the thrombus was already narrowed more than 75 per cent by old atherosclerotic plaques at or distal to the thrombus. The infrequency of coronary thrombi in patients who died of acute cardiovascular collapse without myocardial necrosis, in those in whom necrosis was limited to the subendocardium, in those who died without cardiogenic shock or congestive cardiac failure, and their occurrence at, or proximal to, sites already severely narrowed by old atherosclerotic plaques suggest that coronary thrombi are consequences rather than causes of acute myocardial infarction. The occurrence of components of thrombi, i.e., fibrin and platelets, in old atherosclerotic plaques and the finding of components of old atherosclerotic plaques, i.e., foam cells, cholesterol clefts, pultaceous debris and calcific deposits, in known thrombi (for example, those located in the left atrium of patients with mitral stenosis) strongly suggest, however, that old atherosclerotic plaques are derived, at least in part, from organization of thrombi.

TABLE I   Clinical and Necropsy Data in Fatal Acute Myocardial Infarction (AMI)

Data	Transmural AMI	Subendocardial AMI	Sudden Death	Totals
No. of patients	74	9	24	107
Age range (yr)	26–90	49–83	28–85	26–90
Average	60	69	54	59
Men:Women	52(70%):22(30%)	6(67%):3(33%)	20(83%):4(17%)	78(73%):29(27%)
Old MI*	41 (55%)	7 (78%)	15 (62%)	63 (59%)
Hypertension†	33 (45%)	3 (33%)	11 (46%)	47 (44%)
"Diabetes"‡	26 (35%)	3 (33%)	3 (13%)	32 (30%)
Total no. of major coronary arteries§	222	27	72	327
No. of major coronary arteries	168 (76%)	20 (74%)	56 (78%)	244 (75%)
narrowed >75% by old plaques	(2.3 per patient)	(2.2 per patient)	(2.3 per patient)	(2.3 per patient)
3	41 (55%)	5 (56%)	11 (46%)	57 (53%)
2	17 (23%)	2 (22%)	10 (42%)	29 (27%)
1	11 (15%)	1 (11%)	3 (12%)	15 (14%)
0	5 (7%)	1 (11%)	0	6 (6%)
Coronary artery thrombi	40 (54%)	0	2 (8%)	42 (39%)
Coronary artery hemorrhages	20 (27%)	1 (11%)	5 (21%)	26 (24%)
Heart weight >400 gm	56 (76%)	9 (100%)	15 (63%)	80 (75%)

* Either transmural or subendocardial fibrosis observed at autopsy. This number does not include microscopic-sized microinfarcts.

† Systemic diastolic blood pressure >90 mm Hg.

‡ Includes patients with abnormal fasting blood glucose levels and/or abnormal glucose tolerance tests in addition to patients being treated (by either diet or oral agents or both) for adult onset diabetes mellitus. None of the patients was treated with insulin.

§ Number derived by multiplying number of patients by 3—the number of major coronary arteries (right, anterior descending and left circumflex) per patient.

Acute myocardial infarction (AMI) is generally considered to be the result of thrombotic occlusion of a major extramural coronary artery. Indeed, coronary thrombosis was the name used for years to describe AMI both clinically and pathologically. The inability to find thrombi in major extramural coronary arteries in many patients who died of AMI stimulated us to study the coronary arterial tree systematically in consecutive patients who died from results of extensive myocardial necrosis or from acute cardiovascular collapse in the absence of myocardial necrosis (sudden death). De-scribed here are our observations resulting from the histologic study of the major extramural coronary arteries in 107 such consecutive patients.

PATIENTS STUDIED AND METHODS

The 107 patients (Table I) ranged in age from twenty-six to ninety years (average fifty-nine years); the seventy-eight men ranged in age from twenty-eight to eighty-five years (average fifty-seven years) and the twenty-nine women, twenty-six to ninety years (average sixty-four years). Five patients (four male, one female) were less than forty years old; four had transmural and one had subendocardial infarcts. Of the twenty-six patients (fifteen male, eleven female) more than sixty-nine years of age, nineteen had transmural and five had subendocardial infarcts; two died suddenly. The diagnosis of AMI was established or strongly suggested during life in sixty-six of the seventy-four patients with transmural infarcts and in five of the nine with subendocardial infarcts by history of prolonged substernal chest pain and/or electrocardiographic changes, and usually also elevations in serum enzyme levels. Of the twenty-four patients who died suddenly (less than six hours after onset of symptoms; no myocardial necrosis), fifteen died before and the remainder within three hours after their arrival at the hospital. Of the twelve patients with myocardial necrosis in whom the diagnosis of AMI was not established or strongly sug-

TABLE II   Relationship Between Coronary Arterial Thrombosis and Duration of Survival After AMI

Survival Time	Patients (no.)	Thrombi No.	%
Less than 6 hours	24	2	8
6 hours–3 days	36	18	50
4 days–14 days	31	15	48
15 days–45 days	16	7	44
Totals	107	42	39*

* If the nine patients with subendocardial necrosis and the twenty-four patients who died suddenly (less than six hours) were excluded this percentage would be 54 per cent.

gested during life, five had a sudden worsening of chronic congestive cardiac failure without chest pain (three had complete left bundle branch block) and four had sudden cerebrovascular accidents without chest pain (electrocardiograms were not recorded in two of the four patients).

The interval between the onset of symptoms of AMI and death varied from minutes to forty-five days; the interval was less than six hours in twenty-four patients and more than twenty-one days in six patients (Table II). Each of the latter six patients had clinical evidence of continuing myocardial infarction.

At necropsy, with the exception of the twenty-four patients in whom the interval between onset and death was less than six hours, all had myocardial coagulation necrosis. The infarcts, which involved the left ventricular free wall or ventricular septum or both, were transmural or nearly transmural in seventy-four patients and subendocardial (limited to inner one half of wall) in nine patients (Table I). Patients in whom myocardial necrosis was limited to left ventricular papillary muscles were excluded. At least three sections for histologic study of left ventricular wall were examined in every patient. In ten patients (all with transmural infarcts) the infarcted myocardial wall was aneurysmally dilated at autopsy. In ten other patients a necrotic wall (either left ventricular free wall or ventricular septum) was perforated. In addition to the acute infarcts sixty-three patients had old scars in the left ventricular free walls or ventricular septums, and thirty-five of them had had previous histories of AMI.

Excluding thirteen patients with valvular heart disease (heart weights from 370 to 1,050 gm [average 590 gm]) and one with congenital ventricular septal defect (VSD) (heart weight 730 gm), the hearts in the remaining ninety-three patients weighed from 300 to 800 gm [1] (average 472 gm); in the sixty-nine men without associated valvular heart disease or congenital VSD the average weight was 480 gm and in the twenty-four women, 438 gm. Of the total 107 patients the heart weighed more than 400 gm in eighty (75 per cent). Excluding the fourteen patients with valvular heart disease or congenital VSD, the hearts weighed more than 400 gm in thirty-seven (86 per cent) of forty-three patients with and in twenty-five (64 per cent) of thirty-nine patients without known histories of systemic diastolic hypertension (more than 90 mm Hg). Of thirty men without associated valvular heart disease, congenital VSD or systemic hypertension, the hearts weighed from 300 to 610 gm (average 439 gm) and of nine women, from 300 to 530 gm (average 403 gm). Of thirty men without associated heart disease except for systemic hypertension, the hearts weighed from 360 to 850 gm (average 544 gm) and of thirteen women from 375 to 610 gm (average 459 gm).

The major extramural coronary arteries were sectioned in their entirety in the following manner (Figure

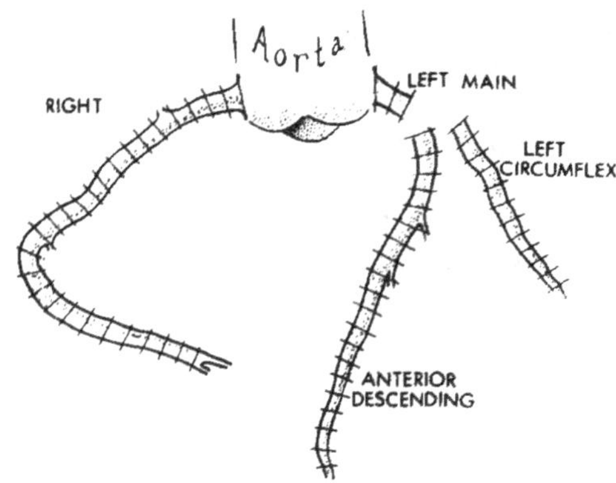

Figure 1. *Method of cutting coronary arteries. Often the left diagonal or marginal vessel also was examined in similar fashion.*

1). Usually before the ventricles or coronary arteries were opened, the right, left main, left circumflex, left anterior descending and posterior descending coronary arteries were excised intact. Each was placed in a separate appropriately labeled container and fixed in 10 per cent buffered formalin. After fixation, each coronary artery was decalcified, its length measured and diagrammatically sketched, and cut transversely at 0.5 cm intervals. Four 0.5 cm segments were placed in a single plastic cricket and decalcified lightly again. The tissues were then dehydrated (alcohols), cleared (xylene), imbedded in paraffin and cut. At least two histologic sections, one stained by hematoxylin and eosin and the other by either Movat's method or elastic Van Gieson or both, were prepared from each 0.5 cm segment. Later, each section was examined by light

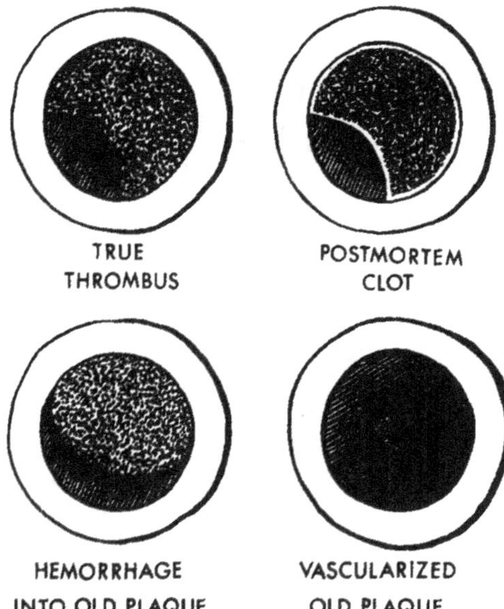

Figure 2. *Diagram illustrating four causes of red lesions in coronary arteries. By gross examination these lesions may be confused with one another. For this reason, histologic examination is essential, and judgments made purely by gross examination are fraught with error.*

microscopy, and the maximal degree of luminal narrowing caused by old atherosclerotic plaques in each vessel was recorded as follows: 0 or none; less than 25 per cent; 26 to 50 per cent; 51 to 75 per cent; and more than 75 per cent. The presence or absence of thrombi, hemorrhage into old atherosclerotic plaques and calcific deposits (graded 0 to 4) were recorded. If thrombus was found, the vessel thrombosed was recorded; the status of the coronary artery at the site of thrombosis was noted, i.e., whether or not the lumen at the site of thrombosis was already narrowed, and to what degree, by old atherosclerotic plaques; the degree of luminal narrowing by old atherosclerotic plaques distal to the thrombus was carefully observed and the components of the thrombus, i.e., erythrocytes, fibrin, platelets and leukocytes, were noted and graded 0 to 4. A

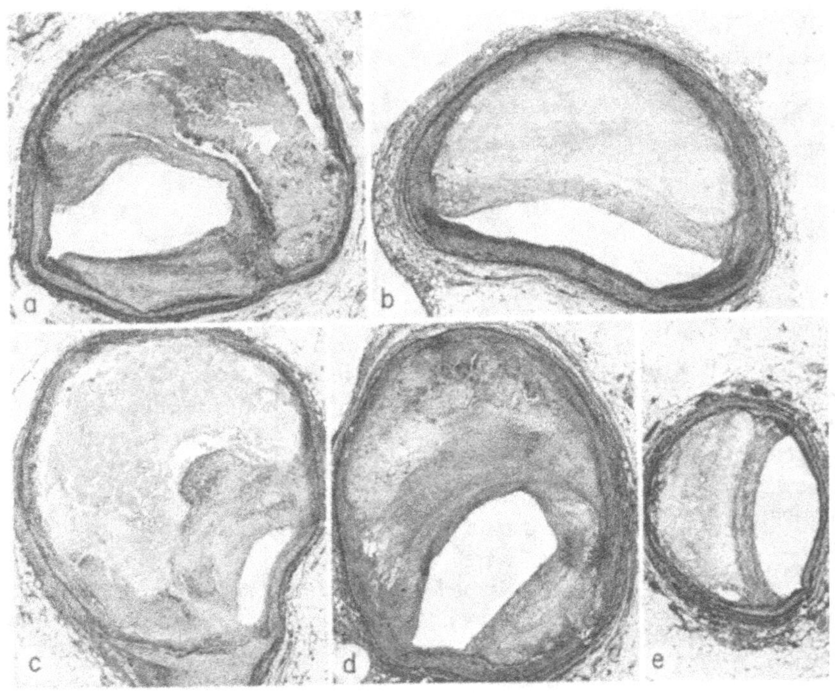

Figure 3. Major extramural coronary arteries in a sixty-three year old woman (A69-262) who died of acute **transmural** myocardial necrosis eight days after onset of symptoms. Death was sudden without antecedent shock or congestive cardiac failure. At necropsy, a large anteroseptal transmural AMI was present, and blood was present in the pericardial space although no discrete focus of myocardial rupture was seen. The heart weighed 375 gm, and no foci of myocardial fibrosis were seen. All extramural coronary arteries were narrowed by old atherosclerotic plaques, and no thrombi or hemorrhages were found in them. **a,** right coronary artery 3 cm from aortic ostium. **b,** left main coronary artery. **c,** left circumflex artery in first 1 cm. **d,** left anterior descending artery in first 1 cm. **e,** left marginal artery. Movat stains; original magnification, each × 16.

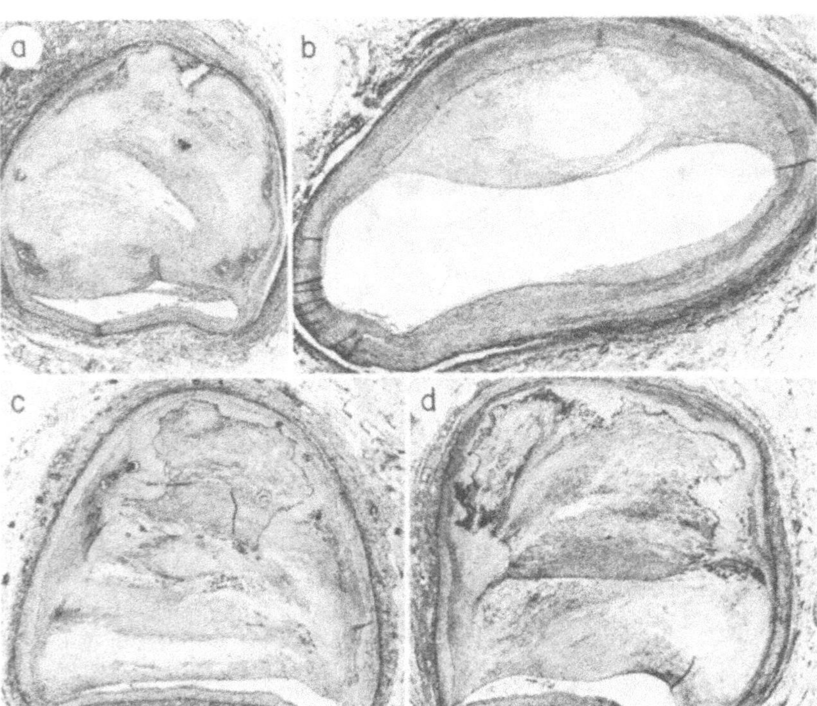

Figure 4. Major extramural coronary arteries at sites of maximal narrowing in a fifty-four year old man (SH No. A4705) who died of acute **subendocardial** myocardial necrosis twelve hours after onset of chest pain. The patient had angina pectoris and adult onset diabetes mellitus but never congestive heart failure or shock. The heart (weight = 430 gm) was severely scarred; left ventricular fibrosis was mainly subendocardial and virtually circumferential from apex to base; rarely, a focus of transmural fibrosis was present. No thrombi or hemorrhages were present in the coronary arteries. **a,** right artery. **b,** left main artery. **c,** left circumflex artery. **d,** left anterior descending artery. All three of the major coronary arteries were narrowed more than 75 per cent by old atherosclerotic plaques. The coronary arteries were heavily calcified, a common observation in patients with diabetes mellitus. Movat stains; original magnification, each × 21.

section of thrombus usually was stained with phosphotungsten-acid hematoxylin to aid in roughly quantitating its various components.

RESULTS

The findings are summarized in Table I and illustrated in Figures 2 to 21. The lumens of one or more of the three major extramural coronary arteries (right, left anterior descending and left circumflex) were narrowed more than 75 per cent by old atherosclerotic plaques in 101 of the 107 patients: in fifteen patients only one of three vessels was narrowed more than 75 per cent; in twenty-nine patients, two vessels; and in fifty-seven patients, the lumens of all three major coronary arteries were narrowed more than 75 per cent (Figures 3 to 6). Excluding three patients with coronary embolism, of the several thousand sec-

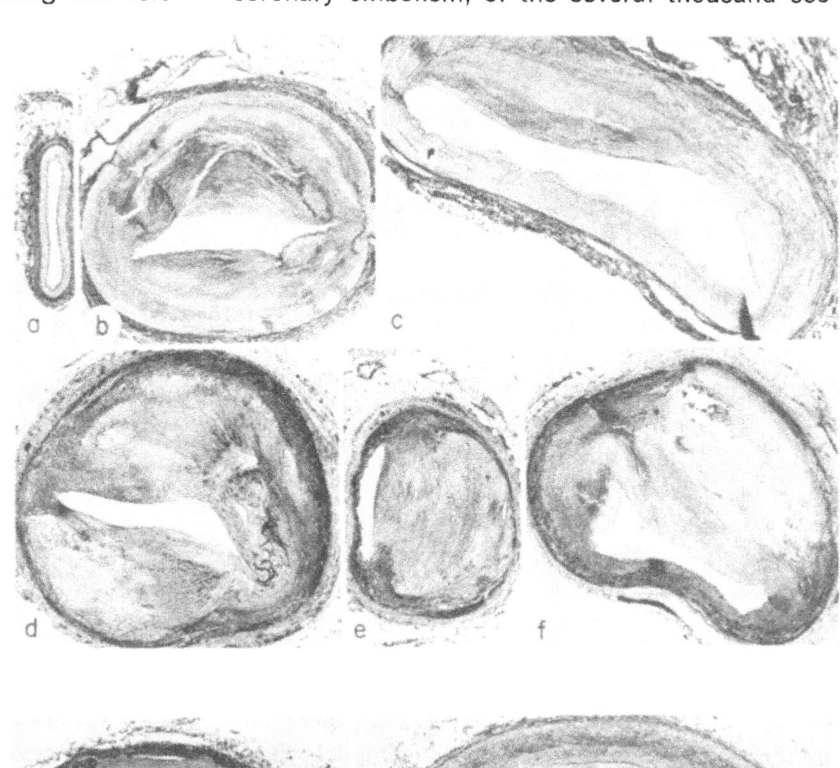

Figure 5. *Extramural coronary arteries in a forty-one year old man (SH No. A4570) who died suddenly and unexpectedly at home (**sudden death**). He apparently had no previous symptoms of cardiac disease. At necropsy, the heart weighed 430 gm and all three major coronary arteries were narrowed more than 75 per cent by old atherosclerotic plaques. No coronary thrombi or hemorrhages were observed. **a**, right posterior descending branch. It is unusual to find a branch of a major coronary artery normal, and this one is, when the major vessels are severely diseased. **b**, right main coronary artery. **c**, left main coronary artery. **d**, left circumflex artery. **e**, left marginal artery. **f**, left anterior descending artery. Movat stains; original magnification, each × 20.*

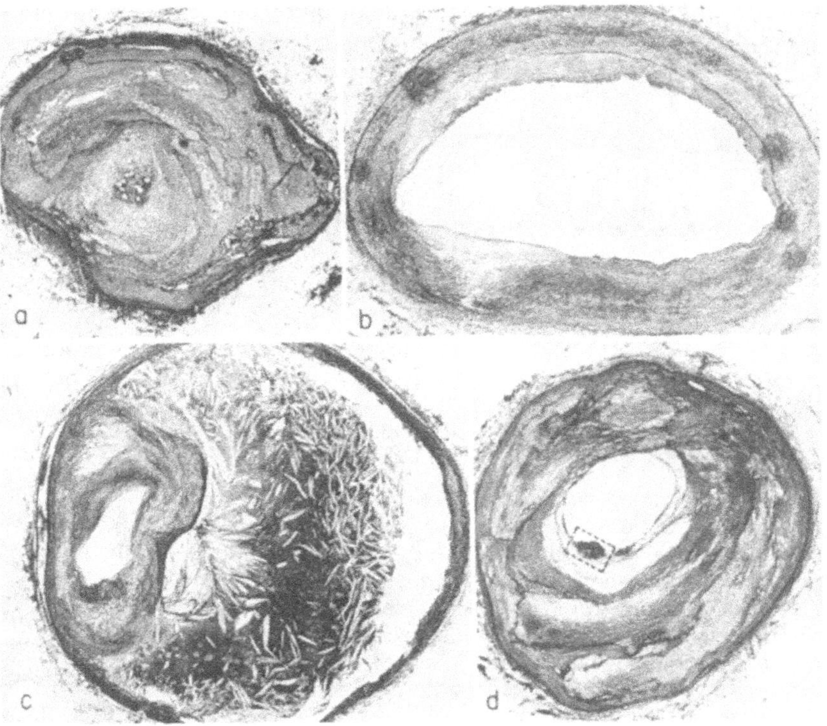

Figure 6. *Major coronary arteries at sites of maximal narrowing in a sixty-five year old man (A71-6) who died three hours after suddenly collapsing while standing. During the final three hours he had multiple arrhythmias, severe shock and congestive cardiac failure. Until this episode he had been asymptomatic, although he was known to have systemic hypertension. At necropsy, the heart weighed 540 gm. The lumens of the right (**a**), left circumflex (**c**) and anterior descending (**d**) arteries were more than 75 per cent narrowed by old plaques. In addition, extravasated blood was present in a plaque in the left circumflex artery (**c**) and a small mural (nonocclusive) platelet thrombus (better seen in Figure 7) was present in the anterior descending branch (**d**). The right artery (**a**) was occluded except for a few recanalized channels. The left main artery (**b**) was wide open. Movat stain (**a**), elastic van Gieson stain (**b**), hematoxylin and eosin stains (**c** and **d**); original magnification, each × 20.*

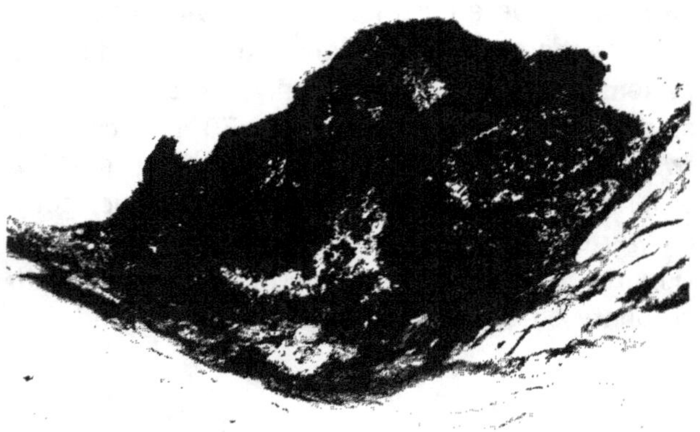

Figure 7. *Platelet thrombus shown in brackets in left anterior descending coronary artery of patient described in Figure 6. This is probably the appearance of an early thrombus and it consists almost entirely of platelets. Hematoxylin and eosin stain, original magnification × 250.*

tions examined only four sections were totally free of old atherosclerotic plaques.

Thrombi or emboli were observed in one of the three major extramural coronary arteries in forty-two (39 per cent) of the 107 patients; thirty-nine had thrombi and three had emboli (Figures 6 to 16). The thrombi in all thirty-nine patients were superimposed on old atherosclerotic plaques, but the emboli in all three patients were not superimposed on old plaques (Figures 18 and 19). The lumens of the coronary arteries distal to antemortem clots were more than 75 per cent narrowed by old atherosclerotic plaques in thirty-seven of the thirty-nine patients with thrombi but in none of the three with emboli. One coronary

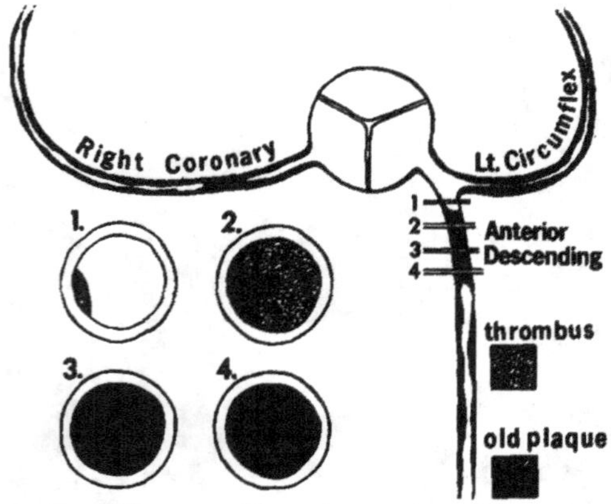

Figure 8. *Diagram illustrating the diffuse nature of coronary atherosclerosis and the usual status of a vessel at and distal to a thrombus. At level 2 in the anterior descending artery the lumen is obstructed primarily by a thrombus. At level 3, however, the major per cent of narrowing is the result of old atherosclerotic plaquing and just distal to the thrombus, the lumen is severely narrowed (more than 75 per cent) or totally obstructed by old plaque only.*

arterial clot was found in thirty-seven of the thirty-nine patients with thrombosis and in each of the three with embolism. The site of myocardial necrosis in each corresponded properly with the artery containing the thrombus or embolus; all patients with antemortem clots in the anterior descending vessel, for example, had anterior wall infarcts. The location of the antemortem clots in the forty patients with single vessel involvement was left anterior descending artery, eighteen patients; right, twelve patients; and left circumflex, ten patients. In the other two patients, each of two coronary arteries contained thrombus. In twenty-nine of the thirty-seven patients with thrombi in a single coronary artery, the lumen was completely closed at the site of thrombosis by combined old arteriosclerotic plaques and recent thrombus. In the other eight patients the lumen was only partially occluded by the recent thrombus. In each of the two patients with thrombi in two coronary arteries the lumen of one artery was completely occluded by thrombus, and the lumen of the second artery was only partially occluded by thrombus. The lumens were completely closed by clot in each of the three patients with embolism. The interval from death to autopsy ranged from two to twenty-three hours (average twelve hours) in the forty-two patients with antemortem clots, and from two to twenty-six hours (average eleven hours) in the sixty-five patients without antemortem clots. There was no sex difference among patients with and without coronary arterial clots; of forty-two with thrombi or emboli, twelve (28 per cent) were women and thirty (72 per cent) were men; of sixty-five patients without thrombi or emboli, seventeen (26 per cent) were women and forty-eight (74 per cent) were men.

None of the three patients with coronary arterial emboli had previous narrowing at the site of embolism by old plaques or luminal narrowing by old plaques distal to the embolus (Figures 18 and 19). Furthermore, none of these three patients had luminal narrowing by old plaques more than 25 per cent in any of the three major coronary arteries. The embolus in each was located in the more distal portion of the coronary artery (left anterior descending in two; right in one) whereas the thrombi in the other thirty-nine patients occurred in the more proximal portions of the coronary arteries. Embolic material in each of these three patients also was present in the small epicardial and in the intramural branches of the coronary arteries. In none of the thirty-nine patients with coronary thrombi was thrombus found in an intramural coronary artery. In one patient with presumed coronary arterial embolism, a thirty-seven year old man with a large congenital VSD, rapid atrial fibrillation suddenly developed, was converted to normal sinus rhythm by electroshock, and was followed four hours later by cardiac arrest. He was resuscitated but never regained consciousness and died three days later. Necropsy disclosed massive necrosis of the caudal portion of the ventricular septum and anterior free wall of left ventricle. The second patient with presumed coronary embolism, a sixty-three year old woman, had rheumatic mitral and aortic valvular stenosis and atrial fibrillation. In this patient severe chest pain suddenly developed and an electrocardiogram showed typical changes of AMI. Necropsy showed extensive necrosis of the anterior portion of the left ventricular free wall and ventricular septum. In the third patient with presumed coronary embolism electrocardiographic features of acute posterior wall myocardial infarction suddenly developed during cardiac catheterization. These changes appeared immediately after flushing the cardiac catheter which lay in the right coronary artery. At necropsy, thirty-one days later, a large embolus was found in the distal right coronary artery and its posterior descending branches, and the posterior wall of the left ventricle was massively necrotic.

Hemorrhages into old atherosclerotic plaques (Figures 6 and 12) were observed in one or more extramural coronary arteries in twenty-six patients, sixteen of whom also had superimposed thrombi. In only one of the twenty-six patients, however, did the extravascular blood in the old plaque appear to actually further narrow the lumen of the vessel.

Of the twenty-seven patients who received anticoagulants during the period of AMI, at necropsy eight had thrombi in a major coronary artery. Three of them also had hemorrhage into an old plaque. and two other patients had hemorrhages into plaques unassociated with thrombosis. Six of the twenty-seven patients receiving anticoagulants had subendocardial infarcts (three patients) or died within six hours (sudden death, three patients).

The intramural coronary arteries (Figures 20 and 21) in the left ventricular free walls and ventricular septums were free of significant luminal narrowing in all 107 patients. Foam cells, cholesterol clefts, calcific deposits or fibrin-platelet thrombi were not observed in any intramural coronary artery, and at least three histologic sections of left ventricular wall were examined in each patient.

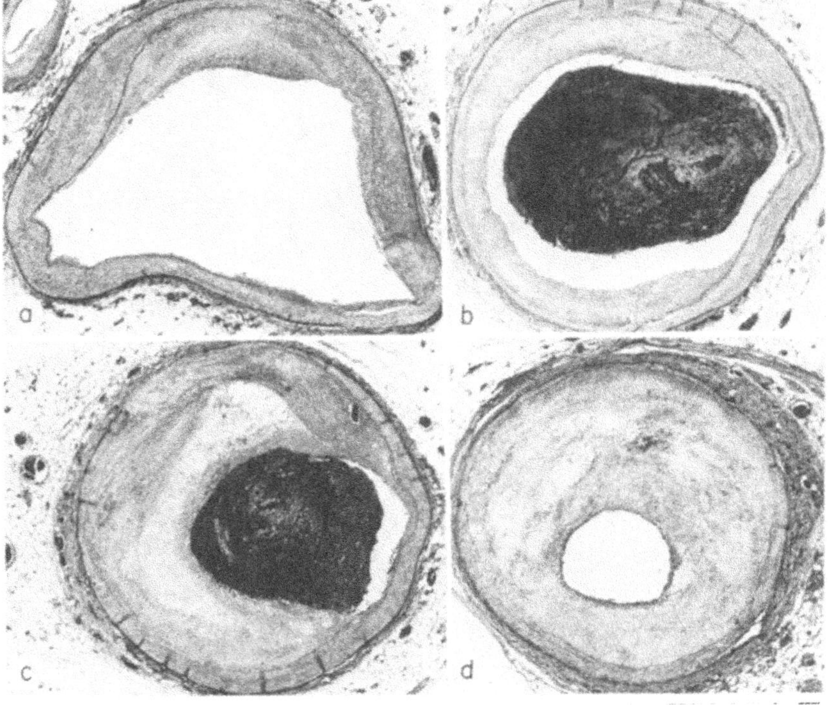

Figure 9. Left circumflex coronary artery in a fifty-seven year old woman (A69-131) who died four days after the onset of transmural AMI. Four levels in the area of the thrombus, as shown in Figure 8, are shown. **a,** proximal to thrombus (level 1). **b,** at this point thrombus is present but it is not attached to the interior lining of the artery (level 2). **c,** now the thrombus is firmly attached. The retraction of the thrombus on one side is an artefact (level 3). **d,** distal to the thrombus (level 4). The lumen is more than 75 per cent narrowed by old plaque. Movat stains; original magnification, each × 21.

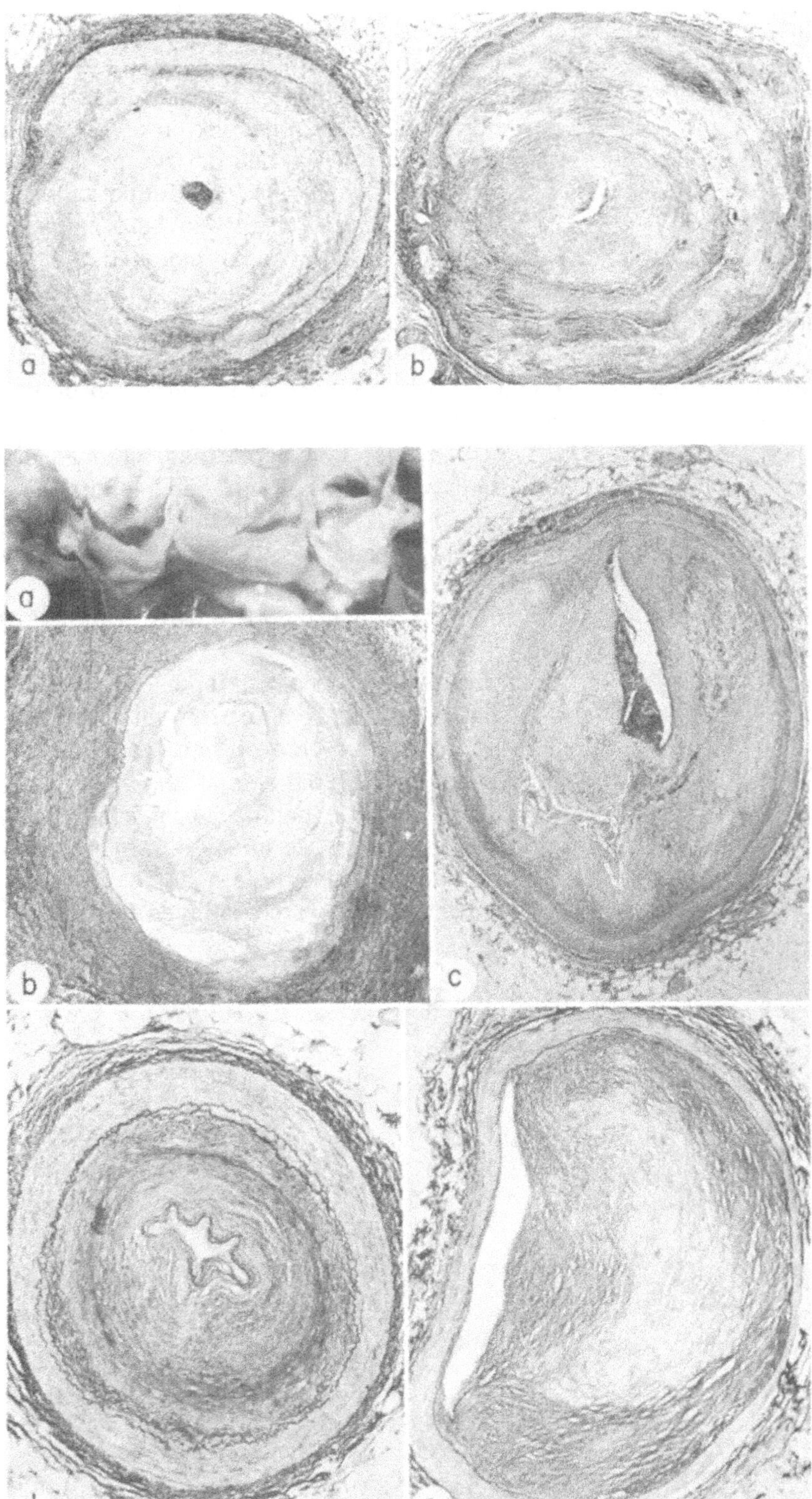

Figure 10. *Anterior descending coronary artery 6 to 7 cm from aortic ostium in a fifty-nine year old woman (A68-285) who had the onset of transmural AMI forty-eight hours before death. She began to have intermittent chest pain two months earlier and had had systemic hypertension for ten years. Her final two days were characterized by shock, pulmonary edema and bradycardia. At necropsy, a "massive" anterior wall infarct, which was aneurysmally dilated, was present. The lumens of all three major coronary arteries were more than 75 per cent narrowed by old plaques. In addition, a small occluding thrombus was present in the left anterior descending vessel (a). The per cent of narrowing caused by the thrombus is small, however, compared to the per cent of narrowing resulting from old atherosclerotic plaques. The lumen both proximal and distal (b) to the thrombus is already severely narrowed by old plaque. Movat stains (a); hematoxylin and eosin stain (b), original magnification, each × 25.*

Figure 11. *Major coronary arteries in a forty-seven year old man (A69-179) who died of an arrhythmia twelve hours after the onset of cardiac ischemic pain. He never had shock or congestive heart failure. He did have systemic hypertension. At necropsy, transmural necrosis was present in the posterolateral left ventricular wall and the aortic ostium of the right coronary artery was severely narrowed (a). A histologic section of the right coronary artery as it arises from the aorta is shown in b. The lumen of the left circumflex just as it arises from the left main coronary artery is shown in c. Its lumen contains a nonoccluding thrombus. The thrombus contains several cholesterol clefts indicating that a plaque may have ruptured upstream. Immediately distal to the thrombus, this artery divided into two branches (d and e) both of which were more than 75 per cent narrowed by old plaques. Movat stains (b and c) and elastic van Gieson stains (d and e); original magnification × 15 (b), × 25 (c), × 60 (d) and × 50 (e).*

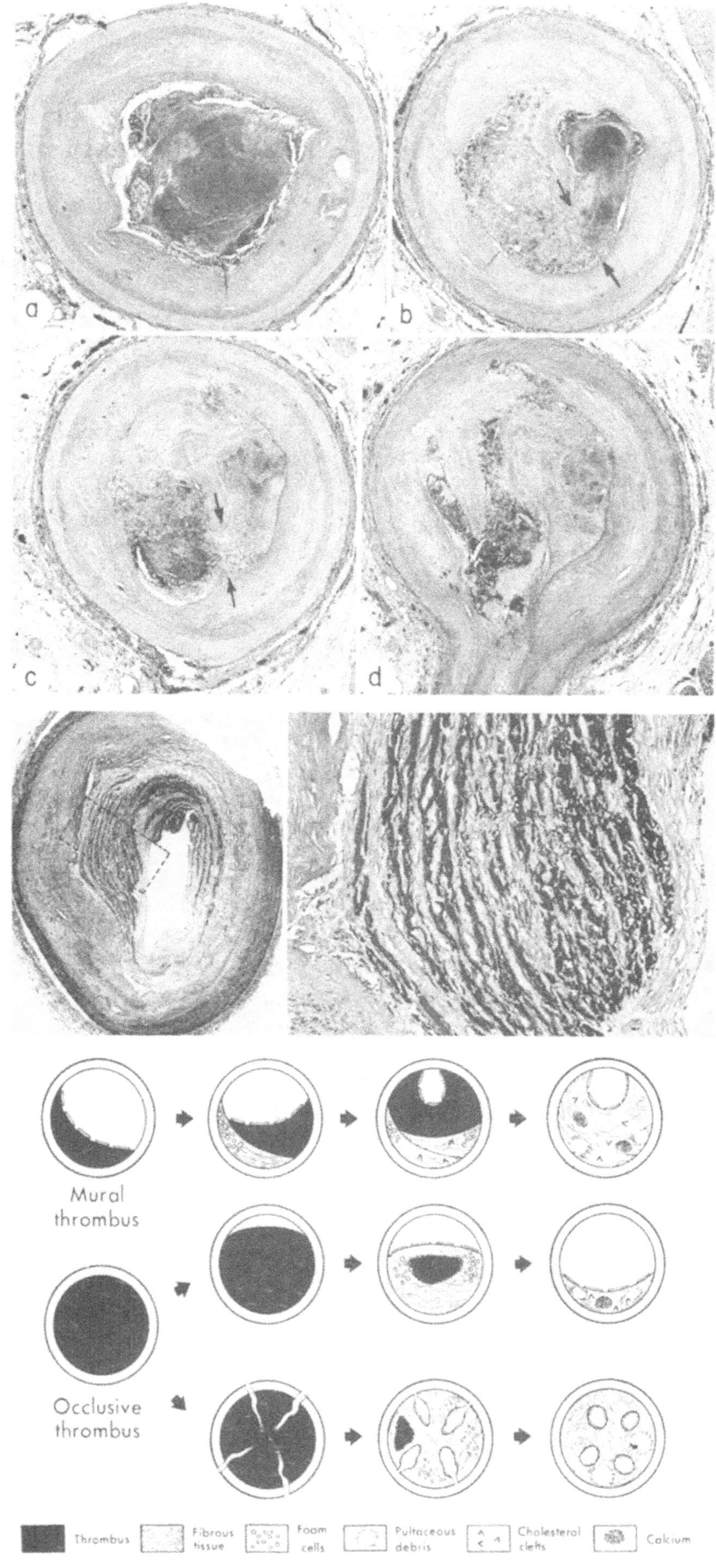

Figure 12. Four sections of anterior descending coronary artery in a forty-seven year old woman (A68-129) who had recurring AMI over a forty-two day period. The sections show a thrombus which is located over a ruptured plaque (between the arrows). Extravasated erythrocytes also are present in the plaque. Serial sections were cut of the area of thrombosis. The four sections shown here were from a segment 360 μ long; **a,** at 12 μ. **b,** at 120 μ. **c,** at 240 μ. **d,** at 360 μ. Movat stains; original magnification, each $\times$ 14.

Figure 13. Right coronary artery in a forty-seven year old man (A70-72) with healed posterior wall left ventricular transmural infarct and rheumatic mitral stenosis. The lumen of the right coronary artery was narrowed more than 75 per cent primarily by fibrous plaques interspersed with fibrin as shown here. The fibrin is dark and the organized fibrous tissue is lighter. A close-up view of the deposits located in the bracket is shown at right. The occurrence of fibrin in atherosclerotic plaques is evidence that thrombosis and atherosclerosis are in some way closely related. Phosphotungstic acid-hematoxylin stain, original magnification $\times$ 23 **(left)** and $\times$ 120 **(right).**

Figure 14. Diagram depicting formation of coronary arterial atherosclerotic plaques from mural and occlusive thrombi. The mural thrombus initially contacts only a portion of the intimal lining. The fibrin-platelet thrombus is covered by endothelial cells and retraction occurs as it organizes into fibrous tissue. Foam cells appear. Another mural thrombus follows, the process of organization is repeated. The lines of demarcation between the separate thrombi gradually fade so that at the final stage histologic study makes recognition of previous components of thrombus difficult. Organization of an occlusive thrombus may occur in two ways. In one, the thrombus retracts from one intimal surface to form a single channel. As it organizes the surface of the thrombus exposed to the lumen is covered by endothelial cells. Organization takes place from the overlying newly grown endothelium and from preexisting intima to encase in fibrous tissue the residual thrombus which may undergo fatty degeneration. Alternatively, organization may occur by capillaries growing into the thrombus at its base. The capillaries may dilate as the thrombus retracts during organization finally leading to the plaque with recanalized channels.

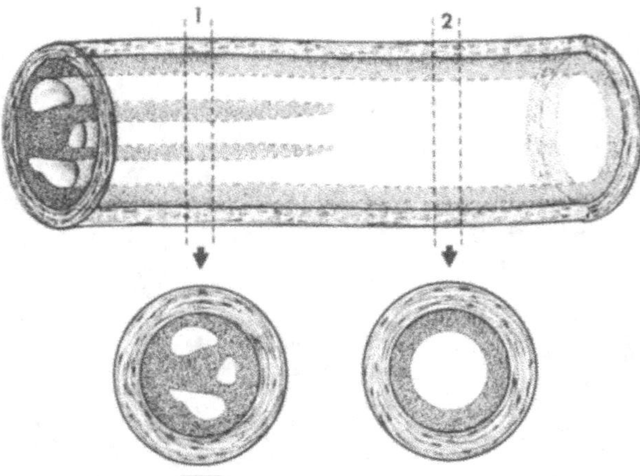

Figure 15. *The multi- and the unichanneled coronary arterial atherosclerotic plaque. Duguid, when studying serial sections of an "organized thrombus," noted that the tissue present between channels in an artery containing multiple revascularized channels was similar to that found in arteries with only one channel. Since the multichannel artery had been recognized as the hallmark of an organized thrombus and since the tissue in both multi- and unichanneled arteries was similar, he reasoned that the causative process also was similar.*

COMMENTS

Although many clinicians and pathologists apparently consider coronary arterial thrombosis the cause of fatal acute myocardial infarction (AMI), the reported frequency of such thrombosis has varied from 21 to 91 per cent [2–22]. Inclusion of cases of subendocardial infarction and sudden death ("acute cardiovascular collapse in the absence of myocardial necrosis") [23] with cases of transmural necrosis is probably the major cause for the variation in frequency.

Coronary arterial thrombi are infrequent in patients who die suddenly with or without previous histories of cardiac disease and in those in whom necrosis is limited to the inner half of the left ventricular wall (subendocardium). Among our twenty-four patients who died suddenly (less than six hours from onset of symptoms), two (8 per cent) had a thrombus in a coronary artery, and of our nine patients with only subendocardial necrosis, none had a coronary arterial thrombus. In contrast, of our seventy-four patients with transmural myocardial necrosis, forty (54 per cent) had a thrombus in a coronary artery.

Although the type of myocardial infarct is probably the most important factor, differing technics of examining coronary arteries at necropsy and differing definitions of what constitutes a true thrombus also may contribute to the varied reported in-cidence of coronary thrombosis in fatal AMI. Studies utilizing only gross inspection of these vessels without confirmation of the presence or absence of thrombus by histologic study are inadequate. Postmortem clots, hemorrhage into old atherosclerotic plaques and even highly vascularized old plaques may be confused with antemortem thrombi (Figure 2). True (antemortem) thrombi are adherent to the luminal surfaces of the arteries and are composed of platelets or fibrin or both, and usually also of erythrocytes and leukocytes. Coronary arterial thrombi are usually about 1 cm in length, and although they are adherent distally they may not be adherent proximally. The composition of a thrombus at varying levels may differ. Distally it is more likely to consist of platelets or fibrin or both (white thrombus), and more proximally it may be composed of erythrocytes, lesser quantities of fibrin, few platelets and some leukocytes (red thrombus). Early thrombi may be composed purely of platelets and are often small and nonocclusive (Figures 6 and 7). The postmortem or false thrombus, in contrast to the true one, is nonadherent and composed mainly of erythrocytes.

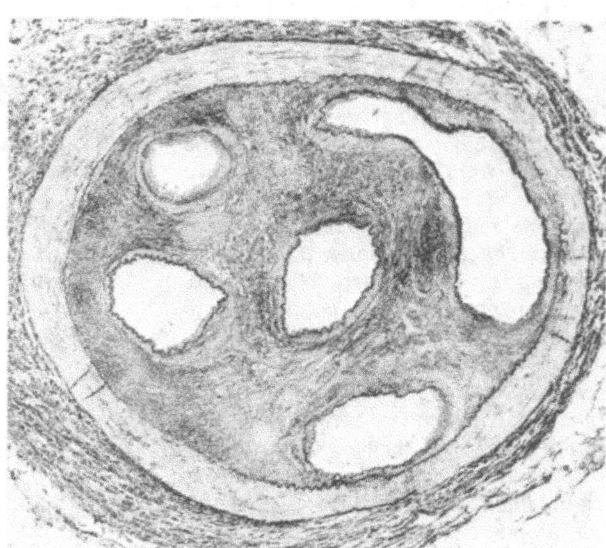

Figure 16. *Recanalized embolus in distal anterior descending coronary artery of a twenty-six year old man (A63-170) in whom a massive anterior wall AMI developed three years before when he had infective endocarditis of the aortic valve. This process clearly resulted from organization of fibrin-platelet-erythrocyte-leukocyte clot, almost surely embolus, and similar lesions are found in patients with extensive coronary arterial atherosclerosis. Note that each recanalized channel has developed its own internal elastic membrane and smooth muscle medial wall. Elastic van Gieson stain, original magnification × 46.*

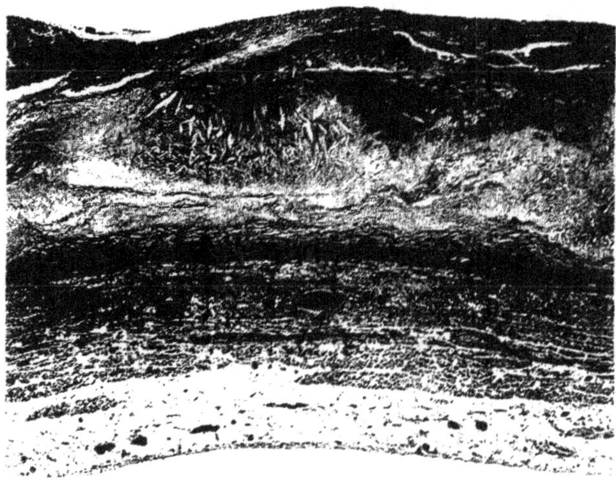

Figure 17. *Left atrial thrombus in a patient with mitral stenosis. Organization of a thrombus may result in plaques which look identical to complicated atherosclerotic plaques. Shown here is a section of left atrial wall from a fifty year old woman (A67-210) with a huge thrombus. Organization of portions of the thrombus led to development of numerous cholesterol clefts, pultaceous debris, calcific deposits as well as fibrous tissue—components of arterial atherosclerotic plaques. Hematoxylin and eosin stain, original magnification × 20.*

Thrombi occurring in patients who died of AMI are, except in cases of embolism, superimposed on old atherosclerotic plaques. Usually the artery containing the thrombus is more than 50 per cent narrowed already by old atherosclerotic plaques, and frequently the degree of luminal narrowing is more than 75 per cent at the distal attachment. In most patients with fatal AMI and coronary arterial thrombi the lumen of the artery distal to the thrombus is more than 75 per cent narrowed by old plaques. In thirty-seven of our forty-two patients with antemortem coronary clots (thrombi in thirty-nine, emboli in three), thrombus was located at or proximal to a site already more than 75 per cent narrowed by old plaque. To reemphasize; in only five of our forty-two patients with coronary arterial thromboembolic material was the vessel containing the clot not narrowed more than 75 per cent by old atherosclerotic plaques, and three of these five had coronary emboli. In a few patients the thrombus occurred in a segment of artery between two sites of extreme narrowing by old plaques. The observation of severe narrowing by old plaques of the coronary artery distal to a thrombus has not been commented on in previous reports to our knowledge. Experimentally, the site of predilection of a

thrombus has been within a "dilated" segment or at the poststenotic luminal expansion [24].

Why fresh thrombi are located at or proximal to sites of narrowing is unclear. Several investigators [4,25–33] have observed thrombi covering cracks in old atherosclerotic plaques, and some [29–31,33] have considered rupture of the innermost layer of plaques the most important precipitating cause of coronary arterial thrombosis. Ruptures occur particularly in fibrous tissue covering deposits of pultaceous debris and lead to discharge of necrotic debris into the arterial lumens or to bleeding into plaques. The break in the plaque exposes collagen to the flowing blood, and this site is said to be a strong stimulus for platelet accumulation [34]. The sudden change in volume of the plaque by discharge of plaque material into the lumen or from hemorrhage into the plaque via the rupture also creates alterations in flow patterns which favor platelet thrombosis [29]. Jørgensen et al. [25] suggested that the pathogenesis of coronary thrombi associated with ruptures of necrotic plaques is different from that unassociated with rupture. That coronary arterial thrombi are related to rupture of necrotic plaques, however, is far from a proved observation. Serial sections are usually necessary to observe cracks in plaques (Figure 12) and even by this means interpretation is often difficult. Cracks in plaques were infrequently observed beneath thrombi in the patients studied by us, and prob-

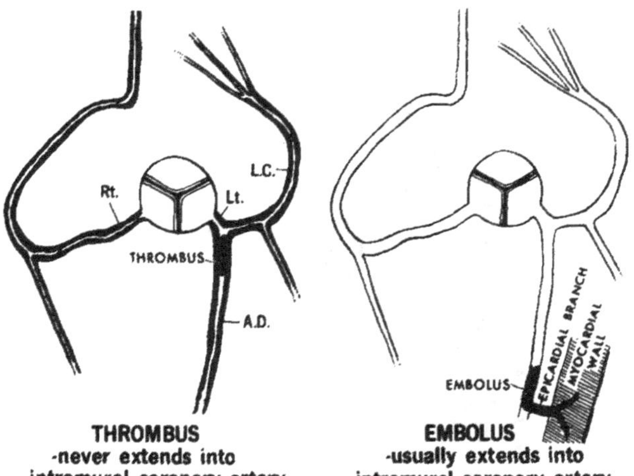

Figure 18. *Diagram depicting differences between coronary arterial embolism and thrombosis. The thrombus is usually proximal and is superimposed on an old plaque. The thrombus does not extend into intramural coronary arteries. The embolus is distal and extends into intramural arteries. The embolus usually occurs in a coronary tree devoid of significant old atherosclerotic plaquing.*

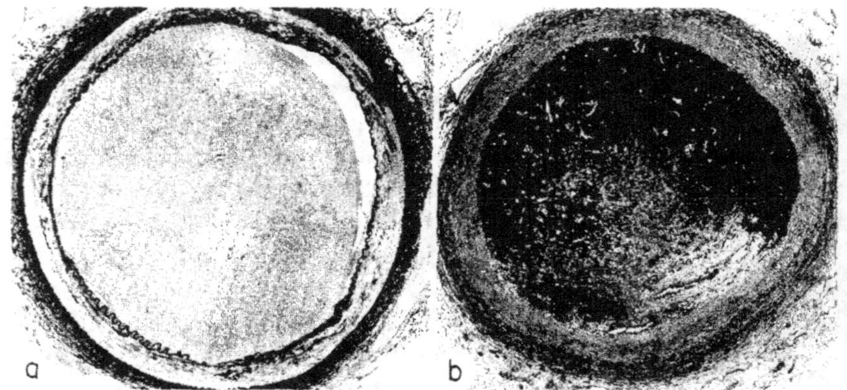

Figure 19. Embolus to right coronary artery in a fifty-six year old man (A70-244). It occurred during cardiac catheterization thirty-one days before death and caused transmural necrosis of the posterior left ventricular wall. Note that the clot has formed in an artery which was previously free of atherosclerotic plaquing. The embolus is showing some evidence of organization distally (b). Elastic van Gieson stain, original magnification × 22 (a); hematoxylin and eosin stain, original magnification × 25 (b).

ably most thrombi form over plaques with intact surfaces [35,36]. Rupture of a plaque may result at times from fixing and cutting an artery without providing prior support of its wall by injection. Fulton [36] injected coronary arteries with a solid supporting medium before sectioning, and in few the intima produced convexity of the lining. In none of his twenty-five patients who died of coronary heart disease (fourteen with AMI) was ulceration of a plaque observed. Interpretation of whether a plaque is cracked or if present, an artefact or real, is fraught with too much difficulty in our opinion to give this possible mechanism of thrombosis undue weight.

The thrombus in fatal AMI is practically always located in the coronary artery which supplies the infarcted myocardium; if the infarct involves the anterior wall of the left ventricle, and if a thrombus occurs, it will be located in the anterior descending coronary artery. Thrombi in either the left anterior descending or circumflex coronary artery generally are located within 2 cm of the bifurcation of the left main coronary artery (or within 4 cm of the left aortic ostium). The left main coronary artery is rarely the site of thrombosis. The proximal portion of the right coronary artery, in contrast, does not appear to be a more frequent site of thrombus formation than does the mid or distal portions. Thrombi are infrequently seen in the small epicardial branches of the major extramural coronary arteries and never occur, other than as platelet aggregates, in intramural coronary arteries.

Not all coronary arterial thrombi produce total luminal occlusion. (The term "occlusion" is not synonymous with "thrombosis" as implied in many reports, since occlusion may be partial as well as complete and since the vessel may be occluded by material other than that which forms a thrombus.) Partially occluding ("mural" or nonocclusive) thrombi were found in seven (18 per cent) and totally occluding (occlusive) thrombi in thirty-three (82 per cent) of our forty patients with thrombi and fatal transmural myocardial necrosis. Pure platelet thrombi, as mentioned earlier, are usually small and infrequently totally occlude lumens. Nonocclusive thrombi, since they are small, may have little functional significance. Even totally occluding thrombi when formed in arteries already more than 90 per cent occluded by old atherosclerotic plaques also may have little functional significance. Thus, it is not enough to know whether or not a coronary artery contains a thrombus. The degree of luminal narrowing by old atherosclerotic plaques at the site of, and distal to, the thrombus, and whether the thrombus is

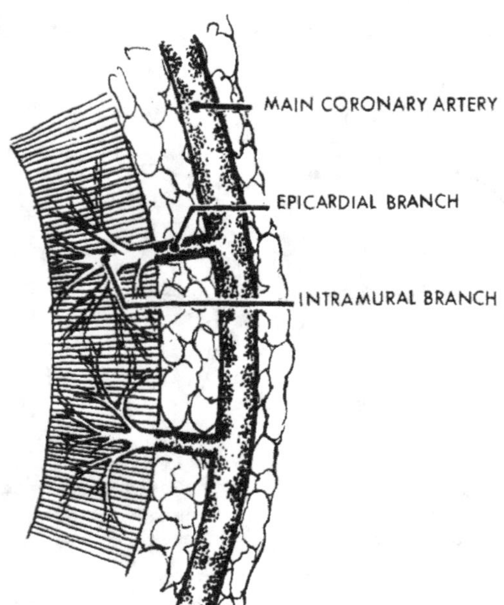

Figure 20. Diagram of a major extramural coronary artery and its epicardial and intramural branches in atherosclerosis. The main artery and its epicardial branches are extensively involved by the atherosclerotic process but the intramural vessels are spared.

totally or only partially occlusive must also be known before the significance of a coronary arterial thrombus can be judged.

The role of coronary thrombosis in AMI is unclear. For several decades coronary thrombosis was considered the cause of AMI. Clinically, AMI represents a sudden change for the patient compared to his preinfarction status. This often dramatic clinical event has been equated at necropsy with the finding of a "fresh" thrombus in a coronary artery. But, only about 50 per cent of the patients with transmural myocardial necrosis and about 10 per cent of the patients with subendocardial necrosis or "sudden cardiovascular collapse without myocardial necrosis" have a thrombus in a coronary artery at necropsy. Thus, nothing new is found in the coronary arteries in the majority of patients who die of cardiac disease. The virtual absence of coronary arterial thrombi in patients who die suddenly of cardiac disease and their presence in only about half of those with myocardial necrosis has given rise to the concept that coronary arterial thrombi are consequences rather than causes of AMI. Comparison of histologic ages of coronary arterial thrombi and of acute myocardial infarcts has indicated to some observers [12] that thrombosis follows rather than precedes myocardial necrosis. Judging the age of a coronary thrombus, however, is difficult and probably inaccurate, and therefore this comparison is unreliable.

An examination of the clinical events during the period of myocardial infarction has provided a possible explanation for the occurrence of coronary arterial thrombi in some patients with AMI and their absence in others. Spain and Bradess [9,20] have shown that the frequency of finding coronary thrombi rises with increasing intervals between the onset of symptoms of myocardial ischemia and death. In their study in 1960 [9] the frequency rose from 16 per cent of 303 patients who survived for less than one hour to 37 per cent of sixty-five patients who survived from one to twenty-four hours, and to 54 per cent of 200 patients who survived for more than twenty-four hours; in their study in 1970 [20] of other patients the frequency rose from 17 per cent of eighty patients who survived for less than one hour to 36 per cent of twenty-two patients who survived from one to eight hours, and to 57 per cent of 100 patients who survived for more than eight hours. Thus, a certain but variable period of survival after the onset of infarction is usually necessary for a thrombus to form.

The presence of coronary arterial thrombi in AMI also has been found to correlate with the presence of the power failure syndrome—a form of shock resulting in "an inability of the myocardium to maintain the level of cardiac output necessary for adequate organ perfusion. There is evidence of underperfusion of one or more organ systems" [22]. In a clinicopathologic study of thirty-seven patients who died of AMI Walston and associates [22] found thrombi in seventeen (71

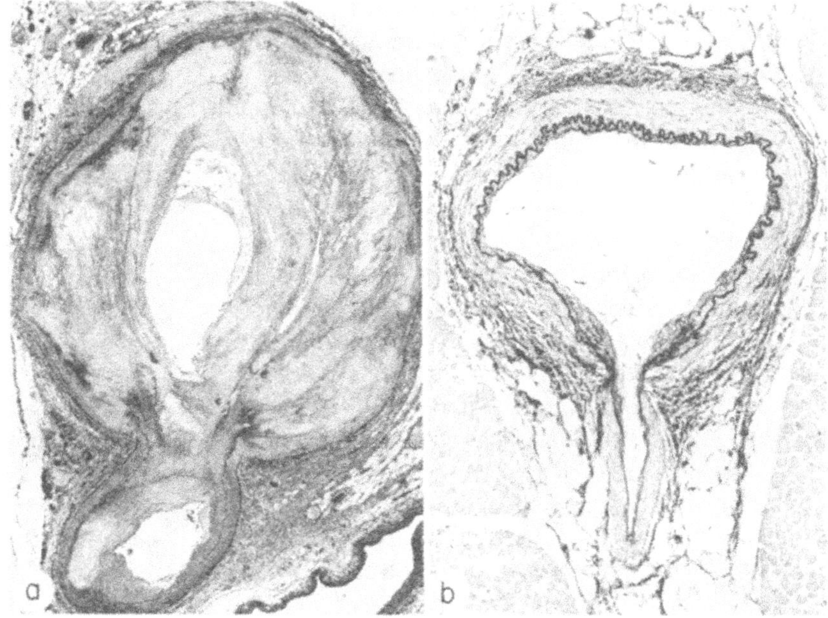

Figure 21. Major coronary artery and its branches in atherosclerosis. a, left anterior descending artery and an epicardial branch from it are severely atherosclerotic in a fifty-four year old man (A70-116) in whom AMI developed eight hours before death. Movat stain, original magnification × 20. b, intramural coronary artery and one of its branches in a fifty-eight year old man (SH No. A4703) with known severe systemic hypertension and angina pectoris. He died three hours after the development of severe chest pain (sudden death). The lumens of the extramural right, left anterior descending, left circumflex and left main coronary arteries were all more than 75 per cent narrowed by old plaque. Despite the severe narrowing of the extramural coronary arteries, the intramural coronary arteries were normal, one of which is seen here. Elastic van Gieson stain, original magnification × 100.

TABLE III   **Types of Activity at Onset of AMI***

Activity	Attacks	
	No.	%
Sleep	198	22†
Rest (lying or sitting)	277	31†
Mild activity	180	20†
Moderate activity (excludes walking)	76	9†
Walking	141	16†
Unusual or severe exertion	18	2†
Totals	890	100

* Adapted from Master, Dack, Jaffe, Amer Heart J 18:434, 1939 [38].
† The percentages for these six activities are very similar to those occurring in the daily lives of most subjects.

per cent) of twenty-four patients with and in only two (15 per cent) of thirteen patients without the power failure syndrome. Of their thirty-seven patients, nineteen had coronary arterial thrombi and seventeen (90 per cent) of these had the power failure syndrome; of their eighteen patients without coronary arterial thrombi, seven (39 per cent) had had the power failure syndrome. Thus a severely diminished cardiac output and consequently slowed coronary arterial blood flow are usually required for a thrombus to form in a coronary artery. It has also been observed at necropsy that the larger the area of myocardial necrosis, the more likely will a thrombus be present in a coronary artery. Of course, the larger the infarct, the more likely will pump failure occur [37].

The type activity experienced by patients at the time of onset of AMI also may reflect slowed blood flow. Master, Dack and Jaffe [38] interviewed 890 patients with AMI and found that symptoms of myocardial infarction appeared in 73 per cent of them during sleep, rest or mild activity (Table III). For myocardial necrosis to begin during inactivity is in direct contrast to angina pectoris, which appears during activity, but is associated with similar degrees of luminal narrowing of the coronary arteries [39–42]. It would appear that decreased coronary arterial blood flow, i.e., relative stasis, is necessary for thrombus to form in a coronary artery and that shock, congestive cardiac failure and inactivity all decrease coronary blood flow. The slow flow concept, however, does not explain the occurrence of coronary arterial thrombi at sites of, and proximal to, severe stenoses caused by old atherosclerotic plaques. Luminal narrowing, however, does introduce points of high velocity gradients which appear to favor

platelet aggregation [43]. A high shearing stress also may damage erythrocytes [44], followed by release of adenosine diphosphate [45] and platelet damage.

Several explanations have been offered for the absence of coronary arterial thrombi in patients who die of AMI or of "acute cardiovascular collapse without myocardial necrosis." Lysis of thrombi before or after death as a result of excessive production of fibrinolysins has not been proved or disproved, although several observations tend to discount the role of postmortem lysis. In fatal AMI or sudden death the major coronary arteries in patients without thrombi are frequently free of blood or blood products. If fresh thrombi had been lysed immediately after death, partially liquefied blood or a remnant of thrombus within the lumen would be expected; this may not be the case. Necropsies performed within fifteen minutes on patients with coronary heart disease who died suddenly have not disclosed evidence of partially lysed thrombi [20]. It is unlikely that postmortem lysis of thrombi could be so selective as to liquefy only those thrombi which allegedly might have been present in patients with subendocardial necrosis and not those associated with transmural necrosis. It is unlikely that postmortem lysis, an artefact, which in a sense occurs by chance, could account for the occurrence of identical percentages of thrombi being present in separate but similar studies carried out a decade apart by the same investigators [9,20].

Inadequate examination of the coronary tree so that thrombi, although actually present, were not observed, is highly unlikely. At least two histologic sections of every 5 mm segment of the entire extramural coronary arterial tree were examined in this study of 107 patients. The chance of missing a thrombus by this technic is unlikely.

The absence of thrombi in coronary arteries of many patients with AMI may partially explain the lack of clear-cut benefits provided to patients with AMI treated with anticoagulants. After twenty years of using these drugs, controversy still continues as to whether or not they are beneficial to patients with AMI. Of factors favoring the use of anticoagulants in patients with AMI, the ability of these drugs to reduce the body's ability to form or extend a thrombus in a coronary artery has been high on the list. This factor, however, has been based on the supposition that AMI is usually caused by coronary thrombosis. The incidence of coronary arterial thrombi in patients with fatal

AMI treated with anticoagulants is similar to that in patients not receiving anticoagulants [25].

Although it may not be the precipitating cause of AMI, thrombosis may still play a major role in causing the underlying coronary atherosclerosis. Indeed, there is little doubt that organization of thrombi contributes to the development of the complicated atherosclerotic plaque. The presence of fibrin and platelets in atherosclerotic plaques strongly connects atherosclerosis with thrombosis. Each has been found in plaques by immuno-fluorescent technics [46,47], and fibrin is commonly found in plaques by histologic (Figure 13) and electron microscopic examination. Histologic evidence that a plaque is derived from thrombus, however, is frequently obscured [48]. As a thrombus is covered by new endothelium, the underlying endothelium is replaced by connective tissue from the intima with resultant obliteration of the original line of demarcation (Figure 14). Thrombi appear to organize by ingrowth of overlying endothelial cells and by connective tissue from the intima [49]. Modified smooth muscle cells [50–52], which are capable of synthesizing collagen, elastin and probably mucopolysaccharides [50,53], and which are present in connective tissue of arterial intima (they also may be derived from endothelium [50]), invade the bases of attached thrombi. Small mural thrombi organize by an avascular process [48,54] whereas larger thrombi become vascularized [55] (Figures 14–16). Capillaries extend from the new overlying endothelium to provide a direct blood supply from the lumen and from vasa vasora to penetrate thrombi at their bases [55,56]. Vascularization is considered the hallmark of an organized thrombus [55]. Capillaries growing into a thrombus have fibrinolytic activity [57] which contributes to resolution of a thrombus as it organizes. These capillaries, which may later atrophy, can be a source of hemorrhage into plaques. Occlusive thrombi, like mural thrombi, may be incorporated into the intima of arteries as atherosclerotic plaques [48]. Occlusive thrombi may retract before endotheliozation is complete and thereby appear later as mural or nonocclusive plaques (Figure 14).

The source of lipids in atherosclerotic plaques is unclear. Fatty degeneration may occur in any thrombus or hematoma; organization of a left atrial thrombus in mitral stenosis, for example, may look identical to an atherosclerotic plaque (Figure 17). Platelets, erythrocytes and plasma all may provide lipids to plaques. When whole blood clots are injected into systemic veins of rabbits, fibrous intimal plaques (containing little lipid) form in pulmonary arteries [58]. Even though the emboli are occlusive they organize by retracting into eccentric plaques. The conversion of thromboemboli to plaques is important evidence for the thrombotic origin of atherosclerosis. When platelet-rich thrombi rather than whole blood clots are injected, typical fatty atherosclerotic plaques containing many foam cells and foci of calcium develop [59]. Erythrocytes contain less lipid than do platelets, but repeated small hemorrhages may lead to accumulation of large amounts of lipid, especially cholesterol [60]. The plasma supplies lipoproteins which are found in both recent and organizing thrombi [61] as well as in old plaques [62].

Atherosclerotic plaques are like fingerprints. No two are alike. In this study of the entire extramural coronary tree of 107 patients with fatal AMI, tremendous variation in the composition of adjacent plaques was noted. Some plaques contained lipid and large quantities of pultaceous debris, whereas others were composed primarily of fibrous tissue. Differences in composition of original thrombi may explain differences in composition of atherosclerotic plaques. Mixed white and red thrombi form plaques that contain some foam cells [63] but not in the quantity found in plaques derived from platelet-rich or white thrombi [59]. The type thrombus, whether mural (nonocclusive) or occlusive, also may affect the composition of a plaque. Occlusive platelet thrombi usually do not accumulate fibrin while undergoing transformation to fibrofatty plaques [59]. Mural platelet thrombi, in contrast, appear to be partially or totally replaced by fibrin before undergoing organization; consequently, the plaques that form are mainly fibromuscular [64–66].

Hemorrhages into old atherosclerotic plaques are common, occurring in twenty-six (24 per cent) of our 107 patients. They probably are of little functional significance. In only one of our twenty-six patients with hemorrhages into plaques did the lumen of the artery appear to have been compromised by the extravasated blood. In contrast to thrombi in coronary arteries in fatal AMI, hemorrhages often occur in coronary arteries unrelated to the areas of necrosis, and they may occur in more than one artery or in multiple sites in the same artery. Hemorrhages appear to form from either breaks in the fibrous capsule covering a plaque or from rupture of a small vascular channel within a plaque. Each of these mechanisms is difficult to prove in the individual patient. Possibly small hemorrhages into old plaques occur chronically and have little to do with AMI. It is possible that some hemorrhages into old plaques may be produced artifactually during cutting and processing of coronary arteries for histologic study. A possible detrimental effect of hemorrhages into plaques is the occurrence of superimposed thrombi. This association, however, may not be as frequent as once supposed. The two may occur together, presumably when a crack in a plaque is the responsible mechanism. Fulton [36] and Jørgensen et al. [25] did not find an association between hemorrhages into plaques and coronary thrombosis, probably because the majority of thrombi were observed over plaques which consisted predominately of fibrous tissue [36]. The incidence of hemorrhages into plaques does not appear to be increased by the use of anticoagulants [25,36].

It is essential to recall that fatal AMI, indeed, nearly all symptomatic ischemic heart disease, is associated with diffuse and severe coronary arterial atherosclerosis. Examination of several thousand histologic sections of coronary arteries in these 107 patients with fatal AMI disclosed atherosclerotic plaquing in all but four sections (excluding those in the three patients with coronary embolism). The degree of luminal narrowing varied, but some plaquing was present on virtually every millimeter of major coronary artery. The lumen of at least one of the three major extramural coronary arteries was narrowed more than 75 per cent by old atherosclerotic plaques in 101 of our 107 patients, and three of the six without this degree of narrowing had coronary emboli. A coronary artery, however, may contain a considerable amount of atherosclerosis and yet be capable of transporting considerable quantities of blood to myocardium. When the degree of coronary narrowing decreases the original lumen by more than 75 per cent, the flow in the vessel is significantly decreased. In the carotid artery, a detectable reduction in flow and pressure does not occur until the degree of luminal narrowing is more than 80 per cent [67]. Among our 107 necropsy patients, the average number of major coronary arteries (three per patient; excludes the left main coronary artery) narrowed more than 75 per cent by old atherosclerotic plaques were: 2.4 in seventy-four patients with transmural necrosis; 2.3 in nine patients with only subendocardial necrosis; and 2.4 in twenty-four patients who died suddenly. Similar observations had been made by Saphir and associates [4], Blumgart et al. [39] and Yater et al. [68] who found "complete occlusions" of usually two major coronary arteries in patients who died with angina pectoris or of AMI. The degree of luminal narrowing of coronary arteries by old atherosclerotic plaques is identical in patients with fatal AMI who have coronary thrombi and in those without coronary thrombi [25].

The sites of maximum narrowing of major extramural coronary arteries are highly variable in a particular patient but certain patterns emerge when large groups of patients with fatal AMI are examined. The lumen of the left main coronary artery is rarely narrowed more than 75 per cent by old atherosclerotic plaques. Maximum narrowing of the left anterior descending and left circumflex coronary arteries is usually within 2 cm of the bifurcation of the left main. The proximal and midportions of the right coronary artery are not predisposed to greater degrees of luminal narrowing by old plaques than is the distal portion. The right coronary artery's main function is to supply the posterior wall of the left ventricle via its posterior descending branches. Thus, narrowing of the right coronary artery at any site promixal to the origins of the posterior descending branches might have similar functional significance. Or, in other words, the left coronary arterial tree begins supplying the left ventricle with oxygen about 2 cm from its origin from the aorta; the right coronary artery does not begin perfusing the left ventricle until it has travelled in the right atrioventricular sulcus for about 12 cm. Thus, severe narrowing of the right coronary artery 11 cm from its aortic ostium might be as significant a lesion as a similar narrowing 2 cm from its ostium. In contrast, severe narrowing of the left anterior descending coronary artery 11 cm downstream without significant proximal narrowing may have less myocardial consequences.

Atherosclerotic lesions generally have been classified into three types [69]: (1) yellow (fatty) streaks or dots, (2) fibrous plaques and (3) complicated plaques. The latter plaques contain calcific deposits, cholesterol clefts, thrombus or all three, and they may ulcerate (into the arterial lumen) or weaken the vessel wall so that it dilates. The atherosclerotic plaques observed in extramural coronary arteries in fatal AMI are of the complicated type. Significant degrees of luminal narrowing of the coronary arteries only by foam cell lesions do not occur with the possible exception of patients with type III hyperlipoproteinemia [70].

In most complicated plaques few foam cells are present, and the luminal narrowing is caused primarily by fibrous tissue, with or without calcific deposits, and pultaceous debris (presumably the end result of the breakdown of foam cells). Why calcific deposits are absent in coronary arteries of some patients with fatal AMI and extensive in others is unknown. Intimal calcific deposits in these vessels increase with age (more than 95 per cent of patients in the United States over eighty years of age have coronary arterial calcific deposits [71] and are more frequent and extensive in patients with systemic hypertension than in normotensive patients [71]. Patients with diabetes mellitus also appear to have larger and more extensive coronary calcific deposits than patients without diabetes.

The occurrence of a clot in the distal portion of a major extramural coronary artery suggests that the cause is embolism rather than thrombosis. This situation occurred in three of our 107 patients. Coronary arterial embolism differs from thrombosis in the following manner (Figure 18): (1) the clot is located distally, not proximally, and is usually in the anterior descending coronary artery; (2) the clot extends into intramural coronary arteries and into the epicardial branches of the major extramural vessel (in thrombosis, no clot is found in intramural coronary arteries and uncommonly in the small epicardial branches of major vessels); and (3) the entire extramural coronary arterial tree is relatively free of old atherosclerotic plaques. (It is difficult to make the diagnosis of embolism anatomically if the lumens of the coronary arteries are more than 50 per cent narrowed by old plaque.) Also, patients with emboli are usually relatively young and have certain predisposing conditions (arrhythmia, infective endocarditis, intracardiac mural thrombosis, etc.) [72–76].

Much has been written about disease of the small coronary arteries. That intramural coronary arteries are narrowed in certain conditions, particularly the neurogenic heart diseases (Friedrich's ataxia, progressive muscular dystrophy, myotonic dystrophy), is now a well established fact [77]. Conditions involving extramural coronary arteries, in our view, have not been shown also to involve the intramural coronary arteries. There are dissenting views, however, on this point [78–81]. Likewise, conditions which clearly involve intramural coronary arteries tend to spare the extramural coronary arteries. With the exception of the small arteries in the left ventricular papillary muscles, which are subjected to maximal systolic intraventricular pressure over the entire circumference of their surfaces, diseases which affect the intramural coronary arteries do not affect the extramural coronary arteries and vice versa. Other than insignificant minimal fibrous intimal proliferation in a rare intramural coronary artery, and that usually in the left ventricular papillary muscles, no abnormality was observed in the intramural coronary arteries in any of our 107 patients. Indeed, the intramural vessels in the heart appear to be protected from intimal proliferation and luminal narrowing by the contracting adjacent myocardium. In coronary atherosclerosis, plaques occur routinely in epicardial branches of major extramural arteries, but as soon as these branches penetrate myocardium, the lumen is suddenly wide open again (Figures 20 and 21). Even in systemic hypertension, the intramural coronary arteries are not affected as are other small systemic arteries in this condition. The coronary arteries are not exposed to the high systolic pressure because they are perfused mainly in diastole. The contracting ventricular myocardium may further lower the intraluminal pressure in these small vessels. Although patients with diabetes mellitus have been reported to have disease of intramural coronary arteries [79], this finding has not been observed by us. Foam cells, cholesterol clefts and pultaceous debris, components of plaques in extramural coronary arteries, are virtually never found in intramural vessels. Thus, significant involvement of intramural coronary arteries does not occur in patients with significant luminal narrowing of extramural coronary arteries.

ACKNOWLEDGMENT

We sincerely thank Dr. Abner Golden, Professor and Chairman, Department of Pathology, Georgetown University, Washington, D.C., Dr. Joseph O'Connell, Pathologist, Suburban Hospital, Bethesda, Maryland, and Dr. Michael Cuadra, Chief of Pathology, District of Columbia General Hospital, Washington, D.C. who allowed us to study the hearts of many patients who had died of acute ischemic heart disease at their respective hospitals. Also, we thank Mrs. Sandra Lewis, Mrs. Louise Holthaus, and Miss Margaret Burk, Section of Pathology, National Heart and Lung Institute, for the several thousand beautifully prepared histologic sections of coronary arteries examined in this study. The photomicrographs were taken by Mr. Walter G. P. Seewald and Mr. Robert W. Nye.

REFERENCES

1. Fortuin NJ, Roberts WC: Congenital atresia of the left main coronary artery. Amer J Med 50: 385, 1971.
2. Barnes AR, Ball RG: The incidence and situation of myocardial infarction in one thousand consecutive postmortem examinations. Amer J Med Sci 183: 215, 1932.
3. Lisa JR, Ring A: Myocardial infarction or gross fibrosis: analysis of 100 necropsies. Arch Intern Med (Chicago) 50: 131, 1932.
4. Saphir O, Priest WS, Hamburger WW, Katz LN: Coronary arteriosclerosis, coronary thrombosis and the resulting myocardial changes. An evaluation of their respective clinical pictures including the electrocardiographic records, based on the anatomical findings. Amer Heart J 10: 567, 1935.
5. Friedberg CK, Horn H: Acute myocardial infarction not due to coronary artery occlusion. JAMA 112: 1675, 1939.
6. Foord AG: Embolism and thrombosis in coronary heart disease. JAMA 138: 1009, 1948.
7. Miller RD, Burchell HB, Edwards JE: Myocardial infarction with and without acute coronary occlusion. A pathologic study. Arch Intern Med (Chicago) 88: 597, 1951.
8. Branwood AW, Montgomery GL: Observations on the morbid anatomy of coronary artery disease. Scot Med J 1: 367, 1956.
9. Spain DM, Bradess VA: The relationship of coronary thrombosis to coronary atherosclerosis and ischemic heart disease. (A necropsy study covering a period of 25 years.) Amer J Med Sci 240: 701, 1960.
10. Kurland GS, Weingarten C, Pitt B: The relation between the location of coronary occlusions and the occurrence of shock in acute myocardial infarction. Circulation 31: 646, 1965.
11. Meadows R: Coronary thrombosis and myocardial infarction. Med J Aust 2: 409, 1965.
12. Ehrlich JC, Shinohara Y: Low incidence of coronary thrombosis in myocardial infarction. A restudy by serial block technique. Arch Path 78: 432, 1964.
13. Mitchell JRA, Schwartz CJ: Arterial Disease, Philadelphia, F.A. Davis, 1965.
14. Baroldi G: Acute coronary occlusion as a cause of myocardial infarct and sudden coronary heart death. Amer J Cardiol 16: 859, 1965.
15. Harland WA, Holburn AM: Coronary thrombosis and myocardial infarction. Lancet 2: 1158, 1966.
16. Kagan A, Livsic AM, Sternby N, Vihert AM: Coronary-artery thrombosis and the acute attack of coronary heart-disease. Lancet 2: 1199, 1968.
17. Chapman I: Relationships of recent coronary artery occlusion and acute myocardial infarction. J Mount Sinai Hosp 35: 149, 1968.
18. Jørgensen L, Hoerem JW, Chandler AB, Borchgrevink CF: The pathology of acute coronary death. Acta Anaesth Scand 29 (suppl): 193, 1968.
19. Hackel DB, Estes EH, Walston A, Koff S, Day E: Some problems concerning coronary artery occlusion and acute myocardial infarction. Circulation 39,40 (suppl): IV-31, 1969.
20. Spain DM, Bradess VA: Sudden death from coronary heart disease. Survival time, frequency of thrombi, and cigarette smoking. Chest 58: 107, 1970.
21. Bouch DC, Montgomery GL: Cardiac lesions in fatal cases of recent myocardial ischemia from a coronary care unit. Brit Heart J 32: 795, 1970.
22. Walston A, Hackel DB, Estes EH: Acute coronary occlusion and the "power failure" syndrome. Amer Heart J 79: 613, 1970.
23. Edwards JE: What is myocardial infarction? Circulation 39,40 (suppl): IV-5, 1969.
24. Jørgensen L: Experimental platelet and coagulation thrombi. A histological study of arterial and venous thrombi of varying age in untreated and heparinized rabbits. Acta Path Microbiol Scand 62: 189, 1964.
25. Jørgensen L, Chandler AB, Borchgrevink CF: Acute lesions of coronary arteries in anticoagulant-treated and in untreated patients. Atherosclerosis 13: 21, 1971.
26. Leary T: Coronary spasm as a possible factor in producing sudden death. Amer Heart J 10: 338, 1935.
27. Clark E, Graef I, Chasis H: Thrombosis of the aorta and coronary arteries with special reference to the "fibrinoid" lesions. Arch Path 22: 183, 1936.
28. Osborn GR: The Incubation Period of Coronary Thrombosis, London, Butterworth & Co., Ltd., 1963.
29. Chapman I: Morphogenesis of occluding coronary artery thrombosis. Arch Path 80: 256, 1965.
30. Constantinides P: Plaque fissures in human coronary thrombosis. J Atheroscler Res 6: 1, 1966.
31. Friedman M, Van den Boverkamp GJ: The pathogenesis of a coronary thrombus. Amer J Path 48: 19, 1966.
32. Jørgensen L: Thrombosis and the complications of atherosclerosis, Atherosclerosis, Proceedings of the Second International Symposium (Jones RJ, ed), New York, Springer-Verlag, 1970, p 94.
33. Friedman M: The coronary thrombus. Its origin and fate. Human Path 2: 81, 1971.
34. Hovig T, Jørgensen L, Packham MA, Mustard JF: Platelet adherence to fibrin and collagen. J Lab Clin Med 71: 29, 1968.
35. Anitschkow N: Morphodynamik der Koronarsklerose des Herzens. Acta Path Microbiol Scand 49: 426, 1960.
36. Fulton WFM: The Coronary Arteries. Arteriography, Microanatomy, and Pathogenesis of Obliterative Coronary Artery Disease, Springfield, Ill., Charles C Thomas, 1965.
37. Page DL, Caulfield JB, Kastor JA, DeSanctis RW, Sanders CA: Myocardial changes associated with cardiogenic shock. New Eng J Med 285: 133, 1971.
38. Master AM, Dack S, Jaffe HL: Activities associated with the onset of acute coronary artery occlusion. Amer Heart J 18: 434, 1939.
39. Blumgart HL, Schlesinger MJ, Davis D: Studies on the relation of the clinical manifestations of angina pectoris, coronary thrombosis, and myocardial infarction to the pathologic findings with particular reference to the significance of the collateral circulation. Amer Heart J 19: 1, 1940.
40. Zoll PM, Wessler S, Blumgart HL: Angina pectoris. A clinical and pathologic correlation. Amer J Med 11: 331, 1951.
41. Lenegre J, Himbert J: Critical study of the relationship between angina pectoris and coronary atherosclerosis. Amer Heart J 58: 539, 1959.

42. Allison RB, Rodriguez FL, Higgins EA Jr, Leddy JP, Abelman WH, Ellis LB, Robbins SL: Clinicopathologic correlations in coronary atherosclerosis. Four hundred thirty patients studied with postmortem coronary angiography. Circulation 27: 170, 1963.

43. Dintenfass L, Rozenberg MC: The influence of the velocity gradient on in vitro blood coagulation and artificial thrombosis. J Atheroscler Res 5: 276, 1965.

44. Nevaril CG, Lynch EC, Alfrey CP Jr, Hellums JD: Erythrocyte damage and destruction induced by shearing stress. J Lab Clin Med 71: 784, 1968.

45. Harrison MJG, Mitchell JRA: The influence of red blood cells on platelet adhesiveness. Lancet 2: 1163, 1966.

46. Woolf N, Crawford T: Fatty streaks in the aortic intima studied by an immuno-histochemical technique. J Path Bact 80:405, 1960.

47. Woolf N, Carstairs KC: Infiltration and thrombosis in atherosclerosis. A study using immunofluorescent techniques. Amer J Path 51: 373, 1967.

48. Duguid JB: Thrombosis as a factor in the pathogenesis of coronary atherosclerosis. J Path Bact 58: 207, 1946.

49. Crawford T, Levene CI: Incorporation of fibrin in the aortic intima. J Path Bact 64: 523, 1952.

50. Haust DM, More RH, Movat HZ: The role of smooth muscle cells in the fibrogenesis of arteriosclerosis. Amer J Path 37: 377, 1960.

51. Geer JC, McGill HC Jr, Strong JP: The fine structure of the human atherosclerotic lesions. Amer J Path 31: 263, 1961.

52. Wissler RW: The arterial medial cell, smooth muscle or multifunctional mesenchyme? J Atheroscler Res 8: 201, 1968.

53. Getz GS, Vesselinovitch D, Wissler RW: A dynamic pathology of atherosclerosis. Amer J Med 46: 657, 1969.

54. Haust MD, More RH, Movat HZ: The mechanism of fibrosis in arteriosclerosis. Amer J Path 35: 265, 1959.

55. Geiringer E: Intimal vascularization and atherosclerosis. J Path Bact 63: 201, 1951.

56. Morgan AD: The Pathogenesis of Coronary Occlusion, Springfield, Ill., Charles C Thomas, 1956.

57. Todd AS: Localization of fibrinolytic activity in tissues. Brit Med Bull 20: 210, 1964.

58. Harrison CV: Experimental pulmonary atherosclerosis. J Path Bact 60: 289, 1948.

59. Hand RA, Chandler AB: Atherosclerotic metamorphosis of autologous pulmonary thromboemboli in the rabbit. Amer J Path 40: 469, 1962.

60. Hartroft WS: Ceroid-like pigments, hemoceroid and hyaloceroid, in atheromatous lesions of human subjects. Amer J Path 28: 526, 1952.

61. Woolf N, Pilkington TRE, Carstairs KC: The occurrence of lipoproteins in thrombi. J Path Bact 91: 383, 1966.

62. Kao VCY, Wissler RW: A study of the immunohistochemical localization of serum lipoproteins and other plasma proteins in human atherosclerotic lesions. Exp Molec Path 4: 457, 1965.

63. Filshie I, Scott GBD: The organization of experimental venous thrombi. J Path Bact 76: 71, 1958.

64. Jørgensen L, Rowsell HC, Hovig T, Mustard JF: Resolution and organization of platelet-rich mural thrombi in carotid arteries of swine. Amer J Path 51: 681, 1967.

65. Woolf N, Bradley JWP, Crawford T, Carstairs KC: Experimental mural thrombi in the pig aorta. The early natural history. Brit J Exp Path 49: 257, 1968.

66. Woolf N, Carstairs KC: The survival time of platelets in experimental mural thrombi. J Path 97: 595, 1969.

67. Brice JG, Dowsett DJ, Lowe RD: The effect of constriction on carotid bloodflow and pressure gradient. Lancet 1:84, 1964.

68. Yater WM, Traum AH, Brown WG, Fitzgerald RP, Geisler MA, Wilcox BB: Coronary artery disease in men eighteen to thirty-nine years of age. Report of eight hundred sixty-six cases; four hundred fifty with necropsy examination. Amer Heart J 36: 334; 481; 683, 1948.

69. Classification of atherosclerotic lesions. Report of a study group. WHO Techn Rep Ser (No. 143), 1958.

70. Roberts WC, Levy RI, Fredrickson DS: Hyperlipoproteinemia. A review of the five types with first report of necropsy findings in type 3. Arch Path 90: 46, 1970.

71. Frink RJ, Achor RWP, Brown AL Jr, Kincaid OW, Brandenburg RO: Significance of calcification of the coronary arteries. Amer J Cardiol 26: 241, 1970.

72. Saphir O: Coronary embolism. Amer Heart J 8: 312, 1933.

73. Hamman L: Coronary embolism. Amer J Med 21: 401, 1941.

74. Shrader EL, Bawell MB, Moragues V: Coronary embolism. Circulation 14: 1159, 1956.

75. Wenger NK, Bauer S: Coronary embolism. Review of the literature and report of fifteen cases. Amer J Med 25: 549, 1958.

76. Oakley C, Yusuf R, Hollman A: Coronary embolism and angina in mitral stenosis. Brit Heart J 23: 357, 1961.

77. James TN: Etiologic concept concerning the obscure myocardiopathies. Progr Cardiovasc Dis 7: 43, 1964.

78. Saphir O, Ohringer L, Wong R: Changes in the intramural coronary branches in coronary arteriosclerosis. Arch Path 62: 159, 1956.

79. Blumenthal HT, Alex M, Goldenberg S: A study of lesions of the intramural coronary artery branches in diabetes mellitus. Arch Path 70: 13, 1960.

80. Donomae I, Matsumoto Y, Kokubu T, Koide R, Kobayashi R, Ikegami H, Ueda E, Fujisawa T, Fujimoto S: Pathological studies of coronary atherosclerosis: especially of sclerosis of intramuscular coronary arteries. Jap Heart J 3: 423, 1962.

81. More BM, Sommers SC: The status of the myocardial arterioles in angina pectoris. Amer Heart J 64: 323, 1962.

Left Ventricular Papillary Muscles

Description of the Normal and a Survey of Conditions Causing them to be Abnormal

By WILLIAM C. ROBERTS, M.D., AND LAWRENCE S. COHEN, M.D.

SUMMARY

The left ventricular papillary muscles appear to be the last portions of the heart to be perfused by coronary arterial blood. As a consequence they are sensitive anatomic markers of myocardial ischemia. Foci of necrosis or fibrosis therefore are commonly seen in these structures, particularly the posteromedial papillary muscle, which has a poorer blood supply than does the anterolateral muscle. Coronary arterial luminal narrowing is the most common cause of necrosis or fibrosis of the left ventricular papillary muscles. Other conditions, all associated with inadequate cardiac output, which may produce these lesions include left ventricular outflow tract obstruction, especially that resulting from congenitally malformed aortic valves, acute valvular regurgitation (infective endocarditis), various cardiomyopathies, and primary endocardial fibroelastosis with or without anomalous origin of one or both coronary arteries from the pulmonary trunk. Various infiltrative diseases, including inflammation (Aschoff bodies, sarcoid, abscesses), amyloid, iron, and neoplasms, also may involve the papillary muscles. Their most common congenital malformation is the parachute or single papillary muscle. Fibrosis or necrosis of adjacent left ventricle free wall without involvement of the papillary muscles themselves may simulate clinically "papillary muscle dysfunction." The anterior papillary muscle of the right ventricle is frequently affected by conditions which also affect the left ventricular papillary muscles. Whether or not necrosis or fibrosis of the right ventricular papillary muscle causes tricuspid regurgitation, however, is unknown at present.

Additional Indexing Words:

Coronary heart disease	Congenital heart disease	Myocardial infarction
Aortic stenosis	Idiopathic cardiomegaly	Cardiac surgery

ONE OF THE MOST significant advances in clinical cardiology during the decade of the 1960's was the appreciation of the importance of the left ventricular papillary muscles to closure of the mitral orifice during ventricular systole. It is now a well-recognized fact that hypoxia, necrosis, or fibrosis of the left ventricular papillary muscles may be associated with varying degrees of mitral regurgitation. Although coronary atherosclerosis is the most common cause of papillary muscle disease, scarred or necrotic papillary muscles have been observed in a number of conditions in which the coronary arteries were normal. Despite our increased awareness of disorders of the papillary muscles, a number of discrepancies have appeared which indicate that our knowledge about these structures is incomplete. For example, a number of patients without precordial murmurs during life have been observed at necropsy to have severe necrosis or fibrosis or both of one or both left ventricular papillary muscles; severe mitral regurgitation during or after acute myocardial infarction has been found at necropsy to be

From the Section of Pathology and the Cardiology Branch, National Heart and Lung Institute, National Institutes of Health, Bethesda, Maryland.

Address for reprints: Dr. William C. Roberts, Section of Pathology, National Heart and Lung Institute, National Institutes of Health, Bethesda, Maryland 20014.

Received January 10, 1972; revision accepted for publication February 7, 1972.

associated with normal papillary muscles, normal mitral leaflets and chordae tendineae, and normal-sized mitral annulae. This report attempts to clarify some of these discrepancies by reviewing some necropsy observations on the cardiac papillary muscles and correlating them with clinical findings.

Normal Left Ventricular Papillary Muscles

Each of the two left ventricular papillary muscles receives chordae tendineae from each mitral valve leaflet (fig. 1). Thus, damage to either papillary muscle may affect both leaflets. Each papillary muscle may be viewed as consisting of a major trunk from which an average of six heads or fingers project (fig. 2). Each papillary muscle has an average of 12 chordae tendineae per head. Each primary or first-order chorda tendinea divides into an average of two secondary or second-order chordae tendineae. Each second-order chorda divides into two or three tertiary or third-order chordae tendineae which attach to the mitral leaflet. Thus, for each primary chorda an average of five tertiary chordae result, and each head of a papillary muscle anchors two first-order and 10 third-order chordae. Consequently, each papillary muscle supports an average of 62 chordae actually attached to mitral leaflets, or both papillary muscles support about 124 third-order chordae or 24 first-order chordae. There is considerable variation, however, in the number of chordae tendineae attached to either papillary muscle or to either mitral leaflet.

Generally in a normal heart the thickness of either papillary muscle is about the same as is that of the left ventricular free wall or ventricular septum. The anterolateral (A-L) papillary muscle normally is slightly larger than the posteromedial (P-M) one. Just as the

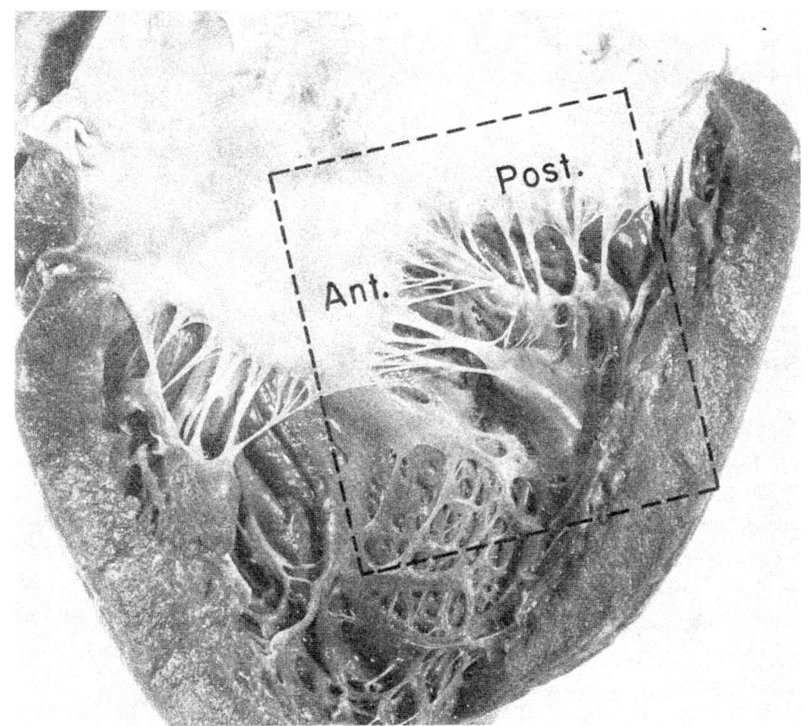

Figure 1

Normal left ventricular papillary muscles. The posteromedial (P-M) papillary muscle, its chordae tendineae, and portions of anterior (Ant.) and posterior (Post.) mitral leaflets attached to it are enclosed by dotted lines. Each papillary muscle receives chordae from both mitral leaflets. Thus, rupture of one head or of the entire trunk of a papillary muscle alters support to both leaflets.

P-M and A-L papillary muscles can differ from each other in the same heart, considerable morphologic variation is observed in comparing either or both muscles from one heart with those of another. The A-L papillary muscle usually (75%) consists of a single major muscle group, whereas the P-M papillary muscle often (65%) consists of two or three major muscle groups.[1] The basal to apex lengths of the papillary muscles also vary considerably. In most individuals the papillary muscles are attached to the left ventricular free walls over a large base and often by several trabecular bridges. Sometimes the site of attachment or anchorage is only slightly larger than the widest circumference of the papillary muscle. Ranganathan and Burch[2] called the former type of papillary muscle *tethered*, in contrast to the *fingerlike* type which protrudes freely into the left ventricular cavity with few or no trabecular attachments. Mixtures of these two types also exist. It is probable that the tethered type has a more abundant blood supply. The axis of orientation of the papillary muscles is generally parallel to the long axis of the left ventricular cavity which is nearly perpendicular to the left atrioventricular valve annulus.[3]

The A-L papillary muscle appears to have a richer blood supply than does the P-M one.[2, 3] Myocardial infarction involving the posterior left ventricular wall usually results in necrosis of the P-M papillary muscle, whereas anterior-wall infarction may spare the A-L papillary muscle.[4] The A-L papillary muscle is supplied by branches from both left anterior descending and left circumflex coronary arteries.[2, 3] The major supply of the P-M papillary muscle is dependent on which coronary artery is dominant. When the right coronary is dominant, and this is the situation in 90% of human hearts, its major supplier is the right coronary artery, and when the left one is dominant the major supplier is the left circumflex. The left circumflex contributes some blood, however, to the P-M papillary muscle no matter which coronary is dominant. The arrangement of the intramural coronary arteries supplying the papillary muscles appears to depend to some

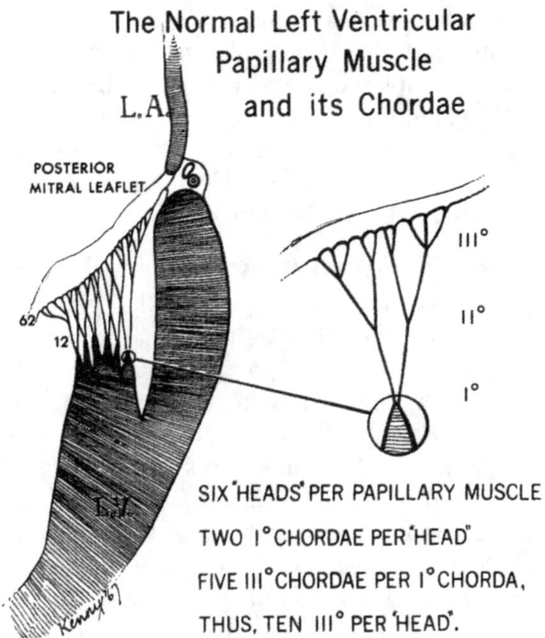

Figure 2

Diagram of a single normal left ventricular papillary muscle and its attached chordae tendineae. Each left ventricular papillary muscle contains an average of six "heads," each of which contains two primary or first-order chordae tendineae. Each primary cord subdivides into two secondary chordae, each of which divides into two or three tertiary or third-order chordae. The number of chordae attached to each left ventricular papillary muscle thus averages 12, and the number of chordae inserting directly into the mitral leaflets from a single papillary muscle averages 62. (These numbers resulted from counting chordae and papillary muscle heads in 12 normal hearts.) Thus, rupture of one papillary muscle head, which contains usually two primary chordae, causes loss of function of at least 10 tertiary chordae.

extent on their gross structure. When they have a fingerlike configuration one or several major intramural vessels (class B arteries of Estes et al.[3, 5]) arise from the epicardial branch, extend through the left ventricular free wall to the bases of the papillary muscles, turn uphill, so to speak, coursing to the apices of the muscles giving off branches along the way. When this artery is single it has been called the "central artery."[2] Papillary muscles or portions of them receiving the central artery usually have few or no anastomotic connections with the extrapapillary subendocardial plexus. The tethered papillary muscles usually do not have a single central artery but many small ones (class A arteries of Estes et al.[3, 5]) with rich anastomotic connections among themselves as well as with the extrapapillary subendocardial plexus.[2, 3]

Although their major blood supply is from intramural coronary arteries, the most peripheral portions of the left ventricular papillary muscles are perfused by intracavitary blood. The actual mechanism by which oxygen diffuses into the immediate subendocardial regions is uncertain. Possibly endocardial pores provide the means.

Abnormal Left Ventricular Papillary Muscles

Types of papillary muscle damage and the causes of the various types are outlined in table 1.

Anatomically Normal Papillary Muscles but Papillary Muscle Dysfunction

Transient ischemia of the papillary muscles is believed to be extremely common and probably results in varying degrees of mitral regurgitation.[6–8] A murmur of mitral regurgitation may occur during an attack of angina pectoris and be absent during pain-free periods.[6–10] Transient systolic murmurs during and after myocardial infarction probably result from papillary muscle ischemia. Arterial perfusion of the left ventricular papillary muscles may be influenced by body position. Brody and Criley[9, 10] documented severe mitral regurgitation and interscapular back pain in a man when he lay supine but both disappeared when he assumed an upright position. Possibly, transient ischemia of the papillary muscles may occur during emotional stress in individuals with normal or nearly normal coronary arteries in a manner similar to that which leads to constriction of the peripheral vascular beds during anxiety or during cigarette smoking.

Left ventricular dilatation of any origin is a frequent cause of papillary muscle dysfunction.[6–8] Under such circumstances the papillary muscles may contract normally, but the spatial relationships between the papillary muscles, the chordae tendineae, and the orifice are altered by the caudal and lateral migration of the left ventricular wall away from the mitral annulus. The valve leaflets are thus pulled downward into the left ventricle, and consequently the mitral orifice becomes incompetent. Also, the axes of the papillary muscles become more oblique with respect to the mitral annulus.

Although it may accompany left ventricular dilatation, mitral annular dilatation is probably a rare cause of mitral regurgitation, and most patients in the past with mitral regurgitation believed to be the result of mitral annular dilatation probably had papillary muscle dysfunction instead. Mitral annular dilatation to the degree capable of causing mitral regurgitation probably does not occur because the surface area of the mitral leaflets is about two times the area of the mitral orifice,[11] and the annulus contracts during ventricular systole.[12] Indeed, the mitral ring has a sphincter-like action since the mitral orifice is smaller during systole than during diastole.[12] In patients with dilated left ventricles, the widest diameter occurs not at the left ventricular base, the area which includes the mitral annulus, but in the midportion of the chamber between apex and base. Indeed, the base of the left ventricle is prevented from dilating freely because the "fibrous skeleton" is attached to it whereas the midportion of the left ventricle is not thus inhibited. Severe left ventricular dilatation may occur without any dilatation of the mitral annulus.

Although it is now well appreciated that mitral regurgitation may occur in patients with dilated left ventricles from any cause without associated left ventricular necrosis or fibrosis, it is less well recognized that necrosis or fibrosis of the left ventricular free wall unassociated with left ventricular dilatation or papillary muscle or mitral tissue lesions also may be associated with mitral regurgitation (fig. 3). Generally, the scarring or necrosis of the myocardium adjacent to the papillary muscles fails to move or moves paradoxically during ventricular systole and the abnormal ventricular contraction may lead to abnormal papillary muscle anchoring with resultant

Table 1

Spectrum of Left Ventricular Papillary Muscle Disease

I.   Anatomically normal papillary muscles but papillary muscle dysfunction:
  A. Transient ischemia
  B. Left ventricular dilatation from any cause
    1. Generalized
    2. Localized
  C. Necrosis or fibrosis in adjacent left ventricular free wall
    1. With coronary arterial narrowing
    2. Without coronary arterial narrowing
  D. Small left ventricular cavity (hypertrophic cardiomyopathy)

II. Necrosis or fibrosis of papillary muscle(s) without rupture:
  A. With coronary arterial narrowing
    1. Acute myocardial infarction
    2. Healed myocardial infarction
  B. Without coronary arterial narrowing
    1. Acute
      a. Shock
      b. Acute valvular regurgitation (infective endocarditis)
    2. Chronic
      a. Anemia
      b. Left ventricular outflow obstruction
        (1) Valvular aortic stenosis
        (2) Discrete and diffuse subaortic stenosis
        (3) Supravalvular aortic stenosis
      c. Systemic hypertension
      d. Origin of left coronary artery or of both coronary arteries from pulmonary trunk
      e. Primary endocardial fibroelastosis of left ventricle
      f. Endomyocardial disease and eosinophilia
        (1) Löffler's fibroplastic parietal endocarditis
        (2) Endomyocardial fibrosis of Davies
      g. Idiopathic cardiomegaly (primary or diffuse myocardial disease)
      h. Focal myocardial disease
        (1) Idiopathic
        (2) "Neurogenic" heart disease
          (a) Progressive muscular dystrophy
          (b) Friedreich's ataxia
          (c) Myotonic muscular dystrophy

III. Necrosis or fibrosis of papillary muscle(s) with rupture:
  A. Acute myocardial infarction from coronary heart disease
  B. Trauma
  C. Miscellaneous
  Types of papillary muscle rupture
    1. Total ("belly or trunk") → rapid death
    2. Partial ("head")
      a. Rapid death
      b. Survival but chronic congestive heart failure

IV. Infiltrative diseases of papillary muscles:
  A. Pyogenic abscess
  B. Granulomas
    1. Aschoff bodies
    2. Sarcoid
  C. Amyloid
  D. Neoplasm
  E. Calcium

      F.   Iron
      G.   Other
V.   Congenital malformations of papillary muscle(s):
      A.   Single papillary muscle (parachute mitral valve syndrome)
      B.   Accessory papillary muscle
      C.   Abnormally large and malpositioned papillary muscles
      D.   Abnormally small and malpositioned papillary muscle
      E.   Insertion of papillary muscle directly into mitral leaflet
VI. Miscellaneous afflictions of papillary muscle(s):
      A.   Excision, partial or complete, during mitral valve replacement
          1.   Atrophy of nonexcised portion of papillary muscle after valve replacement
          2.   Left ventricular aneurysm at site of papillary muscle excision
      B.   Disuse atrophy after excision of mitral leaflets and chordae without excision of
          papillary muscle(s)

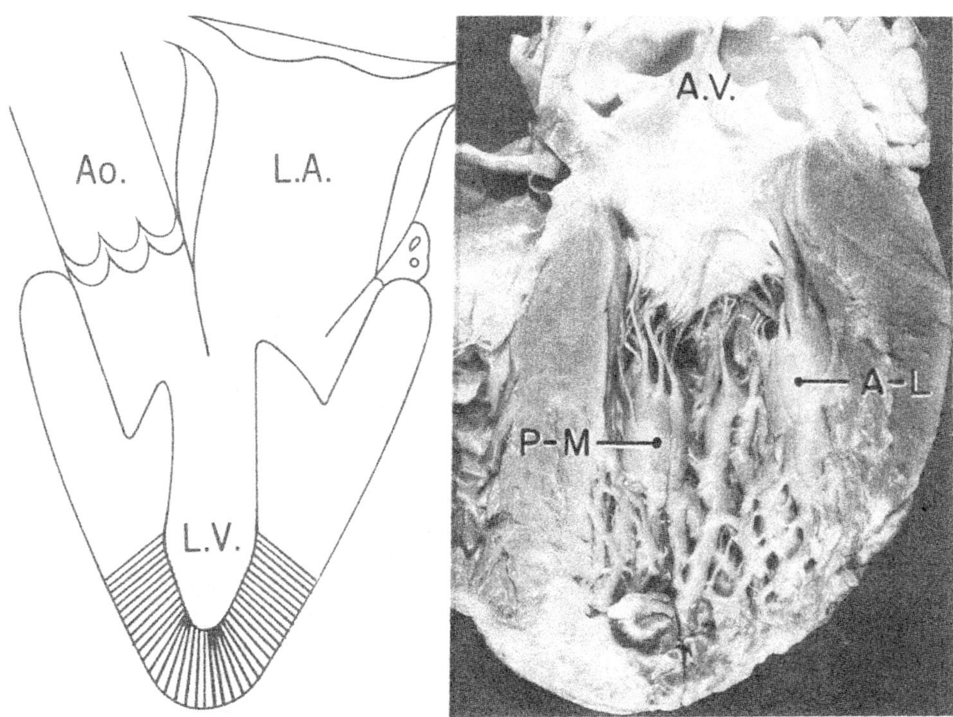

Figure 3

Mitral regurgitation from scarring of the left ventricular free walls but not of the papillary muscles. The heart shows severe scarring of the left ventricular wall from the base of the papillary muscles to the cardiac apex, but the posteromedial (P-M) and anterolateral (A-L) muscles are spared from significant scarring. This 72-year-old man (A68-83) had an acute myocardial infarct at age 60 years. He was well thereafter until age 69 (3 years before death) when mild congestive cardiac failure appeared, but no precordial murmur was heard. On examination 9 months before death a grade I/VI pansystolic apical murmur was heard. Five months later severe congestive heart failure appeared, and cardiac catheterization was performed. The left atrial v waves ranged from 60 to 75 mm Hg and left ventricular cine-angiocardiogram disclosed 3+/4+ mitral regurgitation. Despite this angiographic documentation of mitral regurgitation the precordial murmur was never louder than grade I/VI intensity and located in early and midsystole only. Cardiotomy was performed 3 months before death. The anterior mitral leaflet was found to herniate into the left atrium during ventricular systole but the mitral leaflets and chordae appeared normal. The mitral valve was plicated but congestive cardiac failure, which ultimately was fatal, persisted postoperatively.

mitral regurgitation.[8, 13] Anatomic left ventricular aneurysms unassociated with papillary muscle necrosis or fibrosis may cause mitral regurgitation by the same mechanism (fig. 4).

Abnormal pulling on the papillary muscles unassociated with left ventricular necrosis or fibrosis or with cavity dilatation may occur in patients with hypertrophic cardiomyopathy, and this mechanism may account for the mitral regurgitation in them.[14] The huge thickening of the ventricular septum—the thickest portion is midway between left ventricular base and apex[15]—may distort or bend the anterolateral papillary muscle and prevent proper contraction of this structure during ventricular systole.

Necrosis or Fibrosis of Papillary Muscle(s) without Rupture

Necrosis and fibrosis of one or both left ventricular papillary muscles is extremely common. The necrosis or fibrosis may be either focal or diffuse, involving only one papillary muscle or both, and auscultatory mitral regurgitation may or may not be present. When they are focal, the papillary muscle lesions are generally of two types: (1) involve nearly all the distal or apical portion of the papillary muscle, or (2) involve many areas throughout the entire papillary muscle. The latter lesions usually are small and spare areas adjacent to intramural coronary arteries.[16] When only one papillary muscle contains foci of necrosis or fibrosis it is virtually always

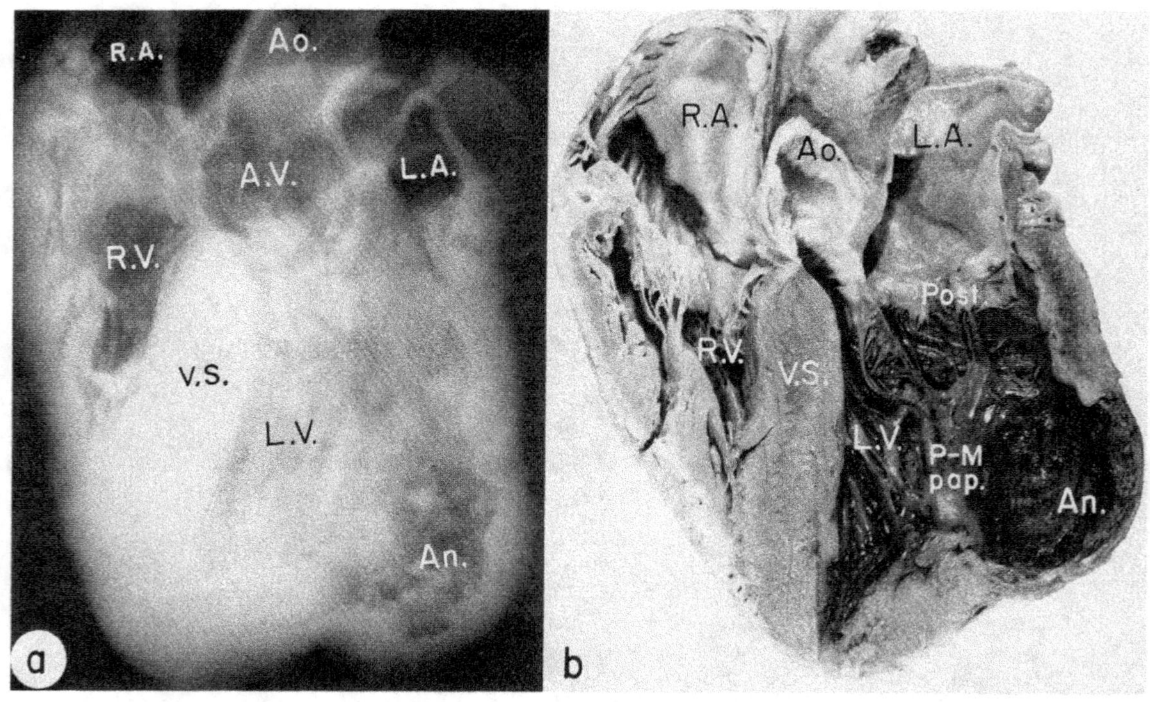

Figure 4

Radiograph of heart specimen (a) and longitudinal section of heart (b) in a 65-year-old man (A67-71) who had an acute myocardial infarct 2 months before death with subsequent development of a left ventricular (L.V.) aneurysm (An.) located in the lateral wall. He developed a murmur consistent with mitral regurgitation. Both left ventricular papillary (pap.) muscles grossly appeared normal but their bases were adjacent to the aneurysm. The mitral regurgitation can probably be attributed to the poor anchorage of the papillary muscles as a result of the aneurysm. R.A. = right atrium; R.V. = right ventricle; V.S. = ventricular septum; L.A. = left atrium; A.V. = aortic valve; Ao. = aorta.

the P-M muscle, since this one has the poorer blood supply.

It is now clear from experimental studies[17-19] that mitral regurgitation is not a consequence of fibrosis involving only papillary muscles themselves. If one or both left ventricular papillary muscles are made fibrotic in the dog, either by injection of formalin or by ligating the base of the muscle, no regurgitation of contrast material from left ventricle to left atrium later occurred on angiographic studies. If, however, the free wall beneath the papillary muscle was made fibrotic at the same time so that ventricular contraction was impaired, mitral regurgitation did result. We have observed a number of patients at necropsy with extensive fibrosis or necrosis of one or both left ventricular papillary muscles, and no precordial murmur had been audible during life. Fibrosis or necrosis of the left ventricular papillary muscles and of the free walls beneath them, however, does not necessarily assure the appearance of a precordial murmur of mitral regurgitation during life. Several patients with silent mitral regurgitation by auscultation have been shown to have mitral regurgitation when left ventricular injection of contrast material also was performed.[20, 21] Necrosis or fibrosis has been observed at necropsy in these patients to involve the papillary muscles extensively and the entire thickness (transmural) of the left ventricular free wall.[21] Silent mitral regurgitation during acute myocardial infarction has been attributed to a diminished flow velocity across the mitral valve secondary to diminished myocardial contractility.[20]

The most common cause of papillary muscle necrosis or fibrosis is narrowing of the coronary arterial lumen by atherosclerosis.[4, 22, 23] The P-M papillary muscle is usually involved in acute posterior myocardial infarction. In anterior-wall infarction, however, the A-L papillary muscle may be spared, presumably because its blood supply is better than that of the P-M muscle. Since infarction limited to the ventricular septum or to the lateral portion of the left ventricular free wall

(i.e. the portions of the left ventricular wall unassociated with papillary muscles) is rare, the papillary muscles are usually involved when myocardial infarction occurs. It, therefore, is surprising that papillary muscle dysfunction is not more frequently observed during or after acute myocardial infarction.

Necrosis or fibrosis of one or both left ventricular papillary muscles is frequent in a number of conditions unassociated with luminal narrowing of the extramural coronary arteries. Inadequate oxygenation of the papillary muscles may occur if the amount of oxygen in the blood is low (i.e., anemia) or if the cardiac output for any reason is inadequate. It is well to keep in mind that the left ventricular papillary muscles are the last portions of the heart to be perfused with coronary arterial blood. To perfuse the apices of the papillary muscles the coronary artery must extend through the entire thickness of the myocardial free wall, turn up hill, and ascend a distance of at least one and often two thicknesses of the free wall. Consequently, it is of little wonder that these structures often show evidences of inadequate oxygenation. Furthermore, the papillary muscles serve as the most sensitive markers of inadequate myocardial oxygenation. Since the P-M papillary muscle is less well perfused than the A-L one, if only one shows foci of necrosis or fibrosis it will nearly always be the P-M muscle. We have observed foci of necrosis in these papillary muscles in patients with anemia from a variety of causes, particularly chronic anemias like sickle-cell disease (fig. 5).

In patients with left ventricular outflow obstruction, lesions are often observed in the papillary muscles. [24-28] Valvular aortic stenosis, whether in infants [24, 25] or in adults, [26-28] when superimposed on a congenitally malformed valve, either unicuspid or bicuspid, is nearly always associated with fibrosis and atrophy of at least the P-M papillary muscle. Rheumatic valvular aortic stenosis combined with organic mitral stenosis or regurgitation, however, infrequently is associated with papillary muscle fibrosis or

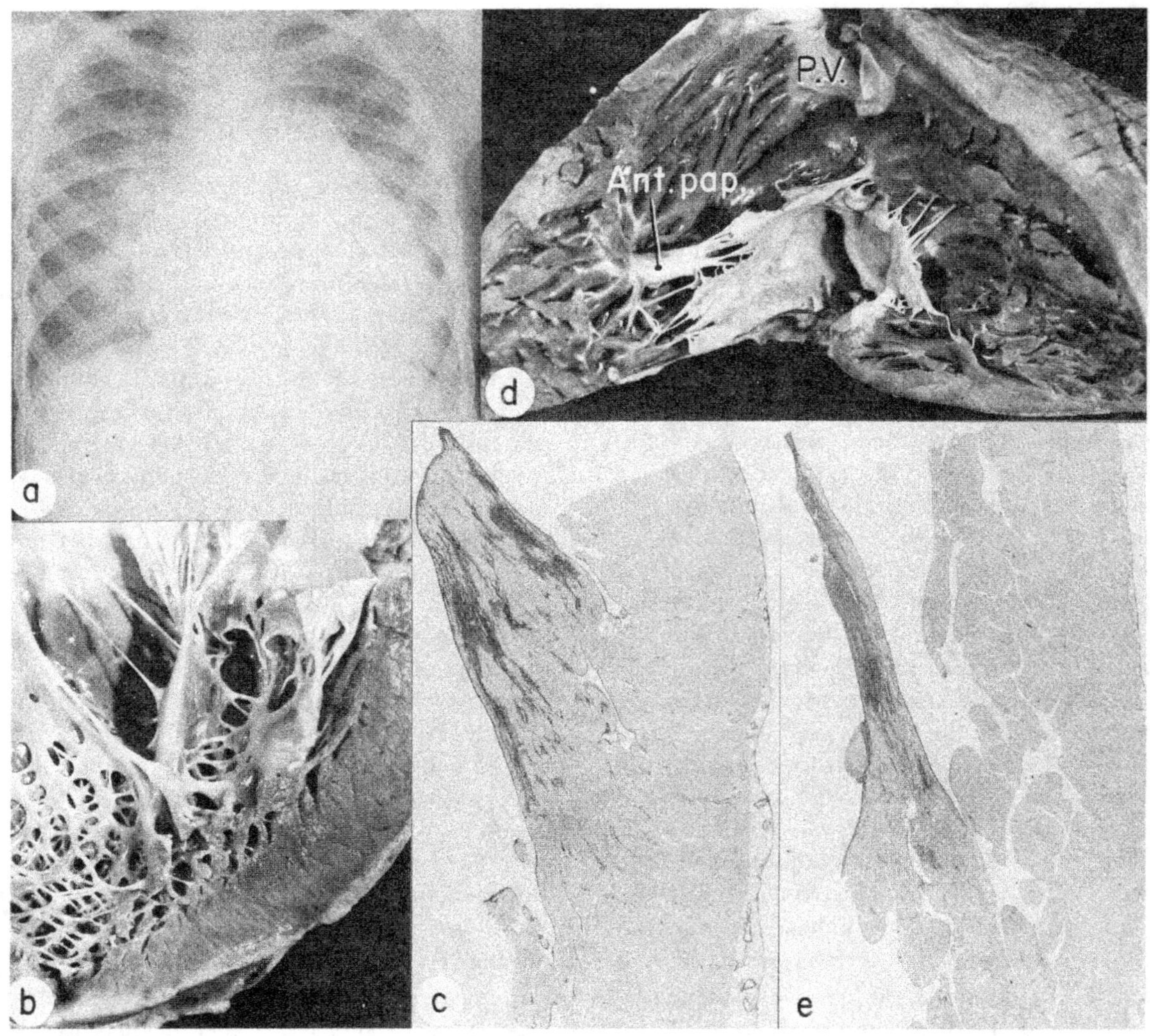

Figure 5

The heart in a 14-year-old girl (A69-13) with sickle-cell disease diagnosed by hemoglobin electrophoresis when she was 4 years old. She had multiple sickle-cell crises and at age 12 years developed congestive cardiac failure. During her last 6 months she had nightly paroxysmal dyspnea and multiple episodes of exertional syncope. She had a grade II/VI systolic murmur over the pulmonic area. Electrocardiogram showed right-axis deviation, right ventricular hypertrophy, and P-pulmonale. The pulmonary arterial pressure was 47/13 mm Hg, and the cardiac output was 6.5 liters/min. (a) Chest roentgenogram. (b) Posteromedial (P-M) left ventricular papillary muscle. (c) Section of P-M papillary muscle showing focal fibrosis. (d) Opened right ventricle showing fibrosis of the anterior (Ant.) papillary (pap.) muscle. P.V. = pulmonic valve. (e) Section of scarred anterior right ventricular papillary muscle. The papillary muscle fibrosis is presumably related to the chronic anemia.

atrophy. Nearly all adult patients with discrete subaortic stenosis or hypertrophic cardiomyopathy with or without diffuse subaortic stenosis have small fibrous scars in both left ventricular papillary muscles, but severe atrophy of one or both muscles is uncommon.

Foci of necrosis also are common in patients with fatal severe valvular regurgitation of recent onset. Among 47 patients dying of active valvular infective endocarditis, 34 (72%) had necrotic lesions in one or both left ventricular papillary muscles, and none had

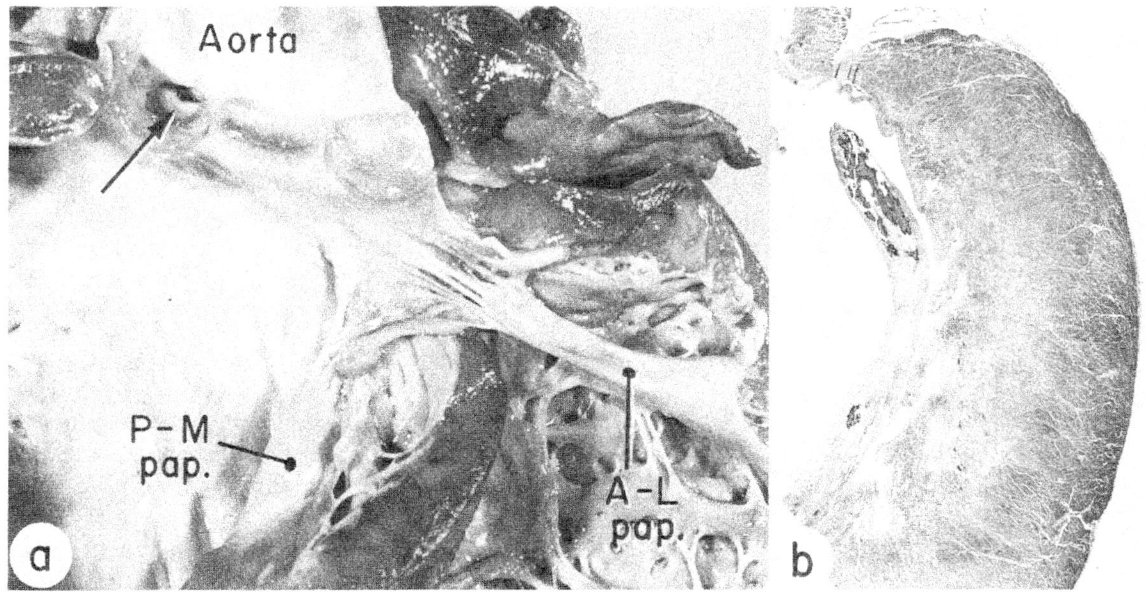

Figure 6

Severe diffuse fibrosis and calcification of the anterolateral left ventricular papillary muscle in a 9-month-old girl (A56-14) in whom the left coronary artery arose anomalously from the pulmonary trunk. She had a grade III/VI systolic precordial murmur. Diffuse endocardial fibroelastosis of the left ventricle and left atrium also was present. (a) Opened left ventricle, aortic valve, and aorta. The ostium of the right coronary artery is designated by the arrow. No left ostium is observed. The distal half of the A-L papillary muscle is severely scarred and calcified. (b) Section of the fibrotic, atrophied, and calcified A-L papillary muscle. (Hematoxylin and eosin stain, × 4.)

significant narrowing of the extramural coronary arteries.[29] Most patients had pure aortic regurgitation, but some had pure mitral regurgitation secondary to the active infective endocarditis. Severely diminished cardiac output with resultant poor myocardial perfusion was believed to be the cause of the papillary muscle necrosis in them.

Small fibrous scars in the papillary muscles are common in patients with systemic hypertension but atrophy of these structures in this condition, unless coronary heart disease also is present, is infrequent. When left ventricular hypertrophy occurs from any cause, the hypertrophy of the papillary muscles probably should be proportional to that of the left ventricular free wall or ventricular septum. This proportional hypertrophy usually exists in cases of systemic hypertension, but infrequently in patients with left ventricular outflow obstruction.

Fibrosis with atrophy of the papillary muscles is to be expected in patients with primary endocardial fibroelastosis of the left ventricle.[30] Histologically, the thickened endocardium in this condition is similar to the media of the aorta, being characterized by the presence of elastic fibrils running parallel to one another and to the surface. Primary left ventricular endocardial fibroelastosis may represent simply an anatomic expression of chronically inadequate coronary arterial perfusion of the left ventricle, and, since the P-M papillary muscle is the least well-perfused portion of the heart, this structure is affected the most. In the congenital condition, origin of the left[31] or both[32] coronary arteries from the pulmonary trunk, diffuse endocardial fibroelastosis of the left ventricle is nearly always an associated lesion. Fibrosis and atrophy of the left ventricular papillary muscles is to be expected in this anomaly, and these patients may present clinically with features of pure mitral regurgitation[33] (fig. 6).

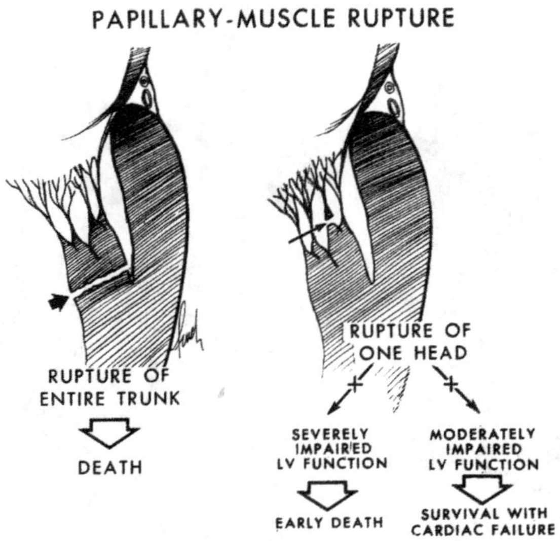

Figure 7

*Diagram depicting two major types of papillary mus-
cle rupture. It is likely that rupture of the entire
trunk (acute myocardial infarction or trauma) (left)
is incompatible with survival since a major portion of
the support to both valve leaflets is destroyed. With
rupture of an apical head (right), survival would
appear to depend upon the extent to which the function of the left ventricle has been impaired by necrosis. With severely impaired ventricular function,
the additional burden of even modest mitral regurgitation may be intolerable, and death is quick. If the
left ventricle is less severely compromised, survival is
possible for weeks or months, but congestive cardiac
failure will almost invariably develop.*

Foci of fibrosis or necrosis in the left
ventricular papillary muscles are infrequent in
patients with the congestive or dilated type of
cardiomyopathy. Severe scarring of one papillary muscle and of the free wall beneath it
was responsible for severe mitral regurgitation
in a patient with primary myocardial disease
studied by Marcus et al.[34] Generally, however,
left ventricular cavity dilatation alone is the
cause of mitral regurgitation in these patients.
Rarely, myocarditis may be localized to
papillary muscle and adjacent left ventricular
free wall.[35] Patients with the neurogenic heart
diseases (Friedreich's ataxia, progressive muscular dystrophy, and myotonic muscular dis-
trophy)[36] generally have scarred left ventricular papillary muscles, especially the P-M one.
The African cardiomyopathy—endomyocar-

dial fibrosis—may be associated with extensive
scarring of the papillary muscles.[37] Usually the
P-M one in this condition is covered by a
thrombus or by dense fibrous tissue which
may represent organization of thrombus.
Likewise, Löffler's fibroplastic parietal endocarditis, which may represent one stage of
endomyocardial fibrosis,[38] is usually associated
with extensive scarring of one or both
papillary muscles.[39]

Necrosis or Fibrosis of Papillary Muscle with Rupture

In contrast to necrosis of a papillary muscle
which occurs in over 50% of patients with fatal
acute myocardial infarction,[4] rupture of a
papillary muscle is rare, occurring in < 1% of
patients with fatal acute myocardial infarction. The rupture may be of two types (fig.
7). One involves the entire central muscle
belly of the papillary muscle and this type
rupture is incompatible with survival since
half the support to each valve leaflet is
destroyed and mitral regurgitation of overwhelming severity results. The second type of
rupture involves only one or two apical heads
of a papillary muscle. The resulting mitral
regurgitation is of lesser magnitude, and
immediate survival is then dependent upon
the degree to which the function of the left
ventricle has been impaired by the infarct. In
patients who survive after papillary muscle
rupture, the functional capacity of the left
ventricle also will govern the extent of clinical
and hemodynamic improvement after mitral
valve replacement.[40]

Although the entire papillary muscle is
usually necrotic, the mitral regurgitation
resulting from rupture of an entire trunk of a
papillary muscle may justifiably be attributed
entirely to the rupture. In contrast, the mitral
regurgitation following rupture of only one
head of a left ventricular papillary muscle
cannot necessarily be attributed entirely to the
rupture since the remainder of the papillary
muscle is nearly always also necrotic. What
percentage of the regurgitant volume is due to
the rupture of a single head and what
percentage to the associated papillary muscle
necrosis is uncertain. Rupture of a single

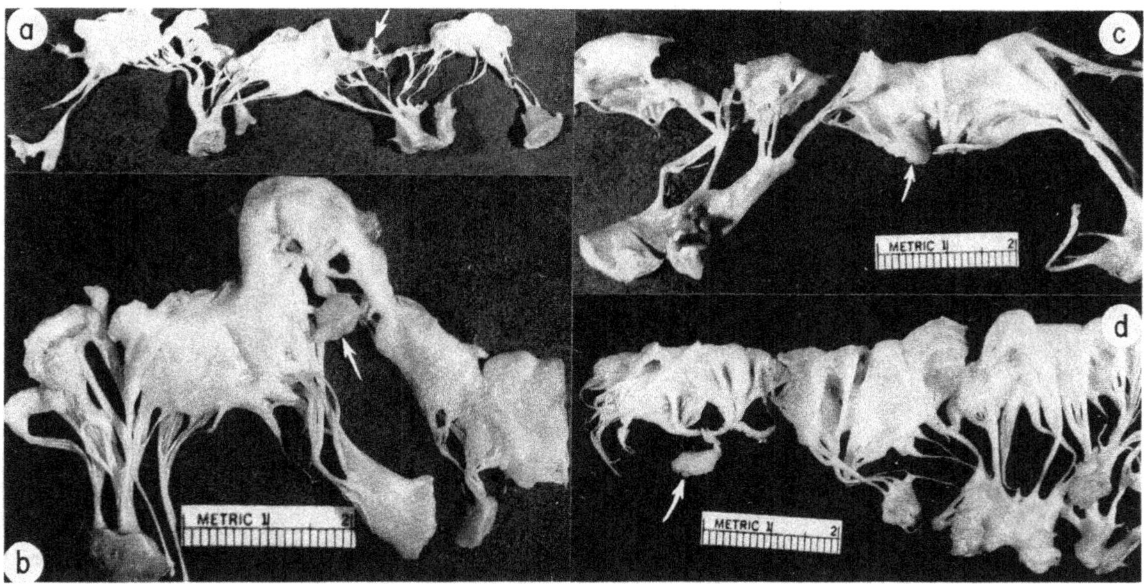

Figure 8

Operatively excised mitral valves in four patients demonstrating rupture of a papillary muscle head in each. Acute myocardial infarction (AMI) had occurred in each 15 months (a), 13 months (b), 3 months (c), and 14 months (d) earlier. All four patients were men, aged 51 to 69 years at the time of operation, and all developed loud (grade III-IV/VI) systolic murmurs typical of mitral regurgitation at the time of AMI. Congestive cardiac failure persisted after AMI. The arrows designate the ruptured papillary muscle heads. All four patients died within 3 years of operation. (The valve replacements were performed by Dr. Andrew G. Morrow.)

primary chorda tendinea in the dog, however, produces immediate severe mitral regurgitation;[41] consequently, rupture of a head, which is equivalent to rupturing two primary chordae tendineae, must in itself be severe. Ruptured papillary muscle heads in four patients are illustrated in figure 8. Each patient was described in detail elsewhere.[40]

Although coronary arterial luminal narrowing by atherosclerosis accounts for most cases of ruptured papillary muscle, trauma may cause either partial or complete rupture of these structures. Blunt trauma, however, when severe enough to cause papillary muscle rupture, is also usually severe enough to rupture the left ventricular free wall. Brock[42] described total rupture of a papillary muscle during mitral commissurotomy, and death ensued in two days.

Infiltrative Diseases of Papillary Muscles

The papillary muscles are subject to various infiltrative processes just like any other portion of myocardium. Pyogenic abscesses, Aschoff bodies, granulomas (fig. 9),[43] neoplasms, amyloid,[44] and iron[45] have all been observed in these structures. Congestive heart failure from severe mitral regurgitation may be the initial symptom of sarcoidosis (fig. 9).

Congenital Malformations of the Left Ventricular Papillary Muscles

The most frequent congenital malformation of these structures is the occurrence of only one papillary muscle (fig. 10). This condition, described as the parachute mitral valve, consists of only one left ventricular papillary muscle to which all mitral chordae tendineae are attached.[46] The resulting mitral valve is usually stenotic,[46] but it may be purely incompetent[47] or it may function normally.[47] The single papillary muscle is usually associated with other malformations including a supramitral valve ring, diffuse subaortic stenosis, and coarctation of the aorta.[46] Other malformations, including valvular aortic stenosis, ventricular septal defect, and valvular

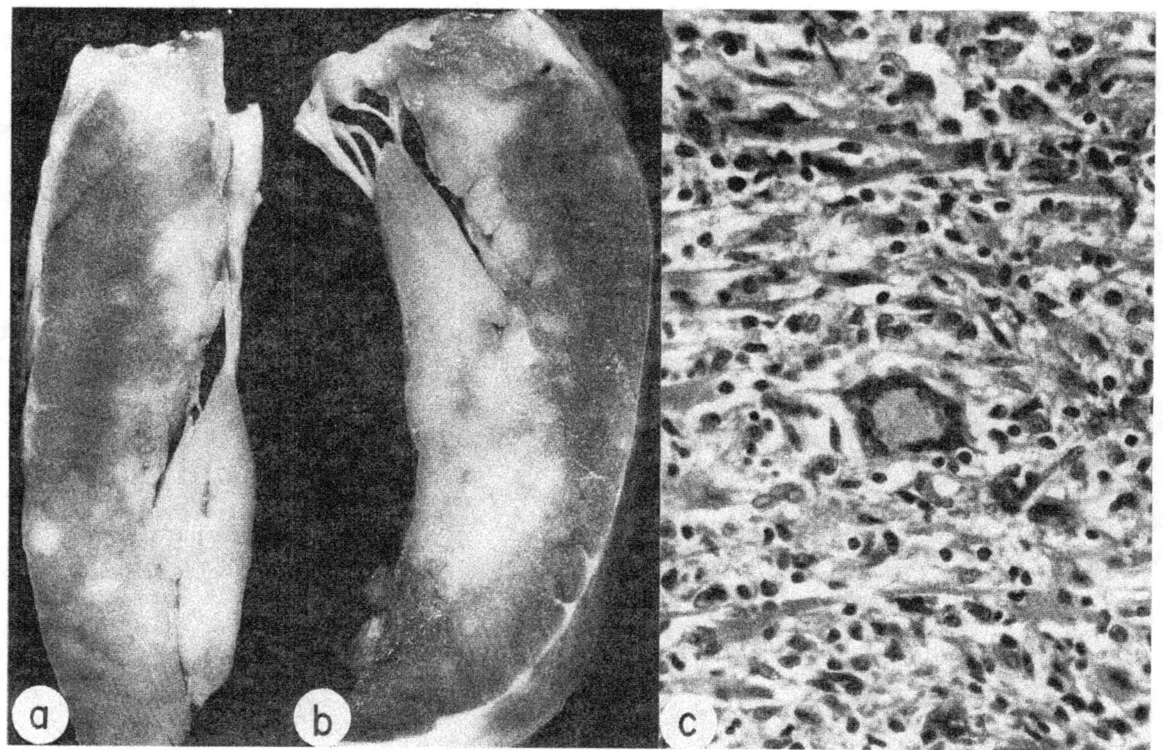

Figure 9

Anterolateral (a) and posteromedial (b) left ventricular papillary muscles in a 26-year-old woman (PGGH A-70-541) who was asymptomatic until 10 days before death when dyspnea appeared. The dyspnea rapidly worsened, and when hospitalized on the day of death she was in acute pulmonary edema. The blood pressure was 80/70 mm Hg, heart rate 160 beats/ min, and a grade III–IV/VI pansystolic blowing apical murmur, which radiated into the axilla, was audible. Chest roentgenogram showed congested lungs, cardiomegaly, and prominent hilar adenopathy. Electrocardiogram showed nonspecific ST-T wave changes and atrial hypertrophy. Several hours after admission ventricular fibrillation occurred, she was resuscitated, but complete heart block appeared. A transvenous pacemaker was inserted, but asystole occurred shortly thereafter. At necropsy, large firm white deposits were present in the walls of all four cardiac chambers and completely replaced both left ventricular papillary muscles (a and b). On histologic section, the firm white areas represented hard granulomas typical of sarcoidosis as seen in (c). (Hematoxylin and eosin stain, × 400.) Similar hard granulomas were present in lymph nodes, liver, spleen, and lung. Stains for acid-fast organisms, other bacteria, and fungi were negative. (Specimen was kindly provided by Dr. James Hutchinson.)

pulmonic stenosis also may occur in association with the single left ventricular papillary muscle.[47] The single papillary muscle malformation may be the most common cause of congenital mitral stenosis.[48]

Not only may one too few papillary muscles occur, but one too many also may occur. An accessory papillary muscle is usually of no functional significance but it has been seen in association with congenital mitral regurgitation.[49] Two papillary muscles may be present and yet one or both still be congenitally malformed. Each of the two papillary muscles may be abnormally large and malpositioned so that the primary orifice of the valve is narrowed.[48, 50] The malpositioning consists of origin of the papillary muscles at sites higher in the left ventricle than normal. Both papillary muscles also may be poorly developed and small. This finding is particularly characteristic of origin of the left coronary artery from the pulmonary trunk. In the latter

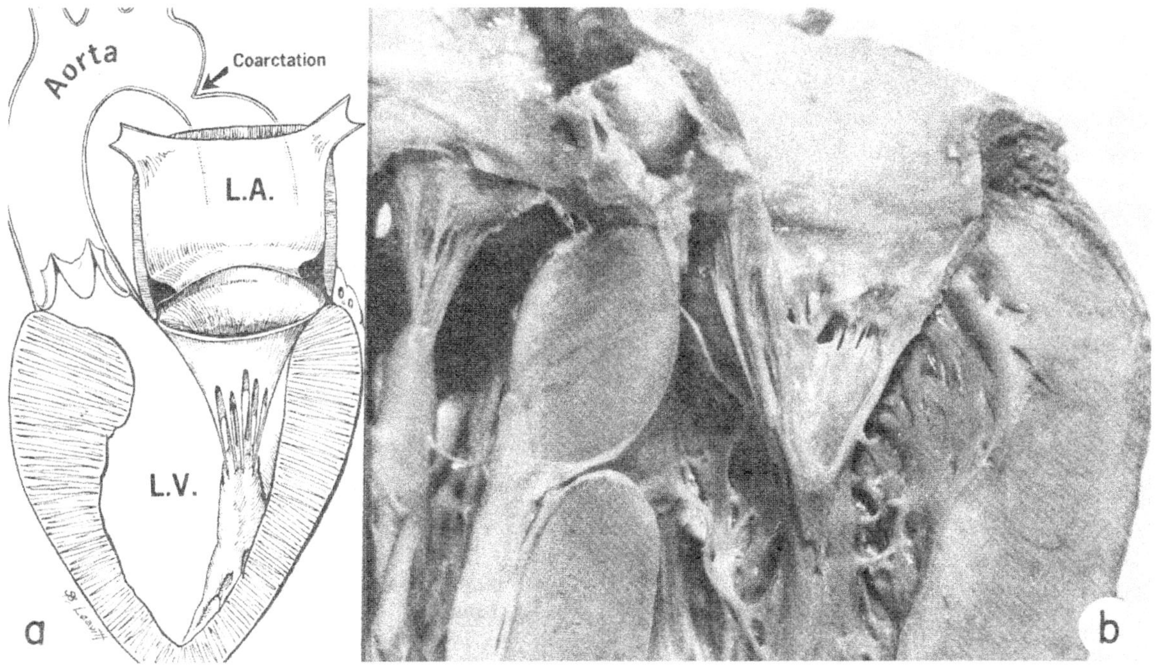

Figure 10

Single left ventricular papillary muscle or parachute mitral valve syndrome. Most patients with a single left ventricular papillary muscle also have a partial or completely circumscribing ring just above the mitral valve or at its annulus, subaortic stenosis, and aortic isthmic coarctation (a). Other anomalies, particularly ventricular septal defect and valvular aortic stenosis, as shown here (b), are also common. A single left ventricular papillary muscle with a parachute mitral valve from a 14-year-old boy (GT#71A-215) is shown in (b). In addition, this child had severe valvular and discrete subvalvular aortic stenosis as well as spontaneous closure of a ventricular septal defect. The aortic valve was congenitally bicuspid. The peak systolic pressure gradient between left ventricle and systemic artery was 80 mm Hg. He died in acute pulmonary edema. He had been asymptomatic until 1 year before death. No abnormality of the mitral apparatus was apparent clinically. (This child was cared for by Dr. Joseph K. Perloff.)

condition the papillary muscles also arise high on the left ventricular wall.[48] Contrasted to the normal heart wherein the papillary muscles arise at the junction of the middle and lower thirds of the left ventricle, in this condition they arise from the upper third of the ventricular wall. Minor functionally insignificant abnormalities of the papillary muscles may occur. A not uncommon one consists of insertion of one papillary muscle directly into one or both mitral leaflets. In acquired rheumatic mitral stenosis, fusion and shortening of the chordae tendineae may be so extensive that it appears that both papillary muscles insert directly into the mitral leaflets.

Consequences of Operative-Excision of the Papillary Muscles at the time of Mitral Valve Replacement

Both left ventricular papillary muscles are excised by most surgeons at the time of mitral valve replacement. The myocardium of the free wall at the sites of excision of these muscles is always infiltrated by inflammatory cells if this area is examined in the early postoperative period.[51] If the papillary muscles are not excised when the mitral leaflets and chordae tendineae are excised during mitral valve replacement, the papillary muscles atrophy and are focally replaced by fibrous tissue.[52]

When the papillary muscles are excised at operation, each is grasped by a clamp extending through the mitral orifice from the left atrium. If the papillary muscles are pulled too vigorously by the clamp when the muscle is excised a portion of left ventricular free wall beneath the left ventricular papillary muscle also may be excised. This may result in perforation of the left ventricular wall, or it may cause severe thinning of the wall at this point with formation of a functioning or anatomic aneurysm or both.

Anterior Papillary Muscle of the Right Ventricle

This structure appears to be susceptible to all the afflictions which affect the left ventricular papillary muscles. This structure in length is usually equivalent to several thicknesses of right ventricular wall, and blood also is required to course "up hill" to perfuse this papillary muscle. This muscle is also most frequently made necrotic or fibrotic by myocardial infarction from coronary arterial atherosclerosis. Its involvement usually indicates "massive" anterior-wall myocardial infarction. Whether or not tricuspid regurgitation is a consequence of necrosis or fibrosis or of infiltrative disease of the right ventricular papillary muscle is uncertain. Necrosis of the distal portion of this papillary muscle is common in coronary heart disease, acute valvular dysfunction as in infective endocarditis, and in chronic anemias (fig. 5).

References

1. RUSTED IE, SCHEIFLEY CH, EDWARDS JE, KIRKLIN JW: Guides to the commissures in operations upon the mitral valve. Mayo Clin Proc 26: 297, 1951
2. RANGANATHAN N, BURCH GE: Gross morphology and arterial supply of the papillary muscles of the left ventricle of man. Amer Heart J 77: 506, 1969
3. ESTES EH JR, DALTON FM, ENTMAN ML, DIXON HB II, HACKEL DB: The anatomy and blood supply of the papillary muscles of the left ventricle. Amer Heart J 71: 356, 1966
4. HEIKKILÄ J: Mitral incompetence as a complication of acute myocardial infarction. Acta Med Scand 182 (suppl 475): 1, 1967
5. ESTES EH JR, ENTMAN ML, DIXON HB II, HACKEL DB: The vascular supply of the left ventricular wall: Anatomic observations, plus a hypothesis regarding acute events in coronary artery disease. Amer Heart J 71: 58, 1966
6. BURCH GE, DE PASQUALE NP, PHILLIPS JH: Clinical manifestations of papillary muscle dysfunction. Arch Intern Med (Chicago) 112: 112, 1963
7. PHILLIPS JH, BURCH GE, DE PASQUALE NP: The syndrome of papillary muscle dysfunction: Its clinical recognition. Ann Intern Med 59: 508, 1963
8. BURCH GE, DE PASQUALE NP, PHILLIPS JH: The syndrome of papillary muscle dysfunction. Amer Heart J 75: 399, 1968
9. BRODY W, CRILEY JM: Functional mitral regurgitation. New Eng J Med 279: 1058, 1968
10. BRODY W, CRILEY JM: Intermittent severe mitral regurgitation: Hemodynamic studies in a patient with recurrent acute left-sided heart failure. New Eng J Med 283: 673, 1970
11. BROCK RC: The surgical and pathological anatomy of the mitral valve. Brit Heart J 14: 489, 1952
12. SMITH HL, ESSEX HE, BALDES, EJ: A study of the movements of heart valves and of heart sounds. Ann Intern Med 33: 1357, 1950
13. SHELBURNE JC, RUBINSTEIN D, GORLIN R: A reappraisal of papillary muscle dysfunction: Correlative clinical and angiographic study. Amer J Med 46: 862, 1969
14. SIMON AL, ROSS J JR, GAULT JH: Angiographic anatomy of the left ventricle and mitral valve in idiopathic hypertrophic subaortic stenosis. Circulation 36: 852, 1967
15. ROBERTS WC, FERRANS VJ: Pathologic aspects of hypertrophic cardiomyopathy: A study of 30 necropsy patients. In preparation
16. BRAND FR, BROWN AL, BERGE KG: Histology of papillary muscles of the left ventricle in myocardial infarction. Amer Heart J 77: 26, 1969
17. MILLER GE JR, COHN KE, KERTH WI, SELZER A, GERBODE F: Experimental papillary muscle infarction. J Thorac Cardiovasc Surg 56: 611, 1968
18. TSAKIRIS AG, RASTELLI GC, AMORIM DD, TITUS JL, WOOD EH: Effect of experimental papillary muscle damage on mitral valve closure in intact anesthetized dogs. Mayo Clin Proc 45: 275, 1970
19. MITTAL AK, LANGSTON M JR, COHN KE, SELZER A, KERTH WJ: Combined papillary muscle and left ventricular wall dysfunction as a cause of mitral regurgitation: An experimental study. Circulation 44: 174, 1971
20. FORRESTER JS, DIAMOND G, FREEMAN S, ALLEN HN, PARMLEY WW, MATLOFF J, SWAN HJC:

Silent mitral insufficiency in acute myocardial infarction. Circulation 44: 877, 1971

21. FALCONE MW, RONAN JA JR, ROBERTS WC: Silent mitral regurgitation complicating silent myocardial infarction: Hemodynamic and morphologic documentation. Chest. In press

22. CEDERQVIST L, SÖDERSTRÖM J: Papillary muscle rupture in myocardial infarction: A study based upon an autopsy material. Acta Med Scand 176: 287, 1964

23. ROBERTS WC, BUJA LM: The frequency and significance of coronary arterial thrombi and other observations in fatal acute myocardial infarction: A study of 107 necropsy patients. Amer J Med 52: 425, 1972

24. MOLLER JH, NAKIB A, EDWARDS JE: Infarction of papillary muscles and mitral insufficiency associated with congenital aortic stenosis. Circulation 34: 87, 1966

25. AROSEMENA E, MOLLER JH, EDWARDS JE: Scarring of the papillary muscles in left ventricular hypertrophy. Amer Heart J 74: 446, 1967

26. ROBERTS WC: The congenitally bicuspid aortic valve: A study of 85 autopsy cases. Amer J Cardiol 26: 72, 1970

27. ROBERTS WC, PERLOFF JK, COSTANTINO T: Severe valvular aortic stenosis in patients over 65 years of age: A clinicopathologic study. Amer J Cardiol 27: 497, 1971

28. FALCONE MW, ROBERTS WC, MORROW AG, PERLOFF JK: Congenital aortic stenosis resulting from a unicommissural valve: Clinical and anatomic features in twenty-one adult patients. Circulation 44: 272, 1971

29. BUCHBINDER NA, ROBERTS WC: Active left-sided valvular infective endocarditis: A study of 45 necropsy patients. Amer J Med. In press

30. MOLLER JH, LUCAS RV JR, ADAMS P JR, ANDERSON RC, JORGENS J, EDWARDS JE: Endocardial fibroelastosis: A clinical and anatomic study of 47 patients with emphasis on its relationship to mitral insufficiency. Circulation 30: 759, 1964

31. NOREN GR, RAGHIB G, MOLLER JH, AMPLATZ K, ADAMS P JR, EDWARDS JE: Anomalous origin of the left coronary artery from the pulmonary trunk with special reference to the occurrence of mitral insufficiency. Circulation 30: 171, 1964

32 ROBERTS WC: Anomalous origin of both coronary arteries from the pulmonary artery. Amer J Cardiol 10: 595, 1962

33. BURCHELL HB, BROWN AL JR: Anomalous origin of coronary artery from pulmonary artery masquerading as mitral insufficiency. Amer Heart J 63: 388, 1962

34. MARCUS FI, GOMEZ L, GLANCY DL, EWY GA, ROBERTS WC: Papillary muscle fibrosis in primary myocardial disease. Amer Heart J 77: 681, 1969

35. ROBERTS WC, ROSS RS, EGGLESTON JC, MASSUMI, RA: Chronic mitral regurgitation of unresolved etiology in the elderly: A clinicopathologic study of two patients. Johns Hopkins Med J 122: 26, 1968

36. PERLOFF JK: Cardiomyopathy associated with heredofamilial neuromyopathic diseases. Mod Conc Cardiovasc Dis 40: 23, 1971

37. DAVIES JNP, BALL JD: The pathology of endomyocardial fibrosis in Uganda. Brit Heart J 17: 337, 1955

38. ROBERTS WC, BUJA LM, FERRANS VJ: Löffler's fibroplastic parietal endocarditis, eosinophilic leukemia, and Davies' endomyocardial fibrosis: The same disease at different stages? Path Microbiol 35: 90, 1970

39. ROBERTS WC, LIEGLER DG, CARBONE PP: Endomyocardial disease and eosinophilia: A clinical and pathologic spectrum. Amer J Med 46: 28, 1969

40. MORROW AG, COHEN LS, ROBERTS WC, BRAUNWALD NS, BRAUNWALD E: Severe mitral regurgitation following acute myocardial infarction and ruptured papillary muscle: Hemodynamic findings and results of operative treatment in four patients. Circulation 38 (suppl II): II-124, II-132, 1968

41. HALLER JA JR, MORROW AG: Experimental mitral insufficiency: An operative method of chronic survival. Ann Surg 142: 37, 1955

42. BROCK RC: Arterial route to aortic and pulmonary valves: Mitral route to aortic valves. Guy Hosp Rep 99: 236, 1950

43. CHISHOLM JC JR: Sarcoid cardiomyopathy. J Nat Med Ass 58: 265, 1966

44. BUJA LM, KHOI NB, ROBERTS WC: Clinically significant cardiac amyloidosis: Clinicopathologic findings in 15 patients. Amer J Cardiol 26: 394, 1970

45. BUJA LM, ROBERTS WC: Iron in the heart: Etiology and clinical significance. Amer J Med 51: 209, 1971

46. SHONE JD, SELLER RD, ANDERSON RC, ADAMS P JR, LILLEHEI CW, EDWARDS JE: The developmental complex of "parachute mitral valve," supravalvular ring of left atrium, subaortic stenosis, and coarctation of aorta. Amer J Cardiol 11: 714, 1963

47. GLANCY DL, CHANG MY, DORNEY ER, ROBERTS WC: Parachute mitral valve. Further observations and associated lesions. Amer J Cardiol 27: 309, 1971

48. DAVACHI F, MOLLER JH, EDWARDS JE: Diseases of the mitral valve in infancy: An anatomic

analysis of 55 cases. Circulation **43**: 565, 1971

49. CARNEY EK, BRAUNWALD E, ROBERTS WC, AYGEN M, MORROW AG: Congenital mitral regurgitation: Clinical, hemodynamic and angiocardiographic findings in nine patients. Amer J Med **33**: 223, 1962

50. CASTANEDA AR, ANDERSON RC, EDWARDS JE: Congenital mitral stenosis resulting from anomalous arcade and obstructing papillary muscles: Report of correction by use of ball valve prosthesis. Amer J Cardiol **24**: 237, 1969

51. ROBERTS WC, MORROW AG: Causes of death and other anatomic observations after cardiac valve replacement: *In* Long-Term Prognosis following Valve Replacement; Advances in Cardiology. Basel, S. Karger, 1972, vol 7, p 226

52. RASTELLI GC, KIRKLIN JW, TITUS JL: Fate of papillary muscles after prosthetic replacement of mitral valve. Mayo Clin Proc **42**: 210, 1967

Left-to-right shunt at atrial level after rupture of papillary muscle from acute myocardial infarction

*Michael R. Nagel, M.D.**
*James A. Ronan, Jr., M.D.***
*William C. Roberts, M.D.****
Washington, D. C.

A systolic murmur may develop during or after acute myocardial infarction from ischemia, necrosis, fibrosis, or rupture of a papillary muscle or from rupture of the ventricular septum. Differentiation of mitral regurgitation from ventricular septal rupture in this setting may be difficult but the distinction is often made by the detection of a high oxygen content of blood in the pulmonary artery, strongly suggesting the presence of a ventricular septal defect. Rarely, mitral regurgitation produces retrograde flow through the pulmonary capillary bed causing elevation of the pulmonary arterial oxygen content.[1] We recently studied a patient who, during acute myocardial infarction, developed increased blood oxygen content in the right side of the heart due to papillary muscle rupture and a newly acquired left-to-right shunt at atrial level. Hemodynamic data indicated that the shunt was located at the atrial level, and necropsy showed that the defect was due to stretching of the fossa ovale region by left atrial dilatation after the acute development of mitral regurgitation. Pertinent clinical and anatomic features of this patient are summarized in this report.

Case report

W. A. (021-39-50), a 65-year-old man who died August 13, 1970, was first seen at Georgetown University Hospital on August 4, 1970. An acute diaphragmatic wall myocardial infarction had occurred 75 days earlier when he had been admitted to another hospital. Six days after the onset of infarction he developed a loud holosystolic apical murmur and severe congestive cardiac failure. Despite bed rest, digitalis, diuretics, and salt restriction during the next 69 days, he remained in chronic heart failure and became cachectic. The electrocardiograms (ECG's) taken by his private physician in previous years specifically showed none of the ECG features of atrial septal defect and his previous chest roentgenograms were normal.

From the Department of Medicine, Division of Cardiology, Georgetown University School of Medicine, Washington, D. C.

This work was supported by grants from the U. S. Public Health Service, the Benjamin May Memorial Fund, and the Special Cardiac Fund.

Received for publication Aug. 14, 1972.

Reprint requests to: Dr. James A. Ronan, Jr., Division of Cardiology, Georgetown University Hospital, 3800 Reservoir Rd., NLW, Washington, D. C. 20007.

*Fellow in Cardiology, Division of Cardiology, Georgetown University Hospital, Washington, D. C. Present address: 15955 Samaritan Dr., San Jose, Calif. 94125.

**Associate Professor of Medicine, Division of Cardiology, Georgetown University School of Medicine, Washington, D. C.

***Chief, Section of Pathology, National Heart and Lung Institute, National Institutes of Health, Bethesda, Md. 20014; and Clinical Associate Professor of Pathology and Medicine (Cardiology), Georgetown University, Washington, D. C.

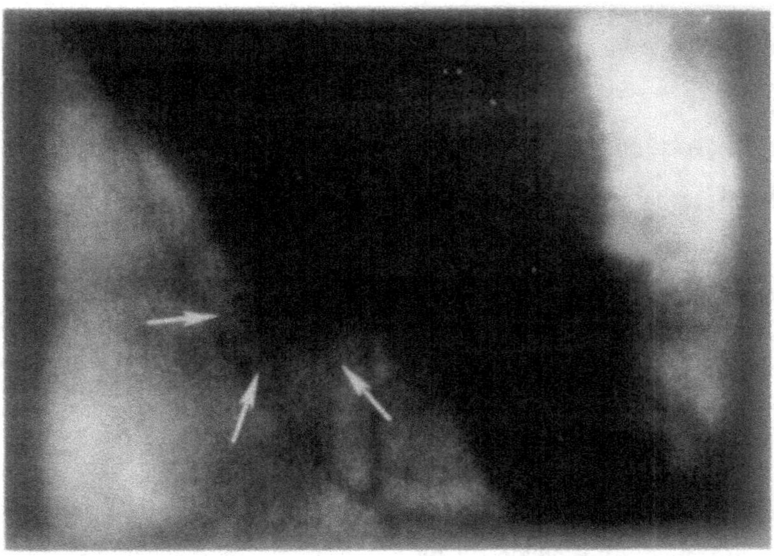

Fig. *1.* Left ventricular cineangiogram in the left anterior oblique view. There is a herniation of the atrial septum (*arrows*) with contrast material crossing from the left to the right atrium. Radiopaque dye can be seen in the left ventricle, aorta, and left atrium. The visible catheter is in the right atrium and right ventricle but the tip in the pulmonary artery is not visible. The left ventricular catheter cannot be seen.

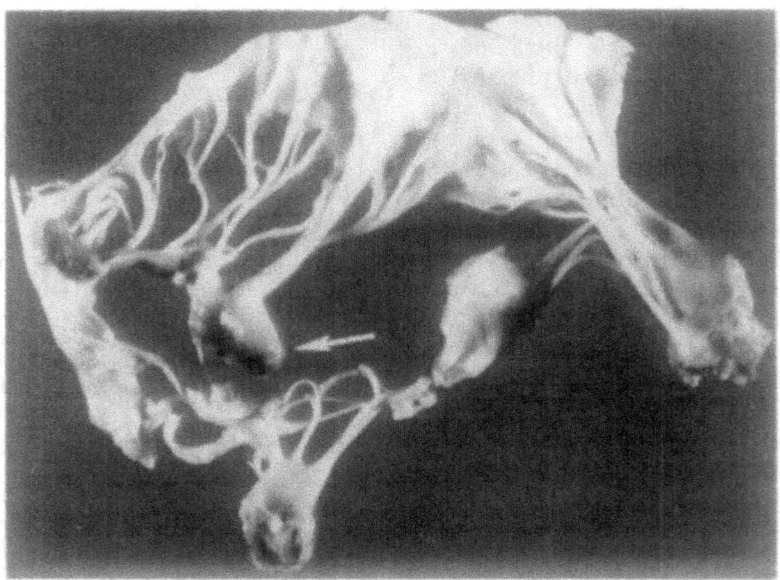

Fig. *2.* Surgical specimen of the mitral valve leaflets and supporting structures. That portion of the posteromedial papillary muscle which had ruptured is smooth and endothelialized (*arrow*).

Right heart catheterization at Georgetown University Hospital showed pulmonary hypertension and disproportionate elevation of the pulmonary arterial wedge "V" waves indicating mitral regurgitation (Table I). The hydrogen inhalation test with the platinum-tipped electrode in the right atrium yielded an appearance time of 3 seconds, documenting a left-to-right shunt at atrial level. Krypton 85 inhalation test with simultaneous blood sampling from pulmonary and left brachial arteries (on two occasions) yielded a calculated pulmonary-to-systemic flow ratio in excess of 4:1. Left ventricular cineangiography disclosed moderately severe mitral regurgitation. A well-defined portion of the atrial septum bulged into the right atrium, and contrast material passed from the left atrium to the right atrium at that position (Fig. 1).

At operation on August 13, 1970, portions of the posteromedial papillary muscle were found detached from its main trunk (Fig. 2). The ruptured

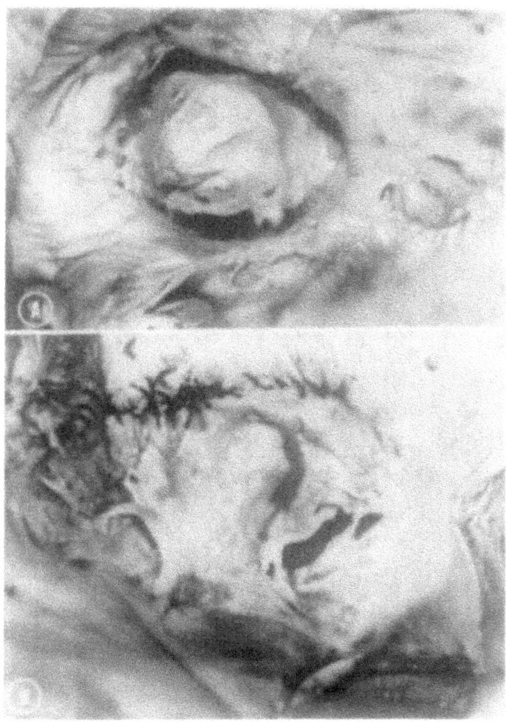

Fig. *3, A* and *B. A*, View of the atrial septum from the right atrium. The fossa ovale is herniating through the atrial septum. *B*, View of the atrial septum from the left atrium. The fossa ovale is bulging into the right atrium, creating the atrial septal defect. Black silk sutures have closed the surgical atriotomy which is in the interatrial groove.

portion contained about half the chordae tendineae attached to the posteromedial muscle. The atrial septum in the area of the fossa ovale was stretched and redundant, thereby bulging into the right atrium, producing a 1.0 cm. sized defect which represented a valvular-incompetent patent foramen ovale. This defect was closed by suture. The mitral valve was excised and was replaced by a size 19 Hufnagel disc prosthesis. The patient could not be weaned from extracorporeal circulation.

At necropsy (70A-376), the left atrium was large and the fossa ovale was aneurysmally dilated. A portion of the fossa ovale herniated into the right atrium enlarging a foramen ovale which had probably been valvular-competent although probe-patent before the rupture of the papillary muscle (Fig. 3).

Discussion

Papillary muscle rupture as a complication of acute myocardial infarction is rare.[2] Two large necropsy series discovered only two out of 6,000 and three out of 14,000 cases, respectively.[3] In 1948, Davison[4] made the first antemortem diagnosis, and in 1957

Sanders and colleagues[5] compiled 56 cases from the literature and added five new ones. Cederquist and Soderstrom[6] reported a four-year necropsy study in 1964, including 569 patients dying of acute myocardial infarction, from a total of 4,741 cases examined. They found a 0.9 per cent incidence of papillary muscle rupture. Mitral valve replacement has been successful in a number of these patients.[7]

The frequency of ventricular septal perforation complicating acute myocardial infarction is probably about 1 per cent.[8,9] Rupture of the ventricular septum classically occurs between 4 and 11 days after acute myocardial infarction and thus overlaps the period during which papillary muscle rupture occurs. The left-to-right shunt may cause biventricular heart failure.[10,11]

Mitral valve disease may be associated with left-to-right shunt at atrial level, but usually it is due to rheumatic mitral stenosis and/or insufficiency, rupture of chordae tendineae, or congenital mitral atresia.[12-14] Following acute myocardial infarction and papillary muscle rupture, our patient developed such a shunt from dilatation of the left atrium so that the foramen ovale which previously had been valvular-competent although patent, was stretched and became valvular incompetent (Fig. 4). Cases of papillary muscle rupture previously reported have not demonstrated interatrial shunting even though shunts were specifically sought.[15,16] In rupture of chordae tendineae, however, either spontaneously or after infective endocarditis, interatrial shunting has occurred.[17,18] Since about 20 to 25 per cent of adults studied at necropsy have valvular-competent but patent foramen ovales[19] as did this patient, it is possible that an interatrial communication might follow acute severe mitral regurgitation of any etiology.

Thus the finding of oxygenated blood in the main pulmonary arteries in patients with acute myocardial infarction and newly-acquired systolic precordial murmurs may be due to left-to-right shunting at atrial level from stretching of the membrane covering the fossa ovale, or from reflux through the capillary bed, or through a shunt at ventricular level. Care should be taken not to diagnose the presence of a

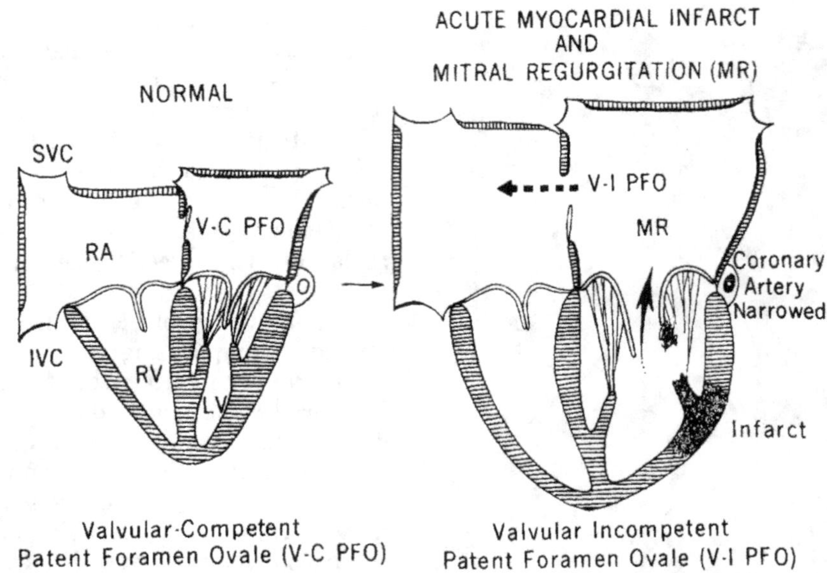

Fig. *4*. Diagrammatic representation of a valvular-competent patent foramen ovale in contrast to a valvular-incompetent patent foramen ovale following myocardial infarction and mitral regurgitation. The left atrial walls have been stretched so that the valve of the patent foramen ovale can no longer cover the defect.

Table I. *Cardiac catheterization data*

Site	Pressure (mm. Hg)	Site	Pressure (mm. Hg)
Right atrium	a = 9 v = 21 mean = 9	Pulmonary artery wedge	a = 25 v = 57 mean = 26
Right ventricle Pulmonary artery	54/8 62/21 mean = 40	Left ventricle Brachial artery	115/29 117/92 mean = 108

ventricular septal perforation on the basis of a step-up in oxygen saturation in the right ventricle unless a left-to-right shunt at atrial level has been excluded.

Summary

Clinical and necropsy observations are described in a patient who developed a large left-to-right shunt at atrial level after rupture of a papillary muscle during acute myocardial infarction. Attention is called to the importance of differentiating this combination from rupture of the ventricular septum and from mitral regurgitation resulting from papillary muscle necrosis with or without rupture.

REFERENCES

1. Tatooles, C. J., Gault, J. H., Mason, D. T., and Ross, J., Jr.: Reflux of oxygenated blood into the pulmonary artery in severe mitral regurgitation, Am. Heart J. **75**:102, 1968.
2. Heikkila, J.: Mitral incompetence complicating acute myocardial infarction, Br. Heart J. **29**:162, 1967.
3. Stevenson, R. R., and Turner, W. J.: Rupture of a papillary muscle in the heart as a cause of sudden death, Bull. Johns Hopkins Hosp. **57**:235, 1935.
4. Davison, S.: Spontaneous rupture of a papillary muscle in the heart; a report of three cases and

a review of the literature, J. Mt. Sinai Hosp. N. Y. **14**:941, 1948.

5. Sanders, R. J., Neubuerger, K. T., and Ravin, A.: Rupture of papillary muscles: Occurrence of rupture of posterior muscle in posterior myocardial infarction, Dis. Chest. **31**:316, 1957.

6. Cederquist, L., and Soderstrom, J.: Papillary muscle rupture in myocardial infarction: a study based upon an autopsy material, Acta Med. Scand. **176**:287, 1964.

7. Morrow, A. G., Cohen, L. S., Roberts, W. C., Braunwald, N. S., and Braunwald, E.: Severe mitral regurgitation following acute myocardial infarction and ruptured papillary muscle: hemodynamic findings and results of operative treatment in four patients, Circulation **37** and **38** (Suppl. II):124, 1968.

8. Bond, V. F., Welfare, C. R., Lide, T. N., and McMillan, R. L.: Perforation of the interventricular septum following myocardial infarction, Ann. Intern. Med. **38**:706, 1953.

9. London, R. E., and London, S. B.: Rupture of the heart: a critical analysis of 47 consecutive autopsy cases, Circulation **31**:202, 1965.

10. Holloway, D. H., Whalen, R. E., and McIntosh, H. D.: Systolic murmur developing after myocardial ischemia or infarction, J.A.M.A. **191**:92, 1965.

11. Selzer, A., Gerbode, F., and Kerth, W. J.: Clinical, hemodynamic, and surgical considerations of rupture of the ventricular septum after myocardial infarction, AM. HEART J. **78**:598, 1969.

12. Demos, N. J., Gerard, F., Sabey, A., Yadusky, R., Timmes, J. J., and Torruella, J. M.: Coexistence of mitral valve disease and atrial septal defect, J. Cardiovasc. Surg. **9**:278, 1968.

13. Espino-Vela, J.: Rheumatic heart disease associated with atrial septal defect: Clinical and pathologic study of twelve cases of Lutembacher's syndrome, AM. HEART J. **57**:185, 1959.

14. Ross, J., Jr., Braunwald, E., Mason, D. T., Braunwald, N. S., and Morrow, A. G.: Interatrial communication and left atrial hypertension–A cause of continuous murmur, Circulation **28**:853, 1963.

15. Austen, W. G., Sokol, D. M., DeSanctis, R. W., and Sanders, C. A.: Surgical treatment of papillary-muscle rupture complicating myocardial infarction, N. Engl. J. Med. **278**:1137, 1968.

16. Breneman, G. M., and Drake, E. H.: Ruptured papillary muscle following myocardial infarction with long survival: Report of two cases, Circulation **28**:862, 1962.

17. Burchell, J. B.: Possibly unrecognized forms of heart disease, Circulation **28**:1153, 1963.

18. Marshall, R. J., and Warden, H. E.: Mitral valve disease complicated by left to right shunt at atrial level, Circulation **29**:432, 1964.

19. Edwards, J. E.: Pathology of the heart, Springfield, Ill., 1960, Charles C Thomas, Publisher, p. 260.

Does Thrombosis Play a Major Role in the Development of Symptom-Producing Atherosclerotic Plaques?

Additional Indexing Words:

Thrombosis   Pathogenesis of atherosclerosis   Fibrin deposition   Atherosclerotic plaques
Mural thrombosis   Coronary artery thrombosis

IN 1852 Rokitansky proposed that atherosclerotic plaques resulted from the organization of thrombi.[1] Virchow[2] disputed this view and since 1913[3] investigations of atherosclerosis, with some exceptions,[4-12] have centered mainly around the role of lipids. Recently, attention has refocused on thrombi.[13-25] Several observations suggest that atherosclerotic plaques result, at least in part, from the organization of thrombi:

1) The presence of known components of thrombi—namely fibrin and platelets—within atherosclerotic plaques (fig. 1).

2) The occurrence of known components of atherosclerotic plaques—namely foam cells, choles-terol clefts, pultaceous debris, calcium—in orga-nized hematomas or known thrombi wherever they occur in the body. An example is the left atrial thrombus in the patient with mitral stenosis.[25] Organization of this thrombus may produce typical complicated atherosclerotic plaques (figs. 2 and 3).

3) The presence of multiple channels in lumens—a recognized consequence of organization of pulmonary arterial thromboemboli.[9] Multilumin-al channels commonly are found in severely atherosclerotic coronary arteries (fig. 4). This observation suggests that thrombi or emboli were at one time present and that they organized. The tissue present between the multiluminal channels is similar to that found in arteries with only one channel (fig. 5). Because the artery with multiple channels has been recognized as the hallmark of an organized thrombus[10] and because the tissue in both multi- and unichanneled arteries is similar,

From the Section of Pathology, National Heart and Lung Institute, National Institutes of Health, Bethesda, Maryland.

Address for reprints: William C. Roberts, M.D., Section of Pathology, National Heart and Lung Institute, National Institutes of Health, Bethesda, Maryland 20014.

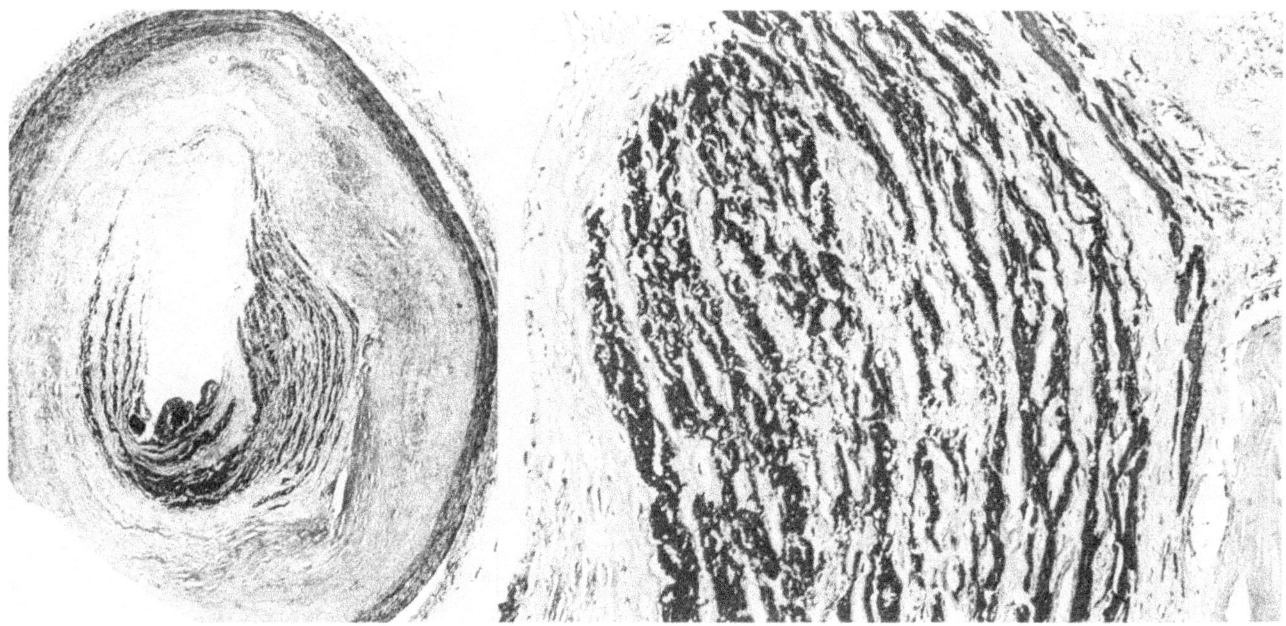

Figure 1

Right coronary artery in a 47-year-old man (A70-72) with healed posterior wall left ventricular transmural infarct and rheumatic mitral stenosis. The lumen of the right coronary artery was narrowed more than 75% primarily by fibrous plaques interspersed with fibrin as shown here. The fibrin is dark and the organized fibrous tissue is lighter. A close-up view of the deposits is shown at right. Phosphotungstic acid-hematoxylin stain; × 23 (left) and × 120 (right). Reproduced from Roberts and Buja.[25]

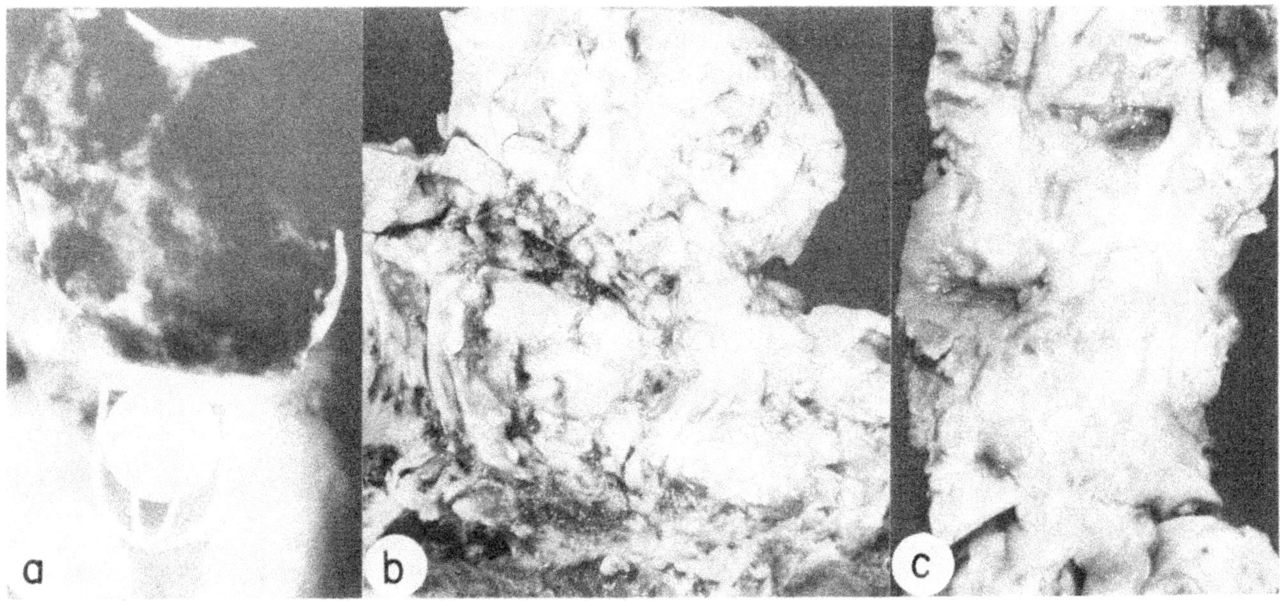

Figure 2

Left atrial atherosclerosis in a 57-year-old woman (A72-192) who died shortly after mitral valve replacement for severe mitral stenosis. A mitral commissurotomy had been done when she was 41 years old. The left atrial wall is heavily calcified (a and b). A close-up of the interior lining of the left atrium (b) shows that it contains plaques similar to those in the aorta (c). Histologic sections of the walls of left atrium and aorta disclosed that each was lined by typical complicated atherosclerotic plaques.

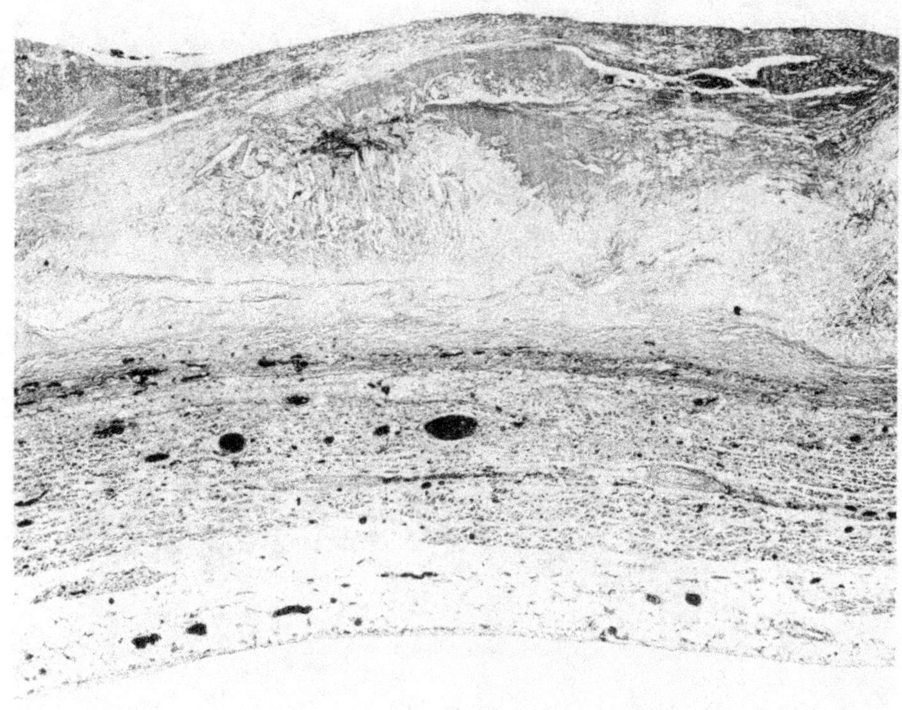

Duguid[6] reasoned that the causative process also was similar.

4) The major component of the complicated atherosclerotic plaque, i.e., those capable of causing significant luminal narrowing, in the coronary arteries of patients with fatal ischemic heart disease is fibrous tissue or collagen, not lipid.[25, 26] This is true whether or not hyperlipidemia is present[26] (fig. 6). Foam cells, actually, are infrequently observed in the coronary arteries in patients with fatal ischemic heart disease. Often the "density" of the fibrous tissue plugging a coronary artery is different in different portions of a plaque and these subunits may be demarcated by distinct elastic lamellae (fig. 7). These subunits suggest that thrombus is deposited at different times and that the "density"

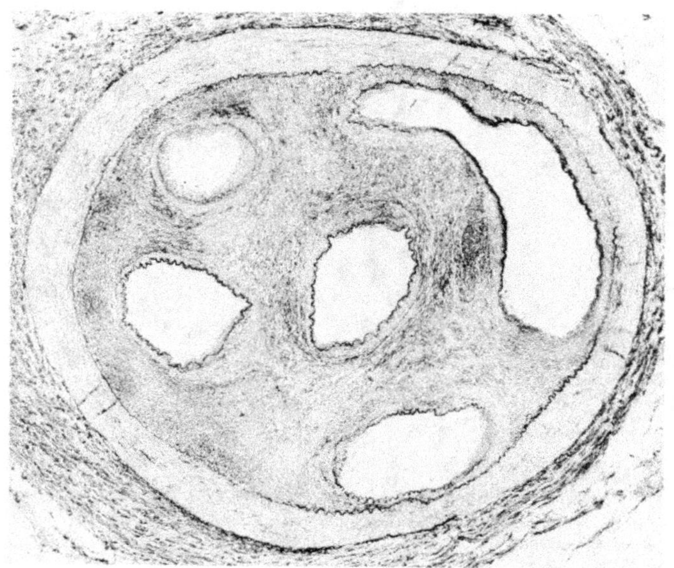

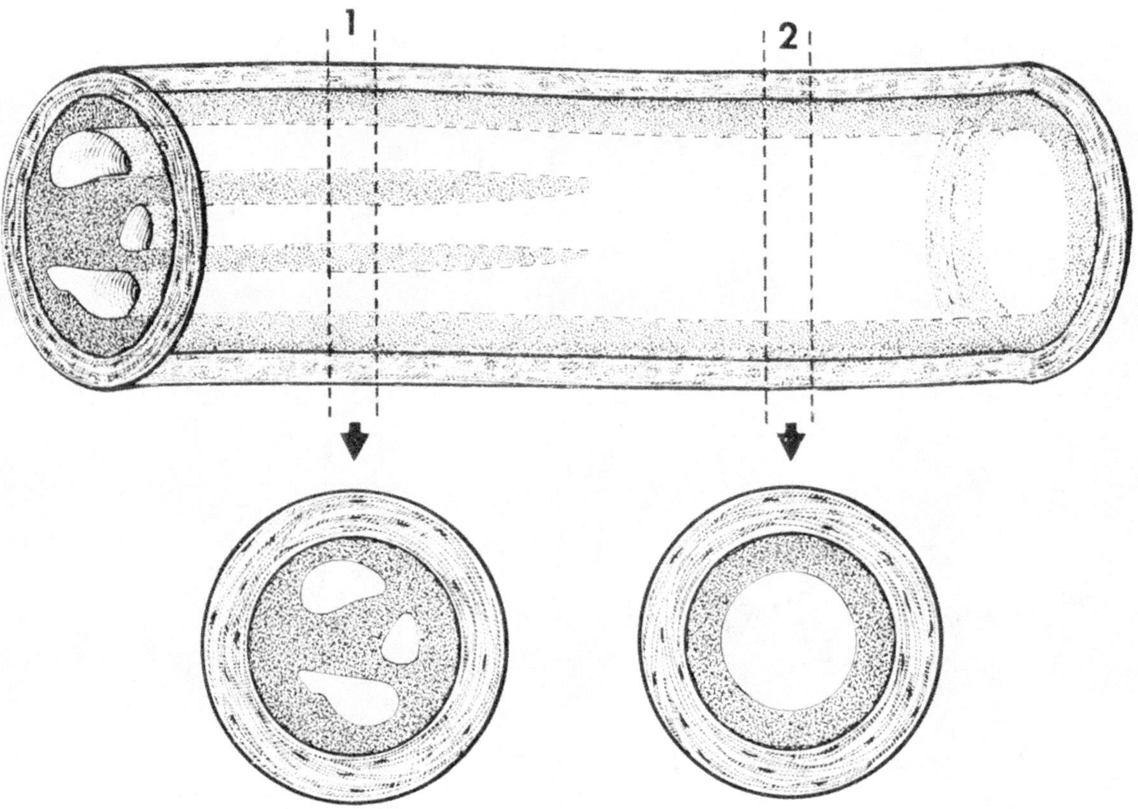

Figure 5

The multi- and unichanneled atherosclerotic coronary artery. The intimal material in each is similar suggesting that the causative process in each is similar. Reproduced from Roberts and Buja.[25]

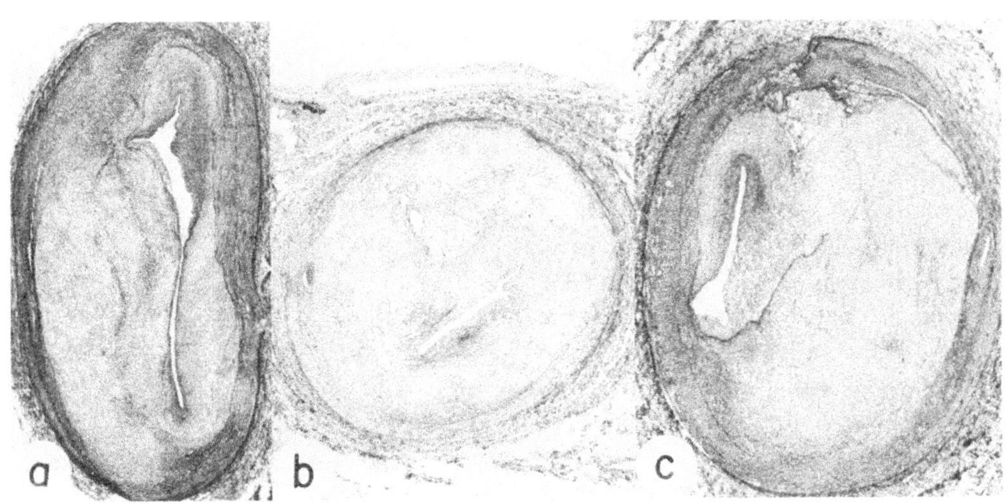

Figure 6

Sections of coronary arteries at sites of maximal narrowing in a 28-year-old man (A70-64) with homozygous type II hyperlipoproteinemia. He died suddenly but had had angina pectoris since age 17. The serum total cholesterol level was 588 mg/100 ml and the triglyceride level, 100 mg/100 ml. During his last years of life he was treated with a low cholesterol diet and cholestyramine. His lowest total serous cholesterol level was 340 mg/100 ml. The luminal narrowing in each of the three major coronary arteries results from fibrous tissue. (a) Right, (b) Left anterior descending, and (c) Left circumflex coronary arteries. Movat stains; each $\times$ 22.

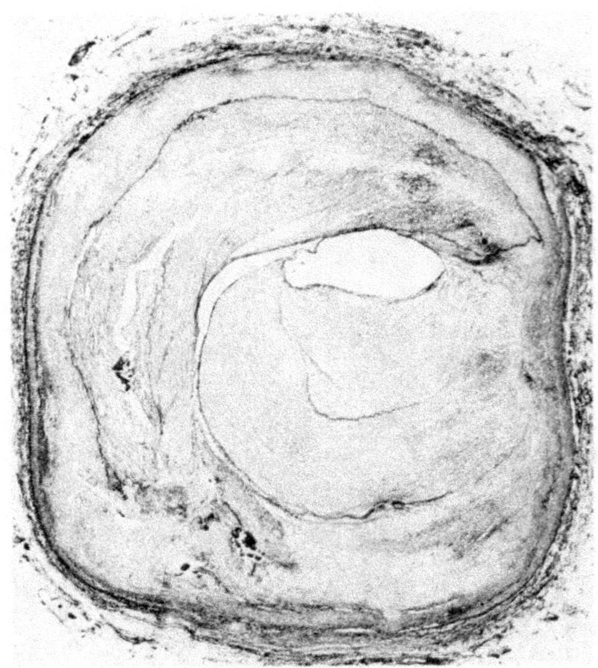

Figure 7

Narrowed coronary artery in a 65-year-old man (A71-6) who died suddenly. Demarcation lines suggest organized thrombi of varying ages.

of the resulting fibrous tissue may be determined by the composition of the initial thrombus, i.e., whether platelets or fibrin predominated.[18]

5) Experimentally-induced thrombi under proper conditions may be transformed into atherosclerotic plaques closely resembling those observed in human coronary arteries.[16, 18]

These factors obviously do not prove that thrombosis is the cause of atherosclerosis, but together they strongly suggest that organization of thrombi plays a major role in the development of the complicated atherosclerotic plaque. Indeed, most serious students of the morphology of the arterial plaque presently support, in whole or in part, the thrombogenic origin of atherosclerosis. Because the clotting factors in the blood appear to be similar in all population groups and because symptomatic atherosclerosis develops only in those population groups with elevated blood lipids, the latter also play a role in the development of the plaque. Lipids may exert their effect, however, more by their ability to alter the clotting mechanism than by their ability to infiltrate the arterial wall.

WILLIAM C. ROBERTS, M.D.

Circulation, Volume XLVIII, December 1973

References

1. ROKITANSKY CA: Manual of Pathological Anatomy, Vol. 4, translated by DAY GE. London, Sydenham Society, 1852, pp 261-272
2. VIRCHOW R: Cellular Pathology. As Based upon Physiological and Pathological Histology. Translated from the Second German edition originally published by J. B. Lippincott and Co., 1863. New York, Dover Publications, 1971
3. ANITSCHOW N, CHALATOW S: Über experimentelle Cholesterinsteatose und ihra Bedeutung für die Entstehung einiger pathologischer Prozesse. Zentralbl Allg Pathol 24: 1, 1913
4. MALLORY FB: The infectious lesions of blood vessels. *In* The Harvey Lectures. Philadelphia, J. B. Lippincott, 1912-1913, pp 150-166
5. CLARK E, GRAEF I, CHASIS H: Thrombosis of the aorta and coronary arteries with special reference to "fibrinoid" lesions. Arch Pathol 22: 183, 1936
6. DUGUID JB: Thrombosis as a factor in the pathogenesis of coronary atherosclerosis. J Pathol Bacteriol 58: 207, 1946
7. DUGUID JB: Thrombosis as a factor in the pathogenesis of aortic atherosclerosis. J Pathol Bacteriol 60: 57, 1948
8. DUGUID JB: Mural thrombosis in arteries. Br Med Bull 11: 36, 1955
9. HARRISON CV: Experimental pulmonary arteriosclerosis. J Pathol Bacteriol 60: 289, 1948
10. GEIRINGER E: Intimal vascularization and atherosclerosis. J Pathol Bacteriol 63: 201, 1951
11. MORGAN AD: The Pathogenesis of Coronary Occlusion. Springfield, Charles C Thomas, 1956
12. HAUST MD, MORE RH, MOVAT HZ: The mechanism of fibrosis in arteriosclerosis. Am J Pathol 35: 265, 1959
13. MITCHELL JRA, SCHWARTZ CJ: Arterial Disease. Philadelphia, F. A. Davis Co., 1965, pp 315-318
14. FULTON WFM: The Coronary Arteries. Arteriography, Microanatomy, and Pathogenesis of Obliterative Coronary Artery Disease. Springfield, Charles C Thomas, 1965
15. PFLEIDERER TH: Thrombosis. *In* Atherosclerosis. Pathology, Physiology, Aetiology, Diagnosis and Clinical Management, edited by SCHETTLER FG, BOYD CS. Amsterdam, Elsevier Publishing Co., 1969, pp 487-529
16. FRIEDMAN M: Pathogenesis of Coronary Artery Disease. New York, McGraw-Hill Book Co., 1969
17. STUDER A: Thrombosis and atherosclerosis. *In* Atherosclerosis. Proceedings of the Second International Symposium, edited by JONES RJ. New York, Springer-Verlag, 1970, pp 20-23
18. CHANDLER AB: Thrombosis and the development of atherosclerotic lesions. *In* Atherosclerosis. Proceedings of the Second International Symposium, edited by JONES RJ. New York, Springer-Verlag, 1970, pp 88-93
19. CHANDLER AB: Thrombosis in the development of coronary atherosclerosis. *In* Atherosclerosis and Coronary Heart Disease, edited by LIKOFF W, SEGAL BL, INSULL W JR, MOYER JH. New York, Grune & Stratton, 1972, pp 28-34

20. FRENCH JE: Formation and fate of a thrombus. *In* Atherosclerosis. Proceedings of the Second International Symposium, edited by JONES RJ, New York, Springer-Verlag, 1970, pp 80-88

21. FRENCH JE: Atherogenesis and thrombosis. Semin Hematol 8: 84, 1971

22. JØRGENSEN L: Thrombosis and the complications of atherosclerosis. *In* Atherosclerosis. Proceedings of the Second International Symposium, edited by JONES RJ. New York, Springer-Verlag, 1970, pp 94-106

23. BORN GVR, CONSTANTINIDES P, FRENCH J, FRIEDMAN M, GRESHAM GA, HAUST MD, LAKI K, SCHWARTZ CJ, SINAPIUS D, SMITH EB, VESTESAEGER M, WERTHESSEN NT, WISSLER RW: Thrombogenic mechanisms in atherosclerosis. *In* The Artery and the Process of Atherosclerosis. Pathogenesis, edited by WOLF S. New York, Plenum Press, 1971, pp 175-184

24. MUSTARD JF, PACKHAM MA: Thrombosis and the development of atherosclerosis. *In* The Pathogenesis of Atherosclerosis, edited by WISSLER RW, GREER JC. Baltimore, Williams & Wilkins, 1972, pp 214-226

25. ROBERTS WC, BUJA LM: The frequency and significance of coronary arterial thrombi and other observations in fatal acute myocardial infarction. A study of 107 necropsy patients. Am J Med 52: 425, 1972

26. ROBERTS WC, FERRANS VJ, LEVY RI, FREDRICKSON DS: Cardiovascular pathology in hyperlipoproteinemia. Anatomic observations in 42 necropsy patients with normal or abnormal serum lipoprotein patterns. Am J Cardiol 31: 557, 1973

Coronary Thrombosis and Fatal Myocardial Ischemia

IN RECENT years the role of coronary thrombosis as a precipitating cause of acute myocardial infarction (AMI) has been questioned. "Which comes first, coronary thrombosis or myocardial necrosis?" Before attempting to answer this question, changes observed routinely in the coronary arteries in fatal ischemic heart disease (IHD) will be reviewed:

1) The coronary arteries are *diffusely* involved by atherosclerotic plaques.[1] Although the lumens of some segments are more severely narrowed than others, *all portions* of the extramural coronary tree are involved by the atherosclerotic process.

2) In fatal IHD, with rare exception, the lumens of at least *two of the three major coronary arteries* are >75% narrowed by old atherosclerotic plaques.[1] The most severe narrowing tends to be in the more proximal portions of the left anterior descending and left circumflex branches; the distal half of the right coronary artery is prone to narrowing that is as severe as that in its proximal portion.

3) The atherosclerotic process is limited to the *epicardial* coronary arteries, i.e., the major trunks and their near right-angle branches. The intramural (intramyocardial) coronary arteries are spared by the atherosclerotic process.

4) The coronary artery responsible for perfusing with oxygen the area of myocardial ischemia is not necessarily the most severely narrowed of the 3 major coronary arteries but its lumen is virtually always >75% narrowed at some point by atherosclerotic plaques.

5) The coronary arterial luminal narrowing in fatal IHD is produced by *complicated* atherosclerotic plaques, as opposed to fatty and fibrous plaques. The latter two types of atherosclerotic plaques are world wide in distribution, but the complicated plaques, i.e., those containing cholesterol clefts, pultaceous debris, calcium, extravasated erythrocytes, etc., are found only in populations which develop symptomatic IHD. The major component of even the complicated atherosclerotic plaque in fatal IHD is fibrous tissue (collagen) and the lipid component is much less evident. Foam cells actually are relatively infrequent in the coronary arteries in fatal IHD, and the lipid which is present is usually extracellular.

Now to coronary thrombosis in fatal IHD. Some observations:

1) Among patients with fatal IHD, thrombi are infrequent (about 10%) in patients dying *suddenly* and in those in whom the necrosis is limited to *subendocardium*. (Sudden death is defined herein as that occurring within 6 hours after onset of symptoms of myocardial ischemia and unassociated with histologic evidence of myocardial necrosis; subendocardium, as the inner one-half of the myocardial wall.)

2) Thrombus is found in a coronary artery in about 55% of patients with fatal *transmural* AMI.[2]

3) Among patients with transmural myocardial necrosis, the major determinant of the presence of coronary thrombosis appears to be the presence or absence of *cardiogenic shock.* At necropsy, >70% of patients with fatal AMI with cardiogenic shock have coronary thrombi whereas only about 15% of patients without the power failure syndrome associated with fatal AMI have coronary thrombi.[3] Tissue necrosis itself, especially in a shock situation, also increases the coagulability of the blood.

From the Section of Pathology, National Heart and Lung Institute, National Institutes of Health, Bethesda, Maryland.

Address for reprints: William C. Roberts, M.D., Building 10A, Room 3E-30, National Heart and Lung Institute, National Institutes of Health, Bethesda, Maryland 20014.

4) The larger the area of myocardial necrosis, the greater the likelihood of coronary thrombosis. The larger the infarcted area, however, the greater the likelihood of cardiogenic shock. The latter generally indicates that >40% of the left ventricular wall is either necrotic or fibrotic or both, whereas shock is infrequently associated with infarcts or scars involving <40% of the left ventricular wall.[4]

5) When coronary thrombosis is associated with AMI, the thrombus is always located in the artery responsible for perfusing the area of myocardial necrosis. Thus, in anterior wall infarction a thrombus, if present, will be located in the left anterior descending coronary artery.

6) Thrombi are found in fatal IHD in coronary arteries which already are severely narrowed by old atherosclerotic plaques. At the distal site of attachment of the thrombus, or just distal to this site, the lumen of the coronary artery is nearly always >75% narrowed by old atherosclerotic plaques.[1] Not infrequently, a thrombus may occur in an area between two sites of severe narrowing, like in a valley between two mountains. If a clot is found in a coronary artery relatively free of old atherosclerotic plaques, embolism rather than thrombosis must be considered.

7) Coronary thrombi in fatal AMI are usually (90%) *single*, usually (80%) *occlusive* (as opposed to mural or non-occlusive), *short* (<2 cm long), and *located entirely in the major trunks* (as opposed to their near right-angle branches or intramural coronary arteries). The thrombus when only a few hours old may consist nearly entirely of platelets, but thereafter is composed primarily of fibrin. By definition, the thrombus is *adherent* to the surface of the arterial wall bordering the lumen.

Since 1912,[5] when Herrick first used the term "coronary thrombosis" to describe the often dramatic clinical event characterized at necropsy by necrosis of portions of left ventricular wall, it has been assumed that the usual cause of AMI is coronary thrombosis. Two factors implicate coronary thrombosis as the *precipitating cause* of AMI: 1) the occurrence of coronary arterial thrombi in many patients with fatal AMI; 2) the location of the thrombus in the coronary artery responsible for supplying the area of myocardial necrosis. Five factors, however, tend to indicate that coronary thrombosis is a *consequence* rather than the precipitating cause of AMI: 1) the very low frequency of thrombi in patients dying suddenly with or without previous evidence of cardiac disease; 2) the increasing frequency of thrombi with increasing intervals between onset of symptoms of AMI and death; 3) the absence of thrombi in fatal transmural AMI nearly as often as they are present; 4) the near absence of thrombi in fatal subendocardial AMI; and 5) the occurrence of thrombi in high percentage only in patients with cardiogenic shock, most of whom have large transmural infarcts.

The key to coronary thrombosis, just as the key to thrombosis occurring anywhere in the body, is *slow blood flow,* or relative stasis, and sufficient *time* for the thrombus to form. The absence of these two factors may explain the absence of coronary thrombosis in the sudden death cases, and the increasing frequency of thrombosis as the interval from onset of symptoms of myocardial ischemia to death increases.[6, 7] There is a marked reduction in blood flow in the coronary artery responsible for supplying the area of myocardial infarction. This observation was made in dogs after inducing AMI, and they had normal, i.e., widely patent, vessels.[8] In fatal AMI in humans, the thrombus is always located in an artery already containing considerable atherosclerotic plaques, and, therefore, the infarct-induced relative coronary stasis is probably even greater. Cardiogenic shock must further diminish coronary flow.

The type activity experienced by patients at the time of onset of AMI may reflect slowed blood flow. Nearly 75% of patients with AMI have the onset of chest pain while sleeping, resting, or performing mild activity.[9] Although inactivity may cause slight diminution in coronary blood flow, considerable stasis of blood (infarction-induced plus cardiogenic shock) is usually necessary for thrombus to form. In contrast to fatal AMI, coronary thrombosis is rarely observed in fatal angina pectoris although the degree of coronary luminal narrowing by atherosclerotic plaques is similar in degree to that observed in AMI. Evidence of thrombus formation is nearly always observed in arteries implanted into left ventricular myocardium, presumably because of poor blood flow.[10] Thrombus formation does not occur in similar arteries implanted into left ventricular myocardium but allowed to drain into right ventricular cavity.[10] Thus, it appears that a period of diminished coronary blood flow is necessary for thrombus to form in a coronary artery. Shock, congestive cardiac failure and inactivity all decrease coronary flow and with time may allow thrombosis.

Further support for the concept that coronary thrombosis is a consequence rather than a precipitating cause of AMI was supplied recently by Erhardt et al.[11] who observed radioactivity at necropsy in coronary arterial thrombi in each of seven patients who had been given radioactive I^{125}-labelled fibrinogen shortly after admission because of AMI. This finding implicates coronary thrombosis as a secondary event occurring sometime after the infarction.

In conclusion, there is substantial evidence that acute thrombus formation does not precipitate acute fatal IHD. The major problem is diffuse generalized coronary atherosclerosis with severe (>75%) luminal narrowing (at least 2 of the 3 major coronary arteries). Six years after Herrick's classic paper in 1919 on coronary thrombosis,[12] the following was written by Nathanson[13] and it may serve as a summary for this piece:

". . . It seems justifiable to conclude from this analysis [review of necropsy reports of 113 cases of severe coronary disease] that coronary disease shows a similar clinical picture irrespective of whether a thrombus is present or not. A prolonged attack, consisting of an initial shock which the patient survives, is more frequent with a thrombus. Such a picture does occur, however, in coronary sclerosis without thrombosis. There does not seem, therefore, to be any justification for drawing any sharp distinction between these conditions. Since coronary thrombosis is constantly associated with sclerosis of the vessels, it is most reasonable to regard a thrombus not as an entity, but merely as one of the end results of coronary disease . . ."

WILLIAM C. ROBERTS

References

1. ROBERTS WC, BUJA LM: The frequency and significance of coronary arterial thrombi and other observations in fatal acute myocardial infarction. A study of 107 necropsy patients. Am J Med 52: 425, 1972
2. ROBERTS WC: The pathology of acute myocardial infarction. Hosp Practice 6: 89, 1971
3. WALSTON A, HACKEL DB, ESTES EH: Acute coronary occlusion and the "power failure" syndrome. Am Heart J 79: 613, 1970
4. PAGE DL, CAULFIELD JB, KASTOR JA, DeSANCTIS RW, SANDERS CA: Myocardial changes associated with cardiogenic shock. N Engl J Med 285: 133, 1971
5. HERRICK JB: Clinical features of sudden obstruction of the coronary arteries. JAMA 59: 2015, 1912
6. SPAIN DM, BRADESS VA: The relationship of coronary thrombosis to coronary atherosclerosis and ischemic heart disease. (A necropsy study covering a period of 25 years). Am J Med Sci 240: 701, 1960
7. SPAIN DM, BRADESS VA: Sudden death from coronary heart disease. Survival time, frequency of thrombi, and cigarette smoking. Chest 58: 107, 1970
8. HELLSTROM HR: Coronary artery stasis after induced myocardial infarction in the dog. Cardiovasc Res 5: 371, 1971
9. MASTER AM, DACK S, JAFFE HL: Activities associated with the onset of acute coronary artery occlusion. Am Heart J 18: 434, 1939
10. YARBROUGH JW, ROBERTS WC, ABEL RM, REIS RL: The cause of luminal narrowing in internal mammary arteries implanted into canine myocardium. Am Heart J 84: 507, 1972
11. ERHARDT LR, LUNDMAN T, MELLSTEDT H: Incorporation of ^{125}I-labelled fibrinogen into coronary arterial thrombi in acute myocardial infarction in man. Lancet 1: 387, 1973
12. HERRICK JB: Thrombosis of the coronary arteries. JAMA 72: 387, 1919
13. NATHANSON MH: Disease of the coronary arteries. Clinical and pathologic features. Am J Med Sci 170: 240, 1925

Steroid Therapy During Acute Myocardial Infarction

A Cause of Delayed Healing and of Ventricular Aneurysm

BERNADINE H. BULKLEY, M.D.
WILLIAM C. ROBERTS, M.D.
Bethesda, Maryland

Clinical and necropsy observations are described in a man who received large doses of corticosteroids for Dressler's syndrome which complicated acute myocardial infarction. Although the patient survived for 63 days, during 53 of which he received corticosteroids, the infarct histologically appeared to be only 10 to 14 days old. Thus, the healing of the infarct was clearly delayed. Experimental studies in dogs were cited in which healing of myocardial infarction was delayed by corticosteroid therapy.

In our patient a large left ventricular aneurysm also developed. Study of previous reports of human subjects receiving corticosteroids during acute myocardial infarction disclosed that aneurysmal formation was also a common complication of corticosteroid therapy for the postmyocardial infarction syndrome.

It is concluded that use of glucocorticosteroids for any reason during acute myocardial infarction may be hazardous, and that their use in patients with the postmyocardial infarction syndrome, a benign and self-limited condition, should be avoided.

It is known that corticosteroids slow or partially inhibit the healing of most wounds. However, the effect of corticosteroids on the healing of an acute myocardial infarction in man has not been determined. Recently, we studied a patient with postmyocardial infarction syndrome at necropsy who had received large doses of corticosteroids during the period of infarction. Our observations in this patient strongly suggest that healing of acute myocardial infarction is delayed by corticosteroid therapy and that this therapy may predispose the patient to ventricular aneurysm.

CASE REPORT

This 64 year old man (T.L., 09-37-82-4), was in good health until 63 days before his death when he had an acute myocardial infarct complicated by congestive heart failure. Ten days later, chest pain appeared in association with a persistent pleuropericardial friction rub and fever, and a diagnosis of Dressler's syndrome was made. For the following 53 days he was given 150 mg of hydrocortisone daily; during that time a large left ventricular aneurysm developed (Figure 1). Six days before his death the patient was transferred to the National Heart and Lung Institute for aneurysmectomy.

From the Section of Pathology, National Heart and Lung Institute, National Institutes of Health, Bethesda, Maryland 20014. Requests for reprints should be addressed to Dr. William C. Roberts, Bldg. 10A, Room 3E30, National Heart and Lung Institute, National Institutes of Health, Bethesda, Maryland 20014. Manuscript accepted September 17, 1973.

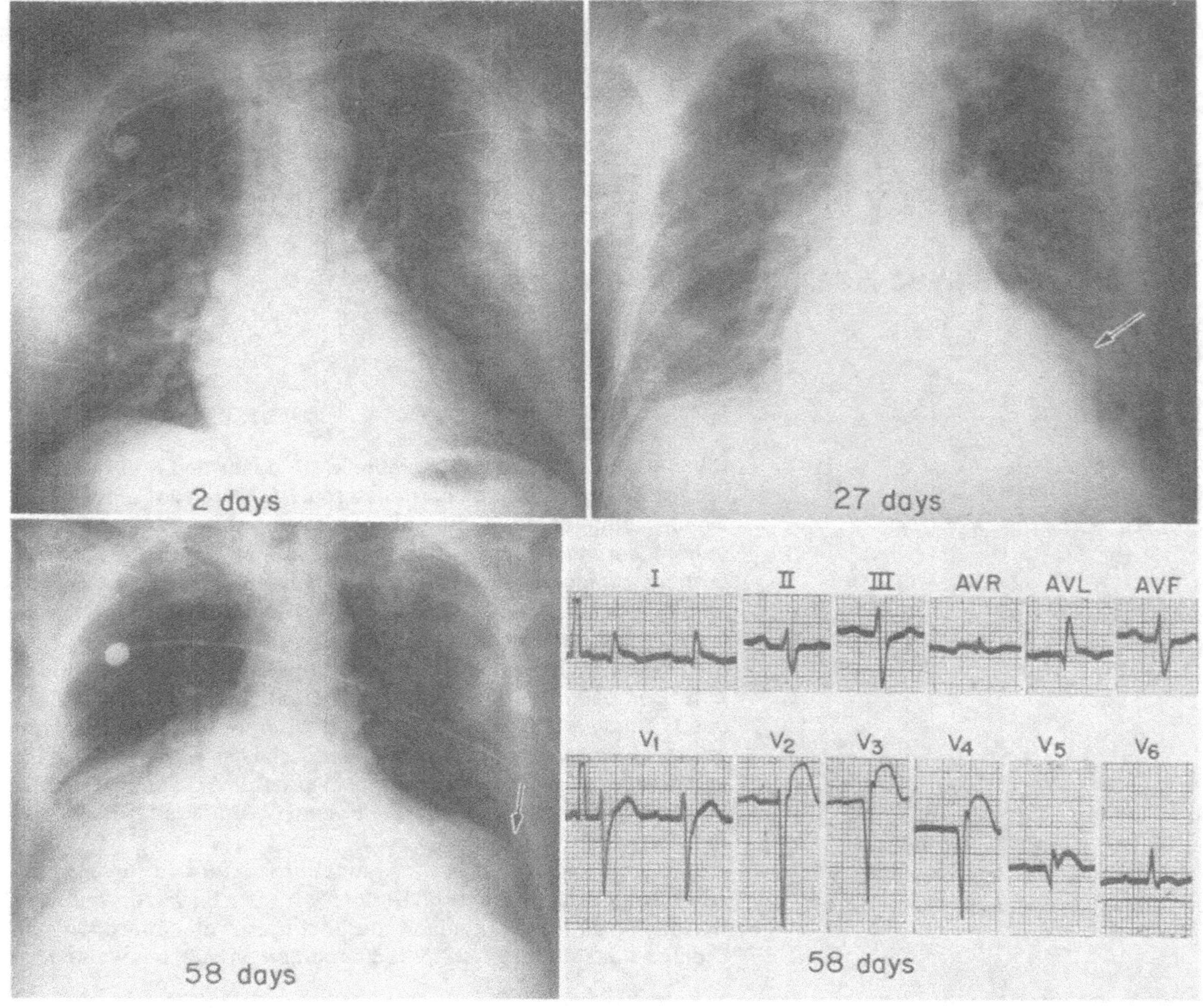

Figure 1. *Roentgenograms and electrocardiogram of the patient who died 63 days after onset of an acute myocardial infarction. The days designate the time from the onset of the infarction. The arrows designate the aneurysm.*

He appeared cachectic. His neck veins were distended, rales were heard in the chest, the liver was enlarged, and there was no subcutaneous edema. No precordial murmur was present, but the apical impulse pulsated paradoxically. Both third and fourth heart sounds were heard. An electrocardiogram (Figure 1) showed a prolonged (0.22 sec) P-R interval, left axis deviation, elevated S-T segments in leads V_2 through V_5, and Q waves in leads I, aVL and V_3 through V_5. At catheterization, the pressure in the left ventricle was 80/24 mm Hg and in the aorta 80/60 mm Hg; cineangiogram confirmed the presence of a large left ventricular aneurysm, which moved paradoxically. At operation, the myocardial infarct, which was aneurysmally dilated, appeared "surprisingly fresh looking" (Andrew G. Morrow, M.D.). "As much of the aneurysm as possible was resected but the patient was unable to be separated from cardiopulmonary bypass. Possibly, an in-

sufficient amount of functional muscle remained to sustain the circulation."

At necropsy (A72-149), the heart weighed 490 g (Figures 2 and 3) and the excised aneurysm another 55 g. The anterior and septal walls, adjacent to the aneurysmectomy incision, were necrotic and covered by organized and recent thrombi. The posterior left ventricular wall was hypertrophied but free of scars and of necrotic myocardium. Histologic sections of the left ventricular wall disclosed large, usually transmural, foci of necrotic myocardium containing few inflammatory cells and only small foci of loose fibrous tissue (Figure 4). The wall of the resected aneurysm consisted primarily of necrotic myocardium bordered by loose fibrous tissue and covered by fibrin thrombus. The entire coronary arterial tree was subserially sectioned. The lumen of the left anterior descending coronary artery was narrowed more than 75 per cent by old ath-

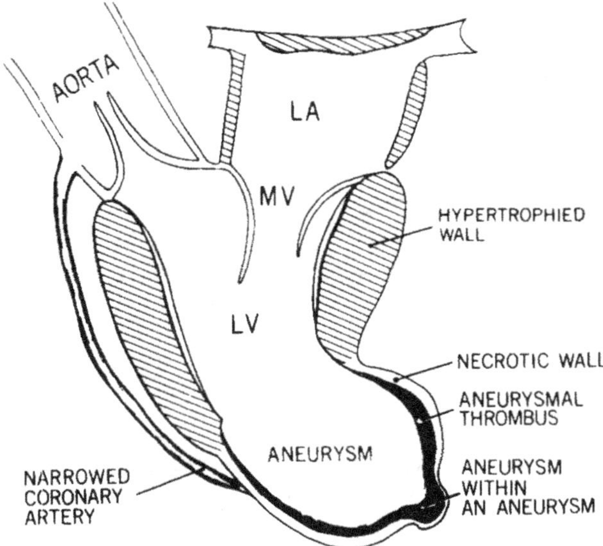

Figure 2. *Diagram summarizing gross observations in the heart.*

erosclerotic plaques, and the lumens of the left circumflex, left main and right coronary arteries were narrowed between 26 and 50 per cent by atherosclerotic plaques (Figure 5). A fibrin thrombus was present in the left anterior descending coronary artery.

COMMENTS

This patient received corticosteroids for 53 days, beginning 10 days after the onset of an acute myocardial infarction. At necropsy, the ventricular wall contained large areas of necrotic myocardium, which histologically was about 10 to 14 days old. Normally, small myocardial infarcts in human subjects heal by 36 days, and large infarcts, by 60 days [1]. Thus, the corticosteroid therapy in our patient clearly impaired healing of his acute myocardial infarct unless he had had a new recent infarct.

Although a controlled study on the effect of steroids on the healing of acute myocardial infarction in human subjects has not been performed, in dogs the administration of glucocorticoids delays this healing process [23]. Normally, an acute myocardial infarct in a dog heals by 21 to 28 days [4], which is considerably faster than in man. In dogs given small (2.5 mg/kg) doses of cortisone after the experimental induction of acute myocardial infarcts, islands of necrotic myocardium still are present at 21 days. When large (10 mg/kg) doses are administered, much larger islands of necrotic myocardium are still present at 21 days [3]. The differences in healing of acute myocardial infarcts in dogs given steroids compared to those not given steroids are also striking when examined at 12 [3] and 14 [2] days after onset. By 60 days, acute myocardial infarcts in dogs are healed irrespective of whether or not steroids have been administered, but the walls of the healed infarcts are thinner in dogs treated with steroids than in those not treated with steroids [3].

Impaired myocardial healing predisposes to the formation of ventricular aneurysm. As already noted, the walls of healed infarcts in dogs receiving corticosteroids are thinner than in dogs not receiving steroids. Of nine patients reported to have the Dressler syndrome in association with a post-infarction ventricular aneurysm [5–7], seven had received corticosteroids [5–8]. Of 10 necropsy patients [10–18] who died of the postmyocardial infarction syndrome, 7 had ventricular aneurysms; 6 of these 7 had been treated with corticosteroids from 10 to 59 days (average 37 days). In contrast, only one of the three with this syndrome in whom an aneurysm did not develop had been treated with corticosteroids, but for only 6 days [12]. The frequency of ventricular aneurysm after myocardial infarction has been reported at necropsy to be as high as 20 per cent [19,20]; this figure is much lower than that suggested by necropsy studies on patients with Dressler's syndrome who have been treated with corticosteroids.

Glucocorticoids have been recommended by some [21–28] for use during the immediate postmyocardial infarction period to control arrhythmias, particularly complete heart block [21,22], to decrease the area of infarction [23,24] and to lower mortality [25–28]. The benefit of this medication in each instance, however, is equivocal [29,30]. The dramatic response of patients with the Dressler's syndrome to corticosteroid therapy has led to the recommendation of a 6 week course of therapy for patients who do not respond to aspirin [10,31]. The postmyocardial infarction syndrome is almost always a benign self-limited disease, however, and the hazards of prolonged corticosteroid treatment may outweigh its usefulness. In our patient, the administration of corticosteroids in large doses was started early after the onset of infarction and continued for a long period (8 weeks). This therapy clearly prevented healing of the infarct and allowed the formation of an aneurysm. Thus, corticosteroids should be used with extreme caution in the early postmyocardial infarction period, and they should not be used at all, except in rare circumstances, in patients with self-limited illnesses, such as Dressler's syndrome.

ACKNOWLEDGMENT

We thank Ms. Sandra J. Lewis, Filippina Giacometti and Linda S. Docks for preparing the histologic sections and Mr. Kenzie L. Edwards for the gross photographs.

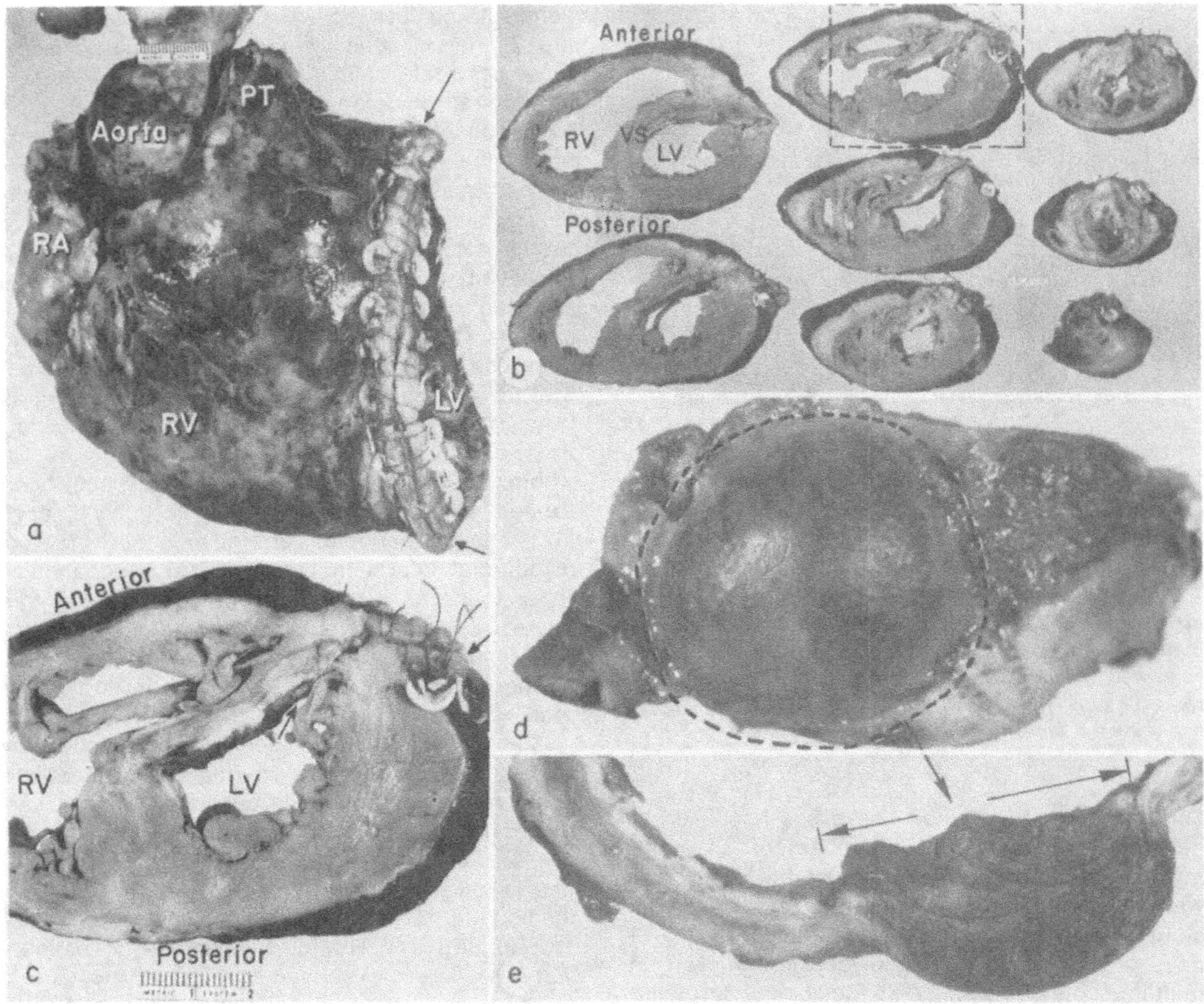

Figure 3. *The heart. **a,** exterior view after aneurysmectomy. The site of resection of the aneurysm is designated by the arrows. LV = left ventricle; PT = pulmonary trunk; RA = right atrium; RV = right ventricle. **b,** transverse sections through the ventricles showing that the anteroseptal infarct extends from base to apex. VS = ventricular septum. **c,** closer view of one of the slices shown in brackets in **b.** The arrows designate the aneurysmectomy incision. The posterior and lateral walls are hypertrophied. **d,** the surface of the excised aneurysm. **e,** longitudinal section through the excised aneurysm showing a small aneurysm (arrows) within the larger aneurysm. The small aneurysm is filled with thrombus. The aneurysmal wall is thin.*

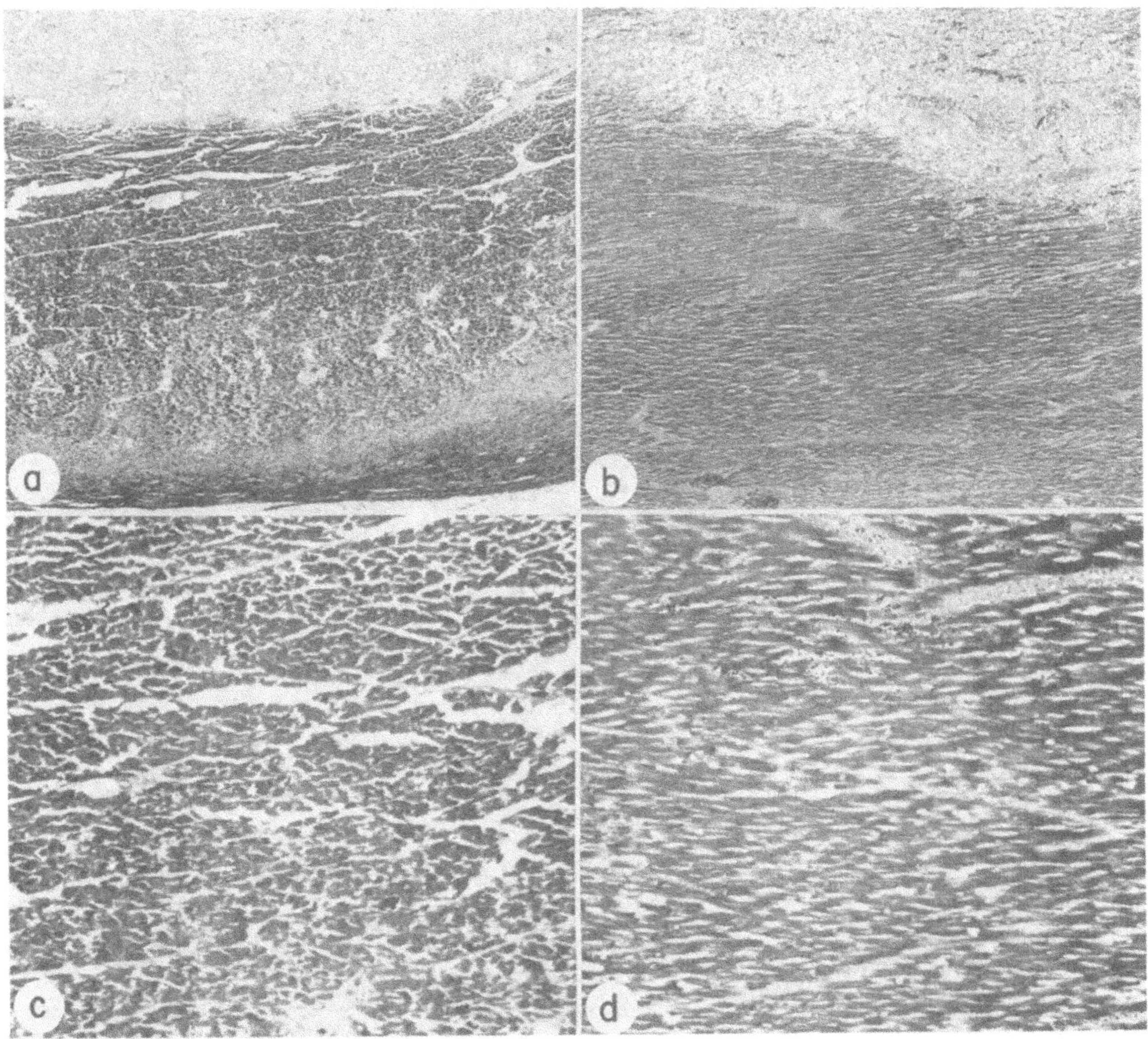

Figure 4. Histologic sections of infarcted left ventricular myocardium from the patient described (a and c) compared to infarcted myocardium in a patient (SH No. A4489) who died 10 days after onset of myocardial infarction (b and d). **a,** large islands of necrotic muscle fibers are surrounded by loose connective tissue. The histologic changes are consistent with a 10 to 14 day infarction and are similar to those in the patient who died 10 days after onset of infarction **(b).** At 10 days large areas of necrotic fibers are present, surrounded by loose connective tissue at the periphery of the infarct. Higher power magnification of the 10 day old infarct **(d)** showed changes similar to those noted in our patient at 63 days **(c).** Hematoxylin and eosin stains; original magnification × 31 (a and b), × 100 (c and d), reduced by 5 per cent.

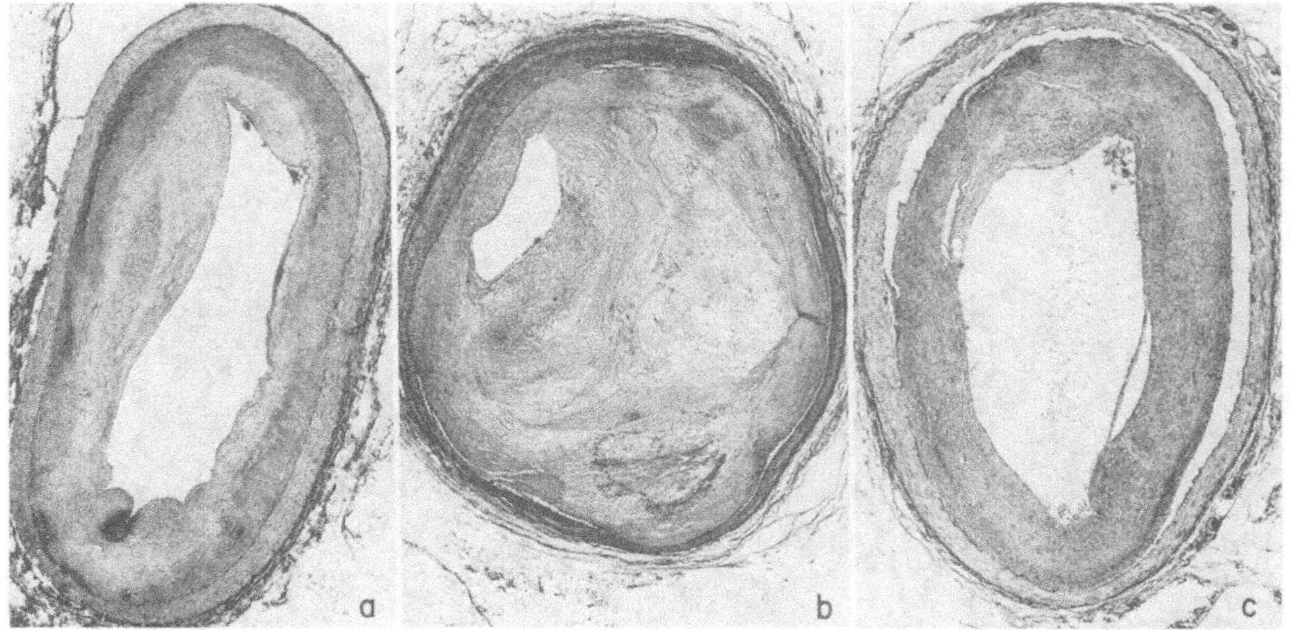

Figure 5. Coronary arteries at sites of maximal narrowing in our patient: **a,** right, **b,** left anterior descending and **c,** left circumflex arteries. Only the left anterior descending coronary artery is severely narrowed. Movat stains; original magnification × 36 (a), × 22 (b) and × 23 (c), reduced by 25 per cent.

REFERENCES

1. Mallory GK, White PD, Salcedo-Salgar J: The speed of healing of myocardial infarction. A study of the pathologic anatomy in seventy-two cases. Am Heart J 18: 647, 1939.
2. Opdyke DF, Lambert A, Stoerk HC, et al.: Failure to reduce the size of experimentally produced myocardial infarcts by cortisone treatment. Circulation 8: 544, 1953.
3. Hepper NGG: The effect of cortisone on healing of experimentally produced myocardial infarction in dogs. Thesis, Mayo Graduate School of Medicine, University of Minnesota, Rochester, 1954.
4. Karsner HT, Dwyer JE Jr: IV. Experimental bland infarction of the myocardium, myocardial regeneration and cicatrization. J Med Res 34: 21, 1916.
5. Bouvrain Y, Fortin P, Perrotin M, et al.: La pleuro-péricardite consécutive à l'infarctus du myocarde. Arch Mal Coeur 53: 134, 1960.
6. Dulac JF, Doury P, Ben-Zenow A: Manifestations péricardiques et infartus du myocarde. A propos de 2 observations. Soc Méd Milit Franc 56: 44, 1962.
7. Berman DA, Grismer JT: Postmyocardial infarction syndrome. Followed by left ventricular aneurysm with papillary muscle dysfunction. Am J Cardiol 25: 349, 1970
8. Tchetchik M, Modai D, Shapiro M: The postmyocardial infarction syndrome and myocardial aneurysm. Harefuah 80: 62, 1971.
9. Curry CL: The relationship between the post-myocardial-infarction syndrome and post-infarction ventricular aneurysm. J Natl Med Assoc 64: 480, 1972.
10. Dressler W: A post-myocardial-infarction syndrome. Preliminary report of a complication resembling idiopathic, recurrent, benign pericarditis. JAMA 160: 1379, 1956.
11. Dressler W: The post-myocardial-infarction syndrome. A report of forty-four cases. Arch Intern Med 103: 28, 1959.
12. Jaffe HL: Pericarditis and pleuritis in acute myocardial infarction. J Mt Sinai Hosp 27: 40, 1960.
13. Luomanmaki K, Helin M, Halonen PI: Postmyocardial infarction syndrome. A review with two case reports. Duodecim 80: 67, 1964.
14. Del Piano E, Lisi B, Balducci R, et al: Considerazioni su alcuni casi di sindrome di Dressler. Policlinico (sez med) 72: 205, 1965.
15. Mertens H, Hüpper G: Herzinfarkt-Spätsyndrom. Bericht über zqei Fälle. Med Klin 61: 838, 1966.
16. Brockel P, Doyran E: Post-myocardial infarction syndrome as a fatal complication. Dtsch Med Wochenschr 91: 1040, 1966.
17. Ravnskov U: Aneurysm of the heart and post-myocardial infarction syndrome. Acta Med Scand 183: 393, 1968.
18. Burchacki J: Myocardial infarction complicated by rupture of an aneurysm of the interventricular septum, Dressler's syndrome and cardiac rupture. Wiad Lek 21: 1317, 1968.
19. Schlichter J, Hellerstein HK, Katz LN: Aneurysm of the heart: A correlative study of one hundred and two proved cases. Medicine 23: 43, 1954.
20. Dubnow MH, Burchell HB, Titus JL: Postinfarction ventricular aneurysm. A clinicomorphologic and electrocardiographic study of 80 cases. Am Heart J 70: 753, 1965.
21. Prinzmetal M, Kennamer R: Emergency treatment of cardiac arrhythmias. JAMA 154: 1049, 1954.
22. Dall JLC, Buchanan J: Steroid therapy in heart-block following myocardial infarction. Lancet 2: 8, 1962.

23. Johnson AS, Scheinberg SR, Gerisch RA, et al.: Effect of cortisone on the size of experimentally produced myocardial infarction. Circulation 7: 224, 1953.
24. Libby P, Maroko PR, Bloor CM, et al.: Reduction of experimental myocardial infarct size by corticosteroid administration. J Clin Invest 52: 599, 1973.
25. Gerisch RA, Compeau L: Treatment of acute myocardial infarction in man with cortisone. Am J Cardiol 1: 535, 1958.
26. Dall JLC, Peel AAF: A trial of hydrocortisone in acute myocardial infarction. Lancet 2: 1097, 1963.
27. Baroody NB, Baroody WG: Adrenocorticosteroids in acute myocardial infarction. Am J Med Sci 250: 402, 1965.
28. Barzilai D, Plavnick J, Hazani A, et al.: Use of hydrocortisone in the treatment of acute myocardial infarction. Summary of a clinical trial in 446 patients. Chest 61: 488, 1972.
29. Semple T, Dall JLC: Steroids in myocardial infarction. Am Heart J 70: 716, 1965.
30. Trial Conducted by the Scientific Subcommittee of the Scottish Society of Physicians. Hydrocortisone in severe myocardial infection. Lancet 2: 785, 1964.
31. Dressler W: Management of pericarditis secondary to myocardial infarction. Progr Cardiovasc Dis 3: 134, 1960.

Coronary Thrombosis in Myocardial Infarction

Report of a Workshop on the Role of Coronary Thrombosis in the Pathogenesis of Acute Myocardial Infarction*

A. BLEAKLEY CHANDLER, MD
Augusta, Georgia

IRVING CHAPMAN, MD
Elmhurst, New York

LEIF R. ERHARDT, MD
Stockholm, Sweden

WILLIAM C. ROBERTS, MD, FACC
Bethesda, Maryland

COLIN J. SCHWARTZ, MD
Hamilton, Ontario, Canada

D. SINAPIUS, MD
Göttingen, West Germany

DAVID M. SPAIN, MD, FACC
Brooklyn, New York

SOL SHERRY, MD, FACC
Philadelphia, Pennsylvania

PAUL M. NESS, MD
Bethesda, Maryland

TOBY L. SIMON, MD
Bethesda, Maryland

*This workshop was held May 21, 1973, at the National Heart and Lung Institute, National Institutes of Health, Bethesda, Md. under the joint sponsorship of the National Heart and Lung Institute Thrombosis Advisory Committee and the American Heart Association Council on Thrombosis. Manuscript accepted June 10, 1974.

Address for reprints: Toby L. Simon, MD, Division of Blood Diseases and Resources, National Heart and Lung Institute, National Institutes of Health, Bethesda, Md., 20014.

In recent years the widely held concept that coronary thrombi cause myocardial infarcts has been seriously questioned. On the basis of pathologic studies, several reports have suggested that coronary thrombi do not cause infarcts but instead are the result of infarction. Should these findings become generally substantiated, the antithrombotic approach to the prevention and therapy of ischemic heart disease must be revised. This workshop was organized to examine more closely this issue and to sort out reasons for such divergent views of the role of thrombosis in the pathogenesis of myocardial infarction.

For many years, "coronary occlusion" or "coronary thrombosis" was a recognized clinicopathologic entity, and myocardial infarction was considered one of the sequelae. But over a period of time the view of this aspect of ischemic heart disease has changed. The entity once known as coronary thrombosis has gradually come to be known as "myocardial infarction." This change in point of view has evolved for a number of reasons.

The evolution of a new perspective on myocardial infarction was furthered by the work of Blumgart et al.,[1-3] who clarified many of the complex relations between coronary thrombi and collateral vessels. They found that thrombotic occlusion could occur without infarction when the collateral circulation appeared adequate, whereas infarcts that did develop usually could be attributed to an occlusive thrombus at a critical location in the coronary arterial tree. At times clinical manifestations were not evident, even in the presence of infarction. These investigators clearly established that thrombotic occlusion can occur with or without infarction, and in either case the event may be clinically silent.

At about the same time Friedberg and Horn[4] published their pivotal work. In contrast to large thrombus-associated myocardial infarcts, small patchy subendocardial infarcts were identified in the absence of coronary occlusion. It was suggested that these subendocardial infarcts developed on the basis of acute relative insufficiency of coronary blood flow. Not only could coronary thrombi occur without infarction; it was now evident that infarcts could occur without thrombosis.

At this stage came a turning point. On the basis of their findings, Friedberg and Horn[4] concluded that the clinical diagnosis of coronary thrombosis was no longer tenable, and that it would be more accurate to regard these cases as instances of myocardial infarction. Miller et al.[5] then drew a sharp distinction between predominantly subendocardial infarcts that were rarely associated with coronary thrombi and predominantly transmural infarcts that were frequently associated with thrombi.

However, as physicians began to think of all types of myocardial infarction as one entity, the role of thrombosis seemed to become less and less well defined. At one extreme, the entire concept of coronary

TABLE I

Coronary Thrombosis in Regional Transmural Infarction

Summary Report	Infarcted Hearts with Coronary Thrombi	Age Limit of In- farcts (wk)	Spatial Relations	Underlying Arterial Lesions	Temporal Relations	Conclusions
Chapman	257/282 (91%)	4*	Occlusion of extramural artery usually subtends infarct and is separated from it by uninvolved segment of artery	Thrombus forms on eroded intimal surface	Not reported	*Thrombus precedes and causes infarct*
Erhardt	7/7†	2‡	Infarcts occur in region supported by occluding artery	Thrombi frequently associated with atherosclerotic stenosis and ulceration	Thrombi incorporate ^{125}I-fibrinogen after onset of clinical manifestations of infarction	*Coronary thrombus may be secondary event*
Roberts	40/74 (54%)	6‡§	Site of myocardial necrosis corresponds properly with artery containing thrombus	All thrombi over old stenosing atherosclerotic plaques	Not reported	*Coronary thrombus follows rather than precipitates acute myocardial infarction*
Schwartz	18/21 (86%)	2*	Thrombi often in two arterial segments. Most thrombi proximal and anatomically subtend infarct	Infarcts related to degree of arterial stenosis	Not reported	*Anatomic dependence of infarcts on coronary thrombi indicates causal relation between thrombi and infarcts*
Sinapius	164/170 (96.5%)	4‡	Constant local relation between thrombosed artery and supported area infarcted	Most thrombi occur over tears in atheromata	Many thrombi have multiple layers of episodic growth. Oldest portion develops before or with onset of symptoms	*Acute infarction caused by complete thrombotic occlusion*
Spain	45/50 (90%)	2‡	Infarcts associated with regional coronary arterial thrombi	Thrombi form at site of well established atherosclerosis	Both infarcts and thrombi have multiple and variable ages that can lead to misinterpretation of temporal relations	*Infarcts are preceded by recent and regional coronary thrombi*

* Age estimated by histologic criteria.
† Cases selected only for study of radioactive thrombi.
‡ Age estimated from time of onset of clinical manifestations of infarction.
§ Only 6 cases had infarcts from 3 to 6 weeks old.

thrombi causing infarcts has been challenged. Branwood and Montgomery[6] tentatively concluded from their study that coronary thrombi are younger than the corresponding infarcts and that thrombosis, rather than the cause, is in fact the final event in infarction. Similar conclusions have been reached by others.[7–11] At the other extreme, some investigators[12–14] have continued strongly to maintain the essential etiologic role of thrombosis in the pathogenesis of acute myocardial infarction.

As reports on this controversial issue continued to appear, a workshop was organized to bring together some of the workers who hold these divergent views, in the hope that an open discussion of their own observations and conclusions would shed some light on the basis of the controversy and give direction for future work.

The Workshop

The participants were in full agreement that the frequency of coronary thrombosis is low in cases of multifocal subendocardial infarcts occurring in the presence of advanced coronary sclerosis or ostial stenosis. There is substantial evidence that lesions of this sort can result from a relative lack of blood supply to this dependent part of the myocardium, either from sudden increased work of the heart or decreased perfusion of the heart from some extrinsic cause. Thrombosis of major arteries as well as thrombotic obstruction of myocardial arteries also may be found in relation to small infarcts. It was recognized that one must search for thrombi or emboli in the small vessels as well as in the epicardial arteries before drawing firm conclusions about the frequency of thrombosis in association with these lesions.

When infarcts that extend beyond the subendocardium were considered, it was evident that coronary thrombosis was frequent, occurring in 86 to 96 percent of the cases in most series, and found in 54 percent in one series (Table I). It is about this type of large, often transmural, infarct that so much controversy has arisen concerning the etiologic role of thrombosis. Granted that thrombosis is commonly associated with these infarcts, the question raised is whether the thrombus is primary and causative, or simply secondary in origin to the infarct itself. Therefore, in preparing summary reports for this paper after the workshop, each investigator placed emphasis on the significance of coronary thrombosis in the pathogenesis of transmural infarction.

Transmural Infarcts

To establish a common basis for evaluation of data, a working definition that encompasses the type of infarcts under consideration by each investigator was sought. The infarcts described in each report generally fall into the group of "transmural" infarcts. Miller et al.,[5] who first introduced the term to convey a sharp contrast with "subendocardial," restricted its use to infarcts that involve at some point the entire thickness of the myocardium.[15] A concept of transmural has been adopted that is not so restrictive, yet is realistic and meaningful in relation to the data in each report. A unifocal and regional infarct that extends through one half or more of the septal or free ventricular wall is considered transmural. This modified concept, although broad, serves to exclude subendocardial infarcts. Although Chapman and Schwartz classify infarcts by size alone and not extent through the wall, their cases clearly belong to this grouping of regional transmural lesions. Thus, all cases in these series can be characterized by this working definition as regional transmural infarcts.

The age of the lesions considered to be acute varies considerably among the series (Table I). Acute infarcts in some series are limited to those less than 2 weeks old; other series include infarcts of 4 to 6 weeks' duration. Roberts notes continued infarction in his cases of 3 to 6 weeks' duration. In these reports, therefore, a wide age range must be taken into account when considering an infarct acute.

Further analysis of Table I reveals that regional transmural infarcts are spatially related to the coronary thrombi in that the occlusions uniformly occur in arteries supplying the infarcted myocardium. The thrombi develop at the site of severe atherosclerotic narrowing, often in association with an acute lesion of an underlying plaque. When temporal relations between the recent thrombi and acute infarcts are considered, unanimity of opinion is lacking. Sinapius and Spain discuss some of the problems encountered in assessing the age of lesions by histologic means alone, and Erhardt introduces a new approach to the dating of thrombi in coronary arteries. These findings and the conclusions concerning the role of coronary thrombosis in transmural myocardial infarction are presented in more detail in the individual reports that follow.

Summary Reports

Chapman

In 1968, I reported on a prospective autopsy study of 292 cases of acute myocardial infarction.[12] Ten of the cases had multiple infarcts of the heart and 282 had a single infarct. A recent coronary artery occlusion by thrombus was associated with 257 (91 percent) of the cases with a single infarct. In another two cases, instead of a thrombus, the occluding mass was a bolus of atheromatous debris extruded from an ulcerated atherosclerotic plaque. Since then I have examined an additional 121 cases of acute myocardial infarction and found a coronary thrombotic occlusion present in 110 (91 percent) (unpublished data). In all but two instances, the occlusion was in an extramural branch of a coronary artery that subtended the infarct. The statistically close association of thrombotic arterial occlusion and acute myocardial infarction and their consistent topographic relation indicate a causal relation.

To determine why my observations were similar to those of some authors and disturbingly different from those of others, I reviewed and analyzed the available reports on the relation of coronary artery occlusion and acute myocardial infarction and concluded that the differences in observations were due to differences in definition and method of examination.[12,16]

I defined an acute myocardial infarction as a well defined zone of necrosis at least 2.5 cm in greatest dimension.[12] The necrosis was usually uniform and the estimated histologic age was less than 1 month. Although this definition is arbitrary, it describes the findings at autopsy of patients with characteristic signs and symptoms of acute myocardial infarction. Small zones of myocardial necrosis, practically always multifocal and subendocardial in distribution, were eliminated from consideration. The infarcts, for the most part, fell into the group of infarcts considered in this workshop as transmural.

Pathogenesis of the coronary thrombus: In a study that demonstrated that coronary thrombi were formed on an eroded intimal surface, I showed that the force that disrupted the intima proceeded from within the vascular wall and was directed toward the lumen.[16,17] I also pointed out that the distal border of a coronary arterial thrombus is separated by 1 to 2 cm of uninvolved artery from the closest margin of an anterior or lateral wall infarct and by 1 to 5 cm from posterior and diaphragmatic wall infarcts.[12] It was apparent from the consistency of these findings that they had pathogenetic significance in the formation of the thrombus and acute myocardial infarction, and the only conclusion these findings would permit was that the coronary thrombus preceded and caused the infarction.

The thrombus precedes and causes the infarct: If the acute myocardial infarction preceded the thrombus, one would have to make the improbable assumption that the infarct consistently caused a force to be generated within the arterial wall, with a vector toward the lumen, which disrupted the intima beneath the thrombus. To accept such an assumption is especially difficult since intimal erosions with and without superimposed thrombi are often seen without associated infarcts. Furthermore, if the acute myocardial infarction caused the thrombus, some of the occlusions would be distributed haphazardly around the periphery and within the confines of the infarct; hence, the consistent presence of the occlusion in a subtending branch of the coronary artery separated from the closest margin of the infarct by a segment of uninvolved artery supports the opinion that the thrombus precedes and causes the infarct.

Erhardt

Study of coronary thrombi by [125]iodine-labeled fibrinogen: In an attempt to clarify the controversial time-relation between the coronary thrombus and necrosis in acute transmural infarction, the incorporation of [125]iodine-labeled fibrinogen into coronary thrombi was studied.[9] Patients admitted to a coro-

nary care unit for suspected acute myocardial infarction were given 100 μc of [125]iodine-labeled fibrinogen. In seven patients who subsequently died of acute myocardial infarction, the coronary thrombus was isolated at autopsy and cut into pieces that were dissolved in a tissue solubilizer. The presence of radioactivity was then measured in a scintillation counter. In five patients the fibrinogen was given within 15 hours from the onset of symptoms. In one patient it was given almost 3 days before clinical evidence of the infarction, and in another not until 47 hours after the onset of symptoms. In all patients except the latter, the entire thrombus was radioactive. In this latter patient only the end parts of the thrombus contained radioactivity, whereas the major central portion was nonradioactive. In five of the seven patients the activity was lowest in the most distal part of the thrombus. Postmortem clots studied as controls contained only trace amounts of radioactivity.

All patients except one had electrocardiographic signs of transmural infarction before the injection of fibrinogen. The subsequent enzyme analysis supported the view that the onset of symptoms corresponded to the onset of myocardial necrosis. All patients died within 2 weeks of the onset of symptoms. At autopsy all patients except one had gross signs of transmural infarction, that is, an infarction extending at any point throughout the ventricular wall from the subendocardium to the epicardium. In the patient without gross signs of fresh myocardial infarction, the subsequent microscopic examination revealed transmural necrosis. The infarcts occurred in the region supported by the occluded coronary artery. Six of the seven patients had severe atherosclerotic stenosis at the site of thrombosis and three of those six patients also had an ulcerated plaque at this site.

The coronary thrombus in myocardial infarction is a secondary event: The results of this study favor the notion that the coronary thrombus in acute transmural infarction is a secondary event. However, the technique used cannot exclude the presence of a small nonradioactive portion. Such a small "primary" thrombus or platelet aggregate, even if not occlusive, might still be the start of the process leading to acute necrosis of the myocardium.

The reduced radioactivity toward the distal end of the thrombus in five of the patients can theoretically be explained in several ways. There might be a different amount of fibrinogen in the distal part of the thrombus when less radioactive fibrinogen was available for incorporation, and this explanation seems most attractive. That a distal growth takes place is best shown by the patient given the fibrinogen 47 hours after the onset of symptoms. Furthermore, as suggested by findings in this patient, thrombus formation might still occur as late as 47 hours from the onset of symptoms. However, this patient had the longest thrombus, 70 mm, and thrombi in the coronary arteries are usually shorter. Consequently, most thrombi might form more rapidly.

It is generally agreed that patients with fatal transmural acute myocardial infarction have extensive and severe coronary atherosclerosis. The reported frequency of superimposed thrombi in these vessels, however, has varied considerably. This presentation summarizes observations on the coronary arteries in 74 patients with fatal transmural acute myocardial infarction.[10]

The 74 patients ranged in age from 26 to 90 years (average 60); 52 (70 percent) were men and 22 (30 percent) women. Systemic hypertension had been known to be present in 33 (45 percent), and 26 (35 percent) were known to have had diabetes of adult onset. None of the latter patients were treated by intramuscularly administered insulin. The maximal interval between onset of symptoms of acute myocardial infarction and death was 45 days. Six patients survived more than 21 days, and each had clinical evidence of continuing myocardial infarction.

Pathologic findings: At necropsy, the major coronary arteries (left main, left anterior descending, left circumflex and right) were excised intact from the hearts. Each artery was put in a separate container of formalin, fixed and decalcified. After decalcification, the coronary arteries were sectioned at 0.5 cm intervals, and all segments were processed for histologic study. At least two histologic sections were examined from each 0.5 cm segment. The hearts were weighed. The ventricles were sectioned transversely and foci of necrosis or fibrosis were recorded. Necrosis was considered transmural if it extended more than 50 percent through the free wall of the left ventricle or ventricular septum beginning at the endocardium. Fortunately, nearly all areas of necrosis involved more than 75 percent of the myocardial wall (from endocardium to epicardium), and usually 100 percent was involved. At least four sections of left ventricular wall also were examined histologically in each patient.

Of 222 major coronary arteries in the 74 patients, the lumen in 168 (76 percent) was narrowed more than 75 percent by old atherosclerotic plaques. An average of 2.3 per patient of the three major arteries (left anterior descending, left circumflex and right coronary) were narrowed more than 75 percent by old atherosclerotic plaques. Thus, in 58 (78 percent) of the patients more than two major coronary arteries were narrowed to this degree by old atherosclerotic plaques. Thrombi were observed in a major coronary artery in 40 (54 percent) of the 74 patients. Hemorrhages into atherosclerotic plaques were found in 20 (27 percent). The heart in 56 (76 percent) weighed more than 400 g.

The thrombi in each of the 40 patients were superimposed on old atherosclerotic plaques. The lumens of the coronary arteries at the site of distal attachment of the thrombus or just distal to the antemortem clots were more than 75 percent narrowed by old atherosclerotic plaques in 38 of the 40 patients with thrombi. Only one coronary thrombus was observed in 37 of the 40 patients. The site of myocardial necrosis in each corresponded properly with the artery containing the thrombus. All patients with antemortem clots in the left anterior descending vessel, for example, had anterior wall infarcts. This vessel was the artery most frequently containing a thrombus. Of the coronary arteries containing thrombi, the residual lumen, that is, the lumen not already obliterated by old atherosclerotic plaques, was totally obliterated in 80 percent, and the thrombi were nonocclusive or mural in the other 20 percent. There were no sex differences among patients with or without coronary arterial thrombi. Anticoagulant agents were given during the period of acute myocardial infarction in 27 patients, and at necropsy 8 of them had a thrombus in a major coronary artery; 3 of them had a hemorrhage into an old atherosclerotic plaque. None of the intramural coronary arteries showed significant luminal narrowing.

The coronary thrombus is consequence rather than cause of acute myocardial infarction: The patients with coronary thrombi usually were those who had had cardiogenic shock. Coronary thrombi were infrequent in patients who died suddenly and in those without evidence of pump failure. Because the arteries were already severely narrowed, the functional significance of the thrombi is uncertain. Furthermore, as previously reported,[10] it was found that patients who died suddenly, with or without previous evidence of ischemic heart disease, and patients with infarcts limited to the subendocardium rarely had coronary thrombi. The infrequency of thrombi in patients who died suddenly, with or without infarction, and their presence for the most part only in patients with transmural infarction strongly suggest that coronary thrombi are consequences rather than causes of acute myocardial infarction.

Schwartz

There would appear to be two distinct populations of myocardial lesions characterized by necrosis or replacement fibrosis, or both—namely, large and small lesions.[18] These have been examined in some detail.[19,20] Large lesions were found to extend over a distance of 4 to 8 cm along the long axis of the heart, with a volume in excess of 8 cc. Most small lesions were found to show no clear relation with the degree of coronary artery stenosis or occlusion, but were more frequent in older patients. Large lesions, on the other hand, which can be considered examples of transmural myocardial infarction, were clearly related both to the degree of coronary artery stenosis, and the presence of coronary artery occlusion.[18–20] It is therefore of more than academic interest to define the size of myocardial lesions in determining the relation of coronary thrombosis to myocardial infarction.

Factors determining frequency of occlusive coronary thrombi: A number of factors are clearly related to the frequency with which one finds occlusive coronary arterial thrombi in the hearts of patients with myocardial infarction.[21,22] These include the definitive histopathologic presence of infarction, infarct size and location, and the histologic age of the infarct. Other factors probably contributing to the current discrepant published results include sample bias, the care and techniques employed at necropsy and the facile inclusion of all cases of sudden cardiac death in the category acute myocardial infarction.[21,22]

Mitchell and Schwartz[18] noted that the frequency of occlusion was significantly less in patients with infarcts histologically more than 4 months of age (66.7 percent) than in patients with more recent infarction (in excess of 90 percent). Moreover, the nature of occlusions found was clearly dependent on infarct age, with a significant decline in the frequency of recent thrombi, and a relatively proportionate increase in the percent frequency of occlusion due to recanalizing thrombi and atheromatous plaques, with increasing infarct age.

The occlusion status of patients with both a classic history of myocardial infarction and electrocardiographic evidence of transmural infarction (the presence of pathologic Q waves) was analyzed.[18] It is clear that in such selected patients the data on frequency and nature of occlusion are similar to findings in a larger series of patients with unequivocal infarction but without electrocardiographic evidence of transmural infarction. Perhaps, therefore, the presence of transmural infarction is merely a reflection of the extent of ischemic necrosis rather than evidence for a different pathogenesis. However, in making this comment one should be aware of the discrepancies that relate to some cases of "infarction," often circumferential and located principally in the subendocardial region, that appear to have a lesser frequency of occlusion.

There is a causal rather than secondary relation between thrombosis and infarction: Myocardial infarction, defined in this presentation with respect to lesions of large size and recent histologic age, is associated with a high, although not universal, frequency of coronary thrombosis. We found recent coronary thrombi in 18 of 21 hearts (86 percent) with single large recent infarcts less than 2 weeks of age histologically.[20] Furthermore, in each case an average of two arterial segments were occluded. In addition, and possibly of critical importance, is the observation that most thrombi occur proximally in the arteries anatomically subtending the areas of infarction. This anatomic dependence is consistent with a causal rather than a secondary relation between thrombosis and myocardial infarction. The occasional case of recent transmural infarction in which no thrombus is found may result from a low cardiac output producing an inadequate regional perfusion in the presence of severe coronary artery stenosis.

Sinapius

Pathologic observations: In a series of 206 autopsy cases of acute myocardial infarction having a duration within 4 weeks of clinical onset, I found 184 occluding or severely narrowing thrombi of the supporting extramural coronary arterial branches.[14] There were 164 thrombi in 170 transmural infarctions (96.5 percent) and 20 thrombi in 36 smaller infarctions (55.5 percent). Transmural infarcts extended through almost the entire thickness of the ventricular wall infarcted and measured at least 4 cm in diameter. There was no evidence that the incidence of thrombosis increased with the duration of survival of the patient after the onset of symptoms. Early infarcts with a patient survival time of 6 to 24 hours were as frequent in the group with coronary arterial thrombosis (24 percent) as in the group without thrombosis (25 percent). Moreover, evidence of pump failure syndrome or congestive heart failure was a little more frequent in cases without thrombosis than in cases with thrombosis.

A study of the size and appositional growth of 91 of the thrombi demonstrated that the average length of thrombi was 16.6 mm in the left anterior descending branch and 24.3 mm in the right coronary artery.[23] Distal apposition was noted in 50 percent and proximal apposition in 22 percent of the thrombi. Proximal apposition was found almost exclusively in the right coronary artery. In two thirds of the thrombi the proximal end was found within the first 3 cm of the main branch.

The oldest portions of 67 of the coronary arterial thrombi, which were cut in transverse sections and studied by serial sections, occurred according to histologic estimation either before or with the onset of clinical symptoms, in no case definitely later. In 33 of these 67 thrombi (49.3 percent) a multilayered structure suggested a recurrent or protracted course. In seven of the cases the thrombi according to histologic estimation must have developed before the onset of clinical symptoms. Most of the occluding coronary arterial thrombi occurred over tears in atheromata.

Temporal and causal relation between thrombus and infarction: The constant local relation between the site of coronary arterial thrombosis and the supported and infarcted area suggests a temporal and causal relation between coronary thrombosis and myocardial infarction. Thrombosis often occurs in two to three episodes beginning with a flat platelet thrombus and completed by further mural thrombi until a terminal thrombus occludes the rest of the lumen. Clinical experience suggests that mural thrombosis without necrosis may produce prodromal symptoms, such as severe attacks of angina pectoris or ischemic signs in the electrocardiogram, even before the real infarction. The acute infarction itself is caused only by the subsequent complete occlusion.

Spain

For several decades it has been generally undisputed that in persons with various degrees of stenotic coronary atherosclerosis, the development of coronary arterial thrombi is the major cause of myocardial infarction. Confusion concerning the role of the thrombus in myocardial infarction occurred in recent years for several reasons. The failure to recognize the fact that coronary thrombi are primarily and almost invariably associated with the transmural (regional, unifocal) infarct involving all or more than half the thickness of the ventricular wall, and only occasionally associated with the subendocardial (nonregional, multifocal) infarct, led to the indiscriminate lumping together of all infarcts and obscured the basic and close statistical relation between coronary thrombi and the transmural infarct.[24]

Myocardial ischemia vs. myocardial infarction: There was also a misinterpretation of the fact that episodes of acute myocardial ischemia terminating in sudden and unexpected death are generally not caused by recent coronary thrombi. This error is probably due to the interchangeable and indiscriminate use of the terms myocardial ischemia and myocardial infarction. Ischemia certainly does not mean infarction. It is but an early step on the road to infarction and need not proceed to the point of cell death. Ischemia is often reversible. An infarct is not reversible. An acute thrombus may not necessarily be the prime initiating event in the precipitation of many ischemic episodes terminating in sudden death. This fact, however, by no means negates the classic view that with few exceptions transmural myocardial infarcts are preceded by the recent formation of thrombi at the site of well established coronary atherosclerosis. The consistent regional anatomic relation between recent coronary thrombi and infarcts is strong evidence of the causative role of thrombosis in infarction.

Frequency of coronary thrombosis in transmural infarction: Recent studies (personal and otherwise) of consecutive autopsies in cases of death due to myocardial infarction derived solely from modern coronary care units and consisting entirely of fatal cases of pump failure and cardiogenic shock reveal that approximately 90 percent of all transmural infarcts are preceded by regional coronary arterial thrombi. We found that 45 of 50 recent transmural infarcts having a clinical age of no more than 2 weeks were associated with recent coronary thrombi (unpublished data). In most previous autopsy studies of patients with myocardial infarction the deaths due to arrhythmia and pump failure have been classified together, and the frequency of coronary thrombi in this overall group ranged from 45 to 70 percent. The elimination of arrhythmia as a cause of death in myocardial infarction by modern therapeutic technique has also eliminated the cases coming to autopsy showing only subendocardial necrosis and no transmural infarction.

Factors leading to misinterpretation of relation of thrombus and infarct: The failure to recognize that the process of ischemia and infarction may be a continuum beginning with ischemia, at first reversible, then in some instances only developing subendocardial necrosis, which may sooner or later be followed by the onset of a thrombus, which in turn produces a transmural infarct, may lead to a misinterpretation of the relative ages of the thrombus and the infarct as determined by histologic examination. The earlier necrotic foci may reveal various degrees of repair. With the appearance of a thrombus, these preexisting areas of necrosis may become incorporated into the new and more extensive transmural infarct. This combination of events can create the mistaken impression that the total area of myocardial necrosis antedated the development of the thrombus.

Infarcts vary in their appearance and state of progression in different areas. Myocardial tissue supplied by the occluded vessel does not consist of homogeneous areas of necrosis. Rather, surrounding a region of central necrosis are patchy areas of abnormal to viable myocardium. These partially altered ischemic areas may enlarge for approximately 18 hours after the initial occlusion. After this period the central area of necrosis expands more rapidly. Therefore, the timing and location of histologic sectioning can profoundly influence the findings and hence the conclusions concerning infarct age. Likewise, thrombi may enlarge after their initial development, and the latest additions may appear younger than the preexisting infarct. Sections taken from such a thrombus may lead to the erroneous conclusion that the entire thrombus developed after the infarct.

The selection and the source of the cases may also influence the frequency of coronary arterial thrombi in autopsy studies on myocardial infarct deaths. In my experience extending over more than 30 years at four major hospitals and covering all categories of hospital populations (city, county, voluntary community and university medical center), the association of coronary thrombi with myocardial infarcts of all types, as seen in consecutive autopsies, has ranged from 45 to 70 percent. In recent years, when the selection of cases no longer included the subendocardial infarcts associated with electrically caused deaths, the frequency of thrombi in the remaining cases (consisting entirely of those with transmural infarcts) was 90 percent.

Discussion

These reports, which summarize the observations and conclusions of each investigator, bring into sharp relief the major points of agreement and disagreement. A recurring question at the workshop was whether there was uniformity in the pathologic criteria used for transmural infarction. It was thought essential to answer this question in order properly to assess the role of thrombosis in myocardial infarction. The working definition of regional transmural infarction adopted in this paper includes each worker's material. Moreover, and equally important, there can be little doubt that the small patchy subendocardial infarcts known to be infrequently associated with coronary thrombi are excluded.

Frequency of Coronary Thrombosis

In these reports a high frequency of coronary

thrombosis is found in acute transmural infarction. The frequency of thrombosis in Roberts' cases, although high, is somewhat lower than that of the other reports. No satisfactory explanation for this disparity emerged during the workshop. The possibility of differences in methodology was thought unlikely. Consideration of other variables such as certain factors relative to the population under study also was unrewarding. For example, in Roberts' cases many of the hearts were hypertrophied, and the question was raised whether this variable could influence the frequency of thrombosis or relative size of the infarcts. This too seems an unlikely basis for the disparity since hypertrophy is a common finding in all series. Spain specifically stated that he finds no difference in frequency of thrombosis in cases with and without hypertension.

Age of the acute lesions: One factor, not heretofore considered in any detail, is the actual age of the acute lesions under study. Even though the size and extent of the infarcts are similar from one series to another, could there be significant differences in the ages of the infarcts? Schwartz presented data at the workshop showing that thrombi decline in frequency as infarcts become older, whereas atherosclerotic plaques increase in number. This observation could signify that incompletely lysed thrombi are transformed into atherosclerotic plaques as they are organized and incorporated into the arterial wall.[18,20] An occlusive thrombus could be organized into an intimal plaque after first retracting to a parietal position.[25,26] The work of Mitchell and Schwartz[18,20] suggests that transformation takes place between the 2nd and 16th weeks after infarction. The rate of change probably depends on thrombus size and stability, thrombolytic activity and the preexisting state of the artery. Occlusive thrombi produced experimentally in previously normal coronary arteries can retract and become converted to sclerotic plaques in as short a period as 3 weeks.[27]

In these reports the age of infarcts was estimated by two equivalent means: either by histologic criteria originally derived from clinical data[28] or by direct estimate from the date of onset of clinical manifestations in each case. There is a fairly wide spread in the age of lesions considered to be acute. The infarcts range in age from up to 2, 4 and, in one series, 6 weeks. It would seem possible therefore that the several series are not closely comparable in terms of the age of lesions, and that this variable could account in part for the recorded differences in frequency of coronary thrombosis. Certainly any future prospective study should have well defined limits for the age as well as topography of the lesions.

Although factors of variance are difficult to identify, the strong influence of case selection is underscored by the repeatedly confirmed observations of coronary thrombosis in cases of spontaneous rupture of an infarcted heart. In this condition infarcts are usually only a few days old. They extend through the entire thickness of the ventricular wall, and coronary thrombosis is found in virtually every case.[29,30]

Thrombosis in absence of infarction: Coronary thrombosis in ischemic heart disease is not confined to its association with infarction; both occlusive and nonocclusive coronary thrombi may occur in the absence of infarction.[1,26] Furthermore, in time the resolution of thrombi and the conversion of residual thrombi to atherosclerotic plaques will obscure the true incidence of coronary thrombosis in any given case.[25] The frequency of coronary thrombosis and the extent of the thrombotic contribution to plaque formation will remain uncertain until more sensitive methods for detecting old and recent thrombi in patients and in pathologic material are developed.

Significance of Coronary Thrombosis

The determination of whether thrombosis plays a causative role in the pathogenesis of infarction depends ultimately, of course, on the evidence that one precedes the other. A number of factors in regard to both spatial and temporal relations bear on this point, but essential to any consideration of evidence must be the recognition that neither thrombi nor infarcts are static in nature. They both take time to develop and evolve. Since the estimation of the age of either an infarct or a thrombus in histologic material is at best crude, comparison of the age of one with the other is made doubly hazardous. Spatial relations between thrombi and infarcts, however, are usually more readily determined.

Spatial relations: The pathologists who hold that coronary thrombi cause infarcts point out that the thrombi are consistently located in a proximal position in the artery or arteries supplying the infarcted myocardium. Chapman further emphasizes that thrombi are never found haphazardly or within the infarcted tissue where they might be considered secondary to necrosis, but are always separated from the infarct by a segment of uninvolved artery. In many cases Schwartz finds multiple thrombotic occlusions that are always in a position subtending the infarct. Even though a thrombus may seem far removed from the site of infarction, the presence of anastomotic collateral vessels may place the remote thrombus at a critical point in the coronary circulation.[1]

The ischemic effect of thrombosis occurring in coronary arteries already severely narrowed by sclerosis is questioned by Roberts, who thinks the functional capacity of such vessels is uncertain. Luminal size in postmortem material, however, may be difficult to equate with true size and capacity in life. As Wissler suggested at the workshop, collapse of the lumen in histologic material may give an unreliable measurement. Experimental flow studies in arteries have consistently shown that no significant reduction in regional flow occurs until the lumen is narrowed by 80 to 90 percent,[31] a finding that has recently been confirmed in the coronary arteries of man.[32] These observations[31,32] tend to support the idea that sclerotic arteries are of functional significance within a wide range of stenosis.

The constant local relation between thrombi and infarcts fits the concept that thrombi play a causal role, but it does not exclude the possibility of a secondary origin. If the thrombus is primary, its localization at any given point in the artery must be explained.[13] Usually there is an explanation. In most cases the thrombi are found to arise at specific sites of rupture or ulceration of atherosclerotic plaques. Therefore, in evaluating the role of coronary thrombosis on the basis of spatial relations, both the constant proximal location of thrombi and the underlying acute arterial lesion must be considered.

Temporal relations: Still, to clarify fully the role of thrombosis in infarction, the time of thrombus formation in relation to the onset of infarction must be known. Thrombus age can be roughly estimated by histologic criteria, but at times even these crude estimates are made less precise when the thrombi have a layered appearance indicating protracted and episodic growth. Sinapius frequently finds histologic evidence of recurrent thrombosis in coronary arteries. He thinks the initial symptoms of myocardial ischemia in some cases may reflect the development of mural thrombi, which then grow to occlude the lumen and produce sufficient ischemia for infarction to occur, an idea similar to that proposed by Feil.[33] In cases now considered to be the "intermediate syndrome,"[34] a mural thrombus, if present, could progress to the point of occlusion or it could cease to grow and regress.

Spain notes that infarcts as well as thrombi may have multiple ages. As a thrombus continues to grow after its initial development, ischemia is intensified and the zone of infarction progressively enlarges. Small older subendocardial infarcts may become incorporated into a developing transmural infarct. This form of protracted thrombus growth and progressive infarction makes the usual histologic criteria for estimating the age of lesions even less reliable, and provides some basis for differences in interpretation.

Erhardt presented a new approach to the estimation of the age of coronary thrombi in cases of infarction by means of administering radioactive ^{125}iodine-tagged fibrinogen.[9,35] Coronary thrombi were shown to incorporate labeled fibrinogen that was administered after the development of clinical evidence of infarction. Although this finding could indicate a secondary origin of a thrombus after infarction, it is also consistent with extension of a preexisting primary thrombus since the technique used cannot exclude the presence of a small nonradioactive portion. However, lack of correlative histologic evaluation of the thrombi in these cases does not permit assessment of propagation or recurrent thrombus growth. Another factor could make interpretation difficult. Sherry and Hirsch suggested that plasma containing radioactive fibrinogen could perfuse a preexisting thrombus. At the workshop, Hirsch described his studies showing that labeled fibrinogen can permeate an experimental venous thrombus after it forms, a finding also recently reported by Kravis et al.[36] Schwartz referred to experiments that suggest fibrinogen could penetrate a thrombus even if endothelialized.[37] Until these factors are taken into account, Erhardt emphasizes that their initial studies must be cautiously interpreted.

In the occasional instances when infarcts develop in association with occlusion of coronary arteries by thromboemboli originating outside the coronary circulation, temporal relations are more clear-cut. In these cases, just as in other organs of the body, it would seem fairly certain that thrombotic occlusion of the arterial lumen precedes the development of infarction.[38,39] Moschos cited experimental evidence that microemboli arising from a thrombus within a coronary artery can enlarge a zone of regional infarction.[40] Microemboli alone may have ischemic effects. After the infusion of a platelet aggregating agent into the coronary circulation, Jörgensen et al.[41] observed the development of myocardial infarcts. These experiments suggest that similar microembolic phenomena recently reported[42] in cases of ischemic heart disease could be a significant factor in producing acute ischemia.

Conclusion

Thrombotic occlusion of coronary arteries frequently is associated with acute regional transmural infarction of the heart. The significance of this association must depend on the evidence that the thrombus either precedes infarction as a primary lesion or follows infarction as a secondary effect. The idea that coronary thrombosis is a secondary event following infarction is provocative and deserves serious consideration. Multiple factors and complex relations involved in thrombus growth and extension of infarcts clearly require further study. Presently, a substantial body of knowledge supports the classic concept of the primary role of thrombosis in the pathogenesis of infarction. Most evidence continues to affirm the basic concept that myocardial infarction can result from acute ischemia produced by thrombotic occlusion of a coronary artery.

This report concerns only a circumscribed aspect of ischemic heart disease, that of acute coronary thrombosis and its relation to acute myocardial infarction. The contribution of thrombosis to the origin and growth of atherosclerotic plaques and to the development of chronic ischemia also must be considered in evaluating the need for antithrombotic measures. Recent work on the ischemic effects of microembolic thrombosis in the myocardial circulation is just beginning to receive attention.

The prevention and treatment of coronary arterial thrombosis and the continued study of its pathogenesis should be stressed in the effort to curtail the morbidity and mortality of ischemic heart disease.

References

1. **Blumgart HL, Schlesinger MJ, Davis D:** Studies on the relation of the clinical manifestations of angina pectoris, coronary thrombosis, and myocardial infarction to the pathologic findings. Am Heart J 19:1–91, 1940

2. **Blumgart HL, Schlesinger MJ, Zoll PM:** Angina pectoris, coronary failure and acute myocardial infarction. JAMA 116: 91–96, 1941

3. **Blumgart HL, Zoll PM, Wessler S:** Angina pectoris. Clinical pathologic study of 177 cases. Trans Assoc Am Physicians 63: 262–267, 1950

4. **Friedberg CK, Horn H:** Acute myocardial infarction not due to coronary artery occlusion. JAMA 112:1675–1679, 1939

5. **Miller RD, Burchell HB, Edwards JE:** Myocardial infarction with and without acute coronary occlusion. Arch Intern Med 88: 597–604, 1951

6. **Branwood AW, Montgomery GL:** Observations on the morbid anatomy of coronary artery disease. Scott Med J 1:367–375, 1956

7. **Baroldi G:** Acute coronary occlusion as a cause of myocardial infarct and sudden coronary heart death. Am J Cardiol 16: 859–880, 1965

8. **Ehrlich JC, Shinohara Y:** Low incidence of coronary thrombosis in myocardial infarction. Arch Pathol 78:432–445, 1964

9. **Erhardt LR, Lundman T, Mellstedt H:** Incorporation of ^{125}I-labelled fibrinogen into coronary arterial thrombi in acute myocardial infarction in man. Lancet 1:387–390, 1973

10. **Roberts WC, Buja LM:** The frequency and significance of coronary arterial thrombi and other observations in fatal acute myocardial infarction. A study of 107 necropsy patients. Am J Med 52:425–444, 1972

11. **Walston A, Hackel DB, Estes EH:** Acute coronary occlusion and the "power failure" syndrome. Am Heart J 79:613–619, 1970

12. **Chapman I:** Relationships of recent coronary artery occlusion and acute myocardial infarction. J Mt Sinai Hosp 35:149–154, 1968

13. **Harland WA:** The pathogenesis of myocardial infarct and coronary thrombosis. In, Thrombosis (Sherry S, Brinkhous KM, Genton E, et al, ed). Washington DC, National Academy of Sciences, 1969, p 126–131

14. **Sinaplus D:** Beziehungen zwischen Koronarthrombosen und Myokardinfarkten. Dtsch Med Wochenschr 97:443–448, 1972

15. **Miller RD:** Personal communication, November 1973

16. **Chapman I:** Morphogenesis of occluding coronary artery thrombosis. Arch Pathol 80:256–261, 1965

17. **Chapman I:** The initiating cause of coronary artery thrombosis. An anatomic study. J Mt Sinai Hosp 36:361–374, 1969

18. **Mitchell JRA, Schwartz CJ:** Arterial Disease. Oxford, Blackwell Scientific Publications, 1965, p 107–114

19. **Schwartz CJ, Mitchell JRA:** The relation between myocardial lesions and coronary artery disease. I. An unselected necropsy study. Br Heart J 24:761–786, 1962

20. **Mitchell JRA, Schwartz CJ:** The relation between myocardial lesions and coronary artery disease. II. A selected group of patients with massive cardiac necrosis or scarring. Br Heart J 25: 1–25, 1963

21. **Schwartz CJ:** On the pathological diagnosis of acute ischaemic heart disease. Atherosclerosis 15:1–4, 1972

22. **Schwartz CJ, Walsh WJ:** The pathologic basis of sudden death. Prog Cardiovasc Dis 13:465–481, 1971

23. **Sinaplus D:** Zur Morphologie verschliessender Koronarthromben. Dtsch Med Wochenschr 97:544–551, 1972

24. **Spain DM:** The pathologic spectrum of myocardial infarction. In, Atherosclerosis and Coronary Heart Disease (Likoff W, Segal BL, Insull W, et al, ed). New York, Grune & Stratton, 1972, p 133–139

25. **Chandler AB:** Thombosis in the development of coronary atherosclerosis. In Ref 24, p 28–34

26. **Duguid JB:** Thrombosis as a factor in the pathogenesis of coronary atherosclerosis. J Pathol Bacteriol 58:207–212, 1946

27. **Pope JT, Chandler AB, Asokan SK, et al:** A morphologic and angiographic study of the evolution of experimental coronary thrombosis in the dog (abstr). Circulation 43: Suppl IV:IV-204, 1973

28. **Mallory GK, White PD, Salcedo-Salgar J:** The speed of healing of myocardial infarction. A study of the pathologic anatomy in 72 cases. Am Heart J 18:647–671, 1939

29. **Benson RL, Hunter WC, Manlove CH:** Spontaneous rupture of the heart. Report of 40 cases in Portland, Oregon. Am J Pathol 9:295–328, 1933

30. **Wessler S, Zoll PM, Schlesinger MJ:** The pathogenesis of spontaneous cardiac rupture. Circulation 6:334–351, 1952

31. **Weale FE:** The haemodynamics of incomplete arterial obstruction. Br J Surg 51:689–693, 1964

32. **Asokan SK, Fraser RC, Kolbeck RC, et al:** Variations in right and left coronary blood flow in man with and without occlusive coronary disease. Br Heart J, in press.

33. **Fell H:** Preliminary pain in coronary thrombosis. Am J Med Sci 193:42–48, 1937

34. **Sawe U:** Early diagnosis of acute myocardial infarction with special reference to the diagnosis of the intermediate coronary syndrome. Acta Med Scand: 545 Suppl:1–76, 1972

35. **Hackel DB, Estes H, Walston A, et al:** Some problems concerning coronary artery occlusion and acute myocardial infarction. Circulation 40: Suppl IV:31–35, 1969

36. **Kravis TC, Shibel EM, Brooks JD, et al:** Incorporation of radio-labelled fibrinogen into venous thrombi induced in dogs. Circulation 49:158–164, 1974

37. **Bell FP, Gallus AS, Schwartz CJ:** Focal and regional patterns of uptake and the transmural distribution of ^{131}I-fibrinogen in the pig aorta in vivo. Exp Mol Pathol 20:281–292, 1974

38. **Hamman L:** Coronary embolism (Lewis A. Conner lecture). Am Heart J 21:401–422, 1941

39. **Wenger NK, Bauer S:** Coronary embolism. Review of the literature and presentation of fifteen cases. Am J Med 25:549–557, 1958

40. **Moschos CB, Lahiri K, Lyons M, et al:** Relation of microcirculatory thrombosis to thrombus in the proximal coronary artery: effect of aspirin, dipyridamole and thrombolysis. Am Heart J 86: 61–68, 1973

41. **Jorgensen L, Rowsell HC, Hovig T, et al:** Adenosine diphosphate-induced platelet aggregation and myocardial infarction in swine Lab Invest 17:616–644, 1967

42. **Jorgensen L:** The role of platelet embolism from crumbling thrombi and of platelet aggregates arising in flowing blood. In Ref 13, p 506–533

IRVING CHAPMAN, MD
Mt. Sinai Medical Services
City Hospital at Elmhurst
Elmhurst, New York

VIRGINIA H. DONALDSON, MD
The Children's Hospital
Research Foundation
Cincinnati, Ohio

LEIF R. ERHARDT, MD
Department of Medicine
Karolinska Institute
Stockholm, Sweden

ANTHONY P. FLETCHER, MD
Department of Medicine
Washington University
School of Medicine
St. Louis, Missouri

WILLIAM T. FRIEDEWALD, MD
Heart and Vascular Division
National Heart and Lung Institute
National Institutes of Health
Bethesda, Maryland

PETER L. FROMMER, MD, FACC
Heart and Vascular Division
National Heart and Lung Institute
National Institutes of Health
Bethesda, Maryland

EDWARD GENTON, MD, FACC
Department of Medicine
University of Colorado
Medical Center
Denver, Colorado

RICHARD GORLIN, MD, FACC
Harvard Medical Unit
Peter Bent Brigham Hospital
Boston, Massachusetts

JAMES W. HAMPTON, MD
Department of Medicine
School of Medicine
University of Oklahoma
Oklahoma City, Oklahoma

FANN HARDING, PhD
Division of Blood Diseases and Resources
National Heart and Lung Institute
National Institutes of Health
Bethesda, Maryland

JACK HIRSCH, MD
Department of Pathology
McMaster University
Hamilton, Ontario, Canada

ALAN J. JOHNSON, MD
Department of Medicine
New York University Medical Center
New York, New York

HAU C. KWAAN, MD
Hematology Section
Veterans Administration Research
Hospital
Chicago, Illinois

CHRISTOS B. MOSCHOS, MD, FACC
Department of Medicine
College of Medicine of New Jersey
Newark, New Jersey

J. FRASER MUSTARD, MD
Department of Pathology
McMaster University
Hamilton, Ontario, Canada

PAUL M. NESS, MD
Division of Blood Diseases and Resources
National Heart and Lung Institute
National Institutes of Health
Bethesda, Maryland

OSCAR D. RATNOFF, MD
Department of Medicine
School of Medicine
Case Western Reserve University
Cleveland, Ohio

WILLIAM C. ROBERTS, MD, FACC
Section on Pathology
National Heart and Lung Institute
National Institutes of Health
Bethesda, Maryland

EDWIN W. SALZMAN, MD
Department of Surgery
Beth Israel Hospital
Boston, Massachusetts

ARTHUR A. SASAHARA, MD, FACC
Cardiopulmonary Section
Veterans Administration Hospital
West Roxbury, Massachusetts

COLIN J. SCHWARTZ, MD
Department of Pathology
McMaster University
Hamilton, Ontario, Canada

ERNEST R. SIMON, MD
Division of Blood Diseases and Resources
National Heart and Lung Institute
National Institutes of Health
Bethesda, Maryland

TOBY L SIMON, MD
Division of Blood Diseases and Resources
National Heart and Lung Institute
National Institutes of Health
Bethesda, Maryland

D. SINAPIUS, MD
Pathologisches Institut der Universitat
Gottingen, West Germany

SHERRILL J. SLICHTER, MD
King County Central Blood Bank
Seattle, Washington

DAVID M. SPAIN, MD, FACC
Brookdale Hospital Medical Center
Brooklyn, New York

JAMES M. STENGLE, MD
Division of Blood Diseases and Resources
National Heart and Lung Institute
National Institutes of Health
Bethesda, Maryland

DONALD G. THERRIAULT, PhD
Division of Blood Diseases and Resources
National Heart and Lung Institute
National Institutes of Health
Bethesda, Maryland

HENRY N. WAGNER, Jr., MD
Department of Radiological Science
Johns Hopkins University
School of Medicine
Baltimore, Maryland

NANETTE K. WENGER, MD, FACC
Department of Medicine
Emory University School of Medicine
Atlanta, Georgia

STANFORD WESSLER, MD
Department of Medicine
The Jewish Hospital of St. Louis
St. Louis, Missouri

WILLIAM J. WILLIAMS, MD
Department of Medicine
Upstate Medical Center
Syracuse, New York

ROBERT W. WISSLER, MD, PhD
Department of Pathology
University of Chicago
Chicago, Illinois

Myocardial Embolus to Coronary Artery*

Result of Rupture of Papillary Muscle During Acute Myocardial Infarction

William J. Hammer, M.D.; Victor J. Ferrans, M.D.; and William C. Roberts, M.D., F.C.C.P.

A patient is described with acute myocardial infarction complicated by rupture of a papillary muscle. A surprise finding at necropsy was a fragment of necrotic myocardium, similar to that at the site of papillary muscle rupture, in one coronary artery. Myocardial embolism to a coronary artery has not been described previously to our knowledge.

Although they are infrequent, emboli to coronary arteries usually consist of fibrin and platelets.[1] Other dislodged materials in coronary arteries have included

*From the Division of Cardiology, Department of Medicine, and the Department of Pathology, Georgetown University, Washington, DC, and the Section of Pathology, National Heart and Lung Institute, National Institutes of Health, Bethesda, Md.
Reprint requests: Dr. Roberts, Bldg 10, Room 3D30, National Institutes of Health, Bethesda 20014*

calcific debris, clumps of neoplastic cells, suture and other foreign materials, and colonies of microorganisms.[2-4] The usual consequence of coronary embolism is acute myocardial infarction.[1] Of over 200 hearts examined systematically[1] at necropsy in patients with fatal coronary heart disease, one was observed to have an embolus of necrotic myocardium in a coronary artery. The patient, a 73-year-old woman, died suddenly ten hours after onset of symptoms (chest pain) of acute myocardial infarction. A precordial murmur was never audible. Necropsy disclosed rupture of one left ventricular papillary muscle and a clump of myocardium in the lumen of the right coronary artery (Fig 1). The embolized myocardium was similar to that observed in the ruptured papillary muscle. Therefore, it appears reasonable to conclude that the embolus to the right coronary artery resulted from dislodgement of myocardium during or shortly following rupture of the left ventricular papillary muscle (Fig 2).

Although observed previously in a carotid artery after splitting of a papillary muscle during mitral commissurotomy,[5] myocardial embolus, to our knowledge, has not been reported previously in a coronary artery. The coronary embolus in the present patient probably would have been missed had not the *entire* major coronary tree been examined histologically, a method used to study the coronary arteries at necropsy in all of our over 200 fatal cases of coronary heart disease.[1] The coronary

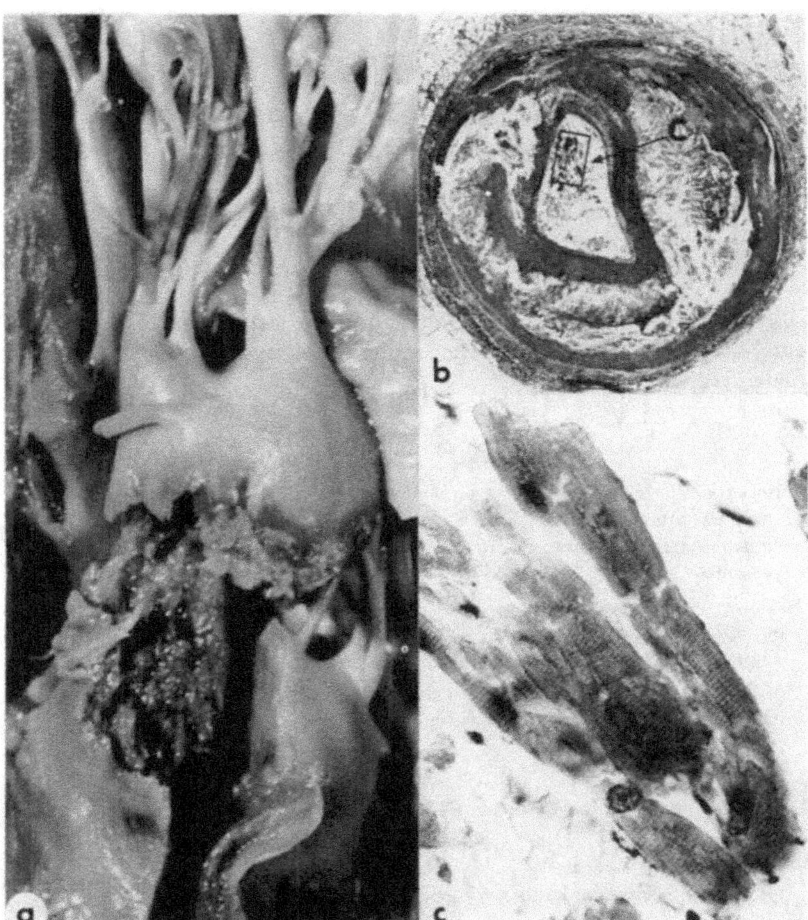

FIGURE 1. Ruptured papillary muscle and myocardial embolus to coronary artery. *a*, Ruptured posteromedial papillary muscle. *b*, Right coronary artery (Movat stain, original magnification × 16). Material enclosed in rectangle is shown in *c*. *c*, Fragment of myocardium (Movat stain, original magnification × 880).

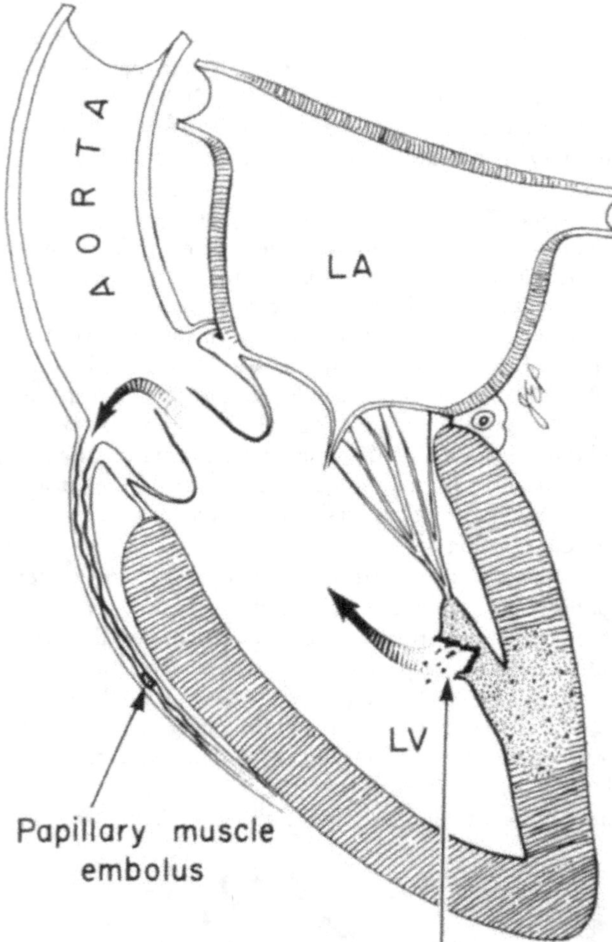

Incomplete rupture of Posteromedial papillary muscle

FIGURE 2. Diagram showing rupture of necrotic papillary muscle with embolization of fragment of myocardium to coronary artery. LA, Left atrium; and LV, left ventricle.

embolus in the present patient obviously represents a complication, rather than a cause, of the acute myocardial infarction.

REFERENCES

1 Roberts WC, Buja LM: The frequency and significance of coronary arterial thrombi and other observations in fatal acute myocardial infarction: A study of 107 necropsy patients. Am J Med 52:425-443, 1972

2 Glotzer DJ, Shaw RS, Scannell JG: Calcific coronary emboli following open valvuloplasty for aortic stenosis. J Thorac Cardiovasc Surg 43:435-440, 1962

3 Morrow AG, Austen WG: A technique for preventing calcific emboli following aortic valvuloplasty. Surg Gynecol Obstet 114:634-635, 1962

4 Buchbinder NA, Roberts WC: Left-sided valvular active infective endocarditis: A study of 45 necropsy patients. Am J Med 53:20-35, 1972

5 Friedman RM, Roberts WC: Myocardial embolus: A complication of mitral valvulotomy. N Engl J Med 272:251-252, 1965

Ruptured Intrathoracic Parathyroid Adenoma*

*Gil H. Santos, M.D., F.C.C.P.;** Che-Lu Tseng, M.D.;† and Robert W. M. Frater, M.D.‡*

A case is presented where hemorrhage into the mediastinum from a ruptured intrathoracic parathyroid adenoma mimicked a dissecting aortic hematoma with acute circulatory collapse demanding emergency volume replacement.

The occurrence of hyperparathyroidism due to an intrathoracically located parathyroid gland is very rare. Parathyroid tumors in the thoracic outlet which are removable by a low cervical incision are also considered as mediastinal tumors by some authorities, who state that the incidence of such tumors can be as high as 21 percent.[1] According to Edwards et al,[2] 10 percent of parathyroid tumors are intrathoracic but can be removed through a cervical approach. The true incidence is more accurately reflected by the Mayo series reported by Scholz et al,[3] in which intrathoracic adenomas removed by sternotomy or found at autopsy constituted only 1.4 percent (14) of 1,000 cases.

Although incidences as high as 21 percent[1] and 10 percent[2] have been reported for intrathoracic parathyroid adenoma, most of these adenomas are, in fact, removable through the cervical approach and should not be considered as mediastinal tumors. Using the previously mentioned criteria, the incidence should, therefore, be in the region of 1 to 2 percent.

CASE REPORT

A 47-year-old woman came to the emergency room with sudden onset of retrosternal pain radiating to both arms and to the back between the scapulae. This was accompanied by dizziness and diaphoresis. Chest x-ray film demonstrated a wide upper mediastinum (Fig 1) compatible with aortic dissection. The medical history revealed that the patient underwent a vagotomy and pyloroplasty four months previously for pyloric obstruction due to duodenal ulcer. Abnormal biochemical findings at that time included a serum calcium level of 12.3 mg/100 ml and a serum phosphate level of 2.7 mg/100 ml. The results of serum parathyroid hormone assay were reported as 994 pg/ml (normal, 500 pg/ml). Skull x-ray films revealed a calvarium with a salt-and-pepper appearance. Hyperparathyroidism was suspected, and the neck was explored surgically. Four normal glands were found, and apart from a biopsy from each gland, they were left undisturbed. Postoperatively the patient's serum calcium level remained elevated, but she refused further work-up. She was then discharged to be followed as an outpatient and was doing well until the present admission. On physical examination the patient was in acute distress, pale and diaphoretic. The blood

*From the Department of Surgery, Albert Einstein College of Medicine, Bronx, NY.
**Instructor in Thoracic Surgery.
†Chief Resident in Thoracic Surgery.
‡Professor of Surgery.
Reprint requests: Dr. Santos, 1825 Eastchester Road, Bronx 10461*

Acute Myocardial Infarction
and Angiographically Normal Coronary Arteries

An Unproven Combination

A NUMBER OF NECROPSY STUDIES have shown that among patients with fatal ischemic heart disease (IHD) at least one and usually two of the three major coronary arteries are greater than 75% narrowed by old atherosclerotic plaque.[1,2] The introduction of selective coronary angiography[3] allowed visualization of these vessels during life, and this technique has demonstrated usually as severe coronary narrowing among patients with *symptomatic* IHD as necropsy has shown among patients with *fatal* IHD.[4-6] Coronary angiography among patients with IHD manifested by acute myocardial infarction (AMI) has disclosed the following: 1) when performed *at the time of AMI*, coronary angiography has always disclosed severe narrowing or complete obstruction of at least one of three major coronary arteries; 2) when performed *at the time of AMI*, coronary angiography has never demonstrated a normal coronary tree; and 3) when performed *after healing of an AMI*, coronary angiography has usually (> 99%) demonstrated severe narrowing of one or more of the three major coronary arteries, and rarely (< 1%), a normal coronary tree.

In recent years much attention has been given to this latter small group of patients with "myocardial infarction and angiographically normal coronary arteries."[7-21] A major implication of most of these reports is that AMI may occur in the presence of normal coronary arteries. This editorial will examine this implication and discuss possible explanations for the occurrence of "myocardial infarction and normal coronary arteriograms."

Of 45 reported patients with "myocardial infarction and angiographically normal coronary arteries" (tables 1 and 2), the AMI was produced at the time of cardiac catheterization in five (table 2); in four of them, coronary angiography was performed at that time and in each an obstructed coronary artery was observed. Repeat catheterization in all five patients at later times, however, disclosed angiographically normal coronary arteries in each. In the other 40 patients (table 1), AMI was unrelated to cardiac catheter-

ization and none of them had coronary angiography at the time of the AMI. In 39 of the 40 patients the interval between the onset of the AMI and the performance of coronary angiography was longer than one month. Thus, the status of the coronary arteries *at the time* of acute myocardial necrosis is uncertain. Indeed, *a normal coronary arterial tree has never been demonstrated by angiography at the time of AMI.*

How then may the coronary tree be entirely normal by angiography after healing of an AMI? At least six explanations need consideration (fig. 1):

1) AMI never occurred. Diagnosis of the myocardial insult, in other words, was incorrect. Documentation of AMI by electrocardiograms and enzyme elevations, however, appeared adequate in all 45 reported patients. Thus, this explanation appears unlikely. It is presumed that the infarcts were transmural.

2) Too large a myocardial mass or too little hemoglobin or too low a perfusion pressure (shock) was present to supply the myocardium by a normal coronary tree. The occurrence of myocardial scars in patients with large hearts and normal coronary arteries is well recognized. Patients with left ventricular outflow obstruction commonly have myocardial scars despite "clean" coronary arteries. The myocardial scars, however, are usually limited to the papillary muscles and to the subendocardium (inner one-half) of the left ventricular free wall or ventricular septum or both. The same applies to subjects with severe chronic anemia such as congenital hemolytic anemia or sickle-cell disease. Likewise, an inadequate coronary perfusion pressure may lead to myocardial necrosis (with later scarring) despite a normal coronary tree, but again the necrosis (or fibrosis) usually is limited to left ventricular papillary muscles and subendocardium.

In contrast to the frequent occurrence of *papillary muscle* and *subendocardial* necrosis or fibrosis in patients with a normal coronary tree but too large a myocardial mass, or too little hemoglobin or too low a perfusion pressure, the occurrence of *transmural* necrosis or fibrosis among these individuals is infrequent. Among 74 necropsy patients with transmural AMI recently studied in our laboratory,[1] only five (7%) had less than 75% luminal narrowing by atherosclerotic plaques of any of the three major coronary arteries

From the Section of Pathology, National Heart and Lung Institute, National Institutes of Health, Bethesda, Maryland.

Address for reprints: Dr. William C. Roberts, Building 10A, Room 3E30, National Institutes of Health, Bethesda, Maryland 20014

TABLE 1. *Clinical Observations in 40 Reported Patients with Acute Myocardial Infarction (AMI) and Subsequently Normal Coronary Arteriograms (Noncatheter Induced)*

First Author	Publication Year	No. Pts.	Age Range (years)	Interval (mo.) From Onset of AMI to Normal Coronary Arteriograms					
				(<1)	(1-2)	(2-3)	(3-6)	(6-12)	(>12)
1. Campeau	1968	5	27-53				1	4	
2. Sidd	1970	1	19				1		
3. Bruschke	1971	4	29-43		1		1		2
4. Glancy	1971	2	34-36						2
5. Nizit	1971	1	17				1		
6. Dear	1971	1	43						1
7. Kimbris	1972	3	16-36	1			2		
8. Schatz	1973	1	14			1			
9. Henderson	1973	1	34						1*
10. Khan	1974	9	22-49			2	3	3	
11. Brest	1974	5	28-40				3	2	
12. Regan	1975	7	34-59		1	3	3		
Totals		40	14-59 (Avg 36)	1	2	6	15	9	7

*This was the second coronary arteriogram. The first study, 31 months earlier or 7 months after AMI, showed mild coronary narrowing. The second study, 38 months after the AMI, was entirely normal.

(table 3). The hearts in each of the five, however, were considerably hypertrophied (avg 780 g) by other cardiac conditions.

Among the 40 reported patients with noncatheter-induced "myocardial infarction and angiographically normal coronary arteries," with rare exception, none had associated cardiac conditions or cardiomegaly by chest roentgenograms or electrocardiogram. Thus, although applicable on occasion, this explanation is not applicable to the patients reported with noncatheter-induced "myocardial infarction and angiographically normal coronary arteries."

3) The coronary arteriograms were misinterpreted. It is well known that angiography tends to underestimate the degree of coronary arterial luminal narrowing.[22, 23] This explanation on occasion may be the proper one but most patients with symptomatic coronary heart disease have some abnormality on angiography of two and often all three of the major extramural coronary arteries.[4-6] Slit-like lumens may account for many of the false negative angiograms (fig. 2).[21] It would be rare, however, to have a severely narrowed slit-like lumen in one major coronary artery without any abnormality by angiography in the other two major coronary arteries.

4) Coronary spasm caused the AMI. Although shown to cause both chest pain and ischemic changes on electrocardiogram, coronary spasm has not been shown to cause myocardial necrosis. The case for spasm is generally considered strongest among patients with Prinzmetal's angina. Of 84 patients with this variant angina reported in English,[24-57] 65 had coronary arteriography (fig. 3),[30, 32-57] and of them, the coronary arteries were severely (> 75%) narrowed in 43 (66%) and normal in 22 (34%). Coronary spasm was

TABLE 2. *Clinical Observations in Five Reported Patients with Acute Myocardial Infarction (AMI) Occurring at Cardiac Catheterization*

First Author	Publication Year	No. Pts.	Age (yrs.)	Interval (mo.) from Catheter-associated AMI to Normal Coronary Arteriogram		
				(<2)	(3-6)	(6-12)
1. Campeau	1968	1	37			1
2. Richardson	1971	1	40	1		
3. Cheng	1972	1	52		1	
4. O'Reilly	1974	2	56 & 64	2		
Totals		5	32-64 (avg 50)	3	1	1

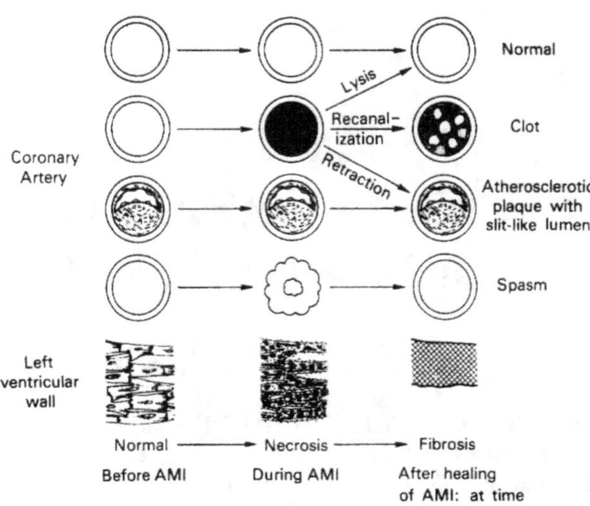

FIGURE 1. *Diagrammatic portrayal of possible appearances of the epicardial coronary arteries and left ventricular myocardium in patients with acute myocardial infarction (AMI) and subsequently normal coronary arteries. The left vertical column indicates the status of the coronary arteries and myocardium before the AMI; the center vertical column, during the AMI; and the right vertical column, after healing of the AMI. If the AMI was caused by a condition affecting only the intramyocardial arteries, by a disproportion between the size of the coronary bed and the amount of myocardium to be oxygenated, the coronary arteries presumably would be normal (top row) at the time of myocardial necrosis as well as before and subsequently. Coronary angiography may show a slit-like eccentric lumen (third row) on occasion to be "normal." If spasm caused the AMI, one or more coronary arteries might be partially obstructed at the time of the AMI (fourth row). If embolism caused the AMI (second row), the clot could subsequently lyse, recanalize, or retract along one side allowing the lumen to be of sufficient size to appear later as "angiographically normal."*

demonstrated in 14 (22%) of the 65 patients: in five of the 43 with narrowed and in nine of the 22 patients with normal coronary arteries. Although it occurred naturally in none of the five patients with both coronary spasm and fixed coronary narrowing, AMI or death occurred after aortocoronary bypass procedures in three of the five patients. None of the 22 patients with angiographically normal coronary arteries had an AMI, but six of them died; none of these, however, were among the nine with demonstrated coronary spasm. Examination of the coronary arteries in five of these six patients (table 4) disclosed severe (> 75%) narrowing of

TABLE 3. *Acute Transmural Myocardial Infarction and Insignificant (<75%) Coronary Narrowing at Necropsy (5 of 74 patients)*

Pts.	Age (Yrs.)	Sex	Associated Condition	Heart Weight (Gms)	Coronary Emboli
1	37	M	VSD	730	+
2	79	F	MS, AS	500	+
3	79	M	AS	730	0
4	56	M	MR	900	+
5	60	M	AS	1050	0
5	37-79 (Avg. 62)	M:F 4:1		500-1050 (avg. 780)	3

Abbreviation: AS = aortic stenosis; MR = mitral regurgitation; MS = mitral stenosis; VSD = ventricular septal defect.

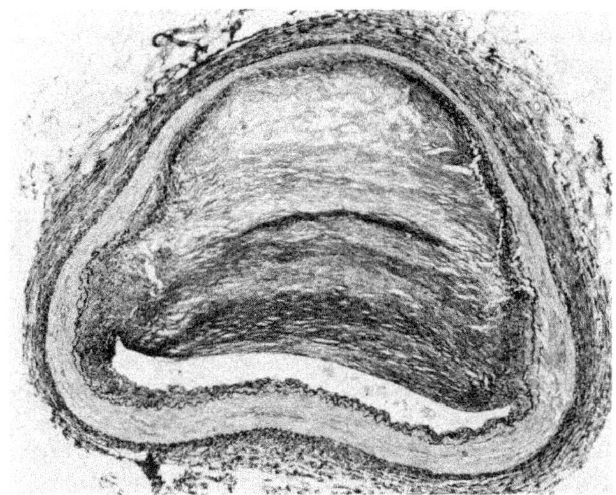

FIGURE 2. *Slit-like eccentric lumen in the left anterior descending coronary artery of a 54-year-old woman (SH #4571) who died suddenly at home. This is the type artery which might be interpreted as normal on coronary angiography. (Elastic van Gieson stain, × 31). Reproduced from Roberts WC: Coronary arteries in fatal acute myocardial infarction (Circulation 45: 215, 1972).*

TABLE 4. *Prinzmetal's Angina: Reported Status of Coronary Arteries at Necropsy in Those with Angiographically Normal Coronary Arteries During Life*

Author	Year	No. Pts	Age	Sex	Status of Coronary Arteries	
					1 of 3 >75% Narrowed	Normal
Gianelly	1968	1	49	F		1**
Cosby	1972	2	46	F	1	
			41	F		1***
Cheng	1973	1	60	M		1
Donsky	1975	1	44	F	1	
Totals		5*			2	3

*All 5 died suddenly.
**Small left coronary artery.
***The right coronary ostium was obstructed by atherosclerotic plaque.

one coronary ostium or artery in three patients and a "small" left coronary artery in a fourth. Thus, only one of the five patients had a "normal" coronary tree at necropsy.

Thus, although it has been shown to cause chest pain and ischemic electrocardiographic changes, coronary spasm has not been shown to cause myocardial necrosis, except possibly in patients with chronic industrial nitroglycerin exposure.[58]

5) *AMI was caused by a condition affecting only the intramural (intramyocardial) coronary arteries without in-* volvement of the extramural coronary arteries. Abnormalities of the intramural coronary arteries have been reported in several conditions (table 5), but to our knowledge, transmural myocardial infarction has never been described as a consequence of disease solely of the intramural coronary arteries. Even in the conditions where observed, involvement of the intramural coronary arteries has been focal, not diffuse, and disease of these small myocardial arteries usually has been associated with a condition affecting other body organs or systems as well.

6) *AMI was caused by an occluding embolus which subsequently lysed or recanalized.* This appears to us the most likely cause of the AMI in patients who subsequently are shown by angiography to have a normal coronary tree. It is reasoned that the coronary arteries were not normal at the time of AMI but that the occlusion resolved between the time of the AMI and the time of coronary angiography. Factors supporting this hypothesis are:

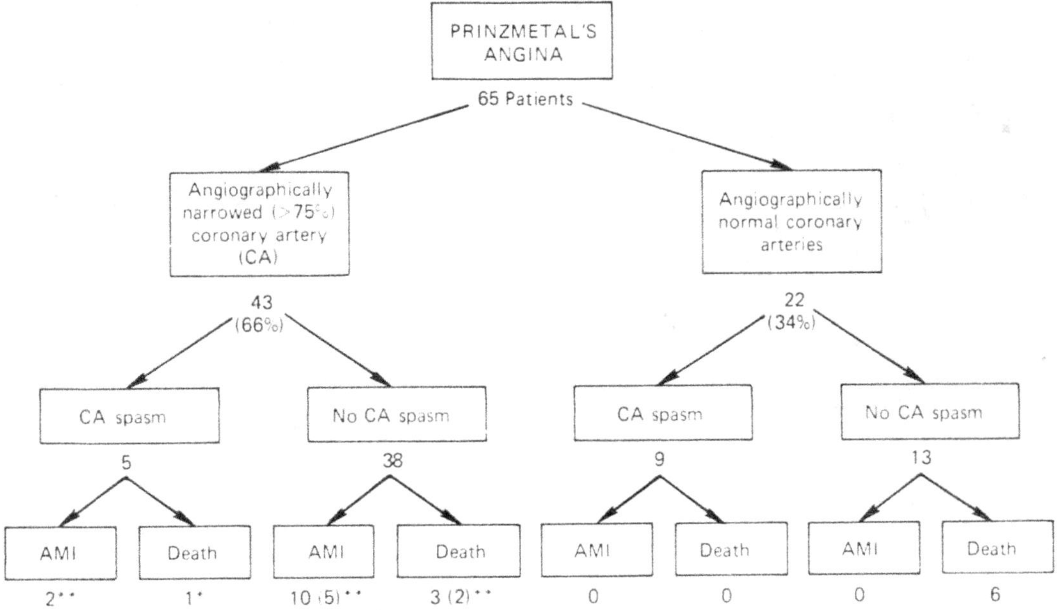

*Death in each followed aorto-coronary bypass operations.

**The non-fatal acute myocardial infarction (AMI) followed aorto-coronary bypass operations.

FIGURE 3. *Frequencies of coronary spasm, acute myocardial infarction, and death in 65 reported patients with Prinzmetal's angina and coronary arteriography.*

TABLE 5. *Conditions Associated with Narrowing of Intramural Coronary Arteries (Excluding Vasculitis)*

1. Atherosclerosis of extramural coronary arteries (limited to vessels in left ventricular papillary muscles)
2. Hypertrophic cardiomyopathy (ASH)
3. Neurogenic cardiac diseases
   A. Friedreich's ataxia
   B. Progressive muscular dystrophy
   C. Progressive myotonic dystrophy
4. Collagen diseases
   A. Systemic lupus erythematosus
   B. Scleroderma
   C. Dermatomyositis
5. Diabetes mellitus
6. Hereditary connective tissue disorders
   A. Marfan syndrome
   B. Hurler syndrome
7. Infiltrative diseases
   A. Amyloid
   B. Neoplasm
8. Emboli
   A. Infective endocarditis
   B. Intracardiac thrombus
   C. Prosthetic valve
   D. Cardiac catheterization
   E. Neoplasm
9. Certain congenital cardiac malformations
   A. Aortic atresia
10. Coagulopathy
    A. Disseminated intravascular coagulation
    B. Thrombotic thrombocytopenic purpura
11. Whipple's disease

A) Arteriographically documented coronary arterial embolic occlusion can completely resolve. Of the five patients with catheter-induced coronary arterial thromboembolic occlusion (table 2), the coronary arteriogram became normal after the AMI in each. In three of the five patients, complete resolution of the occlusion occurred within two months of the onset of the AMI.

B) Conditions associated with an increased risk of arterial thromboemboli were relatively frequent (15%) among the 40 patients (table 1) with noncatheter-induced AMI: three of the four women were taking oral contraceptives; two patients had prosthetic cardiac valves; and one patient had a markedly elevated platelet count.

C) Histologic study of previous known arterial emboli indicates that such lesions may either lyse completely, retract along one side to form an eccentric lumen, or recanalize with multiple luminal channels (figs. 4 and 5).[59] Each of these three means of organization of the clot would be associated with a lumen large enough to produce a normal coronary arteriogram.

D) Among our 74 necropsy patients with transmural AMI, only five had less than 75% luminal narrowing by atherosclerotic plaques of each of their three major coronary arteries (table 4): three of the five had coronary emboli at necropsy[1] and their coronary tree was otherwise normal.

E) Among reported patients with noncatheter-induced AMI, with few exceptions, they were asymptomatic before the occurrence of the AMI and following healing of the AMI they were asymptomatic again without evidence of angina pectoris, congestive cardiac failure, or cardiomegaly. Obviously, an AMI may be the first and only coronary event when the AMI is the result of severe coronary atherosclerosis, but the percentage who return to a totally asymptomatic state is not nearly as high as in the group with "myocardial infarction and angiographically-normal coronary arteries." Acute pulmonary embolism when occurring in previously normal pulmonary arteries and lungs might be analogous (= normal coronary arteries), as opposed to

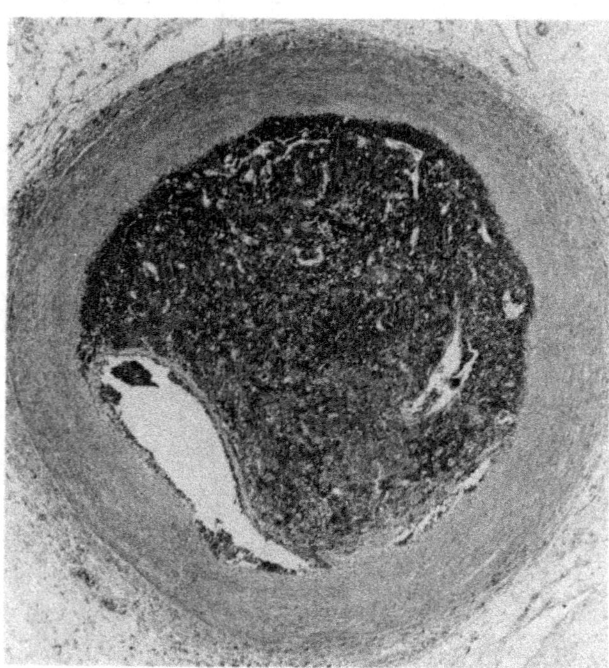

FIGURE 4. *Embolus to right coronary artery in a 56-year-old man (A70-244). Embolism occurred during cardiac catheterization 31 days before death and caused transmural necrosis of the posterior left ventricular wall. The artery before being occluded by the embolus was normal. Partial organization and retraction of the clot have resulted in an eccentric lumen. (Hematoxylin-eosin stain, × 25).*

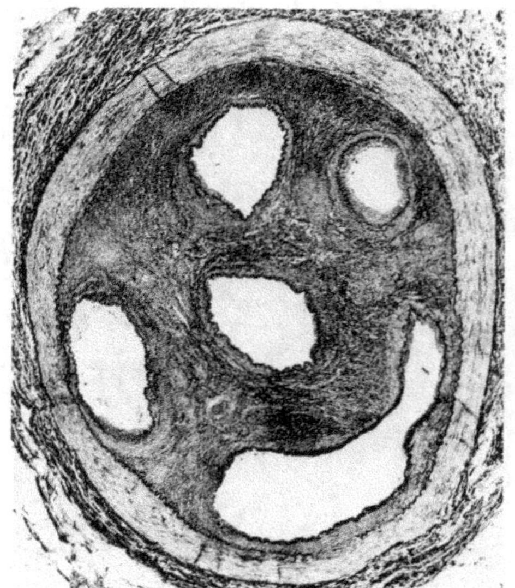

FIGURE 5. *Recanalized embolus in the distal left anterior descending coronary artery of a 26-year-old man (A63-170) who had a transmural acute myocardial infarct three years earlier at the time of active infective endocarditis involving the aortic valve. The anterior descending coronary artery proximal to this site, as well as the other extramural coronary arteries, was normal. (Elastic van Gieson stain, × 46). Reproduced from Roberts WC, Buja LM: The frequency and significance of coronary arterial thrombi and other observations in fatal acute myocardial infarction. A study of 107 necropsy patients. Am J Med 52: 423, 1972*

acute pulmonary embolism superimposed on chronic lung disease (= coronary atherosclerosis).

Thus, *in conclusion,* the following statements may be made concerning reported patients with "myocardial infarction and angiographically normal coronary arteries:" 1) An angiographically normal coronary tree has never been demonstrated at the time of AMI; 2) Among reported patients with "myocardial infarction and angiographically normal coronary arteries," the angiograms were performed after healing, rather than during the AMI; 3) Although there are several explanations for the occurrence of AMI and angiographically normal coronary arteries, and although each may be applicable on occasion, the most reasonable explanation appears to be acute coronary embolism with subsequent clot lysis, retraction, or recanalization, each of which may appear as "angiographically normal."

ERNEST N. ARNETT, M.D.
WILLIAM C. ROBERTS, M.D.

References

1. Roberts WC, Buja LM: The frequency and significance of coronary arterial thrombi and other observations in fatal acute myocardial infarction. A study of 107 necropsy patients. Am J Med 52: 425, 1972
2. Roberts WC, Ferrans VJ, Levy RI, Fredrickson DS: Cardiovascular pathology in hyperlipoproteinemia. Anatomic observations in 42 necropsy patients with normal or abnormal serum lipoprotein patterns. Am J Cardiol 31: 557, 1973
3. Baltaxe HA, Amplatz K, Levin DC: Coronary Angiography. Springfield, Illinois, Charles C Thomas, 1973
4. Hale G, Dexter D, Jefferson K, Leatham A: Value of coronary arteriography in the investigation of ischemic heart disease. Br Heart J 28: 40, 1966
5. Proudfit WL, Shirey EK, Sones FM: Selective cine coronary angiography. Correlation with clinical findings in 1,000 patients. Circulation 33: 901, 1966
6. Ross RS, Friesinger GC: Coronary arteriography. Am Heart J 72: 437, 1966
7. Campeau L, Lesperance J, Bourassa MG, Ashekian PB: Myocardial infarction without obstructive disease at coronary arteriography. Can Med Assoc J 99: 837, 1968
8. Sidd J, Kemp HG, Gorlin R: Acute myocardial infarction in a nineteen-year-old student in the absence of coronary obstructive disease. N Engl J Med 282: 1306, 1970
9. Bruschke AVG, Bruyneel KJJ, Bloch A, van Herper G: Acute myocardial infarction without obstructive coronary artery disease demonstrated by selective cinearteriography. Br Heart J 33: 585, 1971
10. Glancy DL, Marcus ML, Epstein SE: Myocardial infarction in young women with normal coronary arteriograms. Circulation 44: 495, 1971
11. Nizet PM, Robertson L: Normal coronary arteriogram following myocardial infarction in a 17-year-old boy. Am Heart J 28: 715, 1971
12. Dear HD, Russell RO, Jones WB, Reeves TJ: Myocardial infarction in the absence of coronary occlusion. Am J Cardiol 28: 718, 1971
13. Kimbiris D, Segal BL, Munir M, Katz M, Likoff W: Myocardial infarction in patients with normal patent coronary arteries as visualized by cinearteriography. Am J Cardiol 29: 724, 1972
14. Schatz IJ, Mizukami H, Ballagher J, Greenslit FS: Myocardial infarction in a 14-year-old boy with normal coronary arteriograms. Studies of blood oxygen release rate. Chest 63: 963, 1973
15. Henderson RR, Hansing CE, Razavi M, Rowe GG: Resolution of an obstructive coronary lesion as demonstrated by selective angiography in a patient with transmural myocardial infarction. Am J Cardiol 31: 785, 1973
16. Khan AH, Haywood LJ: Myocardial infarction in nine patients with radiographically patent coronary arteries. N Engl J Med 291: 427, 1974
17. Brest AN, Wiener L, Kasparian H, Duca P, Rafter JJ: Myocardial infarction without obstructive coronary artery disease. Am Heart J 88: 219, 1974
18. Richardson PM, Gotsman MS: Angiographic evidence of coronary embolism and resolution. S Afr Med J 45: 805, 1971
19. Cheng TO, Bashour T, Singh BK, Kelser GA: Myocardial infarction in the absence of coronary arteriosclerosis. Result of spasm? Am J Cardiol 30: 680, 1972
20. O'Reilly RJ, Spellberg RD: Rapid resolution of coronary arterial emboli. Myocardial infarction and subsequent normal coronary arteriograms. Ann Intern Med 81: 348, 1974
21. Regan TJ, Wu CF, Weisse AB, Moschos CB, Ahmed SS, Lyons MM: Acute myocardial infarction in toxic cardiomyopathy without coronary obstruction. Circulation 51: 453, 1975
22. Eusterman JH, Achor RWP, Kincaid OW, Brown AL: Atherosclerotic disease of the coronary arteries. A pathologic-radiologic correlative study. Circulation 26: 1288, 1962
23. Vlodaver Z, Frech R, Van Tassel RA, Edwards JE: Correlation of antemortem coronary arteriogram and the postmortem specimen. Circulation 47: 162, 1973
24. Prinzmetal M, Kennamer R, Merliss R, Wada T, Bor N: Angina pectoris. I. A variant form of angina pectoris: Preliminary report. Am J Med 27: 375, 1959
25. Gubbay ER: Prinzmetal's variant angina. Can Med Assoc J 83: 164, 1960
26. Prinzmetal M, Ekmekci A, Kennamer R, Kwoczynski JK, Shubin H, Toyoshima H: Variant form of angina pectoris. Previously undelineated syndrome. JAMA 174: 102, 1960
27. Peretz DI: Variant angina pectoris of Prinzmetal. Can Med Assoc J 85: 1101, 1961
28. Robinson JS: Prinzmetal's variant angina pectoris. Report of a case. Am Heart J 70: 797, 1965
29. Hilal H, Massumi R: Variant angina pectoris. Am J Cardiol 19: 607, 1967
30. Gianelly R, Mugler F, Harrison DC: Prinzmetal's variant of angina pectoris with only slight coronary atherosclerosis. Calif Med 108: 129, 1968
31. Gillilan RE, Hawley RR, Warbasse JR: Second degree heart block occurring in a patient with Prinzmetal's variant angina. Am Heart J 77: 380, 1969
32. Whiting RB, Klein MD, Vander Veer J, Lown B: Variant angina pectoris. N Engl J Med 282: 709, 1970
33. Silverman ME, Flamm MD: Variant angina pectoris. Anatomic findings and prognostic implications. Ann Intern Med 75: 339, 1971
34. Dhurandhar RW, Watt DL, Silver MD, Trimble AS, Adelman AG: Prinzmetal's variant form of angina with arteriographic evidence of coronary arterial spasm. Am J Cardiol 30: 902, 1972
35. Cosby RS, Giddings JA, See JR, Mayo M: Variant angina. Case reports and critique. Am J Med 53: 739, 1972
36. Laks MM, Dahlgren J, Mandel, WJ: Variant angina pectoris. Ann Intern Med 78: 309, 1973
37. Cheng TO, Bashour T, Kelser GA, Weiss L, Bacos J: Variant angina of Prinzmetal with normal coronary arteriograms. A variant of the variant. Circulation 47: 476, 1973
38. Oliva PB, Potts DE, Pluss RG: Coronary arterial spasm in Prinzmetal angina. Documentation by coronary arteriography. N Engl J Med 288: 745, 1973
39. MacAlpin RN, Kattus AA, Alvaro AB: Angina pectoris at rest with preservation of exercise capacity. Prinzmetal's variant angina. Circulation 47: 946, 1973
40. King MJ, Zir LM, Kaltman AJ, Fox AC: Variant angina associated with angiographically demonstrated coronary artery spasm and REM sleep. Am J Med Sci 265: 419, 1973
41. Levi GF, Proto C: Ventricular fibrillation in the course of Prinzmetal's angina pectoris. Report of two cases. Br Heart J 35: 601, 1973
42. MacMillan RM, Rose FD, Flinghoffer JF, Frankl WS: Variant angina pectoris. Cardiol 58: 306, 1973
43. Kristian-Kerin N, Davies B, Macleod CA: Nonocclusive coronary disease associated with Prinzmetal's angina pectoris. Chest 64: 352, 1973
44. Hart NJ, Silverman ME, King SB: Variant angina pectoris caused by coronary artery spasm. Am J Med 56: 269, 1974
45. Gorfinkel HJ, Inglesby TV, Lansing AM, Goodin RR: ST-segment elevation, transient left-posterior hemiblock, and recurrent ventricular arrhythmias unassociated with pain. A variant of Prinzmetal's angina syndrome. Ann Intern Med 79: 795, 1973
46. Betriu A, Solignac A, Bourassa MG: The variant form of angina: Diagnostic and therapeutic implications. Am Heart J 87: 272, 1974
47. Bodenheimer M, Lipski J, Donoso E, Dack S: Prinzmetal's variant angina: A clinical and electrocardiographic study. Am Heart J 87: 304, 1974
48. Schroeder JS, Silverman FJ, Harrison DC: Right coronary arterial spasm causing Prinzmetal's variant angina. Chest 65: 573, 1974
49. Sweet RL, Sheffield LT: Myocardial infarction after exercise-induced electrocardiographic changes in a patient with variant angina pectoris. Am J Cardiol 33: 813, 1974
50. Nevins MA: Variant variant angina pectoris. Ann Intern Med 80: 673, 1974
51. Choquet Y, Proulx J, Primeau R, Lapointe L, Levy R: Coronary hypertonia and angina. Can Med Assoc J 111: 161, 1974
52. Kerin N, Macleod CA: Coronary artery spasm associated with variant angina pectoris. Br Heart J 36: 224, 1974
53. Rose FJ, Johnson AD, Carleton RA: Spasm of the left anterior descending coronary artery. Chest 66: 719, 1974
54. Applefield MM, Ronan JA: Prinzmetal's angina with extensive spasm of the right coronary artery. Chest 66: 721, 1974
55. Donsky MS, Harris MD, Curry GC, Blomqvist CG, Willerson JT,

Mullins CB: Variant angina pectoris: A clinical and coronary arteriographic spectrum. Am Heart J 89: 571, 1975
56. Gaasch WH, Adyanthaya AV, Wang VH, Pickering E, Quinones MA, Alexander JK: Prinzmetal's variant angina: Hemodynamic and angiographic observations during pain. Am J Cardiol 35: 683, 1975
57. Meller J, Conde CA, Donoso E, Dack S: Transient Q waves in Prinzmetal's angina. Am J Cardiol 35: 691, 1975
58. Lange RL, Reid MS, Tresch DD, Keelan MH, Bernhard VM, Coolidge G: Nonatheromatous ischemic heart disease following withdrawal from chronic industrial nitroglycerin exposure. Circulation 46: 666, 1972
59. Harrison CV: Experimental pulmonary atherosclerosis. J Pathol Bacteriol 60: 289, 1948

Atherosclerotic Narrowing
of the Left Main Coronary Artery

A Necropsy Analysis of 152 Patients with Fatal Coronary Heart Disease and Varying Degrees of Left Main Narrowing

BERNADINE H. BULKLEY, M.D., AND WILLIAM C. ROBERTS, M.D.

SUMMARY Histologic sections of the left main (LM) and the other three major coronary arteries were studied in 152 patients. The lumen of the LM in 35 patients was >75% narrowed; in thirty, 50–75%; and in 87, <50% narrowed. The patients with >75% narrowing were younger. Angina pectoris and hyperlipoproteinemia, specifically type II, were more common ($P < 0.02$) and acute transmural and healed subendocardial myocardial infarcts were less frequent ($P < 0.05$) in the patients with >75% LM narrowing than in those with <50% narrowing. Of the three other major coronary arteries, the average number narrowed in the patients with >75% LM narrowing was 2.9; in those with 50–75% LM narrowing, 2.7, and in those with <50% LM narrowing, 2.4. Of the 35 patients with >75% LM narrowing, 33 had >75% luminal narrowing of each of the other three major coronary arteries. Narrowing of the LM, therefore, indicates severe narrowing of usually all major coronary arteries.

SEVERAL ANGIOGRAPHIC STUDIES focusing on the significance of 50% or greater narrowing of the left main (LM) coronary artery have appeared during the past four years.[1-13] None of these studies, however, compared the various cardiac observations in the patients with severe LM coronary narrowing by angiography to observations in patients with lesser degrees of LM narrowing. Necropsy studies focusing on the LM coronary artery in patients with coronary heart disease have not appeared. This report attempts to fill this void by describing certain clinical and morphologic findings in 152 necropsy patients with symptomatic coronary heart disease and varying degrees of narrowing of the LM coronary artery. Observations in the patients with severe (>75%) LM narrowing are compared to those in patients with lesser degrees of LM narrowing.

Methods

In this laboratory the major extramural coronary arteries of patients with ischemic heart disease are subserially sectioned in the following manner.[14] The arteries are excised from the heart intact, fixed in formalin, decalcified, cut at 5 mm intervals, processed in alcohol and xylene, and two histologic sections are prepared from each 5 mm segment. One section is stained by hematoxylin-eosin and the second by Movat's stain. The coronary arteries in approximately 250 patients with ischemic heart disease have been prepared now in this manner. The sections from these 250 patients were re-examined and those patients in whom sections were available for re-examination of all four major coronary arteries were included in this study. On the basis of histologic study of the cross-sections of left main coronary artery, the patients were divided into three groups, each determined by the maximal degree of LM narrowing: 1) >75% cross-sectional area narrowing; 2) 50–75% narrowing; and 3)

<50% narrowing. The clinical and necropsy records of the patients with adequate sections of all four major coronary arteries were then examined. Patients with significant valvular or congenital heart disease or nonatherosclerotic type coronary disease, for example, coronary embolism, were excluded from this study.

A total of 152 patients with adequate sections of each of the four major coronary arteries and without associated heart disease, other than systemic hypertension, were found and form the study group for this analysis.

Results

Of the 152 patients, the cross-sectional area of the lumen of the LM coronary artery was >75% narrowed in 35 patients (23%), 50–75% narrowed in 30 patients (20%), and <50% narrowed in 87 patients (57%) (tables 1 and 2).

Clinical Findings (table 1)

The average age of the 35 patients with >75% LM narrowing was lower (53 years) than in either of the two groups with lesser degrees of LM narrowing (both 59 years). The sex ratio was similar in all three groups (males: females = 3:1). The frequencies of histories of acute myocardial infarcts which healed, congestive cardiac failure and diabetes mellitus were similar in all three groups. The frequency of angina pectoris, however, differed significantly ($P < 0.02$) between those with severe LM narrowing and those without: 66% in the group with >75% and 40% in the group with <50% LM narrowing. Serum cholesterol and triglyceride levels were available in 83 of the 152 patients. (Most of these determinations were done in the Laboratory of the Molecular Disease Branch of the National Heart and Lung Institute formerly under the direction of Doctors Donald S. Fredrickson and Robert I. Levy.) Hyperlipoproteinemia was significantly ($P < 0.01$) more frequent in the patients with >75% LM narrowing than in those with <50% LM narrowing (43% to 16%). Of the 22 patients with type II hyperlipoproteinemia, 11 (50%) had >75% LM narrowing, and of the 12 patients with type IV, three had >75% LM narrowing. Death in all 152 patients was related to ischemic heart disease. Death occurred during or within three days

From the Section of Pathology, National Heart and Lung Institute, National Institutes of Health, Bethesda, Maryland.

Dr. Bulkley's present address is Division of Cardiology, Department of Medicine, The Johns Hopkins Hospital, Baltimore, Maryland.

Address for reprints: Dr. William C. Roberts, Building 10A, Room 3E30, NIH, Bethesda, Maryland 20014.

Received November 18, 1975; revision accepted for publication December 26, 1975.

TABLE 1. *Clinical Observations in Ischemic Heart Disease with Varying Degrees of Left Main Coronary Narrowing (152 Necropsy Patients)*

	Degree of left main narrowing			
	>75%	50–75%	<50%	Totals
Number patients	35	30	87	152
Ages (years); range (avg.)	28–80 (53)	29–91 (59)	26–85 (59)	26–91 (57)
Males: females	25:9	20:10	68:19	113:38
Angina pectoris	23 (66%)*	15 (50%)	35 (40%)*	73 (48%)
Clinical acute MI → healed	16 (46%)	11 (37%)	33 (38%)	60 (40%)
Systemic hypertension	16 (46%)	12 (40%)	55 (62%)	83 (54%)
Diabetes mellitus	8 (23%)	11 (37%)	28 (32%)	47 (31%)
Normal lipoprotein pattern	10 (29%)	7 (23%)	17 (20%)	34 (22%)
Unknown lipoprotein pattern	10 (29%)	15 (50%)	56 (64%)	81 (53%)
Hyperlipoproteinemia	15 (43%)*	8 (27%)	14 (16%)	37 (25%)
Type II	11 (31%)*	3 (10%)	8 (9%)	22 (14%)
Type III	1 (3%)	0	2 (2%)	3 (2%)
Type IV	3 (9%)	5 (17%)	4 (5%)	12 (8%)
Cause of death				
Acute MI	12 (34%)*	13 (43%)	49 (56%)*	74 (49%)
Sudden (coronary)	8 (23%)	7 (23%)	24 (28%)	39 (25%)
Coronary bypass operation	8 (23%)	5 (17%)	4 (5%)	17 (11%)
Congestive heart failure	1 (3%)	3 (10%)	3 (3%)	7 (5%)
LV aneurysmectomy	0	0	3 (3%)	3 (2%)
Cardiac catheterization	3/15 (3%)	0	1/17 (1%)	4/32 (3%)
Non-cardiac	3 (9%)	2 (7%)	3 (3%)	8† (5%)

*Comparison between patients with >75% to those with <50% left main narrowing is significant ($P < 0.05$).
†Seven of these 8 patients had previous clinical evidence of ischemic heart disease.
Note: The percentages refer to the number of patients present in a particular vertical column and they are not applicable horizontally.
Abbreviations: MI = myocardial infarction; LV = left ventricle.

after cardiac catheterization in three (20%) of 15 patients with >75% LM narrowing, and in one (6%) of 17 with <50% narrowing of the LM coronary artery. Of the 17 patients who died during or shortly after a coronary operation, eight had >75% narrowing of the LM coronary artery.

Necropsy Findings (table 2)

The 35 patients with >75% narrowing of the LM had significantly ($P < 0.01$) more narrowing of the other three major coronary arteries than did the patients with <50% narrowing of the LM: an average of 2.9 of the right, left anterior descending and left circumflex compared to 2.4. In the 35 patients with >75% LM narrowing, 94% had >75% narrowing of each of the other three major coronary arteries, whereas 53% of the group with <50% LM narrowing had similarly severe disease. The group with 50 to 75% narrowing of the LM fell midway between the other two groups in severity of atherosclerotic narrowing of the other

TABLE 2. *Necropsy Observations in Ischemic Heart Disease with Varying Degrees of Left Main Coronary Narrowing (152 Necropsy Patients)*

	Degree of left main narrowing			
	>75%	50–75%	<50%	Totals
Number patients	35	30	87	152
Coronary arteries				
LAD >75% narrowed	35 (100%)	30 (100%)	72 (83%)	137 (90%)
LC >75%	33 (94%)*	23 (77%)	66 (76%)*	122 (80%)
Right (Rt) >75%	34 (97%)*	28 (93%)	65 (75%)*	127 (84%)
LAD, LC & Rt >75%	33 (94%)*	23 (77%)	46 (53%)*	102 (67%)
Avg. no. of LAD, LC,				
& Rt >75% narrowed	2.9*	2.7	2.4*	2.5
Myocardium				
Acute MI	15 (43%)*	17 (57%)	56 (64%)*	88 (58%)
Transmural	11 (31%)*	11 (31%)	54 (62%)*	76 (50%)
Subendocardial	4 (11%)	6 (20%)	2 (2%)	12 (8%)
Healed MI	22 (63%)	20 (67%)	52 (60%)	94 (62%)
Transmural	9 (26%)	12 (40%)	36 (42%)	57 (38%)
Subendocardial	13 (37%)*	8 (27%)	16 (18%)*	47 (31%)
Heart weight (g)				
Range	300–600	300–640	300–750	300–750
Average M:F	416:353	489:403	479:423	467:401
M >400	15/25 (60%)	16/21 (76%)	55/66 (83%)	86/112 (77%)
F >350	6/8 (75%)	5/9 (56%)	13/18 (72%)	24/35 (69%)

*Comparison between patients with >75% to those with <50% left main narrowing is significant ($P < 0.05$).
Note: The percentages refer to the number of patients in a particular vertical column and they are not applicable horizontally.
Abbreviations: F = female; M = male; LAD = left anterior descending; LC = left circumflex; MI = myocardial infarction.

three major extramural coronary arteries. No patient had total occlusion (100% narrowing) of the LM coronary artery. The frequency of transmural left ventricular myocardial scars was similar in the three groups; in contrast, subendocardial scars were significantly ($P < 0.05$) more frequent in the 35 patients with >75% LM narrowing compared to the 87 with <50% LM narrowing (37% to 18%). Acute myocardial infarcts of the transmural type (not of the subendocardial type) were significantly ($P < 0.01$) less frequent in the patients with >75% LM narrowing compared to those with <50% LM narrowing (31% to 62%). Sections of the four major coronary arteries in one patient with severe narrowing of the LM are shown in figure 1.

Comments

The first two studies,[1,2] both appearing in 1972, on patients with 50% or greater narrowing of the left main (LM) coronary artery by angiography emphasized a high frequency in these patients of severe angina pectoris, particularly crescendo and rest types, a high frequency of a highly positive exercise test, an increased mortality during or shortly following both cardiac catheterization and aortocoronary bypass procedures, and a generally poor prognosis (table 3). Subsequent studies[3-13] of patients with 50% or greater narrowing of the LM coronary artery by angiography (summarized in table 3) demonstrated a poorer prognosis in the patients with 50% or greater LM narrowing managed medically than in those treated by aorto-coronary bypass operations, but an increased mortality during or shortly after cardiac catheterization has not been confirmed. It is now generally recognized that there are no clinical parameters which indicate "significant" LM coronary narrowing. Indeed, coronary angiography is the only means of clinically diagnosing "significant" LM coronary narrowing.

The observations (summarized in table 3) on patients with 50% or greater narrowing of the LM coronary artery by angiography were not compared to findings in patients with <50% narrowing of the LM coronary artery. Naturally the frequency of angina pectoris was high (94%) (table 3) in these patients because this symptom was the one usually prompting the angiographic study. The present study, however, does show that among necropsy patients with coronary heart disease, the frequency of angina pectoris is significantly ($P < 0.02$) higher in those with >75% LM narrowing than in those with <50% LM narrowing (66% to 40%).

Death during or shortly after cardiac catheterization occurred in three of 15 patients (20%) with >75% LM narrowing in the present necropsy study and in only one of 17 patients (6%) with <50% LM narrowing. In contrast, death during or shortly after cardiac catheterization (angiography) occurred in 18 (3%) of the 561 patients reported with 50% or greater narrowing of the LM by angiography (table 3). More recent studies[6, 8-13] of patients with >50% LM narrowing by angiography have not shown an increased mortality during cardiac catheterization in these patients (table 3).

The mortality during or shortly after aorto-coronary bypass operations in the patients with significant LM narrowing may be higher than in the patients with lesser degrees of LM narrowing. Of the 235 reported patients with 50% or greater narrowing of the LM coronary artery by angiography and in whom this procedure was performed (table 3), 30 (13%) died during or in the early postoperative period. In the present necropsy study, of the 17 patients who underwent aorto-coronary bypass operations, eight had >75% LM narrowing and four had <50% LM narrowing.

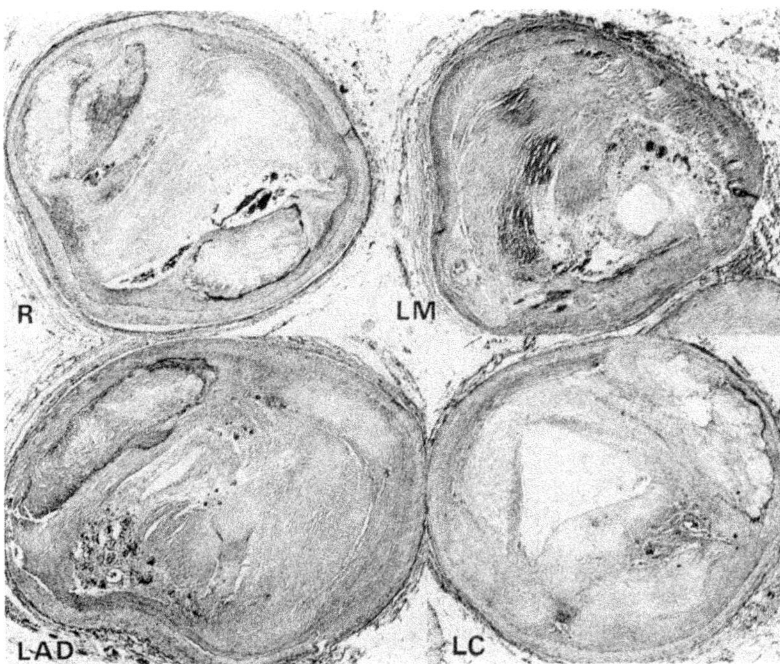

FIGURE 1. *Photomicrographs of histologic sections of coronary arteries in a 57-year-old man (A72-78) who died 24 hours after aorto-coronary arterial bypass operation for severe angina pectoris. All four major coronary arteries were >75% narrowed by atherosclerotic plaques. The section of right (R) coronary artery is approximately 3 cm from its aortic ostium. The sections of the left anterior descending (LAD) and left circumflex (LC) are immediately distal to their origins from the left main (LM). Movat stains (R, LC and LAD); hematoxylin and eosin stain (LM): ×24 (R and LC); ×27 (LM); ×31 (LAD).*

TABLE 3. *Observations in Reported Patients with 50% or Greater Narrowing of the Left Main Coronary Artery by Angiography*

	Cohen and Gorlin[11] (1972 + 1975)	Lavine et al[2] (Dec 1972)	Zeft et al[8] (Jan 1974)	Khaja et al[5] (Aug 1974)	Lim. Proudfit Sones[9] (Aug 1975)	De Mots et al[10] (Aug 1975)	Talano et al[12] (Aug 1975)	Sung et al[13] (Aug 1975)	Totals
Degree of CA narrowing	50% or >	70% or >	75% or >	50% or >*	50% or >	50% or >	>50%	50% or >	—
Number of patients	73	30	56	28	141	58	145	30	561
Angina pectoris	68(93%)	27(90%)	56(100%)	28(100%)	120(85%)	55	141(97%)	30(100%)	525(94%)
Congestive heart failure	4(5%)	—	3(5%)	5(18%)	13(9%)	—	—	—	25/298(8%)
↓LV contractility	43(59%)	24/29(86%)	34(61%)	17(60%)	52/119(44%)	—	110(76%)	27(90%)	327/480(68%)
Abnormality in other 3 CAs									
(Rt., LAD, LC)	49(67%)	29(97%)†		18(64%)	71(50%)	28(49%)		27(90%)	
2 vessel	14(19%)	0	53(95%)‡	10(36%)	41(29%)	18(31%)	140(97%)	2(7%)	540(96%)
1 vessel	4(6%)	1		0	25(18%)	10(17%)			
0 vessel	6(8%)	0	3(5%)	0	4(3%)	2(2%)	5(3%)	1(3%)	21(4%)
% of all patients undergoing CA angiography	4%¶	—	2%	—	6%	2%	—	—	4%
Ages: range (avg.)	32–75(52)	40–70(54)	39–66(55)	34–64(53)	26–72(52)	—	—(55)	40–71(54)	26–75(53)
M:F	61:12	25:5	47:9	22:6	133:8	—	126:19	20:10	434:69(6:1)
Hypertension	—	—	—	—	48(34%)	16	—	9(30%)	73/229(32%)
Hypercholesterolemia	—	13§	—	—	—	23/40	—	10(33%)	46/100(46%)
OMI (history)	—	19(63%)	—	11(39%)	—	14	—		113/332(34%)
OMI (ECG)	26(36%)	19(63%)	—	—	—	11	—	17(57%)	
Normal ECG	—	2(7%)	—	—	40	12	—	—	69/229(30%)
Abnormal stress ECG	34/42(81%)	—	—	14/18(77%)	55	14/19(74%)	—	—	62/79(79%)
Calcium in LM CA	—	7(23%)**	—	—	—	12(21%)	—	—	19/88(22%)
Deaths peri-catheterization	6††	3(10%)	0	0	3‡‡	1¶¶	5(3%)§§	0	18/561(3%)
Deaths peri-CABP	—	2/18(11%)	6(11%)	7/25(28%)***	—	4/28(14%)†††	10/89(11%)	1/19(5%)	30/235(13%)

*75% or greater narrowing in 25 of the 28 patients. †Eight of the 30 had total occlusion of the right coronary artery and > 70% of the left main.‡ > 75% narrowed. ¶Two percent in 1964–71 series and 8% in 1971–73 series.§ > 275 mg/100 ml. **Image intensification fluoroscopy. ††Only 1 death in last 41 studies. ‡‡All before 1967. ¶¶In 83 angiographic procedures. §§No deaths in last 18 months. ***Three of the 7 deaths also had ventricular aneurysmectomy. †††Only 1 death in last 24 patients.

Abbreviations: CA = coronary artery; CABP = coronary-artery-bypass operation; F = female; LAD = left anterior descending; LC = left circumflex; LM = left main; LV = left ventricular; M = male; OMI = old myocardial infarction; Rt = right.

These numbers also suggest that mortality from this procedure is increased in the individuals with greater LM narrowing. Despite its probable higher mortality, this operation has usually achieved striking symptomatic benefit to the patients with both severe and less severe LM narrowing, and also survival is prolonged in the patients with significant LM narrowing by angiography compared to those treated medically.[10-13]

An observation in the present study, not commented on in previous angiographic studies (table 3), is the increased frequency of type II hyperlipoproteinemia among the patients with >75% LM narrowing compared to the patients with <50% LM narrowing. Of our 22 patients with documented type II hyperlipoproteinemia, 11 (50%) had >75% LM narrowing; of the 12 with type IV, 25% had similar LM narrowing, and of the 34 patients with known normal lipoprotein patterns, 29% had >75% LM narrowing. Hypercholesterolemia has been mentioned in three previous studies of patients with LM narrowing by angiography of 50% or greater:[2, 10, 13] of 100 patients with >50% LM narrowing by angiography and serum cholesterol determinations, 46% had elevated (>265 mg/100 ml) levels (table 3). It is likely that most of these 46 patients also had type II hyperlipoproteinemia.

More severe atherosclerosis in the ascending portion than in the descending portion of aorta has been observed in patients with the homozygous variety of type II hyperlipoproteinemia.[15, 16] It is our impression that the amount of atherosclerosis in the ascending aorta also is greater in patients with the heterozygous form of type II hyperlipoproteinemia compared to patients with type IV hyperlipoproteinemia or to patients with normal lipoprotein patterns.[15, 16] In the heterozygous patients, however, the atherosclerosis in the ascending aorta is not nearly as extensive as in the abdominal aorta.[15, 16] Whenever the ascending aorta is involved by atherosclerotic plaques, it would appear reasonable that extension into the proximal portions of the coronary arteries would be more frequent. Of our 22 patients with type II hyperlipoproteinemia, one was a homozygote and both his LM and proximal right coronary arteries were narrowed >75%.[15, 16] Severe (>75%) narrowing of the LM coronary artery also was present in 10 of the 21 patients with the heterozygous form of type II hyperlipoproteinemia.

All previous angiographic studies on patients with >50% LM coronary narrowing have demonstrated extensive disease in one or more of the other three major coronary arteries[1-13] (table 3). Most commonly, significant lesions were demonstrated in the left anterior descending, followed by left circumflex and, lastly, the right coronary artery. It is most unusual for a significant lesion to be present in only one of the other three major coronary arteries when the LM is significantly narrowed, and it is very rare for the LM to be the only major artery significantly involved. Indeed, in only 21 (4%) of the 561 reported patients with 50% or greater LM narrowing by angiography was the LM the only major coronary artery involved (table 3). None of our patients studied at necropsy had severe coronary narrowing limited to the LM. Of our 35 patients with >75% LM narrowing, 94% also had >75% narrowing of the right, left anterior descending

and left circumflex coronary arteries. In contrast, of the 87 patients with <50% LM narrowing, 53% had >75% narrowing of each of the other three major coronary arteries. Thus, marked narrowing of the LM coronary artery is indicative of severe, diffuse coronary atherosclerosis, and may account for the poor prognosis of these patients.[17]

Myocardial damage is frequent in patients with significant LM coronary arterial narrowing. Among the previously reported patients with 50% or greater narrowing of the LM by angiography (table 3), 327 (68%) of the 480 patients with left ventricular angiography had either focal or diffuse abnormalities in left ventricular contraction. Among our 152 necropsy patients, 94 (62%) had subendocardial or transmural left ventricular scars; the percent with transmural scars was not significantly different among the three groups but the percent with subendocardial scars was significantly greater in the patients with >75% LM narrowing compared to the patients with <50% LM narrowing (37% to 18%). In contrast, acute myocardial infarcts (myocardial necrosis contrasted to fibrosis) were observed in 88 (58%) of the 152 patients and the percent with transmural necrosis was significantly less among the patients with >75% LM narrowing contrasted to the patients with <50% LM narrowing. Overt chronic congestive cardiac failure was present in 25 (8%) of the 298 patients previously reported with LM narrowing of 50% or greater by angiography (table 3), and it was severe in 5% of our necropsy patients, not significantly different in any of the three groups.

References

1. Cohen MV, Cohn PF, Herman MV, Gorlin R: Diagnosis and prognosis of main left coronary artery obstruction. Circulation 45 (suppl I): I-57, 1972
2. Lavine P, Kimbiris D, Segal BL, Linhart JW: Left main coronary artery disease. Clinical, arteriographic and hemodynamic appraisal. Am J Cardiol 30: 791, 1972
3. Bruschke AVG, Proudfit WL, Sones FM Jr: Progress study of 590 consecutive nonsurgical cases of coronary disease followed 5–9 years. I. Arteriographic correlations. Circulation 47: 1147, 1973
4. Gotsman MS, Lewis BS, Bakst A: Obstruction of the left main coronary artery — the artery of sudden death. S Afr Med J 47: 641, 1973
5. Khaja F-U, Sharma SD, Easley RM Jr, Heinle RA, Goldstein S: Left main coronary artery lesions. Risks of catheterizations: Exercise testing and surgery. Circulation 49 (suppl II): II-136, 1974
6. Crochet D, Petitclerc R, Campeau L: Left main coronary artery stenosis: Significance of degree of obstruction, associated involvement of other coronary arteries and of status of left ventricular contraction as related to surgery (147 cases). (abstr) Circulation 49 (suppl III): III-111, 1974
7. Saint Pierre A, Amiel M, Jamet Ch, Perrin A: Signification des stenoses atheromateuses du trone commun de la coronaire gauche. Arch Mal Coeur 67: 1305, 1974
8. Zeft HJ, Manley JC, Huston JH, Tector AJ, Auer JE, Johnson WD: Left main coronary artery stenosis. Results of coronary bypass surgery. Circulation 49: 68, 1974
9. Lim JS, Proudfit WL, Sones FM Jr: Left main coronary arterial obstruction: long-term follow-up of 141 nonsurgical cases. Am J Cardiol 36: 131, 1975
10. DeMots H, Bonchek LI, Rösch J, Anderson RP, Starr A, Rahimtoola SH: Left main coronary artery disease. Risks of angiography, importance of coexisting disease of other coronary arteries and effects of revascularization. Am J Cardiol 36: 136, 1975
11. Cohen MV, Gorlin R: Main left coronary artery disease. Clinical experience from 1964–1974. Circulation 52: 275, 1975
12. Talano JV, Scanlon PJ, Meadows WR, Kahn M, Pifarre R, Gunnar RM: Influence of surgery on survival in 145 patients with left main coronary artery disease. Circulation 52 (suppl I): I-105, 1975
13. Sung RJ, Mallon SM, Richter SE, Ghahramani AE, Sommer LS, Kaiser GA, Myerburg RJ: Left main coronary artery obstruction. Follow-up of thirty patients with and without surgery. Circulation 52 (suppl I): I-112, 1975

14. Roberts WC, Buja LM: The frequency and significance of coronary arterial thrombi and other observations in fatal acute myocardial infarction. A study of 107 necropsy patients. Am J Med 52: 425, 1972

15. Roberts WC, Ferrans VJ, Levy RI, Fredrickson DS: Cardiovascular pathology in hyperlipoproteinemia. Anatomic observations in 42 necropsy patients with normal or abnormal serum lipoprotein patterns. Am J Cardiol 31: 557, 1973

16. Roberts WC: The status of the coronary arteries in fatal ischemic heart disease. *In* Innovations in the Diagnosis and Management of Acute Myocardial Infarction, edited by Brest AN, Wiener L, Chung EK, Kasparian H. Philadelphia, FA Davis, 1975, p 1

17. Takaro T, Hultgren HN, Detre KM: VA Cooperative study of coronary arterial surgery. II. Left main disease. (abstr) Circulation 52 (suppl II): II-143, 1975

ANGIOGRAPHICALLY NORMAL ARTERIES AFTER HEALING OF ACUTE MYOCARDIAL INFARCTION

BY ERNEST N. ARNETT, M.D. AND WILLIAM C. ROBERTS, M.D.

During the past eight years there have been reports in the scientific literature of individual patients or small groups of patients who suffered acute myocardial infarctions but in whom subsequent examination by coronary angiography showed what appeared to be normal coronary arteries. The possible occurrence of "myocardial infarction in patients with normal coronary arteriograms" has generated considerable interest and speculation. In this article, Drs. Arnett and Roberts review the published literature and offer their own explanation for this seemingly contradictory phenomenon.

INTRODUCTION

A number of necropsy studies have shown that among patients with fatal coronary heart disease

Dr. Arnett is staff associate, Section of Pathology, National Heart and Lung Institute, Bethesda, Md.

Dr. Roberts is chief, Section of Pathology, National Heart and Lung Institute.

From the Section of Pathology, National Heart and Lung Institute, National Institutes of Health, Bethesda, Md.

(CHD) at least one and usually two of the three major coronary arteries are more than 75 per cent narrowed by old atherosclerotic plaques.[1,2] The introduction of selective coronary angiography[3] allowed visualization of coronary vessels during life, and this technique has demonstrated coronary narrowing in patients with *symtomatic* CHD as severe as that shown by necropsy in patient with *fatal* CHD.[1-6] Coronary angiography in patients with CHD manifested by acute myocardial infarction (AMI) has disclosed the following: (1) when performed at the time of AMI, coronary angiography has always disclosed severe narrowing or complete obstruction of at least one of three major coronary arteries; (2) when performed at the time of AMI, coronary angiography has never demonstrated a normal coronary arterial tree; and (3) when performed after healing of an AMI, coronary angiography has usually (in more than 99 per cent of cases) demonstrated severe narrowing of one or more of the three major coronary arteries and rarely (in less than 1 per cent) a normal coronary arterial tree.

In recent years much attention has been given to this latter small group of patients with "myocardial infarction and angiographically normal coronary arteries.[7-26] A major implication of most of these reports is that AMI may occur in the presence of normal coronary arteries. This article will examine this implication and discuss possible explanations for the occurrence of "myocardial infarction and normal coronary arteriograms."

NORMAL CORONARY ARTERIES and AMI

In 52 reported patients with "myocardial infarction and angiograhically normal coronary arteries" (Tables I and II), the AMI was produced at the time of cardiac catheterization in five (Table II); in four of these, coronary angiography performed at that time demonstrated totally obstructed coronary arteries. Repeat catheterization in all five patients

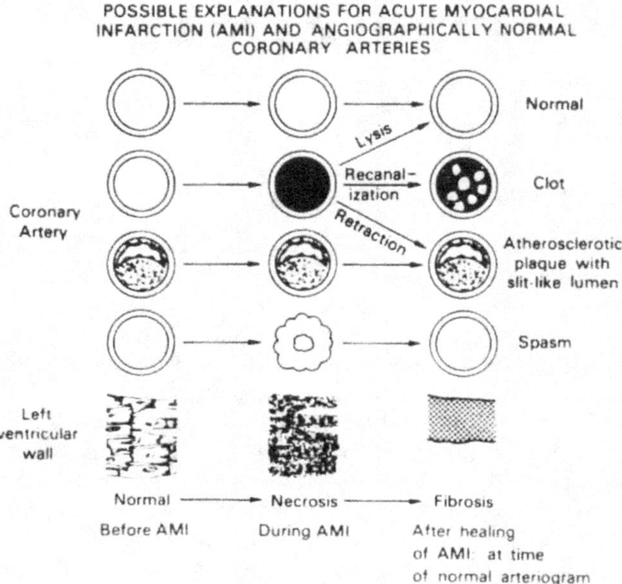

Figure 1. Diagramatic portrayal of possible appearances of the epicardial coronary arteries and left-ventricular myocardium in patients with acute myocardial infarction (AMI) and subsequently normal coronary arteries. The left vertical column indicates the status of the coronary arteries and myocardium before the AMI; the center vertical column, during the AMI, and the right vertical column, after healing of the AMI. If the AMI was caused by a condition affecting only the intramyocardial arteries or by a disproportion between the size of the coronary bed and the amount of myocardium to be oxygenated, the coronary arteries presumably would be normal (top row) at the time of myocardial necrosis as well as before and subsequently. Coronary angiography may show a slitlike eccentric lumen (third row) to be "normal." If spasm caused the AMI, one or more coronary arteries might be partly obstructed at the time of the AMI (fourth row). If embolism caused the AMI (second row), the clot could subsequently lyse, recanalize, or retract along one side, allowing the lumen to be of sufficient size to appear later as "angiographically normal."

at later times, however, disclosed angiographically normal coronary arteries. In the other 47 patients (Table I), AMI was unrelated to cardiac catheterization; none of them had coronary angiography at the time of the AMI. In 46 of the 47 patients the interval between the onset of the AMI and the performance of coronary angiography was longer than one month. Thus, the status of the coronary arteries *at the time of* acute myocardial necrosis is still uncertain. Indeed, *a normal coronary arterial tree has never been demonstrated by angiography at the time of AMI.*

How, then, may the coronary tree be entirely normal at angiography after healing of an AMI? At least six explanations need consideration (Fig. 1):

1. *AMI never occurred.* Diagnosis of the myocardial insult, in other words was incorrect. Documentation of AMI by electrocardiograms and enzyme elevations, however, appeared adequate in all 52 reported patients. Thus, this explanation appears

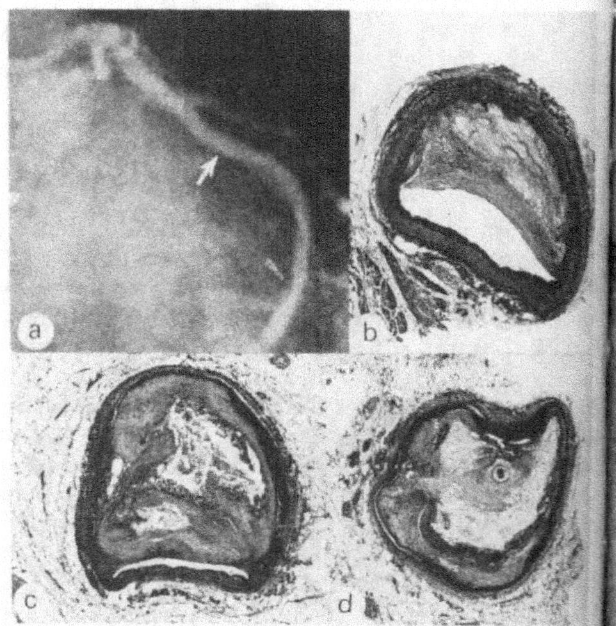

Figure 2. Coronary angiogram two months before death and histologic sections of the coronary arteries in a 61-year-old man (A74-245) who died following aortic valve replacement and insertion of a saphenous vein aortocoronary artery bypass graft. (a) Left circumflex coronary artery, which appeared "normal" angiographically. (b) Histologic section of the narrowed left circumflex coronary artery at the arrow between the atrial and obtuse marginal branches. The lumens of the proximal portions of the left anterior descending (c) and right (d) coronary arteries also were severely narrowed by atherosclerotic plaque. Presumably, the circumflex lesion was missed angiographically because the residual lumen had been viewed only in its widest diameter.

unlikely. It is presumed, however, that the infarcts were transmural rather than nontransmural.

2. Too large a myocardial mass, too little hemo-

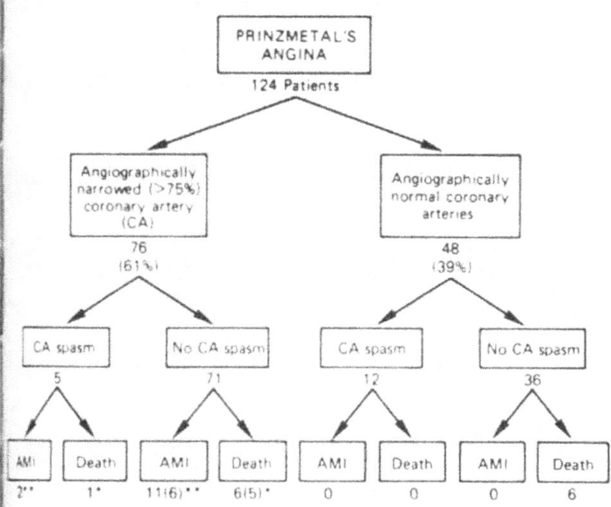

*Death in each followed aorto coronary bypass operations
**The non-fatal acute myocardial infarction (AMI) followed aorto coronary bypass operations

Figure 3. Frequency of coronary spasm, acute myocardial infarction, and death in 124 reported patients with Prinzmetal's angina and coronary arteriography.

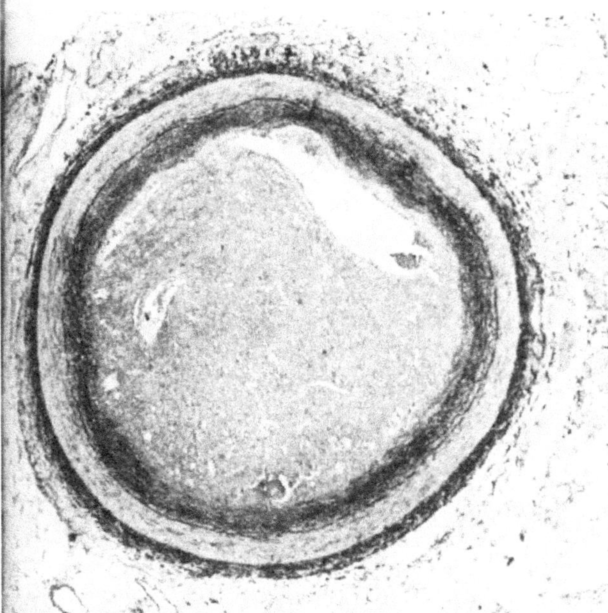

Figure 4. Embolus to right coronary artery in a 56-year-old man (A70-244). Embolism occurred during cardiac catheterization 31 days before death and caused transmural necrosis of the posterior left-ventricular wall. The artery, before being occluded by the embolus, was normal. Partial organization and retraction of the clot have resulted in an eccentric lumen (elastic van Gieson stain x25).

globin, or too low a perfusion pressure (shock) was present to supply the myocardium by a normal coronary tree. The occurrence of myocardial scars in patients with large hearts and normal coronary arteries is well recognized. Patients with left-ventricular outflow obstruction commonly have myocardial scars despite "clean" coronary arteries. The myocardial scars, however, are usually limited to the papillary muscles and to the subendocardium (inner one-half) of the left-ventricular free wall or ventricular septum or both. The same applies to subjects with severe chronic anemia, such as congenital hemolytic anemia or sickle-cell disease. Likewise, an inadequate coronary perfusion pressure may lead to myocardial necrosis (with later scarring) despite a normal coronary tree, but again the necrosis (or fibrosis) is usually limited to left-ventricular papillary muscle and subendocardium.

In contrast to the frequent occurrence of papillary muscle and subendocardial necrosis or fibrosis in patients with a normal coronary tree but too large a myocardial mass, too little hemoglobin, or too low a perfusion pressure, the occurrence of *transmural* necrosis or fibrosis in these persons is infrequent. Among 74 necropsy patients with transmural AMI recently studied in out laboratory,[1] only

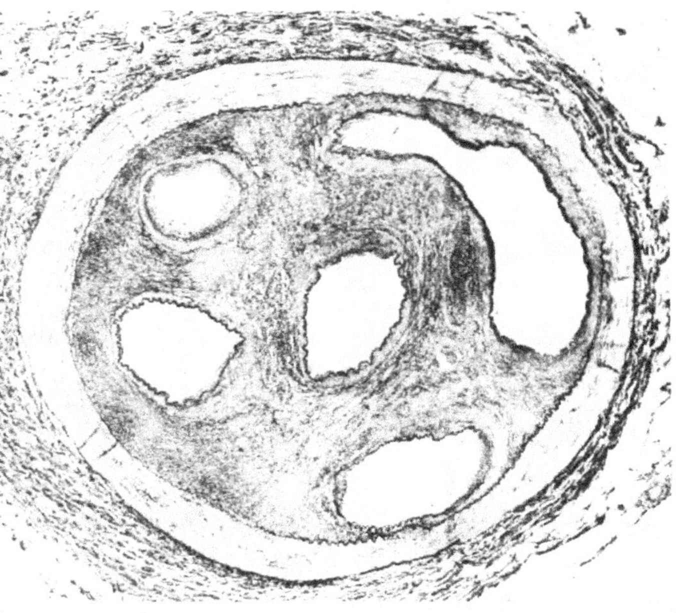

Figure 5. Recanalized embolus in the distal left anterior descending coronary artery of a 26-year-old man (A63-170) who had a transmural acute myocardial infarct three years earlier, at the time of active infective endocarditis involving the aortic valve. The anterior descending coronary artery proximal to this site was normal, as were the other extramural coronary arteries (elastic van Gieson stain, x46). (Reproduced from Roberts WC, Buja LM *Am J Med* 52: 423-443, 1972.)

five (7 per cent) had less than 75 per cent luminal narrowing by atherosclerotic plaques of any of the three major coronary arteries (Table III). The hearts in each of the five, however, were considerably hypertrophied (average: 780 gm) by other cardiac conditions.

Among the 47 reported patients with non-catheter-induced "myocardial infarction and angiographically normal coronary arteries," with rare exception, none had associated cardiac conditions or cardiomegaly by chest roentgenograms or electrocardiogram. Thus, although applicable on occasion, this explanation does not apply to the patients reported with non-catheter-induced "myocardial infarction and angiographically normal coronary arteries."

TABLE I

CLINICAL OBSERVATIONS IN 47 REPORTED PATIENTS WITH ACUTE MYOCARDIAL INFARCTION (AMI) AND SUBSEQUENTLY NORMAL CORONARY ARTERIOGRAMS:
(Non-catheter induced)

First Author	Publication Year	No. Pts.	Age Range (years)	Interval (mo.) From Onset of AMI to Normal Coronary Arteriograms					
				(<1)	(1-2)	(2-3)	(3-6)	(6-12)	(>12)
1. Campeau	1968	5	27–53				1	4	
2. Sidd	1970	1	19				1		
3. Bruschke	1971	4	29–43		1		1		2
4. Glancy	1971	2	34&36						2
5. Nizit	1971	1	17				1		
6. Dear	1971	1	43						1
7. Kimbris	1972	3	16–36	1			2		
8. Potts	1972	2	28&28				1		1
9. DePasquale	1973	1	61						
10. Barcala	1973	1	55			1			
11. Schatz	1973	1	14			1			
12. Henderson	1973	1	34						1
13. Khan	1974	9	22–49			2	3	3	1
14. Brest	1974	5	28–40				3	2	
15. Regan	1975	7	34–59		1	3	3		
16. Sasse	1975	2	16&26				2		
17. Ciraulo	1975	1	40		1				
Totals		47	14–61 (avg 36)	1	3	8	18	9	8

TABLE II

CLINICAL OBSERVATIONS IN 5 REPORTED PATIENTS WITH ACUTE MYOCARDIAL INFARCTION (AMI) OCCURRING AT CARDIAC CATHETERIZATION

First Author	Publication Year	No. Pts.	Age (yrs.)	Interval (mo.) from Catheter-associated AMI to Normal Coronary Arteriogram		
				(<2)	(3-6)	(6-12)
1. Campeau	1968	1	37			1
2. Richardson	1971	1	40	1		
3. Cheng	1972	1	52		1	
4. O'Reilly	1974	2	56&64	2		
Totals		5	37-64 (avg 50)	3	1	1

TABLE III

ACUTE TRANSMURAL MYOCARDIAL INFARCTION and INSIGNIFICANT (<75%) CORONARY NARROWING AT NECROPSY (5 of 74 patients)

Pts.	Age (Yrs.)	Sex	Associated Condition	Heart Weight (Gms)	Coronary Emboli
1	37	M	VSD	730	+
2	79	F	MS, AS	500	+
3	79	M	AS	730	0
4	56	M	MR	900	+
5	60	M	AS	1050	0
5	37-79 (Avg. 62)	M:F 4:1		500-1050 (avg. 780)	3

Abbreviation: AS = aortic stenosis; MR = mitral regurgitation; MS = mitral stenosis; VSD = ventricular septal defect.

3. *The coronary arteriograms were misinterpreted.* It is well known that angiography tends to underestimate the degree of coronary arterial luminal narrowing.[27,28] This explanation may sometimes be the proper one, but most patients with symptomatic coronary atherosclerosis have some abnormality at angiography of two or often all three of the major extramural coronary arteries.[4-6] Slitlike lumens may account for many of the false negative angiograms (Fig. 2).[27] It would be rare, however, to have a severely narrowed slitlike lumen in one major coronary artery without any abnormality at angiography in the other two major coronary arteries.

4. *Coronary spasm caused the AMI.* Although shown to cause both chest pain and ischemic changes on electrocardiogram, coronary spasm has not been shown to cause myocardial necrosis. The case for spasm is generally considered strongest among patients with Prinzmetal's angina (Table IV). Of 143 patients with this variant angina reported in English,[29-67] 124 had coronary arteriography (Fig. 3);[35,37-67] among them, the coronary arteries were severely (more than 75 per cent) narrowed in 76 (61 per cent) and normal in 48 (39 per cent). Coronary spasm was demonstrated in 17 (14 per cent) of the 124 patients—in five of the 76 with narrowed and 12 of the 48 patients with normal coronary arteries. Although it occurred naturally in none of the five patients with both coronary spasm and fixed coronary narrowing, AMI or death

occurred after aortocoronary bypass procedures in three of the five patients. None of the 22 patients with angiograpically normal coronary arteries had an AMI, but six of them died—none, however, among the nine with demonstrated coronary spasm. Examination of the coronary arteries in five of these six patients (Table V) disclosed severe (more than 75 per cent) narrowing of one coronary ostium or artery in three patients and a "small" left coronary artery in a fourth. Only one of the five patients had a "normal" coronary tree at necropsy.

Thus, although it has been shown to cause chest pain and ischemic electrocardiographic changes, coronary spasm has not been shown to cause myocardial necrosis, except possibly in patients with chronic industrial nitroglycerine exposure.[68]

5. *AMI was caused by a condition affecting only the intramural (intramyocardial) coronary arteries without involvement of the extramural coronary arteries.* Abnormalities of the intramural coronary arteries have been reported in several conditions (Table VI), but, to our knowledge, transmural AMI has never been described as a consequence of disease only of the intramural coronary arteries. Even in the conditions where it has been observed, involvement of the intramural coronary arteries has been focal, not diffuse, and disease of these small

TABLE IV

VARIANT ANGINA PECTORIS (PRINZMETAL'S)

1. The chest pain is not related to exertion.
2. The ECG during episodes of pain shows transient S-T segment elevation (rather than depression as in classic angina).
3. Transient coronary spasm is the likely cause of the angina in some patients.
4. Angiography has shown > 75% luminal narrowing of one (rarely more than one) of the 3 major coronary arteries in two-thirds of the patients and normal coronary arteries in the other third.
5. Coronary collaterals usually are absent.
6. Exercise tolerance usually is normal.
7. Left ventricular pressures, cavity size, and ejection fractions, usually are normal.
8. Long-term prognosis is uncertain but probably favorable.

TABLE V

PRINZMETAL'S ANGINA: REPORTED STATUS OF CORONARY ARTERIES AT NECROPSY IN THOSE WITH ANGIOGRAPHICALLY-NORMAL CORONARY ARTERIES DURING LIFE

Author	Year	No. Pts	Age	Sex	Status of Coronary Arteries	
					1 of 3 >75% Narrowed	Normal
Gianelly	1968	1	49	F	~	1**
Cosby	1972	2	46	F	1	
			41	F		1***
Cheng	1973	1	60	M		1
Donsky	1975	1	44	F	1	
Totals		5*			2	3

*All 5 died suddenly
**Small left coronary artery
***The right coronary ostium was obstructed by atherosclerotic plaque

myocardial arteries usually has been associated with a condition affecting other body organs or systems as well.

6. *AMI was caused by an occluding embolus that subsequently lysed or recanalized.* This appears to us the most likely cause of AMI in patients who are subsequently shown by angiography to have a normal coronary arterial tree. It is reasoned that the coronary arteries were not normal at the time of AMI but that the occlusion resolved between the time of the AMI and the time of coronary angiography. Factors supporting this hypothesis are:

A. Arteriographically documented coronary arterial embolic occlusion can completely resolve. In the five patients with catheter-induced coronary arterial thromboembolic occlusion (Table II), the coronary arteriogram became normal after the AMI in each. In three of the five patients, complete resolution of the occlusion occurred within two months of the onset of the AMI.

B. Conditions associated with an increased risk of arterial thromboemboli were relatively frequent (15 per cent) among the 47 patients (Table I) with non-catheter-induced AMI: three of the seven women were taking oral contraceptives,[69,70] two patients had prosthetic cardiac valves, and one patient had a markedly elevated platelet count.

C. Histologic study of previous known arterial

emboli indicates that such lesions may lyse completely, retract along one side to form an eccentric lumen, or recanalize with multiple luminal channels (Figs. 4 and 5).[71]

Each of these three means of organization of the clot almost surely could create a lumen large enough to produce a normal coronary arteriogram.

D. Among our 74 necropsy patients with transmural AMI, only five had less than 75 per cent luminal narrowing by atherosclerotic plaques of each of their three major coronary arteries (Table III): three of the five had coronary emboli at necropsy,[1] and their coronary tree was otherwise normal.

E. With few exceptions, reported patients with non-catheter-induced AMI were asymptomatic before the occurrence of the AMI; after healing of the AMI, they were asymptomatic again and without evidence of angina pectoris, congestive cardiac failure, or cardiomegaly. Obviously, an AMI may be the first and only coronary event when it is the result of severe coronary atherosclerosis, but the percentage of patients who return to a totally asymptomatic state is not nearly as high as that of the group with "myocardial infarction and angiographically normal coronary arteries." Acute pulmonary embolism, when occurring in previously normal pulmonary arteries and lungs, might be analogous (= normal coronary arteries), as opposed to acute pulmonary embolism superimposed on chronic lung disease (= coronary atherosclerosis).

SUMMARY

Thus, in conclusion, the following statements may be made concerning reported patients with "myocardial infarction and angiographically normal coronary arteries": (1) an angiographically normal coronary tree has never been demonstrated *at the time of AMI*; (2) among reported patients with "myocardial infarction and angiographically normal coronary arteries," the angiograms were performed *after healing*, rather than during the AMI; (3) although there are several explanations for the occurence of AMI and angiographically normal coronary arteries and although each may be applicable on occasion, the most reasonable explanation appears to be acute coronary embolism with subsequent clot lysis, retraction, or recanalization—all of which may appear as "angiographically normal." ●

TABLE VI

CONDITIONS ASSOCIATED WITH NARROWING OF INTRAMURAL CORONARY ARTERIES (EXCLUDES VASCULITIS)

1. Atherosclerosis of extramural coronary arteries (limited to vessels in left ventricular papillary muscles)
2. Hypertrophic cardiomyopathy (ASH)
3. Neurogenic cardiac diseases
   A. Friedreich's ataxia
   B. Progressive muscular dystrophy
   C. Progressive myotonic dystrophy
4. Collagen diseases
   A. Systemic lupus erythematosus
   B. Scleroderma
   C. Dermatomyositis
5. Diabetes mellitus
6. Hereditary connective tissue disorders
   A. Marfan syndrome
   B. Hurler syndrome
7. Infiltrative diseases
   A. Amyloid
   B. Neoplasm
8. Emboli
   A. Infective endocarditis
   B. Intracardiac thrombus
   C. Prosthetic valve
   D. Cardiac catheterization
   E. Neoplasm
9. Certain congenital cardiac malformations
   A. Aortic atresia
10. Coagulopathy
    A. Disseminated intravascular coagulation
    B. Thrombotic thrombocytopenic purpura
11. Whipple's disease

Address for reprints: William C. Roberts, M.D.
Building 10A, Room 3E30
National Institutes of Health
Bethesda, Md. 20014

REFERENCES

1. Roberts WC, Buja LM *Am J Med* 52: 425, 1972.
2. Roberts WC, Ferrans VJ, Levy RI, Fredrickson DS *Am J Cardiol* 31: 557, 1973.
3. Baltaxe HA, Amplatz K, Levin DC *Coronary Angiography.* Springfield, Ill., Charles C. Thomas, 1973.
4. Hale G, Dexter D, Jefferson K, Leatham A *Br Heart J* 28: 40, 1966.
5. Proudfit WL, Shirey EK, Sones FM *Circulat* 33: 901, 1966.
6. Ross RS, Friesinger GC *Am Heart J* 72: 437, 1966.
7. Campeau L, Lesperance J, Bourassa MG, Ashekian PB *Can Med Assoc J* 99: 837, 1968.
8. Sidd J, Kemp HG, Gorlin R *N Engl J Med* 282: 1306, 1970.
9. Bruschke AVG, Bruyneel KJJ, Bloch A, van Herper G *Br Heart J* 33: 585, 1971.
10. Glancy DL, Marcus ML, Epstein SE *Circulat* 44: 495, 1971.
11. Nizet PM, Robertson L *Am Heart J* 28: 715, 1971.
12. Dear HD, Russell RO, Jones WB, Reeves TJ *Am J Cardiol* 28: 718, 1971.
13. Kimbiris D, Segal BL, Munir M, Katz M, Likoff W *Am J Cardiol* 29: 724, 1972.
14. Potts KH, Stein PD, Houk PC *Chest* 62: 549, 1972.
15. DePasquale NP, Bruno MS *Chest* 63: 618, 1973.
16. Barcala RP *J Thorac Cardiovasc Surg* 65: 786, 1973.
17. Schatz IJ, Mizukami H, Ballagher J, Greenslit FS *Chest* 63: 963, 1973.
18. Henderson RR, Hansing CE, Razavi M, Rowe GG *Am J Cardiol* 31: 785, 1973.
19. Khan AH, Haywood LJ *N Engl J Med* 291: 427, 1974.
20. Brest AN, Wiener L, Kasparian H, Duca P, Rafter JJ *Am Heart J* 88: 219, 1974.
21. Richardson PM, Gotsman MS *African Med J* 45: 805, 1971.
22. Cheng TO, Bashour T, Singh BK, Kelser GA *Am J Cardiol* 30: 680, 1972.
23. O'Reilly RJ, Spellberg RD *Ann Intern Med* 81: 348, 1974.
24. Regan TJ, Wu CF, Weisse AB, Moschos CB, Ahmed SS, Lyons MM *Circulat* 51: 453, 1975.
25. Sasse L, Wagner R, Murray FE *Am J Cardiol* 35: 448, 1975.
26. Ciraulo DA *Am J Cardiol* 35: 923, 1975.
27. Vlodaver Z, Frech R, Van Tassel RA, Edwards JE *Circulat* 47: 162, 1973.
28. Grondin CM, Dyrda I, Pasternac A, Campeau L, Bourassa MG, Lesperance J *Circulat* 49: 703, 1974.
29. Prinzmetal M, Kennamer R, Merliss R, Wada T, Bor N *Am J Med* 27: 375, 1959.
30. Gubbay ER *Can Med Assoc J* 83: 164, 1960.
31. Prinzmetal M, Ekmekci A, Kennamer R, Kwoczynski JK, Shubin H, Toyoshima H *JAMA* 174: 102, 1960.
32. Peretz DI *Can Med Assoc J* 85: 1101, 1961.
33. Robinson JS *Am Heart J* 70: 797, 1965.
34. Hilal H, Massumi R *Am J Cardiol* 19: 607, 1967.
35. Gianelly R, Mugler F, Harrison DC *Calif Med* 108: 129, 1968.
36. Gillilan RE, Hawley RR, Warbasse JR *Am Heart J* 77: 380, 1969.
37. Whiting RB, Klein MD, Vander Veer J, Lown B *N Engl J Med* 282: 709, 1970.
38. Silverman ME, Flamm MD *Ann Intern Med* 75: 339, 1971.
39. Dhurandhar RW, Watt DL, Silver MD, Trimble AS, Adelman AG *Am J Cardiol* 30: 902, 1972.
40. Cosby RS, Giddings JA, See JR, Mayo M *Am J Med* 53: 739, 1972.
41. Laks MM, Dahlgren J, Mandel WJ *Ann Intern Med* 78: 309, 1973.
42. Cheng TO, Bashour T, Kelser GA, Weiss L, Bacos J *Circulat* 47: 476, 1973.
43. Oliva PB, Potts DE, Pluss RG *N Engl J Med* 288: 745, 1973.
44. MacAlpin RN, Kattus AA, Alvaro AB *Circulat* 47: 946, 1973.
45. King MJ, Zir LM, Kaltman AJ, Fox AC *Am J Med Sci* 265: 419, 1973.
46. Levi GF, Proto C *Br Heart J* 35: 601, 1973.
47. MacMillan RM, Rose FD, Flinghoffer JF, Frankl WS *Cardiol* 58: 306, 1973.
48. Kristian-Kerin N, Davies B, Macleod CA *Chest* 64: 352, 1973.
49. Hart NJ, Silverman ME, King SB *Am J Med* 56: 269, 1974.
50. Gorfinkel HJ, Inglesby TV, Lansing AM, Goodin RR *Ann Intern Med* 79: 795, 1973.
51. Betriu A, Solignac A, Bourassa MG *Am Heart J* 87: 272, 1974.
52. Bodenheimer M, Lipski J, Donoso E, Dack S *Am Heart J* 87: 304, 1974.
53. Schroeder JS, Silverman FJ, Harrison DC *Chest* 65: 573, 1974.
54. Sweet RL, Sheffield LT *Am J Cardiol* 33: 813, 1974.
55. Nevins MA *Ann Intern Med* 80: 673, 1974.
56. Choquet Y, Proulx J, Primeau R, Lapointe L, Levy R *Can Med Assoc J* 111: 161, 1974.
57. Kerin N, Macleod CA *Br Heart J* 36: 224, 1974.
58. Rose FJ, Johnson AD, Carleton RA *Chest* 66: 719, 1974.
59. Applefield MM, Ronan JA *Chest* 66: 721, 1974.
60. Donsky MS, Harris MD, Curry GC, Blomquist CG, Willerson JT, Mullins CB *Am Heart J* 89: 571, 1975.
61. Gaasch WH, Adyanthaya AV, Wang VH, Pickering E, Quinones MA, Alexander JK, *Am J Cardiol* 35: 683, 1975.
62. Meller J, Conde CA, Donoso E, Dack S *Am J Cardiol* 35: 691, 1975.
63. Owlia D, Prabhu R, Pierce JA, Stoughton PV, Shankar KP, Nino A *Chest* 67: 727, 1975.
64. Endo M, Kanda I, Hosoda S, Hayashi H, Hirosawa K, Konno S *Circulat* 52: 33, 1975.
65. Shubrooks SJ Jr, Bete JM, Hutter AM, Block PC, Buckley MJ, Daggett WM, Mundth ED *Am J Cardiol* 36: 142, 1975.
66. Widlansky S, McHenry PL, Corya BC, Phillips JF *Am Heart J* 90: 631, 1975.
67. Haywood LJ, Khan AH, de Guzman M *JAMA* 235: 53, 1976.
68. Lange RL, Reid MS, Tresch DD, Keelan MH, Bernhard VM, Coolidge G *Circulat* 46: 666, 1972.
69. Mann JI, Vessey MP, Thorogood M, Doll R *Br Med J* 2: 241, 1975.
70. Mann JI, Inman WHW *Br Med J* 2: 245, 1975.
71. Harrison CV *J Pathol Bacteriol* 60: 289, 1948.

Site of Myocardial Infarction

A Determinant of the Cardiovascular Changes Induced in the Cat by Coronary Occlusion

Peter B. Corr, Ph.D., David L. Pearle, M.D., John R. Hinton,
William C. Roberts, M.D., and Richard A. Gillis, Ph.D.

SUMMARY   The influence of site of acute myocardial infarction on heart rate, blood pressure, cardiac output, total peripheral resistance (TPR), cardiac rhythm, and mortality was determined in 58 anesthetized cats by occlusion of either the left anterior descending (LAD), left circumflex or right coronary artery. LAD occlusion resulted in immediate decrease in cardiac output, heart rate, and blood pressure, an increase in TPR, and cardiac rhythm changes including premature ventricular beats, ventricular tachycardia, and occasionally ventricular fibrillation. The decrease in cardiac output and increase in TPR persisted in the cats surviving a ventricular arrhythmia. In contrast, right coronary occlusion resulted in a considerably smaller decrease in cardiac output. TPR did not increase, atrioventricular conduction disturbances were common, and sinus bradycardia and hypotension persisted in the cats recovering from an arrhythmia. Left circumflex ligation resulted in cardiovascular changes intermediate between those produced by occlusion of the LAD or the right coronary artery. Mortality was similar in each of the three groups. We studied the coronary artery anatomy in 12 cats. In 10, the blood supply to the sinus node was from the right coronary artery and in 2, from the left circumflex coronary artery. The atrioventricular node artery arose from the right in 9 cats, and from the left circumflex in 3. The right coronary artery was dominant in 9 cats and the left in 3. In conclusion, the site of experimental coronary occlusion in cats is a major determinant of the hemodynamic and cardiac rhythm changes occurring after acute myocardial infarction. The cardiovascular responses evoked by ligation are related in part to the anatomical distribution of the occluded artery.

CLINICAL DATA strongly suggest that cardiovascular changes occurring with human myocardial infarction vary importantly depending on the site of myocardial infarction. For example, second- and third-degree heart block occurs more frequently after posterior wall infarction (usually a consequence of right coronary artery compromise) than after anterior wall infarction (associated with left anterior descending lesions).[1-7] Posterior wall infarcts often are associated with increased parasympathetic activity (sinus bradycardia, transient hypotension, or atrioventricular block), whereas anterior wall infarcts are associated with sympathetic overactivity (sinus tachycardia or transient hypertension.[8] Heart rate and left ventricular filling pressure may be higher and stroke index and stroke work index lower in patients with anterior wall infarctions compared to those with posterior wall infarctions.[9] Some studies suggest a higher mortality rate in patients with anterior wall infarcts than in those with posterior infarcts,[9] although identical mortality rates have also been reported.[10]

From the Departments of Pharmacology and Cardiology, Georgetown University Schools of Medicine and Dentistry, Washington, D.C., and the National Heart and Lung Institute, Bethesda, Maryland.

Supported by grants from the U.S. Public Health Service (HE-13675, RR-5306, and RR-5360).

Dr. Gillis is a recipient of Research Career Development Award HL-70678 from the National Heart and Lung Institute.

Dr. Corr's present address is: Cardiovascular Division, Department of Internal Medicine, Barnes and Wohl Hospitals, 660 South Euclid Avenue, St. Louis, Missouri 63110.

These results were submitted by Peter B. Corr as partial fulfillment of the requirements for the degree of Doctor of Philosophy. A preliminary report was presented at the meeting of the Federation of American Societies for Experimental Biology, April 1974.

Original manuscript received October 20, 1975; accepted for publication August 4, 1976.

These clinical data suggest that the cardiovascular consequences of human myocardial infarction vary dramatically according to the site of infarction. However, experimental evidence for this is almost totally lacking. We are aware of only two studies relevant to this question. In experiments performed in 1918, T wave changes and mortality incidence were compared when each major coronary vessel of the dog was occluded.[11] More recently, the incidence of ventricular fibrillation and mortality were compared after occlusion of each major coronary artery of the dog.[12]

The purpose of our study was to compare systematically the cardiovascular events occurring with occlusion of the three major coronary vessels. Our studies were performed in the cat, since we were able to demonstrate that the coronary distribution in this animal is more nearly analogous to human anatomy than is that of the dog.

Methods

Adult cats unselected as to sex and ranging in weight from 1.5 to 3.9 kg were anesthetized with intravenously administered α-chloralose (70–75 mg/kg). A tracheotomy was performed and mechanical ventilation was instituted with room air, at a tidal volume of 20–25 ml/kg and a rate of 22 breaths/min. Under these conditions, the pH of arterial blood ranged between 7.38 and 7.43. The cats were immobilized with decamethonium bromide (0.25 mg/kg) every 45–60 minutes. Catheters were inserted into the right femoral artery and vein of all cats to permit measurement of blood pressure and administration of drugs. Body temperature was maintained between 37.0°C and 38.0°C by an infrared lamp.

The heart was exposed by excising the 2nd through 5th right ribs. The parietal pericardium was incised and sutured to the chest wall. Coronary occlusion was performed after exposing one of the three major coronary arteries and placing a ligature beneath its most proximal portion. Care was taken to separate the pericoronary nerves from the coronary arteries to prevent their inclusion in the ligature surrounding the vessel. The suture material (no. 4.0) was placed proximal to all branch points of each major vessel. This ligature was tied securely at the moment when occlusion was desired. Only one vessel was occluded in each cat, and the effects were followed visually for 2 hours. At the end of each experiment the ligature was checked to confirm that the vessel had been completely occluded. Systemic arterial pressure, heart rate, and rhythm [lead II of the electrocardiogram (ECG)] were continuously monitored on a Beckman multichannel recorder. "Severe ventricular arrhythmia" was considered to be sustained ventricular tachycardia or fibrillation resulting in a mean arterial pressure of less than 50 mm Hg for at least 5 seconds. Ascending aortic blood flow was measured with a Biotronex BL-610 pulsed-logic flowmeter utilizing a Biotronex electromagnetic flow transducer (BL-6060-E20). The flow probe was calibrated in vitro using saline. The diastolic level of aortic flow obtained from the pulsatile flow trace was used as the zero flow reference point. A Gould-Brush model 260 recorder was used to monitor aortic flow. Total peripheral resistance was calculated as peripheral resistance units (PRU):

$$PRU = \frac{\text{mean arterial blood pressure (mm Hg)}}{\text{mean aortic flow (ml/min)}} \times 60 \ (\text{sec/min})$$

Coronary blood supply to the sinoatrial and atrioventricular nodes was studied in an additional 12 cats. In 10, their major coronary arteries were cannulated and perfused with Vinylite solution using the method described by James.[13] Once the cast had hardened, the two major coronary arteries arising from the aorta were freed from surrounding tissue under direct vision using a dissecting microscope. The sinus node and atrioventricular node arteries were identified[13-15]

Confirmation of the results provided by gross dissection of the coronary arteries was obtained by serially sectioning two additional whole hearts and histologically identifying both the sinoatrial and atrioventricular nodes along with their respective blood supplies. The hearts were excised and placed in buffered formalin. Following fixation, the hearts were processed in alcohol and xylene and embedded in paraffin, and a total of 5,520 sections (2,400 from heart 1 and 3,120 sections from heart 2) were cut at 6-μm intervals. Every fifth section was retained and stained by elastic—van Gieson or Movat methods. The nodal tissue was identified using the criteria described by Lev.[16]

The following drugs were used: α-chloralose (Etablissements Kuhlman, Paris), decamethonium bromide solution (Burroughs Wellcome), and sodium heparin injection (Organon). α-Chloralose was dissolved by heating in distilled water and the solution was cooled to body temperature before use. Doses of drugs were calculated and administered as the respective salt. The vinyl injection solution (blue and red) used to cast the coronary arteries was obtained from Carolina Biological Supply Co.

The data were analyzed by paired comparisons and grouped Student's t-test. Chi-square analysis for 2×2 contingency with the Yates corrections was applied to some of the data and this is indicated under Results. The criterion used for significance was $P < 0.05$.

Results

LEFT ANTERIOR DESCENDING (LAD) OCCLUSION

Data from 30 cats with LAD ligation, 20 of which have been reported previously,[17] are summarized in Table 1. The ECG record of a representative cat is presented as part of Figure 1. With occlusion of the LAD, decreases in cardiac output (measured as aortic flow), heart rate, and blood pressure occurred within minutes (Table 1), and were followed by changes in cardiac rhythm. The decreases in each index were usually maximal within 2 minutes after occlusion and remained constant until the arrhythmia intervened. Therefore, the values in Table 1 were obtained immediately before the development of the arrhythmia. The arrhythmia consisted of unifocal or multifocal premature ventricular beats and occurred in all 30 cats after LAD occlusion. The time to onset of the arrhythmia in the LAD ligation group, as noted by the first ventricular premature beat, was 2.4 minutes. Eleven of the 20 cats developed severe ventricular arrhythmias and six of the 11 died (Table 2), all within 3.5 minutes after coronary occlusion. The other five cats spontaneously recovered and sinus rhythm eventually returned. The average duration of arrhythmia in the 24 surviving cats was 33.5 ± 1.5 minutes.

Total peripheral resistance (TPR) was calculated from the arterial pressure and aortic flow data of five cats (Table 1). Immediately after occlusion and before the arrhythmia, TPR increased significantly, and this increase still was present 1 hour later when the sinus rhythm was reestablished.

Data obtained from 24 surviving cats 1 hour after occlusion, at which time the arrhythmia no longer was present, also are summarized in Table 1. Both heart rate and blood pressure had returned to preocclusion levels. Some restoration of cardiac output had occurred but the difference between the values 1 hour after occlusion and the values before occlusion still were significant.

RIGHT CORONARY ARTERY OCCLUSION

These changes in 14 cats are summarized in Table 1. The ECG record of a representative cat appears as part of Figure 1. Cardiac output decreased only mildly and TPR did not increase significantly. The time to onset of the ventricular arrhythmia was significantly longer than after LAD occlusion. Thirteen of 14 cats developed ventricular arrhythmias, and in one cat this arrhythmia became severe (Table 2). The ventricular arrhythmia consisted of either unifocal or multifocal ventricular beats. The nature of the arrhythmias differed from LAD ligation. Four of the 14 cats developed second- or third-degree heart block, arrhythmias which never occurred after LAD ligation (Table

TABLE 1 *Influence of Site of Coronary Occlusion on Heart Rate (HR), Blood Pressure (BP), Aortic Flow, and Total Peripheral Resistance (PRU)*

| | Before occlusion (control) | | | | Immediately after occlusion and prior to arrhythmia | | | | | 1 hr after occlusion | | | |
Site of occlusion	HR (beats/ min)	Mean BP (mm Hg)	Aortic flow (ml/ min)	PRU	Change in HR (beats/ min)	Change in BP (mm Hg)	Change in aortic flow (ml/ min)	Change in PRU	Onset of ventricular arrhythmia (min)	Change in HR from control (beats/ min)	Change in BP from control (mm Hg)	Change in aortic flow from control (ml/min)	Change in PRU from control
Left anterior descending coronary artery (30)	195.2 ±5.5 (30)	110.5 ±4.7 (30)	284.0 ±9.8 (5)	22.6 ±2.6 (5)	−22.7* ±3.7 (30)	−18.9* ±2.5 (30)	−116.0* ±21.1 (5)	+7.5* ±3.0 (5)	2.4 ± 0.3 (30)	−8.2 ±5.9 (24)	−9.3 ±4.9 (24)	−70.0* ±10.8 (4)	+6.4* ±1.0 (4)
Right coronary artery (14)	203.0 ±4.8 (14)	120.5 ±6.6 (14)	250.0 ±21.0 (7)	24.4 ±1.9 (7)	−31.5* ±6.9 (14)	−25.8* ±6.6 (14)	−24.9† ±19.1 (7)	−0.5 ±1.8 (7)	10.0† ±1.6 (13)	−26.1* ±8.3 (10)	−33.1*† ±8.4 (10)	−47.1* ±11.1 (7)	−0.9 ±2.0 (7)
Circumflex coronary artery (14)	200.5 ±5.6 (14)	103.5 ±5.4 (14)	254.2 ±23.7 (7)	24.0 ±1.9 (7)	−35.0* ±6.6 (14)	−22.7* ±5.3 (14)	−59.1*† +14.3 (7)	+3.2 ±4.5 (7)	6.3†‡ ±1.9 (13)	−7.5 ±7.9 (9)	−19.5* ±4.8 (9)	−37.5 ±23.2 (4)	−1.5 ±4.5 (4)

Results are expressed as mean ± se. Numbers in parentheses indicate number of cats in each group.

* $P < 0.05$ with paired comparisons (comparison was made between data obtained during postocclusion period and data obtained during preocclusion period).

† $P < 0.05$ with group comparisons (comparison was made between data obtained with either circumflex coronary group or right coronary group vs. left anterior descending coronary group).

‡ One cat never developed an arrhythmia; two cats exhibited infrequent premature ventricular beats.

2). The heart block observed in these four cats occurred early after occlusion (1.2 ± 0.3 minutes) and was usually of short duration. Heart block reappeared in two of the four cats after an intervening period of sinus rhythm. In two of the four cats, heart block was followed by a ventricular arrhythmia.

One hour after right coronary artery occlusion there was no increase in TPR, the heart rate and blood pressure remained decreased (in contrast to the LAD results) (Table 1), and the duration of the ventricular arrhythmias was extremely variable, ranging from 6 to 48 minutes in nine of the cats that recovered. Data on the four cats that did not recover from the arrhythmia are not included in Table 1. In the group with LAD occlusion the range was 18–49 minutes and each cat that survived the bouts of ventricular fibrillation or premature ventricular beats recovered from the arrhythmia about 30 minutes after the artery was occluded.

Similarities between the responses that occurred with the two sites of occlusion are as follows: (1) equivalent maximal decreases in heart rate and blood pressure immediately after occlusion (Table 1); (2) equivalent incidence in the occurrence of severe ventricular arrhythmia (Table 2); and (3) significant decreases in cardiac output 1 hour after occlusion (Table 1).

LEFT CIRCUMFLEX CORONARY ARTERY OCCLUSION

This ligation in 14 cats resulted in cardiovascular changes intermediate between those after ligation of the LAD and right coronary arteries. Initially a significant decrease in aortic flow occurred (Table 1), but it was significantly less than that following LAD occlusion. No significant change occurred in TPR. For all three coronary arteries similar decreases in heart rate and blood pressure occurred immediately after occlusion (Table 1). Thirteen of the 14 cats developed an arrhythmia (Table 2), and the

time to onset of the ventricular arrhythmia was significantly longer than that after LAD occlusion (Table 1). The ventricular arrhythmias were similar to those in the two other groups. Death due to ventricular fibrillation occurred in four of 14 cats (Table 2). The incidence of premature ventricular contractions was similar in all three groups (Table 2). As with right coronary artery occlusion, several cats developed heart block (Table 2). Again, this arrhythmia developed early (1.3 ± 0.3 minutes) and before the development of ventricular premature beats. As with LAD occlusion, all cats that did not develop a rhythm disturbance that progressed to fatal ventricular fibrillation eventually returned to sinus rhythm. The mean duration of the ventricular arrhythmia was 19.9 ± 3.2 minutes, and although shorter than the arrhythmia duration with LAD occlusion, the mean value was not significantly different.

The ECG record of a representative cat is presented as part of Figure 1. The summarized data at 1 hour after ligation appears in Table 1. Heart rate returned to preocclusion levels as seen with LAD occlusion. However, as in the case of right coronary ligation, blood pressure remained depressed and TPR was unchanged. Unlike results from either of the other two groups, aortic flow was not significantly reduced at this time.

ARTERIES TO THE SINUS AND ATRIOVENTRICULAR NODES

Twelve hearts were studied. Both the sinus and atrioventricular nodes were supplied primarily from branches of the right coronary artery. In two of the 12 cats a branch of the left circumflex artery provided the blood supply to the sinus node. In three of the 12 cats a branch of the left circumflex artery provided the blood supply to the atrioventricular node. In the cats in which the nodes were supplied by branches of the right coronary artery, the branch to the sinus node appeared as the first major

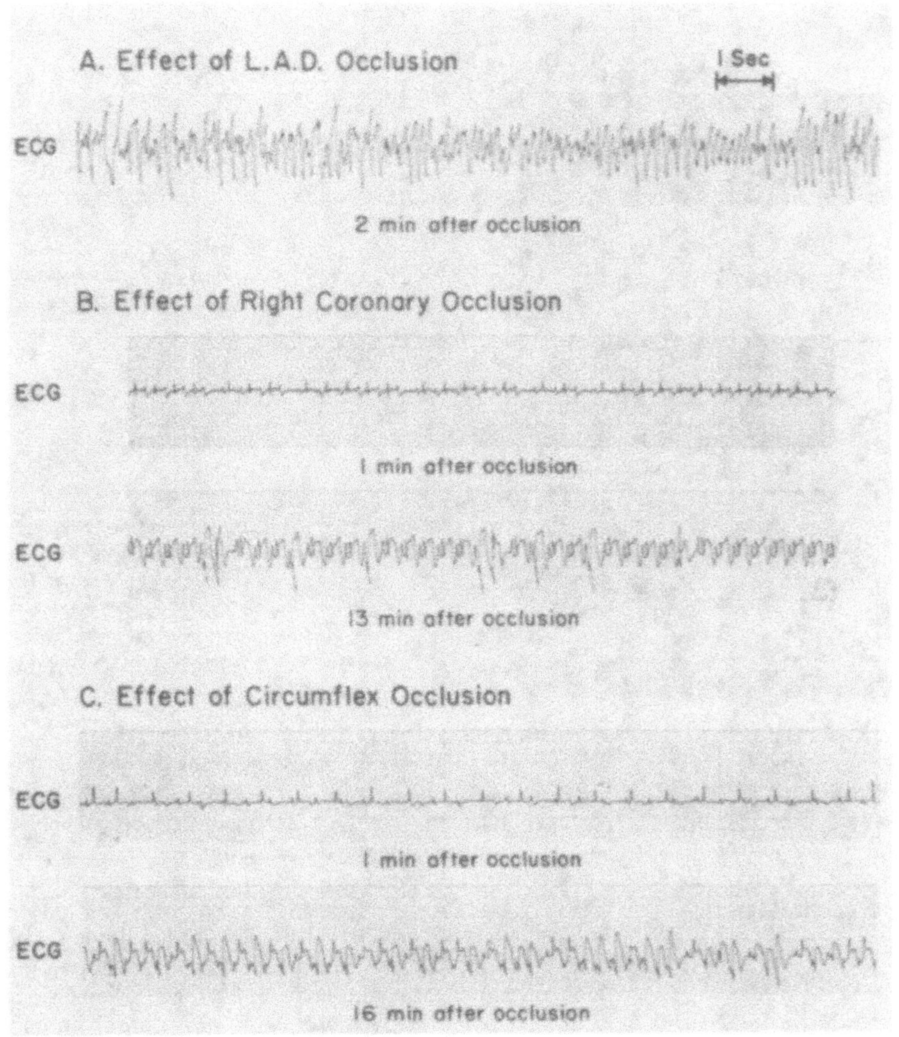

FIGURE 1 *Effect of occlusion of each of the major coronary arteries of the cat on cardiac rhythm as illustrated by the respective electrocardiographic (ECG) tracings. LAD = left anterior descending artery.*

branch off the right coronary artery (Fig. 2), while the branch to the atrioventricular node appeared as the last branch of the right coronary artery just before this major artery became the posterior descending coronary artery (Fig. 3). In the few cats in which the nodes were supplied by the circumflex artery, the artery to the sinus node appeared as the first branch of the left circumflex artery, while the vessel to the atrioventricular node appeared as a branch of the left circumflex artery just before this major artery branched into the posterior descending coronary artery. The origin of the blood supply to the posterior descending artery followed the same pattern as the origin of the atrioventricular node artery. The posterior descending artery was an extension of the right coronary artery in nine (Fig. 3) and an extension of the left circumflex artery in three of the 12 cats studied. (These results confirm earlier findings of Abramson and colleagues,[18] who showed that the majority of cats are right coronary domi-

TABLE 2 *Incidence and Type of Arrhythmia Occurring after Occlusion of Each Major Coronary Artery in the Cat*

Coronary artery occluded	No. of cats	Incidence of arrhythmia (%)	Incidence of premature ventricular contractions (%)	Incidence of 2nd-degree heart block (%)	Incidence of 3rd-degree heart block (%)	Incidence of ventricular tachycardia or ventricular fibrillation of 5-sec duration (%)	Incidence of death due to ventricular fibrillation (%)
Left anterior descending	30	100	100	0	0	40	20
Right	14	100	86	29*	29*	7	7
Circumflex	14	93	93	21*	7	29	29

* $P < 0.05$ with χ^2 distribution test (comparison was made between data obtained with either right coronary group or circumflex coronary group vs. left anterior descending group).

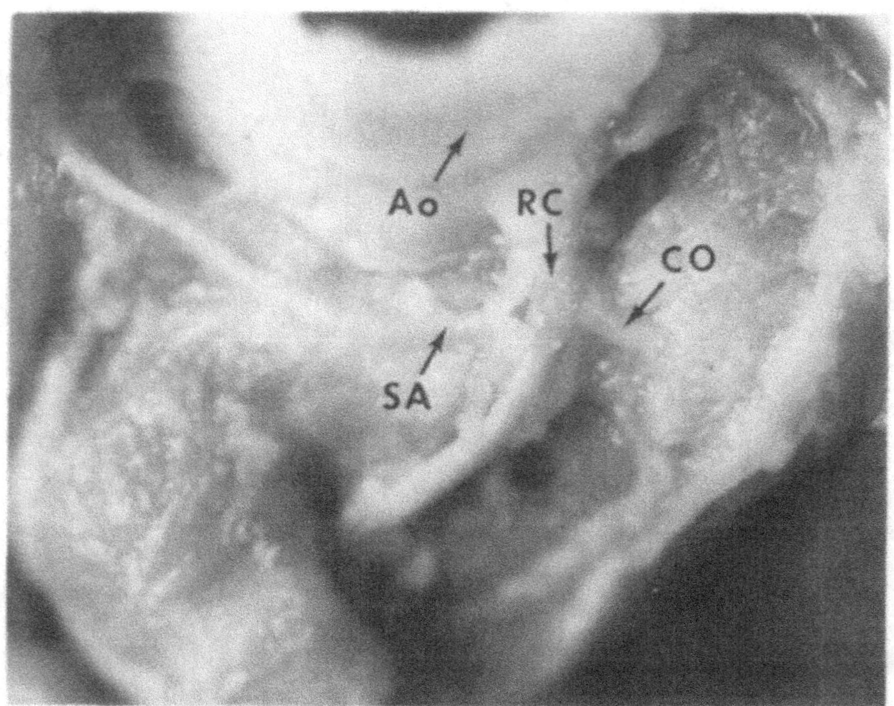

FIGURE 2 *A Vinylite cast of the right coronary artery of the cat viewed from the anterior superior surface of the heart. The right atrial appendage has been retracted. AO, RC, SA, and CO = aorta, right coronary artery, sinus node artery, and conus artery, respectively.*

nant.) Hearts undergoing serial sectioning exhibited the following pattern: One had the sinus node supplied by a branch from the right coronary artery, the other had the sinus node supplied by the left circumflex artery; in both the atrioventricular node was supplied by a branch of the right coronary, and the posterior descending artery appeared as an extension of the right coronary artery (Fig. 4).

Discussion

Occlusion of the three major coronary arteries of the cat produced dissimilar cardiovascular effects. Moreover, the changes after ligation of the feline right coronary artery were similar in many respects to the effects of human posterior infarction, while LAD ligation caused changes analogous to human anterior infarction.

Four major differences in cardiovascular effects were observed and are as follows: (1) occurrence of heart block with right coronary or left circumflex ligation but not with LAD ligation; (2) persistence of sinus bradycardia with right coronary ligation but not with LAD or left circumflex ligation; (3) major decreases in cardiac output initially with LAD occlusion but only minimal decreases in cardiac

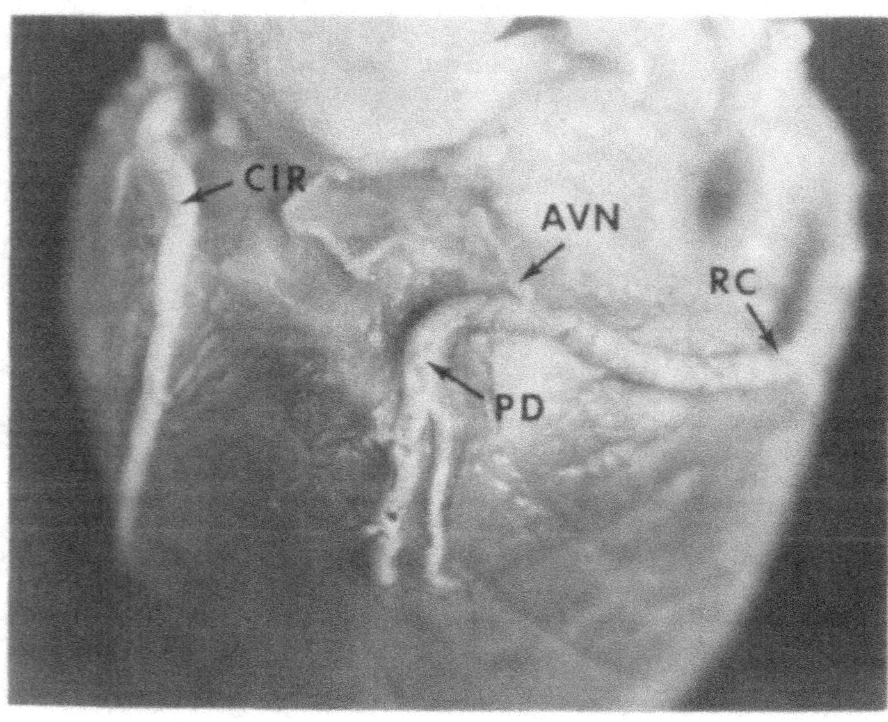

FIGURE 3 *A Vinylite cast of the right and left circumflex coronary arteries of the cat viewed from the posterior surface of the heart. RC = right coronary artery; CIR = left coronary artery; AVN = atrioventricular nodal artery; PD = posterior descending coronary artery. The circumflex artery terminates in the free wall of the left ventricle.*

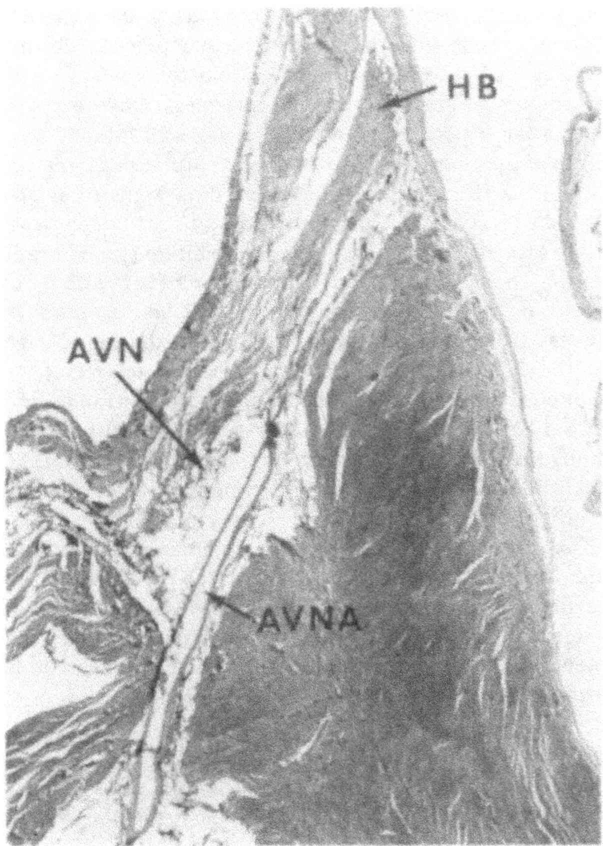

FIGURE 4 *Photomicrograph of a longitudinal section of the atrioventricular node (AVN) region of the cat. The His bundle (HB) is located just cephalad to the portion of the ventricular septum that is just posterior to the membranous septum. The atrioventricular node artery (AVNA) was the last branch of the right coronary just before it became the posterior descending artery. Hematoxylin and eosin stain; 16×.*

output after right coronary ligation; and (4) increase in TPR with LAD ligation but not with right coronary or circumflex ligation.

The occurrence of heart block with right coronary and left circumflex but not with LAD occlusion may be related to the source of the blood supply to the atrioventricular node, to the anatomical location of cholinergic nerve fibers, or to both factors. The artery supplying the atrioventricular node of the cat was shown in the present study to originate from the right coronary artery in nine of 12 cats and from the circumflex in three of 12 cats. Presumably, lack of sufficient oxygen to the atrioventricular node leads to impaired conduction and heart block. Alternatively, numerous cholinergic nerve endings and ganglia have been described between the posterior margin of the atrioventricular node and the anterior wall of the coronary sinus.[19] This area usually is perfused by arterial blood from the right coronary artery. Occlusion would result in ischemia which in turn could cause repetitive firing of these nerves and heart block.

The similarity between our findings relating infarct site with conduction disturbances and the findings of Adgey and colleagues[5] with patients is remarkable. They reported that 23% of the patients with posterior wall infarcts (in the distribution of the right coronary artery) developed atrioventricular block during the 1st hour after the onset of symptoms, whereas none of the patients with anterior wall infarcts (LAD distribution) developed atrioventricular block during this time period.

The persistence of sinus bradycardia with right coronary occlusion also may be related to the source of the blood supply to the sinoatrial node. In the present study, the sinus node artery was shown to be a branch of the right coronary artery in the majority of cats. A study in the rat has shown that sinus rate slows when the sinus node artery is occluded.[20] In addition, part of the slowing may be vagally mediated. Thoren[21] has reported that ligation of the right coronary artery in cats increases the firing of afferent cardiac vagal fibers, and activation of these fibers by electrical stimulation has been shown to produce reflex bradycardia.[22]

The greatest decrease in cardiac output occurred when the LAD was ligated. This was not unexpected since a greater portion of the left ventricular chamber is usually infarcted in occlusion of the LAD as compared to occlusion of the other major vessels.[7] It has been shown that the ischemic region produced by LAD occlusion ceases to contract within 1 minute after occlusion,[23] resulting in a rapid decompensation in ventricular function. Ventricular function then improves within 4–7 minutes by a compensatory increase in diastolic length and tension in the nonischemic portion of the myocardium.[24] Compensation in ventricular function also may be aided by the sympathetic nervous system, since surgical removal of sympathetic ganglia of dogs before LAD occlusion has been shown to prevent the restoration of cardiac output that usually occurs hours after infarction.[25] We found that cardiac output was returning toward preligation levels within 1 hour after infarction.

The degree of hypotension that occurred immediately after occlusion was the same regardless of which artery was occluded. The mechanism for the fall in pressure also seemed to be the same in each group, and presumably was due to the decrease in cardiac output because, in no case, was there a drop in TPR. If TPR had not risen with LAD occlusion, pressure presumably would have reached much lower levels than those seen with right coronary and left circumflex ligation.

The differences in TPR changes seen with occlusion of the various vessels might be explained by the size of the ischemic zone. In our study, we were interested only in the immediate hemodynamic effects of coronary occlusion. During this 1-hour time period, it is extremely difficult to assess quantity of ischemic myocardium, because available techniques do not define clearly the difference between ischemic and normal myocardium.[26]

Alternatively, the variation in TPR response might be related to different reflex responses rather than to quantity of ischemic muscle. The increase in TPR after LAD occlusion is a predictable response. Hypotension immediately after occlusion reduces stretch on sensory elements in the carotid sinus and aortic arch, resulting in excessive discharge of sympathetic efferent nerves to the vasculature. Consequently, TPR should rise. A second factor which might increase TPR is catecholamine release from the adrenal glands. LAD occlusion has been shown experimentally to increase plasma catecholamine levels via a vagal afferent reflex.[27] Such an increase in adrenal medullary hormone could explain the elevated TPR in our cats 1 hour after LAD occlusion, a time when arterial pressure had returned to the preocclusion level.

The unexpected finding, therefore, is the absence of a rise in TPR with right coronary or left circumflex occlusion despite significant hypotension immediately and 1 hour after occlusion. This result suggests that interruption of blood flow in these arteries in some way inhibits the reflex sympathetic vasoconstrictor response that normally occurs when arterial pressure falls. Moreover, the previously mentioned reflex by which LAD occlusion releases catecholamines from the adrenal glands does not appear to be activated by right and left circumflex occlusions.

It is generally accepted that the high incidence of sudden death during acute coronary occlusion results from cardiac arrhythmias.[28] Ventricular fibrillation was the terminal event in all cats dying in our study. Except for one cat in which fibrillation developed 33 minutes after occlusion, this arrhythmia occurred within 4 minutes after occlusion. The frequency of severe arrhythmia and death due to ventricular fibrillation was not significantly different for the three coronary ligations.

The cardiovascular data demonstrated in our study would not be relevant to human myocardial infarction unless the coronary artery distribution is similar in the two species. Our data suggest that the coronary artery anatomy of the cat is similar to that of the human: (1) both species have right coronary dominant systems; (2) in both species the atrioventricular node is perfused primarily by an artery originating from the right coronary artery; and (3) in both species the sinus node is perfused primarily by an artery originating from the most proximal portion of the right coronary artery.[13]

In contrast, the dog (most commonly chosen for studies dealing with acute myocardial infarction) possesses a coronary artery distribution dissimilar to that of the human. In the dog, the atrioventricular node is supplied from a branch of the circumflex artery;[29] the sinus node artery arises not from the proximal portion of the right coronary artery, but most commonly from the distal third of this artery as a terminal branch.[30] Additionally, the crux of the heart usually is supplied from a posterior descending artery originating from the circumflex artery.[29] Compared to the dog, the cat seems to be a better model for assessing the role of the occlusion site in human myocardial infarction.

Functionally, our data suggest that the cardiovascular changes that occur in the cat after experimentally induced coronary occlusion are analogous to those changes that occur in man. Sinus bradycardia and high degrees of atrioventricular block particularly were associated with posterior wall myocardial infarction in both cat and man. One apparent discrepancy between the cat and the human is the finding of Adgey and colleagues[5] that bradycardia does not occur within the first 30 minutes after onset of symptoms of an anterior wall infarction. Bradycardia was a prominent event after LAD occlusion in our study, but was very brief (occurring only over the first 1–3 minutes after occlusion). This short-lived bradycardia may have been missed in even the earliest human studies. Webb and colleagues,[8] observing patients within the 1st hour after symptoms of acute myocardial infarction, have reported that a large percentage with posterior wall infarcts show signs of parasympathetic overactivity, whereas a large percentage with anterior wall infarcts show signs of sympathetic overactivity. This agrees with our findings in cats. Cats with right coronary occlusion exhibited sinus bradycardia, heart block, and hypotension. Cats with LAD occlusion exhibited an increase in TPR and eventual recovery from their early hypotension. Furthermore, eight of the 24 cats with LAD occlusion that recovered exhibited sinus tachycardia at 1 hour after occlusion ($+25.7 \pm 4.8$ beats/min). Finally, we have reported in an earlier study that the ventricular arrhythmia associated with LAD occlusion is maintained by the sympathetic nervous system.[31]

Thus, the differences observed in human infarction sites are mirrored by the contrast between LAD and right coronary ligation in the cat. The different consequences of anterior and posterior infarction might imply different therapy according to infarction site. The cat appears to be a good model to investigate these differences.

Acknowledgments

We thank Drs. Kenneth M. Kent and Ernest N. Arnett for their helpful comments and Filipina Giocometti and Isabel Masket for their technical assistance.

References

1. Cohen DB, Doctor L, Pick A: The significance of atrioventricular block complicating acute myocardial infarction. Am Heart J 55: 215–219, 1958
2. James TN: Arrhythmias and conduction disturbances in acute myocardial infarction. Am Heart J 64: 416–426, 1962
3. Courter SR, Moffat J, Fowler NO: Advanced atrioventricular block in acute myocardial infarction. Circulation 27: 1034–1042, 1963
4. Jackson AE, Bashour FA: Cardiac arrhythmias in acute myocardial infarction. 1. Complete heart block and its natural history. Dis Chest 51: 31–38, 1967
5. Adgey AAJ, Mulholland HC, Geddes JS, Keegan DAJ: Incidence, significance, and management of early bradyarrhythmia complicating acute myocardial infarction. Lancet 2: 1097–1101, 1968
6. Brown RW, Hunt D, Sloman JG: The natural history of atrioventricular conduction defects in acute myocardial infarction. Am Heart J 78: 460–466, 1969
7. Norris RM: Heart block in posterior and anterior myocardial infarction. Br Heart J 31: 352–356, 1969
8. Webb SW, Adgey AAJ, Pantridge JF: Autonomic disturbance at onset of acute myocardial infarction. Br Med J 3: 89–92, 1972
9. Russell RO Jr, Hunt D, Rackley CE: Left ventricular hemodynamics in anterior and inferior myocardial infarction. Am J Cardiol 32: 8–16, 1973
10. Mintz SS, Katz LN: Recent myocardial infarction; an analysis of five hundred and seventy-two cases. Arch Intern Med 80: 205–236, 1947
11. Smith FM: The ligation of coronary arteries with electrocardiographic study. Arch Intern Med 22: 8–27, 1918
12. Pifarre R, Yokoyama T, Ilano AC, Hufnagel CA: Ventricular fibrillation after acute coronary artery occlusion. J Thorac Cardiovasc Surg 53: 335–340, 1967
13. James TN: Anatomy of the Coronary Arteries. New York, Hoeber, 1961
14. James TN: Arrhythmias and conduction disturbances in acute myocardial infarction. Am Heart J 64: 416–426, 1962
15. Lumb G, Singleton HP: Blood supply to the atrioventricular node and bundle of His; a comparative study in pig, dog and man. Am J Pathol 41: 65–75, 1962
16. Lev M: The conduction system. In Pathology of the Heart, ed 3, edited by SE Gould. Springfield, Charles C Thomas, 1968, pp 180–220
17. Corr PB, Gillis RA: Role of the vagus nerves in the cardiovascular

changes induced by coronary occlusion. Circulation **49**: 86–97, 1974

18. Abramson DI, Crawford JH, Roberts GH: The coronary blood supply in the cat. Anat Rec **58**: 25–30, 1933

19. James TN: Pathogenesis of arrhythmias in acute myocardial infarction. Am J Cardiol **24**: 791–799, 1969

20. Baba N, Leighton RF, Weissler AM: Experimental cardiac ischemia, observation of the sinoatrial and atrioventricular nodes. Lab Invest **23**: 168–178, 1970

21. Thoren P: Left ventricular receptors activated by severe asphyxia and by coronary artery occlusion. Acta Physiol Scand **85**: 455–463, 1972

22. Oberg B, Thoren P: Circulatory responses to stimulation of medullated and non-medullated afferents in the cardiac nerve in the cat. Acta Physiol Scand **87**: 121–132, 1973

23. Tennant R, Wiggers CJ: The effect of coronary occlusion on myocardial contraction. Am J Physiol **112**: 351–361, 1935

24. Orias O: The dynamic changes in the ventricle following ligation of the ramus descendens anterior. Am J Physiol **100**: 629–641, 1932

25. Schauer G, Gross L, Blum L: Hemodynamic studies in experimental coronary occlusion. IV. Stellate ganglionectomy experiments. Am Heart J **14**: 669–676, 1937

26. Sobel BE: Salient biochemical features in ischemic myocardium. Circ Res **34/35** (suppl III): 173–180, 1974

27. Staszewska-Barczak J: The reflex stimulation of catecholamine secretion during the acute stage of myocardial infarction in the dog. Clin Sci **41**: 419–439, 1971

28. Lown B, Wolf M: Approaches to sudden death from coronary heart disease. Circulation **44**: 130–142, 1971

29. Lumb G, Shacklett RS, Dawkins WA: The cardiac conduction tissue and its blood supply in the dog. Am J Pathol **35**: 467–487, 1959

30. James TN: Anatomy of the sinus node of the dog. Anat Rec **143**: 251–265, 1962

31. Corr PB, Gillis RA: Effect of autonomic neural influences on the cardiovascular changes induced by coronary occlusion. Am Heart J **89**: 766–774, 1975

Coronary heart disease: a review of abnormalities observed in the coronary arteries

William C. Roberts, M.D.

In this review of the status of the coronary arteries in patients who died of coronary heart disease (CHD), emphasis is placed on the diffuse nature of the atherosclerotic plaquing. Coronary atherosclerosis, for practical purposes, does not become symptomatic heart disease until plaque has narrowed the lumens of two of the three major coronary arteries more than 75% in cross-sectional area. It is suggested that some of this narrowing may be reversed by depletion of the lipid component in plaque; in other words, transient starvation may be effective therapy for symptomatic CHD. Arguments are also presented to support the thrombogenic origin of atherosclerotic plaques and to deemphasize the role of thrombi, if any, in precipitating acute coronary events. The thesis that coronary emboli are the most likely explanation for myocardial infarction with angiographically normal coronary arteries is also supported. Differences in coronary narrowing as observed by angiography and by histologic sectioning are summarized.

Symptoms and signs of coronary heart disease (CHD) are due to abnormal functioning of portions of left ventricular myocardium. The myocardial alterations in turn are consequences of severe narrowing of the lumens of the extramural coronary arteries. Certain changes observed in the coronary arteries at necropsy in patients with fatal CHD will be summarized in this report.

Atherosclerosis has been defined many ways and most definitions include descriptions of the composition of the plaques.[1] The word itself describes the plaque's composition: *sclerosis* = fibrous tissue and *athero* = fatty material. But many "atherosclerotic" lesions contain only fibrous tissue and some contain only fatty material. It seems preferable, therefore, to define atherosclerosis not by the composition of the plaques but by the amount of plaque deposited.

At birth, the intima of the extramural coronary arteries consists of a single layer of endothelium covering the internal elastic membrane. For some years thereafter there is a progressive increase in the thickness of the intima so that by age 20 it is more or less equal to the thickness of the media. This proliferated tissue consists primarily of collagen and elastic fibers. But smooth-muscle cells, some of which contain lipid, are also present. This concentric intimal proliferation occurs in all populations and apparently represents a response to the intra-arterial pressure; it is not considered to be atherosclerosis, which begins only when the thickness of the intima exceeds that of the media (Fig. 1). Atherosclerotic lesions may be concentric or eccentric. Atherosclerosis in contrast to the expected normal intimal proliferation is not worldwide in distribution, occurring only in populations that have an average adult total serum cholesterol level of more than 200 mg%.

Coronary atherosclerosis in fatal coronary heart disease

In patients who have died of CHD, the coronary arteries are diffusely involved with atherosclerotic plaques[2-10] (table). That coronary atherosclerosis is a focal process, as is occasionally observed by coronary angiography, is a myth. Indeed, it is unusual to find any segment of any of the major extramural coronary arteries free of atherosclerotic plaques at necropsy (Fig. 2 and 3). In other words, although the lumens of some segments are narrowed more severely than others, all portions of the extramural coronary tree are involved by the atherosclerotic process.

In fatal CHD, with rare exception, two and commonly three of the major (excluding the left main) coronary arteries are narrowed more than 75% in cross-sectional area by old atherosclerotic plaques. In other words, we need only two of the three major coronary arteries as long as the two are widely patent; we are provided with an extra or "bonus" coronary artery at birth. Thus, with rare exception, if only one of the three is narrowed more than 75%, no evidence of myocardial ischemia occurs — unless, of course, complete obstruction (em-

From the Pathology Branch, National Heart, Lung, and Blood Institute, National Institutes of Health, Bethesda, Md

Address reprint requests to Dr. Roberts, Building 10A, Room 3E-30, NIH, Bethesda, Md 20014

bolus, for example) occurs suddenly in a previously wide-open artery. For practical purposes, such evidence occurs only when at least two of the three major coronaries are more than 75% narrowed in cross-sectional area. The 75% demarcation point is useful because it is at this point that flow of a fluid (blood) through a tube (coronary artery) is decreased. So the major problem is not so much how to eliminate coronary atherosclerosis but simply how to limit it to less than 75% cross-sectional area luminal narrowing. This degree of narrowing is probably present also in patients with symptomatic CHD (Fig. 4) since studies of coronary arteries of patients who died during or shortly after aortocoronary bypass procedures have shown just as much narrowing of their major coronary arteries as in patients with CHD who died of their disease without such intervention.[10,11]

However, the coronary artery responsible for perfusing an area of myocardium that has become necrotic or fibrotic is not necessarily the most severely narrowed of the three major extramural coronary arteries. A patient with an anterior wall infarction may have as much or more luminal narrowing of the right or left circumflex coronary arteries or both as is present in the left descending coronary artery.

The lumens of atherosclerotic coronary arteries are quite variable in shape. The residual lumen may be located centrally or peripherally and its shape may be circular, oval, slitlike, or half-moon. The slitlike lumen, which

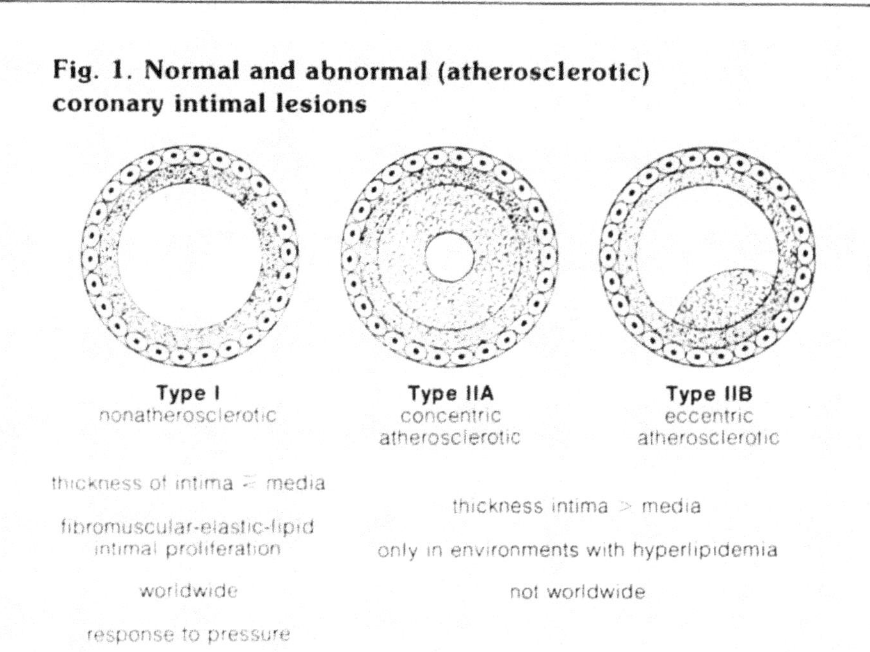

Fig. 1. Normal and abnormal (atherosclerotic) coronary intimal lesions

Status of the coronary arteries and myocardium in fatal ischemic heart disease

	Sudden coronary death (arrhythmia)	Acute myocardial infarction		Angina pectoris
		transmural	subendocardial	
Major coronary arteries				
Diffuse atherosclerosis	+	+	-	+
Luminal narrowing > 75% of 2 of 3 by atherosclerotic plaques	+	+	-	+
Thrombus	10%	60%	0	0
Hemorrhage into plaque	25%	25%	25%	25%
Left ventricular myocardium				
Necrosis	0	+	-	0
Fibrosis (transmural or subendocardial)	50%	50%	50%	50%

extends from one side of the artery to the other, may appear on angiography as a normal-sized orifice.

The initial size of the narrowed artery is also an important factor in determining the amount of coronary arterial area through which blood may flow. Figure 5 shows two arteries, for example, both of which are slightly more than 75% narrowed. Although the percent luminal narrowing by atherosclerotic plaque in each artery is similar, one artery is less than a fourth the size of the other. Thus, the smaller the initial size of the artery, the greater the potential effect of the luminal narrowing. The larger the heart, in general, the greater the cross-sectional area of the coronary arteries and vice versa. Thus, since women have smaller mean heart weights than men, they also have smaller mean cross-sectional areas of coronary arteries.

The atherosclerotic process is limited to the epicardial coronary arteries — the major trunks and their near right-angle branches — and except for those in the papillary muscles,[12] spares the intramyocardial coronary arteries (Fig. 6 and 7).

Certain portions of the coronary tree tend to develop larger atherosclerotic plaques, and therefore more narrowed lumina, than other portions. The most severe narrowing of the left coronary artery is usually within the first 2 cm of the origin of the left anterior descending and left circumflex branches. Calcific deposits nearly always are more extensive in the proximal than in the distal portions of the coronary arteries. It is because of this proximal narrowing that aortocoronary bypass procedures have proved beneficial to many patients with severe angina pectoris and good myocardial function. The right coronary artery, however, is a trap in this regard; its distal third is usually more narrowed than is the proximal or middle third. The distal portions of the coronary arteries also are more difficult than the proximal portions to evaluate by angiography and severe distal narrowings are probably more often missed or underestimated.

Considerable attention has been given to "significant" narrowings — more than 50% reduction in luminal diameter by angiography or more than 75% cross-sectional area narrowing at necropsy — of the left main coronary artery. Severe narrowing of this artery virtually always indicates severe narrowing of each of the other three major coronaries.[9]

Among patients with fatal CHD, those with more than 75% cross-sectional area narrowing of the left main had had a significantly higher frequency of angina pectoris and hyperlipoproteinemia, especially type II, than those with less than 50% cross-sectional narrowing of this artery. The more severely affected patients, however, had had a lower frequency of acute transmural myocardial infarction.[9] Death during cardiac catheterization or coronary angiography, and probably during aortocoronary bypass operations, also appears to occur more frequently among CHD patients with

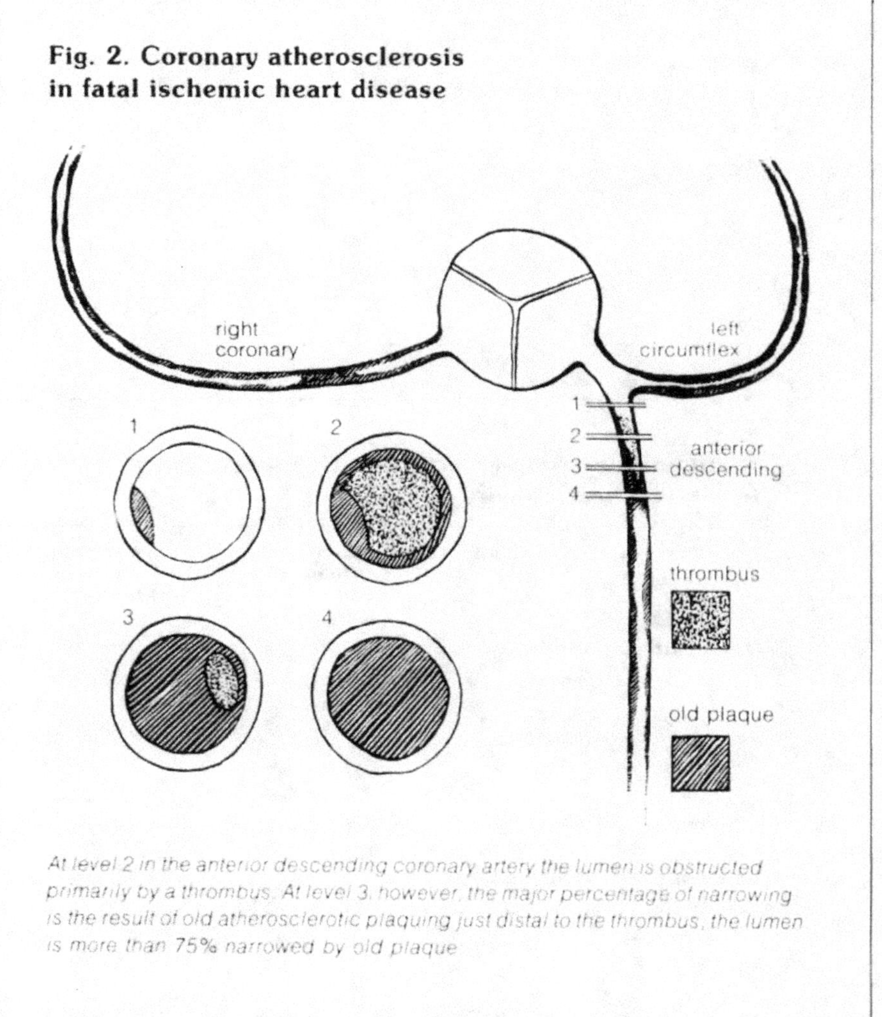

Fig. 2. Coronary atherosclerosis in fatal ischemic heart disease

At level 2 in the anterior descending coronary artery the lumen is obstructed primarily by a thrombus. At level 3, however, the major percentage of narrowing is the result of old atherosclerotic plaquing just distal to the thrombus; the lumen is more than 75% narrowed by old plaque.

more than 75% narrowing of the left main than among the group with less than 50%.

As defined by a World Health Organization committee, the three types of atherosclerotic plaques are lipid, fibrous, and complicated, with only the complicated plaque causing significant (more than 75%) coronary luminal narrowing.[1] Lipid and fibrous plaques are worldwide in distribution while complicated plaque, which contains calcific deposits, cholesterol clefts, pultaceous debris, etc., is found only in populations with total serum cholesterol levels averaging more than 200 mg%. The major component of even the complicated atherosclerotic plaque, however, is fibrous tissue (collagen) with the lipid component much less evident. Foam cells are found infrequently in the coronary arteries of patients who have died of CHD, and the lipid that is present is usually extracellular.

It has been demonstrated in the experimental animal that the lipid component of the plaque is reversible (dissoluble). It is less likely, obviously, that the fibrous component of the atherosclerotic plaque is reversible. Whether or not low-lipid diets or lipid-lowering drugs will cause depletion of lipids in complicated symptom-producing coronary atherosclerotic placques is uncertain. Although fat stores in the body consist predominantly of triglycerides, and atherosclerotic plaque predominantly of cholesterol esters, plaques might decrease in size if caloric intake is low enough to cause a decrease in the size of fat deposits in readily visible portions of the body (anterior panniculus, for example). Emaciated prisoners in World War II apparently had little coronary arterial luminal narrowing. Similar observations have been made in victims of malignant neoplasms. Moreover, the amount of lipid in the atherosclerotic plaque of emaciated patients coming to necropsy appears to be less than that observed in the nonemaciated.

Thus transient starvation may well be a neglected but beneficial form of therapy, possibly also a form of prevention, for symptomatic CHD (Fig. 8). If the lumen of a coronary artery is 90% obliterated by atherosclerotic plaques, for example, about 25% of the plaque generally consists of lipid deposits. So depletion of these lipid deposits in the plaque would reduce the luminal narrowing to less than 75% and the flow of blood would be adequate.

The degree of coronary arterial luminal narrowing by atherosclerotic plaque and the amount of plaque are similar in patients who died of CHD regardless of the fatal coronary event, i.e., acute myocardial infarction (AMI), clinically isolated angina pectoris, sudden coronary death, or progressive congestive cardiac failure after healing of an AMI (ischemic cardiomyopathy) (table).[2-11]

Although the degree of coronary luminal narrowing by atherosclerotic plaque is similar in all four types of coronary events, the myocardial reaction obviously is quite different. Patients with clinically isolated angina pectoris of severe degree usually have near-normal-sized hearts in both weight and ventricular cavity size, little

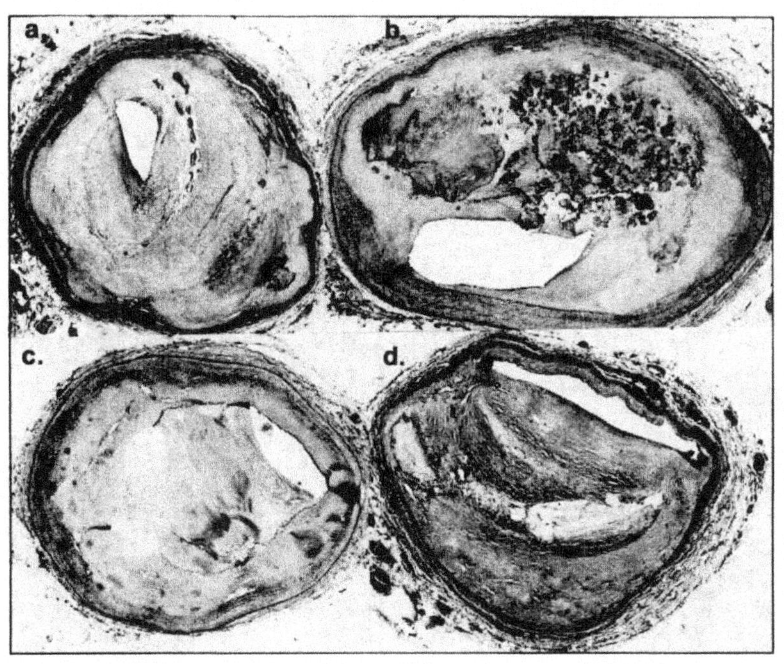

Fig. 3. Coronary arteries in fatal coronary heart disease

These sections represent the sites of maximal narrowing in the right (a), left main (b), left anterior descending (c), and left circumflex (d) coronary arteries of a 41-year-old man who died suddenly after having had angina pectoris for 7 years. Sections a, b, and c are elastic Van Gieson's stain, d, a hematoxylin-eosin stain, each is magnified 25x

if any myocardial fibrosis, and no myocardial necrosis.[10] Patients with ischemic cardiomyopathy usually have large transmural left ventricular scars, large left ventricular cavities, often with aneurysms, and left ventricular mural thrombi.[11] The fatal AMI patients obviously have myocardial necrosis, which usually is transmural. Finally, the patients who die suddenly and unexpectedly usually have hearts like those of patients with clinically isolated angina pectoris. The reasons for the differences in myocardial response to apparently similar degrees of coronary atherosclerosis are uncertain.

The composition of coronary atherosclerotic plaques and the degree of coronary arterial luminal narrowing in patients who died of CHD appear similar whether the blood lipoprotein pattern is normal or abnormal.[6] Patients with types II, III, or IV hyperlipoproteinemia clearly have accelerated atherosclerosis compared with persons of similar age and sex with normal lipoprotein patterns, but hyperlipoproteinemia is not a prerequisite for premature development of severe atherosclerosis. Severe narrowing of the left main coronary artery is more common in patients with type II hyperlipoproteinemia than in patients with types III or IV or in persons with normal lipoprotein patterns.[9] Furthermore, atherosclerosis of the ascending aorta may be prominent in patients with type II hyperlipoproteinemia; this is especially true if the hyperlipoproteinemia is of the homozygous rather than the heterozygous variety.[6] Also, in the homozygous form, the coronary ostia may be narrowed severely by the aortic atherosclerosis, which may involve the aortic valve cusps directly and produce aortic stenosis.[6]

Although advanced age is the number one risk factor in the development of symptomatic atherosclerosis in the Western world, age itself does not necessarily indicate the presence of severe coronary atherosclerosis. Actually, acute myocardial infarction is infrequent in patients over 90 years of age. The explanation probably lies in the fact that the coronary arteries normally dilate with age unless extensive atherosclerotic plaques prevent this "normal" dilatation from occurring (Fig. 9). Obviously, the greater the dilatation, the wider the lumen.

Coronary thrombosis

Up to this point I have considered certain features of old or chronic lesions, namely atherosclerosis, in the coronary arteries in patients with fatal coronary heart disease. No discussion has been presented on what tips the scales in these patients from *adequate* to *inadequate myocardial oxygenation*. Until recently it was thought that a new lesion, usually a thrombus or a

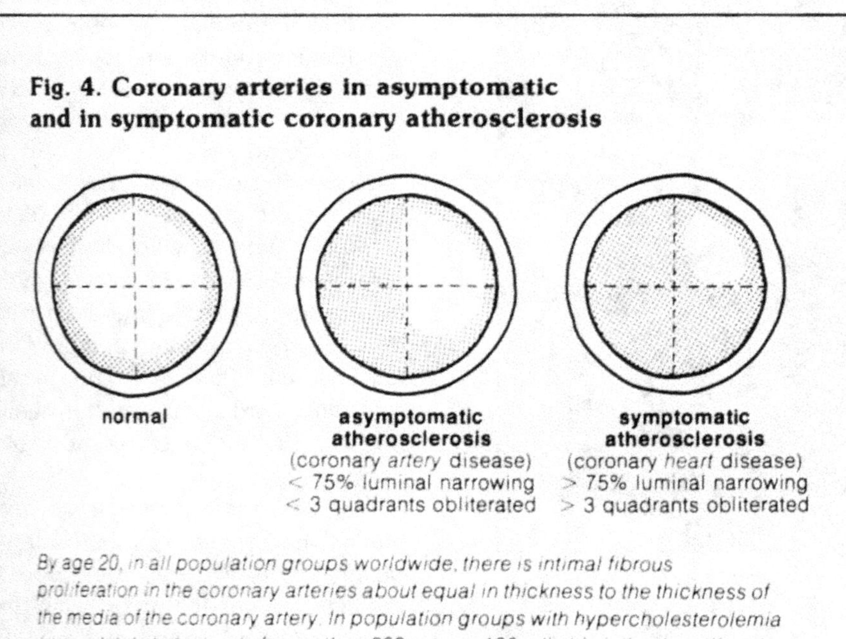

Fig. 4. Coronary arteries in asymptomatic and in symptomatic coronary atherosclerosis

By age 20, in all population groups worldwide, there is intimal fibrous proliferation in the coronary arteries about equal in thickness to the thickness of the media of the coronary artery. In population groups with hypercholesterolemia (serum total cholesterol of more than 200 mg per 100 ml), this intimal proliferative process generally continues. Symptoms of myocardial ischemia rarely occur until the intimal proliferative process obliterates more than 75% of the lumen.

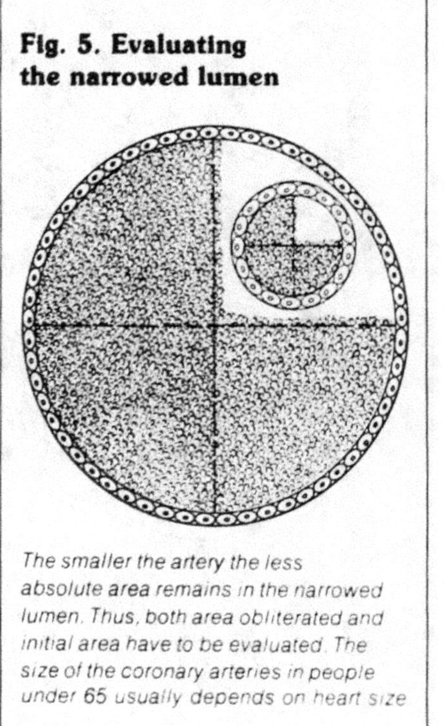

Fig. 5. Evaluating the narrowed lumen

The smaller the artery the less absolute area remains in the narrowed lumen. Thus, both area obliterated and initial area have to be evaluated. The size of the coronary arteries in people under 65 usually depends on heart size.

hemorrhage into an old atherosclerotic plaque, suddenly appeared and this provided a nice anatomic explanation for the usually sudden, dramatic clinical episode of myocardial ischemia, namely acute myocardial infarction or sudden coronary death. Before examining the question as to whether or not a new coronary lesion precipitates a coronary event, a summary of some observations on coronary thrombosis in patients with fatal coronary events appears appropriate:

• Only about 10% of patients who die suddenly of CHD have coronary arterial thrombi.[5] Sudden coronary death is defined herein as that occurring within six hours after onset of symptoms of myocardial ischemia and unassociated with histologic evidence of myocardial necrosis.

• Coronary arterial thrombi are rare in patients in whom myocardial necrosis is limited to the subendocardial region.[5] Subendocardium is defined as the inner one-half of the myocardial wall. Necrosis limited to the subendocardial region is rarely fatal, however, unless the patient has severe cardiomegaly from another condition, such as systemic hypertension or left ventricular outflow tract obstruction.

• A thrombus is found in the lumen of an extramural coronary artery in about 60% of patients with fatal transmural AMI.[5,13] Transmural is defined as that portion of left ventricular wall that includes all of the inner half—subendocardium—and at least some portion of the subepicardial half of the wall.

• Coronary thrombosis was found in 70% of fatal AMI patients who had cardiogenic shock as opposed to only 15% of those who hadn't had the power-failure syndrome.[14-16]

• The larger the area of myocardial necrosis, the greater the likelihood of its having been caused by coronary thrombosis. The larger the infarcted area, however, the greater the likelihood of cardiogenic shock. Shock generally indicates that more than 40% of the left ventricular wall is either necrotic, fibrotic, or both, whereas shock is infrequently associated with infarcts or scars involving less than 40% of the ventricular wall.[15]

• When coronary thrombosis is associated with acute myocardial infarction, the thrombus is always located in the artery responsible for perfusing the area of myocardial necrosis.[5] Thus, in anterior wall infarction a thrombus, if present, will be located in the left anterior descending coronary artery. Thrombi infrequently occur in more than one major coronary artery.

• In fatal CHD thrombi are found in coronary arteries already severely narrowed by old atherosclerotic plaques.[5] At the distal site of attachment of the thrombus, or just distal to this site, the lumen of the coronary artery is nearly always more than 75% narrowed in cross-sectional area by old atherosclerotic plaques (Fig. 2). Not infrequently, a thrombus may occur in an area between two sites at which

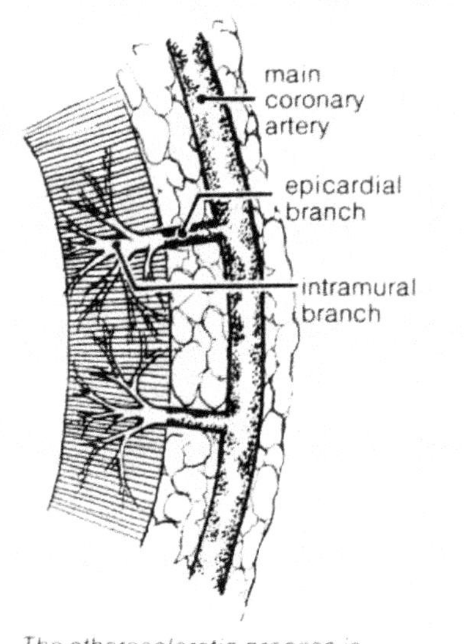

Fig. 6. Where plaque forms

The atherosclerotic process is limited to the epicardial arteries, sparing the intramural portions.

Fig. 7. A papillary muscle in sudden death

Shown here are cross-sectional views of many intramural coronary arteries located in the left ventricular papillary muscle of a 45-year-old man who died suddenly, without previous symptoms, of ischemic heart disease. The arteries have thickened walls and narrowed lumina. This is a common finding in patients with fatal ischemic heart disease.

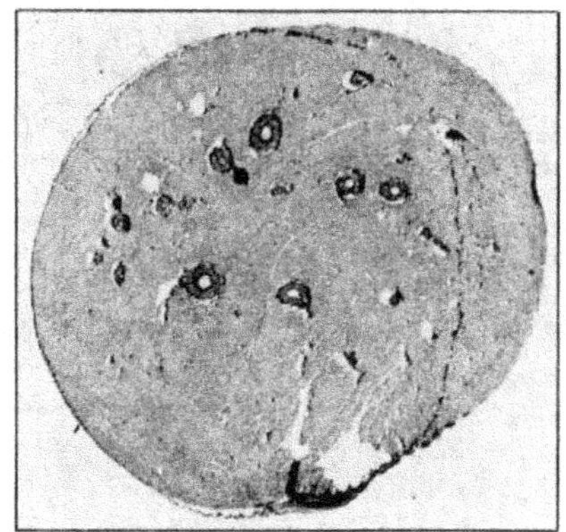

The intramural coronary arteries in the free walls and ventricular system, in contrast, are virtually always normal. At necropsy, this patient's heart weighed only 340 g. The lumina of the left main, left anterior descending, and left circumflex coronary arteries were more than 75% narrowed in cross-sectional area and of the right between 51 and 75% narrowed by atherosclerotic plaques.

severe narrowing has occurred. • In fatal AMI, 90% of coronary thrombi are single and 80% are occlusive. They are usually short (less than 2 cm long) and are located entirely in the major trunks as opposed to their near right-angle branches or the intramural coronary arteries. When only a few hours old the thrombus may consist nearly entirely of platelets, but thereafter it is composed primarily of fibrin. By definition, the thrombus is *adherent* to the surface of the arterial wall bordering the lumen.

The role of thrombosis in fatal coronary heart disease

Since 1912 when Herrick[17] first used the term "coronary thrombosis" to describe the often dramatic clinical event characterized at necropsy by necrosis of portions of left ventricular wall, it has been assumed that thrombosis was the usual cause of acute myocardial infarction. Two factors implicate it as the *precipitating cause* of AMI: the occurrence of coronary arterial thrombi in many patients with fatal AMI and the location of the thrombus in the coronary artery responsible for supplying the area of myocardial necrosis. On the other hand, at least five factors tend to indicate that coronary thrombosis is a *consequence* of AMI: the low frequency of thrombi in patients dying suddenly with or without previous evidence of cardiac disease; the near absence of thrombi in patients with fatal subendocardial AMI; the absence of thrombi in fatal transmural AMI nearly as often as they are present; the increasing frequency of thrombi with increasing intervals between onset of symptoms of AMI and death; and the more common occurrence of thrombi in patients with cardiogenic shock, most of whom have large transmural infarcts.

The key to coronary thrombosis,

and the key to thrombosis occurring anywhere in the body, is *slow blood flow*, or relative stasis, and *sufficient time* for the thrombus to form. The absence of these two factors may explain the absence of coronary thrombosis in the sudden death cases and the increasing frequency of thrombosis as the interval from onset of symptoms of myocardial ischemia to death increases.[18] There is a marked reduction in blood flow in the coronary artery responsible for supplying the area of myocardial infarction. This observation was made in dogs after inducing AMI, and they had normal vessels.[19] In fatal AMI in humans, the thrombus is always located in an artery already containing considerable atherosclerotic plaque and, therefore, the infarct-induced relative coronary stasis is probably even greater. Cardiogenic shock must further diminish coronary blood flow.

Patients' activities at the time of

onset of AMI may reflect slowed blood flow—nearly 75% have the onset of chest pain while sleeping, resting, or performing mild activity.[20] Although inactivity may cause slight diminution in coronary blood flow, infarction-induced stasis plus cardiogenic shock is usually necessary for thrombus to form. In contrast to fatal AMI, coronary thrombosis is rarely observed in fatal angina pectoris, although the degree of coronary luminal narrowing by atherosclerotic plaques is similar in degree to that observed in AMI. Evidence of thrombus formation is nearly always observed in internal mammary arteries implanted into dogs' left ventricular myocardium but if the implant is allowed to drain into right ventricular cavity no thrombus occurs.[21] Thus, it appears that a period of diminished coronary blood flow is necessary for thrombus to form in a coronary artery. Shock, congestive cardiac failure, and inactivity all decrease coronary flow

Fig. 8. The possible effects of lipid lowering in symptomatic coronary heart disease

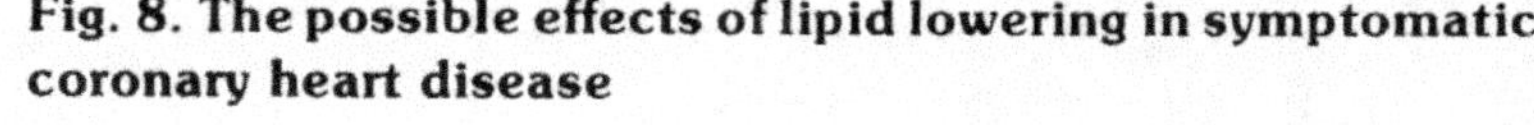

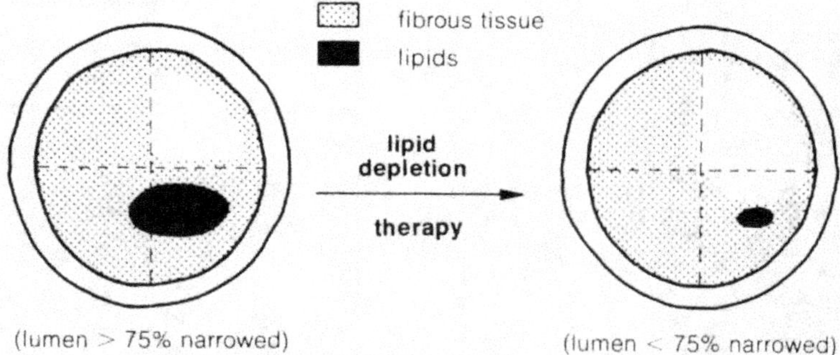

Although the dominant component of atherosclerotic plaque is usually fibrous tissue, lipid deposits form a portion of most plaques. It is likely that the fibrous component of the plaque is nonreversible. In contrast, the lipid component may well be reversible. Transient starvation may cause a diminution in the size of the lipid component and a decrease in luminal narrowing from more than 75%, the amount associated with symptoms, to less than 75%, an amount rarely associated with symptoms.

and with time may allow formation of thrombus.

Additional support for this concept is supplied by Erhardt and associates,[22] who observed radioactivity at necropsy in coronary arterial thrombi in patients who had been given radioactive ^{125}I-labeled fibrinogen shortly after being hospitalized with acute myocardial infarctions. This finding implicates coronary thrombosis as a secondary event occurring some time after the infarction.

Thus, there is substantial evidence that acute thrombus formation does *not* precipitate acute fatal ischemic heart disease. The major problem is diffuse generalized coronary atherosclerosis with more than 75% cross-sectional luminal narrowing of at least two of the three major coronary arteries.

The role of thrombosis in atherosclerosis

Although I have deemphasized the role of coronary thrombosis in precipitating acute myocardial infarction, I would now like to turn the coin over and suggest, as have some other investigators,[23] that thrombosis does play a major role in the development of the atherosclerotic plaques in the first place. Rokitansky[24] in 1852 was the first, to my knowledge, to propose that atherosclerotic plaques resulted from the organization of thrombi. Virchow[25] disputed this view and since 1913, investigations of atherosclerosis, with some exceptions, have centered mainly on the role of lipids. Several observations suggest, however, that atherosclerotic plaques result, at least in part, from the organization of thrombi:

• The presence of known components of thrombi — namely fibrin and platelets — within atherosclerotic plaques (Fig. 10).

• The occurrence of known components of atherosclerotic plaques — namely foam cells, cholesterol clefts, pultaceous debris, and calcium — in organized hematomas or known thrombi wherever they occur in the body. An example is the left atrial thrombus in the patient with mitral stenosis. Organization of this thrombus may produce typical complicated atherosclerotic plaques.[7]

• The presence of multiluminal channels in vessels — a recognized consequence of organization of pulmonary arterial thromboemboli.[26] Multiple luminal channels commonly are found in severely atherosclerotic coronary arteries (Fig. 10), suggesting that thrombi or emboli were at one time present and that they organized. The tissue between the channels is similar to that found in arteries with only one channel (Fig. 11). Because the artery with multiple channels has been recognized as the hallmark of an organized thrombus[27] and because the tissue in multi- and unichanneled arteries is similar, Duguid[23] reasoned that the causative process also was similar.

• The major component of the complicated atherosclerotic plaque, i.e., the one capable of causing fatal CHD, is fibrous tissue or collagen, not lipid.[5] This is true whether or not hyperlipidemia is present.[6] Foam cells are actually infrequent in coronary arteries of patients with fatal CHD. Often the "density" of the fibrous tissue plugging a coronary artery is different in different portions of a plaque and these subunits may be demarcated by distinct elastic lamellae. These subunits suggest that thrombus is deposited at different times and that the density of the resulting fibrous tissue may be determined by the composition of the initial thrombus, i.e., whether platelets or fibrin predominated.[28]

• Experimentally induced thrombi under proper conditions may be transformed into atherosclerotic plaques closely resembling those observed in human coronary arteries.[28]

These factors obviously do not prove that thrombosis is the cause of atherosclerosis, but together they strongly suggest that organization of thrombi plays a major role in the development of the complicated atherosclerotic plaque. Indeed, most serious students of the morphology of the ar-

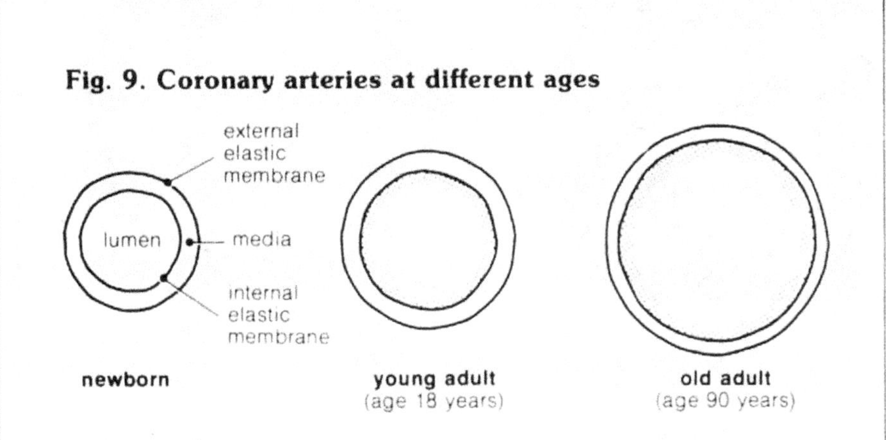

Fig. 9. Coronary arteries at different ages

The dotted area represents the intimal lesion, fibromuscular proliferation, that is presumably a response to intra-arterial pressure and not a form of atherosclerosis

terial plaque currently support, in whole or in part, the thrombogenic origin of atherosclerosis.

Because the clotting factors in the blood appear to be similar in all population groups and because symptomatic atherosclerosis develops only in those population groups with elevated blood lipids (serum cholesterol greater than 200 mg per 100 ml), the latter also play a role in the development of the plaque. Lipids may exert their effect, however, more by their ability to alter the clotting mechanism than by their ability to infiltrate the arterial wall.

Nonthrombotic acute coronary lesions

Hemorrhage into an old atherosclerotic plaque. Hemorrhages into coronary atherosclerotic plaques are observed in about 25% of patients with fatal CHD (table). Even when plaque hemorrhages occur, however, the lumen of the coronary artery is not further narrowed and they have no relationship to the site of myocardial necrosis. In necropsy studies, the anterior wall may have been the site of infarction, but hemorrhages may have involved a plaque in the right coronary artery or all three coronary arteries or multiple sites in a single coronary artery. Plaque hemorrhages may in fact be occurring all through adult life in patients with and without symptomatic CHD. When a coronary thrombus is observed, on the other hand, its location does correspond to the site of necrosis; with anterior wall infarction and coronary thrombosis, the thrombus is located in the left anterior descending coronary artery, and only very rarely are other thrombi found in the right or left circumflex coronary arteries. It appears unlikely, therefore, that plaque hemorrhages are responsible for precipitating acute myocardial ischemia because they do not narrow the lumen and they are not necessarily related to site of myocardial necrosis. **Coronary arterial embolism.** This is a rare cause of fatal coronary heart disease (Fig. 12). Diagnosis of embolism requires identification of the site of dislodgment of the embolus or at least a condition predisposing to development of embolism, such as infective endocarditis, intracardiac mural thrombus, or a coagulopathy. Embolism is extremely difficult to recognize when superimposed on an extensively atherosclerotic coronary arterial tree. Thus, diagnosis of embolism usually requires the occurrence of "clot" in a coronary tree devoid of heavy atherosclerotic plaques. Furthermore, in contrast to coronary thrombosis, which never involves the intramural coronary arteries and infrequently involves the distal portions of the extramural coronary arteries (except for the right one), embolism usually involves both the intra- and extramural arteries, usually the distal portions of the extramural.

Dissecting aneurysm (hematoma) of a coronary artery with and without

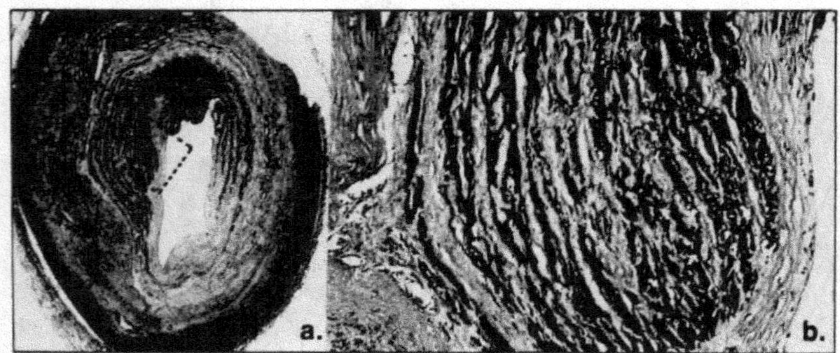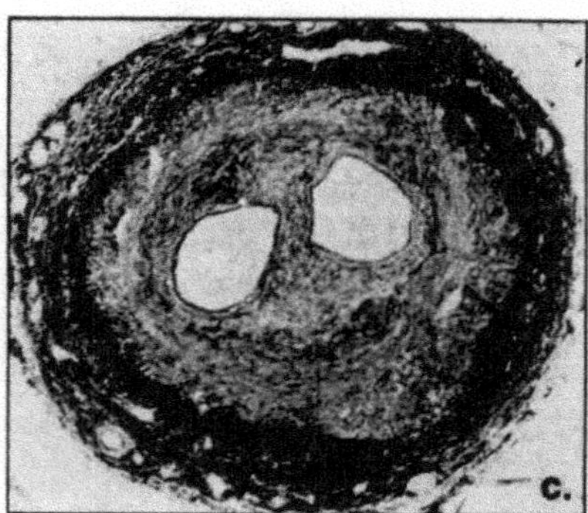

Fig. 10. Evidence implicating clots or emboli in atherogenesis

Fibrin, a known component of thrombi, is seen interspersed in the fibrous plaques that have severely narrowed this right coronary artery of a 47-year-old man with a healed posterior wall left ventricular transmural infarct and rheumatic mitral stenosis. The fibrin is darker (dotted lines, a) than the adjacent organized fibrous tissue. A close-up view of one area of the fibrin deposits is shown in b. The section was stained with phosphotungstic acid–hematoxylin and is magnified 23x (a) and 120x (b).

Multiple luminal channels in the left circumflex coronary artery (c) of a 58-year-old man who had an acute myocardial infarction at age 54 and the onset of symptoms of acute myocardial ischemia one hour before death. These multiple channels suggest organization of clot—either thrombus or embolus. The stain is elastic Van Gieson, magnification 30x.

associated dissection of the aorta. Dissection of one or both coronary arteries with resultant luminal narrowing is commonly associated with dissection of the aorta. The resulting myocardial ischemia in this circumstance may be fatal. Virtually all patients with aortic dissecting aneurysm with or without associated dissection of the coronary arteries have systemic hypertension. Dissection of one or more major coronary arteries, however, may occur, although rarely, in the absence of dissection of the aorta,[28] and when it does, systemic hypertension is infrequent. The underlying precipitating causes of this idiopathic dissection have yet to be identified. Women are more often affected than men, death is usually sudden, and there is no histologic evidence of myocardial necrosis. In addition to the idiopathic variety, isolated coronary dissection may be iatrogenic in origin, a result of either coronary angiography or coronary bypass operations.[29]

MI and angiographically normal coronary arteries

According to coronary angiography, in patients with coronary heart disease manifested by acute myocardial infarction, *at the time of AMI*, there is severe narrowing or complete obstruction of at least one of the three major coronary arteries; *at the time of AMI*, a normal coronary tree has never been demonstrated; and *after healing of an AMI*, more than 99% of patients demonstrate severe narrowing of one or more of the three major coronary arteries and less than 1% have a normal coronary tree. In recent years much attention has been given to this small group of patients with myocardial infarction and angiographically normal coronary arteries.[30] A major implication of most reports on this subject is that AMI may occur in the presence of normal coronary arteries.

There are at least six possible explanations for the occurrence of an angiographically normal coronary arterial tree after healing of an AMI (Fig. 13):

AMI never occurred, an unlikely explanation since AMI was documented in most of the patients reported by both electrocardiographic changes and enzyme elevations.

Too large a myocardial mass or too little hemoglobin or too low a perfusion pressure (shock) was present to supply the myocardium despite a normal coronary tree. The occurrence of myocardial scars in patients with large hearts or severe chronic anemia with or without cardiomegaly and normal coronary arteries is well recognized. Similarly, an inadequate perfusion pressure may lead to myocardial necrosis (with later scarring) despite a normal coronary tree. The necrosis or fibrosis, however, in each of these three circumstances usually is limited to left ventricular papillary muscle and subendocardium of left ventricular free wall.

The coronary arteriograms were misinterpreted. It is well known that coronary angiography tends to underestimate the degree of coronary arterial luminal narrowing. This explanation may on occasion be the proper one but most patients with symptomatic CHD have some abnormality on angiography of two and usually all three of the major extramural coronary arteries.

Coronary spasm caused the AMI. Al-

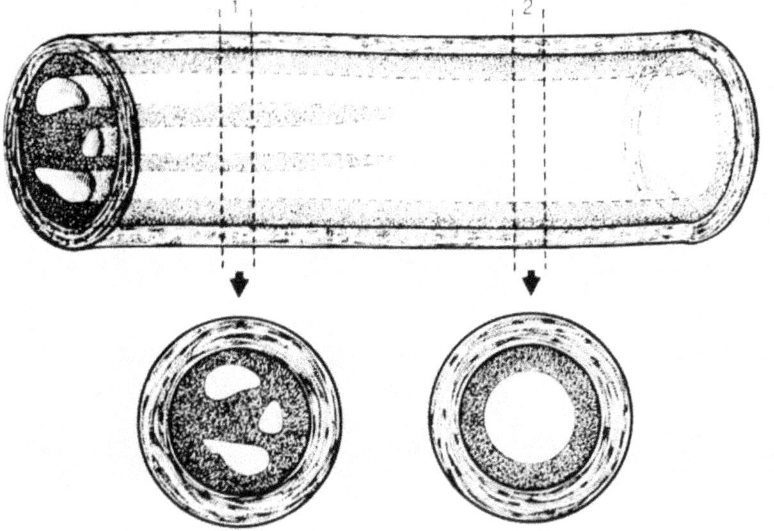

Fig. 11. The multi- and the unichanneled coronary arterial atherosclerotic plaque

The tissue found between channels in an artery containing multiple revascularized channels is similar to that found in arteries with only one channel. Since the multichannel artery has been recognized as the hallmark of an organized thrombus and since the tissues in multi- and unichanneled arteries are similar, it is reasonable to assume that the causative process also is similar.

though shown to cause both chest pain and ischemic changes on electrocardiogram, coronary spasm has not been shown to cause myocardial necrosis. The case for spasm is generally considered strongest among patients with Prinzmetal's angina. Of 143 patients with this variant angina reported in English and summarized by Arnett and Roberts,[31] 124 had coronary arteriography; of these, the coronary arterial luminal diameters were judged to be more than 75% narrowed in 76 or 61% and normal in 48 or 39%. Coronary spasm was demonstrated in 17 (14%) of the 124 patients — in 5 of 76 with narrowed arteries and in 12 of 48 patients with normal coronary arteries. Although neither AMI nor death occurred naturally in any of the 5 patients with both coronary spasm and fixed coronary narrowing, 3 of the 5 had infarctions or died after aortocoronary bypass procedures. None of the 48 patients with angiographically normal coronary arteries had an AMI, and of the 6 who died, none were among the 12 with demonstrated coronary spasm. Examination of the coronary arteries in 5 of these 6 patients at necropsy disclosed more than 75% narrowing of one coronary ostium or artery in 3 patients and a "small" left coronary artery in a fourth; only 1 of the 5 patients, therefore, had a "normal" coronary tree at necropsy. Thus, although it has been shown to cause chest pain and ischemic electrocardiographic changes, coronary artery spasm has not been shown to cause myocardial necrosis.

AMI was caused by a condition affecting only the intramural or intramyocardial coronary arteries, without involvement of the extramural coronary arteries. Abnormalities of the intramural coronary arteries have been reported in a number of conditions but, to our knowledge, transmural AMI has never been described as a consequence of disease of the intramural arteries alone. Even in the conditions where such involvement was observed, it has usually been associated with a condition affecting other body organs or systems as well.

AMI was caused by an occluding embolus that subsequently lysed or recanalized. This appears the most likely cause of acute myocardial infarction in patients subsequently shown by angiography to have normal coronary arterial trees. It is reasoned that the coronary arteries were not really normal at the time of coronary angiography. Facts supporting this hypothesis are as follows:

• Arteriographically documented coronary arterial embolic occlusion can completely resolve. Of five reported patients with catheter-induced coronary arterial thromboembolic occlusion, the coronary arteriogram became normal after the infarction in each.[30] In three of the five patients, complete resolution of the occlusion occurred within two months of the onset of the infarction.

• Conditions associated with an increased risk of arterial thromboemboli are relatively frequent (15%) among reported patients with non-catheter-induced AMI.[30]

• Histologic study of previously known arterial emboli indicates that such lesions may either be lysed completely, retract along one side to form an eccentric lumen, or recanalize with multiple luminal channels.[26] Each of these three means of organization of

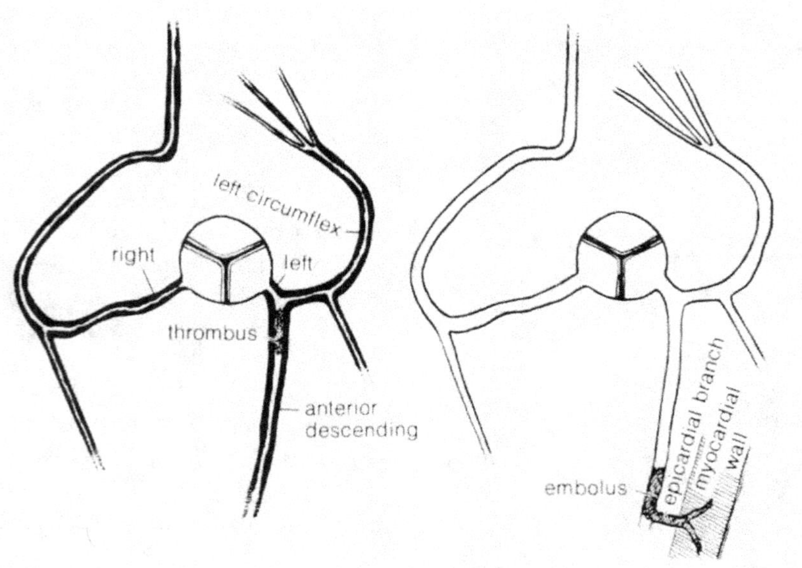

Fig. 12. Differences between coronary arterial thrombosis and embolism

The thrombus (left), which is usually proximal and superimposed on old atherosclerotic plaque, does not extend into intramural coronary arteries. The embolus (right) is distal and usually extends into an intramural artery. Moreover, it usually occurs in a coronary tree devoid of significant old atherosclerotic plaque

the clot almost surely could create a lumen large enough to produce a normal coronary arteriogram.

• Among 74 previously reported necropsy patients with transmural AMI,[5] only 5 had more than 75% luminal narrowing by atherosclerotic plaques in each of their three major coronary arteries; 3 of the 5 had coronary emboli at necropsy and their coronary tree was otherwise normal.

• With few exceptions, patients who have non-catheter-induced AMI were asymptomatic before the occurrence of the infarction and after it had healed they had no evidence of angina pectoris, congestive cardiac failure, or cardiomegaly. Obviously, in patients with severe symptomatic coronary atherosclerosis, an AMI may be the first and only coronary event but the percentage who return to a totally asymptomatic state is not nearly as high. An analogous situation might be acute pulmonary embolism when occurring in previously normal pulmonary arteries and lungs as opposed to acute pulmonary embolism superimposed on chronic lung disease.

Angiographic versus histologic examination

The coronary arteries are examined most commonly today not at necropsy but by selective coronary angiography during life. The observations presented in this report have been based exclusively on those obtained by histologic examination of the coronary arteries. Because angiographic examination of these arteries is now so commonplace, it is appropriate to end this presentation by illustrating differences in these angiographic and histologic means of examination.

Although angiography is the only currently available method of providing information regarding degrees of coronary narrowing during life, it breaks a basic photographic principle that 85% of a photographic frame or negative should be filled with the subject matter. A single site of luminal narrowing on a coronary luminagram may occupy less than 1% of the area of the frame. On histologic examination, in contrast, it is easy to fill 85% of the frame with a cross section of a coronary artery. Thus, true degrees of luminal narrowing are more reliable by histologic examination even though the arteries are not distended by intraluminal pressure. Another obvious difference is that only a longitudinal view of the artery is provided by the angiogram and only the space of the lumen is discernible. By histologic examination, however, cross sections of the coronary artery can be studied, including the lumen, the atherosclerotic plaque, and the original vessel wall.

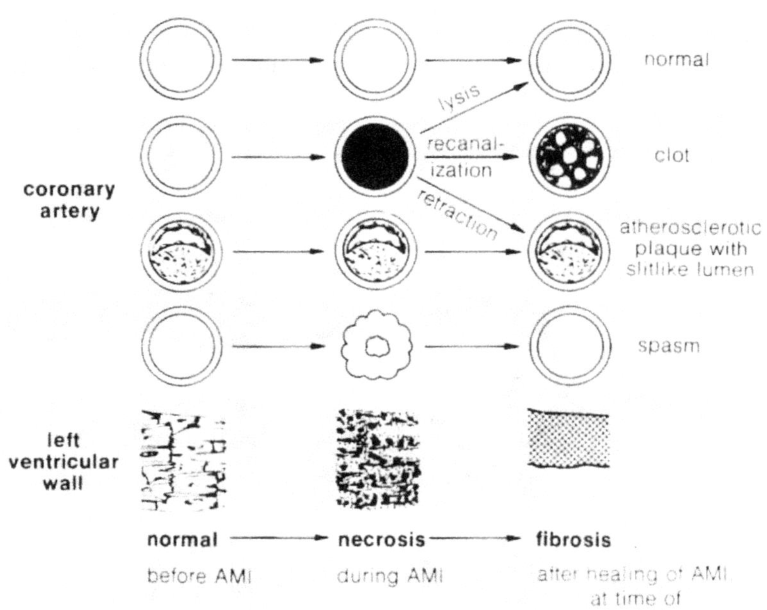

Fig. 13. Why coronary arteries may be angiographically normal after acute myocardial infarction

The left vertical column indicates the status of the coronary arteries and myocardium before the acute myocardial infarction (AMI), the center vertical column, during the AMI, and the right vertical column, after healing of the AMI. If the infarction was caused by a disproportion between the size of the coronary bed and the amount of myocardium to be oxygenated, the coronary arteries presumably would be normal (top row) before, during, and after its event. Coronary angiography may show a slitlike eccentric lumen (third row) on occasion to be "normal," however. If spasm caused the AMI (though this has never been documented), one or more coronary arteries might be partially obstructed at the time of the AMI (fourth row). If embolism caused the AMI (second row), the clot could subsequently lyse, recanalize, or retract along one side allowing the lumen to be of sufficient size to appear later as angiographically normal.

Another difference is the type of luminal narrowing observed. By angiogram, only narrowing of the vessel's *diameter* is discernible. Furthermore, the degree of narrowing is determined by comparing the narrowest areas to adjacent sites, which may also be narrowed by intimal disease but to a somewhat lesser degree. Thus an accurate picture of luminal narrowing can be gained only when the luminal diameter adjacent to the site of narrowing is free of intimal disease, a situation that does not exist in most patients.

As shown in figure 14, a 50% reduction from original luminal *diameter* corresponds to a 75% cross-sectional *area* reduction, and a 75% reduction from original luminal diameter corresponds to a 95% reduction in cross-sectional area. If, however, the lumen adjacent to a site of severe diameter reduction is also already narrowed, the greatest diameter reduction is underestimated. Because coronary atherosclerosis is virtually always diffuse in patients with symptomatic coronary heart disease, the degree of reduction in luminal diameter determined by coronary angiography is nearly always underestimated.

Summary

The coronary arteries in patients with fatal coronary heart disease may be characterized as follows:

• The coronary arteries are *diffusely* involved by atherosclerotic plaques.

• With few exceptions, the lumina of at least two of the three major coronary arteries are reduced more than 75% in cross-sectional area by atherosclerotic plaques.

• The atherosclerosis is limited to the

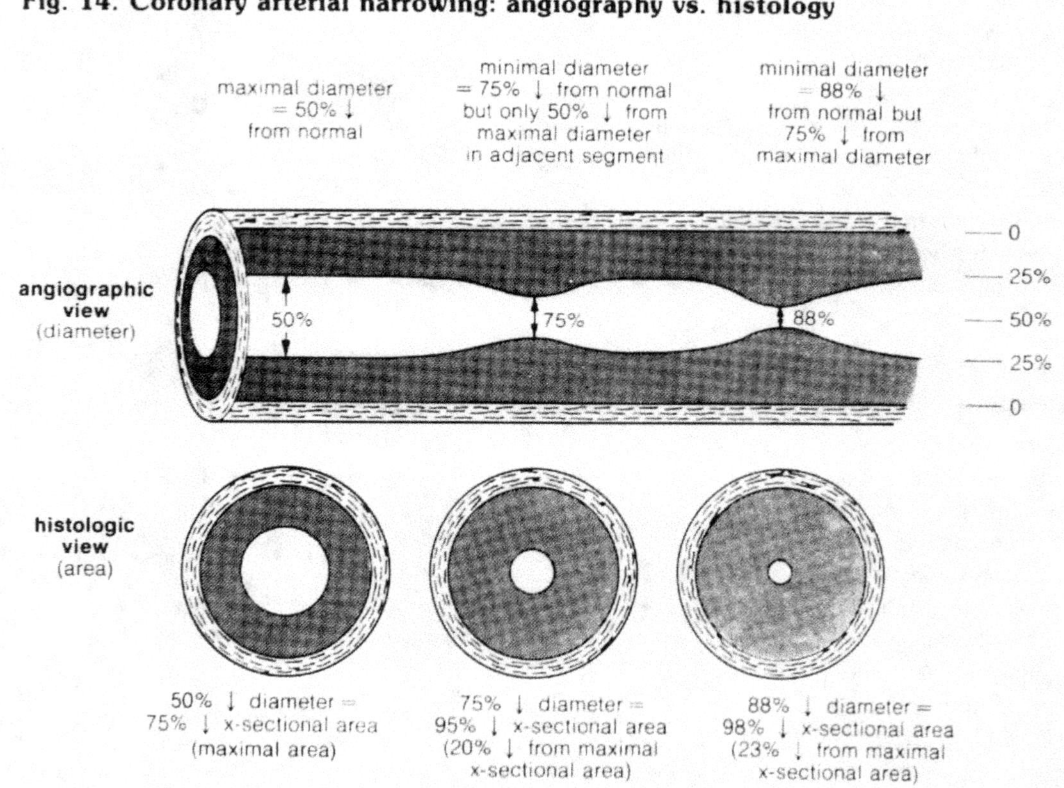

Fig. 14. Coronary arterial narrowing: angiography vs. histology

A 50% reduction in diameter as seen on angiogram, is actually a 75% narrowing on histologic cross section. Similarly, an angiographic reading of 75% becomes 95% on cross section. Moreover, on angiography, narrowing is measured only in relation to the diameter of the adjacent arterial segment, while cross sections permit accurate measurements of plaque formation by comparison with the original vessel wall instead of with adjacent site, which also may be narrowed but to a lesser degree.

epicardial coronary arteries.

• Certain portions of the coronary tree tend to develop larger atherosclerotic plaques and, therefore, more luminal narrowing than other portions.

• Of the three types of atherosclerotic plaques, only the complicated ones cause significant (more than 75%) coronary luminal narrowing.

• The degree of both plaque formation and, in turn, coronary luminal narrowing is similar regardless of the type of fatal coronary event.

• The composition of coronary atherosclerotic plaques and the degree of coronary luminal narrowing appear to be similar whether the blood lipoprotein pattern was normal or abnormal.

• The shapes of lumina of atherosclerotic coronary arteries are quite variable.

• The coronary artery responsible for perfusing an area of myocardium that has become either necrotic or fibrotic is not necessarily the most narrowed (by atherosclerotic plaque) of the three major extramural coronary arteries.

• Advanced age does not necessarily indicate the presence of severe coronary atherosclerosis.

Among patients with fatal CHD certain observations regarding coronary thrombosis are becoming established. For example, coronary thrombi

• are found in only about 10% of patients who die suddenly.

• are rare in patients with isolated subendocardial infarcts.

• occur in about 60% of patients with fatal transmural acute myocardial infarction.

• occur in high percentage only in patients with cardiogenic shock.

• usually occur only in the coronary artery responsible for perfusing the area of myocardial necrosis.

• occur in arteries that already are severely narrowed by old atherosclerotic plaques.

• are usually single, occlusive, short, and located entirely in the major trunks.

• Finally, the larger the area of myocardial necrosis, the greater the likelihood of coronary thrombosis.

Several factors suggest that coronary thrombosis is a consequence of rather than the precipitating cause of AMI. Slow blood flow and sufficient time are prerequisites for thrombus formation.

Several observations suggest that coronary thrombosis plays a major role in the development of coronary atherosclerosis in the first place.

Among the nonthrombotic acute coronary lesions, only hemorrhages into atherosclerotic plaques are common but there is no evidence that they cause coronary narrowing.

Among patients with myocardial infarction and angiographically normal coronary arteries, an angiographically normal coronary arterial tree has never been demonstrated *at the time of AMI*; the angiograms were performed *after healing of*, rather than during, the AMI. Although there are several explanations for the occurrence of AMI with an angiographically normal coronary artery and although each may be applicable on occasion, the most reasonable appears to be acute coronary embolism with subsequent clot lysis, retraction, or recanalization, which leads to a "normal" appearance on angiography.

Comparisons between methods of examining a coronary artery by selective angiography during life and by histology after death indicate that reduction in luminal diameter by angiography is generally underestimated because coronary atherosclerosis is diffuse in patients with symptomatic CHD.

References

1. Classification of atherosclerotic lesions: report of a study group. *WHO Tech Rep Ser* 143:1–20, 1958

2. Roberts WC: The pathology of acute myocardial infarction. *Hosp Prac* 6(12):88–104, 1971

3. Roberts WC: Coronary arteries in fatal acute myocardial infarction. *Circulation* 45:215–230, 1972

4. Roberts WC: Relationship between coronary thrombosis and myocardial infarction. *Mod Concepts Cardiovasc Dis* 41:7–10, 1972

5. Roberts WC, Buja LM: The frequency and significance of coronary arterial thrombi and other observations in fatal acute myocardial infarction: a study of 107 necropsy patients. *Am J Med* 52:425–443, 1972

6. Roberts WC, Ferrans VJ, Levy RI, Frederickson DS: Cardiovascular pathology in hyperlipoproteinemia: anatomic observations in 42 necropsy patients with normal or abnormal serum lipoprotein patterns. *Am J Cardiol* 31:557–570, 1973

7. Roberts WC: Does thrombosis play a major role in the development of symptom-producing atherosclerotic plaques? *Circulation* 48:1161–1166, 1973

8. Roberts WC: Coronary thrombosis and fatal myocardial ischemia. *Circulation* 49:1–3, 1974

9. Bulkley BH, Roberts WC: Atherosclerotic narrowing of the left main coronary artery: a necropsy analysis of 152 patients with fatal coronary heart disease and varying degrees of left main narrowing. *Circulation* 53:823–828, 1976

10. Roberts WC: The coronary arteries and left ventricle in clinically isolated angina pectoris. *Circulation* 54:388–390, 1976

11. Roberts WC, Buja LM, Bulkley BH, Ferrans VJ: Congestive cardiac failure and angina pectoris: opposite ends of the spectrum of symptomatic ischemic heart disease. *Am J Cardiol* 34:870–872, 1974

12. Roberts WC, Cohen LS: Left ventricular papillary muscles: description of the normal and a survey of conditions causing them to be abnormal. *Circulation* 46:138–154, 1972

13. Chandler AB, Chapman I, Erhardt LR, Roberts WC, Schwartz CJ, Sinapius D, Spain DM, Sherry S, Ness PM, Simon TL: Coronary thrombosis in myocardial infarction: report of a workshop on the role of coronary thrombosis in the pathogeneis of acute myocardial infarction. *Am J Cardiol* 34:823–832, 1974

14. Walston A, Hackel DB, Estes EH: Acute coronary occlusion and the "power-failure" syndrome. *Am Heart J* 79:613–619, 1970

15. Page DL, Caulfield JB, Kastor JA, De Sanctis RW, Sanders CA: Myocardial changes associated with cardiogenic shock. *N Engl J Med* 285:133–137, 1971

16. Buja LM, Roberts WC: The coronary arteries and myocardium in acute myocardial infarction and shock, in *Shock in Myocardial Infarction*, ed. RM Gunnar, HS Loeb, SH Rahimtolla. New York: Grune & Stratton, 1974, pp 1–21

17. Herrick, JB: Clinical features of sudden obstruction of the coronary arteries. *JAMA* 59:2015–2020, 1912

18. Spain DM, Bradess VA: Sudden death from coronary heart disease: survival time, frequency of thrombi, and cigarette smoking. *Chest* 58:107–110, 1970

19. Hellstrom HR: Coronary artery stasis after induced myocardial infarction in the dog. *Cardiovasc Res* 5:371–375, 1971

20. Master AM, Dack S, Jaffe HL: Activities associated with the onset of acute coronary artery occlusion. *Am Heart J* 18:434–443, 1939

21. Yarbrough JW, Roberts WC, Abel RM, Reis RL: The cause of luminal narrowing in internal mammary arteries implanted into canine myocardium. *Am Heart J* 84:507–512, 1972

22. Erhardt LR, Lundman T, Mellstedt H: Incorporation of ^{125}I-labeled fibrinogen into coronary arterial thrombi in acute myocardial infarction in man. *Lancet* 1:387–391, 1973

23. Duguid JB: Thrombosis as a factor in the pathogenesis of coronary atherosclerosis. *J Pathol Bacteriol* 58:207–212, 1946

24. Rokitansky CA: *Manual of Pathological Anatomy*, vol. IV. London: Sydenham Society, 1952, pp 261–272

25. Virchow R: *Cellular Pathology as Based upon Physiological and Pathological Histology*. New York: Dover, 1971

26. Harrison CV: Experimental pulmonary arteriosclerosis. *J Pathol Bacteriol* 60:289–293, 1948

27. Geiringer E: Intimal vascularization and atherosclerosis. *J Pathol Bacteriol* 63:201–211, 1951

28. Chandler AB: Mechanisms and frequency of thrombosis in the coronary circulation. *Thromb Res* 4(suppl):3–23, 1974

29. Bulkley BH, Roberts WC: Dissecting aneurysm (hematoma) limited to coronary artery: a clinicopathologic study of six patients. *Am J Med* 55:747–756, 1973

30. Arnett EN, Roberts WC: Acute myocardial infarction and angiographically normal coronary arteries: an unproven combination. *Circulation* 53:395–400, 1976

31. Arnett EN, Roberts WC: Angiographically normal arteries after healing of acute myocardial infarction. *Practical Cardiol* 2:13–19, 1976

The Coronary Arteries in Ischemic Heart Disease: Facts and Fancies

Prof. W. C. Roberts*

Symptoms and signs of ischemic heart disease (IHD) are due to abnormal functioning of portions of left ventricular myocardium. The myocardial alterations in turn are consequences of severe narrowing of the lumens of the extramural coronary arteries. Certain changes observed in the coronary arteries at necropsy in patients with fatal IHD will be summarized in this report.

Definition of coronary atherosclerosis

Atherosclerosis has been defined in many ways and most definitions contain descriptions of the composition of the plaques[7]. The word itself describes the plaque's composition: *sclerosis* = fibrous tissue and *athero* = fatty material. But many 'atherosclerotic lesions' contain only fibrous tissue and some contain only fatty material. It therefore seems preferable to define atherosclerosis not by the composition of the plaques but by the amount of plaque deposited. At birth, the intima of the extramural coronary arteries consists of a single layer of endothelium covering the internal elastic membrane. Thereafter, for some years there is a progressive increase in the thickness of the intima so that, more or less at the age of 20, the thickness of the intima is about the same as that of the media. This proliferated tissue consists primarily of collagen and elastic fibers, but smooth muscle cells, some of which contain lipid, also are present. This concentric intimal proliferation no thicker than that of the media appears to occur in all populations and apparently is simply a response to the intra-arterial pressure; it is not considered to be atherosclerosis, which begins when the thickness of the intima is greater than the thickness of the media (Fig. 1). The lesion may be concentric or eccentric. Atherosclerosis, in contrast to the 'expected normal intimal proliferation' is not

---

* Pathology Branch, National Heart, Lung and Blood Institute, National Institutes of Health, Bethesda, Md. 20014, USA

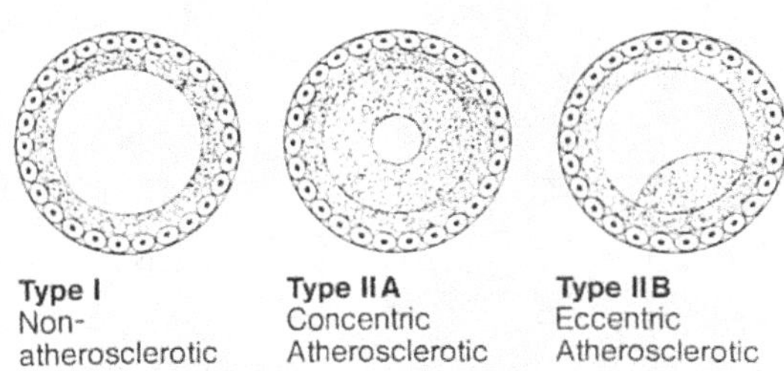

Fig. 1: Diagram showing coronary intimal lesions. In type I, the thickness of the intimal lesion is no more than the thickness of the media, and this lesion is therefore not considered atherosclerotic (see text). Intimal lesions thicker than the equivalent of the media (types IIa and b) are considered atherosclerotic (or arteriosclerotic). These lesions may be concentric or eccentric. (From ROBERTS WC: *Cardiovasc. Med.* 1977, 2, 29; reproduced by kind permission of the publishers)

world wide in distribution but occurs only in populations with hypercholesterolemia (total serum cholesterol > 200 mg per 100 ml).

Extent of coronary atherosclerosis in fatal ischemic heart disease

Among patients with fatal IHD, *the coronary arteries are diffusely involved by atherosclerotic plaques*[3, 17–25] (Table 1). That coronary atherosclerosis is a focal process, as is occasionally observed by coronary angiography, is a myth. Indeed, among patients with fatal IHD, *no segments of any of the major (right, left anterior descending and left circumflex) extramural coronary arteries are free of atherosclerotic plaques at necropsy* (Figs. 2 and 3). Although the lumens of some segments are narrowed more severely than others, all portions of the extramural coronary tree are involved by the atherosclerotic process.

In fatal IHD, with rare exceptions, 2 and commonly all 3 of the 3 major coronary arteries are narrowed > 75 % in cross-sectional area by old atherosclerotic

	SCD	AMI		AP
		TM	SE	
Major coronary arteries				
Diffuse atherosclerosis	+	+	+	+
Luminal narrowing > 75% of 2 of 3 by atherosclerotic plaques	+	+	+	+
Thrombus	10%	60%	0	0
Hemorrhage into plaque	25%	25%	25%	25%
Left ventricular myocardium				
Necrosis	0	+	+	0
Fibrosis (TM or SE)	50%	50%	50%	50%

Abbreviations: AMI = acute myocardial infarction; AP =
angina pectoris; SCD = sudden coronary death; SE = subendocardial; TM = transmural

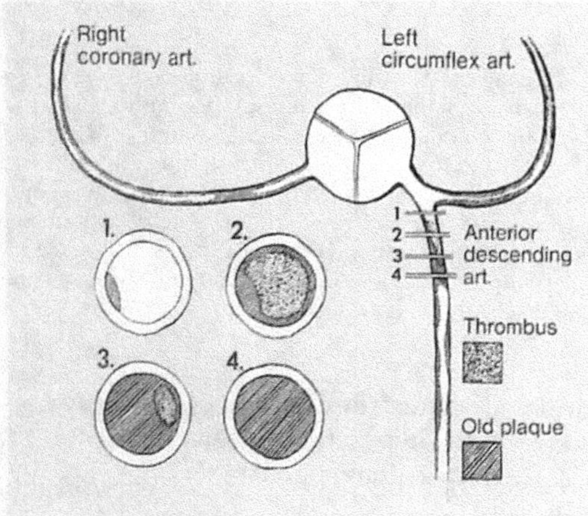

Fig. 2: Diagram illustrating the diffuse nature of coronary
atherosclerosis in fatal ischemic heart disease and the usual
status of a coronary artery at and distal to a thrombus. At
level 2 in the anterior descending coronary artery the lumen
is obstructed primarily by a thrombus. At level 3, however,
the major percentage of narrowing is the result of old
atherosclerotic plaquing. Just distal to the thrombus, the lumen
is severely narrowed (>75%) by old plaque. This situation
occurred in 37 of 39 patients with fatal acute myocardial infarction and coronary thrombosis studied by the author. (From
ROBERTS WC, BUJA LM[20]; reproduced by kind permission of
the publishers)

plaques. Stated another way, we need only 2 of
the 3 major coronary arteries as long as the 2 are
widely patent. In other words, we are provided
with an extra or 'bonus' coronary artery at birth.
Because we need only 2 of the 3 major coronary
arteries, if only one of the 3 is narrowed >75% in

cross-sectional area, no evidence of myocardial
ischemia appears unless, of course, complete obstruction (embolus, for example) occurs suddenly
in a previously wide-open 'normal' artery. Evidence of myocardial ischemia occurs for practical
purposes only when at least 2 of the 3 major coronary arteries are >75% narrowed in cross-sectional area. The 75% demarcation point is useful
because it is here that normal flow is separated
from abnormal flow. Flow of a fluid (blood)
through a tube (coronary artery) is not decreased
until at least 75% of the lumen is obliterated.
Thus, a major challenge is not the elimination of
coronary atherosclerosis but simply the limiting of
coronary atherosclerosis to <75% cross-sectional
area luminal narrowing. Not only is coronary arterial luminal narrowing of >75% observed in
patients with fatal IHD, but this degree is probably
present also in patients with symptomatic IHD
(Fig. 4). Studies of coronary arteries of patients
dying during or shortly after aortocoronary bypass
procedures have shown just as much narrowing of
their major coronary arteries as is present in
patients with IHD who die naturally.

Although the percentage of cross-sectional luminal narrowing of an artery is the major factor in
separating patients with from those without IHD,
the initial size of the artery is also an important
factor in determining the amount of coronary arterial area through which blood may flow. In
Figure 5 are depicted 2 arteries, both of which are
narrowed slightly more than 75% in cross-sectional area. One of the arteries, however, is less
than a fourth the size of the other, although the per
cent luminal narrowing by atherosclerotic plaque
in each is similar. Thus, the smaller the initial size
of the artery, the greater the potential effect of the
luminal narrowing. The larger the heart, in general, the greater the cross-sectional area of the coronary arteries and vice versa. Since women have
lower mean heart weights than men, they also have
smaller mean cross-sectional areas of coronary arteries.

*The atherosclerotic process is limited to the epicar-
dial coronary arteries, ie the major trunks and their
near right-angle branches, and spares the intramyocardial coronary arteries* (Fig. 6). The lumens
of the intramural coronary arteries within the left
ventricular papillary muscles in these patients,
however, are often narrowed by fibrous intimal
proliferation, but this process in these arteries is

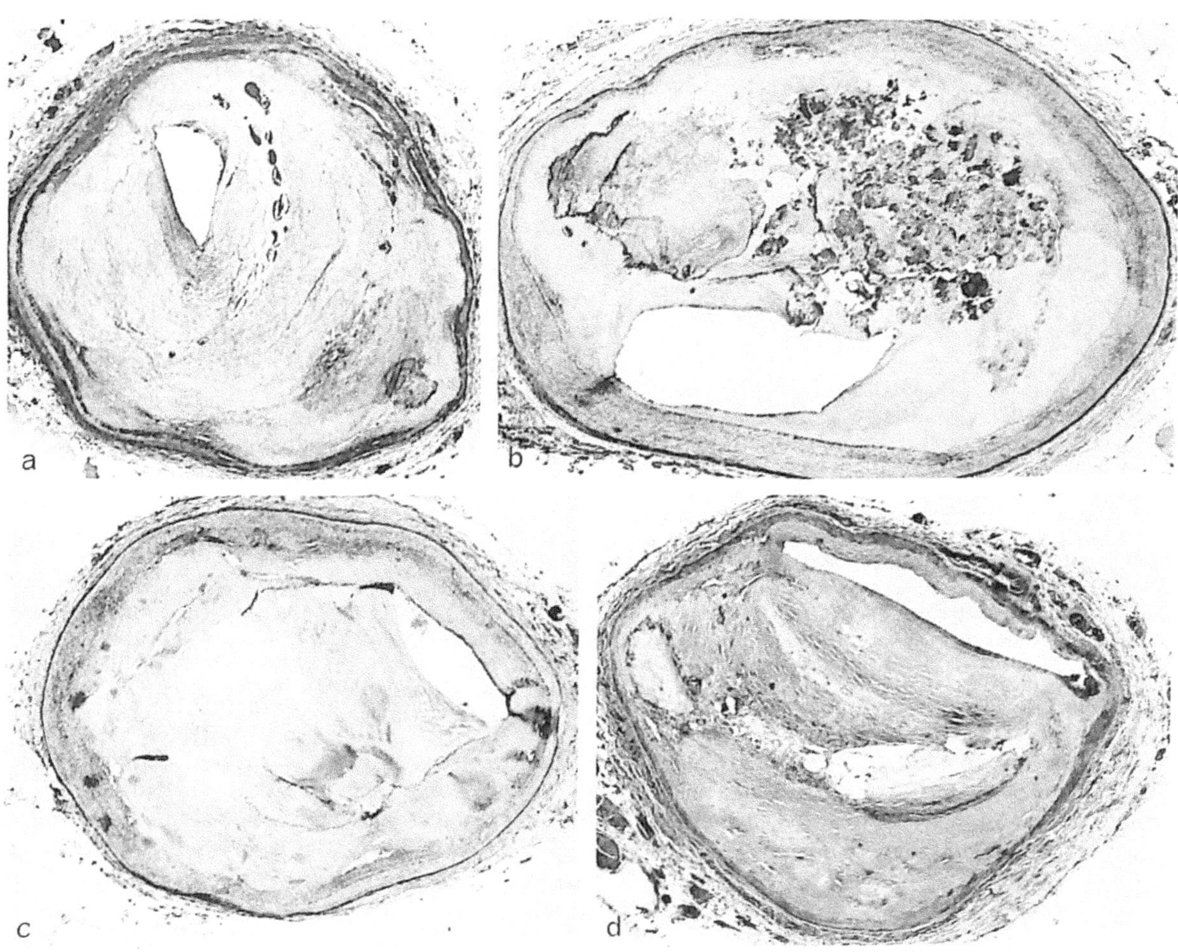

Fig. 3: Major extramural coronary arteries at sites of maximal narrowing in a 41-year-old man who died suddenly after having had angina pectoris for 7 years. a) Right, b) Left main, c) Left anterior descending, d) Left circumflex. a, b, and c = elastic Van Gieson stains, d = hematoxylin and eosin stain; magn. × 27.

really not 'atherosclerotic' in nature and results probably from slowed perfusion to these distal myocardial structures (Fig. 7).

Certain portions of the coronary tree tend to develop larger atherosclerotic plaques, and, therefore, lumens more narrowed than other portions. The most severe narrowing of the left coronary artery is usually within the first 2 cm of the origin of the left anterior descending and left circumflex branches; the distal third of the right coronary artery, in contrast, is usually more narrowed than is the proximal or middle third. Calcific deposits are nearly always more extensive in the proximal than in the distal portions of the coronary arteries. It is

because the narrowing, at least in the left coronary arteries, tends to be greater proximally than distally that aorto-coronary bypass procedures have proved beneficial to many patients with severe angina pectoris and good myocardial function. The right coronary artery, however, is a trap in this regard. The distal portions of the coronary arteries also are more difficult to evaluate by angiography than are the proximal portions, and severe narrowings distally are probably more often missed or underestimated than are severe narrowings in the proximal coronary tree.

Considerable attention has been given to 'significant' narrowings (>50% reduction in luminal

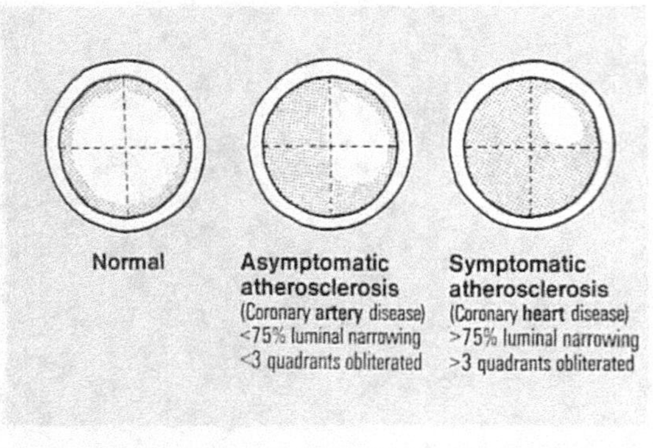

Fig. 4: Differences between degrees of luminal narrowing of coronary arteries in patients with symptomatic and asymptomatic ischemic heart disease. By the age of 20 years, in all population groups world-wide, there is intimal fibrous proliferation in the coronary arteries of about equal thickness to that of the media of the coronary artery. In population groups with hypercholesterolemia (serum total cholesterol > 200 mg per 100 ml), this intimal proliferative process generally continues. Symptoms of myocardial ischemia, with rare exception, do not occur until the intimal proliferative process obliterates > 75% of the lumen. (From ROBERTS WC: *Cardiovasc. Med.* 1977, 2, 29; reproduced by kind permission of the publishers)

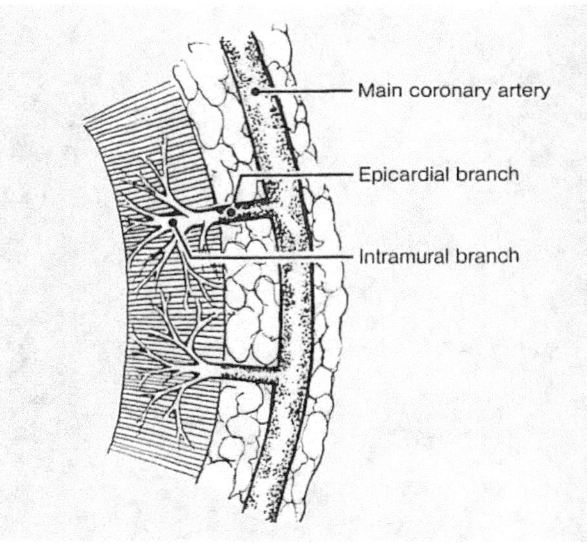

Fig. 6: A main epicardial coronary artery, its epicardial branches, and the intramural branches. The atherosclerotic process is limited to the epicardial arteries and spares the intramural portions. (From ROBERTS WC, BUJA LM[20]; reproduced by kind permission of the publishers)

diameter by angiography or > 75 % cross-sectional area narrowing at necropsy) of the left main coronary artery. Severe narrowing of this artery virtually always indicates severe narrowing of all 3

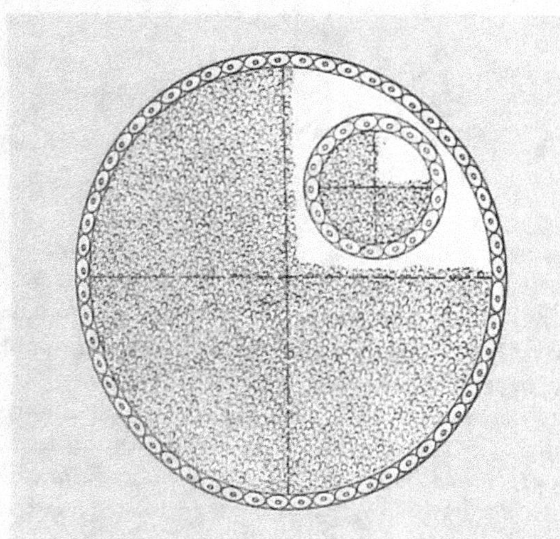

Fig. 5: Cross-section diagram of two theoretical coronary arteries. The lumen of each is slightly more than 75 % narrowed in cross-sectional area. Obviously, however, the absolute area is dependent also on the initial size of the artery. Thus, both area obliterated and initial area have to be evaluated.

major coronary arteries[4]. Among patients with fatal IHD, compared with patients with < 50 % cross-sectional narrowing of the left main coronary artery, patients with > 75 % cross-sectional area narrowing have a significantly higher frequency of angina pectoris and hyperlipoproteinemia, especially type II, but a lower frequency of acute transmural myocardial infarction[4]. Death during cardiac catheterization or coronary angiography and probably during aortocoronary bypass also appears more frequent among the patients with IHD and > 75 % left main narrowing than among the group with < 50 % left main narrowing.

Of the 3 types of atherosclerotic plaques as defined by the World Health Organization Committee[7], namely lipid, fibrous, and complicated, only the complicated plaque causes significant (> 75 %) coronary luminal narrowing. The lipid and fibrous plaques are world wide in distribution. The complicated plaques, ie those containing calcific deposits, cholesterol clefts, pultaceous debris, etc, are found only in populations which develop IHD. The major component of even the complicated atherosclerotic plaque, however, is fibrous tissue (collagen) and the lipid component is much less evident. Foam cells are actually infrequent in the coronary arteries in patients with fatal IHD, and

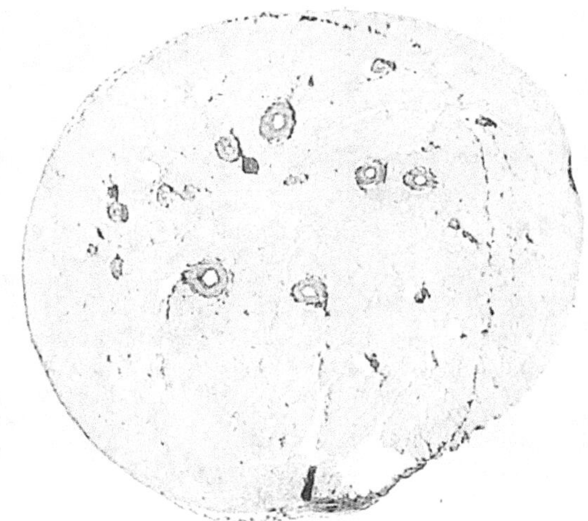

Fig. 7: Cross-section of a left ventricular papillary muscle in a 45-year-old man who died suddenly without previous symptoms of ischemic heart disease. At necropsy, the heart weighed only 340 g. The lumen of the left main, left anterior descending, and left circumflex coronary arteries was > 75 % narrowed in cross-sectional area by atherosclerotic plaques, and the right between 51 and 75 %.
Shown here are cross-sectional views of about 20 intramural coronary arteries located in this papillary muscle. The arteries have thickened walls and narrowed lumens. The intramural coronary arteries in the left ventricular papillary muscles in patients with fatal ischemic heart disease often show these changes. The intramural coronary arteries in the free walls and ventricular system are, in contrast, virtually always normal. (From ROBERTS WC: *Cardiovasc. Med.* 1977, 2, 29; reproduced by kind permission of the publishers)

the lipid which is present is usually extracellular. It has been demonstrated in the experimental animal that the lipid component of the plaque is reversible (dissoluble)[8]. It is less likely, obviously, that the fibrous component of the atherosclerotic plaque is reversible. Whether or not low-lipid diets or lipid-lowering drugs will cause depletion of lipids in complicated symptom-producing coronary atherosclerotic plaques is uncertain. Although fat stores in the body consist predominantly of triglycerides, and atherosclerotic plaques predominantly of cholesterol esters, the latter might nevertheless decrease in size when caloric intake is low enough to cause a decrease in the size of fat deposits in readily-visible portions of the body (anterior panniculus, for example). Emaciated prisoners in World War II apparently had little coronary arterial luminal narrowing. Similar observations have been made in victims of malignant neoplasms. The amount of lipid in atherosclerotic

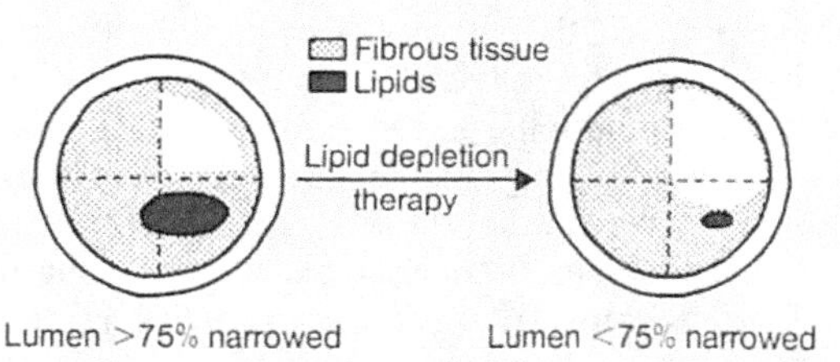

Fig. 8: Composition of atherosclerotic plaque in symptomatic coronary disease and the possible effect of lipid lowering or lipid withdrawal on its composition and luminal size. Although the dominant component of atherosclerotic plaque is usually fibrous tissue, lipid deposits (usually extracellular) form a portion of most plaques. It is likely that the fibrous component of the plaque is nonreversible. In contrast, the lipid component may well be reversible. Transient starvation may possibly cause a diminution in the size of the lipid component and a decrease in luminal narrowing from more than 75 % (the amount associated with symptoms) to less than 75 % (an amount rarely associated with symptoms). (From ROBERTS WC: *Cardiovasc. Med.* 1977, 2, 29; reproduced by kind permission of the publishers)

plaques in emaciated necropsy patients appears to be less than that observed in nonemaciated necropsy patients.

Transient starvation may well be a neglected but beneficial form of therapy (possibly also a form of prevention) for symptomatic IHD (Fig. 8). If the lumen of a coronary artery is 90 % obliterated by atherosclerotic plaques, for example, generally about 25 % of the plaque consists of lipid deposits. Depletion of these lipid deposits in the plaque, consequently, would allow the lumen to be < 75 % narrowed, and, therefore, flow would then be adequate.

The degree of coronary arterial luminal narrowing by atherosclerotic plaques and the extensiveness of the plaques are similar in patients with fatal IHD irrespective of the type of fatal coronary event, ie acute myocardial infarction, clinically-isolated angina pectoris, and sudden coronary death (Table 1)[20-25]. No significant differences in amount of atherosclerotic plaquing have been observed in patients with fatal IHD from transmural acute myocardial infarction (AMI), arrhythmia ('sudden coronary death'), clinically-isolated angina pectoris, or progressive congestive cardiac failure after healing of an AMI ('ischemic cardiomyopathy'). Although the degree of coronary luminal narrowing by atherosclerotic plaques is similar in each of the above 4 types of coronary event, the myocardial reaction is obviously quite different. Patients with clinically-isolated angina pectoris of severe degree usually have hearts which are near-normal in both weight and ventricular cavity size, little if any myocardial fibrosis, and no myocardial necrosis. Patients with ischemic cardiomyopathy usually have large transmural left ventricular scars, large left ventricular cavities, often with aneurysms, and usually left ventricular mural thrombi. The fatal AMI patients obviously have myocardial necrosis, which is usually transmural. The patients with IHD who die suddenly and unexpectedly have hearts close in appearance, as a rule, to those of patients with clinically-isolated angina pectoris. The reasons for the differences in myocardial response to apparently similar degrees of coronary atherosclerosis are uncertain.

The composition of coronary atherosclerotic plaques and the degree of coronary arterial luminal narrowing in patients with fatal IHD appears similar, irrespective of whether or not the blood lipoprotein pattern is normal or abnormal[21]. Patients with type II, III or IV hyperlipoproteinemia clearly have accelerated atherosclerosis compared with persons of similar age and sex with normal lipoprotein patterns, but hyperlipoproteinemia is not a prerequisite for premature development of severe atherosclerosis. Severe narrowing of the left main coronary artery is more common in patients with type II hyperlipoproteinemia than in patients with type III or IV hyperlipoproteinemia or in persons with normal lipoprotein patterns[4]. Furthermore, atherosclerosis of the ascending aorta may be prominent in patients with type II hyperlipoproteinemia; this is especially true if the hyperlipoproteinemia is of the homozygous rather than the heterozygous variety[21]. Also, in the homozygous form, the coronary ostia may be narrowed severely by the aortic atherosclerosis, which may also involve the aortic valve cusps directly.

The shapes of lumens of atherosclerotic coronary arteries are quite variable. The residual lumen may be located centrally or peripherally and its shape may be circular, oval, slit-like, or half-moon. The slit-like lumen, which extends from one side of the artery to the other, may appear on angiography as a normal-sized orifice.

The coronary artery responsible for perfusing an area of myocardium which has become either

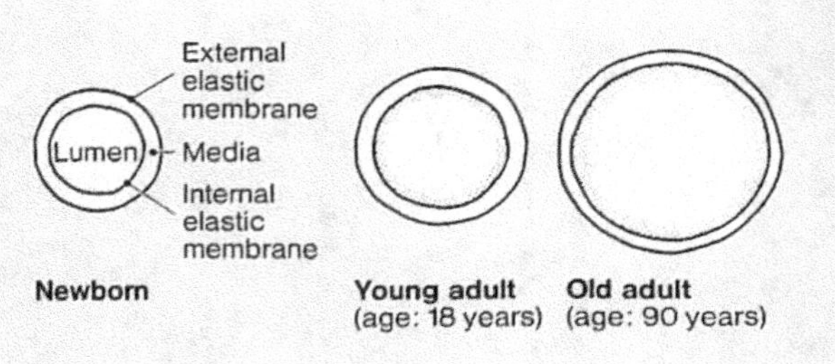

Fig. 9: Diagram showing relative sizes of normal coronary arteries at various ages. The intimal lesion (shaded area) represents fibromuscular proliferation, presumably a response to the intra-arterial pressure and not a form of atherosclerosis. (From ROBERTS WC: *Cardiovasc. Clin.* 1975, 7, No. 2, 1; reproduced by kind permission of the publishers)

necrotic or fibrotic is not necessarily the one of the 3 major extramural coronary arteries most narrowed by atherosclerotic plaques. A patient with an anterior wall infarction may have as much or more luminal narrowing of the right or left circumflex coronary arteries, or both, as is present in the left descending coronary artery.

Although the number one risk factor for development of symptomatic atherosclerosis in the Western World, *advanced age does not necessarily indicate the presence of severe coronary atherosclerosis.* Actually, AMI is infrequent in patients over 90 years of age. The explanation probably lies in the fact that their arteries normally dilate as the years progress, unless extensive atherosclerotic plaques develop within them, and then the plaques prevent this 'normal' dilatation from occurring (Fig. 9). Obviously, the greater the dilatation, the wider the lumen.

Coronary thrombosis

Up to this point this paper has described certain features of old or chronic lesions, namely atherosclerosis, in the coronary arteries of patients with fatal IHD. No discussion has been presented on what 'tips the scales' in these patients from adequate to inadequate myocardial oxygenation. The idea until recently has been that a new lesion, usually a thrombus or a hemorrhage into an old atherosclerotic plaque, has suddenly appeared and this has provided a nice anatomic explanation for the usually sudden, dramatic clinical episode of myocardial ischemia, namely acute myocardial infarction or sudden coronary death. Before examining the question as to whether or not 'a new coronary lesion' precipitates a coronary event, a summary of some observations on coronary thrombosis in patients with fatal coronary events appears appropriate:

Among patients with fatal IHD, *coronary arterial thrombi are infrequent (about 10%) in patients dying suddenly.* ('Sudden coronary death' is defined here as death occurring within 6 hours after onset of symptoms of myocardial ischemia and unassociated with histologic evidence of myocardial necrosis.)

Coronary arterial thrombi are rare (nearly zero per cent) in patients in whom myocardial necrosis is limited to the subendocardial region. ('Subendocardium' is defined as the inner one-half of the myocardial wall.) Necrosis, however, limited to the subendocardial region is rarely fatal unless the patient has severe cardiomegaly from another condition, for example, systemic hypertension or left ventricular outflow tract obstruction.

A thrombus is found in the lumen of an extramural coronary artery in about 60% of patients with fatal transmural AMI[17–20]. ('Transmural' is defined as that portion of left ventricular wall which includes all of the inner half, ie subendocardium, and at least some portion of the subepicardial half of the wall.)

Among patients with fatal transmural myocardial necrosis, coronary thrombosis is far more common among those patients who have had cardiogenic shock than among those who have not (Fig. 10)[3]. At necropsy, over 70% of patients with fatal AMI with cardiogenic shock have coronary thrombi, whereas only about 15% of patients without the power-failure syndrome associated with fatal AMI have coronary thrombi[29].

The larger the area of myocardial necrosis, the greater the likelihood of coronary thrombosis. The larger the infarcted area, however, the greater the likelihood of cardiogenic shock. The latter generally indicates that >40% of the left ventricular wall is either necrotic or fibrotic or both, whereas shock is infrequently associated with infarcts or scars involving <40% of the ventricular wall[16].

When coronary thrombosis is associated with AMI, the thrombus is always located in the artery responsible for perfusing the area of myocardial necrosis[20]. Thus in anterior wall infarction, a thrombus,

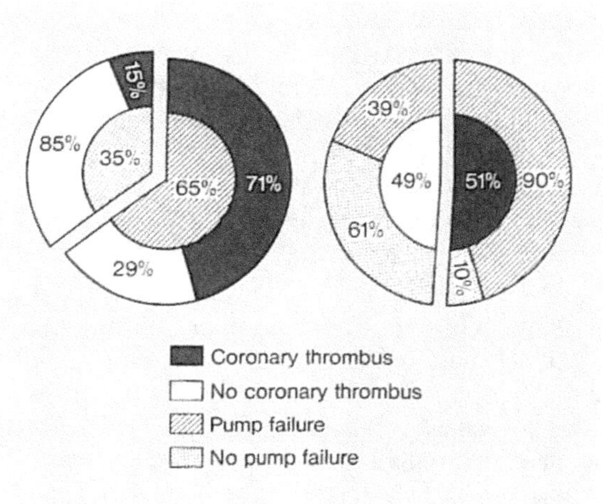

Fig. 10: Diagram showing the close correlation between the presence of cardiogenic shock or pump failure and coronary thrombosis during acute myocardial infarction. (From ROBERTS WC: *Cardiovasc. Clin.* 1975, 7, No. 2, 1: reproduced by kind permission of the publishers)

if present, will be located in the left anterior descending coronary artery. Thrombi infrequently occur in more than one major coronary artery.

Thrombi are found in fatal IHD in coronary arteries which are already severely narrowed by old atherosclerotic plaques[20]. At the distal site of attachment of the thrombus, or just distal to this site, the lumen of the coronary artery is nearly always >75% narrowed already by old atherosclerotic plaques (Fig. 2). Not infrequently, a thrombus may occur in an area between two sites of severe narrowing as in a valley between two mountains.

Coronary thrombi in fatal AMI are usually (90%) single, usually (80%) occlusive (as opposed to mural or non-occlusive), short (<2 cm long), and located entirely in the major trunks (as opposed to their near right-angle branches or intramural coronary arteries). The thrombus when only a few hours old may consist almost entirely of platelets, but thereafter is composed primarily of fibrin. By definition, the thrombus is adherent to the surface of the arterial wall bordering the lumen.

Role of coronary thrombosis in precipitating fatal ischemic heart disease – a negative one

Since 1912 when HERRICK[14] first used the term 'coronary thrombosis' to describe the often dramatic clinical event characterized at necropsy by necrosis of portions of left ventricular wall, it has been assumed that the usual cause of AMI is coronary thrombosis. Two factors implicate coronary thrombosis as the *precipitating cause* of AMI: 1) the occurrence of coronary arterial thrombi in many patients with fatal AMI; 2) the location of the thrombus in the coronary artery responsible for supplying the area of myocardial necrosis. Five factors, however, tend to indicate that coronary thrombosis is a *consequence* rather than the precipitating cause of AMI: 1) the low frequency of thrombi in patients dying suddenly with or without previous evidence of cardiac disease; 2) the near absence of thrombi in patients with fatal subendocardial AMI; 3) the absence, nearly as often as the presence, of thrombi in fatal transmural AMI; 4) the increasing frequency of thrombi, with increasing intervals between onset of symptoms of AMI and death; and 5) the high incidence of thrombi only in patients with cardiogenic shock, most of whom have large transmural infarcts.

The key to coronary thrombosis, just like the key to thrombosis occurring anywhere in the body, is *slow blood flow,* or relative stasis, and *sufficient time* for the thrombus to form. The absence of these two factors may explain the absence of coronary thrombosis in the sudden death cases, and the increasing frequency of thrombosis as the interval from onset of symptoms of myocardial ischemia to death increases[27]. There is a marked reduction in blood flow in the coronary artery responsible for supplying the area of myocardial infarction. This observation was made in dogs after inducing AMI, and they had normal, ie widely patent, vessels[13]. In fatal AMI in humans, the thrombus is always located in an artery already containing considerable atherosclerotic plaques, and therefore the infarct-induced relative coronary stasis is probably even greater. Cardiogenic shock must further diminish coronary flow.

The type of activity in which patients are occupied at the time of onset of AMI may reflect slowed blood flow. Nearly 75% of patients with AMI have the onset of chest pain while sleeping, resting, or engaged in mild activity[15]. Although inactivity may cause slight diminution in coronary blood flow, considerable stasis of blood (infarction-induced plus cardiogenic shock) is usually necessary for thrombus to form. In contrast to fatal AMI, coronary thrombosis is rarely observed in fatal angina pectoris, although the degree of coronary luminal narrowing by atherosclerotic plaques is similar in degree to that observed in arteries implanted into left ventricular myocardium but al-

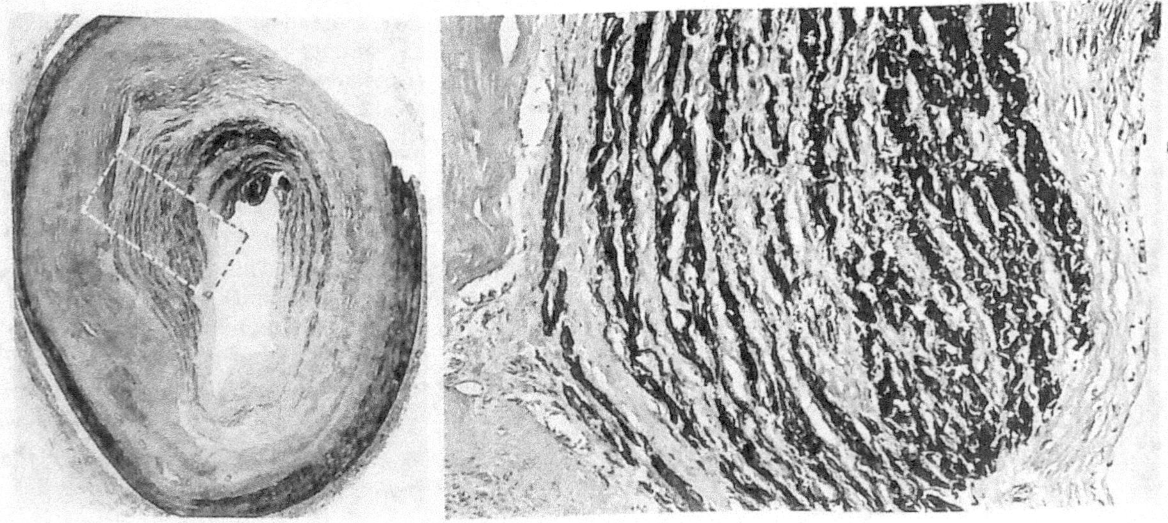

Fig. 11: Right coronary artery in a 47-year-old man with healed posterior wall left ventricular transmural infarct and rheumatic mitral stenosis. The lumen of the right coronary artery was narrowed >75% primarily by fibrous plaques interspersed with fibrin as shown here. The fibrin is dark and the organized fibrous tissue is lighter. A close-up view of one area of the fibrin deposits is shown at right. Phosphotungstic acid hematoxylin stain; magn. × 20 (left), and × 104 (right)

lowed to drain into right ventricular cavity[30]. Thus it appears that a period of diminished coronary blood flow is necessary for thrombus to form in a coronary artery. Shock, congestive cardiac failure and inactivity all decrease coronary flow and with time may allow formation of thrombus.

Further support for the concept that coronary thrombosis is a consequence rather than a precipitating cause of AMI was supplied by ERHARDT and associates[10] who at necropsy observed radioactivity in coronary arterial thrombi in patients who had been given radioactive ^{125}I-labelled fibrinogen shortly after hospitalization because of AMI. This finding implicates coronary thrombosis as a secondary event occurring sometime after the infarction.

Thus there is substantial evidence that acute thrombus formation does not precipitate acute fatal IHD. The major problem is diffuse generalized coronary atherosclerosis with severe (>75%) luminal narrowing of at least 2 of the 3 major coronary arteries.

Role of thrombosis in causing atherosclerosis — a positive one?

Although this paper has de-emphasized the role of coronary thrombosis in precipitating AMI, I would like to 'flip the coin over', and suggest, as have some other investigators[9], that thrombosis plays a major role in the development of the atherosclerotic plaques in the first place. ROKITANSKY[26] in 1852 was the first, to my knowledge, to propose that atherosclerotic plaques resulted from the organization of thrombi. VIRCHOW[28] disputed this view, and since 1913 investigations of atherosclerosis, with some exceptions, have centered mainly on the role of lipids[1]. Several observations suggest, however, that atherosclerotic plaques result, at least in part, from the organization of thrombi:

1) The presence of known components of thrombi (fibrin and platelets) within atherosclerotic plaques (Fig. 11).

2) The occurrence of known components of atherosclerotic plaques (foam cells, cholesterol clefts, pultaceous debris, calcium) in organized hematomas or known thrombi wherever they occur in the body. An example is the left atrial

thrombus in the patient with mitral stenosis[22]. Organization of this thrombus may produce typical complicated atherosclerotic plaques.

3) The presence of multiluminal channels in vessels, a recognized consequence of organization of pulmonary arterial thromboemboli[12]. Multiluminal channels are commonly found in severely atherosclerotic coronary arteries (Fig. 12). This observation suggests that thrombi or emboli were at one time present and that they organized. The tissue present between the multiluminal channels is similar to that found in arteries with only one channel (Fig. 13). Because the artery with multiple channels has been recognized as the hallmark of an organized thrombus[11] and because the tissue in both multi- and unichanneled arteries is similar, DUGUID[9] reasoned that the causative process was also similar.

4) The major component of the complicated atherosclerotic plaque, ie that capable of causing significant luminal narrowing, in the coronary arteries of patients with fatal ischemic heart disease is fibrous tissue or collagen, not lipid[29]. This is true whether or not hyperlipidemia is present[21]. Foam cells, indeed, are infrequently observed in the coronary arteries of patients with fatal ischemic

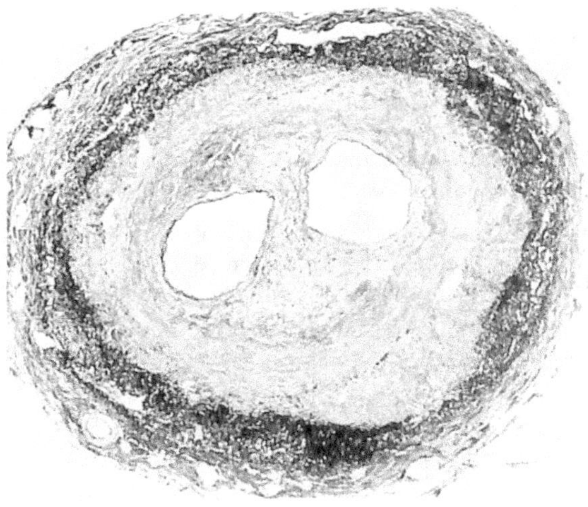

Fig. 12: Multiple luminal channels in the left circumflex coronary artery of a 58-year-old man who had an acute myocardial infarction at the age of 54 and the onset of symptoms of acute myocardial ischemia one hour before death. The occurrence of multiple luminal channels suggests organization of clot, either thrombus or embolus. Elastic van Gieson stain; magn. × 25

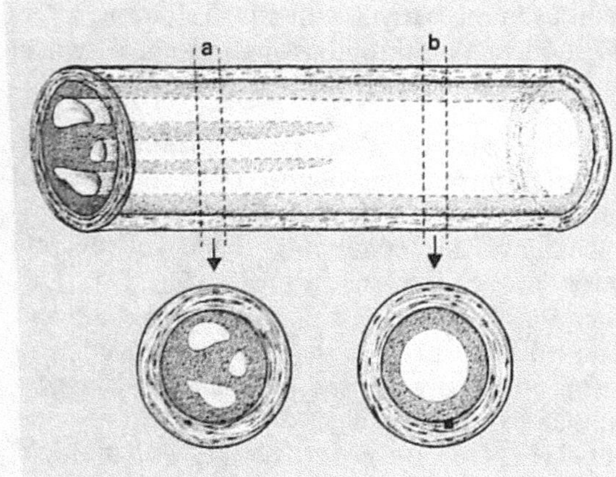

Fig. 13: a) The multi- and b) the unichanneled coronary arterial atherosclerotic plaque. DUGUID[9], when studying serial sections of an 'organized thrombus', noted that the tissue present between channels in an artery containing multiple revascularized channels was similar to that found in arteries with only one channel. Since the multichannel artery has been recognized as the hallmark of an organized thrombus and since the tissue in both multi- and unichanneled arteries was similar, he reasoned that the causative process also was similar. (From ROBERTS WC, BUJA LM[20]; reproduced by kind permission of the publishers)

heart disease. Often the 'density' of the fibrous tissue plugging a coronary artery is different in different portions of a plaque and these subunits may be demarcated by distinct elastic lamellae[20]. These subunits suggest that thrombus is deposited at different times and that the 'density' of the resulting fibrous tissue may be determined by the composition of the initial thrombus, ie whether platelets or fibrin predominated[6].

5) Experimentally-induced thrombi may under proper conditions be transformed into atherosclerotic plaques closely resembling those observed in human coronary arteries[6].

The above factors obviously do not prove that thrombosis is the cause of atherosclerosis, but together they strongly suggest that organization of thrombi plays a major role in the development of the complicated atherosclerotic plaque. Indeed, most current serious students of the morphology of the arterial plaque support, in whole or in part, the thrombogenic origin of atherosclerosis.

Because the clotting factors in the blood appear to be similar in all population groups and because

symptomatic atherosclerosis develops only in those population groups with elevated blood lipids, the last also play a role in the development of the plaque. Lipids may exert their effect, however, more by their ability to alter the clotting mechanism than by their ability to infiltrate the arterial wall.

Non-thrombotic acute coronary lesions

Hemorrhage into an old atherosclerotic plaque. Hemorrhages into coronary atherosclerotic plaques are observed in about 25% of patients with fatal IHD (Table 1). Even when plaque hemorrhages occur, however, the lumen of the coronary artery is not further narrowed. Plaque hemorrhages have no relationship to the site of myocardial necrosis. At least when a coronary thrombus is observed, its location corresponds to the site of necrosis; with anterior wall infarction and coronary thrombosis, the thrombus is located in the left anterior descending coronary artery, and other thrombi, except rarely, are not found in the right or left circumflex coronary arteries. In contrast, when hemorrhages into atherosclerotic plaques occur, they bear no relation to the site of myocardial necrosis. The anterior wall may be the site of infarction, but the hemorrhage may involve a plaque in the right coronary artery, or all 3 coronary arteries, or multiple sites in a single coronary artery. The plaque hemorrhages may be occurring all through adult life in patients with and without symptomatic IHD. It appears unlikely that they are responsible for precipitating acute myocardial ischemia because they do not narrow the lumen and they are not necessarily related to sites of myocardial necrosis.

Coronary arterial embolism (Fig. 14). This is a rare cause of fatal IHD. Diagnosis of embolism requires identification of the site of dislodgment of the embolus or at least a condition predisposing to development of embolism, such as infective endocarditis, intracardiac mural thrombus, or a coagulopathy. Embolism is extremely difficult to recognize when superimposed on an extensively atherosclerotic coronary arterial tree. Thus diagnosis of embolism usually requires the occurrence of 'clot' in a coronary tree devoid of heavy atherosclerotic plaques. Furthermore, in contrast to coronary thrombosis, which never involves the intramural coronary arteries and infrequently the distal portions of the extramural coronary arteries

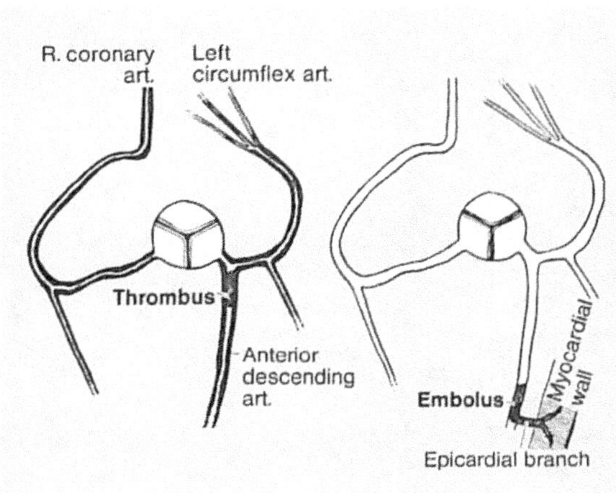

Fig. 14: Diagram depicting differences between coronary arterial thrombosis and embolism. The thrombus is usually proximal to, and superimposed on, old atherosclerotic plaque, and does not extend into intramural coronary arteries. The embolus is distal to and usually extends into an intramural artery. The embolus usually occurs in a coronary tree devoid of significant old atherosclerotic plaque. (From ROBERTS WC, BUJA LM[20]; reproduced by kind permission of the publishers)

(except for the right one), embolism usually involves both the intra- and extramural arteries, usually the distal portions of the latter.

Dissecting aneurysm (hematoma) of a coronary artery with and without associated dissection of aorta. Dissection of one or both coronary arteries with resulting luminal narrowing is commonly associated with dissection of the aorta. The resulting myocardial ischemia in this circumstance may be fatal. Virtually all patients with aortic dissecting aneurysm with or without associated dissection of the coronary arteries have systemic hypertension. Dissection of one or more major coronary arteries, however, may occur, although rarely, in the absence of dissection of the aorta[5]. When isolated to the coronary artery, systemic hypertension is infrequent but other underlying precipitating causes have yet to be identified for this idiopathic dissection. Women are more often affected than men, death is usually sudden, and there is no histologic evidence of myocardial necrosis. In addition to the idiopathic variety, isolated coronary dissection may be iatrogenic in origin, a result of coronary angiography or coronary bypass operations.

Myocardial infarction and angiographically normal coronary arteries

Coronary angiography in patients with IHD manifested by AMI has disclosed the following: 1) when performed *at the time of AMI,* coronary angiography has always disclosed severe narrowing or complete obstruction of at least one of the three major coronary arteries; 2) when performed *at the time of AMI,* coronary angiography has never demonstrated a normal coronary tree; and 3) when performed *after healing of an AMI,* coronary angiography has usually (>99%) demonstrated severe narrowing of one or more of the 3 major coronary arteries, and rarely (<1%) a normal coronary tree. In recent years, much attention has been given to this latter small group of patients with 'myocardial infarction and angiographically normal coronary arteries'[2]. A major implication of most reports on this subject is that AMI may occur in the presence of normal coronary arteries. This section will examine this implication and discuss possible explanations for the occurrence of 'myocardial infarction and normal coronary arteriograms'.

There are at least 6 possible explanations for the appearance of a normal coronary arterial tree on angiography after healing of an AMI (Fig. 15).

AMI never occurred. This explanation is unlikely because most of the reported patients had documentation of the AMI by both electrocardiographic changes and enzyme elevations.

Presence of too large a myocardial mass or too little hemoglobin or too low a perfusion pressure (shock) to supply the myocardium by a normal coronary tree. The occurrence of myocardial scars in patients with large hearts or severe chronic anemia with or without cardiomegaly and normal coronary arteries is well recognized. Likewise, an inadequate perfusion pressure may lead to myocardial necrosis (with later scarring) despite a normal coronary tree. The necrosis or fibrosis in each of these three circumstances is usually limited to left ventricular papillary muscle and subendocardium of left ventricular free wall.

The coronary arteriograms were misinterpreted. It is well known that coronary angiography tends to underestimate the degree of coronary arterial luminal narrowing. This explanation may on occasion be the proper one, but on angiography most

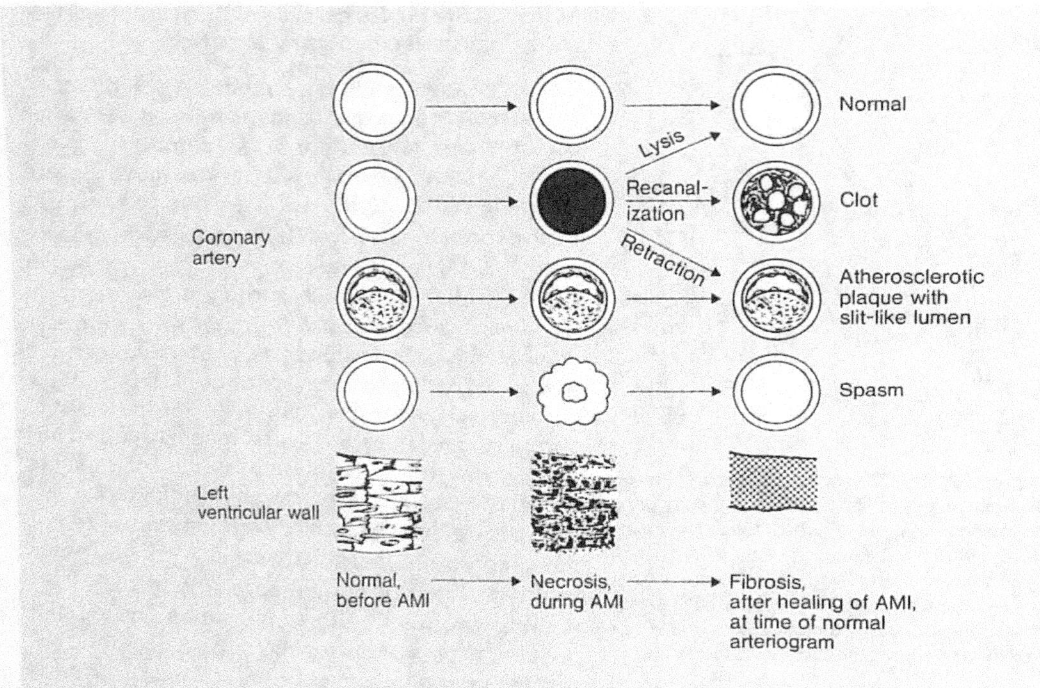

Fig. 15: Diagrammatic portrayal of possible appearances of the epicardial coronary arteries and left ventricular myocardium in patients with acute myocardial infarction (AMI) and subsequently normal coronary arteries. The left column indicates the status of the coronary arteries and myocardium before the AMI; the center column, during the AMI; and the right column, after healing of the AMI. If the AMI was caused by a condition affecting only the intramyocardial arteries, by a disproportion between the size of the coronary bed and the amount of myocardium to be oxygenated, the coronary arteries presumably would be normal (top row) at the time of myocardial necrosis as well as before and subsequently. Coronary angiography may show a slit-like eccentric lumen (third row) on occasion to be 'normal'. If spasm caused the AMI, one or more coronary arteries might be partially obstructed at the time of the AMI (fourth row). If embolism caused the AMI (second row), the clot could subsequently lyse, recanalize, or retract along one side allowing the lumen to be of sufficient size to appear later as 'angiographically normal'. (From ARNETT EA, ROBERTS WC[2]; reproduced by kind permission of the publishers)

patients with symptomatic coronary disease have some abnormality of 2 and usually all 3 major extramural coronary arteries.

Coronary spasm caused the AMI. Although shown to cause both chest pain and ischemic changes on electrocardiogram, coronary spasm has not been shown to cause myocardial necrosis. The case for spasm is generally considered strongest among patients with Prinzmetal's angina. Of 84 patients with this variant angina, reported in English and summarized by ARNETT and ROBERTS[2], 65 had coronary arteriography; among these, the coronary arterial diameters were judged to be severely ($>75\%$) narrowed in 43 (66%) and normal in 22 (34%). Coronary spasm was demonstrated in 14 (22%) of the 65 patients, in 5 of the 43 with narrowed, and in 9 of the 22 with normal coronary arteries. Although it occurred naturally in none of the 5 patients with both coronary spasm and fixed coronary narrowing, AMI or death occurred after aortocoronary bypass procedures in 3 of the 5 patients. None of the 22 patients with angiographically normal coronary arteries had an AMI, but 6 of them died; none, however, were among the 9 with demonstrated coronary spasm. Examination of the coronary arteries at necropsy in 5 of these 6 patients disclosed severe ($>75\%$) narrowing of 1 coronary ostium or artery in 3 patients and a 'small' left coronary artery in a fourth. Thus only 1 of the 5 patients had a 'normal' coronary tree at necropsy. Hence, although it has been shown to cause chest pain and ischemic electrocardiographic changes, coronary spasm has not been shown to cause myocardial necrosis.

AMI was caused by a condition affecting only the intramural (intramyocardial) coronary arteries without involvement of the extramural coronary arteries. Abnormalities of the intramural coronary arteries have been reported in a number of conditions but, to my knowledge, transmural AMI has never been described as a consequence of disease of the intramural coronary arteries only. Even in the conditions where it is observed, involvement of the intramural coronary arteries has usually been associated with a condition affecting other body organs or systems as well.

AMI was caused by an occluding embolus which subsequently lysed or recanalized. This appears the most likely cause of the AMI in patients who are subsequently shown by angiography to have a normal coronary arterial tree. It is reasoned that the coronary arteries were not normal at the time of coronary angiography. Factors supporting this hypothesis are:

a) Arteriographically documented coronary arterial embolic occlusion can completely resolve. In 5 reported patients with catheter-induced coronary arterial thromboembolic occlusion, the coronary arteriogram became normal after the AMI in each[2]. In 3 of the 5 patients, complete resolution of the occlusion occurred within 2 months of the onset of the AMI.

b) Conditions associated with an increased risk of arterial thromboemboli are relatively frequent (15%) among reported patients with non-catheter-induced AMI[2].

c) Histologic study of previously known arterial emboli indicates that such lesions may either lyse completely, retract along one side to form an eccentric lumen, or recanalize with multiple luminal channels[12]. Each of these 3 means of organization of the clot could almost surely create a lumen large enough to produce a normal coronary arteriogram.

d) Among 74 necropsy patients with transmural AMI studied personally[20], only 5 had <75% luminal narrowing by atherosclerotic plaques of each of their 3 major coronary arteries: 3 of the 5 had coronary emboli at necropsy and their coronary tree was otherwise normal.

e) Reported patients with non-catheter-induced AMI, with few exceptions, were asymptomatic before the occurrence of the AMI, and following healing of the AMI they were again asymptomatic without evidence of angina pectoris, congestive cardiac failure or cardiomegaly. Obviously, an AMI may be the first and only coronary event when the AMI is the result of severe coronary atherosclerosis, but the percentage who return to a totally asymptomatic state is not nearly as high as in the group with 'myocardial infarction and angiographically normal coronary arteries'. Acute pulmonary embolism, when occurring in previously normal pulmonary arteries and lungs, might be analogous (= normal coronary arteries), as opposed to acute pulmonary embolism superimposed on chronic lung disease (= coronary atherosclerosis).

Summary

The coronary arteries in patients with fatal ischemic heart disease (IHD) may be characterized as follows: 1) the coronary arteries are diffusely involved by atherosclerotic plaques; 2) with few exceptions, the lumens of at least 2 of the 3 major coronary arteries are >75% narrowed in cross-sectional area by atherosclerotic plaques; 3) the atherosclerosis is limited to the epicardial coronary arteries; 4) certain portions of the coronary tree tend to develop larger atherosclerotic plaques, and therefore more luminal narrowing than other portions; 5) of the 3 types of atherosclerotic plaques, only the complicated ones cause significant (>75%) coronary luminal narrowing; 6) the degree of coronary luminal narrowing by atherosclerotic plaques and the extensiveness of the plaques are similar in patients with fatal IHD, irrespective of the type of fatal coronary event; 7) the composition of coronary atherosclerotic plaques and the degree of coronary luminal narrowing appear to be similar, irrespective of whether the blood lipoprotein pattern was normal or abnormal; 8) the shapes of lumens of atherosclerotic coronary arteries are quite variable; 9) the coronary artery responsible for perfusing an area of myocardium which has become either necrotic or fibrotic is not necessarily the most narrowed (by atherosclerotic plaque) of the 3 major extramural coronary arteries; and 10) advanced age does not necessarily indicate the presence of severe coronary atherosclerosis.

Among patients with fatal IHD, certain observations regarding coronary thrombosis are becoming established: 1) coronary thrombi are infrequent (about 10 %) in patients dying suddenly; 2) coronary thrombi are rare in patients with isolated subendocardial infarcts; 3) coronary thrombi occur in about 60 % of patients with fatal transmural acute myocardial infarction (AMI); 4) coronary thrombi occur in high percentage only in patients with cardiogenic shock; 5) the larger the area of myocardial necrosis, the greater the likelihood of coronary thrombosis; 6) thrombi occur usually only in the coronary artery responsible for perfusing the area of myocardial necrosis; 7) thrombi occur in arteries that are already severely narrowed by old atherosclerotic plaques; and 8) coronary thrombi are usually single, occlusive, short, and located entirely in the major trunks.

Several factors suggest that coronary thrombosis is a consequence rather than the precipitating cause of AMI. Slow blood flow and sufficient time are prerequisites for thrombus formation.

Several observations suggest that coronary thrombosis plays a major role in the development of coronary atherosclerosis in the first place.

Among the non-thrombotic acute coronary lesions, only hemorrhages into atherosclerotic plaques are common, but there is no evidence that they cause coronary narrowing.

Among patients with 'myocardial infarction and angiographically normal coronary arteries', an angiographically normal coronary arterial tree has never been demonstrated at the time of AMI; among reported patients with 'myocardial infarction and angiographically normal coronary arteries', the angiograms were performed after healing, rather than during the AMI; although there are several explanations for the occurrence of AMI and angiographically normal coronary arteries, and although each may be applicable on occasion, the most reasonable explanation appears to be acute coronary embolism with subsequent clot lysis, retraction, or recanalization, all of which may appear as 'angiographically normal'.

References

[1] Anitschkow N, Chalatow S: *Abl. allg. Path. path. Anat.* 1913, 24, 1. – [2] Arnett EA, Roberts WC: *Circulation* 1976, 53, 395. – [3] Buja LM, Roberts WC: *In:* Shock in myocardial infarction. Eds RM Gunnar, HS Loeb, SH Rahimtcola. Grune & Stratton, New York 1974, p. 1. – [4] Bulkley BH, Roberts WC: *Amer. J. Med.* 1973, 55, 747. – [5] Bulkley BH, Roberts WC: *Circulation* 1974, 49/50, Suppl. III, 150. – [6] Chandler AB: *Thromb. Res.* 1974, 4, 3. – [7] Classification of atherosclerotic lesions. Report of a study group. *Wld. Hlth. Org. techn. Rep. Ser.* 1958, No. 143. – [8] Daoud AS, Jarmolych J, Augustyn JM, Fritz KE, Singh JK, Lee KT: *Arch. Pathol. Lab. Med.* 1976, 100, 372. – [9] Duguid JB: *J. Path. Bact.* 1946, 58, 1946. – [10] Erhardt LR, Lundman R, Mellstedt H: *Lancet* 1973, i, 387. – [11] Geiringer E: *J. Path. Bact.* 1951, 63, 201. – [12] Harrison CV: *J. Path. Bact.* 1948, 60, 289. – [13] Hellstrom HR: *Cardiovasc. Res.* 1971, 5, 371. – [14] Herrick JB: *J. Amer. med. Ass.* 1912, 59, 2015. – [15] Master AM, Dack S, Jaffe HL: *Amer. Heart. J.* 1939, 18, 434. – [16] Page DL, Caulfield JB, Kastor JA, de Sanctis RW, Sanders CA: *New Engl. J. Med.* 1971, 285, 133. – [17] Roberts WC: *Hosp. Pract.* 1971, 6, 89. – [18] Roberts WC: *Circulation* 1972, 45, 215. – [19] Roberts WC: *Mod. Conc. cardiovasc. Dis.* 1972, 41, 7. – [20] Roberts WC, Buja LM: *Amer. J. Med.* 1972, 52, 425. – [21] Roberts WC, Ferrans VJ, Levy RI, Fredrickson DS: *Amer. J. Cardiol.* 1973, 31, 557. – [22] Roberts WC: *Circulation* 1973, 48, 1161. – [23] Roberts WC: *Circulation* 1974, 49, 1. – [24] Roberts WC, Buja LM, Bulkley BH, Ferrans VJ: *Amer. J. Cardiol.* 1974, 34, 870. – [25] Roberts WC: *Circulation* 1976, 54, 388. – [26] Rokitansky CA: *In:* Manual of pathologic anatomy. Translated by GE Day. Sydenham Society, London 1952, Vol. 4, p. 261. – [27] Spain DM, Bradess VA: *Chest* 1970, 58, 107. – [28] Virchow R: Cellular Pathology. As bared upon physiological and pathological histology. Translated from the second german edition originally published by J. B. Lippincott and Co., Philadelphia 1863. Dover Publications, New York 1971. – [29] Walston A, Hackel DB, Estes EH: *Amer. Heart J.* 1970, 79, 613. – [30] Yarbrough JW, Roberts WC, Abel RM, Reis RL: *Amer. Heart J.* 1972, 84, 507.

Fatal Coronary Heart Disease–
Is the Coronary Atherosclerosis Focal or Diffuse?

The author reports on his 10-year study of atherosclerosis, which investigated the entire major coronary arterial tree in patients who died of coronary heart disease. Although previous concepts held that coronary atherosclerosis in fatal heart disease was a focal process, the author's study indicates that it is diffuse.

William C. Roberts, M.D.
Chief, Pathology Branch, National Heart, Lung, and Blood Institute; Clinical Professor of Pathology and Medicine (Cardiology), Georgetown University

▶ When I was in medical school, coronary atherosclerosis was thought to be a focal process, that is, that the atherosclerotic plaques were present in some coronary arteries and not in others, and that in any one artery, the plaques were present at some sites and not at others. Later, when attending cardiology conferences and observing coronary angiograms, this concept was reinforced because narrowings were present in some arteries and not in others, and at some sites in a particular artery and not at others. Initially, when I first did necropsies, the focal nature of coronary atherosclerosis was again reinforced because some areas of some arteries by gross examination appeared free of atherosclerotic plaques, or

at least narrowings appeared more severe in some sites than in others.

Beginning in 1968, to investigate coronary atherosclerosis in more detail, the entire major coronary arterial tree was studied in my laboratory, as depicted in Figure 1. A histologic cross-section was examined from each 5-mm long segment of major (right, left main, left anterior descending, left circumflex) coronary artery of patients with fatal coronary heart disease. On an average, the right coronary artery was approximately 12 cm in length, the left main, 1 cm, the

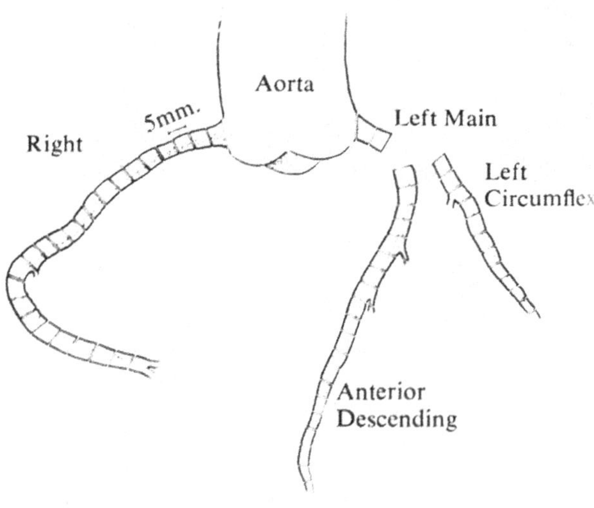

1. Studying the Major Coronary Arteries—The method by which the coronary arteries are examined in the Pathology Branch, National Heart, Lung, and Blood Institute. Each of the major coronary arteries is excised from the heart, fixed in formalin, decalcified, and sectioned at 5-mm intervals. Each 5-mm long segment is processed in alcohol and xylene, embedded in parafin, and at least one histologic section is prepared from each segment and stained by Movat's method.

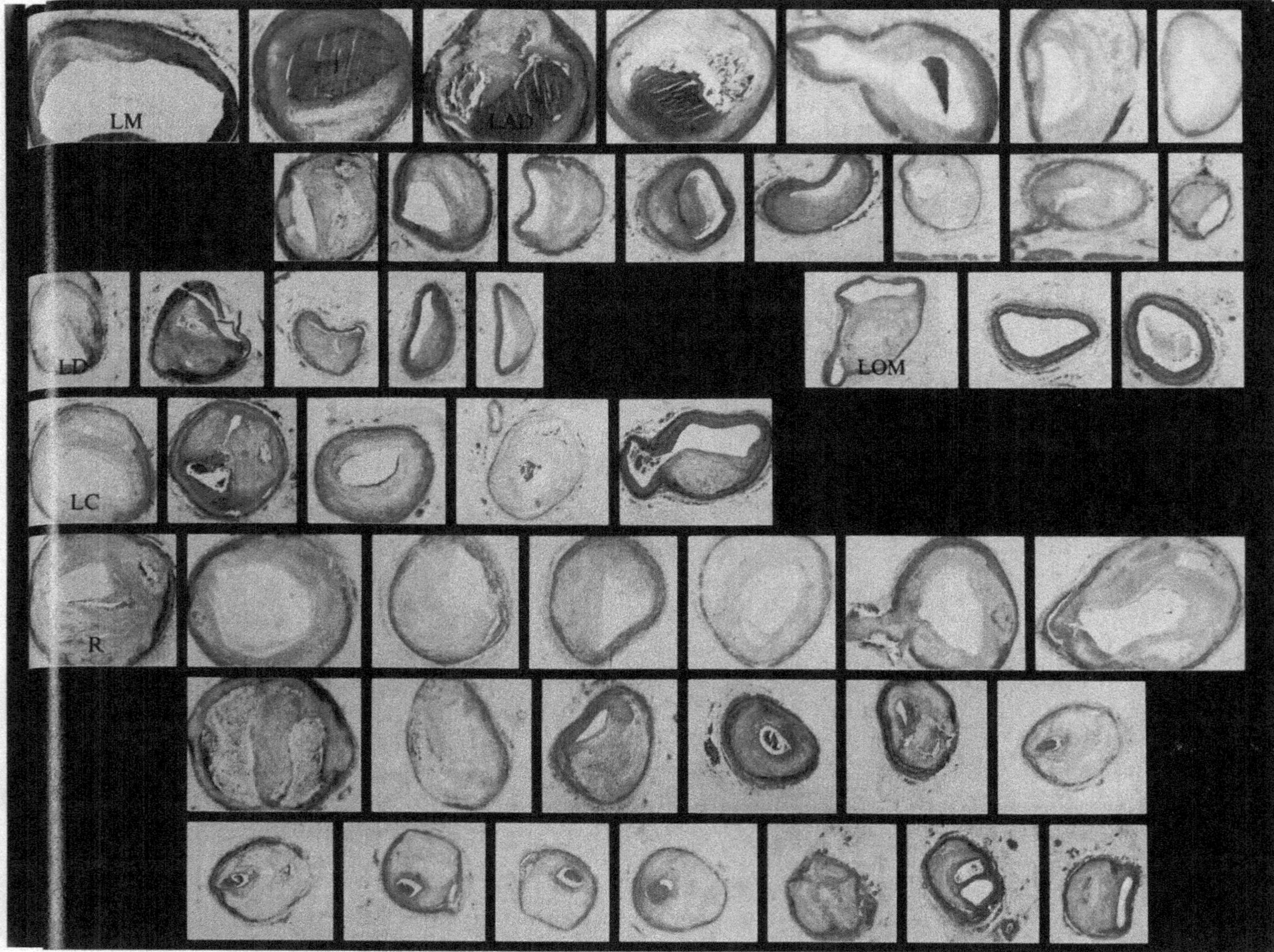

2. Sections of Major Coronary Arteries—Each section was photographed at the same magnification. Shown are two sections of left main (LM); 13 sections of left anterior descending (LAD) coronary artery; five sections of the first left diagonal (LD); three sections of the left obtuse marginal (LOM) coronary artery arising from the left circumflex; five sections of the left circumflex (LC); and 20 sections of the right (R) coronary artery. An antemortum thrombus is present in the distal LM and in the proximal 1 cm of LAD. Save for two sections of LOM, atherosclerotic plaques are present in the lumens of all coronary arteries. Some antemortum thrombus is present in the lumens of some of the coronary arteries, particularly the right one. Each section represents a 5-mm long segment of coronary artery, thus the 48 sections represent 24 cm of coronary artery.

left anterior descending, 14 cm, and the left circumflex, about 6 cm. During these past 10 years, my colleagues and I have studied at necropsy the major coronary arterial tree in over 400 patients with fatal coronary heart disease. These studies unequivocally indicate that coronary atherosclerosis is diffuse and not focal among patients with fatal coronary heart disease. Indeed, the finding of a single normal coronary arterial segment among the many thousands of sections examined in these patients was rare. The

degrees of the coronary arterial narrowing by the atherosclerotic plaques, however, varied considerably. Nevertheless, the atherosclerotic process involved all segments of the major epicardial coronary tree.

There are 38 histologic sections shown in Figure 2, each representing a cross section prepared from a 5-mm long segment of major epicardial coronary artery. Thus, these sections represent 24 cm of coronary artery. The patient was a 52-year-old physician, who died three days after

The Author

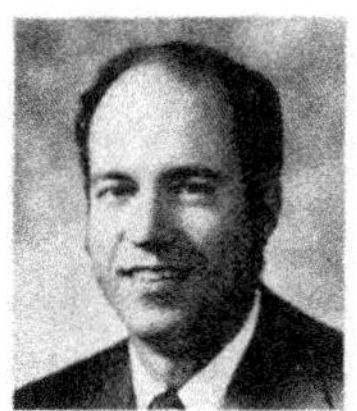

William C. Roberts, M.D.

Dr. Roberts received his M.D. from Emory University in 1958 and did his postgraduate work at Boston City Hospital, the National Institutes of Health, and Johns Hopkins. In addition to serving on the Board of Editors of this journal, Dr. Roberts has contributed extensively to our knowledge of cardiovascular disease in recent years. He received the 1978 Gifted Teacher Award of the American College of Cardiology.

onset of features typical of acute myocardial infarction. A thrombus was present in the proximal portion of the left anterior descending (LAD) and distal portion of the left main (LM) coronary artery. Distal to the coronary thrombus, however, the lumen of the left anterior descending coronary artery was already more than 75% narrowed by atherosclerotic plaque and it was between 50% and 75% narrowed in the cross-sectional area at the site of the thrombus. Both the left circumflex and the right coronary arteries also were more than 75% narrowed by atherosclerotic plaque. In addition, study of Figure 2 indicates that no two coronary arterial sections are alike. Thus, coronary arterial atherosclerotic plaques are like fingerprints—no two are alike when observed in cross-section.

Emphasizing the diffuse nature of coronary atherosclerosis in fatal coronary heart disease appears fatalistic or at least pessimistic about this condition. Fortunately, the most severe narrowing, at least in the branches of the left main coronary artery, is in the proximal half of the vessels. The distal half tends to be less narrowed than the proximal half. This fact is a major reason why coronary bypass surgery has been successful. With the right coronary artery, however, the reverse is true. The severest luminal narrowing tends to be in its distal rather than in its proximal half. Thus, a bypass graft to the right coronary artery, generally is inserted into the proximal portion of a posterior descending branch. An endarterectomy often must be performed in the distal portion of the right coronary artery for the flow through the conduit to have an adequate run-off, which is essential if the graft is to remain patent. ◀

Coronary embolism: a review of causes, consequences, and diagnostic considerations

William C. Roberts, M.D.

Before cardiac catheterization and cardiac surgery—primarily, valve replacement—became feasible, coronary arterial embolism was an extremely rare finding both clinically and at necropsy and was associated primarily with infective endocarditis. Today, coronary embolism is observed at necropsy fairly frequently and its possibility is raised clinically with increasing frequency. Whether or not it produces acute myocardial infarction or sudden death or evidence of cardiac dysfunction is determined primarily by the embolus size, which in turn determines primarily whether it migrates to a small distal coronary artery or becomes impacted in a large trunk. Emboli of minute size—those carried to the very small arteries—are clinically silent but more common than the larger emboli, which obstruct large vessels and usually produce myocardial consequences. Another reason why coronary embolism is of increasing importance is that it appears to be the most reasonable explanation for the phenomenon of acute myocardial infarction followed by angiographically normal coronary arteries.

When a clot is found in the lumen of a pulmonary artery, its cause is usually considered to be embolism. When a clot is found in the lumen of a coronary artery, on the other hand, its cause is usually considered to be in situ thrombosis. Factors supporting an embolic nature of pulmonary arterial clots are their occurrence in apparently previously normal arteries and their extremely common association with an identifiable thrombus in one or more systemic veins or in one or both of the right cardiac chambers. Factors supporting a thrombotic nature of coronary arterial clots are their occurrence in previously abnormal arteries, i.e., those that already contain atherosclerotic plaques, and the absence

of thrombi in a left cardiac cavity (the usual finding) or of a patent foramen ovale in the presence of thrombi in a systemic vein or the right atrium. Occasionally, however, a clot is found in the lumen of a pulmonary artery that contains extensive atherosclerotic plaque or observed in the lumen of a coronary artery that is virtually devoid of atherosclerotic plaque. Under these circumstances, in situ thrombosis is suggested as the mechanism of the clot in the pulmonary artery and embolism is suggested as the mechanism of the clot in the coronary artery.

For many years coronary artery embolism was believed to be a rare phenomenon. During the 100 years following Virchow's description of coronary embolism in 1856, only 62 "well-documented" cases were reported and most of these were isolated case studies.[1] Until 1960, the most

common condition associated with necropsy-diagnosed coronary embolism was active infective endocarditis, which accounted for about 75% of the cases.[1] Most of the remainder were associated with thrombus in the left atrium from mitral stenosis or from thrombus in the left ventricle from either coronary heart disease with myocardial infarction or idiopathic dilated cardiomyopathy. Thus, before the 1960s, coronary embolism was observed most commonly as a consequence of natural disease (Table).

With the introduction of cardiac valve replacement and the more frequent use of cardiac catheterization in the early 1960s, coronary embolism became a more frequent clinical consideration.[2-24] Moreover, the reports beginning in the 1960s of "myocardial infarction with angiographically normal coronary arteries" raised the possibility of coronary embolism as the cause of this phenomenon.[25] Accordingly, coronary embolism has become an important consideration.

Causes of coronary embolism

Summarized in the Table and illustrated in Fig. 1 to 7, the causes of coronary embolism today are more often iatrogenic than natural, although statistics are not available. With few exceptions, the cause of the embolus determines its composition. The nature of embolic materials is varied; the embolus may consist of fibrin-platelet clot, vegetation, neoplasm, bone marrow, shreds of myocardium, calcium,

From the Pathology Branch, National Heart, Lung, and Blood Institute, Bethesda, Md.

Address reprint requests to: Dr. Roberts, Building 10A, Room 3E-30, National Institutes of Health, Bethesda, Md. 20014.

or foreign body materials such as talc, cloth, or silicone rubber.

Consequences of coronary embolism

The consequences of coronary embolism depend on two factors, the size of the embolus and the original size of the artery in which it becomes impacted. The smaller the embolus, the greater the chance that it will migrate distally to a small coronary artery and the less the likelihood of myocardial necrosis or fatal arrhythmia. Conversely, the larger the embolus, the greater the chance that it will impact proximally in a large coronary artery and the greater the likelihood of myocardial necrosis or fatal arrhythmia. An embolus so small that it impacts in a single intramural coronary artery is clinically silent and observed at necropsy only by histologic examination of sections of myocardial wall (Fig. 8).

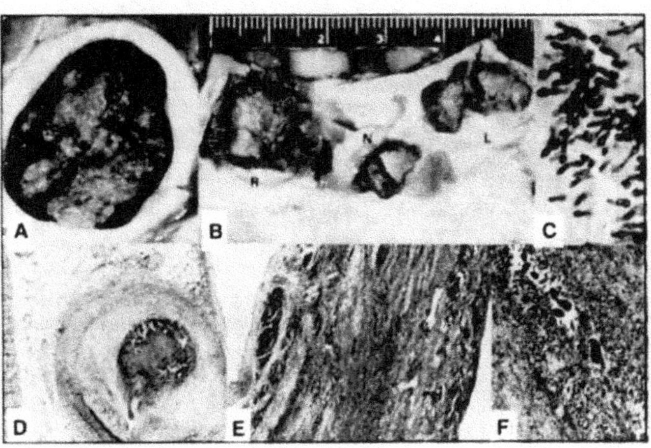

Fig. 1. Embolus to left anterior descending coronary artery from patient with active infective endocarditis affecting aortic valve

Endocarditis was secondary to Candida parapsilosis *infection in 26-year-old opiate addict who experienced sudden excruciating precordial pain 52 days before death. The ECG showed changes characteristic of acute myocardial infarction of the anterior wall. Several days later the left leg suddenly became cold and speech slurred. At necropsy, an embolus was found filling the distal half of the left anterior descending coronary artery and several of its epicardial branches. The right, left circumflex, and left main coronary arteries were normal. Aortic valve (a) shows large vegetations. Opened aortic valve (b) shows vegetation on each of the three cusps; arrow designates ostium of left coronary artery. Material dislodged from one of the* Candida *vegetations (c) had migrated into the left anterior descending coronary artery (d), which is totally occluded by organized and organizing vegetative material. Wall of infarcted left ventricle (e) is seen near its apex; few myocardial fibers remain. Photomicrograph (f) of portion of infarcted left ventricular wall shows giant-cell inflammation reaction to* Candida *organisms. (c—methenamine silver stain, × 775, d—elastic van Gieson's stain, × 21, e—hematoxylin-eosin stain, × 73, f—× 130)*

L = left aortic valve cusp, N = noncoronary aortic valve cusp, R = right aortic valve cusp; scale = centimeters

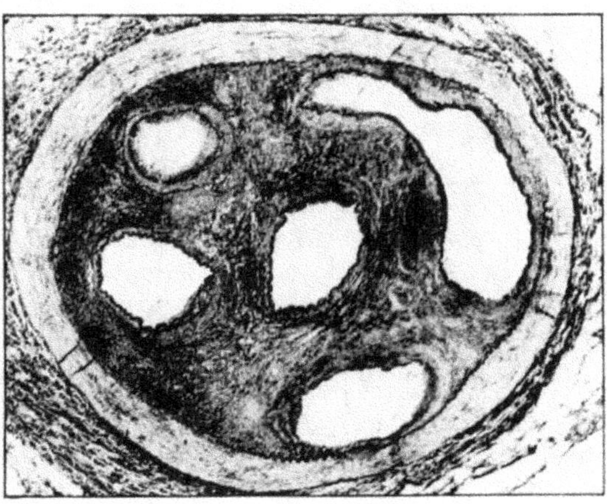

Fig. 2. Distal left anterior descending coronary artery from patient with active infective endocarditis

Thirty-eight months before death, the patient, a 26-year-old man who had been well until five months previously, suddenly developed typical clinical, ECG, and enzyme evidence of acute myocardial infarction of the anterior wall, with recurrent fever. Twelve months before death the left ventricular pressure was 108/30 and the aortic pressure, 108/36 mm Hg. The ECG suggested ventricular aneurysm. One month later, cardiotomy disclosed healed perforations in the congenitally bicuspid aortic valve, which was replaced. Death followed severe congestive cardiac failure that occurred 11 months later. At necropsy, the heart was huge (950 g) and a large transmural left ventricular healed infarct was found. The distal half of the left anterior descending coronary artery contained multiple channels, and tissue between these channels was essentially homogenous. The right, left main, left circumflex, and proximal left anterior descending coronary arteries appeared normal. It is likely that occlusion of the distal left anterior descending coronary artery was caused by vegetative material dislodged 33 months before death (elastic van Gieson's stain, × 46, enlarged from 4×6 to 5×7)

Fig. 3. Right coronary artery from patient who developed clinical and ECG evidence of acute MI during cardiac catheterization

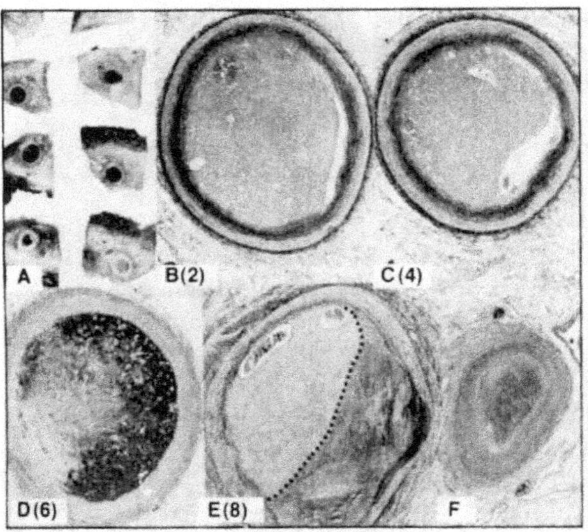

Clinical evidence of mitral regurgitation had been seen for seven years in this 56-year-old man who died 31 days after catheterization. Left ventricular angiography had disclosed severe (4+/4+) mitral regurgitation, and injection of contrast material into the left main coronary artery had shown it and its anterior descending and left circumflex coronary branches to be normal. With placement in the right coronary ostium, the catheter was flushed; chest pain immediately followed. Injection shortly thereafter showed the distal portion of this artery to be occluded, and embolus was suspected. During the next two days, the patient was in shock and severe congestive cardiac failure. Mitral valve replacement was performed. The patient died 27 days later of congestive heart failure. At necropsy, most of the right coronary artery was found filled with organizing and organized clot. In the upper left section (a) are several cross sections of this artery. The photomicrographs labeled b, c, d, and e are of portions of right coronary artery at various sites, specifically at 2, 4, 6, and 8 cm, respectively, from the aortic ostium. In the more distal portions of this artery, the clot is more organized than in the more proximal portions. In section e, about one-half the arterial lumen is obliterated by old plaque. Two recanalized channels are seen in the recent clot. The posterior descending artery (f), a branch of the RCA, is also filled with organizing clot. The lumens by the left main, left circumflex, and left anterior descending coronary arteries were < 25% narrowed by old atherosclerotic plaque, and each was free of clot. (b, c, d, e—elastic van Gieson's stain, × 25; f—hematoxylin-eosin stain, × 25)

Fig. 4. Impaction of large embolus in left main coronary artery during cardiac catheterization in patient with severe coronary atherosclerosis

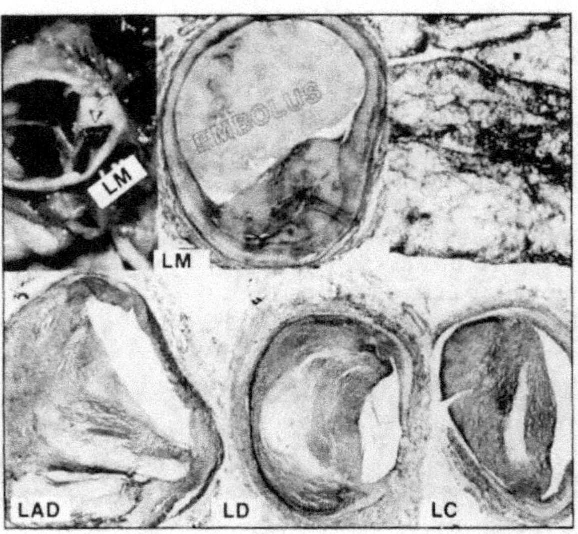

With the catheter tip placed in the left anterior aortic valve sinus, the catheter was flushed. Systemic arterial pressure dropped immediately to shock levels in this patient, a 49-year-old woman, and cardiac arrest occurred. At necropsy, a linear clot (arrow) was found in the left aortic sinus extending into the left main coronary artery (gross specimen, top left). Histology sections showed the embolus to be limited to the left main (LM) coronary artery, which had been narrowed between 25 and 50% in cross-sectional area by old atherosclerotic plaque. The left main coronary artery in this patient gave off three branches: the left anterior descending (LAD), the left diagonal (LD), and the left circumflex (LC); the lumen of each of these three arteries was already obliterated > 75% by old atherosclerotic plaque. The embolus in the left main artery did not extend farther down the coronary tree because it was larger than the residual lumen of any of the three branches of the left main coronary artery. The embolus, shown in photomicrograph at upper right, consists primarily of platelets, and its configuration is suggestive of the lumen of the catheter folded over on itself several times. (LM, LAD, LD, and LC—Movat stain, × 27)

An embolus somewhat larger may occlude multiple intramural coronary arteries in a fingerlike fashion (Fig. 8). When only multiple intramural coronary arteries are obstructed, particularly those located in the inner one-half of the myocardial wall, myocardial necrosis is unlikely to result, probably because of the extensive intramyocardial vascular bed. However, a major danger of obstruction to multiple intramural coronary arteries, particularly those located in the outer one-half of the myocardial wall, is that a "right-angle" epicardial feeding branch may become thrombosed secondarily because of the poor runoff through it (Fig. 8). Occlusion of this branch may in turn lead to secondary thrombosis of the major coronary trunk, and this complication may produce myocardial

Fig. 5. Embolus followed by in situ thrombus in left anterior descending coronary artery from patient with large ventricular septal defect

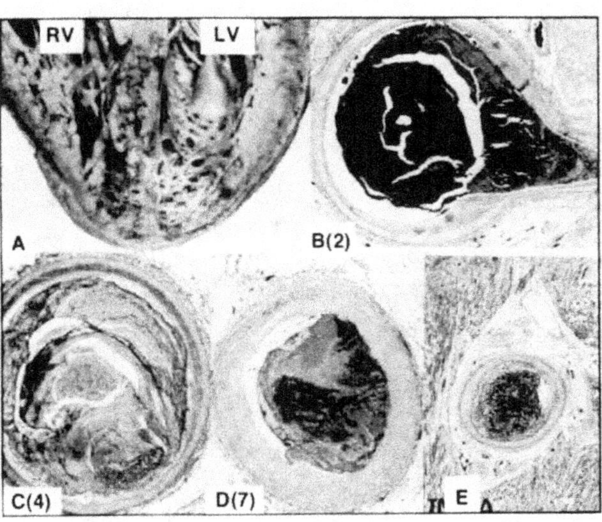

The patient, a 37-year-old man, suddenly developed rapid atrial fibrillation, and cardioversion was applied to restore sinus rhythm. Four hours later he suddenly developed severe chest pain. ECGs showed progressive changes typical of acute myocardial infarction. The patient died three days after onset of chest pain. At necropsy, a large, primarily anteroseptal acute myocardial infarct was found (a). Most of the left anterior descending coronary artery was filled with fibrin-platelet clot. Clot was found not only in the main coronary trunk but also in several right-angle epicardial branches (b, c, and d) and in several intramural coronary arteries (e). The numerals 2, 4, and 7 indicate distance in centimeters from the aortic ostium of the left coronary artery. Note that the left anterior descending coronary artery is virtually free of atherosclerotic plaque. There is evidence of beginning organization of the clot distally, whereas proximally the clot contains large numbers of erythrocytes. This finding suggests that the embolus initially impacted distally and that in situ thrombus later formed more proximally. (b, e—Movat stain, × 22; c—phosphotungstic acid–hematoxylin stain, × 22; d—hematoxylin-eosin stain, × 22)

LV = left ventricle; RV = right ventricle

Fig. 6. Various types of embolic materials found in intramural coronary arteries

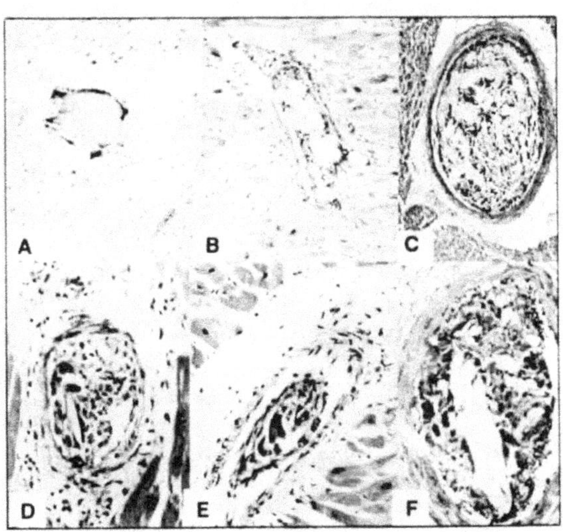

Calcific embolus (a) was found in 60-year-old woman who underwent aortic valve replacement 20 months before death because of severe calcific aortic stenosis. Bone-marrow embolus (b) occurred in man unsuccessfully resuscitated after aortic valve replacement for pure aortic regurgitation. Neoplastic embolus (c) (mucin-producing adenocarcinoma) was found in 24-year-old man. Cholesterol (atherosclerotic) embolus (d) was found in 55-year-old man with extensive atherosclerosis of the extramural coronary arteries (supplied kindly by Michael C. Fishbein, M.D.). Talc (birefringent) embolus (e) occurred in 31-year-old man who could not be separated from cardiopulmonary bypass after aortic valve replacement for severe aortic stenosis. Suture embolus (f) was found in 46-year-old man who died six days after mitral valve replacement for severe regurgitation and mild stenosis. (Hematoxylin-eosin stain, a—× 99; b—× 160; c—× 100; d—× 100; e—× 251; f—× 250)

necrosis. Thus, *secondary thrombosis* of the proximal feeding coronary artery is a potential complication of coronary embolism.

A second, and less important, factor determining the consequence of coronary embolism is the status of the coronary arteries preceding embolism. An embolus to a previously wide-open coronary artery is most likely to migrate quite distally, but because collaterals between the epicardial coronary arteries are relatively poor, myocardial necrosis or ischemia may nevertheless occur (Fig. 9). An embolus of the same size migrating to a previously severely narrowed coronary tree is much more likely to impact proximally and thus lead to sudden death (Fig. 9), despite the collaterals that are likely to be present in this circumstance.

In recent years, much has been written about "myocardial infarction followed by angiographically normal coronary arteries." As has been pointed out recently, the status of the coronary arteries in these patients *at the time of* acute myocardial infarction is rarely known.[25] Coronary angiograms are performed, with rare exception, several months after healing of the acute myocardial infarction. At this later time, the coronary angiograms appear normal, but it is inappropriate to assume that the coronary arteries were normal when acute infarction occurred. It has been reported in at least five patients who had angiographically normal coronary arteries a month or more after acute myocardial infarction occurred that coronary angiograms performed at the time of acute infarction showed at least one of the major extramural coronary arteries to be totally occluded.[25] The mechanism by which a major coronary artery may appear occluded at one time and normal at a later time can only be speculated upon, but embolism appears to be the most likely explanation.[25,26] It is known, for example, that clots injected into systemic veins in animals migrate to the lungs and initially obstruct one or more pulmonary arteries. Several days later, however, a previously obstructed pulmonary artery may become patent because of revascularized channels or retraction of the clot eccentrically, both of which may give a normal appearance angiographically. The same mechanism may occur when embolism involves the coronary arterial system. The embolus may lyse completely, retract along one side, or form "revascularized channels," any of which may give an angiographically normal appearance (Fig. 10). Another factor

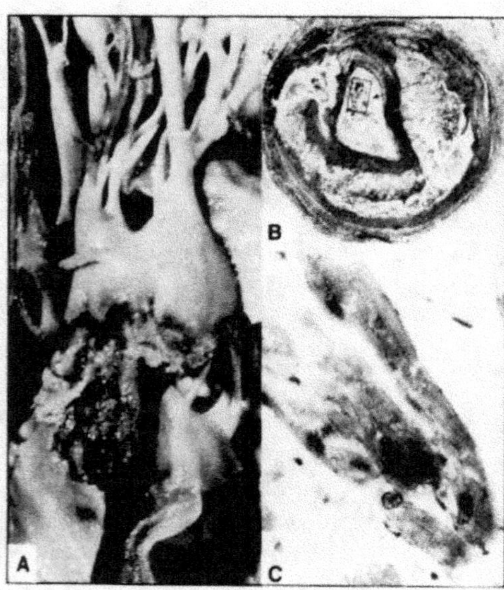

Fig. 7. Myocardial embolus to a major coronary arterial trunk

Embolus migrated after rupture of one left ventricular papillary muscle during acute myocardial infarction (a). At necropsy, fragment of myocardium (arrow) was found in a segment of right coronary artery (b). Photomicrograph of the embolized fragment of myocardium is shown in c. It is presumed that the fragment dislodged from the ruptured papillary muscle and migrated to the coronary artery. (Movat stain, b—×16; c—×830)

Etiology of coronary artery embolism

Natural disease

Infective endocarditis

Noninfective ("marantic") endocarditis

Intracardiac mural thrombus or neoplasm

left ventricle
coronary disease
myocardial disease
valvular disease
miscellaneous

left atrial appendage
any condition associated
with inadequate cardiac output

left atrial body
mitral stenosis only

pulmonary vein(s)
mitral stenosis

Intracardiac, intracavitary neoplasm

primary (myxoma)
secondary (extension from lung
via pulmonary vein)

Iatrogenic disease

Cardiac catheterization, particularly angiography

Cardiac surgery

prosthetic valve
patch closure of septal defect
other

Cardioversion

External cardiac massage

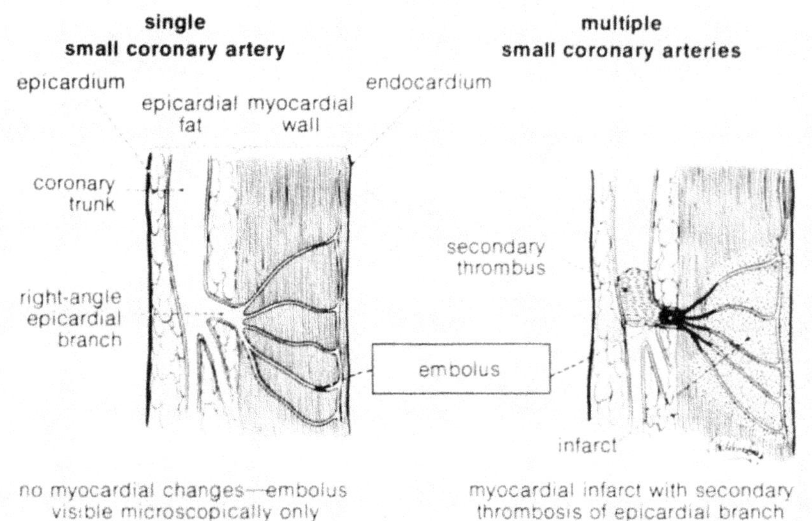

Fig. 8. Effects of embolus size on myocardial consequences of embolus migration

no myocardial changes—embolus visible microscopically only

myocardial infarct with secondary thrombosis of epicardial branch and major coronary trunk

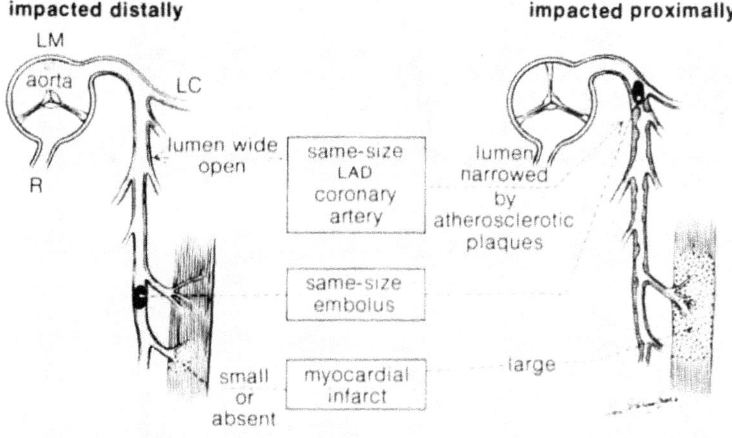

Fig. 9. Effects of atherosclerotic narrowing on myocardial consequences of embolus migration

The embolus impacts proximally in an artery whose lumen is narrowed by atherosclerotic plaque and distally in a nonatherosclerotic artery of identical initial size.

LAD = left anterior descending artery; LC = left circumflex artery; LM = left main coronary artery; R = right coronary artery

suggesting embolism to explain normal coronary angiograms after acute myocardial infarction is the fact that myocardial infarction in all these patients represents the initial coronary event, and after recovery from the infarct, these patients almost always return to an entirely asymptomatic state. Thus, coronary embolism receives additional importance as the most likely explanation.

Diagnostic considerations

Diagnosis of coronary embolism can be suspected clinically when a patient with an appropriate underlying condition (Table) suddenly develops substernal chest pain followed shortly by either cardiac arrest or persistence of pain and development of ECG and enzymatic changes consistent with acute myocardial infarction. Coronary embolism as a cause of angina pectoris has not been demonstrated.

For coronary embolism to cause cardiac arrest or clinically apparent acute myocardial infarction, the embolus must lodge in, or secondary thrombosis must develop in, one of the major epicardial (extramural) coronary arterial trunks. As a rule, a coronary embolus, or any embolus in any artery, migrates distally as far as it can travel, i.e., until its dimensions are larger than those of the arterial lumen. When an embolus becomes impacted in a major epicardial coronary artery with or without extension into one of its near right-angle branches or into the intramural coronary arteries, the clot tends to be located in the distal one-half of the epicardial coronary trunk (Fig. 11), most commonly the left anterior descending coronary artery. This tendency for location of a coronary embolus in the distal half of the coronary trunk is opposite to the situation observed in coronary thrombosis, at least that involving the left coronary artery, in which the clot usually is located in the proximal one-half of the major coronary trunk. In patients who suffer fatal coronary atherosclerosis with thrombosis, the clot is always superimposed on underlying atherosclerotic plaque and no clot is observed in the epicardial branches of the major coronary trunks or in the intramural coronary arteries.[12] In contrast, in patients who suffer coronary embolus with clot in a major coronary trunk, clot usually is also found at necropsy in an epicardial branch of the major trunk and in one or more intramural coronary arteries.

Summary

Coronary embolus, once considered extremely rare, is observed not infrequently at necropsy and should be suspected in any of several circumstances, including acute myocardial infarction with subsequently normal coronary arteries at angiography. Underlying conditions associated with coronary embolism include infective endocarditis, intracardiac thrombus or neoplasm, and iatrogenic disease including cardiac catheterization, cardiac surgery, cardioversion, and external cardiac massage. Embolus should be considered when a patient with one of the associated conditions develops sudden signs of myocardial ischemia or necrosis, and especially when occlusions are demonstrated in the *distal* half of the epicardial coronary tree or extending into intramural coronary arteries. Both findings are less common with coronary thrombus and more characteristic of coronary embolus.

References

1. Wenger NK, Bauer S: Coronary embolism: review of the literature and presentation of fifteen cases. *Am J Med* 25:549–557, 1958

2. Oakley C, Yusuf R, Hollman A: Coronary embolism and angina in mitral stenosis. *Br Heart J* 23:357–369, 1961

3. Hall MRP, Richards WCD: Coronary artery embolism. *Br Heart J* 23:103–106, 1961

4. Jerie P, Poddany V: Coronary embolism in mitral stenosis. *Cardiologia* 40:281–289, 1962

continued on page 710

Fig. 10. Possible explanation for normal coronary angiograms after healing of acute myocardial infarction

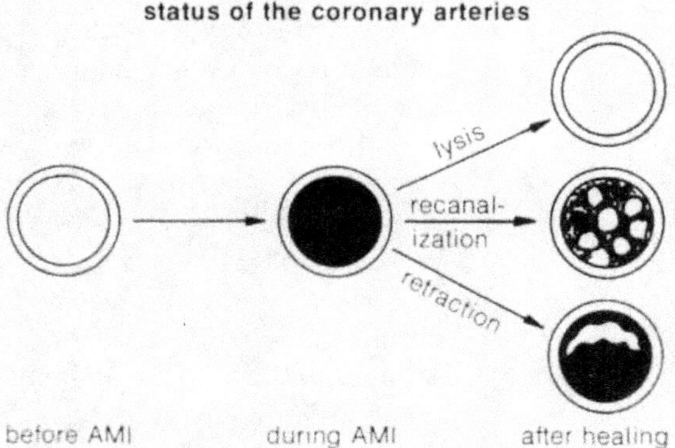

Coronary embolism is the apparent pathogenesis of infarction when the arteries appear normal at subsequent angiography, as may occur if the lumen of each artery affected is restored sufficiently by lysis, recanalization, or retraction of the obstructing clot.

AMI = acute myocardial infarction

Fig. 11. Differences between coronary thrombosis and coronary embolism

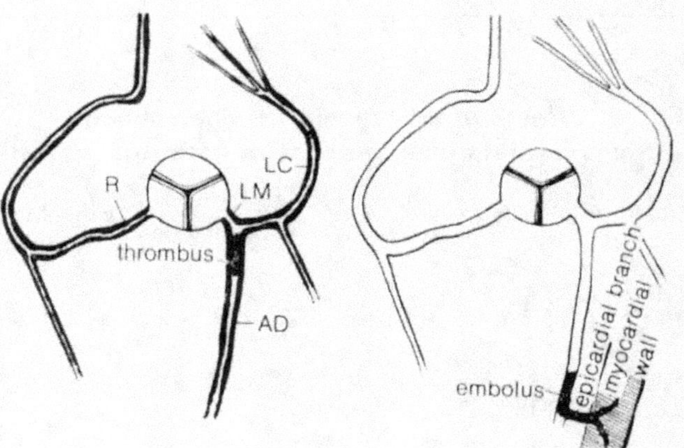

thrombus never extends into intramural coronary artery

embolus usually extends into intramural coronary artery

Usually, a thrombus is located in the more proximal portion of a left coronary artery, superimposed on old atherosclerotic plaque that is extensive in all the major extramural coronary arteries. A coronary embolus is most readily diagnosed when the clot is located in the more distal portion of an epicardial coronary trunk and is continuous with clot in a right-angle epicardial branch, which, in turn, is continuous with clot in the intramural coronary arteries.

AD = anterior descending artery; LC = left circumflex artery; LM = left main artery; R = right coronary artery

5. Holley KE, Bahn RC, McGoon DC, Mankin HT: Spontaneous calcific aortic stenosis. *Circulation* 27 197–202, 1963

6. Rivera R, Tallon R: Coronary embolism in mitral stenosis. *J Cardiovasc Surg* 5 382–385, 1964

7. Cordeiro A, Pimentel C, Laginha F, Ribeiro C, Costa H: Coronary embolism. *Br Heart J* 29 91–95, 1967

8. Oppenheimer EH, Esterly JR: Some aspects of cardiac pathology in infancy and childhood. III. Coronary embolism. *Johns Hopkins Med J* 120 317–325, 1967

9. Gonzalez-Crussi F, Mandy S, Johnson JE, Green JR Jr: Teflon embolism of coronary arteries. *J Thorac Cardiovasc Surg* 54 53–59, 1967

10. Meister SG, Grossman W, Dexter L, Dalen JE: Paradoxical embolism: diagnosis during life. *Am J Med* 53 292–298, 1972

11. Roberts WC, Morrow AG: Causes of death and other anatomic observations after cardiac valve replacement. *Adv Cardiol* 7 226–247, 1972

12. Roberts WC, Buja LM: The frequency and significance of coronary arterial thrombi and other observations in fatal acute myocardial infarction: a study of 107 necropsy patients. *Am J Med* 52 425–443, 1972

13. Price HP, Sollod N, Scott SM, Takaro T: Unusual coronary emboli associated with coronary arteriography. *Chest* 63 698–700, 1973

14. Madden F, Meredith G: Coronary embolism (letter to the editor). *Lancet* 1 665, 1973

15. Sequeira RF, Pomerance A, Green H, Raftery EB: Pathological changes produced by coronary embolization with metallic mercury in the dog. *Br J Exp Pathol* 55 514–518, 1974

16. Cheitlin MD, McAllister HA, de Castro CM: Myocardial infarction without atherosclerosis. *JAMA* 231 951–959, 1975

17. Roberts WC, Fishbein MC, Golden A: Cardiac pathology after valve replacement by disc prosthesis: a study of 61 necropsy patients. *Am J Cardiol* 35 740–760, 1975

18. Hammer WJ, Ferrans VJ, Roberts WC: Myocardial embolus to coronary artery: result of rupture of papillary muscle during acute myocardial infarction. *Chest* 68 843–844, 1975

19. Roberts WC, Hammer WJ: Cardiac pathology after valve replacement with a tilting disc prosthesis (Björk-Shiley type): a study of 46 necropsy patients and 49 Björk-Shiley prostheses. *Am J Cardiol* 37 1024–1032, 1976

20. Smith JM III, Richardson JD, Grover FL, Arom KY, Webb GE, Trinkle JK: Fatal air embolism following gunshot wound of the lung. *J Thorac Cardiovasc Surg* 72 296–298, 1976

21. Steiner I, Hlava A, Prochazka J: Calcific coronary embolization associated with cardiac valve replacement: necropsy x-ray study. *Br Heart J* 38 816–820, 1976

22. Arnett EN, Roberts WC: Active infective endocarditis: a clinicopathologic analysis of 137 necropsy patients. *Curr Probl Cardiol* 1(7) 1–76, 1976

23. Vlodaver Z, Amplantz K, Burchell HB, Edwards JE: *Coronary Heart Disease Clinical, Angiographic and Pathologic Profiles.* New York Springer-Verlag, 1976, p 584

24. Spray TL, Roberts WC: Structural changes in porcine xenografts used as substitute cardiac valves: gross and histologic observations in 51 glutaraldehyde-preserved Hancock valves in 41 patients. *Am J Cardiol* 40 319–330, 1977

25. Arnett EN, Roberts WC: Acute myocardial infarction and angiographically normal coronary arteries: an unproven combination. *Circulation* 53 395–400, 1976

26. Rosenblatt A, Selzer A: The nature and clinical features of myocardial infarction with normal coronary arteriogram. *Circulation* 55 578–580, 1977

Location of Myocardial Infarcts: A Confusion of Terms and Definitions

WILLIAM C. ROBERTS, MD, FACC
JULIUS M. GARDIN, MD[†]

Bethesda, Maryland
Washington, D.C.

Among patients with clinical features suggesting acute myocardial infarction, the standard 12 lead electrocardiogram has been extremely useful during the past 50 years in establishing the diagnosis of myocardial necrosis. In contrast to some previous reports,[1–3] the paper by Sullivan and associates[4] in this issue of the Journal also demonstrates that the electrocardiogram is extremely useful in establishing the diagnosis of healed myocardial infarction. Among their 50 necropsy patients with subendocardial or transmural left ventricular scars, or both, the electrocardiogram showed changes indicative of healed infarction in 47 (94 percent).

Electrocardiogram As Predictor of Infarct Location

Although the electrocardiogram is excellent in detecting the presence of myocardial infarction, many studies have shown that it is not as reliable in pinpointing the exact anatomic location of the myocardial infarct. In the study by Sullivan et al.,[4] for example, the precise electrocardiographic location of the healed myocardial infarct was confirmed at necropsy in only 7 (15 percent) of the 47 patients with an electrocardiographic diagnosis of healed myocardial infarction (Table I). Although the electrocardiogram infrequently predicts the precise location of a myocardial infarct, the study by Sullivan et al.[4] indicates that the electrocardiogram is indeed a good indicator of the general location of a healed myocardial infarct. It is very reliable, for example, in distinguishing between infarcts involving the anterior wall from those involving the pos-

terior wall, but it is unreliable in separating the various subdivisions of anterior and posterior wall infarcts. It is unreliable in sorting out isolated anterior wall infarcts from anterolateral or anteroseptal infarcts or posterolateral from posteroseptal or isolated posterior wall infarcts or in detecting posterior wall infarcts in patients who also have anterior wall infarcts. In addition, it is unreliable in predicting whether an infarct involves the basal or the apical portion of the left ventricle and, as shown by Sullivan et al.,[4] it is a poor predictor of whether a healed infarct is subendocardial or transmural in location.

Although the electrocardiogram is very reliable in predicting the presence of and the general location of a myocardial infarct, it is far less reliable in predicting the extent of an infarct. Among the 47 patients with electrocardiographic evidence of healed myocardial infarction studied by Sullivan et al.,[4] the extent of the fibrosis was accurately predicted by electrocardiogram in only 12 (26 percent); in 33 patients (70 percent), the myocardial infarct was more extensive at necropsy than predicted by electrocardiogram and in only 2 (4 percent) was it less extensive at necropsy than had been predicted by electrocardiogram during life (Table I).

The study by Sullivan et al.[4] reemphasizes the difficulty of making electrocardiographic-morphologic correlative analyses. One problem is the wide range of myocardial lesions in most study populations. Of their 50 patients, 44 (88 percent) had more than one healed myocardial infarct and, indeed, more than half (52 percent) had three or more healed infarcts. In addition, although all 50 patients had a healed myocardial infarct, 10 of them also had acute infarcts that, obviously, also affected the electrocardiographic patterns. Furthermore, nearly one half of their 50 patients (46 percent) had only a subendocardial infarct at necropsy.

Electrocardiographic and Morphologic Terminology

Another problem in these correlative studies is terminology. In the study by Sullivan et al.,[4] the location of the infarct anatomically in the left ventricle was

From the Pathology Branch, National Heart, Lung, and Blood Institute, National Institutes of Health, Bethesda, Maryland and the Division of Cardiology, Department of Medicine, Georgetown University, Washington, D.C. Manuscript received June 22, 1978; revised manuscript received August 15, 1978, accepted August 15, 1978.

† Present address: Division of Cardiology, Department of Medicine, Northwestern University, Chicago, Illinois.

Address for reprints: William C. Roberts, MD, Building 10A, Room 3E30, National Institutes of Health, Bethesda, Maryland 20014.

TABLE I

Location of Healed Myocardial Infarct by Electrocardiogram and at Necropsy. Observations in 47 Necropsy Patients (Data of Sullivan et al.[4])

ECG Location of Healed Myocardial Infarct	Total Patients (no.)	Patients With ECG Infarct Location Confirmed				Patients With Infarct Location Different From That of ECG			
			Extent of Infarct				Extent of Infarct		
		Total	Same as in ECG	Greater Than in ECG	Smaller Than in ECG	Total	Same as in ECG	Greater Than in ECG	Smaller Than in ECG
Inferior	6	3	1	2	0	3	1	2	0
Inferobasal	1	1	1	0	0	0	0	0	0
Inferior + inferobasal	3	2	0	2	0	1	0	0	1
Anteroseptal	10	10	0	10	0	0	0	0	0
Anterolateral	6	4	0	4	0	2	1	1	0
Anteroseptal + anteroseptal	7	2	2	0	0	5	1	3	1
Inferior + anteroseptal	11	9	3	6	0	2	0	2	0
Inferior + anterolateral	3	1	0	1	0	2	2	0	0
Totals	47	32 (68%)	7	25	0	15 (32%)	5	8	2

ECG = electrocardiogram.

categorized into eight separate groups (anteroseptal, anterolateral, anterobasal, inferior, inferobasal, lateral, septal and apical), but there was overlap among groups. For example, the "anterobasal" and "anterolateral" groups included infarcts with involvement of the ventricular septum as did the "anteroseptal" group. There was no "inferoseptal" group so that the "inferior" group included infarcts with involvement of the ventricular septum. The "inferior" group, however, included only the mid 3 cm portion of the left ventricle if viewed on a longitudinal axis, whereas the "inferobasal" group included only involvement of the basal 2 cm of the left ventricle. Sullivan et al.[4] also used the terms "subendocardial" and "transmural," "extensive" and "limited," "apical segment" and "large segment" to describe the locations and extent of myocardial infarcts. With the exception of the "apical segment" (apical 2 cm), these terms were not defined. Thus, a total of 14 terms were utilized to describe the anatomic locations of one or more myocardial infarcts. Applying 14 terms to 50 patients, 88 percent with multiple healed infarcts and 10 with acute infarcts as well, dilutes the figures considerably for each subgroup of patients. Although Sullivan et al.[4] utilized 14 terms to describe the anatomic locations of myocardial infarcts, only 5 terms (anteroseptal, anterolateral, inferior, inferobasal and apical) were used to describe *electrocardiographic* locations of myocardial infarcts.

To diminish confusion between electrocardiographic and anatomic localization of myocardial infarcts, utilization of a common terminology would appear ideal. Certain terms used in electrocardiographic localization of myocardial infarcts are usually not used to designate their location at necropsy. The terms "inferior," "diaphragmatic" and "true posterior," for example, are primarily electrocardiographic terms and are not ideal because they break the principle of parallelism. Their opposites—namely, "superior," "sternal" or "false posterior" (or indeed "true anterior" or "false anterior") —are never used. Therefore, these terms might best be eliminated so that the same terms may be used both electrocardiographically and anatomically. "Inferior" and "diaphragmatic" myocardial infarcts are simply those involving the "posterior" left ventricular wall, primarily the "posteroapical" portion. "True posterior" generally has been considered "posterobasal," but evidence for this is not firm.

Proposed Terminology for Anatomic Location of Infarct

Because the normal left ventricle at necropsy and in ventricular systole during life is in essence a *cone*, proper description of the location of a myocardial infarct of the left ventricle necessitates designation of the portion or portions of involvement of each of the three dimensions of the cone: (1) the *circle*, (2) the *thickness*, and (3) the *length* (top to bottom) (Fig. 1).

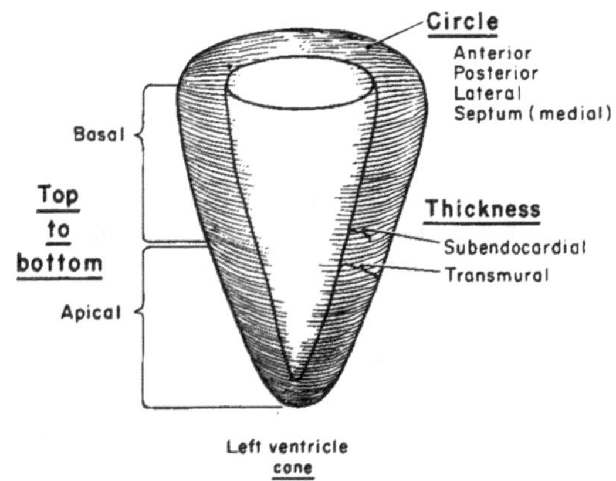

FIGURE 1. Diagram illustrating the three dimensions of the left ventricle as a cone, for localization of infarction.

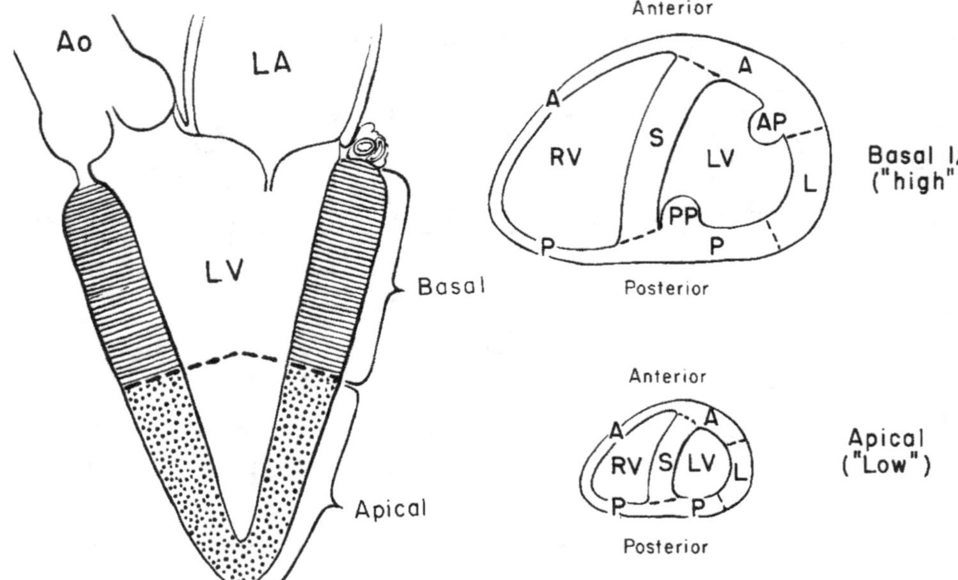

FIGURE 2. Diagrams showing the left ventricle (LV) illustrated as a cone **(left)** and transverse cuts across the right (RV) and left ventricles **(right)**. The length of the ventricle is divided into basal and apical halves. The larger transverse slice **(upper right)** is from the basal half and the smaller transverse slice, from the apical half. The **dotted lines** serve to define the various compartments of the left ventricle. A = anterior wall of the left ventricle and anterolateral wall of the right ventricle; Ao = aorta; AP = anterolateral papillary muscle; L = lateral wall of left ventricle; LA = left atrium; P = posterior wall of the right and left ventricles; PP = posteromedial papillary muscle; S = ventricular septum.

The circle includes the *anterior, posterior* and *lateral* free walls and the *ventricular septum*. The thickness may be designated as *subendocardial,* defined as the inner half, *subepicardial,* defined as the outer half, and *transmural,* defined as involvement of both subendocardium and subepicardium. We prefer using "subendocardium" to designate the inner half, rather than the inner third, of the myocardial wall, because most subendocardial infarcts involve only the inner third, and, therefore, by using the half-way cutoff point, a clear demarcation usually is present between subendocardial and transmural areas. Furthermore, most transmural infarcts involve more than 75 percent of the myocardial wall and, consequently, are clearly separable from infarcts limited to the subendocardium. The length or top to bottom dimension may be divided into basal one-third, mid one-third and apical one-third or simply into *basal one-half* ("high") and *apical one-half* ("low") (Fig. 2). We prefer the latter because there is too much overlap when the ventricles are divided longitudinally into thirds. The specific compartments of the walls of the cardiac ventricles are shown diagrammatically in Figure 2. Designating each of the various compartments of the heart is obviously somewhat arbitrary. We include, for example, the anterolateral papillary muscle of the left ventricle in the anterior compartment, although it could as easily be included in the lateral compartment, or be split in half, in the manner of Sullivan et al.,[4] who included half of this structure in their "anterobasal" compartment and the other half in their "lateral" compartment. The portion of ventricle at each end of the ventricular septum, when viewed transversely, could be included in either the posterior or the anterior compartment or in the ventricular septum. We prefer to include these junction points between right and left ventricular free walls as part of the ventricular septum. We divide the right ventricular free wall into two compartments (anterolateral and poste-

rior) as contrasted to the three free wall compartments of the left ventricle (anterior, posterior and lateral).

To show the portion or portions of the cardiac ventricles involved by myocardial infarcts, the ventricles are divided into basal and apical halves (Fig. 2). Three portions of the *basal* half infrequently are sites of myocardial infarction—namely, the anterior and anteroseptal compartments of the left ventricle and the anterolateral compartment of the right ventricle. "Anterior" myocardial infarction spares the right ventricular free wall, whereas nearly 25 percent of patients with "posterior" left ventricular myocardial infarction have involvement of all or portions of the posterior wall of the right ventricle.[5] Most patients with "posterior" myocardial infarction have involvement of portions of all of the posteromedial papillary muscle of the left ventricle. In contrast, many patients with "anterior" myocardial infarction have no involvement of the anterolateral papillary muscle of the left ventricle.

One problem in designating a myocardial infarct as "anterior" or "posterior" is that each term is usually only partially correct. A large infarct, for example, may be limited to the posterior, posteroseptal or posterolateral portion of left ventricle in its basal half, whereas the area of myocardial involvement may be completely circumferential in much or some of the apical portion of left ventricle. Likewise, an area of myocardial infarction may be entirely subendocardial in one portion and transmural in another.

Correlative Electrocardiographic Patterns

Electrocardiographic patterns for localizing myocardial infarcts in each of the three dimensions of the cone are more often nonspecific than specific. These patterns will be summarized as follows:

Anterior wall of the left ventricle: Myocardial infarction infrequently involves the basal portion of the anterior wall of the left ventricle. In only 3 of the 50 patients (or in only 3 of 78 separate infarcts) with healed myocardial infarction described by Sullivan et al.[4] was the anterobasal segment of the left ventricle the site of infarction, and each of these patients also had infarction involving other segments of the left ventricle. Thus, electrocardiographic "anterior" myocardial infarction nearly always indicates involvement of all or portions of the apical half of the left ventricle and is characterized, in general, by the presence of Q or QS waves of greater than 0.03 second in lead V_1 or V_2, or both.[6] However, infarcts are infrequently limited to just the anterior wall of the left ventricle. None of the 50 patients of Sullivan et al. had isolated anterior wall infarction. The lateral or septal wall (or both) is usually also involved. An *anteroseptal* infarction is usually characterized by Q or QS waves in lead V_3 or V_4, or both[7,8] and an *anterolateral* infarction, by the presence of Q or QS waves in lead V_5 or V_6, or both, and sometimes in leads I or aVL, or both, in addition to the expected Q or QS waves in leads V_3 or V_4, or both.[9–11]

Posterior wall of left ventricle: Although electrocardiographic differences between "true posterior" ("plain posterior") and "inferior" ("diaphragmatic" or "inferoposterior") myocardial infarction have been described,[11] the evidence is not convincing that "posterior" myocardial infarction involving the basal half of the left ventricle can be distinguished electrocardiographically from "posterior" myocardial infarction involving the apical half of this ventricle. ("True posterior" myocardial infarction has been characterized by "tall" [R to S ratio equal to or greater than 1] and "broad" [duration equal to or greater than 0.04 second] R waves in lead V_1 or V_2, or both; "inferior" infarction, by Q waves with a duration of 0.04 second or more in leads II, III and a VF.) Furthermore, although it has been suggested that the additional presence of Q waves in leads V_5 and V_6 denotes involvement (extension) of the "posterolateral" wall,[9] myocardial infarction involving the "posterolateral" wall cannot be reliably differentiated from myocardial infarction involving the "posteroseptal" wall and neither can be reliably delineated from infarction limited to the "posterior" free wall of the left ventricle.[11–13] Thus, "posterior" myocardial infarction with or without involvement of the adjacent septal or lateral walls generally is characterized by Q or QS waves in leads II, III and a VF or the presence of R waves that are broad (0.04 second or more) and tall (R to S ratio more than 1) in lead V_1 or V_2, or both.

Myocardial infarction involving only the ventricular septum, the lateral wall of the left ventricle, the papillary muscle or the right ventricle: In contrast to its ability to distinguish between myocardial infarction involving the "anterior" wall from that involving the "posterior" wall of left ventricle, the electrocardiogram provides no specific pattern to indicate infarction of the ventricular septum,[8,12] the lateral wall of the left ventricle,[14,15] the papillary muscle or the right ventricle.[5,12] However, myocardial infarction is rarely if ever limited to the lateral wall of the left ventricle or to the ventricular septum or the right ventricle. Thus,

whenever the ventricular septum or the left ventricular lateral wall is the site of myocardial infarction, either the anterior or the posterior wall is nearly always involved as well. Moreover, myocardial infarction secondary to coronary arterial narrowing with involvement of the right ventricle is always associated with "posterior" left ventricular infarction, never isolated "anterior" left ventricular infarction.[5] Consequently, the anterolateral wall of the right ventricle is never the site of myocardial infarction unless the entire posterior right ventricular wall is either necrotic or fibrotic, or both. Also, infarction of the posteromedial papillary muscle occurs in most patients with "posterior" infarction; therefore, involvement of this structure can be predicted simply from knowledge that the myocardial infarct is "posterior." In contrast, a high percent of patients with left ventricular "anterior" wall myocardial infarction do not have involvement of the anterolateral papillary muscle; therefore, involvement of this structure cannot be predicted reliably from knowledge that the myocardial infarction involves the "anterior" wall.

Summary

The terminology applicable for describing the location of a myocardial infarct at necropsy is applicable for defining its location by electrocardiogram. Certain terms used primarily electrocardiographically—namely, "inferior," "diaphragmatic" and "true posterior"—should be avoided because their opposites are not used. Ideally, a proper description of the location of a myocardial infarct should include a definition of its involvement in each of the dimensions of the left ventricle (considered as a cone): the portion of the walls of the *circle* involved (anterior, posterior, lateral and septal); the amount of the wall's *thickness* involved (transmural or nontransmural [subendocardial]) and the portions of the wall's *length* involved (basal half or apical half, or both). Certain portions of the walls of both the left and the right ventricles are rare sites of myocardial infarction, and knowledge of these sites helps in more precisely predicting by electrocardiogram the location of the myocardial infarct. Infarction involving the *anterior* wall of the left ventricle rarely is limited to just its basal one-half; therefore, anterior myocardial infarction, for practical purposes, indicates involvement of at least the apical half of this ventricle. In contrast, myocardial infarction involving the basal half of the *posterior* left ventricular wall is common, but the electrocardiogram is not accurate in differentiating posterobasal from posteroapical infarction. Furthermore, the electrocardiogram provides no specific pattern to indicate myocardial infarction of the ventricular septum, the lateral wall of left ventricle, either the posterior or the anterolateral wall of the right ventricle or the papillary muscle. Infarction of the right ventricle virtually never occurs with isolated "anterior" myocardial infarction of the left ventricle. In contrast, nearly 25 percent of patients with "posterior" transmural myocardial infarction also have associated infarction involving at least the posterior wall of the right ventricle.

References

1. **Levine HD, Phillips E:** An appraisal of the newer electrocardiography: correlations in one hundred and fifty consecutive autopsied cases. N Engl J Med 245:833–842, 1951
2. **Achor RWP, Futch WD, Burchell HB, Edwards JE:** The fate of patients surviving acute myocardial infarction. Arch Intern Med 98:162–174, 1956
3. **Woods JD, Laurie W, Smith WG:** The reliability of the electrocardiogram in myocardial infarction. Lancet 2:265–269, 1963
4. **Sullivan W, Vlodaver Z, Tuna N, Long L, Edwards JE:** Correlation of electrocardiographic and pathologic findings in healed myocardial infarction. Am J Cardiol 42:724–732, 1978
5. **Isner JM, Roberts WC:** Right ventricular infarction complicating left ventricular infarction secondary to coronary heart disease. Frequency, location, associated findings, and significance from analysis of 236 necropsy patients with acute or healed myocardial infarction. Am J Cardiol 42, in press
6. **Marriott HJL:** Practical Electrocardiography, fifth edition. Baltimore, Williams & Wilkins, 1972, p 226–253
7. **Myers GB, Klein HA, Stofer BE:** I. Correlation of electrocardiographic and pathologic findings in anteroseptal infarction. Am Heart J 36:535–575, 1948
8. **Rodriquez MI, Anselmi Ch A, Sodi-Pallares D:** The electrocardiographic diagnosis of septal infarctions. Am Heart J 45:525–544, 1953
9. **Wilson FN, Johnston FD, Rosenbaum FF, Erlanger H, Kossmann CE, Hecht H, Cotrim N, Menezes de Oliveira R, Scarsi R, Barker PS:** The precordial electrocardiogram. Am Heart J 27:19–85, 1944
10. **Myers GB, Klein HA, Hiratzka T:** II. Correlation of electrocardiographic and pathologic findings in large anterolateral infarcts. Am Heart J 36:838–881, 1948
11. **Savage RM, Wagner GS, Ideker RE, Podolsky SA, Hackel DB:** Correlation of postmortem anatomic findings with electrocardiographic changes in patients with myocardial infarction. Retrospective study of patients with typical anterior and posterior infarcts. Circulation 55:279–285, 1977
12. **Myers GB, Klein HA, Hiratzka T:** IV. Correlation of electrocardiographic and pathologic findings in infarction of the interventricular septum and right ventricle. Am Heart J 37:720–770, 1949
13. **Myers GB, Klein HA, Hiratzka T:** VI. Correlation of electrocardiographic and pathologic findings in posterolateral infarction. Am Heart J 38:837–862, 1949
14. **Myers GB, Klein HA, Stofer BE:** VII. Correlation of electrocardiographic and pathologic findings in lateral infarction. Am Heart J 37:374–417, 1949
15. **Dunn WJ, Edwards JE, Pruitt RD:** The electrocardiogram in infarction of the lateral wall of the left ventricle. A clinicopathologic study. Circulation 14:540–555, 1956

Right Ventricular Infarction Complicating Left Ventricular Infarction Secondary to Coronary Heart Disease

Frequency, Location, Associated Findings and Significance From Analysis of 236 Necropsy Patients With Acute or Healed Myocardial Infarction

JEFFREY M. ISNER, MD, FACC
WILLIAM C. ROBERTS, MD, FACC

Bethesda, Maryland

From the Pathology Branch, National Heart, Lung, and Blood Institute, National Institutes of Health, Bethesda, Maryland. Manuscript received May 15, 1978; revised manuscript received July 11, 1978, accepted July 12, 1978.

Address for reprints: William C. Roberts, MD, Building 10A, Room 3E-30, National Institutes of Health, Bethesda, Maryland 20014.

Right ventricular infarction associated with left ventricular infarction was identified by gross examination at necropsy in 33 (14 percent) of 236 patients with transmural myocardial infarction. Right ventricular infarction occurred exclusively as a complication of posterior left ventricular infarction. Associated right ventricular infarction occurred in none of the 97 patients with isolated anterior wall infarction of the left ventricle, but in 33 (24 percent) of the 139 patients with posterior left ventricular infarction. Transmural infarction of the posterior ventricular septum was an additional prerequisite for right ventricular infarction. Of the 139 patients with infarction of the posterior left ventricular wall, 74 had no transmural infarction of the ventricular septum and none of these 74 had associated right ventricular infarction. In contrast, of the 65 patients with infarction of the posterior left ventricular wall and transmural infarction of the ventricular septum, 33 (50 percent) had associated right ventricular infarction.

Among the 33 patients with right ventricular infarction, the infarct was limited to the posterior right ventricular free wall in 27 (82 percent); in the other 6 patients (18 percent) it extended to involve the anterolateral right ventricular free wall. Among patients with a posterior left ventricular infarct, those with a right ventricular infarct had right ventricular dilatation nearly three times ($P < 0.05$) more frequently than the patients without a right ventricular infarct. Comparison of the same two groups disclosed no differences in the patients' age, sex, extent of coronary arterial luminal narrowing, right ventricular hypertrophy, right ventricular thrombi or duration of symptoms of myocardial ischemia.

Hemodynamic data in four patients with a right ventricular infarct disclosed previously reported characteristic hemodynamics of right ventricular infarction in only one patient. Recognition of right ventricular infarction is important because it implies specific therapy, namely, aggressive volume administration. Clinical evidence of *posterior left ventricular infarction* and *right ventricular dilatation* should arouse strong suspicion of associated right ventricular infarction.

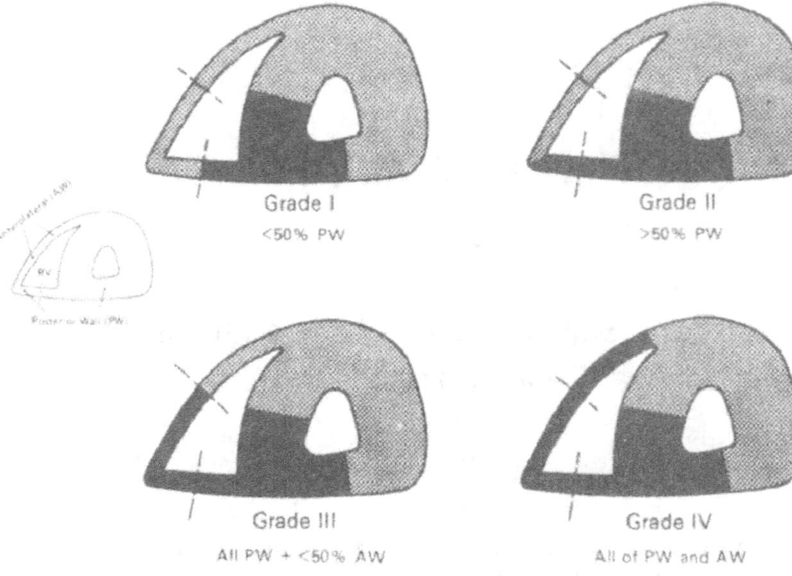

FIGURE 1. Diagram of transverse slices of cardiac ventricles illustrating the scheme used to grade the extent of the right ventricular (RV) infarct. The right ventricular infarct was classified as grade I when it involved less than 50 percent of the posterior wall (PW) of the right ventricle; grade II when it was limited to the posterior wall but involved more than 50 percent of it; grade III when it involved all of the posterior wall and some, but less than 50 percent, of its anterolateral wall (AW); and grade IV when it involved all of the right ventricular posterior wall and more than 50 percent of the anterolateral wall.

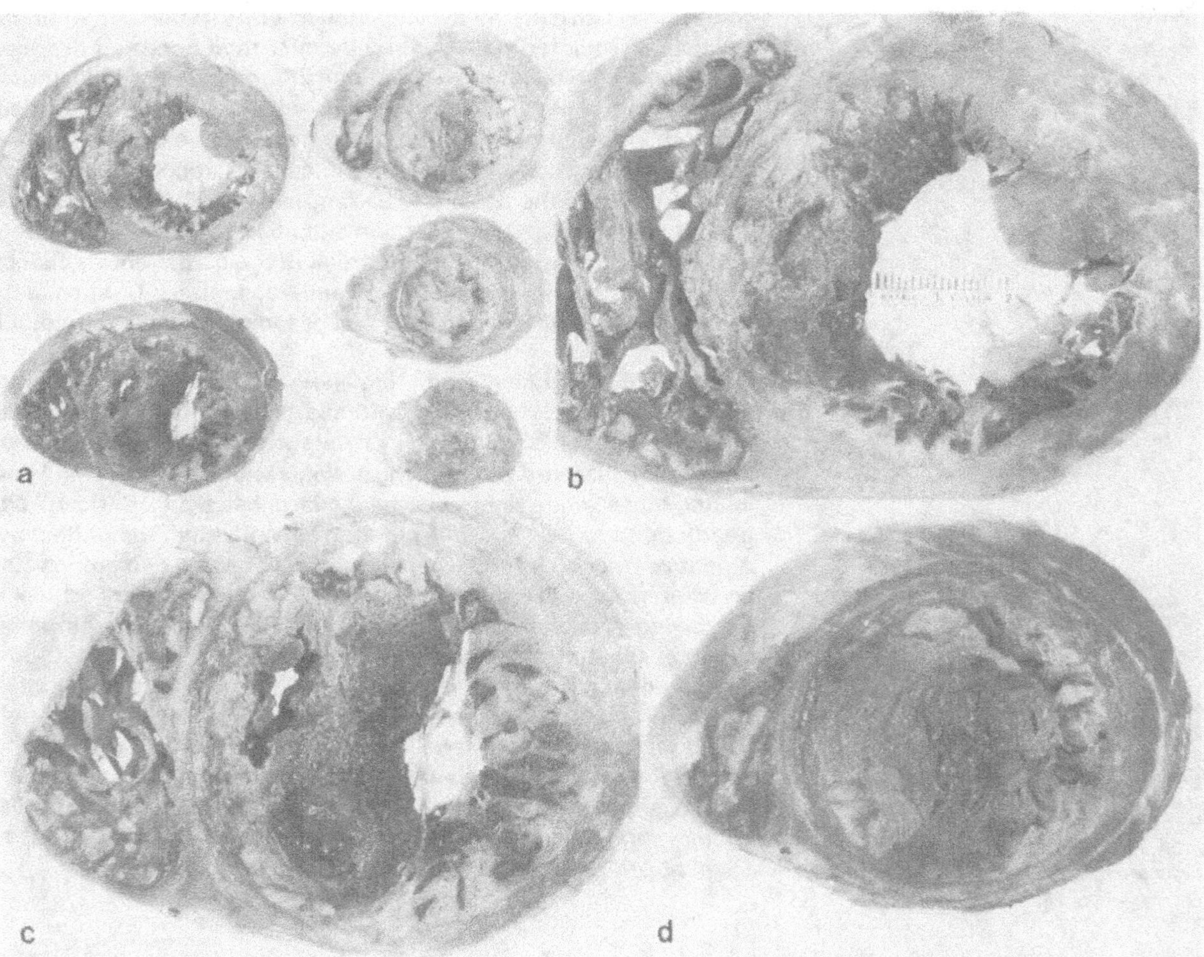

FIGURE 2. Transverse slices of cardiac ventricles illustrating acute myocardial infarction of the right ventricular wall associated with infarction of the ventricular septum and the posterior and anterior walls of the left ventricle in a 66 year old man. The patient had the onset of typical clinical features of acute myocardial infarction beginning 25 days before death. The electrocardiogram showed changes consistent with an acute inferior wall myocardial infarct. Death occurred suddenly. **a,** transverse sections of the cardiac ventricles. **b,** close-up view of the upper left slice in **a,** showing thrombus in both ventricular cavities and necrosis of most of the septum. **c,** close-up view of the bottom left slice in **a,** showing necrosis of the entire septum and all of the posterior right and left ventricular free walls. **d,** close-up view of the upper right slice in **a.** In this slice the infarct is circumferential.

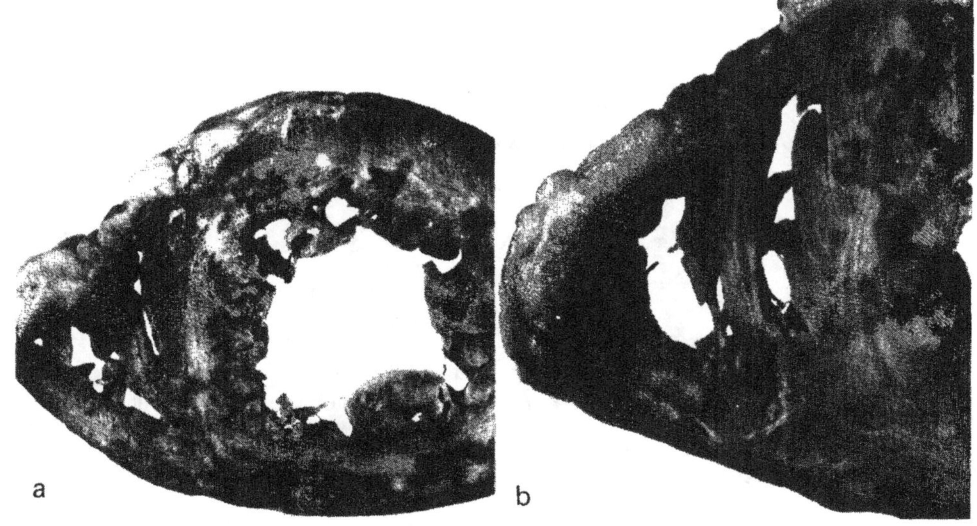

FIGURE 3. Patient 1 (Table IV). Acute right ventricular infarction associated with extensive necrosis of left ventricle in a 57 year old man who died 3 days after the onset of severe chest pain. The electrocardiogram showed changes of acute inferior myocardial infarction. The hemodynamic findings did not suggest associated right ventricular infarction. **a** and **b**, close-up views of two transverse slices of cardiac ventricles showing necrosis of the right ventricle that is limited to but involves more than 50 percent of the posterior wall (grade II). There is associated transmural necrosis of the ventricular septum.

TABLE I

Frequency of Right Ventricular Infarct Among Necropsy Patients With Transmural Left Ventricular Infarction and Relation to Involvement of Ventricular Septum

LV Infarct	no.	Age (yr) Range	Average	Sex M	Sex F	Transmural VS MI	RV MI	No Transmural VS MI	RV MI
Anterior	97	26–90	69	67	30	68	0	29	0
Acute	60	26–90	74	36	24	43	0	17	0
Healed	37	31–80	60	31	6	25	0	12	0
Posterior	139	26–93	62	99	40	65	33 (51%)	64	0
Acute	56	38–93	64	37	19	32	16 (29%)	24	0
Healed	83	26–93	61	62	21	33	17 (20%)	50	0
Totals	236	26	65	166 (70%)	70 (30%)	133	33 (25%)	103	0

LV = left ventricular; MI = myocardial infarct; RV = right ventricular; VS = ventricular septal.

Myocardial infarction secondary to coronary arterial narrowing virtually always involves the left ventricular free wall and often also the ventricular septum. Involvement of the right ventricular free wall secondary to coronary luminal narrowing has until recently rarely been diagnosed clinically, and few morphologic studies have focused on its frequency or extent. The present study examines the frequency of right ventricular infarction in patients with associated transmural left ventricular infarction and determines its extent and relation to the site of the infarction of the left ventricle.

Patients Studied and Methods

All cases of acute or healed myocardial infarction accessioned in the Pathology Branch of the National Heart, Lung, and Blood Institute from January 1969 to February 1978 were reviewed. Patients with acute or healed myocardial infarction who had associated primary valvular heart disease, infiltrative myocardial disease or hypertrophic cardiomyopathy or who had cardiac surgery at any time were excluded. In addition, patients whose myocardial infarct involved only papillary muscle or was limited in all areas to less than 50 percent of the thickness of the left ventricular free wall or ventricular septum (subendocardium) were excluded. A total of 236 patients were accepted for study. By *gross* inspection, transmural (involvement of greater than the inner half of the myocardial wall) infarction of the left ventricular wall was present in each.

On the basis of reexamination of the hearts, the patients were classified into two major groups: (1) those with transmural myocardial necrosis (acute infarct), and (2) those with transmural myocardial fibrosis (healed infarct). When both fibrosis and necrosis were visible grossly in the same heart (34 patients), the group in which the patient was placed was determined by which feature was dominant by visual examination of the heart specimens. The hearts were then further subdivided by location of the left ventricular infarct into two additional groups: (1) anterior wall, and (2) posterior wall. The right ventricular free wall infarcts are shown by the diagrammatic scheme in Figure 1.

The hearts were weighed and the maximal thickness of the free wall of the right ventricle was measured. The size of both ventricular cavities was judged normal or dilated by visual inspection. The presence or absence of ventricular thrombi was recorded.

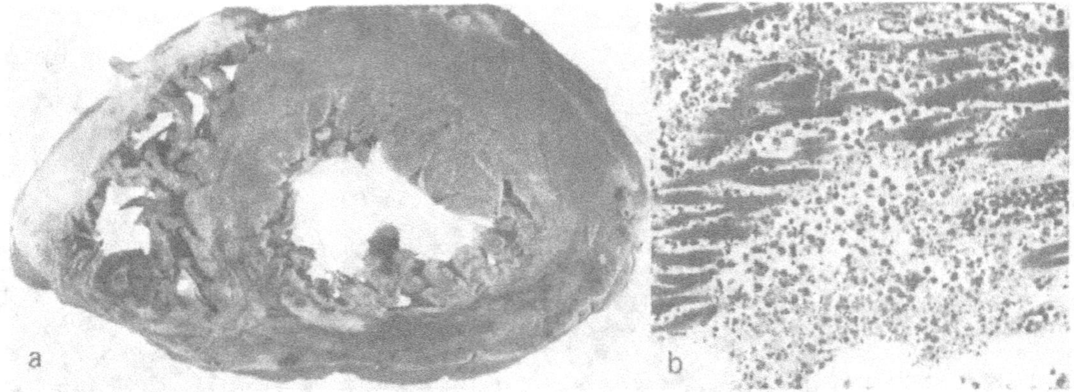

FIGURE 4. Acute right ventricular infarction. **a,** transverse slice of cardiac ventricles illustrating acute infarction of the right ventricle associated with infarction of the posterior wall of the left ventricle in an 82 year old woman who had the onset of typical clinical features of acute infarction 23 days before death. Her last 5 days were complicated by multiple arrhythmias, congestive heart failure and shock. The electrocardiogram was typical of acute myocardial infarction, posterior ("inferior") wall. **b,** photomicrograph of right ventricular wall necrosis from a 68 year old man with acute myocardial infarction involving the right ventricle (grade II), septum and posterior wall of left ventricle. Acute infarction in this patient was complicated by rupture of the ventricular septum 1 day before death. (Phosphotungstic acid hematoxylin stain ×212, reduced by 18 percent.)

The coronary arteries were excised intact and sectioned with a method described elsewhere.[1] Briefly, the excised arteries were cut at 5 mm intervals at right angles to the longitudinal axis of the vessels, and each 5 mm long segment was labeled consecutively, processed in alcohols and xylene, embedded in paraffin and cut. A single Movat-stained histologic section was examined from each 5 mm segment.

The clinical records of each of the 236 patients were reviewed. Hemodynamic data were available in 21 patients.

Results

Incidence and relation to anterior, posterior and septal infarction: Of the 236 patients, 116 had an acute and 120 had a healed left ventricular myocardial infarct.

The findings in these patients are summarized in Table I and various, mainly morphologic, cardiac findings in several patients are illustrated in Figures 1 to 7. The myocardial infarcts in 236 patients involved the anterior wall in 97 patients and the posterior wall in the other 139. The age and sex of patients with anterior and posterior left ventricular myocardial infarcts were similar. Of the 97 patients with an *anterior* left ventricular infarct (acute in 60 [62 percent] and healed in 37 [38 percent]), none had an associated right ventricular infarct; of the 139 patients with a *posterior* left ventricular infarct (acute in 56 [40 percent] and healed in 83 [60 percent]), 33 (24 percent) had an associated

TABLE II

Right Ventricular Infarction: Morphologic Features

RVMI	Patients no.	Patients Age (yr)	RV Features D	RV Features H	RV Features T	Grade of RV MI I	Grade of RV MI II	Grade of RV MI III	Grade of RV MI IV
Acute	16	46–86 (m 65)	2	1	3	6	9	0	1
Healed	17	26–80 (m 56)	10	0	0	3	8	5	1
Totals	33	26–86 (m 62)	12	1	3	9	17	5	2

D = dilatation; H = hypertrophy; M = mean; MI = myocardial infarct; RV = right ventricular; T = thrombus.

TABLE III

Status of Right Ventricle and Coronary Arteries in Patients With Posterior Wall Left Ventricular Myocardial Infarct (MI) With and Without Associated Right Ventricular (RV) Infarct

LVMI	Cases (no.)	D (no. [%])	H (no. [%])	T (no. [%])	Total (no. [%])	With >75% Narrowing* of RCA	With >75% Narrowing* of LAD	With >75% Narrowing* of LCx
With RV MI	33	12[36]	1[3]	3[9]	28[85]	26[93]	20[74]	20[74]
Without RV MI	106	10[9]	5[5]	4[4]	59[56]	50[85]	46[78]	45[76]

* More than 75 percent narrowing of cross-sectional area by plaque. D = dilatation; H = hypertrophy; LAD = left anterior descending coronary artery; LCx = left circumflex coronary artery; RCA = right coronary artery.

right ventricular infarct. Of the total of 236 patients, 133 had transmural infarction of the ventricular septum (Table I), 68 with anterior and 65 with posterior left ventricular infarction. All 33 patients with right ventricular infarction were among the 65 with posterior left ventricular infarction associated with transmural infarction of the ventricular septum. Of the 74 patients with posterior left ventricular infarction without associated transmural infarction of the ventricular septum, none had a right ventricular infarct. None of the patients with an isolated anterior left ventricular infarct had an associated right ventricular infarct whether or not the ventricular septum was involved.

Clinical and morphologic features: Certain clinical and morphologic features of the patients with right ventricular myocardial infarction are summarized in Tables II and III. Only 1 of the 33 patients had hypertrophy of the right ventricular wall (more than 5 mm thick), whereas 12 had right ventricular dilatation. Antemortem thrombus was found in the right ventricle of three patients. The infarct of the right ventricle was limited to its posterior wall (types I and II) (Fig. 2 to 4, 6 and 7) in 36 patients and to both the posterior and anterolateral right ventricular free walls (types III and IV) in the other 7 (Fig. 5 and 9 to 11).

Comparison of the 33 patients with a posterior left ventricular wall infarct and associated right ventricular wall infarction and the 106 patients with a posterior left ventricular wall infarct *without* associated right ventricular wall infarction disclosed no significant differences in the patients' age, sex, length of survival after onset of symptoms of myocardial ischemia (range 1 to 23 days [mean 8] in all groups) or the presence of right ventricular hypertrophy or thrombus (Tables II and III). Right ventricular dilatation, however, was significantly (P <0.05) more frequent among the group with a posterior left ventricular infarct and associated right ventricular wall infarction.

Coronary arterial findings: The three major (right, left anterior descending and left circumflex) coronary

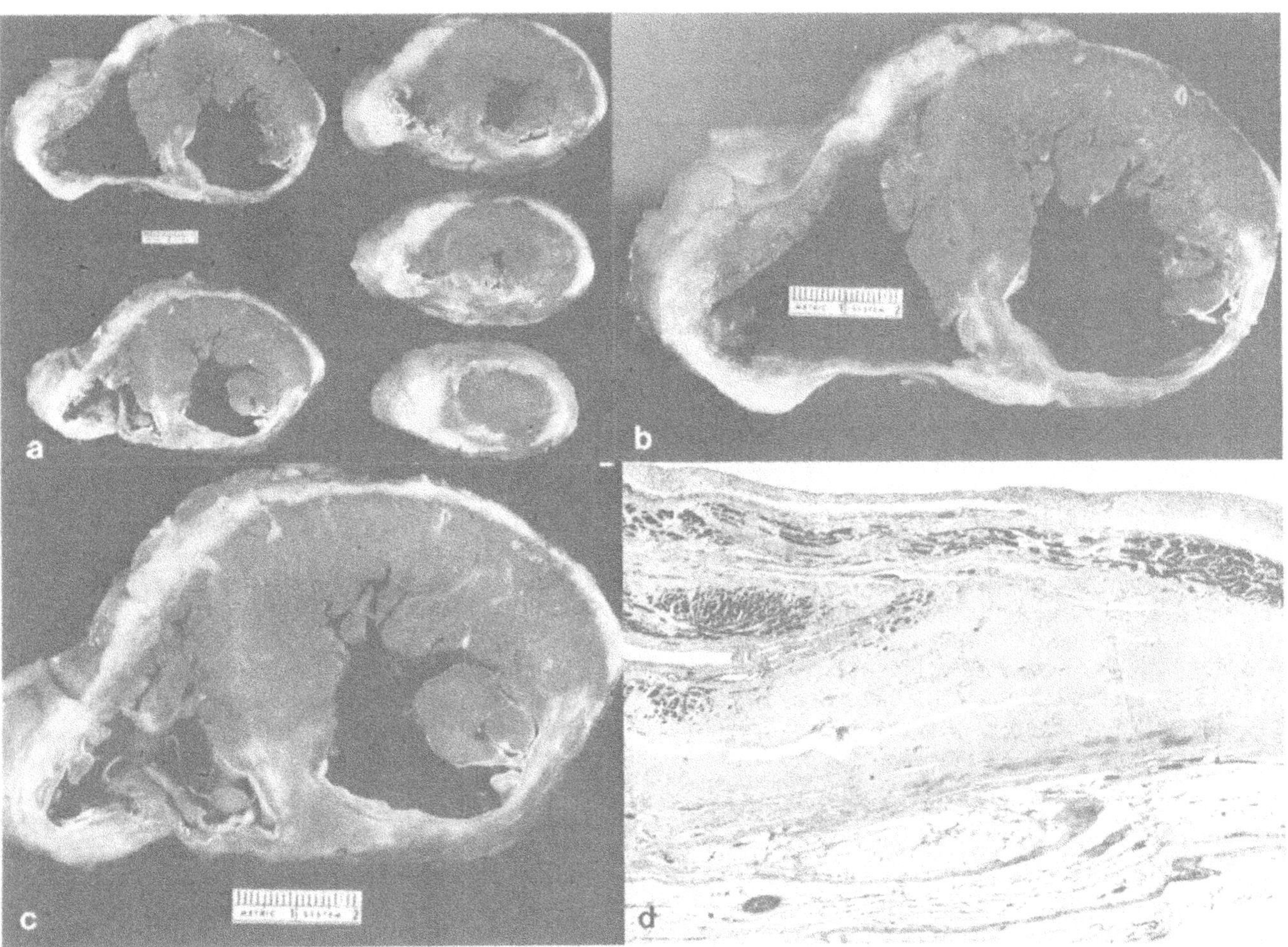

FIGURE 5. Transverse slices of cardiac ventricles **(a, b, c)** and photomicrograph of healed right ventricular infarct **(d)** from a 73 year old man who had had an "inferior" wall myocardial infarct at age 68. The patient was subsequently treated with digoxin and diuretic agents for "mild" congestive heart failure. He died 5 years later from complicatons of eye surgery. **a,** transverse cardiac ventricular slices. **b,** close-up view of slice at upper left in **a**. There are healed posterior right and left ventricular infarcts with thinning of the right (grade II) and left ventricular free walls and the posterior portion of ventricular septum. Both ventricular cavities are dilated. **c,** close-up view of slice at bottom left in **a**, showing additional scarring of the anterolateral wall of the right ventricle. **d,** photomicrograph showing transmural scarring of the right ventricular free wall. (Movat stain ×27, reduced by 25 percent.)

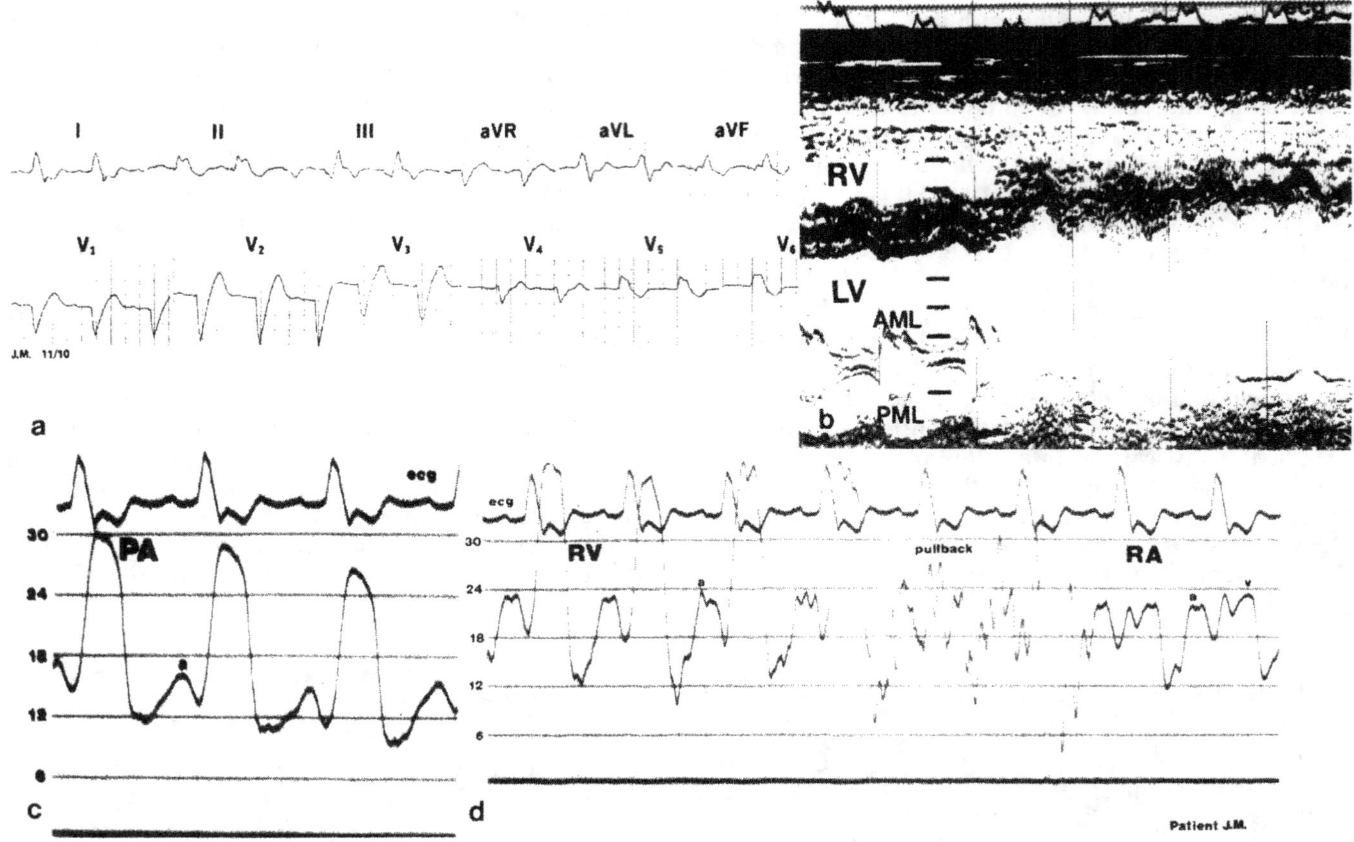

FIGURE 6. Clinical findings recorded in a 48 year old man with healed right ventricular myocardial infarction. The infarction had occurred 7 years before the recordings presented here, and the patient died of progressive congestive heart failure 2 years after the recordings. **a,** electrocardiogram showing S-T segment elevation in lead III, complete left bundle branch block and absent or small R waves in leads V_1 to V_4. **b,** echocardiogram showing biventricular dilatation and abnormal septal motion. AML = anterior mitral leaflet; LV = left ventricle; PML = posterior mitral leaflet; RV = right ventricle. **c,** pulmonary arterial (PA) pressure recording showing a prominent *a* wave. **d,** pullback tracing from the right ventricle (RV) to the right atrium (RA), demonstrating an elevated (18 mm Hg) end-diastolic pressure and prominent *a* waves in the right ventricular pressure tracing.

arteries were examined in detail in 87 (63 percent) of the 139 patients with a left ventricular posterior wall infarct (Table III). Twenty-eight of the 87 had an associated right ventricular infarct and 59 did not. No significant differences were observed among the patients with posterior left ventricular infarcts in the percent of those with and without right ventricular infarction who had more than 75 percent cross-sectional area luminal narrowing by old atherosclerotic plaques in one or more of the three major coronary arteries. The degree of narrowing of the right coronary artery was similar in the patients with and without right ventricular infarction. The percent of patients whose right coronary artery was narrowed more than 75 percent in cross-sectional area by old atherosclerotic plaque was significantly (P <0.05) greater than that of patients whose left anterior descending coronary artery was narrowed to this degree, whether or not infarction involved the right ventricular wall.

Hemodynamic data: Of the 21 patients who had undergone cardiac catheterization, 4 had an associated right ventricular wall infarct (Table IV). In one of the four, the right atrial mean pressure was higher than the mean pulmonary arterial wedge pressure, and both the right ventricular and pulmonary arterial pressure tracings were deformed by a prominent atrial *a* wave (Fig. 6). Hemodynamic data in the other three patients with a right ventricular infarct were consistent with an isolated left ventricular wall infarct with or without left ventricular decompensation.

Comments

Although right ventricular wall infarction secondary to coronary arterial narrowing has recently received attention from the hemodynamic[2-6] and radioisotopic[7,8] standpoints, it has received little attention from a

TABLE IV

Right Ventricular Infarction: Hemodynamic Features

Case no.	State of MI	Grade of RV MI	Pressures (mm Hg)			
			RA Mean	RV(s/d)	PA (s/d)	PAW Mean
1	Acute	II	5	47/10	41/25	24
2	Healed	II	5	35/5	35/15	15
3	Healed	III	7	30/5	28/12	8
4	Healed	III	23	32/23	34/20	20

MI = myocardial infarction; PA = pulmonary arterial; PAW = pulmonary arterial wedge; RA = right atrial; RV = right ventricular; s/d = systolic/diastolic.

morphologic standpoint. Of the eight previous reports mentioning infarction of the right ventricular free wall at necropsy,[2,3,7,9–13] only two[10,11] actually focused on the necropsy diagnosis of right ventricular infarction and, when an associated left ventricular infarct was present, most did not describe its location. Although four reports[7,11–13] showed photographs of infarcts of the right ventricular wall, the extent of the infarcts was rarely described or discernible in the photographs.

Right ventricular infarction: a complication of transmural posteroseptal left ventricular infarction: The present study is based on reexamination of the hearts in 236 necropsy patients with transmural left ventricular myocardial infarction secondary to coronary luminal narrowing. Of the 236 patients, 33 (14 percent) had an infarct involving the right ventricular free wall and all of them had a posteriorly located left ventricular infarct. None of the 97 patients with isolated anterior wall left ventricular infarction had associated right ventricular infarction. Thus, among patients with fatal myocardial infarction secondary to severe coronary arterial luminal narrowing, right ventricular infarction occurred only when the left ventricular infarct involved its posterior wall. Of our 139 patients with a posterior left ventricular infarct, 33 (24 percent) had an associated right ventricular infarct. Even among the patients with a posteriorly located left ventricular infarct, however, transmural infarction of the ventricular septum was a prerequisite for development of right ventricular infarction. Of the 139 patients with a posterior left ventricular infarct, 74 did not have transmural infarction of the ventricular septum and none of the 74 had an associated right ventricular infarct. In contrast, of the 65 with transmural infarction of the ventricular septum, 33 (50 percent) had an associated right ventricular infarct. Thus, *right ventricular infarction among our patients was a complication exclusively of transmural posteroseptal left ventricular infarction.*

The extent of the right ventricular necrosis or fibrosis ranged from less than one half of the posterior right ventricular free wall adjacent to the ventricular septum (nine patients) to involvement of the entire right ventricular free wall (two patients). Among the 33 patients with right ventricular infarction, the infarct was limited to the posterior right ventricular free wall in 26 (79 percent); in the remaining 7 (21 percent), both the posterior and anterolateral walls of the right ventricle were involved.

Role of right ventricular hypertrophy and dilatation: Previous investigators have proposed that right ventricular hypertrophy was either an important predisposing factor[10,14] or an absolute prerequisite[15] for the development of right ventricular myocardial infarction. The results of our study do not confirm this speculation. Right ventricular hypertrophy, in fact, was more frequent among our patients without associated right ventricular infarct. It was observed at necropsy in only 1 (3 percent) of our 33 patients *with* a right ventricular infarct, and in 12 (6 percent) of 203 patients with a left ventricular myocardial infarct unassociated with a right ventricular infarct. Furthermore, although one patient had a history of clinically diagnosed "chronic obstruc-

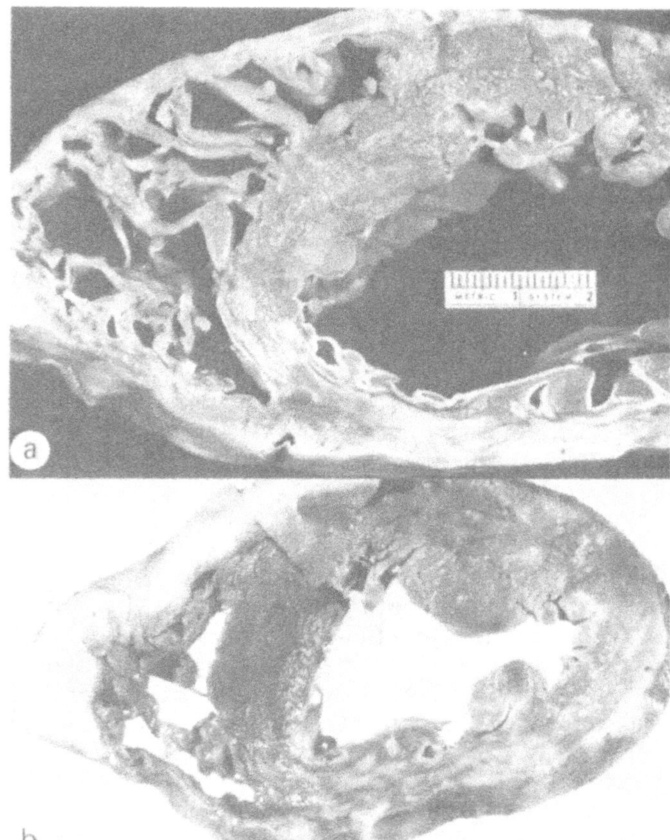

FIGURE 7. Transverse slices of cardiac ventricles showing healed right ventricular infarcts in two patients. **a,** the clinical findings in the patient whose grade III right ventricular wall infarct is shown here are shown in Figure 6. **b,** the posterior right ventricular wall is thinned as is the posterior portion of ventricular septum and posterior portion of left ventricular wall in this 56 year old woman who had an acute myocardial infarct 5 months before death.

tive pulmonary disease," none had necropsy evidence of cor pulmonale. Although extensive right ventricular scarring has been described in various entities associated with right ventricular hypertrophy (including chronic pulmonary emboli[16] and hypertrophic cardiomyopathy[17] in the absence of significant coronary arterial luminal narrowing), such cases were excluded from the present study unless they were associated with left ventricular scarring *and* significant coronary arterial luminal narrowing.

Right ventricular dilatation was the single anatomic feature distinguishing our patients from those without right ventricular myocardial infarction. Among the 139 patients with a posterior wall left ventricular infarct, the right ventricular cavity was dilated in 12 (36 percent) of the 33 patients with and in 10 (9 percent) of 106 patients without an associated right ventricular infarct (Table III). This difference (36 versus 9 percent) is significant (P <0.05). Also, for comparison, right ventricular dilatation occurred in only 16 (16 percent) of the 97 patients with an anterior wall left ventricular infarct, a significantly (P <0.05) lower percent than in our patients with a right ventricular infarct.

Right ventricular mural thrombus: This is another necropsy finding reported to be more frequent among patients with associated right ventricular wall infarction than among patients with an isolated left ventricular wall infarct.[10] However, in our 237 patients with a left ventricular wall infarct, right ventricular thrombus occurred with similar frequency in those with and in those without an associated infarct of the right ventricular wall. Of our 139 patients with a posterior wall left ventricular infarct, right ventricular thrombus occurred in 3 (9 percent) of the 33 patients with and in 4 (4 percent) of the 106 patients without an associated right ventricular infarct; of our 97 patients with an anterior wall left ventricular infarct, right ventricular thrombus occurred in 8 patients (8 percent).

Role of severe right versus left coronary arterial narrowing: Several previous investigators have noted a particularly high frequency of severe luminal narrowing by atherosclerotic plaques of the right coronary artery in patients with a right ventricular infarct associated with a left ventricular infarct. These previous studies, however, did not compare the frequency of severe narrowing of this artery among patients with a right ventricular infarct and those with an isolated left ventricular infarct. Furthermore, the previous studies did not compare the frequency of severe narrowing of the right coronary artery by atherosclerotic plaques with the frequency of severe narrowing of either the left anterior descending or left circumflex coronary artery. Among our patients with posterior wall left ventricular infarction, the percent with greater than 75 percent cross-sectional area luminal narrowing by atherosclerotic plaques of the right coronary artery was similar (about 90 percent) in the patients with and without right ventricular infarction. All our patients with right ventricular infarction had severe (greater than 75 percent cross-sectional area) luminal narrowing of the coronary artery responsible (dominant) for perfusing the posterior ventricular wall (that is, either the right or the left circumflex artery).

Clinical diagnosis: Diagnosis during life of right ventricular infarction in patients with left ventricular infarction secondary to severe coronary arterial luminal narrowing is at best difficult. If the left ventricular infarct is limited to the anterior wall, the chance of an associated right ventricular infarct is minimal. Thus, a *posterior location* of the left ventricular infarction is a prerequisite for right ventricular infarction. Nearly a quarter of all our patients with posterior wall infarction of the left ventricle had associated right ventricular infarction. Thus, if the left ventricular infarct is posterior and transmural, there is a 1 in 4 chance that there will be an associated right ventricular infarct. If, however, the ventricular septum is transmurally infarcted in association with a posterior left ventricular free wall infarction, the chance of an associated right ventricular infarction becomes 1 in 2. But the electrocardiogram is not helpful in distinguishing infarction limited to the posterior left ventricular wall from that involving both posterior and septal walls. The echocardiogram might show diminished motion of the ventricular septum in this circumstance, but the reliability of this technique to determine transmural septal infarction is unproved. One finding suggestive of right ventricular infarction

is right ventricular dilatation, an occurrence nearly 3 times more frequent in our patients with than in those without right ventricular infarction. Right ventricular hypertrophy is rare in patients with right ventricular infarction secondary to coronary narrowing and is therefore not helpful from a diagnostic standpoint.

Hemodynamic findings: role in clinical diagnosis: Before the introduction of newer, noninvasive techniques, the clinical diagnosis of right ventricular myocardial infarction had been limited to cardiac catheterization. The finding of elevated right atrial (or right ventricular end-diastolic) pressure out of proportion to left atrial (or left ventricular end-diastolic) pressure has been suggested as the characteristic hemodynamic profile of right ventricular infarction.[2] Such hemodynamic abnormalities have been confirmed in at least five patients by necropsy.[2,3,7,13] No previous reports, however, have described hemodynamic findings in patients in whom the diagnosis of right ventricular myocardial infarct was first established at necropsy. Three of our four patients with necropsy-confirmed right ventricular myocardial infarction had a hemodynamic profile that was *not* suggestive of associated right ventricular infarction (Table IV). The nondiagnostic hemodynamics in at least one of these three patients were not simply a function of the temporal relation of the catheterization to the infarction because the right-sided cardiac catheterization was performed during the period of acute myocardial infarction. An alternative explanation for the nondiagnostic hemodynamic findings in one or all three of these patients is that they were obscured by relative hypovolemia. Rigo et al.[7] described two patients with cardiogenic shock and a low left ventricular filling pressure in whom the characteristic hemodynamic profile of right ventricular infarction complicating left ventricular infarction was unmasked by volume administration. Thus, it is possible that had our three patients with right ventricular infarction and "nondiagnostic" hemodynamics been stressed with volume or exercise, diagnostic hemodynamic findings might have developed.

Nevertheless, it appears that the hemodynamic profile previously considered characteristic of right ventricular infarction is less diagnostically sensitive than thought and that right ventricular infarction may occur in the presence of normal or near normal intracardiac pressures. Conversely, in the absence of pericardial or valvular heart disease, the hemodynamics described for right ventricular infarction appear to be relatively specific. Hemodynamic findings in 17 other necropsy patients with left ventricular infarction without associated right ventricular infarction disclosed no intracardiac pressure recordings typical of those observed in patients with right ventricular infarction, that is, no false positives.

Simulation of hemodynamics of constrictive pericarditis: The intracardiac pressures characteristic of right ventricular infarction may persist for years after anatomic healing of the infarct, and these pressure tracings may simulate those observed in patients with pericardial heart disease. Our Patient 4 (Table IV) at cardiac catheterization performed 2 years after healing of the acute myocardial infarct still had hemodynamics characteristic of those observed during the period of acute infarction (Fig. 6). Furthermore, the pressure tracings in this patient disclosed prominent *a* waves in both the right ventricle and major pulmonary arteries, findings identical to those described in patients with constrictive pericarditis. Raabe and Chester[13] and Lorell et al.[3] recently pointed out that among patients with acute left ventricular infarction associated with right ventricular infarction the intracardiac hemodynamics could simulate those in patients with pericardial constriction. As in patients with combined acute right and left ventricular wall myocardial infarcts, the characteristic hemodynamic abnormalities in patients with pericardial constriction may not be manifest until the patients are stressed with volume loading or with exercise.[18]

Clinical recognition and determinants of right ventricular dysfunction: Cumulative clinical experience with right ventricular myocardial infarction complicating left ventricular myocardial infarction has clearly established the existence of a specific hemodynamic syndrome of right ventricular dysfunction characterized by underfilling of the left ventricle as a result of impaired right ventricle contractility.[2–8,13] In such patients, right ventricular dilatation is the sole compensatory mechanism by which right ventricular contractility may be augmented. Under such circumstances, volume administration may be critical to maintain a maximal right ventricular filling pressure. Indeed, supplemental volume administration in patients with *elevated* right-sided pressures and a *normal* or near-normal left ventricular filling pressure (that is, patients with right ventricular infarction) has produced marked hemodynamic improvement. Thus, it becomes important to recognize clues to the often occult syndrome of right ventricular dysfunction or right ventricular infarction. Our study suggests that evidence of an "inferior" myocardial infarct combined with evidence of right ventricular dilatation should make one particularly suspicious of the presence of right ventricular infarction.

The amount of hemodynamic data available in patients with proved right ventricular infarction is inadequate to permit conclusions regarding the relation between the extent of the right ventricular infarct and the degree of hemodynamic decompensation. It is likely that the ability of the right ventricle to contribute adequately to left ventricular filling is more a function of the integrity of the ventricular septum than of the integrity of the right ventricular free wall. Starr et al.[19] and others[20,21] have demonstrated in dogs that experimental destruction of the right ventricular free wall does not produce adverse hemodynamic consequences. The contribution of the contracting ventricular septum is apparently great enough to compensate for the loss of participation of the right ventricular free wall. It might be expected that an infarct limited to the juxtaseptal portion of the right ventricular free wall (grade I) or even limited to the entire posterior wall (grade II) would be too small to affect right ventricular function. Yet of our 12 patients with right ventricular dilatation in association with right ventricular infarction, 11 had right ventricular infarction limited to the posterior wall (grade I in 3 and grade II in 8). If right ventricular dilatation constitutes a sign of right ventricular dysfunction, then the latter was not simply a function of the anatomic extent of the right ventricular infarct. It is more likely that the extent of septal involvement (present to a greater degree in all our patients with a right ventricular infarct) was the principal determinant of right ventricular decompensation. In addition, acute myocardial ischemia can in itself lead to acute reduction in ventricular contractility.

Newer, noninvasive methods of diagnosis: Recent reports of echocardiographic and radioisotopic findings in patients with acute myocardial infarction suggest that it may be possible to establish the diagnosis of right ventricular myocardial infarction reliably by noninvasive means. Sharpe et al.[8] demonstrated right ventricular dilatation with M mode echocardiography in five of six patients with acute right ventricular myocardial infarction. Similar results were demonstrated with gated scintigraphy.[7] The frequency of right ventricular dilatation among our patients with right ventricular infarction supports the validity of these noninvasive findings in patients with right ventricular infarction. Additional abnormalities demonstrated on radioisotopic studies in patients with right ventricular infarction include segmental or generalized right ventricular contraction abnormalities and increased right ventricular uptake of technetium pyrophosphate. Of the five patients described by Sharpe et al.[8] with increased uptake of this radionuclide in the right ventricular free wall each had increased uptake in the ventricular septum and posterior left ventricle. This observation is consistent with our finding of consistent involvement of the septum and posterior wall of the left ventricle in patients with right ventricular myocardial infarction.

Role of coronary blood supply to right ventricle: The basis for the apparently exclusive association of right ventricular infarct with infarction of the posterior wall of the left ventricle may be the specific anatomy of the coronary blood supply to the right ventricle. The bulk of the right ventricular myocardium is consistently supplied by numerous branches of the coronary artery supplying the posterior wall of the left ventricle (usually [90 percent[22]] the right coronary artery); with a left dominant system, the circumflex coronary artery supplies both right ventricular and posterior left ventricular branches. Thus, infarction of the right ventricle can result only when the vascular supply to the posterior wall of the left ventricle is compromised as well. In contrast, the anteriormost portion of the right ventricle, including the anterior paraseptal region, has a *dual* blood supply that consists of right ventricular branches from the left anterior descending coronary artery and, most importantly, the conus branch of the right coronary artery. The latter is insurance for the right ventricle in cases of anterior left ventricular infarction; conversely, atherosclerotic narrowing of the right coronary artery proximal to or involving the conus branch probably accounts for most cases of circumferential (type IV) right ventricular myocardial infarction.

References

1. **Roberts WC, Buja LM:** The frequency and significance of coronary arterial thrombi and other observations in fatal acute myocardial infarction. A study of 107 necropsy patients. Am J Med 52:425–443, 1972

2. **Cohn JN, Guiha NH, Broder MI, Limas CJ:** Right ventricular infarction. Clinical and hemodynamic features. Am J Cardiol 33:209–214, 1974

3. **Lorell B, Gold HK, Pohost GM, Dinsmore RE, Leinbach RC, Hutter AM, De Sanctis RW:** Right ventricular infarction: Clinical features, emphasizing its resemblance to cardiac tamponade (abstr). Am J Cardiol 41:409, 1978

4. **Rackley CE, Russell RO:** Right ventricular function in acute myocardial infarction. Am J Cardiol 33:927–929, 1974

5. **Wells DE, Befeler B:** Dysfunction of the right ventricle in coronary artery disease. Chest 66:230–235, 1974

6. **Zone DD, Botti RE:** Right ventricular infarction with tricuspid insufficiency and chronic right heart failure. Am J Cardiol 37:445–448, 1976

7. **Rigo P, Murray M, Taylor DR, Weisfeldt ML, Kelly DT, Strauss HW, Pitt B:** Right ventricular dysfunction detected by gated scintiphotography in patients with acute inferior myocardial infarction. Circulation 57:483–490, 1978

8. **Sharpe DN, Botvinick EH, Shames DM, Schiller NB, Massie BM, Chatterjee K, Parmley WW:** The non-invasive diagnosis of right ventricular infarction. Circulation 57:483–490, 1978

9. **Wartman WB, Hellerstein HK:** The incidence of heart disease in 2,000 consecutive autopsies. Ann Intern Med 28:41–65, 1948

10. **Wade WG:** The pathogenesis of infarction of the right ventricle. Br Heart J 21:545–554, 1959

11. **Laurie W, Woods JD:** Infarction (ischemic fibrosis) in the right ventricle of the heart. Acta Cardiol 18:399–411, 1963

12. **Erhardt LR:** Clinical and pathological observations in different types of acute myocardial infarction. A study of 84 patients deceased after treatment in a coronary care unit. Acta Med Scand [Suppl] 560:7–78, 1974

13. **Raabe DS, Chester AC:** Right ventricular infarction. Chest 73:96–99, 1978

14. **Peter RH, Ramo BW, Ratliff N, Morris JJ:** Collateral vessel development after right ventricular infarction in the pig. Am J Cardiol 29:56–60, 1972

15. **James TN:** The coronary circulation and conduction system in acute myocardial infarction. Prog Cardiovasc Dis 10:410–449, 1968

16. Case Records of the Massachusetts General Hospital (Case 42-1963). New Engl J Med 268:1403–1410, 1963

17. **Roberts WC, Ferrans VJ:** Pathologic anatomy of the cardiomyopathies. Idiopathic dilated and hypertrophic types, infiltrative types, and endomyocardial disease with and without eosinophilia. Hum Pathol 6:287–342, 1975

18. **Bush CA, Stang JM, Wooley CF, Kilman JW:** Occult constrictive pericardial disease. Diagnosis by rapid volume expansion and correction by pericardiectomy. Circulation 56:924–930, 1977

19. **Starr I, Jeffers WA, Mead RH:** The absence of conspicuous increments in venous pressure after severe damage to the right ventricle of the dog and a discussion of the relation between clinical congestive failure and heart disease. Am Heart J 26:291–301, 1943

20. **Bakos ACP:** The question of the function of the right ventricular myocardium: an experimental study. Circulation 1:724–732, 1950

21. **Kagan A:** Dynamic responses of the right ventricle following extensive damage by cauterization. Circulation 5:816–823, 1952

22. **James T:** Anatomy of the Coronary Arteries. New York, Paul B Hoeber, 1961, p 51–60

LOCATION OF ACUTE MYOCARDIAL INFARCTS

By JULIUS M. GARDIN, M.D.,* and WILLIAM C. ROBERTS, M.D.

The electrocardiogram has been invaluable in providing information concerning the presence and, more importantly, the location of acute myocardial infarction (AMI). A major problem is evident, however, in the lack of standardized terminology to be used both electrocardiographically and morphologically. This article focuses on an anatomic approach to establishing such terminology and the ECG patterns to look for when attempting to localize AMI.

INTRODUCTION

Among patients with clinical features suggesting acute myocardial infarction (AMI), the standard 12-lead electrocardiogram (ECG) has been extremely useful during the past 50 years in establishing the diagnosis of myocardial necrosis. In addition to indicating the presence of AMI, the ECG has provided certain information regarding the *location of*

From the Division of Cardiology, Department of Medicine, Georgetown University, Washington, DC, and the Pathology Branch, National Heart, Lung, and Blood Institute, National Institutes of Health, Bethesda, Maryland.

*Present address: Division of Cardiology, Department of Medicine, Northwestern University, Chicago, Illinois.

Address for Reprints:
  William C. Roberts, M.D.
  Bldg 10A, Rm 3E30
  National Institutes of Health
  Bethesda, MD 20014

the AMI. This article reexamines the reliability of the ECG in predicting the anatomic location of AMI and suggests a common terminology for designating the location of AMI, applicable both electrocardiographically and morphologically.

ANATOMIC APPROACH TO TERMINOLOGY FOR LOCALIZATION OF AMI

Because the normal left ventricle at necropsy and in ventricular systole during life, in essence, is a *cone*, proper description of the location of an AMI of the left ventricle necessitates designation of the portion(s) of involvement of each of the three dimensions of the cone, namely, (1) the circle; (2) the thickness; and (3) the length (top to bottom) (Fig. 1).

The circle includes the anterior, posterior, and lateral free walls and the *ventricular septum*. The thickness may be designated as subendocardial, meaning inner one-half; subepicardial, meaning outer one-half; and transmural, meaning involvement of both subendocardium and subepicardium. We prefer defining subendocardium as the inner half of the myocardial wall, rather than just the inner third, because most subendocardial infarcts involve only the inner third, and, therefore, by using the half-way cut-off, a clear demarcation usually is present between subendocardial and transmural. Furthermore, most transmural infarcts involve >75 percent of the myocardial wall, and, consequently, they are clearly separable from infarcts limited to subendocardium. The length or top-to-bottom dimension may be divided into basal third, mid third, and apical third, or simply into basal half ("high") and apical half ("low") (Fig. 2). We prefer the latter because there is too much overlap when the ventricles are divided into thirds. The specific compartments of the walls of the cardiac ventricles are shown diagrammatically in Figure 2. Designating each of the various compartments of the heart, obviously, is somewhat arbitrary. We include, for example, the anterolateral papillary muscle of the left ventricle in the anterior compartment, although it can just as easily be included in the lateral compartment. The portion of ventricle at each end of the ventricular septum, when viewed transversely, could be included in either the posterior or the anterior compartment, or in the ventricular septum. We prefer to include these junction points between right and left ventricular free walls as part of the ventricular septum. We divide the right ventricular free wall into two compartments (anterolateral and posterior) as contrasted to the three free-wall compartments of the left ventricle (anterior, posterior, and lateral).

ANATOMIC COMPARTMENTS OF HEART INVOLVED BY AMI

To show the portion of the cardiac ventricle involved by AMI, the ventricles are divided into basal and apical halves (Fig. 2). Three portions of the basal half infrequently are sites of myocardial necrosis — namely, the anterior and anteroseptal compartments of the left ventricle and the anterolateral compartment of the right ventricle. "Anterior" AMI spares the right ventricular free wall, whereas nearly 25 percent of patients with "posterior" left ventricular AMI have necrosis of all or portions of the posterior wall of the right ventricle. Most patients with "posterior" AMI have necrosis of portions or all of the posteromedial papillary muscle of the left ventricle. In contrast, many patients with "anterior" AMI have no involvement of the anterolateral papillary muscle of the left ventricle.

One of the problems in designating an AMI as "anterior" or "posterior" is that each may be only partially true. A large infarct, for example, may be limited to the posterior, posteroseptal, or posterolateral portion of the left ventricle in its basal half, whereas the area of myocardial necrosis may be completely circumferential in much or some of the apical half of the left ventricle. Likewise, an area of myocardial necrosis may be entirely subendo-

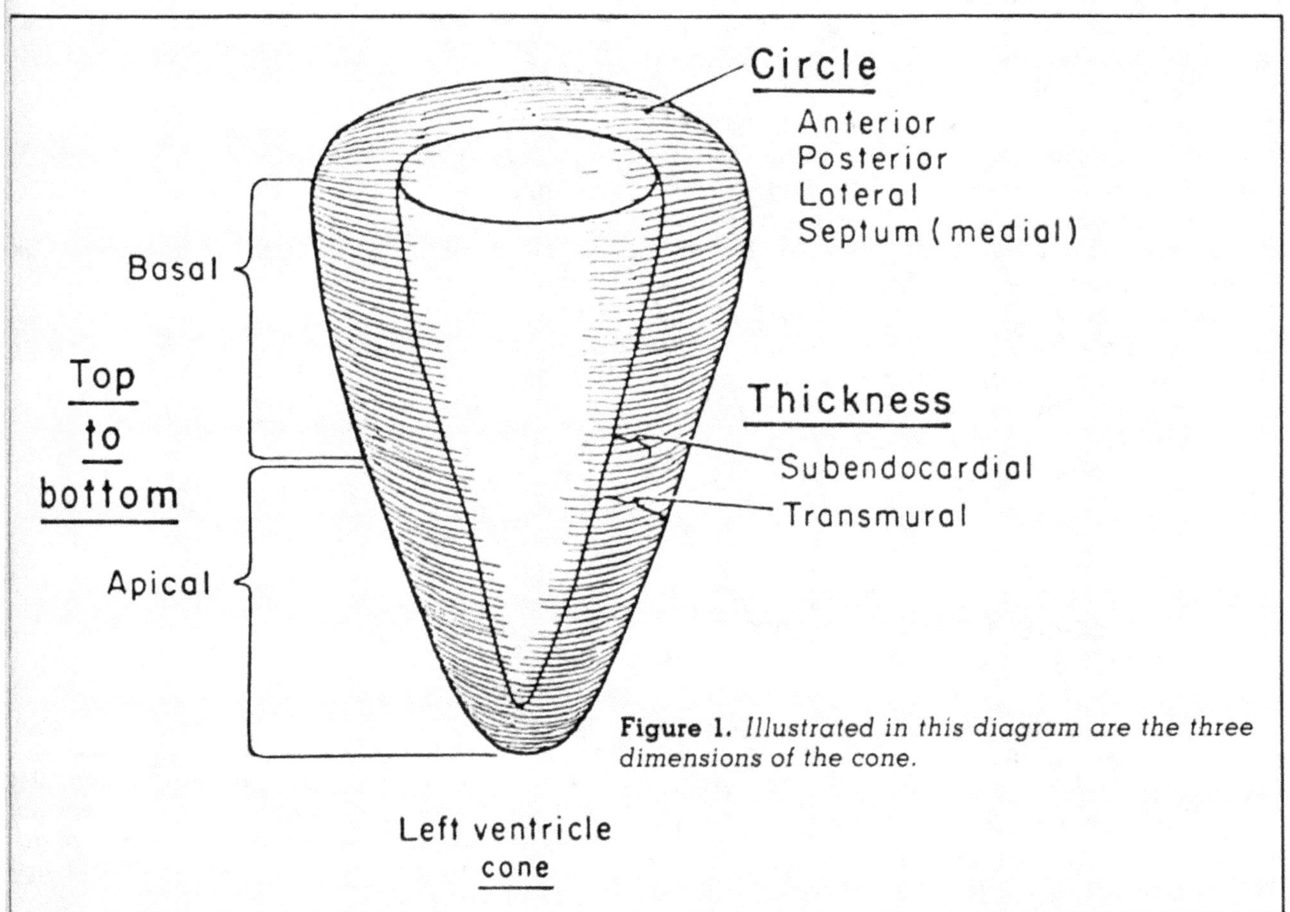

Figure 1. *Illustrated in this diagram are the three dimensions of the cone.*

cardial in one portion and transmural in another. The latter are classified as "transmural."

TERMINOLOGY FOR DESCRIBING SITES OF AMI

Certain terms used in designating AMI by electrocardiogram are not used for designating its location at necropsy. The terms "inferior," "diaphragmatic," and "true posterior," for example, are electrocardiographic terms, and they are poor ones because they break the principle of parallelism. Their opposites, namely, "superior," "sternal," or "false posterior" (or indeed "true anterior" or "false anterior") are never employed. Therefore, these terms might best be eliminated so that the same terms may be used both electrocardiographically and anatomically. "Inferior" and "diaphragmatic" AMI are simply those involving the "posterior" left ventricular wall, possibly primarily the "posteroapical" portion. "True posterior" generally has been considered "posterobasal," but evidence for this is not firm.

ELECTROCARDIOGRAPHIC PATTERNS FOR LOCALIZING AMI IN THE THREE DIMENSIONS OF THE CONE

The focus in this section will center on abnormalities in the QRS complex in AMI. Because *subendocardial* infarcts typically do not cause abnormality of the QRS complex,[2] this section will deal entirely with *transmural* AMI. In addition, fatal AMI limited to the subendocardium, i.e., inner half of the left ventricular wall, is infrequent in our experience and it has been observed by us, wit rare exception, only in patients with left ventricular hypertrophy from another conditio

TABLE I

ELECTROCARDIOGRAPHIC PATTERNS OF TRANSMURAL AMI*

Anatomic Site of Left Ventricular (LV) AMI	Electrocardiographic QRS Changes
Anterior Wall	$Q\,V_3$ and/or V_4
Anteroseptal	QV_3 and/or V_4 + V_1 and V_2
Anterolateral	QV_3 and/or V_4 and V_5 and/or
Posterior Wall	Q II, II, & AVF and/or $R > S$ in
Posteroseptal	V_1 and/or V_2 and ≥ 0.04 sec
Posterolateral	
Ventricular septum	Nothing specific
Lateral Wall	Nothing specific

Papillary muscle
  Anterolateral
  Posteromedial
	Nothing specific

Right ventricle
  With anterior LV
  infarct
	**

With posterior LV infarct	Nothing specific

* *The electrocardiographic pattern shown her can be altered by abnormal cardiac positio cardiomegaly, bundle branch block, previo myocardial infarction and, obviously, incorre lead placement.*

** *Nonexistent or rare*

(systemic hypertension or left ventricular out-flow obstruction) or prolonged shock (of any origin). Thus, opportunity for electrocardiographic-anatomic correlative studies among patients with isolated suben-docardial AMI is limited.[2]

ECG Pattern in Transmural AMI Involving the Anterior Wall of Left Ventricle. AMI at ne-cropsy infrequently involves the more basal portion of the anterior wall of left ventricle. Therefore, "anterior" AMI by ECG nearly always indicates necrosis of all or portions of the apical half, and, in general, is character-ized by the presence of Q waves of greater than 0.03 seconds in leads V_3 and/or V_4[3] (Table 1). AMI, however, infrequently is limited to just the anterior wall of the left ventricle: the lateral or septal wall or both is (are) usually also involved. *Anteroseptal* AMI is character-ized by the presence of Q waves in V_1 and V_2 in addition to the usual presence of Q waves in V_3 and/or V_4[4,5] and *anterolateral* AMI, by the presence of Q waves in V_5 and/or V_6, some-times in leads I and/or AVL, in addition to the expected Q waves in V_3 and/or V_4.[6-8]

ECG Pattern in Transmural AMI Involving Posterior Wall of Left Ventricle. Although dif-ferences by ECG between "true posterior"[3] ("plain posterior"[7]) and "inferior"[3] ("diaphragmatic" or "inferoposterior"[7]) AMI have been described,[3] the evidence is by no means convincing that "posterior" AMI involv-ing the basal half of the left ventricle can be distinguished by ECG from "posterior" AMI involving the apical half of this ventricle. ("True posterior" AMI has been characterized by "tall" [R to S ratio ≥1] and "broad" [≥0.04 second duration] R waves in V_1 and/or V_2; "in-ferior" AMI, by Q waves of ≥0.04 seconds duration in leads II, III, and AVF.) Further-more, although it has been suggested that the additional presence of Q waves in V_5 and V_6 denotes involvement (extension) of the "posterolateral" wall,[3,7] AMI involving the "posterolateral" wall cannot be reliably differentiated from AMI involving the "pos-teroseptal" wall, and neither can be reliably delineated from AMI limited to the "posterior" free wall of the left ventricle.[9,10] Thus, "poste-rior" AMI with or without involvement of the adjacent septal or lateral walls generally is characterized by Q waves in leads II, III, and AVF and/or the presence of broad (≥0.04 sec) and tall (R wave to S wave ratio ≥1) R waves in V_1 and/or V_2.

ECG Pattern in Transmural AMI Involving Only Ventricular Septum, Lateral Wall of Left Ventricle, Papillary Muscle, or Right Ventricle. in contrast to its ability to distin-guish clearly between AMI involving the "anterior" wall from that involving the "posterior" wall of left ventricle, the ECG pro-vides no specific pattern to indicate necrosis of ventricular septum,[4,10] lateral wall of left ventricle,[11,12] papillary muscle, or right ventri-cle.[10] AMI, however, is rarely, if ever, limited exclusively to the lateral wall of the left ven-tricle, to the ventricular septum, or to the right ventricle. Thus, whenever the ventricular sep-tum or the left ventricular lateral wall is the site of AMI, either the anterior or the posterior wall is also involved. Furthermore, as men-tioned, AMI secondary to coronary arterial narrowing and involving the right ventricle is always associated with "posterior" left ven-tricular AMI, never "anterior" left ventricular AMI.[1] Consequently, the anterolateral wall of the right ventricle is never the site of myocardial necrosis unless the entire posterior right ventricular wall is either necrotic or fibrotic or both. Also, necrosis of the posteromedial papillary muscle occurs in most patients with "posterior" AMI; and, therefore, involvement of this structure can be predicted simply by knowing that the AMI is "posterior." In contrast, a high percentage of patients with left ventricular "anterior" wall AMI do not have

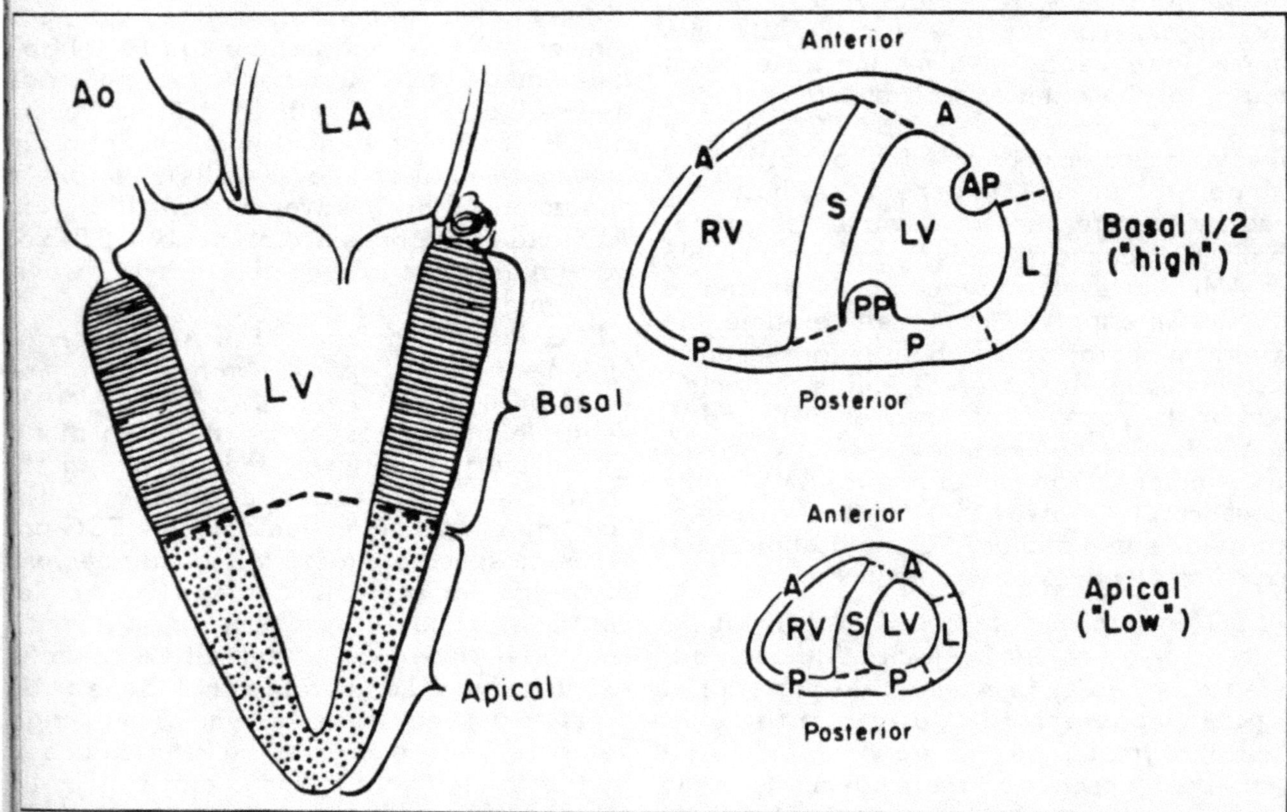

Figure 2. Diagrams showing the left ventricle (LV) illustrated as a cone (left) and transverse cuts across the right (RV) and left ventricles (right). The length of the ventricle is divided into basal and apical halves. The larger transverse slice (upper right) is from the basal half, and the smaller transverse slice, from the apical half. The darker lines serve to define the various compartments of the left ventricle. (A =anterior wall of the left ventricle and anterolateral wall of the right ventricle; Ao =aorta; AP =anterolateral papillary muscle; L =lateral wall of the left ventricle; LA =left atrium; P =posterior wall of both the right and left ventricles; PP =posteromedial papillary muscle; S =ventricular septum.)

involvement of the anterolateral papillary muscle and, therefore, involvement of this structure cannot be predicted reliably by knowing that the AMI involves the "anterior" wall.

SUMMARY

The same terminology applicable for describing the location of an acute myocardial infarct (AMI) at necropsy is applicable for defining its location by electrocardiogram. Certain terms used electrocardiographically, namely "inferior," "diaphragmatic," and "true posterior," should be avoided because their opposites are not used. Ideally, a proper description of the location of an AMI should include defining its involvement in all the dimensions of the left ventricle (considered as a cone): the portion of the walls of the *circle* involved (anterior, posterior, lateral, and septal); the amount of the wall's *thickness* involved (transmural or nontransmural [subendocardial]), and the portions of the wall's *length* involved (basal half or apical half or both). Certain portions of the walls of both the left and right ventricles are rare sites of AMI, and knowing these sites helps in more precisely defining by ECG the location of the AMI. AMI involving the *anterior* wall of the left ventricle rarely is limited to just its basal half; and, therefore, anterior AMI, for practical purposes, indicates involvement of at least the apical half of the ventricle. AMI involving the basal half of the posterior left ventricular wall, in contrast, is common, but the ECG is not accurate in differentiating posterobasal from posteroapical AMI.

Furthermore, the ECG provides no specific pattern to indicate AMI of the ventricular septum, lateral wall of the left ventricle, either posterior or anterolateral walls of the right ventricle, or papillary muscle. AMI of the right ventricle virtually never occurs with "anterior" AMI of the left ventricle. In contrast, nearly 25 percent of patients with "posterior" transmural AMI also have associated AMI involving at least the posterior wall of the right ventricle. ●

REFERENCES

1. Isner JM, Roberts WC *Amer J Card 41*:409, 1978
2. Cook RW, Edwards JE, Pruitt RD *Circulat 18* 603–612, 1958
3. Marriott HJL: *Practical Electrocardiography* 5th edition, Williams & Wilkins, Baltimore 1972, p 226
4. Rodriguez MI, Anselmi ChA, Sodi-Pallares D *Amer Heart J 45*:525–544, 1953
5. Myers GB, Klein HA, Stofer BE *Amer Heart J 36*:535–575, 1948
6. Myers GB, Klein HA, Hiratzka T *Amer Heart J 36*:838–881, 1948
7. Wilson FN, Johnston FD, Rosenbaum FF, Erlanger H, Kossman CE, Hecht H, Cotrim N, Menezes de Oliveira R, Scarsi R, Barker PS *Amer Heart J 27*:19–85, 1944
8. Savage RM, Wagner GS, Ideker RE, Podolsky SA, Hackel DB *Circulat 55*:279–285, 1977
9. Myers GB, Klein HA, Hiratzka T *Amer Heart J 38*:837–862, 1949
10. Myers GB, Klein HA, Hiratzka T *Amer Heart J 37*:720–770, 1949
11. Dunn WJ, Edwards JE, Pruitt RD *Circulat 14* 540–555, 1956
12. Myers GB, Klein HA, Stofer BE *Amer Heart J 37*:374–417, 1949

Quantitation of Coronary Arterial Narrowing at Necropsy in Sudden Coronary Death

Analysis of 31 Patients and Comparison With 25 Control Subjects

WILLIAM C. ROBERTS, MD, FACC
ANCIL A. JONES, MD

Bethesda, Maryland

A quantitative analysis of the degree and extent of coronary arterial narrowing by atherosclerotic plaques in the entire lengths of each of the four major coronary arteries in a group of patients dying suddenly from coronary heart disease ("sudden coronary death") is described at necropsy. Cross sections were examined histologically in a total of 1,564 five mm long segments of the left main, left anterior descending, left circumflex and right coronary arteries in 31 patients with sudden coronary death, and the observations were compared with those from examination of 1,100 five mm segments of the major epicardial coronary arteries in 25 control subjects. An average of 25 cm (50 five mm segments) of coronary artery were examined from each patient and an average of 22 cm (44 five mm segments) from each control subject. Of the 1,564 five mm segments examined in the 31 study patients, 557 (36 percent) were 76 to 100 percent narrowed in cross-sectional area by atherosclerotic plaques (control subjects 3 percent), 536 (34 percent) were 51 to 75 percent narrowed (control subjects 22 percent), 360 (23 percent) were 26 to 50 percent narrowed (control subjects 42 percent) and only 111 segments (7 percent) had 25 percent or less narrowing (control subjects 33 percent). The amount of severe (greater than 75 percent) narrowing of the right, left anterior descending and left circumflex coronary arteries was similar. Additionally, the amount of severe (greater than 75 percent) narrowing in the distal one half of the right, left anterior descending and left circumflex coronary arteries was similar to that in the proximal halves of these three arteries. The number of 5 mm coronary arterial segments narrowed 76 to 100 percent in cross-sectional area in the 31 study patients was not affected by the patient's age at death, sex, presence or absence of previous angina pectoris or myocardial infarction or the weight of the heart.

Although it is recognized that patients who die suddenly from coronary heart disease have considerable narrowing of one or more major epicardial coronary arteries,[1-9] the exact amount of luminal narrowing in any one or in each of the four major epicardial coronary arteries has not been described. Accordingly, we determined the degree of cross-sectional luminal narrowing in each 5 mm segment of each of the four major epicardial coronary arteries in 31 patients who died suddenly from coronary heart disease and compared the findings with those in 25 control subjects.

Methods

Study patients: *Only patients fulfilling the following criteria were included in this study:* (1) Death was known to occur *within 6 hours* of the previously

From the Pathology Branch, National Heart, Lung, and Blood Institute, National Institutes of Health, Bethesda, Maryland. Manuscript received January 16, 1979; revised manuscript received February 27, 1979, accepted February 28, 1979.

Address for reprints: William C. Roberts, MD, Bldg 10A, Rm 3E-30, National Institutes of Health, Bethesda, Maryland 20205.

witnessed usual state of health. (2) Although the patient may have died in a hospital, he or she was not a patient in a hospital at the onset of symptoms suggestive of myocardial ischemia. (3) At necropsy, at least one of the four major (right, left main, left anterior descending, left circumflex) epicardial coronary arteries was more than 75 percent narrowed in cross-sectional area by atherosclerotic plaque. (4) Ventricular myocardial coagulation necrosis was absent at necropsy. (5) A cause of death, either cardiac or noncardiac, other than coronary luminal narrowing was absent. (6) Chronic congestive cardiac failure had never been present. (7) A cardiac operation had never been performed. A review of clinical and necropsy records in the Pathology Branch, National Heart, Lung, and Blood Institute revealed that 31 patients fulfilled these criteria and their hearts and coronary arteries were available for reexamination. Their pertinent clinical and noncoronary cardiac necropsy observations are summarized in Table I.

Control subjects: *Control subjects, similar in age and sex to the study patients, were selected on the basis of the following criteria:* (1) death from a noncardiac condition; (2) absence of symptoms suggesting or indicating myocardial ischemia or cardiac dysfunction during life; (3) absence of systemic hypertension (blood pressure more than 140 mm Hg systolic or more than 90 mm Hg diastolic, or both); (4) absence of therapeutic mediastinal irradiation; and (5) absence of cardiomegaly (heart weight less than or equal to 400 g in men and 350 g in women) at necropsy. A total of 25 subjects who fulfilled these criteria were selected as control subjects: 13 died of carcinoma or sarcoma, 5 of leukemia, 4 of lymphoma and 1 each of heat stroke, gunshot wound and acute infection.

Coronary arterial histologic studies: The coronary arteries in all patients and in control subjects were studied in similar fashion (Fig. 1). The hearts were fixed for at least 1 day in formalin. The four major epicardial coronary arteries then were excised intact, studied roentgenographically and fixed for at least another day. After decalcification (if necessary), each of the four major coronary arteries was cut transversely to its longitudinal axis into approximately 5 mm long segments, and each segment was labeled sequentially from either its aortic ostium or from its origin from the left main coronary artery. The number of 5 mm segments examined in the study patients and control subjects is summarized in Table II. The 5 mm segments were labeled, dehydrated (alcohol and xylene) and embedded in paraffin, and two histologic sections were cut and stained from each paraffin block. The Movat stain was used on one histologic section, and all determinations of luminal narrowing were based on examination of the Movat-stained sections.

The degree of narrowing was determined after histologic examination of each cross section magnified 25 to 50 times. The judgment regarding the degree of luminal narrowing of each 5 mm segment was based on the degree of luminal obliteration within the luminal circle bordered by the internal elastic membrane. The circle was visually subdivided into four equal-sized quadrants, and the degree of cross-sectional area luminal narrowing in each 5 mm segment was graded as 0 to 25, 26 to 50, 51 to 75 or 76 to 100 percent. All sections were examined by one of us, and random sections were examined by the other. In 95 percent of the sections examined by both of us, the degree of grading was similar. In sections from several patients examined independently by two other observers, agreement on degree of severity of narrowing also was greater than 95 percent. (Agreement between degree of narrowing as assessed with magnification during microscopy and with planimetry is also about 95 percent. Comparison of these data is the subject of another study in preparation.)

Myocardial histology: In addition to the sections from the major epicardial coronary arteries, at least three histologic sections extending from the endocardium to the epicardium and at least 2 cm in circumferential dimension were prepared from the left ventricular myocardium of each patient and stained with hematoxylin-eosin. Gross myocardial fibrosis

TABLE I

Quantitation of Coronary Arterial Narrowing in Patients With Sudden Coronary Death and Control Subjects: Clinical Observations and Noncoronary Cardiac Findings

	Patients With Coronary Death (no. = 31)	Control Group (no. = 25)
Age (yr)		
Range	22–85	25–74
Mean	47	49
Sex		
Male	24(77%)	18(22%)
Female	7(23%)	7(28%)
Historical data		
Angina pectoris	16/29(55%)	0/25
Past AMI	0/31	0/25
Chronic CHF	0/31	0/25
Diabetes mellitus	6/29(21%)	0/25
Systemic hypertension	5/19(26%)	0/25
Laboratory data		
Serum cholesterol measured	10/31	21/25
Serum cholesterol >200 mg/dl	9/10*	5/21*
Serum cholesterol values (mg/dl)		
Range	198–700	128–245
Mean	361*	176*
Serum triglyceride measured	9/31	4/25
Serum triglyceride >200 mg/dl	4/9	1/4
Serum triglyceride values (mg/dl)		
Range	86–1,000	106—202
Mean	362	151
Autopsy data		
Heart weight (g)		
Range	260–540	200–400
Mean	420*	288*
Patients with cardiomegaly†	21/31(68%)	0/25
Patients with gross LV scars		
<1/2 wall thickness	6(19%)	0
>1/2 wall thickness	4(13%)‡	0

   * Significant difference between patients and control groups (probability [*P*] <0.05).

   † Heart weight more than 400 g in men or more than 350 g in women.

   ‡ Posterior wall scars in each. These patients never had clinical evidence of acute myocardial infarction.

   AMI = acute myocardial infarct that healed; CHF = congested heart failure; LV = left ventricular.

TABLE II

Number of 5 mm Long Segments of Major Epicardial Coronary Artery Examined Per Patient

Coronary Artery	Number (Range [mean]) of 5 mm Segments per Patient	
	Patients With Sudden Coronary Death (no. = 31)	Control Group (no. = 25)
Right	8–31 (20.0)	12–27 (18.1)
Left main	1–4 (1.8)	1–3 (1.6)
Left anterior descending	13–27 (18.8)	11–26 (15.3)
Left circumflex	4–20 (10.1)	3–27 (9.3)
Total segments of 4 coronary arteries per patient	39–78 (50.5)	31–67 (44.0)

(Table I, 10 patients) and the absence of myocardial coagulation necrosis were confirmed in each patient by histologic examination.

Results

Coronary arterial pathology in study patients versus control subjects: Among the 31 patients with sudden coronary death, a total of 121 major coronary arteries were examined (the left main artery was not examined in 3 patients); among the 25 control subjects, 96 major coronary arteries were examined (the left main artery was not examined in 4 subjects). The *maximal degree* of cross-sectional area of luminal narrowing by atherosclerotic plaque in one or more of the four major coronary arteries in each of the 31 study patients and in each of the 25 control subjects is summarized in Table III. All study patients had 76 to 100 percent cross-sectional area luminal narrowing by atherosclerotic plaque in one or more of the four arteries, and 7 (28 percent) of the 25 control subjects had this degree of narrowing. The *number of arteries* narrowed 76 to 100 percent was quite different in the study patients and control subjects. Of the 31 study patients, 29 (94 percent) had two or more of the four major coronary arteries narrowed 75 percent or more in cross-sectional area by atherosclerotic plaque, whereas only 3 (12 percent) of the 25 control subjects had two or more arteries narrowed to this degree.

Of the study patients, 3 had greater than 75 percent narrowing by atherosclerotic plaque of all four major coronary arteries; 20 patients had three coronary arteries narrowed to this degree; 6 patients had two arteries and 2 patients had a single artery narrowed to this extent. Thus, of the possible 124 major coronary arteries in the 31 study patients (actually only 121 arteries were examined), 86 (67 percent) were more than 75 percent narrowed in cross-sectional area by atherosclerotic plaque for an average of 2.8/4.0 coronary arteries per study patient. If the left main coronary artery was excluded, 83 (89 percent) of the other 93 major (right, left anterior descending and left circumflex) coronary arteries were narrowed more than 75 percent in cross-sectional area by atherosclerotic plaque, for an average of 2.7/3.0 coronary arteries per study patient. Of the

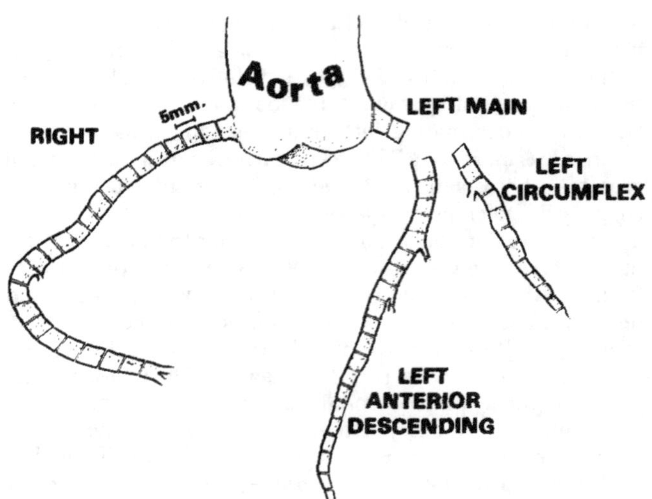

FIGURE 1. Diagram showing the four major coronary arteries and their division into 5 mm segments.

seven control subjects with greater than 75 percent cross-sectional area narrowing by atherosclerotic plaque, one had all four major coronary arteries narrowed to this degree, three had two arteries similarly narrowed and three had only one artery so narrowed. Thus, of the possible 100 major coronary arteries in the 25 control subjects (actually only 96 arteries were examined), a total of 13 (13 percent) were narrowed more than 75 percent in cross-sectional area by atherosclerotic plaque for an average of 0.5/4.0 coronary arteries per control subject. If the left main coronary artery was excluded, 12 (16 percent) of the 75 other major (right, left anterior descending, left circumflex) coronary arteries were narrowed more than 75 percent in cross-sectional area by atherosclerotic plaque for an average of 0.5/3.0 coronary arteries per control patient. Two of the 31 patients had thrombus in one coronary artery. In each the thrombus was superimposed on atherosclerotic plaque, and the calculations of luminal narrowing did not include the amount of luminal obliteration contributed entirely by the thrombus, only that part resulting from atherosclerotic plaque. None of the control subjects had a coronary thrombus.

TABLE III

Number of 31 Patients With Sudden Coronary Death (SCD) and 25 Control Subjects (C) Showing Maximal Luminal Narrowing of One or More Major Epicardial Coronary Arteries by Atherosclerotic Plaque

| Artery | Percent Cross-Sectional Area Luminal Narrowing | | | | | | | | | |
| | 0–25 | | 26–50 | | 51–75 | | 76–100 | | Total | |
	SCD	C	SCD	C	SCD	C	SCD	C	SCD	C
RCA	—	—	0	0	0	3	0	1	0	4
LAD	—	—	0	0	0	1	2	2	2	3
RCA LAD	—	—	0	1	0	4	3	2	3	7
RCA, LCx	—	—	0	0	0	0	3	0	3	0
LAD, LCx	—	—	0	0	0	2	0	1	0	3
RCA, LAD, LCx	—	—	0	2	0	3	20	0	20	5
RCA, LMCA,* LAD, LCx	0	1	0	1	0	0	3	1	3	3
Total no.	0	1	0	4	0	13	31	7	31	25
(%)	(0)	(4)	(0)	(16)	(0)	(52)	(100)	(28)	(100)	(100)

* Sections of left main coronary artery were not examined in three patients with sudden coronary death and four control subjects.

LAD = left anterior descending coronary artery; LCx = left circumflex coronary artery; LMCA = left main coronary artery; RCA = right coronary artery.

TABLE IV

Number and Percent of 5 mm Long Segments of the Four Major Epicardial Coronary Arteries in 31 Patients With Sudden Coronary Death (SCD) and in 25 Control Subjects (C) Showing the Four Grades of Cross-Sectional Luminal Narrowing

| Artery | Percent Cross-Sectional Area Luminal Narrowing | | | | | | | | | |
| | 0–25 | | 26–50 | | 51–75 | | 76–100 | | Total | |
	SCD	C	SCD	C	SCD	C	SCD	C	SCD	C
LMCA										
no.	11	8	19	20	13	3	5	2	48	33
%	(22)	(24)	(40)	(61)	(28)	(9)	(10)	(6)	(100)	(100)
LAD										
no.	55	121	143	154	181	85	205	22	584	382
%	(9)	(32)	(24)	(40)	(31)	(22)	(36)	(6)	(100)	(100)
LCx										
no.	20	90	74	96	104	43	115	3	313	232
%	(6)	(39)	(24)	(44)	(33)	(16)	(37)	(<1)	(100)	(100)
RCA										
no.	25	144	124	200	238	106	232	3	619	453
%	(4)	(32)	(20)	(44)	(38)	(23)	(38)	(<1)	(100)	(100)
Total										
no.	111	363	360	470	536	237	557	30	1564	1100
%	(7)	(33)	(23)	(42)	(34)	(22)	(36)	(3)	(100)	(100)

* Sections not examined in three patients with sudden coronary death and in four control subjects.

LAD = left anterior descending coronary artery; LC = left circumflex coronary artery; LM = left main coronary artery; R = right coronary artery.

Summary of quantitative analysis of coronary arterial narrowing: The results of the *quantitative* analysis of the 5- mm long coronary arterial segments in both study patients and control subjects are summarized in Table IV. Of the 1,564 five mm long segments of major coronary arteries examined in the 31 study patients, 557 segments (36 percent) were 76 to 100 percent narrowed in cross-sectional area by atherosclerotic plaque (control subjects 3 percent), 536 segments (34 percent) were 51 to 75 percent narrowed (control subjects 22 percent), 360 segments (23 percent) were 26 to 50 percent narrowed (control subjects 42 percent) and 111 segments (7 percent) were 0 to 25 percent narrowed (control subjects 33 percent). The mean percent of 5 mm coronary segments narrowed 0 to 25, 26 to 50, 51 to 75 and 76 to 100 percent was sig-nificantly (P <0.05) different between study patients and control subjects at each of the four levels of narrowing (Fig. 2).

The number or percent, or both, of 5 mm long segments narrowed to various degrees in each of the four major coronary arteries also are summarized in Table IV and in Figures 3 and 4. The mean percent of 5 mm segments of left anterior descending, left circumflex and right coronary arteries narrowed was significantly (P <0.05) different between study patients and control subjects at each of the four levels of narrowing. No significant differences were detected in mean percent of segments of left main coronary artery narrowed 0 to 25, 26 to 50, 51 to 75 and 76 to 100 percent between study patients and control subjects. The mean percent of 5 mm segments of right, left anterior descending and left

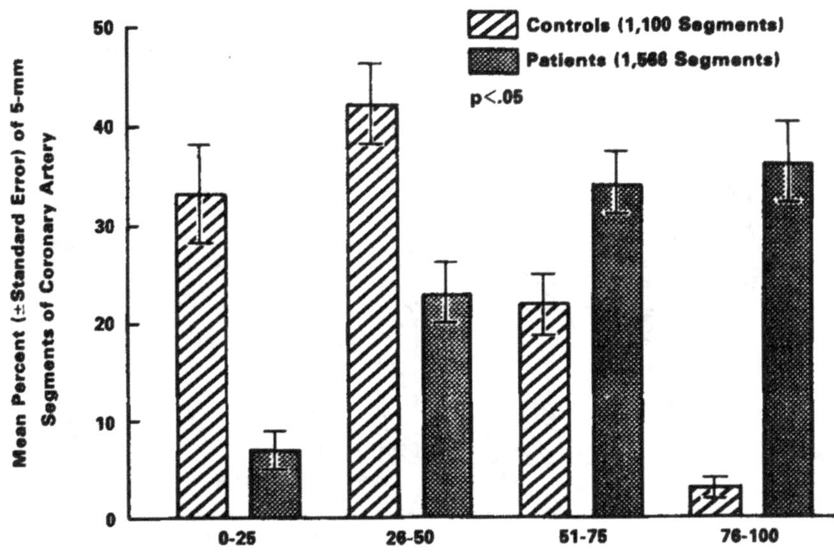

FIGURE 2. Percent of 5 mm segments of all four major coronary arteries narrowed to various degrees in the 31 study patients (aged 22 to 85 years, average 47) and in the 25 control subjects (aged 25 to 74 years, average 49). p = probability.

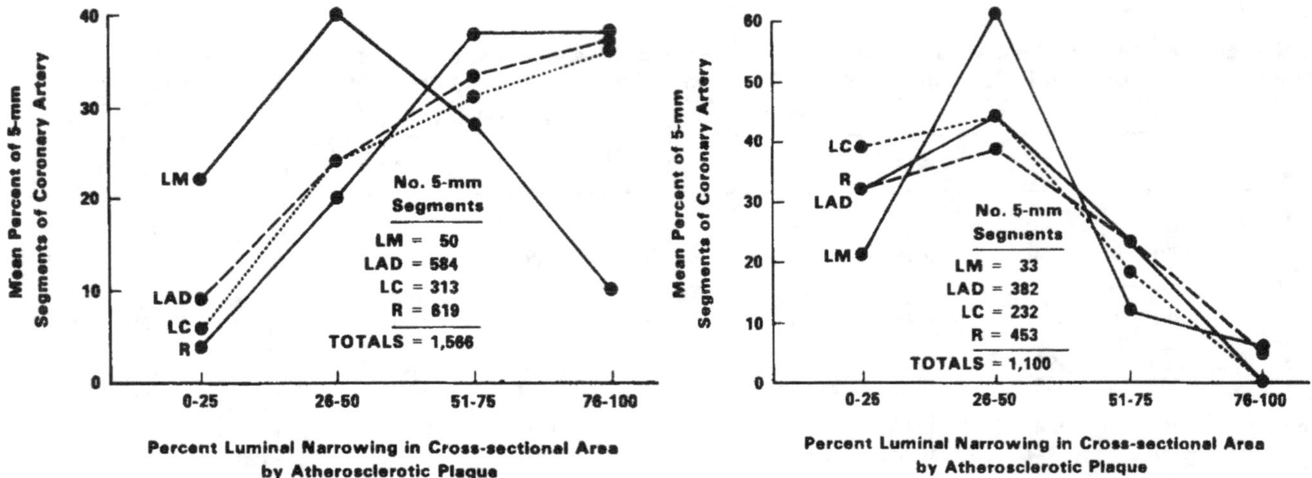

FIGURE 3. Mean percent of 5 mm segments of each of the four major coronary arteries narrowed to various degrees in the 31 patients with sudden coronary death (**left**) and in the 25 control subjects (**right**). The amount of luminal narrowing of the right (R), left anterior descending (LAD), and left circumflex (LC) coronary arteries is similar within each study group. The degree of severe narrowing of the left main (LM) coronary artery is considerably less than that of the other three arteries in the study patients.

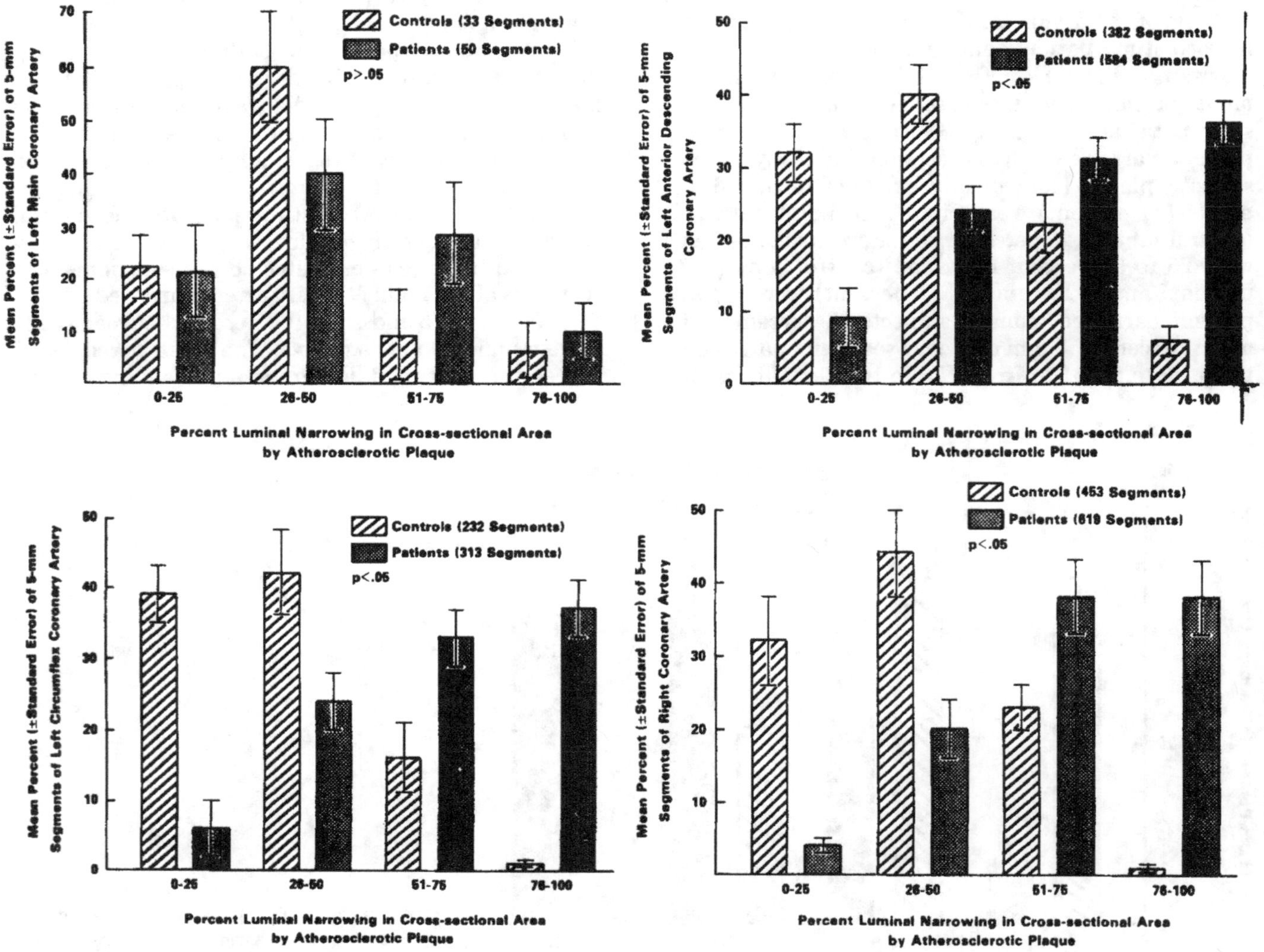

FIGURE 4. Mean percent of 5 mm segments of each of the four major coronary arteries narrowed to various degrees in the 31 patients with sudden coronary death and in the 25 control subjects. **Upper left,** left main artery. **Upper right,** left anterior descending artery. **Lower left,** left circumflex artery. **Lower right,** right coronary artery. p = probability.

circumflex coronary arteries at each of the four levels of narrowing was similar in the study patients. Likewise, the mean percent of segments of each of these three major coronary arteries narrowed to various degrees in the control subjects was similar. The degree of narrowing of the left main artery in both study patients and control subjects was quite different from the mean percent of narrowing of the segments in the other three major coronary arteries.

Proximal versus distal coronary arterial narrowing: The mean percent of 5 mm segments narrowed 76 to 100 percent in cross-sectional area in the proximal half of the right, left anterior descending and left circumflex coronary arteries was similar to the mean percent of 5 mm segments similarly narrowed in the distal half of these arteries (Fig. 5). The mean percent of segments narrowed more than 75 percent was 39 percent in the proximal half of these three arteries and 34 percent in the distal half ($P >0.05$). The distal half of the left anterior descending artery tended to have a smaller proportion of segments narrowed more than 75 percent than did the proximal half of this artery, but the opposite was true in both the right and left circumflex coronary arteries. The percent of 5 mm segments narrowed more than 75 percent in cross-sectional area by atherosclerotic plaque in the first 2 cm of left anterior descending coronary artery also tended to be higher than the percent narrowed more than 75 percent in the remainder of this artery (43 ± 7 percent versus 33 ± 30 [$P >0.05$]). The opposite occurred in the left circumflex coronary artery. The mean percent of 5 mm segments narrowed 76 to 100 percent in cross-sectional area by atherosclerotic plaque in its first 2 cm tended to be less than the mean percent of segments narrowed to this degree distal to that point (32 ± 5 versus 38 ± 6 [$P >0.05$]).

Clinicopathologic correlations: The relation of five clinical or morphologic variables in the study patients to the mean percent of 5 mm coronary segments narrowed more than 75 percent in cross-sectional area is summarized in Table V. Comparison of patients in *three different age groups* (less than or equal to 45, 46 to 65 and more than 65 years) showed no significant differences in mean percent of coronary segments narrowed more than 75 percent. Likewise, no significant differences in mean percent of coronary segments narrowed more than 75 percent in the study patients was apparent when comparing *men with women*, subjects with and subjects without *previous angina pectoris*, subjects with an increased and subjects with a normal *heart weight* and subjects with and subjects without a *healed, transmural left ventricular myocardial infarct* (Table V).

Comments

In many cardiovascular diseases, quantitation of the degree of severity of the condition is commonplace. Examples are the everyday recording of the exact pressure gradients across stenotic valves or the determination, by several means, of the magnitude of a shunt from one side of the circulation to another. Angiography and, more recently, echocardiography, have provided means of measuring cavity size and, the latter, wall thicknesses. Attempts have recently been made to quantitate the size of myocardial infarcts. For years, coronary angiography has demonstrated "narrowing" in one or more epicardial coronary arteries in patients with coronary heart disease, but the exact degree or extent in any one or in all major epicardial coronary arteries has not been precise. Many thousands of au-

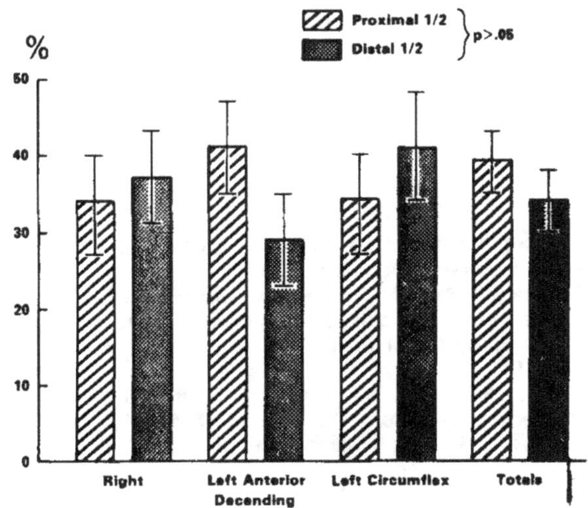

FIGURE 5. Mean percent of 5-mm segments of the right, left anterior descending and left circumflex coronary arteries narrowed more than 75 percent in cross-sectional area by atherosclerotic plaques in the proximal one half compared with the distal one half of each of the three arteries in 31 patients with sudden coronary death. The mean percent of 5 mm segments severely narrowed was similar in both the proximal and distal halves of these three arteries.

TABLE V

Mean Percent of Total 5 mm Segments in the Four Major (Right, Left Main, Left Anterior Descending, and Left Circumflex) Epicardial Coronary Arteries Narrowed >75% in Cross Sectional Area by Atherosclerotic Plaque in 31 Patients With Sudden Coronary Death (SCD): Comparison of Five Clinical or Morphologic Parameters

	Patients (no.)	Mean % (±SE) of 5 mm Coronary Segments Narrowed >75%	P Value
Age (yr)			
<45	15	36 ± 6	
45–65	13	33 ± 5	>0.05
>65	3	36 ± 8	
Sex			
M	24	36 ± 4	
F	7	30 ± 8	>0.05
Angina pectoris			
Present	18	34 ± 8	
Absent	13	35 ± 5	>0.05
Heart weight			
Increased*	21	36 ± 5	
Normal	10	31 ± 5	>0.05
Healed transmural infarct, left ventricle			
Present	4	51 ± 4	
Absent	27	32 ± 4	>0.05

* >400 g in men, >350 g in women.
P = probability; SE = standard error.

topsies during this century have demonstrated severe narrowings in one or more major epicardial coronary arteries of patients with coronary heart disease, but there have been no attempts to quantitate the degree and extent of coronary luminal narrowing at necropsy in these patients.

Quantitative coronary arterial narrowing in sudden coronary death: The present study provides quantitative information on the degree and extent of luminal narrowing in each of the four major epicardial coronary arteries in 31 patients who died suddenly from coronary heart disease. More than 25 cm of the four major (right, left main, left anterior descending and left circumflex) epicardial coronary arteries was examined in each of the 31 patients for a total of nearly 790 cm of major coronary artery. One histologic section was examined from each 0.5 cm segment or a total of 1,564 five mm segments from the 31 patients. Among the 31 patients studied, the lumens in 36 percent of the entire lengths of the four major epicardial coronary arteries were more than 75 percent narrowed in cross-sectional area by atherosclerotic plaque. (A 75 percent cross-sectional area narrowing is equivalent to a 50 percent diameter reduction on luminogram.[10]) The lumens in another 34 percent of the major coronary arteries were narrowed 51 to 75 percent in cross-sectional area. Thus, in the 31 patients with sudden coronary death, 70 percent of the lengths of the four major epicardial coronary arteries were more than 50 percent narrowed in cross-sectional area by atherosclerotic plaque. In contrast to the 36 percent of the lengths of the four major coronary arteries in the study patients with more than 75 percent narrowing of cross-sectional area, only 3 percent of the lengths of the four major coronary arteries in the control subjects were narrowed to this degree.

Not only was severe narrowing widespread in the study patients, but some degree of narrowing was present in virtually every 5 mm segment of coronary artery studied; 93 percent of the coronary tree studied was more than 25 percent narrowed in cross-sectional area, and only 7 percent of the coronary tree was narrowed 25 percent or less in cross-sectional area, and not a single 5 mm segment was entirely normal in any patient. In contrast, one third of the coronary tree in the 25 control subjects was narrowed 25 percent or less in cross-sectional area by atherosclerotic plaque. Thus, coronary atherosclerosis among patients with sudden coronary death is a *diffuse* process, involving, for practical purposes, all segments of all four major epicardial coronary arteries.

Surprisingly, the degree of severe narrowing in the distal half of the right, left anterior descending, and left circumflex coronary arteries in the study patients (also in the control subjects) was just as great as in the proximal half of these arteries. The mean percent of 5 mm segments narrowed more than 75 percent in cross-sectional area by atherosclerotic plaque in the proximal half of each of these three coronary arteries was similar to the mean percent of 5 mm segments similarly narrowed in the distal half of these arteries (Fig. 6). The implications of this observation for aortocoronary bypass grafting are obvious, but it has already been demonstrated that most coronary anastomoses are at sites of atherosclerotic plaques,[11] yet myocardial perfusion apparently is rarely not increased.

The degree of narrowing in the left anterior descending, left circumflex and right coronary arteries was similar; that is, the percent of 5 mm coronary segments narrowed 0 to 25, 26 to 50, 51 to 75 and 76 to 100 in each of these three arteries was similar. The left main coronary artery was considerably less narrowed than the other three major arteries.

Clinical correlations: The amount of severe (greater than 75 percent) coronary arterial narrowing present in the patients with sudden coronary death could not be correlated with their age or sex, the presence or absence of previous angina pectoris, the presence of normal or increased cardiac weight at necropsy or the presence of transmural left ventrical scars at necropsy. Thus, the number of segments of coronary artery narrowed more than 75 percent in cross-sectional area by atherosclerotic plaque among patients with sudden coronary death was similar in the young and old patients, in men and women, in those with and without previous episodes of angina pectoris or myocardial infarction and in those with either a normal-sized or an enlarged heart.

References

1. **Saphir O, Priest WS, Hamburger WW, Katz L:** Coronary arteriosclerosis, coronary thrombosis, and the resulting myocardial changes. An evaluation of their respective clinical pictures including the electrocardiographic records, based on the anatomical findings. Am Heart J 10:567–595, 1935
2. **Blumgart HL, Schlesinger MJ, Davis D:** Studies on the relation of the clinical manifestations of angina pectoris, coronary thrombosis, and myocardial infarction to the pathologic findings with particular reference to the significance of the collateral circulation. Am Heart J 19:1–91, 140
3. **Yater WM, Welsh PP, Stapleton JF, Clark ML:** Comparison of clinical and pathologic aspects of coronary artery disease in men of various age groups: study of 950 autopsied cases from the Armed Forces Institute of Pathology. Ann Intern Med 34:352–392, 1951
4. **Snow PJD, Jones AM, Daber KS:** Coronary disease: a pathological study. Br Heart J 17:503–510, 1955
5. **Kuller L:** Sudden and unexpected non-traumatic deaths in adults. J Chronic Dis 19:1165–1192, 1966
6. **Schwartz CJ, Walsh WJ:** The pathologic basis of sudden death. Prog Cardiovasc Dis 13:465–481, 1971
7. **Roberts WC, Buja LM:** The frequency and significance of coronary arterial thrombi and other observations in fatal acute myocardial infarction. A study of 107 necropsy patients. Am J Med 52:425–443, 1972
8. **Roberts WC:** The coronary arteries and left ventricle in clinically isolated angina pectoris. Circulation 54:388–390, 1976
9. **Vlodaver Z, Amplatz K, Burchell HB, Edwards JE:** Coronary Heart Disease. Clinical, Angiographic, and Pathologic Profiles. New York, Springer-Verlag, 1976, 584
10. **Arnett EN, Isner JM, Redwood DR, Kent KM, Baker WP, Ackerstein H, Roberts WC:** Comparison of degrees of coronary arterial narrowing in coronary heart disease by cineangiography during life to the degree observed histologically at necropsy. Submitted for publication
11. **Spray TL, Roberts WC:** Status of the grafts and the native coronary arteries proximal and distal to coronary anastomotic sites of aorto-coronary bypass grafts. Circulation 55:741–749, 1977

Coronary Artery Narrowing in Coronary Heart Disease: Comparison of Cineangiographic and Necropsy Findings

ERNEST N. ARNETT, M.D.; JEFFREY M. ISNER, M.D.; DAVID R. REDWOOD, M.D.; KENNETH M. KENT, M.D.; WILLIAM P. BAKER, M.D.; HAROLD ACKERSTEIN, M.D.; and WILLIAM C. ROBERTS, M.D.; Bethesda, Maryland

Of 10 patients with fatal coronary heart disease undergoing coronary angiography 0 to 69 d (average, 21) before necropsy, the amount of narrowing in 61 coronary arteries observed angiographically (diameter reduction) during life by three angiographers was compared with that observed histologically (cross-sectional area) at necropsy. No overestimations of the degree of narrowing were made angiographically. Of 11 coronary arteries or their subdivisions narrowed 0 to 50% in cross-sectional area histologically, none were underestimated angiographically; of eight narrowed 51% to 75% histologically, seven had been underestimated, and of 42 narrowed 76% to 100% histologically, 17 were underestimated angiographically. The coronary atherosclerotic plaquing was diffuse ($>$ 25% cross-sectional area narrowing) in 90% of 467 five-millimetre segments of coronary artery examined (24 cm per patient), and this diffuseness of the atherosclerotic process seems to be the major reason for angiographic underestimation of coronary narrowings.

CORONARY ANGIOGRAPHY is at present the only method for ascertaining the presence, location, and degree of coronary arterial narrowing in live patients. The results of coronary angiography generally form the basis of many therapeutic decisions in patients with symptomatic coronary narrowing (1). Despite the liberal indication and enthusiasm for coronary angiography and the ever-increasing application of coronary-bypass surgery (2, 3),

▶ From the Pathology and Cardiology Branches, National Heart, Lung, and Blood Institute, and the Radiology Department, Clinical Center, National Institutes of Health; and the Division of Cardiology, Department of Medicine, National Naval Medical Center; Bethesda, Maryland.

there is relatively little information and that available is conflicting about the accuracy of coronary cineangiography as judged from necropsy study of the coronary arteries of patients who have had coronary angiography shortly before death. Previous studies have relied almost entirely on gross examination of the coronary arteries at necropsy or compared coronary angiograms in life to those done at postmortem examination. This report describes findings in 10 patients (61 coronary arteries or their subdivisions) in whom the degree of coronary narrowing measured by coronary angiography during life was compared with that observed by serial histologic study of the same coronary arteries at necropsy.

Methods

Certain clinical observations in the 10 patients are summarized in Table 1. All had had angina pectoris or an acute myocardial infarction that healed, or both, during life. All 10 underwent aortocoronary-bypass operations; in addition, aortic-valve replacement also was done in three patients because of associated severe aortic valve stenosis in two and pure aortic regurgitation in one. All 10 patients died within 57 days of cardiac operation and within 69 days of coronary angiography. All had more than 75% cross-sectional area narrowing by atherosclerotic plaques of at least one of the major (right, left main, left anterior-descending, left circumflex) coronary arteries found at autopsy.

At necropsy, the major extramural coronary arteries were excised intact from the heart, and diagrams were made of the various branches. Each coronary artery was then placed in a separate container and fixed in 10% buffered formalin. After fixation, radiographs were made of each coronary artery, and if

Table 1. Clinical and Cardiac Morphologic Observations in the Patients Studied*

Patient	Autopsy Number	Age	Sex	Hx AP	Hx AMI → Healed	Interval Cath → Death	Interval Cardiac Op to Death	Heart Weight	Coronary Artery with >75% Cross-Sectional Area Narrowing Histologically						LV T Scar
									R	LM	LAD	LC	LD	LCM	
		yr					*d*	*g*							
1	A74-212	40	F	+	0	20	0	350	+	+	+	+	−	−	+
2	A75-123	40	M	+	0	0	0	400	+	0	0	+	+	+	+
3	A74-266	42	M	+	+	14	0	505	+	0	+	+	+	−	+
4	A75-208	47	F	+	+	2	2	380	−	0	+	0	−	+	+
5	A75-29	52	F	+	0	7	0	310	+	+	+	+	+	+	0
6	A72-208	54	F	+	0	28	0	370	+	+	+	+	−	−	0
7	A72-105	56	M	+	0	39	18	400	+	0	0	0	−	−	+
8	A74-245	61	M	+	+	69	57†	540	−	−	+	0	−	+	+
9	A75-109	66	F	+	0	4	4†	600	+	0	+	+	−	−	0
10	A75-124	69	M	0	+	24	14†	650	0	0	+	+	−	−	+

* AMI = acute myocardial infarct, AP = angina pectoris, cath = catheterization procedure, hx = history of, LAD = left anterior descending, LC = left circumflex, LD = first left diagonal, LM = left main, LOM = left obtuse marginal, LV = left ventricle, Op = aortocoronary-bypass operation, R = right, and T = transmural.
† Also, aortic-valve replacement for stenosis or regurgitation or both.

calcific deposits were present, the artery was decalcified and then cut transversely into 5-mm segments. The tissue was then dehydrated (alcohols), cleared (xylene), embedded in paraffin, and cut. At least two histologic sections, one stained by hematoxylin and eosin and the other by Movat's method, were prepared from each 5-mm segment. The Movat-stained sections were used in ascertaining the degrees of cross-sectional luminal narrowing by atherosclerotic plaque. The judgment of the degree of narrowing of each 5-mm segment was based on the degree of luminal obliteration within the luminal circle bordered by the internal elastic membrane. All sections magnified 25 to 50 times by microscopy were examined independently by three pathologists, and both the intraobserver and interobserver errors were approximately 5%. Furthermore, the degrees of luminal narrowing were checked by planimetry, and a 96% agreement was found between the percent of cross-sectional area narrowing measured by visual inspection under magnification and that by planimetry. This correlative analysis is the subject of a separate report.

In addition to measuring the maximal degree of cross-sectional area narrowing in each of the six epicardial coronary arteries, including both distal and proximal parts in three of them (Table 2), the maximal degree of cross-sectional narrowing by atherosclerotic plaque in each of the 476 five-millimetre segments of coronary artery from the 10 patients was graded from histologic examination as follows: 0 to 25%, 26% to 50%, 51% to 75%, and 76% to 100% (Table 3). When the lumen was eccentric and when the wall of the artery adjacent to the lumen was indented inward, the measurement of the degree of narrowing was made only after visual outward expansion of the collapsed portion of arterial wall. The left anterior-descending, left circumflex, and right coronary arteries were subdivided for recording purposes into proximal and distal parts. The proximal part of both the left anterior-descending and left circumflex arteries consisted of the *first 2 cm*, and the distal parts, distal to that point. The proximal part of the right coronary artery included its proximal *one-half* and the distal part, the distal one-half (to the crux). Thus, a total of nine major coronary arteries or their proximal and distal subdivisions were analyzed in each patient, or a total of 61 coronary arteries or their proximal and distal subdivisions, in the 10 patients (Table 2). The coronary angiograms were reviewed separately by each of three experienced angiographers and the maximal degree of diameter reduction—not cross-sectional area narrowing—was measured for each adequately visualized coronary artery or its proximal and distal subdivisions for which histologic sections were available. The angiographic judgment of the degree of narrowing of a particular coronary artery was always based on examination of multiple angiographic views of the artery. The degree of diameter reduction of each major coronary artery or its proximal and distal subdivisions was graded by each angiographer independently without knowledge of the results of grading by the other two and without knowledge of the maximal degree of narrowing of each coronary artery or its subdivision as ascertained by histologic examination or by previous preoperative angiographic assessment. All three angiographers were aware that they were participating in an angiographic-histologic correlative study. Each of the three angiographers analyzed the same arteries that had been examined histologically. The degree

Table 2. Coronary Angiographic-Histologic Correlations: Coronary Segments Examined and Number Underestimated*

Coronary Artery Examined	Degrees of Histologic XSA Narrowing and (Number Underestimated Angiographically)		
	≤ 50%	51% to 75%	76% to 100%
Left main	3 (0)	3 (3)	2 (2)
LAD proximal	2 (0)	0	8 (1)
LAD distal	1 (0)	2 (2)	4 (2)
LC proximal	1 (0)	2 (2)	6 (3)
LC distal	3 (0)	0	2 (2)
Right proximal	1 (0)	0	7 (2)
Right distal	0	0	6 (2)
First diagonal	0	1 (0)	2 (0)
Left marginal	0	0	5 (3)
Total	11 (0)	8 (7)	42 (17)

*LAD = left anterior descending; LC = left circumflex; XSA = cross-sectional area.

of diameter reduction for each major coronary artery or its proximal and distal subdivisions was graded as follows: 0 to 25%; 26% to 50%; 51% to 75%, and 76% to 100%. The angiographic degree of narrowing was a judgment made by comparing the most-narrowed segment with an adjacent presumably non-narrowed segment. Calipers or other instruments were rarely used to make this measurement. Because for any degree of diameter reduction (by angiography) there is a greater degree of cross-sectional area narrowing (by histology), an *angiographic error* was defined as a difference of more than 25% between the degree of narrowing found by cineangiography during life and that by histology after death.

Coronary angiography in life or at necropsy provides a view of the longitudinal width of the coronary arterial lumen; histologic examination at necropsy, by the method we used, provides a view of the cross-sectional area of the coronary artery. Thus, for any degree of longitudinal narrowing, there is a proportionally greater loss of cross-sectional area. Assuming a central round residual lumen, a 25% reduction in width results in a 44% loss of cross-sectional area. Similarly, a 50% reduction in width results in a 75% obliteration of cross-sectional area; moreover, a 75% reduction in width results in a 95% obliteration of cross-sectional area. In this study, a false-negative angiogram was defined as one that showed less than 50% longitudinal narrowing when histologic examination showed more than 75% obliteration of cross-sectional area.

Results

The amount of cross-sectional area narrowing of the coronary arteries and their proximal and distal subdivisions by histology is summarized in Tables 2 and 3. Of the 61 coronary arteries or their proximal and distal subdivisions examined in the 10 patients, at necropsy the degree of cross-sectional area narrowing by atherosclerotic plaque was 0 to 50% in 11 (18%), 51% to 75% in

Table 3. Number of 5-mm Segments of the Four Major Epicardial Coronary Arteries in the 10 Patients, Studied in Life by Angiography and at Necropsy by Histology, Showing Various Grades of Cross-Sectional Area Luminal Narrowing Found Histologically at Necropsy

Coronary Artery	Cross-Sectional Area Luminal Narrowing				Totals
	0 to 25%	26% to 50%	51% to 75%	76% to 100%	
Left main, *no.*	0	2	16	5	23
Left anterior descending, *no.*	21	27	33	81	162
Left circumflex, *no.*	20	15	32	48	115
Right, *no.*	4	30	58	75	167
Totals, *no.* (%)	45 (10)	74 (16)	139 (29)	209 (45)	467 (100)

eight (13%), and 76% to 100% in 42 (69%) (Table 2). Of the total 467 five-millimetre sections of coronary artery examined histologically in the 10 patients, only 45 sections (10%) were narrowed less than 26% in cross-sectional area by atherosclerotic plaque; 74 (16%) were narrowed 26% to 50%; 139 (29%), 51% to 75%, and 209 (45%), 76% to 100% (Table 3).

As shown in Figure 1, no significant differences in degrees of cross-sectional area narrowing of more than 75% or 51% to 75% by atherosclerotic plaque were observed between the proximal and distal parts of the left anterior-descending, left circumflex, and right coronary arteries in the 10 patients studied.

The number of major coronary arteries or their proximal and distal subdivisions in which the degree of luminal narrowing was significantly underestimated by one or more angiographers is summarized in Table 2. In all 10 patients, a significant narrowing in at least one coronary artery was underestimated by one or more angiographers. Of the 61 major coronary arteries or their proximal and distal subdivisions analyzed, no *overestimations* of the degree of luminal narrowing were made. Furthermore, of the 11 major coronary arteries or their subdivisions narrowed histologically by 50% or less in cross-sectional area, there was a perfect correlation between the degree of narrowing by angiography and that by histology. Of the eight major coronary arteries or their subdivisions that were narrowed by atherosclerotic plaque 51% to 75% in cross-sectional area by histology, however, *underestimation* of the degree of luminal narrowing by one or more angiographers occurred in seven. Of the 42 coronary arteries or their subdivisions 76% to 100% narrowed in cross-sectional area histologically, underestimation by one or more angiographers of the degree of luminal narrowing by angiography occurred in 17. The degree of narrowing was most often underestimated in the left main and proximal left circumflex coronary arteries (Table 2 and 4). The actual degrees of narrowing by angiography and by histology in the 24 coronary arteries or their proximal and distal subdivisions in which errors were made in the degrees of narrowing by angiography and by histology are shown in Table 4. Of the 24 coronary arteries or their subdivisions in which underestimations of the degrees of narrowing were made angiographically, two angiographers erred in nine, and in three arteries or their subdivisions all three angiographers underestimated the degrees of coronary narrowing.

Comments

At least five previously reported studies have compared the degree of coronary arterial luminal narrowing measured by selective coronary cineangiography with that observed at necropsy, and the results have varied widely (4-8). Kemp and associates (4) compared angiographic and postmortem findings in 131 major coronary arteries in 29 patients and concluded that, although the degree of narrowing had been underestimated by angiography in 16 coronary arteries, the degree of underestimation was functionally significant in only three. Vlodaver and associates (5) compared angiographic to necropsy narrowing in 134 coronary arterial segments and found that the degree of luminal narrowing had been significantly underestimated in 44 (33%) of the coronary segments. Grondin and associates (6) compared the angiographic and necropsy findings in 23 patients who died after coronary bypass operations and within 30 days of selective coronary cineangiography: In nine coronary arterial narrowings had been significantly underestimated, and in four of them they had resulted in incomplete myocardial revascularization at operation. Schwartz and associates (7) compared angiographic to necropsy narrowing in 226 coronary segments and found that the degree of narrowing had been significantly underestimated in 34 (15%). Hutchins and associates (8) compared the degree of luminal narrowing in live patients by selective cineangiograms to the degree observed by postmortem angiograms of the coronary arteries of 28 patients who died after cardiac operations. By this method they found that in only 15 (5%) of the 315 coronary arterial segments compared did the cineangiogram underestimate the de-

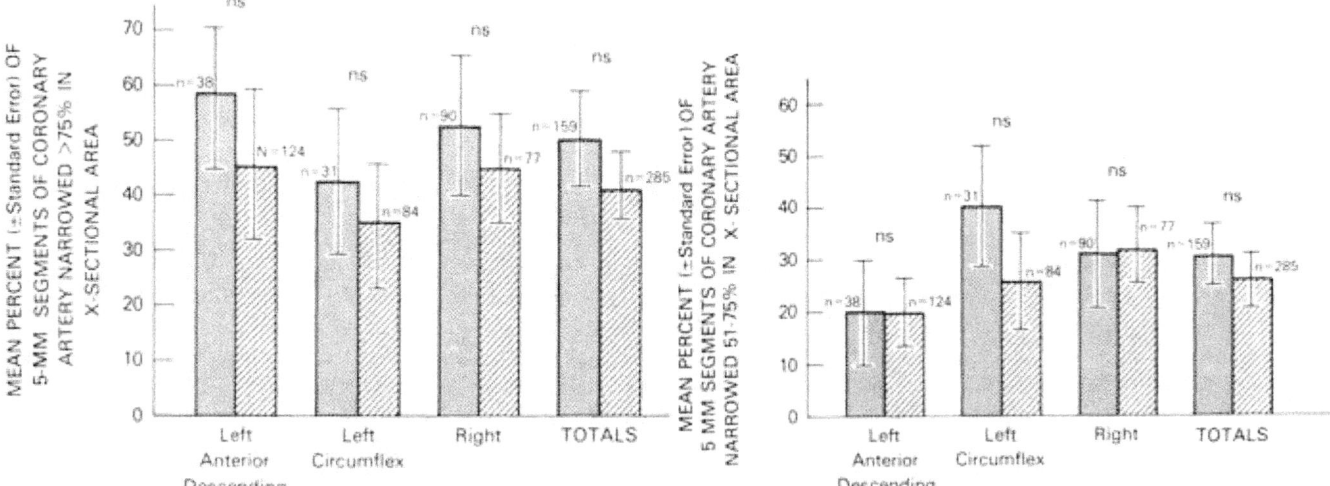

Figure 1. Comparison of the mean percent of 5-mm segments of proximal and distal parts of left anterior-descending, left circumflex, and right coronary arteries narrowed 76% to 100% *(left)* and 51% to 75% *(right)* in cross-sectional area by atherosclerotic plaque in the 10 patients. No significant *(ns)* differences are apparent. X-sectional = cross-sectional; ▨ = proximal, ▨ = distal.

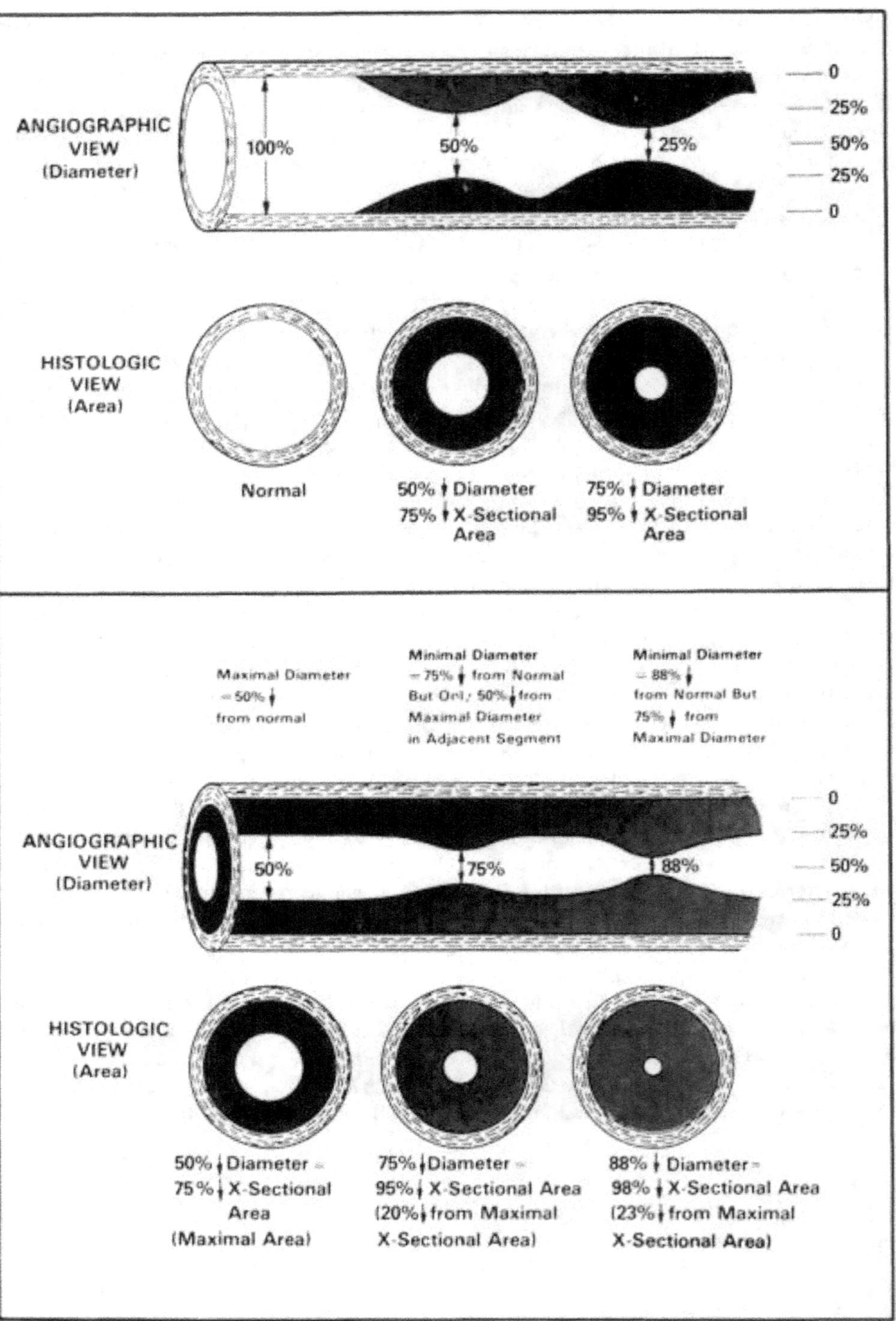

Figure 2. Diagrammatic representation of the relation between longitudinal narrowing (diameter reduction) as seen by coronary angiography and cross-sectional area narrowing as seen by histologic examination of a coronary artery. A coronary arterial segment with a 50% longitudinal width narrowing has a 75% reduction in cross-sectional area. A 75% reduction in longitudinal width corresponds to a 95% reduction in cross-sectional area. The theoretic situation whereby a narrowing is compared with an adjacent perfectly normal segment of artery is shown *above* and the usual real situation is shown *below*. The least-narrowed segment below has a 50% reduction in longitudinal width (= 75% loss of cross-sectional area) and a central-round residual lumen. Because the angiogram is a luminogram and the width of the original arterial lumen is unknown, the least-narrowed segment is often presumed to be normal. The width of more-narrowed segments are compared with that of the least-narrowed, but, nevertheless, narrowed segment. If the least-narrowed segment is itself 50% narrowed, what appears to be a 50% narrowing in an adjacent segment, in fact, is a 75% longitudinal narrowing (= 95% reduction in cross-sectional area); what appears to be a 75% narrowing in an adjacent segment is, in fact, an 88% longitudinal narrowing (= 98% reduction in cross-sectional area).

gree of narrowing by more than 50%. Thus, although each of these five studies, involving a total of 115 patients, showed that coronary cineangiography missed significant coronary arterial narrowings, the frequency of angiographically missed narrowings varied considerably.

Our study shows that selective coronary cineangiography frequently fails to show severe coronary arterial luminal narrowing or greatly underestimates the degree of narrowing. Of 61 coronary arteries or their proximal and distal subdivisions compared angiographically and histologically, at least one of the three angiographers missed a narrowing of more than 75% in cross-sectional area in 17 of 42 segments, and of eight segments narrowed 51% to 75% in cross-sectional area, seven were missed by one or more angiographers. Of the 10 patients studied, all had narrowings missed by at least one angiographer, and in four of the 10, more than one significant (> 75% cross-sectional area) narrowing was missed. Thus, although selective coronary cineangiography is at present the only method for ascertaining their presence, narrowings frequently are missed by this method.

Our study differs from previous studies both in the manner in which the coronary cineangiograms were reviewed and the manner in which the coronary arteries

Table 4. Coronary Arteries Including Their Proximal and Distal Subdivisions Showing Lack of Correlation (Underestimates) by Histologic Degrees of Narrowing

Patient (Number from Table 1)	Autopsy Number	Coronary Artery Involved*	Number of Three Angiographers Making Mistake	Angiographic Narrowing (Diameter Reduction)		
				Angiographic Reader		
				1	2	3
1	A74-212	Left Main	3	0 to 25	26 to 50	0 to 25
		Left Marginal	2	26 to 50	51 to 75	0 to 25
		Proximal LAD	1	> 75	> 75	< 25
		Distal LAD	1	0 to 25	> 75	51 to 75
		Proximal LC	1	> 75	> 75	0 to 25
		Distal LC	1	> 75	> 75	0 to 25
2	A75-123	Left Main	1	0 to 25	26 to 51	51 to 75
		Left Marginal	1	51 to 71	> 75	< 25
3	A74-266	Proximal R	1	26 to 50	51 to 75	> 75
		Distal R	1	0 to 25	> 75	51 to 75
4	A75-208	Left Main	3	0 to 25	0 to 25	0 to 25
		Proximal LC	1	26 to 50	51 to 75	0 to 25
5	A75-29	Distal LAD	3	0 to 25	0 to 25	0 to 25
		Distal LC	2	0 to 25	0 to 25	> 75
		Left Marginal	2	26 to 50	26 to 50	51 to 75
6	A72-208	Left Main	1	51 to 75	51 to 75	0 to 25
		Proximal LC	1	0 to 25	26 to 50	51 to 75
7	A72-105	Left Main	2	0 to 25	0 to 25	26 to 50
		Distal LAD	1	0 to 25	0 to 25	51 to 75
8	A74-245	Proximal LC	2	0 to 25	51 to 75	0 to 25
9	A75-109	Proximal R	2	0 to 25	0 to 25	51 to 75
		Proximal LC	2	0 to 25	51 to 75	26 to 50
10	A75-124	Distal LAD	2	0 to 25	26 to 50	51 to 75
		Distal R	1	51 to 75	26 to 50	51 to 75

Totals, *no.* (%)

* LAD = left anterior descending, LC = left circumflex, R = right.
† For the long coronary subdivision, the length of the severe narrowing was 1.5 cm or greater. When less than 1.5 cm of coronary artery was examined, all 5-mm segments were severely narrowed.

were examined at necropsy. Because observer variability is a major factor in the interpretation of coronary cineangiograms (9-11), it contributes significantly to the accuracy of this method compared with necropsy observations. For this reason, each of our three experienced angiographers independently assessed the degree of longitudinal luminal narrowing (diameter reduction) in each major coronary artery or its proximal and distal subdivisions in which serial histologic sections were available. Thus, unlike previous studies in which the degree of coronary arterial narrowing by angiography was ascertained by consensus among the angiographers, our study incorporated observer variability as a factor influencing accuracy of the method. Using this approach, we were able to find out how often one or more angiographers significantly underestimated the degree of narrowing in each of the 61 coronary arteries or their proximal and distal subdivisions analyzed.

Also different from previous studies in which the degree of coronary arterial narrowing at necropsy was ascertained only by gross examination or by postmortem coronary angiography, our study involved examination of the entire extramural coronary arterial tree by serial histologic sections prepared with special stains to show the location of the elastic laminae. Only when the location of the internal elastic laminae, and thus the boundary of the original coronary arterial lumen, is known can the degree of luminal narrowing caused by atherosclerotic plaque be accurately measured. Thus, gross examination of the transected coronary arteries provides at best only a semiquantitative measure of the degree of luminal narrowing.

Postmortem coronary angiograms have never been found to accurately show the degree of coronary arterial narrowing. Gray and associates (12) in 1962 compared the degree of coronary arterial narrowing seen by postmortem coronary angiograms to the degree found by serial histologic sections of the coronary arteries in 13 autopsied patients. In 36 of the 44 coronary arterial segments

Eccentric Lumen	Diffuse Narrowing†	Number of 5-mm Segments Narrowed to Various Degrees in Cross-Sectional Area at Necropsy by Atherosclerotic Plaque				Patient (Number from Table 1)
		0 to 25%	26% to 50%	51% to 75%	76% to 100%	
+	+	0	0	0	3	1
+ +	0	0	2	8	3	
+	+	0	0	0	4	
0	+	1	1	3	24	
+ +	+	0	0	1	3	
+ +	+	2	2	6	6	
0	+	0	0	2	0	2
+	+	0	0	0	7	
+ +	0	0	1	2	1	3
+	0	0	4	4	1	
0	+	0	0	3	0	4
+	+	0	0	2	0	
+ +	+	0	0	1	10	5
+ +	+	0	0	1	4	
+ +	0	0	0	2	2	
0	+	0	0	0	3	6
+ +	+	0	0	3	0	
0	+	0	0	4	0	7
+	0	7	4	1	0	
0	0	0	1	1	0	8
+ +	+	0	0	3	0	9
+ +	0	0	1	2	1	
+ +	0	0	0	5	3	10
0	0	0	8	10	2	
		10 (6)	24 (14)	64 (36)	77 (44)	Totals, *no.* (%)

narrowed more than 33% of their original area, the postmortem angiogram underestimated the degree of narrowing, and in 20 of the 36 the degree of underestimation was severe. Eusterman and associates (13) compared the degree of luminal narrowing in 479 coronary arterial segments from 50 hearts by postmortem angiogram to the degree found by gross examination. In 73 segments of coronary artery with nonfocal (that is, > 5-mm long) luminal narrowings of more than 50%, the postmortem angiogram underestimated the degree of luminal narrowing in 53 (73%). In 42% of the segments with nonfocal narrowings and in 74% of the segments with focal narrowings in which the postmortem arteriogram had underestimated the degree of narrowing, the error was more than 50%. Thus, the postmortem coronary angiogram seems to grossly underestimate the degree of coronary arterial narrowing, especially when the degree of luminal narrowing is severe, and when the narrowing is produced by a focal lesion.

Because the angiogram is a luminogram, degrees of segmental narrowing are ascertained by comparison with less-narrowed adjacent segments that are presumed to be normal (Figure 2). Coronary atherosclerosis, at least in patients with symptomatic coronary heart disease examined in this study, however, was diffuse, and no truly normal segments of coronary artery were available to compare with the more-severely narrowed segments. Indeed as shown in Table 3, only 45 (10%) of 467 five-millimetre segments of coronary artery examined in our 10 patients were narrowed 25% or less in cross-sectional area, and none of them were entirely normal. The least-narrowed segment, which is presumed to be normal, may itself be considerably narrowed. The result is often that narrowed segments are compared with adjacent less-narrowed but, nevertheless, narrowed segments, and maximal degrees of narrowing are significantly underestimated (Figure 2). If the least-narrowed segment of a coronary artery is in fact 50% narrowed in longitudinal width, an adjacent segment that appears angiographically to be 50% narrowed in width is in fact 75% narrowed. An area that appears to be 75% narrowed in width is in fact 88% narrowed in width. The 75% longitudinal narrowing that appears angiographically to be 50% narrowed results in a 95% obliteration of cross-sectional area. The 88% longitudinal narrowing that appears to be a 75% narrowing results in 98% obliteration of cross-sectional area.

Another problem in interpretation of a coronary angiogram is that the coronary narrowings occupy a small area of the frame. One of the rules of photography is that the subject of interest, in this case a coronary narrowing, should occupy 85% of the frame. Obviously, this ideal situation is not possible with coronary angiography. The actual narrowing may occupy less than 1% of the frame. In contrast, a cross-sectional area photomicrograph of a section of coronary artery can occupy most of the frame of the photograph, and, consequently, the accuracy of the measurement of the degree of cross-sectional area narrowing is very accurate.

Coronary atherosclerosis in the 10 patients with coronary heart disease studied here not only was diffuse (Table 3), but the surfaces of the plaques were irregular and the shapes and positions of the residual lumens were quite variable. Vlodaver and Edwards (14) studied the shapes and positions of the residual lumens in 200 coronary arteries from patients with severe coronary atherosclerosis. In only 30% of the *gross* sections studied were the residual lumens central in location; in 69% the lumens were eccentric and in 29% the eccentric lumens were slitlike. Of our 10 patients, eccentric lumens were found in 17 of the 24 coronary arteries or their proximal and distal subdivisions in which there was a lack of correlation, that is, more than a 25% difference, between the degree of narrowing measured angiographically and that found histologically. Herein is a second major problem with angiography. Unless a coronary artery is viewed in more than one projection, the degree narrowing in any segment with a nonround residual lumen may be greatly underestimated. Although why the coronary cineangiogram had failed to show an area of severe luminal narrowing is not always certain, the presence of diffuse atherosclerosis seems to account for most of the angiographically missed narrowings in our patients.

▶ Requests for reprints should be addressed to William C. Roberts, M.D.; Building 10A, Room 3E30; National Institutes of Health; Bethesda, MD 20205.

Received 7 March 1979; revision accepted 13 June 1979.

References

1. CONTI CR. Coronary arteriography. *Circulation.* 1977;**55**:227-37.
2. BRISTOW JD, BURCHELL HB, CAMPBELL RW, et al. Report of the Ad Hoc Committee on the indications for coronary arteriography: prepared by the Council on Clinical Cardiology of the American Heart Association. *Circulation.* 1977;**55**:969-74A.
3. PICHARD A. Coronary arteriography for everyone? *Am J Cardiol.* 1976;**38**:533-5.
4. KEMP HG, EVANS H. ELLIOTT WC, GORLIN R. Diagnostic accuracy of selective coronary cinearteriography. *Circulation.* 1967;**36**:526-33.
5. VLODAVER Z, FRECH R, VAN TASSEL RA, EDWARDS JE. Correlation of the antemortem coronary anteriogram and the postmortem specimen. *Circulation.* 1973;**47**:162-9.
6. GRONDIN CM, DYRDA I, PASTERNAC A, CAMPEAU L. BOURASSA MG, LESPERANCE J. Discrepancies between cineangiographic and postmortem findings in patients with coronary artery disease and recent myocardial revascularization. *Circulation.* 1974;**49**:703-8.
7. SCHWARTZ JN, KONG Y, HACKEL DB, BARTEL AG. Comparison of angiographic and postmortem finds in patients with coronary artery disease. *Am J Cardiol.* 1975;**36**:174-8.
8. HUTCHINS GM, BULKLEY GH, RIDOLFI RL, GRIFFITH LSC, LOHR FT, PIASIO MA. Correlation of coronary arteriograms and left ventriculograms with postmortem studies. *Circulation.* 1977;**56**:32-7.
9. DETRE KM, WRIGHT E, MURPHY ML, TAKARO T. Observer agreement in evaluating coronary angiograms. *Circulation.* 1975;**52**:979-86.
10. ZIR LM, MILLER SW, DINSMORE RE, GILBERT JP, HARTHORNE JW. Interobserver variability in coronary angiography. *Circulation.* 1976;**53**:627-32.
11. DEROUEN TA, MURRAY JA, OWEN W. Variability in the analysis of coronary arteriograms. *Circulation.* 1977;**55**:324-8.
12. GRAY CR, HOFFMAN HA, HAMMOND WS, MILLER KL, OSEASOHN RO. Correlation of arteriographic and pathologic findings in the coronary arteries in man. *Circulation.* 1962;**26**:494-9.
13. EUSTERMAN JH, ACHOR RWP, KINCAID OW, BROWN AL JR. Atherosclerotic disease of the coronary arteries: a pathologic-radiologic correlative study. *Circulation.* 1962;**26**:1288-95.
14. VLODAVER Z, EDWARDS JE. Pathology of coronary atherosclerosis. *Prog Cardiovasc Dis.* 1971;**14**:256-74.

Thrombocytosis, Coronary Thrombosis and Acute Myocardial Infarction

RENU VIRMANI, M.D.
MARK A. POPOVSKY, M.D.
WILLIAM C. ROBERTS, M.D.
Bethesda, Maryland

From the Pathology Branch, National Heart, Lung, and Blood Institute, The Medical Neurology Branch, National Institute of Neurological and Communicative Disorders and Stroke and the Laboratory of Pathology, National Cancer Institute, National Institutes of Health, Bethesda, Maryland. Requests for reprints should be addressed to Dr. William C. Roberts, Building 10A, Room 3E-30, National Institutes of Health, Bethesda, Maryland 20205. Manuscript accepted January 4, 1979.

Clinical and morphologic findings are described in a 22 year old man with prolonged thrombocytosis, and coronary and splenic arterial thrombi causing myocardial and splenic infarcts. The absence of preexistent extensive coronary atherosclerosis, the presence of thrombus in more than one epicardial artery and in multiple intramural coronary arteries, the presence of arterial thrombosis in a noncoronary artery (splenic) and the absence of another apparent cause of the arterial thromboses are evidences that the intraarterial clotting in this patient was related to the severe thrombocytosis. A review of the reported cases of vascular occlusion associated with thrombocytosis indicates that thrombi have infrequently been confirmed as the mechanism of the vascular occlusion. Although the frequency of vascular thrombi in patients with thrombocytosis has not been established, it is clear that vascular thrombosis can be a consequence of thrombocytosis and, as demonstrated by the present patient, that the coronary artery may be the site of the vascular occlusion, a heretofore unconfirmed event.

Much interest has focused recently on the role of platelets in causing arterial thrombosis and atherosclerosis. Although evidence is lacking that antiplatelet agents, such as aspirin, are effective in preventing or delaying the onset of acute myocardial infarction or other manifestations of coronary heart disease, these agents may be effective in preventing recurrences of transient ischemic attacks [1]. Despite the enormous interest in platelets and their relationship to thrombosis, surprisingly few patients have been described in whom the evidence was convincing that thrombosis was produced by thrombocytosis. Indeed, few patients have been described in whom thrombocytosis was considered the cause of a vascular occlusion which was confirmed to be a thrombus. In this report we describe clinical and necropsy findings in a young man who had prolonged thrombocytosis, and coronary and splenic arterial thrombi, causing myocardial and splenic infarcts, and analyze the reported cases in which vascular occlusion was attributed to thrombocytosis.

CASE REPORT

A 22 year old white man (12-68-78-8), who died on June 6, 1978, had been well until about July 15, 1977 (12 months before death), when, while a student at college, he noted weakness in both legs, especially when climbing stairs. The weakness progressed to involve the arms, and paresthesias appeared in his feet, hands and arms. On August 29, 1977, six weeks after the initial onset of symp-

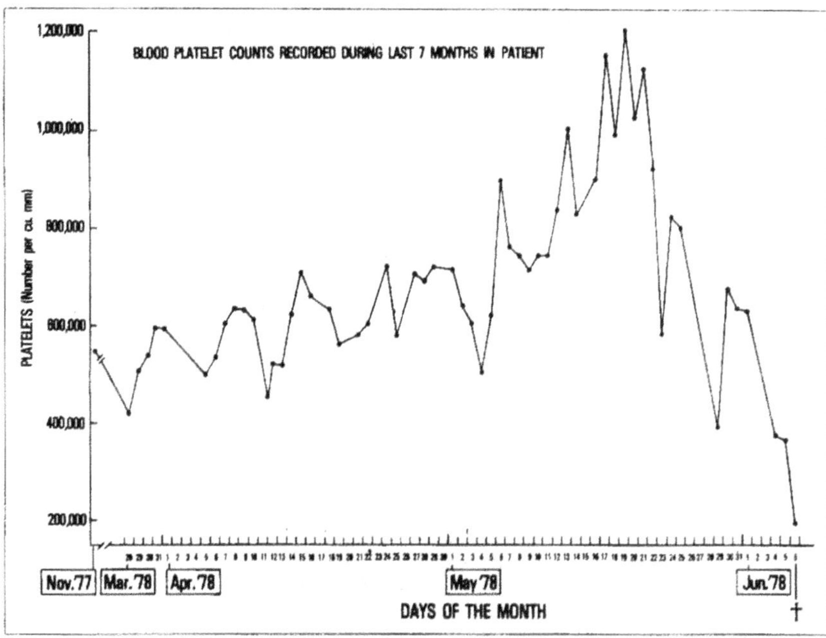

Figure 1. Blood platelet counts recorded in the patient described.

toms, he was hospitalized. The deep tendon reflexes were absent, and the sensory responses in the limbs were markedly reduced. The cerebrospinal fluid protein level was 149 mg/dl with a cell count of 2 cells/mm³; all cells were lymphocytes. The weakness, atrophy, tone and sensation in both arms and legs worsened and became so severe that he was unable to walk. On November 19, 1977, he was rehospitalized. The blood platelet count was 544,000/mm **(Figure 1)**. He was given a total of 7,250 mg of prednisone, or its equivalent, and 1000 U of ACTH during his last 10 months of life without apparent benefit or clinical manifestation of overdose.

Because of progression of his condition to quadriplegia, he was admitted to the National Institute of Neurological and Communicative Disorders and Stroke on March 21, 1978. The limb muscles were severely atrophied. The mental responses were normal as were the test results of cranial nerve function. The blood hematocrit value was 54 per cent (later it decreased to 29 per cent); white blood cell count, 11,500/mm³; platelet count, 466,000/mm³ (Figure 1) and erythrocytic sedimentation rate, 4 mm in 1 hour. The blood glucose was 102 mg/dl; total serum cholesterol, 145 mg/dl; triglyceride, 235 mg/dl; serum total proteins, 5.3 g/dl and serum albumin, 3.0 g/dl. Quantitative immunoglobulins were normal and Bence Jones proteins were absent. Initial chest roentgenogram and electrocardiogram **(Figure 2)** disclosed no abnormalities.

The patient's condition remained unchanged until May 13, 1978, when he complained of abdominal pain. Roentgenograms at that time disclosed multiple areas of increased density in the ileum of the pelvis and in the sacrum. Bone marrow aspiration of the right iliac crest on May 15, 1978, yielded numerous immature and mature plasma cells. The serum total protein was 4.6 with albumin 2.0 g/dl. The serum electrophoretic pattern was normal, and no Bence Jones proteins were detected in the urine. An electrocardiogram on May 22

and May 30 disclosed ischemic changes (Figure 2). The patient's last six days were characterized by evidences of progressively diminishing cardiac output with fluid retention and dyspnea. His weight increased from 72 to 80 kg during his last two months. Also during his hospitalization, the blood pressure, recorded daily, ranged from 90 to 140 mm Hg, systolic, and 64 to 88 mm Hg, diastolic. He was mentally alert to the end and never at any time complained of chest pain.

At necropsy (A78-89), there was 4+/4+ subcutaneous edema. An estimated 500 ml of serous fluid was present in the peritoneal cavity, about 500 ml in each pleural cavity and 180 ml in the pericardial cavity. Grossly, the brain and spinal cord were within normal limits. Histologic study of several branches of the lumbosacral plexus and peripheral nerves disclosed focal absence of myelin and foci of mononuclear cells. Large collections of mature and immature plasma cells, surrounded by sclerotic bone, were found in the ileal and sacral bones but not in any other organ or tissue. These plasma cells stained for immunoglobulin A (IgA) heavy chain and lambda light chain. Megakaryocytes were present in increased numbers in the bone marrow.

A transmural acute and organizing infarct was present in the posterior wall of the left ventricle, involving portions of both apical and basal halves **(Figure 3)**. Histologic study of the myocardial infarct disclosed areas of coagulative necrosis in varying stages of organization (Figure 3). No polymorphonuclear leukocytes were observed in the infarcted area. The major epicardial coronary arteries were excised intact from the heart (weight = 295 g) and cut into 5 mm long segments by a method described elsewhere [2]. Histologic sections from a total of 101 segments (5 mm) of epicardial coronary artery were examined, and the numbers of segments narrowed to various degrees in cross sectional area by atherosclerotic plaques are summarized in **Table I.** Fibrin deposits were found in 20 (20

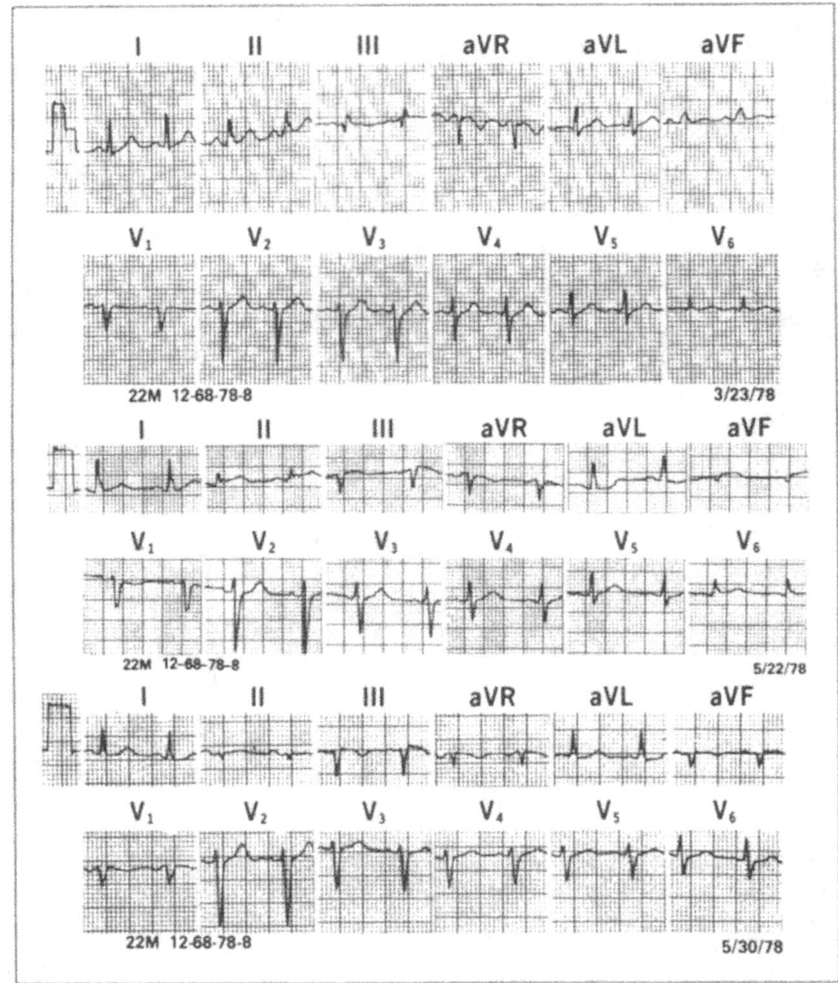

Figure 2. Three electrocardiograms recorded in patient described who died on June 6, 1978. The changes in the electrocardiograms recorded on May 22, 1978, and May 30, 1978, indicate posterior wall, left ventricular damage.

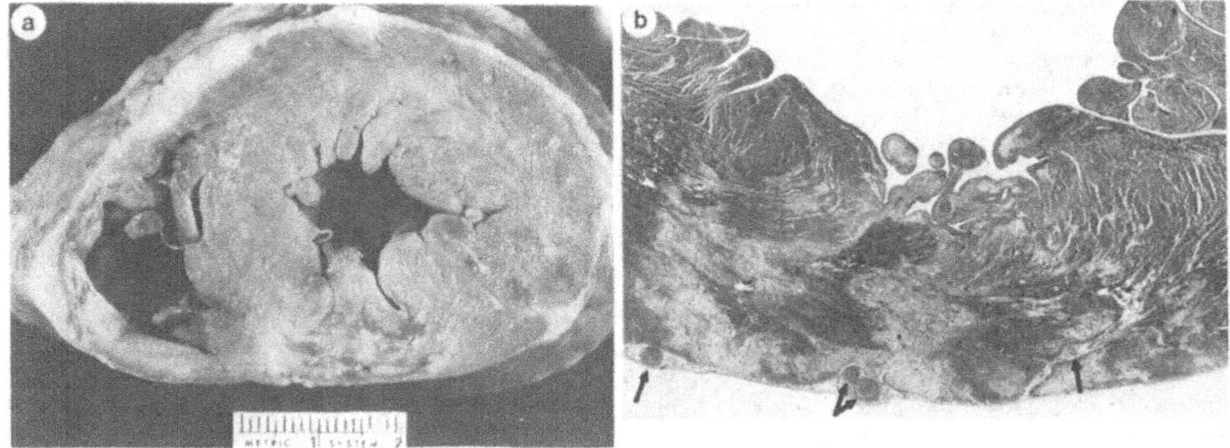

Figure 3. Heart of the patient described. **a,** Transverse slice of the cardiac ventricles disclosing an acute transmural posterior wall infarct. **b,** photomicrograph of area of myocardial necrosis. The arrows designate small coronary arteries occluded by thromboembolic material. Hematoxylin and eosin stain; magnification X 4, reduced by 25 per cent.

TABLE I **Number of 5 mm Long Segments of the Epicardial Coronary Arteries Showing Various Degrees of Cross Sectional Area Luminal Narrowing and Number with Fibrin Deposits in the Patient Described**

Coronary Artery	No. of 5 mm Segments	No. of 5 mm Segments Showing Per Cent of X-Sectional Area Narrowing by Atherosclerotic Plaque				Fibrin in Coronary Arteries				
						In Lumens Only Occlu-sive	Mural	Incorpor-ated in Plaque	In Both Lumen and in Plaque Occlusive	Mural
		0–25	26–50	51–75	76–100					
Right	27	3	15	8	1	1	2	4	1	4
Left main	2	0	1	1	0	0	0	0	0	0
Left anterior descending	20	9	7	4	0	0	0	0	0	0
Left circumflex	7	4	0	3	0	0	0	0	0	0
Right obtuse marginal	6	5	1	0	0	0	0	0	0	0
Left obtuse marginal	11	1	6	3	1	0	0	1	0	0
Left diagonal	8	5	3	0	0	0	0	0	0	0
Posterior descending*	20	19	1	0	0	0	0	0	4	3
Totals	101	46	34	19	2	1	2	5	5	7
		(45)†	(34)	(19)	(2)			20 (20)		

* Includes several branches, all of which arose from the right coronary artery after it passed the crux.
† Figures in parentheses are per cents.

per cent) of these 101 coronary arterial segments (**Figures 4 and 5**, and Table I). Many *intramural* coronary arteries in the posterior left ventricular wall in the area of the myocardial infarct were obstructed by thromboembolic material which was in varying stages of organization (Figure 5). The atrial septum was intact. Thromboembolic material also was present in several small intrapulmonary pulmonary arteries, but no pulmonary infarcts were present. Multiple intrasplenic splenic arteries were occluded by thromboembolic material with resulting infarcts (**Figure 6**). The spleen weighed 650 g. The liver weighed, 2,700 g. Histologically, it was virtually normal.

COMMENTS

The patient we describe had a rare form (about 3 per cent of cases [3–6]) of multiple myeloma (osteoblastic, nonsecretory type with polyneuropathy) and, in addition, had thrombocytosis (for at least seven months) with occlusions by thromboembolic material of several arteries, including coronary, splenic and pulmonary, causing large myocardial and splenic infarcts. The occurrence of multiple arterial thromboses in our young (22 year old) patient when he had marked thrombocytosis suggests that the thrombocytosis initiated the intraarterial clotting. At least seven factors support the view that severe thrombocytosis can cause vascular thrombosis: (1) a number of cases have been reported in which the patients had thrombocytosis and vascular occlusion [7–29]; (2) in a few (namely, six [8,19,23,26,27] reported cases of vascular occlusion and thrombocytosis), thrombosis has been documented anatomically to be the cause of the occlusion; (3) in cases of thrombocytosis and vascular occlusion, more than one vessel frequently (33 per cent) has been confirmed to be the site of thrombosis [7,8,10,11,14–23,25–29]; (4) in a few cases

of thrombocytosis and vascular thrombosis, no significant underlying disease in the vascular wall was demonstrated [8,26,27]; (5) in several cases of vascular occlusions associated with thrombocytosis, symptoms or signs of organ ischemia have disappeared and not recurred after institution of antithrombogenic drug therapy [9,10,14–16,18–22,26–28]; (6) in several cases of thrombocytosis and vascular thrombosis studied in detail, causes of vascular occlusion other than thrombocytosis have been lacking [8,19,23,26,27], and (7) blood withdrawn into citrated syringes or tubes from patients with or without thrombocytosis may contain aggregates of platelets, and aggregates of platelets have been shown to produce vascular thromboses [28,30–32].

At least 96 patients have been described previously in whom one or more vascular occlusions of sudden onset were associated with thrombocytosis (**Table II**) [7–29]: in 61 of the 96 patients, the ages were stated: they ranged from 24 to 81 years (average 54 years); 50 (82 per cent) were more than 40 years old and 11 (18 per cent) were 40 or less; 17 (28 per cent) were more than 65 years of age and only three (5 per cent) were 30 or less. Although vascular obstruction was demonstrated in all 96 patients, evidence that the obstruction was the result of thrombus (or embolus) was provided grossly (either at operation or necropsy) in only 15 (16 per cent) patients, and in only six of them was the thrombus confirmed by histologic examination. Although little or no underlying arterial disease appears to be a near prerequisite for attributing the etiology of a vascular occlusion, i.e., a thrombus (or embolus), to a thrombocytosis, in only three of the 96 previously described patients with thrombocytosis and arterial occlusion without underlying disease has this been reported [8,26,27]. Although our patient had slightly more coronary arterial atherosclerosis than

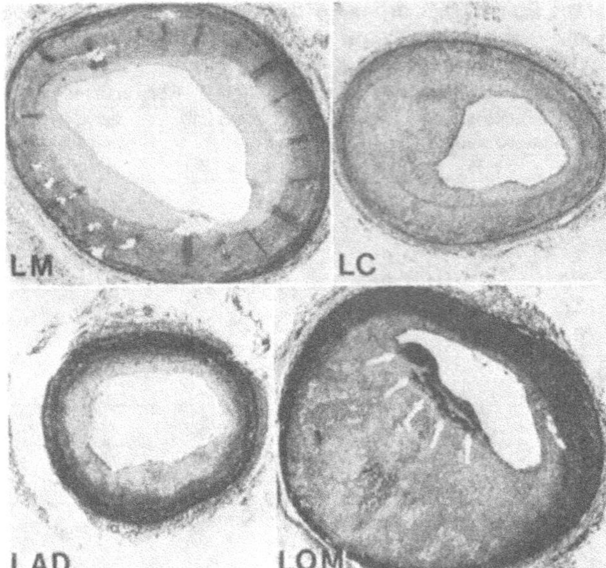

Figure 4. Major epicardial left coronary arteries in the patient at sites of maximal luminal narrowing by atherosclerotic plaque. Fibrin material (arrows) is present within the plaque in the left obtuse marginal (LOM) coronary artery. LM = left main; LC = left circumflex; LAD = left anterior descending. Movat stains; magnification × 20 (LM, LC and LAD); and × 27 (LOM), reduced by 31 per cent.

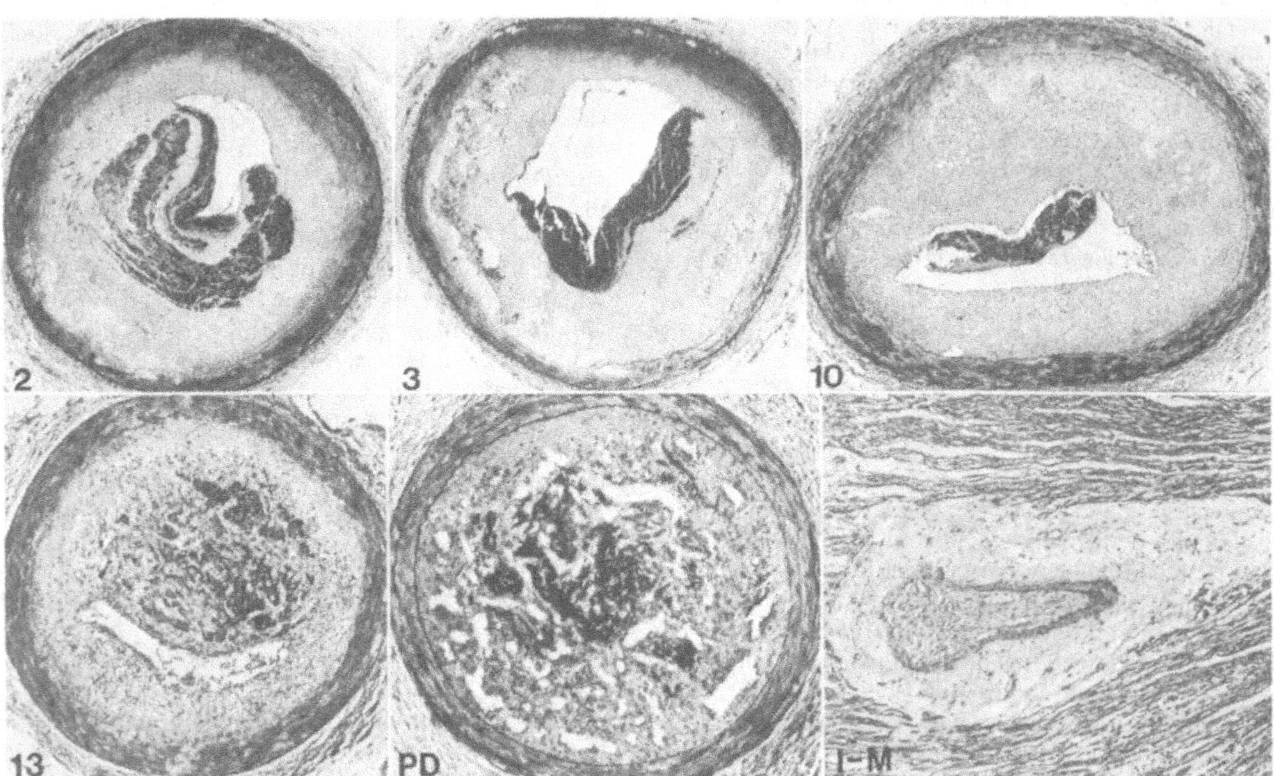

Figure 5. Right (2,3,10,13), posterior descending (PD) and an intramural (I-M) coronary artery of a patient demonstrating fibrin thrombi (dark staining material) in each of the extramural arteries and recanalized channels in obliterative connective tissue in the intramural artery. The fibrin in 3 and 10 is entirely or mainly within the lumen, whereas in 13 and PD the fibrin is incorporated in the plaque. Evidence of organization of the fibrin is evident in 13 and PD. Possibly, some or much of the plaque in all these sections is the result of organization of thrombi. Movat stains (2,3,10,PD) and hematoxylin and eosin stain (13 and IM): magnification × 25 (2,3), × 40 (10), × 80 (13), × 120 (PD) and × 100 (I-M), reduced by 31 per cent.

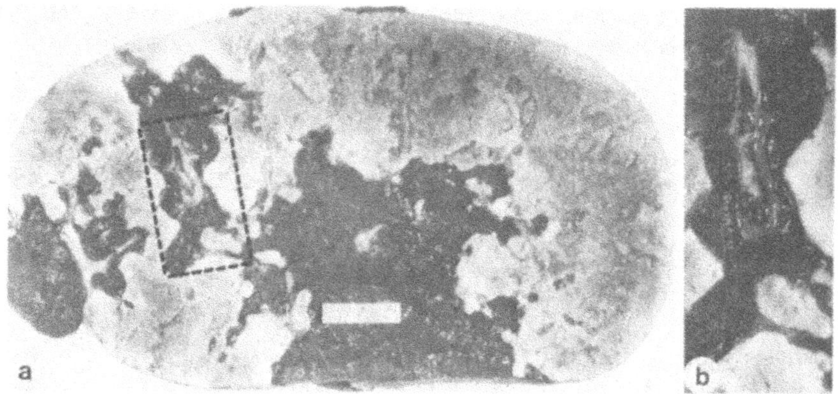

Figure 6. Spleen in patient demonstrating extensive infarction. A close-up of the area within the brackets in **a** is shown in **b**. The intrasplenic artery is totally obstructed by thromboembolic material.

TABLE II   Observations in Reported Cases of Vascular Occlusion and Thrombocytosis ($>$400,000/mm^3)

References	Year of Publication	No. Patients with Thrombocytosis	No. Patients with Vascular Occlusion	Method of Documentation of Vascular Occlusion				No. of Patients with Single or Multiple Vessel(s) Occluded	
				Clinical	Angio	Surg	Necropsy	One	Multiple
Slater, Sherlock [7]	1951	33	3	3	0	0	0	1	2
CPC [8]	1962	1*	1*	0	0	0	1[†]	0	1
Hayes et al. [9]	1963	3	2	2	0	0	0	2	0
Bull et al. [10]	1965	2*	2*	0	0	1	1	1	1
Hirsh, Dacie [11]	1966	25	5	3	0	0	2	2	3
McClure et al. [12]	1966	32	8	8	0	0	0	8	0
Silverstein [13]	1967	15	4	4	0	0	0	3	1
Levine, Swanson [14]	1968	1*	1*	1	0	0	0	0	1
Korenman [15]	1969	7	5	5	0	0	0	4	1
Singer [16]	1969	1*	1*	0	0	1	0	0	1
Dawson, Ogston [17]	1970	17	13	10	0	0	3	11	2
Vreeken, Van Aken [18]	1971	1*	1*	1	0	0	0	0	1
Mundell et al. [19]	1972	1*	1*	0	0	1	0	0	1
Kimbiris et al. [20]	1972	1*	1*	1	0	0	0	1	0
Zucker, Mielke [21]	1972	17	5	5	0	0	0	0	5
Preston et al. [22]	1974	6*	6*	6	0	0	0	2	4
Balz, Minton [23]	1975	2*	2*	0	0	1	1	1	1
Coltheart, Little [24]	1976	47	12	12	0	0	0	12	0
Walsh et al. [25]	1977	22	2	2	0	0	0	1	1
Singh, Wetherley-Mein [26]	1977	27	9	8	0	1	0	8	1
Ehrenfeld et al. [27]	1977	1*	1*	0	0	0	1	0	1
Kun-Yu Wu [28]	1978	39	7	4	3	0	0	4	3
Boxer et al. [29]	1978	239	9	0	8	1	0	7	2
Totals		540	101 (19)[‡]	75 (74)	11 (11)	6 (6)	9 (9)	68 (67)	33 (33)
				101 (100)				101 (100)	

NOTE: Angio = Angiography; Surg = Surgery. Figures in parentheses are per cents.
* Only patients with vascular occlusion with thrombocytosis included in these studies.
[†] Histologic confirmation of thrombus.
[‡] When the 17 patients included in the asterisked studies are excluded, the reported frequency is 16 per cent (84 of 523).

TABLE III   Number of 5 mm Long Segments of the Epicardial Coronary Arteries Showing Various Degrees of Cross Sectional Area Luminal Narrowing by Atherosclerotic Plaque in Control Subjects

Case No.	Autopsy Number	Age (yr) and sex	Cause of Death	No. of 5 mm Segments	No of 5 mm Segments showing % of Cross Sectional Area Narrowing by Atherosclerotic Plaque				Fibrin in Coronary Artery
					0–25	26–50	51–75	76–100	
1	DCMEO 77–852	22,M	Trauma	30	20	10	0	0	0
2	DCMEO 76-12-976	22,M	Trauma	48	12	30	6	0	0
3	A75-16	23,M	Cancer	32	18	13	1	0	0
4	A75-220	23,M	Cancer	58	3	55	0	0	0
5	A74-190	23,M	Cancer	54	54	0	0	0	0
6	A74-204	25,M	Cancer	45	15	19	10	1	0
7	A74-328	26,M	Cancer	27	23	4	0	0	0
	Totals	22–26,M (avg 23)		294*	145 (49)[†]	131 (44)	17 (6)	1 (<1)	0
[‡]A78–89		22,M	Myeloma	56*	16 (29)	23 (41)	16 (28)	1 (2)	12 (21)

* Includes only right, left main, left anterior descending and left circumflex coronary arteries.

[†] Figures in parentheses are per cents.

[‡] The subject of the present report.

was found in seven other men in their 20's who died of trauma or neoplasms (**Table III**), the amount of atherosclerotic plaquing was insignificant compared to that observed in the usual patient with fatal coronary heart disease [2]. Only 2 per cent of the 5 mm long segments of major coronary artery in our patient were more than 75 per cent narrowed in cross sectional area by atherosclerotic plaques, whereas this per cent was less than 1 in the seven control subjects (Table III). In contrast, in 26 patients with clinical evidence of acute fatal myocardial infarction studied in a similar manner, 36 per cent of the 5 mm segments of coronary artery were more 75 per cent narrowed in cross sectional area by atherosclerotic plaque [33]. It is clear that our patient did not have enough coronary atherosclerosis to cause, by itself, an acute myocardial infarction. The infarction in our patient was due to the thrombotic event alone. In the usual patient with coronary thrombosis and fatal acute myocardial infarction, the thrombus is superimposed on an old atherosclerotic plaque which in itself is responsible for severe luminal narrowing [2].

In most patients with sudden onset of symptoms or signs of vascular occlusion, only one vessel is involved. Involvement of more than one vessel, as in our patient, supports a systemic etiology, such as thrombocytosis. Of the 96 previously described patients with thrombocytosis and vascular occlusion, 68 (67 per cent) had only one vessel involved, and 33 (33 per cent) had more than one vessel occluded (Table II). Although both veins and arteries, located in most portions of the body, have been described to be occluded at one time or another, surprisingly, only four patients have been described as having symptoms of myocardial ischemia associated with thrombocytosis [13,20,26], and none have had coronary thrombosis documented anatomically as was the case in our patient. In one patient with symptomatic coronary heart disease and thrombocytosis, a 33 year old woman who had both angina pectoris and gangrenous toes, both the chest pain disappeared, and the color of the toes returned to normal after return of the platelet count to normal [26].

In the typical patient with fatal acute myocardial infarction which is apparent clinically (our patient never had symptoms of myocardial ischemia), coronary thrombus, if it occurs, usually is present in just one of the major epicardial coronary arteries [2]. In our patient, thrombus was present in two epicardial coronary arteries. Furthermore, in the typical patient with acute fatal myocardial infarction, a coronary thrombus, if it occurs, is short, i.e., usually less than 1 cm in length. In our patient, at least 6 cm of the right coronary artery was involved by the thrombotic process. In addition, thrombus was present in virtually all of the posterior descending coronary arteries, an occurrence extremely rare in the usual patient with acute myocardial infarction in whom the thrombus typically is present only in the proximal portion of a major coronary artery [2]. Moreover, the occurrence of clot in the lumen of an intramural coronary artery in the typical patient with fatal acute myocardial infarction is extremely rare except in the circumstance of embolism [2,34]. Our patient, however, had occlusions of multiple intramural coronary arteries by thromboembolic material. An embolic etiology in our patient, however, appears unlikely in view of the lack of a source for an embolus [34].

When vascular occlusion associated with thrombocytosis causes organ or limb ischemia, antithrombogenic or cytotoxic drugs, or both, have, in a number of patients, been associated with relief of the symptoms or signs due to the ischemia. In at least 37 reported cases of thrombocytosis and clinical evidence of organ or limb ischemia, institution of warfarin, heparin, aspirin or cytotoxic drug therapy has allowed relief of ischemic symptoms or signs [9,10,14-16,18-22,26-28]. In six of the 37 cases, near gangrene of one or more toes was present, and in each of the patients normal color returned to the affected toes after the administration of busulfan. In six additional reported cases in which symptoms or signs of limb or organ ischemia were associated with thrombocytosis, the features of ischemia again were reversed by the administration of antithrombogenic or cytotoxic drugs, but the evidences of ischemia recurred after withdrawal of the drugs [18,19,27,28]. Reinstitution of these drugs in each of these six cases, however, again was associated with loss of evidences of organ or limb ischemia, thus confirming the benefit of these drugs in patients with ischemia and thrombocytosis.

If excessive numbers of platelets are considered responsible for the vascular thrombosis in our patient, one might expect to find numerous platelets within the vascular thromboses. Such, however, was not the case in our patient or in any of the six previously described patients with vascular thrombosis (confirmed histologically) associated with thrombocytosis [8,19,23,26,27]. The reason may be that aggregates of platelets rapidly disappear and are replaced by fibrin [35].

To conclude that thrombocytosis is responsible for the vascular thrombosis in our patient, or in any other patient, other real or potential causes of vascular thrombosis must be excluded. Possibly because corticosteroids may exert their effect by causing thrombocytosis, the only other recognized potential or real cause of vascular thrombosis in our patient was corticosteroid treatment [36-41]. He received these drugs over a 10 month period, but during this period he never showed signs indicative of heavy corticosteroid treatment, such as weight gain (our patient lost weight except for the terminal fluid retention), moon face, buffalo hump, cutaneous striae, increase in blood pressure, elevation of serum cholesterol level or glucose intolerance. Although corticosteroid administration for longer than one year has been considered to be responsible for accelerated atherosclerosis in patients with systemic lupus erythematosus, those with considerable atherosclerosis all had clinical evidence of hyperadrenocorticism, increased heart weight and increased epicardial fat, none of which occurred in our patient [41]. Therefore, it appears most reasonable to believe that corticosteroid therapy was not a factor in causing the vascular thromboses in our patient. The actual cause of the thrombocytosis in our patient, however, remains unclear. The increased numbers of megakaryocytes in the bone marrow may represent either a neoplastic or a reactive process, secondary to either multiple myeloma [42,43] or to corticosteroid therapy [36].

REFERENCES

1. Fields WC, Lemak NA, Frankowski RF: Controlled trial of aspirin in cerebral ischemia. Stroke 8: 301, 1977.
2. Roberts WC, Buja LM: The frequency and significance of coronary arterial thrombi and other observations in fatal acute myocardial infarction. A study of 107 necropsy patients. Am J Med 52: 425, 1972.
3. Aguayo A, Thompson DW, Humphrey JG: Multiple myeloma with polyneuropathy and osteosclerotic lesions. J Neurol Neurosurg Pyschiat 27: 562, 1964.
4. Case Records of the Massachusetts General Hospital: Case 29-1972. N Engl J Med 287: 138, 1972.
5. Morley JB, Schwieger AC: The relation between chronic polyneuropathy and osteosclerotic myeloma. J Neurol Neurosurg Psychiat 30: 432, 1967.
6. Azar HA, Zaino EC, Pham TD, et al.: "Non-secretory" plasma cell myeloma. Am J Clin Pathol 58: 618, 1972.
7. Slater PP, Sherlock EC: Splenectomy, thrombocytosis and venous thrombosis. Am Surg 23: 549, 1957.
8. Case Records of Massachusetts General Hospital: Case 66-1962. N Engl J Med 267: 719, 1962.
9. Hayes DM, Spurr CL, Hutaff LW, et al.: Postsplenectomy thrombocytosis. Ann Intern Med 58: 259, 1963.
10. Bull SM, Zikria BA, Ferrer JMI: Mesenteric venous thrombosis following splenectomy: report of two cases. Ann Surg 162: 938, 1965.
11. Hirsh J, Dacie JV: Persistent postsplenectomy thrombocytosis and thromboembolism: a consequence of continuing anemia. Br J Haematol 12: 44, 1966.
12. McClure PD, Ingram GIC, Stacey RS, et al.: Platelet function test in thrombocythaemia and thrombocytosis. Br J Haematol 12: 478, 1966.
13. Silverstein MN: Primary or hemorrhagic thrombocythemia. Arch Intern Med 122: 18, 1968.
14. Levine J, Swanson PD: Idiopathic thrombocytosis. A treatable cause of transient ischemic attacks. Neurology 18: 711, 1968.
15. Korenman G: Neurologic syndromes associated with primary thrombocythemia. J Mt Sinai Hosp 36: 317, 1969.
16. Singer G: Migrating emboli of retinal arteries in thrombocythemia. Br J Ophthal 53: 279, 1969.
17. Dawson AA, Ogston D: The influence of the platelet count on the incidence of thrombotic and haemorrhagic complications in polycythemia vera. Postgrad Med J 46: 76, 1970
18. Vreeken J, Van Aken WG: Spontaneous aggregation of blood platelets as a cause of idiopathic thrombosis and recurrent painful toes and fingers. Lancet 2: 1394, 1971.
19. Mundall J, Quintero P, Kaulla KN, et al.: Transient monocular blindness and increased platelet aggregability treated with aspirin. A case report. Neurology 22: 280, 1972.
20. Kimbiris D, Segal BL, Munirm M, et al.: Myocardial infarction in patients with normal patent coronary arteries as visualized by cinearteriography. Am J Cardiol 29: 724, 1972
21. Zucker S, Mielke CH: Classification of thrombocytosis based on platelet function tests. Correlation with hemorrhagic and thrombotic complications. J Lab Clin Med 80: 385, 1972.
22. Preston FE, Emmanuel IG, Winfield DA, et al.: Essential thrombocythaemia and peripheral gangrene. Br Med J 3: 548, 1974.
23. Blatz J, Minton JP: Mesenteric thrombosis following splenectomy. Ann Surg 181: 126, 1975.
24. Coltheart G, Little JM: Splenectomy. A review of morbidity. Aust N Z J Surg 46: 32, 1976.
25. Walsh PN, Murphy S, Barry WE: The role of platelets in the

pathogenesis of thrombosis and hemorrhage in patients with thrombocytosis. Thrombo Haemostas 38: 1085, 1977.

26. Singh AK, Wetherley-Mein G: Microvascular occlusive lesions in primary thrombocythemia. Br J Haematol 36: 553, 1977.

27. Ehrenfeld M, Penchas S, Eliakim M: Thrombocytosis in rheumatoid arthritis. Recurrent arterial thromboembolism and death. Ann Rheum Dis 36: 579, 1977.

28. Kun-Yu Wu K: Platelet hyperaggregability and thrombosis in patients with thrombocythemia. Ann Intern Med 88: 7, 1978.

29. Boxer MA, Braun J, Ellman L: Thromboembolic risk of post-splenectomy thrombocytosis. Arch Surg 113: 808, 1978.

30. Jørgensen L, Rowsell HC, Horig T, et al.: Adenosine diphosphate-induced platelet aggregation and myocardial infarction in swine. Lab Invest 17: 616, 1967.

31. Haerem JW: Platelet aggregates and mural microthrombi in the early stages of acute, fatal coronary disease. Thromb Res 5: 243, 1974.

32. Chaudhuri S: Platelet adhesiveness in the assessment of ischaemic heart disease. Thromb Res 6: 209, 1975.

33. Roberts WC, Jones AA: Quantitation of coronary arterial narrowing at necropsy in acute myocardial infarction. An analysis of 27 patients and comparison to 22 control subjects. (In preparation.)

34. Roberts WC: Coronary embolism: a review of causes, consequences, and diagnostic considerations. Cardiovasc Med 3: 699, 1978.

35. Jørgensen L: Experimental platelet and coagulation thrombi. A histologic study of arterial and venous thrombi of varying age in untreated and heparinized rabbits. Acta Pathol Microbiol Scand 62: 189, 1964.

36. Cosgriff SW, Diefenbach AF, Vogt W Jr: Hypercoagulability of the blood associated with ACTH and cortisone therapy. Am J Med 9: 752, 1950.

37. Adlersberg D, Schaefer L, Drachman SR: Development of hypercholesteremia during cortisone and ACTH therapy. JAMA 144: 909, 1950.

38. Etheridge EM, Hoch-Legeti C: Lipid deposition in aortas in younger age groups following cortisone and adrenocorticotrophic hormone. Am J Pathol 28: 315, 1952.

39. Skanse B, von Studnitz W, Skoog N: The effect of corticotropin and cortisone on serum lipids and lipoproteins. Acta Encocrinol 31: 442, 1959.

40. Kalbak K: Incidence of arteriosclerosis in patients with rheumatoid arthritis receiving long-term corticosteroid therapy. Ann Rheum Dis 31: 196, 1972.

41. Bulkley BH, Roberts WC: The heart in systemic lupus erythematosus and the changes induced in it by corticosteroid therapy. A study of 36 necropsy patients. Am J Med 58: 243, 1975.

42. Zimelman AP: Thrombocytosis in multiple myeloma (letter to the editor). Ann Intern Med 78: 970, 1973.

43. Kyle RA: Multiple myeloma. Mayo Clin Proc 50: 29, 1975.

Quantification of Coronary Arterial Narrowing in Clinically-Isolated Unstable Angina Pectoris

An Analysis of 22 Necropsy Patients

WILLIAM C. ROBERTS, M.D.
RENU VIRMANI, M.D.
Bethesda, Maryland

A quantitative analysis of the degree and extent of coronary arterial narrowing by atherosclerotic plaques in the entire lengths of each of the four major epicardial coronary arteries in 22 patients with unstable angina pectoris is described at necropsy, and the observations are compared to those in 20 control subjects. All 22 study patients died within three days of an aortocoronary bypass operation, and all 20 control subjects died of malignant neoplasms. Of 1,049 five mm long segments of the left main, left anterior descending, left circumflex and right coronary arteries examined in the 22 patients (average 48 per patient), 497 (47 per cent) were 76 to 100 per cent narrowed in cross-sectional area by atherosclerotic plaques (controls = 1 per cent); 304 (29 per cent) were 51 to 75 per cent narrowed (controls = 29 per cent); 454 (48 per cent) were 26 to 50 per cent narrowed and only 119 (11 per cent) segments were less than 26 per cent narrowed (controls = 22 per cent). The amount of severe (>75 per cent) narrowing of the right, left main, left anterior descending and left circumflex coronary arteries by atherosclerotic plaques was similar. The amount of severe (>75 per cent) narrowing in the distal one half of the right and left anterior descending coronary arteries was significantly (p <0.05) less than in the proximal halves of these two arteries. The per cent of 5 mm segments of coronary artery narrowed 76 to 100 per cent in cross-sectional area in the study patients was not affected by the patients' sex, cardiac weight or by the presence of healed left ventricular infarcts. In the seven younger ($\overline{<}$45 years) patients, however, significantly (p <0.05) more 5 mm segments were narrowed >75 per cent than in the 15 older (>45 years) patients.

From the Pathology Branch, National Institutes of Health, Bethesda, Maryland. Requests for reprints should be addressed to Dr. William C. Roberts, Bldg. 10A, Room 3E30, NHLBI-NIH, Bethesda, Maryland 20205. Manuscript accepted June 7, 1979.

Although it is recognized that patients with angina pectoris usually have considerable narrowing of one or more of their major epicardial coronary arteries [1–4], the exact amount of luminal narrowing in any one or in each of the four major epicardial coronary arteries has not been described. Accordingly, the degree of cross-sectional luminal narrowing in each 5 mm segment of each of the four major epicardial coronary arteries was determined in 22 patients who died shortly after aortocoronary bypass operations for relief of clinically isolated *unstable* angina pectoris; the observations in them were compared to those in 20 control subjects.

PATIENTS STUDIED and METHODS

A total of 22 necropsy patients with clinically-isolated unstable angina pectoris with death within three days of aortocoronary artery bypass operation were included in this study. Certain clinical and cardiac morphologic observations in them are summarized in **Table I. Unstable** angina was defined as anterior thoracic pain of recent onset (less than one month before clinical evaluation) or a recent change in the pattern of the pain in terms of frequency, severity, intensity and ease of provocation. Nocturnal or rest angina or prolonged angina within three months of death was considered unstable. There was no electrocardiographic or enzymatic evidence of recent acute myocardial infarction in any of the hospitalized patients with unstable angina. **Clinically-isolated** was defined as absence of clinical evidence at any time of acute myocardial infarction and of congestive cardiac failure. None of the patients had associated valvular, congenital, primary myocardial (hypertrophic cardiomyopathy) or pericardial heart disease.

Control subjects had the following characteristics: (1) Similar age and sex to that of the study patients. (2) Death from a noncardiac condition. (3) Absence of symptoms suggesting or indicating myocardial ischemia or cardiac dysfunction during life. (4) Absence of systemic hypertension (>140 mm Hg systolic and/or >90 mm Hg diastolic). (5) Absence of therapeutic mediastinal irradiation. (6) Absence of cardiomegaly (>400 g for men and >350 g for women) at necropsy. Twenty subjects, who fulfilled these crtieria, were selected as controls: eight died of carcinoma (breast = three, pancreas = two, ovary = two, tongue = one); four of leukemia, seven of lymphoma and one from multiple myeloma.

The coronary arteries in all patients and in control subjects were studied in similar fashion. The hearts were fixed for at least one day in formalin. The four major epicardial coronary arteries then were excised intact, roentgenograms were taken, and they were fixed for at least another day. Following decalcification (if necessary), each of the four major coronary arteries were cut transversely to their longitudinal axes into approximately 5 mm long segments, and each segment was labeled sequentially from either its aortic ostium or from its origin from the left main. The number of 5 mm segments examined in the study patients and control subjects is summarized in **Table II.** The 5 mm segments were labeled, dehydrated (alcohol and xylene), embedded in paraffin, and two histologic sections were cut and stained from each paraffin block. The Movat stain was used on one histologic section; all determinations of luminal narrowing were based on examination of the Movat stained sections because this stain outlines clearly the internal elastic membrane of the arteries. The degrees of narrowing were based on histologic examination of each cross-section magnified 25 to 50 times. The judgment regarding the degree of luminal narrowing of each 5 mm segment was based on the degree of luminal obliteration within the luminal circle bordered by the internal elastic membrane. The circle was visually subdivided into four equal-sized quadrants, and the per cent of cross-sectional area luminal narrowing in each 5 mm segment was determined as follows: 0 to 26, 26 to 50, 51 to 75 and 76 to 100. All histologic sections from all patients were examined by one of us, and the degrees of narrowing were "spot-checked" by the other. Both the intra- and interobserver errors were approximately 5 per cent. Furthermore, the degrees of narrowing in four of the 22 pa-

tients were checked by planimetry, and a 95 per cent agreement was found between the visual estimation of the per cent of cross-sectional area narrowing and that found by planimetry.

In addition to sectioning the major epicardial coronary arteries, at least three histologic sections extending from endocardium to epicardium and for at least 2 cm in circumferential dimension were prepared from left ventricular myocardium

TABLE I   **Quantification of Coronary Narrowing in Unstable Angina Pectoris. Clinical Observations and Noncoronary Cardiac Findings in 22 Patients and in 20 Controls**

Observations	Patients with Angina	Control Subjects
Patients (no.)	22	20
Age (yr)		
Range	37–59	39–65
Mean	48	51
Sex		
Male	13	11
Female	9	9
Diabetes mellitus (no.)	4	0
Systemic hypertension (no.)	10	0
Duration of angina (mo.)		
Range	2–120	0
Mean	18	0
Total cholesterol determinations		
No. of subjects	19	17
Total cholesterol (>200 mg/dl)	16*	3**
Total cholesterol values (mg/dl)		
Range	148–420	106–245
Mean	266*	171**
Heart weight (g)		
Range	240–520	190–390
Mean	384*	302**
Increased heart weight[†] (no.)	6	0
Left ventricle		
Necrosis (no.)	4‡	0
Fibrosis (no.)	6‡	0

NOTE: Systemic hypertension = systolic blood pressure >140 mm Hg and/or diastolic >90 mm Hg.
* to ** = $p < 0.001$.
[†] Weight >400 g in men and >350 g in women.
‡ None had clinical evidence of acute myocardial infarction.

TABLE II   **Number of 5 mm Long Segments of Major Epicardial Coronary Artery Examined per Patient: 22 Patients with Unstable Angina Pectoris Versus 20 Controls**

Coronary Artery	Angina Pectoris Range	Angina Pectoris Mean	Controls Range	Controls Mean
Left main	1–4	2.1	1–3	1.6
Left anterior descending	6–34	16.0	8–31	17.2
Left circumflex	4–33	12.0	5–19	9.7
Right	9–29	17.7	11–37	19.4
Total segments of 4 coronary arteries per patient	21–75	47.6	28–69	47.7

TABLE III Number of 22 Patients with Unstable Angina Pectoris (AP) and 20 Control Subjects (C) Showing Maximum Luminal Narrowing of One or More Major Epicardial Coronary Arteries by Atherosclerotic Plaques

| | Cross-Sectional Area Luminal Narrowing | | | | | | | | | |
| | 0–25% | | 26–50% | | 51–75% | | 76–100% | | Totals | |
Coronary Artery	AP	C	AP	C	AP	C	AP	C	AP	C
R	0	0	0	0	0	1	1	1	1	2
LAD	0	0	0	0	0	1	0	2	0	3
R, LAD	0	0	0	0	0	4	2	1	2	5
LAD, LM	0	0	0	0	0	0	1	0	1	0
LAD, LC	0	0	0	0	0	2	0	0	0	2
R, LAD, LC	0	0	0	1	0	5	8	1	8	7
R, LM*, LAD, LC	0	0	0	0	0	1	10	0	10	1
Totals										
No.	0	0	0	1	0	14	22	5	22	20
Per cent			0	5	0	70	100	25	100	100

NOTE: R = right, LM = left main; LAD = left anterior descending, LC = left circumflex.
* Sections of LM not examined in three patients with angina and in three control subjects.

from each patient and stained by hematoxylin and eosin. Gross myocardial fibrosis (Table I) was confirmed histologically in six patients (26 per cent) (Table I), and four had transmural left ventricular myocardial coagulation necrosis. No control subjects had either myocardial fibrosis or necrosis by histologic examination.

RESULTS

Among the 22 patients with unstable angina, 85 major coronary arteries were examined (the left main was not examined in three patients); among the 20 control subjects, 77 major coronary arteries were examined (the left main was not examined in three subjects). All 22 study patients had 76 to 100 per cent cross sectional area luminal narrowing by atherosclerotic plaque in at least one of their four major coronary arteries, and five (25 per cent) of the 20 control subjects had this degree of narrowing (**Table III**). Of the 22 study patients, 21 (95 per cent) had two or more of their four major coronary arteries narrowed >75 per cent in cross-sectional area by atherosclerotic plaque, whereas only two (10 per cent) of the 20 control subjects had two or more arteries narrowed to this degree. Of the 22 study patients, 10 (45 per cent) had >75 per cent narrowing by atherosclerotic plaque of all four major coronary arteries; eight (36 per cent) other patients had three arteries narrowed to this degree; three (14 per cent) had two arteries narrowed to this extent, and only one patient had only one of the four arteries >75 per cent narrowed. Thus, of the possible 88 major coronary arteries in the 22 study patients (actually only 85 arteries were examined), 71 (81 per cent) were >75% narrowed in cross-sectional area by atherosclerotic plaque for an average of 3.2/4.0 coronary arteries per study patient. If the left main coronary artery was excluded, 61 (93 per cent) of the other 66 major (right, left anterior descending and left circumflex) coronary arteries were narrowed >75 per cent in cross-sectional area by atherosclerotic plaque, for an average of 2.8/3.0 coronary arteries per study patient.

Of the five control subjects with >75 per cent cross-sectional area narrowing of one or more coronary arteries by atherosclerotic plaque, none had all four major coronary arteries narrowed to this degree, one had three arteries so narrowed, one had two arteries so narrowed, and three had one artery so narrowed. Thus, of the possible 80 major coronary arteries in the 20 control subjects (actually, only 77 arteries were examined), eight (10 per cent) were narrowed >75 per cent in cross-sectional area by atherosclerotic plaque for an average of 0.4/4.0 coronary arteries per control subject. If the left main coronary artery was excluded, eight (13 per cent) of the 60 other major (right, left anterior descending, left circumflex) coronary arteries were narrowed >75 per cent in cross-sectional area by atherosclerotic plaque for an average of 0.4/3.0 coronary arteries per control subject. Thrombus was absent in the coronary arteries in all 22 patients and in all 20 controls.

The results of the **quantitative** analysis of the 5 mm long coronary segments in both study patients and control subjects are summarized in **Figure 1** and in **Table IV**. Of the 1,049 five mm long segments of major coronary arteries examined in the 22 study patients, 497 segments (47 per cent) were 76 to 100 per cent narrowed in cross-sectional area by atherosclerotic plaque (controls = 1 per cent), 304 (29 per cent) were 51 to 75 per cent narrowed (controls = 29 per cent), 129 (12 per cent) were 26 to 50 per cent narrowed (controls = 48 per cent), and 119 (11 per cent) were 0 to 25 per cent narrowed (controls = 22 per cent). The mean per cent of 5 mm coronary segments narrowed 0 to 25, 26 to 50 and 76 to 100 per cent was significantly (p <0.05) different between study patients and control subjects at each of the four levels of narrowing. The mean per cent of 5 mm segments of left main, left anterior descending, left circumflex and right coronary arteries narrowed 0 to 25, 26 to 50, 51 to 75 and 76 to 100 per cent was significantly (p <0.05) different between study patients and control subjects at each of the four levels of narrowing (Figure 1). The

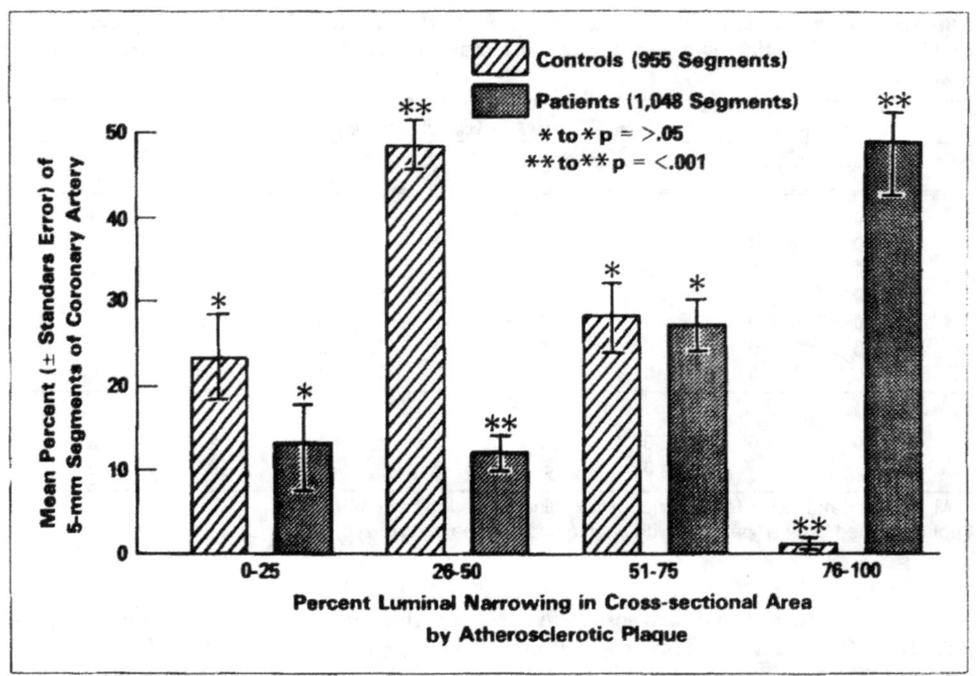

Figure 1. Per cent of 5 mm segments of all four major coronary arteries narrowed to various degrees in the 22 study patients and in the 20 control subjects.

mean per cent of 5 mm segments of the left main, left anterior descending, left circumflex and right coronary arteries at each of the four levels of narrowing was similar in the study patients (**Figure 2**). The mean per cent of segments of each of the four major coronary arteries narrowed to varying degrees in the control subjects was similar (Figure 2).

The mean per cent of 5 mm segments narrowed 76 to 100 per cent in cross-sectional area in the proximal halve of the left anterior descending and right coronary arteries (excluding posterior descending branches) was greater than the mean per cent of 5 mm segments similarly narrowed in the distal halves (**Figure 3**) (p <0.01), but the amount of severe narrowing in the proximal and distal halves of the left circumflex coronary artery was not significantly different (**Figure 4**).

TABLE IV Number and Per Cent of 5 mm Long Segments of the Four Major Epicardial Coronary Arteries in 22 Patients with Unstable Angina Pectoris (AP) and in 20 Control Subjects (C) Showing the Four Grades of Cross-Sectional Luminal Narrowing

Coronary Artery	Cross-Sectional Area Luminal Narrowing								Totals	
	0–25%		26–50%		51–75%		76–100%			
	AP	C	AP	C	AP	C	AP	C	AP	C
Left main*										
No.	0	10	1	13	22	5	17	0	40	28
Per cent		36	2	46	55	18	43		100	100
Left anterior descending										
No.	43	74	58	168	93	94	160	8	354	344
Per cent	12	22	17	49	26	27	45	2	100	100
Left circumflex										
No.	39	59	28	77	82	56	116	2	265	194
Per cent	15	30	10	40	31	29	44	1	100	100
Right										
No.	37	71	42	196	107	119	204	3	390	389
Per cent	9	18	11	50	28	31	52	1	100	100
Totals										
No.	119	214	129	454	304	274	497	13	1,049	955
Per cent	11	22	12	48	29	29	47	1	100	100

* Sections not examined in three patients with angina and in three control subjects.

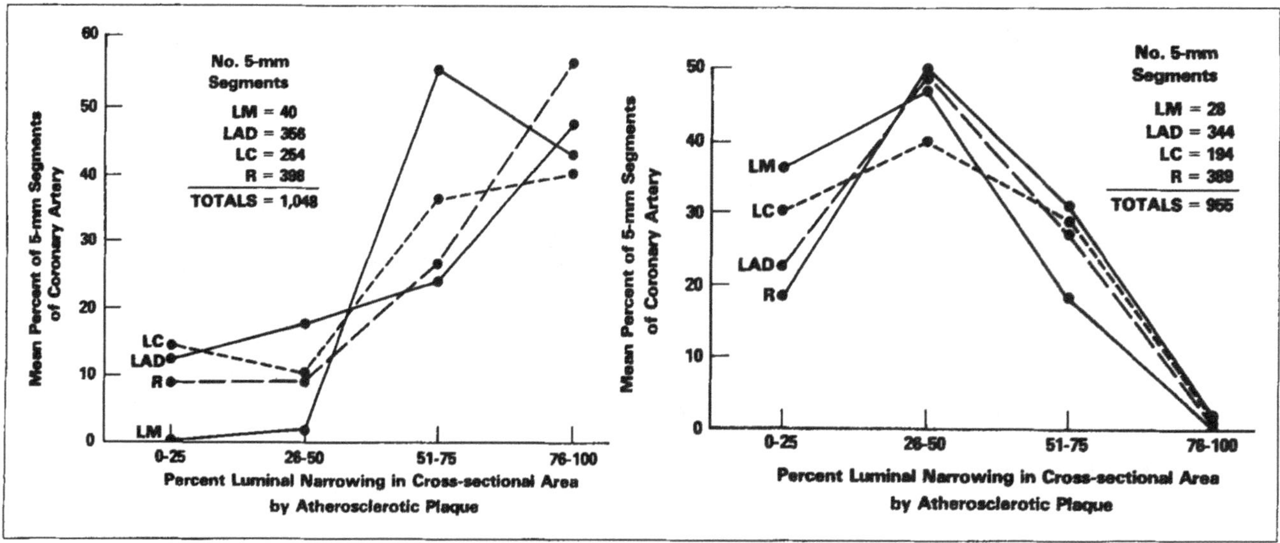

Figure 2. Mean per cent of 5 mm segments of each of the four major coronary arteries narrowed to various degrees in the 22 study patients (**left**) and in the 20 control subjects (**right**). In the study patients the amount of narrowing at each of the four levels of narrowing is similar in each of the four major coronary arteries. The same is true for the control subjects. LM = left main; LAD = left anterior descending; LC = left circumflex; R = right.

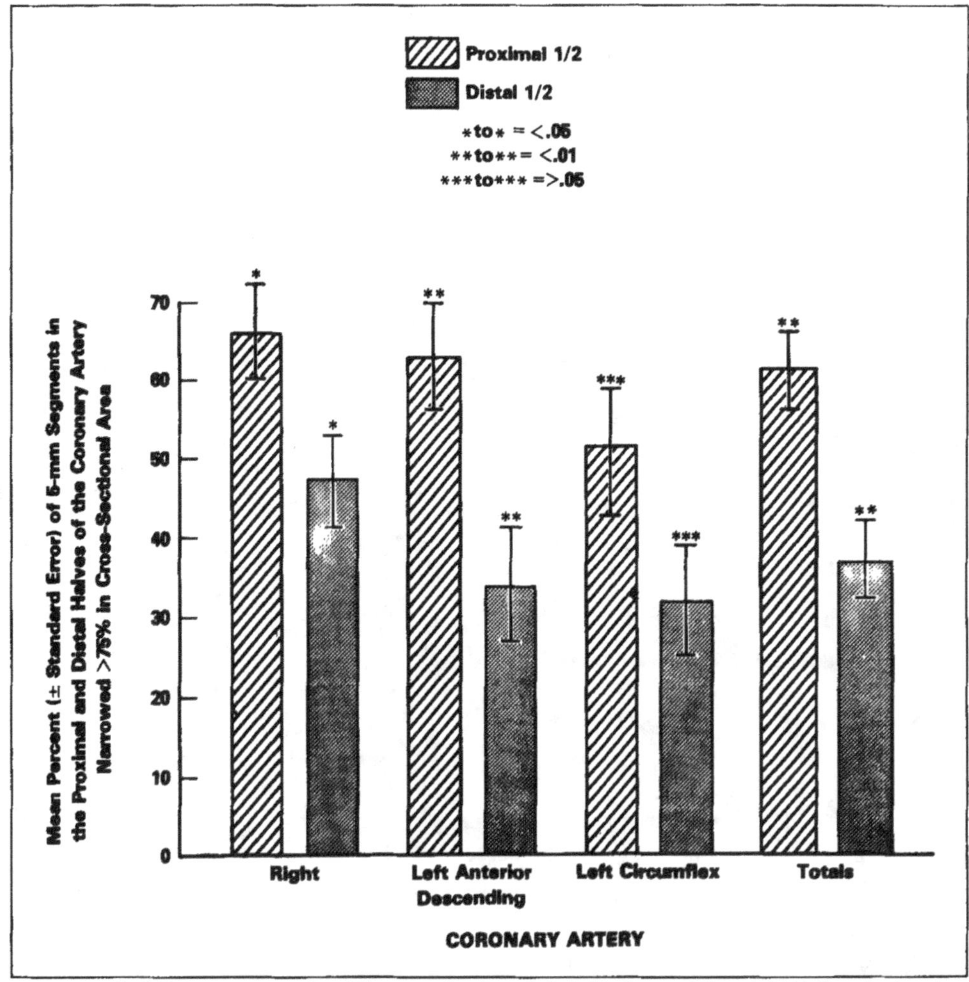

Figure 3. Mean per cent of 5 mm segments of the proximal and distal halves of the right, left anterior descending and left circumflex coronary arteries in the 22 study patients. The mean per cent of 5 mm segments narrowed greater than 75 per cent in cross-sectional area by atherosclerotic plaque in the proximal halves of these three arteries is greater than that in the distal halves of these three arteries.

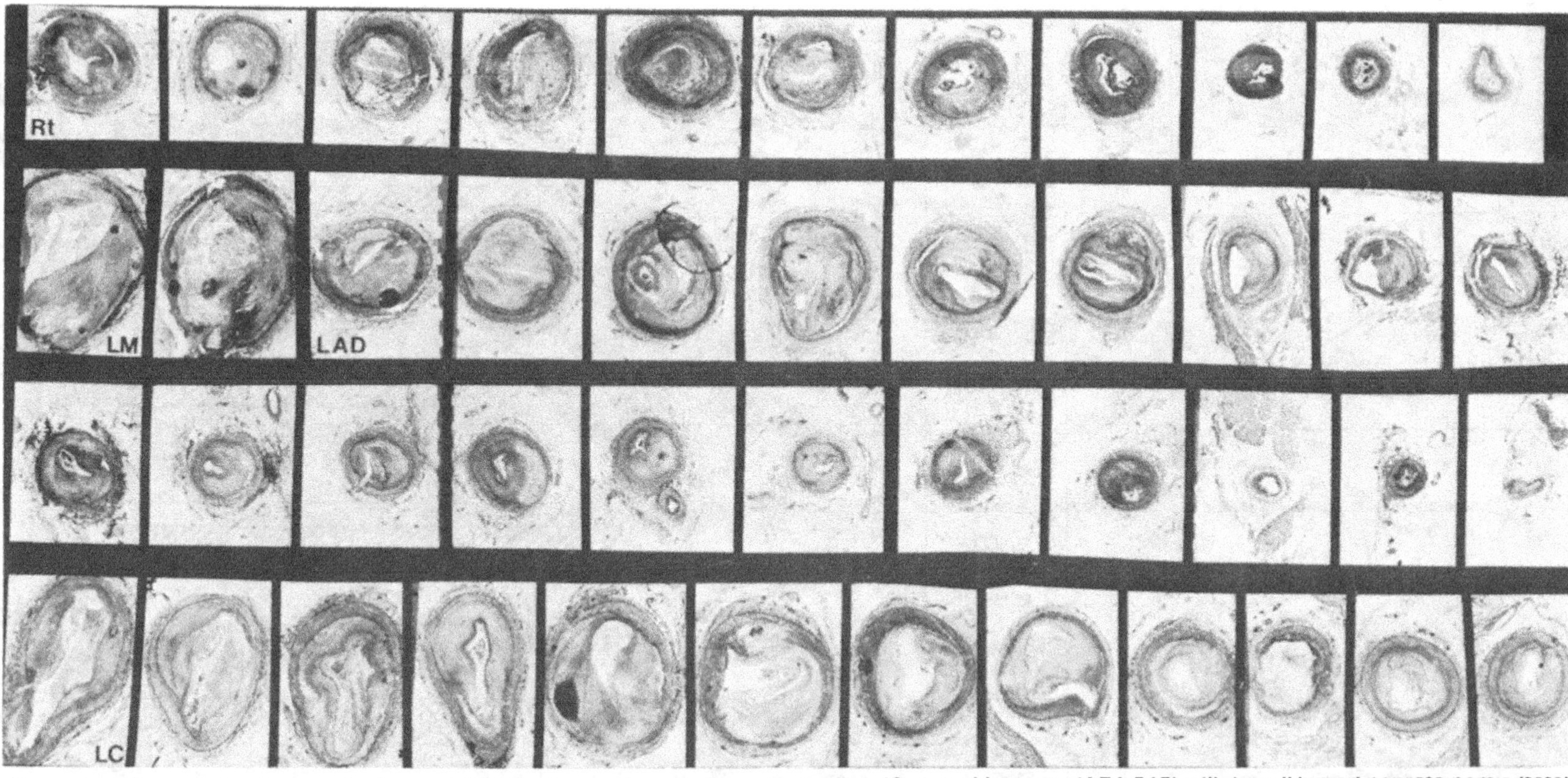

Figure 4. Forty photomicrographs from each of the four major coronary arteries in a 40 year old woman (A74-212) with type II hyperlipoproteinemia (total serum cholesterol = 420 mg/dl) and onset of angina pectoris at age 38 years. During the last few months of life she had worsening angina with 10 to 15 attacks daily provoked by less and less exertion. Finally angina developed at rest and she was occasionally awakened by angina. She had xanthomas on her hands and in her Achilles tendons. Coronary angiography immediately before aortocoronary bypass operation showed severe ($>$70 per cent diameter reduction) narrowing of the left main (LM), left anterior descending (LAD), left circumflex (LC) and right (R) coronary arteries. After anastomosing bypass conduits from aorta to the left anterior descending, right, and left obtuse marginal coronary arteries she could not be weaned from cardiopulmonary bypass and died. Each photomicrograph is from a 5 mm segment of coronary artery, each one is stained by the Movat method and the magnification of each is the same ($\times$25). With one exception, all sections contain atherosclerotic plaques and most show considerable narrowing.

Parameter Analyzed	Patients (no.)	Mean Per cent ($\pm$ Standard Error) of 5 mm Coronary Segments Narrowed >75% in Cross-Sectional Area by Atherosclerotic Plaque	p Value
Age (yr)			
≤45	7	63 ± 6	<0.05
46–65	15	41 ± 6	
Sex			
Men	13	48 ± 6	ns
Women	9	48 ± 8	
Heart weight			
Increased*	6	52 ± 11	ns
Normal	16	48 ± 5	
Healed Infarct[†]			
Left ventricle			
Present	6	48 ± 10	ns
Absent	16	47 ± 6	

* >400 g in men; >350 g in women.
[†] Clinically silent.

The seven patients 45 years of age and younger had a higher percentage of 5 mm segments severely narrowed than did the 15 patients aged 46 to 65 years (63 ± 6 versus 41 ± 6%) (p <0.05) (**Table V**). Sex, heart weight and the presence or absence of a **healed left ventricular infarct** (clinically silent) did not alter the percentage of coronary segments severely (>75 per cent) narrowed.

COMMENTS

Many thousands of autopsies during this century have demonstrated severe narrowings in one or more major epicardial coronary arteries of patients with coronary heart disease, but until recently there has been no attempt to quantify the degree and extent of coronary luminal narrowing in these patients. The present study provides **quantitative** information on the degree and extent of luminal narrowing in each of the four major epicardial coronary arteries in patients with clinically-isolated unstable angina pectoris. Approximately 24 cm (1,049 five mm segments) of the four major (right, left main, left anterior descending and left circumflex) epicardial coronary arteries were examined in each of 22 patients or a total of 525 cm of major coronary artery. Each 1 cm segment was divided into equal-sized halves, and a histologic section was examined from each 5 mm segment. Of the 22 patients studied, in nearly one half (47 per cent) of the entire lengths of the four major epicardial coronary arteries studied, the lumens were >75 per cent narrowed in cross-sectional area by atherosclerotic plaque. In addition, in another 29 per cent of the major coronary arteries luminal narrowing was between 51 and 75 per cent in cross-sectional area. Thus, 76 per cent of the lengths of the four major epicardial coronary arteries in the 22 study patients were >50 per cent narrowed in cross-sectional area by atherosclerotic plaque. (A 75 per cent cross-sectional area narrowing is equivalent to a 50 per cent diameter reduction on luminogram[5]). In contrast, only 30 per cent of the lengths of the four major coronary arteries in the control subjects were narrowed >50 per cent (p <0.001).

Not only was severe narrowing widespread in the study patients, but some degree of narrowing was also present in virtually every 5 mm segment of coronary artery. Of the coronary arterial segments studied, 89 per cent were narrowed over 25 per cent in cross-sectional area, and not a single 5 mm segment in a single patient was entirely normal. Thus, coronary atherosclerosis in necropsy patients with clinically-isolated unstable angina pectoris is **diffuse,** involving, for practical purposes, all segments of all four major epicardial coronary arteries.

Fortunately, from an operative standpoint, the degree of severe (>75 per cent) narrowing in the distal halves of the left anterior descending and right coronary arteries in the 22 study patients was significantly less than in the proximal halves of these two arteries. The distal half of the left circumflex artery was not significantly less narrowed than the proximal half.

Surprisingly, among the study patients, no significant differences were found in the degree of severe narrowing of the left main, left anterior descending, left circumflex or right coronary arteries. In addition, the per cent of 5 mm coronary segments narrowed 0 to 25, 26 to 50 and 76 to 100 per cent in cross-sectional area by atherosclerotic plaque was similar in each of these four arteries. Thus, unstable angina is associated with a high frequency of severe (>75 per cent) narrowing of the left main as well as the other coronary arteries.

The amount of severe (>75 per cent) coronary narrowing present in the study patients was greater in the patients 45 years of age and under than in those over age 45, but the per cent of coronary segments >75 per cent narrowed was similar in men and women, in those with increased compared to those with normal-sized hearts, and in those with compared to those without myocardial scars (healed infarcts).

REFERENCES

1. Zoll PM, Wessler S, Blumgart HL: Angina pectoris. Clinical and pathologic correlations. Am J Med 11: 331, 1951.
2. Lenegre J, Himbert J: Critical study of the relationship between angina pectoris and coronary atherosclerosis. Am Heart J 58: 539, 1959.
3. Guthrie RB, Vlodaver Z, Nicoloff DM, et al.: Pathology of stable and unstable angina pectoris. Circulation 51: 1059, 1975.
4. Roberts WC: The coronary arteries and left ventricle in clinically isolated angina pectoris. A necropsy analysis. Circulation 54: 388, 1976.
5. Arnett EN, Isner JM, Redwood DR, et al.: Coronary arterial narrowing in coronary heart disease: comparison of cinangiographic and necropsy findings. Ann Intern Med 91: 350, 1979.

Structure-Function Correlations in Cardiovascular and Pulmonary Diseases (CPC)

Disappearance of Symptomatic Coronary Heart Disease and Death from a Noncardiac Condition

Clinical Conference from the Pathology Branch, National Heart, Lung, and Blood Institute, National Institutes of Health, Bethesda

Renu Virmani, M.D.; William C. Roberts, M.D., F.C.C.P.

The following contribution inaugurates a new section under the guidance of Dr. William C. Roberts, Bethesda. Although the letters CPC (clinicopathologic conference) serve as a subtitle, the communications in this department offer clinical insights not ordinarily associated with the traditional CPC. Dr. Roberts has indicated by the full title that he considers function, as well as structure, to be vital in these presentations. The Editorial Board and I appreciate the opportunity to present to our readers this new department headed by a distinguished physician.

Alfred Soffer, M.D., F.C.C.P.
Editor-in-Chief

Dr. William C. Roberts: In this conference we will discuss findings in a patient who had had angina pectoris, which disappeared about 18 months before death from a stroke.

Dr. Renu Virmani: A 55-year-old white man, who died Dec 17, 1968, had been well until about September 1963 (just over five years before death) when he noted substernal chest pain without radiation during exertion and relief of the pain with rest. This pain occurred about once or twice a month thereafter until 18 months before death when it disappeared entirely. In December 1966 (two years before death), he had substernal chest pain lasting two hours and unassociated with exertion. The pain on this occasion was more severe than the pain which occurred on exertion, and it was described "as if someone were sitting on my chest." He sought medical care at the time. He was given nitroglycerin and digitalis and kept in bed at home for three weeks. When he returned to activity, he again noted exertional chest pain periodically during the next six months after which it disappeared entirely.

In about March 1967 (21 months before death), he noted soreness in the left side of the mouth and the next month when he returned to his physician to have his "heart medicine" prescription renewed,

a mass was palpated beneath the left mandible. An ulcer in the mouth appeared in August 1967, and biopsy disclosed squamous cell carcinoma. In September 1967, he was admitted to the Clinical Center of the National Institutes of Health. He weighed 74 kg and was 167 cm tall. The blood pressure varied from 150 to 220 mm Hg systolic, and 80 to 110 mm Hg diastolic. Precordial examination revealed a third heart sound and a grade 2/6 systolic murmur along the lower left sternal border and at the apex. The ECG showed voltage criteria of left ventricular hypertrophy and Q waves in leads 2, 3, aVF, V_5, and V_6. The chest roentgenogram showed a normal sized heart. The serum total cholesterol level was 252 mg/100 ml. He had smoked two packs of cigarettes daily for 35 years. He was found to have carcinoma of the floor of the mouth and underwent hemiglossectomy, partial hemiandibulectomy, and bilateral neck dissection on Sept 25, 1967. He never had recurrence of the carcinoma thereafter, and he returned to normal daily activities. In November 1968, he developed evidence of cerebral insufficiency and the next month died shortly after carotid endarterectomy. Electrocardiogram (Fig 1) shortly before death was similar to those recorded during his last five years. Shortly before death, he weighed 69 kg. At necropsy, the heart weighed 380 gm. All four cavities and valves were normal. There was a transmural scar in the pos-

Reprint requests: Dr. Roberts, NIH-NHLBI, Bldg 10A, Room 3E30, Bethesda 20014

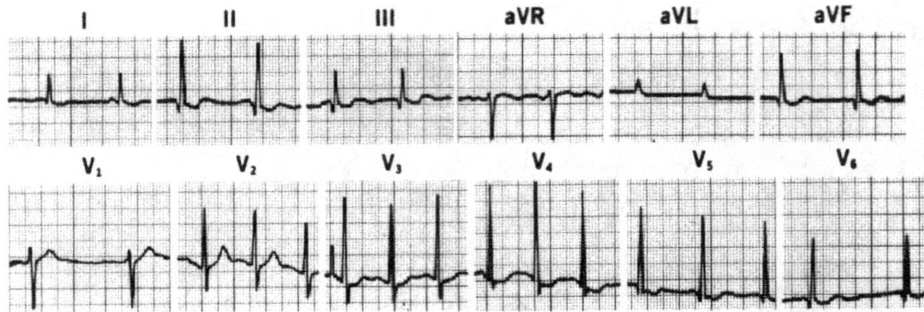

FIGURE 1. Electrocardiogram recorded on Dec 17, 1968, shows voltage criteria of left ventricular hypertrophy and Q waves in leads 2, 3, aVF, V_5, and V_6.

terior wall of left ventricle, and it involved approximately 30 percent of the left ventricular wall including the ventricular septum. The four major coronary arteries were excised, decalcified, and cut into 5-mm segments, and a histologic section was prepared from each 5-mm segment and stained by Movat's method.[1] The amount of luminal narrowing in each section is summarized in Table 1, and the maximum areas of luminal narrowing are shown in Figure 2. The aorta and its branches were severely atherosclerotic; the right internal carotid was totally occluded, and a large cerebral infarct was present. No residual cancer was found.

Dr. Roberts: The patient described above presents the opportunity to examine the coronary arteries in a patient who for nearly four years had angina pectoris which disappeared about 18 months before death from a noncardiac condition. Most patients with angina pectoris with or without associated healed myocardial infarction die suddenly or from acute myocardial infarction. Although we have studied at necropsy several hundred patients with fatal coronary heart disease, the present patient is the first we have encountered who had symptomatic coronary heart disease and died naturally of a non-

cardiac condition after disappearance of angina pectoris. How may angina pectoris disappear in a patient when the angina is secondary to severe coronary atherosclerosis? There are at least seven explanations: (1) the exertion which produced the angina was discontinued; (2) nitroglycerin or other vasodilators were taken before the exertion which in the past had produced angina; (3) acute myocardial infarction which healed occurred and it eliminated the area of myocardial ischemia; (4) successful aortocoronary bypass operation was performed; (5) the coronary lumen was dilated by balloon catheter (coronary angioplasty); (6) the coronary lumen was widened by disappearance of some atherosclerotic plaque; or (7) the patient died. The present patient remained active to nearly his end. There was no aortocoronary bypass operation or angioplasty performed, and he did not take nitroglycerin prophylactically. The patient may have had an acute myocardial infarction about two years before death, but angina pectoris reappeared for another six months after the episode of prolonged chest pain, so in him, the myocardial infarction did not eliminate myocardial ischemia at that time. Our patient did develop carcinoma of the mouth and this was operatively excised, but he never lost more than 5 kg of weight. Thus, massive cachexia, a possible cause of dissolution of atherosclerotic plaques, cannot be a cause of the disappearance of angina in him. Accordingly, the cause of the disappearance of his angina remains obscure.

Despite the disappearance of angina, the amount of coronary arterial luminal narrowing was spectacular! As summarized in Table 1, of 40 5-mm segments of the four major coronary arteries examined, 55 percent of the segments were 76 to 100 percent narrowed in cross-sectional area and another 38 percent were 51 to 75 percent narrowed in cross-sectional area by atherosclerotic plaque alone. Thus, 93 percent of the lumens of the major coronary arteries were > 50 percent narrowed in cross-sectional area. Additionally, only 7 percent of the major coronary arteries were 50 percent or less narrowed

Table 1—*Number and Percent of 5-mm Segments of the Four Major Epicardial Coronary Arteries Showing Four Grades of Cross-Sectional Area Narrowing*

Coronary Artery	No. 5-mm Segments Examined	Percent Cross-Sectional Area Narrowing by Atherosclerotic Plaque			
		0-25	26-50	51-75	76-100
Left main	1	0	0	1	0
Left anterior descending	9	0	0	6	3
Left circumflex	10	0	0	3	7
Right	20	2	1	5	12
Totals No. (percent)	40	2(5)	1(2)	15(38)	22(55)

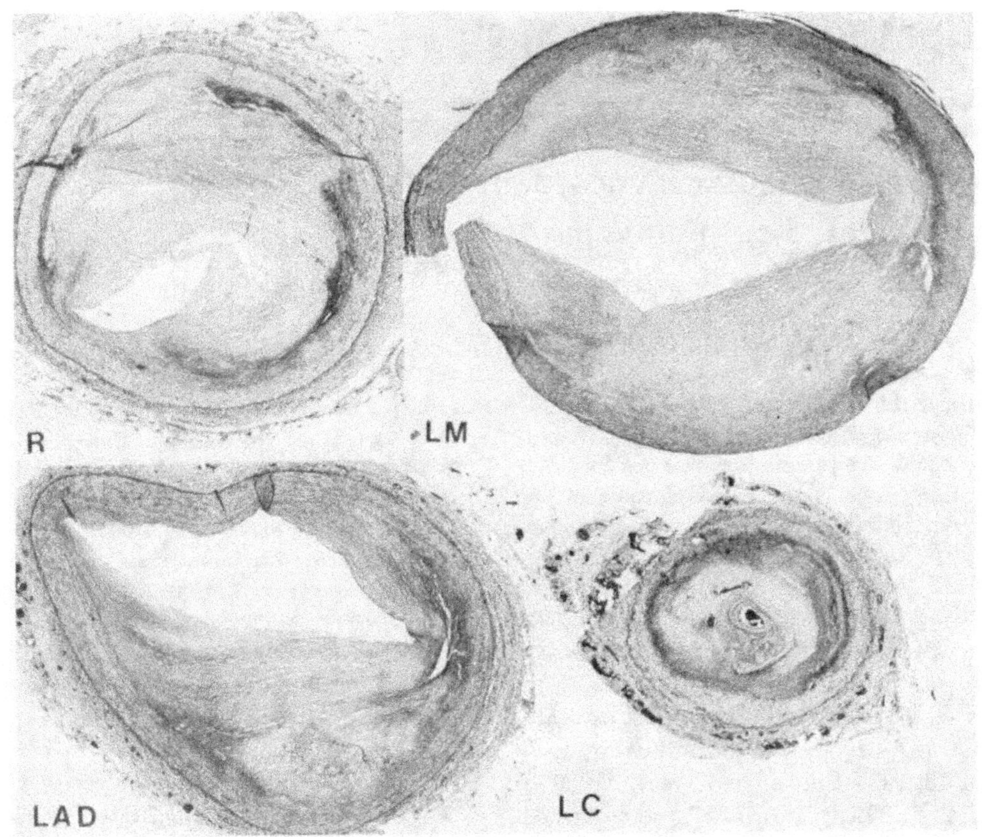

Figure 2. Four photomicrographs from each of the four major coronary arteries(R, right; LM, left main; LAD, left anterior descending; and LC, left circumflex) showing the maximum degrees of cross-sectional area luminal narrowing in each of these arteries (Movat stains, original magnification for each, × 20).

in cross-sectional area.

We have examined several subsets of patients with fatal coronary heart disease,[2-5] including patients with unstable angina pectoris who died within three days after aortocoronary bypass operations, acute myocardial infarction, sudden coronary death, and patients with coronary dilated cardiomyopathy ("ischemic cardiomyopathy"). Among these four subsets of patients, those with unstable angina had the severest coronary narrowing, and the patients with healed myocardial infarcts had the least severe coronary narrowing. The present patient is different from any that we have studied thus far in that the angina disappeared and death was from a noncardiac condition. Yet, the amount of coronary narrowing was severe. Obviously, one cannot appreciate reversal or partial disappearance of portions of some coronary atherosclerotic plaques at necropsy because a necropsy can only be performed once. Reversal of coronary plaquing in the present patient appears unlikely in view of his extensive narrowing by atherosclerotic plaques.

Thus, the present patient emphasizes the point that once symptomatic coronary heart disease oc-
curs, it is indicative of severe coronary narrowing by atherosclerotic plaques and that this principle appears to hold irrespective of whether or not the symptoms of myocardial ischemia disappear or persist.

REFERENCES

1 Roberts WC, Buja LM: The frequency and significance of coronary arterial thrombi and other observations in fatal acute myocardial infarction: A study of 107 necropsy patients. Am J Med 52:425-443, 1972

2 Roberts WC, Virmani R: Quantification of coronary arterial narrowing in clinically-isolated unstable angina pectoris: An analysis of 22 necropsy patients. Am J Med 1979, in press

3 Roberts WC, Jones AA: Quantification of coronary arterial narrowing at necropsy in acute transmural myocardial infarction: An analysis of 27 patients and comparison of findings to those in 22 control subjects. Circulation, in press.

4 Roberts WC, Jones AA: Quantitation of coronary arterial narrowing at necropsy in sudden coronary death: Analysis of 31 patients and comparison with 25 control subjects. Am J Cardiol 44:39-45, 1979

5 Virmani R, Roberts WC: Coronary dilated cardiomyopathy: quantification of coronary arterial narrowing and of left ventricular myocardial scarring in healed myocardial infarction with chronic, eventually fatal congestive cardiac failure. Submitted for publication

Clinical pathologic conference

Left and right ventricular myocardial infarction in idiopathic dilated cardiomyopathy

Jeffrey M. Isner, M.D.
Renu Virmani, M.D.
Samuel B. Itscoitz, M.D.
William C. Roberts, M.D.
Bethesda and Takoma Park, Md.

DR. ROBERTS: Dr. Isner will present the *patient's story* and *clinical findings.*

DR. ISNER: N. S. (Washington Adventist Hospital No. 14403-1), was a 62-year-old woman who died on September 23, 1978. Since age 53 years (1969), she had known of a "heart murmur" and a "large heart." She was asymptomatic until age 60 years when she developed exertional dyspnea and pedal edema. Examination then revealed distended neck veins, basilar pulmonary râles, a large heart, S_3 and S_4 sounds, an apical holosystolic murmur, and another systolic murmur, which increased with inspiration, at the left sternal border. The liver was palpable and both legs were edematous. Electrocardiogram disclosed sinus tachycardia with non-specific ST-T wave changes. The patient was started on digoxin and diuretics. She was hospitalized twice during the subsequent 2 years for overt congestive heart failure. Ten months before death an echocardiogram disclosed a dilated, poorly contracting left ventricle.

Because of increasing congestive cardiac failure she was hospitalized 5 days before death. She denied ever having chest pain. She had drunk alcohol infrequently and never had hypertension to her knowledge. Her blood pressure on admission was 110/90 mm. Hg with a pulsus paradoxus of 20 mm. Hg. Despite distention above the sternal angle of the neck veins, the lung fields

were clear. The right ventricular impulse was more prominent than the left ventricular impulse. The remainder of the precordial examination was unchanged from the findings described 2 years earlier. The liver was enlarged and severe (4+/ 4+) subcutaneous edema was present in the lower legs. The hematocrit was 35 per cent; fasting serum glucose, 109 mg./dl.; serum total cholesterol, 170 mg./dl.; serum glutamic oxalo-acetic transaminase, 61 mU./ml. (normal-7 to 40); lactic dehydrogenase, 302 mU./ml. (normal-100 to 225); creatinine phosphokinase, 208 mU./ml. (normal <145) with cardiac (MB) fraction, 1.9 (nl. $\leq$ 3 per cent). The electrocardiogram (Fig. 1) showed a vertical axis and inverted T waves in Leads III and aV_f, the chest radiograph (Fig. 2) showed marked cardiomegaly, and the echocardiogram (Fig. 3) was similar to the one recorded 10 months earlier. Her course worsened. On the day of death, her skin cooled and became moist, the blood pressure fell, and the electrocardiogram (Fig. 1) showed left bundle branch block. With ambu-bag pulmonary assistance, the arterial pO_2 was 69 mm. Hg; pCO_2, 55 mm. Hg, and pH 7.12. (On admission when breathing room air, the pO_2 had been 85 mm. Hg, pCO_2, 31 mm. Hg, and pH, 7.45.) The patient was intubated, and a Swan-Ganz catheter was inserted. Initial pressures (in mm. Hg) were: right atrial mean, 24; right ventricle, 55/24; pulmonary artery, 55/35; and mean pulmonary capillary wedge, 25. Despite intravenous administration of saline and dopamine, the systemic blood pressure continued to fall. Subxiphoid insertion of a needle ruled out cardiac tamponade. Shortly thereafter, fatal ventricular fibrillation occured.

From the Pathology Branch, National Heart, Lung, and Blood Institute, National Institutes of Health, Bethesda, Maryland, and the Department of Cardiology, Washington Adventist Hospital, Takoma Park, Maryland.

Received for publication Dec. 29, 1978.

Reprint requests: William C. Roberts, M.D., Building 10A, Room 3E30, National Institutes of Health, Bethesda, Md. 20014.

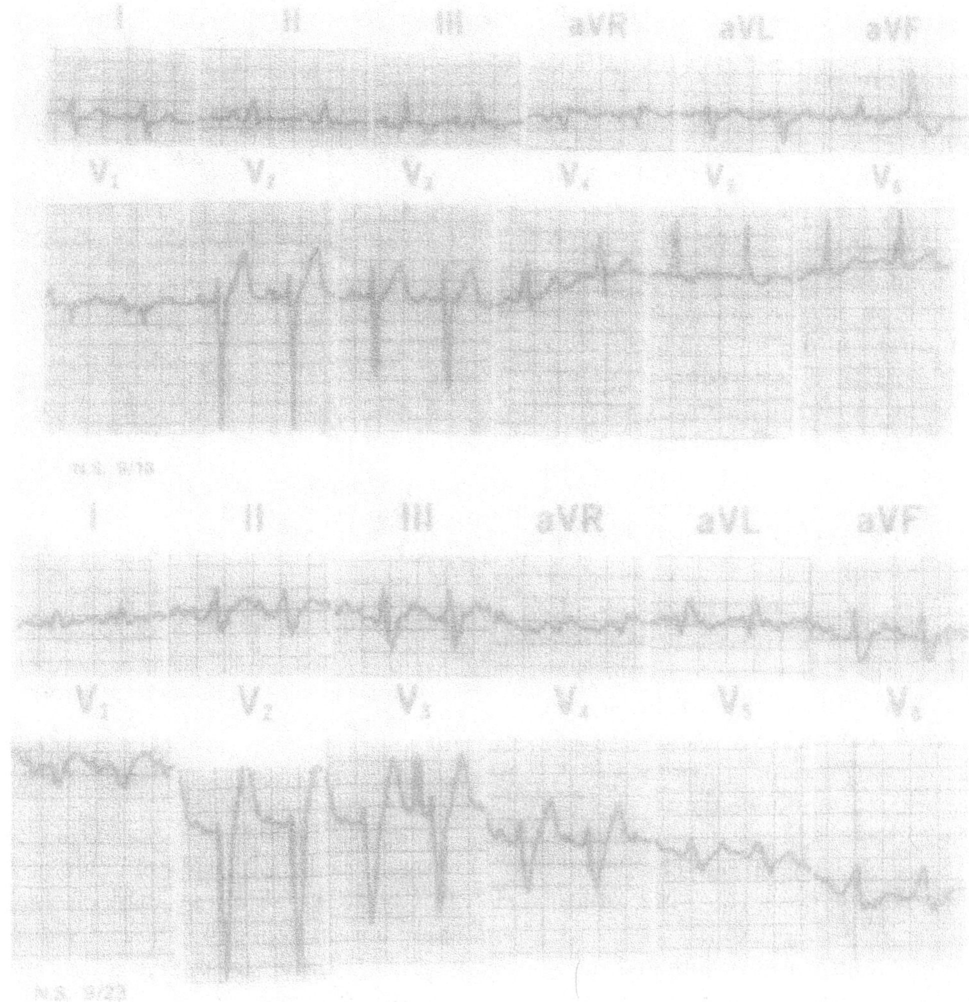

Fig. 1. Electrocardiograms. On admission (9/18), 5 days before death, the T-wave inversions in Leads III and aV$_F$ are the only findings consistent with a scar in the posterior left ventricular free wall. Left bundle branch block appeared on the day of death (9/23).

DR. ROBERTS: Dr. Virmani, would you decribe the *findings at necropsy.*

DR. VIRMANI: At necropsy (WAH No. A7867), about 100 ml. of serous fluid was present in the pericardial sac. The heart weighed 580 grams. All four chambers were markedly dilated. There was transmural scarring of the posterior walls of both left and right ventricles and of the adjacent ventricular septum (Figs. 4 and 5). There were no foci of myocardial necrosis. Thrombi were present in both ventricles, and in the right atrial appendage. The major epicardial coronary arteries were wide open (Fig. 6). At no point were any portions of any epicardial coronary artery >25 per cent narrowed in cross-sectional area. The lungs together weighed 900 grams. Two hemorrhagic infarcts were present: one in the lower lobe of the left lung and the other in the upper lobe of the right lung. Some adjacent pulmonary arteries contained thromboemboli. Small healed infarcts were present in each kidney. The liver weighed 1,450 grams and was congested.

DR. ROBERTS: Thus, we have a patient who was known to have cardiomegaly and an abnormal electrocardiogram for at least 10 years, evidence of chronic congestive heart failure for at least 2 years, never evidence of chest pain, and, at necropsy, very dilated ventricular cavities containing thrombi, large transmural scars involving the free walls of both left and right ventricles and the ventricular septum, and widely patent, virtually normal epicardial coronary arteries. Dr.

Itscoitz, what was your *clinical diagnosis* in this patient?

DR. ITSCOITZ: Three possibilities were considered. One was coronary heart disease, particularly in view of her age (62 years). Against this diagnosis, however, was the absence of chest pain, electrocardiographic absence of clear myocardial damage, and the absence of risk factors for atherosclerosis. Her total serum cholesterol was 170 mg./dl., she did not smoke, her blood pressure had always been normal, and her fasting blood sugar was normal. Idiopathic dilated cardiomyopathy was favored by the history of chronic congestive heart failure, the marked cardiomegaly, and the absence of chest pain, or clear evidence of "organic" valve disease. The third diagnosis considered was pericardial heart disease. This possibility was considered because of the extremely large cardiac silhouette by chest radiograph, the extreme prominence of features of right-sided congestive failure (the neck veins were enormously distended while the lung fields were clear, and she was able to lie flat in bed without distress), and the occurrence of diastolic pressures in the right ventricle and main pulmonary arteries similar to the mean pressures in the right atrium and pulmonary arterial wedge position. The possibility of cardiac tamponade was so high immediately before death that a needle was inserted into the pericardial sac but fluid was not detected.

DR. ROBERTS: Dr. Virmani, your necropsy observations in this patient are consistent with idiopathic dilated cardiomyopathy. What *morphologic criteria make this diagnosis at necropsy?*

DR. VIRMANI: To diagnose idiopathic dilated cardiomyopathy at necropsy, five criteria must be met: (1) both ventricular cavities must be dilated; (2) the heart weight must be increased ($>$ 350 gms. in adult women and $>$ 400 gms. in adult men); (3) the lumens of the major epicardial coronary arteries must be $<$ 75 per cent narrowed in cross-sectional area by atherosclerotic plaque; (4) the four cardiac valves must be anatomically normal or have only minimal focal, small scars; and (5) no associated systemic or other known cardiovascular conditions can be present. In addition, intracardiac thrombi are usually present in one or more cardiac cavities, but this finding is not essential for diagnosis.

DR. ROBERTS: Dr. Itscoitz, although many clinical definitions of idiopathic dilated cardio-

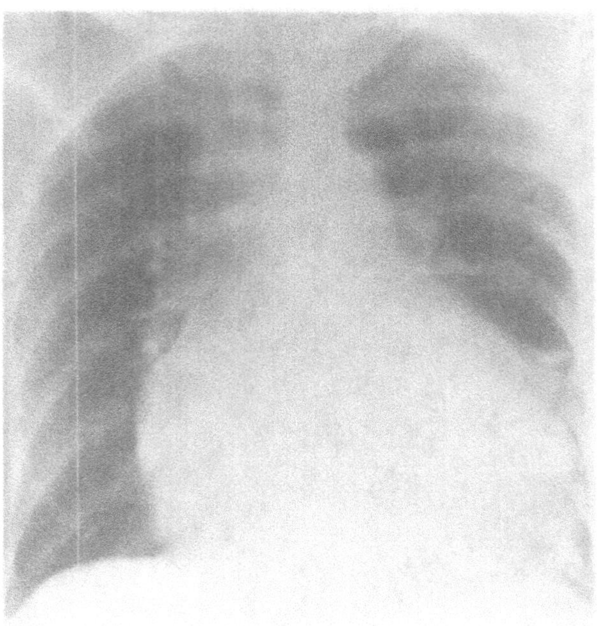

Fig. 2. Posteroanterior chest radiograph on admission 5 days before death The cardiac silhouette is markedly enlarged and the pulmonary vessels are prominent—i.e., "congested."

myopathy include the absence of systemic hypertension and the absence of valvular heart disease, many of these patients have systemic hypertension and most, before the end, have one or more precordial murmurs. *How do you diagnose idiopathic dilated cardiomyopathy in the presence of systemic hypertension or precordial murmurs or both?*

DR. ITSCOITZ: If systemic hypertension is present throughout the entire clinical course, I do not believe the diagnosis of idiopathic dilated cardiomyopathy would then be appropriate. If systemic hypertension were present, however, only at the beginning of the patient's course and was absent in the last few months, the diagnosis of idiopathic dilated cardiomyopathy could still be proper. In other words, if the blood pressure rises progressively and persists throughout the course, diagnosis of idiopathic dilated cardiomyopathy would not be appropriate.

In general, precordial murmurs appear relatively late in the course and the murmurs may get louder as the ventricular cavities get bigger. In the present patient, however, a precordial murmur preceded the presence of overt congestive heart failure, but that is unusual.

DR. ROBERTS: An unusual feature of this

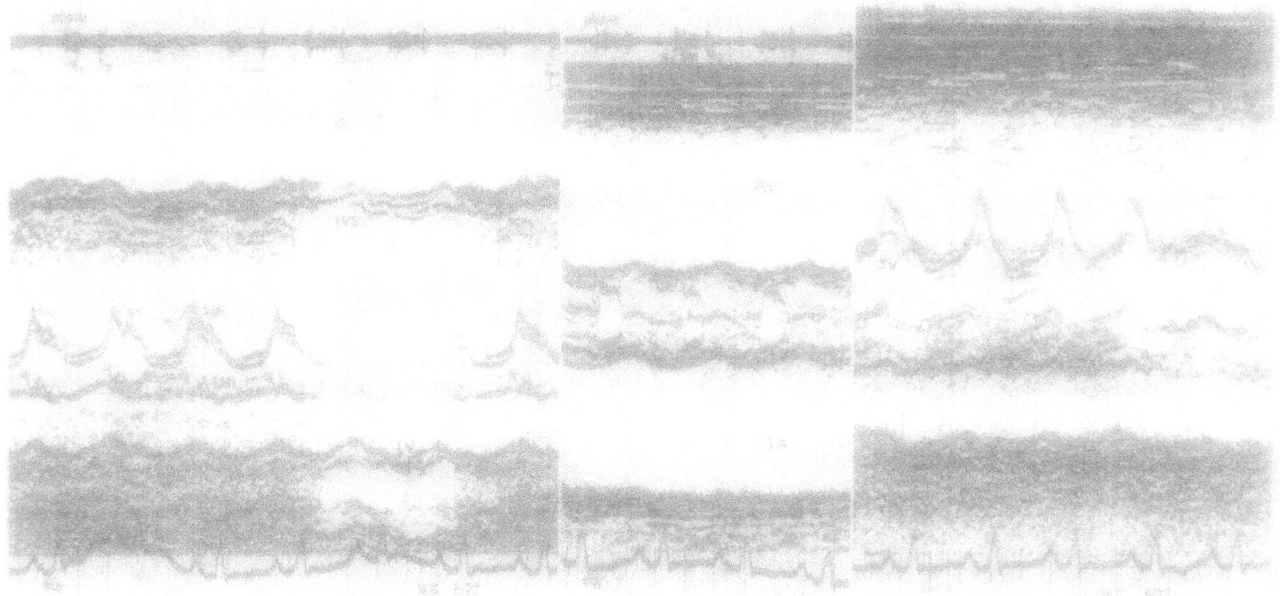

Fig. 3. Echophonocardiograms recorded one day before death. *Left*, ventricular dilatation with diminished excursion of both septum (*IVS*) and left ventricular (*LV*) free wall. There is no evidence of pericardial effusion. *RV* = right ventricle; *AML* and *PML* = anterior and posterior mitral leaflets, respectively. *Middle*, Severely dilated right ventricular outflow tract (*RVOT*). *Ao* = aortic valve within aorta; *LA* = left atrium; *SM* = systolic murmur. *Right*, Another view of the markedly dilated right ventricle at the level of the tricuspid valve (*TV*).

patient morphologically was the presence of a very large cardiac scar involving not only the left ventricular free wall and ventricular septum, but also the right ventricular free wall. I have studied the hearts of 153 necropsy patients with idiopathic dilated cariomyopathy and this patient had the largest ventricular scar of any. In addition, this is one of the few patients with idiopathic dilated cardiomyopathy seen personally at necropsy with extensive right ventricular scarring. Dr. Virmani, *could you enlighten us to the cause of ventricular scarring in patients with idiopathic dilated cardiomyopathy?*

DR. VIRMANI: The cause of cardiac ventricular scarring in patients with idiopathic dilated cardiomyopathy is unclear. By definition, the epicardial coronary arteries cannot be significantly narrowed in this condition, and, therefore, narrowing of these vessels is not a cause of the scarring. Embolism to the coronary arteries from thrombi located within the left side of the heart is a potential cause of left ventricular scarring. In patients with coronary embolism, however, whom we have studied at necropsy, there usually is evidence of occlusion of one or more of the

intramural coronary arteries.[1] Multiple histologic sections of the ventricular walls in the present patient, however, disclosed no abnormality of the intramural coronary arteries and that observation is strong evidence aginst embolism as a cause of scarring. The extremely diminished cardiac output, which occurs in patients with idiopathic dilated cardiomyopathy, generally leads to a "global" myocardial ischemia and not so much to a focal myocardial ischemia. Ventricular scarring is always focal and, therefore, its explanation in these patients is uncertain.

DR. ROBERTS: Recently, Dr. Isner and I reviewed a large number of necropsy patients with coronary heart disease who had both right ventricular and left ventricular myocardial infarction.[2] The present patient, however, shows that right ventricular infarction may occur in the absence of coronary arterial luminal narrowing. Dr. Isner, *what features allow the clinical diagnosis of right ventricular infarction?*

DR. ISNER: From review of clinical and necropsy features of 33 patients with right ventricular myocardial infarction associated with left ventricular infarction, three findings suggest clinical-

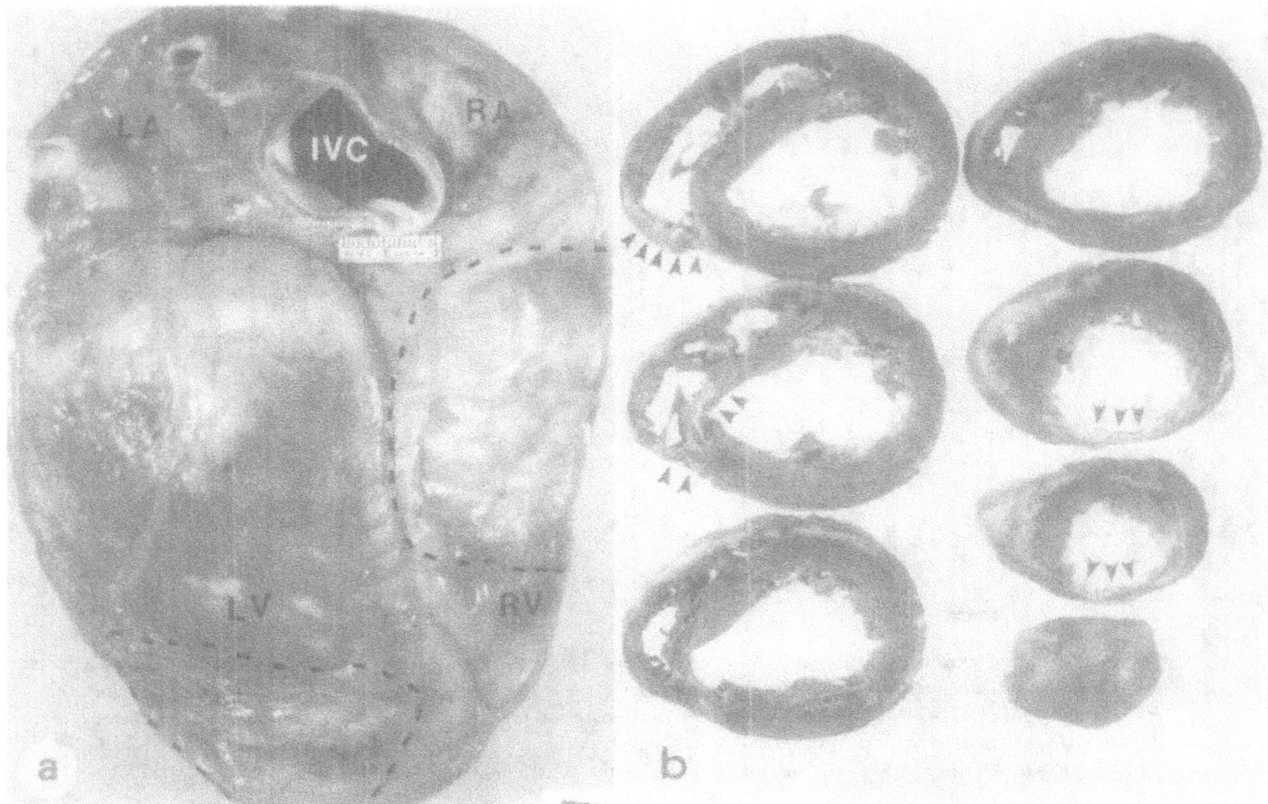

Fig. 4, a and **b.** Transmural ventricular scarring in the patient described. *a*, Posterior view of heart showing external appearance of left ventricular (*LV*) and right ventricular (*RV*) scars (*enclosed by dashed lines*). *b*, Transverse sections of ventricles from base (*upper left*) to apex (*lower right*). *The arrows* designate sites of transmural scarring. *LA* = left atrium; *RA* = right atrium; *IVC* = inferior vena cava.

ly the presence of right ventricular infarction[2]: (1) electrocardiographic evidence of an inferior or posterior left ventricular wall myocardial infarction, (2) evidence of right ventricular dilatation, and (3) a right ventricular filling pressure equal to or out of proportion to the left ventricular filling pressure. Of our 33 patients, all had an associated infarction of the posterior ("inferior") wall of the left ventricle. In contrast, of 97 patients with isolated anterior wall infarction of the left ventricle, none had associated right ventricular myocardial infraction. Furthermore, among the patients with posterior wall left ventricular infarcts, those with right ventricular myocardial infarcts had right ventricular dilatation observed at necropsy nearly three times more frequently than did the patients without right ventricular myocardial infarcts. Comparison of patients with right ventricular myocaridal infarction, however, disclosed no differences in the patient's age, sex, extent of coronary arterial luminal narrowing, presence of right ventricular hypertrophy, or right ventricular thrombi, or the length of symptoms of myocardial ischemia.

Dr. Roberts: Dr. Isner, *what clinical features in the present patient,* in retrospect, *might have suggested the presence of healed right ventricular infarction?*

Dr. Isner: First as Dr. Itscoitz pointed out, the signs of right ventricular failure were out of proportion to those of left ventricular failure. The neck veins were severely distended and yet the patient could lie flat in bed without respiratory distress. Secondly, echocardiograms done at 10 months and at one day before death both demonstrated severe right ventricular dilatation, a finding at least consistent with right ventricular myocardial infarction. Surprisingly, no electrocardiographic evidence of unequivocal infarction of the posterior wall of the left ventricle, however,

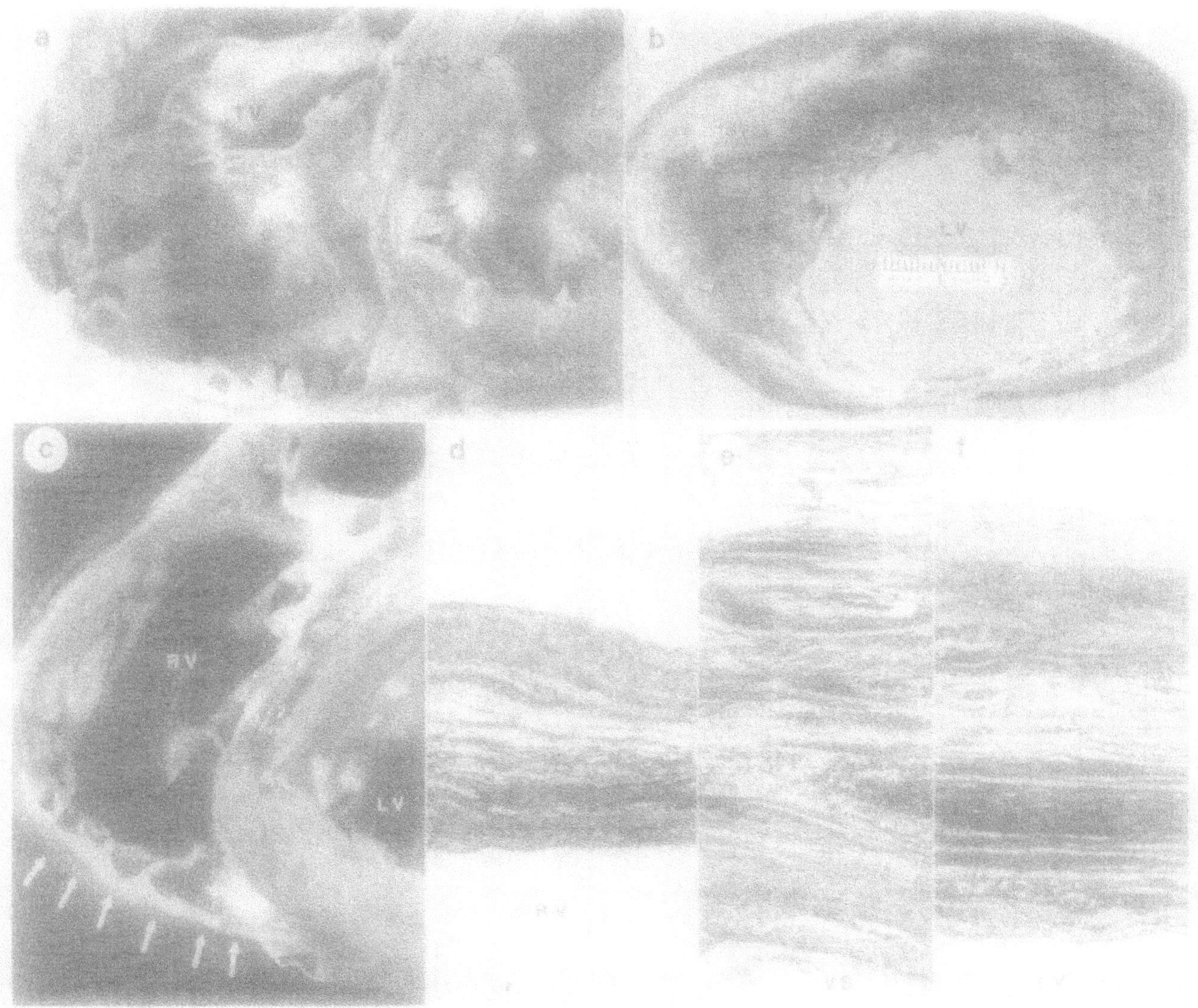

Fig. 5, a through f. Transmural ventricular scarring. *a, Arrows* designate thinning due to healed myocardial infarct of ventricular septum (*VS*) and posterior wall of ventricle (*RV*). *TV* = tricuspid valve. *b,* Posterior wall of left ventricle (*LV*) which is scarred and thinned. *c,* Posterior right ventricular scar (*arrows*) at level approximately 1 cm. caudad to *a. d, e, f,* Photomicrographs of healed transmural infarcts of RV, VS, and LV, respectively. (Movat stains; each original magnification ×36).

was present. The elevation of the pulmonary arterial diastolic pressure to a level of 9 mm. Hg greater than the mean pulmonary capillary "wedge" pressure was a reflection of pulmonary arterial hypertension, in this patient the result of pulmonary emboli. The elevation of right ventricular end-diastolic pressure, however, was out of proportion to both the elevated left ventricular end-diastolic pressure *and* the degree of pulmonary hypertension resulting from the pulmonary emboli. The degree of elevation of right ventricular end-diastolic pressure in this patient would be consistent with an associated right ventricular myocardial infarction.

DR. ROBERTS: Dr. Isner, you[2] and others[3, 4] have mentioned that the signs of right ventricular infarction may mimic those of cardiac constriction or cardiac tamponade. How do you *distinguish the signs emanating from right ventricular infarction from those of pericardial heart disease?*

DR. ISNER: First, electrocardiographic or enzymatic evidence of myocardial infarction certainly would increase suspicion of an associated right

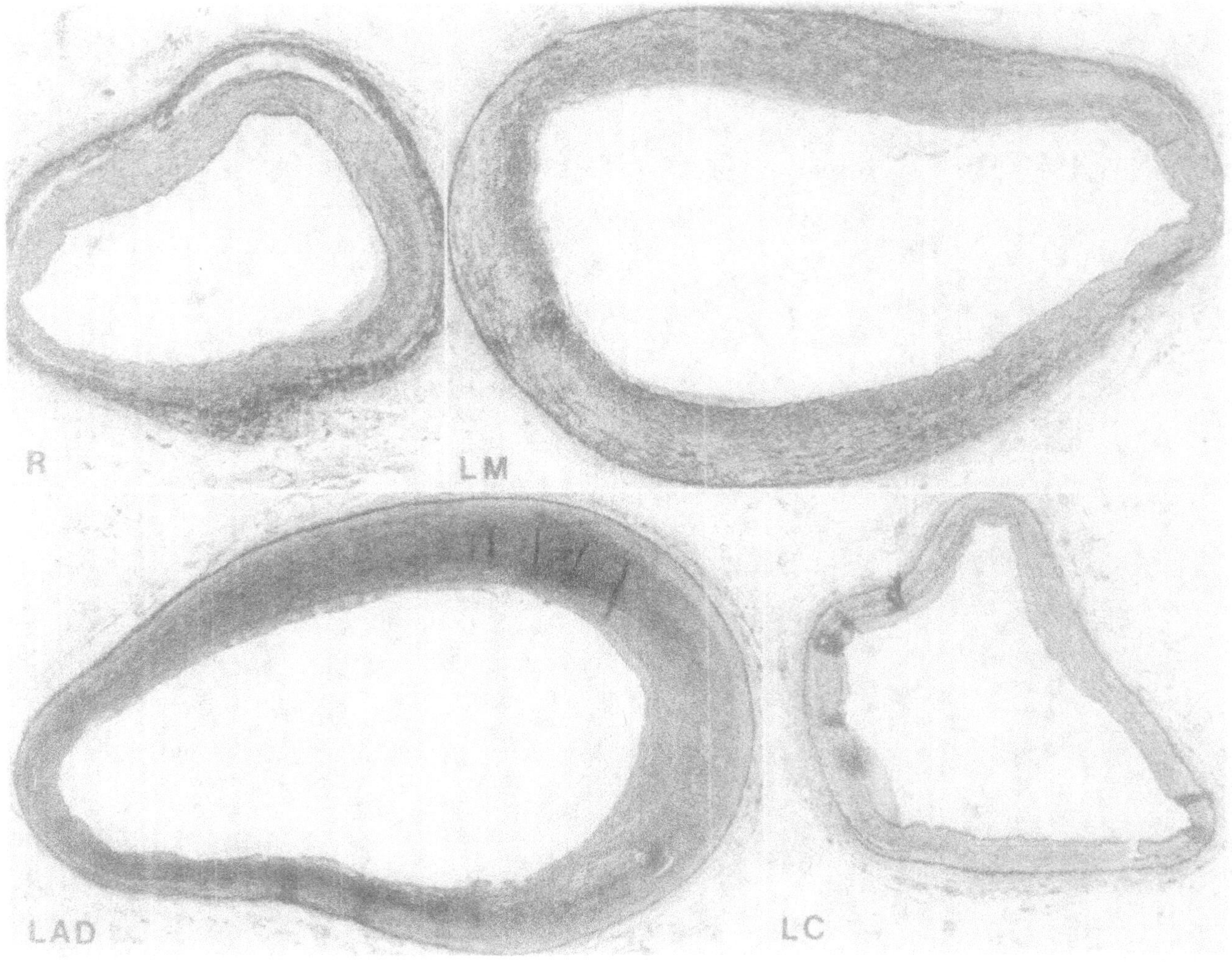

Fig. 6. Photomicrographs of each of the four major (right [R], left main [LM], left anterior descending [LAD], and left circumflex [LC]) coronary arteries at sites of maximal luminal narrowing. None of the coronary arteries were narrowed > 25 per cent in cross-sectional area. (Movat stain; each original magnification ×24).

ventricular infarction as opposed to primary pericardial disease. Secondly, right ventricular dilatation would be most unusual in a patient with impaired cardiac filling due to pericardial heart disease, whereas right ventricular dilatation is commonly present in patients with right ventricular myocardial infarcts. Finally, differentiation between pericardial heart disease and right ventricular myocardial infarction may not be possible on the basis of physical examination alone, and the use of noninvasive tools such as echocardiography and radionuclide angiography or invasive studies may be necessary to determine whether the clinical appearance of the patient is due to pericardial heart disease or to right ventricular myocardial infarction associated with left ventricular infarction.

DR. ROBERTS: The majority of patients with idiopathic dilated cardiomyopathy have mural thrombi in one or more ventricular cavities. The most frequent site is the left ventricle, next the right ventricle, third the right atrial appendage, and fourth, the left atrial appendage. The exact cause of these intracardiac thrombi is unclear, but it seems most reasonable to believe that they result simply from relative blood stasis or inadequate chamber emptying. The danger of intracardiac thrombi, obviously, is that they are sources of systemic and pulmonary emboli. In the present patient, emboli were observed at necropsy in both renal and pulmonary arteries with resulting infarcts of each organ. Dr. Isner, in retrospect, *what features suggested pulmonary embolism as the terminal event in our patient?*

DR. ISNER: The acute drop in blood pressure in spite of longstanding congestive heart failure, the drop in systemic arterial oxygen content, and the appearance of left bundle branch block suggested this possibility."

REFERENCES

1. Roberts, W. C.: Coronary embolism: a review of causes, consequences, and diagnostic considerations, Cardiovasc. Med. **3**:699, 1978.
2. Isner, J. M., and Roberts, W. C.: Right ventricular infarction complicating left ventricular infarction secondary to coronary heart disease. Frequency, location, associated findings, and significance from analysis of 236 necropsy patients with acute or healed myocardial infarction, Am. J. Cardiol. **42**:885, 1978.
3. Lorell, B., Leinbach, R. C., Pohost, G. M., Gold, H. K., Dinsmore, R. E., Hutter, A. M., Pastore, J. O., and De Sanctis, R. W.: Right ventricular infarction. Clinical diagnosis and differentiation from cardiac tamponade and pericardial constriction, Am. J. Cardiol. **43**:465, 1979.
4. Jensen, D. P., Goolsby, J. P., and Oliva, P. B.: Hemodynamic pattern resembling pericardial constriction after acute inferior myocardial infarction with right ventricular infarction, Am. J. Cardiol. **42**:858, 1978.
5. Roberts, W. C., and Ferrans, V. J.: Pathologic anatomy of the cardiomyopathies. Idiopathic dilated and hypertrophic types, infiltrative types, and endomyocardial disease with and without eosinophilia. Hum. Pathol. **6**:287, 1975.
6. Lynch, R. E., Stein, P. D., and Bruce T. A.: Left-ward shift of frontal plane QRS axis as a frequent manifestation of acute pulmonary embolism. Chest **61**:443, 1972.

Quantification of Coronary Arterial Narrowing at Necropsy in Acute Transmural Myocardial Infarction

Analysis and Comparison of Findings in 27 Patients and 22 Controls

WILLIAM C. ROBERTS, M.D., AND ANCIL A. JONES, M.D.

SUMMARY We quantitatively analyzed the degree and extent of coronary arterial narrowing by atherosclerotic plaques in the entire length of each of the four major coronary arteries in 27 necropsy patients with transmural acute myocardial infarction (AMI) and compared the findings with those in 22 control subjects. Of the 1403 5-mm segments examined in the 27 AMI patients, 484 (34%; controls 3%) were 76–100% narrowed in cross-sectional area by atherosclerotic plaques, 528 (38%; controls 25%) were 51–75% narrowed, 319 (23%; controls 44%) were 26–50% narrowed, and only 72 segments (5%; controls 28%) were $\leq 25\%$ narrowed. The amount of severe ($> 75\%$) narrowing of the right, left anterior descending and left circumflex coronary arteries by atherosclerotic plaques was similar, as was the amount of severe narrowing in the distal and proximal halves of these three arteries. The number of severely narrowed 5-mm segments did not correlate significantly with the patient's age at death, the presence or absence of a history of angina pectoris or healed myocardial infarction, or with heart weight. The men, however, had a significantly greater number of severely narrowed 5-mm segments of coronary artery than the women ($p < 0.05$), and the patients with associated transmural left ventricular scars had significantly more severely narrowed segments than did patients without transmural scars.

POSTMORTEM angiographic studies by Blumgart and associates[1] nearly 40 years ago disclosed severe luminal narrowing in usually two of the three major (right, left anterior descending and left circumflex) coronary arteries in patients with fatal acute myocardial infarction (AMI). By histologic study of cross sections of 5-mm segments of the three major coronary arteries in patients with fatal AMI, Roberts and Buja[2] also found that usually at least two of the three major coronary arteries were $> 75\%$ narrowed in cross-sectional area by atherosclerotic plaques. The latter study was qualitative, in that it sought to determine only the number of major coronary arteries narrowed $> 75\%$ in cross-sectional area by atherosclerotic plaque per patient. The present study is quantitative, in that we sought to determine not only if a coronary artery was $> 75\%$ narrowed in cross-sectional area at some point along its course, but also what percentage of its entire length was narrowed to lesser degrees (51–75%, 26–50% and 0–25%). This study is the first attempt to our knowledge to quantitate the degree and extent of narrowing in the major coronary arteries in patients with fatal AMI.

Patients and Methods

We studied 27 necropsy patients with transmural[3] AMI. Clinical and cardiac morphologic observations in these AMI patients are summarized in table 1. In 26 of the 27 patients the ECG was either diagnostic or strongly suggestive of AMI. In all 27 patients, however, AMI was diagnosed clinically. Death appeared to result from cardiogenic shock unassociated with cardiac rupture in 13 patients, from uncontrollable arrhythmias or conduction disturbances in five, from rupture of the left ventricular free wall in two and of the ventricular septum in three, from acute pulmonary edema not associated with shock in two, from intracerebral hemorrhage while on heparin therapy in one and from uncertain cause in one. The interval from onset of symptoms compatible with AMI to death ranged from 12 hours to 38 days (average 8 days), and was less than 24 hours in three patients and over 20 days in two.

Except for two of the three patients who died during the first 24 hours after the onset of AMI, the infarcts were easily visible on gross inspection. The acute infarcts were transmural in all patients, defined as involvement of some portion of the inner half and all or portions of the outer half of the left ventricular wall.[3] In 19 of the 25 patients who had easily discernible infarct margins, the infarcts were large, involving more than 50% of a longitudinal dimension (i.e., from base to apex of left ventricle or involvement of more than one-third of the circumference of at least two of the six or seven ventricular slices cut at 1-cm intervals from apex to base parallel to the posterior atrioventricular sulcus). In the other six patients, the infarcts were of moderate size, involving 20–35% of the circumference of at least two ventricular slices or less than half of the longitudinal dimension of the left ventricle. No patient had a small infarct. At least two histologic sections extending from epicardium to endocardium and at least 2 cm wide from each patient were examined and the presence of coagulative type myocardial necrosis was confirmed in each by histologic examination. Patients

From the Pathology Branch, NHLBI, NIH, Bethesda, Maryland 20205.

Address for correspondence: William C. Roberts, M.D., Building 10A, Room 3E30, National Institutes of Health, Bethesda, Maryland 20205.

Received December 4, 1978; revision accepted September 24, 1979.

Circulation 61, No. 4, 1980.

TABLE 1. *Clinical Observations and Cardiac Morphologic Findings*

| | | Age range (yrs) (mean) | Sex | | Historical data | | | | | Autopsy data | | | |
| | No. of | | M | F | AP | Past AMI | Chronic CHF | DM | SH | Heart weight range (g) | Increased heart | Gross LV scars Wall thickness | |
Group	pts		n	n	n	n	n	n	n	(mean)	weight* n	< ½ n	> ½ n
AMI	27	33–82 (59)	21 (78%)	6 (22%)	11/26 (42%)	6/26 (23%)	5/26 (19%)	8/24 (33%)	13/23 (57%)	310–720 (463)‡	20 (74%)	6 (22%)	5† (19%)
Control	22	29–74 (55)	15 (68%)	7 (32%)	0	0	0	0	0	205–390 (307)‡	0	0	0

*Heart weight > 400 g in men and > 350 g in women.
†Posterior in four patients and anterior in one.
‡$p < 0.05$.
Abbreviations: AP = angina pectoris; AMI = acute myocardial infarction; CHF = congestive heart failure; DM = diabetes mellitus; SH = systemic hypertension; LV = left ventricular.

who had another cardiac disease in addition to coronary heart disease, for example, valvular heart disease or myocardial disease of noncoronary origin, were excluded, as were patients who had had a cardiac operation and those with unequivocal evidence of coronary embolism.

Control subjects were similar in age and sex to the AMI patients and had the following characteristics: 1) death from a noncardiac condition, 2) absence of symptoms of myocardial ischemia or cardiac dysfunction during life, 3) absence of systemic hypertension ($> 140/90$ mm Hg), 4) absence of therapeutic mediastinal irradiation, 5) absence of cardiomegaly (> 400 g for men and > 350 g for women) at necropsy, and 6) absence of left ventricular necrosis and fibrosis. Twenty-two subjects fulfilled these criteria and were selected as controls: 12 died of carcinoma (breast in five, pancreas in three, prostate gland in one, colon in one, ovary in one and tongue in one), four of acute leukemia, three of lymphoma, and one each of heat stroke, gunshot wound and acute infection.

The coronary arteries in all AMI patients and in the control subjects were studied in uniform fashion. The hearts were fixed for at least 1 day in formalin. The four major epicardial coronary arteries then were excised intact, x-rayed and fixed for at least 1 day more. After decalcification (if necessary), each artery was cut transversely to the longitudinal axis into approximately 5-mm segments and each segment was labeled sequentially from either its aortic ostium or from its origin from the left main. The number of segments examined in the AMI patients and control subjects is summarized in table 2. The segments were labeled, dehydrated with alcohol and xylene and embedded in paraffin, and two histologic sections from each paraffin block were cut and stained. The Movat stain was used on one histologic section, which was used for all determinations of luminal narrowing. The degrees of narrowing were based on histologic examination of each cross section magnified 25–50 times. The judgment regarding the degree of luminal narrowing of each 5-mm segment was based on the degree of luminal obliteration within the luminal circle bordered by the internal elastic membrane. The circle

TABLE 2. *Maximal Narrowing of One or More Coronary Arteries by Atherosclerotic Plaques in Patients and Controls*

| | Percent cross-sectional luminal narrowing | | | | | | | | | |
| | 0–25 | | 26–50 | | 51–75 | | 76–100 | | Total | |
Artery	AMI	C	AMI	C	AMI	C	AMI	C	AMI	C
1. R	—	—	0	0	0	2	0	1	0	3
2. LAD	—	—	0	0	0	1	0	3	0	5
3. R, LAD	—	—	0	0	0	3	6	2	6	4
4. R, LC	—	—	0	0	0	0	1	0	1	0
5. LAD, LC	—	—	0	0	0	2	3	1	3	3
6. R, LAD, LC	—	—	0	2	0	3	14	0	14	5
7. R, LM*, LAD, LC	0	0	0	1	0	0	3	1	3	2
Total	0	0	0	3	0	11	27	8	27	22
(%)	(0)	(0)	(0)	(14)	(0)	(50)	(100)	(36)	(100)	(100)

Values not in parentheses refer to number of patients.
*Sections of LM not examined in one AMI patient and in two control subjects.
Abbreviations: R = right coronary artery; LM = left main coronary artery; LAD = left anterior descending coronary artery; LC = left circumflex coronary artery; AMI = acute myocardial infarction; C = control.

was visually subdivided into four equal quadrants, and the percentage of cross-sectional area luminal narrowing in each 5-mm segment was categorized as 0–25%, 26–50%, 51–75% or 76–100%. All histologic sections from all patients were examined by one author and the degrees of narrowing in the sections were "spot-checked" by the other. The intra- and interobserver errors were approximately 5% each. The degrees of narrowing in four of the 27 patients were checked by planimetry and a 95% agreement was found between the visual estimation of the percentage of cross-sectional area narrowing by microscopy (magnified 25–50 times) and that found by planimetry.

Results

Among the 27 AMI patients, 107 major coronary arteries were examined (the left main was not examined in one patient); among the 22 controls, 86 major coronary arteries were examined (the left main was not examined in two subjects). All 27 AMI patients had at least two of the four major coronary arteries narrowed > 75% in cross-sectional area by atherosclerotic plaque, whereas only four of the 22 controls (18%) had two or more arteries narrowed to this degree (table 2). Of the 27 AMI patients, three (11%) had > 75% narrowing by atherosclerotic plaque of all four major coronary arteries; 14 (52%) had three arteries narrowed > 75% and 10 (37%) had two arteries narrowed > 75%. Thus, of the possible 108 major coronary arteries in the 27 AMI patients (actually only 107 arteries were examined), 74 (69%) were > 75% narrowed by atherosclerotic plaque (average 2.7 of four arteries per AMI patient). If the left main coronary artery was excluded, 71 (88%) of the other 81 major (right, left anterior descending and left circumflex) coronary arteries were > 75% narrowed by atherosclerotic plaque (average 2.6 of 3 coronary arteries per study patient). Of the eight control subjects with > 75% narrowing of one or more major coronary arteries, all four arteries were > 75% narrowed in one subject, two arteries were > 75% narrowed in three subjects, and only one artery was > 75% narrowed in four subjects. Thus, of the possible 88 major coronary arteries in the 22 control subjects (only 86 arteries were examined), 14 (16%) were narrowed > 75% in cross-sectional area by atherosclerotic plaque (average 0.6 of four coronary arteries per control). Excluding the left main coronary artery, 13 (20%) of the 66 other major (right, left anterior descending and left circumflex) coronary arteries were narrowed > 75% (average 0.6 of three coronary arteries per control). Fifteen (56%) of the 27 AMI patients had thrombus superimposed on atherosclerotic plaque in one major coronary artery, but only the amount of luminal narrowing resulting from atherosclerotic plaque was considered. No control subject had a coronary thrombus.

The results of the quantitative analysis of the 5-mm coronary segments in both AMI patients and control subjects are summarized in table 3. Of the 1403 segments examined in the 27 AMI patients, 484 (34%; controls 3%) were 100% narrowed in cross-sectional area by atherosclerotic plaque, 528 (38%; controls 25%) were 51–75% narrowed, 319 (23%; controls 44%) were 26–50% narrowed, and 72 (5%; controls 28%) were 0–25% narrowed. The mean percentage of 5-mm coronary segments narrowed was significantly different ($p < 0.05$) between the AMI patients and the control subjects at each of the four levels of narrowing, as were the mean percentages of 5-mm segments of left anterior descending, left circumflex and right coronary arteries ($p < 0.05$) (fig. 1). There were no significant differences between AMI patients and controls in the mean percentage of left main coronary artery segments at each of the four levels of narrowing. The mean percentage of 5-mm segments of right, left anterior descending and left circumflex coronary arteries at each of the four levels of narrowing was similar in the AMI patients, as well as in the control subjects (fig. 1). In contrast, the degree of left main coronary artery narrowing was less in both AMI patients and control subjects.

TABLE 3. *Quantitative Analysis of 5-mm Coronary Artery Segments*

Artery	Percent cross-sectional area luminal narrowing								Total	
	0–25		26–50		51–75		76–100			
	AMI n (%)	C n (%)	AMI n (%)	C n (%)	AMI n (%)	C n (%)	AMI n (%)	C n (%)	AMI n (%)	C n (%)
LM*	11 (24)	6 (19)	18 (40)	20 (62)	12 (27)	4 (13)	4 (9)	2 (6)	45 (100)	32 (100)
LAD	17 (3)	90 (26)	119 (24)	148 (43)	183 (37)	88 (25)	175 (36)	22 (6)	494 (100)	348 (100)
LC	30 (10)	81 (36)	82 (26)	90 (43)	103 (33)	50 (20)	95 (31)	3 (1)	310 (100)	224 (100)
R	14 (3)	108 (27)	100 (18)	179 (45)	230 (41)	108 (27)	210 (38)	4 (1)	554 (100)	399 (100)
Total	72 (5)	285 (28)	319 (23)	437 (44)	528 (38)	250 (25)	484 (34)	31 (3)	1403 (100)	1003 (100)

*LM not examined in one AMI patient and in two control subjects.

Abbreviations: LM = left main coronary artery; LAD = left anterior descending coronary artery; LC = left circumflex coronary artery; R = right coronary artery; AMI = acute myocardial infarction; C = control.

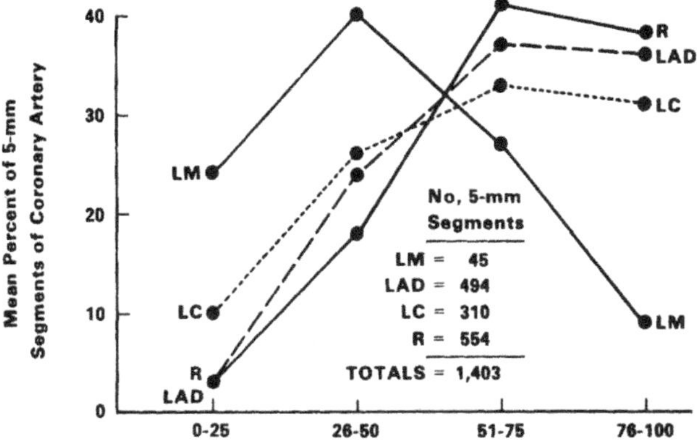

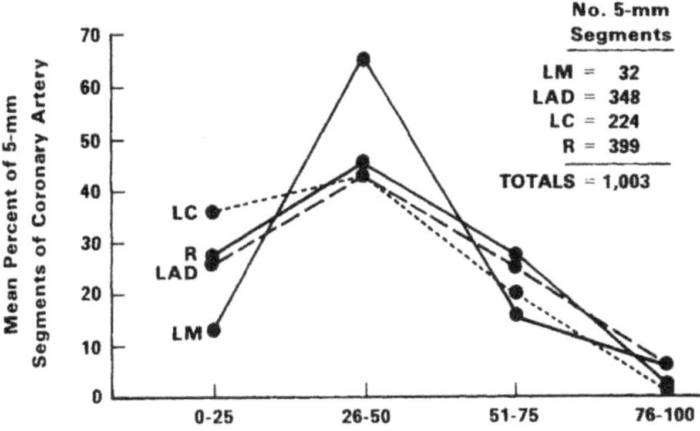

FIGURE 1. *Mean percentage of 5-mm segments of each of the four major coronary arteries narrowed to various degrees in the 27 patients with acute myocardial infarction (A) and in the 22 control subjects (B). The amount of luminal narrowing of the left anterior descending (LAD), left circumflex (LC) and right (R) coronary arteries is similar. The degree of severe narrowing of the left main (LM) coronary artery is considerably less than that of the other three arteries in the study patients.*

The mean percentage of 5-mm segments narrowed > 75% was similar in proximal and distal halves of the right, left anterior descending and left circumflex coronary arteries (fig. 2). The percentage of segments narrowed > 75% in cross-sectional area by atherosclerotic plaque in the first 2 cm of the left anterior descending and right coronary arteries also tended to be higher, but not significantly so, than the percentage narrowed > 75% in the remainder of these arteries (44 ± 6% vs 41 ± 5% and 40 ± 7% vs 38 ± 7%, respectively). The mean percentage of 5-mm segments narrowed > 75% in the first 2 cm of the left circumflex artery was virtually identical to that of more distal segments narrowed > 75% (30 ± 5% vs 30 ± 7%).

The relationship of five clinical or morphologic parameters to the mean percentage of 5-mm coronary segments narrowed > 75% in the AMI patients is summarized in table 4. The men had more severe coronary narrowing than the women, and patients with healed infarcts had more severe narrowing than those without.

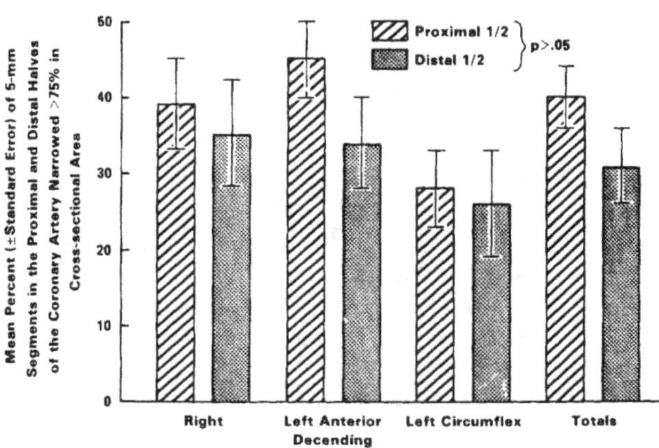

FIGURE 2. *Mean percentage of 5-mm segments of the right, left anterior descending and left circumflex coronary arteries narrowed > 75% in cross-sectional area in proximal and the distal halves of each of the three arteries. The mean percent of 5-mm segments severely narrowed was similar in both proximal and distal halves of these three arteries.*

Discussion

Thousands of autopsies during this century have demonstrated severe narrowing in one or more major epicardial coronary arteries of patients with coronary heart disease, but there has never been an attempt to quantitate the degree and extent of coronary luminal

TABLE 4. *Comparison of Certain Clinical and Morphologic Subgroups*

Parameter	n	Mean (± SEM) of 5-mm coronary segments narrowed > 75% in cross-sectional area (%)	p
Age (years)			
< 45	4	26 ± 10	
45–65	14	33 ± 6	> 0.05
> 65	9	39 ± 6	
Sex			
Male	21	39 ± 7	< 0.05
Female	6	21 ± 16	
Prior clinical CHD AP and/or			
AMI→healed	13	40 ± 5	> 0.05
None	13	32 ± 5	
Heart weight			
Increased*	20	35 ± 5	> 0.05
Normal	6	31 ± 5	
Healed left ventricular transmural infarct			
Present	5	53 ± 8	< 0.05
Absent	22	31 ± 4	

*Heart weight > 400 g in men and > 350 g in women.
Abbreviations: AP = angina pectoris; AMI = acute myocardial infarction; CHD = coronary heart disease.

narrowing in these patients. The present study attempts to fill this void. In 34% of the entire lengths of the four major epicardial coronary arteries in AMI patients (controls 3%), the lumens were > 75% narrowed in cross-sectional area by atherosclerotic plaque and 38% had 50–75% narrowing. Thus, 72% of the lengths of the four major epicardial coronary arteries were > 50% narrowed in cross-sectional area by atherosclerotic plaque in the 27 AMI patients (controls 28%). (A 75% cross-sectional area narrowing is equivalent to a 50% diameter reduction on angiogram.[4])

Severe narrowing was widespread in the AMI patients, and some degree of narrowing was present in virtually every 5-mm segment of coronary artery. In AMI patients, 95% of the lengths of all four major coronary arteries were > 25% narrowed in cross-sectional area, leaving only 5% of the coronary tree narrowed ≤ 25% in cross-sectional area (vs 28% in controls), and not a single 5-mm segment was entirely normal. The degree of severe narrowing in the distal halves of the right, left anterior descending and left circumflex coronary arteries in the 27 AMI patients and in the controls, surprisingly, was just as great as in the proximal halves of these arteries. Similar degrees of narrowing were observed in the left anterior descending, left circumflex and right coronary arteries, but the left main coronary artery was considerably less narrowed. Thus, coronary atherosclerosis among patients with fatal transmural AMI is a diffuse process, involving, for practical purposes, all segments of all four major epicardial coronary arteries.

References

1. Blumgart H, Schlesinger MJ, Davis D: Studies on the relation of the clinical manifestations of angina pectoris, coronary thrombosis, and myocardial infarction to the pathologic findings with particular reference to the significance of the collateral circulation. Am Heart J 19: 1, 1940
2. Roberts WC, Buja LM: The frequency and significance of coronary arterial thrombi and other observations in fatal acute myocardial infarction. A study of 107 necropsy patients. Am J Med 52: 425, 1972
3. Roberts WC, Gardin JM: Location of myocardial infarcts. A confusion of terms and definitions. Am J Cardiol 42: 868, 1978
4. Arnett EN, Isner JM, Redwood DR, Kent KM, Baker WP, Ackerstein H, Roberts WC: Coronary artery narrowing in coronary heart disease: comparison of cineangiographic and necropsy findings. Ann Intern Med 91: 350, 1979

Left Ventricular Aneurysm, Intraaneurysmal Thrombus and Systemic Embolus in Coronary Heart Disease*

Henry Scott Cabin, M.D., and William C. Roberts, M.D., F.C.C.P.

Although left ventricular aneurysm has been reported in association with noncoronary types of cardiac disease, such as hypertrophic cardiomyopathy,[1] congenital deficiencies of myocardium,[2] sarcoidosis,[3] and postoperatively after mitral valve replacement,[4] most occur as a consequence of severe coronary narrowing with myocardial infarction. Most reports on surgical and/or necropsy patients with coronary-induced left ventricular myocardial infarcts and aneurysms have demonstrated a high frequency of thrombi within the aneurysms. Intraaneurysmal thrombi were present in 155 (49 percent) of 314 *necropsy* patients (from five different studies)[5-9] and in 411 (47 percent) of 867 *surgical* patients who underwent left ventricular aneurysmectomy (from ten different studies).[10-19] In contrast to the relative uniform reporting of a high frequency of thrombi within left ventricular aneurysms, the reported frequency of systemic emboli in patients with left ventricular aneurysms has varied considerably. Systemic emboli were described in 100 (32 percent) of the 314 patients with left ventricular aneurysms documented at necropsy,[5-9] but in only 59 (5 percent) of 1,180 reported patients in whom aneurysms were diagnosed by angiography and/or operation.[11-16,18-29] Simpson and associates,[30] examined the frequency of intraaneurysmal thrombi and systemic emboli in patients who underwent left ventricular aneurysmectomy. Mural thrombi were found at operation in 38 (66 percent) of their 58 patients and only two (3 percent) of the 58 had clinical events compatible with systemic emboli. These authors concluded that despite the frequent occurrence of intraaneurysmal thrombi, clinically apparent systemic emboli were rare.

Before accepting the conclusion that systemic emboli are rare in patients with left ventricular aneurysms, it might be useful to examine the definitions used for "left ventricular aneurysm" and "systemic embolus" in several reported studies to determine the uniformity of criteria for diagnosis. Obviously, if definitions of the two items to be analyzed vary from study to study, the results or conclusions may do likewise. *Left ventricular aneurysm* was defined by Simpson and associates[30] as ". . . an abnormally thinned, scarred, or bulging segment of left ventricular free wall noted at the time of surgery;" by Cheng[12] as ". . . a local area of total lack of motion (akinesis) or of paradoxic expansile motion (dyskinesis) during systole of the ventricular wall which may vary in thickness from a paper-thin scar to full-thickness muscle;" by Hines and associates[26] as ". . . a localized area of paradoxically contracting or akinetic ventricle . . .;" by Letac and colleagues[29] as ". . . a sac protruding from the remaining left ventricular contour during both systole and diastole [at angiography] . . .;" by Grondin and associates[27] as ". . . an obvious diastolic bulge with a systolic paradoxical motion [at fluroscopy or angiography] . . .;" by Favaloro and colleagues[19] as ". . . a full-thickness scar tissue replacement of a large segment of the left ventricular wall, usually containing a thrombus and attached to the pericardial sac by adhesions . . . [with] a clear-cut demarcation from the rest of the left ventricle. . . . The absence of a frank bulging mass does not exclude a surgical diagnosis of ventricular aneurysm;" by Loop and associates[15] as ". . . thinned-out transmural scars that have completely lost their trabecular pattern. Although the aneurysm did not always bulge outward, the scar was localized and clearly delineated from surrounding ventricular muscle;" by Phares and colleagues[5] as ". . . defects in the ventricular wall which demonstrate a definite bulge in the external contour of the heart, together with a thinning of the affected region;" by Schlichter and associates[6] as ". . . a

*From the Pathology Branch, National Heart, Lung and Blood Institute, National Institutes of Health, Bethesda.
Reprint requests: Dr. Roberts, Building 10A, Room 3E-30, NIH, Bethesda 20205

localized outpouching of the cavity of a cardiac chamber, with or without outward bulging of the external surface." It is apparent that there is no uniformly accepted definition of left ventricular aneurysm. Consequently, although all the above-cited authors reported findings on patients with "left ventricular aneurysm," their criteria for including and excluding patients varied considerably and, therefore, their findings could also vary considerably.

In clinical studies reporting patients with left ventricular aneurysms, criteria for diagnosis of *systemic* (called by some "peripheral") *emboli* rarely have been defined. Whether the diagnosis of embolism was based entirely on appropriate clinical symptoms and signs or whether confirmation was obtained by angiogram or operation or both has rarely been stated. Reports of necropsy patients with left ventricular aneurysms and systemic emboli usually do not state whether diagnosis was based on the above clinical criteria or on the finding of infarcts in one or more organs at necropsy. Systemic emboli, obviously, might be detected at necropsy, but not during the patient's life and vice versa. Thus, the variability in reported frequency of systemic emboli in patients with left ventricular aneurysms might in part be the result of differing criteria for diagnosis.

Because findings depend to a large extent on the definition of "aneurysm" employed, we have attempted to define left ventricular aneurysm in a way applicable to angiographic, surgical or necropsy studies. We have found it useful to define *left ventricular aneurysm* as a localized cavitary (other than when filled with thrombus) protrusion of left ventricular free wall. Use of the words "anatomic" and "functional" (Fig 1) also is helpful. An *anatomic* aneurysm is a localized protrusion of left ventricular free wall in both ventricular systole and diastole,

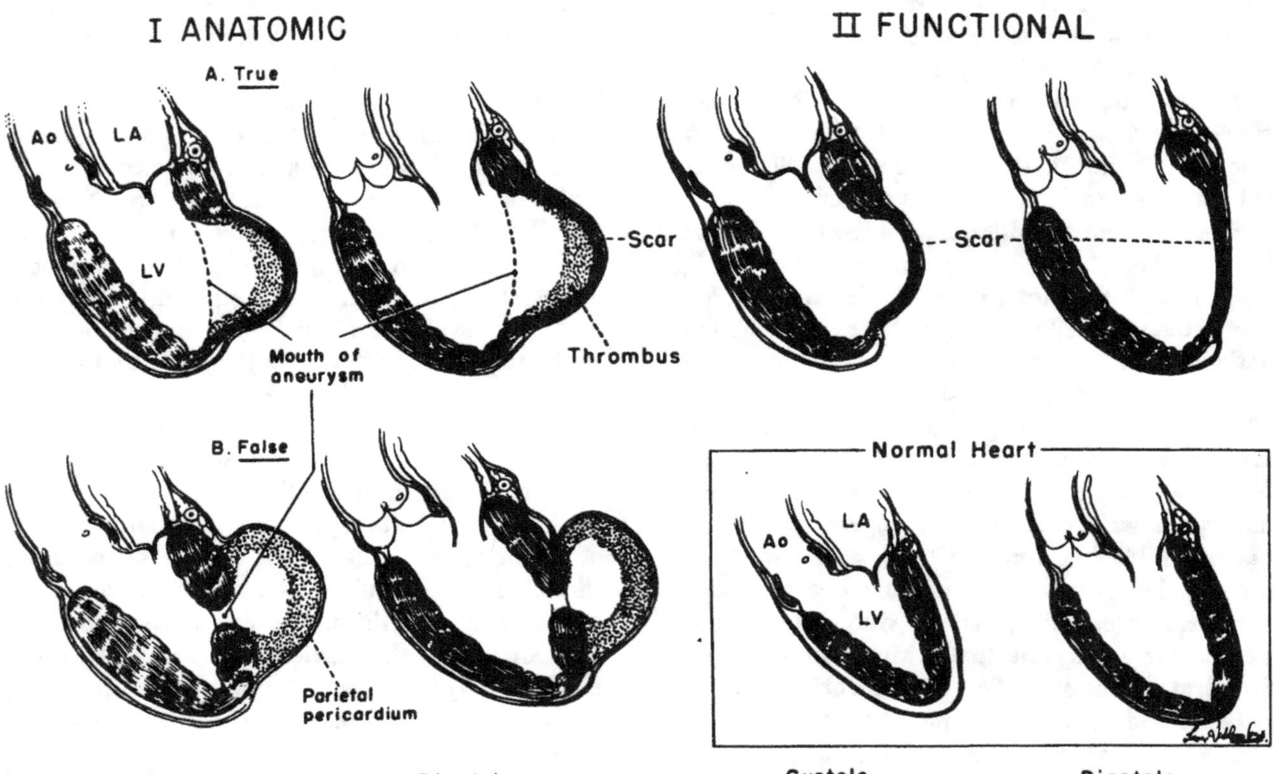

FIGURE 1. Diagrams of hearts in systole and diastole with true and false anatomic, and functional left ventricular aneurysms and healed myocardial infarction. A diagram of a normal heart in systole and diastole is shown for comparison. The true anatomic left ventricular aneurysm protrudes during both systole and diastole, has a mouth that is as wide or wider than the maximal diameter of the aneurysm, has a wall that was formerly the wall of the left ventricle, and is composed of fibrous tissue with or without residual myocardial fibers. A true aneurysm may or may not contain thrombus and almost never ruptures once the wall is healed. The false anatomic left ventricular aneurysm protrudes during both systole and diastole, has a mouth that is considerably smaller than the maximal diameter of the aneurysm and represents a myocardial rupture site, has a wall that is made up of parietal pericardium, virtually always contains thrombus, and often ruptures. The functional left ventricular aneurysm protrudes during ventricular systole, but not during diastole and consists of fibrous tissue with or without myocardial fibers.

whereas a *functional* aneurysm is a protrusion only during ventricular systole. At angiography or at operation, the anatomic aneurysm appears as a localized protrusion of left ventricular free wall during diastole, and during systole the aneurysmal wall may not move at all (akinetic) or may protrude even more than in diastole (dyskinetic or paradoxic movement). A functional aneurysm at angiography or at operation protrudes only during ventricular systole; its wall, therefore, is dyskinetic since it moves outward when the remaining wall moves inward. At necropsy, only an anatomic aneurysm appears aneurysmal. The distinction between anatomic and functional aneurysm is useful because the wall of a functional aneurysm may consist of ischemic (potentially reversible) or necrotic myocardium or mainly fibrous tissue, whereas the wall of an anatomic aneurysm consists of either necrotic or fibrotic tissue or both and neither is reversible. An anatomic left ventricular aneurysm may be either "true" or "false" (Fig 1). A *true* anatomic aneurysm has a mouth that is as wide or wider than the maximal diameter of the aneurysm; its wall was formerly the wall of the left ventricle and consists of necrotic myocardium (acute myocardial infarction) or fibrous tissue (healed myocardial infarction) or both. A *false* anatomic aneurysm, has a mouth that is considerably smaller than the maximal diameter of

the aneurysm and it was the rupture site at the time of the acute myocardial infarction; its wall is composed of parietal pericardium and never contains residual myocardial fibers.

We recently examined the hearts of 28 necropsy patients with true, anatomic left ventricular aneurysms occurring at sites of healed myocardial infarcts. In agreement with most previous studies, we found that intraaneurysmal thrombi were frequent (11 [39 percent] of 28 patients), and histories of clinical signs and symptoms compatible with systemic emboli, infrequent (one [4 percent] patient).

Why are clinical events compatible with systemic emboli infrequent in patients with healed left ventricular infarcts, aneurysms and intraaneurysmal thrombi? For a left ventricular mural thrombus to embolize, a large portion of its surface must be unattached to the underlying wall and exposed to the blood flowing in the ventricular cavity. In patients with *idiopathic dilated cardiomyopathy*, portions of left ventricular mural thrombi frequently embolize because they overly contracting myocardium, have a relatively small area of attachment to left ventricular wall, and protrude into the left ventricular cavity (Fig 2, 3).[1] In patients with left ventricular aneurysms, in contrast, intraaneurysmal thrombi infrequently embolize apparently because they are located in a portion of left ventricle (the

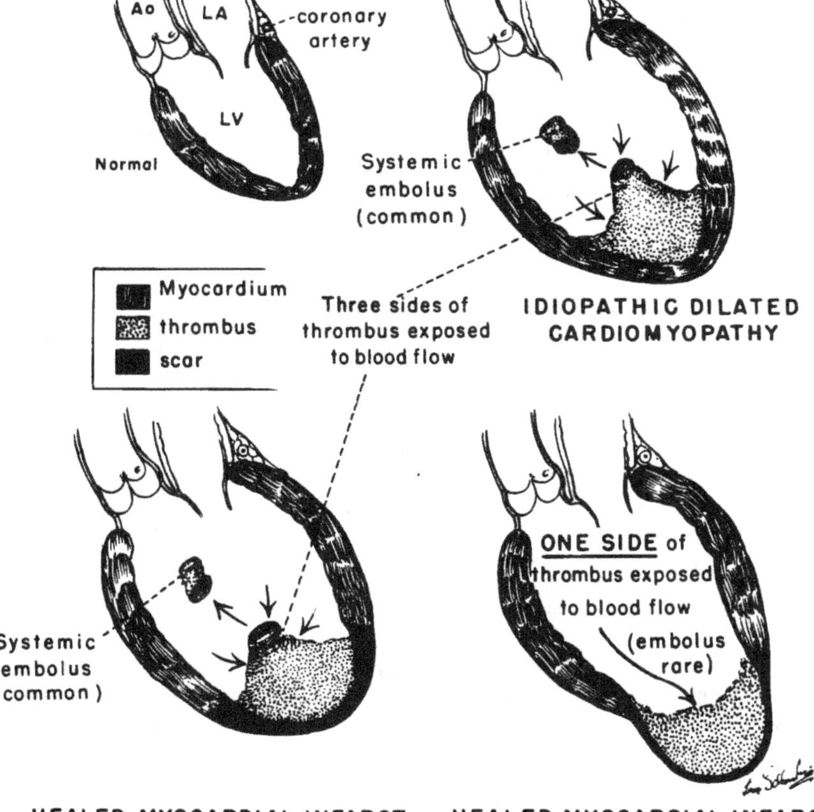

FIGURE 2. Diagram of hearts with *idiopathic dilated cardiomyopathy, healed left ventricular myocardial infarct without aneurysm,* and *healed left ventricular myocardial infarct with aneurysm.* The left ventricle in each contains thrombus. A diagram of a normal heart is shown for comparison. The thrombi in the left ventricular cavities of the hearts with idiopathic dilated cardiomyopathy and healed myocardial infarct without aneurysm are more likely to embolize than is an intraaneurysmal thrombus.

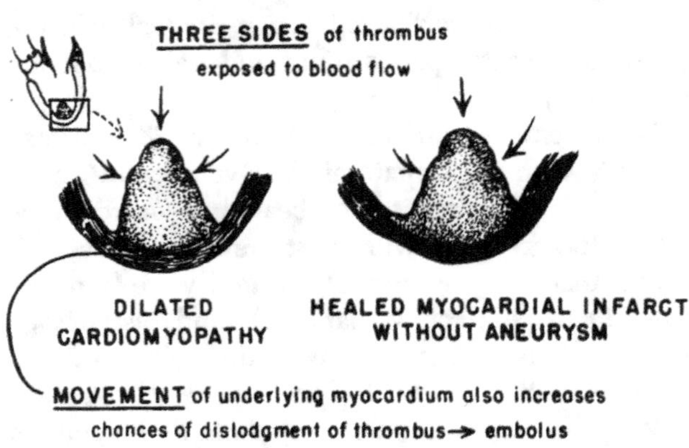

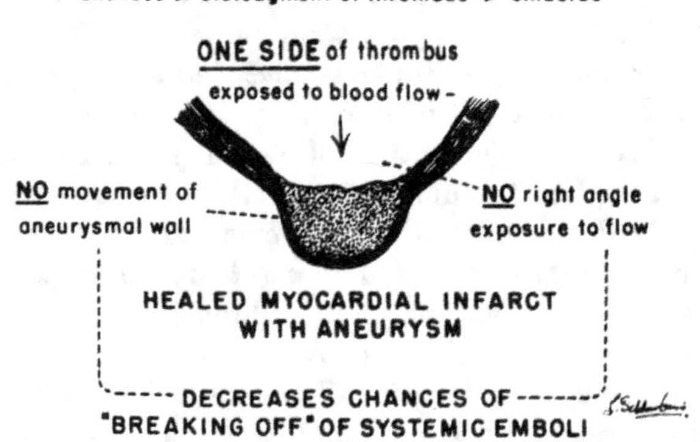

FIGURE 3. Close-up views of the apical portions of the hearts shown in Figure 2. The thrombi in the left ventricles with dilated cardiomyopathy and with healed myocardial infarction without aneurysm are exposed to blood flow on three sides and, therefore, a portion is more likely to dislodge and produce a systemic embolus than is an intraaneurysmal thrombus which is exposed to blood flow on only one side. In addition, the myocardium underlying the thrombus in the heart with dilated cardiomyopathy is contractile, a feature also increasing the likelihood of thrombus dislodgement.

aneurysm) which does not propel its contents in the direction of the outflow tract, the aneurysmal wall underlying the thrombus is virtually devoid of contractile fibers, more of the surface of the thrombus is attached than unattached, and the intraaneurysmal thrombus does not protrude into the left ventricular cavity (Fig 2 and 3).

Should patients with left ventricular aneurysms receive anticoagulants? Simpson and associates[30] found anticoagulants to have no effect on the frequency of intraaneurysmal thrombi or systemic emboli, leading them to suggest that long-term use of anticoagulants is unnecessary in patients with left ventricular aneurysms and "remote" myocardial infarctions. Of their 17 patients receiving anticoagulants, nine had mural thrombi and one of the 17 patients had a clinical event compatible with a systemic embolus; of the 41 patients not receiving anticoagulants, 29 (71 percent) had mural thrombi and 1 (2 percent) of the 41 had a clinical embolic event. The low frequency of clinically apparent systemic emboli in our own 28 patients and in those reported by others[9,11,13,15,16,18-21,23-26,28-30] supports that con-

clusion. In contrast, patients with chronic congestive cardiac failure after healing of acute myocardial infarction but without aneurysm ("ischemic cardiomyopathy" or "coronary dilated cardiomyopathy") commonly have left ventricular thrombi which contact blood on three sides, making dislodgment and embolism a high possibility[31] (Fig 2 and 3). Distinguishing patients with ischemic cardiomyopathy, however, from those with true left venrticular aneurysm after healing of acute myocardial infarction is extremely difficult in the absence of left ventricular angiography. Only two of our 18 patients with left ventricular aneurysm and without left ventricular angiography had the diagnosis of aneurysm made clinically. Thus, in the absence of angiography but in the presence of severe chronic congestive heart failure after healing of acute myocardial infarction, anticoagulants may be warranted in most patients.

In conclusion, a precise definition of "aneurysm" is useful in analyzing patients with "left ventricular aneurysm;" clinical events compatible with systemic emboli are rare despite the frequent presence of intraaneurysmal thrombi in patients with healed myocardial infarcts and anatomic left ventricular aneurysms; the infrequency of systemic emboli probably results from the intraaneurysmal location of the thrombus and the relatively small portion of thrombus exposed to the left ventricular cavity; although it may be reasonable to withhold anticoagulants from patients with left ventricular aneurysm, the difficulty in diagnosing aneurysm in the absence of angiography leads us to suggest their use in most patients with severe, chronic congestive heart failure after healing of acute myocardial infarction.

REFERENCES

1 Roberts WC, Ferrans VJ. Pathologic anatomy of the cardiomyopathies. Idiopathic dilated and hypertrophic types, infiltrative types, and endomyocardial disease with and without eosinophilia. Human Pathol 1975; 6:287-342

2 Swyer AJ, Mauss IH, Rosenblatt P. Congenital diverticulosis of left ventricle. Am J Dis Child 1950; 79:111-114

3 Roberts WC, McAllister HA, Ferrans VJ. Sarcoidosis of the heart. A clinicopathologic study of 35 necropsy patients (group I) and review of 78 perviously described necropsy patients (group II). Am J Med 1977; 63:86-108

4 Rose AG, Losman JG. Subvalvular left ventricular false aneurysm complicating mitral valve replacement. Arch Pathol Lab Med 1978; 102:285-286

5 Phares W, Edwards JE, Burchell HB. Cardiac aneurysms. Clinicopathologic studies. Proc Staff Meet, Mayo Clin 1953; 28:264-271

6 Schlichter J, Hellerstein HK, Katz LN. Aneurysm of the heart. A correlative study of one hundred and two proved cases. Medicine 1954; 33:43-86

7 Abrams DL, Edelist A, Luria MH, Miller AJ. Ventricular

aneurysm. A reappraisal based on study of sixty-five consecutive autopsied cases. Circulation 1963; 27:164-169

8 Dubnow MH, Burchell HB, Titus JL. Postinfarction ventricular aneurysm. A clinicomorphologic and electrocardiographic study of 80 cases. Am Heart J 1965; 70:753-760

9 Davis RW, Ebert PA. Ventricular aneurysm. A clinical-pathologic correlation. Am J Cardiol 1972; 29:1-6

10 Cooley DA, Henly WS, Amod KH, Chapman DW. Ventricular aneurysm following myocardial infarction; results of surgical treatment. Ann Surg 1959; 150-595-612

11 Cooley DA, Hallman GL, Henly WS. Left ventricular aneurysm due to myocardial infarction. Arch Surg 1964; 88:114-121

12 Cheng TO. Incidence of ventricular aneurysm in coronary artery disease. An angiographic appraisal. Am J Med 1971; 50:340-355

13 Kluge TH, Ullal SR, Hill JD, Kerth WJ, Gerbode F. Dyskinesis and aneurysm of the left ventricle. Surgical experience in 36 patients. J Cardiovasc Surg 1971; 12:273-280

14 Graber JD, Oakley CM, Pickering BN, Goodwin, JF, Raphael MJ, Steiner RE. Ventricular aneurysm. An appraisal of diagnosis and surgical treatment. Br Heart J 1972; 34:830-838

15 Loop FD, Effler DB, Navia JA, Sheldon WC, Groves LK. Aneurysms of the left ventricle. Survival and results of a ten-year surgical experience. Ann Surg 1973; 178:399-405

16 Rao G, Zikria EA, Miller WH, Samadani SR, Ford WB. Experience with sixty consecutive ventricular aneurysm resections. Circulation 1974; 50 (suppl 2):149-153

17 Marco JD, Kaiser GC, Barner HE, Codd JE, Willman VL. Left ventricular aneurysmectomy. Arch Surg 1976; 111:419-422

18 Mullen DC, Posey L, Gabriel R, Singh HM, Flemma RJ, Lepley D. Prognostic considerations in the management of left ventricular aneurysms. Ann Thorac Surg 1977; 23:455-460

19 Favaloro RG, Effler DB, Groves LK, Westcott RN, Suarez E, Lozado J. Ventricular aneurysm-clinical experience. Ann Thorac Surg 1968; 6:227-245

20 Gorlin R, Klein MD, Sullivan JM. Prospective correlative study of ventricular aneurysm. Am J Med 1967; 42:512-531

21 Key JA, Aldridge HE, MacGregor DC. The selection of patients for resection of left ventricular aneurysm. J Thorac Cardiovasc Surg 1968; 56:477-483

22 Schattenberg TT, Giuliani ER, Campion BC, Danielson GK. Post-infarction ventricular aneurysm. Mayo Clin Proc 1970; 45:13-19

23 Stoney WS, Alford WC, Burrus GR, Thomas CS. Repair of anteroseptal ventricular aneurysm. Ann Thorac Surg 1973; 15:394-404

24 Cooperman M, Stinson EB, Griepp RB, Shumway NE. Survival and function after left ventricular aneurysmectomy. J Thorac Cardiovasc Surg 1975; 69:321-328

25 Watson LE, Dickhaus DW, Martin RH. Left ventricular aneurysm. Preoperative hemodynamics, chamber volume, and results of aneurysmectomy. Circulation 1975; 52:868-873

26 Hines GL, Rivas J, Epstein H, Delaney T, Mohtashemi M. Surgical treatment of ventricular aneurysms. Seven year experience. NY State J Med 1978; 78:1715-1719

27 Grondin P, Kretz JG, Bical O, Donzeau-Gouge P, Petitclerc R, Campeau L. Natural history of saccular aneurysms of the left ventricle. J Thorac Cardiovasc Surg 1979; 77:57-64

28 Hutchinson JE, III, Green GG, Mekhjian HA, Camunas JL, Habal SM, Parodi EM, Schwartz MJ. Combined left ventricular aneurysm and coronary artery bypass surgery. Arch Surg 1978; 113:1236-1240

29 Letac B, Leroux G, Cribier A, Soyer R. Large ventricular aneurysms occurring after myocardial infarction. Br Heart J 1978; 40:516-522

30 Simpson MT, Oberman A, Kouchoukos NT, Rogers WJ. Prevalence of mural thrombi and systemic embolization with left ventricular aneurysm. Effect of anticoagulation therapy. Chest 1980; 77:

31 Virmani R, Roberts WC: Quantification of coronary arterial narrowing and of left ventricular myocardial scarring in healed myocardial infarction with chronic, eventually fatal, congestive cardiac failure. Am J Med (in press)

Sudden Death While Running in Conditioned Runners Aged 40 Years or Over

BRUCE F. WALLER, MD
WILLIAM C. ROBERTS, MD, FACC

Bethesda, Maryland

Clinical and necropsy observations are described in five white male runners aged 40 to 53 years (average 46 years) who ran 22 to 176 km/week (mean 53 km) for 1 to 10 years (mean 5). None had clinical evidence of cardiac disease before they became habitual runners, and all died while running. At necropsy all had severe atherosclerotic luminal narrowing of their major epicardial coronary arteries. Of the five runners, at least four had hypercholesterolemia, two had systemic hypertension, one had angina pectoris and none had clinical evidence of an acute myocardial infarct. The single symptomatic runner also had an abnormal resting electrocardiogram and a positive exercise stress test. The electrocardiogram (four patients) and exercise stress tests (three patients) in the other four runners were normal. At autopsy, all five men had greater than 75 percent narrowing of cross-sectional area by atherosclerotic plaques of the right, left anterior descending and left circumflex coronary arteries. In three men the entire lengths of these three coronary arteries and also the left main coronary artery were examined histologically (total 5 mm segments = 153); 73 (48 percent) of the segments were narrowed greater than 75 percent in cross-sectional area by atherosclerotic plaques and 32 (21 percent) were narrowed by 51 to 75 percent. Four of the five runners had healed (clinically silent) myocardial infarcts. Thus, coronary heart disease appears to be the major killer of conditioned runners aged 40 years and over who die while running.

The cause of sudden nontraumatic death in conditioned runners (including marathon runners) who died while running has received relatively little attention. At least 17 necropsy patients who died while running have been reported on, but the reported cardiac necropsy information in these patients is limited and incomplete.[1–7] Our study describes clinical and necropsy findings in five additional conditioned runners aged 40 years and over, each of whom died while running and none of whom had clinical evidence of cardiac disease before becoming habitual runners.

Patients Studied

Clinical features (Table I): All five runners were white men aged 40 to 53 years (average 46) and death in each was the result of severe coronary atherosclerosis (Fig. 1 to 9). However, only one (Patient 4) had had clinical evidence of myocardial ischemia. He had had episodes of transient substernal chest pain with radiation to the left arm after he had run about 13 km. After he had walked about 27 meters or so, the pain would disappear. He would then start running again and continue for another 19 to 26 km without further pain. This patient also was the only one of the five with a "positive" exercise stress test result (Fig. 7). However, chest pain did not develop during either of two stress tests, but the S-T segments were markedly depressed (up to 4 mm). When he started running at age 39, however, he had no angina. It appeared when he was 47 years old, 2 years before death. In Patient 3 an echocardiogram taken 2 months before death

From the Pathology Branch, National Heart, Lung, and Blood Institute, National Institutes of Health, Bethesda, Maryland. Manuscript received October 9, 1979; revised manuscript received January 2, 1980; accepted January 9, 1980.

Address for reprints: William C Roberts, MD, Building 10A, Room 3E30, National Institutes of Health, Bethesda, Maryland 20205.

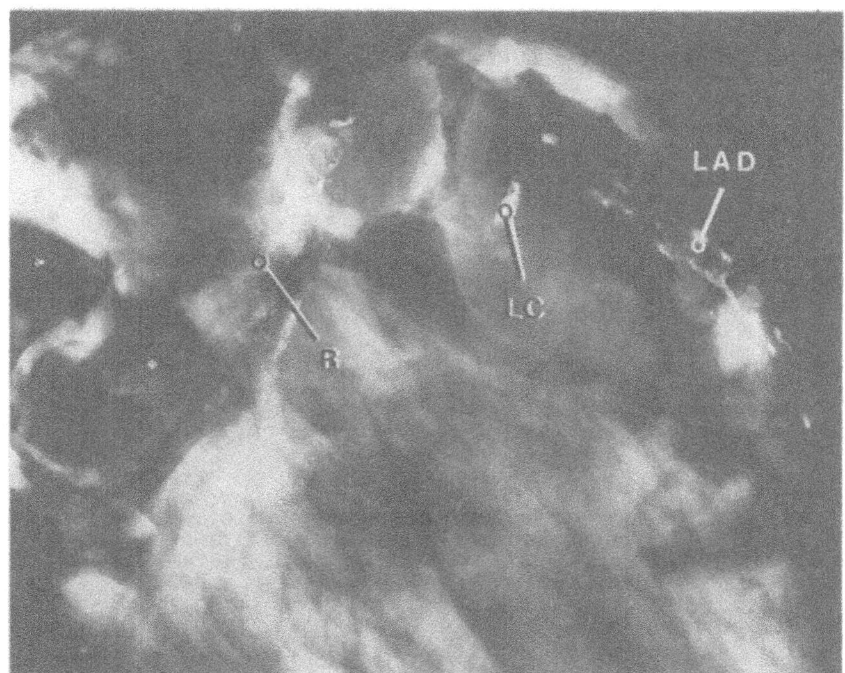

FIGURE 1. Patient 1. Postmortem radiograph showing calcific deposits in the right (R), left anterior descending (LAD) and left circumflex (LC) coronary arteries.

(Fig. 4) revealed a dilated left atrial cavity. During evaluation, a grade 2/6 systolic precordial murmur was heard over the cardiac apex.

Possible risk factors: Three of the five runners had other family members who had had either angina pectoris or acute myocardial infarcts. Total serum cholesterol levels, available in four of the five men, were greater than 300 mg/dl in three and 240 mg/dl in the fourth. In the one man without a cholesterol determination, necropsy disclosed extensive atherosclerotic plaquing in the ascending aorta. (This finding is highly suggestive of an elevated serum cholesterol level and type II hyperlipoproteinemia.[8]) In two of the five men, either the systolic systemic arterial pressure was greater than 140 mm Hg or the diastolic pressure was greater than 90 mm Hg,

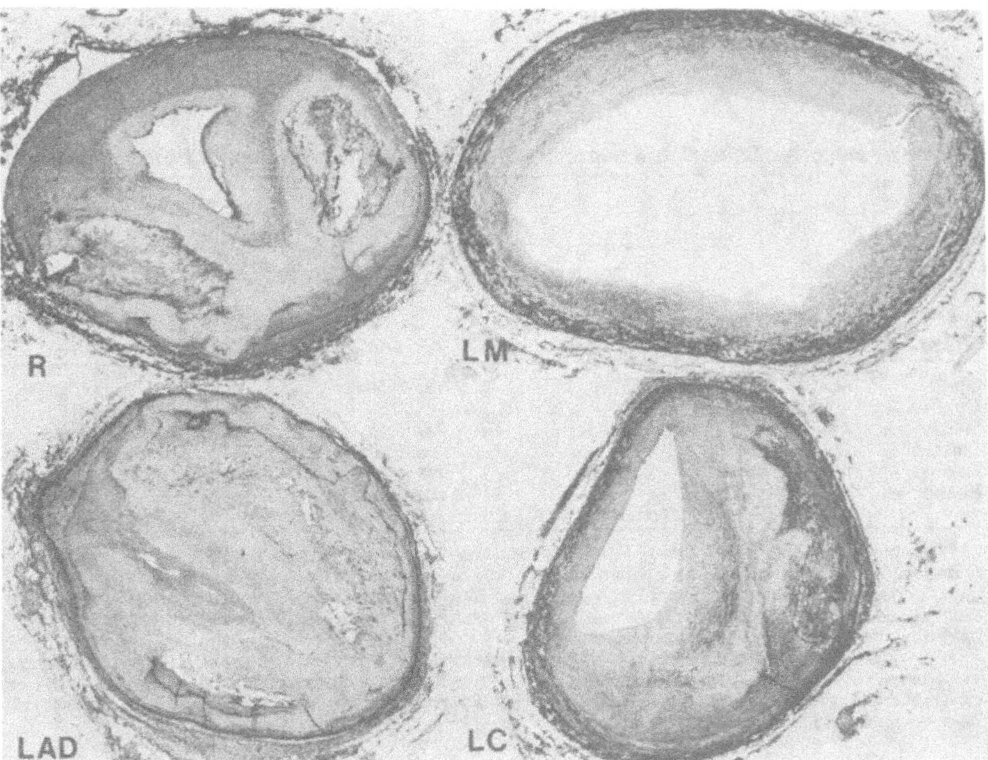

FIGURE 2. Patient 1. Cross sections at sites of maximal narrowing of the right (R), left main (LM), left anterior descending (LAD) and left circumflex (LC) coronary arteries (Movat stain ×20, reduced by 28 percent).

TABLE I

Clinical and Necropsy Observations in Five Conditioned Runners Who Died Suddenly While Running

Case	Age (yr) Race & Sex	Years Run (n)	Average Kilometers Run Weekly (n)	FH of CHD	AP	Interval (days) From Last PE	BW (kg)	Ht (cm)	SAP (mm Hg)	TC (mg/dl)	Abnormal ECG R	E	Interval (days) R and E ECG to Death	HW (g)	LV T Scar	Three Major CA Narrowed >75% in XSA	n Ca 5 mm Segments/ n (%) Narrowed >75%
1 (P.S.)	40WM	5	48	No	No	—	84	71	140/80	—	0	—	182	385	+	3	54/27 (50)
2 (L.W.)	40WM	1	112	Yes	No	90	77	65	130/80	240	0	0	90	460	+	3	. . .
3 (D.W.)	46WM	3	67*	No	No	2	78	68	135/100	310	+	0	60	380	+[†]	3	55/31 (56)
4 (G.B.)	49WM	10	173[‡]	Yes	Yes[§]	320	74	68	160/100	305[‖]	+	+	320	480	+	3	. . .
5 (D.C.)	53WM	5	22	Yes	No	45	79	71	130/70	468	0	0	45	425	0	3	44/15 (34)

* Completed one 42 km race.
[†] Large posterobasal left ventricular aneurysm.
[‡] Completed six 42 km Boston marathon races, seven 80 km JFK races.
[§] Only during running and only during last 2 years of life.
[‖] Initial values of 305 mg/dl 4 years before death; 228 mg/l about 1 year before death when the high density lipoprotein fraction was 41 mg/dl (normal 40 to 80).

AMI = acute myocardial infarction; AP = angina pectoris; BW = body weight; CA = coronary arteries; CHD = coronary heart disease; E = exercise (treadmill test); ECG = electrocardiogram; FH = family history; HW = heart weight; Ht = height; LV = left ventricle; n = number; PE = physical examination; R = resting; SAP = systemic arterial pressure; T = transmural (greater than inner half of wall); TC = total serum cholesterol; XSA = cross-sectional area; 0 = normal; + = abnormal; — = not known or not done.

TABLE II
Number and Percentage of 5 mm Segments of Nine Major Epicardial Coronary Arteries and the Grade of Cross-Sectional Area Luminal Narrowing in Three Conditioned Runners Who Died Suddenly While Running

	Percentage of Cross-Sectional Area Luminal Narrowing				
Major Coronary Artery	0–25 n(%)	26–50 n(%)	51–75 n(%)	76–100 n(%)	Total n(%)
Left anterior descending	6 (6)	10 (18)	13 (24)	28 (52)	54 (100)
Left circumflex	6 (15)	8 (20)	9 (23)	17 (43)	40 (100)
Right	6 (10)	15 (25)	10 (17)	28 (48)	59 (100)
Total	15 (10)	33 (21)	32 (21)	73 (48)	153 (100)

TABLE III
Previously Reported Clinical and Necropsy Observations in Seven Conditioned Runners Who Died Suddenly

First Author	Age (yr) & Sex	Years Run	Average Kilometers Run Daily	Weekly	FH of CHD	AP	History of AMI	Interval (days) From Last PE	SAP (mm Hg)	TC (mg/dl)	Abnormal ECG R	E	HW (gm)	LV T Necrosis	LV T Scar	Major CA Narrowed >75% in XSA (n)	Cause of Death
Opie[1]	46M	. . .	11	. . .	. . .	No	No	. . .	. . .	. . .	. . .	. . .	. . .	. . .	. . .	. . .	?
Opie[2]	. . .M	. . .[a]	. . .	. . .	. . .	. . .	. . .	. . .	. . .	. . .	. . .	. . .	. . .	. . .	. . .	. . .[b]	CHD
Green[3]	44M	8[c]	. . .	80	No	No	No	1	. . .	. . .	No	. . .	350	+[d]	No	0	?
Cantwell[4]	28M	. . .	6	. . .	No	No	No	. . .	. . .	. . .	No	No	. . .	No	No	. . .[e]	?
Noakes[5]	41M	"Many"[f]	. . .	. . .	. . .	No	No	. . .	N[g]	. . .	No	. . .	460	No	No	0	HC
Noakes[6]	41M	3[h]	. . .	. . .	. . .	Yes	Yes	1	. . .	265	+[i]	. . .	345	No	Yes	3	CHD
	44M	3[j]	. . .	46–77	. . .	No	No	78	N[g]	296	. . .	. . .	355	No	Yes	2[k]	CHD

[a] Completed several 32 km runs; [b] "marked" coronary narrowing; [c] completed several 42 km races; [d] resuscitated during race but remained comatose and died 50 days later from infection; [e] only one epicardial coronary artery shown as normal; [f] completed one 84 km and one 42 km race; [g] "normal" but no value given; [h] completed one 80 km race and four 42 km races; [i] acute myocardial infarction 2 yr before death, chest pain during exercise, death during aortocoronary bypass operation; [j] completed eight 42 km marathons, one 56 km race and one 84 km (Comrades) marathon; [k] right coronary artery not described.

AMI = acute myocardial infarction; AP = angina pectoris; CA = coronary arteries; CHD = coronary heart disease; E = exercise; ECG = electrocardiogram; FH = family history; HC = hypertrophic cardiomyopathy; HW = heart weight; LV = left ventricle; n = number; N = normal; PE = physical examination; R = resting; SAP = system arterial pressure; T = transmural (greater than inner half of wall); TC = total serum cholesterol; XSA = cross-sectional area.

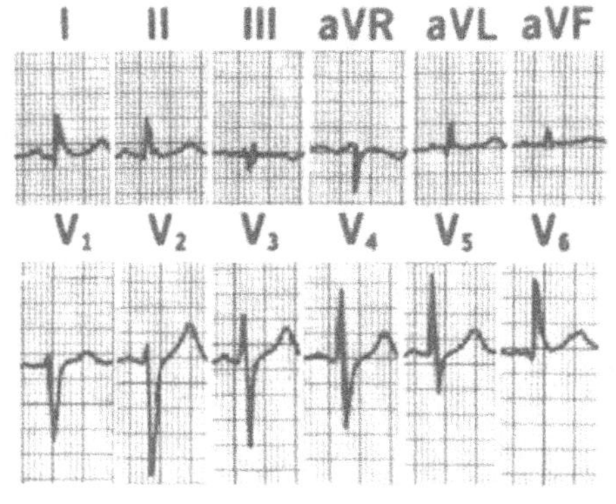

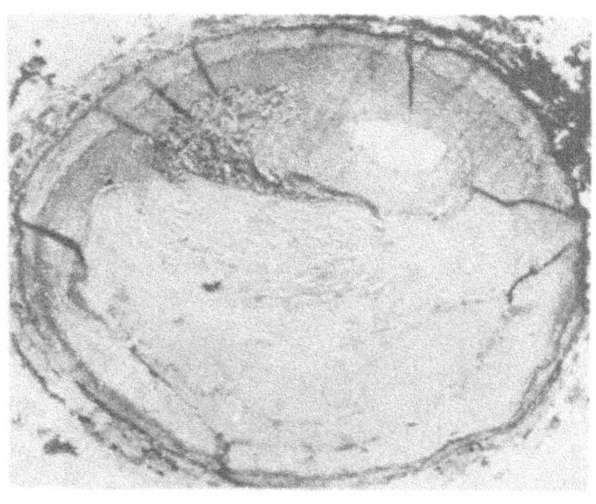

FIGURE 3. Patient 2. Normal resting electrocardiogram obtained 90 days before death (left) and a cross section of the severely narrowed left anterior descending coronary artery (right) (Movat stain × 14, reduced by 26 percent).

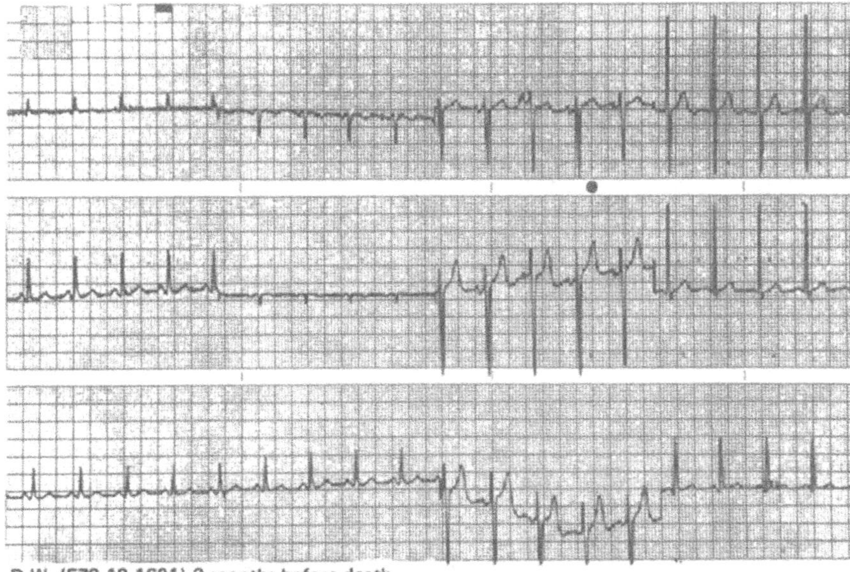

FIGURE 4. Patient 3. Resting electrocardiogram (ECG) (above) obtained 2 months before death showing left ventricular hypertrophy, and echocardiogram (bottom) recorded 2 months before death showing a slightly dilated left atrial (LA) cavity. AML and PML = anterior and posterior mitral leaflets; Ao = ascending aorta; AV = aortic valve; LV = left ventricular cavity; VS = ventricular septum.

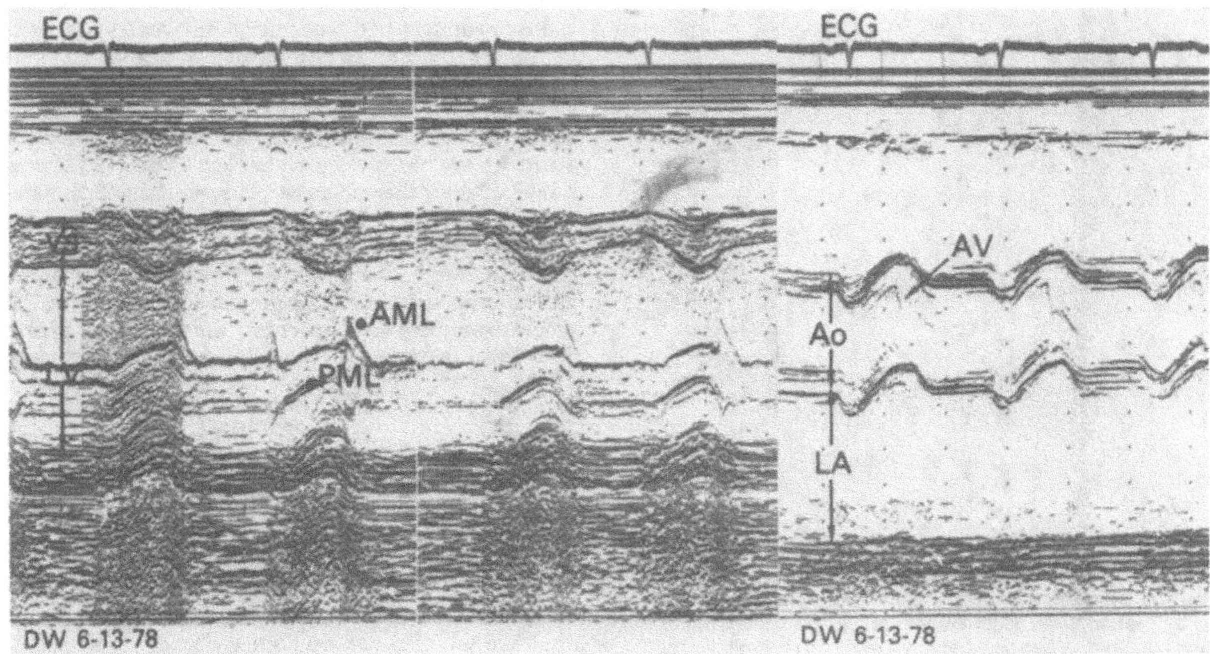

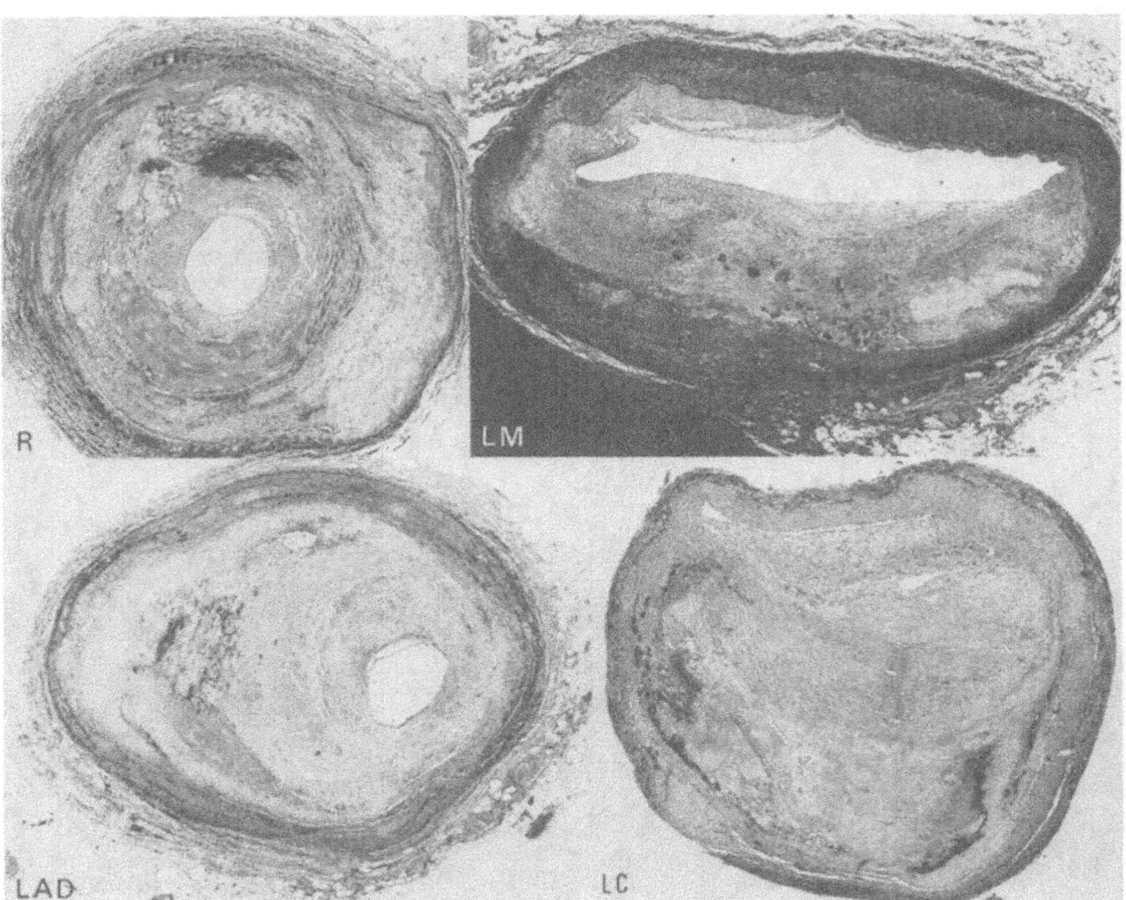

FIGURE 5. Patient 3. The right (R), left main (LM), left anterior descending (LAD) and left circumflex (LC) coronary arteries at sites of maximal narrowing (Movat stain ×22 [R,LM] and ×30 [LAD,LC], reduced by 19 percent).

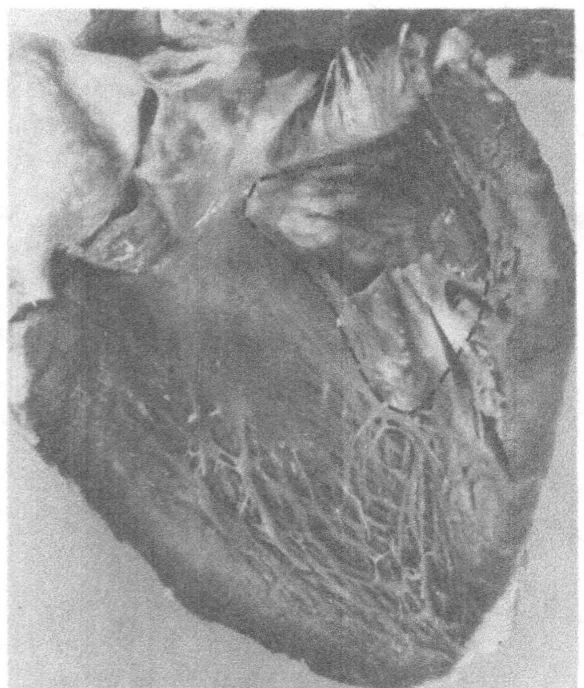

FIGURE 6. Same patient. Opened left ventricle showing an aneurysm at the site of a healed left ventricular basal myocardial infarct (area enclosed by **dashed lines**). Both the infarct and the aneurysm were clinically silent. This patient had a murmur of mitral regurgitation and the posteromedial muscle is severely scarred and atrophied.

or both. However, the heart at necropsy was of increased weight in only one of these two patients; in two of the three patients without recorded elevated systemic arterial pressures, the heart size was increased (over 400 g).

Necropsy findings: Although only Patient 4 had had clinical evidence of myocardial ischemia, at necropsy four of the five runners had transmural left ventricular scars, one (Patient 3) with aneurysm formation (Table I, Fig. 6). Specifically, none of these four men ever had clinical evidence of acute myocardial infarction. In each of the five runners, the right, left anterior descending and left circumflex coronary arteries were narrowed greater than 75 percent in cross-sectional area by atherosclerotic plaques (Fig. 2, 3, 4, 8 and 9). In three of the five patients, the entire lengths of these three arteries were available for examination. Each artery was divided in 5 mm segments and a histologic section was prepared and examined from each segment. Of the 153 five mm segments examined, 73 (48 percent) were narrowed greater than 75 percent in cross-sectional area by atherosclerotic plaques (Table II).

Comments

Of the five conditioned runners described, all died from consequences of severe coronary atherosclerosis. Only one had had clinical evidence of myocardial ischemia, manifested by angina pectoris that occurred only during running and did not appear until the patient's 8th year of running, 2 years before his death. Despite the absence of clinical episodes compatible with acute myocardial infarcts, four of the five runners had transmural left ventricular scars at autopsy. The amount of coronary narrowing in all five runners was severe: In the three in whom the entire lengths of all three major coronary arteries were examined histologically, 34 to 56 percent (average 48 percent) of the segments were narrowed greater than 75 percent in cross-sectional area by atherosclerotic plaques. At least three (and probably four) of the five runners had hypercholesterolemia, three had siblings with clinical evidence of coronary heart disease at a young age and two (possibly three) had systemic hypertension. Thus, these patients were clearly candidates for coronary heart disease.

Marathon running and atherosclerosis: A quick look at the findings in our five runners suggests that Bassler's thesis[9] that marathon running provides "immunity to atherosclerosis" is incorrect.[9] Two of our five men were marathon runners: Patient 3 had completed one 42 km race and Patient 4 had completed six 42 km (Boston marathon) races and seven 83 km (JFK marathon) races. However, Patient 3 did not start running regularly until age 43 when he already had hypercholesterolemia and systemic hypertension. Thus, it is likely that the coronary arteries were already quite narrowed before he began running. Patient 4 started running regularly at age 39 years; he had one brother who had died from acute myocardial infarction at age 32 and a second brother who had two aortocoronary bypass operations performed while in his 40's. In addition, Patient 4 had hypercholesterolemia and systemic hypertension. Thus, this patient may also have had considerable and possibly severe coronary atheroscle-

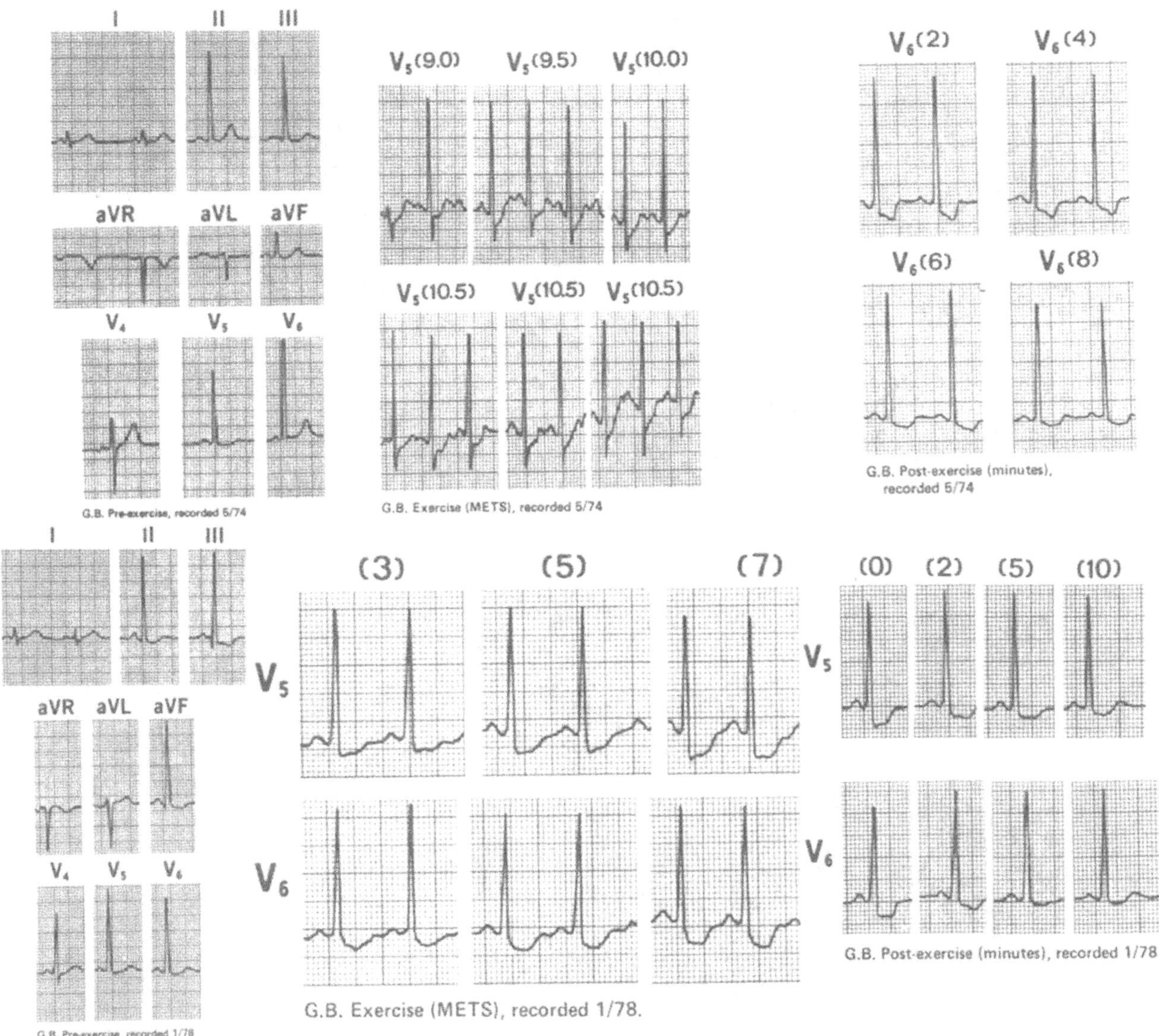

FIGURE 7. Patient 4. **Upper,** electrocardiograms before (**left**), during (**middle**), and after (**right**) an exercise treadmill test performed 4 years before death showing severe S-T segment depression at a maximal speed of 5.5 mph at an 18 percent grade (heart rate = 187 beats/min). **Lower,** another exercise test performed 10 months before death at 3.0 mph at a 10 percent grade (heart rate = 122 beats/min). Both exercise tests, obviously, are strongly positive. METS = metabolic equivalents.

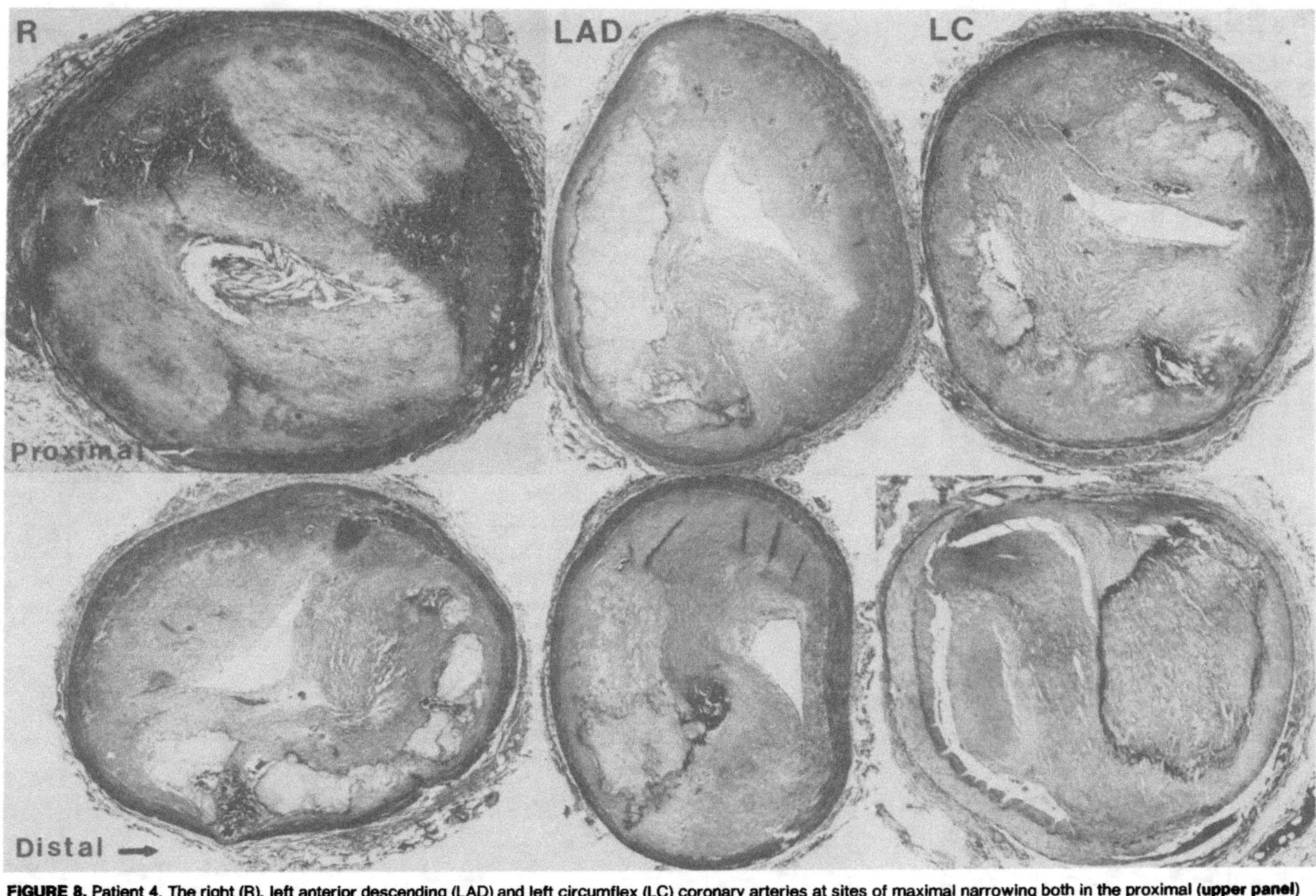

FIGURE 8. Patient 4. The right (R), left anterior descending (LAD) and left circumflex (LC) coronary arteries at sites of maximal narrowing both in the proximal (**upper panel**) and distal (**lower panel**) halves of the respective arteries (Movat stains ×10).

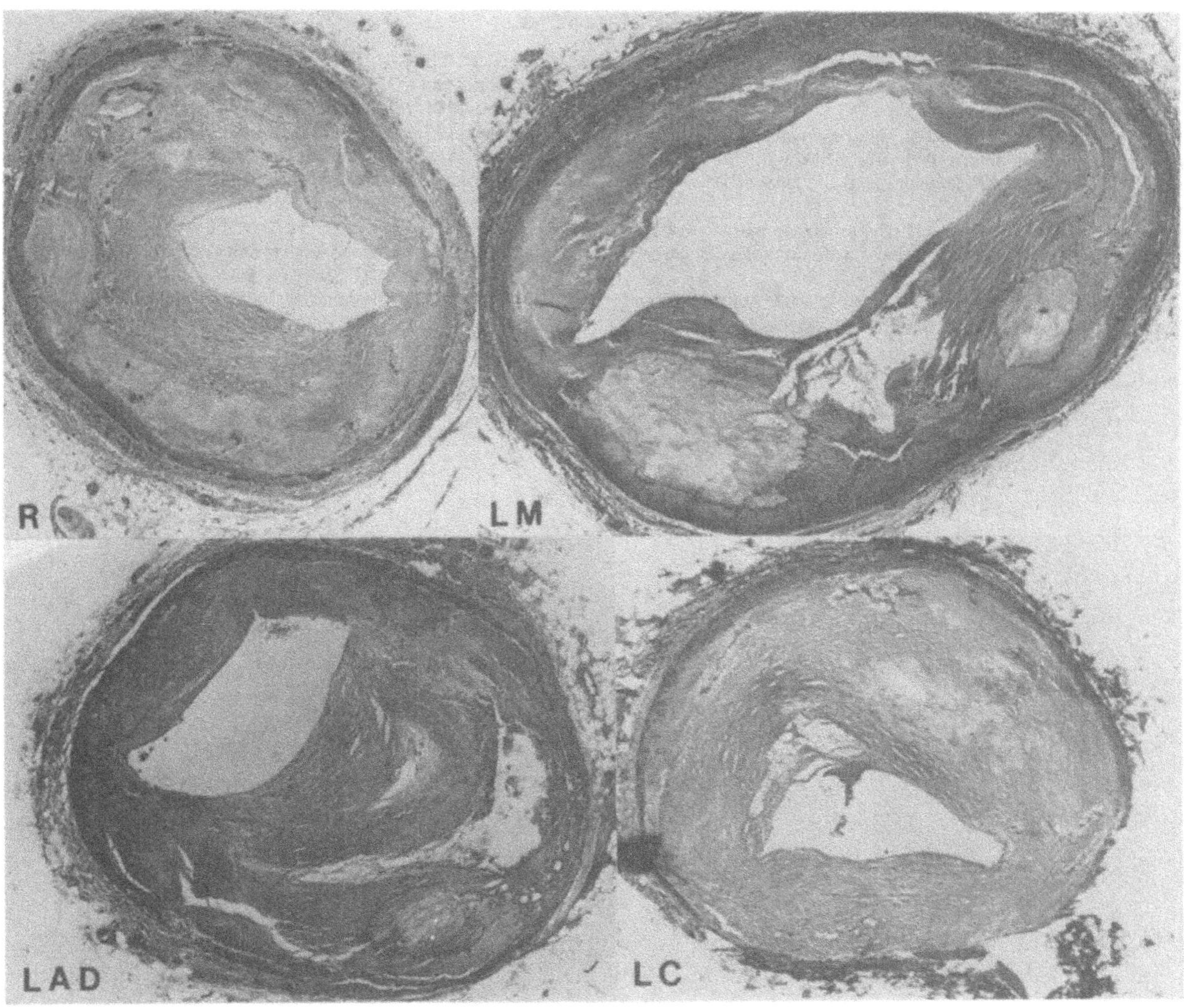

FIGURE 9. Patient 5. The right (R), left main (LM), left anterior descending (LAD) and left circumflex (LC) coronary arteries at sites of maximal narrowing (Movat stains ×12).

rosis by the time he first began to run regularly. Thus, if marathon running is to provide "immunity to atherosclerosis,"[9] the running must start years before the 5th decade of life.

Previously reported studies on coronary artery disease in runners: Our study is not the first to mention severe coronary atherosclerosis as a cause of death in conditioned runners. Although several reports[1–7] have described sudden death in runners, the distance run per week or per day and the length of time that the person had been running regularly is infrequently reported. Findings in seven previously reported runners with some running history are summarized in Table III. Information regarding the serum cholesterol and systemic blood pressure levels and family history of coronary heart disease was supplied in only four patients.[3,5,6] Furthermore, the status of the three major coronary arteries was described in only two patients.[6] Despite the paucity of reported information in the previously reported deaths among conditioned runners, coronary atherosclerosis nevertheless appears to have been the villain in at least three of the seven patients.[2,6]

Thompson et al.[7] recently reported findings in 18 persons who had run periodically from 9 days to 3 or more years, but 4 had run for less than 6 weeks. Fifteen died while running. Data on their 18 subjects were summarized collectively and, therefore, individual clinical and necropsy information was not provided. Additionally, the necropsy information provided was obtained entirely from autopsy protocols, a relatively inaccurate method of obtaining morphologic cardiac information.[10] Of the 18 runners, 13 at necropsy had coronary heart disease, but probably 10 of them had evidence of this diagnosis before they became runners or joggers.

Acknowledgment

We thank Robert L. Flynn, MD, Chevy Chase, Maryland, who graciously supplied the clinical and laboratory information and the results of his 1978 exercise test in Patient 4 (Table I).

References

1. **Opie LH.** Sudden death and sport. Lancet 1975;1:263–6.
2. **Opie LH.** Long distance running and sudden death. N Engl J Med 1975;293:941–2.
3. **Green LH, Cohen SI, Kurland G.** Fatal myocardial infarction in marathon racing. Ann Intern Med 1976;84:704–6.
4. **Cantwell JD, Fletcher GF.** Sudden death and jogging. Phys Sports Med 1978;94–8.
5. **Noakes TD, Rose AG, Opie LH.** Hypertrophic cardiomyopathy associated with sudden death during marathon racing. Br Heart J 1979;41:624–7.
6. **Noakes TD, Opie LH, Rose AG, Kleynhans PHT.** Autopsy-proved coronary atherosclerosis in marathon runners. N Engl J Med 1979;301:86–9.
7. **Thompson PD, Stern MP, Williams P, Duncan K, Haskell WL, Wood PD.** Death during jogging or running. A study of 18 cases. JAMA 1979;242:1265–7.
8. **Roberts WC, Ferrans VJ, Levy RI, Fredrickson DS.** Cardiovascular pathology in hyperlipoproteinemia. Anatomic observations in 42 necropsy patients with normal or abnormal serum lipoprotein patterns. Am J Cardiol 1973;31:557–70.
9. **Bassler TJ.** Marathon running and immunity to atherosclerosis. Ann NY Acad Sci 1977;301:579–92.
10. **Roberts WC.** The autopsy: its decline and a suggestion for its revival. N Engl J Med 1978;299:332–8.

Quantification of Coronary Arterial Narrowing and of Left Ventricular Myocardial Scarring in Healed Myocardial Infarction With Chronic, Eventually Fatal, Congestive Cardiac Failure

RENU VIRMANI, M.D.
WILLIAM C. ROBERTS, M.D.
Bethesda, Maryland

A qualitative and quantitative analysis is described of the amount of ventricular wall myocardial scarring and the degree and extent of coronary arterial narrowing by atherosclerotic plaques in the entire lengths of each of the four major epicardial coronary arteries in 18 necropsy patients with healed transmural myocardial infarcts, and chronic, eventually fatal, congestive heart failure. In all 18 patients, the healed infarcts involved greater than 40 per cent of the left ventricular wall, all had very dilated right and left ventricular cavities, all had hearts weighing more than 450 g (average = 587 g), all had intractable congestive heart failure for longer than three months (average = 2.3 years), and half had intraventricular mural thrombi. Of 1,012 five millimeter segments of the four major epicardial coronary arteries examined in the 18 patients (average 54 segments per patient), 298 segments (29 per cent) were 76 to 100 per cent narrowed in cross-sectional area by atherosclerotic plaques (in 16 control subjects = 6 per cent), 370 (37 per cent) were 51 to 75 per cent narrowed (controls = 35 per cent), 227 (23 per cent) were 26 to 50 per cent narrowed (controls = 43 per cent), and 117 (11 per cent) were 0 to 25 per cent narrowed (controls = 16 per cent). The amount of severe (>75 per cent) narrowing of the right, left anterior descending and left circumflex coronary arteries was similar in the 18 study patients. The left main coronary artery was not severely narrowed in any patient. The amount of severe narrowing in the distal one half of the right, left anterior descending and left circumflex coronary arteries was similar to that in the proximal halves of these three arteries. The per cent of 5 mm segments of coronary artery narrowed 76 to 100 per cent in cross-sectional area in the nine patients was similar to that in the nine patients without left ventricular aneurysm.

Chest pain is a far more frequent functional consequence of severe narrowing of the epicardial coronary arteries than is chronic congestive cardiac failure. Why one patient with severe coronary atherosclerosis has chest pain (angina pectoris or acute myocardial infarction or both) and another has dyspnea (chronic congestive cardiac failure) is unclear. In the present study we focus on a group of patients who at one time had a transmural acute myocardial infarct which healed and either immediately thereafter or at a later time had chronic congestive cardiac failure which became intractable and fatal. Only one patient ever had angina pectoris and that disappeared after the congestive cardiac

From the Pathology Branch, National Heart, Lung, and Blood Institute, National Institutes of Health, Bethesda, Maryland. Requests for reprints should be addressed to Dr. William C. Roberts, Building 10A, Room 3E-30, National Institutes of Health, Bethesda, Maryland 20205. Manuscript accepted November 30, 1979.

failure became severe. In the present study we examine the coronary arteries and the ventricular myocardium in a *quantitative manner* in 18 necropsy patients in whom chronic, eventually fatal, congestive heart failure developed after healing of one or more acute myocardial infarcts. Quantitative studies such as those to be described herein have not been reported previously in patients with healed myocardial infarcts.

PATIENTS STUDIED AND METHODS

The 18 necropsy patients included in the study had the following characteristics: (1) healed infarcts involving at necropsy >75 per cent of the thickness of the left ventricular wall; (2) progressive congestive cardiac failure, eventually fatal, for longer than three months; (3) dilated right and left ventricular cavities; (4) >75 per cent cross-sectional area luminal narrowing by atherosclerotic plaques of one or more of the four major epicardial coronary arteries; (5) absence of left ventricular myocardial necrosis; (6) absence of anatomic valvular lesions capable in themselves of producing valvular dysfunction; (7) absence of a cardiac disease other than coronary heart disease; and (8) absence of a cardiac operation at any time. Certain findings in the 18 study patients are detailed in **Table I**. All but one had a history of acute myocardial infarction in the past, and five had had more than one acute myocardial infarct. Only one patient (Case 15, Table I) had had angina pectoris and that disappeared as the congestive failure worsened.

Observations in the 18 study patients were compared to 16 age- and sex-matched control subjects, all of whom fulfilled the following criteria: (1) death from a noncardiac condition; (2) absence of symptoms suggesting or indicating myocardial ischemia or cardiac dysfunction during life; (3) absence of systemic hypertension (>140 mm Hg systolic and/or >90 mm Hg diastolic); (4) absence of cardiomegaly; (5) absence of left ventricular necrosis or fibrosis; (6) absence of mediastinal irradiation. Of the 16 control subjects, four died of carcinoma (pancreas = two, prostrate gland = one, tongue = one); five of leukemia; six of lymphoma and one of sideroblastic anemia.

The coronary arteries in the 18 study patients and in the 16 control subjects were studied similarly. The hearts were fixed in formalin. The four major epicardial coronary arteries were excised from the heart intact, x-rayed, decalcified (if necessary) and cut transversely to their longitudinal axes into 5 mm long segments. Each segment was labelled sequentially from either its aortic ostium or from its origin from the left main coronary artery. The 5 mm long segments were then dehydrated, embedded in paraffin and at least two histologic sections were cut and stained, one by hematoxylin and eosin and the other by the Movat method. The sections were then analyzed histologically, and the amount of luminal narrowing by atherosclerotic plaques was determined by study of the Movat-stained histologic sections magnified 20 to 50 times. The per cent of cross-sectional area narrowing of each section was graded into four categories: 0 to 25, 26 to 50, 51 to 75 and 76 to 100 per cent.

The location [1] and extent of left ventricular scarring were determined after cutting the ventricles at 1.0 to 1.5 cm intervals beginning at the apex and extending to about 2 cm caudal to the atrioventricular sulcus. All cuts were made parallel to the posterior atrioventricular sulcus. The cutting of the cardiac

TABLE I Clinical and Morphologic Observations in 18 Patients with Coronary Dilated Cardiomyopathy

Pa-tient	Age (yr)	Interval 1st AMI to Death (mo)	Interval Last AMI to Death (mo)	Interval Chronic CHF to Death (mo)	SH	DM	Heart Weight (g)	Per Cent LV Wall Scarred Apical	Basal	LV Throm-bus	No. 4 CA's >75% Narrowed*	No. 5-mm CA Segments Examined*	No. (%) 5-mm Segments >75% Narrowed	WS
							Patients With Left Ventricular Aneurysm							
1	31	36	...	24	0	0	520	100	20	+	2	59	6(10)	0
2	46	88	3	4	+	0	500	67	50	0	2	44	24(55)	+
3	46	48	...	48	0	0	500	67	40	0	3	55	9(16)	+
4	47	48	6	6	0	0	465	67	55	0	3	48	21(43)	0
5	48	144	...	84	0	+	590	100	33	0	3	38	26(68)	0
6	57	204	...	24	+	+	580	100	12	+	3	60	19(32)	0
7	64	132	...	6	+	0	660	67	33	+	3	75	17(23)	0
8	70	24	...	12	+	0	620	100	33	+	3	44	21(48)	0
9	78	72	60	6	+	0	770	100	33	+	1	53	6(11)	0
							Patients Without Left Ventricular Aneurysm							
10	48	108	...	24	0	0	750	33	35	0	3	60	21(35)	0
11	54	96	...	35	0	0	520	50	60	0	3	65	28(43)	0
12	55	72	...	48	0	0	515	67	39	0	1	38	1(3)	0
13	62	144	60	60	0	0	800	10	40	+	2	54	28(52)	0
14	63	48	...	48	0	0	470	100	50	+	2	71	6(8)	+
15	64	48	...	5	0	0	730	50	65	+	2	89	7(8)	0
16	70	180	6	6	+	0	535	100	50	0	2	61	27(44)	0
17	72	96	...	24	0	0	460	33	35	+	2	52	10(20)	0
18	77	72	...	72	+	+	600	100	30	0	3	46	22(48)	0

NOTE: AMI = acute myocardial infarction; AP = angina pectoris; CA = coronary arteries; CHF = congestive heart failure; DM = diabetes mellitus; LV = left ventricle; SH = systemic hypertension (blood pressure systolic >140 mm Hg and diastolic >90 mm Hg); WS = warfarin sodium.

TABLE II Number of 18 Patients (P) with Healed Myocardial Infarction and Chronic Congestive Heart Failure and 16 Control Subjects (C) Showing Maximal Luminal Narrowing of One or More Major Epicardial Coronary Arteries by Atherosclerotic Plaques

Coronary Artery	Per Cent Cross-Sectional Area Luminal Narrowing									
	0–25		26–50		51–75		76–100		Totals	
	P	C	P	C	P	C	P	C	P	C
R	…	…	…	…	0	0	0	1	0	1
LAD	…	…	…	…	0	0	2	3	2	3
LC	…	…	…	…	0	0	0	1	0	1
R,LAD	…	…	…	…	0	1	5	1	5	2
R,LC	…	…	…	…	0	0	1	0	1	0
LAD,LC	…	…	…	…	0	1	1	1	1	2
R,LAD,LC	…	…	…	…	0	5	9	1	9	6
LM,*LAD,LC	…	…	…	…	0	1	0	0	0	1
LM,LAD,LC,R	…	…	…	…	0	0	0	0	0	0
Totals	0	0	0	0	0	8	18	8	18	16
Per cent	0	0	0	0	0	50	100	50	100	100

NOTE: R = right; LM = left main; LAD = left anterior descending; LC = left circumflex.

*Sections of LM not examined in four patients and in one control subject.

ventricles usually resulted in three slices from the apical one half and three from the basal one half of the left ventricle. The amount of left ventricular scarring was determined by measuring circumferentially the amount of scarring in one of the three slices from the apical one half and one from the basal half. The slice chosen for measurement had the maximal degree of scarring in that particular half of the left ventricle. The per cent of basal or apical left ventricular scarring was determined by dividing the total circumference of the left ventricular wall (including ventricular septum) in centimeters into the number of centimeters showing transmural scarring circumferentially.

RESULTS

Of the 18 study patients, 68 major (right, left main, left anterior descending and left circumflex) epicardial coronary arteries were examined. (The left main was not examined in four patients.) The maximal degrees of cross-sectional area narrowing by atherosclerotic plaque in them and in the 16 control subjects are summarized in **Table II.** Of the 18 study patients, 16 (89 per cent) had two or more of their four major epicardial coronary arteries narrowed >75 per cent in cross-sectional area by atherosclerotic plaque, whereas only three (17 per cent)

TABLE III Number and Per Cent of 5 mm Long Segments of the Four Major Epicardial Coronary Arteries Showing the Four Grades of Cross-Sectional Luminal Narrowing in 18 Patients (P) with Healed Myocardial Infarction and Chronic Congestive Heart Failure (CCHF) and in 16 Control Subjects (C)

Coronary Artery	Per Cent Cross-Sectional Area Luminal Narrowing									
	0–25		26–50		51–75		76–100		Totals	
	P	C	P	C	P	C	P	C	P	C
Left main*										
No.	2	6	11	9	18	9	0	0	31	24
Per cent	6	25	36	38	58	37	0	0	100	100
Left anterior descending										
No.	50	41	66	131	113	99	100	25	329	296
Per cent	16	14	19	44	35	34	30	8	100	100
Left circumflex										
No.	40	40	56	54	59	58	53	4	208	156
Per cent	20	26	27	35	29	37	22	2	100	100
Right										
No.	25	39	94	148	180	110	145	15	444	312
Per cent	6	13	21	47	40	35	33	5	100	100
Totals										
No.	117	126	227	342	370	276	298	44	1012	788
Per cent	11	16	23	43	37	35	29	6	100	100

NOTE: LM = left main; LAD = left anterior descending; LC = left circumflex; R = right.

*Sections are not examined in four patients with healed MI + CCHF and in one control subject.

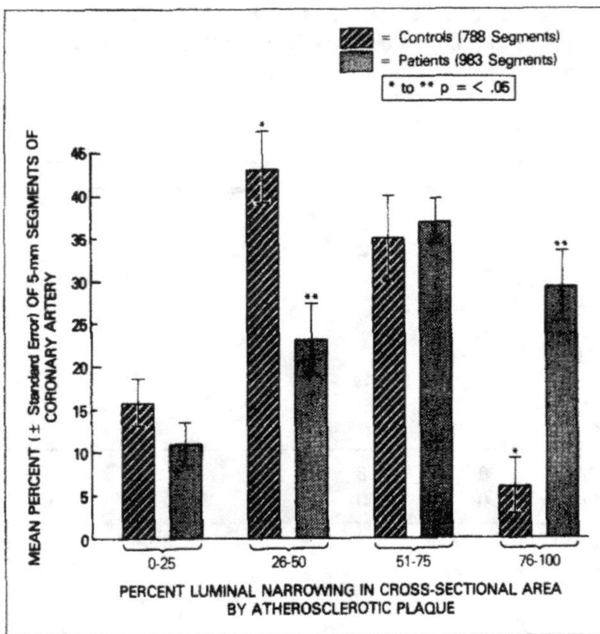

Figure 1. Number and per cent of 5 mm segments of all four major coronary arteries narrowed to various degrees in the 18 study patients and in the 16 control subjects.

of the 16 control subjects had two or more arteries narrowed to this degree. Nine of the 18 study patients had three of their four major coronary arteries narrowed >75 per cent in cross-sectional area by atherosclerotic plaques; seven had two, and two had a single artery narrowed to this extent. Thus, of the possible 72 major coronary arteries in the 18 study patients (actually, only 68 arteries were examined), 43 (63 per cent) were >75

per cent narrowed in cross-sectional area by atherosclerotic plaques for an average of 2.4/4.0 coronary arteries per study patient. The left main coronary artery was not severely (>75 per cent) narrowed in any study patient or in any control subject. If the left main coronary artery was excluded, 43 (80 per cent) of the other 54 major (right, left anterior descending and left circumflex) coronary arteries were narrowed >75 per cent in cross-sectional area by atherosclerotic plaques for an average of 2.4/3.0 coronary arteries per study patient. Of the eight control subjects with >75 per cent cross-sectional narrowing by atherosclerotic plaques of one or more major coronary artery, three (right, left anterior descending and left circumflex) coronary arteries were narrowed to this degree in one subject, two were so narrowed in two subjects, and only one artery was so narrowed in five subjects. Thus, of the possible 64 major coronary arteries in the 16 control subjects (actually, only 63 arteries were examined), 12 (19 per cent) were narrowed >75 per cent in cross-sectional area by atherosclerotic plaques for an average of 0.8/4.0 coronary arteries per control subject. If the left main artery was excluded, 12 (25 per cent) of the 48 other major (right, left anterior descending, left circumflex) coronary arteries were narrowed >75 per cent in cross-sectional area by atherosclerotic plaques for an average of 0.7/3.0 coronary arteries per control subject.

A thrombus was present in one coronary artery, superimposed on atherosclerotic plaque, in two study patients. The amount of luminal obliteration contributed by the thrombus was not included in the calculations of luminal narrowing—only that part contributed by atherosclerotic plaques. No control subject had a coronary thrombus.

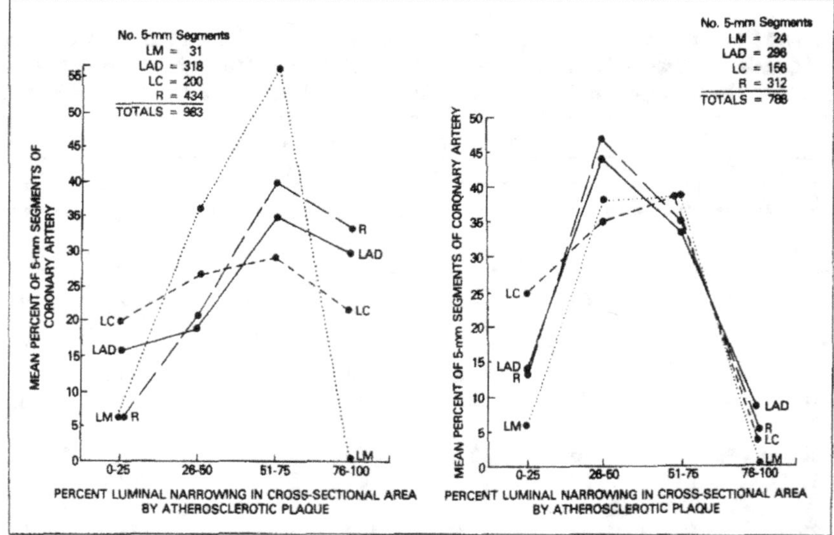

Figure 2. Per cent of 5 mm segments of each of the four major coronary arteries narrowed to various degrees in the 18 study patients (*left*) and in the 16 control subjects (*right*). In the study patients the amount of luminal narrowing of the right (R), left anterior descending (LAD) and left circumflex (LC) coronary arteries is similar. The left main (LM) coronary artery is much less narrowed. The amount of narrowing, or the lack thereof, in each of the four major coronary arteries in the control subjects is similar.

The results of the examination of the 1,012 five millimeter segments in the study patients and in the 788 five millimeter segments in the control subjects are summarized in **Table III** and in **Figure 1**. Of the 5 mm segments of major coronary artery examined in the 18 study patients, 298 segments (29 per cent) were 76 to 100 per cent narrowed in cross-sectional area by atherosclerotic plaques (controls = 6), 370 (37 per cent) were 51 to 75 per cent narrowed (controls = 35 per cent), 227 (23 per cent) were 26 to 50 per cent narrowed (controls = 43 per cent) and 117 (11 per cent) were 0 to 25 per cent narrowed (controls = 16 per cent). The mean per cent of 5 mm coronary segments narrowed 26 to 50 and 76 to 100 per cent was significantly (p <0.05) different between study patients and control subjects. The mean per cent of 5 mm segments of the left anterior descending, left circumflex and right coronary arteries narrowed 76 to 100 per cent was significantly (p <0.05) different between study patients and control subjects (**Figure 2**). No significant difference in mean per cent of segments of left main coronary artery narrowed 0 to 25, 26 to 50, 51 to 75 and 76 to 100 per cent between study patients and control subjects was observed. The mean per cent of 5 mm segments of right, left anterior descending and left circumflex coronary arteries in the study patients was similar at each of the four levels of narrowing (Figure 2). Likewise, the mean per cent of segments of each of these three major coronary arteries narrowed to various degrees in the control subjects was similar (Figure 2). In contrast, the degree of narrowing of the left main coronary artery in both study patients and control subjects was less.

The mean per cent of 5 mm segments narrowed 76 to 100 per cent in cross-sectional area in the proximal one

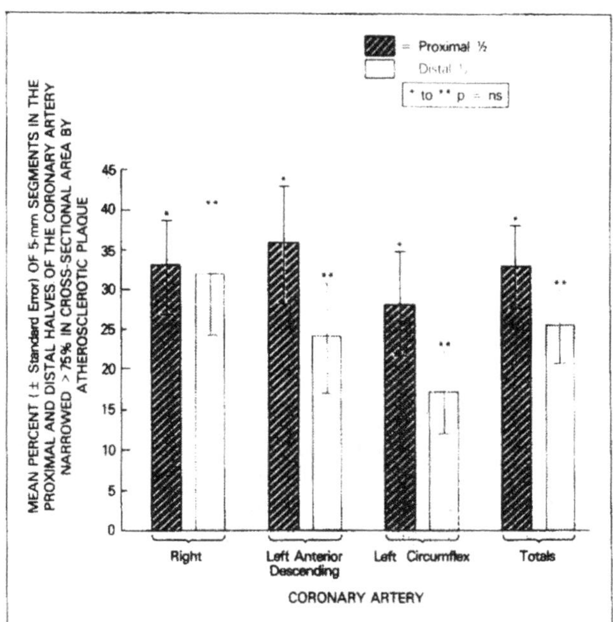

Figure 3. Mean per cent of 5 mm segments of the right, left anterior descending and left circumflex coronary arteries narrowed more than 75 per cent in cross-sectional area in the proximal and distal halves of each of the three arteries. The mean per cent of 5 mm segments severely narrowed was not significantly different in the proximal and distal halves of each of these three arteries.

half of the right, left anterior descending and left circumflex coronary arteries was similar to the mean per cent of 5 mm segments similarly narrowed in the distal one half of these arteries (**Figure 3**).

The mean per cent of 5 mm segments of each of the right, left anterior descending and left circumflex cor-

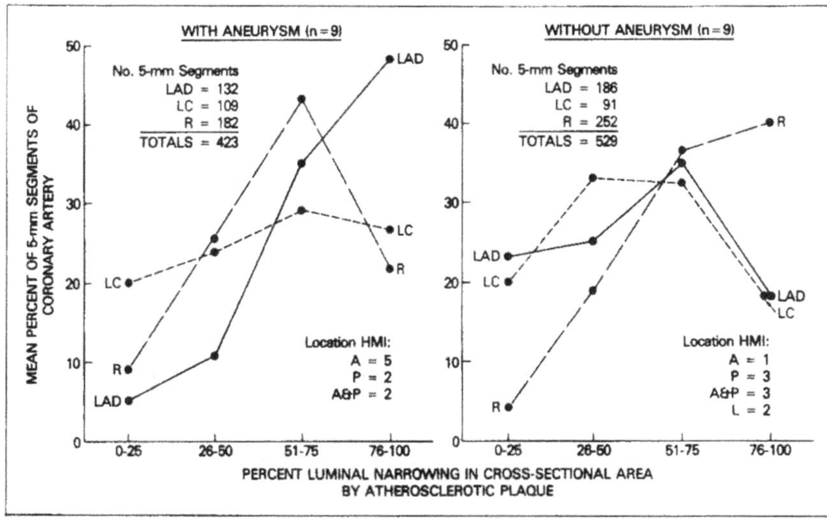

Figure 4. Mean per cent of 5 mm segments of each of the right (R), left anterior descending (LAD), and left circumflex (LC) coronary arteries narrowed to various degrees in the nine study patients with left ventricular aneurysm and in the nine without left ventricular aneurysm. The patients with aneurysm (left) had more narrowing of the left anterior descending artery and the patients without aneurysm (right) had more narrowing of the right coronary artery. A = anterior wall, L = lateral wall and P = posterior wall of left ventricle, HMI = healed myocardial infarct.

TABLE IV   Healed Transmural Myocardial Infarction and Chronic Congestive Heart Failure: Infarct Location

Group	Patients	Location of Transmural Healed MI							
		A*	P*	A+P	L Only	Basal	Apical	Basal + Apical	RV
Healed MI	18	6	5	5	2	2	0	16	2
Aneurysm+	9	5	2	2	0	0	0	9	1
Aneurysm 0	9	1	3	3	2	2	0	7	1
Control subjects	16	0	0	0	0	0	0	0	0

NOTE: A = anterior; L = lateral; P = posterior; RV = right ventricle.
* May or may not include septal and/or lateral walls.

onary arteries narrowed to various degrees was compared in study patients to those without anatomic evidence of left ventricular aneurysm (**Figure 4**). The left anterior descending coronary artery was more narrowed than the right or left circumflex coronary artery in patients with aneurysm, whereas the right coronary artery was most narrowed in the patients without aneurysm (p <0.05).

The location of the healed myocardial infarcts is summarized in **Table IV** and illustrated in **Figures 5, 6 and 7**.

The relationship of four clinical or morphologic parameters in the study patients to the mean per cent of 5 mm coronary segments narrowed >75 per cent in cross-sectional area by atherosclerotic plaque is summarized in **Table V**. Of the four parameters analyzed, significantly greater (p <0.05) coronary narrowing was present in the patients when compared to those without systemic hypertension.

COMMENTS

All 18 study patients described herein were men; all had severe narrowing by atherosclerotic plaques of most of their major epicardial coronary arteries; all had large healed transmural myocardial infarcts (>40 per cent of left ventricular wall); all had very dilated ventricular cavities; all had considerable cardiomegaly (>450 G); all had intractable chronic congestive cardiac failure (average = 2.3 years), and half had intraventricular mural thrombi. Despite the recognized occurrence of chronic congestive cardiac failure in many patients (possibly 25 per cent [2]) after healing of acute myocardial infarcts, we found reports of only four necropsy patients who died of intractable congestive cardiac failure after healing of acute myocardial infarction [3–6]. The current report of 18 patients, therefore, represents a relatively large series and 16 of the 18 patients were observed in a three year period (1976–1978).

The present study provides both qualitative and quantitative information on the degree of narrowing in each of the four major epicardial coronary arteries; in addition, it provides information on the size of the heart and the size of the healed left ventricular infarcts. The amount of coronary narrowing by atherosclerotic plaques in the 18 patients was severe. Although none

had cross-sectional narrowing of >75 per cent of the left main coronary artery, an average of 2.4 of the other three major coronary arteries (right, left anterior descending and left circumflex) were narrowed >75 per cent in cross-sectional area by atherosclerotic plaques (controls = 0.7/3.0). Quantitatively, the amount of coronary narrowing in the study patients was even more impressive. Of the four major epicardial coronary arteries, an average of 27 cm (54 five millimeter segments) of coronary artery were examined in each study patient and an average of 25 cm (49 five millimeter segments) in each control subject. Nearly one third, namely 29 per cent, of the entire lengths of the four major epicardial coronary arteries in the study patients were >75 per cent narrowed in cross-sectional area by atherosclerotic plaques (controls = 6 per cent); another 37 per cent had narrowing between 51 per cent and 75 per cent (controls = 35 per cent), and only 11 per cent had narrowing <26 per cent (controls = 16 per cent). Thus, 66 per cent of the entire lengths of these four coronary arteries were narrowed >50 per cent in cross-sectional area by atherosclerotic plaques (controls = 41 per cent).

Although the amount of narrowing in the left main artery was much less, the amount of narrowing of the right, left anterior descending and left circumflex coronary arteries was similar. Surprisingly, the degree of severe (>75 per cent in cross-sectional area) narrowing in the distal and proximal halves of these three arteries was similar. The amount of severe coronary artery narrowing in the study patients did not correlate with the patient's age, presence or absence of left ventricular aneurysm, or with a history of more than one acute myocardial infarct. The patients with systemic hypertension, however, had more severe coronary artery narrowing than did those with normotension.

Comparison of the observations in our 18 patients with chronic congestive cardiac failure to findings in our previously described 53 patients with fatal coronary heart disease without chronic congestive cardiac failure further emphasizes several unique features of both subsets of coronary patients, neither of whom had myocardial necrosis at necropsy. Patients with *unstable angina pectoris* and *"sudden coronary death"* tend to have much smaller hearts, normal-sized left ventricular cavities, cardiac ventricles devoid of mural thrombi,

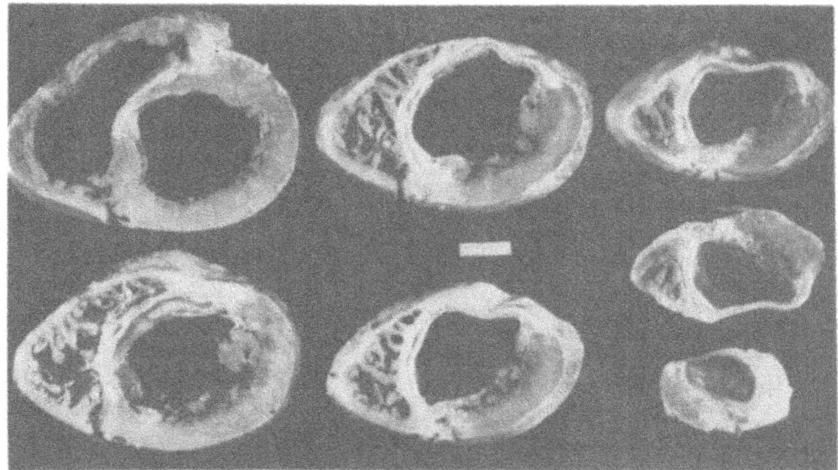

Figure 5. Case 3 (Table I). Transverse slices of the cardiac ventricles illustrating a large transmural healed myocardial infarct. At the base, the anterior and septal walls are scarred and at the apex the entire wall is scarred.

much less ventricular wall scarring (if present) and more extensive coronary arterial luminal narrowing [7,8]. Among 22 personally studied necropsy patients with unstable angina pectoris, 48 per cent of the four major coronary arteries were greater than 75 per cent narrowed in cross-sectional area, including nearly half with narrowing of the left main coronary artery to this extent [7]. Of 31 personally-studied patients with "sudden coronary death," 36 per cent of the four major coronary arteries were greater than 75 per cent narrowed in cross-sectional area, and 10 per cent had narrowing of the left main coronary artery to this extent [8]. Thus, in comparison to patients with unstable angina pectoris

and sudden coronary death, patients with healed myocardial infarcts and chronic congestive cardiac failure tend to have less extensive coronary arterial luminal narrowing but much more extensive left ventricular scarring.

The amount of left ventricular scarring in our 18 patients with chronic congestive cardiac failure after

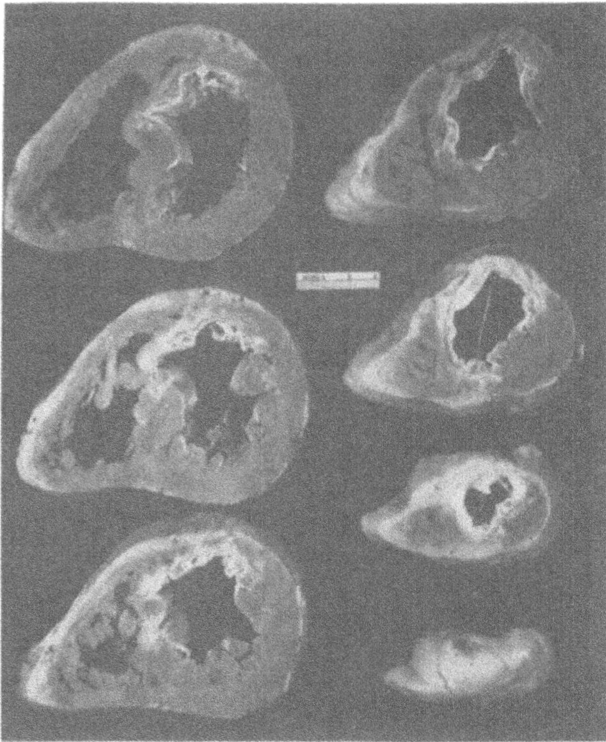

Figure 6. Case 4 (Table I). Transverse slices of the cardiac ventricles showing a transmural, healed myocardial infarct involving the anterior, septal and posterior walls of the left ventricle, and marked dilatation of the left ventricle.

Figure 7. Case 12 (Table I). Transverse slices of cardiac ventricles illustrating healed transmural myocardial infarction of the anteroseptal wall of the left ventricle, extending from base (left three slices) to apex (right four slices).

TABLE V   Mean Per Cent of Total 5 mm Segments in the Four Major (Right, Left Main, Left Anterior Descending and Left Circumflex) Epicardial Coronary Arteries Narrowed >75 Per Cent in Cross-Sectional Area by Atherosclerotic Plaque in 18 Patients with Healed Myocardial Infarction and Chronic Congestive Heart Failure: Comparison of Four Clinical or Morphologic Parameters

Parameters Analyzed	Patients	Mean Per Cent* of 5-mm Coronary Segments Narrowed >75% in Cross-Sectional Area by Atherosclerotic Plaque	p Value
Age (yr)			
<45	1	10	>0.05
45–65	12	28 ± 6	
>65	5	34 ± 8	
Aneurysm			
Present	9	32 ± 7	>0.05
Absent	9	29 ± 6	
>1 AMI			
Present	5	37 ± 8	>0.05
Absent	13	28 ± 6	
Hypertension			
Present	6	42 ± 5	<0.05
Absent	12	25 ± 6	

*± standard error.

healing of acute myocardial infarction is similar to that described in patients dying of cardiogenic shock during the acute phase of myocardial infarction, namely, greater than 40 per cent, of the left ventricular wall [9]. It is obvious that not all patients die during the acute infarction period despite "massive" loss of contracting myocardium. Also, the method used to measure the amount of left ventricular scarring in our patients is different from the technique used by Page and associates [9] who measured the amount of necrotic left ventricular wall in fatal acute myocardial infarction.

And finally, a comment on terminology. Burch [4] has used the term "ischemic cardiomyopathy" to describe patients with chronic congestive cardiac failure secondary to severe coronary narrowing from atherosclerosis. We have no major criticism of this term but prefer the term "coronary dilated cardiomyopathy" to emphasize the coronary origin of the chronic congestive heart failure, ventricular scarring and ventricular dilatation. The latter term contrasts well, for example, with the type of primary myocardial disease best termed "idiopathic dilated cardiomyopathy." Because of differing interpretations of the terms "ischemic cardiomyopathy" and "coronary dilated cardiomyopathy," however, it might be preferable to use neither and use the more descriptive phase of "chronic congestive cardiac failure after healing of acute myocardial infarction."

REFERENCES

1. Roberts WC, Gardin JM: Location of myocardial infarcts: a confusion of terms and definitions. Am J Cardiol 1978; 42: 868–872.
2. Ellis LB, Allison RB, Rodriguez FL, Robbins SL: Relation of the degree of coronary artery disease and of myocardial infarctions to cardiac hypertrophy and chronic congestive heart failure. N Engl J Med 1962; 266: 525–529.
3. Raftery EB, Banks DC, Oram S: Occlusive disease of the coronary arteries presenting as primary congestive cardiomyopathy. Lancet 1969; 2:1147–1150.
4. Burch GE, Giles TD: Ischemic cardiomyopathy: diagnostic, pathophysiologic, and therapeutic considerations. Cardiovasc Clin 1972; 4: 203–220.
5. Case records of the Massachusetts General Hospital, case 51-1970. N Engl J Med 1971; 283: 1392–1401.
6. Burch GE, Giles TD, Martinez E: Echocardiographic detection of abnormal motion of the interventricular septum in ischemic cardiomyopathy. Am J Med 1974; 57: 293–298.
7. Roberts WC, Virmani R: Quantification of coronary arterial narrowing in clinically-isolated unstable angina pectoris: Am J Med 1979; 67: 792–799.
8. Roberts WC, Jones AA: Quantitation of coronary arterial narrowing at necropsy in sudden coronary death. Analysis of 31 patients and comparison with 25 control subjects. Am J Cardiol 1979; 44: 39–45.
9. Page DL, Caulfield JB, Kastor JA, DeSanctis RW, Sanders CA: Myocardial changes associated with cardiogenic shock. N Engl J Med 1971; 285: 133–137.

Status of the Coronary Arteries at Necropsy in Diabetes Mellitus with Onset After Age 30 Years

Analysis of 229 Diabetic Patients With and Without Clinical Evidence of Coronary Heart Disease and Comparison to 183 Control Subjects

BRUCE F. WALLER, M.D.

Bethesda, Maryland

PASQUALE J. PALUMBO, M.D.

J. T. LIE, M.D.

Rochester, Minnesota

WILLIAM C. ROBERTS, M.D.

Bethesda, Maryland

From the Departments of Medicine and Pathology, Mayo Clinic and Mayo Foundation, Rochester, Minnesota; and the Pathology Branch, National Heart, Lung, and Blood Institute, National Institutes of Health, Bethesda, Maryland. Requests for reprints should be addressed to Dr. Bruce F. Waller, Bldg. 10A, Room 3E-30, National Institutes of Health, Bethesda, Maryland 20205. Manuscript accepted March 31, 1980.

Clinical and morphologic observations were made in 229 necropsy patients with diabetes mellitus (DM) with onset of diabetes mellitus after 30 years of age—65 without (DM−CHD) and 164 with (DM+CHD) clinical evidence of coronary heart disease (CHD). These observations were compared to those in 183 age-sex-matched nondiabetic control subjects who died from a fatal coronary event (CHD−DM). The average number of three major (right, left anterior descending, left circumflex) coronary arteries per patient narrowed >75 percent in cross-sectional area by atherosclerotic plaques was identical in the 229 diabetic patients (DM−CHD and DM+CHD) and in the control subjects (CHD−DM), namely, 2.5/3.0. This similarity in the amount of coronary arterial narrowing was present irrespective of the age at onset (after 30 years) or duration of diabetes mellitus. The DM+CHD patients had more severe narrowing of the three major coronary arteries than did the DM−CHD patients (p < 0.01). The amount of severe narrowing in the proximal halves of each of these three arteries was similar to that in the distal halves. The amount of severe (>75 percent in cross-sectional area) narrowing of the left main coronary artery was greater in the patients with diabetes mellitus than in the nondiabetic controls: 13 percent versus 6 percent (p < 0.01). The type of treatment received by the patients with diabetes mellitus or their adherence to the therapeutic program as measured by the level of random fasting blood sugar did not alter the amount of severe coronary narrowing observed at necropsy.

Although each has been recognized as a distinct entity for many decades, both diabetes mellitus and coronary heart disease were not recognized in the same patient until 1870 [1]. In 1883, Vergely [2] was so impressed with the frequency of angina pectoris in patients with diabetes mellitus that he urged the examination of the urine of all patients with angina to search for sugar. The frequency of angina in patients with diabetes mellitus was soon further emphasized by others [3–6]. Naunyn [7] in 1906 appears to have been the first to discuss atherosclerosis as a cause of death in patients with diabetes mellitus. Among 49 necropsy patients with diabetes mellitus (average duration of diabetes mellitus = 2.6 years) described by him, four (8 percent) died from consequences of coronary atherosclerosis. Brunton [8] also emphasized the presence of coronary atherosclerosis in patients with diabetes mellitus. Cardiovascular disease, however, was an infrequent cause of death among patients with diabetes mellitus in the pre-insulin era. Of 1,164 patients with diabetes mellitus studied at the Joslin Clinic and who died between 1897 and 1922, coronary heart disease was the cause of death in only 22 (2 percent), whereas *diabetic coma* was fatal in 555 (48 percent) of them [9]. After insulin was introduced in 1922, Warren and Root [10,11] reported "coronary sclerosis" as a "striking pathologic finding" in 11 of 17 necropsy patients with diabetes mellitus over 40 years of age. Wilder [12] found "coronary sclerosis" in 17 (34 percent) of 49 necropsy patients with diabetes mellitus, and Strauss [13] found "extensive" cerebral or coronary sclerosis in 21 (38 percent) of 54 patients with diabetes mellitus. Many subsequent studies in the post-insulin period demonstrated a high frequency of fatal and nonfatal cardiovascular disease among patients with diabetes mellitus.

Of 24 necropsy studies of diabetic patients (with onset >age 30 years) reported in the post-insulin period [10-12,14-34], 19 [10-12,17-28] indicated the percent of patients with coronary arterial narrowing by atherosclerosis or by thrombus; of them, only 12 [10-12, 15,17-28,30,31,33] compared their observations to those in nondiabetic control subjects. Of 5,484 patients with diabetes mellitus described in these 19 studies [10-12,15,17-28], 2,087 (28 percent) had "coronary narrowing" by atherosclerotic plaques compared to 3,240 (6 percent) of 50,154 nondiabetic subjects. Although these studies indicate that patients with diabetes mellitus have more coronary atherosclerosis than subjects without diabetes mellitus, they have several deficiencies: (1) the data with two exceptions [23,31] were obtained exclusively from autopsy protocols, not from reexamination of the hearts themselves; (2) the coronary narrowings by atherosclerotic plaques were described only in general terms, such as "mild, moderate, severe, marked or significant"; (3) the subjects used as controls were generally not matched for age and sex and, with the exception of three studies [16,19,26], were picked irrespective of the presence or absence of clinical evidence of coronary heart disease; and (4) the amount of coronary atherosclerosis at necropsy was not correlated to the age at onset or duration of diabetes mellitus.

To correct some deficiencies of these earlier studies, we examined the degree of cross-sectional area narrowing by atherosclerotic plaques in the four major epicardial coronary arteries in 65 patients with diabetes mellitus without clinical evidence of coronary heart disease (hereafter called "DM−CHD"), in 164 necropsy patients with diabetes mellitus and clinical evidence of coronary heart disease (hereafter called "DM+CHD"), and in 183 necropsy patients with clinical evidence of coronary heart disease but without diabetes mellitus (hereafter called "CHD−DM"). In all 229 patients with diabetes mellitus (65 + 164), the onset of diabetes mellitus occurred after age 30 years. The answers to three major questions were sought: (1) Do necropsy patients with DM+CHD have more, less or similar amounts of coronary narrowing by atherosclerotic plaques than patients with CHD−DM? (2) Do necropsy patients with DM+CHD have more, less or similar amounts of coro-

nary narrowing by atherosclerotic plaques than patients with DM−CHD? (3) Among patients with onset of diabetes mellitus after age 30 years, does the age at onset or the duration of the diabetes mellitus correlate with the amount of coronary narrowing by atherosclerosis?

PATIENTS STUDIED AND METHODS

A computer print-out was obtained on all patients studied in the Diabetic Section of the Metabolic Division of the Department of Medicine at the Mayo Clinic from 1945 through 1975. All patients had to fulfill the following criteria: (1) the patient was seen on at least three occasions in the Diabetic Section from 1945 through 1975; (2) the patient was a resident of Olmsted County, the area which includes Rochester, Minnesota, the location of the Mayo Clinic; (3) the patient died and an autopsy was performed during the period 1945 through 1975; (4) associated organic valvular, pulmonary, primary and secondary (other than the result of coronary narrowing) myocardial heart diseases were lacking, and (5) a cardiac operation had never been performed. The print-out included a list of 314 patients. Because of (1) deficiencies in historic medical information, or (2) presence of diabetes mellitus for less than one year, or (3) incomplete fulfillment of our definition of diabetes mellitus, or (4) onset of diabetes mellitus before the age 30 years, or (5) presence of noncoronary cardiac disease or (6) unavailability of the heart specimen, 85 (27 percent) of the 314 patients were eliminated. Thus, 229 necropsy patients with diabetes mellitus constitute the study patients.

In this study, diabetes mellitus was defined either as fasting blood sugar >120 mg/dl (Folin-Wu) or >110 mg/dl (Autoanalyzer®) on two consecutive determinations, or increases in both 1- and 2-hour blood glucose values corrected for age in a glucose tolerance test [35]. The date on which a blood glucose value was first abnormally increased was considered the date of diagnosis of diabetes mellitus, irrespective of whether or not glycosuria or symptoms (polyuria and/or polydipsia) had been present earlier. Coronary heart disease was defined as the presence of a fatal coronary event; the patient may or may not have had one or more nonfatal coronary events before the fatal one.

In the clinical records, the presence or absence of the following parameters was sought: age at diagnosis of diabetes mellitus; age at diagnosis (if present) of coronary heart disease; age at death; sex; duration of diabetes mellitus; presence of obesity (>25 percent increase in predicted body weight by age and height); cigarette smoking (>20 cigarettes daily for >10 years); leg claudication and/or dermal ulcers; stroke (sudden fatal or nonfatal motor deficit); systemic hypertension (systolic systemic pressure >140 mm Hg and/or diastolic pressure >90 mm Hg on three separate days); diabetic retinopathy (included both *nonproliferative* [microaneurysms, hemorrhages, exudates] and *proliferative* changes (nonproliferative changes plus vitreous hemorrhages, new vascular channels, blindness]); and the highest serum total cholesterol level recorded. In addition, the immediate cause of death and the type of treatment received for diabetes mellitus at various times during the study period were recorded.

The heart specimens in each of these 229 patients were reexamined. The degree of cross-sectional area narrowing by atherosclerotic plaques of each of the four major (right, left main, left anterior descending and left circumflex) epicardial

TABLE I   Observations in Necropsy Patients with Diabetes Mellitus (DM) (onset > age 30 years) or Clinical Coronary Heart Disease (CHD), or Both[1]

Parameter	DM−CHD	DM+CHD	CHD−DM
Patients (no.)	65	164	183
Age at death (yr)			
Range	45–90	40–97	40–90
Mean	69	69	69
Sex (%)			
Male	58	58	56
Female	42	42	44
Age at diagnosis of CHD (yr)[1]			
Range	. . .	40–93	40–88
Mean	. . .	67	66
Age at diagnosis of DM (yr)			
Range	31–88	33–93	. . .
Mean	61	60	. . .
Duration of DM (yr)			
Range	1–33	1–34	. . .
Mean	9	10	. . .
Angina pectoris	0	91 (55)*	79 (43)*
Cigarette smokers[2]	21 (32)*	78 (48)*	127 (69)*
Systemic hypertension[3]	17 (26)*	86 (52)*	95 (52)
Mean TC (mg/dl)[4]	260	255*	285*
Obesity[5]	0	30 (18)*	10 (5)*
Stroke	0	16 (10)	13 (8)
Claudication and/or DU	0	42 (26)	34 (19)
Retinopathy[6]	10 (15)*	64 (39)*	0
Cardiac weight (g)			
Range	212–440	280–690	385–670
Mean	380*	450**	460**
Acute MI—transmural[7]	0	91 (55)*	79 (43)*
Healed MI—transmural[7]	14 (22)[8]*	146 (89)*	88 (48)*
Cause of death			
AMI	0	91 (55)*	79 (43)*
SCD	0	50 (31)*	104 (57)*
Chronic CHF	0	23 (14)	0
Rupture LV wall	0	20 (12)	18 (10)
Average no. of 3 major (R, LAD, LC)	2.4 / 3.0	2.6 / 3.0	2.5 / 3.0
CA per patient narrowed >75% in cross-sectional area by AP divided by no. of CA per patient			
No. patients in whom none, 1, 2 or 3 major (R, LAD, LC) CA narrowed >75% by AP.			
0	6 (9)	0	0
1	5 (8)	17 (10)	26 (14)
2	13 (20)	32 (20)	42 (23)
3	41 (63)	115 (70)	115 (63)
No. patients with LMCA narrowed 75% by AP	7 (11)	23 (14)*	11 (6)**

NOTE: AMI = acute myocardial infarction; AP = atherosclerotic plaque; CA = coronary arteries; CHF = congestive heart failure; DU = dermal ulcer; LAD = left anterior descending; LC = left circumflex; LM = left main; LV = left ventricle; MI = myocardial infarction; SCD = sudden coronary death; TC = total serum cholesterol. Figures in parentheses are percents. On the same horizontal line *—* or *—** = p <0.01 and **—** = p <0.05

[1] Clinical coronary heart disease includes patients with angina pectoris, myocardial infarction, or both, and who died with acute myocardial infarction, chronic congestive heart failure, or both, or suddenly.

[2] Smoked > 20 cigarettes daily for > 10 years.

[3] Systolic pressure > 140 mm Hg and/or diastolic pressure > 90 mm Hg on three separate days.

[4] Total serum cholesterol values at the time of diagnosis of coronary heart disease, diabetes mellitus, or available values on patients who died suddenly.

[5] > 25 percent increase in predicted body weight by age and height (Dubois' Body Surface Chart, Boothby and Standford).

[6] Includes both nonproliferative (microaneurysms, hemorrhages, exudates) and proliferative changes (nonproliferative changes plus vitreous hemorrhages, new vascular channels and/or blindness).

[7] Involvement of inner one half of left ventricular wall.

[8] Clinically silent events.

arteries was sought. Each artery was cut at 3 to 5 mm intervals perpendicular to its longitudinal axis, and the maximal degree of cross-sectional area narrowing by atherosclerotic plaques, as determined by visual inspection, of the left main and the proximal and distal halves of the right, left anterior descending and left circumflex coronary arteries was recorded as follows: 0 to 25; 26 to 50; 51 to 75 and 76 to 100. The left ventricular myocardium was examined for the presence or absence of transmural (involvement of more than the inner one half of the left ventricular wall—usually >75 percent of the wall was involved) necrosis or fibrosis, or both, and for the presence of free wall rupture. In addition, the autopsy protocols were examined to record the original heart weight. The presence of transmural left ventricular wall necrosis was always confirmed by examination of appropriate histologic sections.

Control subjects for the study patients were selected as follows. Information from patients with fatal coronary heart disease examined at autopsy at the Mayo Clinic from 1948 onward was available in the computer "bank." The ages and sexes of the described study patients with diabetes mellitus were matched with necropsy patients with fatal coronary events but without diabetes mellitus and the matched nondiabetic patients became the control subjects. Nonfatal coronary events may or may not have been present before the fatal coronary event in the control subjects. All control subjects, just as the study patients, had resided in and died in Olmsted County, Minnesota. The same clinical data sought in the study patients also were gathered in the control subjects. Likewise, the hearts of the control subjects were reexamined in the same fashion as were those of the study patients. The hearts of both the study patients and control subjects were examined without knowledge by the examiner of whether the cardiac specimen had belonged to a study patient or to a control subject.

RESULTS

The clinical and morphologic cardiac findings in both the study patients and in the control subjects are summarized in **Table I**. The 229 patients with diabetes mellitus were divided into two groups: 65 who died of noncardiac conditions and without clinical evidence of myocardial ischemia during life (DM−CHD); and 164 who had fatal coronary heart disease (acute transmural myocardial infarction in 91 [55 percent], sudden coronary death in 50 [30 percent] or chronic congestive heart failure after healing of acute transmural myocardial infarction in 23 [14 percent]) (DM+CHD). All 183 control subjects (CHD−DM) had fatal coronary events with and without preceding clinical evidence of myocardial ischemia, but none had clinical evidence of diabetes mellitus.

Of the three major (right, left anterior descending, left circumflex) coronary arteries per patient in each of the three study groups, an average of 2.4 (DM+CHD), 2.6 (DM+CHD) and 2.5 (CHD−DM) per patient, respectively, was narrowed >75 percent in cross-sectional area by atherosclerotic plaques (Table I). The patients with DM+CHD had more coronary narrowing than did the patients with DM−CHD, but in the group with DM−CHD the amounts of severe (>75 percent) coronary narrowing were similar to those in the patients with CHD−DM. Irrespective of whether diabetes mellitus appeared from ages 31 to 45 years, 46 to 60 years or after 60 years of age, no significant difference was observed in the average number of three major coronary arteries per patient narrowed >75 percent: 31 to 45 years = 2.4/3; 46 to 60 years = 2.4/3 and >60 years = 2.5/3. Moreover, no significant differences in the average number of three major coronary arteries per patient narrowed to this degree were noted in these age-at-onset categories between either of the two study groups with diabetes mellitus and the control subjects. In each age-of-onset group the average age at death was similar. There were no major differences between the combined diabetic study patients (DM+CHD and DM−CHD) and control subjects (CHD−DM) in the amount of severe (>75 percent) coronary narrowing by atherosclerotic plaque when the effects of duration of diabetes mellitus were considered. Irrespective of whether diabetes mellitus was present one to five, six to 10, 11 to 25 or 26 to 40 years, the average number of three major coronary arteries per patient narrowed to this severity was similar (2.5 or 2.6/3.0). The average age at death also was similar in each group. Among the two subgroups of patients with diabetes mellitus, the duration of diabetes mellitus altered the severity of coronary narrowing only in the one to five year duration category. The patients with DM−CHD had significantly less severe coronary narrowing than either the patients with DM+CHD or the patients with CHD−DM (p < 0.01). Thus, after five years' duration of diabetes mellitus no significant differences in severe coronary narrowing were observed among the patients with either DM−CHD, DM+CHD or CHD−DM. Furthermore, the types of treatment prescribed for management of diabetes mellitus did not significantly alter the degree of severe (>75 percent) coronary narrowing observed at necropsy in each of the four major epicardial coronary arteries. Likewise, when the frequency of occurrence of random fasting blood glucose levels observed in the study patients with diabetes mellitus as less than, equal to or greater than 150 mg/dl was correlated with the number of coronary arteries per patient narrowed >75 percent in cross-sectional area by atherosclerotic plaques, no significant differences were found.

Among the 229 diabetic patients with (164 patients) and without (65 patients) clinical coronary heart disease (DM+CHD and DM−CHD), there were no significant differences in the amount of severe (>75 percent in cross-sectional area) narrowing by atherosclerotic plaques of none, one, two or three major (right, left circumflex and left anterior descending) coronary arteries (**Figure 1**). Of the 164 patients with DM+CHD, 147 (90 percent) had two or three coronary arteries narrowed >75 percent by atherosclerotic plaques, and of the 65 patients with DM−CHD, 54 (83 percent) (p > 0.05) had two or three coronary arteries so narrowed (Figure 1). The presence or absence of symptoms of coronary heart disease among these 229 patients with diabetes mellitus, therefore, did not alter the number of major coronary arteries severely narrowed by atherosclerotic plaques

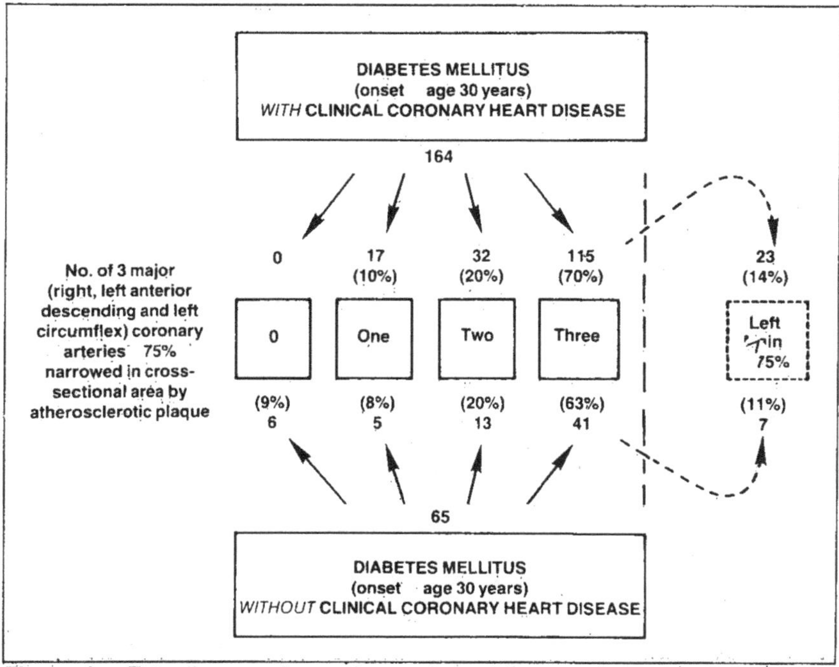

Figure 1. This diagram shows the number of three major epicardial coronary arteries narrowed >75 percent in cross-sectional area by atherosclerotic plaques in 229 necropsy patients with diabetes mellitus, 164 of whom had a fatal coronary event and 65 of whom did not. The number of patients with three coronary arteries narrowed >75 percent, and who also had the left main coronary artery narrowed to this degree, is represented by the dashed-line box.

at necropsy. All 164 patients with DM+CHD had at least one coronary artery narrowed >75 percent in cross-sectional area by atherosclerotic plaques, and 59 (91 percent) of the 65 patients with DM−CHD had similar narrowing (Figure 1). Six (9 percent) patients with DM−CHD had no major arteries narrowed >75 percent in cross-sectional area but all six had at least one of these major arteries narrowed 51 to 75 percent. These six patients did not differ significantly in the number of "risk factors" they had compared to those in the remaining 59 patients with DM−CHD. Of the 347 patients with coronary heart disease, the 164 with and the 183 without diabetes mellitus had a similar number of coronary arteries narrowed >75 percent in cross-sectional area (**Figure 2**): 17 (10 percent) of the 164 patients with diabetes mellitus had a single artery narrowed to this extent, and 26 (14 percent) of the 183 subjects without diabetes mellitus had only one artery so narrowed. In contrast, 147 (90 percent) of the 164 patients with DM+CHD and 157 (86 percent) of the 183 patients with CHD−DM had two or three of the major coronary arteries narrowed to this degree (Figure 2). In all 347 patients with coronary heart disease, irrespective of whether or not diabetes mellitus was present, at least one of the four major coronary arteries was narrowed >75 percent in cross-sectional area by atherosclerotic plaque (Figure 2).

Among the 230 patients with clinical coronary heart disease and narrowing of >75 percent in cross-sectional area of each of the three major coronary arteries, 23 (14 percent) of the 164 patients with DM+CHD and 11 (6 percent) of the 183 control subjects with CHD−DM also had the left main coronary artery narrowed by atherosclerotic plaques to this degree (p <0.01) (Figure 2). Of the 156 patients with diabetes mellitus who had narrowing of >75 percent in cross-sectional area of each of the three major coronary arteries, 23 (14 percent) of the 164 with and seven (11 percent) of the 65 without clinical coronary heart disease had similarly severe narrowing of the left main coronary artery (p < 0.05) (Figure 1). Each of the 30 patients with diabetes mellitus (Figure 1) and each of the 11 control subjects without diabetes mellitus (Figure 2) who had severe (>75 percent) narrowing of the left main coronary artery also had similar degrees of narrowing in each of the three other major coronary arteries. The amount of severe (>75 percent) narrowing of the left main coronary artery among the 229 diabetic patients did not vary with the age of onset of the diabetes mellitus when it was divided into two age categories (31 to 45 and 46 to 60 years) or with the duration of diabetes mellitus when it was divided into four categories (1 to 5, 6 to 10, 11 to 25 and 26 to 40 years). The amount of severe (>75 percent) narrowing of the left main coronary artery, however, was significantly greater among the 99 patients with diabetes mellitus in whom the onset of diabetes mellitus was after age 60 years

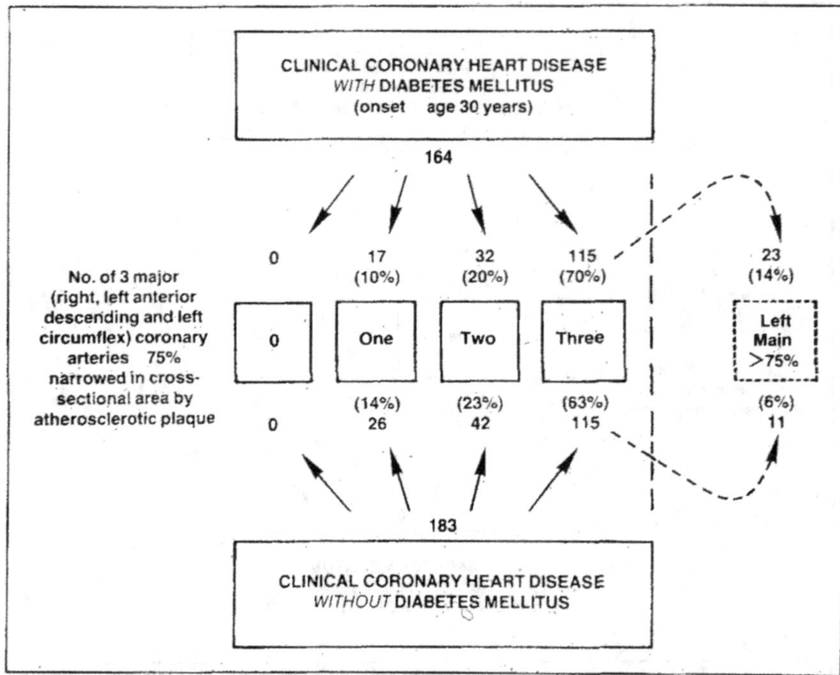

Figure 2. This diagram compares the number of three major epicardial coronary arteries narrowed >75 percent in cross-sectional area by atherosclerotic plaques in 347 patients with fatal coronary events, 164 of whom had diabetes and 183 of whom did not. The number of patients with three coronary arteries narrowed >75 percent, and who also had severe narrowing of the left main coronary artery, is represented by the dashed-line box.

compared to that in their 85 age-sex matched control subjects without diabetes: 10 (12 percent) of the 78 patients with DM+CHD and three (14 percent) of the 21 patients with DM−CHD whose onset of diabetes mellitus was after age 60 years had severe (>75 percent) narrowing of the left main coronary artery whereas only three (3 percent) of their 85 age and sex matched nondiabetic control subjects (CHD−DM) had this degree of narrowing (p < 0.01). No significant differences in percent with severe left main narrowing were present in the 130 patients with diabetes mellitus whose onset of diabetes mellitus was between 31 and 60 years of age compared to their 98 age and sex matched control subjects without diabetes mellitus (13 percent versus 8 percent).

In contrast to the left main coronary artery, no significant difference in the amount of severe (>75 percent) narrowing of the left anterior descending, left circumflex or right coronary arteries was present between the two groups of diabetic patients (DM+CHD and DM−CHD) and the nondiabetic control subjects (CHD−DM). Furthermore, the patients with DM−CHD and the patients with CHD−DM had similar amounts of severe narrowing of all four major coronary arteries, and both groups had less narrowing than the patients with DM+CHD (Table I). The amount of severe (>75 percent) narrowing by atherosclerotic plaques in the *proximal* and *distal* halves of the left anterior de-

scending, left circumflex and right coronary arteries also was similar in both diabetic groups (DM+CHD and DM−CHD) and in the control group (CHD−DM) (**Figure 3**).

Significant differences in the type of fatal coronary events occurred in the 164 patients with DM+CHD compared to the 183 subjects with CHD−DM. The patients with DM+CHD had a higher frequency of fatal acute myocardial infarcts (91 [55 percent] versus 79 [43 percent], p < 0.01) and fatal chronic congestive heart failure (23 [14 percent] versus 0), but a *lower* frequency of sudden coronary death (50 [31 percent] versus 104 [57 percent], p < 0.01) (Table I). All patients with sudden coronary death had out of hospital deaths. When viewing the three types of fatal coronary events with respect to age at onset (after age 30 years) and duration of diabetes mellitus, acute myocardial infarction remained the most frequent, and sudden coronary death was the second most common, fatal coronary event, regardless of the age at onset of diabetes mellitus. Chronic congestive heart failure, however, became the second most frequent event in the patients who had had diabetes mellitus for more than 25 years. Thus, irrespective of the patient's age at appearance of diabetes mellitus (after age 30 years) or the duration of diabetes mellitus, the most common fatal and nonfatal coronary event was acute myocardial infarction. The frequency of transmural left ventricular scarring differed between

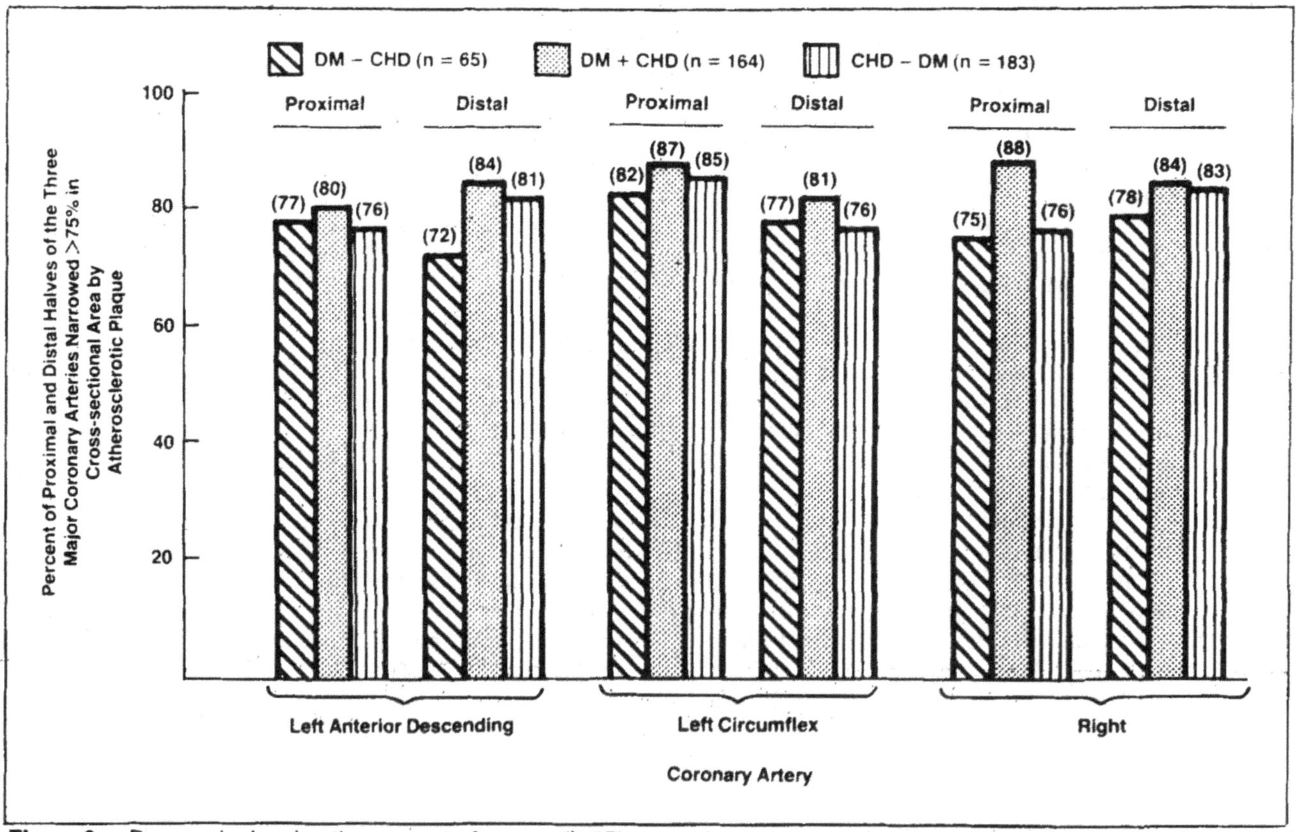

Figure 3. Bar graph showing the amount of severe (>75) narrowing by atherosclerotic plaques of the proximal and distal halves of the three major coronary arteries: in 65 necropsy patients with diabetes mellitus (DM) without clinical coronary heart disease (CHD), in 164 with DM+CHD, and in 183 with CHD−DM (onset of diabetes mellitus after age 30 years).

each of the two diabetic study groups (DM+CHD and DM−CHD) and the control subjects (CHD−DM) (Table I). One or more transmural (involvement of > inner one half of wall) left ventricular scars were present in 14 (22 percent) of the 65 patients with DM−CHD, in 146 (89 percent) of the 164 patients with DM+CHD and in 88 (48 percent) of the 183 subjects with CHD−DM (p < 0.01).

COMMENTS

In the study described three groups of necropsy patients were examined to determine, by a qualitative approach, if patients with onset of diabetes mellitus after age 30 years and in whom death occurred between 40 and 97 years (average 69 years) had more, less or a similar amount of severe (>75 percent cross-sectional area) narrowing of one or more of the four major epicardial coronary arteries by atherosclerotic plaques than did patients of similar age and sex without diabetes mellitus but with fatal coronary heart disease. The hearts in each of the 229 diabetic necropsy patients and in each of the 183 control subjects were reexamined. In contrast to some previous studies based entirely on interpretations of descriptions in autopsy protocols [10–12,17–28], our

study disclosed similar degrees of severe narrowing by atherosclerotic plaques of the right, left anterior descending and left circumflex coronary arteries in the diabetic patients with (DM+CHD) or without (DM−CHD) clinical evidence of coronary heart disease and in the patients with fatal coronary heart disease but without diabetes mellitus (control subjects = CHD−DM group). No significant differences were observed in the degree of severe narrowing by atherosclerotic plaques between the proximal and distal halves of these three coronary arteries in either diabetic group or in the controls. The average percents of the proximal and distal halves of the three major coronary arteries narrowed >75 percent in cross-sectional area were: left anterior descending, 78 and 79 percent; left circumflex, 84 and 78 percent; and right, 80 and 81 percent. A significantly (p < 0.01) higher frequency of severe narrowing of the left main coronary artery occurred in the 229 patients with diabetes mellitus (DM+CHD and DM−CHD) than in the patients without (CHD−DM). Additionally, a significantly (p < 0.01) higher frequency of severe narrowing of the left main coronary artery was present in the patients with DM+CHD than in those with CHD−DM. Although the patients with DM−CHD had less narrowing of the coronary artery at necropsy than the patients with DM+CHD, the patients with DM−CHD and CHD−DM had similar amounts of narrowing by atherosclerotic plaques in all four major coronary arteries.

Previously reported necropsy studies [10–12,14–34] vary tremendously in the percent of diabetic patients with narrowed coronary arteries [10–12,15,17–28]. Only one earlier necropsy report [32], to our knowledge, compared the amount of narrowing among the three major coronary arteries, and in this study each major coronary artery of 32 patients was narrowed, on the average, 62 percent (+2.5 on a scale of 1 to 4). The amount of proximal versus distal coronary arterial narrowing by atherosclerosis has not been described previously in diabetic patients examined at autopsy. Dortimer and associates [36], however, reported angiographic coronary narrowing (*diameter reduction*) in diabetic and in nondiabetic patients using a scoring system involving proximal and distal coronary segments: in 16 (43 percent of the 37 with diabetes mellitus) patients, 82 (74 percent) of 111 segments were narrowed >70 percent in diameter (2.2 segments/patient) whereas in 20 (25 percent) of 79 control subjects, 128 of 237 (54 percent) segments (1.6 segments/patient) were so narrowed; in 17 (22 percent) of 76 coronary arteries in the 37 patients with diabetes mellitus, three of every five segments ("diffuse disease") were narrowed >70 percent in diameter compared to 31 (28 percent) of the 110 arteries in the control subjects (p = ns).

Our necropsy observations support some recent observations in patients with diabetes mellitus undergoing aortocoronary saphenous vein bypass procedures [37–41]. Chychota and associates [37], Verska and Walker [38], and Draskoczy and associates [39] reported no significant differences in the "mean luminal diameter of grafted coronary arteries," operative coronary "graft flow rates" or operative mortality between diabetic and nondiabetic patients with angina pectoris undergoing aortocoronary saphenous vein bypass operations.

In none of the previously reported necropsy studies years of age separated into categories by age at onset. Only two [27,29] of the 21 earlier necropsy studies described duration of diabetes mellitus and neither mentioned the amount of coronary narrowing by atherosclerotic plaques. Warren and Le Compte [27] reported causes of death in 115 patients with diabetes mellitus for 15 to 25 years (mean 19 years) and in 15 patients with diabetes mellitus for 26 to 40 years (mean = 30 years). The percent of patients with fatal acute myocardial infarction in each group was similar (15 of 41 (36 percent) versus five of 15 (33 percent)).

The type of treatment for diabetes mellitus in our diabetic patients did not alter the degree of severe (>75 percent) coronary narrowing observed at necropsy. Likewise, the degree of adherence to the diabetic diets by the diabetic patients, as reflected by the number of random fasting blood sugar levels less than, equal to, or greater than 150 mg/dl, did not significantly effect the degree of severe coronary narrowing observed in our diabetic patients.

Acute myocardial infarction appears to be the most frequent fatal coronary event in diabetic patients studied at necropsy. This finding was the case in our diabetic patients and it also was the case in 10 previously reported studies when cause of death was mentioned [10,11,15,17,20,22,23,27–29]. "Sudden coronary death," was the second most common fatal coronary event among our diabetic patients and the most common among our control subjects. If it can be assumed that patients who die of "angina" or "coronary insufficiency" represent "sudden coronary death," only 218 (15 percent) of 1,456 previously described patients in eight [10,11,17,18,20,23,27,29] studies died suddenly. Of the 1,245 diabetic patients described in five [10,18,22,27,30] of 20 previously reported studies, 162 (13 percent) died from chronic congestive heart failure, a percent similar to that in our patients. In our patients, the frequency of the three types of fatal coronary events (acute myocardial infarction, sudden coronary death and chronic congestive cardiac failure) did not appear to be altered by the patient's age at onset (after age 30 years) of diabetes mellitus or by the duration of diabetes mellitus.

Healed transmural left ventricular scars were found at autopsy more frequently in our diabetic patients (160 of 229 (70 percent)) than in our nondiabetic controls (88 of 183 (48 percent)) (p < 0.01). Among our two diabetic groups, healed transmural left ventricular scars occurred in only 14 (22 percent) of the 65 patients with DM−CHD and in 146 (89 percent) of the 164 patients with DM+CHD. Of 1,634 previously described diabetic necropsy patients the presence of healed myocardial infarcts was noted in only 187 (11 percent) [14,22,23,27,30,31].

The frequency of left ventricular free wall rupture complicating acute myocardial infarction has been reported to be more frequent in diabetic than in nondiabetic patients. At least seven previously reported necropsy studies of diabetic patients have mentioned the frequency of left ventricular free wall rupture [11,14,17,20,27,29,30]. The frequency has ranged from 2 percent (four of 175) [20] to 7 percent (one of 15) with an average of 3 percent (23 of 776) compared to an average of 1 percent (33 of 2,986) in two groups of nondiabetic controls [29,30]. In contrast, a similar frequency of cardiac rupture occurred in our patients with and without diabetes mellitus. Left ventricular rupture occurred in 20 (9 percent) of our 229 diabetic patients (including the 65 with a noncardiac cause of death) and in 18 (10 percent) of our 183 nondiabetic controls (Table I). The 9 percent frequency of left ventricular rupture in our diabetic patients is three times higher than that reported previously at autopsy in patients with diabetes mellitus [11,14,17,20,27,29,30].

REFERENCES

1. Seegen J: Der Diabetes Mellitus auf Grundlage Zahlreicher Beobachtungen dargestellt. Leipzig: J. O. Wiegel. 1870; 182.
2. Vergely P: De l'angine de poitrine dans ses rapports avec le diabvete. Gaz hedb de ned (series 2) 1883; 20: 364.
3. Dreyfous F: Pathogenie et accidents nerveux du diabete sucre. Paris: Delahaye & Lecrrosnier 1883; 81.
4. Huchard H: Des manifestations cardiagues et de l'angina de potrine chez les diabetiques. Bull Mem Soc Therap Paris (series 2) 1888; 15: 1.
5. Mayer J: Ueber den Zusammenhang des Diabetes Mellitus mit Erkrankungen des Herzens. Ztschr f Klin Med 1888; 14: 212.
6. Ord WM: A clinical lecture on diabetes. Clin J 1893; 2: 193.
7. Naunyn B: Der Diabetes Mellitus, 2nd edn. Wein: Holder, 1906; 260.
8. Brunton L: On the heart in relation to diabetes. Practitioner 1907; 79: 42.
9. Marks HH, Krall LP: Onset, course, prognosis, and mortality in diabetes mellitus. In: Marble A, White P, Bradley RF, Krall LP, eds. Joslin's Diabetes Mellitus, 11th ed. Philadelphia: Lea & Febiger, 1971; 225.
10. Warren S, Root HF: The pathology of diabetes with special reference to pancreatic regeneration. Am J Pathol 1925; 1: 415.
11. Root HF, Warren S: A clinical and pathologic study of twenty-six cases of diabetes. Boston Med Surg 1926;194: 45.
12. Wilder RM: Necropsy findings in diabetes. South Med J 1926; 19: 241.
13. Strauss H: Über Änderungen in den Finalzuständen der Diabetiker. Klin Med 1928; 24: 1378.
14. Ophüls W: A statistical survey of 3000 autopsies. San Francisco: Stanford University Press, 1926; 131.
15. Gibb WF, Logan VW: Diabetes mellitus: a study of 147 autopsied diabetics. Arch Intern Med 1929; 43: 376.
16. Levine SA: Coronary thrombosis. Medicine (Baltimore) 1929; 8: 253.
17. Blotner H: Coronary disease in diabetes mellitus. N Engl J Med 1930; 203: 709.
18. Nathanson MH: Coronary disease in 100 autopsied diabetics. Am J Med Sci 1932; 183: 495.
19. Enklewitz M: Diabetes and coronary thrombosis. An analysis of cases which came to necropsy. Am Heart J 1934; 9: 386.
20. Root HF, Sharkey TP: Coronary arteriosclerosis in diabetes mellitus. N Engl J Med 1936; 215: 605.
21. Root HF, Bland EF, Gordon WH, et al.: Coronary atherosclerosis in diabetes mellitus. JAMA 1939; 113: 27.
22. Pollack H, Dolger HA, Ellenberg M: An analysis of the diabetic morbidity and mortality in a general hospital. Am J Med Sci 1941; 202: 246.
23. Stearns S, Schlesinger MJ, Rudy A: Incidence and clinical significance of coronary artery disease in diabetes mellitus. Arch Intern Med 1942; 80: 463.
24. Lisa JR, Magiday M, Galloway I, et al.: Arteriosclerosis with diabetes mellitus. A study of the pathologic findings in 193 diabetic and 2,250 nondiabetic patients. JAMA 1942; 120: 192.
25. Millard EB, Root HF: Degenerative vascular lesions and diabetes mellitus. J Digest Dis 1948; 15: 41.
26. Clawson BJ, Bell ET: Incidence of fatal coronary disease in nondiabetic and in diabetic persons. Arch Pathol 1949; 48: 105.
27. Warren S, LeCompte PM: The pathology of diabetes mellitus, 3rd ed, Philadelphia: Lea & Febiger, 1952; 218.
28. Feldman M, Feldman M Jr: The association of coronary occlusion and infarction with diabetes mellitus. A necropsy study. Am J Med Sci 1954; 28: 53.
29. Thomas WA, Lee KT, Rabin ER: Fatal acute myocardial infarction in diabetic patients. A comparative study of 94 autopsied diabetics with acute myocardial infarction and 406 autopsied non-diabetics with acute myocardial infarction, with special reference to age and sex distributions. Arch Intern Med 1956; 98: 489.
30. Goldenberg S, Alex M, Blumenthal HT: Sequelae of arteriosclerosis of the aorta and coronary arteries. A statistical study in diabetes mellitus. Diabetes 1958; 7: 98.
31. Goodale AS, Daoud AS, Florentin R, et al.: Chemical-anatomic studies of arteriosclerosis and thrombosis in diabetes. I. Coronary arterial wall thickness, thrombosis, and myocardial infarcts in autopsied North Americans. Exp Mol Pathol 1962; 1: 353.
32. Moses C: Atherosclerosis. Mechanisms as a guide to prevention. Philadelphia: Lea & Febiger, 1963; 74–90.
33. Warren S, LeCompte PM, Legg MA: The Pathology of Diabetes Mellitus, 4th edition. Philadelphia: Lea & Febiger. 1966; 188–199, 357–361, 521–515.
34. Ingelfinger JA, Bennett PH, Liebow IM, et al.: Coronary heart disease in the Pima Indians. Electrocardiographic findings and postmortem evidence of myocardial infarction in a population with a high prevalence of diabetes mellitus. Diabetes 1976; 25: 561.
35. Palumbo PC, Elveback LR, Chu Chu-Pin, Connolly DC, Kurland LT: Diabetes mellitus: incidence, prevalence, survivorship, and causes of death in Rochester, Minnesota (1945–1970). Diabetes 1976; 25: 566.
36. Dortimer AC, Shendy PN, Shiroff RA, et al.: Diffuse coronary artery disease in diabetic patients. Fact or fiction? Circulation 1978; 57: 133.
37. Chychota MN, Gau GT, Pluth JR, et al.: Myocardial revascularization. Comparison of operability and surgical results in diabetic and non-diabetic patients. J Thorac Cardiovasc Surg 1973; 65: 856.
38. Verska JJ, Walker WJ: Aortocoronary bypass in the diabetic patient. Am J Cardiol 1975; 35: 774.
39. Draskoczy SP, Leland OS, Bradley RF: Aorto-coronary bypass in the diabetic patient. Kidney Int 1974; 6: 537.
40. Hamby RI, Sherman L, Mehta J, et al.: Reappraisal of the role of the diabetic state in coronary artery disease. Chest 1976; 70: 251.
41. Barner HB, Kaiser GC, et al.: Coronary graft flow and glucose tolerance: evidence against the existence of myocardial microvascular disease. Vasc Surg 1975; 9: 220.

True Left Ventricular Aneurysm and Healed Myocardial Infarction

Clinical and Necropsy Observations Including Quantification of Degrees of Coronary Arterial Narrowing

HENRY S. CABIN, MD
WILLIAM C. ROBERTS, MD, FACC

Bethesda, Maryland

Clinical and necropsy observations are described in 28 patients (24 men) aged 31 to 85 years (mean 62) with healed myocardial infarction and a true left ventricular aneurysm. In contrast to findings in other subsets of necropsy patients with fatal coronary heart disease, chronic congestive heart failure was frequent (22 patients); angina pectoris was infrequent (4 patients) and, when present, never severe; recurrence of acute myocardial infarction (2 patients), sudden death (2 patients) and clinically evident systemic emboli (1 patient) were infrequent; survival for more than 5 years after healing of the acute infarction was infrequent (in 3 of 21 patients with clinically diagnosed acute myocardial infarcts); and survival for longer than 1 year after aneurysmectomy was lacking (0 of 7 patients). Additionally, 23 of the 28 patients had a large heart (greater than 400 g [mean 523], 26 had dilated nonaneurysmal portions of the left ventricle, and all but 1 had a large (greater than 30 percent of the left ventricular wall) myocardial infarct. In 25 of the 28 patients, two or more of the four major epicardial coronary arteries were greater than 75 percent narrowed in cross-sectional area by atherosclerotic plaques. In 992 segments (each 5 mm long) of a major coronary artery examined in 22 patients (45 segments/patient), narrowing was greater than 75 percent in 323 segments (33 percent) and ranged from 51 to 75 percent in 419 (42 percent), from 26 to 50 percent in 210 (21 percent) and from 0 to 25 percent in 40 (4 percent). Thus, the scarred, hypertrophied and aneurysmally dilated left ventricle infrequently produces chest pain or fatal arrhythmia despite diffuse, severe coronary narrowing.

Although ventricular aneurysm is a relatively frequent consequence of acute myocardial infarction, surprisingly few clinicopathologic studies are available that include more than five patients with left ventricular aneurysm and healed myocardial infarction[1-5] (Table I). Consequently, we analyzed clinical and morphologic findings in 28 necropsy patients with healed myocardial infarction and left ventricular aneurysm (Table II), focusing on the amounts of coronary narrowing present, because precise anatomic information in this area is lacking. Also, we call attention to certain clinical features in these patients that distinguish them from other subsets of patients with coronary heart disease.

Methods

Study patients: *All 28 patients fulfilled the following criteria:* (1) presence of a left ventricular free wall (endocardium, myocardium and epicardium) convex protrusion, the wall of which consisted of dense fibrous tissue with or without an occasional "island" of myocardial fibers; (2) absence of myocardial necrosis within the wall of the left ventricular aneurysm; (3) diameter of the mouth of the left ventricular aneurysm larger than or similar to that of the aneurysm itself; (4) absence of associated noncoronary heart disease; and (5) examination of all hearts by both authors.

From the Pathology Branch, National Heart, Lung, and Blood Institute, National Institutes of Health, Bethesda, Maryland. Manuscript received February 19, 1980; revised manuscript received April 24, 1980, accepted April 29, 1980.

Address for reprints: William C. Roberts, MD, Building 10A, Room 3E-30, National Institutes of Health, Bethesda, Maryland 20205.

Certain Clinical and Cardiac Necropsy Observations from 5 Previously Reported Studies in English Comprising More Than 20 Necropsy Patients With Left Ventricular Aneurysm

First author (year)	Phares (1953)	Schlichter (1954)	Abrams (1963)	Dubnow (1965)	Davis (1972)
Years covered	1916–1951	1930–1945	1956–1961	1952–1963	1946–1968
LV aneurysm defined	+[a]	+[b]	—	+[c]	—
Patients (n)	40	102	65	80	27[d]
Age (yr) range (mean)	37–85; (74)	36–85 (—)	— (68)	43–96 (68)	42–89 (59)
Male/female ratio	27:13	80:22	52:13	65:15	35:5
Pts (n) with aneurysm at site of MI	—	102 (100%)	63 (97%)	80 (100%)	—
Pts (n) with aneurysmal wall healed	—	61 (60%)	39 (60%)	"Most"	—
Pts (n) with associated noncoronary heart disease	—	27 (28%)	—	—	—
Angina pectoris	5 (13%)	—	—	—	25 (63%)
Chronic CHF	24 (60%)	71 (71%)	"Infrequent"	61[e] (75%)	35 (88%)
Clinical events compatible with systemic emboli	2[e] (5%)	36[e] (35%)	—	10[e] (13%)	2 (5%)
Clinical diagnosis of acute MI	20 (50%)	66 (65%)	45 (69%)	58 (73%)	36 (90%)
Pts (n) surviving 5 yr after acute MI	—	8/66 (12%)	33/45 (69%)	13/48 (27%)	—
Clinical diagnosis of aneurysm	—	—	4 (6%)	13 (16%)	6/27 (22%)
Modes of death					
Chronic CHF	16 (40%)	—	7 (11%)	—	5/27 (19%)
Acute MI	7 (18%)	—	32 (49%)	34 (43%)	16/27 (59%)
Sudden	6 (15%)	0	0	—	0
Rupture of aneurysm	0	0	2 (3%)	1 (1%)	1/27 (4%)
Thromboemboli	2 (5%)	—	0	7 (9%)	0
Noncardiac	7 (18%)	18 (18%)	23 (35%)	9 (11%)	5/27 (19%)
Rupture of nonaneurysmal wall	1 (3%)	0	0	0	0
Systemic hypertension	19 (48%)	69 (68%)	14 (22%)	23 (29%)	—
Diabetes mellitus	4 (10%)	23 (23%)	24 (37%)	—	—
Pts (n) with LV aneurysmectomy	0	0	0	0	4 (10%)
Heart weight increased	33 (83%)[f]	—	—	66[f] (83%)	—
Pts (n) with LV cavity dilated	—	—	—	—	—
Amount of coronary narrowing	Severe	Severe	—	Severe	Severe
Size of MI	—	Large	—	—	—
Intraaneurysmal thrombus	—	55 (54%)	9/65 (14%)	52 (65%)	12/27 (44%)
Pts (n) in whom heart illustrated	2 (5%)	3 (3%)	0	2 (3%)	0

[a] "...defects in the ventricular wall which demonstrate a definite bulge in the external contour of the heart, together with a thinning of the affected region"; [b] "...a localized outpouching of the cavity of a cardiac chamber, with or without outward bulging of the external surface"; [c] "...a protrusion of a localized portion of the external aspect of the ventricle accompanied by a corresponding protrusion of the ventricular cavity"; [d] Study included 40 patients with necropsies in 27. Data refers to all 40 patients unless specified. [e] minimal number; [f] heart weight >100 g above expected normal.

CHF = congestive heart failure; LV = left ventricular; MI = myocardial infarct; Pts = patients; — = no information.

The 28 patients (Table II) ranged in age from 31 to 85 years (mean 62); 13 were aged 65 years or older, and 24 were men. Chronic congestive heart failure occurred in 22 patients (79 percent), angina pectoris in 4 (14 percent) and clinical episodes compatible with systemic emboli in 1 (4 percent). A history of systemic hypertension, before the acute myocardial infarction, was present in 13 patients, and 5 had diabetes mellitus. Clear documentation of acute myocardial infarction was present in 21 patients and only 3 of them survived for as long as 5 years (Fig. 1). Aneurysmectomy (with coronary bypass in three patients) was performed in seven patients: in six for chronic congestive heart failure and in one for refractory arrhythmias; none of the seven was alive 1 year after operation.

Acute myocardial infarction recurred in two patients and was fatal in one. Thirteen patients died of refractory congestive heart failure; two died suddenly; six from noncardiac causes and one from rupture of the left ventricular aneurysm. In the latter patient a septic process involved the aneurysmal wall. Five of the seven patients undergoing aneurysmectomy died as a direct consequence of the operation, and the other two, from persistent chronic congestive heart failure.

The aneurysm was diagnosed clinically in 12 patients (43 percent): in 6 patients (21 percent), the electrocardiogram was consistent with aneurysm and in 3 (11 percent) the chest radiograph suggested aneurysm; the aneurysm was diagnosed with angiography in each of the 10 patients in whom this procedure was performed.

Examination of coronary arteries: The four major coronary arteries were examined in all 28 patients. In addition, in 22 patients in whom the entire lengths of the right, left main, left anterior descending and left circumflex coronary arteries were available, each of these four arteries was cut transversely into 5 mm long segments and each segment was labeled, processed for histologic study, and a histologic section stained by the Movat method[6] was prepared and examined.

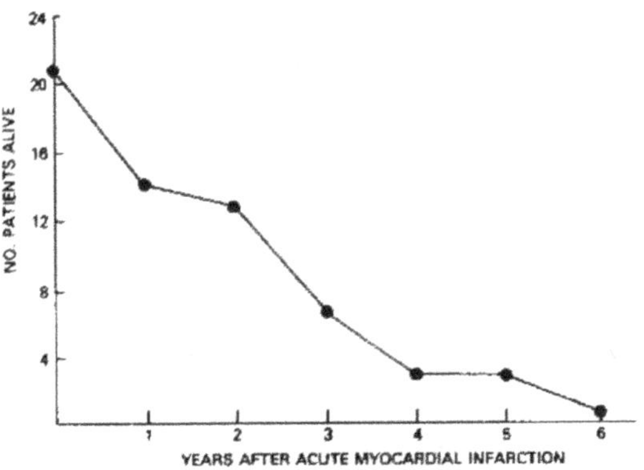

FIGURE 1. Length of survival after acute myocardial infarction in 21 necropsy patients with left ventricular aneurysm and unequivocal history of acute myocardial infarction.

TABLE II

Clinical and Cardiac Necropsy Observations in the 28 Patients

Case	Age (yr) & Sex	Clinically Diagnosed AMI	Interval (mo) AMI to Death	AP After AMI	Chronic CHF After AMI	Clinical Episode Compatible With SE	LV Angiogram	Clinical Diagnosis of Aneurysm	History SH Before AMI	SAP >149/90 mm Hg After AMI	DM
Patients Without Left Ventricular Aneurysmectomy											
1	31M	+	36	0	+	0	+	+	−	0	0
2	39M	+	36	0	+	0	+	+	−	0	0
3	45M	+	3	0	+	0	0	0	+	0	0
4	46M	0	—[a]	0	0	0	0	0	+	0	0
5	46M	+	36	0	+	0	0	0	−	0	0
6	47M	+	6	0	+	0	0	0	+	+	0
7	57M	+	24	+	0	0	0	0	+	0	+
8	60F	+	7	0	+	0	+	+	+	0	0
9	61M	+	3	0	+	0	0	0	−		0
10	62M	0	—[a]	0	0	0	0	0	−	0	0
11	65M	+	3	0	+	+	0	0	+	0	0
12	68M	0	—[a]	0	+	0	0	0	−	0	+
13	69M	+	24	+	+	0	0	0	+	0	+
14	70M	+	23	0	+	0	0	+	+	+	0
15	71M	+	36	0	+	0	0	0	+	0	0
16	75M	0	—[a]	0	+	0	0	0	+	+	0
17	77M	+	6	0	+	0	0	0	−	0	0
18	78M	+	60	0	+	0	0	+	+	0	0
19	80M	0	—[a]	+	+	0	0	0	−	0	0
20	84M	0	—[a]	0	0	0	0	0	−	0	0
21	85F	0	—[a]	0	0	0	0	0	−	0	0
Patients With Left Ventricular Aneurysmectomy											
22	49M	+	60	0	+	0	+	+	−	0	0
23	55F	+	24	0	+	0	+	+	+	+	0
24	55M	+	24	+	+	0	+	+	−	0	+
25	56M	+	120	0	+	0	+	+	−	0	+
26	64M	+	8	0	0	0	+	+	−	0	0
27	67F	+	24	0	+	0	+	+	−	0	0
28	77M	+	26	0	+	0	+	+	+	0	0
Totals (or range)	31–85 24M, 4F	21	3–120	4	22	1	10	12	13	4	5
Percent	86M, 14F	75		14	79	4	36	43	46	14	18
Mean	62		28								

[a] Clinically silent acute myocardial infarction; [b] heart weight does not include operatively excised specimen.

AMI = acute myocardial infarct; AP = angina pectoris; CA = coronary arteries; CHF = congestive heart failure; DM = diabetes mellitus; LV

The degree of narrowing in all 5 mm long segments was determined by examination of the histologic sections magnified 25 to 50 times. *The percent of cross-sectional area narrowing* by atherosclerotic plaque was divided into four categories of narrowing: 0 to 25, 26 to 50, 51 to 75 and 76 to 100. The accuracy of these determinations was verified by random evaluations by other observers and by videoplanimetry, and both the intra- and interobserver error was less than 5 percent.[7]

Results

The ventricular aneurysm: The hearts in the 28 patients (Table II) weighed from 330 to 705 g (mean 523) and in 23 patients the weight was over 400 g. In 20 patients the aneurysm involved the *anterior* (11 patients) (Fig. 2), *posterior* (6 patients) (Fig. 2) or *lateral* (3 patients) (Fig. 3 and 4) walls of the *mid or basal third,* or both, of the left ventricle, with or without involvement of the apical third. In the other eight patients, the aneurysm was designated as *apical* because it involved mainly or only the apical third of the left ventricle, involving in each the entire wall in this portion of the heart (Fig. 5 and 6).

The coronary arteries: Among the 28 study patients (Table II), a total of 112 major (right, left main, left anterior descending and left circumflex) epicardial coronary arteries were examined. At least one of the four major epicardial coronary arteries was narrowed greater than 75 percent in cross-sectional area by atherosclerotic plaques in all 28 patients (Table III). Of the 112 major coronary arteries in the 28 patients, 71 (63 percent) were greater than 75 percent narrowed in cross-sectional area by atherosclerotic plaques, an average of 2.5 of 4.0 coronary arteries/patient. The left main coronary artery was narrowed greater than 75 percent in cross-sectional area in two patients.

Analysis of the 992 five mm long coronary arterial segments in 22 patients disclosed atherosclerotic narrowing of cross-sectional area of 76 to 100 percent in 323 segments (33 percent) 7 of 51 to 75 percent in 419 (42 percent), of 26 to 50 percent in 210 (21 percent) and of 0 to 25 percent in 40 (4 percent) (Table IV). The left anterior descending coronary artery was significantly ($p < 0.05$) more severely narrowed than the other three

| Case | Mode of Death | | | | | | Heart Weight (g) | Site of LV Aneurysm | Thrombus in LV Aneurysm | LV Dilated | Number of 4 Major CA Narrowed 76–100% in XSA | Number of 5 mm Segments of CA Studied | Number (%) of 5 mm Segments Narrowed 76–100% in XSA |
	SCD	AMI	Chronic CHF	Cardiac Op	Non-Cardiac Cause	LV Aneurysm Rupture							
							Patients Without Left Ventricular Aneurysmectomy						
1	0	0	+	0	0	0	520	Apical	0	+	2	56	8(14)
2	0	0	+	0	0	0	520	Apical	+	+	3	40	12(30)
3	0	0	+	0	0	0	500	Anterior	0	+	2	43	24(56)
4	+	0	0	0	0	0	380	Posterior	0	+	3	56	27(48)
5	0	0	+	0	0	0	500	Anterior	0	+	3	51	5(10)
6	0	0	+	0	0	0	465	Anterior	0	+	3	35	13(37)
7	0	+	0	0	0	0	575	Posterior	0	+	3	58	35(60)
8	0	0	+	0	0	0	530	Anterior	0	+	3	49	25(51)
9	0	0	+	0	0	0	530	Apical	+	+	2	—	—
10	0	0	0	0	+	0	500	Posterior	0	+	2	45	7(16)
11	0	0	+	0	0	0	430	Lateral	+	+	3	—	—
12	0	0	0	0	+	0	600	Posterior	0	+	3	—	—
13	0	0	+	0	0	0	430	Anterior	0	+	3	59	33(56)
14	0	0	+	0	0	0	618	Anterior	+	+	3	41	18(44)
15	0	0	0	0	+	0	360	Anterior	0	+	3	31	8(26)
16	+	0	0	0	0	0	670	Apical	+	0	3	63	27(43)
17	0	0	0	0	0	+	585	Lateral	+	+	3	43	7(16)
18	0	0	+	0	0	0	705	Apical	+	+	1	50	5(10)
19	0	0	0	0	+	0	330	Lateral	+	+	1	30	1(3)
20	0	0	0	0	+	0	390	Apical	0	0	3	—	—
21	0	0	0	0	+	0	380	Apical	+	+	2	13	8(61)
							Patients With Left Ventricular Aneurysmectomy						
22	0	0	+	0	0	0	650[b]	Anterior	0	+	1	53	12(23)
23	0	0	0	+	0	0	500[b]	Posterior	0	+	3	—	—
24	0	0	0	+	0	0	700[b]	Anterior	+	+	3	54	6(11)
25	0	0	0	+	0	0	550[b]	Anterior	0	+	2	—	—
26	0	0	0	+	0	0	572	Anterior	0	+	2	29	15(51)
27	0	0	+	0	0	0	500[b]	Apical	0	+	2	48	6(13)
28	0	0	0	+	0	0	658	Posterior	+	+	4	45	21(47)
Totals (or range)	2	1	13	5	6	1	330–700			11	26	71	992	323
Percent	7	4	46	18	21	4				39	93			
Mean							523					2.5	45	15(33)

= left ventricular; mo = months; Op = operation; SAP = systolic arterial pressure; SCD = sudden coronary death; SE = systemic embolus; SH = systemic hypertension; Th = thrombus; XSA = cross-sectional area; + = present or positive; 0 = absent or negative; − = no information available.

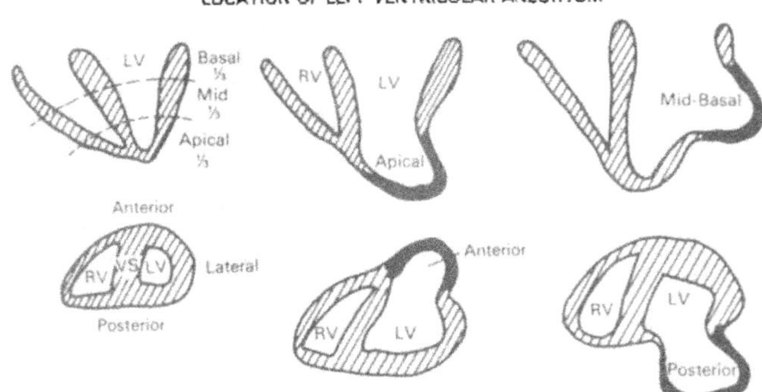

FIGURE 2. Locations of left ventricular aneurysms. The locations of apical (**top middle**) and mid-basal (**top right**) aneurysms are shown. The anterior, lateral and posterior walls of a transverse cardiac ventricular slice (**bottom left**) and the locations of anterior (**bottom middle**) and posterior (**bottom right**) wall aneurysms are shown. An aneurysm is considered anterior, posterior or lateral if it involves the anterior, posterior or lateral walls of the mid or basal third, or both, of the left ventricle with or without involvement of the apical third. An aneurysm is considered apical if it is limited to the apical third of the left ventricle. LV = left ventricle; RV = right ventricle; VS = ventricular septum.

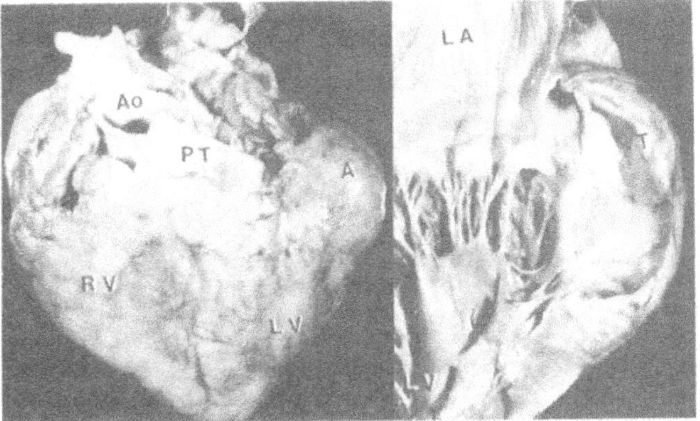

FIGURE 3. Patient 19 (Table II). Exterior view (**left**) and longitudinal section (**right**) of the heart from an 80 year old man (GT 72A-233) without a history of acute myocardial infarction but with angina pectoris and congestive heart failure. He died from carcinoma of the bladder. A lateral wall left ventricular aneurysm (A) that contains thrombus (T) is present. Ao = aorta; LA = left atrium; LV = left ventricle; PT = pulmonary trunk; RV = right ventricle.

major coronary arteries (Fig. 7). The mean percent of 5 mm segments severely narrowed in the proximal half of the right, left anterior descending and left circumflex coronary arteries was similar to that in the distal half of each of these arteries (Fig. 8).

Of the 22 patients in whom the amount of coronary arterial narrowing was quantified, 10 had an anterior, 6 an apical, 4 a posterior and 2 a lateral left ventricular aneurysm. In the 10 patients with an *anterior* left ventricular aneurysm, 79 (60 percent) of 132 five mm segments of the left anterior descending, 61 (34 percent) of 179 segments of the right and 19 (17 percent) of 115 segments of the left circumflex coronary artery were narrowed greater than 75 percent in cross-sectional area. In the 6 patients with an *apical* aneurysm, 35 (50 percent) of 70 segments of the left anterior descending, 17 (13 percent) of 130 segments of the right and 12 (20 percent) of 61 segments of the left circumflex coronary artery were narrowed greater than 75 percent. In the four patients with a *posterior* aneurysm, 26 (37 percent)

of 71 segments of the left anterior descending, 40 (50 percent) of 80 segments of the right and 24 (50 percent) of 48 segments of the left circumflex coronary artery were narrowed greater than 75 percent. In the two patients with a *lateral* aneurysm, 1 (4 percent) of 26 segments of the left anterior descending, 1 (3 percent) of 34 segments of the right and 6 (55 percent) of 11 segments of the left circumflex coronary artery were narrowed greater than 75 percent.

Comments

Clinical versus anatomic definition of ventricular aneurysm: Our study included only patients with a localized convex protrusion of the entire thickness of the left ventricular wall at necropsy. The wall of the aneurysm formerly was the wall of left ventricle, and the mouth of the aneurysm was larger than or as large as the maximal diameter of the aneurysm. These patients therefore had a *true anatomic* left ventricular aneurysm. When a localized left ventricular protrusion is

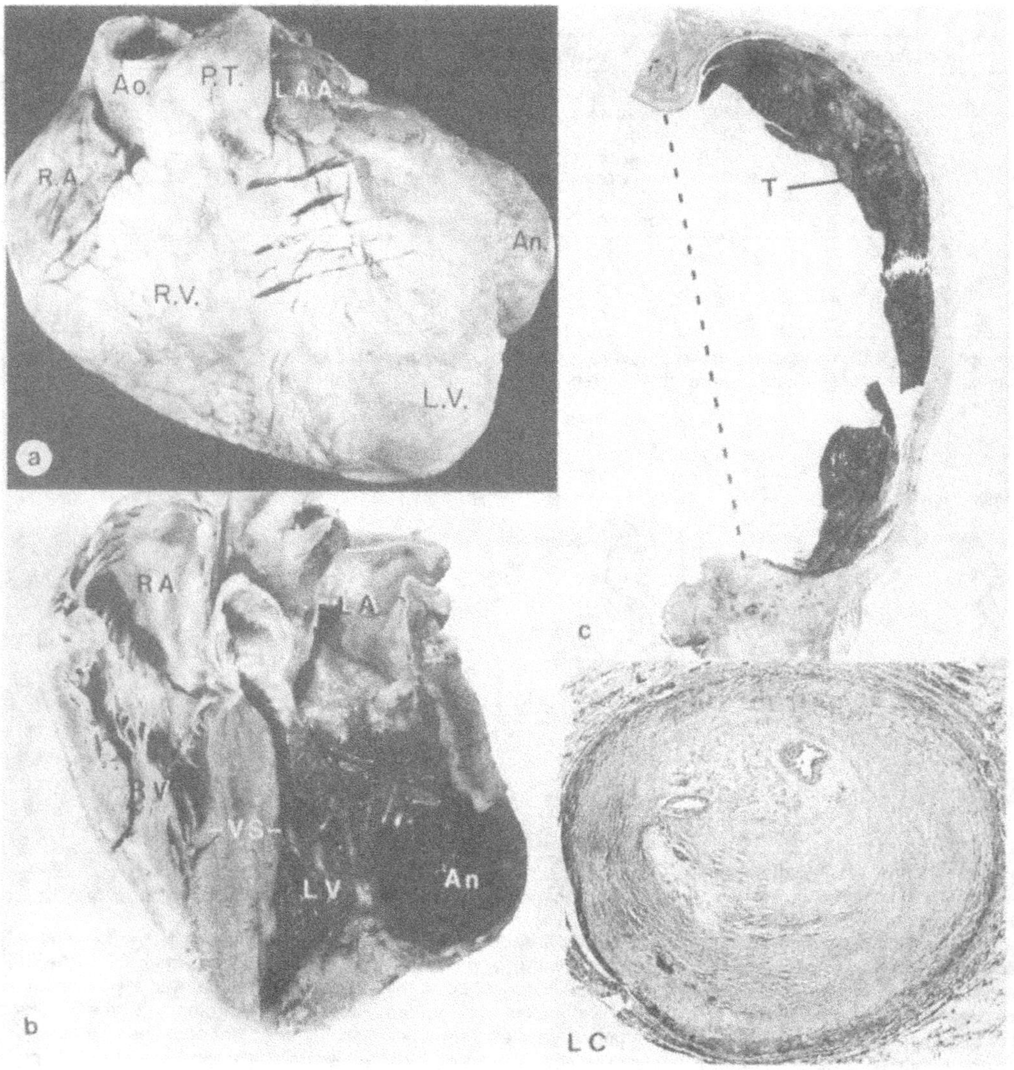

FIGURE 4. Patient 11 (Table II). Exterior view (a) and longitudinal section (b) of the heart and photomicrograph of the aneurysmal wall (c) and of the left circumflex (LC) coronary artery at point of maximal narrowing from a 65 year old man (A67–71) with no history of acute myocardial infarction or angina pectoris who died of progressive congestive heart failure. a, exterior view of the anterior surface of the heart showing the lateral wall left ventricular (L.V.) aneurysm (An.). b, longitudinal section of the heart showing the lateral wall left ventricular aneurysm and the dilated nonaneurysmal portion of the left ventricular cavity. VS = ventricular septum. c, histologic section of the scarred aneurysmal wall, the thrombus (T) adherent to its wall, and the mouth of the aneurysm (dashed line) (Movat stain ×2, reduced by 25 percent). ×2 LC, left circumflex coronary artery at its point of maximal narrowing. (Hematoxylin–eosin ×26, reduced by 25 percent. Ao = aorta; LA = left atrium; L.A.A. = left atrial appendage; P.T. = pulmonary trunk; R.A. = right atrium; R.V. = right ventricle; VS = ventricular septum.

present at necropsy, the protrusion must have been present during life in both ventricular systole and diastole. Patients in whom a localized protrusion is observed only during ventricular systole (*functional aneurysm*) would not have a protrusion at necropsy, and therefore such patients are not included in this analysis. Because the wall of the left ventricular aneurysm in our patients contained few if any myocardial fibers, the anatomic aneurysm could have been either akinetic or dyskinetic during life but not hypokinetic. Thus, clinical studies that have defined left ventricular aneurysm by hypokinetic wall motion abnormality or by akinetic or dyskinetic portions of wall,[8–16] without specifying protrusion during both phases of the cardiac cycle,[17–19] have included many patients without an anatomic aneurysm.

A precise definition of left ventricular aneurysm is crucial, in our view, because the findings to a large extent are dependent on the definition of aneurysm. In contrast to previous necropsy studies of patients with left ventricular aneurysm,[1,5,20] in our study all our patients had an aneurysm at the site of *healed* myocardial infarction and patients with an aneurysm at the sites of acute infarction were excluded. Additionally, our study excluded patients with associated noncoronary types of heart disease. Furthermore, in contrast to previous studies,[2,3,5] our study is based on personal examination of all the hearts of the patients included, rather than on examination of autopsy protocols, a recognized relatively inaccurate method of obtaining cardiovascular information.[21]

Pathologic Features

Characteristics of the aneurysm: In 27 of our 28 patients, the *left ventricular scars* involved more than 30 percent of the left ventricular wall. In none of five previously reported necropsy studies in English involving more than 20 patients[1–5] (Table I) was the size of the myocardial infarcts (which healed) quantified. However, in the study by Schlichter et al.,[2] the infarcts

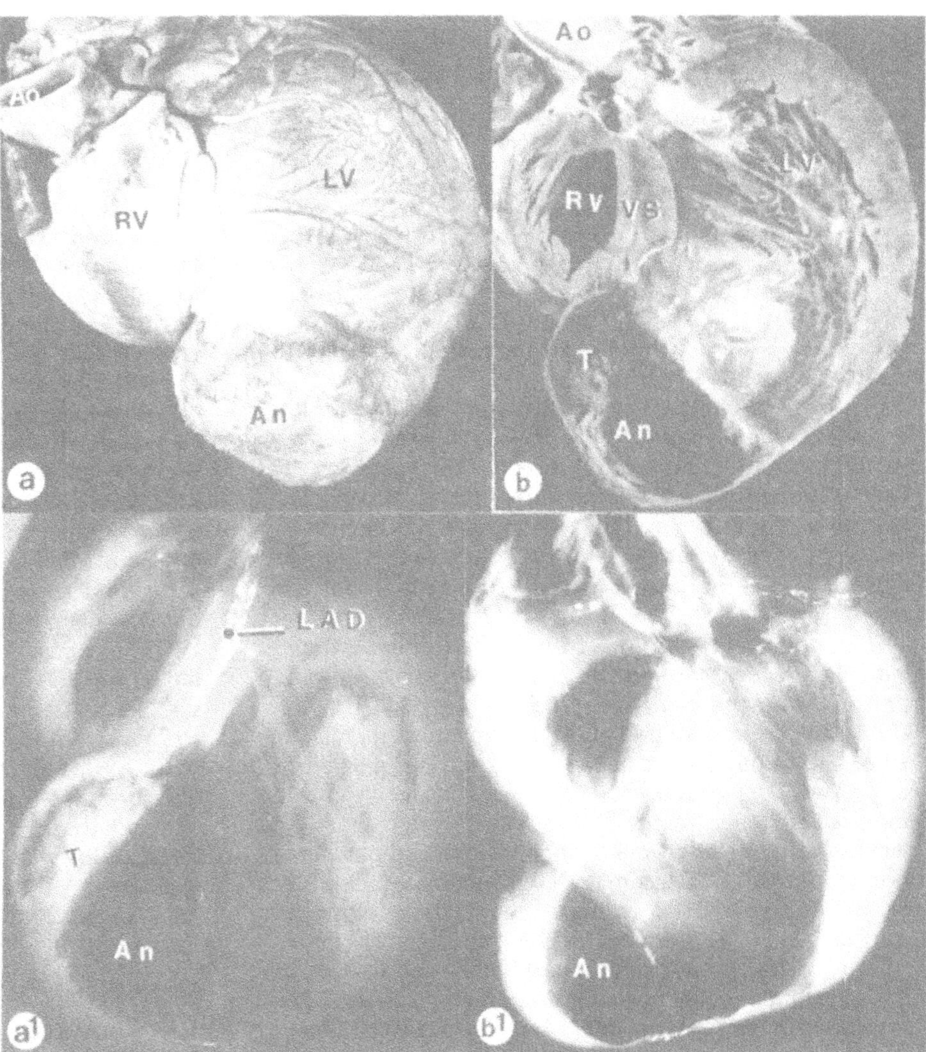

FIGURE 5. Patient 18 (Table II). Unopened heart and roentgenogram (a and a¹) and after a longitudinal cut (b, b¹) from a 78 year old man (GT 76A-171) who died of congestive heart failure 5 years after an acute myocardial infarction. a, exterior view of the heart showing a large apical wall left ventricular (LV) aneurysm (An). a¹, roentgenogram of a showing calcific deposits in the left anterior descending (LAD) coronary artery and in the wall of the aneurysm. The intraaneurysmal thrombus (T) also is seen. b, longitudinal section of the heart showing the apical aneurysm and the markedly dilated nonaneurysmal portion of the left ventricular cavity. b¹, roentgenogram of b showing calcific deposits in the coronary arteries and in the wall of the aneurysm. Ao = aorta; RV = right ventricle; VS = ventricular septum.

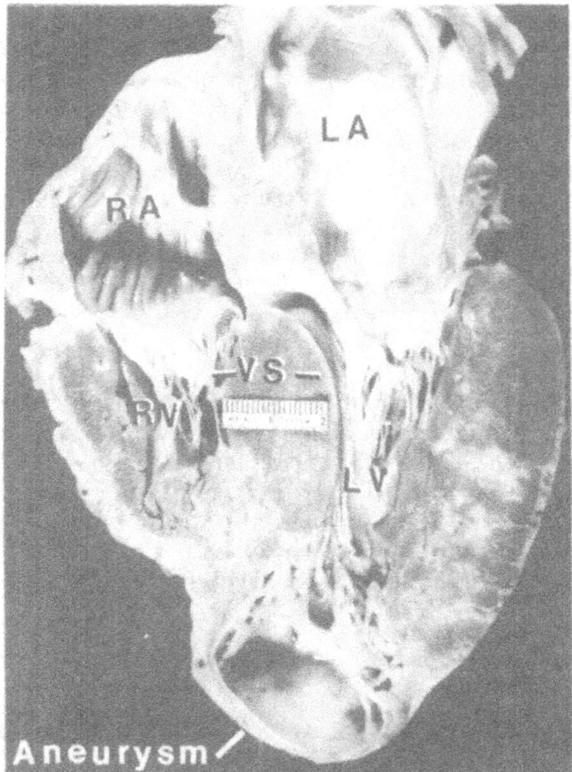

FIGURE 6. Patient 20 (Table II). Longitudinal section of the heart from an 80 year old man (GT 72A-219) who had no clinical evidence of coronary heart disease and died of acute pneumonia. An apical left ventricular (LV) aneurysm is present. The nonaneurysmal wall is hypertrophied and the left ventricular cavity is not dilated. LA = left atrium; RA = right atrium; RV = right ventricle; VS = ventricular septum.

TABLE III

Number of 28 Patients With Severe* Narrowing of One or More Major Coronary Arteries and Number of 112 Major Coronary Arteries With Such Narrowing

Number of Coronary Arteries With Severe Narrowing	Number of Patients	Total Number of Coronary of Arteries (4/patient)	Total Number of Coronary Arteries With Severe Narrowing
1	3	12	3
2	8	32	16
3	16	64	48 } 2.5/4.0
4	1	4	4
Totals	28	112	71 (63%)

* 75 percent or greater narrowing of cross-sectional area.

were described as "large," apparently in most patients.

Scarring in portions of the left ventricular wall not involved in or adjacent to the aneurysm was absent in our 28 patients. This finding was not reported in previous studies[1–5,20,22–24] of necropsy patients with left ventricular aneurysm. The significance of this observation is that the aneurysm represents, with few exceptions, the only myocardial infarction that occurred.

The nonaneurysmal portion of the left ventricular wall was hypertrophied in 24 (86 percent) of our 28 patients and the *heart weight was increased* (greater than 350 g in women and greater than 400 g in men). In 20 of the 24 patients, the heart weighed 500 g or more. Only two of five previous necropsy studies (Table I) mentioned heart weight. Phares et al.[1] found the heart weight to be "100 grams or more above the predicted normal" in 33 (83 percent) of 40 patients and Dubnow et al.,[4] found it "100 grams or more above expected normal" in 66 (83 percent) of their 80 patients.

The portion of left ventricular cavity uninvolved by aneurysm was dilated in 26 (93 percent) of our 28 patients. Information on left ventricular cavity size is lacking in previous necropsy studies of patients with left ventricular aneurysm[1–5,20,22–24] (Table I).

Characteristics of the coronary arteries: *The degree of narrowing of the epicardial coronary arteries* in necropsy patients with healed left ventricular aneurysm was recognized as "severe" in previous studies (Table I)[1,2,4,5] as well as in our patients. Phares et al.[1] mentioned "severe" narrowing of the left anterior descending coronary artery in a "majority" of their 40 patients. Schlichter et al.[2] described "severe" coronary narrowing in an unspecified number of their 102 patients. Dubnow et al.[4] described "occlusive lesions" in one or more coronary arteries in all of their 80 patients, and Davis and Ebert[5] reported greater than 50 percent luminal narrowing (whether cross-sectional area or diameter reduction not specified) in two or more of the three major (left anterior descending, left circumflex and right) coronary arteries in 20 of their 24 necropsy patients. In 25 of our 28 patients, two or three of the three major coronary arteries were narrowed greater than 75 percent in cross-sectional area by atherosclerotic plaques, and in the other 3 patients, only one artery was similarly narrowed.

Although several previous studies have superficially mentioned degrees of coronary narrowing in necropsy patients with left ventricular aneurysm, *quantitative information on the extent and distribution of the narrowing in each of the four major coronary arteries* has not been reported previously. In 22 of our 28 patients, an average of 33 percent (range 3 to 61) of the lengths of the four major arteries were narrowed 76 to 100 percent and another 42 percent were narrowed 51 to 75 percent in cross-sectional area by atherosclerotic plaque. The left anterior descending artery had significantly more 5 mm long segments narrowed severely (greater than 75 percent) than did the other major arteries. This was true for the patients with an anterior wall or apical aneurysm (16 patients) but not in the patients with a posterior or lateral wall aneurysm (6 patients).

Clinical Features

Sex and age: It is well recognized that coronary heart disease is more frequent in men than in women by a ratio of about 2:1. Among necropsy patients with left

Number and Percent of 5 mm Long Segments of the Four Major Epicardial Coronary Arteries With the Four Grades of Cross-Sectional Area Luminal Narrowing*

Coronary Artery	Percent Cross-Sectional Area Luminal Narrowing				
	0–25	26–50	51–75	76–100	Totals
Left main					
n	1	14	18	2	35
%	(3)	(40)	(51)	(6)	(100)
Left anterior descending					
n	11	45	102	141	299
%	(4)	(15)	(34)	(47)	(100)
Left circumflex					
n	17	54	103	61	235
%	(7)	(23)	(44)	(26)	(100)
Right					
n	11	97	196	119	423
%	(3)	(23)	(46)	(28)	(100)
Totals					
n	40	210	419	323	992
%	(4)	(21)	(42)	(33)	(100)

* Data based on 22 patients.

ventricular aneurysm, this sex difference is more pronounced. Of our 28 patients, 24 were men and 4 were women (Table II), yielding a man to woman ratio of 6:1. Of the 287 necropsy patients with left ventricular aneurysm reported on in four previous studies[1-4] (Table I), 224 (78 percent) were men and 63 (22 percent) were women. Of necropsy patients with fatal coronary heart disease, those with compared to those without left ventricular aneurysm tend to be older. The mean age of 185 necropsy patients with left ventricular aneurysm from three previously reported studies[1,3,4] was 69 years. The mean age of our 28 patients was 62 years (range 31 to 85), and 17 (61 percent) were 60 years of age or older (Table II).

Heart failure and angina: *Chronic congestive heart failure* was the most frequent manifestation of cardiac dysfunction in our patients, occurring in 22 (79 percent) of the 28. In contrast, angina pectoris was present in only 4 (14 percent) of the 28 patients and in each of them it was infrequent (Table II). Other investigators have also noted a high frequency of chronic congestive heart failure in their patients: in 24 (60 percent) of 40 patients[1]; in 71 (71 percent) of 102 patients[2]; in at least 61 (75 percent) of 80 patients[4]; and in 35 (88 percent) of 40 patients[5] (Table I). The frequency of angina pectoris in necropsy patients with left ventricular aneurysm has rarely been mentioned. Davis and Ebert[5] recorded angina in 25 (63 percent) of their 40 patients reported

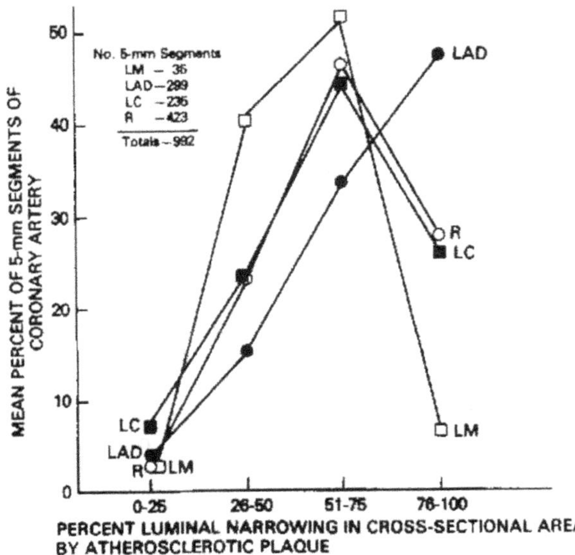

FIGURE 7. Mean percent of 5 mm long segments of the left main (LM), left anterior descending (LAD), left circumflex (LC), and right (R) coronary arteries narrowed to various degrees in 22 study patients with healed myocardial infarction and left ventricular aneurysm.

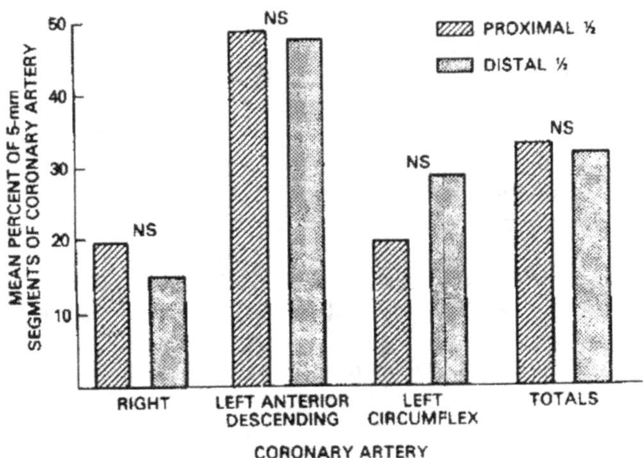

FIGURE 8. Mean percent of 5 mm long segments of the right, left anterior descending and left circumflex coronary arteries narrowed more than 75 percent in cross-sectional area by atherosclerotic plaques in the proximal and distal halves of each artery in 22 study patients with healed myocardial infarction and left ventricular aneurysm. NS = no significant difference.

to have left ventricular aneurysm, but the criteria for diagnosis of aneurysm in their patients were imprecise. Phares et al.[1] found severe angina in 5 (13 percent) of their 40 patients. All our patients with chronic congestive heart failure had dilated nonaneurysmal portions of left ventricle, in general a fairly reliable anatomic indicator for the presence of chronic congestive heart failure in patients without valvular heart disease or intercirculatory shunts. It appears that the dilated left ventricle even in patients with severely narrowed coronary arteries infrequently causes angina pectoris, and when it does, the angina is mild and infrequent.

Systemic hypertension: This was present in at least 13 of our 28 patients before the acute myocardial infarction and in the remaining 15 patients information regarding the level of the systemic blood pressure before the infarction was inadequate. Only four patients had systemic hypertension after healing of the acute infarction (Table II). Thus, systemic hypertension is infrequent in patients with healed myocardial infarction and true left ventricular aneurysm. It seems likely that the explanation for the considerable cardiomegaly in most of our patients was the presence of systemic hypertension, undiagnosed in most, before the acute myocardial infarction. Also, it is likely that the poorly contracting aneurysmally dilated left ventricle after healing of the acute infarction was incapable of creating sufficient cardiac output to allow elevation of the systemic arterial pressures. The frequency of systemic hypertension in previously described necropsy patients with left ventricular aneurysm has ranged from 22 percent (14 of 65 patients)[3] to 68 percent (69 of 102 patients).[2] It is not apparent from these previous studies[1–4] (Table I) whether the systemic hypertension was present before or after the acute myocardial infarction, or both, or whether the information was derived by history or by actual blood pressure recording.

Thromboembolism: Although left ventricular aneurysms frequently contain thrombi, the frequency of *clinical events compatible with systemic emboli* is quite variable. Of our 28 patients, 11 (39 percent) had intraaneurysmal thrombi but only 1 had an event compatible with a systemic embolus; none of the 17 patients without intraaneurysmal thrombi had a compatible event (Table II). Of 102 patients with left ventricular aneurysm reported by Schlichter et al.,[2] 55 (54 percent) had intraaneurysmal thrombi; and at least 36 (35 percent) of their 102 patients had a clinical event compatible with a systemic embolus. Of the 80 patients reported on by Dubnow et al.,[4] 52 (65%) had intraaneurysmal thrombi, and 10 (minimum) had a clinical embolic event. Only 9 (14 percent) of the 65 patients described by Abrams et al.[3] had intraaneurysmal thrombi, and the frequency of clinical systemic emboli was not mentioned (Table I). Despite the variability in the reported frequency of clinical events compatible with systemic emboli in patients with left ventricular aneurysm and healed myocardial infarction, intraaneurysmal thrombus formation is frequent and it would, therefore,

appear reasonable to use anticoagulant agents in these patients.

Clinical diagnosis: Surprisingly, clinical diagnosis of left ventricular aneurysm by means other than left ventricular angiography is infrequent. The diagnosis of left ventricular aneurysm was made in each of our 10 patients who underwent left ventricular angiography but among the other 18 patients, diagnosis by chest radiograph or electrocardiogram was made in only 2. Persistent S-T elevation in the electrocardiogram after healing of the acute myocardial infarction was observed in only 6 (21 percent) (4 of whom also had angiography) of our 28 patients. In previous studies clinical diagnosis of left ventricular aneurysm was made in only 4 (6 percent) of 65 necropsy patients,[3] in 13 (16 percent) of 80 necropsy patients,[4] and in 6 (22 percent) of 27 necropsy patients[5] (Table I).

Prognosis: *Survival* in patients who manifest a left ventricular aneurysm after a clinically documented acute myocardial infarction is clearly diminished compared with that in patients with healed myocardial infarction unassociated with aneurysm. Of our 21 patients whose acute infarction was diagnosed clinically, only 3 lived 60 months or longer thereafter (Fig. 1). In previous studies of patients with left ventricular aneurysm and earlier clinical documentation of acute myocardial infarction, only 8 (12 percent) of 66[2] and 13 (27 percent) of 48[4] survived 5 years or longer after infarction (Table I).

Causes of death: It is well recognized that most patients with severe coronary arterial narrowing from atherosclerosis either die suddenly, from so-called sudden coronary death or from acute myocardial infarction. This situation holds whether the coronary event is a first or a subsequent one. Such, however, was not the situation among our patients with left ventricular aneurysm and healed myocardial infarction (Table II). Only 2 of our 28 patients died suddenly, and only 1 had a fatal acute myocardial infarction. Thirteen of our 28 patients died from intractable congestive heart failure and 5 from consequences of left ventricular aneurysmectomy. It is likely that congestive heart failure would have proved fatal in at least four of these latter five patients. Rupture of a healed true left ventricular aneurysm is an extremely rare occurrence. Rupture did occur, however, in one of our patients but only because septicemia developed and a septic process invaded the aneurysmal wall. Chronic congestive heart failure was not as frequent a fatal event, and fatal acute myocardial infarction was more frequent in previous necropsy studies[1,3–5] (Table I). "Sudden coronary death" was noted to be an infrequent mode of death in previous reports (6 [15 percent] of 40 patients,[1] none of 102 patients,[2] none of 65 patients[3] and none of 24 patients).[5]

Conclusions: Thus, from our study of 28 necropsy patients with true anatomic left ventricular aneurysm and healed myocardial infarction, the following conclusions appear justified: The myocardial infarct is large; the heart weight is increased and the nonscarred left ventricular wall is hypertrophied; the nonaneurysmal portions of the left ventricular cavities are dilated; the major epicardial coronary arteries are severely narrowed; chronic congestive heart failure is frequent and is the most common cause of death; angina pectoris is infrequent; recurrence of acute myocardial infarction is infrequent; clinical events compatible with systemic emboli are infrequent despite frequent intraaneurysmal thrombus; the long-term prognosis is poor; sudden death is infrequent; and clinical diagnosis of the left ventricular aneurysm without left ventricular angiography is infrequent.

References

1. **Phares W, Edwards JE, Burchell HB.** Cardiac aneurysms: clinicopathologic studies. Mayo Clin Proc 1953;28:264–71.
2. **Schlichter J, Hellerstein HK, Katz LN.** Aneurysm of the heart. A correlative study of one hundred and two proved cases. Medicine 1954;33:43–86.
3. **Abrams DL, Edelist A, Luria MH, Miller AJ.** Ventricular aneurysm. A reappraisal based on study of sixty-five consecutive autopsied cases. Circulation 1963;27:164–9.
4. **Dubnow MH, Burchell HB, Titus JL.** Postinfarction ventricular aneurysm. A clinicomorphologic and electrocardiographic study of 80 cases. Am Heart J 1965;70:753–60.
5. **Davis RW, Ebert PA.** Ventricular aneurysm. A clinical-pathologic correlation. Am J Cardiol 1972;29:1–6.
6. **Movat HZ.** Demonstration of all connective tissue elements in a single section. Pentachrome stains. Arch Pathol Lab Med 1955;60:289–95.
7. **Isner JM, Wu M, Virmani R, Jones AA, Roberts WC.** Comparison of degrees of coronary arterial luminal narrowing determined by visual inspection of histologic sections under magnification among three independent observers and comparison to that obtained by video planimetry: an analysis of 559 five-mm segments of 61 coronary arteries from eleven patients. Lab Invest 1980;42:566–70.
8. **Gorlin R, Klein MD, Sullivan JM.** Prospective correlative study of ventricular aneurysm. Mechanistic concept and clinical recognition. Am J Med 1967;42:512–31.
9. **Cheng TO.** Incidence of ventricular aneurysm in coronary artery disease. An angiographic appraisal. Am J Med 1971;50:340–55.
10. **Kitamura S, Echevarria M, Kay JH, et al.** Left ventricular performance before and after removal of the noncontractile area of the left ventricle and revascularization of the myocardium. Circulation 1972;45:1005–17.
11. **Bruschke AVG, Proudfit WL, Sones FM, Jr.** Progress study of 590 consecutive nonsurgical cases of coronary disease followed 5–9 years. II. Ventriculographic and other correlations. Circulation 1973;47:1154–63.
12. **Hines GL, Rivas J, Epstein H, Delaney T, Mohtashemi M.** Surgical treatment of ventricular aneurysms. Seven year experience. NY State J Med 1978;78:1715–9.
13. **Hutchinson JE III, Green GG, Mekhjian HA, et al.** Combined left ventricular aneurysm and coronary artery bypass surgery. Arch Surg 1978;113:1236–40.
14. **Kapelanski DP, Al-Sadir J, Lamberti JJ, Anagnostopoulos CE.** Ventricular features predictive of surgical outcome for left ventricular aneurysm. Circulation 1978;58:1167–74.
15. **Walker WE, Stoney WS, Alford WC, et al.** Techniques and results of ventricular aneurysmectomy with emphasis on anteroseptal repair. J Thorac Cardiovasc Surg 1978;76:824–31.
16. **Buda AJ, Stinson EB, Harrison DC.** Surgery for life-threatening ventricular tachyarrhythmias. Am J Cardiol 1979;44:1171–7.
17. **Letac B, Leroux G, Cribier A, Soyer R.** Large ventricular aneurysms occurring after myocardial infarction. Br Heart J 1978;40:516–22.
18. **Grondin P, Kretz GJ, Bical O, Donzeau-Gouge P, Petitclerc R, Campeau L.** Natural history of saccular aneurysms of the left ventricle. J Thorac Cardiovasc Surg 1979;77:57–64.
19. **Burton NA, Stinson EB, Oyer PE, Shumway NE.** Left ventricular aneurysm. Preoperative risk factors and long-term postoperative results. J Thorac Cardiovasc Surg 1979;77:65–75.
20. **Moyer JB, Hiller GI.** Cardiac aneurysm: clinical and electrocardiographic analysis. Am Heart J 1951;41:340–58.
21. **Roberts WC.** The autopsy: its decline and a suggestion for its revival. N Engl J Med 1978;299:332–8.
22. **Ball D.** Aneurysm of the heart. The clinical recognition of aneurysm of the left ventricle. Am Heart J 1938;16:203–18.
23. **Parkinson J, Bedford PE, Thomson WAR.** Cardiac aneurysm. Q J Med 1938;7:455–78.
24. **Dressler W, Pfeiffer R.** Cardiac aneurysm. A report of ten cases. Ann Intern Med 1940;14:100–21.

Cross-sectional Area of the Proximal Portions of the Three Major Epicardial Coronary Arteries in 98 Necropsy Patients with Different Coronary Events

Relationship to Heart Weight, Age and Sex

CHARLES S. ROBERTS AND WILLIAM C. ROBERTS, M.D.

SUMMARY   The cross-sectional area (the portion enclosed by the internal elastic membrane) of histologic sections from the first 5-mm long segments of the right, left anterior descending and left circumflex coronary arteries was determined by videoplanimetry in 98 necropsy patients with coronary heart disease and in 46 control subjects who did not have significant coronary narrowing. Significant ($p < 0.001$) differences were observed in the mean cross-sectional area of each of the three major coronary arteries in the subgroups of coronary patients and among and between the control subjects. These differences resulted primarily from differences in heart weight and, to a slight extent, in age. Difference in sex was not significant. The 20 patients with angina pectoris had the smallest coronary arteries (mean cross-sectional area of each of the 60 arteries 6.0 mm^2) and the smallest hearts (mean weight 386 g). The 18 patients with healed myocardial infarcts and intractable congestive heart failure had the largest coronary arteries (mean area 8.6 mm^2) and the largest hearts (mean weight 588 g). The 23 patients with acute transmural myocardial infarcts and the 19 with sudden coronary death had similar-sized coronary arteries (mean area 7.6 mm^2) and similar-sized hearts (mean weight 471 g). The 18 patients with healed myocardial infarcts, subsequently asymptomatic courses and noncardiac deaths had slightly enlarged arteries (mean area 6.9 mm^2) and hearts (mean weight 430 g). The 31 control subjects with cancer and normal or near-normal-sized hearts (mean weight 309 g) had the smallest coronary arteries (mean area 5.0 mm^2). The 16 controls with aortic valve disease had the largest hearts (mean weight 730 g) and the largest coronary arteries (mean area 9.6 mm^2). When heart weights were equalized (450 g), older patients had larger coronary arteries than younger patients (mean area $\leq$ 40 years 6.5 mm^2, 41–60 years 6.8 mm^2 and $>$ 60 years 7.6 mm^2).

DEGREES of coronary arterial luminal narrowing in patients with symptomatic or fatal coronary heart disease have been studied extensively in recent years. The degrees of coronary narrowing in necropsy patients with fatal coronary heart disease are usually recorded in terms of cross-sectional area. Studies from this laboratory and others indicate that patients with fatal coronary heart disease at necropsy usually have narrowing by atherosclerotic plaques of more than 75% in cross-sectional area of at least two of the three major (right, left anterior descending and right) epicardial coronary arteries, and that over 30% of the entire lengths of these three major arteries are narrowed to this extent.[1-7] Although degrees of cross-sectional area narrowing at necropsy of the major epicardial coronary arteries have demonstrated certain differences among subsets of patients with fatal coronary heart disease,[3-7] cross sectional area does not provide complete anatomic information. A large artery and a small artery, for example, can be similarly narrowed in cross-sectional area and yet the area through which blood can flow in the large artery obviously is greater than the area through which blood

can flow in the smaller artery (fig. 1). In the present study, therefore, we describe the sizes of the three major coronary arteries in necropsy patients with clinical evidence of coronary heart disease and in control subjects and examine whether the sizes of these arteries are similar or different in various subgroups of coronary patients and, if different, why.

Patients and Methods

Ninety-eight necropsy patients were included in this study. Twenty patients had clinically isolated angina pectoris[4] (table 1). Each died within 3 days of an aortocoronary bypass procedure, and during life their only evidence of myocardial ischemia was angina pectoris; none had had clinical evidence (historical and electrocardiographic) of acute myocardial infarction or chronic congestive heart failure. Twenty-three patients had fatal transmural (involving greater than the inner half of the left ventricularwall) acute myocardial infarcts[5] which by history and by histologic examination were 24 hours to 30 days old. Nineteen patients died suddenly and unexpectedly, and this subgroup hereafter will be referred to as sudden coronary death.[3] Each died within 6 hours after the onset of chest pain, which, if present, began outside the hospital. None ever had evidence of congestive heart failure. At necropsy, at least one of the three major epicardial coronary arteries was greater than 75% narrowed in cross-sectional area by atherosclerotic plaques. None of these 19 patients at necropsy had ventricular wall myocardial coagulation

From the Pathology Branch, National Heart, Lung, and Blood Institute, National Institutes of Health, Bethesda, Maryland.

Address for correspondence: William C. Roberts, M.D., Building 10A, Room 3E-30, National Institutes of Health, Bethesda, Maryland 20205.

Received November 5, 1979; revision accepted March 31, 1980.

Circulation 62, No. 5, 1980.

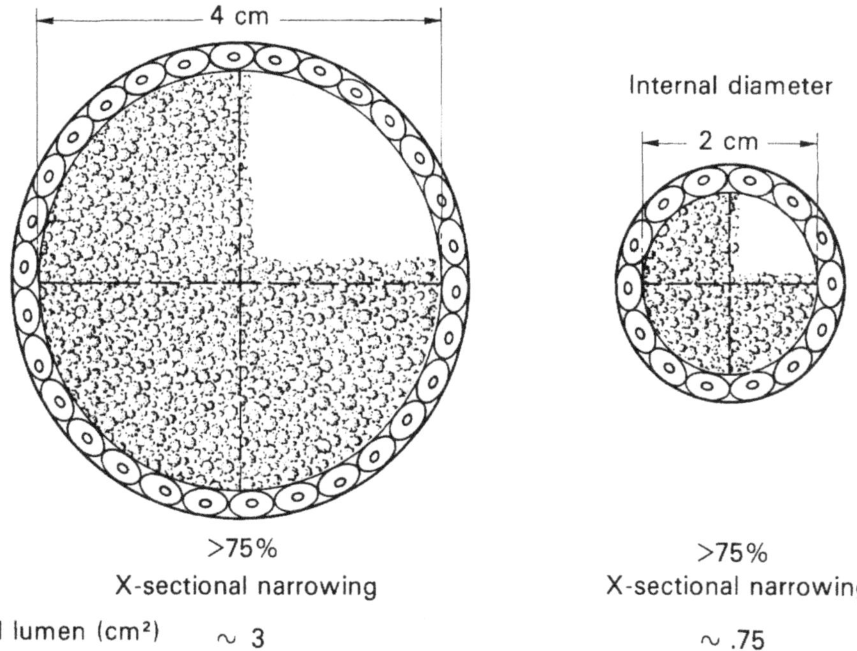

FIGURE 1. *Diagram of transverse sections of two coronary arteries, both of which are narrowed greater than 75% in cross-sectional area. Although both are similarly narrowed in cross-sectional area, one can accommodate a much larger blood flow because it is much larger.*

necrosis. At necropsy, 36 patients had healed transmural myocardial infarcts. These 36 patients were divided into two groups: 18 with nonfatal healed myocardial infarcts,[7] i.e., patients who had had acute myocardial infarcts that healed and who subsequently died of noncardiac conditions, and 18 with fatal healed myocardial infarcts,[6] i.e., patients who had had transmural acute myocardial infarcts that healed and either immediately or later developed chronic congestive cardiac failure that became intractable and

TABLE 1. *Mean Cross-sectional Area of the Right, Left Anterior Descending, and Left Circumflex Coronary Arteries, Heart Weight, Age and Sex in the Five Groups of Coronary Patients and in the Two Groups of Control Subjects*

Group	Pts	Sex M	Sex F	Age (years), range and mean	Heart weight (g), range and mean	Mean XSA (mm²) of R, LAD, LCCA, range and mean
				Coronary patients		
1—Angina pectoris	20	12	8	37–59 (49)	240–520 (386)	2.7–13.1 (6.0)
2—Healed MI (noncardiac death)	18	15	3	25–80 (63)	310–540 (430)	3.3–12.3 (6.9)
3—Acute MI	23	17	6	33–82 (58)	310–720 (482)	3.6–11.9 (7.6)
4—Sudden coronary death	19	17	2	28–85 (54)	300–670 (459)	5.2–14.9 (7.7)
5—Healed MI (cardiac death)	18	18	0	31–78 (58)	450–800 (588)	5.3–13.4 (8.6)
				Control subjects		
1—Cancer	31	17	14	26–74 (51)	135–470 (309)	2.04–9.07 (5.0)
2—Aortic valve	15	13	2	34–81 (56)	550–1050 (730)	7.1–14.9 (9.6)

Abbreviations: XSA = cross-sectional area; R = right coronary artery; LAD = left anterior descending coronary artery; LCCA = left circumflex coronary artery; MI = myocardial infarction.

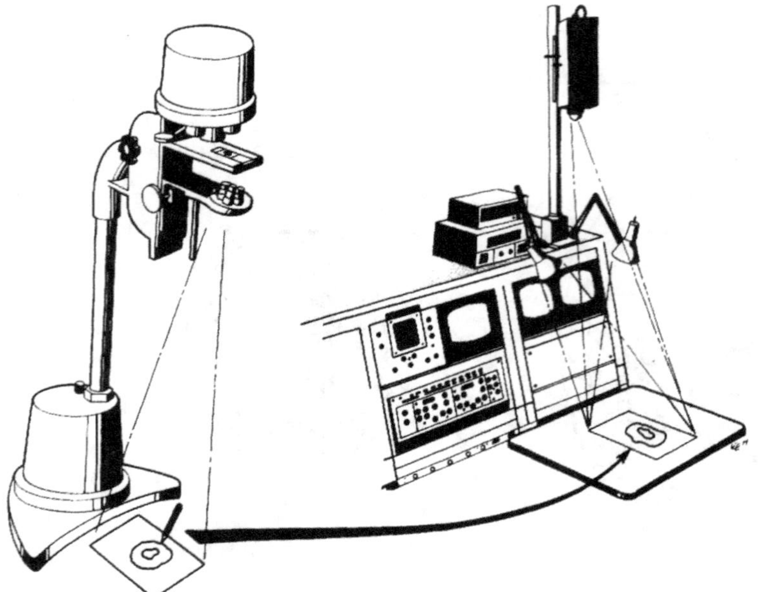

fatal. Patients with associated valvular, congenital or pericardial heart diseases or hypertrophic cardiomyopathy or myocardial diseases not secondary to coronary disease were excluded from these coronary subgroups.

The hearts in all 98 patients were studied in similar fashion. The hearts were cleaned of postmortem clots, all portions of parietal pericardium were excised, the aorta and pulmonary trunk were excised about 2 cm cephalad to their sinotubular junctions and the hearts were carefully weighed. After fixation in 10% buffered formalin for at least 24 hours, the major epicardial coronary arteries were excised intact from the hearts and fixed again for at least another 24 hours. They were then x-rayed and if calcific deposits were present the arteries that contained calcium were decalcified. The right, left main, left anterior descending, and left circumflex coronary arteries were then cut into 5-mm-long segments at right angles to the longitudinal axes of the arteries and each segment was numbered chronologically beginning at its origin from the aorta (right and left main coronary arteries), or in the case of the left anterior descending and left circumflex arteries, from their origin from the left main. Each 5-mm segment was processed and dehydrated in alcohols and xylenes, embedded in paraffin, cut, and stained by Movat's pentachrome method. The latter was used because it clearly delineates the artery's internal elastic membrane.

We studied three histologic sections of coronary artery from each patient, for a total of 294 sections. From each patient, one Movat-stained section of the right, left anterior descending and left circumflex coronary arteries was examined. Each section was prepared from the first 5-mm long segment — the artery's most proximal portion — of the respective artery.

The cross-sectional areas of the coronary arteries were determined by planimetry (KE-compensating polar planimeter) (fig. 2). Each histologic section was positioned on the stage of a projection-light microscope that magnified the image 650 times (fig. 2). The circumference of the internal elastic membrane was then traced on white paper. Although all sections examined had atherosclerotic plaques in the lumens, this study concerned the total area enclosed by the artery's internal elastic membrane irrespective of the presence or absence of superimposed atherosclerotic plaque. Where the internal elastic membrane was artifactually indented, the lumen was extrapolated to a circular form. Each tracing then was placed under a focused camera and the resultant video signal was passed through an electronic integrator and displayed on a television monitor (fig. 2).[8] The threshold level of the television monitor was adjusted so that the area of opacification estimated by video planimeters activated by the video signal corresponded to the original lumen (area enclosed by the internal elastic membrane). The analog output voltages of the video planimeters, calibrated on a grid system, provided on-line measurements of the cross-sectional area.

The area of each artery enclosed by the internal elastic membrane provided by videoplanimetry was converted into actual area in the following manner. A slide containing a 2-mm scale was projected onto tracing paper and recorded via the projection microscope in the same manner in which histologic sections of coronary arteries were projected and traced. The traced scale was converted into a square box, which was placed under the focused camera of the video planimeter console. The scale of the video-planimeter was then set to read 4 mm^2 because the original length of one side of the box had been projected and traced from a 2-mm long scale. The actual cross-sectional areas of the right, left anterior descending and left circumflex coronary arteries were added together to obtain the sum of the cross-sectional area of each patient. This number was divided by 3 to obtain the mean cross-sectional area for each patient.

For comparison with the 98 coronary patients, 46 subjects served as controls. During life none of them had clinical evidence of coronary heart disease and at necropsy none had any of their major coronary arteries narrowed greater than 75% in cross-sectional area by atherosclerotic plaques. The control subjects consisted of two major groups: 31 patients died of various cancers and 15 died of complications of aortic valve disease. Of the 31 control subjects with cancer, 26 had hearts that weighed 400 g or less and the other five had hearts that weighed 410–470 g. Of the 15 patients with aortic valve disease, 11 had stenosis with peak systolic pressure gradients between left ventricle and a systemic artery of 12–155 mm Hg (average 74 mm Hg), and the remaining four patients had pure aortic regurgitation of severe degree. The reason for selecting these two groups of control subjects was to obtain both normal and near-normal-sized hearts and also very large hearts. The coronary arteries in the 46 control subjects were examined in the same manner as in the 98 study patients.

Results

The findings in this study are summarized in tables 1–4. Except for similar values in the acute myocardial infarct and sudden coronary death subgroups, the mean values of the mean cross-sectional areas of each of the three major coronary arteries in each of the subgroups of coronary patients differed significantly ($p < 0.0001$), and also, these values differed significantly ($p < 0.0001$) from those of the control subjects. The 20 patients with angina pectoris had the smallest coronary arteries (mean cross-sectional area of each of the 60 arteries 6.0 mm²) and the 18 patients with healed myocardial infarcts with progressive and eventually fatal congestive heart failure had the "largest" coronary arteries (mean cross-sectional area of each of the 54 arteries 8.6 mm²). The 23 patients with acute myocardial infarcts and the 19 with sudden cardiac death had similar-sized coronary arteries (mean cross-sectional area of each of the 126 arteries 7.6 mm²) and the 18 patients with healed myocardial infarcts and subsequently asymptomatic courses and noncardiac causes of death had relatively small coronary arteries (mean cross-sectional area of each of the 54 arteries 6.9 mm²). The 31 control subjects with cancer had the smallest coronary arteries of any group (mean cross-sectional area of each of the 93 arteries 5.0 mm²) and the 15 patients with aortic valve disease had the largest coronary arteries (mean area of each of the 45 arteries 9.6 mm²) ($p < 0.0001$).

The differences in cross-sectional area of the coronary arteries among the subsets of 98 coronary patients and between and among the 46 control subjects is attributable primarily to differences in heart weight (tables 1–3). The coronary subgroup with angina pectoris had the smallest hearts (average 386 g); the subgroups, with healed myocardial infarction with chronic congestive cardiac failure, had the largest hearts (average 588 g). The other three groups were intermediate. The cancer control subjects, who had the smallest coronary arteries, had the smallest hearts

TABLE 2. *Relation of Mean Cross-sectional Area of the Right, Left Anterior Descending and Left Circumflex Coronary Arteries to the Heart Weight in the 98 Coronary Patients and in the 46 Control Subjects*

Parameter	Heart weight (gs)						Totals
	≤ 300	301–400	401–500	501–600	601–700	> 700	
Coronary patients							
1—No. patients	2	36	26	22	7	5	98
2—Age (years), range and mean	43–54 (49)	25–82 (52)	36–85 (58)	31–77 (59)	49–78 (61)	48–78 (61)	25–85 (56)
3—Male:female ratio	0:2	23:13	24:2	21:1	6:1	5:0	79:19
4—Heart weight (g), range and mean	240–300 (270)	310–400 (360)	420–500 (465)	510–600 (546)	610–670 (635)	720–800 (754)	240–800 (468)
5—Mean XSA (mm²) of R, LAD and LCCA, range and mean	3.2–5.6 (4.4)	2.7–10.6 (5.9)	4.4–14.9 (7.2)	5.6–13.3 (8.9)	6.2–13.4 (9.7)	5.7–12.8 (10.3)	2.7–14.9 (7.4)
Control subjects							
1—No. subjects	16	10	5	4	3	8	46
2—Age (years), range and mean	26–67 (47)	27–67 (52)	56–74 (64)	54–66 (61)	34–69 (56)	45–81 (54)	26–81 (53)
3—Male:female ratio	7:9	6:4	4:1	3:1	3:0	7:1	30:16
4—Heart weight (g), range and mean	135–300 (243)	310–400 (352)	410–470 (436)	550–600 (568)	620–700 (660)	720–1050 (838)	135–1050 (447)
5—Mean XSA (mm²) of R, LAD and LCCA, range and mean	2.0–6.3 (3.8)	3.0–9.1 (5.9)	5.8–9.0 (7.0)	7.1–10.4 (8.4)	7.7–8.8 (8.2)	8.2–14.9 (10.8)	2.0–14.9 (6.5)

Abbreviations: XSA = cross-sectional area; R = right coronary artery; LAD = left anterior descending coronary artery; LCCA = left circumflex coronary artery.

TABLE 3. *Relation of Mean Cross-sectional Area of the Right, Left Anterior Descending and Left Circumflex Coronary Arteries to Sex with Actual and Equalized Heart Weights in the 98 Coronary Patients and in the 46 Control Subjects*

	No. patients	Heart weight (g), range and mean	Mean XSA (mm²) of R, LAD, and LCCA, range and mean	Equalized mean heart weight	Mean XSA (mm²) for R, LAD and LCCA
			Coronary patients		
Men	79	310–800 (490)	2.7–14.9 (7.7)	450	7.1
Women	19	240–610 (376)	3.2–11.4 (5.9)	450	7.1
			Control subjects		
Men	30	200–1050 (509)	2.0–14.9 (7.7)	450	6.8
Women	16	135–750 (329)	2.0–8.6 (4.4)	450	6.0

Abbreviations: XSA = cross-sectional area; R = right coronary artery; LAD = left anterior descending coronary artery; LCCA = left circumflex coronary artery.

(average 309 g) and the aortic valve control subjects, who had the largest coronary arteries, had the largest hearts (average 730 g). When the heart weights for each of the seven groups (five subgroups of coronary patients and two control groups) were equalized by using the same regression coefficient, no significant differences ($p = 0.63$) were found among the mean values of cross-sectional area of the coronary arteries (table 3).

The mean values of cross-sectional areas of the coronary arteries in the women were significantly ($p < 0.0001$) different from the values in the men (mean cross-sectional area of each of the 19 women's 57 coronary arteries was 5.9 mm² [range 3.2–11.4 mm²] and of the 79 men's 237 arteries, 7.7 mm² [2.7–14.9 mm²]) (table 3). These mean differences, however, resulted from differences in heart weight. The heart weights of the 19 women ranged from 240–610 g (mean 376 g) and those of the 79 men, 310–800 g (mean 490 g). When the heart weights for the women and men with coronary heart disease were equalized by using the same regression equation, no significance differences in mean areas of the coronary arteries between the sexes was apparent (table 3). Similar findings regarding sex were observed in the control subjects (16 women and 30 men). Of the 31 cancer control subjects, 14 were women (mean coronary cross-sectional area 3.9 mm² and mean heart weight 280 g) and 17 were men (mean coronary cross-sectional area 6.0 mm² and mean heart weight 334 g); of the 15 aortic valve disease control subjects, two were women (mean coronary cross-sectional area 7.9 mm² and mean heart weight 675 g) and 13 were men (mean coronary cross-sectional area 9.9 mm² and mean heart weight 738 g).

Age had a small independent effect on the mean cross-sectional area of the coronary arteries in the study patients. The younger patients had smaller coronary arteries than the older patients. The mean cross-sectional area of the 33 coronary arteries in the 11 patients ages 40 years or younger was 5.7 mm²; in the 150 arteries in the 50 patients ages 41–60 years, the mean area was 6.8 mm², and in the 111 arteries of the 37 patients over 60 years of age, the mean area was 8.5 mm² ($p < 0.0001$) (table 4). Most of the difference in cross-sectional area among the age groups resulted from differences in heart weights. The younger patients had smaller hearts, on the average, than the older patients. The mean heart weight in the 11 patients ages 40 years and younger was 395 g; in the 50 patients ages 41–60 years, 456 g, and in the 37 patients older than 60 years, 506 g ($p < 0.0001$). When heart weight was equalized among the 98 coronary patients after dividing them into five age groups (≤ 40, 41–50, 51–60, 61–70 and > 70 years), the mean cross-sectional areas were significantly ($p > 0.001$) different except in the age groups 41–60 years (table 4). Thus, aging itself among the coronary patients increased the cross-sectional areas of the three major coronary arteries. The nature of selecting the control subjects, i.e., those with normal- or near-normal-sized hearts (cancer victims) and those with huge hearts (aortic valve disease victims), prevented adequate numbers of patients in each of the five age-group divisions to determine if age per se caused the coronary arteries of the control subjects to enlarge.

Discussion

Our findings indicate that there are significant differences in the mean cross-sectional areas of the three major coronary arteries in patients with various coronary events, but that these differences are nearly all accounted for by differences in heart weight and, to a slight extent, age. Thus, the size of the coronary artery (the area enclosed by the internal elastic membrane, irrespective of the degree of luminal narrowing by atherosclerotic plaque) is unimportant in determining whether a person develops evidence of myocardial ischemia. Although the area through which blood

TABLE 4. *Relation of Mean Cross-sectional Area of the Right, Left Anterior Descending and Left Circumflex Coronary Arteries to Age in the 98 Coronary Patients and in the 46 Control Subjects*

Parameter	Age (years)					Totals
	≤ 40	41–50	51–60	61–70	> 70	
Coronary patients						
1—No. patients	11	25	25	23	14	98
2—Age (years), range and mean	25–40 (35)	41–50 (47)	51–60 (55)	61–70 (65)	72–85 (78)	25–85 (56)
3—Heart weight (g) range and mean	340–520 (392)	240–750 (480)	300–720 (433)	310–800 (503)	330–770 (510)	240–800 (468)
4—Mean XSA of R, LAD and LCCA, range and mean	2.7–10.6 (5.7)	3.2–13.1 (7.1)	4.2–13.3 (6.6)	3.3–13.4 (8.1)	5.0–14.9 (9.2)	2.7–14.9 (7.4)
Control subjects						
1—No. patients	7	13	10	14	2	46
2—Age (years), range and mean	22–39 (32)	42–50 (46)	51–60 (56)	61–69 (65)	74–81 (78)	26–81 (53)
3—Heart weight (g), range and mean	135–700 (306)	230–810 (405)	250–1050 (633)	210–660 (401)	410–770 (590)	135–1050 (447)
4—Mean XSA of R, LAD and LCCA, range and mean	2.0–8.8 (4.5)	2.1–14.9 (5.8)	5.0–14.6 (8.3)	3.5–10.5 (6.6)	9.0–9.3 (9.2)	2.0–14.9 (6.5)

Abbreviations: XSA = cross-sectional area; R = right coronary artery; LAD = left anterior descending coronary artery; LCCA = left circumflex coronary artery.

might flow in a large artery narrowed greater than 75% in cross-sectional area by atherosclerotic plaque is greater than that of a small artery with a similar degree of cross-sectional area narrowing, the larger artery is large because the myocardial mass that it must perfuse is large and vice versa. Consequently, a 75% cross-sectional area narrowing in a large coronary artery has the same effect on myocardial perfusion as a similar degree of narrowing in a small coronary artery. The patients with angina pectoris had the smallest coronary arteries because they had the smallest hearts. The patients with healed myocardial infarcts who are left with chronic congestive heart failure that becomes intractable and fatal had the largest coronary arteries because they had the largest hearts. However, patients with healed myocardial infarcts who recovered completely, never had further evidence of myocardial ischemia, and died from noncardiac causes tended to have relatively small hearts (just larger, on the average, than those of the pure angina pectoris group) and, therefore, relatively small coronary arteries. The patients with sudden coronary death and those with acute myocardial infarcts had similar-sized hearts, and, therefore, similar-sized coronary arteries. Previous findings revealed similar degrees of cross-sectional narrowing throughout the entire lengths of the coronary arteries in patients with sudden coronary death and acute myocardial infarction.[3,5] In both groups, 35% of the four major coronary arteries were narrowed greater than 75% in cross-sectional area. Also of note is the previous observation[4] that the angina patients had the most severe degrees of cross-sectional area narrowing (48% of their four major coronary arteries were narrowed

more than 75% in cross-sectional area) and the patients with healed myocardial infarcts irrespective of whether or not they died from cardiac or noncardiac causes had the least degree of severe cross-sectional area narrowing (30% of their major coronary arteries were greater than 75% narrowed in cross-sectional area by atherosclerotic plaque).[6,7]

This study also demonstrated that sex did not have an independent effect on the size of the coronary arteries. Women, on the average, however, had smaller coronary arteries than men, but this difference is entirely accountable for by differences in heart weight. This sex difference in heart size might explain why the early mortality after aortocoronary bypass operations, as reported by Hall and associates,[9] is higher in women than in men. Women have smaller hearts, on the average, than men, and most of the bypass operations are performed for angina, which in itself is associated on the average with the smallest hearts of any of the various coronary events. The combination of pure angina and womanhood, in general, makes for relatively small hearts and, therefore, relatively small coronary arteries. The smaller the coronary artery, the greater the difficulty in inserting a conduit and the greater the likelihood after the coronary anastomosis that the runoff via the conduit into the native coronary artery will not be good. When coronary bypass fails to result in an adequate increase in myocardial oxygenation, the greater the likelihood of early death.[10,11]

Age affected the cross-sectional area of the coronary arteries. This observation may suggest that it takes less cross-sectional area narrowing in younger persons to produce myocardial ischemia than it does in older persons, heart weight and other factors being equal. Elderly persons are known to have larger and more tortuous coronary arteries than younger adults. This "senile dilatation" comes about through both transverse widening and longitudinal lengthening. The present study indicates that this so-called senile dilatation, which occurs as a more-or-less normal event in insignificantly narrowed coronary arteries, also occurs, but probably to a lesser extent, in coronary arteries that are significantly narrowed by atherosclerotic plaques. Because arteries tend to be larger in older adults than in younger adults, coronary bypass anastomoses may be more readily accomplished in the old than in the young. From a technical standpoint, the young woman with pure angina pectoris may be at a greater risk of early mortality or lesser improvement than the elderly woman with similar symptoms and a similar-sized heart.

Acknowledgment

We thank Margaret C. Wu, Ph.D., Biometrics Branch, National Heart, Lung, and Blood Institute, National Institutes of Health, for providing the statistical analyses of the data presented.

References

1. Roberts WC, Buja LM: The frequency and significance of coronary arterial thrombi and other observations in fatal myocardial infarction. A study of 107 necropsy patients. Am J Med 52: 425, 1972
2. Roberts WC: The coronary arteries and left ventricle in clinically isolated angina pectoris. Circulation 54: 388, 1976
3. Roberts WC, Jones AA: Quantitation of coronary arterial narrowing at necropsy in sudden coronary death. Analysis of 31 patients and comparison with 25 control subjects. Am J Cardiol 44: 39, 1979
4. Roberts WC, Virmani R: Quantitation of coronary arterial narrowing in clinically isolated unstable angina pectoris. An analysis of 22 necropsy patients. Am J Med 67: 792, 1979
5. Roberts WC, Jones AA: Quantification of coronary arterial narrowing at necropsy in acute transmural myocardial infarction. Analysis and comparison of findings in 27 patients and 22 controls. Circulation 61: 786, 1980
6. Virmani R, Roberts WC: Quantification of coronary arterial narrowing and of left ventricular myocardial scarring in healed myocardial infarction with chronic eventually fatal, congestive cardiac failure. Am J Med 68: 831, 1980
7. Virmani R, Roberts WC: Non-fatal healed transmural myocardial infarction and fatal non-cardiac disease. Qualification and quantification of coronary arterial narrowing and of left ventricular scarring in 18 necropsy patients. Br Heart J. In press
8. Dvorak JA, Schuette WH, Whitehouse WC: A simple video method for the quantification of microscopic objects. J Microscopy 102: 71, 1974
9. Hall RJ, Garcia E, Wukasch DC, Hallman GL, Cooley DA: Aortocoronary bypass (CAB): long-term follow-up. (abstr) Circulation 52 (suppl II): II-90, 1975
10. Spray TL, Roberts WC: Status of the grafts and the native coronary arteries proximal and distal to coronary anastomotic sites of aortocoronary bypass grafts. Circulation 55: 741, 1977
11. Spray TL, Roberts WC: Changes in saphenous veins used as aortocoronary bypass grafts. Am Heart J 94: 500, 1977

Amount of Narrowing by Atherosclerotic Plaque in 44 Nonbypassed and 52 Bypassed Major Epicardial Coronary Arteries in 32 Necropsy Patients Who Died Within 1 Month of Aortocoronary Bypass Grafting

BRUCE F. WALLER, MD
WILLIAM C. ROBERTS, MD, FACC

Bethesda, Maryland

In 32 necropsy patients who died within 30 days of an aortocoronary bypass operation performed for relief of angina pectoris, the lumens in 42 (95 percent) of 44 nonbypassed and in 52 (100 percent) of 52 bypassed arteries were narrowed 76 to 100 percent in cross-sectional area by atherosclerotic plaque. Of 616 five mm segments of the 44 nonbypassed arteries examined histologically, 292 (47 percent) were narrowed 76 to 100 percent in cross-sectional area by atherosclerotic plaque; of 728 segments examined in the 52 bypassed arteries, 375 (52 percent) were similarly narrowed. Thirty-two (73 percent) of the 44 nonbypassed coronary arteries (in 23 patients) had been judged to be narrowed 50 percent or less in diameter on preoperative coronary angiography, but at necropsy 31 (97 percent) of these arteries were narrowed 76 to 100 percent in cross-sectional area and the other artery was narrowed 51 to 75 percent. Thus, significant amounts of atherosclerotic plaque tend to be present at necropsy in all three major coronary systems of patients with angina pectoris who die early after an aortocoronary bypass operation.

In patients undergoing aortocoronary bypass operations, one, two or three or more bypass conduits are inserted. The decision to bypass one major coronary artery and not another is usually determined by the degree and location of the narrowing or the size of the coronary artery on preoperative angiography. The accuracy of angiographic judgment or the status of the nonbypassed coronary artery has, to our knowledge, not been evaluated at necropsy in patients who died early after aortocoronary bypass operations. Thus, 44 nonbypassed coronary arteries were examined in 32 necropsy patients who died within 30 days of an aortocoronary bypass operation carried out for relief of angina pectoris, and the observations on the nonbypassed arteries were compared with those on the bypassed arteries.

Methods

Study patients: In the Pathology Branch of the National Heart, Lung, and Blood Institute, from 1972 through July 1979, we examined at necropsy the hearts of 117 patients who died after aortocoronary bypass procedures; 75 patients (64 percent) died within 60 days of the operation and 42 (36 percent) died later. Of the 75 patients who died within 60 days of operation, 43 (57 percent) had three or more aortocoronary bypass conduits inserted. The remaining 32 patients, all of whom died within 30 days of the bypass operation, had one (13 patients) or two (19 patients) bypass conduits inserted. This paper concerns only the latter 32 patients, whose ages ranged from 34 to 70 years (mean 55); 22 were men and 10 were women. All 32 patients had angina pectoris preoperatively, which was stable in 6 (19 percent) and unstable in 26 (81 percent). (Unstable angina pectoris was defined as anterior thoracic pain of recent onset [less than 1 month before clinical evaluation] or a recent change in the pattern of the pain

From the Pathology Branch, National Heart, Lung, and Blood Institute, National Institutes of Health, Bethesda, Maryland. Manuscript received November 26, 1979; revised manuscript received June 24, 1980, accepted June 27, 1980.

Address for reprints: William C. Roberts, MD, Building 10A, Room 3E30, National Heart, Lung, and Blood Institute, National Institutes of Health, Bethesda, Maryland 20205.

in terms of frequency, severity, intensity and ease of provocation. Nocturnal angina or angina at rest or prolonged angina within 3 months of death was considered unstable.)

In addition to coronary heart disease, six patients (all with stable angina pectoris) also had valvular heart disease: isolated aortic-valve stenosis in two, isolated mitral stenosis in one, pure mitral regurgitation secondary to papillary muscle dysfunction in one and combined aortic and mitral stenosis in two. These six patients also had replacement of the mitral or aortic valve, or both, with a prosthesis in addition to the aortocoronary bypass procedure. In these six patients with associated valvular heart disease, 12 of the 18 major coronary arteries received a bypass conduit, or one major coronary artery was not bypassed in each. Excluding the 6 patients with associated valvular heart disease, none of the other 26 patients had had clinical evidence of congestive cardiac failure and none of the total 32 patients had had a clinical event compatible with acute myocardial infarction. However, at necropsy 4 of the 32 patients had one or more transmural left ventricular scars, and 7 other patients had relatively small subendocardial foci of left ventricular necrosis.

Eighteen of the 32 patients died in the operating room because of inability to be separated from cardiopulmonary bypass. The remaining 14 patients died after varying periods of shock (low cardiac output syndrome). The interval from the end of the operation to death in these 14 patients ranged from 2 hours to 24 days; in 4 patients, 12 hours or less; in 3 patients, from 16 to 24 hours; in 4 patients, from 2 to 4 days; and in 3 patients, from 6, 14 and 24 days, respectively. None of the 18 patients who died in the operating room had left ventricular myocardial necrosis detected histologically at necropsy. Of the remaining 14 patients who died later, 4 had one or more foci of left ventricular myocardial necrosis (that is, acute myocardial infarction) at necropsy.

Examination of coronary arteries: This report focuses on the status of the 44 major nonbypassed and the 52 bypassed epicardial coronary arteries in the 32 patients. The major arteries analyzed were the right, left anterior descending and left circumflex (Table I). However, if a conduit had been

TABLE I

Summary of Coronary Arterial Findings in 32 Patients With Angina Pectoris Who Died Within 30 Days of Aortocoronary Bypass

Nonbypassed coronary arteries		
Left anterior descending (LAD) only	1	20 patients
Left circumflex (LCx) only	9	(single artery)
Right (RCA) only	10	
LAD and LCx	2	12 patients
LAD and RCA	1	(two arteries)
LCx and RCA	9	
Nonbypassed coronary arteries and (number of arteries) narrowed more than 75% in cross-sectional area by atherosclerotic plaque		
LAD	4 (4)	44 arteries
LCx	20 (19)	(42 > 75%)
RCA	20 (19)	
Number of 5 mm segments in 44 nonbypassed coronary arteries and (number of arteries) [%] narrowed more than 75% in cross-sectional area by atherosclerotic plaque	616 (292) [47%]	
Bypassed coronary arteries		
LAD only	9	12 patients
LCx only	1	(single artery)
RCA only	2	
LAD and LCx	10	20 patients
LAD and RCA	9	(two arteries)
LCx and RCA	1	
Bypassed coronary artery and number of arteries narrowed more than 75% in cross-sectional area by atherosclerotic plaque		
LAD	28 (28)	52 arteries
LCx	12 (12)	(52 > 75%)
RCA	12 (12)	
Total number of 5 mm segments in 52 bypassed coronary arteries and (number of arteries) [%] narrowed more than 75% in cross-sectional area by atherosclerotic plaque	728 (375) [52%]	

TABLE II

Angiographic and Histologic Comparison of Amount of Coronary Arterial Narrowing by Atherosclerotic Plaque in 32 of 44 Nonbypassed Major Epicardial Coronary Arteries With Less Than 50 percent Diameter Reduction on Preoperative Angiography

Histologic Finding at Necropsy	Preoperative Angiographic Narrowing (diameter reduction)		
	0–30%	31–50%	Total
LAD			
Number of arteries	1	2	3
Number narrowed >75% *	1	2	3
Number of 5 mm segments	14	29	43
Number (%) narrowed >75% *	6 (43)	13 (45)	19 (44)
LCx			
Number of arteries	1	14	15
Number narrowed >75% *	1	14	15
Number of 5 mm segments	5	133	138
Number (%) narrowed >75% *	1 (20)	65 (49)	66 (48)
RCA			
Number of arteries	2	12	14
Number narrowed >75% *	2	11	13
Number of 5 mm segments	46	216	262
Number (%) narrowed >75% *	20 (43)	106 (49)	126 (48)
Totals			
Number of arteries	4	28	32
Number (%) narrowed >75% *	4 (100)	27 (96)	31 (97)
Number of 5 mm segments	65	378	443
Number (%) narrowed >75% *	27 (42)	184 (49)	211 (48)

* Cross-sectional area.

placed to the left obtuse marginal coronary artery, the left circumflex system then was considered to have been bypassed. If neither the left obtuse marginal nor the left circumflex coronary artery had been bypassed, only the status of the left circumflex artery was included in our analysis. Of the 44 nonbypassed coronary arteries, preoperative coronary angiograms showed some degree of narrowing in 43: diameter reduction 10 to 30 percent in 3 arteries, 31 to 50 percent in 28 arteries, 51 to 75 percent in 1 artery and 76 to 100 percent in 11 arteries (Table II). In the latter 12 arteries, either coronary bypass grafting had not been planned (six cases) or at operation the artery was not found or was deemed too small to bypass (six cases). In all 52 bypassed coronary arteries, preoperative selective angiograms disclosed greater than 50 percent narrowing in diameter.

The nonbypassed and bypassed coronary arteries were examined at necropsy in similar fashion. Each artery was excised intact from the heart and subjected to X-ray examination. If calcific deposits were present radiographically the artery was decalcified. The arteries were then cut transversely to the longitudinal axes into 5 mm long segments. The 5 mm segments were labeled, dehydrated and embedded in paraffin; several histologic sections were cut and one was stained by the Movat method and examined. All determinations of luminal narrowing were based on examination of the Movat-stained sections because this stain clearly outlines the artery's internal elastic membrane. The degree of narrowing was based on histologic examination of each cross section magnified 25 to 50 times. The judgment regarding the degree of luminal narrowing of each 5 mm segment was based on the degree of luminal obliteration within the luminal circle bordered by the internal elastic membrane. This method has been demonstrated[1] to be almost as accurate as videoplanimetry and the intra- and interobserver errors to be less than 5 percent. The percent cross-sectional area luminal narrowing by atherosclerotic plaque in each 5 mm segment was determined as follows: 0 to 25, 26 to 50, 51 to 75, 76 to 95 and 96 to 100. In arteries with eccentric lumens and walls indented artifactually

into them, the judgment of degrees of narrowing at necropsy was determined only after visual expansion of the collapsed portion of wall.

Results

Nonbypassed versus bypassed coronary arteries: At necropsy, the lumens in 42 (95 percent) of the 44 nonbypassed coronary arteries and the lumens in all 52 bypassed coronary arteries were narrowed 76 to 100 percent in cross-sectional area by atherosclerotic plaques (Table I). (A 75 percent narrowing of cross-sectional area [necropsy] is equivalent to a 50 percent reduction in diameter [angiogram].[2]) The results of the examination of each 5 mm long segment of the 44 nonbypassed and the 52 bypassed coronary arteries are summarized in Table III and in Figure 1. Of the 616 five mm segments in the 44 nonbypassed arteries, 292 (47 percent) were narrowed 76 to 100 percent in cross-sectional area by atherosclerotic plaque; 143 (23 percent) were narrowed, 51 to 75 percent; 109 (18 percent) were narrowed 26 to 50 percent; and 72 (12 percent) were narrowed 0 to 25 percent. Of the 728 five mm segments in the 52 bypassed arteries 375 (52 percent) were narrowed 76 to 100 percent in cross-sectional area by atherosclerotic plaques; 215 (29 percent) were narrowed 51 to 75 percent; 123 (17 percent) were narrowed 26 to 50 percent, and 15 (2 percent) were narrowed 0 to 25 percent. The amount of severe (more than 75 percent cross-sectional area) narrowing by atherosclerotic plaques in the proximal and distal halves of the nonbypassed and bypassed left anterior descending and right coronary arteries was similar (Fig. 2). The proximal half of the nonbypassed left circumflex coronary artery had a higher proportion of 5 mm segments narrowed 76 to 100 percent than did the distal half of this

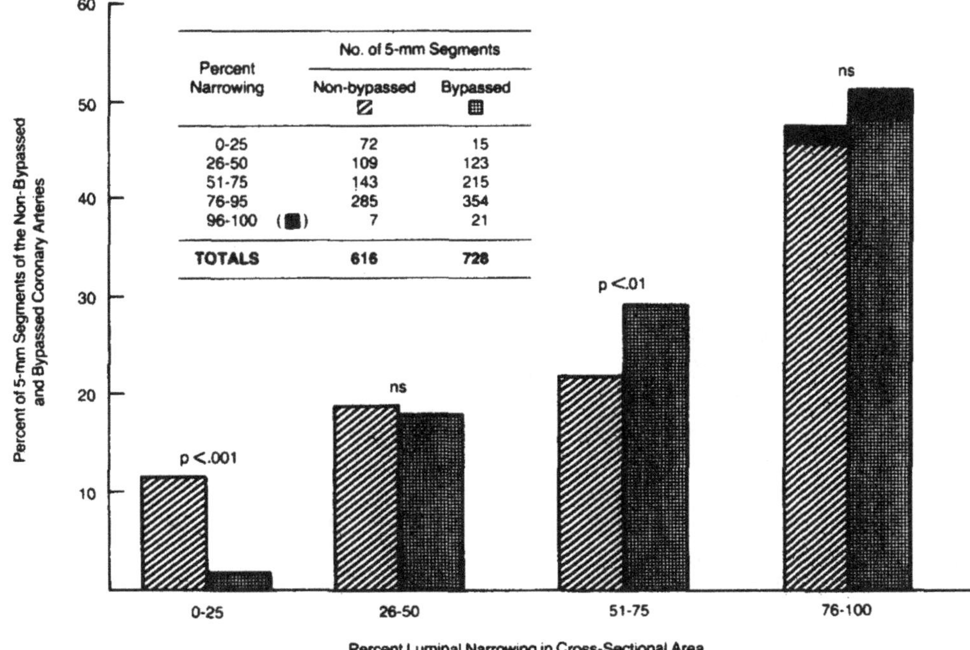

Percent Narrowing	No. of 5-mm Segments	
	Non-bypassed	Bypassed
0-25	72	15
26-50	109	123
51-75	143	215
76-95	285	354
96-100	7	21
TOTALS	**616**	**728**

FIGURE 1. Bar graph showing percent of 5 mm segments of 44 nonbypassed and 52 bypassed major epicardial coronary arteries narrowed to various degrees in 32 necropsy patients with angina pectoris who died within 30 days of an aortocoronary bypass operation.

Number and Percent of 5 mm Segments of 44 Nonbypassed (N) and 52 Bypassed (B) Major Epicardial Coronary Arteries and Grade of Cross-Sectional Area Luminal Narrowing

Coronary Artery	Percent Cross-Sectional Area Luminal Narrowing											
	0–25		26–50		51–75		76–95		96–100		Total	
	N	B	N	B	N	B	N	B	N	B	N	B
LAD												
n	6	12	6	72	16	117	25	195	2	8	55	404
%	(11)	(3)	(11)	(18)	(29)	(29)	(45)	(48)	(4)	(2)	(100)	(100)
LCx												
n	28	2	34	28	41	40	95	63	2	4	200	137
%	(14)	(2)	(17)	(20)	(21)	(29)	(47)	(46)	(1)	(3)	(100)	(100)
RCA												
n	38	1	69	23	86	58	165	96	3	9	361	187
%	(11)	(1)	(18)	(12)	(24)	(31)	(46)	(51)	(2)	(5)	(100)	(100)
Total	72	15	109	123	143	215	285	354	7	21	616	728
	(12)[†]	(2)[†]	(18)	(17)	(23)*	(29)*	(46)	(49)	(1)	(3)	(100)	(100)

* $p < 0.01$. [†] $p < 0.001$.
LAD = left anterior descending, LCx = left circumflex, RCA = right coronary artery.

artery but the proportions were similar in the bypassed artery.

Preoperative coronary angiographic versus autopsy findings: Of the 32 nonbypassed coronary arteries (in 23 patients) judged to have a diameter reduction of 50 percent or less on preoperative coronary angiography, at necropsy 31 (97 percent) were narrowed 76 to 100 percent in cross-sectional area by atherosclerotic plaque (211 [48 percent] of 443 five mm segments) and 1 (3 percent) was narrowed 51 to 75 percent in cross-sectional area (Table II). Figures 3 and 4 show, respec-

tively, a cross section from each 5 mm segment of the right coronary artery and the angiogram of this artery in 1 of the 23 patients with one or more major coronary arteries that were not bypassed because of insignificant reduction in diameter. Of the 12 nonbypassed coronary arteries (in nine patients) judged to be either "severely narrowed" or "too small to bypass" on preoperative coronary angiography, at necropsy 11 were narrowed 76 to 100 percent in cross-sectional area by atherosclerotic plaque (81 [47 percent] of 173 five mm segments) and 1 was narrowed 51 to 75 percent.

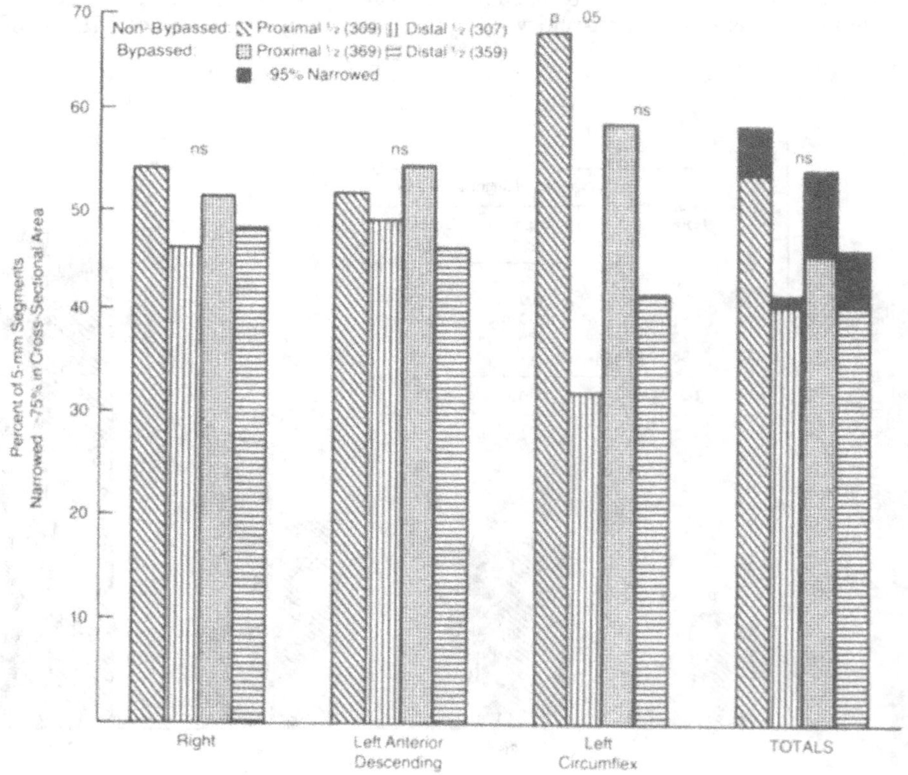

FIGURE 2. Bar graph showing percent of 5 mm segments of the proximal and distal halves of the 44 nonbypassed and 52 bypassed major epicardial coronary arteries narrowed more than 75 percent in cross-sectional area by atherosclerotic plaque in 32 necropsy patients who died within 30 days of aortocoronary bypass grafting.

Comments

Autopsy findings in fatal coronary artery disease:
This study demonstrates that our necropsy patients with angina pectoris who died soon after aortocoronary bypass operations had *diffuse* coronary atherosclerosis and that their preoperative angiograms frequently underestimated the severity of the coronary narrowing.

Other studies from this laboratory and elsewhere have also shown that among patients with fatal coronary heart disease (irrespective of the type of coronary event), coronary atherosclerosis in the major epicardial coronary arteries is diffuse and severe and that it is unusual to find a normal 5 mm long segment in any of the three major (right, left anterior descending and left

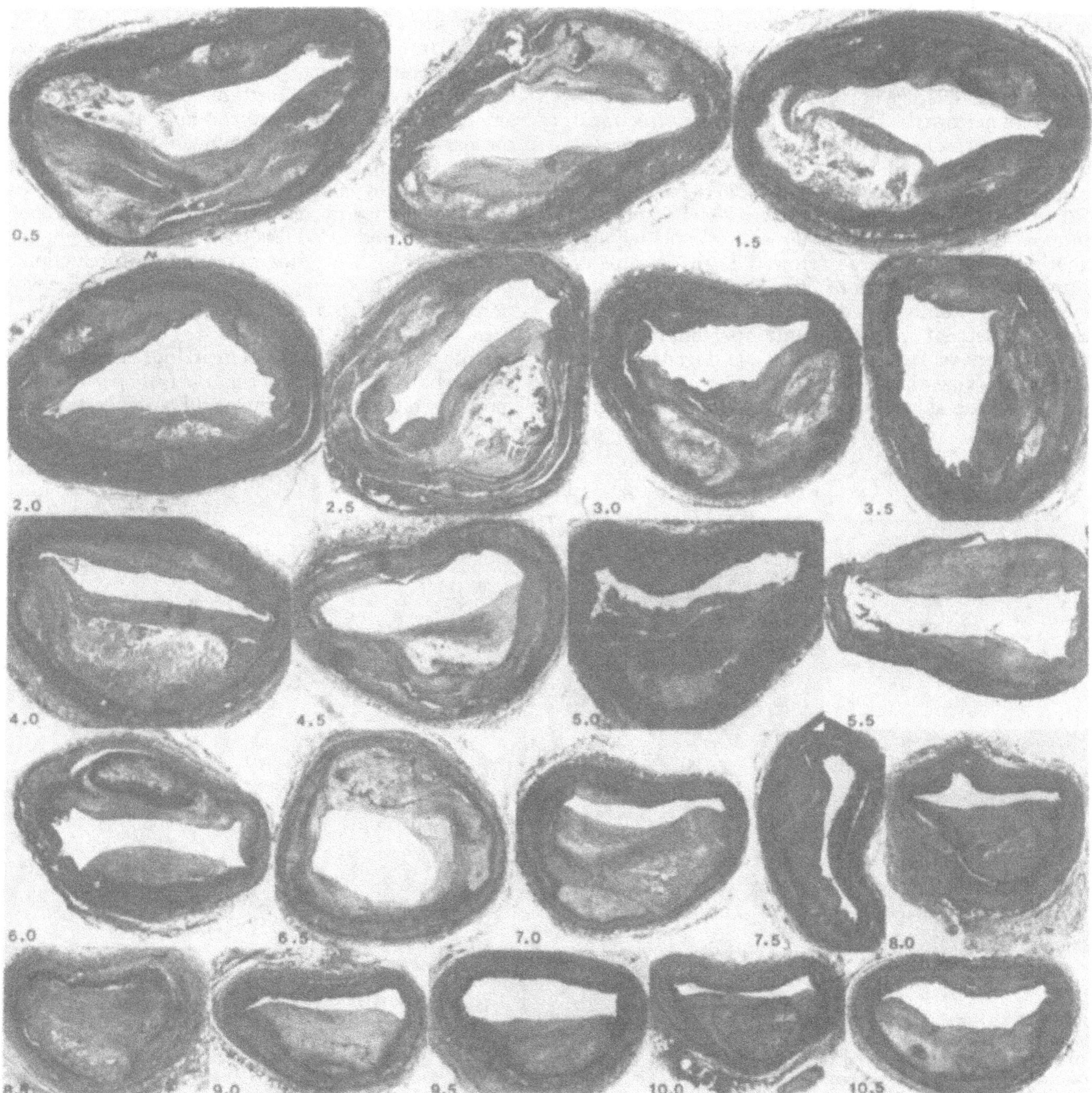

FIGURE 3. Cross-sections from each of 21 five mm segments of the right coronary artery in 1 of the 32 patients in whom one or more major coronary arteries were not bypassed because the preoperative angiogram indicated 50 percent or less diameter reduction. The histologic sections begin with the first 5 mm segment of the right coronary artery (0.5 cm) and extend to the origin of the posterior descending branch (10.5 cm). The amount narrowing of cross-sectional area of the lumen by atherosclerotic plaque (determined with videoplanimetry) in these 21 histologic sections was as follows: 76 to 100 percent in 10 (48 percent), 51 to 75 percent in 6 (28 percent) and 50 percent or less in 5 (24 percent).

circumflex) coronary arteries.[3–8] Among necropsy patients studied in our laboratory with unstable angina pectoris,[4] acute myocardial infarction,[5] sudden coronary death[6] and healed myocardial infarction with either cardiac[7] or noncardiac[8] death, the lumens of at least 30 percent of the three major coronary arteries were narrowed 76 to 100 percent in cross-sectional area by atherosclerotic plaque and about 70 percent of the lengths of these three arteries were narrowed more than 50 percent in cross-sectional area. Additionally, the lumens in only about 10 percent of the lengths of these three arteries were narrowed 25 percent or less in cross-sectional area. Among the 44 nonbypassed coronary arteries in our 32 patients, 292 (47 percent) of 616 five mm segments (an average of 20/artery) of nonbypassed artery were narrowed 76 to 100 percent in cross-sectional area by atherosclerotic plaque and another 23 percent were narrowed 51 to 75 percent. Of the 52 bypassed coronary arteries in our 32 patients, 375 (52 percent) of 728 five mm segments were narrowed 76 to 100 percent in cross-sectional area by atherosclerotic plaque and another 29 percent were narrowed 51 to 75 percent. Furthermore, only 12 percent of the 5 mm long segments of the nonbypassed coronary arteries were narrowed 25 percent or less, and only 2 percent of the bypassed arteries were so narrowed. Thus, the odds appear to favor the view that all three major coronary arteries will be considerably narrowed in necropsy patients with angina pectoris who died early after an aortocoronary bypass operation.

Coronary angiographic versus autopsy findings: Several studies among patients with symptomatic coronary heart disease have emphasized that coronary angiograms tend to underestimate the amount of coronary luminal narrowing. Among 61 coronary arteries examined with angiography during life and subsequently at necropsy in our laboratory,[2] in 17 (40 percent) of the 42 vessels narrowed 76 to 100 percent in cross-sectional area at necropsy, the narrowing was underestimated by two or three angiographers; and in 7 of 8 arteries narrowed 51 to 75 percent in cross-sectional area at necropsy, the narrowing was underestimated by one or more of the three angiographers. Thus, among patients with severe coronary atherosclerosis, coronary angiography tends to underestimate the actual degrees of luminal narrowing. Among 32 (76 percent) of the 44 nonbypassed coronary arteries (from 23 patients) described in this study, preoperative coronary angiography indicated less than 50 percent reduction in diameter in 21 arteries and 50 percent reduction in 11. However, at necropsy 31 of these 32 arteries were narrowed more than 75 percent in cross-sectional area.

Role of coronary bypass grafting: Several clinical studies have demonstrated that the early postoperative mortality rates and the frequency of postoperative acute

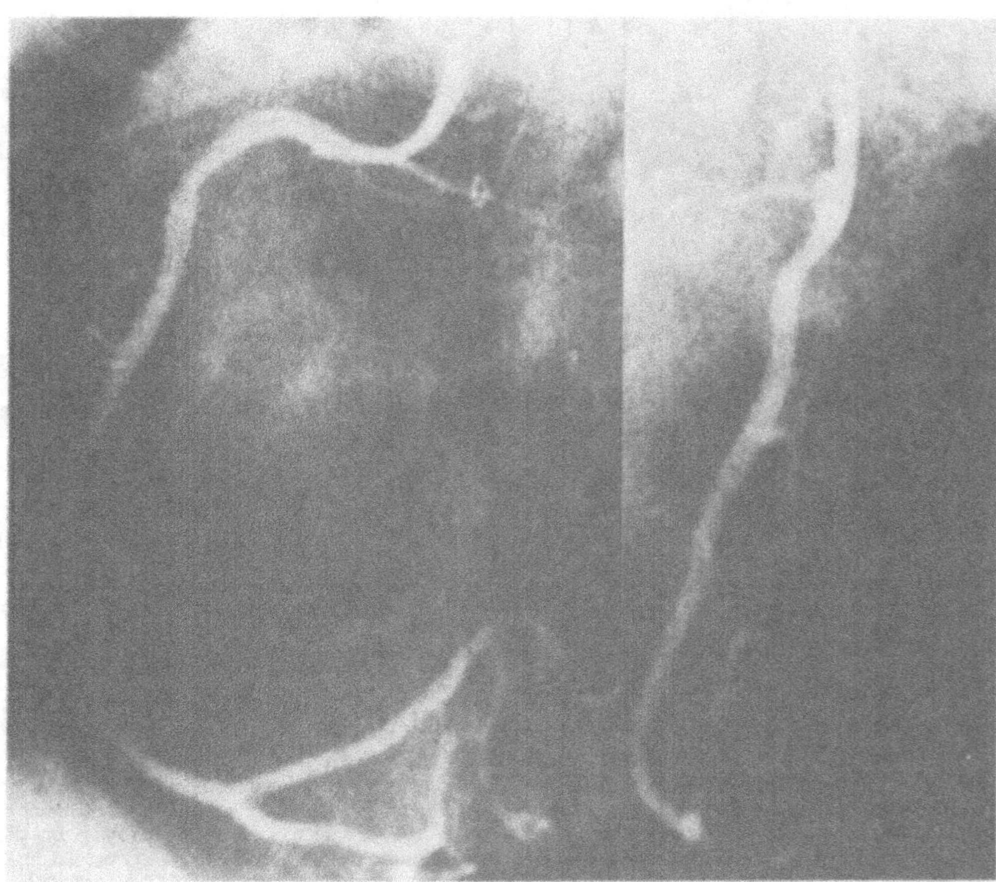

FIGURE 4. Same patient. Two views of the preoperative selective coronary arteriogram of the right coronary artery in the patient whose right coronary artery is shown histologically in Figure 3. The maximal diameter reduction in both right (**right**) and left (**left**) anterior oblique views was judged to be between 40 and 50 percent.

myocardial infarction are lower, and the frequency of disappearance of angina pectoris and improvement in exercise tolerance are greater in patients having three or more aortocoronary grafts than in those with two grafts and less in patients having two grafts than in those having only one. Stiles et al.[9] found the combined immediate and 6 month mortality rate to be 4 percent in 445 patients receiving three grafts, 9 percent in the 416 patients receiving two grafts and 21 percent in the 85 patients receiving a single graft. Sheldon et al.[10] observed clinical evidence of acute myocardial infarction early postoperatively in only 6 (3 percent) of 187 patients having multiple grafts and in 49 (17 percent) of 286 patients having a single graft. Of 58 patients followed up 13 to 36 months by Assad-Morell et al.,[11] 21 (80 percent) of 26 receiving three or more grafts had no angina pectoris compared with 12 (63 percent) of 19 patients receiving two grafts and only two (16 percent) of 13 patients with a single graft. Sheldon et al.[10] reported similar results. Consequently, the frequency of a second coronary bypass operation for recurrence of

angina pectoris also is much greater in patients having one or two grafts inserted in the first aortocoronary bypass procedure compared with those having three or more grafts inserted in the first operation.[12–17] Assad-Morell et al.[11] found "positive" ischemic exercise responses with the exercise (stress) treadmill test in only 2 (9 percent) of 23 patients with three or more grafts, in 23 (70 percent) of 30 patients with two grafts and in 23 (96 percent) of 24 patients with only one graft.

Finally, progression of the atherosclerotic process in nonbypassed coronary arteries appears to be the major cause of recurrence of myocardial ischemia late after aortocoronary bypass operation. Seides et al.[18] restudied 22 patients 53 to 84 months after aortocoronary bypass grafting who had had at least one graft patent 3 to 9 months after the bypass operation. At the late study, 31 of 33 grafts were patent, but angina pectoris had reappeared in 11 of 16 patients who had become asymptomatic early after operation. Progression of narrowing in ungrafted coronary arteries accounted for the clinical deterioration in 9 of these 11 patients.

References

1. **Isner JM, Wu M, Virmani R, Jones A, Roberts WC.** Comparison of degrees of coronary arterial luminal narrowing determined by visual inspection of histologic sections under magnification among independent observers and comparison to that obtained by videoplanimetry: an analysis of 559 five-mm segments of 61 coronary arteries from eleven patients. Lab Invest 1980;42:566–70.

2. **Arnett EN, Isner JM, Redwood DR, et al.** Coronary artery narrowing in coronary heart disease: comparison of cineangiographic and necropsy findings. Ann Intern Med 1979;91:350–6.

3. **Roberts WC, Buja LM.** The frequency and significance of coronary arterial thrombi and other observations in fatal acute myocardial infarction. A study of 107 necropsy patients. Am J Med 1972;52:425–43.

4. **Roberts WC, Virmani R.** Quantification of coronary arterial narrowing in clinically-isolated unstable angina pectoris. An analysis of 22 necropsy patients. Am J Med 1979;67:792–8.

5. **Roberts WC, Jones AA.** Quantitation of coronary arterial narrowing at necropsy in acute transmural myocardial infarction: analysis and comparison of findings in 27 patients and 22 control. Circulation 1980;61:789–90.

6. **Roberts WC, Jones AA.** Quantitation of coronary arterial narrowing at necropsy in sudden coronary death: an analysis of 31 patients and comparison of findings to those in 25 control subjects. Am J Cardiol 1979;44:39–45.

7. **Virmani R, Roberts WC.** Quantification of coronary arterial narrowing and of left ventricular myocardial scarring in healed myocardial infarction with chronic, eventually fatal, congestive heart failure. Am J Med 1980;68:831–8.

8. **Virmani R, Roberts WC.** Non-fatal healed myocardial infarction and fatal non-cardiac disease: qualification and quantification of coronary arterial narrowing and of left ventricular scarring in 18 necropsy patients. Br Heart J, in press.

9. **Stiles QR, Lindesmith GG, Tucker BL, Hughes RK, Meyer BW.** Long-term follow-up of patients with coronary artery bypass grafts. Circulation 1976;54:Suppl III:III-33–4.

10. **Sheldon WC, Rincon G, Pichard AD, Razavi M, Cheanvechai C, Loop FD.** Surgical treatment of coronary artery disease: pure graft operations, with a study of 741 patients followed 3–7 years. Prog Cardiovasc Dis 1975;18:237–53.

11. **Assad-Morell JL, Frye RL, Connolly DC, et al.** Aorto-coronary artery saphenous vein bypass surgery. Clinical and angiographic results. Mayo Clin Proc 1975;50:379–86.

12. **Stiles QR.** Reoperation for myocardial revascularization. Cleve Clin Q 1978;45:136–8.

13. **Johnson WD, Hoffman JF Jr, Flemma RJ, Tector AJ.** Secondary surgical procedure for myocardial revascularization. J Thorac Cardiovasc Surg 1972;64:524–9.

14. **Thomas CS, Alford WC, Burrus GR, Frist RA, Stoney WS.** Results of reoperation for failed aortocoronary bypass grafts. Arch Surg 1976;111:1210–3.

15. **Irarrazaval MJ, Cosgrove DM, Loop FD, Ennix CL Jr, Groves LK, Taylor PC.** Reoperation for myocardial revascularization. J Thorac Cardiovasc Surg 1977;73:181–8.

16. **Winkle RA, Alderman EL, Shumway NE, Harrison DC.** Results of reoperation for unsuccessful coronary artery bypass surgery (abstr). Circulation 1975;51:Suppl I:I-62.

17. **Culliford AT, Girdwood MD, Isom OW, Krauss KR, Spencer FC.** Angina following myocardial revascularization. Does time of recurrence predict etiology and influence results of operation? J Thorac Cardiovasc Surg 1979;77:889–95.

18. **Seides SF, Borer JS, Kent KM, Rosing DR, McIntosh CL, Epstein SE.** Long-term anatomic fate of coronary-artery bypass grafts and functional status of patients five years after operation. N Engl J Med 1978;298:1213–7.

Quantification of amounts of coronary arterial narrowing in patients with types II and IV hyperlipoproteinemia and in those with known normal lipoprotein patterns

The amount of cross-sectional area narrowing by atherosclerotic plaques in each 5 mm long segment of the left main, left anterior descending, left circumflex, and right coronary arteries was analyzed at necropsy in 15 patients with type II hyperlipoproteinemia (HLP), in 13 with type IV HLP, and in 10 with known normal lipoprotein patterns. All 38 study patients had clinical evidence of coronary heart disease. Of the 2593 five mm segments examined histologically, narrowing of 76% to 100% in cross-sectional area by atherosclerotic plaques was as follows: type II = 39%, type IV = 67%, and normal lipoprotein pattern = 35% (controls = 4%). Utilizing a scoring system of 1 to 4 for the four categories of narrowing (0% to 25%, 26% to 50%, 51% to 75%, 76% to 100%), the mean score per 5 mm segment for the patients with type IV HLP was significantly higher (3.5) than that for the patients with type II HLP (3.0), normal lipoprotein patterns (3.0), and the controls (2.3). Thus, our patients with type II HLP and those with normal lipoprotein patterns had similar amounts of severe coronary narrowing and significantly less severe coronary narrowing than the patients with type IV HLP. (AM HEART J 101:52,1981.)

Henry Scott Cabin, M.D., and William C. Roberts, M.D. *Bethesda, Md.*

Surprisingly few morphologic studies on the coronary arteries in patients with known hyperlipoproteinemia (HLP) have been reported. An earlier study from this laboratory[1] examined the number of four major coronary arteries narrowed 76% to 100% in cross-sectional area by atherosclerotic plaques in 40 necropsy patients with type II, IV, or normal lipoprotein patterns, 26 of whom had symptomatic coronary heart disease. That study, purely a qualitative one, showed no differences in the number of coronary arteries severely narrowed among the three groups of patients analyzed. The present study extends the previous study by examining the entire lengths of each of the four major coronary arteries (an average of 26 cm per patient) in 38 necropsy patients with type II, IV, or normal lipoprotein patterns, all of whom had symptomatic coronary heart disease, and determines the amount of cross-sectional area narrowing by atherosclerotic plaques in each 5 mm segment of each artery. This type analysis, which might be considered a quantitative

one, was undertaken to determine if this more precise technique might reveal differences in degrees of coronary narrowing among patients with type II, IV, or normal lipoprotein patterns.

METHODS

Study patients. All 38 study patients fulfilled the following two criteria. (1) Serum cholesterol and triglyceride determinations and lipoprotein phenotyping were performed at the National Institutes of Health (31 patients) or at an outside institution (seven patients) with results diagnostic for type II HLP (15 patients) (homozygous type II HLP was excluded), type IV HLP (13 patients), or normal lipoprotein patterns (10 patients). (2) There was clinical evidence of coronary heart disease (history of myocardial infarction, angina pectoris, chronic congestive heart failure, and/or sudden coronary death). The clinical findings and noncoronary artery necropsy findings in the 38 patients are summarized in Table I. Patients with noncoronary types of cardiac disease, other than systemic hypertension, were excluded from this study.

The mean age at death of the patients with normal lipoprotein patterns was higher than that of patients with types II or IV HLP (58 years vs 51 years and 48 years, respectively [$p < 0.05$]). All three study groups had a similar proportion of men and women; no significant differences among the three groups were present in the frequency of past or fatal acute myocardial infarction, angina pectoris, systemic hypertension, diabetes mellitus,

From the Pathology Branch, National Heart, Lung and Blood Institute, National Institutes of Health.

Received for publication Sept. 18, 1980; accepted Sept. 25, 1980.

Reprint requests: William C. Roberts, M.D., Building 10A, Room 3E30, National Institutes of Health, Bethesda, MD 20205.

Table I. Observations on 15 type II HLP, 13 type IV HLP, and 10 normal lipoprotein pattern patients and on 15 control subjects

	Type II (15)	Type IV (13)	Normal (10)	Controls (15)
Age (yr), range (mean)	29-58(51)	31-65(48)	31-78(58)	25-69(48)
Male:female	13:2	11:2	9:1	13:2
Angina pectoris	12	11	5	0
Past Hx of acute MI	7	7	5	0
Chronic CHF	1	2	4	0
Family Hx of CHD[a] (HLP)	7(6)	4(0)	2(0)	0(0)
Systemic hypertension[b]	6	6	2	0
Diabetes mellitus	2	5	2	0
Total cholesterol (mg/dl), range (mean)	280-591(409)	140-735 (323)	121-233(168)	128-245(176)
Triglyceride (mg/dl), range (mean)	86-442(241)	210-2820(878)	76-150(104)	106-202(151)
Mode of death				
Sudden	9	4	1	0
AMI	3	2	2	0
Chronic CHF	0	0	2	0
Unstable angina pectoris	2	0	0	0
CABG	0	6	4	0
CC	1	1	1	0
Noncardiac	0	0	0	15
Heart weight (gm), range (mean)	300-640(425)	380-650(487)	320-890(571)	200-400(288)
Transmural LV F(N)	10(4)	10(5)	9(3)	0(0)

Abbreviations and symbols: [a] = onset before age 55; [b] = >140/90 mm Hg; CABG = coronary artery bypass grafting; CC = cardiac catheterization; CHD = coronary heart disease; CHF = congestive heart failure; F = fibrosis; HLP = hyperlipoproteinemia; Hx = history; LV = left ventricular; MI = myocardial infarct; N = necrosis.

Table II. Numbers of each major epicardial coronary artery narrowed 76% to 100% in cross-sectional area (XSA) by atherosclerotic plaques in 15 patients with type II HLP, 13 with type IV HLP, and 10 with normal lipoprotein patterns and in 15 control subjects

Lipoprotein pattern	No. of patients	Total No. of CA	Numbers of CA narrowed 76%-100% in XSA					Mean No. of 4 CA per patient narrowed >75% in XSA
			LM	LAD	LC	R	Totals	
Type II	15	59[a]	9	13	12	14	48 (81%)	3.2
Type IV	13	51[a]	6	13	13	13	45 (88%)	3.5
Normal	10	40	1	9	8	8	26 (65%)	2.6
Totals	38	150	16	35	33	35	119 (79%)	3.2
Controls	15	59[a]	1	6	1	4	12 (20%)	0.8

Abbreviations: LAD = left anterior descending; LC = left circumflex; LM = left main; R = right coronary arteries; CA = coronary arteries.
[a] = left main CA not examined in one type II patient, one type IV patient, and one control subject.

or family history of onset of clinical evidence of coronary heart disease before age 55. Compared to the patients with normal lipoprotein patterns, the type II patients had a lower frequency of chronic congestive heart failure ($p < 0.05$) and a higher frequency of sudden coronary death ($p < 0.05$).

Control subjects. The control subjects were selected on the basis of the following criteria: (1) absence of clinically evident coronary heart disease, (2) absence of systemic hypertension (blood pressure > 140 mm Hg systolic or > 90 mm Hg diastolic or both), (3) absence of therapeutic mediastinal irradiation, and (4) heart weight at necropsy ≤ 400 gm in men and ≤ 350 gm in women. Fifteen age- and sex-matched subjects were selected (Table I): seven

died of carcinoma, three died of leukemia, three died of lymphoma, and one each died of heat stroke and cryptococcal meningitis.

Coronary artery disease quantification. In the 38 study patients and 15 control subjects the entire lengths of the right, left main, left anterior descending, and left circumflex coronary arteries were removed from the heart and were cut transversely into 5 mm long segments. Each segment was labeled, processed for histologic study, and a histologic section stained by the Movat method[2] was prepared and examined. The degree of narrowing in all 5 mm segments was determined by examination of the histologic sections magnified 25 to 50 times. The percent of cross-sectional area narrowing by atherosclerotic plaques

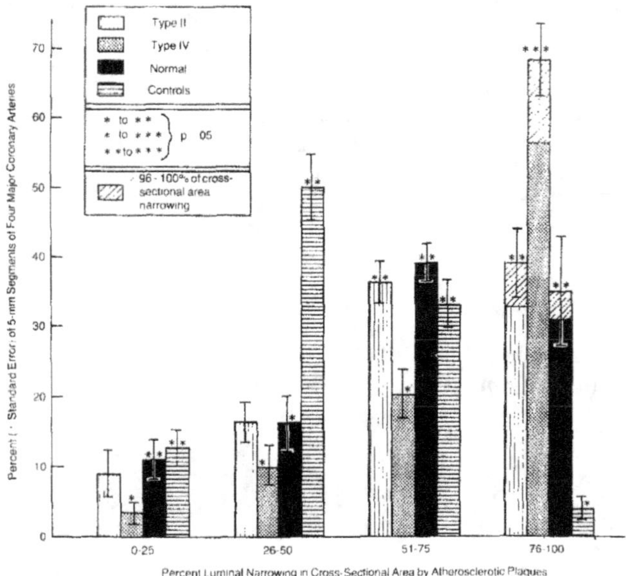

Fig. 1. Percent of 5 mm segments of all four major coronary arteries narrowed to various degrees in 15 patients with type II HLP, 13 patients with type IV HLP, and 10 patients with normal lipoprotein patterns and symptomatic coronary heart disease, and in 15 control subjects without symptomatic coronary heart disease.

was divided into five categories of narrowing: 0% to 25%, 26% to 50%, 51% to 75%, 76% to 95%, and 96% to 100%. The accuracy of these determinations was verified by random evaluations by other observers and by videoplanimetry, and both the intra- and interobserver error was < 5%.[3]

RESULTS

Coronary disease in study patients. Among the 38 study patients, a total of 150 major (right, left main, left anterior descending, and left circumflex) epicardial coronary arteries were examined (the left main coronary artery was not examined in one type II and in one type IV patient), and the results are summarized in Tables II and III. At least two of the four major arteries were narrowed severely (76% to 100% in cross-sectional area) by atherosclerotic plaques in all study patients with the exception of one type II HLP patient who had severe narrowing of only the left main coronary artery. A significantly ($p < 0.01$) greater number of the four major epicardial coronary arteries per patient were narrowed severely in the type IV HLP group than in the normal lipoprotein pattern group. Otherwise the number of four coronary arteries per patient narrowed severely in the three study groups was similar. The percent of patients with severe narrowing of the left main coronary artery was significantly ($p < 0.05$) greater in both type II and IV HLP groups than in the normal lipoprotein pattern group.

Coronary disease in control subjects. Of 59 major epicardial coronary arteries examined in the 15

control subjects (the left main coronary artery was not examined in one subject), significantly fewer arteries per subject were narrowed 76% to 100% in cross-sectional area by atherosclerotic plaques than in the patients with type II, IV, or normal lipoprotein patterns ($p < 0.001$) (Tables II and III). In one control subject, the left main coronary artery was severely narrowed.

Quantitative comparison of coronary disease in study and control individuals. The results of the quantitative analysis of the 2593 five-millimeter long coronary arterial segments in both study patients and control subjects are summarized in Table IV and in Figs. 1 to 5. The type IV HLP group had a significantly higher percent of 5 mm coronary segments narrowed 76% to 100% in cross-sectional area by atherosclerotic plaques than the type II and normal lipoprotein pattern groups ($p < 0.005$), both of which had similar amounts of severe narrowing. All three study groups had a greater percent of segments narrowed severely than did the control group ($p < 0.001$). In addition, the type IV HLP group had a greater percent of 5 mm segments narrowed 96% to 100% than the normal lipoprotein pattern group ($p < 0.05$), had less 51% to 75% cross-sectional area narrowing than the other two study groups and the controls ($p < 0.01$), and had less 0% to 25% narrowing than the normal lipoprotein pattern and control groups ($p < 0.05$). The percent of 5 mm segments narrowed for each of the five categories of narrowing was similar in the type II and normal lipoprotein pattern patients.

Index of cross-sectional vessel narrowing. Each 5 mm segment of coronary artery in every study patient and control subject was given a score of 1 to 4 based on the amount of cross-sectional area narrowing, as follows: $1 = 0\%$ to 25% narrowing,

---

Table III. Number of patients with type II HLP, type IV HLP, or normal lipoprotein patterns and number of control subjects with one to four of four major coronary arteries (CA) narrowed 76% to 100% in cross-sectional area by atherosclerotic plaques

Total no. CA narrowed 76%-100%	Type II[a]	Type IV[a]	Normal	Controls
4	7	6	0	0
3	5	7	6	1
2	2	0	4	2
1	1[b]	0	0	5
0	0	0	0	7
Totals	15	13	10	15

[a] = left main coronary artery not examined in one type II and in one type IV patient.
[b] = left main coronary artery.

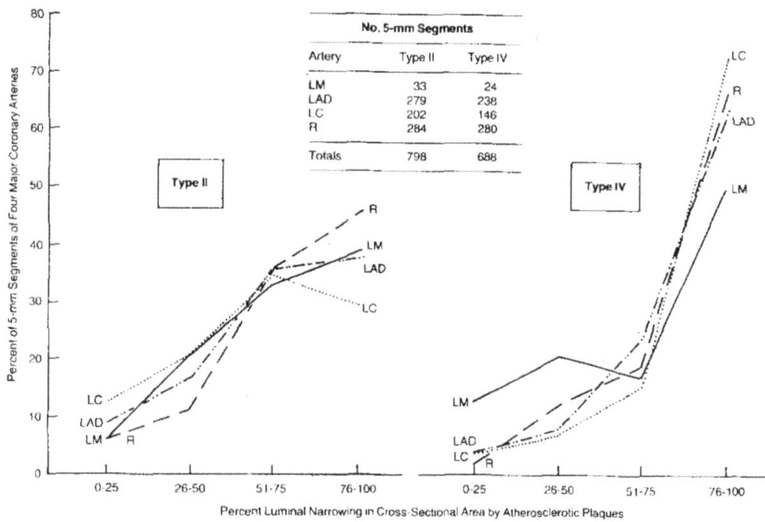

Fig. 2. Percent of 5 mm segments of the right *(R)*, left main *(LM)*, left anterior descending *(LAD)*, and left circumflex *(LC)* coronary arteries narrowed to four categories of narrowing in 15 patients with type II and 13 with type IV HLP and symptomatic coronary heart disease.

Table IV. Amounts of cross-sectional area luminal narrowing in the 5 mm segments of the four major epicardial coronary arteries in the 15 patients with type II HLP, 13 with type IV HLP, 10 with normal lipoprotein patterns, and in the 15 control subjects

Lipoprotein pattern	No. (%) 5 mm coronary segments in each of four categories of narrowing					No. 5 mm segments per group	Score* per group	Mean score per pt	Mean no. 5 mm segments per pt	Mean score† per 5 mm segment
	0%-25%	*26%-50%*	*51%-75%*	*76%-95%*	*96%-100%*					
Type II	73(9)	130(16)	284(36)	262(33)	49(6)	798	2429	162	53	3.0
Type IV	24(3)	67(10)	138(20)	383(56)	76(11)	688	2408	185	53	3.5
Normal	49(11)	75(16)	179(38)	143(31)	20(4)	466	1388	139	47	3.0
Controls	82(13)	322(50)	209(33)	28(4)	0(0)	641	1465	98	43	2.3

*Sum derived by assigning a number to each 5 mm segment in each of four categories of cross-sectional area narrowing as follows: 1 = 0%-25% narrowing; 2 = 26%-50%; 3 = 51%-75%; and 4 = 76%-100%.
†Number derived by dividing either the total number of 5 mm coronary segments per group into the total score per group, or by dividing the number of 5 mm segments per patient (pt) into the score per patient.

2 = 26% to 50%, 3 = 51% to 75%, and 4 = 76% to 100%. The score per 5 mm segment (obtained by dividing the score per patient by the number of 5 mm segments of coronary artery examined per patient) for the type II HLP patients ranged from 1.8 to 3.8 (mean 3.0); the score for the type IV HLP patients ranged from 2.6 to 3.9 (mean 3.5); the score for the patients with normal lipoprotein patterns ranged from 2.4 to 3.7 (mean 3.0), and the score for the control subjects ranged from 1.9 to 3.0 (mean 2.3) (Table IV). The mean score per 5 mm segment was significantly greater in the type IV HLP group than in the type II ($p < 0.01$) and normal lipoprotein pattern groups ($p < 0.02$), and was significantly greater in the three study groups than in the control group ($p < 0.001$).

Evaluation of individual coronary arteries. The percent of 5 mm long segments narrowed to various degrees in each of the four major coronary arteries in each study group and in the control group is shown in Figs. 2 and 3. The percent of 5 mm segments narrowed 76% to 100% in cross-sectional area in the left anterior descending, left circumflex, and right coronary arteries was significantly greater in the type IV patients than in the type II and normal lipoprotein pattern patients and control subjects ($p < 0.05$). The left main coronary artery in the type II and IV patients had a similar percent of segments narrowed 76% to 100%, which was greater than that for the normal lipoprotein pattern patients and control subjects. Within each study group there were no significant differences among the amounts of severe narrowing in the left anterior descending, left circumflex, and right coronary arteries.

Evaluation of proximal vs distal vessel disease. The percent of 5 mm segments narrowed 76% to 100% in

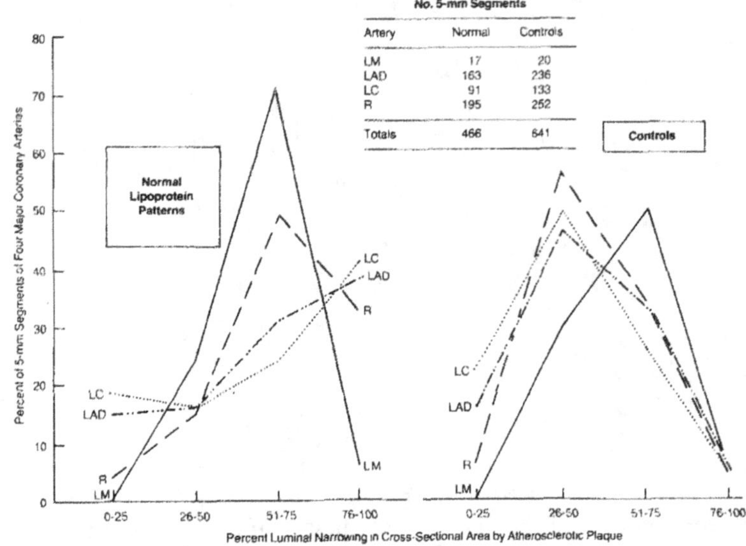

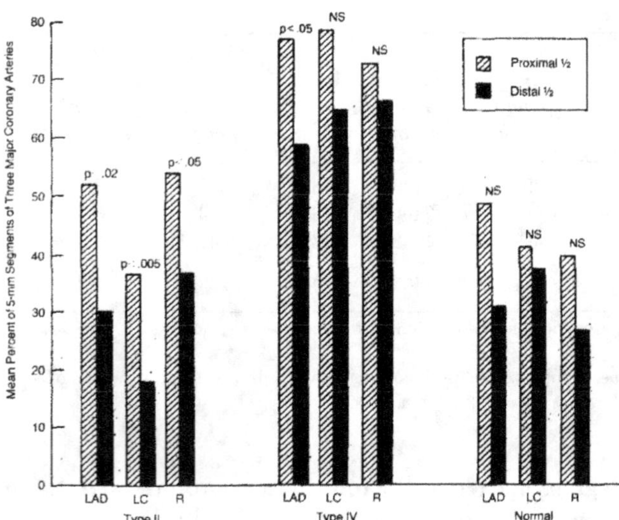

Fig. 3. Percent of 5 mm segments of the right *(R)*, left main *(LM)*, left anterior descending *(LAD)*, and left circumflex *(LC)* coronary arteries narrowed to four categories of narrowing in 10 patients with normal lipoprotein patterns and symptomatic coronary heart disease and in 15 control subjects without symptomatic coronary heart disease.

Fig. 4. Mean percent of 5 mm segments of the right *(R)*, left anterior descending *(LAD)*, and left circumflex *(LC)* coronary arteries narrowed 76% to 100% in cross-sectional area by atherosclerotic plaques in the proximal and distal halves of each artery in 15 patients with type II HLP, 13 with type IV HLP, and 10 with normal lipoprotein patterns and symptomatic coronary heart disease.

cross-sectional area by atherosclerotic plaques was significantly greater in the proximal than in the distal halves of the left anterior descending ($p < 0.02$), left circumflex ($p < 0.005$), and right ($p < 0.05$) coronary arteries in the type II patients and in the left anterior descending artery ($p < 0.05$) in the type IV patients (Fig. 4).

DISCUSSION

Qualitative evaluation of coronary disease. In the present study, two or more of the four major coronary arteries were narrowed severely (76% to 100% in cross-sectional area) by atherosclerotic plaques in 27 (96%) of 28 patients with type II or IV HLP, and no significant difference was observed between the two groups in the number of four coronary arteries per patient so narrowed. Additionally, the left main coronary artery frequently was severely narrowed—in nine of 15 patients with type II and in six of 13 patients with type IV HLP.

These qualitative coronary necropsy studies can be compared to coronary angiographic studies performed during life. One of the first angiographic studies to examine the relationship of coronary narrowing to HLP was by Heinle et al.,[4] who found no significant difference in the percent of the four major coronary arteries that were totally occluded between patients with type II and type IV HLP. Murray et al.[5] and Bloch et al.[6] later reported a higher percent of major epicardial coronary arteries narrowed $> 50\%$ in diameter in patients with type II than in those with type IV HLP. Bloch et al.[6] also found a higher frequency of significant narrowing of the left main coronary artery in their type II patients (10 of 24) than in their type IV patients (1 of 22). In contrast, Heinle et al.[4] reported narrowing of the left main coronary artery in none of 36 patients with type II HLP and in only three of 32 patients with type IV HLP. A more recent study by

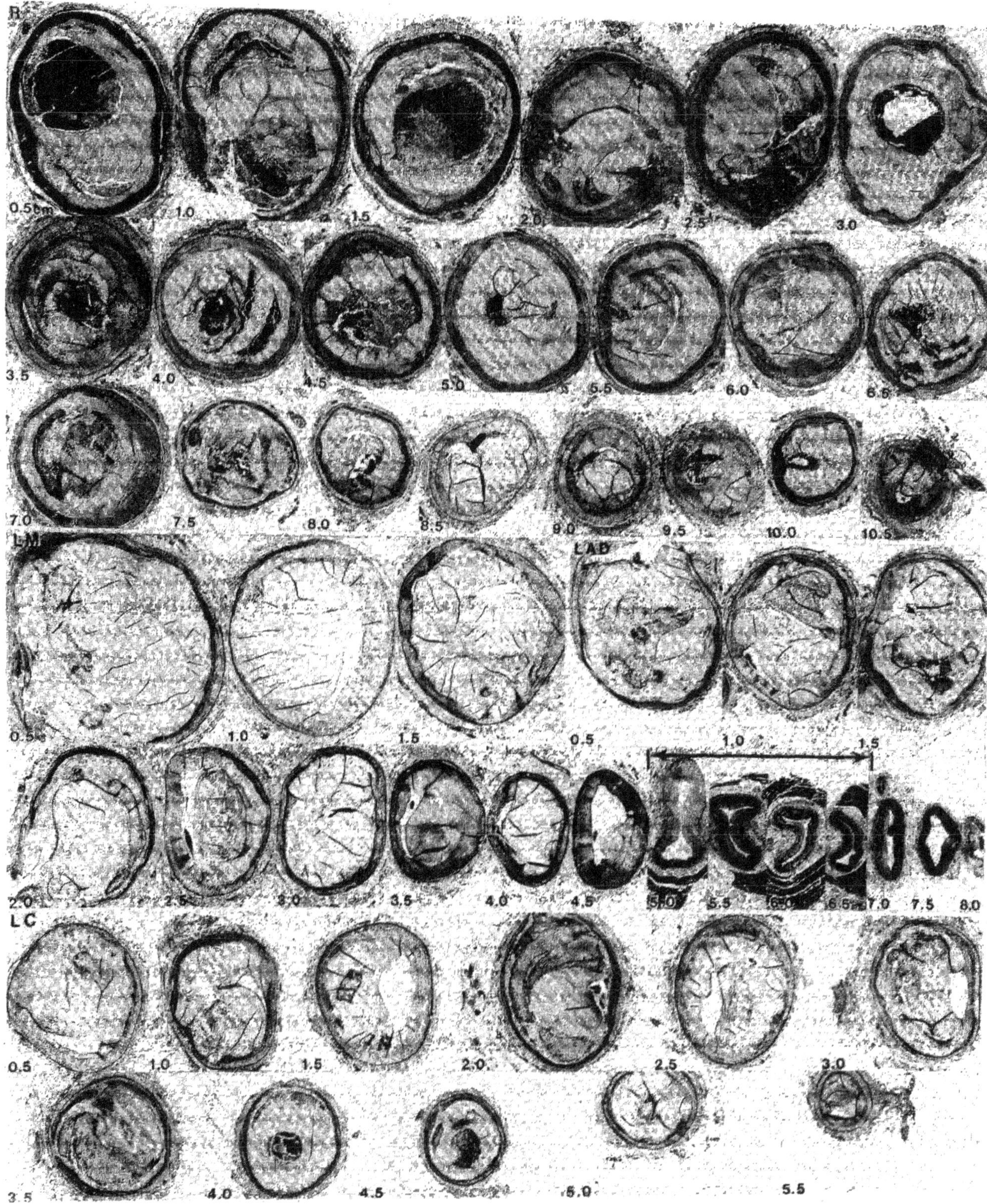

Fig. 5. Photomicrographs of each 5 mm segment of the right *(R)*, left main *(LM)*, left anterior descending *(LAD)*, and left circumflex *(LC)* coronary arteries from a 54-year-old man (No. A71-67) with type IV HLP (triglyceride = 465 mg/dl, total cholesterol = 186 mg/dl) who had angina pectoris and died during cardiac catheterization. The numbers in the *lower left* of each photomicrograph indicate the distance in centimeters from the coronary artery ostia or from the bifurcation of the left main coronary artery. Every 5 mm segment has severe narrowing by atherosclerotic plaques except for the distal left anterior descending coronary artery which includes a portion of artery that is intramyocardial (indicated by the *arrows*). (Movat stain; original magnification ×14.)

Gotto et al.[7] reported no significant differences in the number of four major coronary arteries narrowed $> 25\%$ in diameter between patients with type II and those with type IV HLP.

Quantitative evaluation of coronary disease. Analysis of the number of the four major epicardial coronary arteries severely narrowed in our patients disclosed no significant differences between the type II and type IV HLP groups, and results from angiographic studies are conflicting. A quantitative approach, however, whereby the amount of narrowing of each 5 mm long segment of each of the four major coronary arteries was determined, disclosed significantly more severe narrowing in our patients with type IV than in those with type II HLP or in those with normal lipoprotein patterns. Although previous studies have emphasized the frequency of type IV HLP in patients with significant coronary arterial narrowing,[7-9] no previous study of patients with symptomatic coronary heart disease, to our knowledge, has reported more severe coronary arterial narrowing in patients with type IV than in those with type II HLP.

The percent of 5 mm coronary segments narrowed 76% to 100% in cross-sectional area by atherosclerotic plaques in our patients with type IV HLP (67%) also far exceeded that found in other subsets of necropsy patients with coronary heart disease studied in this laboratory by the quantitative technique: sudden coronary death = 557 (36%) of 1564 segments[10]; clinically isolated unstable angina pectoris = 497 (47%) of 1049 segments[11]; acute transmural myocardial infarction = 484 (34%) of 1403 [12]; healed myocardial infarction with chronic, eventually fatal congestive heart failure without aneurysm = 150 (28%) of 536 segments[13]; nonfatal healed transmural myocardial infarction with fatal noncardiac disease = 292 (32%) of 924 segments[14]; and true left ventricular aneurysm and healed myocardial infarction = 323 (33%) of 992 segments.[15]

REFERENCES

1. Roberts WC, Ferrans VJ, Levy RI, Fredrickson DS: Cardiovascular pathology in hyperlipoproteinemia: Anatomic observations in 42 necropsy patients with normal or abnormal serum lipoprotein patterns. Am J Cardiol **31**:557, 1973.
2. Movat HZ: Demonstration of all connective tissue elements in a single section: Pentachrome stains. Arch Pathol **60**:289, 1955.
3. Isner JM, Wu M, Virmani R, Jones AA, Roberts WC: Comparison of degrees of coronary arterial luminal narrowing determined by visual inspection of histologic sections under magnification among three independent observers and comparison to that obtained by video planimetry: An analysis of 559 five mm segments of 61 coronary arteries from eleven patients. Lab Invest **42**:566, 1980.
4. Heinle RA, Levy RI, Fredrickson DS, Gorlin R: Lipid and carbohydrate abnormalities in patients with angiographically documented coronary artery disease. Am J Cardiol **24**:178, 1969.
5. Murray RG, Tweddel A, Third JLHC, Hutton I, Hillis WS, Lorimer AR, Lawrie TDV: Relation between extent of coronary artery disease and severity of hyperlipoproteinaemia. Br Heart J **37**:1205, 1975.
6. Bloch A, Dinsmore RE, Lees RS: Coronary arteriographic findings in type-II and type-IV hyperlipoproteinaemia. Lancet **1**:928, 1976.
7. Gotto AM, Gorry AG, Thompson JR, Cole JS, Trost R, Yeshurun D, De Bakey ME: Relationship between plasma lipid concentrations and coronary artery disease in 496 patients. Circulation **56**:875, 1977.
8. Salel AF, Riggs K, Mason DT, Amsterdam EA, Zelis R: The importance of type IV hyperlipoproteinemia as a predisposing factor in coronary artery disease. Am J Med **57**:897, 1974.
9. Hamby RI: Clinical-anatomical correlates in coronary artery disease. Mount Kisco, NY, 1979, Futura Publishing Co.
10. Roberts WC, Jones AA: Quantitation of coronary arterial narrowing at necropsy in sudden coronary death: Analysis of 31 patients and comparison with 25 control subjects. Am J Cardiol **44**:39, 1979.
11. Roberts WC, Virmani R: Quantification of coronary arterial narrowing in clinically-isolated unstable angina pectoris: An analysis of 22 necropsy patients. Am J Med **67**:792, 1979.
12. Roberts WC, Jones AA: Quantification of coronary arterial narrowing at necropsy in acute transmural myocardial infarction: Analysis and comparison of findings in 27 patients and 22 controls. Circulation **61**:786, 1980.
13. Virmani R, Roberts WC: Quantification of coronary arterial narrowing and of left ventricular myocardial scarring in healed myocardial infarction with chronic, eventually fatal, congestive cardiac failure. Am J Med **68**:831, 1980.
14. Virmani R, Roberts WC: Non-fatal healed transmural myocardial infarction and fatal non-cardiac disease. Qualification and quantification of coronary arterial narrowing and of left ventricular scarring in 18 necropsy patients. Br Heart J. (In press)
15. Cabin HS, Roberts WC: True left ventricular aneurysm and healed myocardial infarction: Clinical and necropsy observations including quantification of degrees of coronary arterial narrowing. Am J Cardiol **46**:754, 1980.

Running to Death*

Bruce F. Waller, M.D.; Robert S. Csere, M.D.; William P. Baker, M.D.; and William C. Roberts, M.D., F.C.C.P.

Herein we will discuss findings in a conditioned runner who died suddenly, shortly after completing a 5-km run.

A 51-year-old man had been healthy until his sudden death in March 1980. In 1975 (aged 46 years), he started jogging and quickly began averaging about 19 km (12 mi) weekly (4.8 km four times a week). At that time, his blood pressure was 140/95 mm Hg, and he began taking a diuretic daily. The total serum cholesterol was 273 mg/dl. In 1976, he began lifting weights and doing other types of calisthenics regularly. The total serum cholesterol level in 1978 was 250 mg/dl, and his systemic arterial pressure was 130/80 mm Hg. In November 1979 (four months before death), he noted "tiredness in one arm" while running, and went to a hospital emergency room, where the ECG shown in Figure 1 was recorded. The heart rate was 55 beats/min, and the blood pressure

120/80 mm Hg. A chest roentgenogram (Fig 2) was normal. He continued to run 19 km weekly thereafter without chest pain or "arm tiredness." He collapsed and died in his bathroom while preparing to shower shortly after completing a 5 AM, 5-km run. Clinical manifestations of cardiac disease were absent in other family members.

At necropsy the heart weighed 390 g. Transverse ventricular sections showed a healed transmural myocardial infarct extending from base to apex and involving primarily the ventricular septum (Fig 3). The left anterior descending and left circumflex coronary arteries were narrowed 76 to 100 percent in cross-sectional area by atherosclerotic plaques (Fig 4). Of 53 five-mm coronary segments of the left main, left anterior descending, left circumflex, and right coronary arteries, 9 (17 percent) on histologic examination were narrowed 76 to 100 percent in cross-sectional area by atherosclerotic plaques, including one segment narrowed

*From the Pathology Branch, National Heart, Lung, and Blood Institute, National Institutes of Health, and the Pathology and Cardiology Departments, National Naval Medical Center, Bethesda, Md.
Reprint requests: Dr. Roberts, Building 10A, Room 3E30, National Institutes of Health, Bethesda 20205*

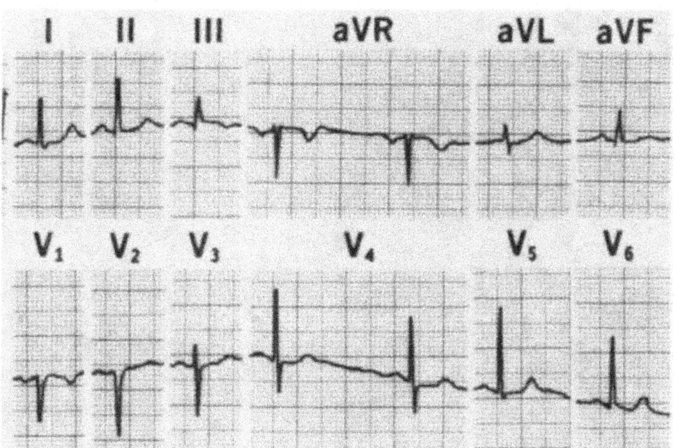

FIGURE 1. ECG recorded four months before death. Absence of R wave in V₂ and nonspecific ST-T segment and T waves changes.

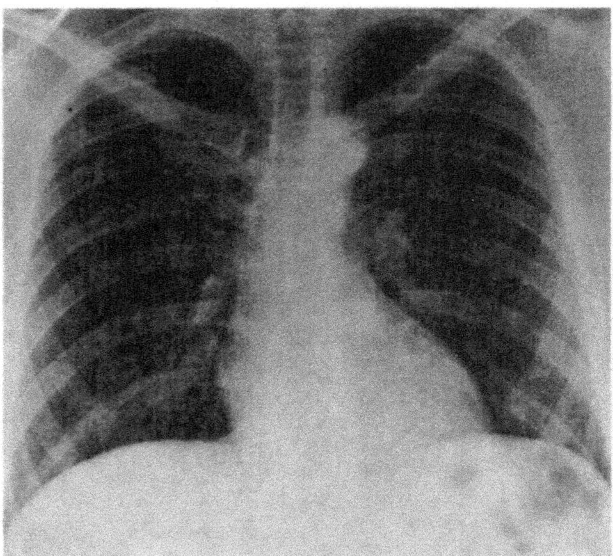

FIGURE 2. Posteroanterior chest roentgenogram obtained four months before death.

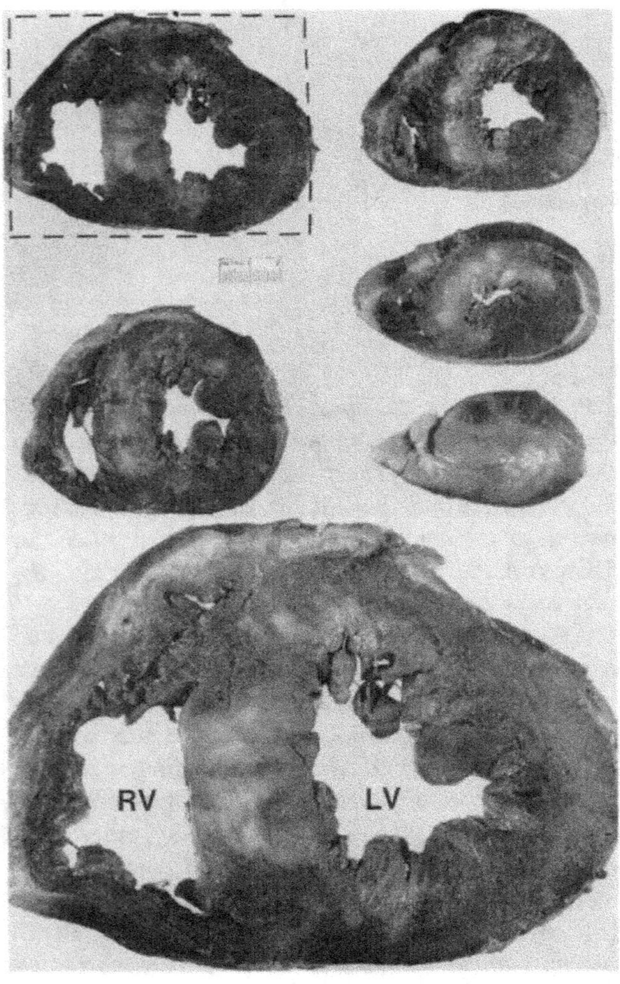

FIGURE 3. Transverse ventricular myocardial sections *(upper)*. Healed transmural infarct extending from base to apex and involving primarily ventricular septum; close-up *(lower)* of bracketed section. LV = left and RV = right ventricular cavities, respectively.

95 to 100 percent (Fig 5); 15 (28 percent) were narrowed 51 to 75 percent; 25 (47 percent), 26 to 50 percent; and 4 (8 percent), 0 to 25 percent. Thus, 34 (64 percent) of the 53 five-mm segments were narrowed >50 percent in cross-sectional area by plaques. By assigning a number for the category of narrowing for each 5-mm coronary segment (4 = 76 to 100 percent narrowing; 3 = 51 to 75 percent; 2 = 26 to 50 percent, and 1 = 0 to 25 percent), a total score of 135 was found for the 53 five-mm segments, giving each segment a mean score of 2.5 (135 ÷ 53). Thus, the lumen of each 5-mm coronary segment was narrowed on the average about 63 percent in cross-sectional area by atherosclerotic plaques. None of the coronary arteries contained fibrin or platelet thrombus or extravasated erythrocytes into atherosclerotic plaques.

Running appears to be the most efficient regular exercise, and it is estimated to be done regularly by about 25 million Americans. Few conditioned runners smoke cigarettes, are overweight, or go to psychiatrists. Nearly all "feel better" and perform their tasks better than they did before they began running regularly. Although unproved, running is believed to dilate previously normal or relatively normal coronary arteries (one of the means to increase the amount of blood perfusing myocardium is to dilate the coronary arteries), but it is uncertain whether dilation is possible in runners with

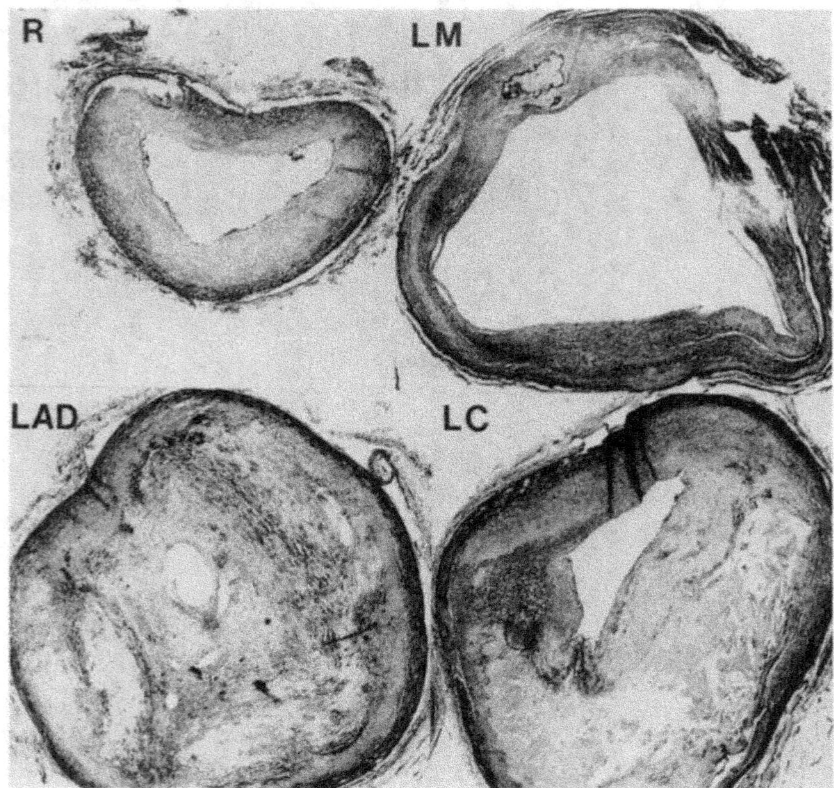

FIGURE 4. Cross-sections of sites of maximal narrowing of right (R), left main (LM), left anterior descending (LAD), and left circumflex (LC) coronary arteries (Movat stain, orginal magnification ×26).

COLLECTED REPRINTS

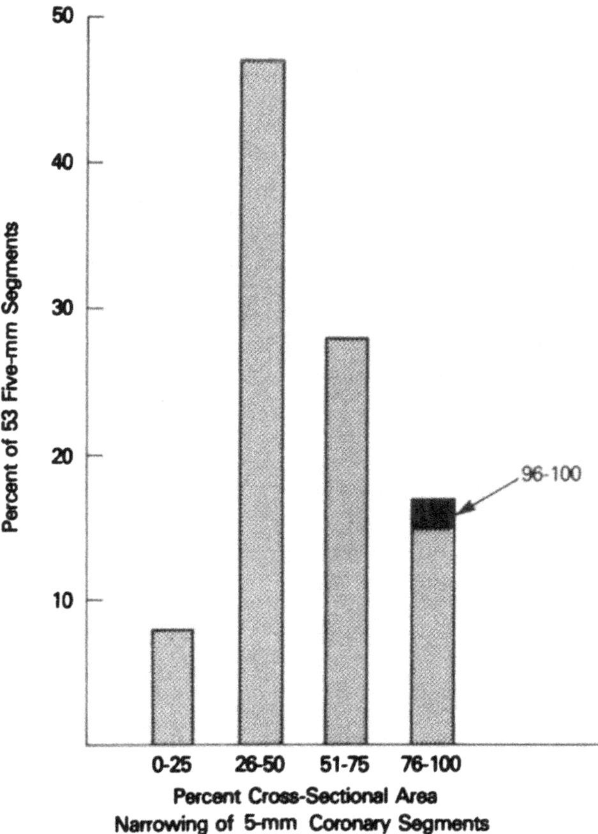

FIGURE 5. Percent of 5-mm segments of right, left main, left anterior descending, and left circumflex coronary arteries narrowed to four categories of cross-sectional area narrowing.

previous coronary events, *ie*, patients with known coronary atherosclerotic narrowing. Although reason dictates that it must, regular running has not been shown to increase longevity compared with not running.

Recently we reported cardiac findings in five men, aged 40 to 53 years (average, 46 years) who ran 22 to 176 km weekly (mean, 53 km) for one to ten years (mean, five years).[1] None had had clinical evidence of cardiac disease before they became habitual runners, and all died while running. After running regularly for several years, one showed an abnormal resting ECG and a positive exercise stress test; he also had angina pectoris while running. At necropsy all five had 76 to 100 percent cross-sectional area narrowing by atherosclerotic plaques of the right, left anterior descending, and left circumflex coronary arteries. In three, who had the entire lengths of these three arteries plus the left main coronary artery available for examination, 73 (48 percent) of the 153 five-mm segments were narrowed 76 to 100 percent in cross-sectional area by atherosclerotic plaques.

In comparison with the previously described five runners,[1] the present patient had less severe coronary narrowing; only 17 percent of the 5-mm seg-

ments of his four major arteries were narrowed 76 to 100 percent, compared with 34, 50, and 56 percent, respectively, in the three previously described runners studied quantitatively. Although severe, the amount of narrowing in our patient is not as great (range, 30 to 48 percent) as that usually observed in patients with fatal coronary heart disease.[2-6] The present patient also had hypercholesterolemia and systemic hypertension. He had not started to run regularly until aged 46 years, and died at the age of 51. He probably had considerable coronary atherosclerosis by the time he first began to run regularly. Bassler[7] stated that marathon running provides "immunity to atherosclerosis." Although the present patient was not a marathon runner, three of our five previously described runners were marathoners; none began running regularly, however, until aged 39 years, and all died by the age of 50.[1] It is likely, therefore, that they also had considerable coronary atherosclerosis before they became conditioned runners.

Our patient had a relatively large transmural left ventricular scar. Four of the five runners previously described by Waller and Roberts[1] also had transmural left ventricular scars, all of which were clinically silent events, as in our patient. Whether acute myocardial infarcts are more commonly clinically inapparent in conditioned runners compared with nonrunners is uncertain.

Several reports have described sudden death in runners, but few have provided the distance run per week (or per day) or the length of time that the person ran regularly.[8-14] Furthermore, these reports often lack information regarding the serum cholesterol and systemic blood pressure levels and whether other family members had coronary heart disease. Despite the scarcity of reported information in reported deaths among conditioned runners,[8-14] coronary atherosclerosis nevertheless appears to have been the villain in most of the previously described patients.

REFERENCES

1 Waller BF, Roberts WC. Sudden death while running in conditioned runners aged 40 years or over. Am J Cardiol 1980; 45:1292-1300

2 Roberts WC, Jones AA. Quantitation of coronary arterial narrowing at necropsy in sudden coronary death: analysis of 31 patients and comparison with 25 control subjects. Am J Cardiol 1979; 44:39-45

3 Roberts WC, Virmani R. Quantification of coronary arterial narrowing in clinically-isolated unstable angina pectoris: an analysis of 22 necropsy patients. Am J Med 1979; 67:792-98

4 Roberts WC, Jones AA. Quantification of coronary arterial narrowing at necropsy in acute transmural myocardial infarction: analysis and comparison of findings in

27 patients and 22 controls. Circulation 1980; 61:786-90

5 Virmani R, Roberts WC. Quantification of coronary arterial narrowing and of left ventricular myocardial scarring in healed infarction with chronic and eventually fatal, congestive heart failure. Am J Med 1980; 68:831-38

6 Virmani R, Roberts WC. Non-fatal healed transmural myocardial infarction and fatal non-cardiac disease: qualification and quantification of coronary arterial narrowing and of left ventricular scarring in 18 necropsy patients. Br Heart J (in press)

7 Bassler TJ. Marathon running and immunity to atherosclerosis. Ann NY Acad Sci 1977; 301:579-92

8 Opie LH. Sudden death and sport. Lancet 1975; 1:263-66

9 Opie LH. Long distance running and sudden death. N Engl J Med 1975; 293:941-42

10 Green LH, Cohen SI, Kurland G. Fatal myocardial infarction in marathon racing. Ann Intern Med 1976; 84:704-06

11 Cantwell JD, Fletcher GF. Sudden death and jogging. Phys Sports Med 1978; 94-198

12 Noakes TD, Rose AG, Opie LH. Hypertrophic cardiomyopathy associated with sudden death during marathon racing. Br Heart J 1979; 41:624-27

13 Noakes TD, Opie LH, Rose AG, Kleynhans PHT. Autopsy-proved coronary atherosclerosis in marathon runners. N Engl J Med 1979; 301:86-89

14 Thompson PD, Stern MP, Williams P, Duncan K. Haskell WL, Wood PD. Death during jogging or running: a study of 18 cases. JAMA 1979; 242:1265-67

Significance of Coronary Arterial Thrombus in Transmural Acute Myocardial Infarction

A Study of 54 Necropsy Patients

FRANK C. BROSIUS III, M.D., AND WILLIAM C. ROBERTS, M.D.

SUMMARY In 54 necropsy patients with transmural acute myocardial infarction (AMI) and coronary arterial thrombi, histologic sections of coronary arteries that contained the thrombi were examined by videoplanimetry to determine if the amount of luminal narrowing caused by thrombi was comparable to that produced by underlying atherosclerotic plaques, and to determine the amount of luminal narrowing by plaques immediately proximal and distal to the thrombi. The 54 coronary arteries in the 54 patients were narrowed 33–98% (mean 81%) by atherosclerotic plaque alone in cross-sectional area at the site of the thrombus (occlusive in 47 and nonocclusive in seven), from 26–98% (mean 75%) within the 2-cm segment proximal to the thrombus, and from 43–98% (mean 79%) within the 2-cm segment distal to the thrombus. Of the 54 arteries, 52 (96%) were narrowed 76–98% in cross-sectional area by atherosclerotic plaque alone at or immediately proximal or distal to the thrombus and 26 (48%) were narrowed 91–98% by plaque alone. The thrombi were 0.1–6.0 mm² (mean 1.4 mm²) in cross-sectional area and the underlying atherosclerotic plaques were 3.0–21.0 mm² (mean 8.7 mm²). Thus, among necropsy patients with transmural AMI, coronary thrombi occur at sites already severely narrowed by atherosclerotic plaques.

THROMBI in coronary arteries of necropsy patients with transmural acute myocardial infarction (AMI) have been observed in numerous studies. Herrick, in 1912[1] and 1919,[2] found them in four patients with fatal AMI, and for many decades thrombi were believed to have precipitated AMI. They were considered so important in causing this acute event that the term "coronary thrombosis" was used for years to describe the event that most physicians now call "acute myocardial infarction."[3] In recent years the primary role of coronary thrombus in precipitating AMI has been questioned.[4-20] To evaluate the significance of

coronary thrombus in AMI, we examined in detail the coronary arteries containing thrombi in 54 necropsy patients with transmural AMI. Several previously undescribed observations on coronary thrombi resulted, which clarify the significance of coronary thrombi in AMI.

Patients and Methods

All necropsy patients with transmural AMI accessioned in the Pathology Branch, National Heart, Lung, and Blood Institute, were reviewed. Of 235 such patients, 99 had histologic sections available from each 5-mm segment of each of the four major coronary arteries (right, left main, left anterior descending and left circumflex). Movat-stained histologic sections, approximately 55 per patient, were reviewed, and a thrombus was found in one of the four major coronary arteries in 54 patients (55%). These 54 patients constitute the study group.

In each patient, the coronary artery that contained the thrombus was examined. The maximal degree of

From the Pathology Branch, National Heart, Lung, and Blood Institute, National Institutes of Health, Bethesda, Maryland.

Dr. Brosius's present address: Department of Medicine, University Hospital, Ann Arbor, Michigan 48109.

Address for correspondence: William C. Roberts, M.D., Building 10A, Room 3E-30, National Institutes of Health, Bethesda, Maryland 20205.

Received February 15, 1980; revision accepted August 12, 1980.

Circulation 63, No. 4, 1981.

cross-sectional area narrowing by atherosclerotic plaque was determined at the site of the thrombus, in the 2-cm portion of artery proximal to the proximal portion of the thrombus, and in the 2-cm segment of coronary artery distal to the distal site of attachment of the thrombus (fig. 1). The length of the thrombus was determined by the number of 5-mm-long segments of coronary artery that contained thrombus. Thus, if three sections prepared from three 5-mm-long coronary segments contained thrombus, the thrombus was judged to be 1.5 cm long.

A coronary arterial thrombus was defined as a collection of fibrin (with or without engulfed eryth-rocytes) or platelets or both within the residual lumen and attachment of the fibrin/platelets to the luminal surface of the artery (fig. 2). Among the 54 patients with fatal AMI, this luminal surface always was the surface of an underlying atherosclerotic plaque. The thrombus was always attached to the intimal surface in its distal portion, but in a few patients it was not attached in its most proximal portion. The thrombus was considered occlusive when it occupied the residual lumen of the artery, i.e., the portion not occupied by atherosclerotic plaque (fig. 2). In many patients, the occlusive thrombi were detached from the surface of the underlying plaque in some areas, but this detachment was considered artifactual, the result

of processing the artery through dehydrating solutions (alcohol and xylene) during the processing of the tissues for histologic sectioning. The thrombus was considered nonocclusive when it filled a relatively small portion of the residual lumen, with no evidence of previous circumferential attachment to the surface of the underlying atherosclerotic plaque (fig. 2).

The maximal degrees of cross-sectional area narrowing by atherosclerotic plaque were determined at the site of the coronary thrombus and within the 2-cm portions of the artery proximal and distal to the thrombus by means of a video-based, computer-linked system described elsewhere.[21, 22] Briefly, Movat-stained sections of coronary artery were positioned on the stage of a projection-light microscope. The image was then magnified × 650 onto opaque white paper and a pencil tracing was made of the artery's original lumen (denoted by the black-staining internal elastic membrane), the area occupied by atherosclerotic plaque, and, in the case of nonocclusive thrombi, the area occupied by the thrombus (fig. 2). The area of the occlusive thrombus was the difference between the area of the original lumen and the area of the atherosclerotic plaque. In the case of nonocclusive thrombus, the area of the thrombus was determined directly by tracing the borders of its projected image. Also, in the case of nonocclusive thrombus, the

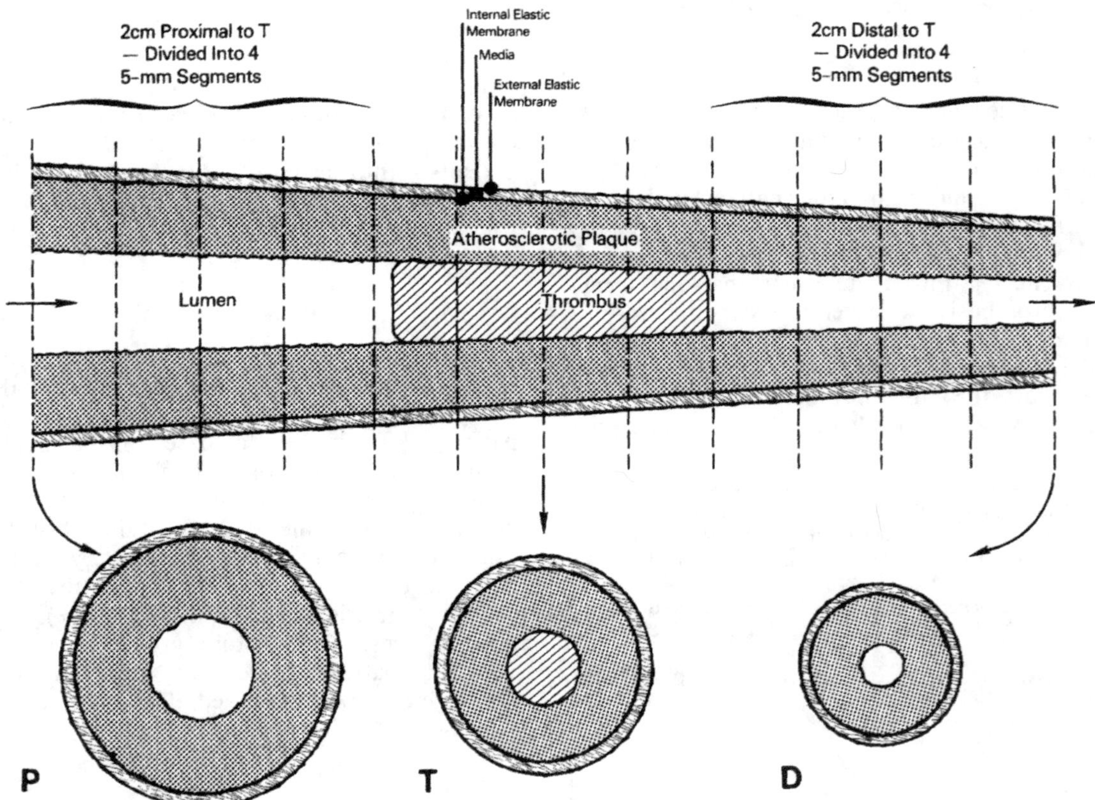

FIGURE 1. *Diagram of an "average" coronary artery with an occlusive thrombus. The four 5-mm segments of coronary artery proximal (P) to the thrombus (T) were narrowed an average of 75% in cross-sectional area by atherosclerotic plaque (AP), the four segments with an occlusive thrombus were narrowed an average of 81% by plaque, and the four segments distal (D) to the thrombus were narrowed an average of 79% by plaque.*

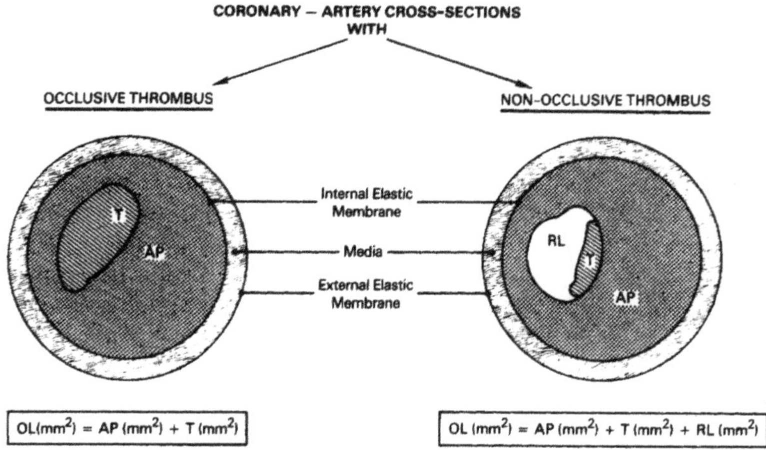

FIGURE 2. *Diagram of cross sections of coronary arteries with occlusive and non-occlusive thrombi and the method of calculating the cross-sectional area of the atherosclerotic plaque (AP), thrombus (T) and residual lumen (RL). OL = original lumen (area enclosed by internal elastic membrane).*

residual lumen was the difference between the artery's original lumen and the sum of the area occupied by atherosclerotic plaque plus the area occupied by the nonocclusive thrombus (fig. 2). In the sections of coronary artery proximal and distal to the thrombus, the residual lumen was the difference between the artery's original lumen and the area occupied by atherosclerotic plaque. The percent of cross-sectional area narrowed by atherosclerotic plaques and by thrombi (in the case of nonocclusive thrombi) was calculated. The area of each artery enclosed by the internal elastic membrane (original lumen), the area of the atherosclerotic plaque and that of the nonocclusive throm-

bus provided by videoplanimetry were converted into actual area.

All patients had had AMIs that involved the entire inner half of the left ventricular wall and a portion or all of the outer half of the left ventricular wall. In addition to these acute left ventricular infarcts, 20 patients had one or more transmural scars. The 54 patients ranged in age from 38–92 years (mean 62 years); 41 were men and 13 were women.

Results

The major morphologic findings in the 54 coronary arteries containing thrombi are summarized in tables

TABLE 1. *Data in the 54 Autopsy Patients: Coronary Thrombi*

Coronary artery with T	No. of pts	Dominant posterior artery	Distance (cm) of T from origin of coronary artery	Length (cm) of T	Duration (days) from clinical onset of AMI to death	Maximal narrowing (%) of coronary artery containing T			
						Proximal 2 cm to T	At site of T		Distal 2 cm to T
							By AP only	By T only	
Occlusive									
Right	19	19	0.5–15.5 (4.8)	0.5–10.0 (2.4)	1–18 (5.7)	56–98 (79)	33–98 (80)	2–67 (20)	51–96 (80)
Left anterior descending	19	—	0.0–6.0 (2.1)	0.5–5.0 (1.4)	1–25 (6.9)	26–94 (68)	64–97 (82)	3–36 (18)	43–97 (78)
Left circumflex	9	6	0.0–5.0 (2.3)	0.5–1.5 (1.1)	1–45 (9.6)	59–90 (75)	69–97 (80)	3–31 (20)	51–98 (80)
Subtotals	47	25	0.0–15.5 (3.2)	0.5–10.0 (1.8)	1–45 (6.9)	26–98 (74)	33–98 (81)	2–67 (19)	43–98 (79)
Nonocclusive									
Right	0	—	—	—	—	—	—	—	—
Left anterior descending	3	—	0.5–2.0 (1.2)	0.5–1.0 (0.7)	1–7 (4.3)	50–91 (72)	79–85 (82)	2–5 (4)	47–88 (63)
Left circumflex	4	1	0.5–3.0 (1.5)	0.5–1.0 (0.8)	1–28 (8.0)	82–92 (88)	59–96 (79)	2–24 (10)	67–92 (81)
Subtotals	7	1	0.5–3.0 (1.4)	0.5–1.0 (0.7)	1–28 (6.4)	50–92 (80)	59–96 (80)	2–24 (7)	47–92 (73)
Totals	54	26	0.0–15.5 (2.9)	0.5–10.0 (1.6)	1–45 (6.8)	26–98 (75)	33–98 (81)	2–67 (18)	43–98 (79)

Abbreviations: T = thrombus; AMI = acute myocardial infarction; AP = atherosclerotic plaque.

TABLE 2. *Total Numbers of the Three Major Coronary Arteries Showing Five Categories of Narrowing*

Site	Number of coronary arteries with maximal narrowing (%) by atherosclerotic plaque alone					Totals
	(0–25)	(26–50)	(51–75)	(76–90)	(91–100)	
Proximal 2 cm to thrombus	0	5 (12%)	10 (24%)	20 (48%)	7 (16%)	42
				(64%)		
At site of thrombus	0	2 (4%)	11 (20%)	27 (50%)	14 (26%)	54
				(76%)		
Distal 2 cm to thrombus	0	3 (6%)	15 (28%)	22 (41%)	13 (25%)	53
				(66%)		
Either at, or proximal or distal to thrombus	0	0	2 (4%)	26 (48%)	26 (48%)	54 (100%)
				(96%)		

1–3 and illustrated in figures 1 and 2. The thrombi were occlusive in 47 patients (87%) and nonocclusive in seven (13%). The coronary arterial systems containing thrombi were left anterior descending in 22 (41%), right in 19 (35%), and left circumflex in 13 (24%). In one of the 19 patients with a thrombus in the right coronary system, the thrombus was present only in the posterior descending branch of the right coronary artery. In one of the 13 patients with a thrombus in the left circumflex system, the thrombus was present in the left obtuse marginal branch rather than the left circumflex proper. Of the 13 patients with a thrombus in the left circumflex system, this artery was the dominant posterior perfusing artery in seven: in six of nine

TABLE 3. *Areas of Minimal Residual Lumen of Coronary Artery*

Site	Number of coronary arteries with minimal residual luminal area* at site			Total
	>2 mm²	>1–2 mm²	≤1 mm²	
Proximal 2 cm to thrombus	18 (42%)	12 (29%)	12 (29%)	42
At site of thrombus	14 (26%)	20 (37%)	20 (37%)	54
Distal 2 cm to thrombus	6 (11%)	15 (28%)	32 (61%)	53
Either at, or proximal or distal to thrombus	1 (2%)	12 (22%)	41 (76%)	54 (100%)

*Represents area not occupied by atherosclerotic plaque; ignores further occlusion by thrombus.

patients with occlusive thrombi and in one of four with nonocclusive thrombi (table 1).

The coronary thrombi ranged from 0.5–10 cm long (mean 1.6 cm) (table 1). The occlusive thrombi were 0.5–10 cm long (mean 1.8 cm) and the nonocclusive thrombi were 0.5–1.0 cm long (mean 0.7 cm). The mean lengths of occlusive thrombi in the right coronary artery were longer than the mean lengths of occlusive thrombi in the left anterior descending and left circumflex coronary arteries ($p < 0.025$) (table 1). In the case of the right coronary artery, the length of the thrombus increased directly as the intervals increased between onset of AMI and death; such was not the case, however, with thrombi in the left anterior descending and left circumflex coronary arteries.

The distance from the origin of a coronary artery (aorta for the right and left main for the left anterior descending and left circumflex) to the most proximal portion of a coronary thrombus ranged from 0–15.5 cm (mean 2.9 cm). This mean distance was 3.2 cm (range 0–15.5 cm) for the occlusive thrombi and 1.4 cm (range 0.5–3.0 cm) for the nonocclusive thrombi (NS). The mean distance of an occlusive thrombus from the aorta in the right coronary artery, however, was significantly ($p < 0.01$) greater than the mean distance of either an occlusive or nonocclusive thrombus from the left main in either the left anterior descending or left circumflex coronary arteries.

The amount of luminal narrowing by atherosclerotic plaques and by thrombus proximal, at, and distal to the coronary thrombus is summarized in tables 1–3. The maximal luminal narrowing by atherosclerotic plaques alone at the site of the thrombus varied from 33–98% (mean 81%); the maximal coronary luminal narrowing by thrombus alone varied from 2–67% (mean 19%) in the 47 patients with occlusive thrombi and from 2–24% (mean 7%) in the seven patients with nonocclusive thrombi. The maximal luminal narrowing by atherosclerotic plaques in the 2 cm of coronary artery proximal to the thrombus ranged from 26–98% (mean 75%), and in the 2 cm distal to the distal site of attachment of the thrombus from 43–98% (mean 79%). No significant differences were noted in the amount of maximal luminal narrowing at, proximal, or distal to the thrombus between the 47 patients with occlusive thrombi and the seven with nonocclusive thrombi (table 1). Likewise, no significant differences were observed in the amount of maximal luminal narrowing at, proximal or distal to the coronary thrombus in the three major coronary arteries (table 1).

The absolute area occupied by atherosclerotic plaques, the area occupied by thrombus, and the area of the residual coronary lumens for the sites of maximal narrowing at, proximal and distal to coronary artery thrombi were as follows. At the site of maximal luminal narrowing of the coronary artery at the site of the thrombus, the area occupied by atherosclerotic plaque ranged from 1.5–15.0 mm² (mean 7.2 mm²); the area occupied by occlusive thrombus, from 0.1–6.0 mm² (mean 1.5 mm²); and that occupied by nonocclusive thrombus, from 0.1–1.5 mm² (mean 0.5 mm²). The area of the original coronary lumen (that enclosed by internal elastic membrane) at the site of the thrombus ranged from 3–21 mm² (mean 8.7 mm²); proximal to the thrombus, from 2.8–13.6 mm² (mean 8.7 mm²); and distal to the thrombus, from 0.8–13.5 mm² (mean 5.1 mm²). The maximal area occupied by atherosclerotic plaque proximal to the thrombus ranged from 2.2–12.1 mm² (mean 6.5 mm), and distal to the thrombus, from 0.4–11.8 mm² (mean 4.0 mm²). No significant differences in mean areas between the 47 patients with occlusive and nonocclusive coronary thrombi were observed in the original size of the coronary artery or in the amount of lumen obliterated by atherosclerotic plaque proximal, at or distal to the coronary thrombus. Likewise, we found no differences in mean areas among the three major coronary arteries in the 47 patients with occlusive thrombi or in the seven with nonocclusive thrombi.

The amount of coronary luminal narrowing in cross-sectional area by atherosclerotic plaques in five categories of narrowing at, proximal and distal to thrombi are summarized in table 2. In 52 (96%) of the 54 coronary arteries with thrombi, the lumens of the arteries at, proximal or distal to the thrombi were already narrowed 76–100% in cross-sectional area by atherosclerotic plaques: in 27 of 42 arteries (64%) examined proximal to the thrombus (in 12 arteries the thrombi began at or virtually at the origin of the coronary artery from the aorta or left main coronary artery), in 35 (66%) of 53 arteries examined distal to the distal site of attachment of the thrombus, and in 41 (76%) of the 54 coronary arteries (or patients) at the site of attachment of the thrombus. Furthermore, in 26 (48%) of the 54 coronary arteries, the lumens of the arteries at, proximal or distal to the thrombi were

narrowed 91–98% in cross-sectional area by atherosclerotic plaques. In 16 (30%) of 54 coronary arteries with thrombi, the site of most severe narrowing by atherosclerotic plaque in the portion of artery examined was within the 2 cm proximal to the thrombus: in 25 of 54 (46%) it was at the site of the thrombus and in 13 of 54 (24%) it was in the 2-cm segment distal to the thrombus. The site of most severe narrowing in coronary arteries was not significantly different between occlusive and nonocclusive thrombi.

The areas in three categories of the coronary arteries not occupied by atherosclerotic plaques proximal and distal to and at the site of attachment of the thrombus are summarized in table 3.

At the site of attachment of thrombi, the underlying atherosclerotic plaques contained extravasated erythrocytes in 21 (39%) of the 54 patients: in 18 (38%) of 47 with occlusive thrombi and in three of seven with nonocclusive thrombi. In none of the 21, however, did the hemorrhage into the pultaceous debris of the plaque appear to compromise the lumen.

Discussion

The relationship of coronary thrombi to AMI has received considerable attention in recent years. Some investigators believe that thrombi precipitate transmural AMI,[1-3, 23-33] primarily because coronary thrombi are frequently found in patients with fatal AMI and, when found, they are located in the artery that perfuses the area of infarcted left ventricular myocardium. Others believe that coronary thrombi follow the AMI, resulting from the slowed flow (in the coronary artery) produced by the infarct itself.[5-15, 17-20] This view is based primarily on the absence of coronary thrombi in a significant percentage of patients with fatal transmural AMI,[4-10, 13, 14, 18] their absence in patients with fatal coronary events other than transmural AMI (sudden coronary death,[15, 34, 35] subendocardial infarcts[14] and angina pectoris[36]), their increased frequency in patients with relatively longer durations of survival after AMI,[5, 10] and their high frequency in patients with severe congestive heart failure or cardiogenic shock with AMI.[11, 12, 37, 38] However, surprisingly little detailed information is available on the status of a coronary artery containing a thrombus in patients with fatal AMI.

The results of the present study raise questions regarding the importance of coronary thrombi in patients with fatal transmural AMI. The major finding in our study is that among patients with fatal AMI, thrombi are found in major coronary arteries that already are severely narrowed by old atherosclerotic plaques at, immediately proximal and/or immediately distal to the site of thrombosis. The lumen of the coronary artery containing the thrombus was already narrowed an average of 79% (range 26–98%) in cross-sectional area by atherosclerotic plaque alone at and within 2 cm proximal and distal to the thrombus; i.e., an "average" coronary artery with a thrombus was severely narrowed (79% in cross-sectional area) at three sites (at, proximal and distal to the thrombus). The "average" coronary arterial narrowing at the site of thrombus, however, actually underestimates the true severity of the narrowing in the vicinity of the thrombus. The site of most severe narrowing in the approximately 6-cm portion of artery examined was within the 2 cm proximal to the thrombus in 16 of 54 (30%) coronary arteries, at the site of thrombus in 25 (46%), and within the 2-cm segment distal to the thrombus in 13 (24%). At the site of most severe narrowing, 96% of the coronary arteries were narrowed 76–98% in cross-sectional area by atherosclerotic plaque, and half were narrowed 91–98%. In contrast, the percent of coronary lumen narrowed by thrombus alone averaged 19% of the original cross-sectional area of the artery (range 2–67%) in the 47 patients with occlusive thrombi, and 7% (range 2–24%) in the seven patients with nonocclusive thrombi. Thus, if thrombus were the only luminal material, the amount of thrombus within the coronary artery, with a few exceptions, probably would not by itself diminish or slow blood flow. A corollary to this statement is that among necropsy patients with fatal AMI, the coronary thrombus, when present, is always superimposed on an atherosclerotic plaque. The exception is coronary embolism, when clot may be present without underlying atherosclerotic plaque.[14, 39] (Patients with coronary emboli, however, an infrequent cause of fatal AMI, were excluded from our study.)

Others[15, 25, 29] have reported that thrombi, when present in a coronary artery in necropsy patients with AMI, most often are found in the more proximal portions of the major coronary arteries. Our study confirmed this observation, at least in regard to the two major branches of the left main coronary artery; but we also found thrombi to be more proximal in the case of nonocclusive than occlusive thrombi. Among the 47 patients with occlusive thrombi, the distance from the origin of the coronary artery to the proximal portion of the thrombus averaged 3.2 cm (range 0–15.5 cm), and among the seven patients with nonocclusive thrombi, 1.4 cm (range 0.5–3 cm). Of the 28 patients with occlusive thrombi in either the left anterior descending or left circumflex coronary artery, this distance averaged 2.1 cm (range 0–6 cm) and with the right coronary artery, 4.8 cm (range 0.5–15.5 cm). Thus, thrombi in the right coronary artery tend to be in its middle third more often than the proximal third.

The length of coronary thrombi in necropsy patients with fatal AMI has been described previously.[19, 28] Of 91 patients studied by Sinapius,[28] the average coronary thrombus was 2.0 cm long. Of 12 patients studied by Erhardt and colleagues,[19] the average coronary thrombus was 2.7 cm long (range 0.4–8.5 cm). Among our 54 study patients, the average coronary thrombus was 1.6 cm long (range 0.5–10 cm); the occlusive thrombi were longer than the nonocclusive thrombi, 1.8 vs 0.7 cm. Also, occlusive thrombi in the right coronary arteries tended to be longer than those in the left anterior descending and left circumflex coronary arteries (2.4 vs 1.4 and 1.1, $p < 0.025$). Because the right and left anterior descending coronary

arteries in adults are over 10 cm long and the left circumflex is usually about 6 cm long, the actual length of a coronary artery occupied by thrombus is small, and in no patient was the entire length of a coronary artery occupied by thrombus. In the right coronary artery, there was a weak, but significant, positive correlation between the length of an occlusive thrombus and the duration of survival of a patient between the time of AMI and death ($p < 0.05$). This relation suggests that thrombi may lengthen or "grow" with time. This finding supports the work of Erhardt and associates,[15, 19] who demonstrated growth of thrombi after AMI by their uptake of ^{125}I-labeled fibrinogen.

In seven of 13 patients, the left circumflex coronary artery with a thrombus was also the dominant posterior artery (i.e., the artery that crossed the crux of the heart and supplied the artery to the atrioventricular node). The left circumflex coronary artery is the dominant posterior artery in only about 12% of a random sample from a large population.[40] The left circumflex appears to be more prone to thrombosis when it is the dominant posterior artery.

Finally, not all thrombi occupy the entire residual lumen of a coronary artery. In seven of our 54 patients (13%), the coronary thrombus was nonocclusive. It occupied on an average only 7% of the cross-sectional area of the coronary artery (range 2–24%) and was an average of 0.7 cm long (range 0.5–1.0 cm). These nonocclusive thrombi probably have little, if any, capacity to interfere with coronary arterial blood flow.

References

1. Herrick JB: Clinical features of sudden obstruction of the coronary arteries. JAMA **59**: 2015, 1912
2. Herrick JB: Thrombosis of the coronary arteries. JAMA **72**: 387, 1919
3. Levine SA, Brown CL: Coronary thrombosis: its various clinical features. Medicine **8**: 245, 1929
4. Branwood AW, Montgomery GL: Observations on the morbid anatomy of coronary artery disease. Scott Med J **1**: 367, 1956
5. Spain DM, Bradess VA: The relationship of coronary thrombosis to coronary atherosclerosis and ischemic heart disease (A necropsy study covering a period of 25 years). Am J Med Sci **240**: 701, 1960
6. Ehrlich JC, Shinohara Y: Low incidence of coronary thrombosis in myocardial infarction. A restudy by serial block technique. Arch Pathol **78**: 432, 1964
7. Meadows R: Coronary thrombosis and myocardial infarction. Med J Aust **2**: 409, 1965
8. Baroldi G: Acute coronary occlusion as a cause of myocardial infarct and sudden coronary heart death. Am J Cardiol **16**: 859, 1965
9. Baroldi G: Lack of correlation between coronary thrombosis and myocardial infarction or sudden 'coronary' heart death. Ann NY Acad Sci **156**: 504, 1969
10. Spain DM, Bradess VA: Sudden death from coronary heart disease. Survival time, frequency of thrombi, and cigarette smoking. Chest **58**: 107, 1970
11. Walston A, Hackel DB, Estes EH: Acute coronary occlusion and the "power failure" syndrome. Am Heart J **79**: 613, 1970
12. Hellstrom HR: Coronary artery stasis after induced myocardial infarction in the dog. Cardiovasc Res **5**: 371, 1971
13. Roberts WC: Coronary arteries in fatal acute myocardial infarction. Circulation **45**: 215, 1972
14. Roberts WC, Buja LM: The frequency and significance of cor-

onary artery thrombi and other observations in fatal acute myocardial infarction. A study of 107 necropsy patients. Am J Med **52:** 425, 1972

15. Erhardt LR, Lundman T, Mellstedt H: Incorporation of ^{125}I-labeled fibrinogen into coronary arterial thrombi in acute myocardial infarction in man. Lancet **1:** 387, 1973

16. Roberts WC: Does thrombosis play a major role in the development of symptom-producing atherosclerotic plaques? Circulation **48:** 1161, 1973

17. Roberts WC: Coronary thrombosis and fatal myocardial ischemia. Circulation **49:** 1, 1974

18. Baroldi G, Radice F, Schmid G, Leone A: Morphology of acute myocardial infarction in relation to coronary thrombosis. Am Heart J **87:** 65, 1974

19. Erhardt LR, Unge G, Boman G: Formation of coronary artery thrombi in relation to onset of necrosis in acute myocardial infarction in man. A clinical and autoradiographic study. Am Heart J **91:** 592, 1976

20. Branwood AW: The development of coronary thrombosis following myocardial infarction. Lipids **13:** 378, 1978

21. Marcus ML, Schuette WH, Whitehouse WC, Baily JJ, Douglas MA, Glancy DL: Use of a video system in the study of ventricular function in man. Am J Cardiol **32:** 175, 1973

22. Dvorak JA, Schuette WH, Whitehouse WC: A simple video method for the quantification of microscopic objects. J Microsc **102:** 71, 1974

23. Schwartz CJ, Mitchell JRA: The relation between myocardial lesions and coronary artery disease. I. An unselected necropsy study. Br Heart J **24:** 761, 1962

24. Mitchell JRA, Schwartz CJ: Arterial Disease. Philadelphia, FA Davis, 1965

25. Harland WH, Holburn AM: Coronary thrombosis and myocardial infarction. Lancet **2:** 1158, 1966

26. Chapman I: Relationships of recent coronary artery occlusion and acute myocardial infarction. J Mt Sinai Hosp **35:** 149, 1968

27. Jørgensen L, Hoerem JW, Chandler AB, Borchgrevink CF: The pathology of acute coronary death. Acta Anaesthesiol Scand **29:** 193, 1968

28. Sinapius D: Beziehungen zwischen koronarthrombosen und myokardinfarkten. Dtsch Med Wochenschr **97:** 443, 1972

29. Sinapius D: Zur morphologie verschliefsender koronarthromben. Lokalisation, länge, zusammensetzung, wachstum. Dtsch Med Wochenschr **97:** 544, 1972

30. Chapman I: The cause-effect relationship between recent coronary artery occlusion and acute myocardial infarction. Am Heart J **87:** 267, 1974

31. Davies MJ, Woolf N, Robertson WB: Pathology of acute myocardial infarction with particular reference to occlusive coronary thrombi. Br Heart J **38:** 659, 1976

32. Rifoldi RL, Hutchins GM: The relationship between coronary artery lesions and myocardial infarcts: ulceration of atherosclerotic plaques precipitating coronary thrombosis. Am Heart J **93:** 468, 1977

33. Horie T, Sekiguchi M, Hirosawa K: Coronary thrombosis in pathogenesis of acute myocardial infarction. Histopathological study of coronary arteries in 108 necropsied patients using serial sections. Br Heart J **40:** 153, 1978

34. Kagan A, Livsic AM, Sternby N, Vihert AM: Coronary-artery thrombosis and the acute attack of coronary heart-disease. Lancet **2:** 1199, 1968

35. Roberts WC, Jones AA: Quantitation of coronary arterial narrowing at necropsy in sudden coronary death. Analysis of 31 patients and comparison with 25 control subjects. Am J Cardiol **44:** 39, 1979

36. Roberts WC, Virmani R: Quantification of coronary arterial narrowing in clinically-isolated unstable angina pectoris. An analysis of 22 necropsy patients. Am J Med **67:** 792, 1979

37. Blumgart HL, Schlesinger MJ, Zoll PM: Multiple fresh coronary occlusions in patients with antecedent shock. Arch Intern Med **68:** 181, 1941

38. Kurland GS, Weingarten C, Pitt B: The relation between the location of coronary occlusions and the occurrence of shock in acute myocardial infarction. Cicrculation **31:** 646, 1965

39. Roberts WC: Coronary embolism: a review of causes, consequences, and diagnostic considerations. Cardiovasc Med **3:** 699, 1978

40. James TN: Anatomy of the Coronary Arteries. New York, PB Hoeber, 1961

Coronary Arterial Disease in Systemic Lupus Erythematosus

Quantification of Degrees of Narrowing in 22 Necropsy Patients (21 Women) Aged 16 to 37 Years

YASMEEN S. HAIDER, M.D.
WILLIAM C. ROBERTS, M.D.
Bethesda, Maryland

The degrees of cross-sectional area luminal narrowing by atherosclerotic plaques of each 5 mm long segment of each of the four major (right, left main, left anterior descending and left circumflex) epicardial coronary arteries in 22 necropsy patients (age 16 to 37 years, 21 women) with systemic lupus erythematosus (SLE) was determined, and the findings were compared to those in 13 control subjects. Of 623 coronary segments (5 mm long) in the patients with SLE, 80 (13 percent) were narrowed 76 to 100 percent (controls = 0 of 431 segments); 125 (20 percent), 51 to 75 percent (controls = 6 percent); 273 (44 percent), 26 to 50 percent (controls = 63 percent) and 145 (23 percent), 0 to 25 percent (controls = 31 percent). Of the 22 patients with SLE, 10 had one or more of the four major coronary arteries narrowed 76 to 100 percent in cross-sectional area, and 12 patients had lesser degrees of narrowing similar to that in the 13 control subjects. The 10 patients with SLE and severe coronary narrowing compared to the 12 patients with SLE and no severe (>75 percent) coronary narrowing had significantly higher (1) mean values of total serum cholesterol (382 versus 290 mg/dl), (2) mean systolic/diastolic systemic arterial pressures (175/119 versus 151/93 mm Hg), (3) frequencies of mitral valvular disease (seven of 10 patients versus none of 12 patients) and (4) frequencies of pericardial adhesions (seven of 10 patients versus three of 12 patients).

Involvement of the heart in systemic lupus erythematosus (SLE) is well established [1–6], and, in patients not treated with corticosteroids, affects the pericardium ("pericarditis"), endocardium ("Libman-Sacks endocarditis") and myocardium ("myocarditis"). After institution of corticosteroid therapy, systemic hypertension with resulting left ventricular hypertrophy became a frequent occurrence in patients with SLE [6]. Additionally, a number of patients with SLE treated with corticosteroids clinically have had manifestations of coronary heart disease and, at necropsy, narrowing of one or more major epicardial coronary arteries. The extent of the coronary narrowing in patients with SLE, however, has not been described in detail. To fill this deficiency, we studied quantitatively at necropsy the four major epicardial coronary arteries in 22 young adult patients with SLE.

PATIENTS STUDIED AND METHODS

The files of the Pathology Branch, National Heart, Lung, and Blood Institute, and those of the Laboratory of Pathology, National Cancer Institute, were reviewed for necropsy patients aged 16 to 40 years with SLE. A total of 22 patients, 21 women and one man (Patient 8, Table I) were found, and they form the basis

From the Pathology Branch, National Heart, Lung, and Blood Institute, National Institutes of Health, Bethesda, Maryland. Requests for reprints should be addressed to Dr. William C. Roberts, Building 10A, Room 3E-30, National Institutes of Health, Bethesda, MD 20205. Manuscript accepted October 2, 1980.

TABLE I Clinical and Necropsy Observations in 10 Necropsy Patients with Systemic Lupus Erythematosus (SLE) and Significant (Group I) Coronary Arterial Narrowing

	Patient										Mean
	1	2	3	4	5	6	7	8	9	10	
Age (yr)	18	21	22	23	24	28	31	32	33	36	27
Race	B	W	W	B	B	W	W	W	B	B	
Age (yr) at onset of SLE	17	18	18	22	20	19	20	25	28	31	22
Duration of SLE (mo)	12	30	48	13	38	100	123	75	53	60	55
Arterial pressure (mm Hg)											
Systolic	210	180	180	150	210	230	210	170	120	90	175
Diastolic	140	130	120	110	130	150	140	105	100	60	118
Prednisone therapy											
Duration (mo)	9	23	40	10	38	31	16	36	53	22	28
Dose (mg/day)	15	12.5	50	40	30	60	30	15	10	90	35
Cushing's syndrome	0	+	+	0	+	+	0	+	0	+	
Subcutaneous edema	+	+	+	+	+	+	0	+	0	+	
Total cholesterol* (mg/dl)	470	445	376	230	560	441	334	408	...	176	382
Urea nitrogen* (mg/dl)	164	116	126	13	120	13	43	115	72	27	81
Creatinine* (mg/dl)	10.0	4.8	...	1.0	9.7	0.7	1.1	...	...	1.2	4
Serum protein total* (g/dl)	5.0	4.7	4.0	5.3	3.8	5.4	4.9	5.1	...	8.3	5
Serum albumin* (g/dl)	1.7	2.0	1.9	2.0	1.4	1.4	2.1	1.7	...	3.4	2
Total urinary protein* (g/day)	29.5	4.0	†	4.4	7.4	3.8	8.0	7.4	...	2.1	8
Hematocrit (%)	30	23	29	29	26	30	28	34	33	30	29
Heart weight (g)	280	350	300	280	500	420	530	780	300	310	405
Body weight (kg)	41	54	55	59	97	37	58	65	35	47	55
Pericardial adhesions	0	+	+	+	0	+	0	+	+	+	
Abnormal mitral valve	0	+	+	+	0	+	+	+	+	0	
5-mm coronary artery segments (no.)	24	21	26	35	27	37	22	38	29	39	30
Segments narrowed (no.)											
51–75%	4	14	8	11	9	3	8	6	5	9	8
76–100%	2	1	3	3	1	31	2	26	1	1	7
Four coronary arteries >75% ↓ (no.)	2	1	2	2	1	3	1	4	1	1	1.8

* Highest value recorded.
† 4+/4+ by qualitative analysis.

of this report. All 22 patients died between 1959 and 1978. Certain clinical and morphologic observations in them are summarized in **Table I and II.** Their ages at death ranged from 16 to 37 years (mean 25 years). Their ages at the time of diagnosis of SLE ranged from 11 to 31 years (mean 21 years). The duration from diagnosis of SLE to death ranged from four to 123 months (mean 51 months). All had positive lupus erythematosus preparations. All were treated with prednisone in varying doses from four to 88 months (mean 34 months), and shortly before death 14 of the 22 patients had typical clinical features of exogenous Cushing's syndrome. None received other immunosuppressant agents. The usual blood hematocrit in the last year of life was less than 37 percent in all 22 patients (mean 30 percent). The highest serum total cholesterol levels (19 patients) ranged from 116 to 560 mg/dl (mean 331 mg/dl); in three, this level was <180 mg/dl and in 12 patients >300 mg/dl. The lowest serum total protein values (20 patients) ranged from 3.8 to 8.3 mg/dl (mean 5.3 mg/dl) and the lowest serum albumin values ranged from 1.3 to 3.7 mg/dl (mean 2.2 mg/dl); in 16 patients the value was <2.5 mg/dl. The highest blood urea nitrogen levels (21 patients) ranged from 8 to 230 mg/dl (mean 81 mg/dl); in 14 patients this value was >40 mg/dl. The highest serum creatine values (18 patients) ranged from 0.3 to 10.0 mg/dl; in eight patients this value was >1.5 mg/dl. Excessive amounts of protein were present in the urine in 20 of 21 patients; in 14, the amount of protein excreted in the urine in 24 hours ranged from 2.1 to 29 g. The following criteria for the nephrotic syndrome were fulfilled by 16 patients: (1) serum total protein >6.0 g/dl; (2) serum albumin <3.0 g/dl; (3) urinary protein >3.5 g/24 hours; (4) serum total cholesterol >240 mg/dl and (5) "pitting" subcutaneous edema. Systemic hypertension (systolic blood pressure >140 mm Hg or diastolic pressure >90 mm Hg or both) at least during the last few months of life occurred in 17 of the 22 patients.

None of the 22 patients had angina pectoris or a clinical event compatible with acute myocardial infarction. By electrocardiogram, none had evidence of "myocardial ischemia" or "damage;" one (Patient 7, Table II), however, had complete right bundle branch block. Neither the parents nor the siblings of the 22 patients with SLE had histories of symptomatic or fatal coronary events while aged 50 years or under.

At necropsy, the hearts weighed from 270 to 780 g (mean 358 g); in seven, the weight was >350 g. Fibrous pericardial adhesions were present in 10 patients; anatomically abnormal mitral valves, of the type seen in SLE [6], occurred in seven patients, one (Patient 8, Table I) of whom also had a thickened aortic valve. None had grossly visible foci of myocardial fibrosis or necrosis.

Each of the four major (left main, left anterior descending, left circumflex and right) epicardial coronary arteries were examined in similar fashion. The hearts were fixed in 10 percent formaldehyde. The four major coronary arteries then were excised intact and following decalcification, if necessary, were cut transversely to their longitudinal axes into 5-mm long

	Patient												Mean
	1	2	3	4	5	6	7	8	9	10	11	12	
Age (yr)	16	16	16	17	18	23	25	28	28	33	35	37	24
Race	B	W	W	W	W	W	B	W	W	W	W	W	
Age at onset SLE (yr)	11	14	12	14	15	23	23	20	21	28	29	31	20
Duration SLE (mo.)	43	25	39	31	36	4	24	89	77	58	72	72	48
Arterial pressure (mm Hg)													
Systolic	160	110	190	140	85	115	185	150	200	125	180	180	151
Diastolic	100	70	110	100	50	80	115	105	100	100	80	110	93
Prednisone therapy													
Duration (mo)	40	19	39	4	13	2	. . .	88	87	4	72	63	39
Dose (mg/day)	60	15	10	50	12.5	250	. . .	10	20	40	10	20	45
Cushing's syndrome	+	+	+	+	+	0	+	+	+	0	+	0	
Subcutaneous edema	0	0	+	+	+	0	0	+	0	0	0	+	
Total cholesterol (mg/dl)*	350	124	278	420	. . .	116	262	328	258	420	233	400	290
Urea nitrogen (mg/dl)*	49	8	165	26	. . .	11	84	95	96	61	67	230	81
Creatinine (mg/dl)*	2.6	0.3	3.1	10.0	1.3	0.8	. . .	1.8	1.0	1.3	9.3	9.0	3.7
Serum protein total (g/dl)	5.2	7.5	5.0	4.0	6.4	6.8	4.4	3.9	5.8	5.0	7.4	4.2	5.5
Serum albumin (g/dl)*	2.0	3.7	2.7	1.6	2.8	2.0	1.3	1.5	2.3	2.0	3.6	2.1	2.3
Total urinary protein (g/day)	6.4	0	. . .†	19.1	. . .	. . .	. . .†	7.1	3.5	7.0	2.5	3.5	6.1
Hematocrit (%)	28	36	41	35	34	29	27	29	25	32	25	33	31
Heart weight (g)	270	270	300	280	285	220	280	420	380	270	575	290	320
Body weight (kg)	77	51	48	52	57	41	. . .	76	. . .	41	54	56	55
Pericardial adhesions	0	0	0	0	0	+	+	+	0	0	0	0	
Abnormal mitral valve	0	0	0	0	0	0	0	0	0	0	0	0	
5-mm coronary artery segments (no.)	21	21	26	19	26	19	23	54	28	21	32	35	27
Segments narrowed (no.)													
51–75%	0	0	1	0	11	0	2	16	0	10	2	6	4
76–100%	0	0	0	0	0	0	0	0	0	0	0	0	0
Four coronary arteries >75% ↓ (no.)	0	0	0	0	0	0	0	0	0	0	0	0	0

* Highest value recorded.

† 4+/4+ by qualitative analysis.

segments. Each segment was labelled sequentially from either its aortic ostium or from its origin from the left main. The number of 5-mm segments examined in each study patient is presented in Tables I and II. The 5-mm segments were labelled, dehydrated, embedded in paraffin, and two histologic sections were cut and stained from each paraffin block. The Movat stain was used on one histologic section. All determinations of luminal narrowing were based on examination of the Movat stained sections because this stain outlines clearly the internal elastic membrane of the arteries. The degree of narrowing was based on histologic examination of each cross section magnified 25 to 50 times. The judgment regarding the degree of luminal narrowing of each 5-mm segment was based on the degree of luminal obliteration within the luminal circle bordered by the internal elastic membrane. The percent of cross-sectional area luminal narrowing was categorized into five separate groups: 0 to 25, 26 to 50, 51 to 75, 76 to 95 and 96 to 100. All histologic sections from all patients were examined by one of us, and the degrees of narrowing were confirmed in several patients by others. (Both the intra- and interobserver errors of this method are approximately 5 percent [7].) The degrees of narrowing of all sections judged by visual inspection under microscopy to be narrowed >75 percent in cross-sectional areas were checked by videoplanimetry. A 95 percent agreement was found between the percent of luminal narrowing by visual inspection under microscopy and that found by planimetry [7].

The narrowing of the epicardial coronary arteries in the 22 study patients was compared to that in 13 control subjects whose coronary arteries were examined in a similar fashion. These subjects ranged in age from 19 to 39 years (mean 31 years), and 12 were women. All died from noncardiac conditions (cancer, eight; suicide, four; acute pancreatitis, one). None had clinical evidence at any time of symptoms of cardiac dysfunction or evidence of myocardial ischemia. All had recorded systolic and diastolic blood pressures <140/90 mm Hg. None received mediastinal irradiation, and only one received prednisone and that for less than two months. The serum total cholesterol values (nine patients) ranged from 130 to 260 mg/dl (mean 186 mg/dl); in four patients, the level was >200 mg/dl. Serum total protein, serum albumin, blood urea nitrogen, serum creatine and urinary protein (five patients) values were normal in each. The hearts ranged in weight from 200 to 375 g (mean 265 g) and the body weights (10 patients) from 35 to 74 kg (mean 57 kg). None had pericardial adhesions, grossly visible foci of myocardial fibrosis or necrosis or mitral valve disease.

RESULTS

Of the 22 patients with SLE, 10 (hereafter called group I) had at least one (total 18; mean 1.8) of their 40 major epicardial coronary arteries narrowed 76 to 100 percent in cross-sectional area by atherosclerotic plaques, and the other 12 patients (hereafter called group II) had none

Patient	5-mm Coronary Segments Narrowed to Various Degrees (no.)				Total 5-mm S/Pt	Total Score*	Mean Score†
	0–25%	26–50%	51–75%	76–100%			
Group I. SLE With Significant Coronary Narrowing							
1	8 (33)	10 (42)	4 (17)	2 (8)	24	48	2.00
2	1 (5)	5 (24)	14 (67)	1 (5)	21	57	2.71
3	5 (19)	10 (38)	8 (31)	3 (12)	26	61	2.35
4	4 (11)	17 (49)	11 (31)	3 (9)	35	83	2.37
5	3 (11)	14 (52)	9 (33)	1 (4)	27	62	2.30
6	0 (0)	0 (0)	3 (8)	34 (92)	37	145	3.92
7	2 (9)	10 (45)	8 (36)	2 (9)	22	54	2.45
8	0 (0)	0 (0)	6 (16)	32 (84)	38	146	3.84
9	10 (35)	13 (45)	5 (17)	1 (3)	29	55	1.90
10	11 (28)	18 (46)	9 (23)	1 (5)	39	78	2.00
Mean	4 (15)	10 (34)	8 (28)	8 (23)	30	79	2.58
Group II. SLE Without Significant Coronary Narrowing							
1	12 (57)	9 (43)	0 (0)	0 (0)	21	30	1.43
2	13 (62)	8 (38)	0 (0)	0 (0)	21	29	1.38
3	14 (54)	11 (42)	1 (4)	0 (0)	26	39	1.50
4	8 (42)	11 (58)	0 (0)	0 (0)	19	30	1.58
5	2 (8)	13 (50)	11 (42)	0 (0)	26	61	2.35
6	6 (32)	13 (68)	0 (0)	0 (0)	19	32	1.68
7	11 (48)	10 (43)	2 (9)	0 (0)	23	37	1.61
8	5 (9)	33 (61)	16 (30)	0 (0)	54	119	2.20
9	11 (39)	17 (61)	0 (0)	0 (0)	28	45	1.61
10	0 (0)	11 (52)	10 (48)	0 (0)	21	52	2.48
11	6 (19)	24 (75)	2 (6)	0 (0)	32	60	1.87
12	13 (37)	16 (46)	6 (17)	0 (0)	35	63	1.80
Mean	8 (34)	15 (53)	4 (13)	0 (0)	27	50	1.79
Control Subjects							
1	5 (31)	11 (69)	0 (0)	0 (0)	16	27	1.69
2	1 (4)	22 (92)	1 (4)	0 (0)	24	48	2.00
3	12 (43)	14 (50)	2 (7)	0 (0)	28	58	2.07
4	5 (12)	25 (58)	13 (30)	0 (0)	43	81	1.88
5	9 (26)	25 (74)	0 (0)	0 (0)	34	59	1.73
6	13 (32)	27 (66)	1 (2)	0 (0)	41	70	1.71
7	21 (47)	24 (53)	0 (0)	0 (0)	45	69	1.53
8	14 (41)	18 (53)	2 (6)	0 (0)	34	56	1.65
9	28 (70)	12 (30)	0 (0)	0 (0)	40	52	1.30
10	0 (0)	25 (81)	6 (19)	0 (0)	31	68	2.19
11	8 (36)	12 (54)	2 (1)	0 (0)	22	38	1.73
12	10 (30)	22 (67)	1 (3)	0 (0)	33	57	1.73
13	9 (22)	31 (77)	0 (0)	0 (0)	40	71	1.77
Mean	10 (31)	21 (63)	2 (6)	0 (0)	33	58	1.77

NOTE: Figures in parentheses are percents. S/Pt = coronary segments per patient.

* Sum derived by assigning a number to each segment in each of the 4 categories of cross-sectional area narrowing as follows: 1 = 0–25% narrowing; 2 = 26–50%; 3 = 51–75% and 4 = 76–100%.

† Number derived by dividing the total number of 5-mm coronary segments per patient into the total score.

of their 48 major coronary arteries narrowed to this extent. Of the 10 study patients in group I, one had all four major coronary arteries narrowed 76 to 100 percent, one had three arteries so narrowed, three had two arteries so narrowed, and five had one artery severely narrowed. All 52 major coronary arteries in the 13 control subjects were narrowed <75 percent in cross-sectional area. The number of 5-mm coronary segments narrowed 76 to 100 percent in cross-sectional area in the 10 patients in group I ranged from one (4 percent) (in four patients) to 34 (92 percent) (mean 23 percent) of the total 5-mm segments per patient (mean = 30/patient) (**Table III**).

The amount of cross-sectional area narrowing in each 5-mm segment of coronary artery in each patient was given a score of 1 to 4 as follows (Table III): 1 = 0 to 25

TABLE IV   Number and Percent of 5-mm Segments of Each of Four Major Coronary Arteries Narrowed (to five Categories) in 22 Necropsy Patients with Systemic Lupus Erythematosus (SLE) and in 13 Necropsy Control Subjects (CS)

Segments Narrowed	Left Main (no.)	Left Anterior Descending (no.)	Left Circumflex (no.)	Right (no.)	Totals (no.)
0–25%					
SLE-I	1 (7)	19 (17)	17 (25)	7 (7)	44 (15)
SLE-II	9 (43)	37 (34)	18 (28)	37 (29)	101 (31)
CS	8 (53)	58 (34)	23 (30)	46 (27)	133 (31)
26–50%					
SLE-I	8 (53)	40 (36)	19 (27)	30 (30)	97 (32)
SLE-II	10 (47)	57 (52)	41 (63)	68 (52)	176 (54)
CS	7 (47)	101 (60)	50 (65)	110 (65)	266 (63)
51–75%					
SLE-I	4 (27)	23 (20)	12 (17)	38 (37)	77 (26)
SLE-II	2 (10)	15 (14)	6 (9)	25 (19)	48 (15)
CS	0	11 (6)	4 (5)	23 (8)	28 (6)
76–95%					
SLE-I	2 (13)	29 (26)	14 (20)	26 (26)	71 (24)
SLE-II	0	0	0	0	0
CS	0	0	0	0	0
96–100%					
SLE-I	0	1 (<1)	8 (11)	0	9 (3)
SLE-II	0	0	0	0	0
CS	0	0	0	0	0
Totals					
SLE-I	15 (100)	112 (100)	70 (100)	101 (100)	298 (100)
SLE-II	21 (100)	109 (100)	65 (100)	130 (100)	325 (100)
CS	15 (100)	170 (100)	77 (100)	169 (100)	431 (100)

NOTE: Figures in parentheses are percents.

percent narrowing, 2 = 26 to 50 percent, 3 = 51 to 75 percent, and 4 = 76 to 100 percent. The number of 5-mm segments of coronary artery examined per patient averaged 30 for each patient in group I, 27 for each patient in group II and 33 for each control subject; the *total score* averaged 79 for each patient in group I, 50 for each patient in group II and 58 for each control subject; the *mean score* was 2.58 ± 0.13 (range 1.90 to 3.90) for each patient in group I, 1.79 ± 0.10 (range 1.38 to 2.48 for each patient in group II and 1.77 ± 0.08 (range 1.30 to 2.19) for each control subject (Table III). The differences in mean scores between the patients in groups I and II and between the patients in group I and the controls was highly significant ($p < 0.005$). Likewise, the mean score for all 22 patients with SLE was 2.15 ± 0.14, a significant difference from the mean score of the 13 control subjects ($p < 0.02$).

In **Table IV** and in **Figure 1** the numbers and percents of 5-mm segments of coronary artery narrowed to each of the five categories of narrowing for the patients with SLE in groups I and II and for the control subjects are summarized. Of the 298 segments of coronary artery examined in the 10 patients in group I, nine (3 percent) were narrowed 96 to 100 percent, and 71 (24 percent) were narrowed 76 to 95 percent. None of the 325 seg-

ments in the 12 patients in group II and none of the 431 segments in the 13 control subjects were narrowed to this degree. Among the coronary segments narrowed 51 to 75 percent in cross-sectional area, the percentage in the patients in group I was 28; in the patients in group II, 13, and in the control subjects, 6. These differences were significant ($p < 0.05$).

None of the 22 patients with SLE had active coronary arteritis or definite histologic evidence of healed coronary arteritis.

COMMENTS

These findings demonstrate that our young adult necropsy patients with SLE on the whole had more extensive and more severe coronary arterial narrowing by atherosclerotic plaques than did our control subjects of similar age and sex. Of the 623 five-millimeter segments of the four major (right, left main, left anterior descending and left circumflex) coronary arteries in the 22 patients with SLE, 80 (13 percent) were narrowed 76 to 100 percent in cross-sectional area by plaques whereas none of the 431 five-millimeter coronary segments in the 13 control patients was narrowed to this degree. Although over-all the 22 patients with SLE had more coronary narrowing than did the control subjects,

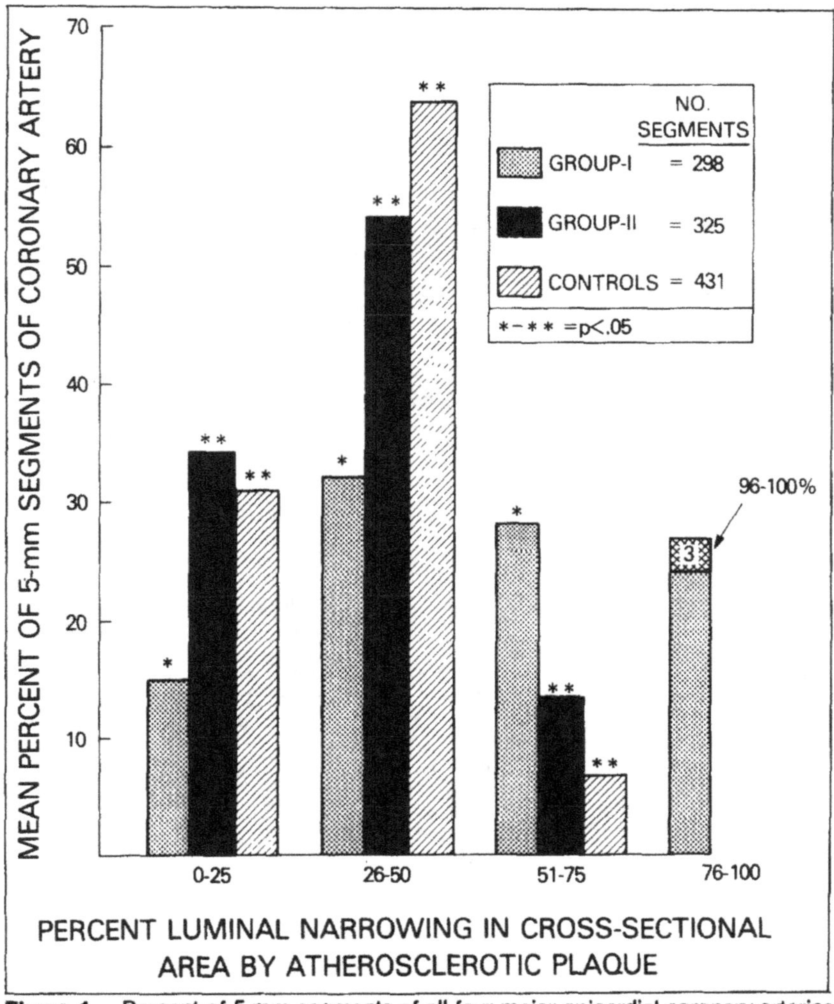

Figure 1. Percent of 5 mm segments of all four major epicardial coronary arteries narrowed to various degrees in 22 necropsy patients (group 1 and group II with systemic lupus erythematosus) and in 13 control subjects.

over half of the patients with SLE had degrees of coronary narrowing similar to the control subjects. Of the 22 patients with SLE, 10 (group I) had 76 to 100 percent narrowing of at least one (average 1.8 of 4.0) major epicardial coronary artery and the other 12 (group II) patients with SLE and all 13 control subjects had lesser degrees of narrowing. By applying a point score to the category of narrowing for each 5-mm segment of coronary artery (Table III), the mean score for the 10 group I patients with SLE was 2.6 and for both the 12 patients with SLE in group II and the controls, 1.8. Thus, some patients with SLE clearly have accelerated coronary atherosclerosis and others do not.

Comparison of a number of clinical parameters between the 10 patients with SLE and severe (>75 percent) coronary narrowing to the 12 patients with SLE and lesser degrees of narrowing disclosed two significant differences. The patients with SLE in group I compared to those in group II had higher mean levels of serum total cholesterol (382 versus 290 mg/dl) and higher mean levels of systemic systolic/diastolic arterial pressures (175/118 mm Hg versus 151/93 mm Hg). Before attributing the accelerated coronary atherosclerosis in the patients with SLE in group I to higher levels of serum total cholesterol and systemic arterial pressures, however, it should be noted that the mean serum total cholesterol (186 mg/dl) and mean systemic systolic/diastolic arterial pressures (118/77 mm Hg) in the control subjects were much lower than those in patients with SLE in either group I or group II and that the patients with SLE in group II and the control subjects had similar degrees of coronary narrowing. Thus, the cause of the accelerated coronary atherosclerosis in the patients with SLE remains unclear, although it seems reasonable to believe that hypercholesterolemia and systemic hypertension are at least contributing factors.

Coronary atherosclerosis, just like systemic hypertension, was rarely described in patients with SLE who died before the introduction of *corticosteroid therapy* for this condition [6,8]. All of our 22 patients with SLE received corticosteroid treatment, but the mean daily dose of prednisone in the 10 patients with SLE in group I was similar to that in the 12 patients with SLE in group II (15 versus 14 mg).

The *nephrotic syndrome* is another factor believed to accelerate coronary atherosclerosis [9]. In our patients with SLE, however, this syndrome was nearly as frequent in group II (eight of 12 patients) as in group I (eight of 10 patients).

Two noncoronary cardiac findings at necropsy were different in the two groups of patients with SLE. Compared to the patients in group II those in group I had a significantly higher frequency of pericardial adhesions (seven of 10 patients versus three of 12 patients) and of mitral valvular disease (seven of 10 patients versus none of 12 patients). The much higher frequency of pericardial and valvular involvement in the patients with SLE and considerable coronary narrowing suggests an immunologic factor as a possible cause of the coronary disease.

REFERENCES

1. Sacks LE: A hitherto undescribed form of valvular and mural endocarditis. Arch Intern Med 1924; 33: 701.
2. Baehr G, Klemperer P, Shifrin A: A diffuse disease of the peripheral circulation (usually associated with lupus erythematosus and endocarditis). Trans Assoc Am Physicians 1935; 50: 139–155.
3. Gross L: The cardiac lesion in Libman-Sacks disease with a consideration of its relationship to acute diffuse lupus erythematosus. Am J Pathol 1940; 16: 375–406.
4. Klemperer P, Pollock AD, Baehr G: Pathology of disseminated lupus erythematosus. Arch Pathol 1941; 32: 569–631.
5. Humphries EM: The cardiac lesions of acute disseminated lupus erythematosus. Ann Intern Med 1948; 28: 12–14.
6. Bulkley BH, Roberts WC: The heart in systemic lupus erythematosus and the changes induced in it by corticosteroid therapy. A study of 36 necropsy patients. Am J Med 1975; 58: 243–264.
7. Isner MJ, Wu M, Virmani R, Jones A, Roberts WC: Comparison of degrees of coronary arterial luminal narrowing determined by visual inspection of histologic sections under magnification among three independent observers and comparison to that obtained by video planimetry. An analysis of 559 five-mm segments of 61 coronary arteries from eleven patients. Lab Invest 1980; 42: 566–570.
8. Jensen G, Sigurd B: Systemic lupus erythematosus and acute myocardial infarction. Chest 1973; 64: 653.
9. Curry CR, Roberts WC: Status of the coronary arteries in the nephrotic syndrome. Analysis of 20 necropsy patients aged 15–35 years to determine if coronary atherosclerosis is accelerated. Am J Med 1977; 63: 183–192.

Transmural Myocardial Infarction in Hypertrophic Cardiomyopathy

A Cause of Conversion from Left Ventricular Asymmetry to Symmetry and from Normal-Sized to Dilated Left Ventricular Cavity

Bruce F. Waller, M.D.; Barry J. Maron, M.D.; Stephen E. Epstein, M.D.; and William C. Roberts, M.D., F.C.C.P.

Herein we will discuss a woman with hypertrophic cardiomyopathy who had an acute myocardial infarction which healed.

CASE REPORT

A 30-year-old woman who died on Oct 8, 1978, first had a precordial murmur noted at age 15 years (1963). At age 17, she was studied at the National Heart Institute. Her mother and father were healthy and free of known cardiac disease. Each of three brothers had precordial murmurs of apparently undetermined etiology, but none had symptoms of cardiac dysfunction. The peripheral arterial pulse had a rapid upstroke and down-stroke. A loud fourth heart sound (S_4), an intermit-tent third heart sound (S_3), and a grade 3/6 systolic ejection-type murmur, which was loudest along the left sternal border and which increased in in-tensity with the Valsalva maneuver, were audible. The ECG (Fig 1) disclosed sinus rhythm, QRS axis of about $-35°$, and voltage changes indicative of severe left ventricular hypertrophy. Chest roentgenogram disclosed an enlarged cardiac silhou-ette and cardiac catheterization (Table 1), a 12-mm Hg peak left ventricular-to-brachial arterial systolic pressure gradient at rest and a 32-mm Hg gradient with the Valsalva maneuver. Left ven-tricular angiography disclosed a small- to normal-sized left ventricular cavity.

At age 18 years, mild exertional dyspnea and fatigue appeared, and a second cardiac catheteriza-tion was performed (Table 1). At age 21, the dys-pnea and fatigue worsened, and the pulmonary

*From the Pathology and Cardiology Branches, National Heart, Lung, and Blood Institute, National Institutes of Health, Bethesda, Md.
Reprint requests: Dr. Roberts, Building 10A, Room 3E30, National Institutes of Health, Bethesda 20205

vascular markings on roentgenogram were more prominent. Propranolol, digoxin, and diuretic ther-apy was begun, and the dyspnea lessened. Elec-trocardiogram (Fig 1) now disclosed sinus rhythm, QRS axis of about $-40°$, and left ventricular hyper-trophy with a "strain" pattern. At age 22, she noted exertional substernal chest pain that disappeared quickly with rest, and the pain recurred intermit-tently during the next eight years. Now on ECG, the QRS axis was about $-60°$; the P-R interval, 0.16 sec.

At age 26, she had two episodes of dizziness. Precordial examination now disclosed a grade 5/6 systolic ejection murmur with a thrill over the left sternal border. Chest roentgenogram (Fig 2) showed an increased cardiothoracic ratio. The ECG (Fig 1) was unchanged from four years earlier. Intracardiac electrophysiologic studies disclosed a normal H-V interval. On M-mode echocardiogram (Fig 3 [9-3-

Table 1—Hemodynamic Data on Patient Studied*

	Age 17 (1965)	Age 18 (1966)
Left ventricle, s/d	112/28	95/20
Brachial artery, s/d	100/66 (70)	95/57 (65)
LV-BA peak systolic gradient, Rest ×Valsalva	12×32	0×20
Left atrium, a:v:m	—	13:20:15
Pulmonary arterial wedge, m	18	—
Pulmonary artery, s/d	40/22	26/13
Right ventricle, s/d	40/22	32/3
Right atrium, a:v:m	—	5:2:2
Cardiac index, L/min/m²	2.8	2.4

*Pressure measurements in mm Hg.

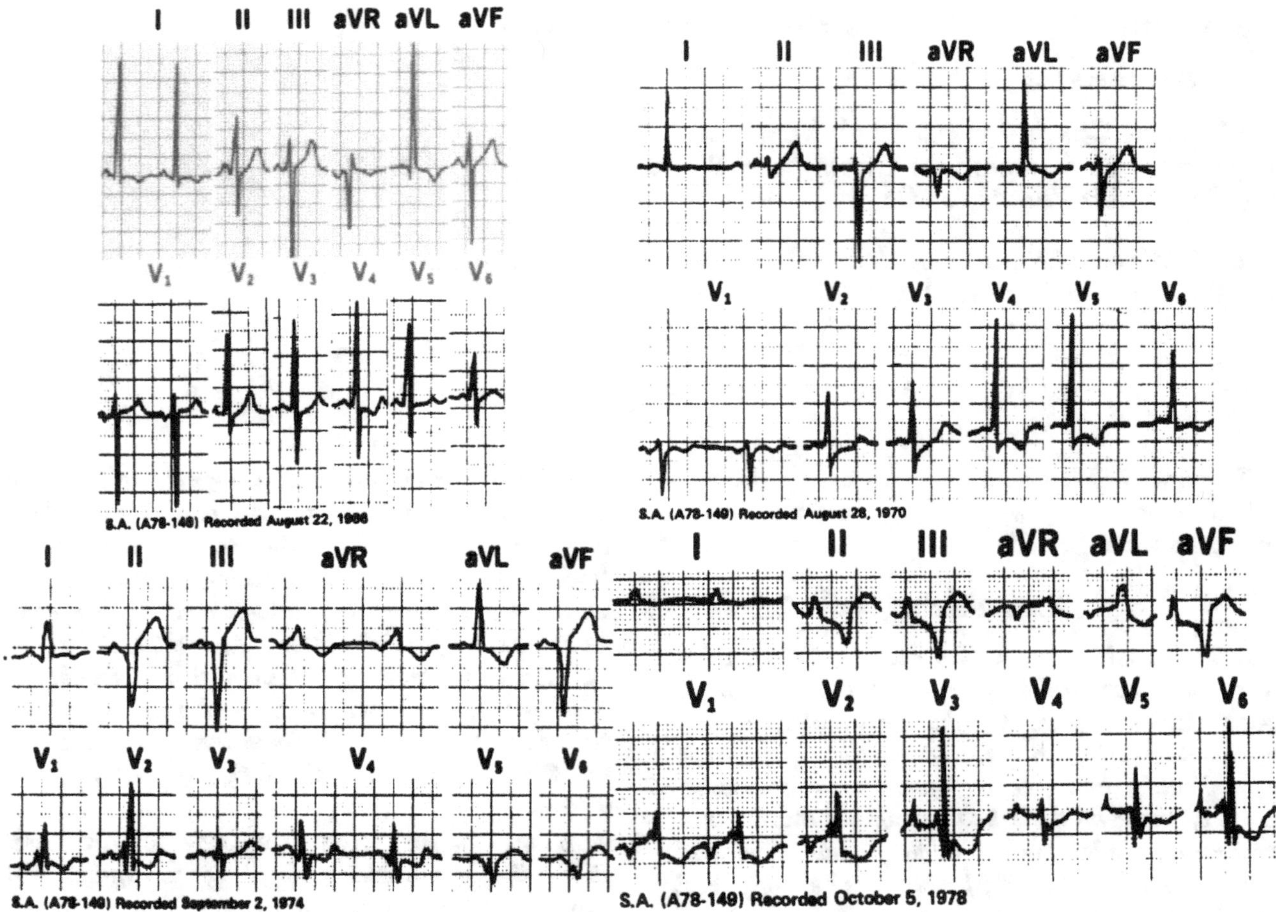

FIGURE 1. Four ECGs from our patient recorded over a 14-year period. During this time, the P-R interval lengthened, the QRS axis became more leftward, the QRS duration widened, and the QRS voltage lessened.

74]), *the ventricular septum was 23 mm in thickness in both diastole and peak systole; the left ventricular free wall measured up to 13 mm in thickness in diastole and 27 mm in peak systole; the left ventricular cavity was about 38 mm in transverse dimension in end-diastole and 23 mm in peak systole. The left ventricular ejection fraction was 50 percent.*

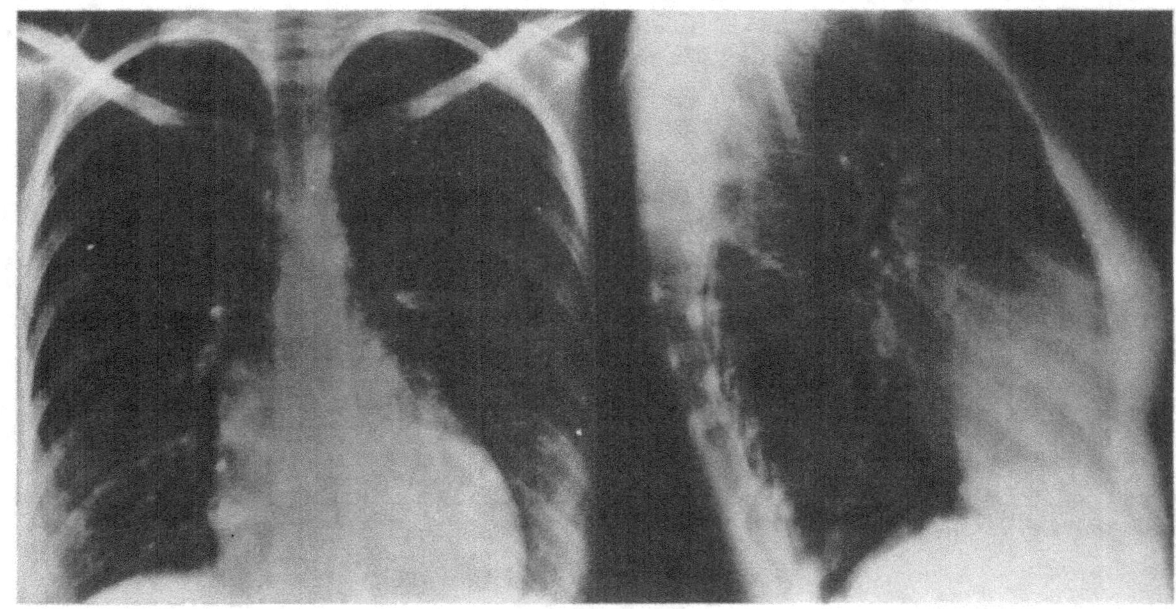

FIGURE 2. Posteroanterior and lateral chest roentgenograms obtained September 1974. The cardiac silhouette is enlarged.

At age 30 (nine months before death), in January 1978, the exertional chest pain became more frequent, and the patient had the first of three episodes of sudden severe dyspnea diagnosed as acute pulmonary edema. In July 1978, an episode of hemoptysis prompted another hospitalization, and repeated ECG disclosed atrial fibrillation. On Sept 9, 1978, while sitting, she had chest pain associated with nausea and sweating. After about two hours of progressive worsening of the pain, she arose and collapsed. The rescue squad arrived a few minutes later and began cardiopulmonary resuscitation, which continued until arrival at the local hospital about 20 minutes later. On ECG after arrival at the hospital, no R waves were present in the precordial leads. Her heart contractions shortly thereafter were adequate to sustain adequate pressure. Later that day, an episode of ventricular tachycardia was documented. During the 20 days in the local hospital, she gradually regained consciousness, and although able to speak, she was unable to speak in sentences or recall past events.

Cardiac enzymes were elevated.

On Sept 28, 1978, she was transferred to the National Heart Institute. Her mental status was unchanged. The systemic blood pressure was 90/62 mm Hg, and the jugular veins were mildly distended. Now no precordial murmur was audible at rest; with straining, a grade 2/6 systolic ejection murmur was heard along the left sternal border. An S₃ also was present. No subcutaneous edema was present, and the liver was not palpable. Chest roentgenogram showed bilateral pleural effusions and a left basilar pulmonary infiltrate, which prevented evaluation of cardiac size. On M-mode echocardiogram (Fig 3 [9-28-78]), the ventricular septum was about 13 mm in thickness in both diastole and peak systole; the left ventricular free wall measured up to 10 mm in thickness in diastole and 14 mm in peak systole; the left ventricular cavity was 50 mm in transverse dimension in diastole and 46 mm in peak systole. The left ventricular ejection fraction was about 10 percent. On Sept 29, 1978, Mobitz II heart block was noted, and a temporary pacemaker

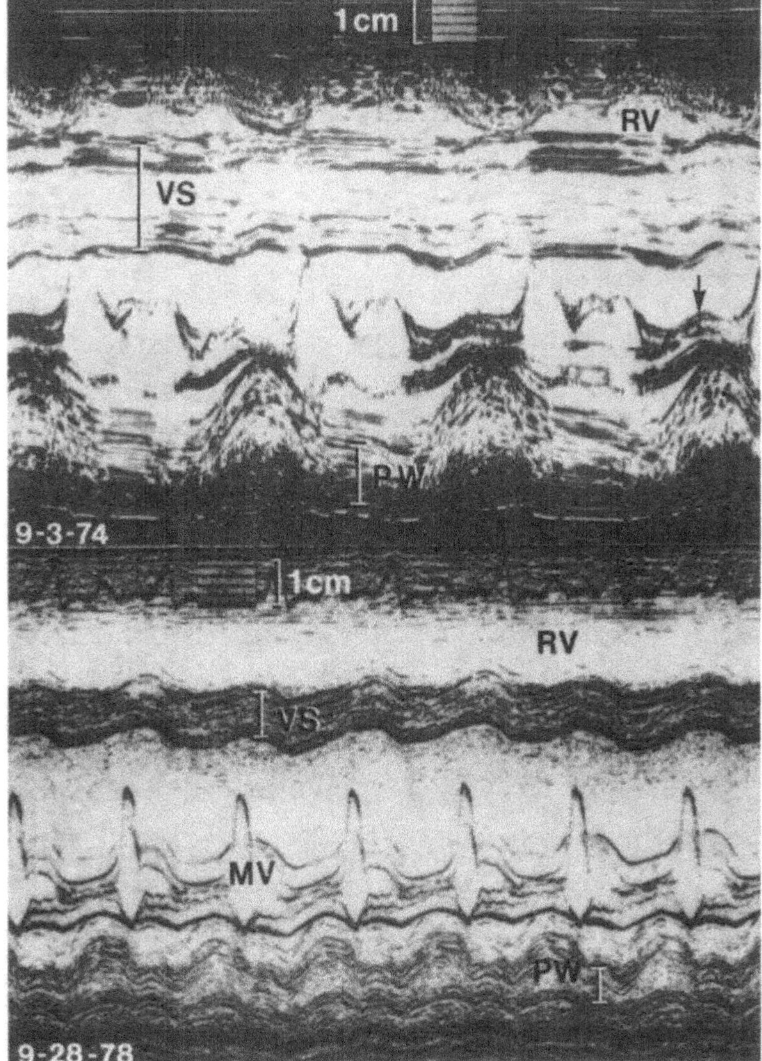

Figure 3. M-mode echocardiograms. The ventricular septum (VS) is much thicker than left ventricular free wall (PW); anterior mitral leaflet moves slightly anteriorly (*arrow*) during ventricular systole, and right (RV) and left ventricular cavities are of normal size. On 9-28-78, VS and PW are of similar thickness, and both are much thinner than on 9-3-74. Anterior mitral leaflet (MV) no longer moves anteriorly during ventricular systole, and left ventricular (LV) cavity is dilated.

was inserted. During the next two days, she became hypotensive, acidotic, febrile, and was intubated. Ventricular fibrillation occurred six days before death, and she was resuscitated. An ECG obtained three days before death (Fig 1) showed a QRS axis of about −75°, widened QRS complexes, and a P-R interval of 0.20 sec. Fatal ventricular fibrillation occurred on Oct 8, 1978.

At necropsy (A78-149), the heart weighed 510 g (Fig 4 and 5). A healed transmural infarct involved the left ventricular free wall and ventricular septum (Fig 4). The ventricular septum measured up to 15 mm in thickness, and the left ventricular free wall up to 20 mm in thickness. Both ventricular and both atrial cavities were dilated. A small fibrous

plaque was present in the left ventricular outflow tract in apposition to the anterior mitral leaflet. The lumens of the major epicardial coronary arteries were narrowed less than 25 percent in cross-sectional area (Fig 5). Some intramural coronary arteries in the ventricular septum had thickened walls and a few had narrowed lumens (Fig 5). On quantitative examination by a method described elsewhere,[1] 53 percent of the area of the ventricular septum (where a transverse section was examined) and 5 percent of the area of the left ventricular free wall were occupied by disorganized myocardial fibers.

COMMENTS

The 30-year-old patient described converted from a nondilated (hypertrophic cardiomyopathy) to a dilated type of cardiomyopathy, and this conversion probably took place about two months before death. When first seen at age 17, she had left

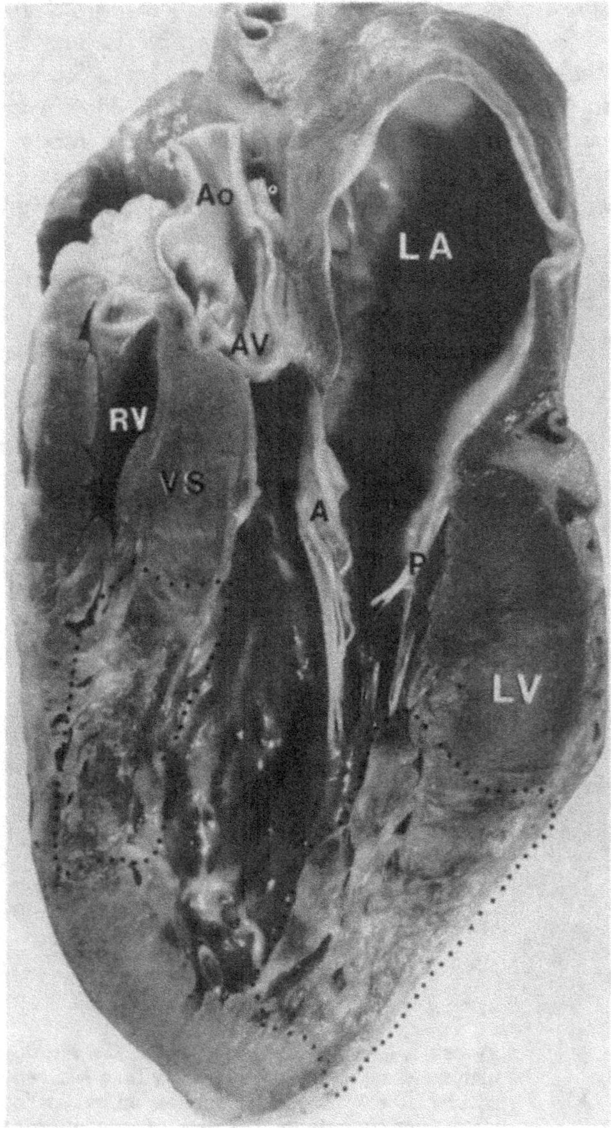

FIGURE 4. Anteroposterior healed transmural infarct (*dotted area*) present in left ventricular free wall (LV) and ventricular septum (VS). Both left ventricular and left atrial (LA) cavities dilated. A = anterior and P = posterior mitral valve leaflets; Ao = ascending aorta; AV = aortic valve; RV = right ventricular cavity.

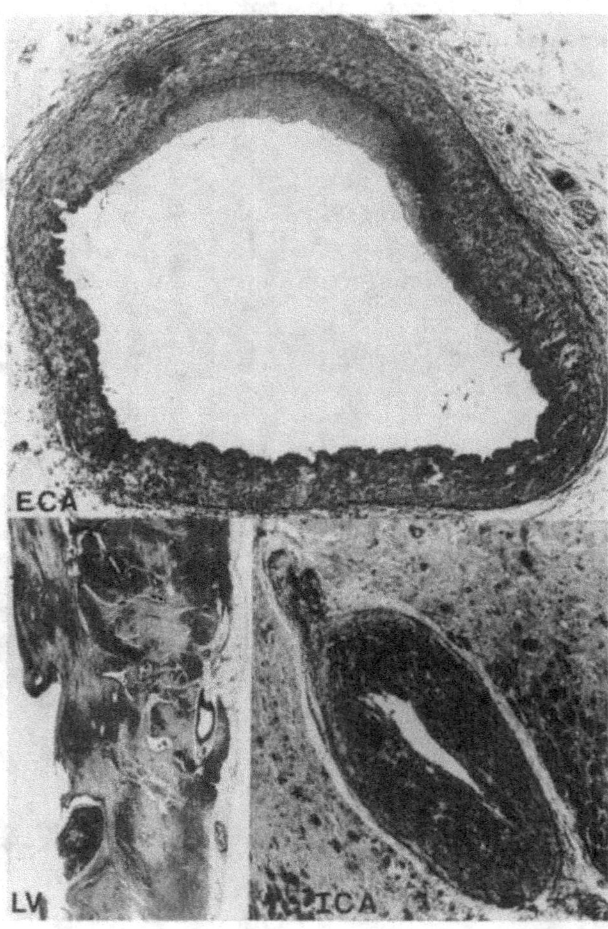

FIGURE 5. The lumens of the major epicardial (E) coronary arteries were virtually normal. (*Upper*): Left anterior descending coronary artery (CA) (original magnification × 14). (*Lower left*): Longitudinal section of wall of left ventricle (LV) which has a transmural scar partially covered by thrombus (original magnification × 4). (*Lower right*): An intramural (1) CA from infarcted ventricular septum has thickened walls and a narrowed lumen (original magnification × 150; all Movat stains).

ventricular hypertrophy by ECG and a normal- to small-sized left ventricular cavity by angiography.

At age 26 the left ventricular cavity was still of normal size by echocardiogram, but by age 30 it was considerably dilated. From ages 17 to 30, the intensity of the precordial murmur, ECG findings, and ventricular wall thicknesses also changed. At age 17, the systolic precordial murmur was of grade 2-3/6 in intensity; at age 26, it was grade 5/6 and associated with a thrill, and by age 30 it was absent. The ventricular septum by echocardiogram at age 26 during both peak systole and end-diastole measured about 23 mm in thickness, but at age 30 was only 15 mm in thickness; the left ventricular free wall at age 26 was 27 mm in thickness during peak systole and 14 mm four years later. The left ventricular ejection fraction (by echocardiogram) diminished from 50 percent at age 26 to 10 percent at age 30.

The cause of the transformation of the left ventricular cavity from a nondilated to a dilated one appears to have been the occurrence of transmural left ventricular infarction. Two months before death this patient had severe substernal chest pain associated with nausea and sweating, and approximately two hours after onset, the heart arrested. Although cardiac resuscitation was successful, the mental processes thereafter were slowed. At necropsy, a considerable portion of left ventricular free wall and ventricular septum was transmurally scarred, yet the epicardial coronary arteries were virtually free of atherosclerotic plaques. Thus, hypertrophic cardiomyopathy is a cause of transmural myocardial infarction in the absence of significant narrowing of the epicardial coronary arteries. Although the occurrence of myocardial infarction in hypertrophic cardiomyopathy is established,[2] the cause of the infarction usually is not discernible. Although usually not apparent clinically, transmural myocardial infarction appears to be the most common cause of ventricular cavity dilation in patients with hypertrophic cardiomyopathy. We have previously studied seven patients with hypertrophic cardiomyopathy in whom transmural left ventricular scars were present at necropsy.[2] Severe chronic congestive heart failure and supraventricular arrhythmias were present in six, left ventricular outflow obstruction under basal conditions was absent or minimal in all seven, angina pectoris was absent in all seven, clinical evidence of acute myocardial infarction was present in only one, and significant narrowing of the major epicardial coronary arteries was present in only one. Transmural myocardial infarction has been present at necropsy in 15 percent of the patients with hypertrophic cardiomyopathy we studied.[2]

SUMMARY

Transmural myocardial infarction in the absence of epicardial coronary arterial narrowing is fairly common at necropsy in patients with hypertrophic cardiomyopathy. Although difficult to diagnose clinically in patients with hypertrophic cardiomyopathy, acute myocardial infarction occasionally has a typical presentation, as in the patient presented in this report. More often, however, transmural acute myocardial infarction in patients with hypertrophic cardiomyopathy is not associated with classic signs and symptoms, but leads to production of, or worsening of, congestive cardiac failure which thereafter usually rapidly progresses. Thus, transmural myocardial infarction is a major complication of hypertrophic cardiomyopathy.

REFERENCES

1 Maron BJ, Roberts WC. Quantitative analysis of cardiac muscle cell disorganization in the ventricular septum of patients with hypertrophic cardiomyopathy. Circulation 1979; 59:689-706

2 Maron BJ, Epstein SE, Roberts WC. Hypertrophic cardiomyopathy and transmural infarction without significant atherosclerosis of the extramural coronary arteries. Am J Cardiol 1979; 43:1086-1102

Non-fatal healed transmural myocardial infarction and fatal non-cardiac disease

Qualification and quantification of coronary arterial narrowing and of left ventricular scarring in 18 necropsy patients

RENU VIRMANI, WILLIAM C ROBERTS

From Pathology Branch, National Institutes of Health, Bethesda, Maryland, USA

SUMMARY   A qualitative and quantitative analysis of the amount of myocardial scarring and the degree and extent of coronary arterial narrowing by atherosclerotic plaque in the entire lengths of each of the four major epicardial coronary arteries is described in 18 necropsy patients with healed transmural myocardial infarcts and death from a non-cardiac condition. An average of 30 per cent of the basal half and 38 per cent of the apical half of the left ventricular wall was scarred. The nine patients with clinical evidence of previous acute myocardial infarction tended to have larger left ventricular scars than the nine patients without such evidence but the difference was not significant. An average of 26 cm (51 5 mm segments) of coronary artery were examined from each patient and 25 cm (49 5 mm segments) from each of 19 control subjects. Of 924 segments examined in the 18 patients, 292 (32%) were 76 to 100 per cent narrowed in cross-sectional area (controls=5); 321 (35%) were 51 to 75 per cent narrowed (controls= 34%); 210 (23%) were 26 to 50 per cent narrowed (controls=44 %), and 101 (11%) were 0 to 25 per cent narrowed (controls=17%). The extent of severe narrowing of 75 per cent or more was similar (25%) in the left anterior descending and left circumflex coronary arteries; the right was the most severely narrowed artery and the left main was not severely narrowed in any patient. Excluding, then, the left main artery, the amount of severe narrowing in the proximal and distal halves of the other three vessels was similar. The amount of severe narrowing was not related to the age at death or to heart weight, but was greater in patients with hypertension or with a history of acute myocardial infarction.

Much is now known about the amount of left ventricular damage and the extent of coronary arterial narrowing present in patients dying either suddenly, or with acute myocardial infarction, or with chronic congestive cardiac failure after the healing of an acute infarction, but information on these two points is lacking in patients with old healed infarcts who subsequently die of non-cardiac conditions. The present report attempts to fill this void by describing the findings in 18 such patients, all of whom died at least two years after their acute myocardial infarction.

Patients and methods

Eighteen patients were studied. All fulfilled the

Received for publication 28 November 1979

following criteria: (1) death from a non-cardiac cause; (2) a previous healed myocardial infarction involving at some point >50 per cent of the thickness of the left ventricular wall; (3) an absence of left ventricular myocardial necrosis; (4) no clinical evidence of congestive cardiac failure; (5) normal sized right and left ventricular cavities; (6) no cardiac surgery having been undertaken; and (7) no other cardiac disease present. Clinical details are set out in Table 1. Nine had a history of acute myocardial infarcts in the past, four of them (cases 2, 3, 6, and 9) having had two acute infarcts documented clinically. Three patients had had angina pectoris. Nineteen age and sex matched control subjects were also studied. All fulfilled the following criteria: (1) death from a non-cardiac condition; (2) no symptoms suggesting myocardial ischaemia

Table 1 *Clinical and morphological observations in 18 patients with non-fatal healed transmural myocardial infarcts and fatal non-cardiac conditions*

Case no.	Age (y)	Sex	Interval (years) 1st AMI to death	Angina pectoris	Hyper-tension	Diabetes	Total serum cholesterol (mg/100 ml)*	Heart weight (g)	Percentage LV wall scarred Apical	Basal	No. 5 mm CA segments examined	No. (%) 5 mm segments > 75% narrowed	No. CA > 75% narrowed	Cause of death
Clinically apparent acute myocardial infarct														
1	60	M	22	0	+	0	325	540	0	30	56	17 (30)	3	Hodgkin's disease
2	62	M	13	0	+	0	—	520	25	20	63	6 (9)	1	Bowel infarct
3	63	M	8	0	0	0	—	420	35	30	37	14 (38)	2	Trauma
4	63	M	10	0	–	0	—	510	100	35	57	16 (28)	3	Trauma
5	65	M	14	0	0	0	—	310	25	30	55	6 (11)	1	Carcinoma, lung
6	73	F	2	0	–	+	—	535	45	25	42	25 (59)	3	Carcinoma, colon
7	78	M	5	+	+	0	—	475	35	50	43	11 (26)	1	Renal failure
8	78	M	6	0	0	+	—	430	35	30	64	36 (56)	3	Carcinoma, pancreas
9	80	M	16	0	+	0	—	420	100	60	44	17 (39)	2	Carcinoma, lung
Clinically silent acute myocardial infarct														
10	50	M	—	+	+	0	—	510	100	60	75	21 (28)	3	Acute pancreatitis
11	55	M	—	+	+	0	252	380	0	35	40	22 (55)	3	Carcinoma, mouth
12	57	M	—	0	0	0	180	310	20	15	40	5 (13)	2	Hodgkin's disease
13	62	M	—†	0	0	0	—	500	25	25	48	10 (21)	2	Carcinoma, lung
14	64	F	—	0	+	+	—	360	0	15	73	21 (29)	2	Stroke
15	65	M	—	0	+	0	220	365	20	25	49	24 (49)	3	Carcinoma, lung
16	66	M	—	0	0	0	185	370	25	20	57	10 (18)	2	Carcinoma, pancreas
17	69	F	—	0	0	0	—	310	100	20	50	9 (18)	2	Carcinoma, mouth
18	72	M	—	0	0	+	—	490	0	25	31	4 (13)	1	Stroke

Abbreviations: AMI, acute myocardial infarction; CA, coronary arteries. Hypertension = > 140 systolic or > 90 mmHg diastolic.
*For conversion to SI units multiply by 0·0259 to arrive at mmol/l.
†Electrocardiogram 19 years before death showed changes typical of a healed myocardial infarct.

or cardiac dysfunction; (3) no systemic hypertension (blood pressure > 140 mmHg systolic and/or > 90 mmHg diastolic); (4) no cardiomegaly; (5) no left ventricular fibrosis or necrosis; and (6) no history of mediastinal irradiation. Seven of the 19 had died of carcinoma (pancreas two, ovary two, prostate two, tongue one); five of leukaemia; six of lymphoma; and one of sideroblastic anaemia.

The coronary arteries in the 18 patients and 19 control subjects were studied in a similar fashion. The hearts were fixed in 10 per cent formalin for at least one day. The four major epicardial coronary arteries (right, left main, left anterior descending, and left circumflex) were removed intact, x-rayed (Fig. 1), decalcified, and then cut transversely to their longitudinal axes into segments 5 mm in length. Each segment was labelled sequentially either from its aortic ostium or from its origin from the left main coronary artery. The segments were dehydrated and embedded in paraffin, and at least two histological sections were cut from each and stained, one by haematoxylin and eosin and the other by the Movat method. The degree of luminal narrowing within the internal elastic membrane by atherosclerotic plaque was based on histological examination of the Movat stained cross-sections magnified 25 to 50 times. The percentage of cross-sectional area luminal narrowing of each section was graded into four categories: 0 to 25, 26 to 50, 51 to 75, and 76 to 100. As a check, the degree of cross-sectional narrowing in three of the 18 patients was measured by planimetry and a 96 per cent agreement was found between this and the visual estimation on microscopy.

The location and the extent of left ventricular scarring was determined after cutting the ventricles at approximately 1 cm intervals beginning at the left ventricular apex and extending to about 2 cm caudal to the posterior atrioventricular sulcus. The ventricular incisions were made parallel to the posterior atrioventricular sulcus. In most cases six slices of the ventricles were examined, including three from the basal half and three from the apical half. The extent of left ventricular scarring was determined by circumferential measurement of it in one of the three apical slices and in one of the three basal slices, choosing the one with the maximal amount of scarring in each group. The percentage of scarring was determined by dividing the circumferential length of the transmural scar by the total circumference of the slice (including the ventricular septum).

Results

In the 18 patients, 71 major epicardial coronary arteries were examined (right, left main, left anterior descending, and left circumflex). The left

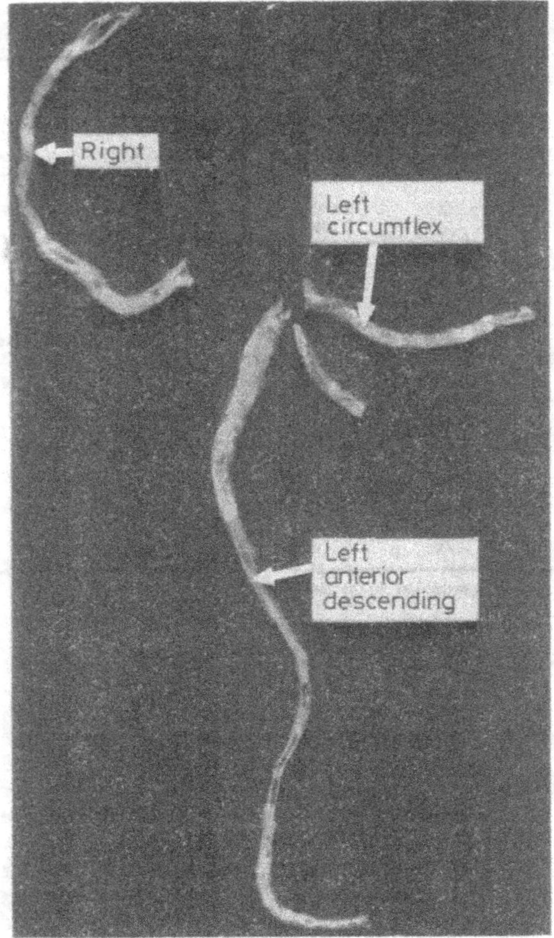

Fig. 1 *Radiograph of the major epicardial coronary arteries after removing them from the heart at necropsy. Calcific deposits are present in all of them. The short segment is the left main coronary artery.*

Table 2 *Summary of number of 5 mm long segments of major epicardial coronary artery examined*

Coronary artery	Number (range [mean]) of 5 mm segments per patient	
	Patients (18)	Controls (19)
Right	6–28 (16·7)	11–37 (19·7)
Left main	1– 6 (2·0)	1– 3 (1·6)
Left anterior descending	8–39 (19·4)	10–32 (18·1)
Left circumflex	3–24 (11·4)	3–29 (10·1)
Total segments of four coronary arteries per patient	24–67 (49·5)	27–75 (49·4)

and six had one. Thus, of 74 major coronary arteries studied, 15 (20%) were narrowed to this extent, an average of 0·8 per control subject. If the left main is excluded, the percentage rises to 27, that is 15 of the 55 other major coronary arteries studied.

None of the patients or the control subjects had a thrombus in any of the four major coronary arteries.

The numbers of 5 mm long segments of coronary arteries examined are summarised in Tables 2 and 3, and in Fig. 2. Of the 924 segments examined in the 18 patients, 292 segments (32%) were 76 to 100 per cent narrowed in cross-sectional area (controls =5%, $p < 0.005$), 321 (35%) were 51 to 75 per cent narrowed (controls =34%), 210 (23%) were 26 to 50 per cent narrowed (controls =44% $p < 0.005$), and 101 (11%) were 0 to 25 per cent narrowed (controls =17%). In the patients the percentage

main was not examined in one patient. In the 19 control subjects 74 major coronary arteries were examined (the left main was not examined in two subjects). Four patients had one, seven had two, and seven had three of their four major coronary arteries narrowed 76 to 100 per cent in cross-sectional area by atherosclerotic plaque. Thus, of the possible 71 major coronary arteries studied, 39 (55%) were narrowed to this extent, an average of 2·2 per patient. If the left main coronary artery is excluded the percentage rises to 72, that is 39 of the 54 other major coronary arteries. In the 10 control subjects one had three arteries narrowed by >75 per cent in cross-sectional area, three had two,

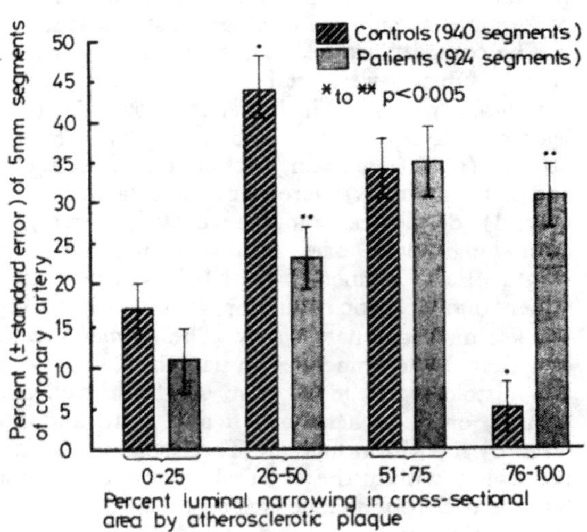

Fig. 2 *Number and percentage of 5 mm segments of all four major coronary arteries narrowed to various degrees in the 18 study patients and in the 19 control subjects.*

Table 3 *Number and percentage of 5 mm segments of four major epicardial coronary arteries showing the four grades of cross-sectional luminal narrowing*

| Coronary artery | | Per cent cross-sectional area luminal narrowing | | | | | | | | | |
| | | 0–25 | | 26–50 | | 51–75 | | 76–100 | | Totals | |
		P	C	P	C	P	C	P	C	P	C
Left main*	No.	5	7	13	12	17	9	0	0	35	28
	%	(14)	(25)	(37)	(43)	(49)	(32)	0	0	(100)	(100)
Left anterior	No.	58	49	92	157	123	111	92	27	365	344
descending	%	(16)	(14)	(25)	(46)	(34)	(32)	(25)	(8)	(100)	(100)
Left circumflex	No.	24	51	56	63	74	75	62	4	216	193
	%	(11)	(26)	(26)	(33)	(34)	(39)	(29)	(2)	(100)	(100)
Right	No.	14	50	49	181	107	127	138	17	308	375
	%	(5)	(13)	(16)	(48)	(35)	(34)	(45)	(5)	(100)	(100)
Totals	No.	101	157	210	413	321	322	292	48	924	940
	%	(11)	(17)	(23)	(44)	(35)	(34)	(32)	(5)	(100)	(100)

*Sections not examined in one patient and in two control subjects.
Abbreviations: P, patients; C, control subjects.

of segments narrowed was similar at all levels of severity in the left anterior descending and left circumflex coronary arteries, the right coronary artery showed the highest incidence of severe narrowing, and the left main was not severely narrowed in any patient. In the control subjects the incidence of narrowing in each of the four major coronary arteries was similar at the four categories of narrowing and was not significantly different at any level (Fig. 3). The percentage of segments narrowed 76 to 100 per cent in cross-sectional area was significantly higher in the proximal half of the right and left anterior descending coronary arteries than it was distally (Fig. 4).

The weight of the heart, the location of the healed myocardial infarcts, and the amount of left ventricular scarring are summarised in Tables 1 and 4 and illustrated in Fig. 5 to 8. The heart weight was normal (<400 g in men and <350 g in women) in six and increased in 12 patients. The

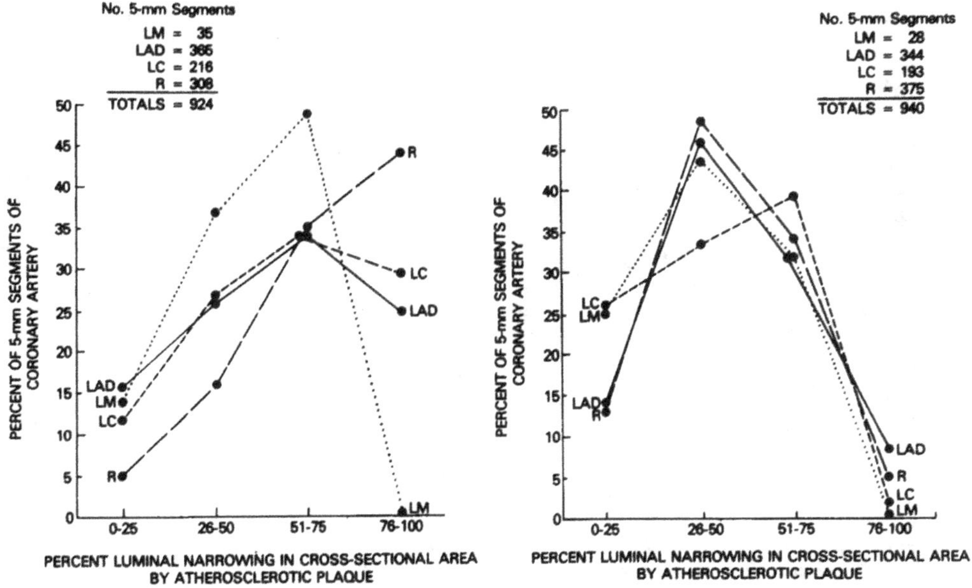

Fig. 3 *Percentage of 5 mm segments of each of the four major coronary arteries narrowed to various degrees in the 18 patients (left) and in the 19 control subjects (right).*

Table 4 *Location of transmural left ventricular scar and percentage of 5 mm segments of four major coronary arteries narrowed 51 to 75 per cent and 76 to 100 per cent in cross-sectional area by atherosclerotic plaque*

Case no.*	Percentage LV wall scarred		Dominant posterior coronary artery	No. 5 mm segments	Percentage 5 mm segments narrowed 51–75 per cent in cross-sectional area				Percentage 5 mm segments narrowed 76 to 100 per cent in cross-sectional area			
	Apical half	Basal half			R	LM	LAD	LC	R	LM	LAD	LC
Posterior wall												
14	0	15	R	73	21	37	19	30	79	0	6	0
18	0	25	LC	31	86	100	92	64	0	0	0	36
1	0	30	R	56	29	0	38	40	59	0	12	40
11	0	35	R	40	15	100	71	30	62	0	20	70
12	20	15	R	40	22	—	42	23	22	0	0	54
16	25	20	R	57	62	0	22	0	0	0	28	0
13	25	25	R	48	39	0	17	45	33	0	0	36
5	25	30	R	55	36	100	45	33	27	0	0	0
3	35	30	R	37	19	100	80	48	81	0	0	12
8	35	30	R	64	36	50	23	42	54	0	77	34
6	45	25	R	42	33	0	13	55	44	0	87	45
7	35	50	R	43	10	0	23	0	90	0	0	0
4	100	35	R	57	65	100	33	58	25	0	29	33
9	100	60	R	44	54	100	43	70	81	0	0	12
Anterior wall												
2	25	20	LC	63	6	0	14	17	0	0	27	0
15	20	25	R	49	39	100	26	30	61	0	32	70
17	100	20	LC	50	33	50	33	33	17	0	33	0
10	100	60	R	75	29	0	46	28	48	0	18	72

Abbreviations: LAD, left anterior descending coronary artery; LC, left circumflex coronary artery; LM, left main coronary artery; LV, left ventricular; R, right coronary artery.
*The case number corresponds to the case number in Table 1. The patients are listed in order of progressively increased amounts of left ventricular scarring.

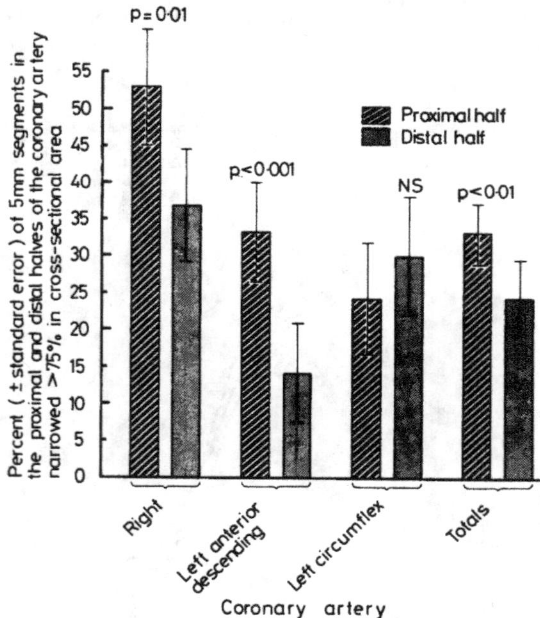

Fig. 4 *Percentage of 5 mm segments of the right, left anterior descending, and left circumflex coronary arteries narrowed 76–100% in cross-sectional area in the proximal and distal halves of each of the 3 arteries in the 18 patients.*

most frequent location of the transmural infarcts was the posterior wall of the left ventricle (14 patients). In four patients the infarct involved only the basal half of the left ventricle. One patient (case 10, Table 1) had a small left ventricular thrombus (about 1 cm in diameter) and he had been in septic

Table 5 *Mean percentage of segments in four major coronary arteries narrowed > 75 per cent in cross-sectional area in 18 patients: comparison of four clinical or morphological indices*

Indices analysed	No. of patients	Mean percentage (±standard error) of coronary segments narrowed > 75% in cross-sectional area	p value
Age (y)			
46–65	10	27 ±4	> 0·05
> 65	8	33 ±7	
History of acute myocardial infarction			
Present	9	35 ±6	< 0·05
Absent	9	24 ±4	
Systemic hypertension			
Present	8	38 ±5	< 0·05
Absent	8	25 ±5	
Heart weight			
Increased*	12	31 ±4	> 0·05
Normal	6	26 ±8	

* > 400 g in men and > 350 g in women.

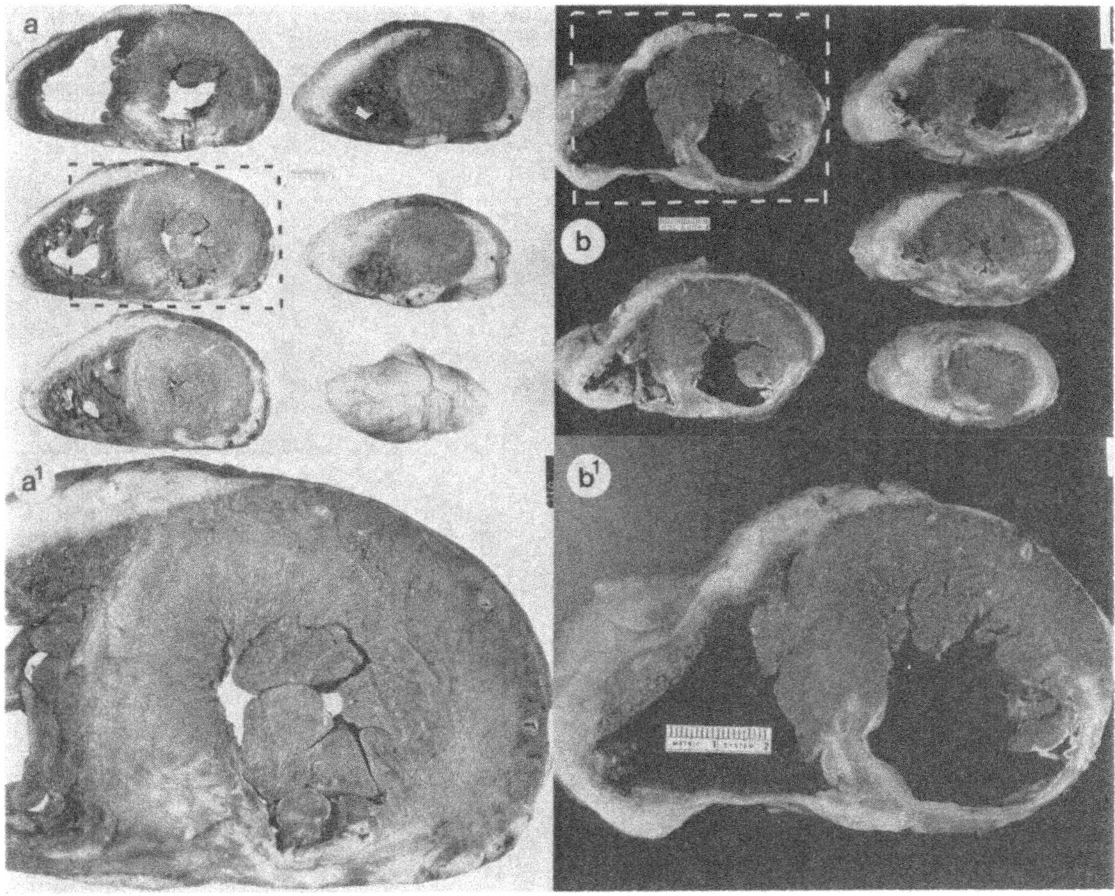

Fig. 5   *Transverse slices of the cardiac ventricles in case 1 (a and a¹) and in case 7 (Table 1) (b and b¹).*
Transverse slices of the cardiac ventricles illustrating transmural healed posterior wall myocardial infarcts.
a¹ and b¹ are close-up views of the slices from a and b enclosed by the interrupted line. The most apical portion of
the heart in b is not shown.

shock for several days before death from acute pancreatitis.

The relation between the site of the left ventricular transmural scar and the amount of coronary narrowing in each of the 18 patients is tabulated in Table 5. In nine of the 14 with *posterior* wall scars, the dominant posterior perfusing coronary artery (right in 13; left cirumflex in one) had a higher percentage of segments severely narrowed ($>75\%$) than the left anterior descending coronary artery. In two of the four patients with *anterior* wall scars, the left anterior descending coronary artery had a higher percentage of segments severely narrowed ($>75\%$) than the dominant posterior perfusing coronary artery (right in two, left circumflex in

two). The location of the transmural scar, therefore, did not necessarily indicate which of the coronary arteries was most narrowed.

Table 5 shows the relation of age, hypertension, a history of infarction, and heart weight in the 18 patients to the mean percentage of coronary segments severely narrowed ($>75\%$). The second and third of these were significantly correlated ($p < 0.05$).

Comments

Although none of the 18 patients died from coronary heart disease, and only three had angina, the

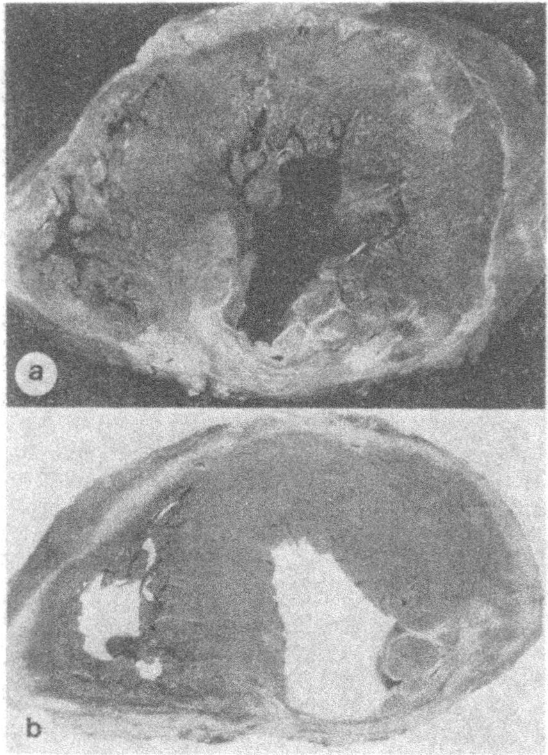

Fig. 6   *Single transverse slices of cardiac ventricles in case 3 (a) and in case 5 (Table 1) (b), showing transmural posterior wall healed myocardial infarcts in each.*

amount of coronary narrowing they had was extensive. Two or three of the four major epicardial coronary arteries examined were narrowed by more than 75 per cent in cross-sectional area by atherosclerotic plaques in 14 of them. In none, however, was the left main coronary artery narrowed to this extent. Furthermore, the total length of these major arteries so severely narrowed was considerable—292 of the 924 5 mm long segments of artery examined (32%) compared with 5 per cent in the control subjects. Another 321 segments (35%) were narrowed in cross-sectional area to between 51 and 75 per cent. Thus, 61 per cent of the total length of the four major coronary arteries were more than 50 per cent narrowed in cross-sectional area by atherosclerotic plaque. Only 11 per cent of the segments were 25 per cent narrowed or less.

Even in the four patients in whom only one major coronary artery was more than 75 per cent narrowed, plaque was extensive, with that degree of narrowing being present in between 27 and 90 per cent of

segments examined. Such extensive coronary narrowing is similar to that observed in patients with fatal acute myocardial infarcts[1] and sudden coronary death[2] but less than that found in patients with unstable angina pectoris.[3]

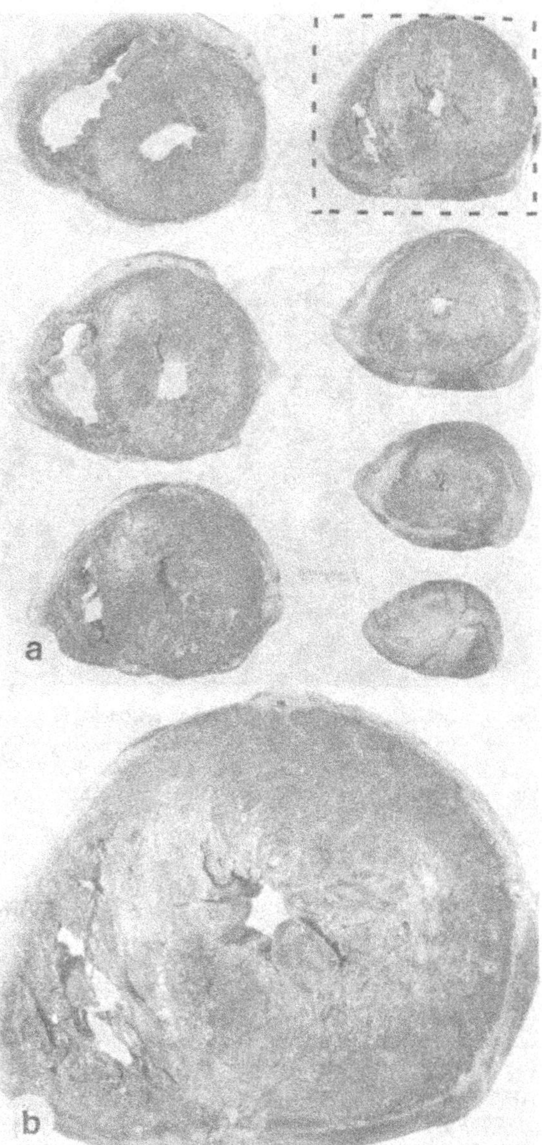

Fig. 7   *Transverse slides (a) of the cardiac ventricles in case 15 (Table 1); this patient has a healed transmural anteroseptal myocardial infarct. The close-up (b) is of the slice enclosed by the interrupted line in a.*

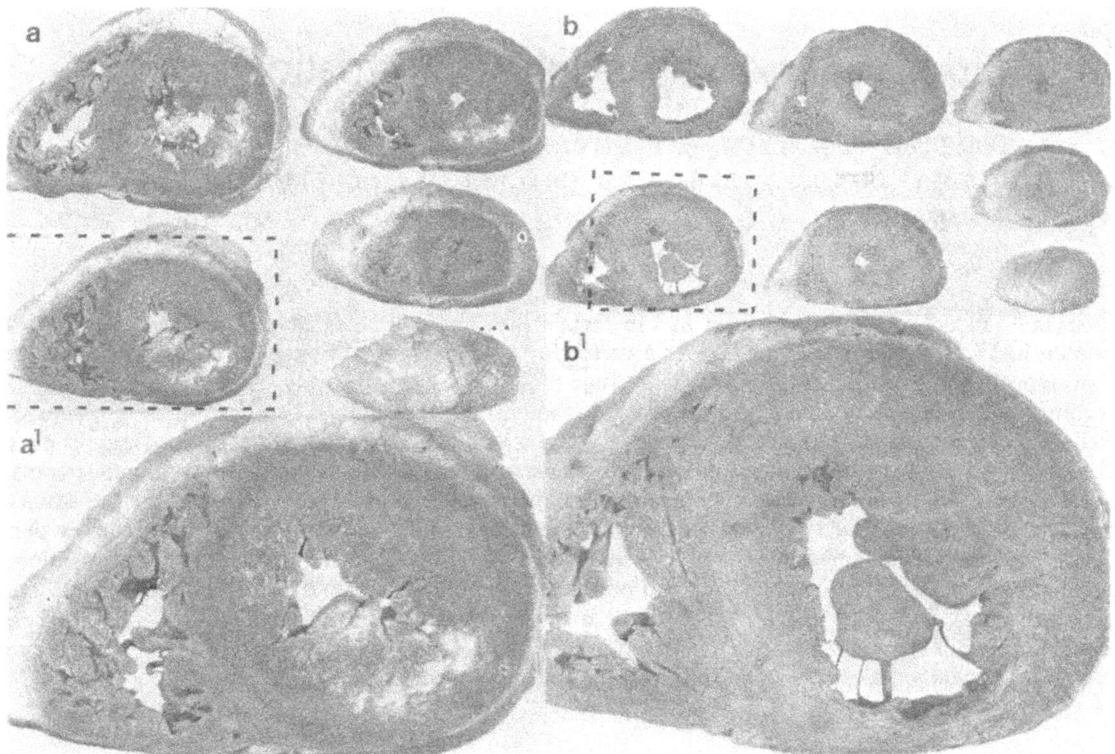

Fig. 8 *Transverse slices of the cardiac ventricles in case 16 (a and a¹) and in case 18 (Table 1) (b and b¹) showing healed posterior wall transmural myocardial infarcts. a¹ and b¹ are close-up slices of the slices in a and b enclosed by the interrupted line.*

Comparison of the two groups of patients with and without a previous clinical history of acute myocardial infarction disclosed a significant difference between them. Severe narrowing ($> 75\%$) was more extensive in the former, 35 per cent ± 6 of the 5 mm segments compared with 24 ± 4.

Although none of our patients died from cardiac disease, the sizes of the left ventricular scars at necropsy were surprisingly large. With the left ventricle arbitrarily divided into two halves, apical and basal, the amount of scarring in the basal half ranged from 15 to 60 per cent (mean 30) and that in the apical half, from 0 to 100 per cent (mean 38%). The nine patients with an overt previous acute myocardial infarction also had larger myocardial scars on average than the nine without this history, but the difference was not significant.

References

1 Roberts WC, Jones AA. Quantitation of coronary arterial narrowing at necropsy in acute transmural myocardial infarction: an analysis of 27 patients and comparison of findings to those in 22 control subjects. *Circulation* (In press).
2 Roberts WC, Jones AA. Quantitation of coronary arterial narrowing at necropsy in sudden coronary death. Analysis of 31 patients and comparison with 25 control subjects. *Am J Cardiol* 1979; **44**: 39–45.
3 Roberts WC, Virmani R. *Quantification* of coronary arterial narrowing in clinically-isolated *unstable angina* pectoris: an analysis of 22 necropsy patients. *Am J Med* 1979; **67**: 792–9.

Requests for reprints to Dr William C Roberts, Pathology Branch, National Heart, Lung and Blood Institute, National Institutes of Health, Bethesda, Maryland 20014, USA.

Accuracy of Angiographic Determination of Left Main Coronary Arterial Narrowing

Angiographic–Histologic Correlative Analysis in 28 Patients

JEFFREY M. ISNER, M.D., JOAN KISHEL, M.D., KENNETH M. KENT, M.D., JAMES A. RONAN, JR., M.D., ALLAN M. ROSS, M.D., AND WILLIAM C. ROBERTS, M.D.

SUMMARY To evaluate the accuracy of coronary angiography in identifying severe narrowing of the left main coronary artery (LMCA), the degree of narrowing observed by angiography was compared to that observed at necropsy in 28 patients with symptomatic coronary heart disease in whom angiography had been performed within 40 days of death. The angiograms were evaluated independently by three experienced angiographers. In 20 of the 28 patients (71%), the degree of narrowing of the LMCA was either under-estimated (13 patients) or overestimated (10 patients) by two or three of three angiographers; of 84 angiographic judgments made by the three angiographers in the 28 patients, 54 (64%) were underestimates (33 judgments, 39%) or overestimates (21 judgments, 25%) of the degree of LMCA narrowing. Of 12 LMCAs narrowed 76–100% in cross-sectional area at necropsy, six were underestimated at preoperative angiography by two or three of three angiographers; of 12 LMCAs narrowed 51–75% in cross-sectional area at necropsy, all 12 were either under- or overestimated angiographically by two or three of three angiographers; of four LMCAs narrowed 26–50% in cross-section at necropsy, two were overestimated by two of three angiographers. Thus, angiographic determination of degrees of narrowing of the LMCA during life is subject to considerable error. The angiographic errors appear to have resulted primarily from the presence of atherosclerotic plaque in the LMCA and an insufficient number of angiographic projections.

CORONARY BYPASS SURGERY appears to increase longevity in patients with significant stenosis of the left main coronary artery (LMCA), so identification of "significant" narrowing in this artery generally is considered to be an indication for the bypass operation regardless of the symptomatic status of the patient.[1] Accurate identification of the degree of LMCA narrowing, therefore, is of paramount importance. Although coronary angiography is the most reliable means of identifying patients with significant stenosis of the LMCA, the accuracy of this technique has not been subjected to critical analysis. In the present report we examine the accuracy of coronary angiography in evaluating the LMCA by comparing the results of antemortem angiography to histologic observations at necropsy.

Patients and Methods

Review of hearts accessioned in the Pathology Branch of the National Heart, Lung, and Blood Institute from 1972 through January 1979 yielded 28 patients who had had coronary angiograms performed within 40 days of death and in whom the coronary angiograms were available for review. Clinical observations in these patients are summarized in table 1. The patients were 31–72 years old (average 55 years). Twenty were men and eight were women. All 28 patients had had angina pectoris; eight also had associated mitral or aortic valve disease or both. The coronary angiograms were performed in six institutions by the Judkins technique (24 patients) or the Sones technique (four patients).

At necropsy, the major extramural coronary arteries, including the LMCA, were excised intact from the heart, fixed in 10% buffered formalin, x-rayed, decalcified (if necessary), and cut transversely into 5-mm-long segments. (We did not use pressure perfusion of the coronary arteries before fixation.) The tissue was then dehydrated (alcohols), cleared (xylene), embedded in paraffin and cut. One section was stained by Movat's pentachrome method from each 5-mm segment. In addition, the original paraffin-embedded blocks of LMCA from six patients were recut at 6-μ intervals. Of the 1160 sections cut, every twentieth section was stained by Movat's method and examined. Histologic evaluation of the degrees of cross-sectional area narrowing by atherosclerotic plaques was performed by visual inspection of each Movat-stained section magnified 20–50 times by light microscopy. The judgment regarding the degree of cross-sectional area narrowing of each section was based on the degree of luminal obliteration within the luminal circle bordered by the internal elastic membrane and was graded as 0–25%, 26–50%, 51–75% and

From the Pathology and Cardiology Branches, National Heart, Lung, and Blood Institute, National Institutes of Health, Bethesda, Maryland; the Cardiology Division, Department of Medicine, Washington Adventist Hospital, Takoma Park, Maryland; and the Cardiology Division, Department of Medicine, George Washington University, Washington, D.C.

Dr. Kishel's present address: Department of Pathology, University of Pennsylvania, School of Medicine and Hospital, Philadelphia, Pennsylvania.

Dr. Isner's present address and address for correspondence: Tufts University School of Medicine, New England Medical Center Hospital, 171 Harrison Avenue, Boston, Massachusetts 02111.

Received March 18, 1980; revision accepted September 5, 1980.

Circulation 63, No. 5, 1981.

TABLE 1. *Clinical, Necropsy and Angiographic Data*

Pt no.	Sex	Age (years)	Interval (days), cath to death	VHD	% CSA narrowing at necropsy	% DR LMCA on Angio			Total no. ang correct	Total no. ang under	Total no. ang over	Views	Angio Q	Cath
						Ag 1	Ag 2	Ag 3						
1	M	31	1*	0	3	1	1	1	0	3	0	AP	AAB	Jud
2	F	35	14	0	4	1	1	3†	1	2	0	LAO	AAA	Jud
3	M	40	0	0	3	3	3	3	0	0	3	—	AAA	Jud
4	F	40	20	0	4	1	1	1	0	3	0	LAO	ABA	So
5	M	42	14	0	2	1	3	3	1	0	2	RAO	ABA	So
6	M	45	15	0	4	4	4	4	3	0	0	Retro only	ABA	Jud
7	F	47	1*	0	3	1	1	Ab	0	2	0	RAO AP	AII	Jud
8	M	49	5	0	4	4	4	4	3	0	0	—	AAA	Jud
9	M	51	38	0	4	3	3	3	3	0	0	RAO LAO	AAA	Jud
10	F	52	7	0	3	1	1	3	0	2	1	RAO	AAA	So
11	M	54	21	0	3	1	1	1	0	3	0	RAO LAO	AAA	Jud
12	M	54	2	0	4	4	4	4	3	0	0	LAO	AAA	Jud
13	M	56	39	0	3	3	3	3	0	0	3	RAO LAO	ABA	Jud
14	M	57	39	0	2	1	3	2	1	0	2	LAO	AAA	Jud
15	F	57	15	0	4	1	1	1	0	3	0	—	ABA	Jud
16	M	58	1	0	4	1	2	1	0	3	0	—	AAA	Jud
17	M	59	15	0	3	1	4	1	0	2	1	—	AAA	Jud
18	F	65	15	0	3	1	1	1	0	3	0	LAO	AAA	Jud
19	M	66	8	0	4	4	4	4	3	0	0	RAO LAO	AAA	Jud
20	M	67	2*	0	4	4	4	4	3	0	0	Retro only	AAA	Jud
21	M	58	15	AR	4	1	3	1	1	2	0	RAO LAO	ABA	Jud
22	M	60	29	AS	3	3	3	4	0	0	3	RAO LAO	ABA	So
23	M	63	8	MR	3	3	3	3	0	0	3	RAO LAO	AIB	Jud
24	M	64	29	AR	2	1	1	1	3	0	0	LAO	AAA	Jud
25	F	66	29	MS	2	1	1	1	3	0	0	LAO	AAA	Jud
26	F	66	4	AS	3	1	3	1	0	2	1	RAO LAO	AAA	Jud
27	M	69	27	AR	3	2	3	3	1	0	2	LAO	AAA	Jud
28	M	72	8	AS	4	1	1	1	0	3	0	RAO LAO	AAA	Jud

*Catheterization-related death.

†Angiographer diagnosed LMCA ostial narrowing 51–75%; at necropsy, ostium was not narrowed.

Abbreviations: A = adequate; Ab = angiographer abstained; Angio = angiogram; Ang = angiographer; AP = anteroposterior; AR = aortic regurgitation; AS = aortic stenosis; B = borderline; Cath = type catheter used; DR = diameter reduction (1 = 0–25%, 2 = 26–50%, 3 = 51–75%, 4 = 76–100%); I = inadequate; Jud = Judkins; LAO = very shallow left anterior oblique; LMCA = left main coronary artery; MR = mitral regurgitation; MS = mitral stenosis; NC = no call; over = overestimated; Q = quality of angiogram as evaluated by Ang 1, Ang 2, Ang 3; RAO = very shallow right anterior oblique; retro only = LMCA filling visualized only by collaterals from right coronary artery; So = Sones; under = underestimated; VHD = valvular heart disease; CSA narrowing = cross-sectional area narrowing (2 = 26–50%, 3 = 51–75%, 4 = 76–100%); — = LMCA not studied in AP, very shallow RAO or very shallow LAO projections.

76–100%. The judgment made by light microscopy was confirmed and specifically quantified for each section of LMCA with a video-based, computer-linked, planimetry system.[2] When the walls of the artery adjacent to the lumen were indented inward, determination of the degree of narrowing was made only after visual outward expansion of the collapsed portion of the arterial wall. Histologic determination of the degree of cross-sectional area narrowing was performed without knowledge of the results of angiographic interpretation.

The coronary angiograms were reviewed separately by each of three experienced angiographers without knowledge of the results of the grading by the other two and without knowledge of the results of either preoperative angiographic assessment or postmortem histologic evaluation. All three angiographers were aware that they were participating in an angiographic-correlative study; none was aware that this study was limited to an analysis only of the angiographic accuracy of LMCA narrowing. None of the three angiographers had performed any of the angiograms. Each judged the degree of narrowing of the LMCA as well as the degrees of narrowing of the other major coronary arteries. The maximal percent of diameter reduction — not cross-sectional area narrowing — was determined for each major coronary artery as follows: 0–25%, 26–50%, 51–75%, and 76–100%. All three angiographers used calipers or similar measuring devices. Each angiographer was asked to evaluate the quality of the angiograms (adequate, borderline or inadequate) and whether the number of views was adequate to evaluate each of the four major coronary arteries; if for any reason the angiographer considered the cineangiograms to be of borderline or inadequate quality, he was given the option of abstaining from making a judgment.

Coronary angiography in life or at necropsy provides a view of the longitudinal dimension of the coronary arterial lumen; histologic examination at necropsy, by the method we used, provides a view of the cross-sectional area of the coronary artery. For any degree of longitudinal narrowing there is a proportionately greater loss of cross-sectional area (table 2). Assuming a central round residual lumen, a 25% reduction in diameter results in a 44% loss of cross-sectional area. Thus, because for any degree of diameter reduction (by angiography) there is a greater degree of cross-sectional area narrowing (by histology), an angiographic underestimation was defined as an angiographic judgment that underestimated the degree of cross-sectional area narrowing by an absolute difference of > 25% or more. Because there is a smaller degree of diameter reduction (by angiography) for any given degree of cross-sectional area narrowing (by histology), an angiographic overestimation was defined as an angiographic estimate that was at least as great as the degree of cross-sectional area narrowing observed at necropsy. For example, an estimate by the angiographer that the LMCA was narrowed 51–75% in diameter (angiography) when in fact histologic evaluation disclosed that it was narrowed 51–75% in cross-sectional area would be an angiographic overestimation.

TABLE 2. *Corresponding Reduction in Cross-sectional Area for a Given Degree of Diameter Reduction*

Diameter reduction (angiography)		Cross-sectional area reduction (histology)	
%	Code*	%	Code*
0.10		19%	
0.15	1	28%	2
0.20		36%	
0.25		44%	
0.30		51%	
0.35		58%	
0.40	2	64%	3
0.45		70%	
0.50		75%	
0.55		80%	
0.60		84%	
0.65	3	88%	4
0.70		91%	
0.75		94%	
0.80		96%	
0.85		98%	
0.90	4	99%	
0.95		100%	
1.00		100%	

*"Code" here refers to the numbers used in table 1 to denote the quartile of diameter reduction and cross-sectional area narrowing, respectively (1 = 0–25%, 2 = 26–50%, 3 = 51–75%, 4 = 76–100%).

Results

Cross-sectional Area Narrowing Observed Histologically at Necropsy

The degree of cross-sectional area luminal narrowing of the LMCA at necropsy in our 28 patients is

TABLE 3. *Left Main Coronary Artery: Accuracy of Antemortem Cineangiography Compared to Postmortem Histology in 28 Necropsy Patients*

No. LM (No. angiographic errors)	% LM narrowing by histology			Totals	
	26–50	51–75	76–100		
No. LM (No. underestimated [U])	4 (0)	12 (7)	12 (6)	28 (13)	[46%]
No. LMX3A (No. underestimated)	12 (0)	36 (17)	36 (16)	84 (33)	[39%]
No. LM (No. overestimated [0])	4 (2)	12 (8)	12 (0)	28 (10)	[36%]
No. LMX3A (No. overestimated)	12 (4)	36 (17)	36 (0)	84 (21)	[25%]
Totals					
No. LM (No. either U or 0)	4 (2)	12 (12)	12 (6)	28 (20)	[71%]
No. LMX3A (No. either U or 0)	12 (4)	36 (34)	36 (16)	84 (54)	[64%]

Abbreviations: LMX3A = total judgments by three angiographers concerning the left main coronary artery.

listed in tables 1 and 3. In 12 patients, the LMCA at necropsy was narrowed > 75% in cross-sectional area (corresponding to > 50% in diameter reduction by angiography); in 12 patients it was narrowed 51–75% (corresponding to 26–50% diameter reduction by angiography), and in four patients it was narrowed 26–50% in cross-sectional area (corresponding to ≤ 25% diameter reduction by angiography).

Angiographic Underestimation of the LMCA Narrowed > 75% in Cross-sectional Area at Necropsy (fig. 1)

Of the 12 patients in whom the LMCA was narrowed 76–100% in cross-sectional area, angiography underestimated the degree of LMCA narrowing in six (patients 2, 4, 15, 16, 21, 28; table 1). Of the 18 estimates in these six patients, 16 represented angiographic errors (table 1). In 15 of the 16 errors, the angiographer judged the LMCA to be < 25% narrowed when it was narrowed > 75% in cross-sectional area. In four of the six patients, all three angiographers concurred in their underestimation, and in the other two, two of three angiographers concurred. The cineangiograms of three patients were cited as borderline in quality by one angiographer; in another patient, the same angiographer made a "low-confidence" call because the LMCA was too short to evaluate. Otherwise, the quality of the films was judged to be adequate, and the angiographers were satisfied that the available views allowed satisfactory evaluation of the LMCA. Nevertheless, review of the cineangiograms disclosed that in only two of the six patients was a very shallow right anterior oblique view obtained; in only four of the six patients was a very shallow left anterior oblique view obtained, and in none of the six patients was a flat anteroposterior view recorded. In five of six patients, both the proximal left anterior descending and the proximal left circumflex coronary arteries were narrowed > 75% in cross-sectional area by atherosclerotic plaque.

TABLE 4. *Left Main Coronary Narrowing at Necropsy Determined by Video Planimetry of Histologic Sections*

Cross-sectional area narrowing at necropsy		No. of pts	
26–50%	26–30%	0	
	31–35%	1	
	36–40%	0	(4)
	41–45%	1	
	46–50%	2	
51–75%	51–55%	2	
	56–60%	1	
	61–65%	2	(11)
	66–70%	2	
	71–75%	4	
76–100%	76–80%	4	
	81–85%	2	
	86–90%	2	(12)
	91–95%	2	
	96–100%	2	

Angiographic Underestimation of the LMCA Narrowed 51–75% in Cross-sectional Area (fig. 2)

In the 12 patients in whom the LMCA was narrowed 51–75% in cross-sectional area at necropsy (corresponding to 26–50% diameter reduction), angiography underestimated the degree of LMCA narrowing in seven (patients 1, 7, 10, 11, 17, 18 and 26; table 1). In 17 of 21 judgments in these seven patients, the LMCA was called < 25% diameter reduction by angiography. All three angiographers concurred in three of the seven patients, while two of the three concurred in the other four patients. Two underestimates by one angiographer were "low-confidence calls" due to inadequate quality of the films in one patient and a very short LMCA in a second patient. Two other underestimations occurred in association with "borderline" quality films. In two of the seven patients anteroposterior projections had been obtained, including one patient in whom all three angiographers underestimated the degree of narrowing. In two of the seven patients neither an anteroposterior view nor a projection at a very shallow obliquity was obtained. The proximal branches of the LMCA were each narrowed > 50% in cross-sectional area in all seven patients, including two in whom each was narrowed > 75% in cross-sectional area.

Angiographic Overestimates (fig. 3)

Angiography overestimated the degree of LMCA narrowing in 10 patients (patients 3, 5, 10, 13, 14, 17, 22, 23, 26 and 27; table 1). In two patients in whom the LMCA was narrowed 26–50% cross-sectional area by histologic examination, two of three angiographers overestimated the corresponding degree of angiographic narrowing (diameter reduction): in one patient, the two angiographers judged the LMCA narrowing to be 51–75% diameter reduction (corresponding to > 75% cross-sectional area narrowing); in the second patient, the two angiographers estimated the diameter reduction to be 51–75% and 26–50% (corresponding to 76–100% and 51–75% narrowing, respectively, in cross-sectional area). Of the two cineangiograms, one was judged to be of "borderline" quality by one angiographer in one patient. Angiographic views of the LMCA included one very shallow obliquity in each of the two patients. In both patients there was > 75% cross-sectional area narrowing of the proximal left anterior descending and left circumflex coronary arteries. The remaining overestimates involved eight patients with 51–75% cross-sectional area narrowing of the LMCA at necropsy. In six of the 10 patients in whom angiographic overestimates occurred, serial step sections were cut at 6-μ intervals from the original paraffin block of LMCA and confirmed in each that the initial assessment of the LMCA by histology at necropsy was valid.

Effect of Angiographic Projection on LMCA Foreshortening

The cineangiograms were also reviewed to determine which projection resulted in maximal foreshortening of the LMCA. All projections resulted in

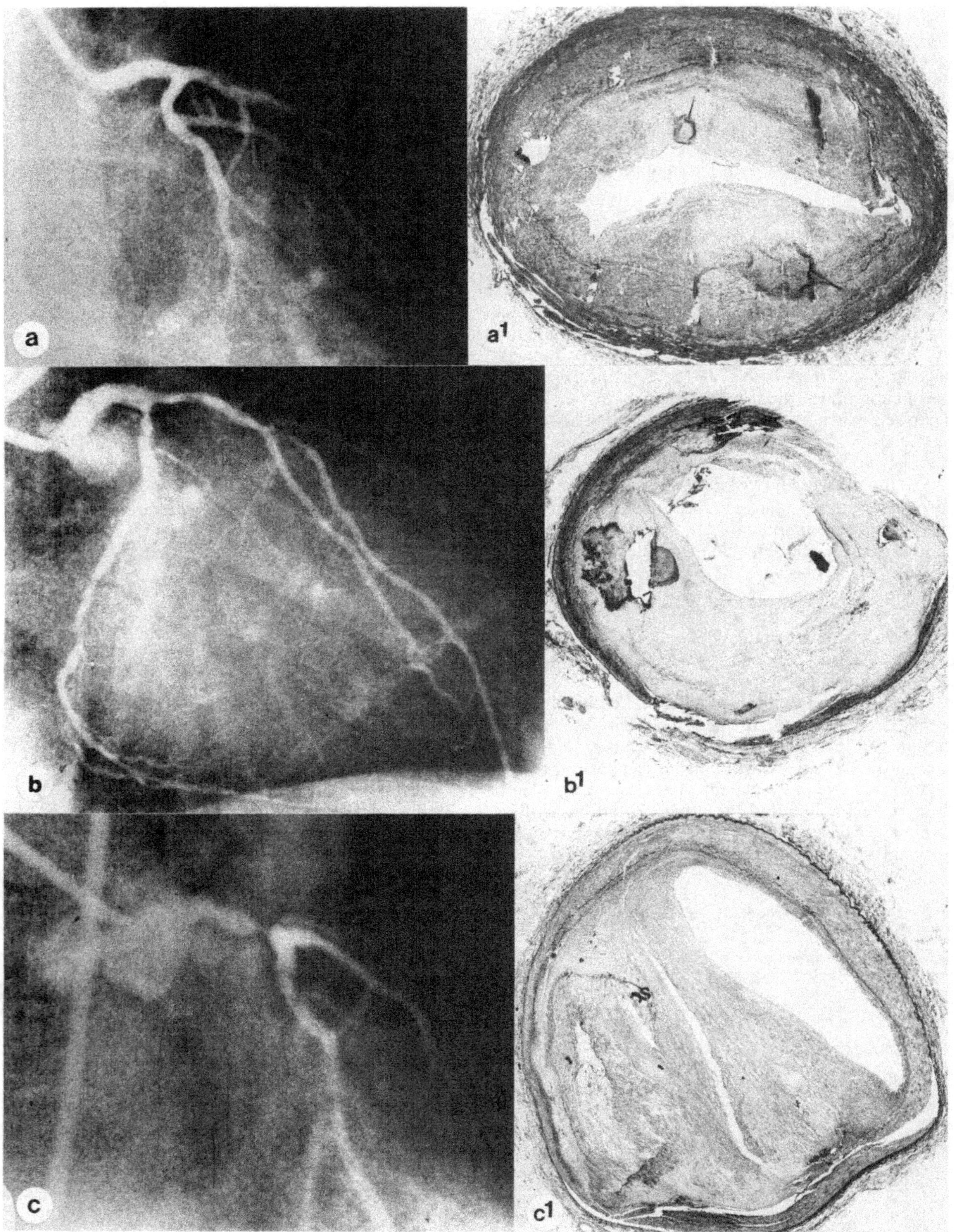

FIGURE 1. *Cineangiogram frames (a, b, and c) showing maximal diameter reduction and corresponding histologic sections (a¹, b¹ and c¹) showing greater than 75% cross-sectional area narrowing of the left main coronary artery (LMCA) in three patients. In figures a and a¹ (patient 16, table 1), LMCA narrowing by angiography was estimated as < 25%, 26–50% and < 25% respectively. In b and b¹ (patient 28, table 1), the LMCA was called "normal" (< 25% narrowed) by all three angiographers. In c and c¹ (patient 12, table 1), although the degree of cross-sectional area narrowing at necropsy of the LMCA is similar in this patient to the two above patients, angiographic narrowing is much more apparent (diameter reduction was correctly estimated as > 75% by all three angiographers). Movat stains; magnifications × 27 (a¹ and c¹), × 16 (b¹).*

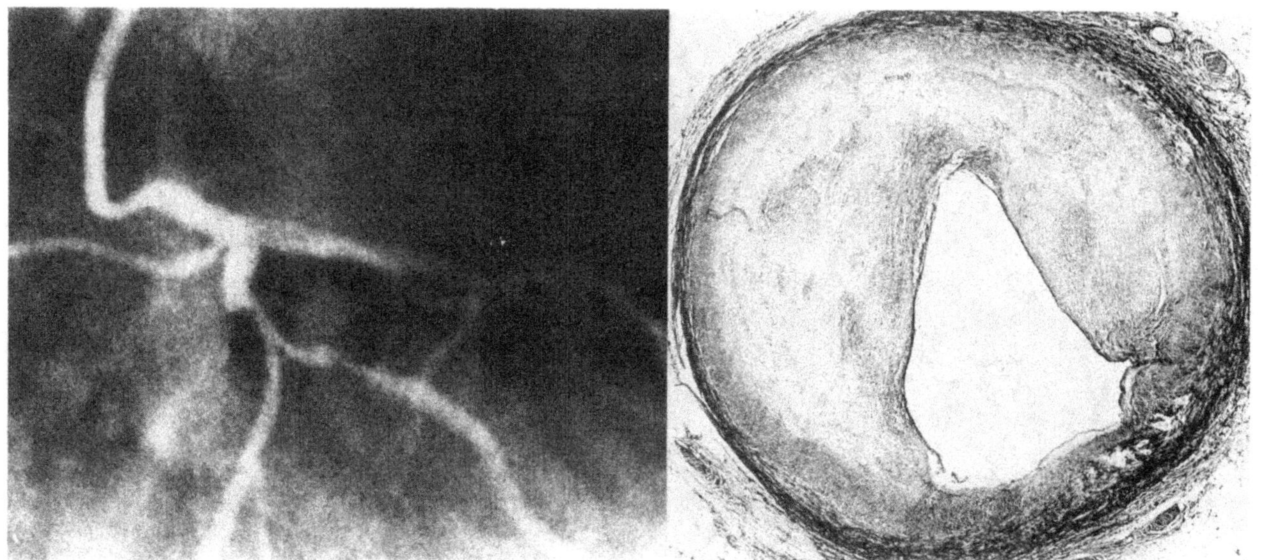

FIGURE 2. *Cineangiographic frame showing maximal diameter reduction and photomicrograph of histologic section showing 51–75% cross-sectional area narrowing of the left main coronary artery (LMCA) in patient 17 (table 1). The LMCA was judged to be normal (< 25% narrowed) by two of the three angiographers.*

apparent foreshortening of the LMCA in at least one patient. The steeper obliquities, however, consistently produced the greatest degree of foreshortening; the shallow obliquities (particularly the right anterior oblique) produced less consistent foreshortening. An anteroposterior projection was obtained in only two patients; in one, it provided the maximum angiographic length of LMCA of the available views, while in the second the angiographic length was shorter in the anteroposterior view than in the right anterior oblique projection (i.e., foreshortened).

Discussion

The limitations of noninvasive methods in the identification of narrowing of the LMCA are well known.[3][7] Coronary angiography has consequently been acknowledged as the only accurate means of identifying patients with significant narrowing of the LMCA.[8] Since the suggestion of Cohen et al.[9] in 1972 that patients with LMCA disease be arbitrarily separated into angiographic subsets of moderate (51–74%) and severe (≥ 75%) degrees of narrowing (diameter reduction), the concept has persisted that the degree of LMCA stenosis (e.g., 51–74% vs > 75%) could be accurately judged by coronary angiography. The present study, however, suggests that accurate angiographic identification of LMCA narrowing may be more difficult, and that quantification of less than extremely severe (i.e., ≥ 90% luminal diameter reduction) degrees of LMCA narrowing often may be impossible.

In only nine patients did all three angiographic interpretations correspond to what was observed in the LMCA at necropsy (including two patients with total occlusion in whom the LMCA was opacified only by retrograde filling from the right coronary artery). In six of the 12 patients in whom the LMCA was narrowed > 75% in cross-sectional area (corresponding to ≥ 50% narrowing in angiographic luminal diameter), the LMCA was called 0–25% diameter reduction in 15 of 18 estimates. In seven of 12 patients in whom the LMCA was narrowed 51–75% in cross-sectional area (corresponding to 26–50% diameter reduction), the LMCA was called 0–25% diameter reduction by angiography; although underestimations in this group have less serious implications, the extent of underestimations (17 of 21 judgments) confirms the difficulties involved in precise determination of angiographic narrowing. Finally, in 10 patients, at least one angiographer overestimated the degree of coronary narrowing: despite < 75% cross-sectional area narrowing in all 10 patients (corresponding to < 50% diameter reduction by angiography), all 10 were estimated by at least one angiographer to have > 50% stenosis of the LMCA.

The extent of interobserver agreement among the three angiographers in this study was strong. This finding is in contrast to what has been reported in studies designed to evaluate interobserver variability in interpreting coronary angiograms.[10][12] However, in one such study,[10] interobserver variability was least (i.e., interobserver agreement was greatest) in evaluating the right coronary artery and the LMCA. The inaccuracies in the angiographic evaluation of the LMCA appear to be more a function of the technique of recording the LMCA on film than a variation in observer acuity involved in viewing the same cineangiogram.

Interpretation of the angiographic appearance of the LMCA is subject not only to problems that complicate coronary angiography in general, but to spe-

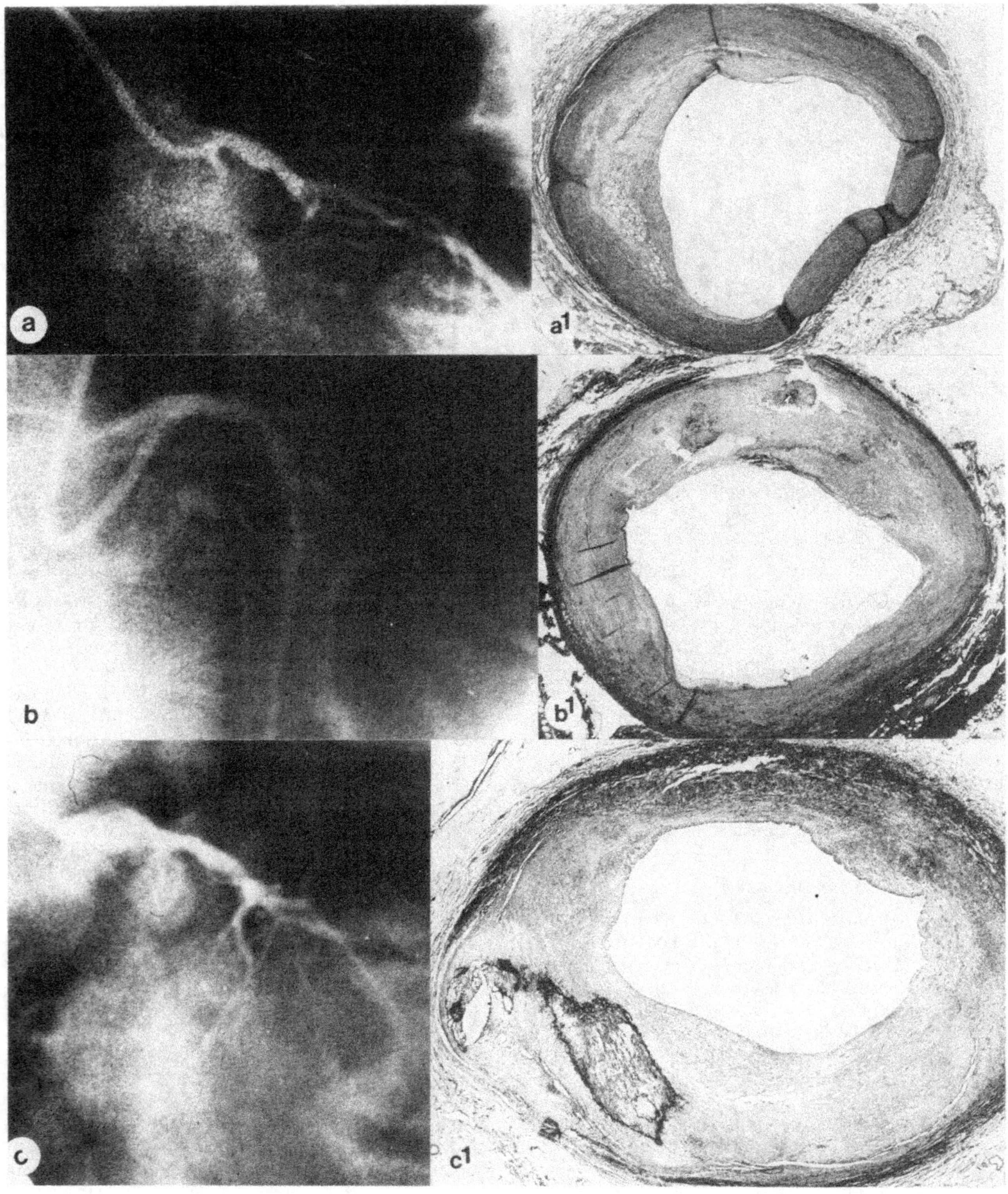

FIGURE 3. *Cineangiogram frames (a, b and c) showing maximal diameter reduction and photomicrographs (a^1, b^1 and c^1) of histologic sections that show 26–50% cross-sectional area narrowing (a^1) and 51–75% narrowing (b^1 and c^1) of the left main coronary artery (LMCA) in three patients. In a and a^1 (patient 14, table 1), the LMCA narrowing was overestimated by two of three angiographers. In b and b^1 (patient 22, table 7), the LMCA narrowing was overestimated by all three angiographers. In c and c^1 (patient 27, table 1), the LMCA narrowing was overestimated by two of three angiographers.*

cific problems deriving from the special anatomy of the LMCA. Underestimation of coronary arterial narrowing by coronary angiography has been documented in at least six studies,[13-18] and the frequency of angiographically missed severe narrowings (> 75% in cross-sectional area) has been determined to be as high as 39%.[18] Quantitative histologic examination of the coronary arteries at necropsy has indicated that two morphologic features in particular account for the tendency to underestimate degrees of coronary narrowing: the coronary atherosclerotic process is diffuse, rather than focal, and the residual nonoccluded lumen is usually eccentric in location and often slit-like in shape.[18, 19] Diffuse narrowing forces the angiographer to compare sites of maximal narrowing to adjacent sites that may be less, but still severely narrowed; rarely, then, does the angiographer have a truly normal, uncompromised luminal diameter on which to base estimates of percent coronary luminal diameter reduction.

In contrast, histologic examination allows identification of the original "true" lumen as indicated by the internal elastic membrane. Eccentric, slit-like lumens pose no problem in estimating the degree of narrowing at necropsy, but may be a source of angiographic error when they allow the entire diameter of the artery to be opacified with contrast material. In the case of the LMCA, the hazards posed by these two morphologic characteristics are exacerbated by its short length and unpredictable course. The LMCA is the shortest of the four major epicardial coronary arteries. For atherosclerotic narrowing to involve the LMCA diffusely, it need only extend over a length of 3–12 mm; such narrowing would obliterate any portion of "normal" or relatively unobstructed lumen for comparison. If the proximal left anterior descending and left circumflex coronary arteries are severely narrowed as well (as was the case in five of seven patients with > 75% cross-sectional area narrowing of the LMCA in whom angiography underestimated the degree of narrowing), the angiographer may be deprived of any reasonable standard for comparison. Furthermore, the LMCA is the only major epicardial coronary artery without a "fixed anchorage." The left anterior descending artery, for example, generally follows the course of the ventricular septum, while the proximal left circumflex and right coronary arteries lie within the subepicardial adipose tissue of the atrioventricular grooves. Although the lengths of these arteries may be variable, their locations are relatively constant. In contrast, the LMCA may arise at an unpredictable angle from the aorta and may follow one of three axes in each of the horizontal and frontal planes before bifurcating into the left anterior descending and left circumflex branches.[20]

The problems of diffuse narrowing, eccentric, slit-like lumens, short lengths and varying courses of the LMCA make the routine use of multiple obliquities particularly critical for proper angiographic evaluation. The lack of an adequate number of projections perhaps contributed as much as any other factor to the number of angiographic underestimates in our patients. Of the six patients in whom LMCA narrowing of > 75% in cross-sectional area (at necropsy) was underestimated, none was viewed in the anteroposterior projection and only three patients were examined in very shallow obliquities. Of the seven patients in whom the LMCA was narrowed 51–75% in cross-sectional area and was underestimated angiographically, only two were viewed in the anteroposterior projection and only five in a very shallow obliquity. None of the 13 patients in whom the LMCA was narrowed > 50% in cross-sectional area were studied in all three projections (anteroposterior, very shallow right anterior oblique and very shallow left anterior oblique). Although recommendations have varied widely regarding the number of views necessary for satisfactory angiographic evaluation of the LMCA, more recent experience suggests that all three projections are mandatory for complete examination of the LMCA. Lipton and co-workers[21] found that when these three views were routinely used, the angiographic frequency of LMCA stenosis was considerably higher (74 of 500 cases, 15%) than that reported in most studies. Nath and associates[22] performed 120 consecutive coronary arteriograms of the LMCA in all three views and found eight patients with LMCA stenosis, five of whom were recognized only in the anteroposterior projection. Both these studies and the present one demonstrate that any one of the three views may result in angiographic foreshortening of the LMCA, depending on its course. It seems prudent, then, to accept the recommendation that all three views need be used routinely for adequate angiographic analysis of the LMCA.

In the 10 patients in whom angiography overestimated the degree of LMCA narrowing, the discrepancies between angiography and necropsy were not as wide as in those patients in whom angiography underestimated the degree of narrowing. In all 10 patients, for example, there was at least 26–50% cross-sectional area narrowing and in nine of the 10 patients the LMCA was narrowed 51–75% in cross-sectional area. Even this degree of cross-sectional area narrowing, however, results in less than 50% diameter reduction. Angiographic estimates of > 50% diameter reduction in such patients, although not widely discrepant, may be troublesome from a practical standpoint because such patients are likely to be recommended for coronary bypass surgery. In some patients overestimation may be inconsequential (depending on their symptomatic status and the status of their remaining coronary arteries), but in others angiographic overestimation of the degree of LMCA narrowing could result in an inappropriate decision for operative therapy.

Many factors may contribute to angiographic overestimation of LMCA narrowing. Inadequate filling of the LMCA with contrast material clearly can lead to angiographic overestimation of the degree of narrowing. The funnel-shaped origin of the LMCA as it arises from the aorta often makes adequate filling of the proximal portion of the LMCA difficult,[21] and this may have been the basis for overestimation in one patient. Aortic valve disease represents another potential cause of underfilling of the LMCA. Retrograde coronary blood flow has been demonstrated in patients with aortic stenosis at end-systole and aortic regurgitation at end-diastole.[23] Four of our patients in whom angiography overestimated the degree of LMCA narrowing had aortic valve disease (stenosis in two, pure regurgitation in two). In reviewing the angiograms of these four patients retrospectively, underfilling of the LMCA due to aortic regurgitation was considered the likely cause of overestimation in one patient. Technical problems, such as injecting an inadequate amount of contrast material, or injecting the contrast material too slowly or through a catheter with excessive length, may prevent optimal visualization of the LMCA.[24] The possibility that these technical considerations contributed to overestimation in our patients cannot be ruled out, because this information was not available to us in most patients. Spasm, specifically LMCA spasm, is another potential explanation for angiographic overestimation. At least five patients with spasm (apparently catheter-induced) of the LMCA near the ostium have been reported.[17, 25-27] Furthermore, there was no evidence that nitroglycerin had been given to any of our patients before or after injection of contrast material into the LMCA in an attempt to relieve or rule out LMCA spasm. Nevertheless, the experience of others suggests that LMCA spasm is rare, even after provocation with ergonovine.[5]

The results of this study demonstrate that angiographic evaluation of the LMCA is subject to significant error. Because critical narrowing of the LMCA is presently considered to be a prima facie indication for coronary artery bypass surgery, regardless of the symptomatic status of the patients, accurate angiographic evaluation of the LMCA is essential. Angiographic data from this and other studies suggest that this can best be achieved by the use of multiple (at least three) angiographic projections.

References

1. Epstein SE, Kent KM, Goldstein RE, Borer JS, Rosing DR: Strategy for evaluation and surgical treatment of the asymptomatic or mildly symptomatic patient with coronary artery disease. Am J Cardiol 43: 1015, 1979
2. Dvorak JA, Schuette WH, Whitehouse WC: A simple video method for the quantification of microscopic objects. J Microsc 102: 71, 1974
3. Plotnick GD, Greene HL, Carliner NH, Becker LC, Fisher ML: Clinical indicators of left main coronary artery disease in unstable angina. Ann Intern Med 91: 149, 1979
4. Dash H, Massie BM, Botvinick EH, Brundage BH: The non-invasive identification of left main and three-vessel coronary artery disease by myocardial stress perfusion scintigraphy and treadmill exercise electrocardiography. Circulation 60: 276, 1979
5. Conti CR, Selby JH, Cristie LG, Pepine CJ, Curry RC Jr, Nichols WW, Conetta DG, Feldman RL, Mehta J, Alexander JA: Left main coronary artery stenosis: clinical spectrum, pathophysiology, and management. Prog Cardiovasc Dis 22: 73, 1979
6. Stone PH, Goldschlager N: Left main coronary artery disease: review and appraisal. Cardiovasc Med 4: 165–178, 1979
7. Iskandrian AS, Tuma-Aid JR, Owens JS, Kimbiris D, Bemis CE, Segal BL: Left main coronary artery disease: experience with 94 patients and review of the literature. Cardiology 61: 360, 1976
8. Epstein SE: Importance of identifying left main coronary artery narrowing in subsets of patients with coronary artery disease. Ann Intern Med 91: 308, 1979
9. Cohen MV, Cohn PF, Herman MV, Gorlin R: Diagnosis and prognosis of main left coronary artery obstruction. Circulation 45 (suppl I): I-57, 1972
10. Detre KM, Wright E, Murphy ML, Takaro T: Observer agreement in evaluating coronary angiograms. Circulation 52: 979, 1975
11. DeRouen TA, Murray JA, Owen W: Variability in the analysis of coronary arteriograms. Circulation 55: 324, 1977
12. Zir LM, Miller SW, Dinsmore RE, Gilbert JP, Harthorne JW: Interobserver variability in coronary angiography. Circulation 53: 627, 1976
13. Kemp HG, Evans H, Elliott WC, Gorlin R: Diagnostic accuracy of selective coronary cinearteriography. Circulation 36: 526, 1967
14. Frech R, Van Tassel RA, Edwards JE: Correlation of the antemortem coronary arteriogram and the postmortem specimen. Circulation 47: 162, 1973
15. Grondin CM, Dydra I, Pasternac A, Campeau L, Bourassa MG, Lespérance J: Discrepancies between cineangiographic and postmortem findings in patients with coronary artery disease and recent myocardial revascularization. Circulation 49: 703, 1974
16. Schwartz JN, Kong Y, Hackel DB, Bartel AG: Comparison of angiographic and postmortem findings in patients with coronary artery disease. Am J Cardiol 36: 174, 1975
17. Hutchins GM, Bulkley BH, Ridolfi RL, Griffith LSC, Lohr FT, Piasio MA: Correlation of coronary arteriograms and left ventriculograms with postmortem studies. Circulation 56: 32, 1979
18. Arnett EN, Isner JM, Redwood DR, Kent KM, Baker WP, Ackerstein H, Roberts WC: Coronary artery narrowing in coronary heart disease: comparison of cineangiographic and necropsy findings. Ann Intern Med 91: 350, 1979
19. Vlodaver Z, Edwards JE: Pathology of coronary atherosclerosis. Prog Cardiovasc Dis 14: 256, 1971
20. McAlpine WA: Heart and Coronary Arteries. Berlin, Springer-Verlag, 1975, pp 144–145
21. Lipton MJ, Pfeifer JF, Murphy ML, Hultgren HN: Dangers of left main coronary artery lesions: angiographic technique and evaluation. Invest Radiol 12: 447, 1977
22. Nath PH, Velasquez G, Castaneda-Zuniga WR, Zollikofer C, Formanek A, Amplatz K: An essential view in coronary arteriography. Circulation 60: 101, 1979
23. Carroll RJ, Falsetti HL: Retrograde coronary artery flow in aortic valve disease. Circulation 54: 494, 1976
24. Pepine CJ, Feldman RL, Nichols WW, Conti CR: Coronary angiography: potentially serious sources of error in interpretation. Cardiovasc Med 2: 747, 1977
25. Murphy ES, Rösch J, Boicourt OW, Rahimtoola SH: Left main coronary artery spasm. A potential cause for angiographic misdiagnosis of severe coronary artery disease. Arch Intern Med 136: 350, 1976
26. Tzivoni D, Merin G, Milo S, Gotsman MS: Spasm of left main coronary artery. Br Heart J 38: 104, 1976
27. Vlodaver Z, Amplatz K, Burchell HB, Edwards JE: Coronary Heart Disease. Clinical, Angiographic, and Pathologic Profiles. Berlin, Springer-Verlag, 1976, p 234

Fatal Cardiac Arrest During Cardiac Catheterization for Angina Pectoris: Analysis of 10 Necropsy Patients

HENRY SCOTT CABIN, MD
WILLIAM C. ROBERTS, MD, FACC

Bethesda, Maryland

Data on 10 patients with angina pectoris and fatal cardiac arrest during cardiac catheterization were analyzed to determine the circumstances of death and the severity and distribution of the coronary arterial narrowing. Nine patients died during attempted coronary angiography, and the remaining patient during right-sided cardiac catheterization. At least three of four major epicardial coronary arteries were narrowed 76 to 100 percent in cross-sectional area by atherosclerotic plaques in all 10 patients. Seven of these patients had this degree of narrowing of the left main coronary artery by plaque, and two additional patients had severe (more than 75 percent) narrowing of the left main coronary artery by thromboembolic material superimposed on small atherosclerotic plaques. Among 354 five mm long segments of the left main, left anterior descending, left circumflex and right coronary arteries in eight patients, the percent narrowing to various degrees in cross-sectional area by atherosclerotic plaques was as follows: 96 to 100 percent, 9; 76 to 95 percent, 49; 51 to 75 percent, 23; 26 to 50 percent, 13; and 0 to 25 percent, 6. With use of a scoring system of 1 to 4 for the amount of narrowing in each 5 mm segment (1 = 0–25 percent, 2 = 26 to 50 percent, 3 = 51 to 75 percent and 4 = 76 to 100 percent), the mean score per 5 mm segment for the group was 3.34. Thus, patients with angina pectoris who die during cardiac catheterization have particularly severe and diffuse coronary atherosclerosis and usually severe narrowing of the left main coronary artery.

Death during cardiac catheterization is rare, and the opportunity to study at necropsy a patient who died during this procedure is even rarer. During the past 11 years we studied at necropsy 10 patients with angina pectoris who died during cardiac catheterization at eight hospitals. This report describes our observations.

Patients Studied and Methods

Patients: Clinical and necropsy findings in the 10 patients are summarized in Table I. Their ages ranged from 35 to 62 years (mean 47); seven were men and three women. All 10 patients had angina pectoris; in 8, it was the only manifestation of myocardial ischemia; in the remaining 2 patients (Cases 6 and 7), a clinical event diagnostic of acute myocardial infarction also had occurred 4 and 3 years, respectively, before death. Angina pectoris was stable in two patients

From the Pathology Branch, National Heart, Lung, and Blood Institute, National Institutes of Health, Bethesda, Maryland. Manuscript received December 22, 1980; revised manuscript received February 10, 1981, accepted February 13, 1981.

Address for reprints: William C. Roberts, MD, Building 10, Room 3E30, National Institutes of Health, Bethesda, Maryland 20205.

TABLE I

Clinical and Necropsy Observations in 10 Study Patients With Angina Pectoris and Fatal Cardiac Arrest During Cardiac Catheterization

Case	Age (yr) & Sex	Year of CC	Heart Weight (g)	THMI	Four Major CA Narrowed 76 to 100% in XSA by AP (n)	5 mm Segments of CA (n)	Number of 5 mm Segments Narrowed 76 to 100% in XSA by AP (%)	Coronary Score per Patient[*]	Coronary Score per 5 mm Segment[†]
1	35M	1978	340	0	3	—	—	—	—
2	38M	1979	430	0	4	53	34 (64)	176	3.32
3	40M	1969	370	0	4	39	26 (67)	143	3.66
4	40M	1975	400	+	4	39	22 (56)	127	3.26
5	42F	1975	340	0	4	54	24 (44)	172	3.19
6	45M	1973	540	+	3[§]	—	—	—	—
7	49F	1970	260	+	3[‖]	24	16 (67)	83	3.46
8[‡]	57F	1976	350	0	4	40	25 (63)	132	3.30
9	57M	1977	310	+	4	52	35 (67)	187	3.60
10	62M	1980	500	0	3[‖]	53	22 (42)	155	2.92

[*] Derived by assigning a number to each 5 mm segment of coronary artery based on the amount of narrowing of cross-sectional area by atherosclerotic plaques (1 = 0 to 25 percent narrowing; 2 = 26 to 50 percent; 3 = 51 to 75 percent; and 4 = 76 to 100 percent). [†] Derived by dividing the coronary score per patient by the number of 5 mm segments examined from that patient. [‡] Patient died during right-sided cardiac catheterization. [§] Left main coronary artery not examined. [‖] Left main coronary artery narrowed less than 75 percent by atherosclerotic plaques but occluded by thromboembolic material.

AP = atherosclerotic plaques; CA = coronary arteries; CC = cardiac catheterization; THMI = transmural healed myocardial infarct; XSA = cross-sectional area.

(Cases 9 and 10) and unstable in eight. Unstable angina was defined as chest pain of recent onset (less than 3 months), nocturnal pain or pain at rest or a change in frequency, severity, intensity or ease of provocation of the pain within the past 3 months. No patient had evidence of congestive heart failure, associated valvular heart disease or hypertrophic cardiomyopathy. Four patients had known type II hyperlipoproteinemia; two patients (Cases 6 and 7) had diabetes mellitus and one (Case 9) had systemic hypertension. No patient had electrocardiographic or enzymatic evidence of myocardial necrosis immediately before cardiac catheterization.

Circumstances of the cardiac arrest: In 5 of the 10 patients the cardiac arrest occurred while the catheter was in the left sinus of Valsalva, and in 3 while it was in the right sinus; in 2 patients no contrast material had been injected into a coronary artery. In three patients cardiac arrest occurred after injection into the left main but before injection into the right coronary artery; in one patient, after injection into the right and before injection into the left main artery, and in two patients after injection into the left main and right coronary arteries. In one patient arrest occurred during right-sided cardiac catheterization before introduction of the catheter into a systemic artery or into the left side of the heart; in another patient no information about the circumstances of the arrest was available. The Judkins technique was utilized in eight patients and the Sones technique in one (Case 1) of the nine patients who died during attempted coronary angiography. In nine patients medical means of resuscitation were unsuccessful, and in one patient (Case 6) cardioversion from ventricular fibrillation was successful but the patient remained hypotensive with pulmonary edema and died 2 hours later. In Cases 1 and 4 closed chest massage and mechanical ventilation were continued while the patients were transported to the operating room and aortocoronary bypass performed, but neither patient could be weaned from cardiopulmonary bypass after insertion of the conduits.

Autopsy procedures: In 8 of the 10 patients, the entire lengths of the right, left main, left anterior descending and left circumflex coronary arteries were removed from the hearts and cut transversely into segments 5 mm long; each segment was labeled, processed for histologic study and a histologic section prepared, stained by the Movat method[1] and exam-

ined. The degree of narrowing in each 5 mm segment was determined by examination under the microscope magnified 25 to 50 times. The percent of narrowing of cross-sectional area by atherosclerotic plaques was divided into five categories: 0 to 25, 26 to 50, 51 to 75, 76 to 95 and 96 to 100 percent. The accuracy of these determinations was verified by videoplanimetry and shown to have an error of less than 5 percent.[2]

Left ventricular myocardial necrosis was noted at necropsy in two patients, both of whom underwent coronary bypass operations after prolonged unsuccessful resuscitative efforts; in Patient 1, the necrosis was transmural and in Patient 4, it was limited to subendocardium (inner half). Four patients (two of whom had had a clinically diagnosed acute myocardial infarct) had grossly visible transmural left ventricular scars.

Control subjects: We selected nine control subjects similar in age (mean 47 years) and sex (six men and three women) to the study patients. All had angina pectoris (unstable in seven) and underwent uncomplicated cardiac catheterization with coronary angiography within 1 month of death; each died during or within 3 days after aortocoronary arterial bypass grafting. The four major epicardial coronary arteries were removed in their entirety from all nine hearts, processed and examined as described for the study patients. At necropsy, no subject had foci of myocardial necrosis, but six had foci of transmural myocardial fibrosis. Five of the latter six subjects had had a clinical event typical of acute myocardial infarction.

TABLE II

Number of Study Patients and Control Subjects With One to Four of Four Major Coronary Arteries Narrowed 76 to 100 Percent in Cross-Sectional Area by Atherosclerotic Plaque

Coronary Arteries Narrowed 76 to 100 Percent (n)	Study Patients	Control Subjects
4	6	2
3	4	6
2	0	1
1	0	0
0	0	0
Totals	10	9

TABLE III

Number of Each Major Epicardial Coronary Artery Narrowed 76 to 100 Percent and Total Number of Coronary Arteries Narrowed 96 to 100 Percent In Cross-Sectional Area by Atherosclerotic Plaques (AP) In 10 Study Patients and 9 Control Subjects

| | | | Coronary Arteries | | | | | | |
| | | | Number Narrowed 76 to 100 Percent | | | | | Number (%) Narrowed 96 to 100% | Mean Number per Patient Narrowed 76 to 100% |
Group	Persons (n)	Total	LM	LAD	LC	R	Total		
Study	10	39*	7	10	10	9	36 (92%)	12 (31%)	3.6
Control	9	34*	2	9	8	9	28 (82%)	10 (29%)	3.1

* Left main coronary artery not examined in one study patient and In two control subjects.
CA = coronary arteries; LAD = left anterior descending; LC = left circumflex; LM = left main; R = right coronary.

Results

Study Patients

Among the 10 study patients, a total of 39 major (right, left main, left anterior descending and left circumflex) epicardial coronary arteries were examined (the left main coronary artery was not examined in one patient) and the results are summarized in Tables I to III. In all study patients at least three of the four major coronary arteries were narrowed severely (76 to 100 percent of cross-sectional area) by atherosclerotic plaques. The left main coronary artery was severely narrowed by atherosclerotic plaques in seven patients (Fig. 1), and was narrowed 26 to 75 percent by atherosclerotic plaques in two (but the residual lumen was occluded by thromboembolic material [Fig. 2]). Thus, the left main coronary artery was narrowed 76 to 100 percent in cross-sectional area by atherosclerotic plaques or thrombus, or both, in 9 of the 10 study patients.

The results of the quantitative analysis of the 5 mm long segments of coronary artery from eight study patients are summarized in Tables I and IV and in Figures 3 to 5. Of 354 such segments, 30 (9 percent) were narrowed 96 to 100 percent in cross-sectional area by atherosclerotic plaques; 173 segments (49 percent) were narrowed 76 to 95 percent; 83 segments (23 percent) 51 to 75 percent; 45 segments (13 percent) 26 to 50 percent, and 23 segments (6 percent) 0 to 25 percent.

A scoring system was utilized to indicate both the severity and the extent of coronary arterial narrowing. Every 5 mm long segment of coronary artery from each patient was assigned a score of 1 to 4 based on the amount of cross-sectional area narrowing by atherosclerotic plaques as follows: 1 = 0–25 percent, 2 = 26 to 50 percent, 3 = 51 to 75 percent and 4 = 76 to 100 percent narrowing. A total score was obtained for each patient and the score per 5 mm segment was then calculated by dividing the total score per patient by the number of segments examined from that patient. The total scores for the study patients ranged from 83 to 187 (mean 147) and the scores per 5 mm segment from 2.92 to 3.66 (mean 3.34) (Table I).

The percent of 5 mm segments narrowed to various degrees in each of the four major coronary arteries in the study patients is shown in Figure 4. There was no significant difference in the amount of severe narrowing among the four arteries. The mean percent of 5 mm segments narrowed 76 to 100 percent in cross-sectional area was significantly greater in the proximal than in the distal halves of the left anterior descending (p <0.01) and right (p <0.005) coronary arteries in the study patients (Fig. 5).

Control Subjects

Eight of the nine control subjects had severe narrowing of at least three major epicardial coronary arteries but only two patients had severe narrowing of all four arteries (Table II). Significantly more major coronary arteries were severely narrowed in the study patients than in the control subjects (p <0.01, Table II) and there was severe narrowing of the left main coronary artery in more study patients than in control subjects

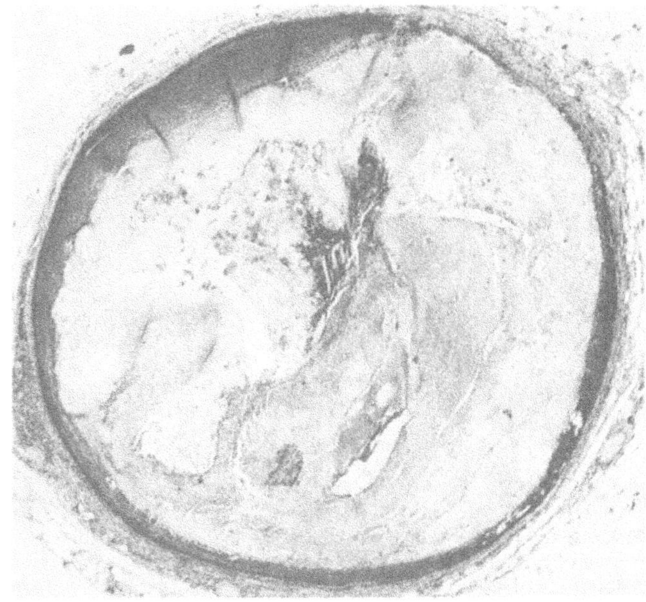

FIGURE 1. Patient 2. Photomicrograph of a cross section of the left main coronary artery in a 38 year old man who had unstable angina pectoris and fatal cardiac arrest during cardiac catheterization. The other three major epicardial coronary arteries were similarly narrowed. (Movat stain ×20, reduced by 7 percent.)

(p <0.05, Table III). The results of the quantitative analysis of the 5 mm coronary arterial segments from the nine control subjects are summarized in Table IV and Figures 4 and 5. The percent of segments from all four coronary arteries narrowed in each category did not differ significantly from that in the study group; however, the percent of segments of the left anterior descending coronary artery narrowed 76 to 100 percent was significantly less than in the study patients (p <0.02). The mean score per 5 mm segment was significantly greater for the study patients than for the control subjects (p <0.025).

Comments

Results of previous studies: Relatively little anatomic information is available on the amount, location and extent of coronary arterial narrowing in patients with angina pectoris who died during cardiac catheterization. Several[3–10] but not all[11–15] investigators suggested that patients with, compared with those without, severe narrowing of the left main coronary artery are at a greater risk of dying during cardiac catheterization. Among patients with angina pectoris who died during or up to 5 days after coronary angiography, severe narrowing of the left main coronary artery

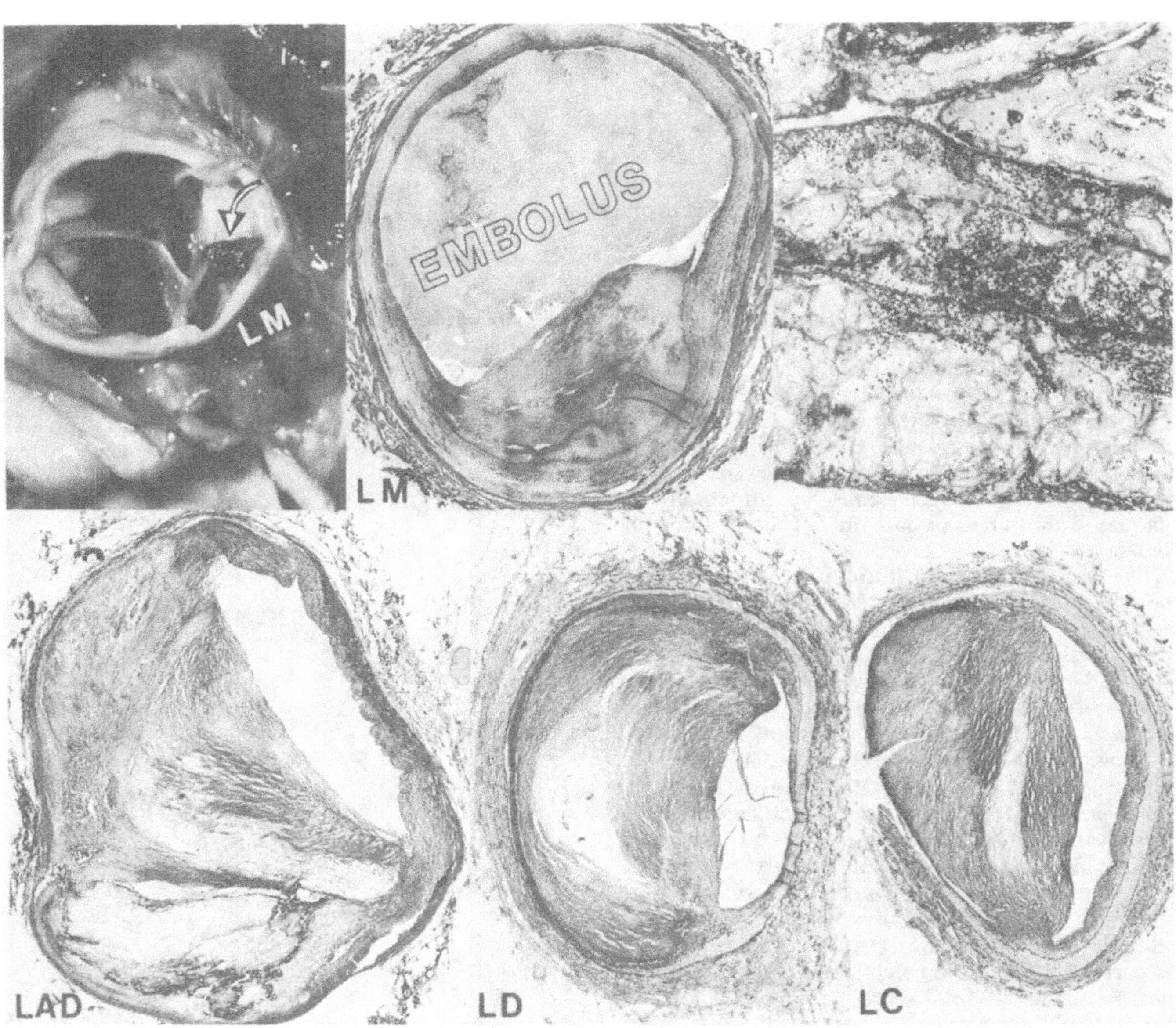

FIGURE 2. Patient 7. With the catheter tip placed in the left sinus of Valsalva the catheter was flushed. Systemic arterial pressure decreased immediately to shock levels in this 49 year old woman, and cardiac arrest occurred. At necropsy, a linear clot (**arrow**) was found in the left aortic sinus extending into the left main coronary artery (gross specimen, **top left**). Histologic sections showed the embolus to be limited to the left main (LM) coronary artery, which had been narrowed between 26 and 50 percent in cross-sectional area by old atherosclerotic plaque. The left main coronary artery in this patient gave off three branches: the left anterior descending (LAD), the left diagonal (LD) and the left circumflex (LC); the lumen of each of these three arteries was already obliterated more than 75 percent by old atherosclerotic plaque. The embolus in the left main artery did not extend farther down the coronary tree because it was larger than the residual lumen of any of the three branches of the left main coronary artery. The embolus, shown in the photomicrograph at **upper right**, consisted primarily of platelets, and its configuration is suggestive of the lumen of the catheter folded over on itself several times. (Movat stain ×27, reduced by 7 percent.)

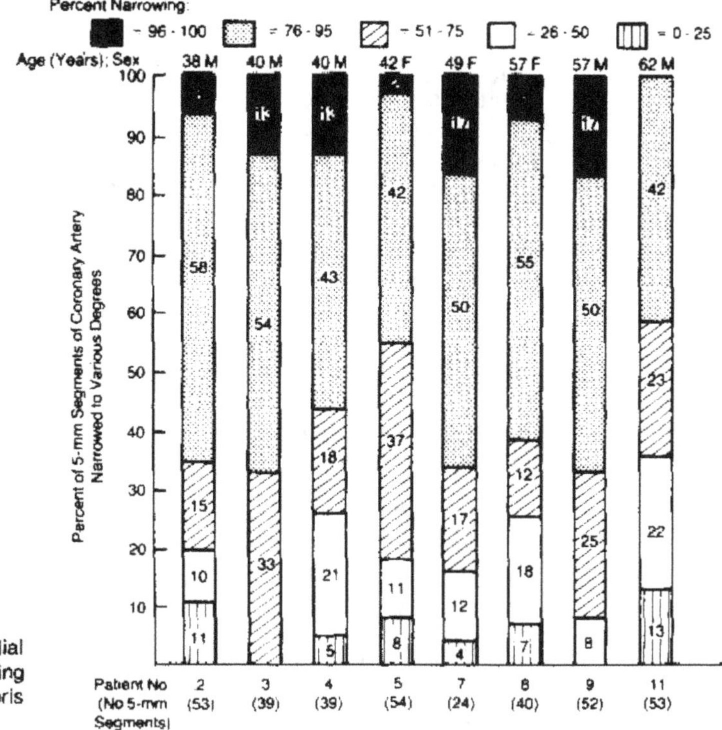

FIGURE 3. Percent of 5 mm segments of the four major epicardial coronary arteries with five categories of cross-sectional area narrowing by atherosclerotic plaques in eight study patients with angina pectoris who died during cardiac catheterization.

was found on angiography in 8 of 11 patients studied by Bourassa and Noble,[6] in 4 of 7 studied by Wolfson et al.[7] and in 5 of 12 studied by Davis et al.[9] Furthermore, at least three of the four major coronary arteries were severely narrowed in 9 of the 11 patients studied by Bourassa and Noble,[6] in 6 of the 7 reported on by Wolfson et al.[7] and in 11 of 12 reported on by Davis et al.[9] Thus, in 17 (57 percent) of the 30 patients (10 of whom died *during* the catheterization procedure) studied by these three groups of investigators, the lumen of the left main coronary artery was narrowed more than 50 percent in diameter, and in 26 (87 percent) at least three of the four major epicardial coronary arteries were severely narrowed.

Characteristics of the 10 study patients: All of our 10 patients with angina pectoris had cardiac arrest *during* cardiac catheterization. None had had chronic congestive heart failure or clinical evidence of acute myocardial infarction immediately before the catheterization. Nine died during attempted coronary angiography and one during right-sided cardiac catheterization. At necropsy, at least three of the four major

TABLE IV

Number and Percent of 5 mm Segments of the Four Major Epicardial Coronary Arteries in Eight Study Patients (P) Who Died During Cardiac Catheterization and in Nine Control Subjects (C) Who Died During or Shortly After Aortocoronary Bypass Operations Showing the Five Grades of Cross-Sectional Area Luminal Narrowing by Atherosclerotic Plaques

| | Percent Cross-Sectional Area Luminal Narrowing | | | | | | | | | |
| | 0–25 | | 26–50 | | 51–75 | | 76–95 | | 96–100 | |
Coronary Artery	P	C	P	C	P	C	P	C	P	C
LM										
n	0	2	2	3	4	7	6	2	1	1
(%)	(0)	(13)	(15)	(20)	(31)	(47)	(46)	(13)	(8)	(7)
LAD										
n	10	31	19	42	27	36	57	47	2	6
(%)	(9)	(19)	(16)	(26)	(23)	(22)	(50)	(29)	(2)	(4)
LC										
n	12	14	9	16	18	13	49	53	12	4
(%)	(12)	(14)	(9)	(16)	(18)	(13)	(49)	(53)	(12)	(4)
R										
n	1	13	15	22	34	42	61	79	15	14
(%)	(1)	(8)	(12)	(13)	(27)	(25)	(48)	(46)	(12)	(8)
Total										
n	23	60	45	83	83	98	173	181	30	25
(%)	(6)	(13)	(13)	(19)	(23)	(22)	(49)	(40)	(9)	(6)

LAD = left anterior descending coronary artery; LC = left circumflex coronary artery; LM = left main coronary artery; R = right coronary artery.

epicardial coronary arteries in all 10 patients were narrowed 76 to 100 percent in cross-sectional area by atherosclerotic plaques, and the left main coronary artery in 9 of the 10 patients was narrowed to this degree (by plaque only in 7 and by thromboembolic material superimposed on plaque in 2). The appearance of the clot in these last two patients indicated that it had originated in the catheter (Fig. 2).[16]

Examination of each 5 mm segment from the entire lengths of the four major epicardial coronary arteries in 8 of our 10 patients disclosed that a mean of 58 percent of segments were narrowed 76 to 100 percent in cross-sectional area, an amount substantially higher than the mean percent in other groups of necropsy patients previously studied in this laboratory: sudden coronary death (36 percent),[17] acute transmural myocardial infarction (34 percent),[18] healed myocardial infarction with chronic, eventually fatal congestive heart

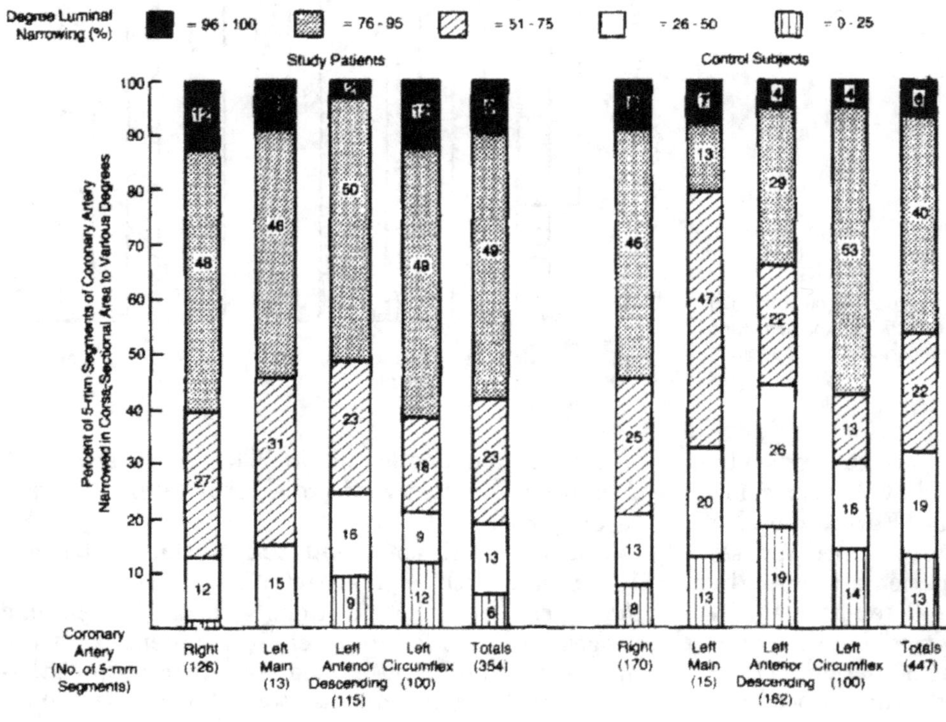

FIGURE 4. Percent of 5 mm segments in each of the four major epicardial coronary arteries with five categories of cross-sectional area narrowing by atherosclerotic plaques from eight study patients dying during cardiac catheterization and in nine control subjects.

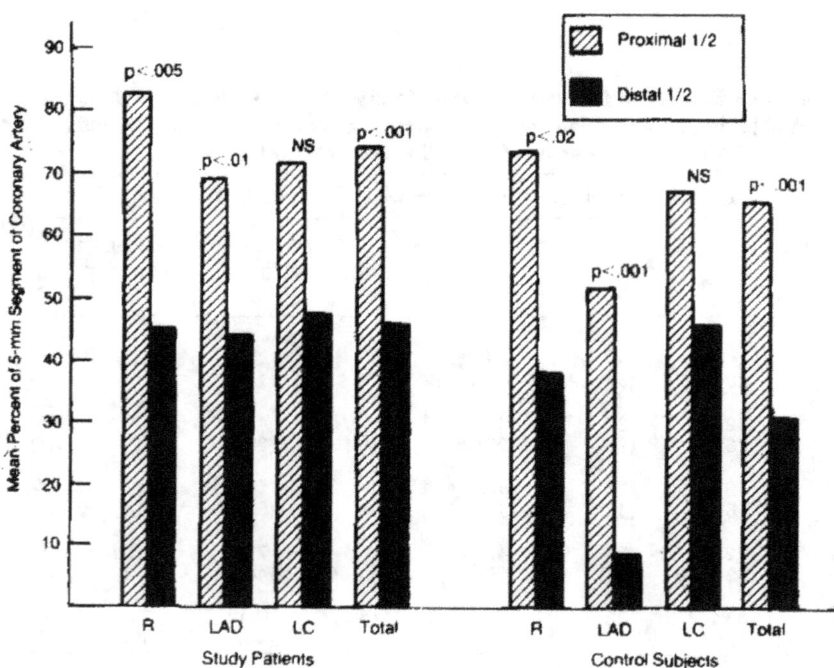

FIGURE 5. Mean percent of 5 mm segments in the proximal and distal halves of the right (R), left anterior descending (LAD) and left circumflex (LC) coronary arteries narrowed 76 to 100 percent in cross-sectional area by atherosclerotic plaques in eight study patients who died during cardiac catheterization and in nine control subjects.

TABLE V

Comparison of Certain Cardiac Observations Including Amounts of Coronary Narrowing by Atherosclerotic Plaques at Necropsy in 10 Study Patients and Nine Control Subjects With Findings in Five Other Subgroups of Necropsy Patients With Coronary Heart Disease

Subgroup (reference)	Patients (n)	Age Range (mean) (yr)	Number (%) of Patients With LMCA Narrowed >75% in XSA	Number (%) of 5 mm Segments Narrowed >75% in XSA	Mean Score*	Number (%) of Patients With LV T F	Number (%) of Patients With LV T N	Number (%) of Patients With AP	Number (%) of Patients With CCHF
Sudden coronary death[17]	31	22–85 (47)	3 (10)	557 (36)	2.98	4 (13)	0	16 (52)	0
Acute myocardial infarct[18]	27	33–82 (59)	3 (11)	484 (34)	3.01	5 (19)	27 (100)	11 (41)	5 (19)
HMI → Fatal CCHF without LV aneurysm[19]	9	48–77 (63)	0	150 (28)	2.78	9	0	1 (11)	9
HMI → LV aneurysm[20]	28	31–85 (62)	2 (7)	323 (33)	3.03	28 (100)	1 (4)	4 (14)	22 (79)
HMI → noncardiac death[21]	18	50–80 (66)	0	292 (32)	2.87	18 (100)	0	3 (17)	0
AP → CABP Death	9	32–65 (47)	2	206 (46)	3.01	6	0	9	0
AP → CC Death	10	35–62 (47)	7	203 (58)	3.32	4	2	10	0

* Mean score is derived by assigning a number to each 5 mm segment based on the amount of cross-sectional area narrowing by atherosclerotic plaques (1 = 0 to 25 percent narrowing; 2 = 26 to 50 percent; 3 = 51 to 75 percent; 4 = 76 to 100 percent) and then by dividing the total score for the group by the number of 5 mm segments examined in that group.

AP = angina pectoris; CABP = coronary artery bypass; CC = cardiac catheterization; CCHF = chronic congestive heart failure; F = fibrosis; HMI = healed myocardial infarct; LM = left main; LV = left ventricular; N = necrosis; T = transmural; XSA = cross-sectional area.

failure without ventricular aneurysm (29 percent),[19] healed myocardial infarction with true left ventricular aneurysm (33 percent),[20] and nonfatal healed transmural myocardial infarction with fatal noncardiac disease (32 percent)[21] (Table V). In addition, comparison of our 10 study patients with a group of patients with angina pectoris who died during or shortly after aortocoronary bypass operation (preceded by uncomplicated cardiac catheterization) disclosed more severe coronary narrowing (as assessed by a coronary scoring system) in the 10 study patients than in the 9 control subjects.

Surgical implications: In a patient with angina pectoris who cannot be resuscitated from cardiac arrest during cardiac catheterization, emergency aortocoronary bypass grafting appears warranted. Our study suggests that in such patients, the surgeon can assume that at least three and usually all four major epicardial coronary arteries are narrowed 76 to 100 percent in cross-sectional area. Furthermore, although the atherosclerotic process is diffuse, the amount of severe luminal narrowing is usually greater in the proximal than in the distal halves of the major coronary arteries, and, therefore, each would usually be suitable for grafting.

References

1. **Movat HZ.** Demonstration of all connective tissue elements in a single section: pentachrome stains. Arch Pathol 1955;60:289–95.
2. **Isner JM, Wu M, Virmani R, Jones AA, Roberts WC.** Comparison of degrees of coronary arterial luminal narrowing determined by visual inspection of histologic sections under magnification among three independent observers and comparison to that obtained by video planimetry: an analysis of 559 five-mm segments of 61 coronary arteries from eleven patients. Lab Invest 1980;42:566–70.
3. **Cohen MV, Cohn PF, Herman MV, Gorlin R.** Diagnosis and prognosis of main left coronary artery obstruction. Circulation 1972;45:Suppl I:I-57–65.
4. **Lavine P, Kimbiris D, Segal BL, Linhart JW.** Left main coronary disease: clinical, arteriographic and hemodynamic appraisal. Am J Cardiol 1972;30:791–6.
5. **Lim JS, Proudfit WL, Sones FM Jr.** Left main coronary arterial obstruction: long-term follow-up of 141 nonsurgical cases. Am J Cardiol 1975;36:131–5.
6. **Bourassa MG, Noble J.** Complication rate of coronary arteriography: a review of 5250 cases studied by a percutaneous femoral technique. Circulation 1976;53:106–14.
7. **Wolfson S, Grant D, Ross AM, Cohen LS.** Risk of death related to coronary arteriography: role of left coronary arterial lesions. Am J Cardiol 1976;37:210–6.
8. **Bulkley BH, Roberts WC.** Atherosclerotic narrowing of the left main coronary artery: a necropsy analysis of 152 patients with fatal coronary heart disease and varying degrees of left main narrowing. Circulation 1976;53:823–8.
9. **Davis K, Kennedy JW, Kemp HG Jr, Judkins MP, Gosselin AJ, Killip T.** Complications of coronary arteriography from the collaborative study of coronary artery surgery (CASS). Circulation 1979;59:1105–12.
10. **Hamby RI.** Clinical-Anatomical Correlates in Coronary Artery Disease. Mount Kisco: Futura, 1979:79–171.
11. **Zeft HJ, Manley JC, Huston JH, Tector AJ, Auer JE, Johnson WD.** Left main coronary artery stenosis: results of coronary bypass surgery. Circulation 1974;49:68–76.
12. **Rösch J, De Mots H, Antonovic R, Rahimtoola SH, Judkins MP, Dotter CT.** Coronary arteriography in left main coronary artery

disease. Am J Roentgenol 1974;121:583–90.

13. **Khaja FU, Sharma SD, Easley RM, Heinle RA, Goldstein S.** Left main coronary artery lesions: risks of catheterization; exercise testing and surgery. Circulation 1974;50:Suppl II:II-136–40.

14. **Demots H, Bonchek LI, Rösch J, Anderson RP, Starr A, Rahimtoola SH.** Left main coronary artery disease: risks of angiography, importance of coexisting disease of other coronary arteries and effects of revascularization. Am J Cardiol 1975;36:136–41.

15. **Sung RJ, Mallon SM, Richter SE, et al.** Left main coronary artery obstruction: follow-up of thirty patients with and without surgery. Circulation 1975;51, 52:Suppl I:I-112–8.

16. **Takaro T, Pifarre R, Wuerflein RD, et al.** Acute coronary occlusion following coronary arteriography: mechanisms and surgical relief. Surgery 1972;72:1018–29.

17. **Roberts WC, Jones AA.** Quantitation of coronary arterial narrowing at necropsy in sudden coronary death: analysis of 31 patients and comparison with 25 control subjects. Am J Cardiol 1979;44: 39–45.

18. **Roberts WC, Jones AA.** Quantification of coronary arterial narrowing at necropsy in acute transmural myocardial infarction: analysis and comparison of findings in 27 patients and 22 controls. Circulation 1980;61:786–90.

19. **Virmani R, Roberts WC.** Quantification of coronary arterial narrowing and of left ventricular myocardial scarring in healed myocardial infarction with chronic, eventually fatal, congestive cardiac failure. Am J Med 1980;68:831–8.

20. **Cabin HS, Roberts WC.** True left ventricular aneurysm and healed myocardial infarction: clinical and necropsy observations including quantification of degrees of coronary arterial narrowing. Am J Cardiol 1980;46:754–63.

21. **Virmani R, Roberts WC.** Non-fatal healed transmural myocardial infarction and fatal non-cardiac disease. Qualification and quantification of coronary arterial narrowing and of left ventricular scarring in 18 necropsy patients. Br Heart J, in press.

Survival for 20 years or longer after transmural acute myocardial infarction: Analysis of eight well-documented necropsy patients

Clinical and necropsy findings are described in eight patients who lived 20 to 31 years (mean 24 years) after healing of a transmural acute myocardial infarct. Two had left ventricular aneurysms and one had both right and left ventricular infarcts. Survival for 2 decades or more after healing of a transmural acute myocardial infarct has rarely been documented and descriptions of hearts at necropsy in patients with well-documented infarcts 20 years or more earlier are virtually nonexistent. (AM HEART J 102:176, 1981.)

Bruce M. McManus, M.D., Ph.D., and William C. Roberts, M.D. *Bethesda, Md.*

Although many reports are available describing follow-up of patients for up to 5 years after acute myocardial infarction (AMI), only 10 reports to our knowledge have described follow-up for longer than 10 years AMI.[1-10] Of these reports which provide clinical data in 3769 patients, 11 patients (six reported by Richards et al.[5] and five by Sigler[10]) lived 20 years or longer. Single case studies also are available in at least 14 other patients who lived 20 years or longer (the longest survivor was 38 years[15]) after AMI.[11-15] Of these 25 reported patients (11 plus 14), 15 died and necropsy information was reported in three.[12, 13, 15] Because the morphologic and clinical data on patients surviving 20 years or longer without operative intervention after AMI are lacking, we describe our observations in an additional eight patients.

METHODS AND RESULTS

Patients studied. Certain clinical and morphologic features (Figs. 1 to 7) in the eight men are summarized in Table I. The AMI occurred at ages 28 to 57 years (mean 42 years) and death at ages 51 to 78 years (mean 66 years). The AMI in each was well documented by typical clinical and ECG features, by confirmation of hospitalization, by review of medical records, and by discussion with the spouse and/or family.

From the Pathology Branch, National Heart, Lung, and Blood Institute, National Institutes of Health.

Received for publication March 6, 1981; accepted Apr. 3, 1981.

Reprint requests: William C. Roberts, M.D., Pathology Branch, Bldg. 10A, Room 3E-30, National Heart, Lung and Blood Institute, National Institutes of Health, Bethesda, MD 20205.

Post-AMI clinical features. Following the AMI, patients No. 6 (Figs. 5 and 6) and No. 7 (Fig. 7) (Table I) never again had clinical symptoms of myocardial ischemia or dysfunction. Patient No. 1 remained asymptomatic until 18 years after the initial AMI when mild angina pectoris and congestive heart failure (CHF) appeared, and he later had a second and fatal AMI (Fig. 1). Patient No. 4 had evidence of CHF from the time of healing of the AMI and it progressed slowly during the subsequent 23 years until his death while sleeping (Fig. 3). Patients No. 2, 3, and 5 had angina pectoris without CHF; patients No. 2 and 3 died from a second AMI (Fig. 2), and patient No. 5 died suddenly (Fig. 4). Selective coronary angiography in patient No. 1, performed 2 years before death, disclosed total obstruction of the left anterior descending artery proximally, severe (> 75% decrease in diameter) stenosis of the right coronary and mild (< 50% decrease in diameter) narrowing of the left circumflex artery, and left ventricular angiography revealed a large left ventricular aneurysm[19] with reduced (25%) ejection fraction.

Necropsy findings. At necropsy, patients No. 1 and 4 had large healed anterior wall myocardial infarcts (Figs. 1 and 3) which were aneurysmally dilated; patient No. 6 had a relatively small posterior wall healed left ventricular (LV) infarct and a large healed right ventricular (RV) infarct (Fig. 6). Patient No. 2 had a healed anterior wall infarct and an acute posterolateral LV infarct (Fig. 2). Patients No. 5 (Fig. 4), 7, and 8 each had posteroseptal healed LV infarcts. All eight patients had at least two of the four major (right, left main, left anterior descending, left circumflex) epicardial coronary arteries narrowed > 75% in cross-sectioned area by atherosclerotic plaques (Figs. 1 and 6). In patients No. 5 and 6, a histologic section of each 5 mm long segment of each of the four major coronary epicardial coronary arteries was prepared and the findings are summarized in Tables II and III.

Fig. 1. Patient No. 1 (Table I). ECG recorded 4 days before death showing left bundle branch block. *a*, Nearly totally occluded right coronary artery (Movat stain; original magnification ×30) *b*, Transverse section of ventricles showing large healed transmural anterior wall infarct and recent posterior infarct.

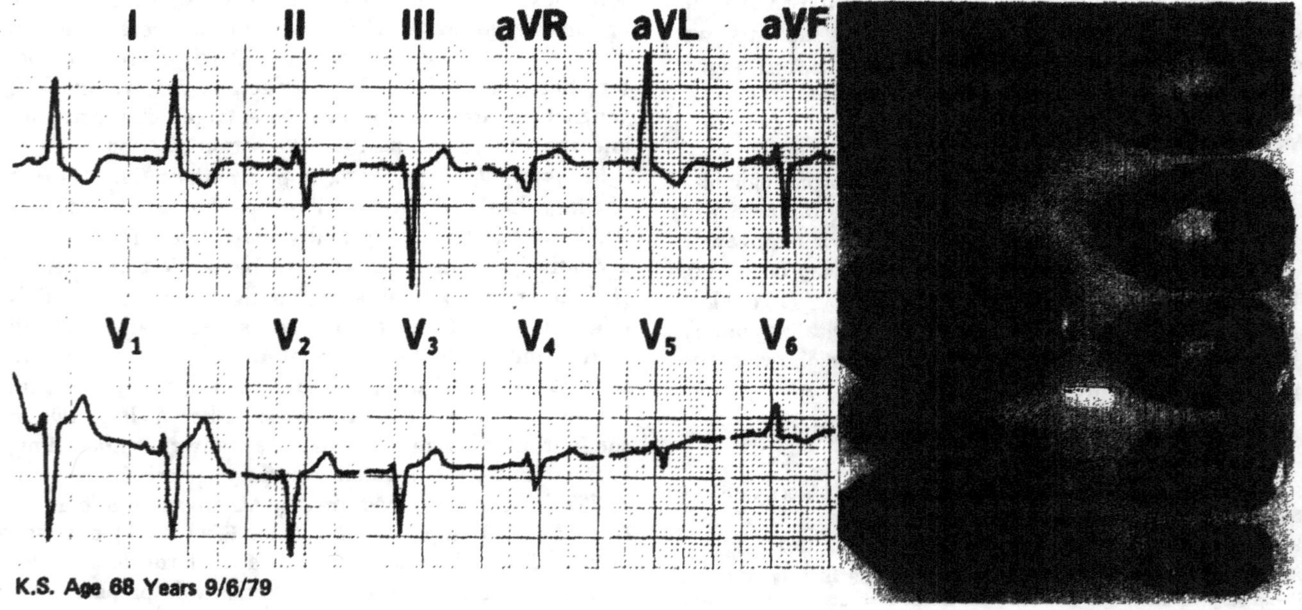

Fig. 2. Patient No. 2 (Table I). ECG recorded 6 days before death showing left bundle branch block. The transverse ventricular slices show extensive anterior wall and septal scarring from apex to base, focal posterior wall scarring, and a dilated left ventricular cavity.

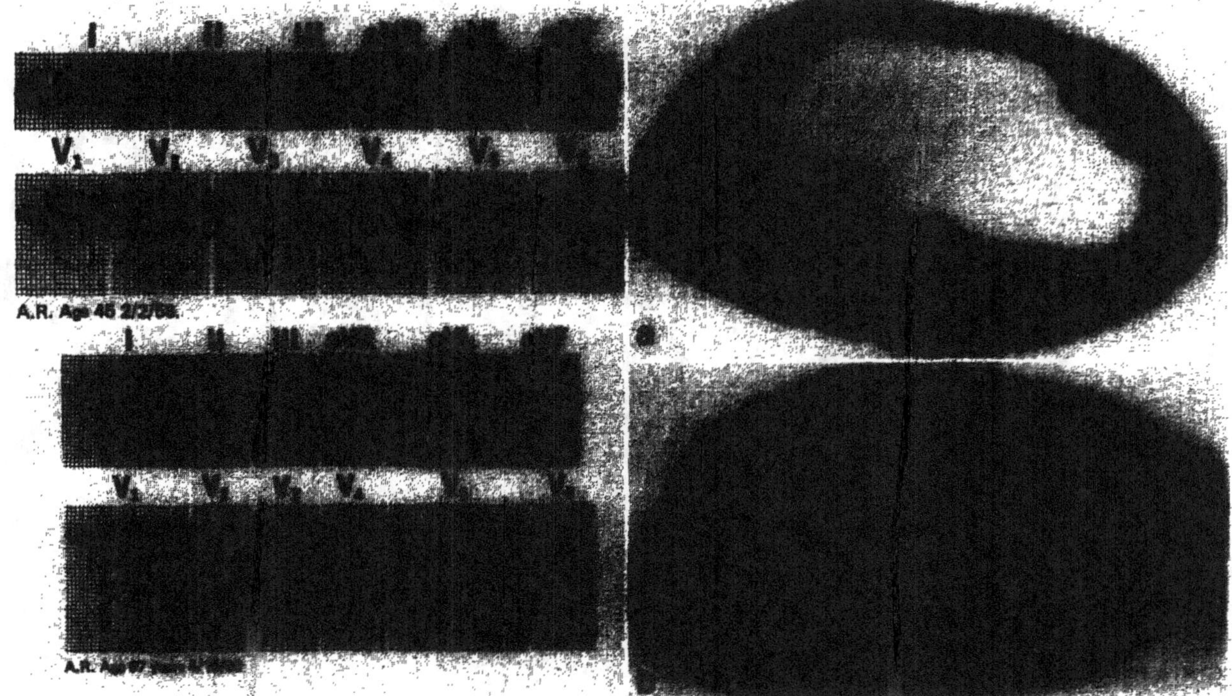

Fig. 3. Patient No. 4 (Table I). ECGs recorded at the time of the AMI in 1958 and 4.5 months before death in 1980. Transverse sections of the ventricle aneurysm (*a*) with calcific deposits (*b*).

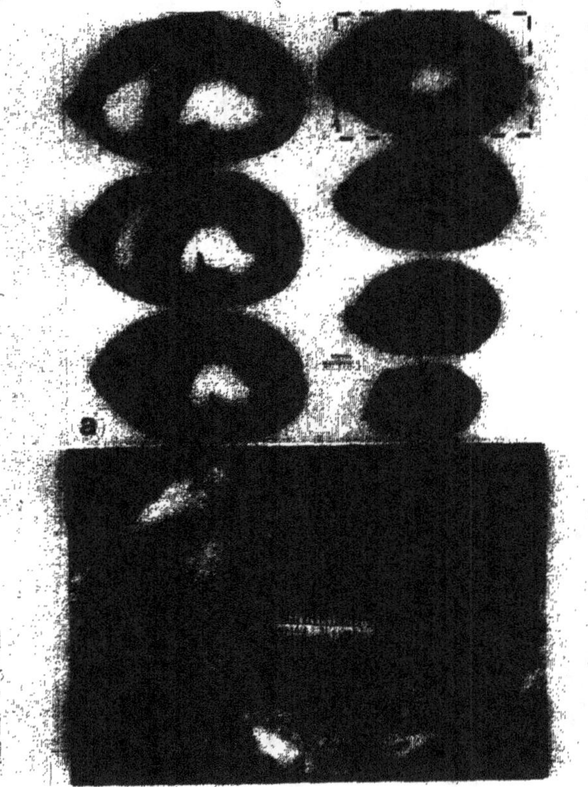

Fig. 4. Patient No. 5 (Table I). *a*, Transverse sections of ventricles showing extensive healed transmural infarct of the posterior left ventricular wall extending from apex to base and dilated cavities. *b*, Close-up of bracketed section from *a*.

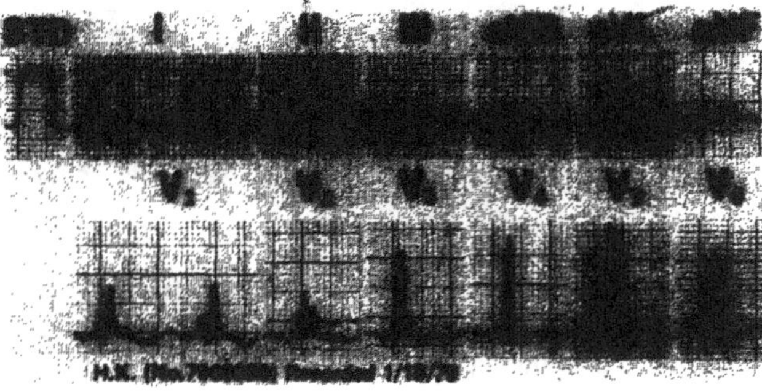

Fig. 5. Patient No. 6 (Table I). ECG recorded 8 months before death showing Q waves in leads II, III, and aV_F and right bundle branch block.

DISCUSSION

Consideration of factors related to prolonged survival post-AMI. Each of the eight above-described patients lived 20 years or longer after healing of a transmural AMI which in two patients was large and aneurysmal and in one was associated with a large RV healed infarct. Despite the large sizes of the infarcts in the patients with aneurysms, one was asymptomatic for 18 of his surviving 20 years, and the second lived an active life (jogged, golf) for 23 years after the AMI, despite some signs of CHF which later progressed. The patient with the associated RV infarct never had symptoms of myocardial ischemia or dysfunction during the entire 25-year postinfarct period.

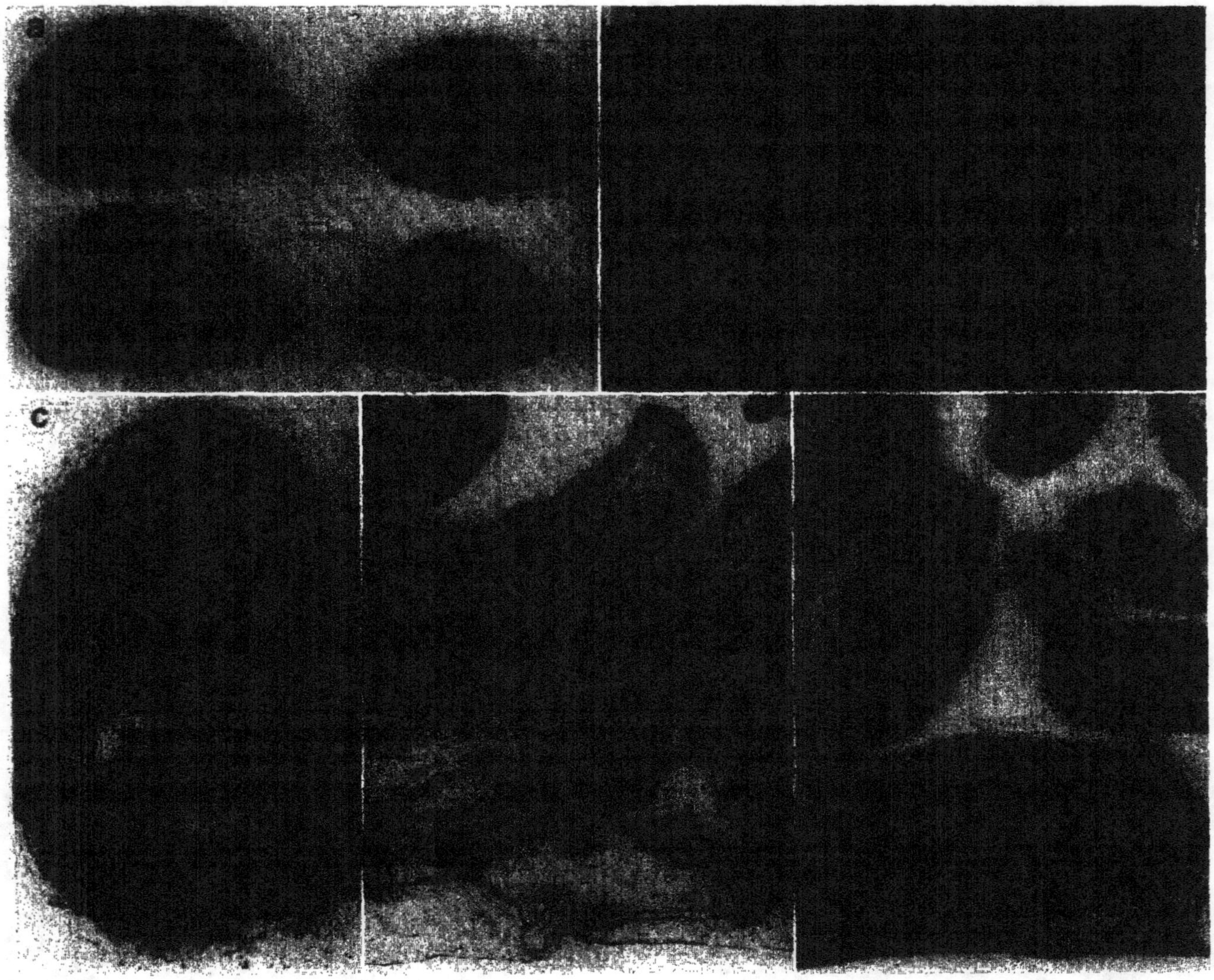

Fig. 6. Patient No. 6 (Table I). Transverse sections of the ventricles (*a*) showing infarct of both left and right (*b*) ventricular walls posteriorly. Photomicrographs of posterior left (*d*) and right (*e*) ventricular walls showing extensive scarring of each. (Hematoxylin and eosin stains; original magnifications ×12). Severe narrowing by atherosclerosis of right coronary artery (*c*). (*c*, Movat staining; original magnification ×28).

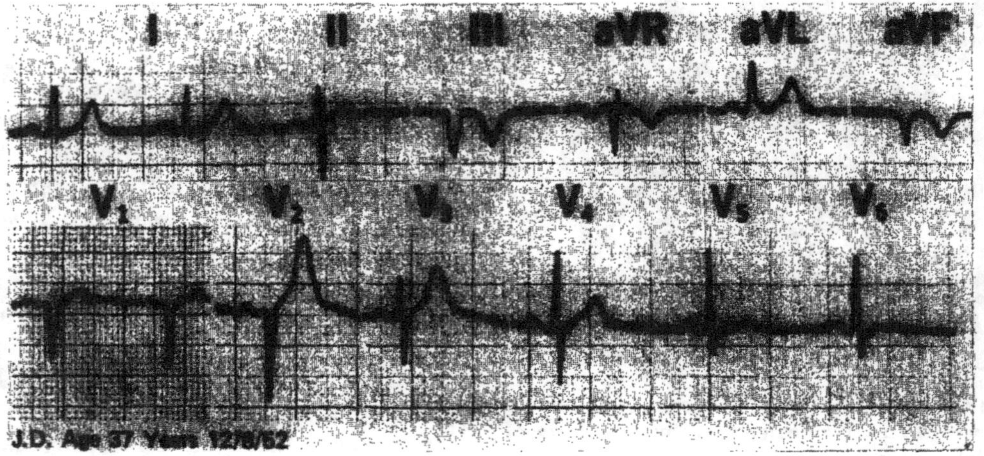

Fig. 7. Patient No. 7 (Table I). ECG recorded at the time of the AMI 28 years before death.

Table I. Clinical and necropsy features of eight patients who lived 20 years or longer after their first acute myocardial infarction (AMI)

Pt.	Age (yrs) at death	Age (yrs) at AMI	Inter-val (yrs) AMI to death	Mode of death	SH Before AMI	SH After AMI	AP[a]	AMI[a]	CHF[a]	CS Pre AMI	CS Post AMI
1	59	39	20	AMI	−	0	+[b]	+	+[b]	+	+
2	68	47	21	AMI	+	0	+	+	0	0	0
3	78	57	21	AMI	−	−	+	+	0	−	−
4	67	45	22	Sudden	+	0	0	0	+	0	0
5	51	28	23	Sudden	0	+	+	0	0	+	+
6	73	48	25	GI	0	0	0	0	0	+	0
7	65	37	28	Sudden	+	+	0	0	0	+	+
8	68	37	31	CHF	−	0	0	0	+	+	−

[a]After initial acute myocardial infarction.
[b]Appeared at age 57 years.
[c]Mean of two values (200 and 240 mg/dl).
[d]Mean of two values (190 and 310 mg/dl).
[e]Mean of 10 values during last 15 years (range 266 to 405 mg/dl) despite a low cholesterol diet.
[f]Periodic atrial fibrillation.
[g]Blood pressure normal with patient on diuretic therapy.
[h]Mean of two values (235 and 254 for TC and 182 and 393 for TG).
[i]Single value obtained on day of death during the acute gastrointestinal illness.
[j]Mean of two values (239 and 270 mg/dl).

AMI = acute myocardial infarct; An = aneurysm; AP = angina pectoris; APB = atrial premature beats; BBB = complete bundle branch block; BP = systemic blood pressure; CHF = congestive heart failure; CS = cigarette smoker; GI = gastrointestinal disorder; LV = left ventricle; N = normal; RV = right ventricle; s/d = systolic/diastolic; SH = systemic hypertension; SR = sinus rhythm; TC = total serum cholesterol; TG = serum triglyceride; VPB = ventricular premature beats.

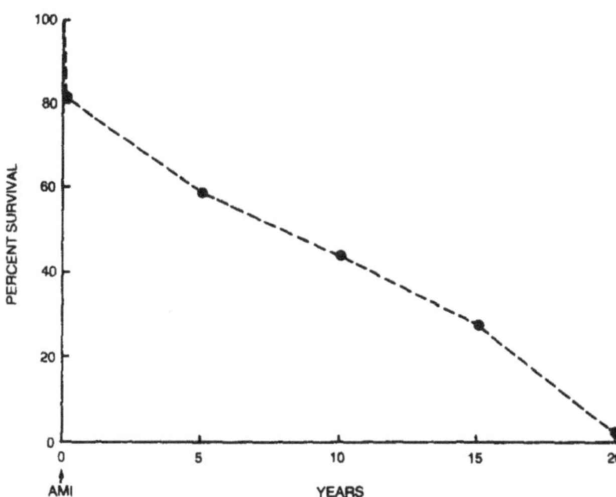

Fig. 8. Approximate cumulative survival (%) at selected year periods of published reports[2, 3, 5, 7] of nonoperated patients followed at least 15 years after their first nonfatal acute myocardial infarction (AMI).

Extended long-term survival post-AMI; a unique and largely unpredictable phenomenon in young adult males. Review of reported studies of patients followed for at least 10 years after AMI disclosed that about 40% survived 10 years but less than 1% survived for longer than 20 years (Fig. 8).[2, 3, 5, 7] Little detailed information, however, is available on the patients who lived 20 years or longer after AMI.[2, 5, 8-15] Obviously, to live longer than 20 years after AMI, the AMI must occur at a relatively young age and death must occur at a relatively late age. Of the six patients in whom this information was available,[2, 11-13, 15] the mean age at the time of the AMI was 47 years and the mean age of death was 78 years. The interval from the first AMI to death in 25 reported patients ranged from 20 to 38 years (mean 27 years). Information regarding myocardial dysfunction and ischemia was available in 7 of the 25 patients[5, 10, 13, 15]; four were asymptomatic during the entire postinfarction period (28, 28, 30, and 38 years), one was asymptomatic for 27 of his 37 year postinfarction period, and only two had clear evidence of cardiac dysfunction or ischemia and one of these had a clinically silent LV aneurysm and persistent systemic hypertension. Information regarding location and size of the AMI and the status of the epicardial coronary arteries was provided in only 3 of the 11 patients.[12, 14, 15] Thus, from analysis of the previously reported patients surviving > 20 years after AMI factors which allowed their prolonged survival are not clear. Evidence of myocar-

| BP[a] s/d (mm Hg) | TC[a] | TG[a] | Electrocardiogram[a] | | | | | | Heart weight (gm) | Location, LV healed infarct | LV An |
| | | | SR | Axis | BBB | Q Waves | APB | VPB | | | |
	(mg/dl)										
125/80	220[c]	250[d]	+	Left	Left	+	+	+	480	anterior	+
115/80	–	–	+	Left	Left	0	0	0	475	anterior	0
130/80	–	–	+	N	0	0	0	0	460	anterior	0
110/70	338[e]	165	+[f]	N	Left	+	0	+	430	anterior	+
125/80[g]	245[h]	238[h]	+	N	0	+	0	0	550	posterior	0
140/80	101[i]	–	+	N	Right	+	0	+	405	posterior	0
145/90	255[j]	82	+	N	0	+	0	0	450	posterior	0
100/65	–	–	+	N	Right	–	0	+	550	posterior	0

Table II. Number and percent of 5 mm segments of the four major epicardial coronary arteries narrowed to various degrees in cross-sectional area (XSA) by atherosclerotic plaques in patient No. 5

| Coronary artery | No. of 5 mm segments examined | No. of 5 mm segments narrowed in percent to various degrees in XSA | | | | |
		0-25	26-50	51-75	76-95	96-100
Left main	2	0	0	1	1	0
Left anterior descending	12	0	0	0	5	7
Left circumflex	12	0	0	0	6	6
Right	17	0	0	3	11	3
Totals: No.	43	0	0	4	23	16
(%)		(0)	(0)	(9)	(54)	(37)

Table III. Number and percent of 5 mm segments of the four major epicardial coronary arteries narrowed to various degrees in cross-sectional area (XSA) by atherosclerotic plaques in patient No. 6

| Coronary artery | No. of 5 mm segments examined | No. of 5 mm segments narrowed in percent to various degrees in XSA | | | | |
		0-25	26-50	51-75	76-95	96-100
Left main	1	0	1	0	0	0
Left anterior descending	20	3	5	7	5	0
Left circumflex	4	1	1	2	0	0
Right	18	1	4	3	5	5
Totals: No.	43	5	11	12	10	5
(%)		(12)	(26)	(28)	(23)	(12)

dial ischemia after healing of the AMI was absent or minimal in most of the 25 patients.

RV infarction and LV aneurysm. The finding of a healed RV infarct in patient No. 6 provides evidence that this complication of LV infarction is not necessarily of deleterious prognostic significance. Survival for such long periods after AMI—long enough to form an aneurysm as occurred in our patients Nos. 1 and 4 also—is of course unusual.[14, 17] None of the 28 patients with true aneurysm formation at sites of healed myocardial infarction reported previously from this laboratory survived longer than 5 years.[18, 19]

REFERENCES

1. Billings FT Jr, Kalstone BM, Spencer JL, Ball COT, Meneely GR: Prognosis of acute myocardial infarction. Am J Med **7**:356, 1949.
2. Smith C: Length of survival after myocardial infarction. JAMA **151**:167, 1953.
3. Cole DR, Singian EG, Katz LN: The long-term prognosis following myocardial infarction, and some factors which affect it. Circulation **9**:321, 1954.
4. Master AM, Jaffe HL, Teich EM, Brinberg L: Survival and rehabilitation after coronary occlusion. JAMA **156**:1552, 1954.
5. Richards DW, Bland EF, White PD: A completed twenty-five-year follow-up study of 200 patients with myocardial infarction. J Chronic Dis **4**:415, 1956.
6. Weiss MM: Ten-year prognosis of acute myocardial infarction. Am J Med Sci **231**:9, 1956.
7. Zukel WJ, Cohen BM, Mattingly TW, Hrubec Z: Survival following first diagnosis of coronary heart disease. Am Heart J **78**:159, 1969.
8. Sigler LH: Prognosis of angina pectoris and coronary occlusion. Followup of 1,700 cases. JAMA **146**:998, 1951.
9. Sigler LH: Prognosis of angina pectoris and myocardial infarction. Further report. Am J Cardiol **6**:252, 1960.
10. Sigler LH: Long survival following myocardial infarction. Report on 255 patients living ten years or longer after the first attack. Am J Cardiol **9**:547, 1962.
11. Palmer JH: The prognosis following recovery from coronary thrombosis, with special reference to the influence of hypertension and cardiac enlargement. QJ Med **6**:49, 1937.
12. White PD: A new record in longevity after coronary thrombosis. JAMA **108**:1796, 1937

13. Drake EH: Long survival following coronary thrombosis. Am Heart J 20:634, 1940.
14. Master AM, Jaffe HL: Complete functional recovery after coronary occlusion and insufficiency. JAMA 147:1721, 1951.
15. White PD, Donovan H: Hearts: Their long follow-up. Philadelphia, 1967, W.B. Saunders Co, p 175.
16. Isner JM, Roberts WC: Right ventricular infarction complicating left ventricular infarction secondary to coronary artery disease: Frequency, location, associated findings and significance from analysis of 236 necropsy patients with acute and healed myocardial infarction. Am J Cardiol 42:885, 1978.
17. Penner SL, Peters M: Longevity with ventricular aneurysm: Report of a case with a survival period of fifteen years. N Engl J Med 234:523, 1946.
18. Cabin HS, Roberts WC: Left ventricular aneurysm, intraaneurysmal thrombus and systemic embolus in coronary heart disease. Chest 77:586, 1980.
19. Cabin HS, Roberts WC: True left ventricular aneurysm and healed myocardial infarction. Clinical and necropsy observations including quantification of degrees of coronary arterial narrowing. Am J Cardiol 46:754, 1980.

Comparison of Degree and Extent of Coronary Narrowing by Atherosclerotic Plaque in Anterior and Posterior Transmural Acute Myocardial Infarction

FRANK C. BROSIUS III, M.D., AND WILLIAM C. ROBERTS, M.D.

SUMMARY   The percentage of cross-sectional area narrowing by atherosclerotic plaques in each 5-mm-long segment of the right, left main, left anterior descending and left circumflex coronary arteries was determined at necropsy in 50 patients who died of a first acute transmural myocardial infarction (AMI). The amount and extent of the coronary narrowing were compared in the 22 patients with anterior wall AMI and in the 28 patients with posterior wall AMI. Although the percentage of coronary arteries narrowed 76–100% was similar in the anterior and posterior wall AMI patients (74% vs 75%; average 3.0 of 4 coronary arteries per patient), the patients with anterior wall AMI had less severe narrowing of each of the 5-mm segments of the four major coronary arteries than did the patients with posterior wall AMI. Of the 1166 5-mm coronary segments examined in the 22 anterior wall AMI patients, 23% were narrowed 76–100% in cross-sectional area by atherosclerotic plaque, and of the 28 patients with posterior wall AMI, 39% of the segments were 76–100% narrowed ($p < 0.001$). Among the anterior AMI patients, a higher percentage of the 5-mm segments of the left anterior descending coronary artery was severely ($> 75\%$) narrowed than either posterior perfusing coronary artery. The percentage of segments narrowed 76–100% for each of the major coronary arteries in the posterior AMI patients, however, was similar. Thus, our necropsy patients with posterior wall AMI had more extensive and severe coronary artery narrowing than did our patients with anterior wall AMI. If the coronary arteries had not been examined quantitatively, this difference in severity would not have been apparent.

PATIENTS with acute myocardial infarction (AMI), with rare exception, have severe narrowing by atherosclerotic plaques of at least one and usually two or more of the four major epicardial coronary arteries.[1-6] Little information is available on the amount of coronary narrowing in patients who have anterior compared with those who have posterior ("inferior"[6]) wall left ventricular infarcts. Little information is also available on the amount of narrowing by atherosclerotic plaques in the four major coronary arteries in patients with either anterior or posterior left ventricular infarcts.[7] AMI of the anterior left ventricular wall is believed by many to indicate a severe "lesion" in the left anterior descending coronary artery and absent or lesser degrees of narrowing of the dominant posterior coronary artery. Similarly, a posterior AMI is generally considered to indicate a severe "lesion" in the right or left circumflex coronary arteries and absent or lesser degrees of narrowing of the left anterior descending coronary artery.[8] We examined both qualitatively and quantitatively at necropsy each of the four major epicardial coronary arteries in 50 patients who died during their first transmural AMI.

Patients and Methods

At the Pathology Branch, National Heart, Lung, and Blood Institute, 209 patients with transmural AMI unassociated with valvular heart disease, congenital cardiovascular anomalies, coronary emboli, major systemic disease or aortocoronary bypass operation have been studied. One hundred forty-nine patients were excluded from this analysis because the four major epicardial coronary arteries were unavailable for detailed histologic examination or

From the Pathology Branch, National Heart, Lung, and Blood Institute, National Institutes of Health, Bethesda, Maryland.

Address for correspondence: William C. Roberts, M.D., Building 10A, Room 3E-30, National Institutes of Health, Bethesda, Maryland 20205.

Received July 8, 1980; revision accepted February 19, 1981.

Circulation 64, No. 4, 1981.

because one or more grossly visible left ventricular free wall scars were present. Ten patients were excluded because the transmural AMI involved both anterior and posterior left ventricular free walls equally or was limited to the lateral or septal walls of the left ventricle. The remaining 50 patients form the basis of this study. In all 50 patients, the fatal AMI was the patient's first; none had grossly visible subendocardial (inner half) or transmural left ventricular free wall scars at necropsy.

The transmural AMI involved the anterior wall in 22 patients and the posterior wall in 28 patients, with or without involvement of the adjacent lateral wall or ventricular septum (fig. 1). In many patients, the AMI involved only the anterior or posterior wall in the basal portion of left ventricle but was circumferential, or nearly so, in the apical portion of left ventricle. The designation of "anterior" or "posterior" location of the AMI in these circumstances was determined by which wall was involved in the basal half of the ventricle.

Cardiac findings in the 50 patients are summarized in tables 1 and 2. Thirty-four men and 16 women, ages 33–82 years (mean 63 years), were studied. The interval from onset of symptoms compatible with AMI to death ranged from 24 hours to 42 days (mean 6 days): in two patients the interval was greater than 21 days; in five patients, 15–21 days; and in 43 patients, 14 days or less. No significant differences in age, sex or interval from onset of AMI to death were present between the 22 patients with anterior and the 28 patients with posterior wall AMI.

The four major coronary arteries — right, left main, left anterior descending and left circumflex — were examined. Each was excised intact, fixed, x-rayed, decalcified (if necessary) and cut transversely to its longitudinal axis into approximately 5-mm segments. Each segment was labeled sequentially from either its aortic ostium or from its origin from the left main. The 5-mm segments were labeled, dehydrated with alcohol and xylene, embedded in paraffin, and two histologic sections were cut and stained from each paraffin block. The Movat stain was used on one histologic section and all determinations of luminal narrowing were based on examination of the Movat-stained sections. The degree of narrowing by atherosclerotic plaque alone was determined by histologic examination of each cross-section magnified 25–50 times. The judgment regarding the degree of luminal narrowing of each 5-mm segment was based on the degree of luminal obliteration within the luminal circle bordered by the internal elastic membrane. The circle was visually subdivided into four equal-sized quadrants, and cross-sectional area luminal narrowing in each 5-mm segment was categorized as follows: 0–25%, 26–50%, 51–75% and 76–100%. The latter category of narrowing was subdivided into 76–95% and 96–100% to determine the number of segments totally occluded or nearly so. For recording purposes, the "dominant posterior coronary artery" was considered the artery that coursed to the crux of the heart and gave origin to the artery to the atrioventricular node and to one or more posterior descending coronary arteries. In 45 patients, the right coronary artery was the dominant posterior and in five patients, the left circumflex was the dominant posterior. The nondominant posterior coronary artery (the "other posterior artery") was the left circumflex in 45 patients and the right circumflex in five patients. When only three major coronary arteries (left anterior descending, dominant posterior and other posterior) were tabulated for each patient, the degree of narrow-

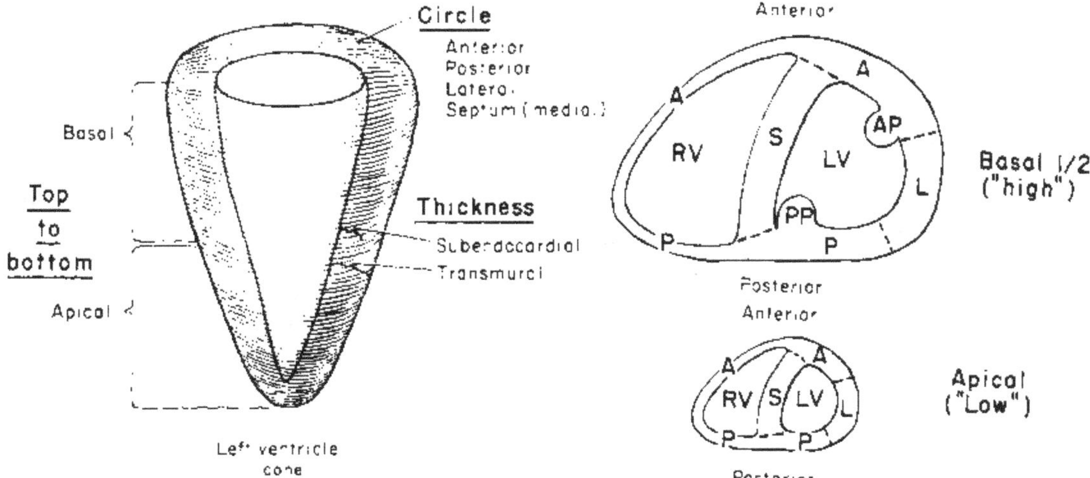

FIGURE 1. *Diagrams showing the left ventricle (LV) as a cone (left) and transverse cuts across the right ventricle (RV) and the LV (right). The length of the ventricle is divided into basal and apical halves. The larger transverse slice (upper right) is from the basal half and the smaller transverse slice is from the apical half. The dotted lines define the various compartments of the left ventricle. A = anterior wall of the left ventricle and anterolateral wall of the right ventricle; Ao = aorta; AP = anterolateral papillary muscle; L = lateral wall of left ventricle; LA = left atrium; P = posterior wall of the right and left ventricles; PP = posteromedial papillary muscle; S = ventricular septum.*

TABLE 1. *Selected Cardiac Findings in 22 Necropsy Patients with Fatal Acute Transmural Anterior Wall Myocardial Infarction*

Pt	Age (years)	Sex	Heart weight (g)	Necrosis VS	Necrosis Lat	No. of LAD, DP, & OP narrowed > 75% by AP	Narrowing of 5-mm segments of four coronary arteries Totals	Percentages of totals	No. LAD	No. DP	No. OP	Location of CA thrombus	
1	33	F	370	+	0	3	47(5) [1]	(11)[2]	17(3)[0]	19 (1) [0]	11(1) [1]	+	LAD
2	46	M	540	+	+	3	59(17)[1]	(29)[2]	24(6)[0]	20 (6) [0]	15(5) [1]	+	LAD
3	50	F	380	+	+	3†	56(16)[1]	(29)[2]	23(8)[0]	19 (3) [0]	14(5) [1]	0	—
4	53	M	390	+	0	3	54(33)[3]	(61)[6]	15(8)[0]	19*(15)[2]	20(10)[1]	0	—
5	54	M	350	+	+	3	55(19)[0]	(35)[0]	15(6)[0]	26 (5) [0]	14(8) [0]	0	—
6	54	M	380	+	0	3†	47(19)[3]	(40)[6]	15(3)[0]	17 (10)[2]	15(6) [1]	+	LAD
7	55	M	415	+	0	2	71(9) [0]	(13)[0]	25(4)[0]	21 (5) [0]	25(0) [0]	+	LAD
8	58	M	450	+	0	3	37(7) [1]	(19)[3]	12(3)[1]	16 (3) [0]	9(1) [0]	0	—
9	58	M	500	+	+	2	55(6) [0]	(10)[0]	19(5)[0]	24 (1) [0]	12(0) [0]	+	LAD
10	59	M	580	+	+	3†	55(16)[0]	(29)[0]	17(7)[0]	21 (7) [0]	17(2) [0]	+	LAD
11	62	M	335	+	+	3	57(9) [1]	(16)[2]	23(6)[1]	15 (1) [0]	19(2) [0]	+	LAD
12	63	M	350	+	0	1	50(2) [0]	(4) [0]	25(2)[0]	18 (0) [0]	7(0) [0]	+	LAD
13	64	M	375	+	0	2	57(16)[1]	(28)[2]	21(7)[1]	28 (9) [0]	8(0) [0]	+	LAD
14	65	M	350	0	+	3	38(5) [1]	(13)[3]	13(2)[0]	20*(1) [0]	5(2) [1]	+	LAD
15	66	M	360	+	0	2	33(5) [0]	(15)[0]	11(4)[0]	16 (1) [0]	6(0) [0]	+	LAD
16	68	F	560	0	0	3†	49(20)[3]	(41)[6]	12(5)[1]	22*(8) [0]	15(7) [2]	+	LAD
17	69	M	490	+	+	3†	67(11)[0]	(17)[0]	17(9)[0]	31 (1) [0]	19(1) [0]	0	—
18	71	F	630	+	0	3†	64(16)[1]	(25)[2]	17(6)[1]	35 (4) [0]	12(6) [0]	+	LAD
19	71	F	350	+	+	3	55(10)[0]	(18)[0]	16(5)[0]	27 (4) [0]	12(1) [0]	0	—
20	73	M	370	+	0	3	47(12)[0]	(26)[0]	14(2)[0]	25 (9) [0]	8(1) [0]	+	LAD
21	81	F	400	+	0	3†	40(15)[0]	(38)[0]	10(6)[0]	17 (6) [0]	13(3) [0]	0	LAD
22	81	F	420	+	0	2	76(5) [0]	(7) [0]	25(4)[0]	30 (0) [0]	17(2) [0]	0	—
Total		15 M		20	9		1166(273)[17]	4-61 0-6	385(110)[5]	486(100)[4]	295(63)[8]	14	
Mean	62		425			2.7/3.0	52(12)[0.8]	(24)(1.6)	17(5)[0.2]	22(4)[0.2]	14(3)[0.4]		

Numbers in parentheses represent number of segments narrowed > 75%; numbers in brackets represent number of segments narrowed > 95%.

*Dominant posterior artery was the left circumflex.

†In addition, the left main was narrowed > 75%. Thus, seven of the 22 patients had severe narrowing of all four major coronary arteries (see text).

Abbreviations: AP = atherosclerotic plaques; CA = coronary artery; DP = dominant posterior; LAD = left anterior descending; Lat = lateral wall; OP = other posterior coronary artery; VS = ventricular septum; + = present; 0 = absent.

ing of the left main coronary artery was included in the tabulations of both the left anterior descending and the left circumflex (whether dominant posterior or other posterior) coronary arteries of all 50 patients (table 3). Because the left main coronary artery was usually only 1 cm long, an average of only two 5-mm segments was added to the total numbers of segments examined in each of the 50 patients.

In 45 of the 50 patients, the infarcts involved portions of the lateral wall or ventricular septum or both in addition to the anterior or posterior left ventricular free walls (fig. 1). In 21 of the 22 patients with anterior infarcts who had involvement of other left ventricular quadrants, portions of the lateral wall were infarcted in nine patients and portions of the ventricular septum were infarcted in 20 patients (table 1). In addition, portions of the posterior wall in the apical halves of the left ventricle were infarcted in nine of the 22

patients with predominantly anterior wall infarcts. Division of the left ventricular wall into four quadrants (fig. 1) in the 22 patients with anterior wall infarcts disclosed that six had necrosis in all four quadrants, six in three, nine in two and one in one. In 24 of the 28 patients with posterior infarcts who had involvement of other quadrants, portions of the lateral wall also were infarcted in 10 patients and portions of the ventricular septum in 17 patients (table 2). In addition, portions of the anterior wall in the apical halves of the left ventricle were infarcted in three of these 28 patients. Division of the left ventricle into four quadrants in the 28 patients with posterior infarcts disclosed that one had some necrosis in all four quadrants, four in three, 19 in two, and four in one quadrant.

The sizes of the left ventricular infarcts in 27 of the 50 patients were quantitated by determining the per-

TABLE 2. Selected Cardiac Findings in 28 Necropsy Patients with Fatal Acute Transmural Posterior Wall Myocardial Infarction

Pt	Age (years)	Sex	Heart weight (g)	Necrosis VS	Necrosis Lat	No. of LAD, DP, & OP narrowed >75% by AP	Totals	Percentages of totals	No. LAD	No. DP	No. OP	Location of CA thrombus	
1	38	F	340	-	0	2	33(10)[2]	(30)[6]	14(2) [0]	15 (8) [2]	4(0) [0]	+	R
2	43	M	400	+	-	3	31(22)[4]	(71)[13]	12(10)[3]	12*(5) [1]	7(7) [0]	-	LC
3	43	M	540	+	0	3	31(6) [0]	(19)[0]	14(4) [0]	13 (1) [0]	4(1) [0]	+	R
4	45	M	575	+	0	3	57(32)[3]	(56)[5]	20(9) [2]	20 (13)[1]	17(10)[0]	+	R
5	49	M	545	0	+	3	69(27)[2]	(39)[3]	16(5) [1]	37 (14)[0]	16(8) [1]	+	R
6	56	F	410	+	0	3	54(22)[3]	(41)[6]	22(12)[1]	20 (5) [1]	12(5) [1]	+	R
7	57	M	490	-	0	2	47(19)[1]	(40)[2]	21(11)[1]	15 (8) [0]	11(0) [0]	+	LAD
8	57	M	400	0	+	2	39(7) [0]	(18)[0]	11(5) [0]	16*(2) [0]	12(0) [0]	0	—
9	58	M	550	0	0	3	78(27)[1]	(35)[1]	29(10)[0]	31 (7) [0]	18(10)[1]	0	—
10	61	M	450	0	+	3	37(19)[6]	(51)[16]	10(8) [4]	22 (8) [0]	5(3) [2]	+	LC
11	61	M	810	-	0	3	67(17)[1]	(25)[1]	28(1) [0]	25 (15)[1]	14(1) [0]	+	R
12	65	M	700	0	0	3	41(18)[2]	(44)[5]	15(4) [0]	17 (10)[2]	9(4) [0]	0	—
13	65	M	450	-	0	3	53(22)[2]	(42)[4]	19(7) [1]	25 (14)[1]	9(1) [0]	-	R
14	66	F	300	0	+	3	37(23)[0]	(62)[0]	13(10)[0]	12 (8) [0]	12(5) [0]	0	—
15	68	M	450	-	0	3	56(37)[1]	(66)[2]	18(9) [0]	27 (20)[1]	11(8) [0]	+	R
16	68	F	390	0	0	3	42(10)[1]	(25)[2]	18(3) [0]	14 (4) [0]	10(3) [1]	0	—
17	68	M	460	0	0	3	74(22)[1]	(30)[1]	32(7) [0]	30 (12)[1]	12(3) [0]	-	R
18	70	F	310	-	-	3	48(18)[0]	(38)[0]	17(10)[0]	18 (6) [0]	13(2) [0]	0	—
19	72	M	510	+	-	3+	59(24)[3]	(41)[5]	26(15)[3]	24 (5) [0]	9(4) [0]	-	R
20	73	M	400	0	·	3	47(9) [0]	(19)[0]	24(6) [0]	17 (2) [0]	6(1) [0]	+	LAD
21	74	M	650	+	0	3+	79(22)[0]	(28)[0]	27(7) [0]	32 (9) [0]	20(6) [0]	+	R
22	77	M	300	0	·	3	47(27)[5]	(57)[11]	17(9) [4]	21 (14)[0]	9(4) [1]	+	LC
23	77	F	440	·	0	3	59(11)[0]	(19)[0]	22(6) [0]	19 (3) [0]	18(2) [0]	0	—
24	77	M	530	+	0	3	46(15)[1]	(33)[2]	16(4) [0]	18 (6) [1]	12(5) [0]	0	—
25	77	M	560	-	0	3	54(37)[5]	(69)[9]	22(16)[1]	19 (14)[3]	13(7) [1]	0	—
26	80	F	380	-	0	3	45(15)[0]	(33)[0]	11(3) [0]	29 (9) [0]	5(3) [0]	0	—
27	80	F	380	-	0	3+	41(26)[1]	(63)[2]	10(7) [0]	21 (15)[1]	10(4) [0]	0	—
28	82	F	300	0	-	3	49(11)[0]	(22)[0]	17(3) [0]	22 (4) [0]	10(4) [0]	0	—
Total		19 M		17	10		1420(555)[45]	18-71 0-16	521(203)[21]	591(241)[16]	308(111)[8]	16	
Mean	65		452			2.9/3.0	51(20)[1.6]	(40)[3.5]	19(17)[0.8]	21(9)[0.6]	11(4)[0.3]		

Numbers in parentheses represent number of segments narrowed > 75%; numbers in brackets represent number of segments narrowed > 95%.

*Dominant posterior artery was the left circumflex.

†In addition, the left main was narrowed > 75%. Thus, three of the 28 patients had severe narrowing of all four major coronary arteries.

Abbreviations: LC = left circumflex; R = right coronary artery. Other abbreviations as in table 1.

centage of grossly visible necrotic myocardium in each of the five or six transverse slices (each about 1 cm thick) of the left ventricle by a videoplanimetry system described elsewhere.[9] The sum of the area of necrosis in all ventricular slices (fig. 1) divided by the sum of the total left ventricular myocardial area in all slices provided the percentage of necrotic myocardium in each patient. The percentage of necrotic left ventricular wall was 18–69% (mean 33%) in the 12 patients with anterior infarcts and 19–49% (mean 27%) in the 15 patients with posterior infarcts (NS).

The data were analyzed using the t test for paired and unpaired data. A difference between groups was considered statistically significant when $p < 0.05$.

Results

Of the 88 major epicardial coronary arteries in the 22 patients with anterior wall AMI, 65 (74%) were narrowed 76–100% in cross-sectional area at some point by atherosclerotic plaques alone (average 3.0 arteries/patient). Of the 112 major epicardial coronary arteries in the 28 patients with posterior wall AMI, 84 (75%) were narrowed 76–100% (average 3.0 arteries/patient) (table 3). Thus, the percentage of

TABLE 3. *Major Epicardial Coronary Arteries Narrowed > 75% in Cross-sectional Area in 50 Necropsy Patients with Fatal Initial Acute Myocardial Infarction*

Location of AMI	No. of pts	Total CA	LM	LAD	LC	RCA	Total	LAD	DP	OP	Total
Anterior	22	88	7	22	16	20	65/88 (74%)	22	20	17	59/66* (89%)
Posterior	28	112	3	28	26	27	84/112 (75%)	28	28	25	81/84* (96%)
Total	50	200	10 (20%)	50 (100%)	42 (84%)	47 (94%)	149/200 (74%)	50 (100%)	48+ (96%)	42+ (84%)	140/150 (93%)

139/150 (93%)

*The left main coronary artery is included as part of both the LAD and LC in each of the 50 patients. Nine of the 10 patients with severe (> 75%) narrowing of the left main coronary artery also had similar degrees of narrowing of both the LAD and LC, and the remaining patient had severe narrowing of the LAD but not of the LC.

+The RCA was the dominant posterior coronary artery in 45 of the 50 patients and the left circumflex was the DP in five patients (10%). The other posterior coronary artery, therefore, was the left circumflex in 45 patients and the RCA in five patients.

Abbreviations: CA = coronary artery; LM = left main coronary artery; LAD = left anterior descending coronary artery; LC = left circumflex; RCA = right coronary artery; DP = dominant posterior artery; OP = other posterior artery.

coronary arteries narrowed 76–100% in cross-sectional area by atherosclerotic plaques was qualitatively similar in the patients with anterior and posterior AMI.

The number of arteries per patient that were narrowed 76–100% by atherosclerotic plaques is given in table 4. Narrowing of more than 75% in individual coronary arteries is given in table 3.

The results of the quantitative analysis of the 5-mm coronary segments from each of the four major coronary arteries in the 50 patients are summarized in figures 2 and 3. The numbers and percentages of coronary segments severely narrowed for individual patients are given in tables 1 and 2. Of the 2586 5-mm coronary segments examined histologically in the 50 patients, 1166 segments were from the 22 patients with anterior AMI and 1420 were from the 28 patients with posterior AMI. Two hundred seventy-three segments (23%) were narrowed 76–100% in the anterior AMI group; 17 of these segments (1.5%) were narrowed

TABLE 4. *Severe Narrowing by Atherosclerotic Plaques in the Four Major Coronary Arteries in 50 Necropsy Patients with Acute Transmural Myocardial Infarction*

No. of coronary arteries narrowed > 75% XSA	Location of AMI		Total	
	Anterior wall (n = 22)	Posterior wall (n = 28)	n	%
4*	6 (27%)	3 (11%)	9	(18)
3	10+ (45%)	22 (78%)	32	(64)
2	5 (23%)	3 (11%)	8	(16)
1	1 (5%)	0	1	(2)
Total	22 (100%)	28 (100%)	50	(100)

*Includes left main, left anterior descending, left circumflex and right coronary arteries.

+The left main coronary artery was severely narrowed (> 75%) in one of these 10 patients. Thus, 10 patients, seven with anterior and three with posterior AMI, had severe narrowing of the left main artery.

Abbreviations: AMI = acute myocardial infarction; XSA = cross-sectional area.

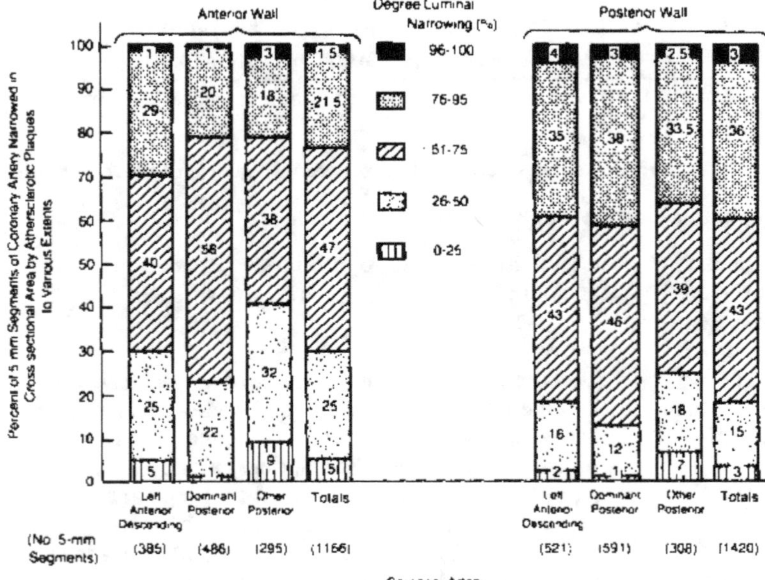

FIGURE 2. *Percentages of 5-mm segments of each of three major epicardial coronary arteries narrowed by atherosclerotic plaques in 22 patients with anterior and 28 patients with posterior transmural acute myocardial infarction.*

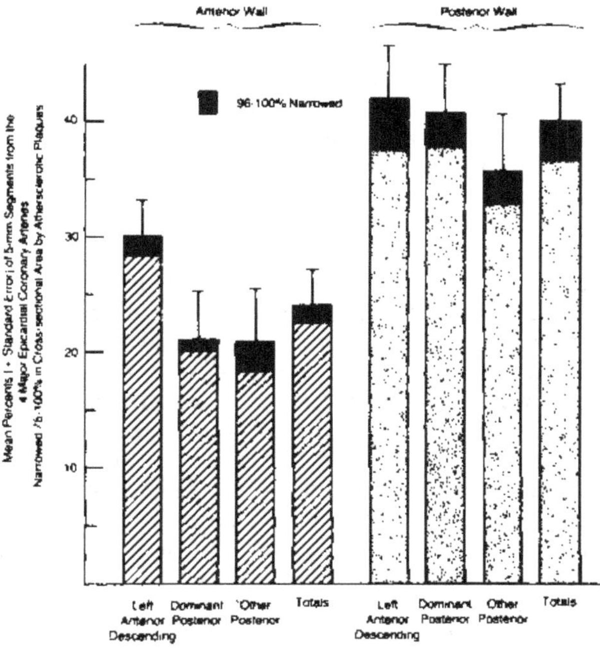

FIGURE 3. *Mean percentages of 5-mm segments of the four major epicardial coronary arteries narrowed 76–100% in cross-sectional area by atherosclerotic plaques in 22 patients with anterior and in 28 patients with posterior transmural acute myocardial infarction.*

96–100%. In the posterior AMI group, 559 segments (39%) were narrowed 76–100% ($p < 0.001$); 45 of these segments (3.2%) were narrowed 96–100%. Five hundred forty-one segments (47%) were narrowed 51–75% in the anterior AMI group and 612 (43%) in the posterior AMI group (NS). Two hundred ninety-seven segments (25%) in the anterior AMI group and 212 segments (15%) in the posterior AMI group were narrowed 26–50% ($p < 0.02$). Fifty-five segments (5%) in the anterior AMI group and 41 segments (3%) in the posterior AMI group were narrowed 0–25% (NS) (fig. 2).

The mean percentages of segments narrowed 76–100% in the four major coronary arteries in the two groups are shown in figure 3. A larger percentage of 5-mm segments of major coronary arteries were narrowed 76–100% in the posterior AMI group than in the anterior AMI group ($p < 0.001$). The frequency of severe (76–100%) narrowing of the left anterior descending, the dominant posterior and the other posterior coronary arteries was significantly ($p < 0.05$, < 0.005, and < 0.01, respectively) greater in the patients with posterior AMI than in those with anterior AMI.

Among the 22 patients with anterior AMI, the mean percentage of severely narrowed segments of the left anterior descending coronary artery was significantly ($p < 0.05$) greater than the mean percentage of segments of either the dominant posterior or other posterior artery so narrowed. No significant differences in the mean percentages of severely narrowed 5-mm segments of left anterior descending, dominant

posterior and other posterior coronary arteries were found in the 28 patients with posterior AMI.

The percentage of 5-mm segments narrowed 76–100% in each of the major coronary arteries in each of the 50 patients is shown in tables 1 and 2. Among the 22 patients with anterior AMI, 4–61% (mean 24%) of the 5-mm coronary segments were narrowed 76–100%, of which 0–6% (mean 1.6%) of the segments were narrowed 96–100% in cross-sectional area by atherosclerotic plaque. Among the 28 patients with posterior AMI, 18–71% (mean 40%) of the 5-mm segments were narrowed 76–100%, of which 0–16% (mean 3.5%) were narrowed 96–100%.

Discussion

The purposes of this study were to determine the degree and extent of narrowing in each of the four major epicardial coronary arteries in patients with their first anterior AMI compared with those in patients with their first posterior wall AMI, and to determine whether the left anterior descending coronary artery was more narrowed in anterior AMI, and whether the dominant posterior coronary artery was more narrowed in posterior AMI. Attempts to answer the first question by determining the number of major (right, left main, left anterior descending and left circumflex) epicardial coronary arteries that were severely (76–100% in cross-sectional area) narrowed by atherosclerotic plaque showed no differences between the two groups. Sixty-five of the 88 major coronary arteries (74%) in the 22 patients with anterior AMI were narrowed 76–100% and 84 of the 112 arteries (75%) in the 28 patients with posterior AMI were similarly narrowed (table 3).

One qualitative difference between the two AMI groups was the frequency of severe narrowing of the left main coronary artery. Seven of the 22 anterior AMI patients (32%) and three of the 28 posterior AMI patients (11%) ($p = 0.06$) had severe narrowing of the left main coronary artery.

The quantitative analysis showed distinct differences between the two AMI groups. The 28 patients with posterior AMI had significantly more extensive narrowing of the major coronary arteries by this approach than did the 22 patients with anterior AMI. Of the 1166 5-mm segments in the 22 anterior AMI patients, 273 (23%) were narrowed 76–100% by atherosclerotic plaques, and of the 1420 5-mm coronary segments in 28 patients with posterior AMI, 555 (39%) were similarly narrowed ($p < 0.001$). However, the extent of the coronary narrowing varied greatly among the individual patients in each group (tables 1 and 2). Among the 22 patients with anterior AMI, 4–61% of the 5-mm coronary segments were narrowed 76–100%; among the 28 patients with posterior AMI, 18–71% of the segments were narrowed 76–100%. Although the patients with posterior AMI had more extensive, severe coronary narrowing than did the patients with anterior AMI, the atherosclerotic plaques in both groups were extensive. Among the patients with anterior AMI, only 5% (55 of 1166) of the segments were narrowed 25% or less and among the posterior AMI patients, only 3% (41 of 1420) of the segments were narrowed 25% or less. No segment in either group was normal.

Comparison of the percentages of 5-mm segments narrowed 76–100% showed that all three major coronary arteries were more narrowed in the posterior AMI patients than in the anterior AMI patients (fig. 3). Also, the narrowing of the left anterior descending coronary artery was more severe in the 28 patients with posterior AMI than in the 22 patients with anterior AMI.

Some physicians believe that patients with anterior wall AMI have severe narrowing of the left anterior descending coronary artery with less severe narrowing of the dominant posterior coronary artery and that patients with posterior wall AMI have severe narrowing of the right or left circumflex coronary artery (or both) with less narrowing of the left anterior descending coronary artery. Our data do not support this belief. In all 22 patients with anterior AMI, the left anterior descending artery was narrowed 76–100% by atherosclerotic plaques, but in 20 of these patients, the dominant posterior coronary artery, which was the right coronary artery in 86%, was also severely narrowed. In all 28 patients with posterior AMI, both the dominant posterior (right in 93%) and the left anterior descending coronary arteries were narrowed 76–100%. However, the mean percentage of segments of the left anterior descending coronary artery narrowed 76–100% was significantly greater than that of either the dominant posterior or other posterior coronary artery in the 22 patients with anterior AMI (30% vs 21%, $p < 0.05$). Among the 28 patients with posterior AMI, however, the percentages of segments narrowed 76–100% did not differ between the left anterior descending, dominant posterior (right in 93%) and other posterior (left circumflex in 93%) coronary arteries.

Although the left anterior descending coronary artery was more extensively narrowed than the dominant or other posterior coronary artery in the anterior AMI group, 10 of these 22 patients had more extensive, severe narrowing in one or both posterior coronary arteries (dominant or other) than in the left anterior descending coronary artery. Although no significant differences in the percentage of coronary segments severely narrowed was noted between one or both posterior supplying coronary arteries and the left anterior descending coronary artery in the 28 posterior AMI patients as a group, in nine of these 28 patients, the percentage of severely narrowed 5-mm segments of the left anterior descending coronary artery was greater than that of either posterior coronary artery.

In this study, we determined that the location of a fatal first transmural AMI in a patient with extensive coronary atherosclerosis does not necessarily indicate which of the major coronary systems is most narrowed by atherosclerotic plaque. We do not know whether this finding is applicable to patients who survive AMI.

This finding, however, clearly does not apply to an AMI caused by an embolus[10] or ligation of a previously normal coronary artery.[11, 12] In this situation, the resulting AMI corresponds to the artery suddenly occluded. Further, thrombi superimposed on coronary atherosclerotic plaques are nearly always located in the coronary artery that supplies the necrotic area. Thirty of our 50 patients (60%) had a coronary thrombus, and in 28, the thrombus was located in the artery subtending the area of infarction. Coronary artery thrombi occurred in 14 of the 22 patients (64%) with anterior wall AMI and in 16 of the 28 patients (57%) with posterior wall AMI (NS). There was a similar percentage of 5-mm segments of coronary artery narrowed 76–100% by atherosclerotic plaque in the 30 patients with and in the 20 patients without coronary thrombi. Also, the frequency of hemorrhages into coronary atherosclerotic plaques was similar in both anterior and posterior AMI patients. In none of the coronary segments did a hemorrhage into a plaque appear to narrow the lumen of a coronary artery.

In conclusion, among necropsy patients with fatal first AMI, most have severe and extensive narrowing of at least three major coronary arteries, irrespective of whether the infarct involves the anterior or the posterior left ventricular wall. Patients with anterior AMI, however, have a greater likelihood of having more than 75% narrowing of the left main coronary artery than patients with posterior AMI, whereas patients with posterior AMI have more extensive, severe narrowing of the right, left anterior descending and left circumflex coronary arteries. The individual variation in severe coronary narrowing is great among patients in both groups; therefore, our findings are not necessarily applicable to the individual patient but are applicable to groups of patients who had a fatal first AMI. Our observations do not explain why some patients with severe coronary atherosclerosis have anterior wall AMI and others have posterior wall AMI, nor why a thrombus occurs in one coronary artery and not in another, similarly narrowed coronary artery.

References

1. Barnes AR, Ball RG: The incidence and situation of myocardial infarction in one thousand consecutive postmortem examinations. Am J Med Sci 183: 215, 1932
2. Saphir O, Priest WS, Hamburger WW, Katz LN: Coronary arteriosclerosis, coronary thrombosis and the resulting myocardial changes. An evaluation of their respective clinical pictures including the electrocardiographic records, based on the anatomical findings. Am Heart J 10: 567, 1935
3. Blumgart HL, Schlesinger MJ, Davis D: Studies on the relation of the clinical manifestations of angina pectoris, coronary thrombosis and myocardial infarction to the pathological findings. Am Heart J 19: 1, 1940
4. Roberts WC, Buja LM: The frequency and significance of coronary artery thrombi and other observations in fatal acute myocardial infarction. A study of 107 necropsy patients. Am J Med 52: 425, 1972
5. Jones AA, Roberts WC: Quantification of coronary arterial narrowing at necropsy in acute transmural myocardial infarc-

tion. Analysis and comparison of findings in 27 patients and 22 controls. Circulation **61**: 786, 1980

6. Roberts WC, Gardin JM: Location of myocardial infarcts. A confusion of terms and definitions. Am J Cardiol **42**: 868, 1978

7. Penther P, Boschat J, Blanc JJ, Granatelli P, Germa D: Les lésions myocardiques et coronariennes dans l'infarctus myocardique antérieur et postérieur. Etude anatomique macroscopique comparative. Nouv Presse Med **5**: 2223, 1976

8. Spain DM: Coronary atheromatous disease — clinical pathological correlations. Cardiovasc Clin **4**: 53, 1972

9. Dvorak JA, Schuette WH, Whitehouse WC: A simple video method for the quantification of microscopic objects. J Microsc **102**: 71, 1974

10. Roberts WC: Coronary embolism: a review of causes, consequences, and diagnostic considerations. Cardiovasc Med **3**: 699, 1978

11. Karsner HT, Dwyer JE Jr: Studies in infarction. IV. Experimental bland infarction of the myocardium, myocardial regeneration and cicatrization. J Med Res **34**: 21, 1916

12. Jennings RB, Wartman WB: Reactions of the myocardium to obstruction of the coronary arteries. Med Clin North Am **41**: 3, 1957

Type III hyperlipoproteinemia:Quantification, distribution, and nature of atherosclerotic coronary arterial narrowing in five necropsy patients

The amount of cross-sectional area (XSA) narrowing in each 5 mm long segment of each of the four major epicardial coronary arteries was determined in each of five patients with type III hyperlipoproteinemia (HLP) and symptomatic, fatal atherosclerotic coronary disease (CAD). Four had angina pectoris; two had acute myocardial infarcts which healed, and two died suddenly. Of the four major epicardial coronary arteries, all four were narrowed 76% to 100% in XSA by atherosclerotic plaques in two patients, three were narrowed to this degree in two patients, and two were so narrowed in one patient. Three patients had severe narrowing of the left main coronary artery. The percent of 5 mm long segments of coronary artery narrowed to various degrees was as follows: 96% to 100%, 0 to 37 (mean 14); 76% to 95%, 14 to 61 (mean 35); 51% to 75%, 9 to 41 (mean 24); 26% to 50%, 0 to 42 (mean 16), and 0% to 25%, 0 to 27 (mean 11). Utilizing a scoring system of 1 to 4 for the four categories of narrowing (1 = 0% to 25%, 2 = 26% to 50%, 3 = 51% to 75% and 4 = 76% to 100% XSA narrowing), scores per 5 mm segment for each patient ranged from 2.5 to 3.9 (mean 3.1). Thus these five type III HLP patients had severe diffuse coronary narrowing by atherosclerotic plaques. (AM HEART J 102:830, 1981.)

Henry Scott Cabin, M.D., David E. Schwartz, M.D., Renu Virmani, M.D., H. Bryan Brewer, Jr., M.D., and William C. Roberts, M.D. *Bethesda, Md.*

From the Pathology and Molecular Disease Branches; National Heart, Lung and Blood Institute; National Institutes of Health.

Received for publication June 23, 1981; accepted July 6, 1981.

Reprint requests: William C. Roberts, M.D., Pathology Branch, NHLBI–NIH, Bldg. 10A, Room 3E-30, Bethesda, MD 20205.

It is well recognized that patients with type III hyperlipoproteinemia (HLP) have a high frequency of symptomatic coronary heart disease (CHD) and peripheral vascular disease.[1-4] No systematic analy-

Table I. Clinical and necropsy findings in five type III hyperlipoproteinemia patients

	Patient 1	Patient 2	Patient 3	Patient 4	Patient 5
Age (yrs)	49	51	52	54	75
Race	W	W	W	W	W
Sex	F	M	F	F	M
FH type III	+	+	0	0	0
Diabetes mellitus	+	0	+	0	+
Systemic SAP/DAP (mm Hg)	190/105	162/94	160/100	110/66	180/100
Cigarette smoker	+	+	+	0	0
Peak serum Tg (mg/dl)	2367	870	429	825	700
Peak serum TC (mg/dl)	610	382	338	660	500
Body weight (kg)	60	91	69	85	50
Height (cm)	157	—	168	155	—
AP (yrs present)	0	+ (6)	+ (3)	+ (5)	+ (24)
CHF (yrs present)	0	0	+ (2)	+ (0.5)	+ (3)
C (yrs present)	0	+ (18)	+ (5)	0	+ (22)
AMI (yrs before death)	0	+ (23)	+ (3)	0	0
Mode of death	Sudden	Sudden	AMI	CABG	CHF
Heart weight (gm)	350	550	480	370	410
LV fibrosis	0	+	+	+	+
LV necrosis	0	0	+	0	0
Spleen weight (gm)	200	280	350	—	—
Liver weight (gm)	2200	1900	2285	—	—

Abbreviations: AMI = acute myocardial infarct; AP = angina pectoris; C = claudication; CABG = coronary artery bypass grafting; CHF = congestive heart failure; DAP = diastolic arterial pressure; FH = family history; LV = left ventricular; SAP = systolic arterial pressure; TC = total cholesterol; Tg = triglyceride; yrs = years.

sis, however, of the status of the epicardial coronary arteries in this relatively rare form of HLP has been described. Accordingly, we examined histologically each 5 mm long segment of each of the four major coronary arteries in five patients with type III HLP and fatal CHD.

METHODS

Clinical and serum lipid features. The five study patients had serum cholesterol and triglyceride determinations and lipoprotein phenotyping performed at the National Heart, Lung and Blood Institute by methods described elsewhere,[5] and in each the results were diagnostic for type III HLP. All five patients had a very low density lipoprotein cholesterol/triglyceride ratio greater than 0.30. The clinical findings and noncoronary artery necropsy findings in the five patients are summarized in Table I. The initial manifestation of CHD was angina pectoris in two patients, acute myocardial infarction in two, and sudden coronary death in one. The interval from symptoms of myocardial ischemia to death ranged from 0 to 24 years (mean 11 years). Three patients (No. 3, 2, and 5, Table I) had leg claudication for 5, 18, and 22 years, respectively, before death. Patients No. 1 and 2 (Table I) were habitual alcoholics. Peak serum triglyceride levels in the five patients ranged from 429 to 2367 mg/dl (mean 1038), and peak total serum cholesterol from 338 to 660 mg/dl (mean 498).

Coronary artery necropsy exam technique. The entire lengths of the right (R), left main (LM), left anterior descending (LAD), and left circumflex (LC) coronary arteries were removed from each heart intact and cut transversely into 5 mm long segments. Each segment was labelled, processed for histologic study, and a histologic section from each segment was prepared and stained by the Movat method.[6] The degree of narrowing in all 5 mm segments was determined by examination of the histologic sections magnified 25 to 50 times. The percent of cross-sectional area (XSA) narrowing by atherosclerotic plaques was divided into five categories: 0 to 25, 26 to 50, 51 to 75, 76 to 95, and 96 to 100. The accuracy of these determinations was verified by random evaluations by other observers and by videoplanimetry, and both the intra- and interobserver error was less than 5%.[7] The patient with type III HLP previously reported in detail[8] from this laboratory was not included in the present analysis because the entire lengths of the four major epicardial coronary arteries were not available for reexamination.

RESULTS

Patients with multivessel stenoses. Of the four major arteries, all four were narrowed 76% to 100% in XSA by atherosclerotic plaque in two patients (Fig. 1), three arteries were so narrowed in two patients, and two arteries were so narrowed in one

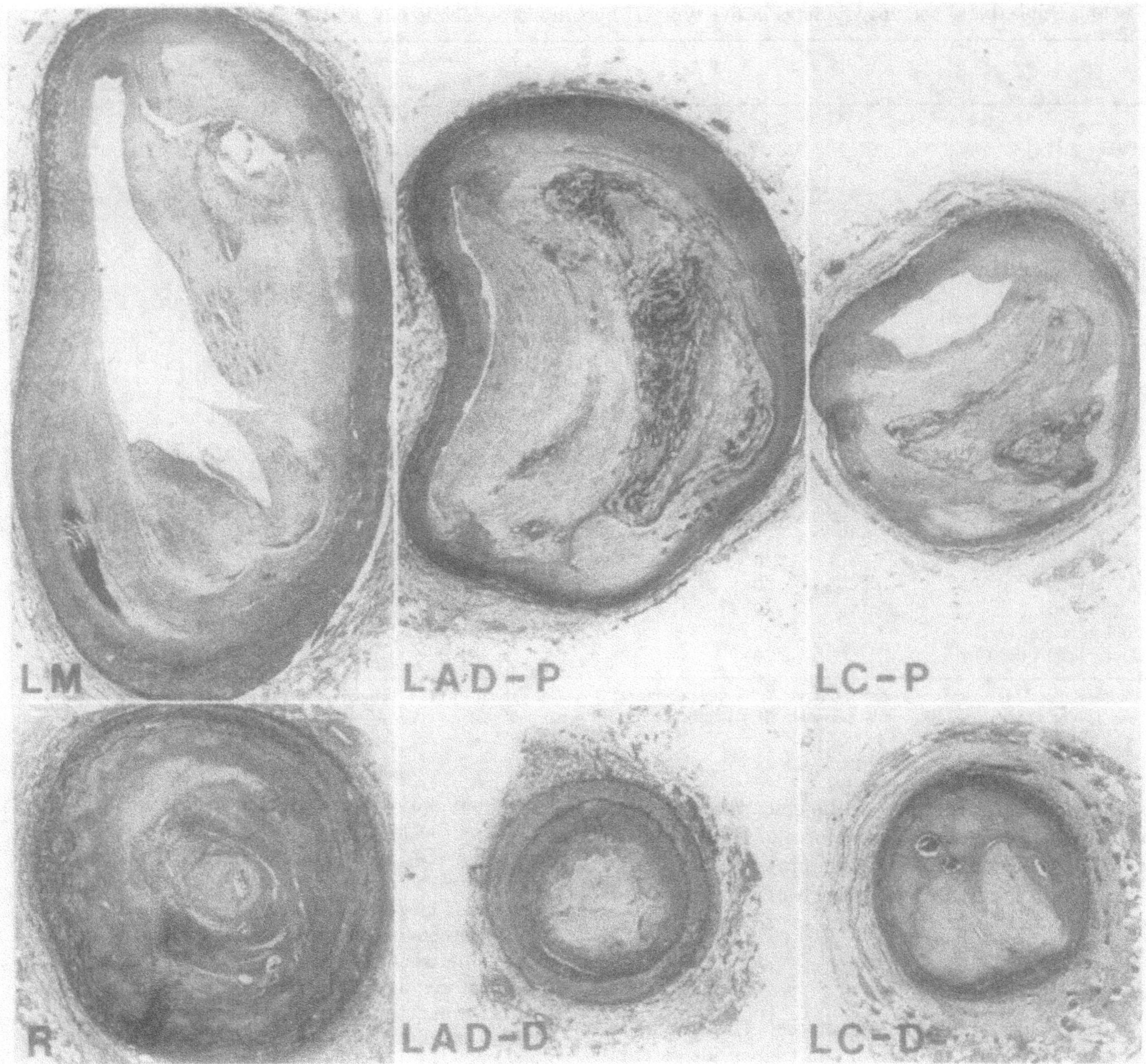

Fig. 1. Photomicrographs of sections of left main *(LM)*, right *(R)*, left anterior descending *(LAD)* (proximal *[P]* and distal *[D]*) and left circumflex *(LC)* (*P* and *D*) coronary arteries at their points of maximal narrowing in patient No. 2 (Table I). Each section is narrowed severely by atherosclerotic plaque. (Movat stain; original magnification ×21.)

patient. Three patients had severe narrowing of the LM coronary artery.

Extent and location of coronary disease. The results of the analysis of the 257 five mm long segments of the four coronary arteries from the five study patients are shown in Figs. 2 to 4 and in Table II. The percent of 5 mm segments narrowed 96% to 100% ranged from 0 to 37 (mean 14); 76% to 95%, from 14 to 61 (mean 35); 51% to 75%, from 9 to 41 (mean 24); 26% to 50%, from 0 to 42 (mean 16), and 0% to 25%, from 0 to 27 (mean 11) (Fig. 2 and Table II). Although the mean percent of segments nar-

rowed 76% to 100% was greater in the R (63%) than in the LAD (40%) and LC (45%) coronary arteries (Fig. 3), the differences were not statistically significant. No significant difference was observed between the mean percent of 5 mm segments narrowed 76% to 100% in XSA in the proximal and distal halves of the R, LAD, and LC coronary arteries (Fig. 4). Every 5 mm segment of coronary artery in each of the five patients was given a score of 1 to 4 based on the amount of XSA narrowing as follows: 1 = 0% to 25% narrowing; 2 = 26% to 50%; 3 = 51% to 75%, and 4 = 76% to 100%. The scores per 5 mm segment

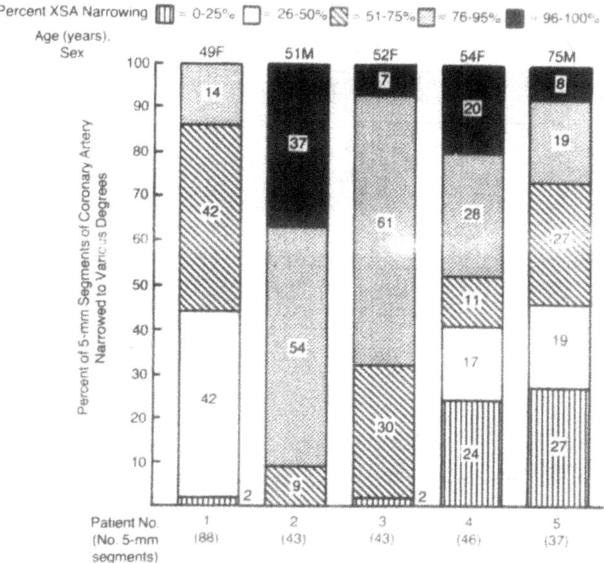

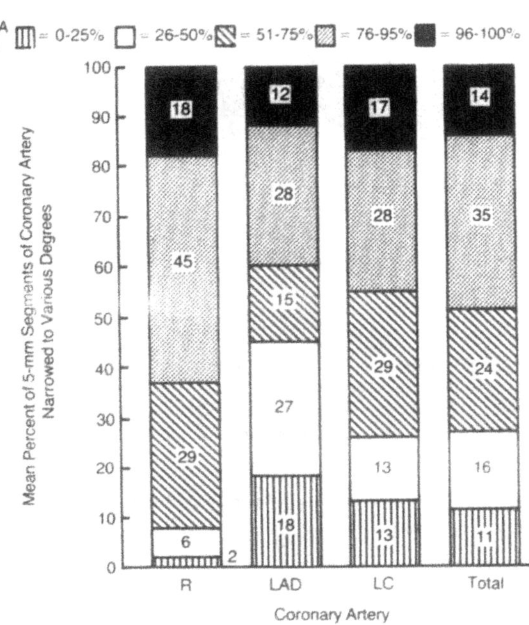

Fig. 2. Percent of 5 mm long segments of the four major epicardial coronary arteries with five categories of cross-sectional area *(XSA)* narrowing by atherosclerotic plaques in each of the five patients with type III hyperlipoprotein-emia.

Fig. 3. Mean percent of 5 mm long segments of the right *(R)*, left anterior descending *(LAD)*, and left circumflex *(LC)* coronary arteries narrowed to five categories of cross-sectional area *(XSA)* narrowing in five patients with type III hyperlipoproteinemia.

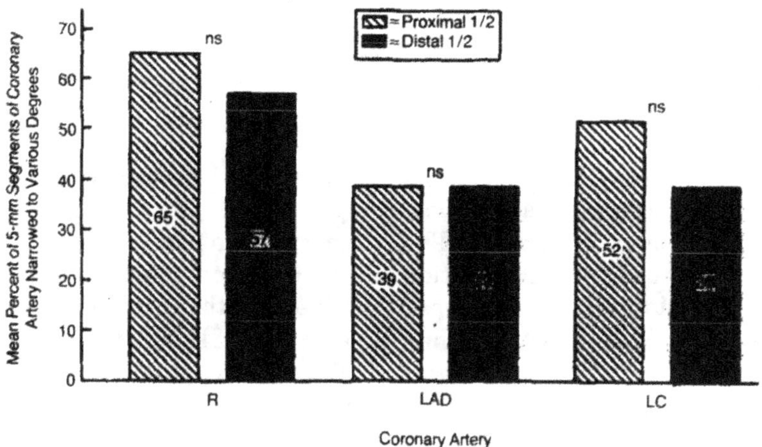

Fig. 4. Mean percent of 5 mm long segments from the proximal and distal halves of the right *(R)*, left anterior descending *(LAD)*, and left circumflex *(LC)* coronary arteries narrowed 76% to 100% in cross-sectional area by atherosclerotic plaques in five patients with type III hyperlipoproteinemia.

(obtained by dividing the total score per patient by the number of 5 mm segments of coronary artery examined per patient) ranged from 2.5 to 3.9 (mean 3.1) (Table II).

Histologic nature of coronary atherosclerosis. The coronary arterial atherosclerotic plaques in each patient were composed primarily of fibrous tissue with only rare foam cells (Fig. 1). Thus, the plaques were indistinguishable from those seen in patients with type II or IV HLP or known normal lipoprotein patterns (Table III). Sections of liver were available for examination in two patients (No. 1 and 3), and

sections of spleen in three patients (No. 1, 3, and 5). In one patient (No. 1), foam cells were present in the liver, and in one patient (No. 1) the spleen. Foam cells also were present in left atrial endocardium[8] in one patient (No. 2).

DISCUSSION

Multivessel coronary stenoses present in all type III HLP patients studied. Three necropsy patients with type III HLP have been reported[8-10] previously and each had symptomatic CHD. In two the LAD, LC, and R coronary arteries were narrowed 76% to 100%

Table II. Coronary artery necropsy observations in five type III hyperlipoproteinemia patients

Pt.	CA's narrowed 76%-100% in XSA by AP				No. 5 mm segments of CA	No. (%) segments of CA with various degrees of XSA narrowing					Coronary[a] score per 5 mm segment
	LM	LAD	LC	R		0%-25%	26%-50%	51%-75%	76%-95%	96%-100%	
1	0	0	+	+	88	2(2)	38(42)	36(41)	12(14)	0	2.7
2	+	+	+	+	43	0	0	4(9)	23(54)	16(37)	3.9
3	0	+	+	+	43	1(2)	0	13(30)	26(61)	3(7)	3.6
4	+	+	+	+	46	11(24)	8(17)	5(11)	13(28)	9(20)	2.8
5	+	+	0	+	37	10(27)	7(19)	10(27)	7(19)	3(8)	2.5
Totals (mean)	3	4	4	5	257(51)	24(11)	53(16)	68(24)	81(35)	31(14)	3.1

Abbreviations: AP = atherosclerotic plaque; CA = coronary artery; LAD = left anterior descending; LC = left circumflex; LM = left main; R = right; XSA = cross-sectional area. [a]See results section for explanation of coronary scoring system.

Table III. Comparison of CAD extent and distribution in five present type III HLP patients to CAD necrospy findings in 38 previously reported symptomatic type II/IV HLP/normal LP patients

	No. of Patients	No of patients with 76%-100% XSA narrowing of each major CA				No. 5 mm segments of CA	Range (mean) of percent 5 mm segments narrowed 76%-100% in XSA per patient	Range (mean) of coronary score[b] per 5 mm segment
		LM	LAD	LC	R			
Type II HLP	15	9[a]	13	12	14	798	3-84 (40)*	1.8-3.8 (3.0)*
Type IV HLP	13	6[a]	13	13	13	688	25-92 (68)**	2.6-3.9 (3.5)**
Normal	10	1	9	8	8	466	8-71 (36)*	2.4-3.7 (3.0)*
Type III HLP	5	3	4	4	5	257	14-91 (49)	2.5-3.9 (3.1)

Abbreviations: CAD = coronary artery stenosis; HLP = hyperlipoproteinemia; LAD = left anterior descending; LC = left circumflex; LM = left main; R = right; XSA = cross-sectional area; LP = lipoprotein pattern; [a]left main CA not examined in one type II and one type IV HLP patient; [b]see Results section for explanation of coronary scoring system. * to ** = $p < 0.02$.

in XSA by atherosclerotic plaques[8, 10] and in the third patient "the coronary arteries were almost completely occluded by grumous material."[9] The present study analyzed the amount and distribution of coronary arterial narrowing in five necropsy patients with type III HLP. All five patients had severe narrowing of at least two of the four major epicardial coronary arteries and four had severe narrowing of three or four of the four arteries. The LM coronary artery was narrowed severely in three patients.

Comparison of CAD extent in type III HLP to types II/IV HLP. Examining each 5 mm segment from the entire lengths of the four major epicardial coronary arteries in these patients revealed that, on the average, 49% of all the segments were narrowed severely. In an earlier report,[11] such an approach was used to study the amounts of coronary narrowing (CAD) in 38 necropsy patients with type II or IV HLP or normal lipoprotein patterns and symptomatic CHD (Table III). The 13 patients with type IV had a greater mean percent of coronary artery segments narrowed severely (68%) than the 15 patients with type II (40%) ($p < 0.005$) or 10

patients with normal lipoprotein patterns (36%) ($p < 0.005$). The LM coronary artery was severely narrowed in 9 of 15 type II, 6 of 13 type IV, and in 1 of 10 patients with normal lipoprotein patterns. Although the relatively small number of patients with type III HLP in the present study does not allow meaningful statistical comparisons with these previously studied patients, our data suggest that patients with type III have a frequency of severe narrowing of the LM coronary artery similar to that in the type II and IV patients and have at least as much overall severe coronary artery narrowing as the type II patients.

Reversibility of type III atherosclerosis dependent on disease process stage. An earlier report indicated that when serum cholesterol and triglyceride levels were lowered by diet and drug therapy in patients with type III HLP, peripheral blood flow improved and claudication as well as angina pectoris, when present, decreased in severity or disappeared entirely.[2] This concept of the reversibility of the arterial narrowing was supported by the observation, in the first necropsy report of a type III patient, that the primary component of the atherosclerotic plaque was lipid-laden foam cells.[8] In the five additional necropsy patients with type III HLP (analyzed in this report), however, the atherosclerotic plaques contained minimal or no foam cells and were composed primarily of fibrous tissue. Thus at least at the end-stage of the atherosclerotic process, there is little morphologic evidence to suggest that the atherosclerotic plaques are more likely to be reversible through lowering of serum lipid levels than in patients with type II, type IV, or normal lipoprotein patterns.

REFERENCES

1. Fredrickson DS, Levy RI, Lees RS:Fat transport in lipoproteins—An integrated approach to mechanisms and disorders. N Engl J Med **276**:215, 1967.
2. Zelis R, Mason DT, Braunwald E, Levy RI:Effects of hyperlipoproteinemias and their treatment on the peripheral circulation. J Clin Invest **49**:1007, 1970.
3. Morganroth J, Levy RI, Fredrickson DS:The biochemical, clinical, and genetic features of type III hyperlipoproteinemia. Ann Intern Med **82**:158, 1975.
4. Fredrickson DS, Goldstein JL, Brown MS:The familial hyperlipoproteinemias. *In* Stanbury JB, Wyngaarden JB, Fredrickson DS, editors: The metabolic basis of inherited disease. 4th ed. New York, 1978, McGraw-Hill Book Co, Inc, p 604.
5. Fredrickson DS, Morganroth J, Levy RI:Type III hyperlipoproteinemia: An analysis of two contemporary definitions. Ann Intern Med **82**:150, 1975.
6. Movat HZ:Demonstration of all connective tissue elements in a single section. Pentachrome stains. Arch Pathol Lab Med **60**:289, 1955.
7. Isner JM, Wu M, Virmani R, Jones AA, Roberts WC: Comparison of degrees of coronary arterial luminal narrowing determined by visual inspection of histologic sections under magnification among three independent observers and comparison to that obtained by video planimetry: An analysis of 559 five-mm segments of 61 coronary arteries from eleven patients. Lab Invest **42**:566, 1980.
8. Roberts WC, Levy RI, Fredrickson DS:Hyperlipoproteinemia: A review of the five types with first report of necropsy findings in type 3. Arch Pathol **90**:46, 1970.
9. Holimon JL, Wasserman AJ: Autopsy findings in type 3 hyperlipoproteinemia. Arch Pathol **92**:415, 1971.
10. Roberts WC, Ferrans VJ, Levy RI, Fredrickson DS:Cardiovascular pathology in hyperlipoproteinemia: Anatomic observations in 42 necropsy patients with normal or abnormal serum lipoprotein patterns. Am J Cardiol **31**:557, 1973.
11. Cabin HS, Roberts WC: Quantification of amounts of coronary arterial narrowing in patients with types II and IV hyperlipoproteinemia and in those with known normal lipoprotein patterns. Am Heart J **101**:52, 1981.

Sudden death while playing professional football

William C. Roberts, M.D., and Barry J. Maron, M.D.
Bethesda, Md.

A recent study of 29 competitive athletes aged 13 to 31 years dying suddenly disclosed that 28 of them died from cardiovascular conditions, the most common being hyper-

From the Pathology and Cardiology Branches, National Heart, Lung and Blood Institute, National Institutes of Health.

Received for publication June 25, 1981; accepted July 10, 1981.

Reprint requests: William C. Roberts, M.D., Pathology Branch, NHLBI-NIH, Bldg. 10A, Room 3E-30, Bethesda, MD 20205.

trophic cardiomyopathy.[1] Atherosclerotic coronary heart disease was the cause of death in three. Recently we studied the heart in a young man who died while walking back to the huddle after having run a pass pattern in a professional football game. He had been well until September 5, 1971 (six weeks before death), when at about 10 P.M. he developed intense upper abdominal pain, which also was associated with "aching" in his shoulders, brief syncope, severe sweating, and bradycardia. Several hours later he was hospitalized by the team surgeon. On admission, the pain was still present, blood pressure was 140/90 mm Hg, and heart rate was 90 beats per minute (bpm) and regular. No precordial murmurs were present. Neither the liver nor the spleen was palpable. The chest roentgenogram was normal.

By the next day, the pain had nearly disappeared without the patient's having received any medicines, and

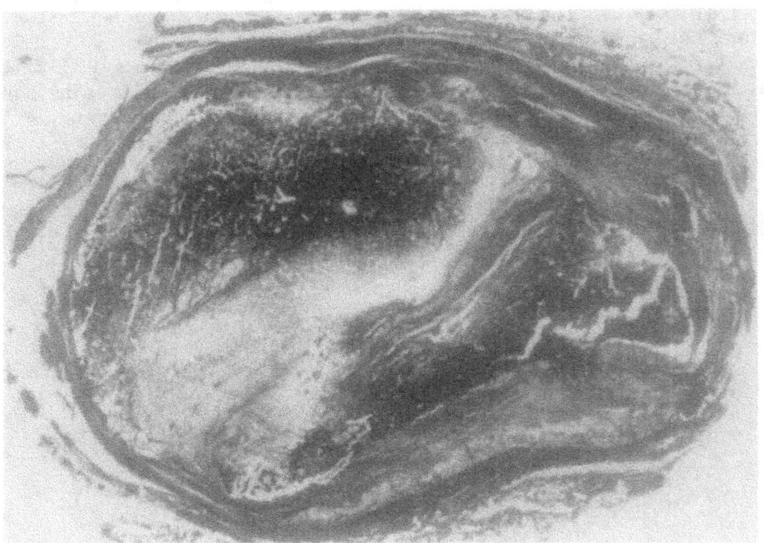

Fig 1. Photomicrograph of section of left anterior descending coronary artery showing total occlusion of the lumen by atherosclerotic plaque which contains large numbers of extravasated erythrocytes. (Movat stain; original magnification ×15.)

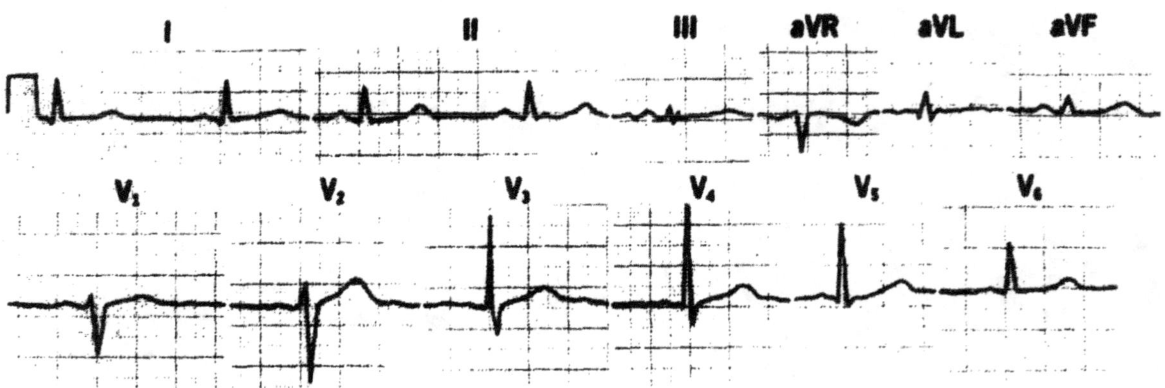

Fig 2. Electrocardiogram recorded slightly less than 4 months before death at the beginning of the patient's last football season.

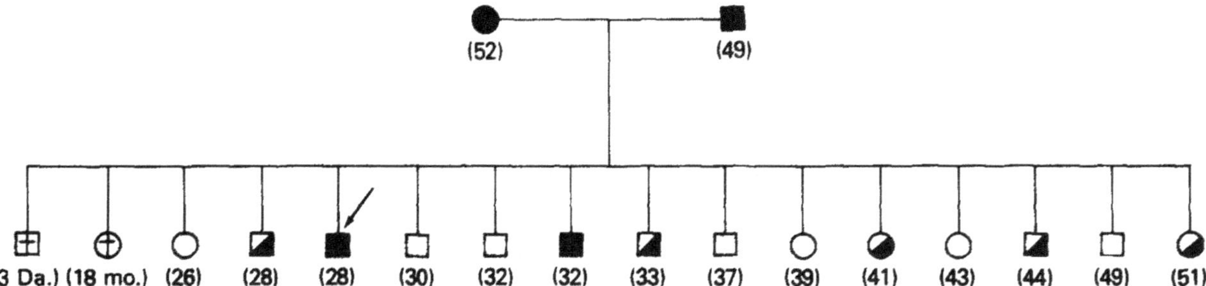

Fig 3. Family tree in the patient described, who is indicated by the *arrow. Numbers* represent ages in years. *Squares* symbolize males and *circles* females. *Symbols in black* are the family members with known type II hyperlipoproteinemia: *solid black* indicates fatal coronary heart disease. *Da* = days and *mo* = months for ages of the two family members in whom lipid data were unavailable.

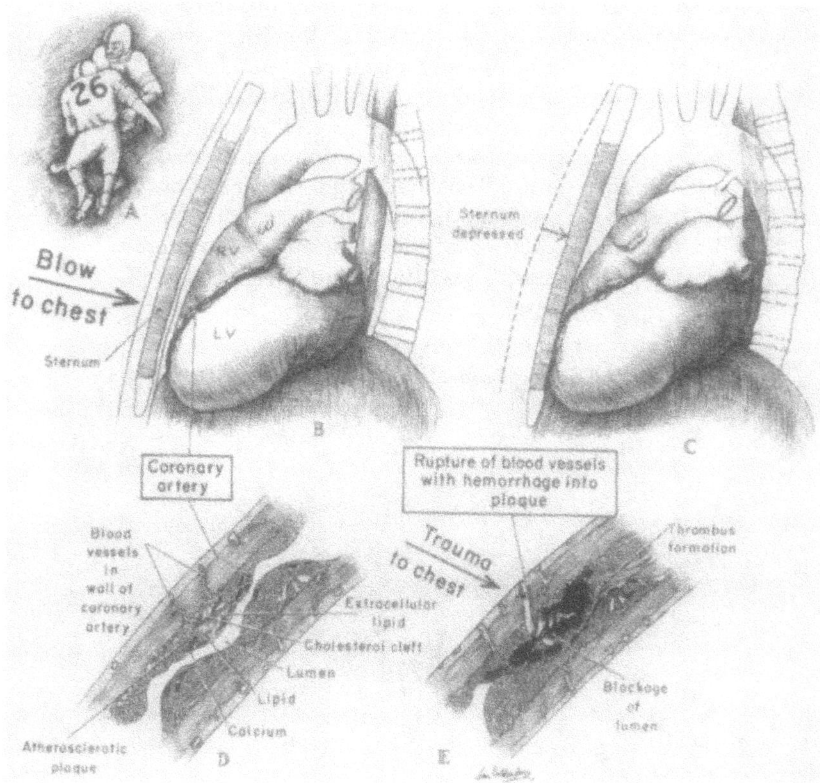

Fig 4. Drawing showing probable mechanism of hemorrhages into atherosclerotic plaques in the coronary arteries in the patient described. *RV* = right ventricle; *LV* = left ventricle.

on September 7 he was discharged. Because of fever at home, he was rehospitalized on September 9. The serum lactic dehydrogenase was elevated. The results of intravenous pyelogram, selective splenic and renal angiograms, and studies of renal function (to rule out splenic rupture) were normal. The pain did not recur and he was discharged on September 12, 1971. He resumed football practice and was apparently asymptomatic until October 28, 1971, when during the course of a professional football game, he suddenly died. At necropsy, the heart weighed 410 gm and its posterolateral wall was the site of a large transmural healing infarct, consistent with a 6-week duration. The right, left anterior descending, and left circumflex coronary arteries were diffusely atherosclerotic and

severely narrowed by atherosclerotic plaques, many of which contained extravasated erythrocytes (Fig. 1). A small thrombus with underlying plaque hemorrhage was present in the right coronary artery. Both the liver (2200 gm) and spleen (640 gm) were enlarged.

Reexamination of the clinical features after death in this patient make it clear that he had an acute myocardial infarction 6 weeks before death, and that the "left upper quadrant" pain almost surely was pain of acute myocardial infarction. Although no electrocardiogram or family historical information was recorded in his last 6 weeks of life, interview and examination on July 1, 1971 (less than 4 months before death—at the beginning of football practice) had disclosed that his total serum cholesterol was elevated (350 mg/dl), that his electrocardiogram (Fig. 2) was within normal limits, and that many members of his family had documented type II hyperlipoproteinemia with or without symptomatic or fatal coronary heart disease (Fig. 3).

The unusual anatomic feature about the epicardial coronary arteries in this patient was the extensiveness of the hemorrhages into the atherosclerotic plaques. Tackling and blocking, such as the present patient did, almost surely caused contact of the anterior surface of the heart with the underlying sternum. As long as the coronary arteries are normal or near normal, as is presumably the usual situation in professional football players, the arteries absorb these "blows" without consequence since they are freely pliable. When these arteries are heavily atherosclerotic, as in the present patient, their pliability is lost and then contact of the surface of the heart with the underlying sternum logically might result in "cracking" of the atherosclerotic plaques, allowing hemorrhage into them in the manner shown in Fig. 4. The crack in the plaque in turn may lead to intraluminal thrombosis. Additionally, "jarring" without actual contact of heavily atherosclerotic coronary arteries, such as the left circumflex or posterior portion of the right, might also produce cracks in plaques with resulting plaque hemorrhage.

REFERENCE

1. Maron BJ, Roberts WC, McAllister HA, Rosing DR, Epstein SE: Sudden death in young athletes. Circulation **62**:218, 1980.

Coronary Narrowing in Types II, III, and IV Hyperlipoproteinemia and in Known Normal Lipoprotein Patterns

HENRY SCOTT CABIN, MD, WILLIAM C. ROBERTS, MD

Numerous epidemiologic and angiographic studies have analyzed the association of serum cholesterol, serum triglyceride, and hyperlipoproteinemia with coronary artery disease. Little morphologic information, however, is available concerning the status of coronary arteries in patients with hyperlipoproteinemia. In this paper, previous studies are reviewed and results of coronary artery studies in 43 necropsy patients with types II, III, or IV hyperlipoproteinemia or with normal lipoprotein patterns are presented.

EPIDEMIOLOGIC STUDIES

The role of cholesterol as a risk factor for the development of symptomatic and eventually fatal coronary heart disease is generally accepted. Several studies have provided considerable epidemiologic information that suggests the risk of developing coronary heart disease is directly related to the serum total cholesterol level.[1-16] In the Framingham study,[6] the risk of developing cardiovascular disease in men of all ages and in women under age 50 was found to be proportional to the antecedent serum cholesterol level. The serum total cholesterol level was, however, of little use in predicting the development of coronary heart disease in women over age 50 at the time of entry into the study. Many studies[8,11,15,17-27] also have reported a higher mean serum total cholesterol level among patients with coronary heart disease compared with age-matched controls.

Although most reports have shown a direct correlation of serum triglyceride level with risk for developing coronary heart disease,[5-9,11,13,16] some have not found this relationship to persist when adjusted for cholesterol, obesity, or diabetes mellitus.[6,8,14,28] In the Stockholm prospective study,[7,16] however, which followed 3,168 men for nine years, the risk of developing myocardial infarction or sudden coronary death was independently related to both the fasting serum cholesterol and triglyceride level at the time of entry into the study. Similarly, Pelkonen and associates[13] studied 1,648 middle-age Finnish men and found that both serum triglyceride and cholesterol concentrations were independently associated with cardiovascular mortality. In addition, several studies have shown that hypertriglyceridemia is more frequent than is hypercholesterolemia among patients with coronary heart disease (Table I).[9,24,26-32]

Some investigators have stressed the importance of lipoprotein analysis, in addition to cholesterol and triglyceride determinations, in evaluating the role of lipid abnormalities in the development of coronary heart disease. Plasma lipoproteins are complexes of lipid, protein, and carbohydrate, and their basic function is to solubilize lipids and transport them in plasma.[33-34] They are divided into five classes, based on differences in density (determined by ultracentrifugation) or mobility (determined by electrophoresis), and are designated chylomicrons, very low density (prebeta) lipoproteins (VLDL), intermediate density (broad-beta) lipoproteins (IDL), low density (beta) lipoproteins (LDL), and high density (alpha) lipoproteins (HDL).[35] Elevations of chylomicrons, LDL, IDL, and

From the Pathology Branch, National Heart, Lung, and Blood Institute, National Institutes of Health, Bethesda, Maryland.

Address for reprints: Henry Scott Cabin, MD, Section of Cardiology, Yale University School of Medicine, 333 Cedar St, New Haven, CT 06504

TABLE I

PERCENTAGE OF PATIENTS WITH HYPERCHOLESTEROLEMIA ($\uparrow$TC) OR HYPERTRIGLYCERIDEMIA ($\uparrow$Tg) OR BOTH AMONG PATIENTS UNDERGOING CORONARY ANGIOGRAPHY OR WITH CLINICALLY DIAGNOSED CORONARY HEART DISEASE

Study	Year	Patients (N)	$\uparrow$TC (upper limit of normal in mg/100 ml)	$\uparrow$Tg (upper limit of normal in mg/100 ml)
Albrink et al[31]	1959	82	18% (269)	70% (175)
Hayes et al[26]	1964	151	32% (279)	37% (167)
Carlson et al[29]	1966	100	25% (322)	40% (195)
Cramer et al[32]	1966	135	44% (280)	32% (160)
Leren et al[30]	1971	420	71% (275)	21% (200)
Goldstein et al[27]	1973	500	16% (284)	24% (164)
Dolder et al[9]	1975	240	25% (279)	35% (199)
McLaughlin et al[45]	1977	99	19% (249)	51% (149)
Hamby[24]	1979	962	11% (300)	35% (166)

VLDL are referred to as types I, II, III, and IV hyperlipoproteinemias (HLP), respectively. A combined increase of chylomicrons and of VLDL constitutes type V HLP, and type II HLP has been subdivided into IIA (increased LDL) and IIB (increased LDL and VLDL). Although all five groups of HLP are associated with hypercholesterolemia or hypertriglyceridemia or both, only types II, III, and IV have been associated with an increased risk of developing coronary heart disease. Elevated levels of HDL have been associated with a decreased risk of coronary heart disease.[15,34,36] Type III HLP is rare, but its association with coronary heart disease is generally accepted.[33,35,37-42] Type II HLP has been well established as a risk factor for the development of coronary heart disease,[35,43] as has hypercholesterolemia. Stone and associates[43] studied 1,403 adult relatives of 116 patients followed at the National Institutes of Health for type II HLP and compared the frequency of symptomatic coronary heart disease in relatives with type II HLP and in those with normal lipoprotein patterns (NLPP). Angina pectoris occurred in 22% of type II and 6% of NLPP relatives ($P < .001$), and acute myocardial infarction in 6% of type II and 1% of NLPP relatives ($P < .002$). The cumulative probability of developing symptomatic coronary heart disease by age 60 was 52% in male and 33% in female type II relatives, compared with 13% and 9%, respectively, in NLPP relatives.

Although most studies show that type IV HLP is frequent in patients with coronary heart disease (Table II),[17,18,20,30,44-46] whether the relation of type IV HLP or VLDL levels to the risk of developing coronary heart disease persists when adjusted for other factors is controversial. In the Framingham study,[6] the risk of developing coronary heart disease was proportional to levels of beta (LDL) and prebeta (VLDL) lipoproteins. When adjusted for cholesterol level, however, VLDL had no independent effect on the risk of developing coronary heart disease in men of all ages and in young women (<54 years). In older women (≥54 years), however, an independent effect of VLDL on the risk of coronary heart disease was discernible.

ANGIOGRAPHIC STUDIES

In addition to information regarding the significance of cholesterol and triglyceride levels and of types II, III, and IV HLP as risk factors for the de-

TABLE II

PERCENTAGES OF PATIENTS WITH TYPE II OR IV HYPERLIPOPROTEINEMIA (HLP) AMONG PATIENTS UNDERGOING CORONARY ANGIOGRAPHY OR WITH CLINICALLY DIAGNOSED CORONARY HEART DISEASE

Study	Year	Patients (N)	Type II HLP	Type IV HLP
Heinle et al[46]	1969	126	29%	25%
Leren et al[30]	1971	420	59%	12%
Salel et al[44]	1974	105	20%	46%
Murray et al[17]	1975	133	22%	27%
McLaughlin et al[45]	1977	99	14%	46%
Gotto et al[18]	1977	496	11%	26%
Dick et al[20]	1978	233	26%	22%

velopment of coronary heart disease, considerable information is also available on the relation of these various lipid disorders to the amount and extent of coronary arterial narrowing. This information has been primarily derived from coronary angiography in patients with symptoms of coronary heart disease. Cramér and associates[32] reported angiographic findings in 135 men and 41 women (91 with chest pain or previous myocardial infarct) and found that severe coronary arterial changes (luminal narrowing resulting in delayed filling of peripheral vessels) occurred significantly more frequently among patients with hypertriglyceridemia (>160 mg/100 ml) than among those with normal triglyceride levels (≤160 mg/100 ml). The frequency of severe coronary narrowing in patients with hypercholesterolemia (>280 mg/100 ml), however, was similar to that in patients with cholesterol ≤280 mg/100 ml. Fuster and associates[47] found no difference in the number of coronary arteries with >50% diameter reduction or in the distribution or degree of coronary narrowing among 61 patients with hypercholesterolemia (>300 ml/100 ml) or hypertriglyceridemia (>150 mg/100 ml) or both, compared with 239 patients with normal lipids (all studied less than one year after onset of "typical" symptoms of coronary heart disease). Similarly, Nitter-Hauge and Enge[48] found no correlation between serum cholesterol or triglyceride levels and amount or extent of coronary narrowing among 71 patients with a history of myocardial infarction or angina pectoris. Proudfit and associates[49] found an increasing frequency of abnormal coronary arteriograms (any amount of coronary narrowing) correlated with increasing serum cholesterol levels among 147 men under age 40. Gotto and colleagues[18] studied 496 patients who underwent coronary angiography for evaluation of chest pain and found that both cholesterol and triglyceride levels were correlated with the frequency and extent (number of vessels involved) of coronary artery disease (>25% diameter reduction).

Analyses of the relation of types II and IV HLP to coronary angiographic findings have also been conflicting. Heinle and associates[46] reported findings in 192 patients who underwent coronary angiography for suspected coronary or valvular heart disease. Types II and IV HLP occurred significantly more frequently in those with any degree of coronary narrowing, as compared with those with normal coronary arteries, but the lipoprotein pattern was not related to the type of coronary lesion ("occlusion, single stenosis, multiple stenoses, or diffuse narrowing"), the vessel involved, or the presence of collaterals. Murray and colleagues,[17] however, studied 133 male patients with chest pain (those with noncoronary heart disease were excluded) and found that type II HLP was associated more often than was type IV HLP with severe narrowing (>50% diameter reduction) of two or three coronary arteries. Similar findings were reported by Bloch and associates[50] who studied 46 patients with known type II or type IV HLP, of whom all but four had angina pectoris prior to catheterization. They also found severe (>50%) narrowing of the left main coronary artery and severe narrowing of both the proximal and distal portions of the other three major coronary arteries more frequently in type II than in type IV HLP patients. In contrast, Gotto and associates[18] studied 496 patients with chest pain and found a larger number of coronary arteries narrowed by more than 25% in diameter among the type IV HLP compared with the normal lipoprotein pattern (NLPP) patients; there was no significant difference between the type II and type IV HLP or NLPP patients. The difference between the type IV HLP and NLPP patients did not persist when patients without coronary artery disease were excluded.

The conflicting results in these angiographic studies may in part be explained by differing patient populations, variability in definitions of hyperlipoproteinemia, and varying methods of interpretation of coronary arteriograms.

MORPHOLOGIC STUDIES

We have studied 43 necropsy patients who had symptomatic coronary heart disease during life and who had type II, III, or IV HLP or NLPP.[42,51] Little morphologic information was previously available on the status of the coronary arteries in HLP,[39–41] and the studies described here are the first quantitative analyses and comparisons of the amounts and locations of coronary narrowing by atherosclerotic plaques in necropsy patients with HLP or NLPP. Previous necropsy studies reported only the maximal amounts of narrowing in each of the four major epicardial coronary arteries and had found no differences among patients with symptomatic coronary disease and with type II, III, or IV HLP or NLPP.[41]

The 43 study patients (35 men, 8 women) ranged in age from 29 to 78 years (mean, 52 years). Certain clinical findings in the 15 patients with type II HLP, 5 with type III HLP, 13 with type IV HLP, and 10 with NLPP are summarized in Table III. The mean age at death of the NLPP patients was significantly higher than that of the type II or IV HLP patients (P < .05). The proportion of men and women was similar in the type II and IV HLP and NLPP patients, but there were significantly more women in the type III HLP group than in the type II HLP group (P < .05). No significant difference among the four groups was found for frequency of angina pectoris or past or fatal acute myocardial infarction. Chronic congestive heart failure was more frequent in the type III HLP and NLPP groups than it was in the type II group (P < .05). The mean serum total cholesterol level was higher in the type

TABLE III
CLINICAL FINDINGS IN 15 PATIENTS WITH TYPE II HYPERLIPOPROTEINEMIA, 5 WITH TYPE III, 13 WITH TYPE IV, AND 10 WITH NORMAL LIPOPROTEIN PATTERNS (NLPP)

Finding	Type II (N = 15)	Type III (N = 5)	Type IV (N = 13)	NLPP (N = 10)
Age range in years (mean)	29−58 (51)*	49−75 (56)	31−65 (48)*	31−78 (58)**
Male:female	13:2**	2:3*	11:2	9:1
Angina pectoris	12	4	11	5
AMI by history	7	2	7	5
Chronic CHF	1**	3*	2	4*
Systemic hypertension	6	4*	6	2**
Diabetes mellitus	2**	3*	5	2
TC (mg/100 ml), range (mean)	280−591 (409)*	338−660 (498)*	140−735 (323)***	121−233 (168)**
Tg (mg/100 ml), range (mean)	86−442 (241)*	429−2367 (1038)**	210−2820 (878)**	76−150 (104)***
Mode of death				
Sudden	9*	2	4	1**
AMI	3	1	2	2
CHF	0	1	0	2
Unstable angina pectoris	2	0	0	0
CABG	0*	1	6**	4**
Cardiac Catheterization	1	0	1	1

Note: Comparison of * to **, ** to ***, and * to *** = $P < .05$.
AMI = acute myocardial infarction; CABG = coronary artery bypass grafting; CHF = congestive heart failure; TC = total cholesterol; Tg = triglyceride.

II and III HLP patients than in the type IV or NLPP patients ($P < .05$), and the mean serum triglyceride level was higher in the type III and IV patients than in the type II or NLPP patients ($P < .05$). The mean serum triglyceride and cholesterol levels were significantly lower in the NLPP group than in any of the HLP groups.

Among the 43 study patients, a total of 172 major epicardial coronary arteries (right, left main, left anterior descending, and left circumflex) were examined, and the results are summarized in Tables IV and V. At least two of the four major arteries were narrowed severely (76%−100% in cross-sectional area) by atherosclerotic plaques in all study patients, except for one type II HLP patient who had severe narrowing of only the left main coronary artery. Significantly more patients in the types II, III, and IV HLP groups had severe narrowing of all four major coronary arteries than did those in the NLPP group ($P < .05$). The type IV HLP patients had a greater mean number of the four coronary arteries narrowed severely per patient than did the NLPP patients (3.5/4.0 versus 2.6/4.0, respectively; $P < .01$). Severe narrowing of the left main coronary artery occurred more frequently in the three HLP groups than in the NLPP group. Thus analysis of only the maximal amounts of narrowing in each major epicardial coronary artery in the 43

TABLE IV
NUMBER OF PATIENTS WITH TYPE II, III, OR IV HYPERLIPOPROTEINEMIA OR NORMAL LIPOPROTEIN PATTERNS WITH MAJOR CORONARY ARTERIES NARROWED 76%−100% IN CROSS-SECTIONAL AREA BY ATHEROSCLEROTIC PLAQUES

Total Number of Coronary Arteries Narrowed	Lipoprotein Pattern			
	II	III	IV	Normal
4	7	2	6	0
3	5	2	7	6
2	2	1	0	4
1	1	0	0	0
0	0	0	0	0
Total	15	5	13	10

study patients revealed significant differences between the HLP and the NLPP patients, but not among the HLP groups.

A more precise quantitative approach was then utilized to determine if there were any differences in amount or location of coronary artery narrowing by atherosclerotic plaque among the HLP groups and between each of the HLP groups and the NLPP

TABLE V

NUMBER OF PATIENTS WITH EACH OF THE FOUR MAJOR CORONARY ARTERIES NARROWED 76%–100% IN CROSS-SECTIONAL AREA BY ATHEROSCLEROTIC PLAQUES

	Patients (N)	Patients with Each Coronary Artery Narrowed > 75%				Mean Number of Four Coronary Arteries per Patient Narrowed > 75%
		LM	LAD	LC	R	
Type II HLP	15	9	13	12	14	3.2
Type III HLP	5	3	4	4	5	3.2
Type IV HLP	13	6	13	13	13	3.5
Normal	10	1	9	8	8	2.6

$P < .01$ (for Type IV HLP and Normal)

HLP = hyperlipoproteinemia; LAD = left anterior descending; LC = left circumflex; LM = left main; R = right.

group. The entire lengths of the four major epicardial coronary arteries were removed in their entirety from each of the 43 hearts, cut transversely into 5-mm segments, and the amount of narrowing in each segment was determined by histologic examination. The mean percentage of 5-mm segments of coronary artery with severe narrowing was far greater in the type IV (67%) than in the type II (39%) HLP or NLPP (35%) groups ($P < .005$) (Figure 1). The difference in amounts of severe narrowing between the type II HLP and NLPP groups was not significant. The mean percentage of 5-mm segments narrowed severely in the type III HLP patients was 44%, but the small number of type III patients did not allow meaningful statistical comparison. The percentage of 5-mm segments narrowed 76%–100% in cross-sectional area by atherosclerotic plaques was significantly greater in the proximal than in the distal halves of the left anterior descending (52% versus 30%, respectively; $P < .02$), left circumflex (37% versus 18%, respectively; $P < .005$), and right (53% versus 37%,

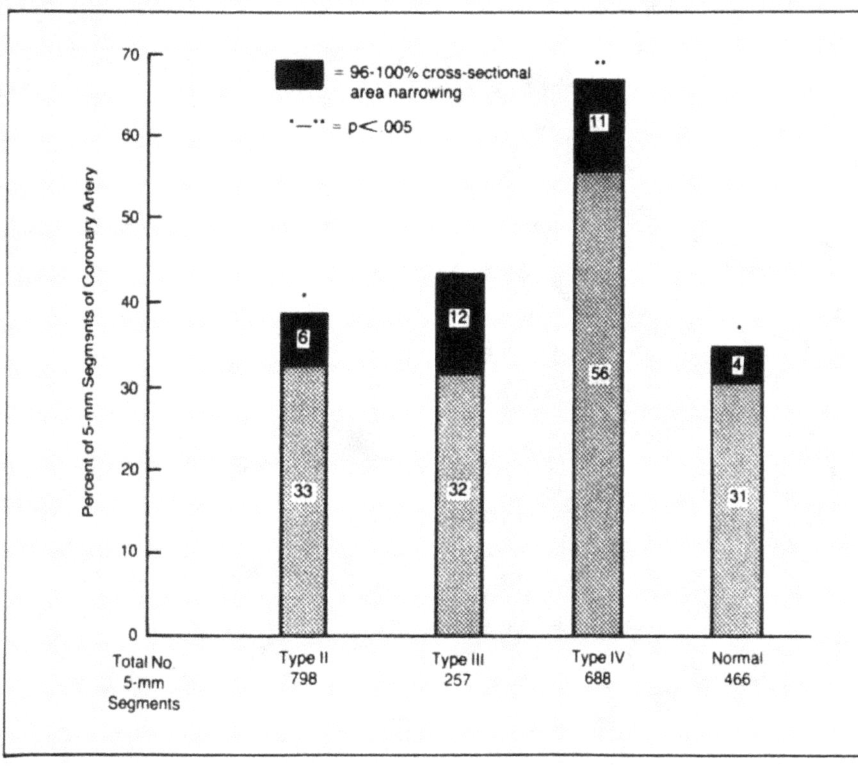

Figure 1. Percentage of 5-mm segments of all four major coronary arteries narrowed 76%–95% (cross-hatched area) and 96%–100% (solid area) in cross-sectional area by atherosclerotic plaques in 15 patients with type II HLP, 5 with type III HLP, 13 with type IV HLP, and 10 with normal lipoprotein patterns and symptomatic coronary heart disease.

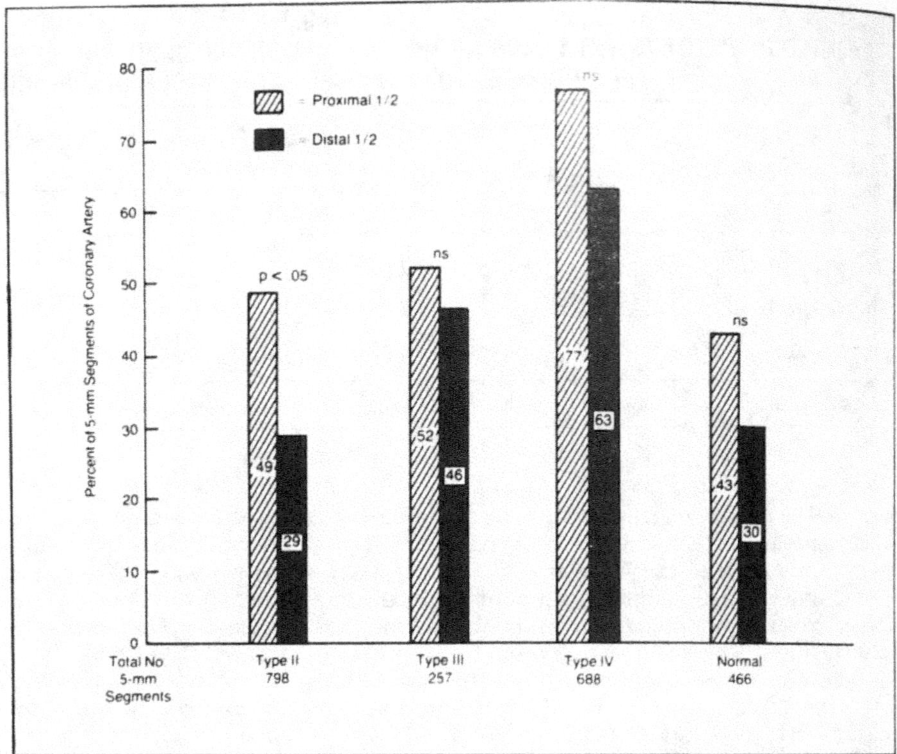

Figure 2. Percent of 5-mm segments in the proximal and distal halves of all four major coronary arteries narrowed 76%–100% in cross-sectional area by atherosclerotic plaques in each of the four groups of patients

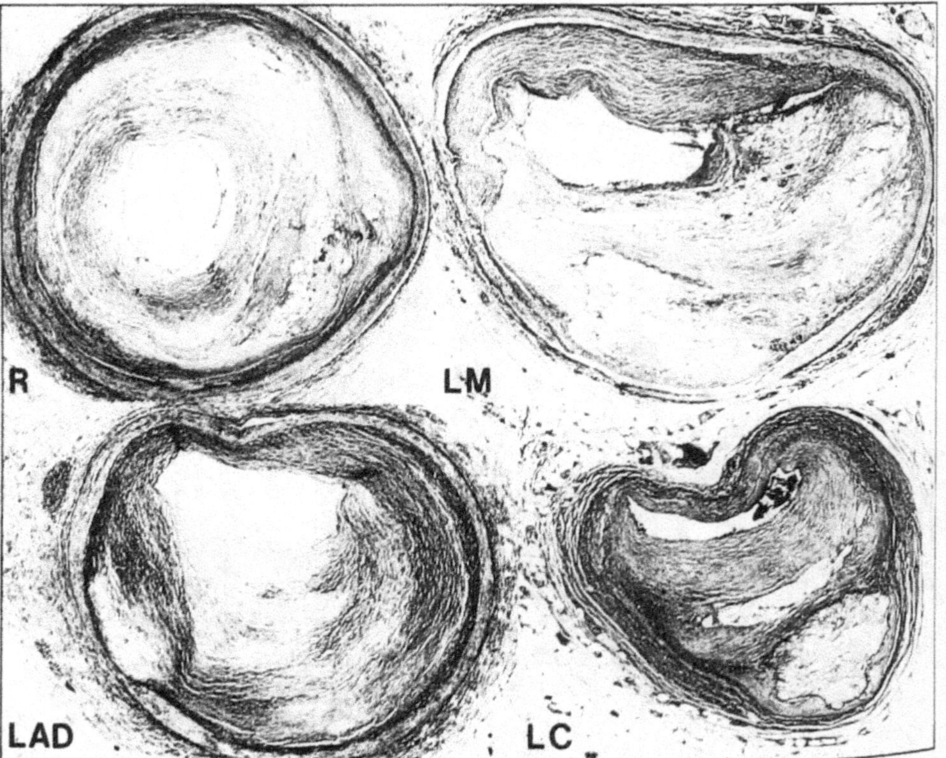

Figure 3. Photomicrographs of the right (R), left main (LM), left anterior descending (LAD), and left circumflex (LC) coronary arteries at points of maximal narrowing in a 51-year-old man with type II hyperlipoproteinemia. He had angina pectoris and died of acute myocardial infarction. The fasting serum total cholesterol was 348 mg/100 ml and triglyceride, 126 mg/100 ml. Each coronary artery is narrowed severely by atherosclerotic plaques, composed primarily of fibrous tissue (Movat stain, ×29)

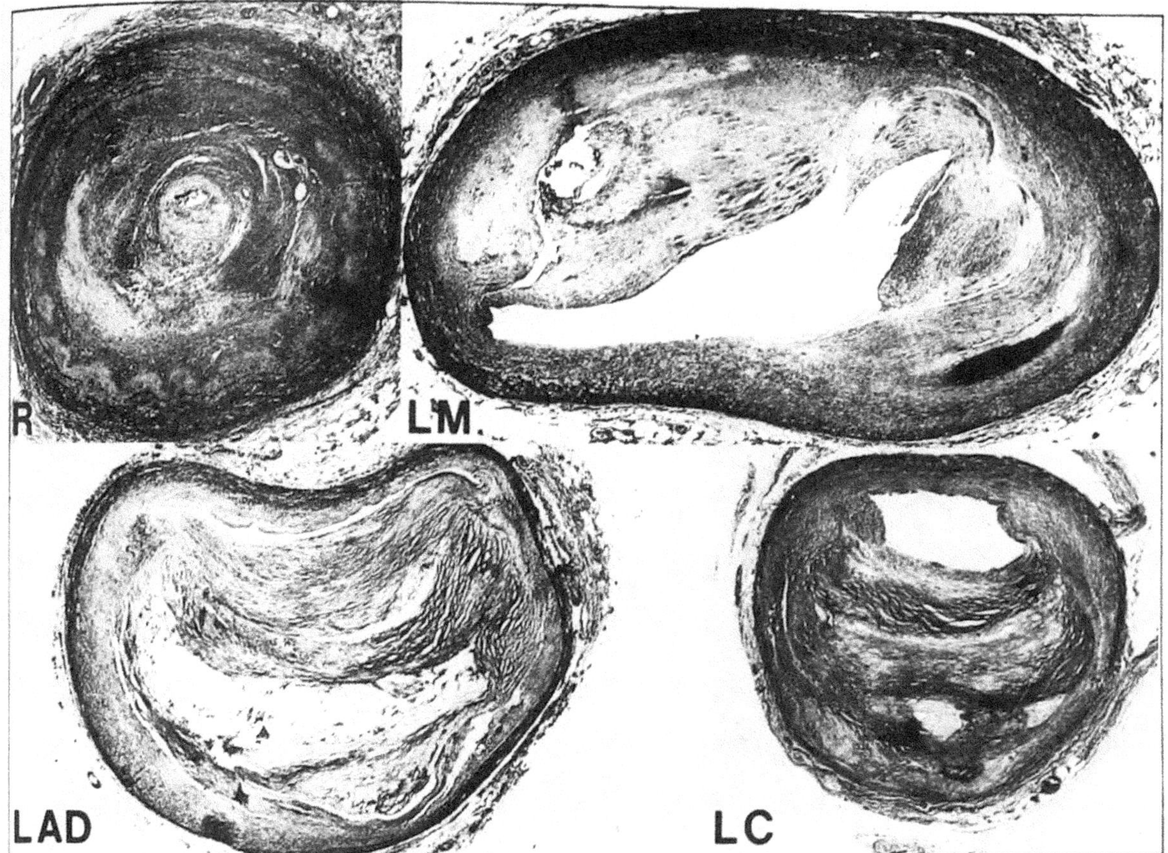

Figure 4. Photomicrographs of the right (R), left main (LM), left anterior descending (LAD), and left circumflex (LC) coronary arteries at sites of maximal narrowing in a 51-year-old man with type III HLP who died suddenly and had previous acute myocardial infarction and angina pectoris. His fasting serum total cholesterol was 382 mg/100 ml, and triglyceride, 870 mg/100 ml. Each coronary artery is narrowed severely by atherosclerotic plaques composed primarily of fibrous tissue. (Movat stain, ×21).

respectively; $P < .05$) coronary arteries in the type II patients, in the left anterior descending (76% versus 59%, respectively; $P < .05$) in the type IV patients, and in none of the major arteries in the type III and NLPP patients. Overall, only the type II patients had more severe narrowing in the proximal than in the distal halves of the major coronary arteries (Figure 2).

The atherosclerotic plaques in all four groups of patients were composed primarily of fibrous tissue and were indistinguishable, regardless of the presence or type of HLP (Figures 3 through 6). Although the first necropsy report of the coronary arteries in type III HLP[39] suggested that in many areas the plaques contained predominantly foam cells, this observation has not been substantiated by subsequent study of five necropsy patients with type III HLP[42] (Figure 4).

CONCLUSION

Hypercholesterolemia and type II hyperlipoproteinemia (HLP) are well-established risk factors for premature development of coronary heart disease. Hypertriglyceridemia and type IV HLP, although common in patients with coronary heart disease, are not uniformly accepted as independent risk factors for the development of coronary heart disease. In patients with symptomatic coronary heart disease, angiographic studies have provided conflicting information regarding the relation of increased serum cholesterol or triglyceride levels or of HLP to the severity and extent of coronary narrowing. In recent necropsy studies in our laboratory, we have quantitated the amount and extent of coronary artery narrowing by atherosclerotic plaque in 43 patients with fatal coronary heart disease and with types II, III, or IV HLP or normal

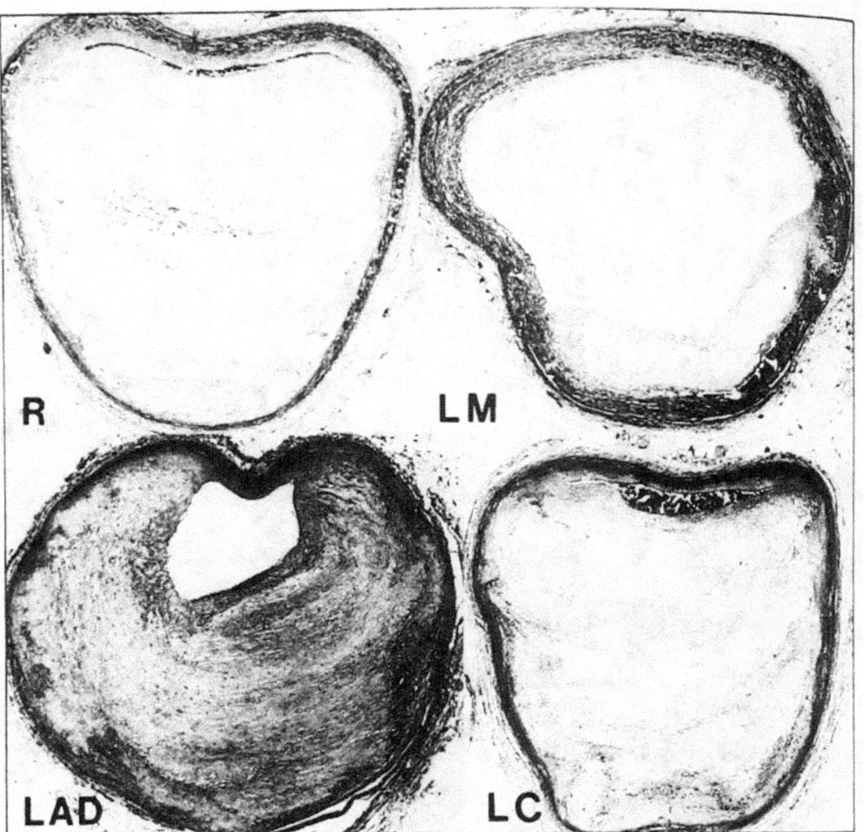

Figure 5. Photomicrographs of the right (R), left main (LM), left anterior descending (LAD), and left circumflex (LC) coronary arteries at points of maximal narrowing in a 33-year-old man with type IV HLP. He had angina pectoris and acute myocardial infarction and died during coronary artery bypass surgery. The fasting serum total cholesterol was 260 mg/100 ml, and triglyceride, 410 mg/100 ml. The R, LAD, and LC arteries are narrowed severely by atherosclerotic plaques. (Movat stain, ×20)

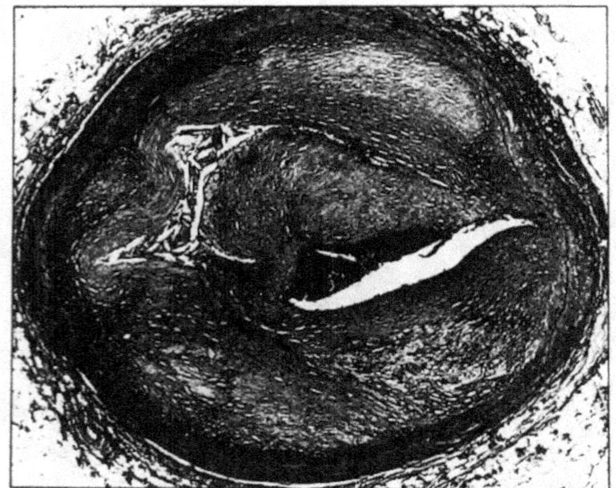

Figure 6. Photomicrograph of the left circumflex coronary artery at its point of maximal narrowing in a 47-year-old man with a normal lipoprotein pattern and angina pectoris and who died from acute myocardial infarction. The fasting serum total cholesterol was 136 mg/100 ml, and triglyceride, 76 mg/100 ml. The left circumflex coronary artery is severely narrowed by atherosclerotic plaques, as were the right and left anterior descending coronary arteries, and a small superimposed mural thrombus is present. (Movat stain, ×35)

lipoprotein patterns. All three HLP groups had more-frequent, severe (76%–100% in cross-sectional area) narrowing of the left main coronary artery than did the NLPP group. The type IV HLP patients had 67% (mean value) of the entire lengths of the four major coronary arteries narrowed severely, compared with 39%, 44%, and 35% for types II and III HLP and NLPP patients, respectively. Thus, these data suggest that among patients with symptomatic coronary heart disease, those with type IV HLP have more-extensive severe coronary narrowing than do those with other forms of HLP or NLPP.

REFERENCES

1. Kannel WB, Dawber TR, Kagan A, et al: Factors of risk in the development of coronary heart disease—Six-year follow-up experience. The Framingham study. Ann Intern Med 1961; 55:33–50

2. Keys A, Taylor HL, Blackburn H, et al: Coronary heart disease among Minnesota business and professional men followed fifteen years. Circulation 1963; 28:381–395

3. Chapman JM, Massey FJ Jr: The interrelationship of

serum cholesterol, hypertension, body weight, and risk of coronary disease. Results of the first ten years follow-up in the Los Angeles heart study. *J Chronic Dis* 1964; 17:933–949.

4. Jensen J, Blankenhorn DH, Kornerup V: Coronary disease in familial hypercholesterolemia. *Circulation* 1967; 36:77–82.

5. Tibblin G: Risk factors in coronary heart disease. *Adv Cardiol* 1970; 4:123–130.

6. Kannel WB, Castelli WP, Gordon T, et al: Serum cholesterol lipoproteins and the risk of coronary heart disease: The Framingham study. *Ann Intern Med* 1971; 74:1–12.

7. Carlson LA, Böttiger LE: Ischaemic heart-disease in relation to fasting values of plasma triglycerides and cholesterol: Stockholm prospective study. *Lancet* 1972; 1:865–868.

8. Wilhelmsen L, Wedel H, Tibblin G: Multivariate analysis of risk factors for coronary heart disease. *Circulation* 1973; 48:950–958.

9. Dolder MA, Oliver MF: Myocardial infarction in young men: Study of risk factors in nine countries. *Br Heart J* 1975; 37:493–503.

10. Thomas CB, Ross DC, Duszynski KR: Youthful hypercholesterolemia: Its associated characteristics and role in premature myocardial infarction. *Johns Hopkins Med J* 1975; 136:193–206.

11. Rosenman RH, Brand RJ, Jenkins CD, et al: Coronary heart disease in the western collaborative group study: Final follow-up experience of 8½ years. *JAMA* 1975; 233:872–877.

12. Rhoads GG, Gulbrandsen CL, Kagan A: Serum lipoproteins and coronary heart disease in a population study of Hawaii Japanese men. *N Engl J Med* 1976; 294:293–298.

13. Pelkonen R, Nikkila EA, Koskinen S, et al: Association of serum lipids and obesity with cardiovascular mortality. *Br Med J* 1977; 2:1185–1187.

14. Costas R Jr, Garcia-Palmieri MR, Nazario E, et al: Relation of lipids, weight and physical activity to incidence of coronary heart disease: The Puerto Rico heart study. *Am J Cardiol* 1978; 42:653–658.

15. Kannel WB, Castelli WP, Gordon T: Cholesterol in the prediction of atherosclerotic disease: New perspectives based on the Framingham study. *Ann Intern Med* 1979; 90:85–91.

16. Carlson LA, Böttiger LE, Ahfeldt PE: Risk factors for myocardial infarction in the Stockholm prospective study: A 14-year follow-up focussing on the role of plasma triglycerides and cholesterol. *Acta Med Scand* 1979; 206:351–360.

17. Murray RG, Tweddel A, Third JLHC, et al: Relation between extent of coronary artery disease and severity of hyperlipoproteinemia. *Br Heart J* 1975; 37:1205–1209.

18. Gotto AM, Gorry GA, Thompson JR, et al: Relationship between plasma lipid concentrations and coronary artery disease in 496 patients. *Circulation* 1977; 56:875–883.

19. Hatch FT, Reissell PK, Poon-King TMW, et al: A study of coronary heart disease in young men: Characteristics and metabolic studies of the patients and comparison with age-matched healthy men. *Circulation* 1966; 33:679–702.

20. Dick TBS, Stone MC: Prevalence of three major risk factors in random sample of men and women, and in patients with ischaemic heart disease. *Br Heart J* 1978; 40:617–626.

21. Walker WJ, Gregoratos G: Myocardial infarction in young men. *Am J Cardiol* 1967; 19:339–343.

22. Gertler MM, Garn SM, Lerman J: The interrelationships of serum cholesterol, cholesterol esters and phospholipids in health and in coronary artery disease. *Circulation* 1950; 2:205–214.

23. Oliver MF, Boyd GS: The plasma lipids in coronary artery disease. *Br Heart J* 1953; 15:387–392.

24. Hamby RI: *Clinical-Anatomical Correlates in Coronary Artery Disease.* New York, Futura Publishing Company, 1979, pp 217–284.

25. Lawry EY, Mann GV, Peterson A, et al: Cholesterol and beta lipoproteins in the serums of Americans: Well persons and those with coronary heart disease. *Am J Med* 1957; 22:605–623.

26. Hayes D, Neill DW: Serum cholesterol and trigylcerides in ischaemic heart disease. *Clin Sci* 1964; 26:185–192.

27. Goldstein JL, Hazzard WR, Schrott HG, et al: Hyperlipidemia in coronary heart disease: I. Lipid levels in 500 survivors of myocardial infarction. *J Clin Invest* 1973; 52:1533–1543.

28. Hulley SB, Rosenman RH, Bawol RD, et al: Epidemiology as a guide to clinical decisions: The association between triglyceride and coronary heart disease. *N Engl J Med* 1980; 302:1383–1389.

29. Carlson LA, Wahlberg F: Serum lipids, intravenous glucose tolerance and their interrelation studied in ischaemic cardiovascular disease. *Acta Med Scand* 1966; 180:307–315.

30. Leren P, Haabrekke O: Blood lipids in patients with coronary heart disease. Acta Med Scand 1971; 189:505–509.

31. Albrink MJ, Man EB: Serum triglycerides in coronary artery disease. *Arch Intern Med* 1959; 103:4–8.

32. Cramer K, Paulin S, Werko L: Coronary angiographic findings in correlation with age, body weight, blood pressure, serum lipids and smoking habits. *Circulation* 1966; 33:888–900.

33. Fredrickson DS, Levy RI, Lees RS: Fat transport in lipoproteins: An integrated approach to mechanisms and disorders (5 pts). *N Engl J Med* 1967; 276:34–44, 94–103, 148–156, 215–225, 273–281.

34. Gofman JW, Young W, Tandy R: Ischemic heart disease, atherosclerosis, and longevity. *Circulation* 1966; 34:679–697.

35. Fredrickson DS, Goldstein JL, Brown MS: The familial hyperlipoproteinemias, in Stanbury JB, Weingaarden JB, Fredrickson DS (eds): *The Metabolic Basis of Inherited Disease,* 4th ed. New York, McGraw-Hill, 1978, pp 604–655.

36. Gordon T, Castelli WP, Hjortland MC, et al: High density lipoprotein as a protective factor against coronary heart disease: The Framingham study. *Am J Med* 1977; 62:707–714.

37. Zelis R, Mason DT, Braunwald E, et al: Effects of hyperlipoproteinemias and their treatment on the peripheral circulation. *J Clin Invest* 1970; 49:1007–1015.

38. Morganroth J, Levy RI, Fredrickson DS: The biochemical, clinical, and genetic features of type III hyperlipoproteinemia. *Ann Intern Med* 1975; 82:158–174.

39. Roberts WC, Levy RI, Fredrickson DS: Hyperlipoproteinemia: A review of the five types with first report of necropsy findings in type 3. *Arch Pathol* 1970; 90:46–56.

40. Holimon JL, Wasserman AJ: Autopsy findings in type 3 hyperlipoproteinemia. *Arch Pathol* 1971; 92:415–417.

41. Roberts WC, Ferrans VJ, Levy RI, et al: Cardiovascular pathology in hyperlipoproteinemia: Anatomic observations in 42 necropsy patients with normal or abnormal serum lipoprotein patterns. *Am J Cardiol* 1973; 31:557–570.

42. Cabin HS, Schwartz DE, Virmani R, et al: Type III hyperlipoproteinemia: Quantification of amounts of coronary arterial narrowing in 5 necropsy patients. *Am Heart J* 1981; 102:830–835.

43. Stone NJ, Levy RI, Fredrickson DS, et al: Coronary artery disease in 116 kindred with familial type II hyperlipoproteinemia. *Circulation* 1974; 49:476–488.

44. Salel AF, Riggs K, Mason DT, et al: The importance of type IV hyperlipoproteinemia as a predisposing factor in coronary artery disease. *Am J Med* 1974; 57:897–903.

45. McLaughlin PR, Berman ND, Morton BC, et al: Long-term angiographic assessment of the influence of coronary risk factors on native coronary circulation and saphenous vein aortocoronary grafts. *Am Heart J* 1977; 93:327–333.

46. Heinle RA, Levy RI, Fredrickson DS, et al: Lipid and carbohydrate abnormalities in patients with angiographically documented coronary artery disease. *Am J Cardiol* 1969; 24:178–186.

47. Fuster V, Frye RL, Connolly DC, et al: Arteriographic patterns early in the onset of the coronary syndromes. *Br Heart J* 1975; 37:1250–1255.

48. Nitter-Hauge S, Enge I: Relation between blood lipid levels and angiographically evaluated obstructions in coronary arteries. *Br Heart J* 1973; 35:791–795.

49. Proudfit WL, Shirey EK, Sones FM Jr: Selective cine coronary arteriography: Correlation with clinical findings in 1,000 patients. *Circulation* 1966; 33:901–910.

50. Bloch A, Dinsmore RE, Lees RS: Coronary arteriographic findings in type-II and type-IV hyperlipoproteinemia. *Lancet* 1976; 1:928–930.

51. Cabin HS, Roberts WC: Quantification of amounts of coronary arterial narrowing in patients with types II and IV hyperlipoproteinemia and in those with known normal lipoprotein patterns. *Am Heart J* 1981; 101:52–58.

Comparison of Amount and Extent of Coronary Narrowing by Atherosclerotic Plaque and of Myocardial Scarring at Necropsy in Anterior and Posterior Healed Transmural Myocardial Infarction

Henry Scott Cabin, M.D., and William C. Roberts, M.D.

SUMMARY   The amount of cross-sectional area narrowing by atherosclerotic plaque in each 5-mm-long segment from the entire lengths of the right, left main, left anterior descending and left circumflex coronary arteries and the size, predominant location and extent of myocardial scarring were determined in 59 necropsy patients with a healed transmural myocardial infarct (MI). The mean number of the four major epicardial coronary arteries narrowed severely (76–100% in cross-sectional area) was 3.0 in the 37 patients with posterior MI and 2.6 in the 22 patients with anterior MI ($p < .025$). The mean percent of severely narrowed 5-mm segments from all four major coronary arteries was similar in the anterior and posterior MI groups, 38% vs 46%. The patients with anterior MI, however, had a higher percentage of severely narrowed 5-mm segments of the left anterior descending than of the left circumflex but not the right coronary artery, 46% vs 25% ($p < 0.001$) and 40% (NS). The patients with posterior MI had a higher percentage of severely narrowed segments of the right and left circumflex coronary arteries than of the left anterior descending artery, 55% and 51% vs 32% ($p < 0.05$). The anterior MI group had, on the average, larger left ventricular scars than the posterior MI group (20% vs 9%, $p > 0.002$) and more frequent scarring of the ventricular septum, 16 patients (73%) vs six patients (16%) ($p < 0.001$).

IN A RECENT REPORT,[1] the amount and extent of coronary narrowing at necropsy were determined in a quantitative fashion in 22 patients with an acute anterior myocardial infarct (MI) and in 28 patients with an acute posterior ("inferior"[2]) MI. In the present study, the amount and extent of coronary arterial narrowing and of myocardial scarring at necropsy in 22 patients with a healed anterior MI were compared with those in 37 patients with a healed posterior MI.

Patients and Methods

Of the 59 patients with a healed transmural MI, 37 had a posterior left ventricular scar and 22 an anterior scar, with or without involvement of the adjacent lateral wall or ventricular septum. In some of the patients the MI involved only the anterior or posterior wall in the basal portion of left ventricle, but involved most or all of the left ventricle at the apex. The designation of anterior or posterior was determined by examining the basal half of the heart. Certain clinical and necropsy findings for each of the two groups of patients are summarized in tables 1 and 2. The ages and sex distribution were similar in the two groups. An acute MI was clinically diagnosed in 17 patients (77%) with an anterior MI and in 15 (41%) with a posterior MI ($p < 0.05$); one anterior MI patient (5%) and four posterior MI patients (11%) had two clinical episodes of acute MI (NS). The interval from the first clinical episode of acute MI to death was 2–204 months (mean 37 months) in the anterior MI patients and 4–276 months (mean 76 months) in the posterior MI patients (NS).

There was no significant difference between the two groups in the frequency of angina pectoris, chronic congestive heart failure, systemic hypertension, diabetes mellitus, sudden coronary death, fatal acute MI or noncardiac modes of death.

In each of the 59 patients, the entire lengths of the right, left main, left anterior descending and left circumflex coronary arteries were removed from the heart intact, fixed in an unpressurized state in formalin for about 48 hours, radiographed, and decalcified if calcific deposits were present. Then, each of the four major arteries were cut transversely into 5-mm segments, processed in alcohol and xylene and cut. At least one 6-μ-thick section from each 5-mm segment was prepared for histologic study; it was stained by the Movat method,[3] which stains the internal elastic membrane black, fibrous tissue tan, mucoid material light green, smooth muscle red, erythrocytes red and nuclei black. The degree of luminal narrowing in each 5-mm segment was determined by examination under the microscope (magnification $\times$ 25–50). The percent of cross-sectional area narrowing by atherosclerotic plaque was separated into five categories: 0–25%, 26–50%, 51–75%, 76–95% and 96–100%. The accuracy of these determinations was verified by video planimetry and had an error of less than 5%.[4]

The amount of myocardium replaced by scar was determined by tracing the grossly visible areas of scar and the total left ventricular area, including ventricular septum, from the apical surfaces of each of five or six 1-cm-thick transverse ventricular slices cut from apex to base. The area of scar and the total left ventricular area were then determined by a video planimetry system. The sum of the areas of fibrosis from each slice divided by the sum of the left ventricular areas from all the slices provided the MI size, expressed as a percent of the total left ventricular area.

From the Pathology Branch, National Heart, Lung, and Blood Institute, National Institutes of Health, Bethesda Maryland.

Address for correspondence: William C. Roberts, M.D., Pathology Branch, National Heart, Lung, and Blood Institute, National Institutes of Health, Bethesda, Maryland 20205.

Received August 3, 1981; revision accepted November 20, 1981.

Circulation 66, No. 1, 1982.

TABLE 1. *Clinical and Necropsy Findings in Each of 22 Necropsy Patients with a Healed Anterior Wall Myocardial Infarct*

Pt	Age (years)	Sex	Hx AMI	Inter-val (mo) AMI to death	AP	CHF	Mode of death	Heart weight (g)	MI location VS	MI location L	MI size (%)
1	25	M	0	—	0	0	NC	350	+	0	20
2	27	M	+	12	0	0	SCD	490	+	+	28
3	44	M	0	—	0	+	AMI	450	+	+	8
4	46	M	+	36	0	+	CHF	500	+	0	25
5	49	F	+	36	+	0	CC	260	+	0	35
6	52	F	+	36	+	+	AMI	480	0	0	20
7	54	F	+	4	0	+	SCD	—	+	+	55
8	54	M	+	24	+	+	AMI	430	+	+	20
9	55	F	+	3	0	0	SCD	480	+	0	21
10	56	M	+	2	0	0	AMI	450	+	+	12
11	59	M	+	—	0	0	SCD	320	0	+	13
12	62	M	0	—	0	+	NC	640	0	0	16
13	64	M	+	8	0	0	Op*	572	+	0	21
14	67	M	+	3	0	+	CHF	370	0	0	40
15	68	F	0	—	+	+	AMI	420	+	0	12
16	72	M	+	204	+	−	CABG	540	+	0	7
17	72	M	+	36	+	+	SCD	—	+	0	5
18	73	F	+	12	0	+	NC	535	+	0	5
19	74	M	0	—	+	+	SCD	410	0	+	23
20	76	F	+	72	+	0	AMI	330	0	+	10
21	78	M	+	50	0	−	NC	430	+	0	18
22	80	M	+	60	0	+	NC	615	+	0	18

*Left ventricular aneurysmectomy.

†LM narrowed > 75%.

‡Dominant posterior is the LC.

§See Results section for explanation of scoring system.

Abbreviations: AMI = acute MI; AP = angina pectoris; Ath = atherosclerotic plaque; CA = coronary arteries; CABG = coronary artery bypass grafting; CC = cardiac catheterization; CHF = chronic congestive heart failure; Hx = history of; L = lateral wall; LAD = left anterior descending; LC = left circumflex; LM = left main; MI = myocardial infarct; NC = noncardiac; Op = operation; R = right; SCD = sudden coronary death; VS = ventricular septum.

Results

Among the 59 patients, 236 major epicardial coronary arteries were examined (tables 3 and 4). Of the 88 arteries from the anterior MI group, at least one 5-mm segment in 57 arteries (65%) was narrowed severely (76–100% in cross-sectional area) by atherosclerotic plaque, an average of 2.6 coronary arteries per patient; of the 148 major epicardial coronary arteries examined in the posterior MI group, 112 (76%) were severely narrowed, an average of 3.0 coronary arteries per patient ($p < 0.05$).

All four arteries were severely narrowed in one of 22 anterior MI patients (4%) and in eight of 37 posterior MI patients (22%) (NS); three arteries were severely narrowed in 12 anterior MI patients (55%) and in 24 posterior MI patients (65%) (NS); two arteries were severely narrowed in eight anterior MI patients (36%) and in three posterior MI patients (8%) ($p < 0.05$); one artery was severely narrowed in one anterior MI patient (4%) and in two posterior MI patients (5%) (NS).

The left main coronary artery was severely narrowed in four of 22 anterior MI patients (18%) and in nine of 37 posterior MI patients (24%) (NS); the left anterior descending was severely narrowed in 21 of 22 anterior MI patients (95%) and in 33 of 37 posterior MI patients (89%) (NS); the left circumflex was severely narrowed in 11 of 22 anterior MI patients (50%) and in 33 of 37 posterior MI patients (89%) ($p < 0.001$); the right circumflex was severely narrowed in 21 of 22 anterior MI patients (95%) and in all 37 posterior MI patients (NS).

The results of the quantitative analysis of the amount of narrowing in each of the 2608 5-mm segments of right, left anterior descending and left circumflex coronary arteries from the 59 patients are summarized in figures 1 and 2. Of the 895 5-mm segments from the 22 anterior MI patients, 67 (7%) were narrowed 96–100% in cross-sectional area by atherosclerotic plaque; 273 (31%) were narrowed 76–95%; 303 (34%), 51–75%; 173 (19%), 26–50%; and 79 (9%), 0–25%. Of the

No. of CAs narrowed > 75% by Ath	5-mm segments of 3 CAs (LM excluded)						Mean score CA§
	No.	Totals		No. LAD, LC or R (No. 76–95%) [No. 96–100%]			
		No. (%) 76–95%	No. (%) 96–100%	LAD	LC	R	
3†	63	12 (19)	2 (3)	30 (8) [2]	12 (0) [0]	21 (4) [0]	2.6
2	41	2 (5)	0 (0)	15 (1) [0]	11 (0) [0]	15 (1) [0]	2.4
3	43	27 (63)	0 (0)	12 (10) [0]	8 (4) [0]	23 (13) [0]	3.5
3	48	5 (10)	0 (0)	14 (2) [0]	10 (1) [0]	24 (2) [0]	2.9
3	22	12 (55)	4 (18)	7 (5) [0]	3 (1) [0]	12 (6) [4]	3.5
3	42	26 (62)	3 (7)	13 (10) [0]	12 (7) [1]	17 (9) [2]	3.6
1†	32	0 (0)	0 (0)	14 (0) [0]	10 (0) [0]‡	8 (0) [0]	1.8
3	25	14 (56)	7 (28)	8 (6) [0]	7 (1) [6]	10 (7) [1]	3.8
2	54	15 (28)	12 (22)	19 (7) [1]	8 (0) [0]	27 (8) [11]	3.2
2	41	7 (17)	0 (0)	10 (2) [0]	8 (0) [0]	23 (5) [0]	2.9
3	38	7 (18)	4 (11)	15 (5) [0]	7 (1) [4]	16 (1) [0]	2.9
2	33	9 (27)	0 (0)	10 (7) [0]	9 (0) [0]	14 (2) [0]	2.9
2	30	11 (37)	5 (17)	13 (5) [4]	7 (0) [0]	10 (6) [1]	3.3
3	30	10 (33)	1 (3)	5 (4) [0]	10 (4) [0]	15 (2) [1]	3.1
4†	45	26 (58)	6 (13)	13 (9) [2]	8 (3) [0]	24 (14) [4]	3.6
3	50	15 (30)	5 (10)	18 (7) [4]	11 (4) [0]	21 (4) [1]	3.0
2	58	4 (7)	0 (0)	19 (2) [0]	13 (0) [0]	26 (2) [0]	2.4
3	36	16 (44)	3 (8)	16 (6) [3]	11 (6) [0]‡	9 (4) [0]	3.3
3†	35	6 (17)	3 (9)	19 (2) [0]	7 (0) [0]	9 (4) [3]	2.5
2	26	4 (15)	0 (0)	10 (3) [0]	4 (0) [0]	12 (1) [0]	2.8
3	62	36 (58)	9 (15)	23 (15) [6]	14 (6) [0]	25 (15) [3]	3.6
2	41	9 (22)	3 (7)	16 (4) [2]	10 (0) [0]	15 (5) [1]	2.9

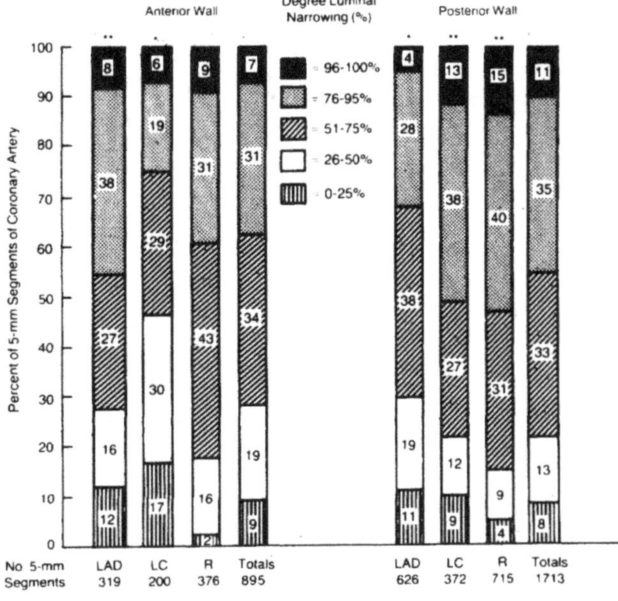

FIGURE 1. *Percent of 5-mm segments of the right (R), left anterior descending (LAD), and left circumflex (LC) coronary arteries narrowed to various degrees by atherosclerotic plaques in 22 patients with an anterior and 37 with a posterior wall transmural healed myocardial infarct (MI).*

1713 5-mm segments of coronary artery from the 37 posterior MI patients, 186 (11%) were narrowed 96–100%; 604 (35%), 76–95%; 560 (33%), 51–75%; 229 (13%), 26–50%; and 134 (8%), 0–25%. There were no significant differences between the two groups of pa-

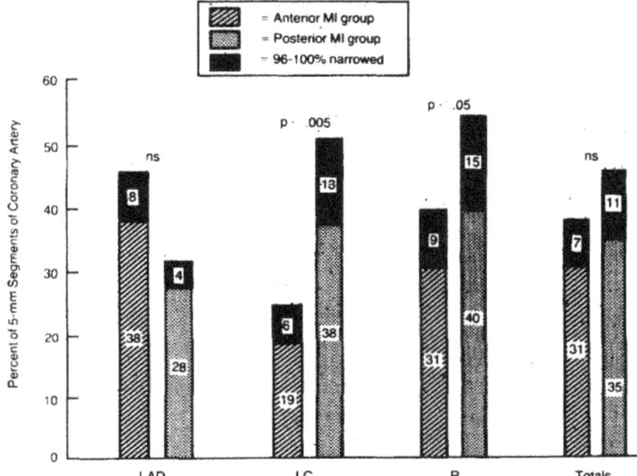

FIGURE 2. *Percent of 5-mm segments of the right (R), left anterior descending (LAD), and left circumflex (LC) coronary arteries narrowed 76–100% in cross-sectional area by atherosclerotic plaques in 22 patients with an anterior and 37 with a posterior wall transmural healed myocardial infarct (MI).*

TABLE 2. *Clinical and Necropsy Findings in Each of 37 Necropsy Patients with a Healed Posterior Wall Myocardial Infarct*

Pt	Age (years)	Sex	Hx AMI	Interval (mo) AMI to death	AP	CHF	Mode of death	Heart weight (g)	MI location VS	L	MI size (%)
1	43	F	0	—	0	0	SCD	330	0	0	4
2	46	M	+	60	0	0	SCD	460	0	+	7
3	47	F	0	—	+	0	CABG	480	+	0	3
4	49	F	0	—	+	0	CABG	450	0	0	2
5	51	M	0	—	0	+	AMI	550	0	+	—
6	51	M	+	10	+	0	SCD	520	0	+	21
7	51	M	+	276	+	0	SCD	550	0	0	22
8	52	M	0	—	0	0	SCD	310	0	+	2
9	52	M	0	—	0	0	AMI	510	+	0	6
10	54	M	+	120	+	+	CC	505	0	+	5
11	57	M	0	—	0	0	NC	310	0	0	8
12	57	M	0	—	+	0	CC	450	0	0	—
13	59	M	+	96	+	0	AMI	430	0	0	4
14	60	M	+	60	+	0	SCD	460	0	0	3
15	61	M	+	120	0	+	CHF	—	0	0	29
16	61	F	+	72	0	+	SCD	540	0	0	11
17	62	M	+	144	0	+	CHF	800	0	+	4
18	62	M	0	—	+	+	NC	540	0	0	—
19	62	M	0	—	0	0	NC	500	0	0	4
20	63	M	0	—	0	0	NC	450	+	0	2
21	64	M	0	—	0	0	AMI	550	0	0	1
22	64	F	0	—	0	0	NC	—	+	0	7
23	64	F	0	—	0	+	SCD	500	0	0	1
24	65	M	0	—	0	0	SCD	540	0	0	12
25	65	M	+	10	0	0	NC	430	0	+	16
26	65	M	0	—	0	0	NC	—	+	+	3
27	67	M	0	—	0	0	NC	390	0	+	1
28	68	M	0	—	0	0	NC	480	0	0	6
29	69	F	+	96	0	+	AMI	470	0	0	14
30	69	M	+	4	+	0	AMI	390	0	+	17
31	75	M	0	—	0	0	AMI	525	0	+	6
32	77	M	0	—	0	+	CHF	600	0	+	12
33	77	M	+	6	0	+	CHF	585	0	+	48
34	78	M	0	—	0	0	AMI	400	0	+	17
35	81	F	+	24	0	0	AMI	400	0	0	9
36	82	F	0	—	0	+	NC	495	0	0	2
37	—	—	+	48	+	0	SCD	645	+	0	3

*LM narrowed > 75%.
†Dominant posterior CA is the LC.
‡See results section for explanation of CA scoring system.
Abbreviations: See table 1.

tients in any of the five categories of cross-sectional area narrowing.

A scoring system was used to indicate both the severity and extent of coronary arterial narrowing. Every 5-mm segment of coronary artery from each patient was assigned a score of 1–4, based on the amount of cross-sectional area narrowing by atherosclerotic plaque: 1 = 0–25% narrowing; 2 = 26–50%; 3 = 51– 75%; and 4 = 76–100%. A total score was obtained for each patient and the score per 5-mm segment was then calculated by dividing the total score per patient by the number of 5-mm segments examined from that patient. The scores were 1.8–3.8 (mean 3.0) in the anterior MI group and 1.9–3.9 (mean 3.2) in the posterior MI group (NS).

The mean percent of 5-mm segments narrowed 76–

| No. of CAs narrowed > 75% by Ath | 5-mm segments of 3 CAs (LM excluded) | | | | | | Mean score CA‡ |
| | Totals | | | No. LAD, LC or R (No. 76–95%) [No. 96–100%] | | | |
	No.	No. (%) 76–95%	No. (%) 96–100%	LAD	LC	R	
3	19	7 (37)	4 (21)	9 (5) [0]	3 (1) [0]	7 (1) [4]	3.2
3	40	18 (43)	2 (5)	17 (7) [0]	8 (4) [2]	15 (7) [0]	3.5
3*	43	12 (28)	2 (5)	6 (4) [1]	11 (0) [0]	26 (8) [1]	2.3
3	38	7 (18)	4 (11)	15 (5) [0]	7 (1) [4]	16 (1) [0]	2.9
3	54	21 (39)	13 (24)	17 (4) [3]	19 (12) [1]	18 (5) [9]	3.6
3	64	18 (28)	7 (11)	18 (9) [1]	15 (2) [0]	31 (7) [6]	3.3
4*	41	22 (54)	16 (39)	12 (5) [7]	12 (6) [6]	17 (11) [3]	3.9
2	60	9 (15)	1 (2)	27 (0) [0]	10 (4) [1]	23 (5) [0]	2.7
4*	35	24 (69)	3 (9)	12 (6) [0]	5 (4) [0]	18 (14) [3]	3.7
4*	50	1 (2)	43 (86)	15 (1) [8]	11 (0) [11]	24 (0) [24]	3.7
3	37	10 (27)	2 (5)	18 (3) [0]	12 (6) [1]†	7 (1) [1]	2.7
4*	51	25 (49)	9 (18)	18 (11) [0]	19 (12) [3]†	14 (2) [6]	3.6
3	45	26 (58)	6 (13)	18 (11) [1]	4 (2) [0]	23 (13) [5]	3.6
4*	54	15 (28)	4 (7)	22 (2) [0]	12 (5) [3]	20 (8) [1]	3.3
3	40	6 (15)	5 (13)	16 (1) [0]	7 (1) [5]	17 (4) [0]	2.6
3	35	16 (46)	4 (11)	14 (5) [0]	8 (3) [1]	13 (8) [3]	3.4
4*	39	15 (38)	10 (26)	8 (4) [0]	6 (2) [0]	25 (9) [10]	3.6
1	34	1 (3)	0 (0)	9 (0) [0]	14 (0) [0]	11 (1) [0]	1.9
2	44	7 (16)	0 (0)	18 (0) [0]	9 (3) [0]	17 (4) [0]	2.5
3	47	7 (15)	0 (0)	28 (1) [0]	8 (2) [0]	11 (4) [0]	2.1
3	47	19 (40)	3 (6)	20 (5) [0]	4 (2) [1]	23 (12) [2]	3.3
3	54	21 (39)	1 (2)	27 (2) [0]	6 (1) [0]	21 (18) [1]	2.9
3	54	21 (39)	6 (11)	21 (3) [2]	12 (7) [1]	21 (11) [3]	3.0
3	62	33 (53)	5 (8)	21 (12) [0]	16 (6) [0]	25 (15) [5]	3.5
3	50	9 (18)	0 (0)	21 (2) [0]	10 (3) [0]	19 (4) [0]	2.9
3	46	20 (43)	5 (11)	18 (7) [0]	9 (5) [1]	19 (8) [4]	3.5
4	30	20 (67)	2 (7)	6 (5) [0]	9 (5) [2]	15 (10) [0]	3.7
1	36	11 (31)	1 (3)	16 (0) [0]	2 (0) [0]	18 (11) [1]	2.7
3	32	12 (38)	2 (6)	5 (4) [0]	10 (1) [0]	17 (7) [2]	3.2
3	85	36 (42)	6 (7)	36 (10) [0]	11 (9) [1]	38 (17) [5]	3.4
4*	72	24 (33)	2 (3)	20 (5) [0]	26 (9) [1]	26 (10) [1]	3.1
3	43	25 (58)	3 (7)	8 (4) [0]	13 (7) [1]	22 (14) [2]	3.6
3	42	7 (17)	0 (0)	18 (1) [0]	6 (5) [0]	18 (1) [0]	3.0
3	51	22 (43)	4 (8)	19 (8) [2]	9 (2) [2]	23 (12) [0]	3.4
3	52	33 (63)	5 (10)	20 (11) [0]	11 (8) [0]	21 (14) [5]	3.8
2	42	16 (38)	3 (7)	17 (6) [1]	9 (0) [0]	16 (10) [2]	3.1
3	45	8 (18)	3 (7)	16 (5) [1]	9 (1) [2]	20 (2) [0]	2.7

100% in cross-sectional area by atherosclerotic plaque in the right, left anterior descending and left circumflex coronary arteries for each of the two study groups is shown in figure 2. The right ($p < 0.05$) and left circumflex ($p < 0.005$) coronary arteries had a greater mean percentage of segments narrowed 76–100% in the posterior MI patients than in the anterior MI patients; the left anterior descending coronary artery had a similar percentage of severe narrowing in both groups. Within the anterior MI group, the left anterior descending had a greater mean percentage of severely narrowed segments than the left circumflex coronary artery ($p < 0.001$) and a mean percentage similar to that in the right coronary artery. Within the posterior MI group, the left anterior descending had less severe narrowing than the right ($p < 0.001$) and left circumflex ($p < 0.05$) coronary arteries.

The amount of left ventricular (including ventricular septum) myocardium replaced by fibrous tissue was 5–55% (mean 20%) in the anterior MI patients and 1–48% (mean 9%) in the posterior MI patients ($p < 0.002$). The ventricular septum was included in the

TABLE 3. *Number of 22 Patients with an Anterior and 37 with a Posterior Transmural, Healed Myocardial Infarct (MI) with One to Four Major Coronary Arteries Narrowed 76–100% in Cross-sectional Area*

No. narrowed 76–100%	Anterior		Posterior		p	Totals	
4	1	(5%)	8	(22%)	NS	9	(15%)
3	12	(55%)	24	(65%)	NS	36	(61%)
2	8	(36%)	3	(8%)	< 0.05	11	(19%)
1	1	(5%)	2	(5%)	NS	3	(5%)
0	0		0				
Total	22	(100%)	37	(100%)		59	(100%)

The "Location of MI" heading spans the Anterior and Posterior columns.

area of MI in 16 of 22 anterior MI patients (73%) and in six of 37 posterior MI patients (16%) ($p < 0.001$). The lateral wall was involved in eight anterior MI patients (36%) and in 14 posterior MI patients (38%) (NS). Portions of the posterior wall (predominantly in the apical half of the heart) were replaced by fibrous tissue in eight of 22 anterior MI patients (36%), and areas of the anterior wall (predominantly apical half) were scarred in four of 37 posterior MI patients (11%). Division of the left ventricle into four quadrants (anterior, septal, posterior and lateral) revealed that on the average, 2.5 quadrants contained areas of scarring in the anterior MI patients, compared with 1.6 quadrants in the posterior MI patients ($p < 0.05$).

Discussion

Although it is often assumed that patients with an anterior wall myocardial infarct (MI) have severe coronary narrowing primarily in the anterior circulation (left anterior descending coronary artery) and those with a posterior wall (inferior) MI have severe narrowing in the posterior circulation (right or left circumflex coronary arteries),[5] little anatomic information is available to determine the validity of this hypothesis. In a recent report,[1] the amount and location of coronary arterial narrowing by atherosclerotic plaque was determined in patients whose first acute MI was fatal. The patients with a posterior acute MI had more overall severe (76–100% cross-sectional area) narrowing, as well as more severe narrowing in the left anterior descending, right and left circumflex coronary arteries, than the patients with an anterior acute MI. Although

there was quantitatively more severe narrowing in these arteries in the posterior MI patients, all but one patient in both groups had severe narrowing of at least two of the three arteries and there was no significant difference between the two groups in the number of arteries with severe narrowing. Thus, the location of severe coronary artery narrowing by atherosclerotic plaques did not appear to determine the location of the acute MI.

We performed a similar type of quantitative analysis of coronary arterial narrowing in patients who died up to 23 years after healing of an anterior or posterior MI. In contrast to the findings in the study of patients with fatal first acute MI, the patients with a healed posterior or anterior MI had a similar overall percentage of 5-mm segments of coronary artery narrowed 76–100% (46% and 38%), but the posterior MI patients had significantly more coronary arteries per patient severely narrowed. Additionally, the posterior compared to the anterior MI patients had a similar number of segments of left anterior descending coronary artery narrowed severely but more segments narrowed severely in the left circumflex and right coronary arteries. Thus, although most patients in both groups had at least two major coronary arteries narrowed severely, the patients with a posterior healed MI had more severe narrowing in the posterior circulation than those with an anterior MI, but the anterior and posterior MI patients had a similar amount of severe narrowing in the "anterior" circulation. Both groups of patients with a healed MI had a far greater percentage of 5-mm segments severely narrowed than previously reported control subjects[6] who had no symptoms of myocardial ischemia and died from noncardiac conditions (46% and 38% vs 4%).

In the previously reported patients with an anterior, fatal, first acute MI, there was quantitatively more severe narrowing of the left anterior descending than of the right or left circumflex coronary arteries, but in those with a posterior MI there was a similar amount of narrowing in all three arteries. Of our patients with healed MI, however, those with anterior MI had similar amounts of severe narrowing in the left anterior decending and right coronary arteries but less severe narrowing in the left circumflex than in the left anterior descending coronary artery. Those with a posterior healed MI had more severe narrowing in the right and

TABLE 4. *Numbers of Each Major Epicardial Coronary Artery Narrowed 76–100% in Cross-sectional Area by Atherosclerotic Plaques in 22 Patients with an Anterior and 37 with a Posterior Wall Transmural Healed Myocardial Infarct*

Location of MI	No. of pts	Total no. of CAs	LM	LAD	LC	R	Totals	Mean no. of CAs per patient narrowed 76–100%
Anterior	22	88	4 (18%)	21 (95%)	11 (50%)	21 (95%)	57 (65%)	2.6
Posterior	37	148	9 (24%)	33 (89%)	33 (89%)	37 (100%)	112 (76%)	3.0
p			NS	NS	< 0.001	NS	NS	< 0.05

The "No. of pts with CA narrowed 76–100%" heading spans the LM, LAD, LC, R and Totals columns.

Abbreviations: MI = myocardial infarction; CA = coronary artery; LAD = left anterior descending; LC = left circumflex; LM = left main; R = right.

left circumflex than in the left anterior descending coronary artery.

Although these results suggest that the location of the MI and the location of the most severe coronary arterial narrowing for patients with healed posterior MI are related, exceptions were frequent: eight of the 37 posterior MI patients (22%) had a greater percentage of severely narrowed segments in the left anterior descending than in the dominant posterior artery (right coronary artery in all but two patients). For the anterior MI group, seven of the 22 patients (32%) had a greater percentage of severely narrowed segments in the dominant posterior artery (right coronary in all but two patients) than in the left anterior descending coronary artery.

The patients with an anterior MI had significantly larger areas of scarring and more frequent involvement of the ventricular septum and of the opposite wall (posterior for those with anterior MI) than patients with a posterior healed MI. Despite the larger, more extensive infarcts in patients with a healed anterior MI, the anterior MI compared with the posterior MI patients had significantly fewer severely narrowed coronary arteries and less severe narrowing in the right and left circumflex coronary arteries, and a similar amount of severe narrowing in the left anterior descending and left main coronary arteries.

References

1. Brosius FC III, Roberts WC: Comparison of degree and extent of coronary narrowing by atherosclerotic plaque in anterior and in posterior transmural acute myocardial infarction. Circulation **64:** 715, 1981
2. Roberts WC, Gardin JM: Location of myocardial infarcts. A confusion of terms and definitions. Am J Cardiol **42:** 868, 1978
3. Movat HZ: Demonstration of all connective tissue elements in a single section: pentachrome stains. Arch Pathol **60:** 289, 1955
4. Isner JM, Wu M, Virmani R, Jones AA, Roberts WC: Comparison of degrees of coronary arterial luminal narrowing determined by visual inspection of histologic sections under magnification among three independent observers and comparison to that obtained by video-planimetry: an analysis of 559 five-mm segments of 61 coronary arteries from eleven patients. Lab Invest **42:** 566, 1980
5. Spain DM: Coronary atheromatous disease — clinical pathological correlations. Cardiovasc Clin **4:** 53, 1972
6. Cabin HS, Roberts WC: Quantification of amounts of coronary arterial narrowing in patients with types II and IV hyperlipoproteinemia and in those with known normal lipoprotein patterns. Am Heart J **101:** 52, 1981

Sudden Death in Prinzmetal's Angina With Coronary Spasm Documented by Angiography

Analysis of Three Necropsy Patients

WILLIAM C. ROBERTS, MD, FACC*
R. CHARLES CURRY, Jr., MD, FACC†
JEFFREY M. ISNER, MD, FACC*
BRUCE F. WALLER, MD*
BRUCE M. McMANUS, MD*
RENATO MARIANI-CONSTANTINI, MD‡
ALLAN M. ROSS, MD, FACC‡

Bethesda, Maryland
Gainesville, Florida
Washington, D.C.

Clinical and necropsy findings are described in three patients who had angina pectoris at rest, S-T segment elevation on electrocardiography during chest pain, coronary arterial spasm on angiography and sudden death. Although significant "fixed" coronary narrowing (that is, narrowing due to atherosclerotic plaques) was appreciated by angiography in only one of the three patients, necropsy disclosed in all three patients severe fixed coronary narrowings involving particularly the artery in which spasm had been demonstrated during life. Additionally, examination of each 5-mm long segment of the coronary artery that had been spastic during life (two patients) disclosed several focally spastic segments at necropsy, indicating that spasm persisted after death. Although most previously described necropsy patients with Prinzmetal's angina had some fixed coronary narrowing, underlying fixed narrowing may be difficult to identify angiographically as demonstrated by the three patients in this study.

Coronary arterial narrowing by spasm has been extensively documented as a cause of myocardial ischemia.[1][12] Although myocardial ischemia due to dynamic coronary narrowing may cause angina pectoris, acute myocardial infarction and even sudden death, necropsy information in such patients is sparse.[13-23] In this report we describe clinical and necropsy findings in three patients with angina pectoris at rest, transient episodes of S-T segment elevation during chest pain, angiographically documented coronary arterial spasm and sudden death.

Patients Studied

Clinical Observations

Certain clinical and necropsy observations in the three patients are summarized in Table I and illustrated in Figures 1 to 7. Each patient had substernal chest pain at rest that, at least initially, was relieved by nitroglycerin. In Patient 1, the pain had occurred almost daily for 6 months, each episode lasting about 2 minutes. Patient 2 had chest pain up to 10 times weekly, the episodes typically lasted 5 to 15 minutes and had begun about 11 years before he died. He had been hospitalized more than 20 times because of chest pain or syncope. In Patient 3 the chest pain was usually precipitated by exercise and relieved by rest, and it occurred rarely at rest.

The electrocardiogram at rest in all three patients was usually normal. Each patient had S-T segment elevation documented by continuous electrocardiographic recordings (Patients 1 and 2) or by administration of ergonovine maleate (0.2 mg) (Patients 2 and 3), but not by exercise stress testing; the S-T elevation was associated with substernal nonexertional chest pain. Patient 2 had both brady- and tachyarrhythmias with attacks of angina at rest. Atrial pacing (160 beats/min) in Patients 2 and 3 resulted in S-T depression in lead V_5. In Patient 3, pacing produced occasional ventricular premature complexes; with administration of 0.2 mg of ergonovine maleate pacing produced typical chest pain, S-T segment elevation and a marked increase in left ventricular end-diastolic pressure. All were resolved after administration of nitroglycerin sublingually.

Left ventricular angiograms in all three patients disclosed a normal sized cavity without wall motion abnormalities or mitral regurgitation. The ejection fraction was normal in each patient.

From the Pathology Branch, National Heart, Lung, and Blood Institute, Bethesda, Maryland*; the Department of Medicine, University of Florida School of Medicine and the Veterans Administration Hospital, Gainesville, Florida†; and the Departments of Pathology and Medicine (Cardiology), George Washington University, Washington, D.C.‡ Manuscript received October 21, 1981; revised manuscript received December 22, 1981, accepted December 23, 1981.

Address for reprints: William C. Roberts, MD, Building 10A, Room 3E30, National Institutes of Health, Bethesda, Maryland 20205.

TABLE I

Clinical and Necropsy Observations In Three Patients With Coronary Arterial Spasm

	Patient		
	1	2	3
Age (yr) at death	32	57	61
Race	Black	White	White
Sex	Woman	Man	Man
Angina pectoris			
Rest (duration)	+(6 mo)	+(11 yr)	+(30 yr)
Exertional	0	0	+
Cigarette smoker	0	+(40 pack yr)	+(80 pack yr)
Total serum cholesterol (mg/dl)	146	124	297
Interval (days) from last cardiac catheterization to death	78	730	30
Pressures (s/d) (mm Hg)			
Left ventricle	182/24	92/7	115/12
Aorta	182/90	92/75	115/70
Coronary narrowing on angiography (% diameter reduction)			
LM	0	<25	15
LAD fixed → (spasm)	25 → (80)	25 → (90)	50
LC	25	<25	50
R	0	<15	30 → (100)
Interval (hours) death to necropsy	30	6	
Heart weight (gm)	400	400	320
Body weight (kg)	64	65	76
Coronary narrowing at necropsy (% cross-sectional area)			
LM	0–25	0–25	51–75
LAD	76–95	76–100	76–100
LC	25–50	0–25	51–75
R	76–95	51–75	76–100

d = diastole; LAD = left anterior descending coronary artery; LC = left circumflex coronary artery; LM = left main coronary artery; R = right coronary artery; s = systole.

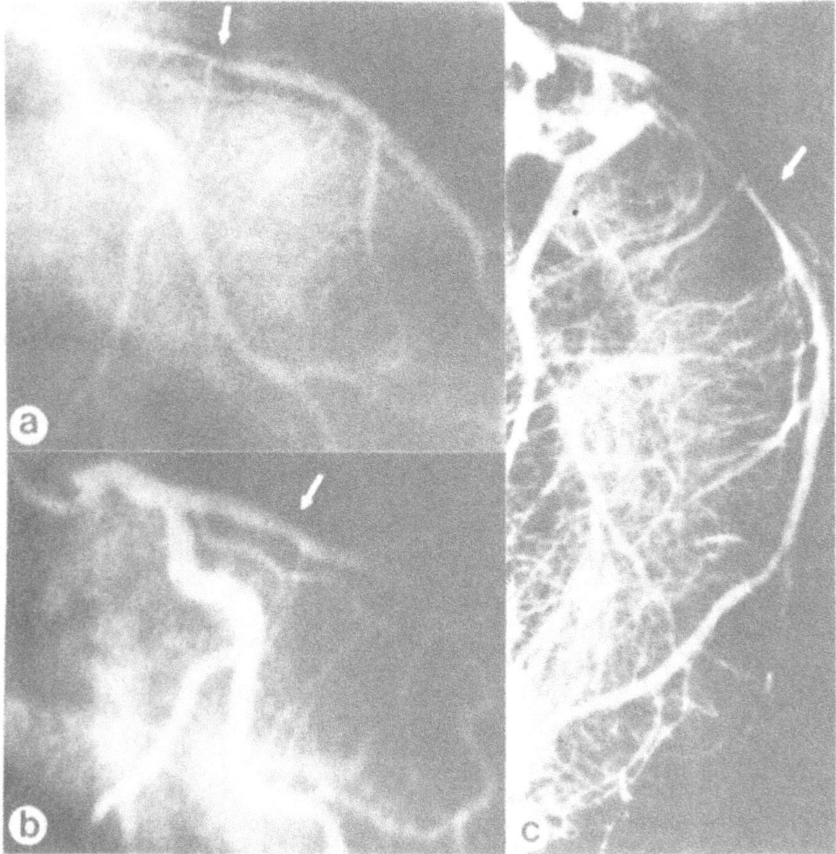

FIGURE 1. Patient 1. **a** and **b**, premortem and **c**, postmortem angiograms. **a**, coronary angiogram during pain 4 months before death showing severe reduction in diameter (**arrow**) of the left anterior descending artery. **b**, coronary angiogram after administration of nitroglycerin showing partial resolution of the narrowing in the left anterior descending artery. **c**, postmortem angiogram of the left anterior descending coronary artery showing severe reduction in diameter (**arrow**) near the site of fixed diameter narrowing in the premortem angiogram.

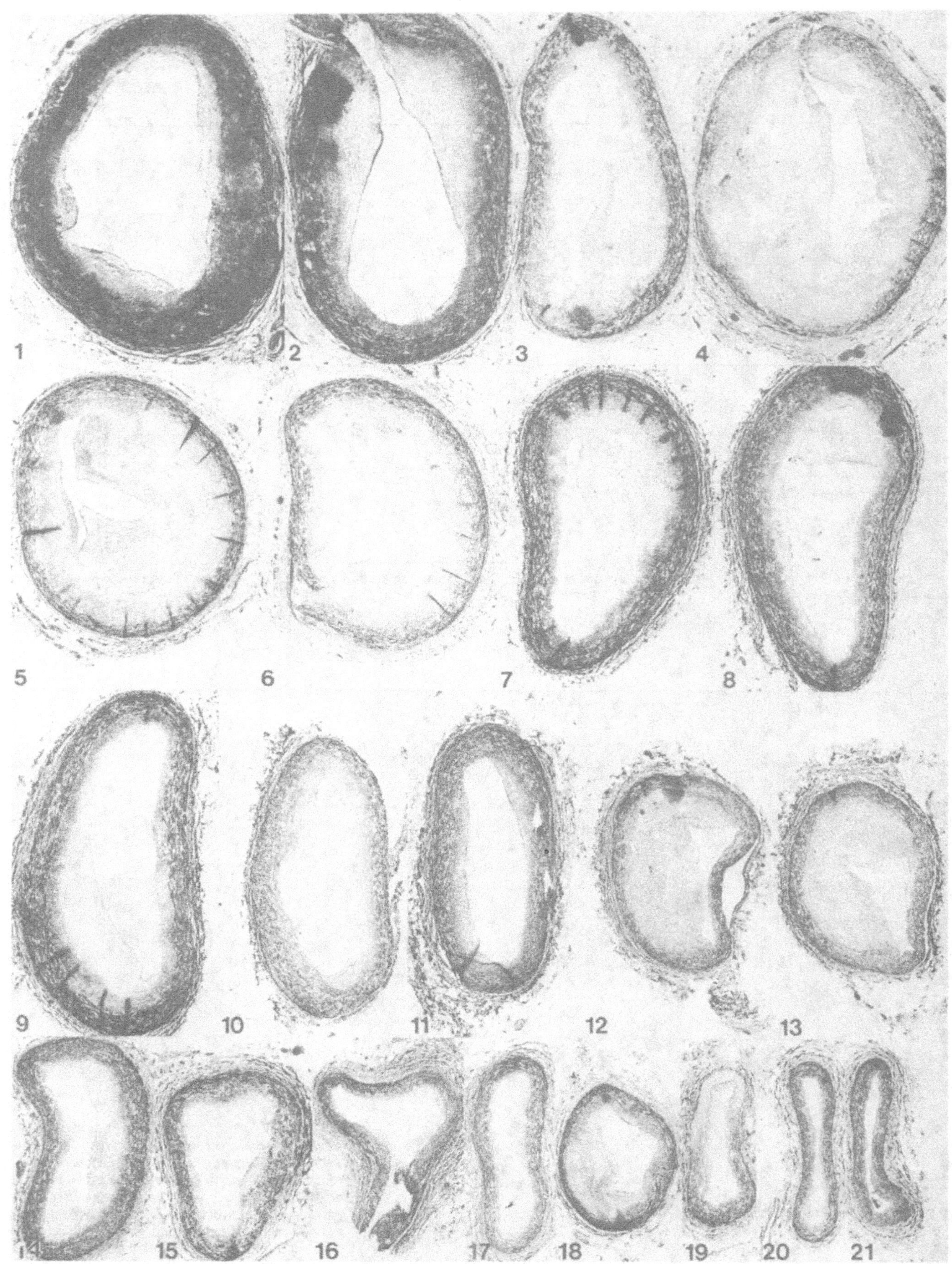

FIGURE 2. Patient 1. Photomicrographs of cross sections of 21 of the 24 five-mm segments of the left anterior descending coronary artery, which had documented spasm. The histologic sections begin with the first 5 mm segment of the left anterior descending artery (1) and extend to the most distal portion (21). The amount of narrowing of cross-sectional area was as follows: 76 to 100 percent in 3 segments (14 percent); 51 to 75 percent in 3 (14 percent); 26 to 50 percent in 10 (48 percent) and 0 to 25 percent in 5 (24 percent). The spasm, as shown in Figure 1, involved segments 3 to 7. The degrees of narrowing in the distorted or squashed segments were determined only after visually expanding the exterior border of the arterial segment in this patient and in the other two patients. (Movat stain ×25, reduced by 35 percent.)

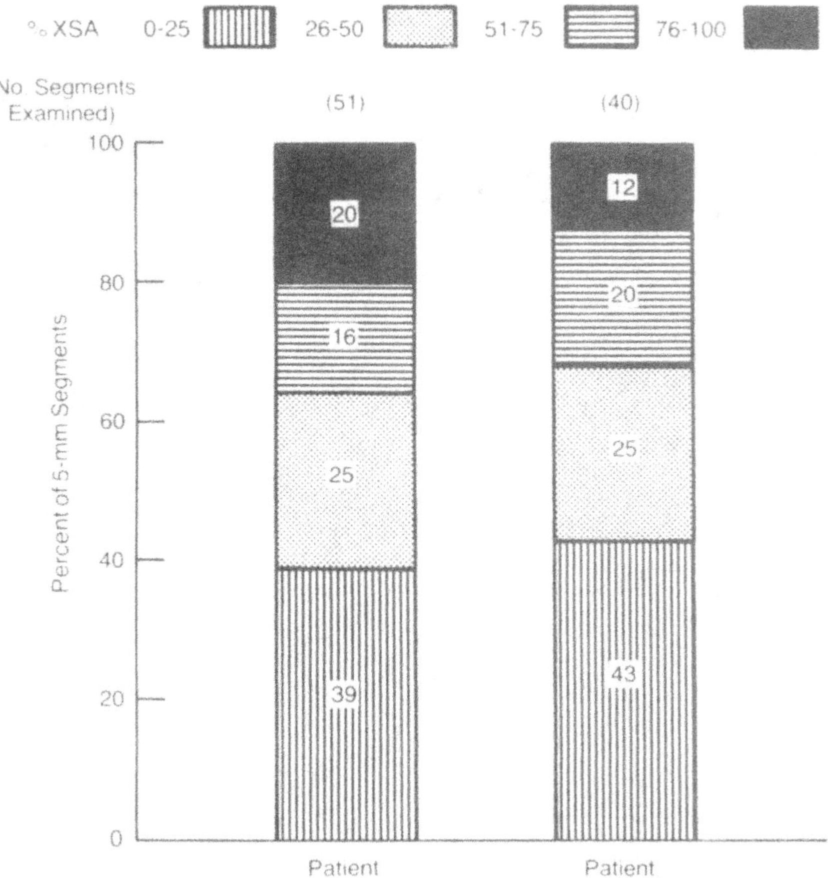

FIGURE 3. Patients 1 and 3. Number and percent of 5 mm segments of the right, left main, left anterior descending and left circumflex coronary arteries narrowed to various degrees in cross-sectional area (XSA) by atherosclerotic plaques.

Coronary angiography: Angiography disclosed no significant fixed narrowing (that is, narrowing produced by atherosclerotic plaques) in Patients 1 and 2 (Fig. 1 and 4) but up to 50 percent narrowing in the diameter of the left anterior descending and left circumflex coronary arteries in Patient 3 (Fig. 6). Spasm occurred spontaneously in the left anterior descending coronary artery in Patients 1 and 2, decreasing the lumen in each from about a 25 percent reduction in diameter from fixed lesions to about an 80 to 90 percent reduction in diameter by the superimposed spasm. In Patient 3, spasm occurred only after administration of ergonovine maleate and involved the right coronary artery, increasing its reduction in luminal diameter from 30 percent (produced by a fixed lesion) to total occlusion. The angiographically demonstrated spasm in each of the three patients was associated with typical substernal chest pain and S-T segment elevation. After sublingual nitroglycerin, the observed spontaneous or ergonovine-induced chest pain, S-T segment elevation and coronary arterial narrowing resolved in each patient within 10 minutes.

Each patient died suddenly out of the hospital during an attack of chest pain unresponsive to nitroglycerin.

Morphologic Observations

At necropsy, no foci of myocardial fibrosis or necrosis was present. The four cardiac valves and the sizes of the four cardiac cavities were normal. In Patients 1 and 3, the four major epicardial coronary arteries were excised intact from the heart, cut transversely into 5 mm segments, and a Movat-stained histologic section was prepared and examined from each 5 mm segment. The hearts had been fixed in a nonpressurized state before being submitted to the Pathology Branch. The results of these quantitative studies in these two patients are summarized in Figure 3. In Patient 2, five histologic sections of the coronary arteries were available for examination (Fig. 5).

In each of the three patients at least one of the four major epicardial coronary arteries was narrowed 76 to 100 percent in cross-sectional area by atherosclerotic plaque—the left descending artery in all three patients and the right also in Patients 1 and 3. In the coronary artery that was shown to develop spasm by angiography during life in Patients 1 and 3, histologic sections of the same artery at necropsy disclosed considerable fixed narrowing as well as "spasm" in the area of the artery where spasm had been demonstrated during life (Fig. 2 and 7). Additionally, in Patient 1, angiography at necropsy with injection of contrast material selectively in a syringe under "hand pressure" demonstrated "spasm" in the left anterior descending coronary artery similar to that which had been observed during life. The left anterior descending coronary artery did not have an intramyocardial portion (that is, "tunneled" coronary artery or myocardial bridge) in any of the three patients.

Discussion

Angiographic-morphologic discrepancies in estimation of fixed coronary arterial narrowing superimposed on spasm: Each of our three patients had angina pectoris at rest, documented S-T segment elevation in the electrocardiogram during chest pain, documented spasm of a major epicardial coronary artery during selective angiography and sudden death. Addi-

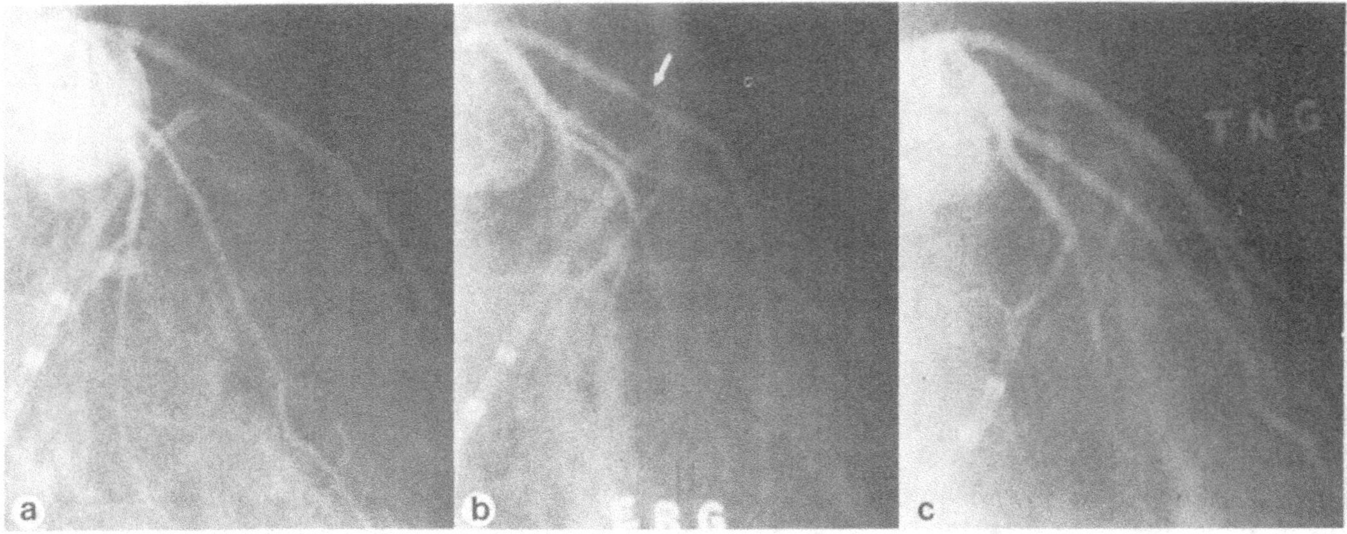

FIGURE 4. Patient 2. Coronary arteriogram of the left coronary system showing mild fixed narrowing of the proximal left anterior descending artery (**a**), marked dynamic narrowing at the same site after administration of ergonovine maleate (ERG) (**arrow**) (**b**), and relief of spasm with nitroglycerin (NTG) (**c**).

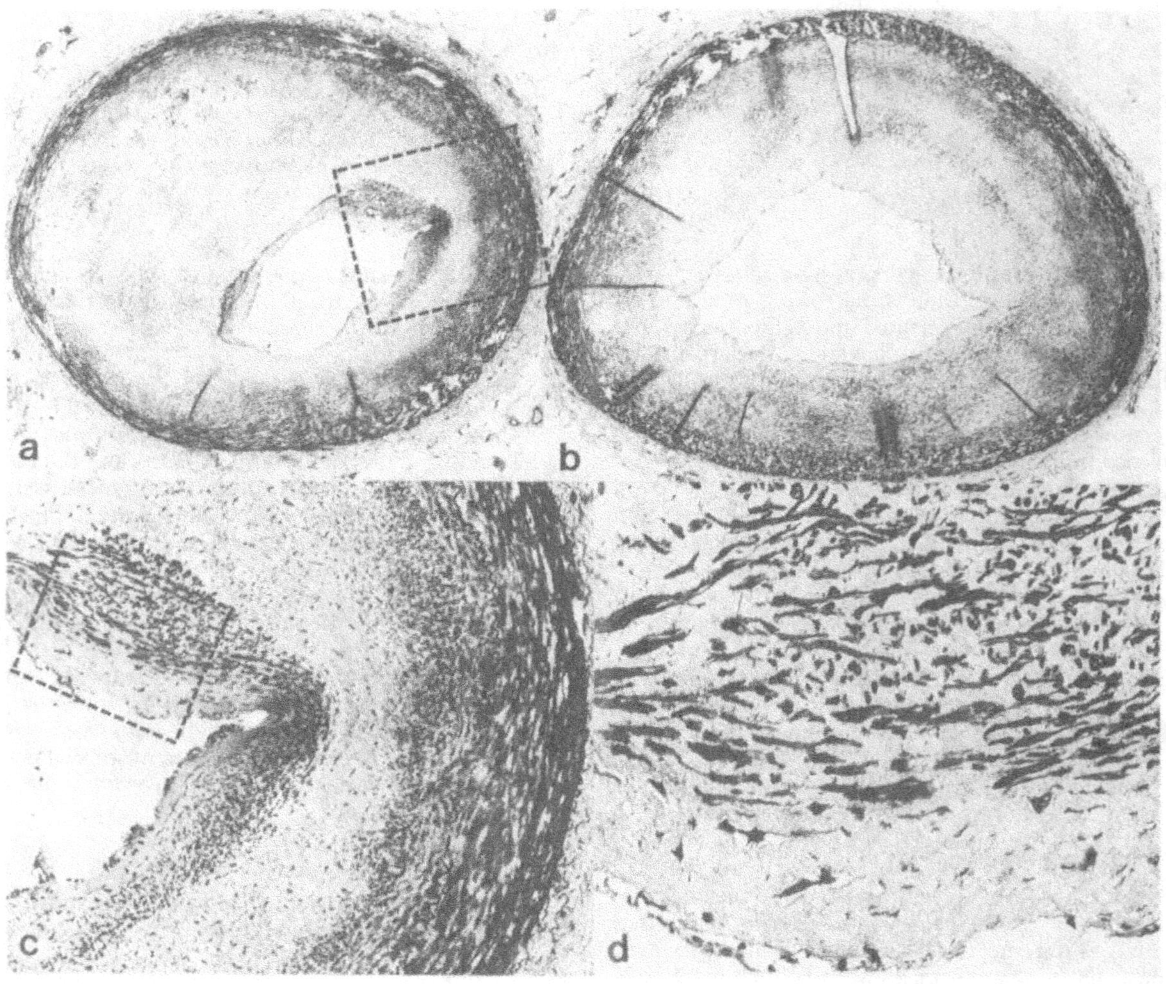

FIGURE 5. Patient 2. **a** and **b**, transverse histologic sections of the left anterior descending coronary artery at the approximate site of spasm showing marked narrowing of cross-sectional area. **c** and **d**, higher magnifications of the internal plaque showing a predominance of smooth muscle cells (**dark**). (Movat stain: **a** and **b** ×38, (**c**) ×107, (**d**) ×330, all reduced by 19 percent.)

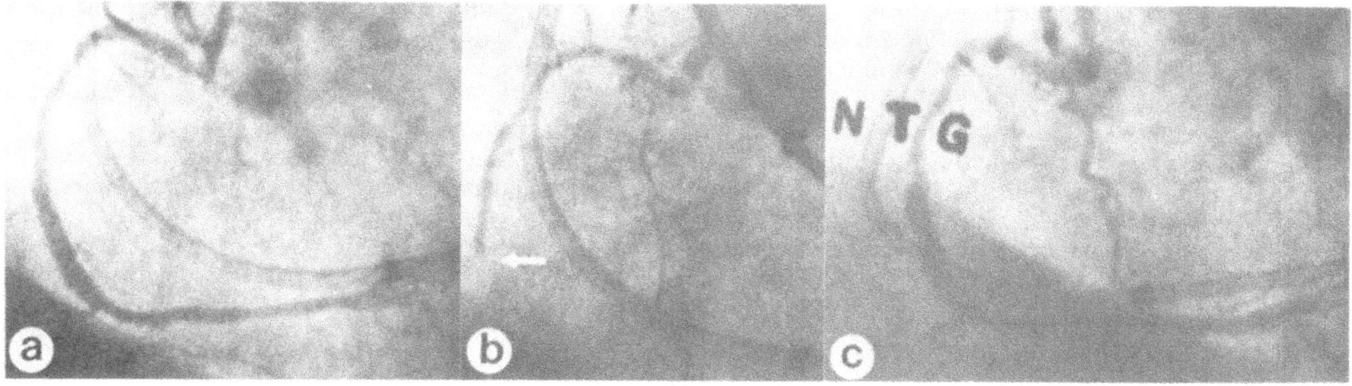

FIGURE 6. Patient 3. Coronary arteriogram of the right coronary artery showing moderate fixed narrowing (**a**), ergonovine maleate-induced spasm with complete occlusion (**arrow**) (**b**) and nitroglycerin-induced (NTG) dilation with residual fixed narrowing near the site of ergonovine-induced spasm (**c**).

tionally, only one of the three patients had significant fixed coronary narrowing by angiography. However, a surprise finding at necropsy was considerable fixed luminal narrowing in the major coronary artery in which severe spasm had been demonstrated. Thus, had necropsy not been performed in each of these three patients, angina pectoris and sudden death in each might reasonably have been attributed entirely or nearly entirely to coronary spasm rather than to the combination of both fixed and dynamic coronary narrowing. Although it is now well recognized that selective angiography during life tends to underestimate the actual degrees of luminal narrowing because areas of severest narrowing are simply compared with areas of less severe narrowing rather than with areas without narrowing,[24,25] the discrepancies observed in our patients were striking. In Patients 1 and 3 the maximal degree of fixed narrowing in the left anterior descending coronary artery on angiography was judged to be a 25 percent reduction in diameter, but at necropsy, the cross-sectional area narrowing was 76 to 95 percent. In all three patients the lumen of the right coronary artery was judged on angiography to be narrowed by 25 percent or less in diameter, but at necropsy the cross-sectional area narrowing was 76 to 95 percent in Patients 1 and 2 and 51 to 75 percent in Patient 3. The coronary arteries in Patients 1 and 3 were devoid of calcific deposits and consequently it is likely that the arteries were more distensible in life because the intraluminal pressure at necropsy obviously was zero. Nevertheless, the angiographic-morphologic discrepancies in degrees of luminal narrowing in one or more major coronary arteries, and particularly in the artery where spasm had been demonstrated, were striking in each patient. In Patient 1, the coronary angiogram performed at postmortem examination corresponded identically with the angiogram obtained during chest pain before administration of nitroglycerin during life—providing evidence that the narrowing observed at necropsy was a combination of both fixed narrowing by atherosclerotic plaques plus that produced by superimposed spasm.

Necropsy evidence of coronary arterial narrowing in patients with spasm: Necropsy information is limited on the status of the major epicardial arteries and left ventricular myocardium in patients in whom angina pectoris at rest with S-T-segment elevation had been documented during life. We found data on only 13 patients,[13–23] but detailed necropsy information on the amount of coronary narrowing was limited in all of them. In one of the original patients described by Prinzmetal et al.,[13] ". . . both major coronary arteries were . . . markedly sclerotic . . ." and the ". . . posterior coronary artery" was 80 percent narrowed. Subsequently, at least 12 additional patients have been studied at necropsy and reported on.[14–23] All 13 (including the patient of Prinzmetal et al.[13]) had transient S-T segment elevation during angina at rest and 6 also had crescendo type angina. Of the 10 with coronary angiograms,[15,17–23] nondrug-induced transient reduction in diameter (spasm) was documented in 5[17,21,23] (1 of whom may have had catheter-induced spasm). Of the 13 patients, 3 died after aortocoronary bypass operations[17,21,22]; of the other 10 patients, 6 died suddenly out of the hospital[14–16,18,20,21]—1 died of chronic congestive heart failure,[13] 2 died shortly after cardiac catheterization procedures[19,23] and 1 died of complications of acute myocardial infarction.[23] In at least 9 of the 13 patients[13,14,16–18,20,22,23] significant fixed narrowing also appeared to be present at necropsy in at least one of the four major epicardial coronary arteries. Additionally, 6 of the 13 patients[13–16,20,21,23] had one or more foci of left ventricular scarring. Thus, most (at least 9 of 13) previously described patients with clinical evidence (S-T segment elevation on electrocardiography during angina at rest) of coronary spasm had significant fixed coronary narrowing by atherosclerotic plaques and most (9 of 12) had some left ventricular myocardial damage (either necrosis[14,21,23] or fibrosis,[13,15,16,20,23] or both[21]).

Necropsy evidence of coronary spasm: In addition to its demonstration at necropsy in two of our three patients with Prinzmetal's angina, coronary "spasm" was demonstrated at necropsy in a 25 year old man reported on by El-Maraghi and Sealey.[26] In contrast to our three patients and to the 13 with Prinzmetal's angina just described, the patient described by El-Maraghi and Sealey did not have angina either at rest or on exertion during life or S-T segment elevation except during the period of documented acute myocardial infarction. Nevertheless, this patient had evidence of spasm in both the left anterior descending and right coronary arteries on postmortem coronary angiography and "contraction rings" in the right coronary artery when it was opened longitudinally at necropsy. Thus, it would appear from this described patient[26] and from the coronary findings at necropsy in two of our patients that spasm in a coronary artery may persist after death, just as the contracted state of the cardiac ventricles persists after death.[27] The other unique feature of the case reported by El-Maraghi and Sealey is the absence of atherosclerotic plaques or other fixed lesions in the epicardial coronary arteries of their patient. Thus, coronary spasm without associated fixed narrowings on rare occasion can produce acute myocardial infarction and, as reported by others,[8,9,14-16,18,20,21] sudden cardiac arrest.

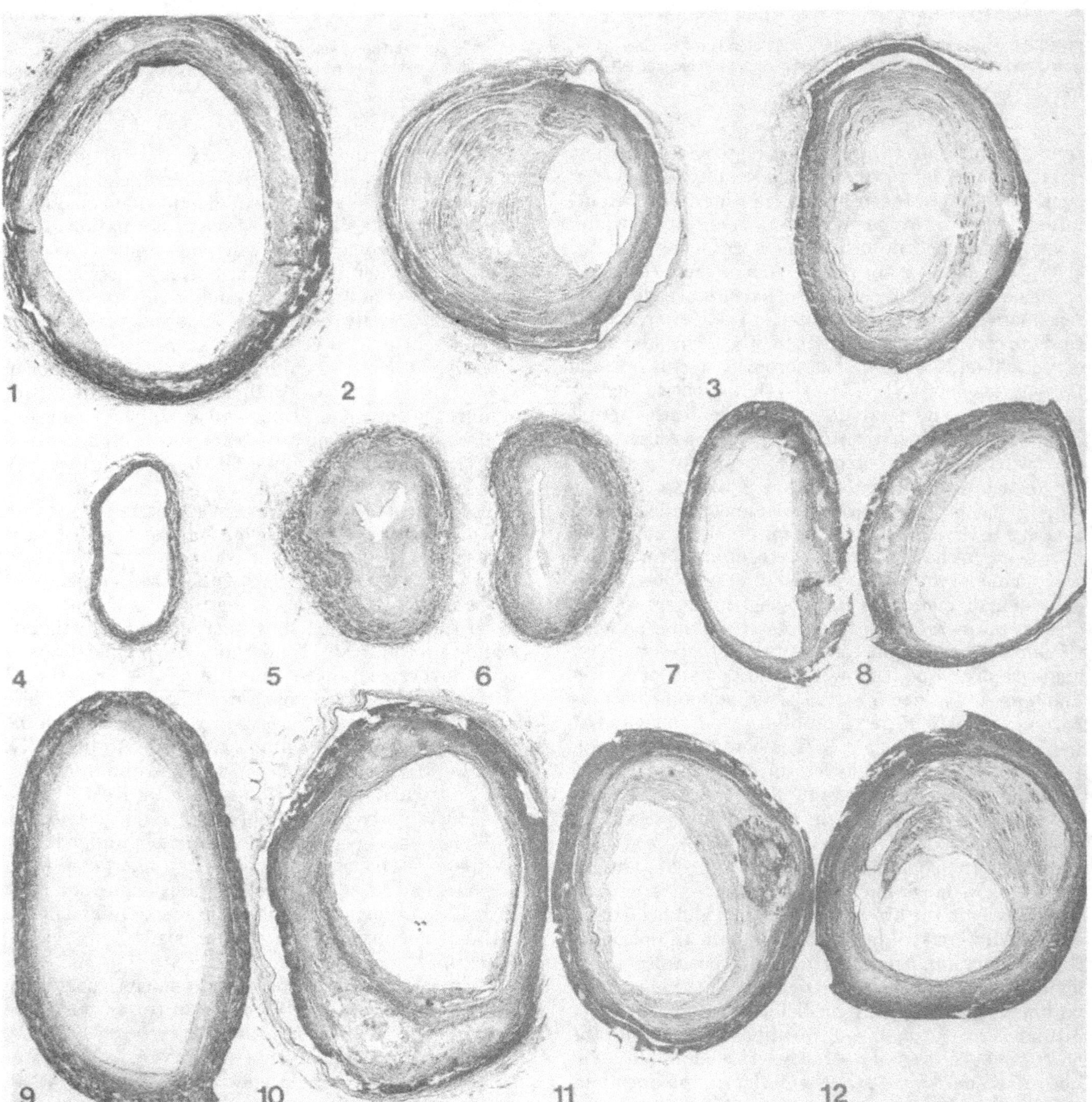

FIGURE 7. Patient 3. Photomicrographs of cross sections of each of the 5 mm sections of the right coronary artery showing diffuse moderate to severe narrowing of cross-sectional area in most segments. The sites of severest narrowing (5 and 6) correspond to the sites of ergonovine-induced spasm and they were taken at the same magnification as were all the other photomicrographs. (Movat ×25, all reduced by 34 percent.)

References

1. **Oliva PB, Potts DE, Pluss RG.** Coronary arterial spasm in Prinzmetal angina: documentation by coronary arteriography. N Engl J Med 1973;288:745–51.

2. **MacAlpin RN, Kattus AA, Alvaro AB.** Angina pectoris at rest with preservation of exercise capacity. Prinzmetal variant angina. Circulation 1973;47:946–58.

3. **Higgins CB, Wexler L, Silverman JF, Schroeder JS.** Clinical and arteriographic features of Prinzmetal's variant angina: documentation of etiologic factors. Am J Cardiol 1976;37:831–9.

4. **Selzer A, Langston M, Ruggeroli C, Cohn K.** Clinical syndrome of variant angina with normal coronary arteriogram. N Engl J Med 1976;295:1343–7.

5. **Oliva PB, Breckinridge JC.** Arteriographic evidence of coronary arterial spasm in acute myocardial infarction. Circulation 1977;56:366–74.

6. **Johnson AD, Stroud HA, Vieweg WVP, Ross J Jr.** Variant angina pectoris. Clinical presentations, coronary angiographic patterns, and the results of medical and surgical management in 42 consecutive patients. Chest 1978;73:786–94.

7. **Hillis LD, Braunwald E.** Coronary-artery spasm. N Engl J Med 1978;299:695–702.

8. **Conti CR, Pepine CJ, Curry RC Jr.** Coronary artery spasm: an important mechanism in the pathophysiology of ischemic heart disease. Curr Probl Cardiol 1979;4:1–70.

9. **Conti CR, Curry RC Jr.** Coronary artery spasm and myocardial ischemia. Mod Concepts Cardiovasc Dis 1980;49:1–6.

10. **Yasue H, Omote S, Takizawa A, Nagao M, Miwa K, Tanaka S.** Exertional angina pectoris caused by coronary arterial spasm: effects of various drugs. Am J Cardiol 1979;43:647–52.

11. **Cipriano PR, Koch FH, Rosenthal SJ, Schroeder JS.** Clinical course of patients following the demonstration of coronary artery spasm by angiography. Am Heart J 1981;101:127–34.

12. **Amsterdam EA, Mason DT.** Coronary spasm: old problem, new questions. Am Heart J 1981;101:242–3.

13. **Prinzmetal M, Kennamer R, Merliss R, Wada T, Bor N.** Angina pectoris. I. A variant form of angina pectoris. Preliminary report. Am J Med 1959;27:375–88.

14. **Peretz DI.** Variant angina pectoris of Prinzmetal. Can Med Assoc J 1961;85:1101–2.

15. **Gianelly R, Mugler F, Harrison DC.** Prinzmetal's variant of angina pectoris with only slight coronary atherosclerosis. California Med 1968;108:129–32.

16. **Silverman ME, Flamm MD Jr.** Variant angina pectoris. Anatomic findings and prognostic implications. Ann Intern Med 1971;75:339–43.

17. **Dhurandhar RW, Watt DL, Silver MD, Trimble AS, Adelman AG.** Prinzmetal's variant form of angina with arteriographic evidence of coronary arterial spasm. Am J Cardiol 1972;30:902–5.

18. **Cosby RS, Giddings JA, See JR, Mayo M.** Variant angina. Case reports and critique. Am J Med 1972;53:739–42.

19. **Cheng TO, Bashour T, Kelser GA Jr, Weiss L, Bacos J.** Variant angina of Prinzmetal with normal coronary arteriograms. A variant of the variant. Circulation 1973;47:476–85.

20. **Donsky MS, Harris MD, Curry GC, Blomqvist CG, Willerson JT, Mullins CB.** Variant angina pectoris: a clinical and coronary arteriographic spectrum. Am Heart J 1975;89:571–8.

21. **Wiener L, Kasparian H, Duca PR, et al.** Spectrum of coronary arterial spasm. Clinical, angiographic and myocardial metabolic experience in 29 cases. Am J Cardiol 1976;38:945–55.

22. **Bharati S, Dhingra RC, Lev M, Towne WD, Rahimtoola SH, Rosen KM.** Conduction system in a patient with Prinzmetal's angina and transient atrioventricular block. Am J Cardiol 1977;39:120–5.

23. **Maseri A, L'Abbate A, Baroldi G, et al.** Coronary vasospasm as a possible cause of myocardial infarction. A conclusion derived from the study of "preinfarction" angina. N Engl J Med 1978;299:1271–7.

24. **Arnett EN, Isner JM, Redwood DR, et al.** Coronary artery narrowing in coronary heart disease: comparison of cineangiographic and necropsy findings. Ann Intern Med 1979;91:350–6.

25. **Isner JM, Kishel J, Kent KM, Ronan JA Jr, Ross AM, Roberts WC.** Accuracy of angiographic determination of left main coronary arterial narrowing. Angiographic-histologic correlative analysis in 28 patients. Circulation 1981;63:1056–64.

26. **El-Maraghi NRH, Sealey BJ.** Recurrent myocardial infarction in a young man to coronary arterial spasm demonstrated at autopsy. Circulation 1980;61:199–207.

27. **Maron BJ, Henry WL, Roberts WC, Epstein SE.** Comparison of echocardiographic and necropsy measurements of ventricular wall thickness in patients with and without disproportionate septal thickening. Circulation 1977;55:341–6.

Relation of healed transmural myocardial infarct size to length of survival after acute myocardial infarction, age at death, and amount and extent of coronary arterial narrowing by atherosclerotic plaques: Analysis of 70 necropsy patients

The percent of left ventricular wall (including ventricular septum) replaced by scar was determined in 70 necropsy patients with a healed transmural myocardial infarct (MI). The MI involved from 1% to 55% (mean 13%) of the left ventricular wall. The ages at death of the patients ranged from 25 to 82 years (mean 62) and did not signficantly correlate with MI size ($r = -0.12$). Of the 70 patients, 41 (59%) had unequivocal histories of an acute MI: the interval from the MI to death in them ranged from 2 to 276 months (mean 50) and correlated negatively with MI size ($r = -0.32$, $p < 0.05$), and the age at the MI ranged from 26 to 79 years (mean 58) and did not correlate with MI size ($r = -0.05$). The four major epicardial coronary arteries were examined quantitatively in 56 patients; the number of coronary arteries with severe narrowing ranged from one to four (mean 2.9) and did not correlate with MI size ($r = -0.24$). The mean MI size in the 12 patients with and in the 44 without severe narrowing of the left main coronary artery was identical (each 13%). The entire lengths of the right, left anterior descending, and left circumflex coronary arteries in the 56 patients were divided into 5 mm long segments and the amounts of cross-sectional area narrowing in each of the resulting 2489 segments were determined by histologic examination. The percent of 5 mm segments with severe (cross-sectional area narrowing 76% to 100%) narrowing by atherosclerotic plaques in each patient ranged from 3% to 93% (mean 44%) and did not correlate with MI size ($r = -0.20$). When the 28 patients with an MI involving > 10% of the left ventricular wall were compared to those with an MI involving ≤ 10%, a similar overall percentage of 5 mm segments of coronary artery was severely narrowed (43% vs 42%). In addition, a similar percentage of segments was narrowed severely in each of the three major epicardial coronary arteries. Thus in our necropsy patients with a healed transmural MI, the MI size correlated with length of survival after an acute MI (in patients with definite histories of an acute MI) but not with age at death or with the amount, location, or extent of coronary arterial narrowing by atherosclerotic plaques. (Am Heart J 104:216, 1982.)

Henry Scott Cabin, M.D., and William C. Roberts, M.D. *Bethesda, Md.*

The amount of left ventricular (LV) myocardium involved in an acute myocardial infarct (MI) is one of the determinants of survival during the acute event. Among survivors of acute MI, the amount of LV myocardium replaced by scar has not been examined in relation to the duration of life after the acute MI, the age of the patient at the time of the acute MI and at the time of death, and the amount,

extent, and location of coronary narrowing by atherosclerotic plaques at necropsy. To answer these questions, we analyzed findings in 70 necropsy patients with healed transmural MI.

METHODS

Determination of MI size. All 70 patients had a healed transmural (involving more than the inner one half of the thickness of the LV wall at any point[1]) MI at necropsy. The percent of LV myocardium replaced by scar was determined in each patient by tracing the grossly visible areas of LV scar and the total LV area, including ventricular septum, from the apical surfaces of each of five or six 1 cm thick transverse ventricular slices cut from apex to base parallel to the posterior atrioventricular sulcus. The

From the Pathology Branch, National Heart, Lung and Blood Institute, National Institutes of Health.

Received for publication Feb. 9, 1982; accepted March 10, 1982.

Reprint requests: William C. Roberts, M.D., Bldg. 10A, Room 3E-30, NIH, Bethesda, MD 20205.

Table I. Clinical observations in 39 necropsy patients with healed transmural myocardial infarction (MI) involving $\leq 10\%$ and in 31, $> 10\%$ of the left ventricular (LV) wall

	MI size		
	< 10% of LV wall *(39 pts)*	*> 10% of LV wall* *(31 pts)*	p *value*
Ages (years): range (mean)	39-82 (62)	25-80 (62)	NS
Male: Female	29:10	23:8	NS
History of acute MI	18 (46%)	23 (74%)	< 0.05
Angina pectoris	16 (41%)	8 (26%)	NS
Chronic congestive heart failure (CHF)	10 (26%)	17 (55%)	< 0.05
Systemic hypertension	16 (41%)	10 (32%)	NS
Diabetes mellitus	8 (21%)	10 (32%)	NS
Mean interval (mo) acute MI to death	75	36	< 0.05
Modes of death			
Sudden	11 (28%)	10 (32%)	NS
Acute MI	10 (26%)	6 (19%)	NS
Chronic CHF	2 (5%)	6 (19%)	NS
Cardiac operation	3 (8%)	1 (3%)	NS
Noncardiac	12 (31%)	7 (23%)	NS

Table II. Numbers of patients in each study group with the left main, left anterior descending, left circumflex, and right coronary arteries narrowed 76% to 100% in cross-sectional area by atherosclerotic plaque

MI *size*	*No.* *pts.*	*Total no.* *of CA*	*Number (%) of pts with* *CA narrowed 76%-100%*					*Mean No.* *4 CA per* *pt narrowed* *> 75%*
			LM	*LAD*	*LC*	*R*	*Totals*	
$\leq 10\%$ LV wall	28	112	7(25)	25(89)	23(82)	28(100)	83(74)	3.0
$> 10\%$ LV wall	28	112	5(18)	27(96)	19(68)	27(96)	78(70)	2.8
p			NS	NS	NS	NS	NS	NS

CA = coronary arteries; LAD = left anterior descending; LC = left circumflex; LM = left main; pts = patients; R = right.

area of LV scar and the total LV area were then determined by a videoplanimetry system. The sum of the LV areas provided the MI size expressed as a percent of total LV area.

Determination of degree of coronary atherosclerosis. In 56 of the 70 patients the entire length of the right (R), left main (LM), left anterior descending (LAD), and left circumflex (LC) coronary arteries was removed from the heart intact, fixed in an unpressurized state in 10% formalin for about 48 hours, radiographed, and if calcific deposits were present, decalcified. Then each of the four major arteries were cut transversely into 5 mm long segments, processed in alcohol and xylene, and cut. At least one 6 μm thick section from each 5 mm segment was prepared for histologic study and stained by the Movat method.[2] The degree of luminal narrowing in each 5 mm long segment was determined by microscopic examination at a magnification of 25 to 50 times. The percent of cross-sectional area narrowing by atherosclerotic plaques was divided into five categories of narrowing: 0% to 25%, 26% to 50%, 51% to 75%, 76% to 95%, and 96% to 100%. The accuracy of these determinations was verified by videoplanimetry and was shown to have an error of < 5%.[3]

RESULTS

Correlation of CHF and acute MI to healed MI size. In 39 patients the MI involved $\leq 10\%$ and in 31 it involved $> 10\%$ of the LV wall. Clinical findings in these two groups of patients are summarized in Table I. Compared to the patients with a smaller MI ($\leq 10\%$), those with a larger MI ($> 10\%$) more frequently had chronic congestive heart failure (CHF) (55% vs 26%) and clinical diagnoses of the acute MI (74% vs 46%).

Relation of survival to headed MI size. The age at death of the 70 patients did not correlate with the size of the healed MI at necropsy, which ranged from 1% to 55% (mean 13%) ($r = -0.12$). The age at the time of acute MI in the 41 patients with unequivocal histories of acute MI ranged from 26 to 79 years (mean 58) and did not correlate with the size of the

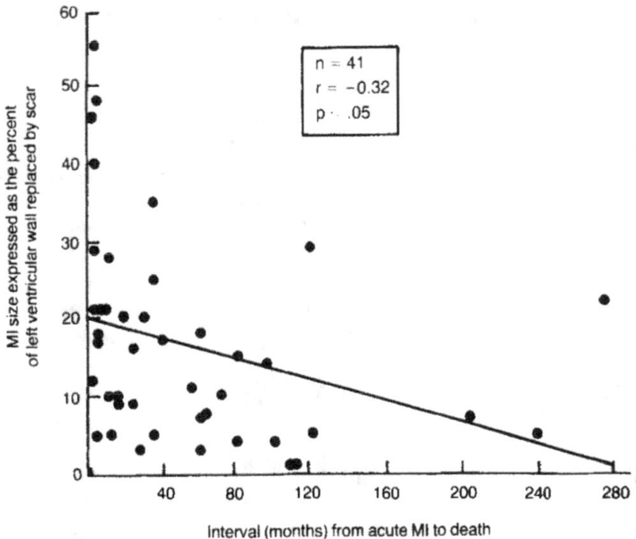

Fig. 1. Relationship of myocardial infarct *(MI)* size to length of survival after acute MI in 41 necropsy patients with unequivocal histories of acute MI and healed transmural MI at necropsy.

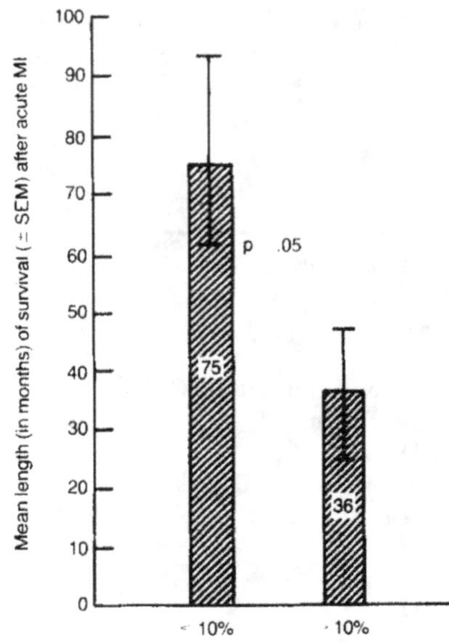

Fig. 2. Mean length of survival after acute myocardial infarction *(MI)* in 23 necropsy patients with healed MI involving > 10% and in 18 patients with MI involving ≤ 10% of the left ventricular wall.

healed MI ($r = -0.05$). The interval from acute MI to death in the 41 (54%) patients with unequivocal histories of acute MI ranged from 2 to 276 months (mean 50 months) and correlated negatively with the size of the healed MI ($r = -0.32$, $p < 0.05$) (Fig. 1). In addition, mean survival was significantly longer in the patients in whom the MI involved ≤ 10% of the LV wall (75 months) compared to those in whom it involved > 10% of the LV wall (36 months) ($p < 0.05$) (Fig. 2).

Relation of degree of coronary narrowing to healed MI size. Among 28 patients with MI involving ≤ 10% and in 28 with MI involving > 10% of the LV wall, a total of 224 major (R, LM, LAD, and LC) epicardial coronary arteries were examined and the results are summarized in Table II. Of the 112 arteries examined in the patients with MI size ≤ 10%, 83 (74%) were narrowed severely (76% to 100% in cross-sectional area) by atherosclerotic plaques, an average of 3.0/4.0 coronary arteries per patient; of the 112 arteries examined in the patients with MI size ≤ 10%, 78 (70%) were narrowed severely, an average of 2.8/4.0 coronary arteries per patient ($p = $ NS). The number of major coronary arteries severely narrowed did not correlate with the extent of the MI size ($r = -0.24$).

All four arteries were severely narrowed in six (21%) of the 28 patients with MI size ≤ 10% and in two (7%) of the 28 patients with MI size > 10% ($p = $ NS). Three arteries were severely narrowed in 16 (57%) and 19 (68%) patients, respectively ($p = $ NS); two arteries were so narrowed in five

(18%) and six (21%) patients, respectively ($p = $ NS); and one artery was severely narrowed in one (4%) and one (4%) patient, respectively ($p = $ NS). The LM coronary artery was severely narrowed in seven (25%) patients with MI size ≤ 10% and in five (18%) with MI size > 10% ($p = $ NS) (Table II). Additionally, the mean MI size in the 12 patients with severe narrowing of the LM coronary artery was the same as the MI size in the 44 patients without severe narrowing of the LM (13% in each group).

The results of the quantitative analysis of the 2489 five mm segments of the R, LAD, and LC coronary arteries are summarized in Fig. 3. No correlation was observed between the percent of 5 mm segments of coronary artery narrowed severely and the MI size ($r = -0.20$) (Fig. 4). Of the 1260 five mm segments from the 28 patients with MI involving ≤ 10% of the LV wall, 76 (6%) were narrowed 96% to 100% in cross-sectional area by atherosclerotic plaques; 459 (36%) were narrowed 76% to 95%; 394 (31%), 51% to 75%; 195 (15%), 26% to 50%, and 136 (11%) were narrowed 0% to 25%. Of the 1229 five mm segments from the 28 patients with MI involving > 10% of the LV wall, 111 (9%) were narrowed 96% to 100%; 413 (34%) were narrowed 76% to 95%; 443 (36%), 51% to 75%; 186 (15%), 26% to 50% and 76 (6%) were narrowed 0% to 25%. No significant differences were observed between the two groups of patients in any of the five

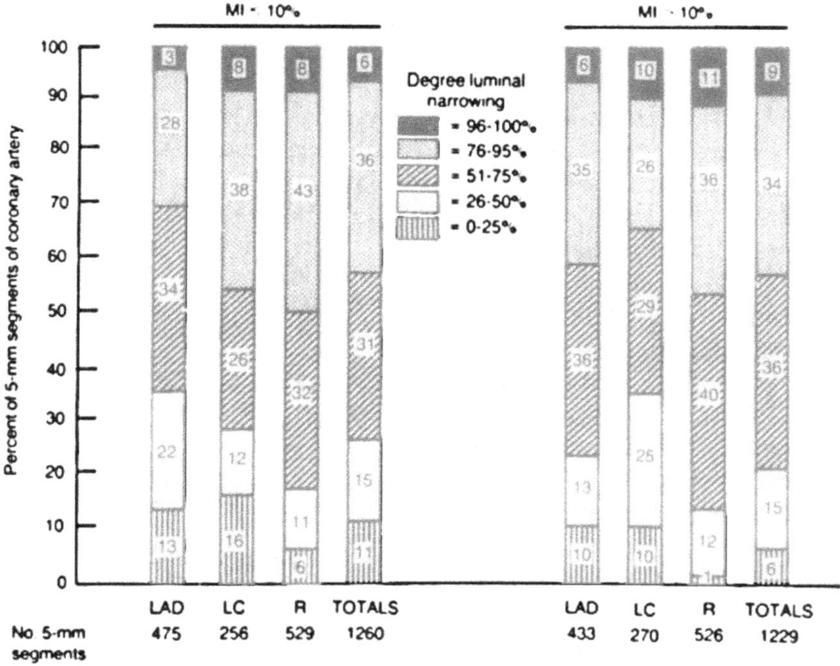

Fig. 3. Percent of 5 mm segments of the right *(R)*, left anterior descending *(LAD)*, and left circumflex *(LC)* coronary arteries narrowed to various degrees by atherosclerotic plaques in the 28 patients with the myocardial infarct *(MI)* involving ≤ 10% and in the 28 and the MI involving > 10% of the left ventricular wall.

categories of narrowing. Additionally, no significant differences occurred between the two groups in the percent of segments narrowed severely in the LAD, LC, or R coronary arteries.

A scoring system was utilized to indicate both the severity and extent of the coronary narrowing. Every five mm long segment from each patient was assigned a score of 1 to 4 based upon the amount of cross-sectional area narrowing by atherosclerotic plaques as follows: 1 = 0% to 25% narrowing; 2 = 26% to 50%; 3 = 51% to 75%; 4 = 76% to 100%. A total score was obtained for each patient and the score per 5 mm segment was then calculated by dividing the total score per patient by the number of 5 mm segments examined from that patient. The score for each 5 mm segment for the group with MI size ≤ = 10% ranged from 2.1 to 3.8 (mean 3.1) and for the group with MI size > 10%, from 2.4 to 3.9 (mean 3.1) (p = NS).

DISCUSSION

Although considerable interest exists in interventions directed at limiting myocardial infarct (MI) size, little information is available on the relation of the size of an MI to the clinical course and length of survival after healing of an acute MI. In addition, it is not known whether MI size is related to the age of the patient at the time of the acute MI or at death,

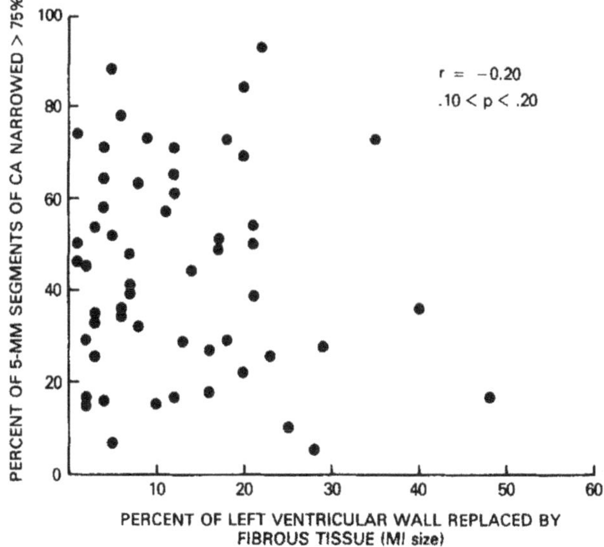

Fig. 4. Relation of myocardial infarct *(MI)* size to percent of 5 mm segments of coronary artery *(CA)* narrowed 76% to 100% in cross-sectional area by atherosclerotic plaque in 56 necropsy patients with healed transmural MI.

the mode of death, or to the amount and extent of coronary arterial narrowing by atherosclerotic plaques. In previous reports from this laboratory, we examined the relation of the size of a healed MI to the location of the MI[4] and to the presence or absence of a clinically documented acute MI.[5] We found that an MI located primarily in the LV anterior wall was significantly larger than those located primarily in the LV posterior wall, and that patients with a clinically recognized MI had significantly larger areas of scarring than those without a clinically recognized MI.

In the present study, we found that the size of the healed MI at necropsy did not correlate with the age of the patient at the time of the acute MI or at death, with the frequency of angina pectoris after healing of the acute MI, or with the frequency of sudden coronary death or fatal acute MI, or with the amount, location, and extent of coronary arterial narrowing by atherosclerotic plaques at necropsy. Patients with an MI involving $\leq 10\%$ of the LV wall compared to those with an MI involving $> 10\%$ had a similar number of major coronary arteries with severe (76% to 100% in cross-sectional area) narrowing, a similar frequency of severe narrowing of the left main coronary artery, and a similar overall percent of 5 mm segments of coronary artery severely narrowed. In addition, the amount of severe narrowing in the LAD, LC, and R coronary arteries was similar between the two groups of patients. The size of the healed MI, however, did correlate with the *frequency of chronic congestive heart failure* and with the *length of survival after the acute MI*.

Although there was considerable variability in length of survival in patients with an MI involving $< 20\%$ of the LV wall, only 2 of 15 patients with MI involving $\geq 20\%$ survived for more than 3 years after the acute MI. Thus prolonged survival after healing of an acute MI is infrequent in patients with a large MI.

REFERENCES

1. Roberts WC, Gardin JM: Location of myocardial infarcts: A confusion of terms and definitions. Am J Cardiol **42**:868, 1978.
2. Movat HZ: Demonstration of all connective tissue elements in a single section: Pentachrome stains. Arch Pathol **60**:289, 1955.
3. Isner JM, Wu M, Virmani R, Jones AA, Roberts WC: Comparison of degrees of coronary arterial luminal narrowing determined by visual inspection of histologic sections under magnification among three independent observers and comparison to that obtained by video planimetry: An analysis of 559 five-mm segments of 61 coronary arteries from eleven patients. Lab Invest **42**:566, 1980.
4. Cabin HS, Roberts WC: Comparison of amount and extent of coronary narrowing by atherosclerotic plaque and of myocardial scarring at necropsy in anterior-vs-posterior *healed* transmural myocardial infarction. Analysis of 59 necropsy patients. Circulation (In press)
5. Cabin HS, Roberts WC: Quantitative comparison of extent of coronary narrowing and size of healed myocardial infarct in 33 necropsy patients with clinically *recognized* and in 28 necropsy patients with clinically *unrecognized* ("silent") previous acute myocardial infarction. Am J Cardiol (In press)

Relation of Serum Total Cholesterol and Triglyceride Levels to the Amount and Extent of Coronary Arterial Narrowing by Atherosclerotic Plaque in Coronary Heart Disease

Quantitative Analysis of 2,037 Five mm Segments of 160 Major Epicardial Coronary Arteries in 40 Necropsy Patients

HENRY SCOTT CABIN, M.D.
WILLIAM C. ROBERTS, M.D.

Bethesda, Maryland

The amount of cross-sectional area narrowing by atherosclerotic plaques was determined histologically in each 5 mm segment of the entire lengths of the right, left main, left anterior descending, and left circumflex coronary arteries in 40 patients with fatal coronary heart disease and known fasting serum total cholesterol and triglyceride levels. The patients were divided into four groups based upon the serum total cholesterol and triglyceride levels: group I, total cholesterol of 250 mg/dl or less, triglyceride of 170 mg/dl or less; group II, total cholesterol of 250 or less, triglyceride of more than 170; group III, total cholesterol of more than 250, triglyceride of 170 or less; group IV, total cholesterol of more than 250, triglyceride of more than 170. The number of 5 mm segments of coronary artery narrowed severely (76 to 100 percent in cross-sectional area) by atherosclerotic plaques in each group was as follows: 172 of 505 (34 percent) 5 mm segments from group I; 242 of 353 (69 percent) segments from group II; 120 of 295 (41 percent) from group III and 425 of 884 (48 percent) segments from group IV. The mean percentage of 5 mm segments narrowed severely was significantly greater in group II than in group I (p $<$0.005) or group III (p $<$0.01). Additionally, the mean number of four coronary arteries per subject severely narrowed and the number of subjects with severe narrowing of the left main coronary artery were significantly greater in groups II and III than in group I. The percentages of 5 mm segments narrowed severely correlated significantly with the serum triglyceride level (p $<$0.03). Although it correlated with the number of severely narrowed coronary arteries per subject, the serum total cholesterol level did not correlate with the percentage of 5 mm segments of coronary artery with severe narrowing.

Earlier studies [1–4] from this laboratory described the status of the coronary arteries at necropsy in patients with known types II, III, and IV hyperlipoproteinemia, but they did not analyze quantitatively the relation between the serum total cholesterol and triglyceride levels

From the Pathology Branch, National Heart, Lung and Blood Institute, National Institutes of Health, Bethesda, Maryland. Reprint requests should be addressed to Dr. William C. Roberts, Building 10A, Room 3E-30, National Institutes of Health, Bethesda, Maryland 20205. Manuscript accepted on January 20, 1982.

and the amount and extent of coronary arterial narrowing by atherosclerotic plaque. Consequently, we determined the amount of narrowing in each 5 mm segment of the entire lengths of the four major coronary arteries in 40 patients with known serum total cholesterol and triglyceride levels and symptomatic coronary heart disease, and by dividing the subjects into various groups, according to the cholesterol and triglyceride levels, determined if these levels were related to the amounts of coronary narrowing.

SUBJECTS AND METHODS

All 40 patients had fasting serum total cholesterol and triglyceride determinations by the enzymatic method during life and fatal coronary heart disease. The cholesterol and triglyceride levels reported were measured when the patients were clinically stable, not within two months of acute myocardial infarction, acute decompensation of chronic congestive heart failure, or an operative procedure. When more than one level was available, the initial value was utilized, as subsequent levels were often obtained after initiation of diet and/or drug therapy to lower serum lipid levels. Of the 40 subjects, 37 also had lipoprotein determinations and were classified as having type II (15 patients) or IV (12 patients) hyperlipoproteinemia or normal lipoprotein patterns (ten patients). Group I included 11 patients with total cholesterol of 250 mg/dl or less and triglyceride of 170 mg/dl or less; group II (six patients) had total cholesterol of 250 or less and triglyceride of more than 170; group III (six patients) had total cholesterol of more than 250 and triglyceride of 170 or less; group IV (17 patients) had total cholesterol of more than 250 and triglyceride of more than 170. Certain clinical findings in the 40 study subjects are summarized in **Table I.** Eighteen (45 percent) of the 40 patients died suddenly: six (15 percent) from acute myocardial infarction, two (5 percent) from chronic congestive heart failure, ten (25 percent) shortly after aortocoronary bypass grafting, and four (10 percent) during cardiac catheterization. No significant differences were observed among the four groups in mean age at death, or frequency of clinical history of acute myocardial infarction, diabetes mellitus, or systemic hypertension. Angina pectoris occurred more frequently in groups III and IV than in group I (p <0.05); chronic congestive heart failure, more frequently in group I than in group IV (p <0.05); and sudden coronary death, more frequently in group IV than in group I.

For each of the 40 study patients, the entire lengths of the right, left main, left anterior descending, and left circumflex coronary arteries were removed from the heart and were cut transversely into 5 mm segments. Each segment was labeled and processed for histologic study, and a histologic section stained by the Movat method [5] was prepared and examined. The degree of narrowing in each 5 mm segment was determined by examination under the microscope magnified 25 to 50 times. The percentage of cross-sectional area narrowing by atherosclerotic plaques alone was determined in five categories of narrowing: 0 to 25, 26 to 50, 51 to 75, 76 to 95, and 96 to 100 percent. The accuracy of these determinations was verified by video planimetry and shown to have an error of less than 5 percent [6].

RESULTS

Results of the analysis of the maximal amounts of narrowing in each major epicardial coronary artery are summarized in **Tables II** and **III.** The mean number of four coronary arteries per subject narrowed at any point 76 to 100 percent in cross-sectional area by atherosclerotic plaque was greater in groups II (3.7/4.0), III (3.7/4.0), and IV (3.1/4.0) than in group I (2.6/4.0) (p <0.001, p <0.001, and p <0.05, respectively). Additionally, the number of patients with severe (76 to 100 percent) narrowing of the left main coronary artery was greater in groups II and III (four of six in both) than in group I (one of 11) (p <0.05). There was no significant difference in the frequency of severe narrowing of the left anterior descending, left circumflex, and right coronary arteries among the four study groups.

The results of the quantitative analysis of the amounts of narrowing in each of the 2,037 five mm long segments of coronary artery are summarized in **Table IV** and in **Figure 1.** The mean percentage of 5 mm segments narrowed 76 to 100 percent in cross-sectional area was greater in group II (70 percent) than in group I (35 percent) (p <0.005) or group III (44 percent) (p <0.01), but no significant differences were observed between group IV (49 percent) and each of the other three groups. In every 5 mm segment from all 40 patients, the severe narrowing, if present, was produced by atherosclerotic plaques except for two 5 mm segments from two subjects (27 and 40, Table I), which had 51 to 75 percent cross-sectional area narrowing by atherosclerotic plaque and severe narrowing produced by thrombus. The amount of narrowing produced by thrombus was not included in this analysis.

A scoring system was utilized in which each 5 mm segment of coronary artery in each subject was given a score of 1 to 4 based on the amount of cross-sectional area narrowing as follows: 1 for 0 to 25 percent narrowing; 2 for 26 to 50 percent; 3 for 51 to 75 percent; 4 for 76 to 100 percent. The score per 5 mm segment for each subject was obtained by dividing the total score per subject by the number of 5 mm segments examined from that subject. The mean score per 5 mm segment (Table IV) was greater in group II (3.55) than in groups I (2.95) (p <0.01), III (3.13) (p <0.10), or IV (3.11) (p <0.02).

The serum triglyceride level in the 40 patients correlated significantly (p <0.03) with the percentage of 5 mm segments narrowed 76 to 100 percent in cross-sectional area by atherosclerotic plaques (**Figure 2**),

TABLE I Certain Clinical and Necropsy Findings in the 40 Study Subjects

Subject No.	Age (yr)	Sex	History AMI	History AP	History CHF	TC	Tg	Study Group	SH	DM	HW (g)	LV F	LV N	No. of Four CA Narrowed >75% by Ath	No. of 5 mm Segments	No. (%) of 5 mm Segments 76–100%	No. (%) of 5 mm Segments 96–100%	Mean* Score CA
1	29	F	0	+	0	430	86	III	0	0	300	0	0	4	73	10 (14)	0	2.3
2	31	M	+	0	+	170	101	I	0	0	520	+	0	2	56	7 (13)	1 (2)	2.5
3	31	F	0	+	+	245	497	II	+	+	380	+	+	4	57	32 (56)	4 (7)	3.1
4	33	M	+	+	0	260	410	IV	+	0	380	+	0	3	57	43 (75)	9 (16)	3.5
5	40	M	0	+	0	233	112	I	0	0	370	+	+	3	39	26 (67)	5 (13)	3.7
6	40	M	+	+	0	229	80	I	0	0	550	+	0	2	39	9 (23)	4 (10)	2.3
7	44	M	0	0	+	140	264	II	0	0	500	+	0	4	53	36 (68)	6 (11)	3.6
8	45	M	+	+	0	261	800	IV	+	+	430	+	0	4	52	41 (79)	8 (15)	3.8
9	45	M	0	+	0	370	280	IV	0	0	410	0	0	3	54	15 (28)	0	2.7
10	47	M	+	+	0	136	76	I	+	0	460	+	+	3	41	29 (71)	2 (5)	3.7
11	47	M	+	+	0	572	253	IV	0	0	330	+	0	4	66	28 (42)	2 (3)	3.1
12	48	M	+	+	0	285	405	IV	0	0	430	0	0	3	58	27 (47)	2 (3)	3.3
13	49	F	0	+	0	423	1,462	IV	+	+	450	+	0	3	46	27 (59)	4 (9)	3.2
14	49	M	+	+	0	591	388	IV	+	0	420	+	+	4	32	27 (84)	2 (7)	3.8
15	49	M	+	+	+	426	112	III	+	0	565	+	0	3	38	11 (29)	1 (3)	2.9
16	49	F	+	+	0	320	127	III	0	0	260	+	0	3	24	16 (67)	4 (17)	3.5
17	50	M	+	+	0	244	600	II	0	0	480	+	+	3	37	27 (73)	2 (5)	3.6
18	51	M	0	+	0	348	126	III	0	0	400	+	+	4	38	17 (45)	4 (11)	3.2
19	51	M	0	0	0	335	191	IV	0	0	400	+	+	4	66	29 (44)	4 (6)	3.0
20	51	M	0	+	0	420	274	IV	0	+	490	0	0	2	58	20 (34)	9 (16)	3.1
21	51	M	+	+	0	436	338	IV	+	0	380	+	0	3	33	22 (67)	0	2.5
22	52	M	+	0	0	362	241	IV	0	+	430	+	0	3	70	28 (40)	4 (6)	3.2
23	52	M	0	+	0	350	442	IV	+	0	420	0	0	3	52	19 (37)	3 (6)	3.3
24	54	F	+	+	+	373	195	IV	+	0	400	+	0	1	33	1 (3)	1 (3)	1.8
25	54	M	+	+	0	186	465	II	0	+	505	+	+	4	55	48 (87)	19 (35)	3.7
26	55	M	+	+	0	400	1,500	IV	0	0	490	+	0	3	49	12 (25)	2 (4)	2.6
27	56	M	+	+	0	735	2,820	IV	0	+	450	+	+	3	47	43 (91)	8 (17)	3.9
28	57	M	0	+	0	520	168	III	0	0	570	+	0	4	70	33 (47)	1 (1)	3.3
29	57	M	0	+	0	280	124	III	+	0	360	+	0	4	52	33 (63)	9 (17)	3.6
30	58	M	0	+	0	357	263	IV	+	0	640	+	0	3	59	21 (36)	9 (15)	3.3
31	59	M	0	+	0	183	228	II	+	0	640	+	0	4	58	47 (81)	3 (5)	3.8
32	59	M	+	0	0	180	150	I	0	0	320	+	0	3	39	11 (28)	4 (10)	2.8
33	60	M	0	+	0	325	215	IV	0	0	390	+	0	3	52	22 (42)	12 (23)	2.8
34	62	M	0	+	0	160	136	I	0	0	840	+	+	3	47	7 (15)	0	2.8
35	63	M	0	+	+	175	148	I	+	0	890	+	0	3	62	41 (66)	4 (6)	3.7
36	64	M	+	+	+	146	150	I	0	+	730	+	0	2	72	17 (24)	3 (4)	2.6
37	64	M	+	0	0	170	82	I	0	0	570	+	0	2	29	15 (51)	1 (3)	3.3
38	65	M	0	0	0	193	210	II	+	0	540	+	0	3	93	52 (56)	5 (5)	3.5
39	71	M	0	0	+	121	116	I	0	0	650	+	0	2	50	4 (8)	0	2.4
40	78	F	0	0	0	187	121	I	0	+	360	0	0	3	31	6 (19)	0	2.6

* See results section for explanation of scoring system.
AMI = acute myocardial infarction; AP = angina pectoris; CHF = congestive heart failure; TC = total cholesterol; Tg = triglyceride; SH = systemic hypertension; DM = diabetes mellitus; HW = heart weight; LV = left ventricular; F = fibrosis; N = necrosis; CA = coronary arteries; Ath = atherosclerotic plaque.

TABLE II

TABLE II   **Number of Subjects in Each Study Group with One to Four of the Four Major Epicardial Coronary Arteries (CA) Narrowed 76–100% in Cross-Sectional Area (XSA) by Atherosclerotic Plaque**

	Study Group			
	I	II	III	IV
No. CA Narrowed	Tg ≤ 170	Tg > 170	Tg ≤ 170	Tg > 170
76–100% in XSA	TC ≤ 250	TC ≤ 250	TC > 250	TC > 250
4	0	4	4	4
3	6	2	2	11
2	5	0	0	1
1	0	0	0	1
0	0	0	0	0
Totals	11	6	6	17

Tg = triglyceride; TC = total cholesterol.

TABLE III   **Numbers of Four Major Epicardial Coronary Arteries (CA) Narrowed 76–100% in Cross-Sectional Area by Atherosclerotic Plaque in the Four Study Groups**

Study Group	No. Subjects	Total No. CA	No. of Subjects with Narrowing >75%					Mean No. of CA per Subject Narrowed >75%
			LM	LAD	LC	R	Totals	
I Tg ≤ 170 TC ≤ 250	11	44	1*	10	10	7	28 (64%)	2.6*
II Tg > 170 TC ≤ 250	6	24	4***	6	6	6	22 (92%)	3.7**
III Tg ≤ 170 TC > 250	6	24	4***	6	6	6	22 (92%)	3.7**
IV Tg > 170 TC > 250	17	68	6	15	15	16	52 (76%)	3.1***

* to ** = p <0.001.   * to *** = p <0.05.   ** to *** = p <0.05.
LM = left main; LAD = left anterior descending; LC = left circumflex; R = right; Tg = triglyceride; TC = total cholesterol.

TABLE IV   **Amounts of Cross-Sectional Area (XSA) Luminal Narrowing in the 5 mm Segments of the Four Major Coronary Arteries (CA) in the Four Study Groups**

Study Group	No. (%) of 5 mm Segments of CA in Categories of XSA Narrowing by Ath					No. of 5 mm Segments per Group	Mean Score per 5 mm Segment
	0–25%	26–50%	51–75%	76–95%	96–100%		
I Tg ≤ 170 TC ≤ 250	57 (11)	94 (19)	182 (36)	148 (29)	24 (5)	505	2.95*
II Tg > 170 TC ≤ 250	11 (3)	19 (5)	81 (23)	203 (58)	39 (11)	353	3.55**
III Tg ≤ 170 TC > 250	28 (9)	49 (17)	98 (33)	101 (34)	19 (6)	295	3.13
IV Tg > 170 TC > 250	62 (7)	146 (17)	251 (28)	346 (39)	79 (9)	884	3.11***
Totals	158 (8)	308 (15)	612 (30)	798 (39)	161 (8)	2037	3.19 (mean)

* to ** = p <0.01.   ** to *** = p < 0.02.   † See results section for explanation of scoring system.
Ath = atherosclerotic plaque; Tg = triglyceride; TC = total cholesterol.

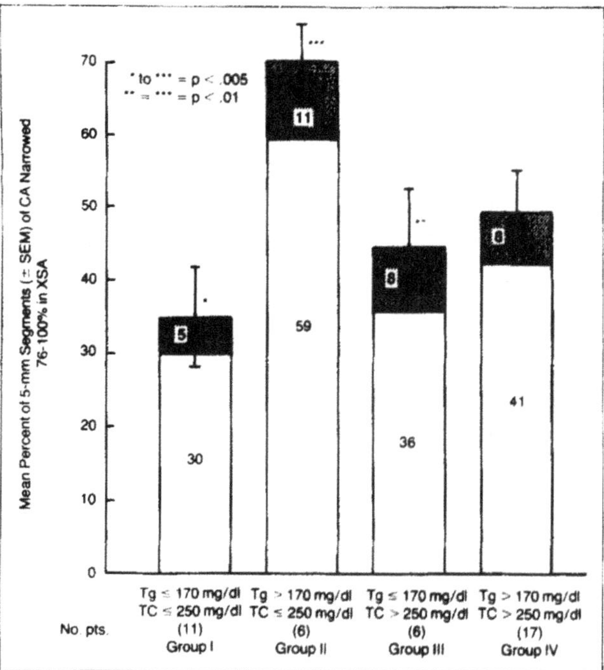

Figure 1. Mean percentage of 5 mm segments of all four major epicardial coronary arteries (CA) narrowed 76 to 100 percent in cross-sectional area (XSA) by atherosclerotic plaques in the four study groups. The **shaded portion** of each bar indicates the mean percentage of 5 mm segments narrowed 96 to 100 percent and the **open portion,** the mean percentage narrowed 76 to 95 percent.

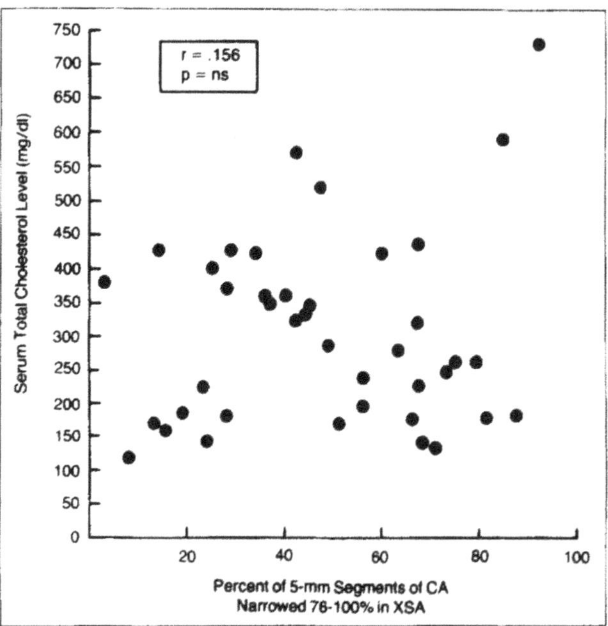

Figure 2. Relation between serum triglyceride level and percentage of 5 mm segments of coronary artery (CA) narrowed 76 to 100 percent in cross-sectional area (XSA) by atherosclerotic plaque. Each **dot** represents a single subject.

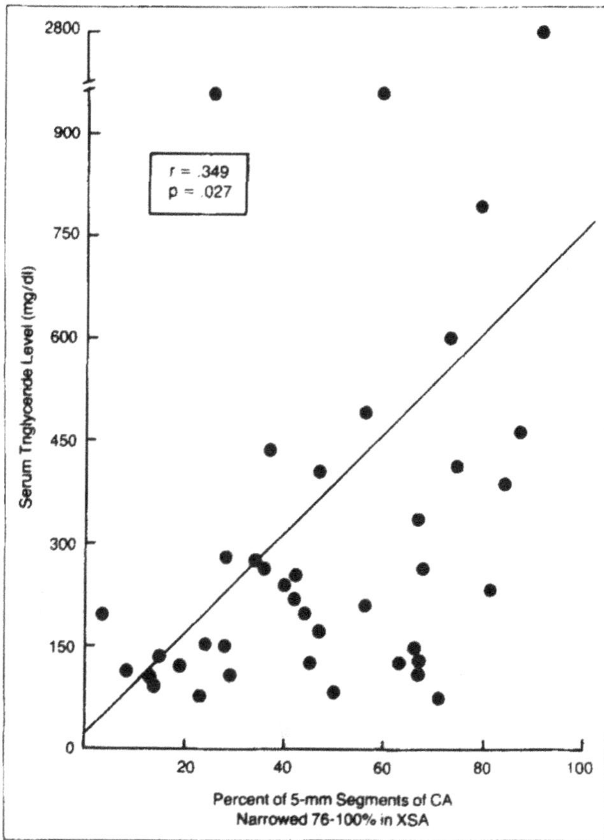

Figure 3. Relation between serum total cholesterol level and percentage of segments of coronary artery (CA) narrowed 76 to 100 percent in cross-sectional area (XSA) by atherosclerotic plaque. Each **dot** represents a single subject.

but the level of serum total cholesterol did not correlate significantly (**Figure 3**).

The 40 patients also were divided into three groups based on either the serum total cholesterol or triglyceride levels (**Figures 4** and **5**) (total cholesterol or triglyceride of less than 200 mg/dl; total cholesterol or triglyceride of more than 300. The patients with triglyceride of less than 200 mg/dl and triglyceride between 201 and 300 mg/dl had a significantly lower mean percentage of 5 mm segments narrowed severely than those with triglyceride of more than 300 mg/dl (37 percent and 47 percent versus 65 percent, p <0.005 and 0.05, respectively) (Figure 4). When the 40 patients were divided into three groups based on the serum total cholesterol level, no significant differences were found in the mean percentage of 5 mm segments of coronary artery narrowed severely among those with total cholesterol of less than 200 mg/dl, total cholesterol between 201 and 300 mg/dl, and total cholesterol of more than 300 mg/dl (Figure 5).

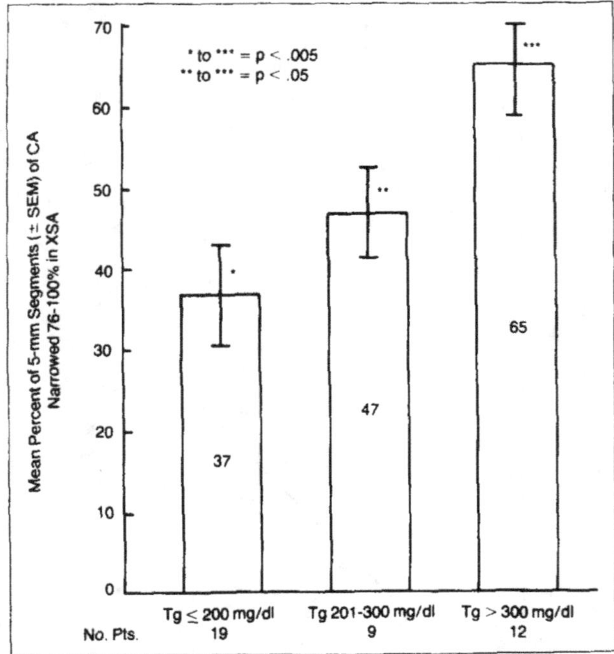

Figure 4. Mean percentage of 5 mm segments of coronary artery (CA) narrowed 76 to 100 percent in cross-sectional area (XSA) by atherosclerotic plaque in the 40 study subjects divided into three groups according to the serum triglyceride (Tg) level.

Figure 5. Mean percentage of 5 mm segments of coronary artery (CA) narrowed 76 to 100 percent in cross-sectional area (XSA) by atherosclerotic plaque in the 40 study subjects divided into three groups according to the serum total cholesterol (TC) level.

COMMENTS

Several reports have examined the relation between serum total cholesterol and triglyceride levels and the presence, degree, and/or extent of coronary arterial narrowing as determined angiographically [7–15], and the results are conflicting. Cramér and associates [7] performed coronary angiography on 224 patients (119 with symptomatic coronary heart disease) and found a significant relation between hypertriglyceridemia (more than 160 mg/dl) but not hypercholesterolemia (more than 280 mg/dl) and "severe" coronary arterial narrowing. Fuster and colleagues [11] studied 300 patients with symptomatic coronary heart disease and found no relation between hypertriglyceridemia (more than 150 mg/dl) or hypercholesterolemia (more than 300 mg/dl) and the number or distribution of coronary arteries narrowed or the degree of narrowing. Nitter-Hauge and Enge [9] found no correlation between total cholesterol and triglyceride levels and a calculated coronary score in 71 patients with angina pectoris or myocardial infarct who underwent angiography. Proudfit and co-workers [8] found an association between total cholesterol level and frequency of "abnormal" coronary angiographic findings in 147 men younger than 40 years, and Gotto and associates [14] found a significant correlation between total cholesterol and triglyceride levels and the frequency of angiographically diagnosed coronary heart disease and the number of arteries involved in 496

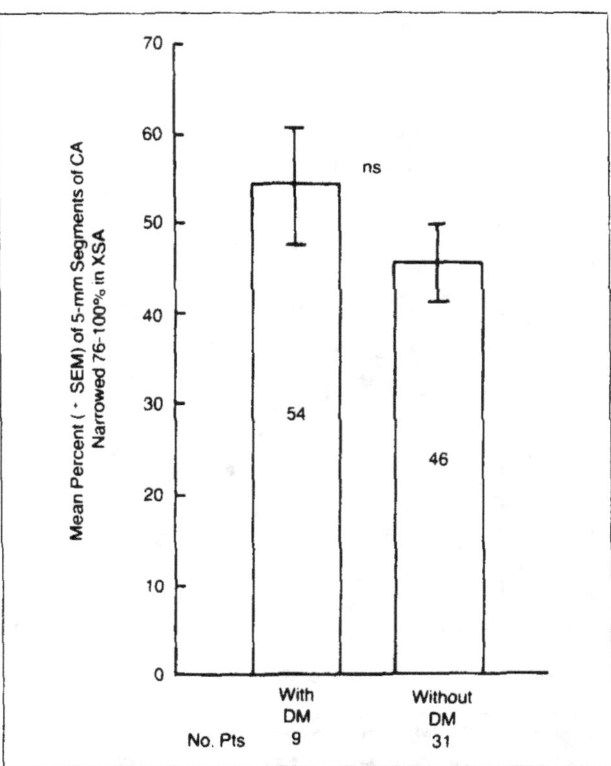

Figure 6. Mean percentage of 5 mm segments of coronary artery narrowed 76 to 100 percent in cross-sectional area (XSA) by atherosclerotic plaque in 31 study subjects without and in nine with diabetes mellitus (DM).

patients with chest pain. Murray and colleagues [10] observed a significant relation between total cholesterol and triglyceride levels and the extent of coronary arterial narrowing in 133 men studied angiographically for chest pain.

In the present study, the entire lengths of the four major epicardial coronary arteries from 40 patients with fatal coronary heart disease were studied at necropsy. The subjects were divided into groups determined by the level of the serum total cholesterol and triglyceride. Although all but one of the 40 patients had at least two of four major coronary arteries narrowed severely (76 to 100 percent in cross-sectional area), the subjects with "normal" total cholesterol and triglyceride levels (group I) had significantly fewer major coronary arteries narrowed severely by atherosclerotic plaque than did the subjects with hypercholesterolemia and/or hypertriglyceridemia (groups II, III, and IV). Additionally, the left main coronary artery was severely narrowed significantly more frequently in subjects with hypercholesterolemia (group II) or hypertriglyceridemia (group III) than in those with normal levels (group I). Thus, analysis of the number of the four major coronary arteries with severe narrowing revealed a similar relation of total cholesterol and triglyceride levels to coronary arterial narrowing.

When a more precise technique, however, was utilized to determine the amount of coronary narrowing, a significant relation was found between triglyceride levels and amounts of severe coronary narrowing but none between total cholesterol levels and amounts of severe narrowing. The amount of cross-sectional area narrowing by atherosclerotic plaque was determined in each 5 mm segment of coronary artery from the 40 patients, and those in groups I and III had a significantly lower mean percentage of segments narrowed severely than those in group II. No significant difference was observed in the mean percentage of coronary segments narrowed severely between the subjects with hypercholesterolemia and a "normal" serum triglyceride level (group III) and those in whom both levels were "normal" (group I). Utilizing linear regression analysis to compare serum triglyceride and total cholesterol levels with percentage of coronary segments severely narrowed, the serum triglyceride level but not the serum total cholesterol level was correlated significantly with the amount of severe narrowing. Although diabetes mellitus was slightly more frequent in the subjects with hypertriglyceridemia (seven of 23 [30 percent]) than in those without (four of 17 [24 percent]), the difference was not significant. Additionally, the mean percentages of 5 mm segments of coronary artery with severe narrowing in the nine diabetic and in the 31 nondiabetic patients were similar (**Figure 6**).

It is often assumed that coronary heart disease is unlikely to develop in persons with serum total cholesterol levels below 160 mg/dl, and such levels of serum total cholesterol are the norm in societies with little or no coronary heart disease. Five (13 percent) of our 40 study patients, however, had serum total cholesterol levels of 121 to 160 mg/dl (mean 141) and each had at least two of the four major epicardial coronary arteries narrowed severely, with 8 to 68 percent (mean 37) of the 5 mm segments of the four major coronary arteries so narrowed. In four of the five subjects, the serum triglyceride level was 150 mg/dl or less. Thus, although the amount of severe coronary arterial narrowing, in general, correlates with triglyceride levels, severe extensive narrowing may still occur with low serum total cholesterol and triglyceride levels.

Although it suggests that in patients with fatal coronary heart disease the serum triglyceride level correlates more strongly with the amount of severe coronary narrowing than does the serum total cholesterol level, our study does not allow any conclusion about the relative importance of serum total cholesterol and triglyceride levels as *risk factors* for coronary heart disease. Our 40 patients, like those in most previously discussed angiographic studies, had symptomatic and/or fatal coronary heart disease. Thus, our findings are only applicable to patients who already have symptoms of coronary heart disease and retrospectively to patients without symptoms who have sudden coronary death.

REFERENCES

1. Roberts WC, Levy RI, Fredrickson DS: Hyperlipoproteinemia: a review of the five types with first report of necropsy findings in type 3. Arch Pathol 1970; 90: 46.
2. Roberts WC, Ferrans VJ, Levy RI, Fredrickson DS: Cardiovascular pathology in hyperlipoproteinemia: anatomic observations in 42 necropsy patients with normal or abnormal serum lipoprotein patterns. Am J Cardiol 1973; 31: 557.
3. Cabin HS, Roberts WC: Quantification of amounts of coronary arterial narrowing in patients with types II and IV hyperlipoproteinemia and in those with known normal lipoprotein patterns. Am Heart J 1981; 101: 52.
4. Cabin HS, Schwartz DE, Virmani R, Brewer HB Jr, Roberts WC: Type III hyperlipoproteinemia: quantification, distribution and nature of atherosclerotic coronary arterial narrowing in five necropsy patients. Am Heart J 1981; 102: 830–835.
5. Movat HZ: Demonstration of all connective tissue elements in a single section: pentachrome stains. Arch Pathol 1955; 60: 289.
6. Isner JM, Wu M, Virmani R, Jones AA, Roberts WC: Comparison of degrees of coronary arterial luminal narrowing determined by visual inspection of histologic sections under magnification among three independent observers and comparison to that obtained by video planimetry: an analysis of 559 five-mm segments of 61 coronary arteries from

eleven patients. Lab Invest 1980; 42: 566.

7. Cramér K, Paulin S, Werkö L: Coronary angiographic findings in correlation with age, body weight, blood pressure, serum lipids, and smoking habits. Circulation 1966; 33: 888.

8. Proudfit WL, Shirey EK, Sones FM Jr: Selective cine coronary arteriography. Correlation with clinical findings in 1,000 patients. Circulation 1966; 33: 901.

9. Nitter-Hauge S, Enge I: Relation between blood lipid levels and angiographically evaluated obstructions in coronary arteries. Br Heart J 1973; 35: 791.

10. Murray RG, Tweddel A, Third JLHC, Hutton I, Hillis WS: Relation between extent of coronary artery disease and severity of hyperlipoproteinemia. Br Heart J 1975; 37: 1205.

11. Fuster V, Frye RL, Connolly DC, Danielson MA, Elveback LR, Kurland LT: Arteriographic patterns early in the onset of the coronary syndromes. Br Heart J 1975; 37: 1250.

12. McLaughlin PR, Berman ND, Morton BC, et al.: Long-term angiographic assessment of the influence of coronary risk factors on native coronary circulation and saphenous vein aortocoronary grafts. Am Heart J 1977; 93: 327.

13. Salel AF, Fong A, Zelis R, Miller RR, Borhani NO, Mason DT: Accuracy of numerical coronary profile. Correlation of risk factors with arteriographically documented severity of atherosclerosis. N Engl J Med 1977; 296: 1447.

14. Gotto AM, Gorry GA, Thompson JR et al.: Relationship between plasma lipid concentrations and coronary artery disease in 496 patients. Circulation 1977; 56: 875.

15. Hamby RI: Clinical correlates of coronary angiography. In: Clinical-anatomical correlates of coronary artery disease. New York: Futura Publishing, 1979: 285–341.

Embolus to the Left Main Coronary Artery

BRUCE F. WALLER, MD*
DOUGLAS S. DIXON, MD
RAK W. KIM, MD
WILLIAM C. ROBERTS, MD

Washington, D.C.

The consequences of coronary embolism depend on 2 factors, the *size of the embolus* and the *size of the lumen of the artery in which it becomes impacted.* The smaller the embolus, the greater the chance that it will migrate distally to a small coronary artery and the less the likelihood of myocardial necrosis or fatal arrhythmia. Conversely, the larger the embolus, the greater the chance that it will impact proximally in a large coronary artery and the greater the likelihood of myocardial necrosis or fatal arrhythmia. An embolus so small that it impacts in a single intramural coronary artery is clinically silent and observed at necropsy only on histologic examination of sections of myocardial wall (Fig. 1). An embolus somewhat larger may occlude multiple intramural coronary arteries in a fingerlike fashion (Fig. 1). When only multiple intramural coronary arteries are obstructed, particularly those located in the inner one half of the myocardial wall, myocardial necrosis is unlikely to result, probably because of the extensive intramyocardial vascular bed. A major danger of obstruction to multiple intramural coronary arteries, however, particularly those located in the outer one half of the myocardial wall, is that a "right angle" epicardial feeding branch may become thrombosed secondarily

From the Pathology Branch, National Heart, Lung, and Blood Institute, Bethesda, Maryland and the District of Columbia Medical Examiners Office, Washington, D.C.

* Present address: Indiana University Medical Center, Indianapolis, Indiana.

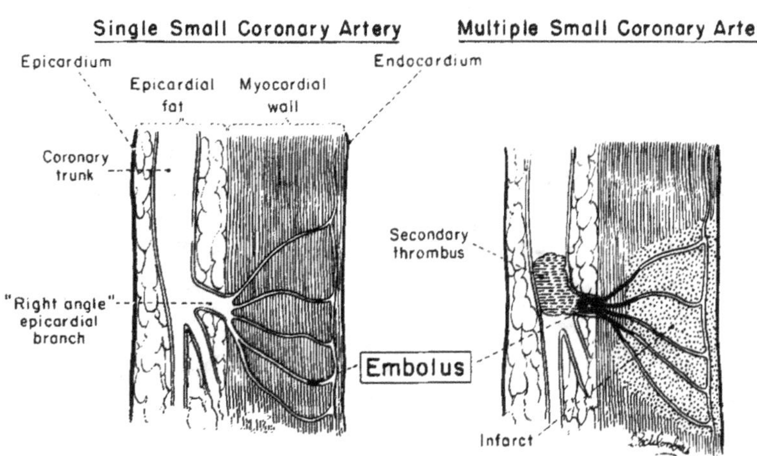

FIGURE 1. Diagram showing the effects of embolus size on left ventricular myocardium. (Reproduced with permission.[1]) **Left panel,** no myocardial changes; embolus visible microscopically only. **Right panel,** myocardial infarct with secondary thrombosis of epicardial branch and major coronary trunk.

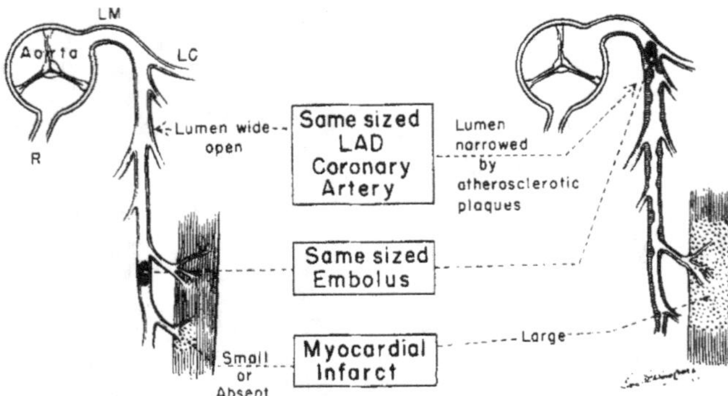

FIGURE 2. Diagram showing the effects of atherosclerotic narrowing on myocardial consequences of coronary embolus. The embolus may impact proximally in an artery whose lumen is narrowed by atherosclerotic plaque (**right**) and distally in a nonatherosclerotic artery of identical initial size (**left**). Arteries: LAD = left anterior descending; LC = left circumflex; LM = left main; R = right. (Reproduced with permission.[1])

because of the poor runoff through it (Fig. 1). Occlusion of this branch may in turn lead to secondary thrombosis of the major coronary trunk, and this complication may produce myocardial necrosis. Thus, secondary thrombosis of the proximal feeding coronary artery is a potential complication of coronary embolism.

A second and less important factor determining the consequence of coronary embolism is the status of the coronary arteries before embolism. An embolus to a previously wide-open coronary artery is most likely to migrate distally, but because collateral vessels between the epicardial coronary arteries are relatively poor, myocardial necrosis or ischemia may nevertheless occur (Fig. 2).[1] An embolus of the same size migrating to a previously severely narrowed coronary tree is much more likely to impact proximally and thus lead to sudden death (Fig. 2), despite the collateral vessels that are likely to be present in this circumstance.[2]

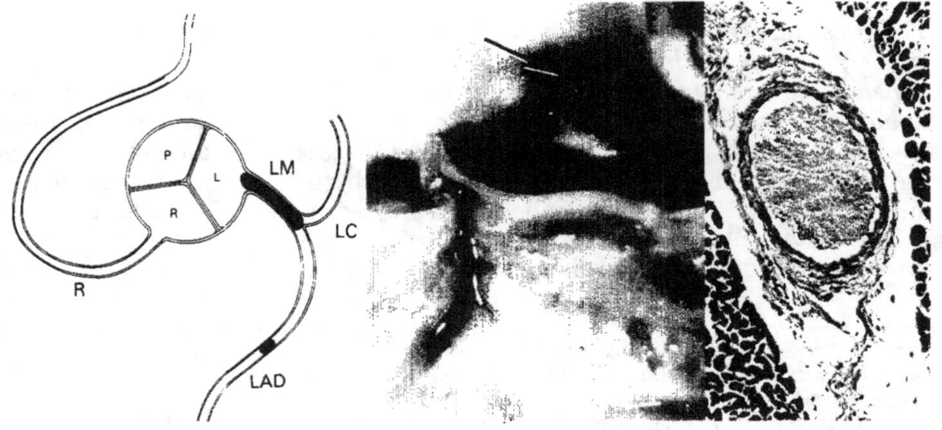

FIGURE 3. Left main (LM) coronary embolus in a 37 year old man (DCMEO #82-03-337) who was found dead in his hotel room. **Left,** diagram of coronary tree. The left anterior descending (LAD), left circumflex (LC), and right (R) coronary arteries are free of atherosclerotic plaque. **Center,** embolus (**arrow**) in the ostium of the LM coronary artery. **Right,** fragment of fibrin-platelet embolus in the lumen of an intramural coronary artery. Microinfarcts were present in the left ventricular wall. L = left, P = posterior, and R = right aortic sinuses. Movat stain; magnification ×150, reduced 32 percent.

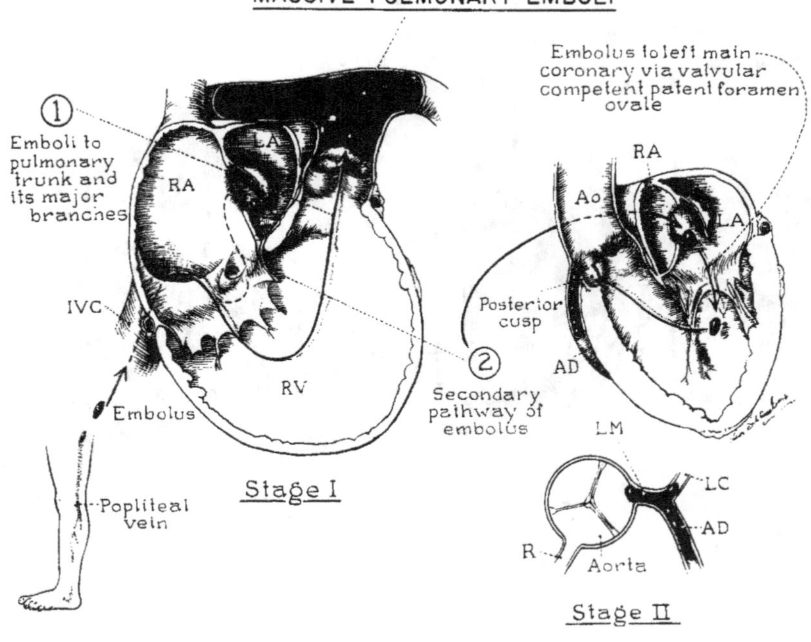

FIGURE 4. Diagram showing an embolus to the left main (LM) coronary artery via a valvular-competent patent foramen ovale after presumed elevation of the right atrial (RA) pressure from massive pulmonary emboli in a 48-year-old chronic schizophrenic man (DCMEO #81-04-261) who died suddenly while hospitalized for gastrointestinal bleeding of undetermined cause. AD = anterior descending; Ao = aorta; IVC = inferior vena cava; LA = left atrium; LC = left circumflex artery; R = right coronary artery; RV = right ventricle.

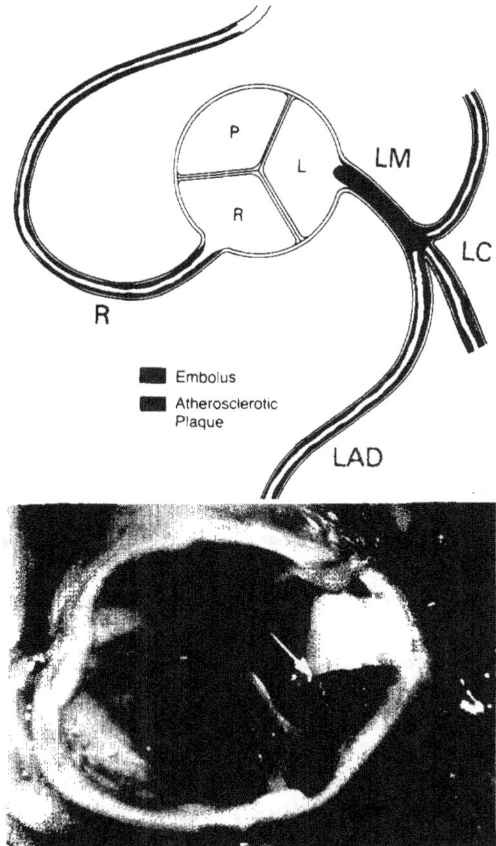

FIGURE 5. Left main (LM) coronary embolus in a 49 year old man (A70-205) who died during cardiac catheterization. **Top,** diagram of coronary tree with severe narrowing by atherosclerotic plaque of the left anterior descending (LAD), left circumflex (LC), and right (R) coronary arteries. **Bottom,** fibrin-platelet embolus (**arrow**) protruding from the ostium of the LM coronary artery. Aortic sinuses: L = left; P = posterior; R = right.

Embolus to the left main coronary artery is extremely rare, and no previous report has focused on fibrin-platelet emboli to this artery. One report[3] described a myocardial embolus to this artery. During the past 2 years, we studied 2 men, aged 37 and 48 years, who had fibrin-platelet emboli to the left main coronary artery, causing sudden death in each. In both, the major coronary arteries were essentially free of atherosclerotic plaque. The source of the embolus in 1 was unknown; in the second, the source was peripheral venous thrombi which crossed the atrial septum (paradoxic embolus) (Fig. 3 and 4). A third patient, a 49 year old woman studied in 1970, had an embolus to the left main coronary artery during left-sided cardiac catheterization[2,4] (Fig. 5). The latter patient had severe narrowing by atherosclerotic plaque of all the major epicardial coronary arteries.

Thus, embolus to the left main coronary artery is *rare* but usually *fatal*.

References

1. **Roberts WC, Buja LM.** The frequency and significance of coronary arterial thrombi and other observations in fatal acute myocardial infarction. A study of 107 necropsy patients. Am J Med 1972;52: 425–443.
2. **Roberts WC.** Coronary embolism: a review of causes, consequences, and diagnostic considerations. Cardiovasc Med 1978;3: 699–710.
3. **Loisance D, Aubry P, Heulin A, Di Matteo J.** Embolism of a fragment of the mitral papillary muscle to the left main coronary artery. A rare complication of valve replacement. Arch Mal Coeur 1979;72: 1029–1033.
4. **Cabin HS, Roberts WC.** Fatal cardiac arrest during cardiac catheterization for angina pectoris: analysis of 10 necropsy patients. Am J Cardiol 1981;48:1–7.

Quantitative Comparison of Extent of Coronary Narrowing and Size of Healed Myocardial Infarct in 33 Necropsy Patients With Clinically Recognized and in 28 With Clinically Unrecognized ("Silent") Previous Acute Myocardial Infarction

HENRY SCOTT CABIN, MD and WILLIAM C. ROBERTS, MD

Clinical and necropsy observations are described in 61 patients with a healed transmural myocardial infarction, 33 with and 28 without a clinical history of acute myocardial infarction. There were no significant differences between the 2 groups of patients in mean age, sex, or frequency of angina pectoris, chronic congestive heart failure, systemic hypertension, sudden coronary death, or fatal acute myocardial infarction. Compared with the patients with clinically recognized acute myocardial infarction, the patients with clinically unrecognized (silent) infarction had a significantly (p <0.05) higher incidence of diabetes mellitus (43 versus 15%), death from noncardiac causes (39 versus 9%), posterior (inferior) wall infarcts (82 versus 55%), and smaller infarcts (mean size 7 versus 17% of left ventricular wall). The patients with and without clinically recognized infarction had similar numbers of the 4 major coronary arteries severely (76 to 100% in cross-sectional area) narrowed (mean 2.8 versus 2.9/4.0 per patient), insignificant differences in incidence of severe narrowing of the left main coronary artery (18 versus 29%), similar overall percents of 5 mm segments of the 4 major coronary arteries severely narrowed (43 versus 42%), and similar percents of severely narrowed 5 mm segments of the right (46 versus 55%), left anterior descending (39 versus 33%), and left circumflex (41 versus 41%) coronary arteries.

Some patients with acute myocardial infarction have symptoms and signs indicative of coagulation necrosis of a portion of the left ventricular myocardial wall, and others apparently have no clinical manifestations caused by the myocardial necrosis, that is, the event is clinically silent. Indeed, possibly as many as 50% of acute myocardial infarcts are not recognized clinically.[1-11] Although several previous studies[1-11] have focused on clinically unrecognized acute myocardial infarction, none have compared at necropsy the degrees of coronary arterial narrowing and the extent of the myocardial damage in patients with clinically *recognized* versus those with clinically *unrecognized* acute myocardial infarction that healed. The present study compares the amount of coronary arterial narrowing and left ventricular myocardial scarring in 33 patients with a clinically unrecognized with that in 28 patients with a clinically recognized transmural acute myocardial infarct that healed.

Methods

Study patients: All 61 study patients had a healed transmural myocardial infarct defined as a left ventricular scar involving more than the inner one half of the thickness of the left ventricular wall at any point.[12] For each patient the medical records were reviewed in detail by at least one of us and the patients were divided into 2 groups according to the presence (33 patients) or absence (28 patients) of a clinical history of acute myocardial infarction. Patients were included in the clinically recognized myocardial infarction group (hereafter referred to as the recognized infarct group) if there was a record of hospitalization for acute myocardial infarction with subsequent confirmation of the diagnosis by established electrocardiographic and enzymatic criteria. All 33 patients

From the Pathology Branch, National Heart, Lung and Blood Institute, National Institutes of Health, Bethesda, Maryland.

Address for reprints: William C Roberts, MD, Building 10A, Room 3E30, National Institutes of Health, Bethesda, Maryland 20205.

TABLE I Clinical Findings in 33 Patients With Clinically Recognized and in 28 With Clinically Unrecognized Acute Myocardial Infarction (MI) and Healed Transmural Infarction at Necropsy

	Clinically Recognized Acute MI (33 Patients)		Clinically Unrecognized Acute MI (28 Patients)		p Value
	n	%	n	%	
Age (yr)					
Mean	61	. .	60	. . .	NS
Range	27–81	. . .	25–82	. . .	
Male:female ratio	25:8	. . .	21:7	. .	NS
Angina pectoris	14	42	6	21	NS
Chronic congestive heart failure	14	42	9	32	NS
Systemic hypertension	11	33	12	43	NS
Diabetes mellitus (adult onset)	5	15	12	43	<0.05
Mode of death					
Sudden	13	39	6	21	NS
Acute MI	8	24	7	25	NS
Chronic congestive heart failure	5	15	1	4	NS
Cardiac operation	2*	6	2†	7	NS
Cardiac catheterization	2	6	1	4	NS
Noncardiac	3	9	11	39	<0.01

* Coronary artery bypass grafting in 1 and left ventricular aneurysmectomy in 1.
† Coronary artery bypass grafting in both.

TABLE II Myocardial Infarct (MI) Size and Location in 33 Patients With and in 28 Without a Clinical History of Acute MI and a Healed Transmural MI at Necropsy

Clinical History of Acute MI	Patients (n)	MI Size (%)		Number of Patients With Major (Minor)* Involvement of Each Left Ventricular Wall by MI			
		Range	Mean	Anterior	Posterior	Septal	Lateral
+	33	1–55	17	16 (1)	15 (3)	1 (12)	1 (14)
0	28	1–23	7	5 (1)	22 (1)	1 (8)	0 (9)
p value	. .	<0.001		<0.01	<0.025	NS	NS

* For each patient, major involvement refers to the left ventricular wall with the most scarring and minor involvement refers to 1 or more additional walls with scarring. In all but 3 patients the anterior or posterior wall of left ventricle was the site of major involvement.

TABLE III Number of Major Epicardial Coronary Arteries (CA) Narrowed 76 to 100% in Cross-Sectional Area (XSA) by Atherosclerotic Plaque in 33 Patients With and 28 Without a History of Acute Myocardial Infarction (MI) and a Healed Transmural MI at Necropsy

Clinical History Acute MI	Patients (n)	Total CA (n)	Patients With CA Narrowed 76–100% in XSA										Mean CA per Patient Narrowed 76–100%
			LM		LAD		LC		R		Totals		
			n	%	n	%	n	%	n	%	n	%	
+	33	132	6	18	32	97	23	70	32	97	93	70	2.8
0	28	112	8	29	24	86	21	75	28	100	81	72	2.9
p value	. . .	. .		NS		NS		NS		NS		NS	NS

LAD = left anterior descending; LC = left circumflex; LM = left main; R = right.

had prolonged chest pain at rest. Patients were included in the clinically unrecognized acute myocardial infarction group (hereafter referred to as the unrecognized infarct group) if detailed medical records were available and there was no report of hospitalization for acute myocardial infarction or record of unstable angina pectoris, prolonged chest pain at rest, acute worsening of congestive heart failure or syncope (except within the final 2 months of life). In the patients with unrecognized acute myocardial infarction, electrocardiograms never indicated a pattern consistent with acute myocardial infarction except in the 7 (of 28) patients in whom this event was fatal; all 28 patients, of course, had transmural left ventricular scars. Patients with an equivocal or inadequate history

were excluded as were patients with symptoms suggestive of acute myocardial infarction who did not seek hospitalization or who were hospitalized but did not have laboratory confirmation of the diagnosis of acute infarction.

Pathologic examination: In each patient, the heart was cut into 5 or 6 one cm thick transverse ventricular slices from apex to base parallel to the posterior atrioventricular sulcus. The major location of the infarct was determined by identifying the portion of left ventricular wall with the greatest amount of scar. When the infarct was circumferential at the apex, the basal portion of the heart was used to determine the predominant location of the infarct. In all but 3 of the 61 patients the infarct was located predominantly in the anterior or posterior wall with or without involvement of the ventricular septum or lateral wall (defined as that portion of left ventricular wall between the lateral borders of the anterolateral and posteromedial papillary muscles).

The percent of myocardium replaced by scar was determined by tracing the grossly visible areas of scar and the total left ventricular area including ventricular septum (with compensation for wall thinning in areas of scar) from photographs of the apical surfaces of each transverse ventricular slice. The area of scar and the total left ventricular area were then determined by a videoplanimetry system. The sum of the areas of scarring divided by the sum of the left ventricular areas provided the infarct size expressed as a percent of total left ventricular area.

In each of the 61 patients, the entire lengths of the right, left main, left anterior descending, and left circumflex coronary arteries were removed from the heart intact, fixed in an unpressurized state in 10% formalin for about 48 hours, radiographed, and if calcific deposits were present, decalcified. Then each of the 4 major arteries was cut transversely into 5 mm long segments, processed in alcohol and xylene and cut. At least one 6 μm thick section from each 5 mm segment was prepared for histologic study and stained by the Movat method.[13] The degree of luminal narrowing in each 5 mm long segment was determined by microscopic examination at a magnification of 25 to 50 times. The percent of cross-sectional area narrowing by atherosclerotic plaque was divided into 5 categories of narrowing: 0 to 25, 26 to 50, 51 to 75, 76 to 95, and 96 to 100. The accuracy of these determinations was verified by videoplanimetry and shown to have an error of less than 5 percent.[14]

Statistical analysis: The unpaired and paired Student's *t* test was employed for the quantitative comparisons of coronary narrowing. Chi-square analysis was utilized for comparison of clinical variables and for comparison of amounts of coronary narrowing by qualitative means.

Results

Clinical findings (Table I): Angina pectoris occurred in 14 (42%) of the 33 patients in the recognized infarct group (after the infarct in each) and in 6 (21%) of the 28 patients in the unrecognized infarct group (p <0.10). Diabetes mellitus of adult onset occurred more frequently in the unrecognized than in the recognized infarct group (12 [43%] versus 5 [15%]) (p <0.05). Among the 17 patients with diabetes mellitus, angina pectoris was present in 4 of the 12 patients with clinically unrecognized infarcts and in 2 of the 5 patients with recognized infarcts. Death from noncardiac causes occurred more often in the unrecognized infarct group (11 [39%] versus 3 [9%]) (p <0.01).

Location and size of infarct (Table II): The predominant location of the healed myocardial infarct was the anterior wall of the left ventricle in 16 (48%) of 33 patients from the recognized infarct group and in 5 (18%) of 28 from the unrecognized infarct group (p <0.01); posterior wall in 15 (45%) and 22 (79%), respectively (p <0.025); lateral wall in 1 (3%) and none, respectively (p = NS); and ventriculum septum in 1 (3%) and 1 (4%), respectively (p = NS). The percent of left ventricular myocardium (including ventricular septum) infarcted ranged from 1 to 55 (mean 17) in the recognized infarct group and from 1 to 23 (mean 7) in the unrecognized infarct group (p <0.001).

TABLE IV Number of 33 Patients With and 28 Without a Clinical History of Acute Myocardial Infarction (MI) and a Healed Transmural MI at Necropsy with 0 to 4 of 4 Major Coronary Arteries (CA) Narrowed 76 to 100% in Cross-Sectional Area (XSA) by Atherosclerotic Plaque

CA (n) Narrowed 76–100% in XSA	Clinical History of Acute MI				p Value
	+		0		
	n	%	n	%	
4	5	15	5	18	NS
3	20	61	17	61	NS
2	7	21	4	14	NS
1	1	3	2	7	NS
0	0		0		NS
Totals	33	100	28	100	

Incidence of severe coronary narrowing (Tables III and IV): Of the 132 major (right, left main, left anterior descending, and left circumflex) epicardial coronary arteries examined in the 33 patients in the recognized infarct group, at least one 5 mm segment in 93 (70%) arteries was narrowed severely (76 to 100% in cross-sectional area) by atherosclerotic plaques, an average of 2.8 of 4.0 coronary arteries per patient; of the 112 major coronary arteries examined in the 28 patients in the unrecognized infarct group, 81 (72%) were so narrowed, an average of 2.9 of 4.0 coronary arteries per patient (p = NS). No significant difference was observed in the numbers of patients with severe narrowing of any of the 4 major arteries, or in the numbers of patients with 0 to 4 of the 4 major coronary arteries severely narrowed.

Quantitative analysis of amount of narrowing in 2,705 five mm long segments of the right, left anterior descending, and left circumflex coronary arteries (Fig. 1 and 2): Of the 1,443 five mm segments in the 33 patients in the recognized infarct group, 167 (12%) were narrowed 96 to 100% in cross-sectional area by atherosclerotic plaque; 444 (30%) were narrowed 76 to 95%; 519 (36%), 51 to 75%; 230 (16%), 26 to 50%; and 84 (6%), 0 to 25%. Of the 1,262 five mm segments of coronary artery in the 28 patients in the unrecognized infarct group, 91 (7%) were narrowed 96 to 100%; 461 (36%) were narrowed 76 to 95%; 374 (30%), 51 to 75%; 197 (16%), 26 to 50%; and 139 (11%), 0 to 25% (Fig. 1). There was no significant difference between the 2 groups in any of the 5 categories of cross-sectional area narrowing.

Within the recognized infarct group there was no significant difference in the percent of 5 mm segments of coronary artery with severe narrowing among the left anterior descending, left circumflex, or right coronary arteries (39, 41, and 46%, respectively) (Fig. 2). In the unrecognized infarct group, however, the right coronary artery had a significantly greater percent of 5 mm segments narrowed severely than the left anterior descending (p <0.02) and left circumflex coronary arteries (p <0.03) (55, 33, and 41%, respectively). There was no significant difference between the 2 groups in the per-

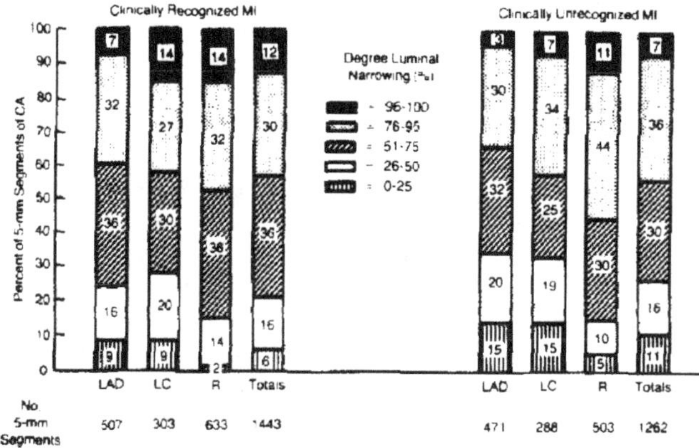

FIGURE 1. Percent of 5 mm segments of the right (R), left anterior descending (LAD), and left circumflex (LC) coronary arteries (CA) narrowed to various degrees by atherosclerotic plaque in 33 patients with clinically recognized and in 28 patients with clinically unrecognized acute myocardial infarction (MI) and healed transmural infarction at necropsy.

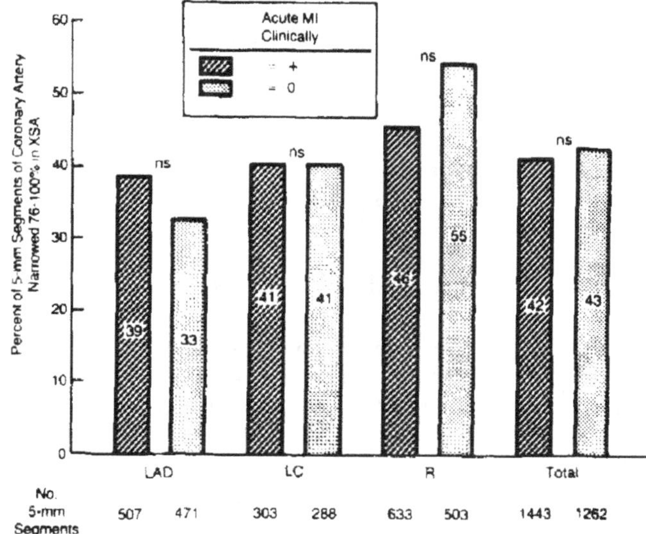

FIGURE 2. Percent of 5 mm segments of the right (R), left anterior descending (LAD), and left circumflex (LC) coronary arteries narrowed 76 to 100% in cross-sectional area (XSA) by atherosclerotic plaque in 33 patients with and in 28 patients without a clinical history of acute myocardial infarction (MI) and a healed transmural infarction at necropsy.

cent of 5 mm segments narrowed severely in each of the 3 major coronary arteries.

A scoring system was utilized to indicate both the severity and extent of coronary narrowing. Every 5 mm long segment of coronary artery from each patient was assigned a score of 1 to 4 based on the amount of cross-sectional area narrowing by atherosclerotic plaque as follows: 1 = 0 to 25% narrowing; 2 = 26% to 50%; 3 = 51 to 75%; and 4 = 76 to 100%. A total score was obtained for each patient and the score per 5 mm segment was then calculated by dividing the total score per patient by the number of 5 mm segments examined from the patient. The scores per 5 mm segment ranged from 1.8 to 3.9 (mean 3.2) in the recognized infarct group and from 1.9 to 3.7 (mean 3.1) in the unrecognized infarct group (p = NS).

Comments

Considerable controversy exists regarding the incidence and, in fact, the very existence of the entity that has been variously referred to as *unrecognized silent, undiagnosed, painless, asymptomatic,* or *inapparent* myocardial infarction. Some investigators[11,15] have suggested that a careful history taken within a short time of the acute myocardial infarct from a "... nonpsychotic, nonsenile, and nonmedicated ..." individual will always disclose some symptom that in retrospect indicates that infarction had occurred. Necropsy studies have been particularly questioned because of the utilization of historic material obtained by nonprimary physicians who usually had not carefully questioned the patient about symptoms referable to the cardiovascular system.

Because of these difficulties, in the present analysis necropsy patients with healed transmural myocardial infarct were divided into clinically recognized and clinically unrecognized infarct groups by asking the question: was there a clinical history of hospitalization for suspected acute myocardial infarction with subsequent laboratory confirmation? Patients in whom this was the case were included in the recognized infarct group. The history of the remaining patients was further analyzed to exclude from the unrecognized infarct group those patients who reported some clinical event with or without hospitalization (such as change in pattern of chest pain, or acute worsening of congestive heart failure or syncope) that occurred more than 2 months before death that might have represented an atypical yet symptomatic acute myocardial infarction. Obviously, the latter analysis is still subject to variability in history-taking and history-giving abilities, patient recall, and variability in a patient's symptom threshold and does not exclude the stoic patient who for whatever reason does not report his symptoms or seek hospitalization. With these reservations in mind and by excluding all patients with an equivocal or inadequate history, we believe it valid to determine whether the 2 groups of patients just defined differed in clinical or necropsy findings, with particular emphasis on infarct size and location and amount and extent of coronary narrowing.

Clinical differences between clinically recognized and unrecognized infarct group: Previous studies have suggested that patients with clinically unrecognized compared with those with clinically recognized acute myocardial infarction have angina pectoris less frequently and that patients with angina pectoris rarely have clinically unrecognized infarcts.[2,3,5–7] In the present study, 21% of the patients in the unrecognized infarct group had typical angina pectoris compared with 42% of those in the recognized infarct group. This difference approached but did not achieve statistical significance (0.05 <p <0.10). In addition, the incidence of fatal acute myocardial infarction was similar in both groups (25 and 24%, respectively). Thus, patients with a clinically unrecognized acute myocardial infarction that healed had an incidence of symptomatic myocardial ischemic events (fatal acute infarction or angina pectoris) which did not differ significantly from that in patients in whom the acute myocardial infarction was clinically recognized.

Some [5,7,16,17] but not all [2] investigators have reported an association between diabetes mellitus and clinically unrecognized or painless acute myocardial infarction. The present study supports that relationship by showing a significantly increased incidence of diabetes mellitus among the patients in the unrecognized infarct group (43%) compared with those in the recognized infarct group (15%).

Differences in location and extent of infarction: Johnson et al. [2] reported that subendocardial infarcts were less often clinically recognized than transmural infarcts. In addition, they found that among patients with subendocardial infarcts, those in the lateral and posterior walls of the left ventricle were less often recognized than those involving the anterior wall, and among patients with transmural infarcts, those in the lateral wall were less often clinically recognized than those in the anterior or posterior walls. These results are difficult to compare with those in the present study because of differing definitions of the terms *subendocardial* and *transmural* and differing methods of describing infarct locations. The present study includes only patients with healed transmural myocardial infarcts (involving greater than 50% of the thickness of the left ventricular wall at any point), which includes many patients who according to the definitions used by Johnson et al. [2] would be considered to have subendocardial infarcts (involving "... predominantly [*but not exclusively*] the endocardial half of the left ventricle"). In our necropsy experience, healed myocardial infarction limited to the endocardial half of the left ventricular wall is unusual, and if the infarct involves any portion of the epicardial half of the wall in addition to involvement of the subendocardial half, we consider it transmural. In addition, all but 3 of our 61 patients had infarction predominantly involving the anterior or posterior wall of the left ventricle with or without involvement of the lateral wall or the ventricular septum. Anterior wall infarction was significantly more common in the patients with recognized than unrecognized infarcts (48 versus 18%), while posterior wall infarction was more common in patients with unrecognized than in those with recognized infarcts (79 versus 45%). Among patients with clinically recognized infarction, the incidence of anteriorly and posteriorly located infarcts was similar (48 and 45%), while among those with clinically unrecognized infarction, posteriorly located scars were far more common than anteriorly located scars (79 versus 18%).

The size of the myocardial infarct in patients with unrecognized versus those with recognized infarct has not been previously reported. The mean percentage of left ventricular wall replaced by scar was significantly

smaller in our patients with unrecognized than in those with recognized infarction (7 versus 17%).

Severity and extent of coronary artery narrowing: The amount and extent of coronary narrowing by atherosclerotic plaque in the entire lengths of the 4 major epicardial coronary arteries were examined qualitatively and quantitatively in all 61 patients, and no significant difference between the 2 study groups was observed. The patients with unrecognized or recognized infarcts had a similar mean number of coronary arteries narrowed severely (76 to 100% in cross-sectional area) (2.9 versus 2.8 of 4.0), a similar incidence of severe narrowing of the left main coronary artery (29 versus 18%), a similar overall percent of severely narrowed 5 mm coronary segments (43 versus 42%), and a similar percent of severely narrowed 5 mm segments of the left anterior descending, left circumflex, and right coronary arteries. To our knowledge, this information on clinically unrecognized infarct patients is not available elsewhere.

In summary, our necropsy patients with clinically unrecognized compared with those with clinically recognized healed transmural infarcts had similar incidences of angina pectoris and fatal acute myocardial infarction and higher incidences of diabetes mellitus and noncardiac causes of death, smaller infarcts more often located in the posterior wall of left ventricle, and similarly severe and extensive coronary narrowing by atherosclerotic plaque.

References

1. **Roseman MD.** Painless myocardial infarction: a review of the literature and analysis of 220 cases Ann Intern Med 1954;41:1–8
2. **Johnson WJ, Achor RWP, Burchell HB, Edwards JE.** Unrecognized myocardial infarction A clinicopathologic study Arch Intern Med 1959;103. 253–261
3. **Stokes J III, Dawber JR.** The "silent coronary" the frequency and clinical characteristics of unrecognized myocardial infarction in the Framingham study Ann Intern Med 1959;50 1359–1369
4. **Lindberg HA, Berkson DM, Stamler J, Poindexter A.** Totally asymptomatic myocardial infarction: an estimate of its incidence in the living population Arch Intern Med 1960, 5.628–633
5. **Melichar F, Jedlicka V, Havlik L.** A study of undiagnosed myocardial infarctions Acta Med Scand 1963;174 761–768
6. **Kannel WB, McNamara PM, Feinleib M, Dawber TR.** The unrecognized myocardial infarction. Fourteen-year follow-up experience in the Framingham study Geriatrics 1970;25.75–87
7. **Margolis JR, Kannel WB, Feinbeib M, Dawber TR, McNamara PM.** Clinical features of unrecognized myocardial infarction—silent and symptomatic Eighteen year follow-up the Framingham study Am J Cardiol 1973;32 1–7
8. **Medalie JH, Goldbourt U.** Unrecognized myocardial infarction: five-year incidence, mortality, and risk factors Ann Intern Med 1976;84:526–531.
9. **Kannel WB, Sorlie P, McNamara PM.** Prognosis after initial myocardial infarction: the Framingham study Am J Cardiol 1979;44:53–59
10. **Rosenman RH, Friedman M, Jenkins CD, Straus R, Wurm M, Kositchek R.** Clinically unrecognized myocardial infarction in the Western collaborative group study Am J Cardiol 1967,19 776–782.
11. **Schweizer W.** Silent myocardial infarction. Geriatrics 1968;23.96–98.
12. **Roberts WC, Gardin JM.** Location of myocardial infarcts· a confusion of terms and definitions Am J Cardiol 1978;42 868–872
13. **Movat HZ.** Demonstration of all connective tissue elements in a single section: pentachrome stains Arch Pathol 1955;60:289–295
14. **Isner JM, Wu M, Virmani R, Jones AA, Roberts WC.** Comparison of degrees of coronary arterial luminal narrowing determined by visual inspection of histologic sections under magnification among three independent observers and comparison to that obtained by video planimetry an analysis of 559 five-mm segments of 61 coronary arteries from eleven patients Lab Invest 1980,42:566–570
15. **Halberstam MJ.** Sharpening your ears for "silent" MIs. Mod Med 1980; 48:62–68.
16. **Bradley RF, Schonfeld A.** Diminished pain in diabetic patients with acute myocardial infarction. Geriatrics 1962;17 322–326.
17. **Faerman I, Faccio E, Milei J, Nunez R, Jadzinsky M, Fox D, Rapaport M.** Autonomic neuropathy and painless myocardial infarction in diabetic patients Histologic evidence of their relationship Diabetes 1977;26: 1147–1158

Status of the Major Epicardial Coronary Arteries 80 to 150 Days After Percutaneous Transluminal Coronary Angioplasty

Analysis of 3 Necropsy Patients

BRUCE F. WALLER, MD, BRUCE M. McMANUS, MD, PhD, H. JOEL GORFINKEL, MD, JOAN C. KISHEL, MD, EDWARD C. H. SCHMIDT, MD, KENNETH M. KENT, MD, and WILLIAM C. ROBERTS, MD

Certain clinical and necropsy cardiac findings are described in 3 men who had percutaneous transluminal coronary angioplasty (PTCA) of the left anterior descending (LAD) coronary artery 80, 90, and 150 days before sudden death. Each patient had a decrease in the mean transstenotic coronary gradient (17, 38, and 43 mm Hg) and an angiographic increase in the LAD luminal diameter (55, 60, and 65%). At necropsy, the LAD coronary artery in the area of the PTCA in each patient was narrowed 76 to 95% in cross-sectional area by atherosclerotic plaques. No cracks in plaques or other lesions which may have resulted from the PTCA procedure were identified histologically in the LAD coronary artery of any patient.

Several studies have described morphologic changes early ($\leq$60 days) in coronary arteries in humans[1-3] and in animals[4-6] after PTCA. Although several reports[7-10] have described angiographic appearances of coronary arteries late (>60 days) after PTCA, morphologic observations have not been reported in coronary arteries subjected to PTCA >60 days before death. In this report, clinical and necropsy cardiac findings are described in 3 men who died suddenly 80, 90, and 150 days, respectively, after PTCA.

Patients Studied

Clinical observations: Each patient had exertional angina pectoris for only 1 to 2 months before PTCA. Coronary angiography and PTCA performed 80, 90, and 150 days, respectively, before death disclosed severe (76 to 95% diameter reduction) luminal narrowing of the LAD coronary artery and insignificant (<50% diameter reduction) narrowing of the left main, left circumflex, and right coronary arteries (Table I, Fig. 1 to 3). At PTCA, the LAD in each patient was dilated 55, 60, and 65%, respectively (Table I), and the mean coronary pressure gradient fell 17, 38, and 43 mm Hg, respectively, in the 3 patients. Exercise treadmill testing in each patient 1 to 11 days after PTCA disclosed electrocardiographic changes of J point depression in 2 patients (Patients 2 and 3) and no changes in the third patient. No patient developed angina pectoris during or within an hour of the exercise test.

Angina pectoris did not recur after PTCA in Patients 1 and 2. Patient 3 remained pain-free for the first 105 days after PTCA, but during the last 45 days he had 3 episodes of mild exertional angina relieved promptly by nitroglycerin. After PTCA, all 3 patients thereafter received long-term administration of dipyridamole; 2 (Patients 1 and 2) received salicylates; 2 (Patients 2 and 3) received isosorbide dinitrate; and 1 patient each received verapamil (Patient 1) and nifedipine (Patient 2). Two patients (Patients 2 and 3) died suddenly at home or work without apparent chest pain. Patient 1 was killed during an automobile accident while intoxicated (alcohol).

Morphologic observations: At necropsy, no foci of myocardial fibrosis or necrosis were present. In all 3 patients, the 4 major epicardial coronary arteries were excised from the heart and cut transversely into 5-mm segments; a Movat-stained histologic section was prepared from each segment and examined. The results of the quantitative studies, representing the consensus of 3 observers (BFW, BMM, JCK), are summarized in Figure 4.

From the Pathology and Cardiology Branches, the National Heart, Lung, and Blood Institute, National Institutes of Health, Bethesda, Maryland; the Department of Medicine (Cardiology), Mt. Carmel Medical Center, Columbus, Ohio; and the Department of Pathology, Memorial Hospital, Easton, Maryland. Manuscript received July 16, 1982, accepted July 16, 1982.

Address for reprints: William C. Roberts, MD, Building 10A, Room 3E-30, National Institutes of Health, Bethesda, Maryland 20205.

TABLE I Observations In 3 Necropsy Men Who Died >60 Days After Percutaneous Transluminal Coronary Angioplasty (PTCA)

Observation	Patient 1	Patient 2	Patient 3
Age (yr) at death	33	48	57
Systemic pressure (mm Hg)	135/90	110/80	150/90
Interval (days) from PTCA to death	80	90	150
Maximal coronary narrowing by angiography (% diameter reduction)			
LM	0	0	0
LAD	80	85	85
LC	≤50	≤25	≤25
R	≤50	0	≤25
Change (% diameter reduction) in LAD	80 → 25	85 → 25	85 → 20
Mean intracoronary pressure (mm Hg) before → after dilation			
Proximal	104 → 85	. . .	80 → 80
Distal	52 → 50	. . .	25 → 68
Gradient	52 → 35	50 → 12	55 → 12
Maximal coronary narrowing at necropsy (% cross-sectional area)			
LM	26–50	0–25	0–25
LAD	76–95	76–95	76–95
LC	76–95	26–50	51–75
R	76–95	76–95	51–75
Cororary narrowing at necropsy at site of PTCA (% cross-sectional area)	76–95	76–95	75–95
Heart weight (g)	450	490	415

LAD = left anterior descending; LC = left circumflex; LM = left main; R = right.

The site of the PTCA was determined from the area of maximal diameter reduction on the pre-PTCA coronary angiogram (Fig. 1). The catheter diameter just proximal to its tip was measured (in millimeters) on a black and white glossy print of 1 frame of the cineangiogram. A right anterior oblique angiographic view was used to view the bifurcation of the LAD and left circumflex coronary arteries. A magnification correction factor was determined by dividing the angiographic catheter diameter by the actual catheter diameter (provided by the manufacturer). The angiographic distance (in millimeters) from the origin of the LAD from the left main coronary artery to the site of maximal diameter reduction was measured. To locate this area of the LAD at necropsy, the distance measured on the angiogram was divided by the magnification correction factor. The LAD length was then measured at necropsy starting at the origin of the LAD from the left main coronary artery. The 5-mm coronary artery segment containing this area was recorded.

In each patient, at least 1 of the 4 major coronary arteries was narrowed 76 to 95% in cross-sectional area by atherosclerotic plaques: the LAD in all 3 patients, the right in Patients 1 and 2, and the left circumflex in Patient 1. The site of the PTCA in the LAD coronary artery in each patient was narrowed 76 to 95% in cross-sectional area by atherosclerotic plaque. The 5-mm segment of LAD containing the site of PTCA in each patient was serially sectioned at 10 μm intervals; every fifth section was stained. A total of 72 histologic sections in the area of PTCA was examined (26 in Patient 1, 34 in Patient 2, and 12 in Patient 3). Of the total 153 5-mm coronary segments from the 3 patients, none was narrowed 96 to 100%, 14 (9%) were narrowed 76 to 95%, and 34 (22%) were narrowed 51 to 75% in cross-sectional area by athero-

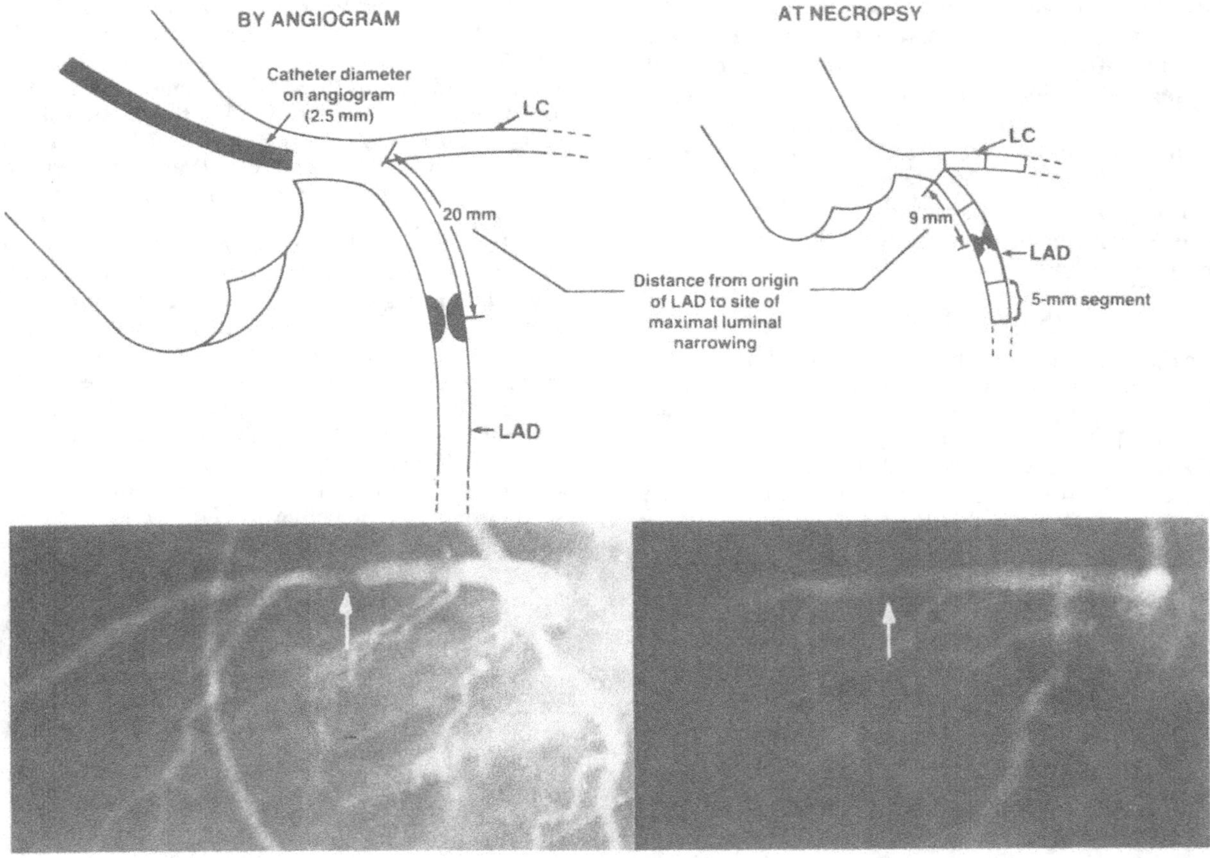

FIGURE 1. Patient 1. **Top panel,** diagram illustrating method of determining at necropsy the site of PTCA during life. **Bottom panels,** frames of coronary angiogram showing an increase in diameter of the left anterior descending (LAD) artery after PTCA (**arrows**). LC = left circumflex coronary artery.

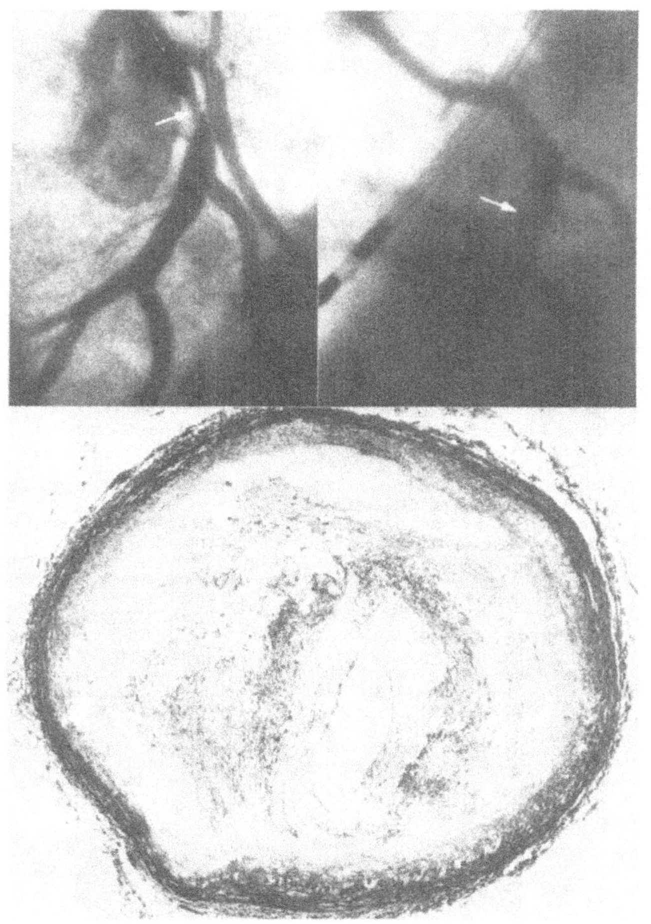
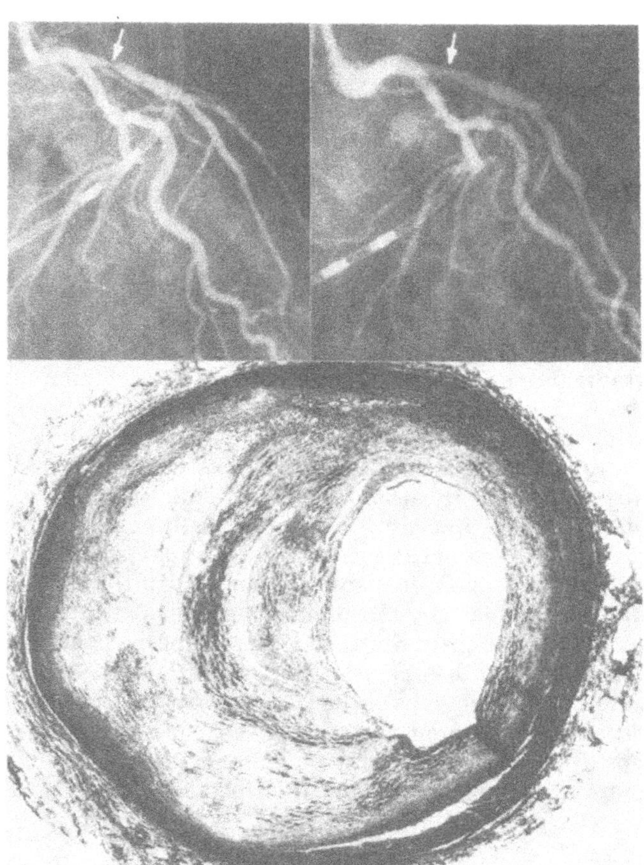

FIGURE 2. Patient 2. **Top panels,** frames of coronary angiogram 90 days before death showing an increase in diameter of the LAD artery after PTCA (**arrows**). **Bottom panel,** histologic section of the LAD artery at the site of previous PTCA procedure, showing severe luminal narrowing by atherosclerotic plaque (Movat stain; magnification X22).

FIGURE 3. Patient 3. **Top panels,** frames of coronary angiogram 150 days before death showing an increase in diameter of the LAD artery after PTCA (**arrows**). **Bottom panel,** histologic section of the LAD artery at the site of a previous PTCA procedure, showing severe luminal narrowing by atherosclerotic plaque (Movat stain; magnification X23).

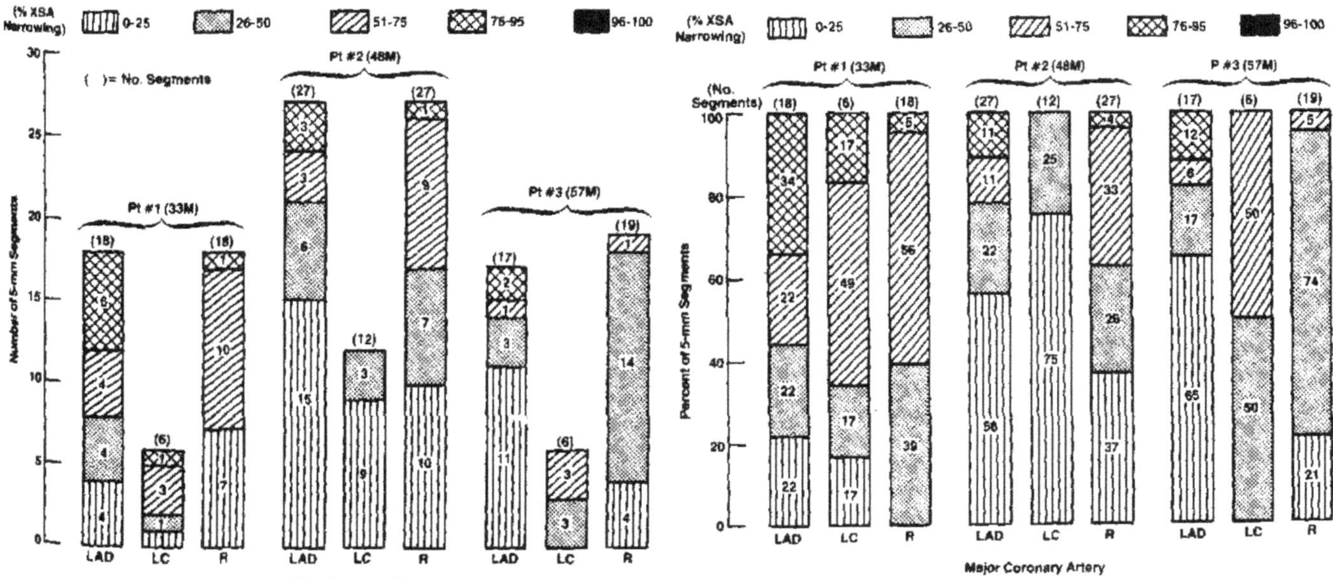

FIGURE 4. Number (**left panel**) and percent (**right panel**) of 5-mm segments of the LAD, left circumflex (LC), and right (R) coronary arteries narrowed to various degrees in cross-sectional area (XSA) by atherosclerotic plaques in the 3 necropsy patients.

sclerotic plaques (Fig. 4). In each patient, the LAD coronary artery had the most segments narrowed 76 to 95%: 6 of 8 in Patient 1, 3 of 4 in Patient 2, and 2 of 2 in Patient 3. Histologic assessment of the atherosclerotic plaque in the area of the PTCA compared with other areas of atherosclerotic plaque in the same artery or other coronary arteries in the same patient disclosed no distinctive morphologic difference.

Comments

The 3 men described above had PTCA of the LAD coronary artery 80, 90, and 150 days before death; each had a decrease in the mean transstenotic coronary gradient and an angiographic increase in the lumen of the LAD coronary artery. Only 1 had angina pectoris after the PTCA procedure, and each died suddenly. At necropsy, each patient had 76 to 95% cross-sectional area narrowing by atherosclerotic plaques in the area of the PTCA procedure. Despite examination of numerous sections of the coronary artery, histologic study of the atherosclerotic plaques in the area of the PTCA did not disclose any morphologic lesions attributable to the PTCA procedure. Indeed, comparison of the composition of the plaques at the site of the PTCA with plaques in other areas of the LAD and with those in the other major coronary arteries in the same patient did not disclose any distinctive differences. While splits, tears, and breaks have been described histologically in coronary arteries of humans and in animals immediately after the PTCA procedure,[1-6] these distinctive morphologic lesions were not recognized late in our 3 patients.

References

1. **Lee G, Ikeda RM, Joye JA, Bogren HG, DeMaria AN, Mason DT.** Evaluation of transluminal angioplasty of chronic coronary artery stenosis. Value and limitations assessed in fresh human cadaver hearts. Circulation 1980; 61:77–83.
2. **Block PC, Myler PK, Stertzer S, Fallon JT.** Morphology after transluminal angioplasty in human beings. N Engl J Med 1981;305:382–385.
3. **Baughman KL, Pasternak RC, Fallon JT, Block PC.** Transluminal coronary angioplasty of postmortem human hearts. Am J Cardiol 1981;48:1044–1047.
4. **Block PC.** Histological and ultrastructural studies in animals. In: Proceedings of the Workshop on Percutaneous Transluminal Coronary Angioplasty. Hyattsville, MD: DHEW publication no. (NIH)80–2030, March 1980:155–156.
5. **Block PC, Baughman KL, Pasternak RC, Fallon JT.** Transluminal angioplasty: correlation of morphologic and angiographic findings in an experimental model. Circulation 1980;61:778–785.
6. **Block PC, Fallon JT, Elmer D.** Experimental angioplasty: lessons from the laboratory. Am J Radiol 1980;135:907–912.
7. **Gruntzig AR, Senning A, Siegenthaler WE.** Nonoperative dilatation of coronary artery stenosis. N Engl J Med 1979;301:61–68.
8. **Cowley MJ, Vetrovec GW, Wolfgang TC.** Efficacy of percutaneous transluminal angioplasty: technique, patient selection, salutary results, limitations and complications. Am Heart J 1981;101:272–280.
9. **Kent KM, Bonow RD, Rosing DR, Ewels CJ, Lipson LC, McIntosh CL, Bacharach S, Green M, Epstein SE.** Improved myocardial function during exercise after successful percutaneous transluminal angioplasty. N Engl J Med 1982;306:441–446.
10. **Kent KM, Bentivoglio LG, Block PC, Cowley MJ, Dorros G, Gosselin AJ, Gruntzig A, Myler RK, Simpson J, Stertzer SH, Williams DO, Fisher L, Gillespie MJ, Detre K, Kelsey S, Mullin SM, Mock MB.** Percutaneous transluminal coronary angioplasty: report from the registry of the National Heart, Lung, and Blood Institute. Am J Cardiol 1982;49:2011–2020.

Cardiovascular Disease in the Very Elderly

Analysis of 40 Necropsy Patients Aged 90 Years or Over

BRUCE F. WALLER, MD and WILLIAM C. ROBERTS, MD

Clinical and necropsy observations are described in 40 patients (29 women) aged 90 years and older. The majority (21 patients [57%]) died during the 4 coldest months, and 12 (30%), during the 4 warmest months. At necropsy, 39 had ≥1 major cardiac abnormalities, the most frequent being calcific deposits in the major epicardial coronary arteries in 37 (92%). In 28 patients (70%), 1 or more of the 4 major arteries was narrowed 76 to 100% in cross-sectional area (XSA) by atherosclerotic plaques, an average of 1.9/4.0 per patient: the 12 patients with clinical events compatible with myocardial ischemia (angina pectoris or myocardial infarction) had an average of 2.2/4 and the other 28 patients an average of 1.0/4.0. In 36 patients, a histologic section was examined from each 5 mm long segment from each of the 4 major coronary arteries: of the 1,789 segments, only 6 (<1%) were narrowed 96 to 100% in XSA by plaques; 147 (8%), 76 to 95%; 339 (19%), 51 to 75%; 930 (52%), 26 to 50%, and 367 (21%), 0 to 25%. The average amount of XSA narrowing for the 1,789 segments was about 42%. In 10 patients with clinical evidence of myocardial ischemia, the average amount of narrowing per segment was approximately 55%; in the 26 patients without clinical ischemia, the average was about 38%. Of the 40 patients, 18 (45%) had left ventricular transmural foci of fibrosis or necrosis or both. Of 14 patients with transmural scars, only 1 had a clinical event compatible with acute myocardial infarction; of the 10 with acute myocardial infarction at necropsy, only 4 had typical clinical features of infarction.

Calcific deposits were present in ≥1 aortic valve cusps in 22 patients (55%), causing aortic valve stenosis in 2, and in the mitral anulus in 19 (47%), probably causing mitral valve stenosis in 1.

Amyloid deposits were present in the heart in at least 9 patients; they were grossly visible and caused fatal cardiac dysfunction in 4, and microscopically visible only in 5, causing no cardiac dysfunction. Eight patients (20%) had chronic congestive heart failure; 27 of 39 (69%) had either a history of systemic hypertension or blood pressure >140/90 mm Hg during their final year of life. Precordial murmurs were recorded in 25 (62%) patients—systolic only in 24 and both systolic and diastolic in 1. Data from electrocardiograms were available in 30 patients: 12 (40%) had atrial fibrillation; 12 (40%), abnormal axis; 12, complete bundle branch block; 1, criteria for left ventricular hypertrophy (despite increased cardiac mass in 67%); and 1, low voltage.

All patients had fairly extensive atherosclerosis of the aorta, with aneurysmal formation in 5 with fatal rupture in 3. Five had strokes, which were fatal in 4. At least 5 had leg claudication. Two had massive pulmonary emboli superimposed on chronic obstructive pulmonary disease.

Thus, cardiovascular disease was present at necropsy in 39 of our 40 patients, but frequently it was not diagnosed clinically.

Although the average age at death has increased dramatically during this century, the maximal length of life has not changed.[1] The percentage of individuals surviving for 90 years and beyond, however, is increasing.[2] In 1980, about 1% of the population in the United States was aged 90 years or older.[2] Very few necropsies are performed in patients dying after age 90 years (frequency about 4%)[3] and, therefore, little attention has been focused on the clinical and morphologic frequencies and types of cardiovascular disease observed in these very elderly persons. This report describes the types of cardiovascular disease found at necropsy in 40 patients aged 90 years or over.

Patients

General observations: Clinical and morphologic observations in the 40 patients are detailed in Table I. The patients died and underwent necropsy at 12 different hospitals (10 in the Washington, D.C. area [37 patients]); subsequently the heart and frequently the aortas were examined in all 40 patients by 1 of us (WCR). The year of death in 37 patients was between

From the Pathology Branch, National Heart, Lung, and Blood Institute, National Institutes of Health, Bethesda, Maryland. Manuscript received and accepted September 24, 1982.

Address for reprints: William C. Roberts, MD, Building 10A, Room 3E-30, National Institutes of Health, Bethesda, Maryland 20205.

TABLE I   Clinical and Morphologic Observations in 40 Necropsy Patients Aged 90 to 103 Years

Case	Age (yr) & Sex	Race	CP	AP	AMI	AD	CCHF	DM	Hx SH	SAP (mm Hg)	S	AF	BBB R	BBB L	QRS Axis R	QRS Axis L	TC (mg/100 ml)
1	90F	W	+	0	+	0	0	0	+	145/70	0	+	0	+	0	+	—
2	90F	W	+	+	+	0	0	+	0	120/80	0	0	—	—	—	—	—
3	90M	B	+	0	+	+	0	0	+	140/70	0	+	0	+	0	0	236
4	90M	B	0	0	0	+	+	0	0	110/70	0	+	0	+	0	+	250
5	90F	W	+	0	+	+	0	+	+	118/80	0	+	0	+	0	0	—
6	90F	W	0	0	0	0	0	0	0	118/70	0	0	0	0	0	0	—
7	90F	W	0	0	0	0	0	0	+	170/90	0	0	0	0	0	0	223
8	90F	W	0	0	0	0	0	0	+	80/60	0	0	0	0	0	0	—
9	91F	B	0	0	0	0	0	+	+	84/—	0	0	0	0	0	0	—
10	91M	B	0	0	0	0	0	0	+	140/90	0	+	0	0	0	0	—
11	91F	B	0	0	0	0	0	0	+	95/60	0	0	0	0	0	0	—
12	91M	W	0	0	0	0	0	0	+	116/85	+	+	0	0	0	0	—
13	91F	W	+	0	+	+	0	0	+	120/60	0	—	—	—	—	—	283
14	92F	W	+	+	0	+	+	0	0	110/70	0	+	+	0	+	0	—
15	92F	W	0	0	0	0	0	0	+	230/110	0	0	0	0	0	+	—
16	92F	W	+	0	+	0	0	0	0	...	0	—	—	—	—	—	—
17	92F	W	0	0	0	+	+	0	+	100/50	0	+	0	0	0	0	—
18	93F	W	0	0	0	+	0	0	+	...	0	—	—	—	—	—	—
19	93M	W	+	0	+	+	0	0	+	170/60	0	—	—	—	—	—	—
20	93F	B	+	0	+	+	0	+	+	135/60	0	—	—	—	—	—	243
21	93F	W	0	0	0	+	+	0	+	120/70	0	0	0	+	0	+	—
22	93F	W	0	0	+	+	+	0	+	125/80	0	—	—	—	—	—	273
23	95F	W	+	0	+	+	0	0	0	110/70	0	—	—	—	—	—	—
24	95F	W	0	0	0	0	0	0	0	140/60	0	0	0	0	0	0	—
25	95F	W	+	0	0	0	0	+	+	125/100	0	0	0	0	0	+	—
26	95M	B	+	0	0	+	0	0	+	120/115	0	+	+	0	+	+	—
27	96M	W	0	0	0	+	+	0	+	90/70	0	+	+	0	0	+	—
28	95M	W	0	0	0	0	0	0	0	130/70	0	0	0	+	0	+	181
29	95F	W	0	0	0	0	0	0	+	...	0	+	+	0	+	0	235
30	96F	B	0	0	0	+	+[†]	0	+	140/90	+	—	—	—	—	—	108
31	97F	W	0	0	0	0	0	0	+	118/75	+	+	0	0	0	0	—
32	97F	W	0	0	0	+	0	0	0	140/60	0	0	0	0	0	0	—
33	97F	W	0	0	0	0	0	0	0	...	+	0	0	0	0	0	—
34	97M	W	0	0	0	+	+	0	+	...	0	0	0	0	0	0	—
35	98F	W	0	0	0	0	0	0	0	130/85	0	0	0	0	0	0	—
36	98F	W	0	0	0	0	0	0	0	170/80	0	0	0	+	0	+	165
37	99M	W	+	+	0	0	0	0	+	130/85	+	0	0	0	0	0	—
38	100F	W	0	0	0	0	0	0	0	170/80	0	—	—	—	—	—	—
39	100M	W	0	0	0	0	0	0	0	...	0	0	0	0	0	0	—
40	103F	B	0	0	0	0	0	0	0	110/70	0	0	+	0	0	+	—
Total or mean	(94)		13 (32%)	3 (7%)	10 (25%)	17 (42%)	7 (17%)	5 (12%)	25 (62%)	...	4 (10%)	12 (40%)	5 (17%)	7 (23%)	3 (7%)	10 (33%)	220 ...

* Aortic valve stenosis.

† Idiopathic dilated cardiomyopathy.

A = cardiac amyloidosis (++ = massive, grossly visible deposits; + = minute, visible on microscope only); AD = abnormal dyspnea; AF = atrial fibrillation; AMI = acute myocardial infarction clinically; AP = angina pectoris; AV = aortic valve cusp; BBB = bundle branch block; BW = body weight; C = cardiac; CA = coronary artery; CCHF = chronic congestive heart failure; CP = chest pain; DM = diabetes mellitus; F = fibrosis; FAAA = fusiform abdominal aortic aneurysm; HW = heart weight; Hx = history; L = left; LAD = left anterior descending; LC = left circumflex; LV = left ventricular; MCS = mean coronary score; MVA = mitral valve anulus; N = necrosis; O = other; PHD = pericardial heart disease; R = right; S = stroke; SAP = systemic arterial pressure; SH = systemic hypertension; TC = total serum cholesterol; V = vascular.

TABLE I (continued)

Case	Mode of Death			BW (kg)	HW (g)	Calcific Deposits			(%) 5 mm Segments Narrowed to Various Degrees				MCS	Transmural LV			PHD	FAAA
	C	V	O			CA	MVA	AV	0–25	26–50	51–75	76–100		N	F	A		
1	+	0	0	55	550	3+	3+	4 + a	0	17(39)	21(49)	5(12)	2.72	+	0	0	0	0
2	+	0	0	41	340	2+	0	0	. . .	. . .	. . .	. . .	. . .	+	0	0	0	0
3	+	0	0	50	450	2+	0	2+	9(18)	16(31)	12(24)	13(27)	2.58	+	+	0	0	0
4	+	0	0	—	520	1+	3+	1+	29(53)	24(44)	2(3)	0	1.51	0	0	++	0	0
5	+	0	0	45	400	2+	2+	1+	16(26)	24(39)	11(18)	10(17)	2.25	+	0	0	0	0
6	0	0	+	45	220	1+	1+	2+	16(37)	13(30)	11(26)	3(7)	1.89	0	0	0	0	0
7	0	0	+	47	270	1+	0	1+	6(16)	25(68)	5(13)	1(3)	2.03	0	0	0	0	0
8	0	+	0	50	505	2+	0	0	0	19(40)	15(32)	12(28)	2.85	0	+	0	0	+
9	0	0	+	60	480	2+	0	0	. . .	. . .	. . .	. . .	. . .	0	0	+	0	0
10	0	+	0	—	490	1+	0	1+	33(72)	13(28)	0	0	1.28	0	0	0	0	0
11	0	+	0	46	375	4+	4+	0	9(14)	40(64)	12(19)	2(3)	2.11	0	0	0	0	0
12	+	0	0	65	390	2+	0	1+	16(26)	24(39)	11(18)	10(17)	2.25	0	+	0	0	0
13	+	0	0	—	520	2+	0	0	11(17)	24(37)	16(25)	13(21)	2.48	+	+	0	0	+
14	+	0	0	49	380	1+	1+	1+	10(25)	17(43)	8(20)	5(12)	2.20	0	+	0	+	0
15	0	0	+	50	400	1+	1+	1+	19(33)	39(67)	0	0	1.67	0	0	0	0	0
16	+	0	0	85	280	2+	3+	1+	0	30(70)	8(18)	5(12)	2.42	+	0	0	0	0
17	+	0	0	55	525	2+	4+	4+	3(7)	37(80)	6(13)	0	2.07	0	0	0	0	0
18	0	0	+	—	500	3+	1+	2+	15(23)	46(72)	2(3)	1(2)	1.83	0	+	0	0	0
19	+	0	0	66	470	2+	0	1+	6(14)	14(33)	15(35)	8(18)	2.58	+	+	0	0	0
20	+	0	0	—	510	1+	0	0	0	18(24)	18(42)	18(34)	3.08	+	+	0	0	0
21	+	0	0	—	380	1+	0	0	22(48)	20(43)	4(9)	0	1.61	0	0	++	0	0
22	+	0	0	67	560	3+	3+	2+	7(15)	12(26)	14(31)	12(28)	2.69	+	+	0	0	0
23	+	0	0	—	490	1+	0	0	. . .	. . .	. . .	. . .	. . .	+	+	0	0	0
24	0	0	+	58	350	1+	4+	1+	3(6)	31(65)	12(25)	2(4)	2.27	0	0	0	0	0
25	0	+	0	—	460	2+	0	0	18(49)	19(51)	0	0	1.51	0	0	0	0	+
26	0	+	0	47	580	2+	0	0	5(8)	36(59)	19(31)	1(2)	2.26	0	0	0	0	0
27	+	0	0	50	660	3+	2+	2+	9(12)	44(59)	15(20)	7(9)	2.27	0	+	++	0	0
28	0	0	+	—	385	2+	0	1+	12(19)	32(52)	16(26)	2(3)	2.13	0	0	0	0	0
29	0	0	+	52	440	2+	2+	1+	2(3)	48(69)	15(22)	4(6)	2.30	0	+	+	0	0
30	+	0	0	50	630	0	0	0	15(31)	33(69)	0	0	1.69	0	0	0	0	0
31	0	+	0	45	300	2+	4+	1+	11(29)	17(45)	9(24)	1(2)	2.00	0	0	0	0	0
32	0	0	+	55	360	2+	3+	0	19(36)	29(55)	3(5)	2(4)	1.77	0	0	0	0	0
33	0	+	0	41	320	2+	3+	0	8(18)	29(66)	7(16)	0	1.98	0	0	0	0	0
34	+	0	0	68	600	3+	1+	1+	2(5)	24(62)	8(20)	5(13)	2.41	0	0	++	+	+
35	0	0	+	53	360	0	0	0	. . .	. . .	. . .	. . .	. . .	0	0	0	0	0
36	0	0	+	52	320	1+	0	0	8(27)	21(70)	1(3)	0	1.77	0	0	0	0	0
37	+	0	0	50	510	2+	0	0	5(11)	22(47)	15(32)	5(10)	2.43	0	+	0	0	0
38	0	+	0	45	280	4+	2+	2+	0	23(58)	12(30)	4(12)	2.51	0	0	+	0	0
39	0	0	+	—	335	2+	0	1+	18(32)	21(37)	16(28)	2(3)	2.04	0	+	+	0	0
40	0	0	+	55	345	0	0	0	5(11)	41(89)	0	0	1.89	0	0	+	0	0
Total	19	8	13	(53)	431	37	19	22	367	930	339	153	2.15	10	14	4	2	4
(Mean)	(47%)	(20%)	(32%)	. . .	. . .	(92%)	(47%)	(55%)	(21%)	(52%)	(19%)	(8%)	. . .	(25%)	(35%)	(10%)	(5%)	(10%)

1967 and 1982; the other 3 patients had been studied both clinically and at necropsy at the National Institutes of Health in 1954, 1966, and 1967, respectively. The month of death was known in 37 patients: death occurred during 4 cold months (November to February) in 21 (57%); during 4 warm months (June to September) in 11 (30%), and during intermediate weather months in 5 (13%) (p <0.05). (The data throughout this study were analyzed using the t test for paired and unpaired data and linear regression tests to determine correlation coefficients.) The ages of death in the 40 patients ranged from 90 to 103 (mean 94); 29 (72%) were women and 11 (28%) were men; 31 (78%) were white and 9 (22%) were black.

Heart weights and body weights: The weight of the heart was increased (>350 g in women and >400 g in men) in 27 (67%) patients. The hearts in the 29 women ranged from 220 to 630 g (mean 408), and those in the 11 men, from 335 to 660 g (mean 490). The body weights in the 23 women ranged from 41 to 85 kg (mean 52) and the heart weight-body weight ratio, from 0.003 to 0.013 (mean 0.007). Thus, the mean heart weight was 0.7% of the body weight (normal value for younger women is approximately 0.4%[4]). The body weights in 7 men ranged from 47 to 68 kg (mean 50) and the heart weight-body weight ratios, from 0.006 to 0.013 (mean 0.009). Thus, the mean heart weight was 0.6% of the mean body weight (the normal value for younger men is approximately 0.45%[4]).

Necropsy observations (Table II): *Coronary arterial calcification (Fig. 1 to 6):* Calcific deposits within atherosclerotic plaques were observed grossly in the epicardial coronary arteries in 37 (92%) patients. In 28 patients, radiograms of the heart or of the excised coronary arteries were performed; all patients had calcific deposits in the coronary arteries: 23 (82%), in the left anterior descending, left circumflex, and right coronary arteries, and the other 5 patients, in 2 of these 3 major

TABLE II Morphologic Cardiac Observations in 40 Necropsy Patients Aged 90 to 103 Years

	Patients	
	n	%
Coronary arterial disease		
Calcium	37	92
Luminal narrowing 76 to 100% in XSA by atherosclerotic plaques of ≥1 major coronary arteries	28	70
Acute myocardial infarction	10	25
Healed myocardial infarction	14	35
Aortic valve disease		
Calcium	22	55
Stenosis	2	5
Mitral anular disease		
Calcium	19	47
Cardiac amyloidosis (fatal)	4	10
Dilated cardiomyopathy	1	3
Obliterative pericardial disease		
Idiopathic	1	5
Iatrogenic	1	5

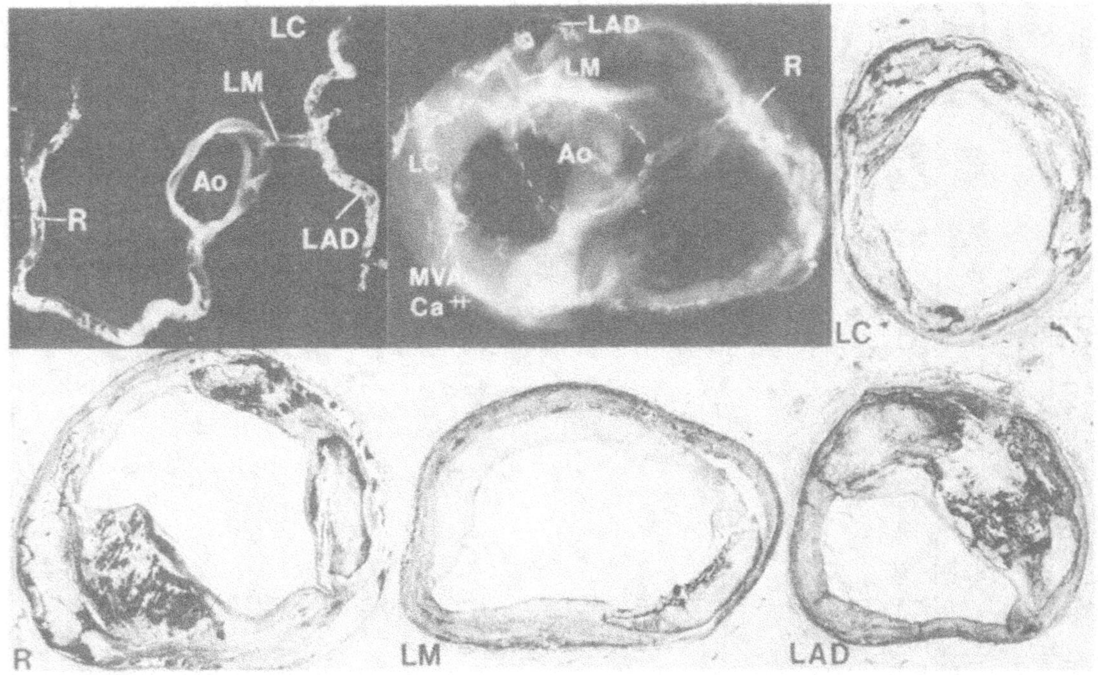

FIGURE 1. Patient 29 (SH #A80-74). Tortuous and heavily calcified coronary arteries in a 95-year-old woman who never had symptoms of cardiac dysfunction and who died from a perforated gastric ulcer. **Top left,** postmortem radiogram of the excised right (R), left main (LM), left anterior descending (LAD), and left circumflex (LC) coronary arteries. **Top center,** radiogram of a portion of the heart after removing the walls of the atria and most of the walls of the ventricles. MVA = mitral valve anulus. **Top right and lower panels,** photomicrographs of coronary arteries at sites of maximal narrowing by calcified atherosclerotic plaques. (Movat stains; magnification ×17, reduced 40%.) This case illustrates extensive calcific deposits in the coronary arteries without significant luminal narrowing.

coronary arteries. In 23 of the 28 patients, the left main coronary artery was studied radiographically: 18 (78%) had calcific deposits. Thus, of 112 major epicardial coronary arteries studied radiographically in 28 patients, 97 (87%) were seen to contain calcific deposits. Of the 37 patients with demonstrated calcific deposits in the epicardial coronary arteries, 26 (70%) also had calcific deposits in either aortic valve cusps or mitral anulus or both. Of the 3 patients without calcium in the coronary arteries, none had calcific deposits in either aortic valve cusps on mital anulus (Fig. 7 and 8).

Coronary arterial atherosclerosis (qualitative studies): At necropsy, 39 of the 40 patients had ≥1 significant cardiac conditions on *gross* examination. One or more of the 4 major (right, left main, left anterior descending, left circumflex) epicardial coronary arteries was narrowed 76 to 100% in XSA by atherosclerotic plaques in 28 (70%) patients; 37 (92%) had grossly palpable calcific deposits in ≥1 major coronary arteries. None of the 28 patients had significant (>75% in XSA) narrowing in the left main coronary artery. Of the other 3 major coronary arteries, 1 was significantly narrowed in 8 patients (29%), 2 were narrowed 76 to 100% by plaques in 15 patients (53%), and 3 arteries were so

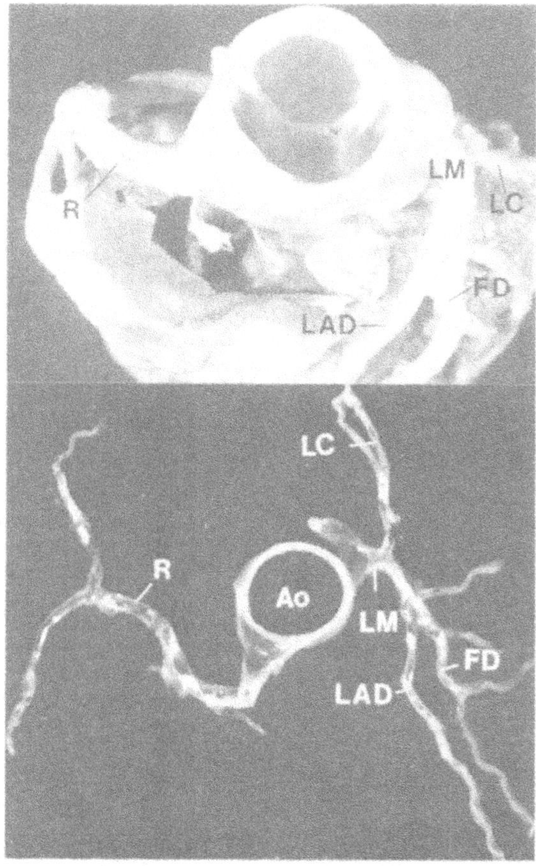

FIGURE 2. Patient 28 (SH #A79-77). Coronary arteries in a 95-year-old man who never had symptoms of cardiac dysfunction and who died from cancer. **Top,** aorta and coronary arteries from above. **Bottom,** radiograms of aortic root (Ao) and excised coronary arteries which contain calcific deposits. FD = first diagonal; LAD = left anterior descending; LC = left circumflex; LM = left main; R = right.

narrowed in 5 patients (18%). Of the 112 major coronary arteries in these 28 patients, 53 were significantly narrowed, an average of 1.9/4 major coronary arteries per patient. Of the 160 major coronary arteries in the 40 patients, the average number narrowed per patient was 1.3.

Of the 12 patients *with clinical evidence of myocardial ischemia* (angina pectoris or a clinical event diagnosed as or compatible with acute myocardial infarction or both), at least 1 of the 4 major coronary arteries was narrowed 76 to 100% in XSA by plaques: in 10 patients, 2 arteries (right, left anterior descending, or left circumflex) were so narrowed and in the other 2 patients, 3 arteries. Thus, of the 48 major coronary arteries (4 per patient) in these 12 patients, 26 arteries were significantly narrowed, an average of 2.2/4.0 per patient.

Of the 28 patients *without clinical evidence of myocardial ischemia*, at least 1 of the 4 major coronary arteries was narrowed 76 to 100% in XSA by atherosclerotic plaques in 16 patients (57%): in 8 patients, only 1 artery was so narrowed; in 5 patients, 2 arteries; and in 4 patients, 3 arteries. In 12 patients (43%), none of the 4 major coronary arteries was significantly narrowed. Thus, of the 112 major coronary arteries in these 28 patients, 27 (24%) were significantly narrowed, an average of 1.0/4.0 per patient.

Coronary arterial atherosclerosis (quantitative studies): In 36 patients, including 26 of the 28 in whom 1 or more of the 4 major coronary arteries were significantly narrowed and in 10 of the 12 in whom none of the 4 arteries was significantly narrowed, each of the 4 major coronary arteries was decalcified and cut into 5 mm long segments. Each segment was processed in alcohols and xylene, and imbedded in paraffin. At least 1 histologic section was cut and stained by the Movat method from each segment. Of the 1,789 5 mm segments from the 36 patients (an average of 49 segments per patient [range 30 to 75]), 6 (<1%) were narrowed 96 to 100% in XSA by atherosclerotic plaques; 147 (8%), 76 to 95%; 339 (19%), 51 to 75%; 930 (52%), 26 to 50%; and 367 (21%), 0 to 25%.

A scoring system was utilized to indicate the severity of the coronary narrowing. Every 5 mm long segment was assigned a score of 1 to 4 based on the amount of XSA narrowing by atherosclerotic plaques as follows: 1 = 0 to 25%, 2 = 26 to 50%, 3 = 51 to 75%, and 4 = 76 to 100% narrowing. A total score was obtained for each patient. The mean score per 5 mm segment was then calculated by dividing the total score per patient by the number of segments examined. The total scores for the 36 patients ranged from 53 to 170 (average 107) and the mean score per 5 mm segment, from 1.28 to 3.08 (average 2.15) (Fig. 9). This mean score indicates that each of the 1,789 5 mm segments was narrowed on an average of about 42% in XSA (Fig. 9).

Of the 40 patients, 12 had clinical evidence of myocardial ischemia. Of these 12 patients, the 4 major epicardial coronary arteries were available in their entirety for quantitative studies in 10. Of 467 5 mm coronary segments in these 10 patients, 2 (<1%) were narrowed 96 to 100% in XSA by atherosclerotic plaques; 90 (19%), 76 to 95%; 135 (29%), 51 to 75%; 198 (43%), 26 to 50%;

and 42 (9%), 0 to 25% (Fig. 10). The total score for each of the 10 patients ranged from 88 to 159 (average 120) and the mean score per 5 mm segment of coronary artery, from 2.20 to 3.08 (average 2.59), indicating that each 5 mm segment was narrowed an average of approximately 55% in XSA.

Of the 28 patients without clinical evidence of myocardial ischemia, the 4 major coronary arteries were available for quantitative studies in 26. Of 1,322 5 mm coronary segments examined in these patients, 4 (<1%) were narrowed 96 to 100% in XSA by atherosclerotic plaques; 63 (5%) were narrowed 76 to 95%; 206 (16%), 51 to 75%; 727 (55%), 26 to 50%; and 322 (24%), 0 to 25% (Fig. 10). The total score for each patient ranged from 53 to 170 (average 98) and the mean score per 5 mm segment, from 1.28 to 2.85 (average 2.01) (Fig. 9), indicating that each of the 1,322 5 mm segments was narrowed an average of about 38% in XSA. Of these 26 patients, ≥1 of the 4 major coronary arteries was significantly narrowed in 16. Of the 857 5 mm coronary segments examined in the 26 patients, 4 segments (<1%) had lumens narrowed 96 to 100% in XSA by plaques; 63 (7%), 76 to 95%; 183 (22%), 51 to 75%; 464 (54%), 26 to 50%; and 143 (17%), 0 to 25%. The total score for each of the 16 patients ranged from 56 to 170 (average 111) and the mean score per 5 mm segment, from 1.77 to 2.85 (mean 2.20). Thus, each of the 857 5 mm segments was narrowed an average of approximately 44% in XSA. In

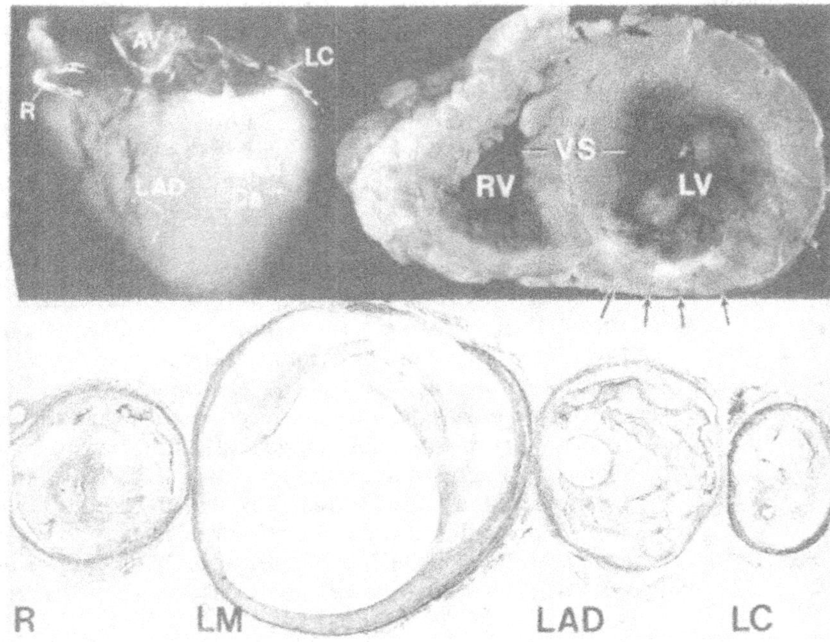

FIGURE 3. Patient 22 (LRC #5). Heart and coronary arteries in a 93-year-old woman who was hospitalized with worsening chronic congestive heart failure. **Top left,** postmortem radiogram showing calcific deposits in the right (R), left anterior descending (LAD), and left circumflex (LC) coronary arteries and in the mitral valve anulus (MVA) and aortic valve. **Top right,** view of right (RV) and left (LV) ventricles and ventricular septum (VS) showing a transmural scar (**arrows**). **Bottom,** coronary arteries at sites of maximal narrowing. LM = left main. (Movat stains; magnification ×17, reduced 40%.)

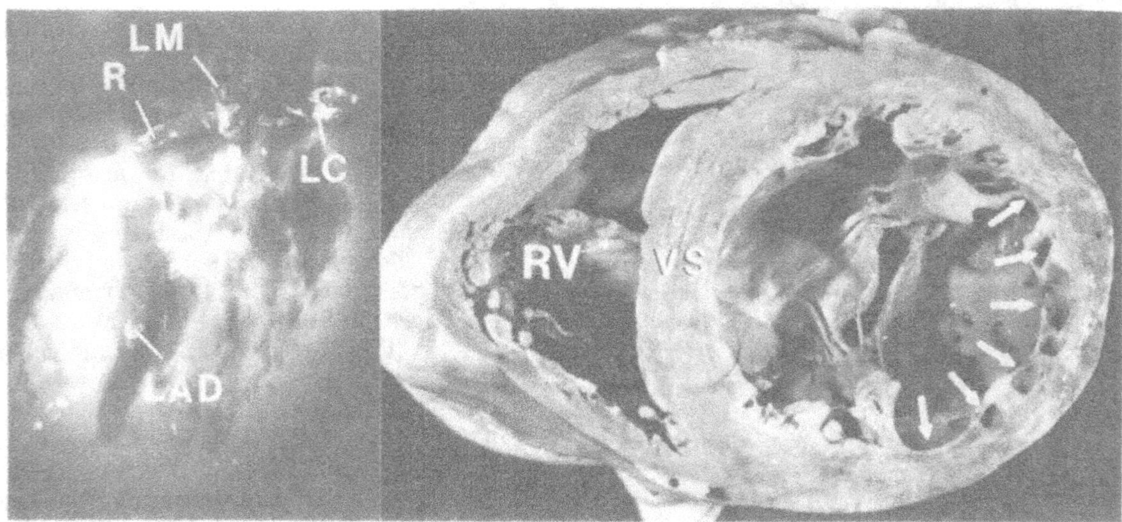

FIGURE 4. Patient 13 (LRC #3). This 91-year-old woman had a "typical" clinical acute myocardial infarct, which was fatal. **Left,** postmortem radiogram showing calcific deposits in the right (R), left main (LM), left anterior descending (LAD), and left circumflex (LC) coronary arteries. **Right,** view of left and right (RV) ventricles showing transmural necrosis and fibrosis (**arrows**) and dilated ventricles. VS = ventricular septum.

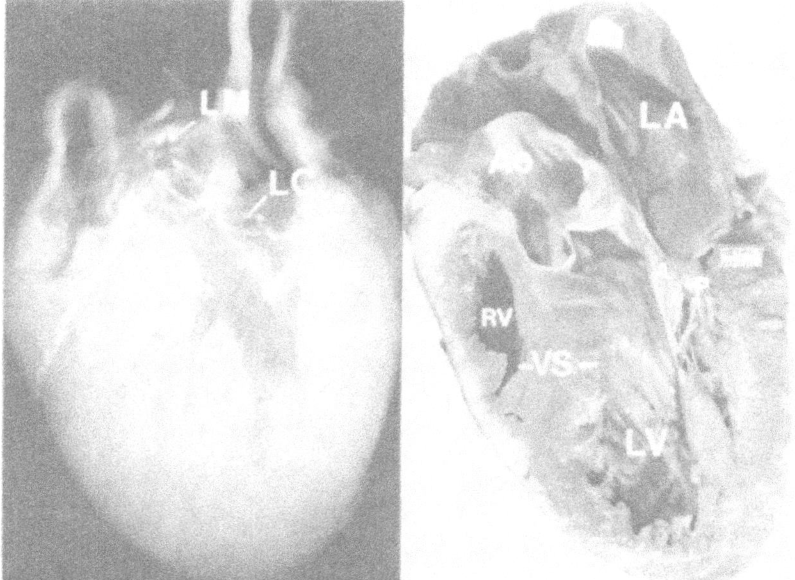

FIGURE 5. Patient 8 (SH #A82-1). This 90-year-old woman had no symptoms of cardiac dysfunction and died from a ruptured fusiform abdominal aortic aneurysm. **Left,** postmortem radiogram of the entire heart showing calcific deposits in the left anterior descending (LAD), left circumflex (LC), and left main (LM) coronary arteries. **Right,** view of heart cut in an anteroposterior fashion (M-mode or long-axis 2-dimensional echocardiographic view) showing a dilated left atrium (LA) and left ventricle (LV). A and P = anterior and posterior mitral valve leaflets; Ao = aorta; RV = right ventricle; VS = ventricular septum.

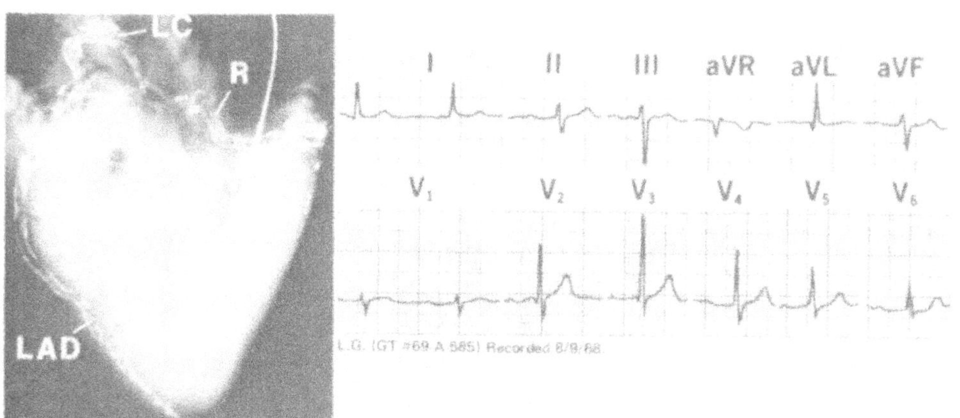

FIGURE 6. Patient 34 (GT #69A-585). This 97-year-old man had complete heart block and had a pacemaker inserted when he was 91 years old. **Left,** radiogram of heart at necropsy showing calcific deposits in the left anterior descending (LAD), left circumflex (LC), and right (R) coronary arteries, and a pacemaker wire in the right ventricle (RV). LV = left ventricle. **Right,** electrocardiogram.

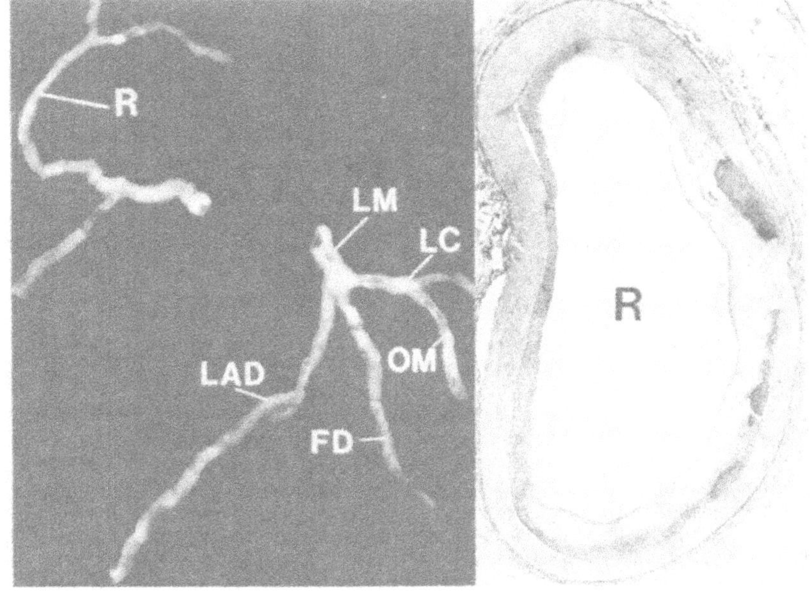

FIGURE 7. Patient 30 (DCGH #68A80). This 96-year-old woman had chronic congestive heart failure from dilated cardiomyopathy. Her total serum cholesterol level was 108 mg/dl. **Left,** postmortem radiogram of the right (R), left main (LM), left anterior descending (LAD), left circumflex (LC), first diagonal (FD), and left obtuse marginal (OM) coronary arteries showing no calcific deposits. **Right,** right coronary artery section devoid of calcium or narrowing. (Movat stain; magnification ×16, reduced 23%.)

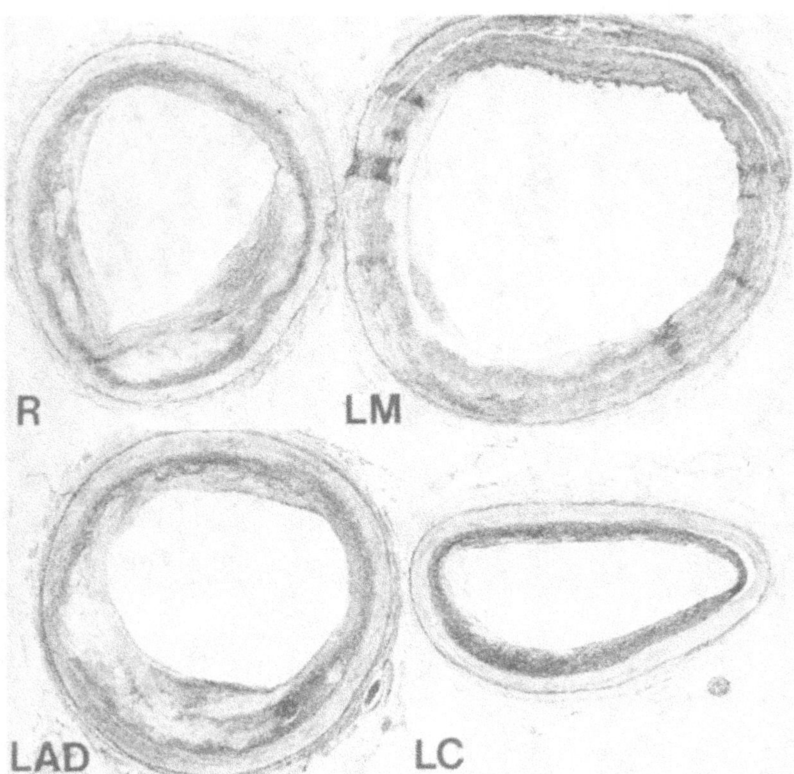

FIGURE 8. Patient 40 (GT #70A301). Right (R), left main (LM), left anterior descending (LAD), and left circumflex (LC) coronary arteries at sites of maximal narrowing in a 103-year-old woman. She never had evidence of cardiac dysfunction and died from complications of a duodenal ulcer. The coronary arteries are devoid of calcium and of significant narrowing. (Elastic van Gieson's stain; magnification ×16, reduced 31%.)

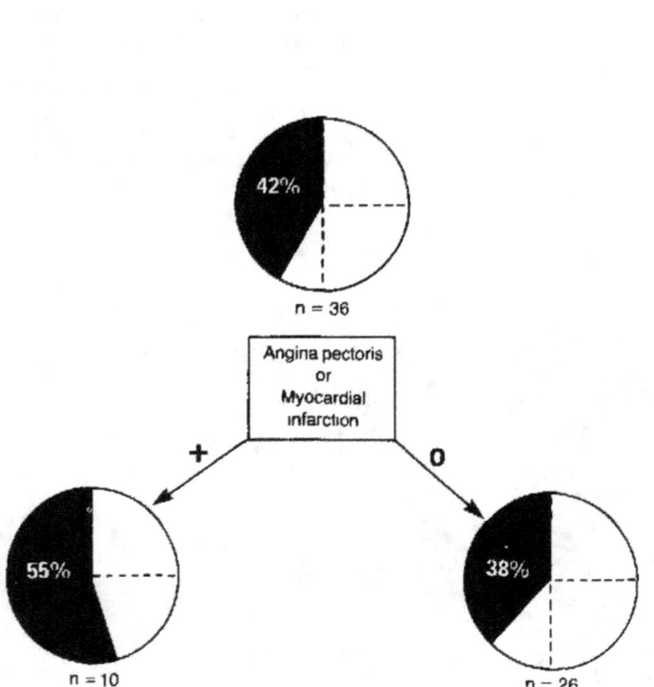

FIGURE 9. Mean percent cross-sectional area narrowing by atherosclerotic plaques in 1,789 5 mm segments of the 4 major epicardial coronary arteries in 36 necropsy patients aged 90 years and older, 10 of whom had angina pectoris or acute myocardial infarction or both and 26 of whom did not. The mean percentage of narrowing for each 5 mm segment differs significantly in the group with clinical evidence of myocardial ischemia (55%) and the group without such evidence (p <0.05).

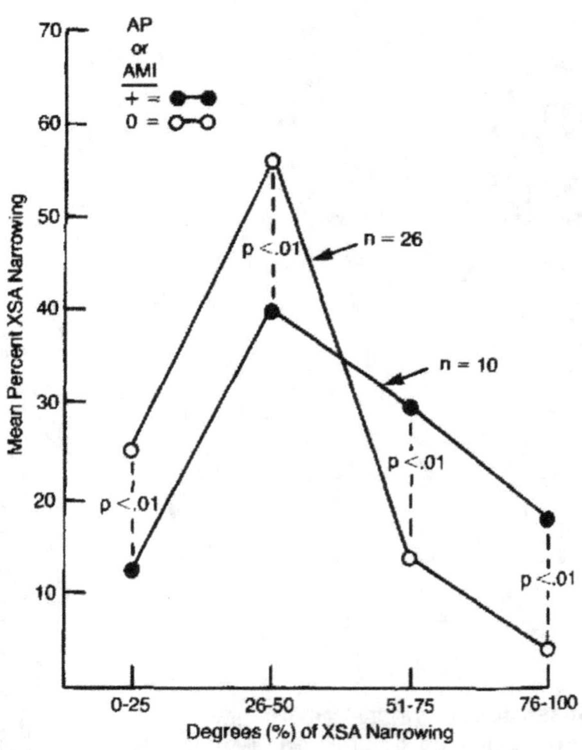

FIGURE 10. Mean percent cross-sectional area (XSA) narrowing by atherosclerotic plaques in the 5 mm segments of the right, left main, left anterior descending, and left circumflex coronary arteries in the 36 patients in whom the 4 major coronary arteries in their entirety were available for examination. The 36 patients were classified into 10 with and 26 without clinical evidence of myocardial ischemia. For each of the 4 categories of narrowing, a highly significant (p <0.01) difference in the amount of narrowing was observed.

the 10 patients without significant narrowing, 465 5 mm segments were examined: 23 (5%) were narrowed 51 to 75% in XSA by plaque; 263 (57%), 26 to 50%; and 179 (38%) ≤25%. The total score for each of these 10 patients ranged from 53 to 138 (average 85) and the mean score per 5 mm segment, from 1.28 to 2.07 (average 1.66). Thus, each of the 465 segments was narrowed an average of approximately 29%.

Left ventricular fibrosis or necrosis or both: Of the 40 patients, 18 (45%) had ≥1 grossly visible foci of transmural (involvement of all the inner one half and a portion of or all of the outer one half of left ventricular wall) sites of necrosis or fibrosis or both (Fig. 3 and 4). Of the 18 patients, 5 had foci of transmural necrosis only, 8 had transmural scars only, 4 had transmural foci of necrosis and fibrosis, and 1 had transmural fibrosis and subendocardial (involvement of less than the inner one half of the left ventricular wall) necrosis. Of the 23 transmural infarcts in 18 patients, 11 (2 acute, 11 healed [10 patients]) were "small"; 9 (7 acute, 2 healed [8 patients]) were "large"; and 2 (both healed [2 patients]) were "intermediate" in size. All 18 patients had narrowing of 76 to 100% in XSA by atherosclerotic plaque of ≥1 of the 4 major epicardial coronary arteries. None of the 10 patients with fatal acute myocardial infarction had a thrombus in a major coronary artery at necropsy.

Valvular and anular calcification (Fig. 11 to 16): Grossly visible calcific deposits were present in ≥1 of the 3 aortic valve cusps (on their aortic surfaces) in 22 patients (55%): in 20 patients, the amount of calcium on the cusps was mild (graded 1+ or 2+/4+) and valvular function was considered normal; in the other 2 patients (Cases 1 and 17) (Fig. 11), the cuspal calcific deposits were extensive (4+/4+) and cuspal mobility was limited, and the orifice in each appeared severely stenotic.[5]

Of the 40 patients, 19 (47%) had grossly visible *mitral anular calcific deposits:* graded 1+ in 5 patients (26%), 2+ in 5 (26%), 3+ in 5 (26%), and 4+ in 4 (22%).[6] In 1 of the 4 patients with 4+ mitral anular calcium (Patient 11), the mitral orifice appeared stenotic (Fig. 13). Of the 40 patients, 26 (65%) had calcific deposits in the aortic valve or mitral anulus or both: in both aortic valve and mitral anulus in 16 (62%), in aortic valve only in 7 (27%), and in mitral anulus only in 3 (11%).

Cardiac amyloidosis (Fig. 17): Four patients had extensive amyloid deposits detected grossly in the walls of all 4 cardiac chambers and in many other body organs.[8] The extent of the deposits in each patient produced symptoms and signs of cardiac dysfunction,

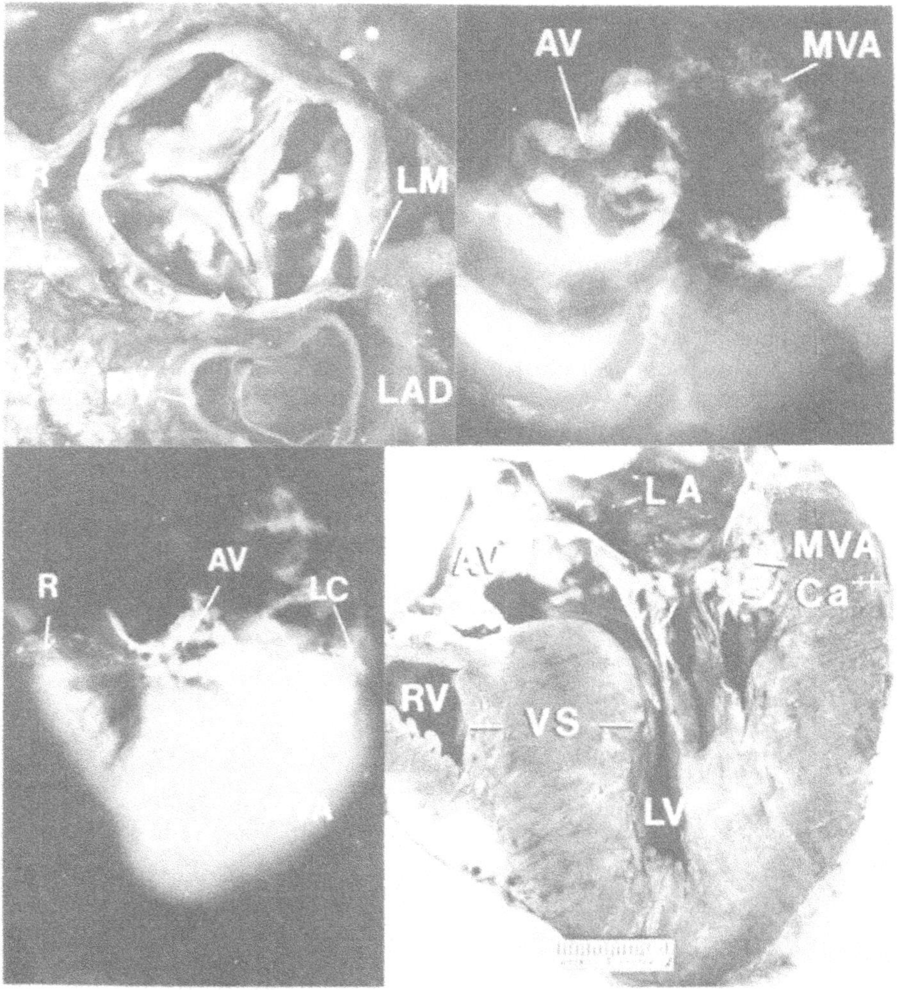

FIGURE 11. Patient 17 (GT #78A58). A 92-year-old woman with clinically recognized and eventually fatal aortic valve stenosis. **Top left,** stenotic aortic valve from above. PV = pulmonic valve; R = right; LM = left main; LAD = left anterior descending coronary arteries. **Top right,** postmortem radiogram showing heavy calcific deposits in the aortic valve (AV) and in mitral valve anular (MVA) region. **Bottom left,** radiogram of the heart at necropsy showing calcific deposits in the coronary arteries, in the aortic valve, and in the mitral anular region. **Bottom right,** long-axis view of heart (M-mode or 2-dimensional long-axis view) showing a small left ventricular (LV) cavity, a thickened and "sigmoid-shaped" ventricular septum (VS), and the stenotic aortic valve just above the right ventricular (RV) outflow tract. LA = left atrium.

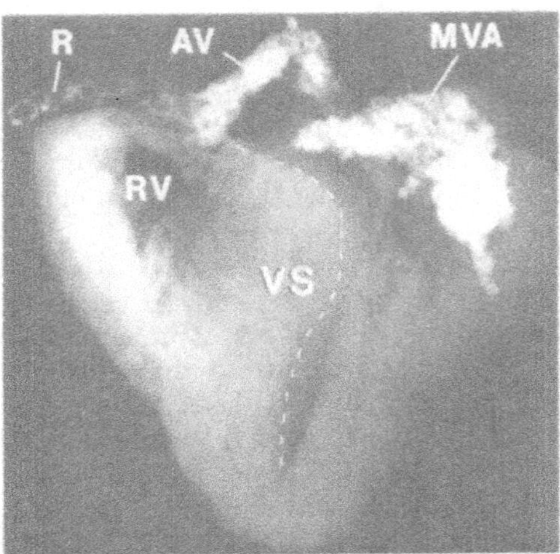

FIGURE 12. Patient 31 (GT #68A-367). Radiogram of the heart showing heavy calcific deposits in the aortic valve (AV), mitral valve anulus (MVA), and right (R) coronary artery. The ventricular septum (VS) has a *S* or sigmoid shape (**dashed line**). RV = right ventricle.

manifested primarily by chronic congestive cardiac failure. The presence of extensive amyloidosis was confirmed by histologic examination. At least 5 other patients also had amyloid deposits. The extent of the cardiac amyloid deposits in these 5 patients, however, was minimal and detectable only by histologic examination. Among the 40 patients, histologic sections (1 to 8 per patient [mean 3]) of left ventricular myocardium extending from endocardium to epicardium were examined in 37: 9 of the 37 patients (24%) had amyloid deposits, which were "massive" in 4 and minimal in 5.

Idiopathic dilated cardiomyopathy: One patient (Case 30) had a large heart (700 g), dilated ventricular cavities without foci of myocardial fibrosis or necrosis, normal valves and pericardia, epicardial coronary arteries virtually free of atherosclerotic plaques, and chronic congestive heart failure. Although a history of systemic hypertension was absent, the blood pressure in the last month of life was recorded as 140/90 mm Hg.

The kidneys, however, were near normal. This patient, therefore, fulfills criteria for diagnosis of idiopathic dilated cardiomyopathy. The patient apparently had habitually consumed excessive quantities of alcohol.

Obliterative "pericarditis": Two patients (Cases 14 and 34) had obliterated space between visceral and parietal pericardia by adhesions, some calcified. One (Patient 14) had had talcum powder sprinkled on the epicardium 29 years before death at operation (Beck procedure) for relief of angina pectoris.[9] This patient was the only 1 of the 40 who had undergone a cardiovascular operation. The cause of the obliterative pericardial disease in the other patient was not determined.

Disease of aorta: In 34 of the 40 patients, the status of the aorta was known. In all 34, the aorta was dilated in both its transverse and longitudinal dimensions. The latter produced varying degrees of tortuosity. Some degree of atherosclerotic plaquing was present in the aorta in all 34 patients. The most extensive plaquing involved the abdominal portion. Three patients (Cases 8, 13, and 34) had atherosclerotic fusiform abdominal aortic aneurysms with intraaneurysmal thrombus; death in 1 (Patient 8) was secondary to aneurysmal rupture. One patient (Case 25) had an atherosclerotic fusiform aneurysm of the descending thoracic aorta which ruptured, and 1 patient (Case 11) had a dissection limited to descending thoracic aorta; death was due to rupture of the aneurysm into the esophagus.[10]

Cerebrovascular disease: Extensive cerebral arterial atherosclerosis was described in the necropsy reports in each of the 4 patients (Cases 30, 31, 33, and 38) with clinical strokes.

Pulmonary embolism: Massive pulmonary embolism, that is, thromboembolic material in 1 or both major right and left main pulmonary arteries, was observed at necropsy in 2 patients (Cases 10 and 26). Both had underlying chronic obstructive pulmonary disease.

Clinical observations: *Evidence of coronary heart disease:* Of the 40 patients, 12 (30%) had definite or probable clinical evidence of coronary heart disease as manifested by angina pectoris or acute myocardial infarction or both: 1 patient (Case 14) had angina only, 1

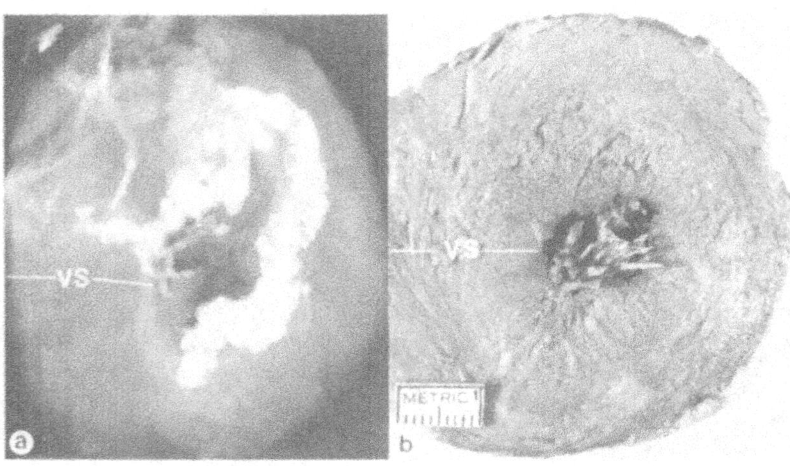

FIGURE 13. Patient 11 (GT #80-A-126). A 90-year-old woman with heavy mitral valve anular calcific deposits which reduced the mitral valve orifice to <1 cm in diameter (**a**). The unusual feature of the mitral calcium in this patient was that it not only was located behind the posterior mitral leaflet (mitral anular region) but it also extended across the anterior mitral leaflet nearly producing a letter *O*, as has been described previously.[7] She died from rupture of a descending thoracic aortic aneurysm. VS = ventricular septum. **b**, view of the left ventricle at the level of the tips of the mitral leaflets showing a very small cavity.

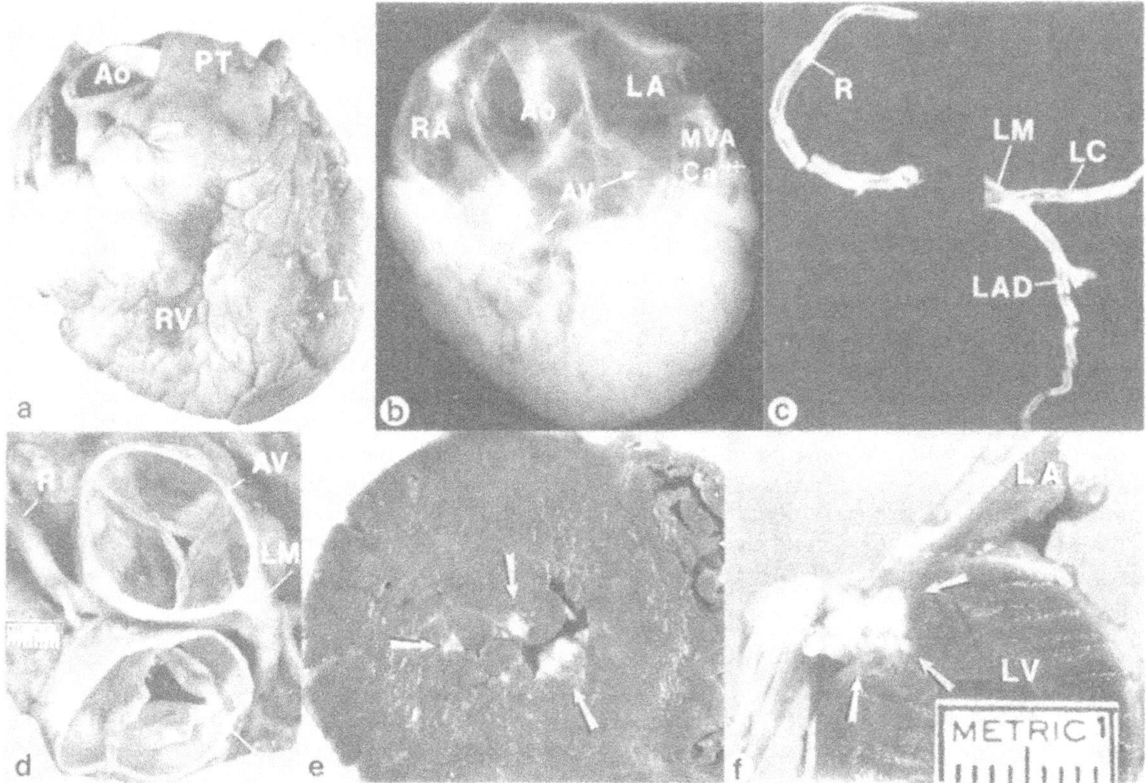

FIGURE 14. Patient 32 (SH #A81-62). A 97-year-old woman who never had clinical evidence of cardiac dysfunction and who died from cancer. **a,** external view of anterior surface of the heart showing an increased amount of subepicardial fat. Ao = aorta; LV = left ventricle; PT = pulmonary trunk; RV = right ventricle. **b,** postmortem radiogram showing calcific deposits in the mitral valve anulus (MVA) and aortic valve (AV). LA = left atrium; RA = right atrium. **c,** radiogram of the excised coronary arteries showing a few calcific deposits. LAD = left anterior descending; LC = left circumflex; LM = left main; R = right. **d,** view of aortic valve (AV) and pulmonic valve (PV) from above. **e,** view of left ventricle showing calcific deposits (**arrows**) in the papillary muscles. **f,** calcific deposits in mitral anular region.

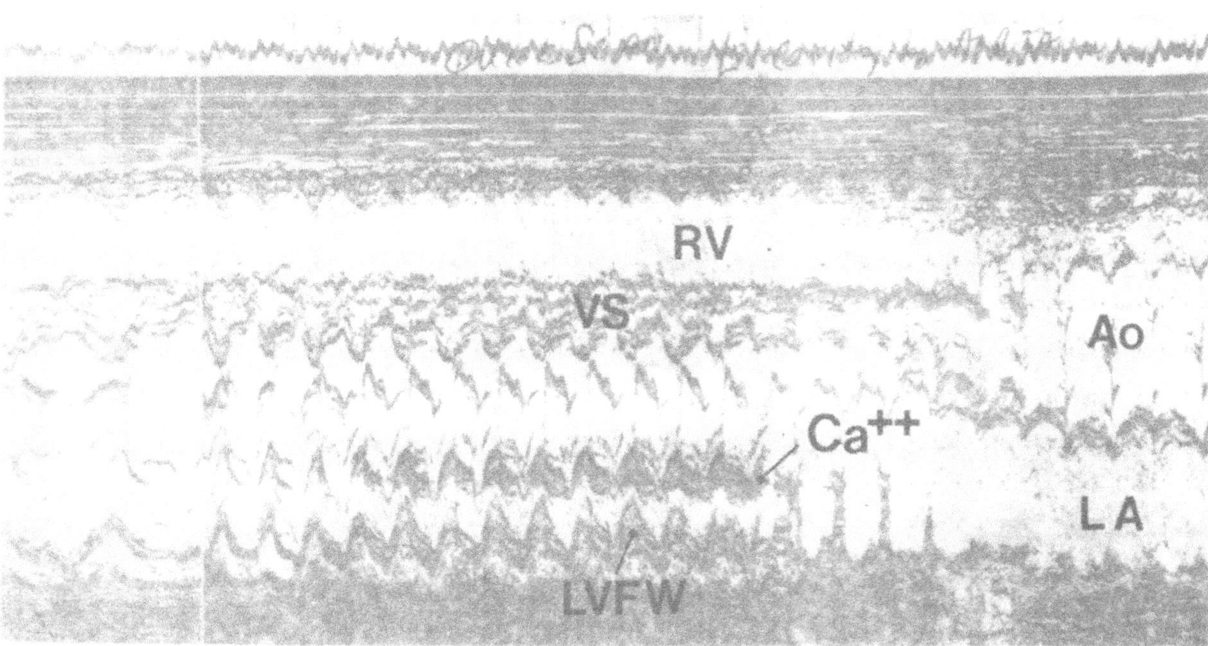

FIGURE 15. Patient 32 (SH #80-18). M-mode echocardiogram obtained 10 months before death from the patient whose heart is shown in Figure 14. The ascending aorta (Ao) has a larger diameter than does the left atrium (LA). The left ventricular (LV) cavity is small. Calcium is present in the mitral anular region. (We thank Dr. Robert Montgomery, Bethesda, Maryland, for allowing us to show this echocardiogram from his patient.)

(Case 37) had angina and a nonfatal acute myocardial infarct 2 years before death. (This patient died 24 hours after onset of increased dyspnea and vague chest pain but at necropsy no myocardial necrosis was visible histologically.) One patient (Case 2) had angina and a fatal acute myocardial infarct, and 9 patients had fatal acute myocardial infarcts which in each was the first one seen clinically. The clinical records regarding anginal attacks in the 3 patients are deficient in details: 2 patients (Cases 2 and 37) were stated to have had angina for "many years" and the third patient (Case 14) had angina for 29 years (since age 63). In none of the 3 patients was there information regarding the frequency of the anginal attacks and only 1 (Patient 37) was known to have taken nitroglycerin tablets.

Ten patients had deaths compatible with acute myocardial infarction. Of these 10 patients, however, only 3 (Cases 13, 16, and 23) had typical "crushing" substernal chest pain associated with typical electrocardiographic changes and enzyme elevations. The remaining 7 patients all were hospitalized because of some acute change in their status; however, acute myocardial infarction was never clearly established in these patients until necropsy. Only 5 of the 7 had chest pain, and it was atypical and not severe. Four had acute worsening of dyspnea. None had typical electrocardiographic features of acute myocardial infarction, but 5 had complete left bundle branch block at admission to the hospital. In 5 of these 7 patients in whom serum enzymes (creatine phosphokinase, lactic dehydrogenase, serum glutamic-oxaloacetic transaminase) were determined, the values were elevated in 4. Of the 14 patients with transmural left ventricular scars, only 1 had a clinical event diagnosed as acute myocardial infarction.

Chronic congestive heart failure was described in 8 patients (20%). In 4 patients (Cases 4, 21, 27, and 34) its cause, as determined initially by necropsy, was diffuse cardiac amyloidosis: in 1 patient (Case 17), its cause was aortic valve stenosis, which was diagnosed clinically; 1 patient (Case 14) had obliterative pericardial disease from the Beck procedure 25 years earlier[9]; 1 patient (Case 30) had cardiomegaly (660 g heart) of uncertain cause clinically (at necropsy the condition was considered idiopathic dilated cardiomyopathy); 1 patient (Case 22) also had congestive heart failure of uncertain cause clinically but at necropsy had a transmural left ventricular scar and severe narrowing of all 3 major epicardial coronary arteries. Of the 8 patients with chronic congestive heart failure, all had cardiomegaly at necropsy and 6 had histories of systemic hypertension during life.

Systemic hypertension: Information regarding "a history of hypertension" or an actual indirect systemic arterial blood pressure recording in the last year of life was available in 39 of the 40 patients: 19 (51%) had "a history" of systemic hypertension; of the 34 patients with actual blood pressure recordings, only 7 had systolic pressures >140 mm Hg or diastolic pressures >90 mm Hg. Of the 39 patients on whom information was available, 27 (69%) had either "a history of hypertension" or a recorded elevated blood pressure in the last year of life. Of the other 12 patients, only 1 (Case 23) had unequivocal cardiomegaly without explanation.

Diabetes mellitus: Five patients, all women, had diabetes mellitus. In 2, its duration was known: 20 years (Patient 5) and 40 years (Patient 20). One patient (Case 5) was treated with insulin; 1 (Case 9) with diet alone; 1 (Case 2) with diet plus tolbutamide; in 2 patients the type therapy received was unknown. Although 3 patients (Cases 2, 5, and 20) had transmural left ventricular scars, none had clinical events compatible with acute myocardial infarction.

Precordial murmurs: Of the 40 patients, 25 (62%) had had precordial murmurs. In all 25, the murmur was

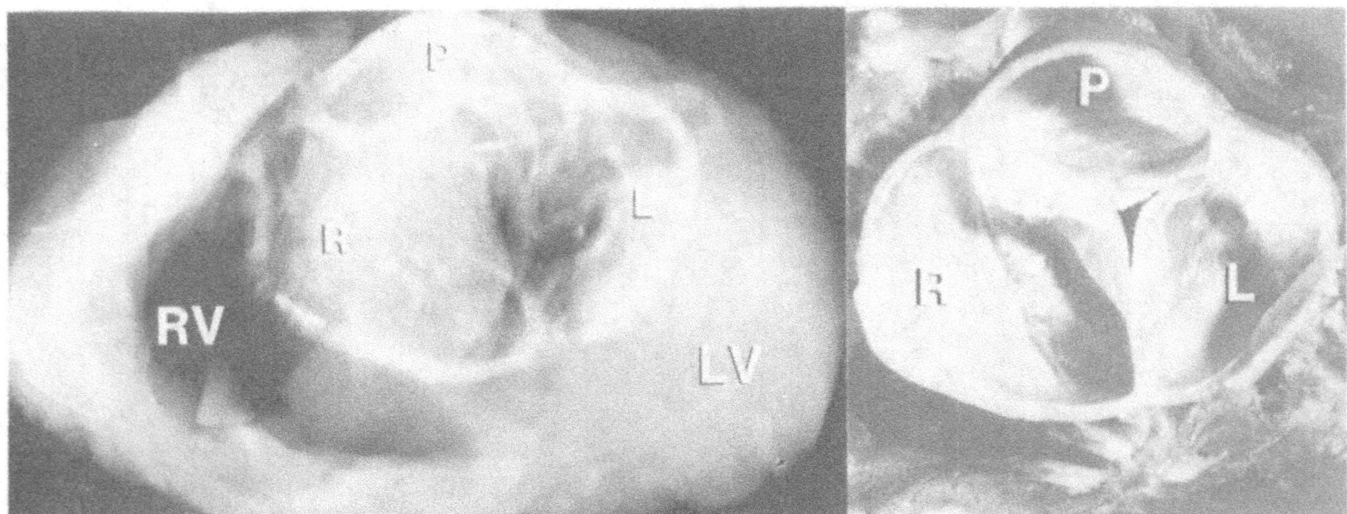

FIGURE 16. Patient 28 (SH #79-77). A 95-year-old man who never had symptoms of cardiac dysfunction and died from sarcoma. The coronary arteries are shown in Figure 2. **Left,** radiogram of heart at necropsy showing considerable enlargement of the aorta in comparison to the ventricles. LV = left ventricle; RV = right ventricle; R = right, L = left, and P = posterior sinuses of Valsalva. **Right,** aortic valve from above. The coronary arteries had been excised before the radiogram and photographs were taken.

described as systolic: apical only in 6; left sternal border only in 8; basal only in 2; all 3 locations in 3; and unspecified in 6. Only 1 (Case 9) of the 25 patients had both diastolic and systolic precordial murmurs. The diastolic murmur appeared to represent mild aortic regurgitation from systemic hypertension. The intensity of the murmur in the 24 patients with purely systolic murmurs was grade 1/6 in 2 patients, grade 2/6 in 5, grade 3/6 in 8, grade 4/6 in 4, and unspecified in 5. The cause of the precordial systolic murmurs was variable and often unclear. Of the 24 patients, 17 (71%) had calcific deposits in either the mitral valve anulus or aortic valve cusps or both: in mitral anulus only in none, in aortic valve only in 4, and in both mitral anulus and aortic valve in 13. In only 4 of the 17 patients, however, was the extent of calcium grade 3 to 4/6. In contrast, of the 15 patients without precordial murmurs recorded, 8 (53%) had calcific deposits in either mitral anulus or aortic valve cusps or both: in 3, the extent of the calcific deposits was either grade 3 or 4/6, but 4 of these 8 patients underwent precordial examination while in severe respiratory distress (3 patients) or in coma (1 patient). The blood hematocrit level ranged from 29 to 46% (mean 39) in the 18 patients with precordial murmurs and known hematocrit values, and from 30 to 57%

(mean 38) in the 10 without precordial murmurs but known hematocrit values.

Noncardiac vascular disease: Five patients had strokes, which were fatal in 4 (Cases 12, 31, 33, and 38) and nonfatal in 1 (Case 30). Of the 3 patients with fusiform abdominal aortic aneurysms, only the 1 (Case 8) which ruptured was diagnosed during life. Neither the patient (Case 25) with a ruptured fusiform aneurysm of thoracic aorta nor the patient (Case 11) with rupture of the descending thoracic aorta into the esophagus had the condition diagnosed during life.[10] Five patients (Cases 1, 3, 9, 20, and 25) had leg claudication, requiring amputations in 2 (Cases 3 and 9) for gangrene. In the 2 patients with massive pulmonary embolism, this condition was suspected clinically.

Electrocardiographic data (Fig. 18 and 19) (Tables III and IV): Information on electrocardiograms recorded at age 90 years or later was available in 30 of the 40 patients. In 24 patients, the electrocardiograms were available for reexamination but in the other 6 patients, only the electrocardiographic reports were available. Of the 30 patients, 3 (Cases 1, 3, and 5) had electrocardiograms recorded during the acute illness (recordings 4, 9, and 7 days, respectively, before death). The illnesses, although not diagnosed clinically, were seen at necropsy

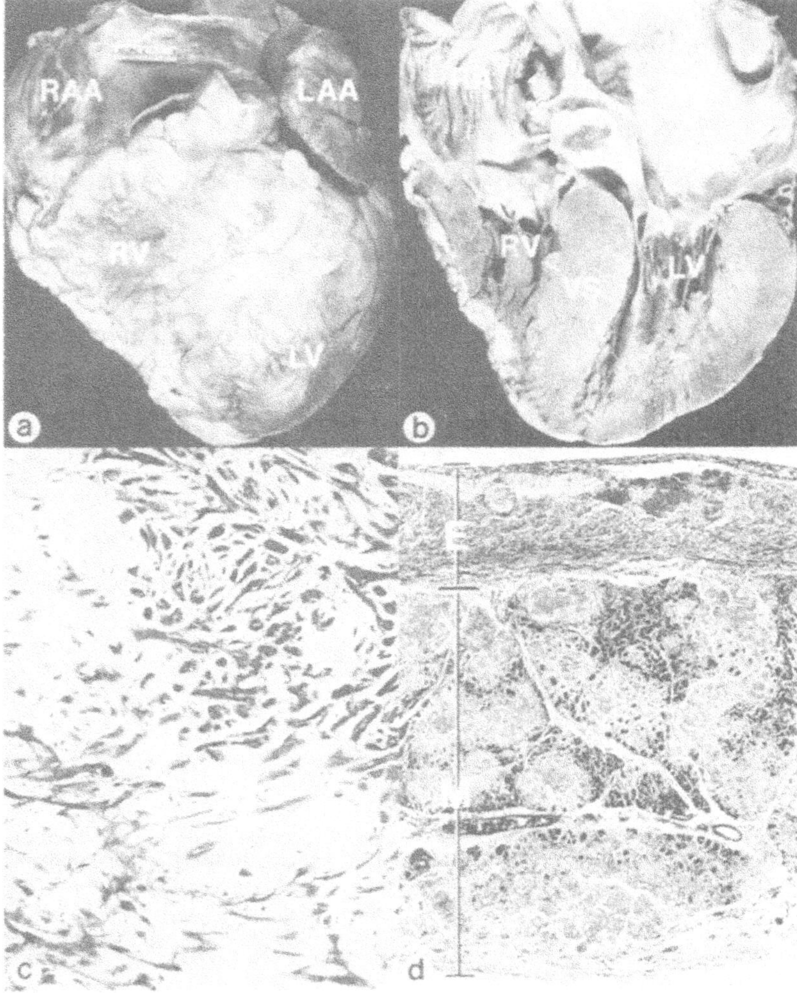

FIGURE 17. Patient 4 (DCGH #69A391), a 90-year-old man with chronic, eventually fatal congestive heart failure from clinically unrecognized cardiac amyloidosis. **a,** external view of the heart showing a prominent left ventricle (LV) and left atrial appendage (LAA). PT = pulmonary trunk; RAA = right atrial appendage; RV = right ventricle. **b,** right-to-left longitudinal cut of the heart (4-chamber, 2-dimensional echocardiographic view) showing thickened ventricular walls and dilated right (RA) and left (LA) atria. VS = ventricular septum. **c,** photomicrograph of a portion of the left ventricle showing extensive amyloid deposits. **d,** photomicrograph of LA wall showing amyloid deposits in endocardium (E) and in myocardium (M). (Hematoxylin-eosin stains; magnification ×100 (c) and ×25 (d), both reduced 35%.)

to clearly result from acute myocardial infarction. The electrocardiograms in all 3, however, disclosed only atrial fibrillation and complete left bundle branch block and these findings in all 3 patients were known to be present before the fatal acute myocardial infarction. The electrocardiograms in the other 27 patients were not recorded during periods of acute myocardial ischemia. Of the 30 patients on whom electrocardiographic information was available, 8 had clinical evidence of heart disease and 22 did not; the findings are summarized in Table III.

The QRS voltage in all 12 leads in each of 24 patients is summarized in Table IV (Fig. 19). The total 12-lead QRS voltage ranged from 82 to 251 mm (mean 151) (10 mm = 1 mV). In the 19 women, the total voltage ranged from 82 to 251 mm (mean 158), and in the 5 men, from 105 to 154 mm (mean 101) (p <0.05). The total 12-lead QRS voltage did not correlate with either heart (r = −0.01) or body weight (r = −0.2). The 24 patients in whom the total 12-lead QRS voltage was measured were separated into 2 groups: 8 patients in whom clinical evidence of cardiac dysfunction was present (coronary heart disease in 5, massive cardiac amyloid in 2, aortic valve stenosis in 1) and 16 patients without such evidence. Comparison of the total QRS voltage in the 8 patients with and in the 16 patients without clinical evidence of heart disease disclosed no significant difference (mean 147 mm versus mean 152 mm). Breakdown on the 8 patients with cardiac dysfunction did show some differences: the total 12-lead QRS voltage in the 5 patients with angina pectoris or acute myocardial infarction (Patients 1, 3, 5, 14, and 37) ranged from 123 to 163 mm (mean 143); in the 2 patients with massive cardiac amyloidosis (Patients 21 and 27) it was 102 and 117 mm (mean 109); and in the 1 patient with aortic valve stenosis (Patient 17) it was 238 mm.

Of 29 patients on whom information was available, 18 (62%) received *digitalis* and only 2 appeared to have evidence of digitalis toxicity.

Blood hematocrit levels in the last month of life, known in 29 patients, ranged from 29 to 57% (mean 38).

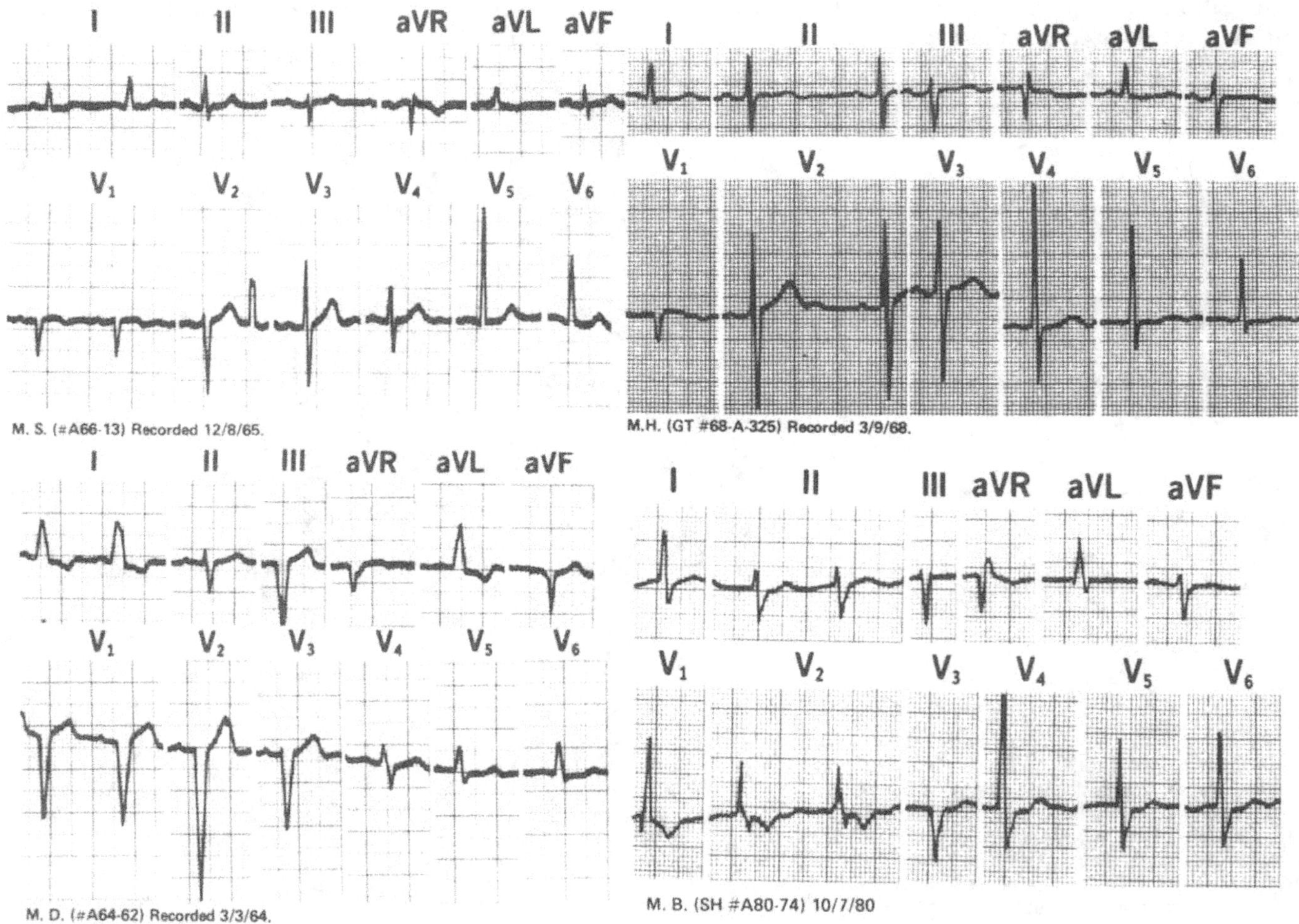

FIGURE 18. Electrocardiograms in 4 patients, each recorded at age 90 years or older. None ever had symptoms of cardiac dysfunction and each died from noncardiac conditions. **Top left,** Patient 7 (A66-13). The electrocardiogram was recorded 43 days before death and it is normal (heart weight 270 g). **Top right,** Patient 15 (GT #68A325). The electrocardiogram was recorded 11 days before death and it shows left QRS axis deviation and a slightly prolonged P-R interval (heart weight 400 g). **Bottom left,** Patient 36 (A64-62). This electrocardiogram was recorded 28 days before death and it shows left-axis deviation and complete left bundle branch block (heart weight 320 g). **Bottom right,** Patient 29 (SH #A80-74). This electrocardiogram was recorded 128 days before death and it shows atrial fibrillation, left-axis deviation, and complete right bundle branch block (heart weight 440 g).

Total serum cholesterol levels recorded at age 90 years or older, available in 10 patients, ranged from 108 to 283 mg/100 ml (mean 220).

Total serum protein values, available in 18 patients, ranged from 5.2 to 8.1 g/100 ml (mean 6.8). Serum albumin values, available in 19 patients, ranged from 2.0 to 4.5 g/100 ml (mean 3.3).

Blood urea nitrogen values, available in 27 patients, ranged from 7 to 70 g/100 ml (mean 33). Most values were obtained during the last month of life and some patients were clearly dehydrated at the time.

Modes of death: Of the 40 patients, 18 (45%) appeared to have died from consequences of cardiac disease, 7 (17%) from noncardiac but vascular problems, and 15 (38%) from noncardiac and nonvascular problems.

Of the 18 patients with cardiac causes of death, 10 had acute transmural myocardial infarcts, 1 (Case 14) had chronic congestive cardiac failure after healing of acute transmural myocardial infarcts, and 1 (Case 37) died in ventricular fibrillation after 24 hours of chest pain and at necropsy was shown to have severe coronary atherosclerosis without myocardial necrosis. Fatal congestive heart failure was due to aortic valve stenosis in 1 (Patient 17), to cardiac amyloidosis in 4 (Patients 4, 21, 27, and 34), and to idiopathic dilated cardiomyopathy in 1 (Patient 30). Of the 7 patients with noncardiac and nonvascular causes of death, 4 (Patients 12, 31, 33, and 38) died from complications of strokes, and the other 3, from rupture of aortic aneurysms (Patients 8, 11, and 25). Of the 15 patients with noncardiac and nonvascular

causes of death, 7 (Cases 6, 7, 9, 28, 32, 35, and 36) died from various malignant neoplasms; 3 from nonneoplastic gastrointestional problems (bowel obstruction from adhesions in 1 [Patient 15], perforated gastric ulcer in 1 [Patient 29], and active duodenal ulcer in 1 [Patient 40]); 2 (Patients 24 and 39) from complications of bone fractures after falls; 2 (Patients 10 and 26) from massive pulmonary emboli superimposed on chronic obstructive pulmonary disease; and 1 (Patient 18) from uncertain cause. Of the 7 patients with fatal malignant neoplasms, 3 (Cases 6, 7 and 28) had 2 neoplasms and 4 (Cases 9, 32, 35, and 36) had 1 neoplasm.

Discussion

As in any body organ or tissue, certain changes take place in the cardiovascular system as life progresses. Some of these changes allow easy identification of the very elderly heart when examining cardiac specimens as unknowns. The "normal" elderly heart has relatively small ventricular cavities and relatively large atria and great arteries (Fig. 20). The ascending aorta and left atrium, in comparison with the relatively small left ventricular cavity, appear particularly large. The cor-

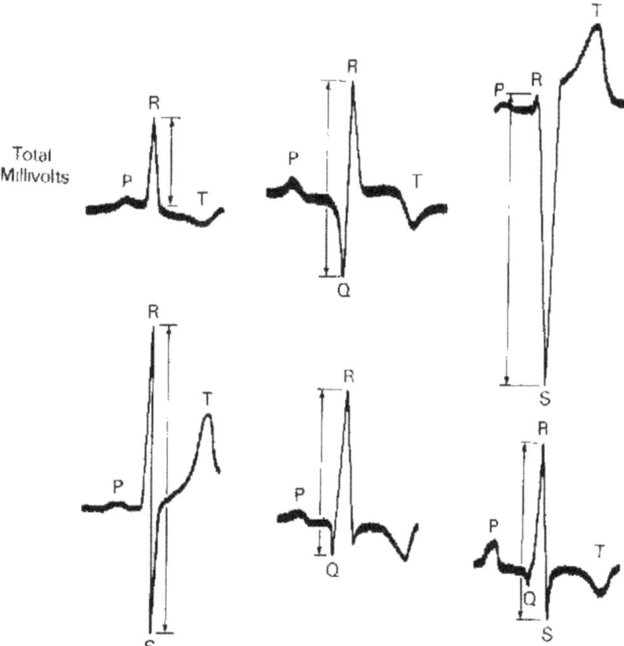

FIGURE 19. Various QRS complexes, and how each was measured. (Reproduced with permission from Siegel RJ, Roberts WC: Electrocardiographic observations in severe aortic valve stenosis: correlative necropsy study to clinical, hemodynamic, and ECG variables demonstrating relation of 12-lead QRS amplitude to peak systolic transaortic pressure gradient. Am Heart J 1982;103:210–221.)

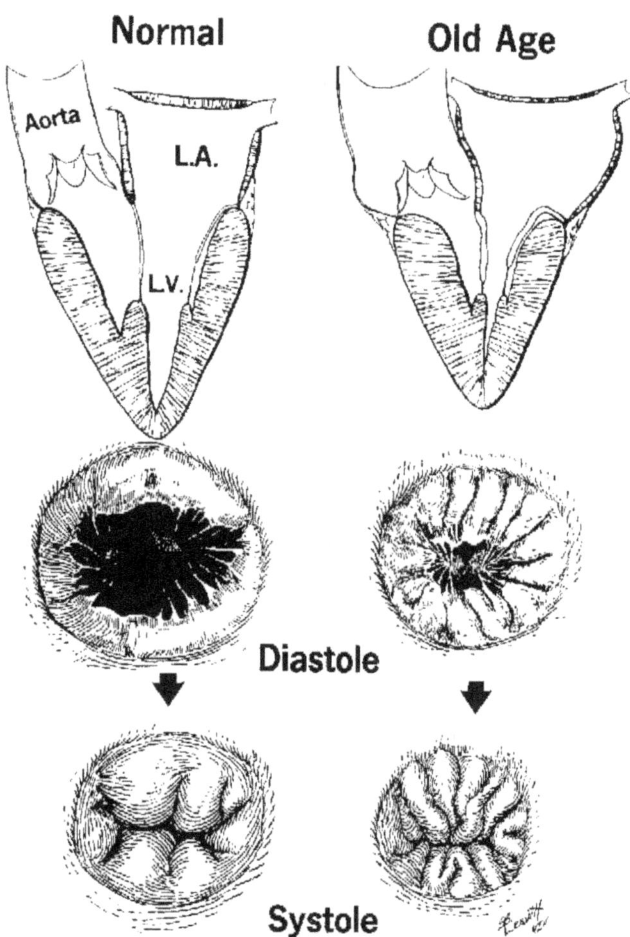

FIGURE 20. Diagram summarizing cardiac changes in the very elderly. The left atrial (LA) cavity enlarges and the left ventricular (LV) cavity becomes smaller. The amount of space available for the mitral leaflets decreases with aging, and consequently the number of scallops in the leaflets appears to increase.

onary arteries increase in both length and width and the former, particularly in association with the decreasing sizes of the cardiac ventricles, results in tortuosity. (The young river is straight and the old one, winding.) The subepicardial adipose tissue increases in amount with aging. The leaflets of each of the 4 cardiac valves thicken with age, particularly the atrioventricular valves, which have a smaller area to occupy in the ventricles because of the diminishing size of the latter. Histologic examination discloses large quantities of lipofuscin pigment in myocardial cells; some contain mucoid deposits ("mucoid degeneration"). These changes appear to affect all population groups of elderly individuals irrespective of where they reside on this earth and irrespective of their level of serum lipids. An elevated systemic arterial pressure appears to both accelerate and amplify these "normal" expected aging cardiac changes.

Both the aorta and its branches and the major pulmonary arteries and their branches enlarge with age. Because the enlargement is in both longitudinal and transverse dimensions, the aorta, like the coronary arteries, tends to become tortuous. This process also is amplified as the vertebral bodies become smaller and the height, somewhat shorter. The major pulmonary arteries appear to be too short and to have too low a pressure to dilate longitudinally.

Although several reports have described cardiovascular finding at necropsy in aged persons, old age was defined as >55,[11] >65,[12] or >75[13] years, and consequently findings in those aged 90 years and over could not be separated from those occurring in the "younger" older persons. The present study appears to be the first to focus entirely on a group of necropsy patients aged 90 years or older. A major finding in our study is the high frequency of calcific deposits in the heart. Of the 40 patients, 37 (92%) had calcific deposits in the epicardial coronary arteries. In most, the deposits were extensive. Although the calcific deposits were located entirely in atherosclerotic plaques, which are located in the intima, the presence of calcific deposits in the coronary arteries in this very elderly population did not necessarily indicate the presence of significant (>75% XSA) luminal narrowing. In contrast, the presence of calcific deposits in epicardial coronary arteries in persons aged <65 years generally indicates the presence of significant luminal narrowing.[14] The calcific deposits tended to occur in each of the 4 major (right, left main, left anterior descending, and left circumflex) epicardial arteries and were always larger in the proximal than in the distal halves of the right, left anterior descending, and left circumflex arteries or, if small, limited to their proximal halves.

Calcific deposits occurred with near equal frequency (55% and 47%) in the aortic valve cusps and in the mitral anular region. The deposits in the aortic valve were located on the aortic aspects of 1 or more of the 3 cusps and usually were unassociated with commissural fusion. The presence or absence of aortic valve stenosis was determined by the quantity of calcium deposited. In 2 patients, the extent of the calcific deposits imparted an immobility to the cusps resulting in aortic valve stenosis. The mitral "anular" calcific deposits, of course, were not limited to the anulus but included the space between the ventricular aspect of the posterior mitral leaflet and the mural endocardium of left ventricular free wall behind posterior mitral leaflet. Often this "anular" calcium extended into the adjacent left ventricular myocardium. Most patients with aortic valve calcium had mitral "anular" calcium and vice versa and all with aortic valvular or mitral "anular" calcium had coronary arterial calcific deposits.

The presence of calcium in the 3 locations in the heart, namely the coronary artery, the aortic valve, and

TABLE III   Electrocardiographic Observations in 30 Patients Aged 90 to 103 Years

| | Clinical Heart Disease | | Total | |
Abnormality	Present* (n = 8)	Absent (n = 22)	n	%
Atrial fibrillation	5	7	12	40
Abnormal QRS axis			12	40
Left (−30 to −90°)	4	6		
Right (+111 to +210°)	1	1		
Complete (QRS ≥0.12 second) BBB			12	40
Left	6	1		
Right	1	4		
Ventricular premature complexes	4	6	10	33
Atrial premature complexes	1	2	3	10
Heart Block			8	27
P-R interval >0.20 second	3	3		
Second degree	0	1		
Third degree (complete)	1†	0		
Q-wave abnormality without BBB			4	13
Q II, III, aV_f	0	1		
Q-S V_1–V_3	0	1		
Both	0	2		
Left ventricular hypertrophy without BBB (R in V_5 or V_6 + S in V_1 ≥35 mm)	1	0	1	3
Low voltage (QRS ≤15 mm in I + II + III)	0	1	1	3

* Coronary heart disease = 3; cardiac amyloidosis = 4; aortic valve stenosis = 1.
† Pacemaker inserted 6 years before death.
BBB = bundle branch block.

TABLE IV Total QRS Voltage in 24 Necropsy Patients Aged ≥90 Years: 8 With (Angina Pectoris [AP] or Acute Myocardial Infarction [AMI] in 5, Amyloid in 2, Aortic Valve Stenosis [AS] in 1) and 16 Without Symptoms of Cardiac Dysfunction

| Pt | Age (yr) & Sex | Clinical Heart Disease | Body Wt (Kg) | Heart Wt (g) | QRS (mm) | | | | | | | | | | | | Sum 1 + 11 +111 | Sum R + L +F | Sum 1 − 111 +R − F | Sum $V_1 - V_6$ | Total |
					I	II	III	R	L	F	V_1	V_2	V_3	V_4	V_5	V_6					
							Patients (n = 8) With Symptoms of Cardiac Dysfunction														
5	90F	AMI	100	400	8	5	6	6	7	5	11	28	21	12	7	15	19	18	37	94	131
1	90F	AMI + AS	120	540	6	7	8	5	6	6	15	20	14	14	11	11	21	17	38	85	123
3	90M	AMI	110	450	5	8	9	5	6	10	12	24	26	19	11	10	22	21	43	102	145
14	92F	AP	107	380	7	8	9	7	7	8	14	12	20	40	16	15	24	22	46	117	163
17	92F	As	120	525	16	15	14	17	13	12	16	25	34	35	25	16	45	42	87	151	238
21	93F	Amyloid	...	380	10	6	12	5	10	10	9	10	11	14	14	6	28	25	53	64	117
27	96M	Amyloid	126	660	6	5	11	2	8	8	7	18	12	11	9	5	22	18	40	62	102
37	99M	AMI	110	510	7	11	7	8	6	7	22	22	6	18	22	18	25	21	46	108	154
Range (mean)	(93)	...	(137)	(481)	...	...	...	...	...	...	...	...	...	...	...	...	19–45 (26)	17–42 (23)	37–87 (49)	62–151 (98)	102–238 (147)
							Patients (n = 16) Without Symptoms of Cardiac Dysfunction														
6	90F	0	100	220	10	12	8	10	8	8	10	24	27	28	22	14	30	26	56	125	181
7	90F	0	104	270	7	10	6	10	4	7	10	22	30	38	32	17	23	21	44	149	193
8	90F	0	110	505	9	7	13	5	9	9	12	16	13	3	4	7	29	23	52	55	107
11	91F	0	99	375	10	10	6	10	5	6	22	21	25	21	18	14	26	21	47	121	168
15	92F	0	109	400	8	8	9	6	8	8	25	27	33	31	20	13	25	22	47	149	196
24	95F	0	128	350	6	7	4	6	7	5	7	6	5	6	10	13	17	18	35	47	82
29	95F	0	120	440	5	10	10	10	10	8	19	15	33	32	22	20	25	18	43	141	184
25	95F	0	...	460	14	11	12	6	12	10	12	17	18	15	5	4	37	28	65	71	136
28	95M	0	...	385	4	13	10	8	4	11	3	8	11	14	11	8	27	23	50	55	105
31	96F	0	100	300	7	15	10	11	4	11	9	16	17	22	29	28	32	26	58	121	179
32	97F	0	120	360	9	5	3	8	12	5	10	19	16	14	15	10	17	25	42	84	126
33	97F	0	90	320	10	6	10	7	9	6	7	16	15	23	28	23	26	22	48	112	160
35	98F	0	117	360	5	10	8	7	3	8	8	15	14	12	8	5	23	18	41	62	103
36	98F	0	115	320	10	9	15	6	10	10	20	34	18	10	8	9	34	26	60	99	159
39	100M	0	...	335	6	6	1	6	2	3	14	11	2	24	24	12	13	11	24	87	111
40	103F	0	120	345	13	25	37	20	22	13	26	19	16	25	23	12	75	55	130	121	251
Range (mean)	(95)	...	(110)	(359)	...	...	...	...	...	...	...	...	...	...	...	...	13–75 (28)	11–55 (24)	24–130 (52)	47–149 (100)	82–251 (152)

Pt = patient; Wt = weight.

the mitral "anulus," might be termed *the senile cardiac calcification syndrome* and strongly suggests that the etiology of the calcific deposits in each of the 3 locations is similar. It is well appreciated, as already mentioned, that the calcific deposits in the coronary arteries are located in atherosclerotic plaques and, therefore, that the calcific deposits in both aortic valve and mitral anular regions might be viewed as anatomic expressions of the atherosclerotic process. All 3 appear to occur only in populations where the total serum cholesterol level is >150 mg/100 ml. Of our 40 patients, total serum cholesterol levels were available in 10: in only 1 (Patient 30) was the level <150, and in 2 the level was 150 to 200 mg/100 ml. In Patient 30, whose value was 108 mg/100 ml, no calcific deposits were present in any of the 3 sites; in Patient 36 whose level was 165 mg/100 ml, minimal calcific deposits were present only in the coronary arteries; and in Patient 28, whose level was 181 mg/100 ml, small calcific deposits were present in the aortic valve (Fig. 16) and coronary arteries. In contrast, of the 7 patients in whom the total serum cholesterol level was >200 mg/100 ml, calcific deposits were present in either aortic valve or mitral anulus or both in 5 patients and in the coronary arteries in all 7 patients; in each the deposits were larger. Calcific deposits in the coronary artery, aortic valve cusp, and mitral anulus are extremely rare in populations where total serum cholesterol levels are <150 mg/100 ml and, of course, clinical evidence of coronary heart disease in these population groups is extremely rare[15] despite a high prevalence of systemic hypertension.

Of the 40 patients, 28 had narrowing of >75% in XSA of ≥1 of the 4 major epicardial coronary arteries. Of the 28 patients, 17 had transmural foci of left ventricular fibrosis or necrosis (myocardial infarction) and of the 12 with insignificant coronary narrowing, none had grossly visible acute or healed myocardial infarcts. Of the 14 patients with healed myocardial infarcts, only 1 had a clinical event compatible with acute myocardial infarction which healed. Of the 10 patients with acute myocardial infarcts at necropsy, only 3 had typical clinical features of acute myocardial infarction; the other 7 had acute changes in their clinical course and acute myocardial infarction was either suspected or compatible with the acute illness. Angina pectoris was described in 3 patients, 1 of whom was among the 10 with fatal acute myocardial infarcts, and 1 of whom had had a nonfatal acute infarct. Thus, 12 patients had clinical features compatible with coronary heart disease and each was among the 28 with significant narrowing of ≥1 of the major coronary arteries. Conversely, of the 28 patients with significant coronary narrowing at necropsy, 16 (57%) never had either angina pectoris or acute myocardial infarction. Of the total 40 patients, only 12 (30%) had clinical events compatible with coronary heart disease and only in 6 were the clinical events really typical.

In 36 of the 40 patients, each of the 4 major coronary arteries were divided into 5 mm long segments and the degree of XSA narrowing by atherosclerotic plaque was determined for each segment. Of the 1,789 5 mm segments in the 36 patients, the average amount of XSA narrowing by atherosclerotic plaques/segment was 42% (range 19 to 69). Of the 467 5 mm segments in the 10 patients with clinical evidence of coronary heart disease, the average amount of XSA narrowing/segment was 55% (range 43 to 69), and 1,322 segments in the 26 patients without clinical evidence of coronary heart disease, 38% (range 19 to 40) (p <0.01). Among 129 patients aged 22 to 85 years (mean 56), the amount of XSA narrowing by atherosclerotic plaques/segment averaged 67%; in the control subjects, that is, those without symptomatic coronary heart disease, XSA narrowing averaged 32%. The mean percent of 5 mm coronary segments narrowed 76 to 100% in XSA in the 36 patients was 13% (range 2 to 89); of the 10 patients with symptomatic coronary heart disease, the mean was 19% (range 10 to 34); and of the 26 patients without symptomatic coronary heart disease, the mean was 7% (range 2 to 28) (p <0.05). The mean of 19% in patients with symptomatic coronary heart disease aged ≥90 was half that observed in patients aged ≤85 years (mean 56) with fatal coronary heart disease and the mean of 8% was nearly 3 times that observed in the younger patients without fatal coronary heart disease.[16-21]

These detailed morphologic studies of the coronary arteries in these very elderly persons suggest that the degree of severe coronary narrowing necessary to have a fatal or near-fatal coronary event is considerably less than that necessary to have a coronary event in younger patients. Moreover, these studies indicate that these very elderly patients without symptoms of coronary heart disease have distinctly more coronary luminal narrowing by atherosclerotic plaques that do control subjects who are younger, (mean age 52 years).[16 21] The latter observation suggests that coronary heart disease may be underdiagnosed clinically in the very elderly.

Clinical diagnosis of cardiac and other conditions in patients aged 90 years and over appears more difficult than in younger persons. Historic information may be difficult to obtain because of impaired intellect on the part of the patient and an impaired diagnostic pursuit on the part of the physician. Physicians caring for these very elderly persons may focus primarily on the prevention of suffering and only secondarily on accurate diagnosis or longer-term therapy. Patients aged 90 years and over generally have outlived their spouses and private physicians, and often are "inherited" by nursing-home physicians who may have limited access to earlier medical records.

Angina pectoris appears particularly difficult to diagnose in the very elderly because they may not be able to describe this symptom. Acute myocardial infarction also is difficult to diagnose clinically but it is often fatal in the very elderly. Of 11 clinical acute infarcts at or after age 90 years in our patients, 10 were fatal. Only 4 of the 11 acute infarcts were clearly diagnosed clinically; most others were manifest as more dyspnea. Furthermore, the electrocardiogram is not as useful in diagnosis of acute myocardial infarction in the very elderly because left bundle branch block is frequent and it, of course, prevents the appearance of typical changes. Serial recordings of electrocardiograms also appear to be quite infrequent in the very elderly. Only

2 of our 10 patients with fatal acute myocardial infarction had as many as 2 electrocardiograms recorded during the final illness.

Physical examination in the very elderly may be both difficult and misleading. The lack of mobility may prevent proper positioning of the elderly patient for proper examining. Precordial murmurs, although very common (25 of our 40 patients), infrequently indicate significant functional abnormality. Although 22 of our 40 patients had calcific deposits in the aortic valve, only 2 appeared to have actual aortic valve stenosis. Likewise, although 19 of the 40 patients had mitral anular calcific deposits, in only 1 patient did the calcific deposits appear to actually narrow the mitral orifice.

Electrocardiographic abnormalities are common in elderly persons. Of our 30 patients with electrocardiograms available, all had ≥ 1 abnormalities recorded, the most frequent ones being abnormal axis, atrial fibrillation, and complete bundle branch block. Although 15 of the 30 patients had cardiomegaly (>350 g in women, >400 g in men) at necropsy, only 1 had voltage criteria for left ventricular hypertrophy shown by electrocardiography. Likewise, only 1 had low voltage. Measurement of the QRS amplitude in each of the 12 leads was performed in 24 patients; these measurements have never been recorded previously in elderly individuals. The total QRS voltage was similar in the 8 patients with and in the 16 patients without clinical evidence of cardiac disease (mean 147 mm versus mean 152 mm [10 mm = 1 mV]). Although normal amplitudes of the QRS complexes in all 12 leads in elderly patients are lacking, Simonson[22] provided data on the upper and lower limits of amplitude of the QRS complexes in each of the 12 leads in normal men and women aged 20 to 59 years (means not available). The upper and lower limits of normal for men aged 50 to 59 years was 277 and 36 mm, and for the women 248 and 27 mm, respectively.

Acknowledgment: We thank Filippina Giacometti, Barbara Winterrowd, Margaret Moore, Mary McMahon, Alvado Campbell, and Exa Murray for assistance far beyond the call of duty in the completion of this project.

References

1. **Fries JF.** Aging, natural history, and the compression of morbidity. N Engl J Med 1980;303:130-135.
2. **Siegel JS.** Recent and prospective demographic trends for the elderly population and some implications for health care In: Haynes SG, Feinleib M, eds. Second Conference on the Epidemiology of Aging. U.S. Department of Health and Human Services. Washington DC, NIH Publication No. 80-969, 1980;293.
3. **Kohn RR.** Cause of death in very old people JAMA 1982;247:2793-2797.
4. **Eckner FAD, Brown BW, Davidson DL, Glagov S.** Dimensions of normal hearts after standard fixation by controlled pressure coronary perfusion Arch Pathol Lab Med 1969;88:497-507.
5. **Roberts WC, Perloff JK, Constantino T.** Severe valvular aortic stenosis in patients over 65 years of age. A clinicopathologic study. Am J Cardiol 1971;27:497-506.
6. **Roberts WC, Perloff JK.** Mitral valve disease A clinico-pathologic survey of the conditions causing the mitral valve to function abnormally. Ann Intern Med 1972;77:939-975
7. **Roberts WC, Waller BF.** Mitral valve "anular" calcium forming a complete circle or "O" configuration: clinical and necropsy observations. Am Heart J 1981;101:619-621.
8. **Buja LM, Khoi NB, Roberts WC.** Clinically significant cardiac amyloidosis. Clinicopathologic findings in 15 patients Am J Cardiol 1970;26:394-405.
9. **Beck CS.** Coronary artery disease. A report to William Harvey 300 years later Am J Cardiol 1958;1:38-45
10. **Roberts WC.** Aortic dissection: anatomy, consequences and causes. Am Heart J 1981;101:195-214.
11. **Surgiura M, Hiraoka K, Ohkawa S, Shimada H.** A clinicopathologic study on the heart diseases in the aged. The morphologic classification of 1,000 consecutive autopsy cases. Jpn Heart J 1975;16:526-537.
12. **Pomerance A.** Cardiac pathology in the elderly. In: Noble RJ, Rothbaum DA, eds. Geriatric Cardiology. Philadelphia: FA Davis, 1981· 9-54
13. **Pomerance A.** Pathology of the heart with and without cardiac failure in the aged. Br Heart J 1965,27:697-710.
14. **Aldrich RF, Brensike JF, Battaglini JW, Richardson JM, Loh IK, Stone NJ, Passamani ER, Ackerstein H, Seningen R, Borer JS, Levy RI, Epstein SE.** Coronary calcifications in the detection of coronary artery disease and comparison with electrocardiographic exercise testing. Results from the National Heart, Lung, and Blood Institute's Type II Coronary Intervention Study. Circulation 1979;59:1113-1124.
15. **Gelfand M.** Heart disease in the elderly African. Br Heart J 1961;23:387-392.
16. **Roberts WC, Jones AA.** Quantitation of coronary arterial narrowing at necropsy in sudden coronary death. Analysis of 31 patients and comparison with 25 control subjects. Am J Cardiol 1979;44:39-45
17. **Roberts WC, Virmani R.** Quantification of coronary arterial narrowing on clinically-isolated unstable angina pectoris. An analysis of 22 necropsy patients. Am J Med 1979;67:792-799.
18. **Roberts WC, Jones AA.** Quantification of coronary arterial narrowing at necropsy in acute transmural myocardial infarction: analysis and comparison of findings in 27 patients and 22 controls. Circulation 1980;61:786-790.
19. **Virmani R, Roberts WC.** Quantification of coronary arterial narrowing and of left ventricular myocardial scarring in healed myocardial infarction with chronic, eventually fatal, congestive heart failure Am J Med 1980;68:831-838.
20. **Cabin HS, Roberts WC.** True left ventricular aneurysm and healed myocardial infarction. Clinical and necropsy observations including quantification of degrees of coronary arterial narrowing. Am J Cardiol 1980;46:754-763
21. **Virmani R, Roberts WC.** Non-fatal healed transmural myocardial infarction and fatal non-cardiac disease. Qualification and quantification of coronary arterial narrowing. Br Heart J 1981;45:434-441.
22. **Simonson F.** Differentiation Between Normal and Abnormal in Electrocardiography. St Louis· CV Mosby, 1961:328.

Coronary Arterial Rupture During Coronary Angioplasty

JEFFREY E. SAFFITZ, MD, PhD,*
THOMAS E. ROSE, MD, JOHN B. OAKS, MD,
and WILLIAM C. ROBERTS, MD

Although percutaneous transluminal coronary angioplasty (PTCA) appears to be a relatively safe and effective procedure, reported complications include cor-

From the Pathology Branch, National Heart, Lung, and Blood Institute, National Institutes of Health, Bethesda, Maryland. Manuscript received November 4, 1982, accepted December 6, 1982.

* On leave of absence from the Department of Pathology, Washington University, St. Louis, Missouri.

onary occlusion and dissection with or without acute myocardial infarction.[1,2] Herein, a hitherto unreported complication of PTCA is described.

A 77-year-old man with unstable angina pectoris by coronary angiography had focal severe stenosis of a dominant right coronary artery (Fig. 1a), a normal left coronary system, and normal left ventricular function. PTCA of the right coronary artery was performed. The tight stenosis prevented appropriate placement of a 2-mm Gruntzig catheter; therefore, the narrowing was dilated initially by multiple inflations of a Simpson catheter advanced across a guide wire, and subsequently by a 3-mm Gruntzig catheter at 4 atm (Fig. 1b). Post-PTCA angiograms demonstrated mild residual stenosis (Fig. 1c). Coronary angiography 3 months later disclosed significant stenosis again at the site of the previous dilatation procedure (Fig. 1d). Repeat PTCA was performed. Multiple inflations of a 3-mm Gruntzig catheter at a maximal pressure of 9 atm reduced the stenosis to about 60% diameter reduction. A 3.7-mm Gruntzig catheter was then positioned and inflated 5 times at a maximal pressure of 10

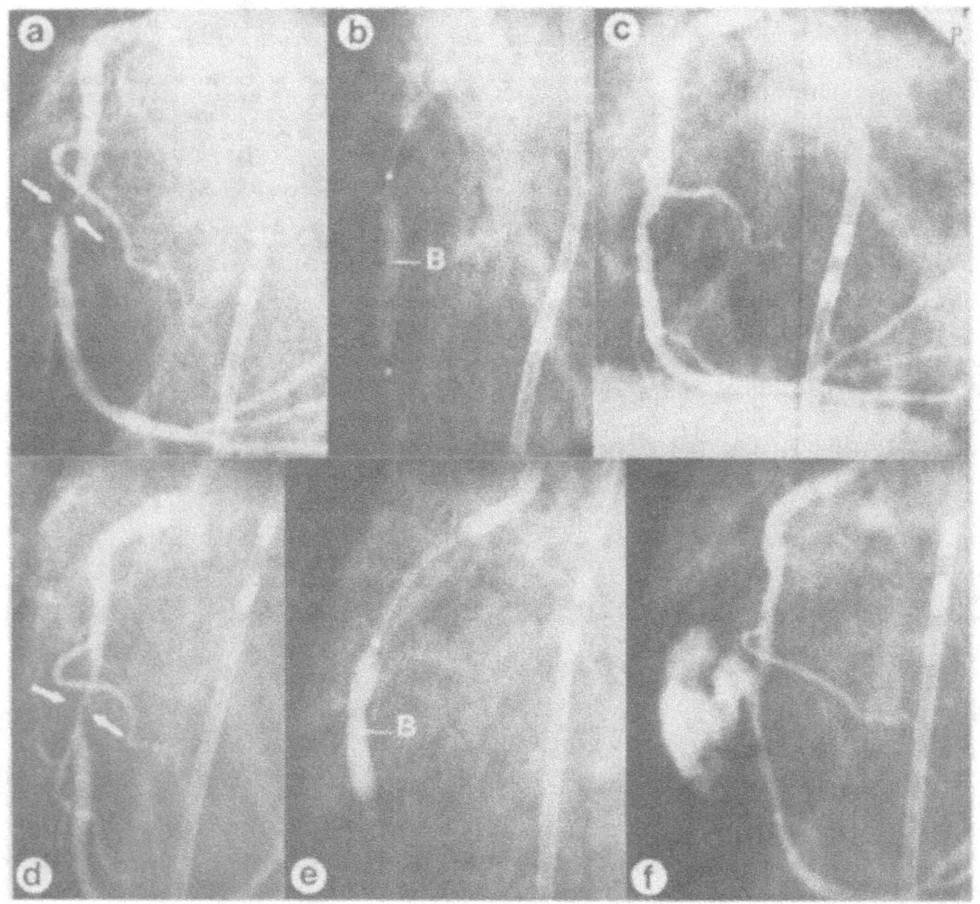

FIGURE 1. Right coronary arteriograms before (**a** and **d**), during (**b** and **e**), and after (**c** and **f**) percutaneous transluminal coronary angioplasty (PTCA). **a,** a discrete severe narrowing is present (**arrows**). **b,** the stenosis was dilated by a 3-mm Gruntzig balloon (B) catheter. **c,** mild residual narrowing remained after the first PTCA procedure. **d,** the previously dilated area was again severely narrowed (**arrows**) 3 months after the first PTCA procedure. **e,** the narrowing was dilated by a 3.7-mm Gruntzig balloon (B) catheter. **f,** arteriography after PTCA showed leakage of contrast material into the epicardial tissues. The luminal diameter immediately proximal and distal to the narrowing is approximately equal to that of the pacing catheter (**d**). The diameter of the inflated balloon (**e**) is larger than that of the pacing catheter and thus exceeds the diameter of the nonstenotic arterial lumen.

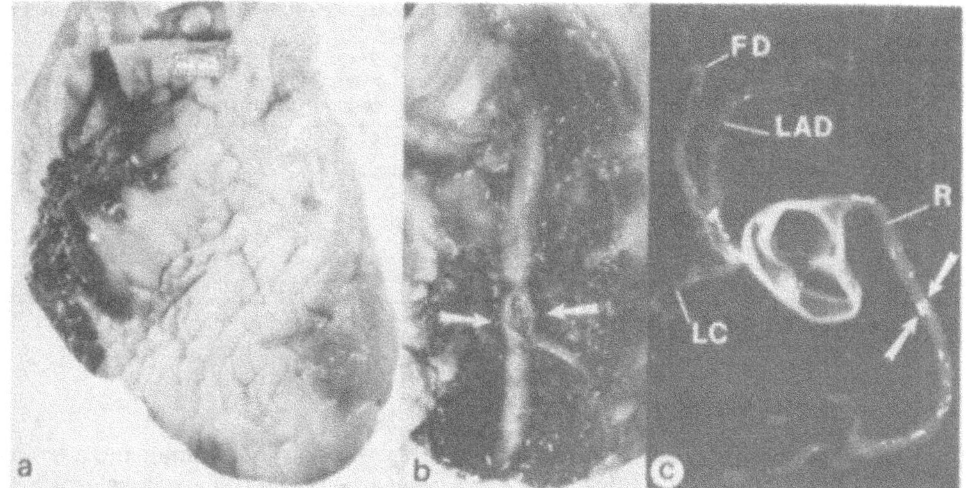

FIGURE 2. a, Photograph of heart showing hemorrhage in the right atrioventricular sulcus which contains the right coronary artery. **b,** a rupture site (**arrows**) in the right coronary artery 3.5 cm from the aortic ostium. **c,** radiograph of the major epicardial coronary arteries demonstrating focal calcific deposits. **Arrows** designate the site of rupture of the right (R) coronary artery. FD = first diagonal; LAD = left anterior descending; LC = left circumflex. (Photographs by M. M. M. Moore.)

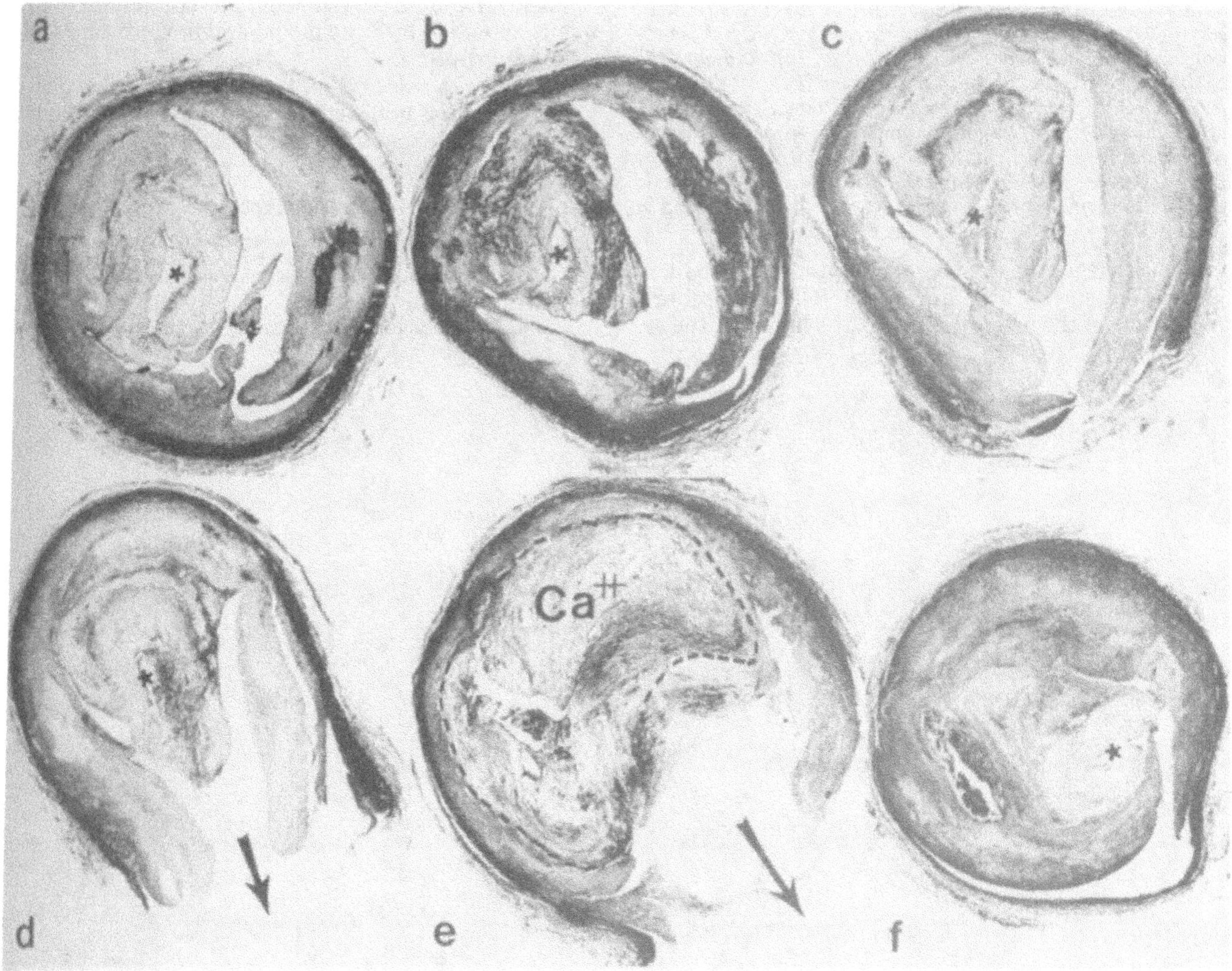

FIGURE 3. Photomicrographs of cross-sections of the right coronary artery in the vicinity of the rupture site. Proximal to the rupture site (**a**) the atherosclerotic plaque is split. This split communicates with the original lumen, indicated by the **asterisks.** The split extends through the media (**b**) and adventitia (**c**) until through-and-through rupture (**arrows**) occurs (**d,e**). Rupture occurred opposite a large calcified (Ca^{++}) plaque (outlined by **dashed line**). Distal to the rupture site (**f**), additional splitting of the intimal plaque is seen communicating with the original lumen.

TABLE I   Number of 5-mm Segments of the 4 Major Epicardial Coronary Arteries Showing the 4 Grades of Cross-Sectional Area Narrowing

Coronary Artery	Length (cm)	5-mm Segments (n)	5-mm Segments (n) Narrowed to Each of 4 Categories of Cross-Sectional Area Narrowing			
			0–25%	26–50%	51–75%	76–100%
R	8.5	17	1	. . .	9	7
LM	0.5	1	. . .	1	. . .	. . .
LAD	9.0	18	2	11	5	. . .
LC	4.5	9	3	6	. . .	. . .
Totals	22.5	45	6 (13%)	18 (40%)	14 (31%)	7 (16%)

LAD = left anterior descending, LC = left circumflex, LM = left main, and R = right coronary artery.

atm (Fig. 1e). On the fifth inflation, the proximal end of the balloon ruptured. Angiography then demonstrated extravasation of contrast material into the epicardial tissue plus run-off into the distal right coronary artery (Fig. 1f). The heart rate and arterial blood pressure quickly decreased; blood was drained from the pericardial sac, but fatal cardiac arrest ensued.

At necropsy, the heart weighed 265 g. The epicardial adipose tissue surrounding the right coronary artery was hemorrhagic (Fig. 2a) and an elliptical rupture site measuring 0.6 cm in the long axis was present in the right coronary artery 3.5 cm from the ostium (Fig. 2b). Radiographs of the major epicardial coronary arteries (Fig. 2c) disclosed focal calcific deposits. The results of histologic examination of 5-mm segments of the major epicardial coronary arteries are shown in Table I. A 1.7-cm segment of right coronary artery containing the rupture site was subserially sectioned and photomicrographs of several sections are illustrated in Figure 3.

It is clear that the right coronary artery in the patient just described ruptured during the PTCA procedure. At the site of the arterial rupture, the lumen of the ar-tery was extremely small and a large amount of calcium was present in the atherosclerotic plaque. In addition, the artery itself was quite small. (The patient weighed only 105 pounds and the heart weighed only 265 g.) The presence of a *small, rigid (calcified) artery* and the use of a *balloon larger than the artery* itself caused the arterial rupture in this patient. Balloon dilatation was successful in enlarging the lumen by splitting the plaque. However, the splitting was not limited to plaque but extended into the media and adventitia, resulting in fatal rupture.

To our knowledge, rupture of a coronary artery during PTCA has not been reported previously. The lesson of this case is that angioplasty balloons larger than the artery to be dilated should not be employed.

References

1. **Dorros G, Cowley M, Simpson J.** Members of Executive Committee of NHLBI-PTCA Registry. National Heart, Lung, and Blood Institute registry report of complication of percutaneous transluminal angioplasty (abstr). Am J Cardiol 1981;47:396.
2. **Bourassa MG.** Percutaneous transluminal coronary angioplasty—still an investigational procedure. Mayo Clin Proc 1981;56:334–335.

Extravasated erythrocytes, iron, and fibrin in atherosclerotic plaques of coronary arteries in fatal coronary heart disease and their relation to luminal thrombus: Frequency and significance in 57 necropsy patients and in 2958 five mm segments of 224 major epicardial coronary arteries

The presence of extravasated erythrocytes (EE), iron (I), and fibrin (F) within coronary atherosclerotic plaques and their relation to intraluminal coronary thrombus was determined in 2958 five-mm segments of 224 major epicardial coronary arteries in 57 patients with fatal coronary heart disease and in 1290 five-mm segments of 103 coronary arteries in 27 control (c) subjects. Intraplaque EE were present in 10% of the segments (controls [c] = 1%), in 35% of the arteries (c = 5%), and in 84% of the patients (c = 19%); I was present in 4% of the segments (c = < 1%), in 14% of the arteries (c = 4%), and in 57% of the patients (c = 22%); intraplaque F was present in 2% of the segments (c = < 1%), in 17% of the arteries (c = 3%), and in 63% of the patients (c = 7%). Intraluminal thrombus, present only in the patients with acute myocardial infarction and in none of the controls, occurred in 3% of the segments, in 8% of the arteries and in 26% of the patients. Intraplaque hemorrhage or EE occurred usually in the absence of intraluminal thrombus and conversely intraluminal thrombus occurred more frequently without than with underlying plaque hemorrhage. The frequency of intraplaque EE, I, and F was proportional to the amount of coronary atherosclerotic plaque present. Intraplaque I and F infrequently were observed in the absence of EE. The significance of extravasated erythrocytes, iron, and fibrin in atherosclerotic plaques remains unclear. (AM HEART J 105:788, 1983.)

Renu Virmani, M.D., and William C. Roberts, M.D. *Bethesda, Md.*

Extravasation of erythrocytes into coronary atherosclerotic plaques has been the subject of many reports.[1-17] The observations in most reports were based on microscopic examination of histologic sections of portions of coronary arteries which on gross examination had changes consistent with hemorrhage into a plaque or intraluminal thrombus. At least two reports[18, 19] have discussed iron (hemosiderin) deposition within atherosclerotic plaques, but no reports (to our knowledge) have described the frequency of fibrin deposits within coronary atherosclerotic plaques. To determine the frequency of extravasated erythrocytes, iron, and fibrin deposits within coronary atherosclerotic plaques, we examined microscopically 2958 five-mm segments of 224 major epicardial coronary arteries in 57 patients with fatal coronary heart disease and in 1290 five-mm segments of 103 major epicardial coronary arteries in 27 control subjects. Additionally, we correlated their presence to the degrees of cross-sectional area luminal narrowing produced by the atherosclerotic plaques and to the presence of intraluminal thrombus.

METHODS

Patients. Of the 57 patients with coronary heart disease, 20 died from transmural *acute myocardial infarction* diagnosed both clinically and at necropsy,[20] 20 died suddenly *(sudden coronary death)* (i.e., usually in less than 5 minutes but all within 6 hours from onset of an acute change in clinical state[21]), and 17 died within 3 days

From the Pathology Branch, National Heart, Lung and Blood Institute, National Institutes of Health.

Received for publication Sept. 22, 1982; accepted Oct. 15, 1982.

Reprint requests: William C. Roberts, M.D., National Institutes of Health, Bldg. 10A, Room 3E-30, Bethesda, MD 20205.

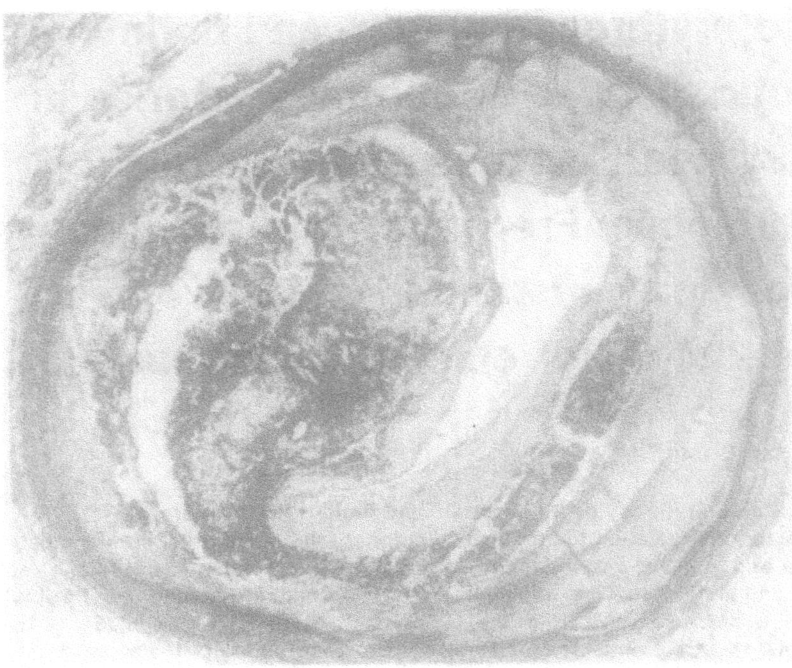

Fig. 1. *Extravasated erythrocytes* in an atherosclerotic plaque of the right coronary artery in a 61-year-old man with acute myocardial infarct. (Movat stain; original magnification ×23.)

of an aortocoronary bypass operation performed for *clinically isolated angina pectoris*[22] (Table I). None of the 20 patients with acute myocardial infarction or sudden coronary death had had an aortocoronary bypass operation. These 57 patients were compared to 27 age- and sex-matched control subjects who had the following characteristics: (1) death from a noncardiac condition; (2) absence of symptoms suggesting or indicating myocardial ischemia or cardiac dysfunction during life; (3) absence of systemic hypertension (>140 mm Hg systolic and/or >90 mm Hg diastolic); (4) absence of cardiomegaly (>400 gm [men] and >350 gm [women]); and (5) absence of left ventricular fibrosis or necrosis.

Histologic examination. The epicardial coronary arteries in all 57 patients and in the 27 control subjects were studied in a similar fashion. In four patients and in five control subjects the left main coronary artery was not available for examination. The four major epicardial coronary arteries were excised intact, x-rayed, and fixed for at least 2 days. After decalcification (if the radiograph had shown calcific deposits), each of the four major coronary arteries was cut transversely to its longitudinal axes into 5-mm long segments and each segment was labelled sequentially from either its aortic ostium or from its origin from the left main. The 5-mm segments were labelled, dehydrated (alcohol and xylene), embedded in paraffin, and three histologic sections were cut and stained from each paraffin block. The hematoxylin and eosin stained sections were used to determine the presence of extravasated erythrocytes and fibrin within atherosclerotic plaques and the presence of intraluminal thrombus; the Prussian blue stain was used to determine the presence or absence of iron within atherosclerotic plaques; and the Movat stain was used for determining the amount of cross-sectional area luminal narrowing of the four major extramural coronary arteries by atherosclerotic plaque. The Movat stain also delineated clearly extravasated erythrocytes and fibrin deposits. The degree of narrowing was based on histologic examination of each cross section magnified 25 to 50 times. The judgment regarding the degree of luminal narrowing of each 5-mm segment was based on the degree of luminal obliteration within the luminal circle bordered by the internal elastic membrane. The percent of cross-sectional area luminal narrowing in each 5-mm segment was determined as follows: 0-25, 26-50, 51-75, and 76-100.

The location of the intraplaque extravasated erythrocytes, iron, and fibrin was designated as occurring in pultaceous debris, fibrous tissue, or in mucoid material. The relation of intraplaque extravasated erythrocytes, iron, and fibrin to each other and to intraluminal thrombus was recorded. Additionally, the presence of each of these four components was correlated with the amount of cross-sectional area luminal narrowing by atherosclerotic plaque.

RESULTS

Intraplaque erythrocytes, iron, and fibrin, and intralumen thrombus. The frequency of intraplaque extravasated erythrocytes (Fig. 1), iron (Fig. 2) and fibrin (Fig. 3), and of intraluminal thrombus (Fig. 4) in the coronary arteries is summarized in Tables II to V. Of the 57 *patients,* 48 (84%) had extravasated erythro-

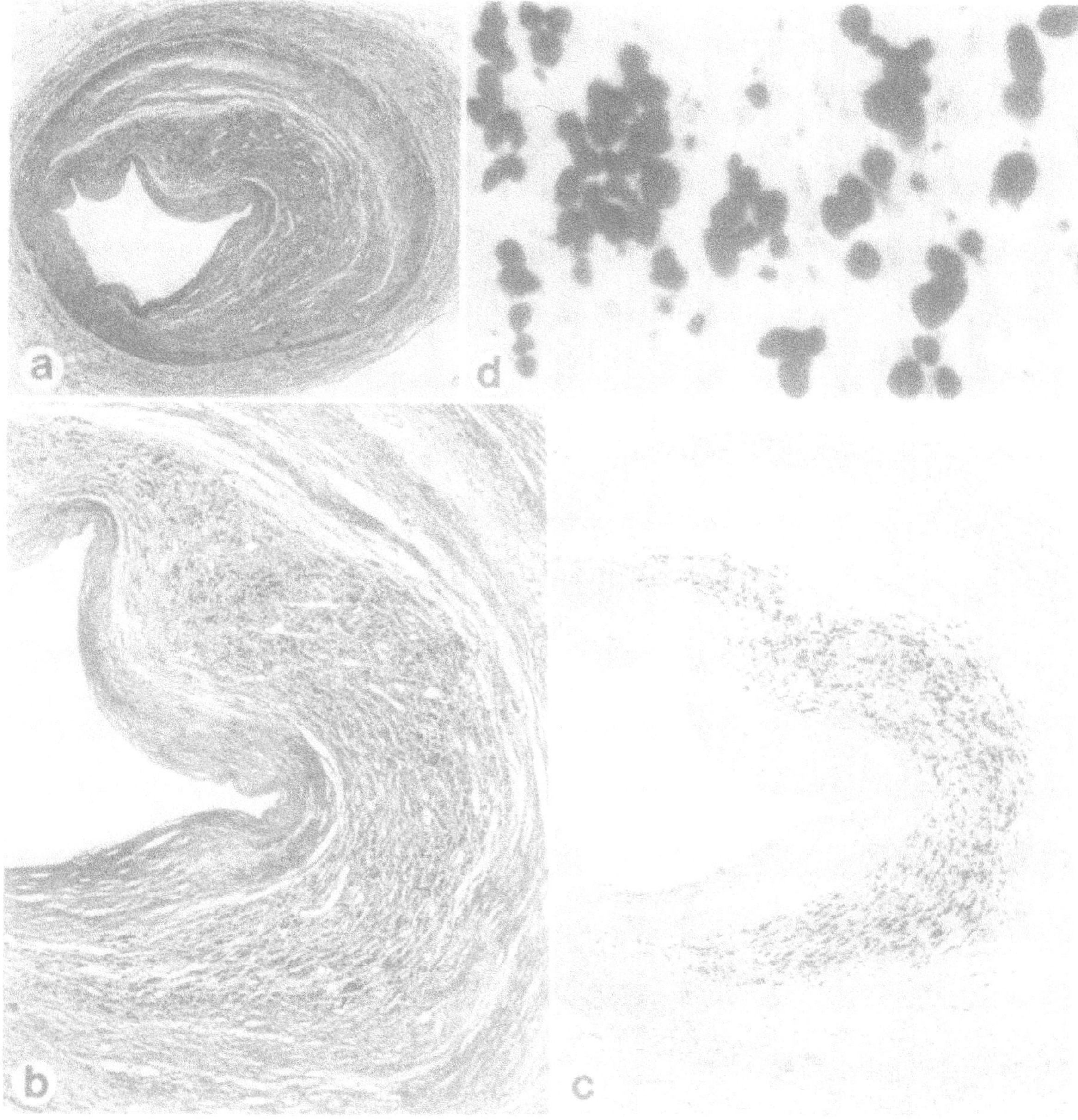

Fig. 2. *Intraplaque iron* in the right coronary artery of a 40-year-old man who died suddenly from severe coronary heart disease. *a,* First centimeter of right coronary artery. *b,* Close-up of iron deposits. *c,* Same portion as *b* but stained for iron. *d,* Close-up of iron deposits from *c.* (Hematoxylin-eosin stains: original magnifications ×23 [*a*], ×55 [*b*]; Prussian blue stains: original magnifications ×45 [*c*], ×400 [*d*].)

cytes (controls = 5 [19%] of 27); 32 (56%), iron (controls = 6 [22%]); and 36 (63%), fibrin (controls = 2 [7%]) within atherosclerotic plaques. Intraluminal thrombus was present in 15 (26%) of the 57 patients and in none of the 27 control subjects. No differences in frequency of intraplaque extravasated erythrocytes, or iron or fibrin was present among the three subgroups of coronary patients (acute myocardial infarction, sudden coronary death, or isolated angina pectoris). In contrast, intraluminal thrombi were found only in the patients with acute myocardial infarction, two of whom, however, were in the angina pectoris group with acute infarction immediately after aortocoronary bypass operations.

Epicardial coronary arteries. Of the 224 *major coronary arteries* in the 57 patients, 79 (35%) had extravasated erythrocytes (controls = 5 [5%] of 103 arteries); 32 (14%) had iron (controls = 4 [4%]), and 39 [17%] had fibrin (controls = 3 [3%]) within

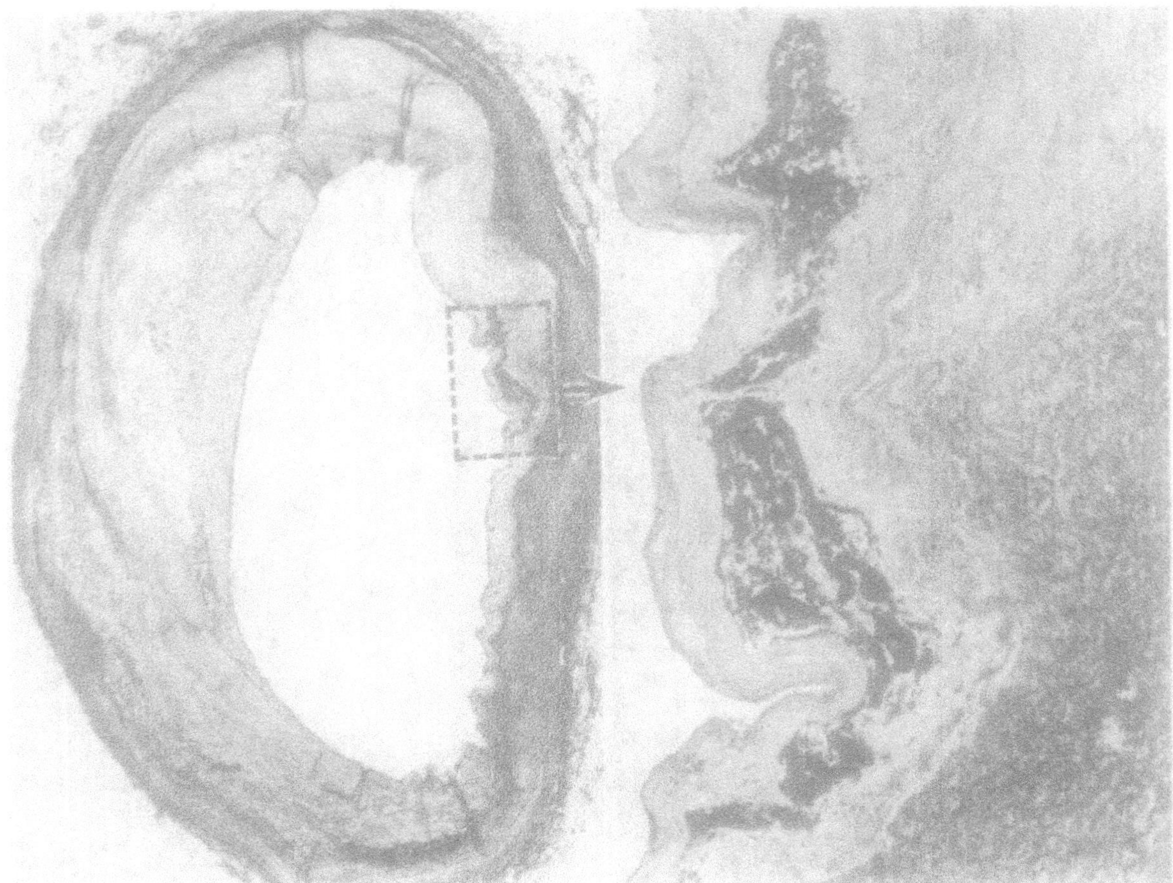

Fig. 3. *Intraplaque fibrin* (brackets) in right coronary artery in a 61-year-old man with acute myocardial infarction. (Movat stain; original magnifications ×23 [*left*], original magnifications ×135 [*right*].)

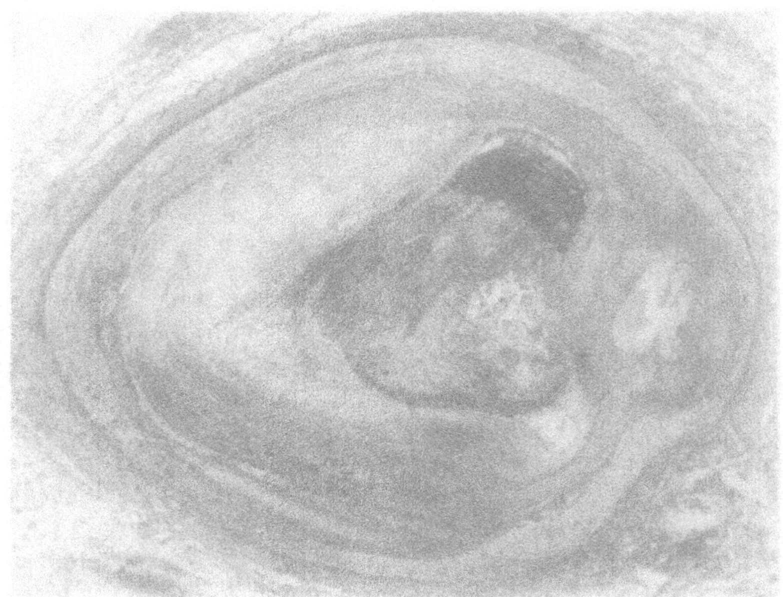

Fig. 4. *Intraluminal thrombus* in the right coronary artery of a 65-year-old man who had been asymptomatic until 6 days before death when he had an acute myocardial infarct complicated by rupture of both the ventricular septum and left ventricular free wall. (Movat stain; original magnification ×27.)

Table I. Clinical and morphologic observations in the 57 coronary patients and in the 27 control subjects

Group	No. pts	Age (yr) Range (m)	Sex		Clinical findings [No. (%)]					
			M	F	AP	AMI	SH	CHF	DM	H
Coronary	57	28-82 (58)	42 (74)	15 (26)	41 (72)	14 (25)	23 (40)	6 (10)	13 (25)	14 (25)
AMI	20	43-82 (63)	14	6	15	8	8	1	6	1
SCD	20	28-78 (53)	16	4	9	6	7	5	2	6
AP	17	40-69 (49)	12	5	17	0	8	0	3	7
Controls	27	41-78 (54)	19 (67)	9 (33)	0	0	0	0	0	0

Abbreviations: AMI = acute myocardial infarction; AP = unstable angina pectoris; CA = coronary arteries; CHF = congestive heart failure; DM = diabetes mellitus; F = female; H = hyperlipoproteinemia; LV = left ventricle; (m) = mean; M = male; pts = patients; S = subendocardial; SCD = sudden coronary death; SH = systemic hypertension; T = transmural.

Table II. Number (%) of 57 coronary patients and 27 control subjects containing at least 1 coronary atherosclerotic plaque, extravasated erythrocytes (EE), iron (I), and/or fibrin (F) and in at least 1 coronary lumen and thrombus (T)

Group	No pts	Intraplaque							
		EE only	I only	F only	EE + I	EE + F	I + F	EE + I + F	None
Coronary	57	7 (12)	1 (2)	3 (5)	9 (16)	11 (19)	1 (2)	21 (37)	4 (7)
AMI	20	2	1	2	2	5	0	7	1
SCD	20	1	0	1	3	6	0	6	3
AP	17	4	0	0	4	0	1	8	0
Controls	27	1 (4)	4 (15)	0	2 (7)	2 (7)	0	0	18 (67)

Abbreviations as in Table I.

*Both patients had acute transmural myocardial infarcts shortly after aortocoronary bypass operations.

atherosclerotic plaques, which were located entirely within the intima. Intraluminal thrombus was present in 18 (8%) of the 224 arteries and in none of the 103 arteries in the 27 controls. The frequency of intraplaque extravasated erythrocytes was similar (about 35%) in all major coronary arteries in the three subgroups of coronary patients. Intraplaque iron was more frequent in the subset of patients with angina pectoris (16 [24%] of 66 arteries) than in the subset with either acute myocardial infarction (7 [9%] of 79 arteries) or sudden coronary death (9 [11%] of 79 arteries). Intraplaque fibrin was less frequent in the coronary arteries in the subset of coronary patients with sudden coronary death than in the subsets with either acute myocardial infarction or angina pectoris.

Coronary segments. Of the 2958 *five-mm segments* of the 224 coronary arteries in the 57 patients, 287 (10%) had extravasated erythrocytes (controls = 15 [1%] of 1290 segments), 133 (4%) had iron (controls = 10 [<1%]), and 67 (2%) had fibrin (controls = five [<1%]) within atherosclerotic plaques. Intraluminal thrombus was present in 94 (3%) of the 2958 coronary segments in the patients, all of

| | Morphologic observations [No. (%)] | | | | | | | |
| Heart weight (gm) (m) | Fibrosis, LV | | Necrosis, LV | | No. (%) CA narrowed > 75% in X-sectional area | | | |
	T	S	T	S	1	2	3	4
300-680 (425)	19 (33)	12 (21)	20 (35)	3 (5)	5 (9)	8 (14)	32 (56)	12 (21)
310-680 (434)	8	2	18	2	2	3	13	2
300-670 (465)	9	4	0	0	2	3	12	3
330-520	2	6	2	1	1	2	7	7
210-390 (308)	0	0	0	0	4 (15)	3 (11)	0	0

| Intraluminal | | | | |
T + EE	T + F	T + EE + F	T + EE + I + F	0/T
1 (2)	2 (3)	5 (9)	7 (12)	42 (74)
1	2	5	5	7
0	0	0	0	20
0	0	0	2*	15
0	0	0	0	0

whom had transmural acute myocardial infarcts, and in none of the 1290 five-mm coronary segments in the control subjects.

The relation between intraplaque extravasated erythrocytes, iron, and fibrin and intraluminal thrombus to the degree of luminal narrowing of each 5-mm segment of the 224 coronary arteries in the 57 patients (and in the controls) is summarized in Table VI. The larger the atherosclerotic plaque (or the greater the degree of luminal narrowing by plaque), the greater the frequency of intraplaque extravasated erythrocytes, iron, and fibrin.

The mean percent of 5-mm segments containing intraplaque extravasated erythrocytes, iron, and fibrin was similar in the right, left anterior descending, and left circumflex coronary arteries. No segments of the left main coronary artery contained intraplaque iron or intraluminal thrombus. The predominant location of the extravasated erythrocytes in the atherosclerotic plaques was as follows: in pultaceous debris in 136 (47%) five-mm segments; in fibrous tissue in 91 (32%) segments; and in mucoid material in 60 (21%) segments.

DISCUSSION

Previous studies. The reported frequency of intraplaque hemorrhages into atherosclerotic plaques of coronary arteries in patients with coronary heart disease has ranged from 17%[13] to 100%.[4] Combining a total of 777 patients so studied from seven previously published reports,* 290 patients (37%) had extravasated erythrocytes in coronary atherosclerotic plaques. In addition, the frequency of coronary intraplaque hemorrhage has been described in nine other studies in which the types of patients analyzed were not clear to us or were not mentioned.† Combining these nine studies yielded an additional 1343 patients of whom 362 (27%) had extravasated erythrocytes into coronary atherosclerotic plaques. The range from the nine studies varied from 5% to 100%; the 27% would have been considerably higher if the study by Paterson,[3] in which the author

*Refs. 1, 4, 9, 10, 13, 15, and 17.
†Refs. 2, 3, 5-9, 11, 14, and 16.

Table III. Number and percent of 224 coronary arteries in 57 coronary patients and 103 coronary arteries in 27 control subjects containing extravasated erythrocytes (EE), iron (I), and fibrin (F) in atherosclerotic plaques and thrombus (T) in coronary lumens

Group	No pts	No. CA examined	No. (%) with EE	No. (%) CA with EE				No. (%) with I
				1	2	3	4	
Coronary	57	224	79 (35)	15	19	6	2	32 (14)
AMI	20	79	25 (32)	4	6	3	0	7 (9)
SCD	20	79	28 (35)	6	9	0	1	9 (11)
AP	17	66	26 (39)	5	4	3	1	16 (24)
Controls	27	103	5 (5)	1	2	0	0	4 (4)

Abbreviations as in Table I.

Table IV. Number (%) of 2958 five-mm segments of 224 major coronary arteries in 57 coronary patients and number (%) of 1290 five-mm segments of 103 major coronary arteries in 27 control subjects containing extravasated erythrocytes (EE), iron (I), and/or fibrin (F) in atherosclerotic plaques and thrombus (T) in coronary lumens

		Intraplaque									
		EE		I		F		Number (%) with:			
Group	Number segments	Total	Isolated	Total	Isolated	Total	Isolated	EE + I	EE + F	I + F	E + I + F
Coronary	2958	287(10)	191(6)	133(4)	61(2)	67(2)	42(1)	69(2)	17(<1)	7(<1)	3(<1)
AMI	1037	109(11)	79(8)	34(3)	15(1)	25(2)	14(1)	17(1)	9(<1)	2(<1)	2(<1)
SCD	1094	90(8)	56(5)	41(4)	15(1)	21(2)	13(1)	26(2)	4(<1)	3(<1)	2(<1)
AP	827	88(11)	56(5)	58(7)	31(4)	21(3)	15(2)	26(3)	4(<1)	2(<1)	0
Controls	1290	15(1)	10(>1)	10(<1)	5(<1)	5(<1)	3(<1)	5(<1)	0	0	0

Abbreviations as in Table I.

Table VI. Relation between the presence of extravasated erythrocytes (EE), iron (I), and fibrin (F) in atherosclerotic plaques and of thrombus (T) in lumina in each 5-mm segment of the 4 major epicardial arteries to the degree of luminal narrowing by atherosclerotic plaques in each 5-mm segment

		No. (%) of 5-mm coronary segments with EE, I, F, and T in each of 4 categories									
		0-25%					26-50%				
Group	Number segments	Sub-total	EE	I	F	T	Sub-total	EE	I	F	T
Coronary	2950	260 (9)	0	0	0	0 / 0	452 (15)	6 (1)	4 (1)	3 (1)	18 (4)
AMI	1037	69	0	0	0	0	198	2	0	2	16
SCD	1094	100	0	0	0	0	173	1	2	1	0
AP	827	91	0	0	0	0	81	3	2	0	2
Controls	1290	358 (28)	0	0	0	0	502 (39)	3	2	1	0

Intraplaque							Intraluminal		
No. (%) CA with I			No. (%) with F	No. (%) CA with F			No. (%) with T	No. (%) CA	
1	2	3		1	2	3		1	2
13	5	3	39 (17)	15	9	2	18 (8)	12	3
4	0	1	18 (23)	4	4	2	16 (20)	10	3
2	2	1	9 (11)	5	2	0	0	0	0
7	3	1	12 (18)	6	3	0	2* (3)	2	0
4	0	0	3 (3)	3	0	0	0	0	0

Intraluminal				
T				
Total	Isolated	T + EE	T + EE + I	T + F
94(8)	54(2)	31(40)	3/40	6/40
85(8)	50(59)	30(35)	2/35	3/35
0	0(0)	0	0	0
9(1)	4(<1)	1/5	1/5	3/5
0	0	0	0	0

of cross-sectional area narrowing by atherosclerotic plaques									
51-75%					76-100%				
Sub-total	EE	I	F	T	Sub-total	EE	I	F	T
1044 (35)	68 (7)	17 (2)	6 (1)	25 (2)	1202 (41)	213 (18)	112 (9)	58 (5)	51 (4)
420	32	2	5	25	350	75	32	18	44
362	19	6	1	0	459	70	33	19	0
262	17	9	0	0	393	68	47	21	7
356 (28)	4	2	3	0	74 (6)	8	6	1	0

Table V. Summary of frequency in any combination of intraplaque extravasated erythrocytes (EE), iron (I), and fibrin (F) and of intraluminal thrombus (T)

	No.	EE	I	F	T
Per person					
Patient	57	48 (84)	32 (56)	36 (63)	15 (26)
Control	27	5 (19)	6 (22)	2 (7)	0
Per artery					
Patient	224	79 (35)	32 (14)	39 (17)	18 (8)
Control	103	5 (5)	4 (4)	3 (3)	0
Per segment					
Patient	2958	287 (10)	133 (4)	67 (2)	94 (3)
Control	1290	15 (1)	10 (<1)	5 (<1)	0

found only 32 of 700 adults with coronary plaque hemorrhages, had been excluded.

Present study. In contrast to the previous studies, the present investigation examined the frequency of intraplaque extravasated erythrocytes and also that of iron and fibrin within coronary arteries of patients with fatal coronary heart disease and in control subjects, and it examined their frequency *per patient, per coronary artery,* and *per 5-mm segment of all four major coronary arteries.* Frequency of intraplaque hemorrhage, iron, and fibrin was determined by histologic examination irrespective of whether or not an intraplaque hemorrhage or intraluminal thrombus was suspected from the gross examination of the coronary arteries. As summarized in Table V, the frequency of coronary intraplaque extravasated erythrocytes, iron, and fibrin, and of intraluminal thrombus in both patients and controls was always highest when the frequency category analyzed was the percent per patient, intermediate when it was the percent per major coronary artery, and least when it was the percent of 5-mm segments of coronary artery. Thus the frequencies of coronary intraplaque extravasated erythrocytes in our study were considerably higher on the average than that previously reported in patients with fatal coronary heart disease. In addition, their frequency in control subjects of similar age and sex was determined, and the frequencies of intraplaque iron and fibrin in the coronary arteries in both coronary patients and control subjects are here reported for the first time.

Plaque hemorrhage vs intraluminal thrombus. The frequency of coronary intraplaque hemorrhage was always higher than that of iron and fibrin, in which the frequency was similar, and much higher than intraluminal thrombus in all three categories analyzed (patients, arteries, segments). This observation suggests that the intraplaque hemorrhage precedes the iron and fibrin deposition and also that plaque hemorrhage does not necessarily play an important role in the development of the intraluminal thrombus. Indeed, plaque hemorrhage usually occurred in the absence of intraluminal thrombus, and conversely intraluminal thrombus occurred more frequently without underlying plaque hemorrhage than with it. In only a third of the 5-mm coronary segments did plaque hemorrhage and intraluminal thrombus coexist.

Plaque hemorrhage related to plaque extent. The frequency of intraplaque hemorrhage, iron, and fibrin also were proportional to the amount of coronary atherosclerotic plaque (or to the degree of cross-sectional luminal narrowing by plaque). Thus if the plaques were small, the frequency of the three intraplaque elements was small, and vice versa. Accordingly, the control subjects who as a group had small plaques, had a low frequency of extravasated erythrocytes, iron, and fibrin. The frequency of intraluminal thrombus, however, was not proportional to the size of the underlying atherosclerotic plaque.

Plaque iron and fibrin related to plaque hemorrhage. Although intraplaque hemorrhage was observed in the absence of intraplaque iron or fibrin, the latter two rarely occurred in the absence of intraplaque hemorrhage. The frequency of intraplaque hemorrhage and fibrin was roughly similar in all four major coronary arteries; intraplaque iron and intraluminal thrombus were absent in the left main coronary artery but they too were roughly similar in the other three major coronary arteries.

Location of plaque elements. The predominant location of the intraplaque elements varied. Extravasated erythrocytes were most likely to occur in pultaceous debris, but they also were found in loose fibrous tissue and mucoid material; iron and fibrin, in contrast, were located mainly in the fibrous tissue components of the plaques. The fibrin deposits were located close to the surface of the plaque bordering the lumen.

Conclusions. With the exception of intraplaque iron and angina pectoris, no relation was observed between intraplaque extravasated erythrocytes, iron, and fibrin and the type of fatal coronary event, namely acute myocardial infarction, sudden coronary death, or angina pectoris. The significance of the relation between intraplaque iron and angina is unclear. Perhaps small intraplaque hemorrhages, almost surely the precursor of the iron deposits, in some way trigger anginal attacks. In contrast to the overall poor relation between the intraplaque hemorrhage, iron, and fibrin to the type of coronary event, intraluminal thrombus was found only in patients with acute myocardial infarction.

REFERENCES

1. Boyd AN: An inflammatory basis for coronary atherosclerosis. Am J Pathol **4**:159, 1928.
2. Paterson JC: Vascularization and hemorrhage of intima of arteriosclerotic coronary arteries. Arch Pathol **22**:13, 1936.
3. Paterson JC: Capillary rupture with intimal hemorrhage as a causative factor in coronary thrombosis. Arch Pathol **25**:474, 1938.
4. Wartman WB: Occlusion of the coronary arteries by hemorrhage into their walls. Am Heart J **15**:459, 1938.
5. Horn H, Finkelstein LE: Atherosclerosis of the coronary arteries and the mechanism of their occlusion. Am Heart J **19**:655, 1940.
6. Paterson JC: Some factors in the causation of intimal haemorrhages and in the precipitation of coronary thrombi. Can Med Assoc J **44**:114, 1941.
7. Nelson MG: Intimal coronary artery haemorrhage as a factor in the causation of coronary occlusion. J Pathol Bacteriol **53**:105, 1941.
8. English JP, Willius FA: Hemorrhagic lesions of the coronary arteries. Arch Intern Med **71**:549, 1943.
9. Durlacher SH, Fisk AJ, Fisher RS, Lovitt WV: Coronary artery lesions in sudden death. Circulation **8**:446, 1953.
10. Drury RAB: The role of intimal hemorrhage in coronary occlusion. J Pathol Bacteriol **67**:207, 1954.
11. Hamilton JD, Mowbray JH: The significance of intramural hemorrhage in coronary atherosclerosis (abstr). Circulation **14**:486, 1956.
12. Chapman I: Morphogenesis of occluding coronary artery thrombosis. Arch Pathol **80**:256, 1965.
13. Baroldi G: Acute coronary occlusion as a cause of myocardial infarct and sudden coronary heart death. Am J Cardiol **16**:859, 1965.
14. Constantinides P: Plaque fissures in human coronary thrombosis. J Atheroscler Res **6**:1, 1966.
15. Friedman M, Van Den Bovenkamp G: The pathogenesis of coronary intramural hemorrhages. Br J Exp Pathol **47**:347, 1966.
16. Friedman M: Pathogenesis of coronary thrombosis, intramural and intraluminal hemorrhage. Adv Cardiol **4**:20, 1970.

17. Roberts WC, Buja LM: The frequency and significance of coronary arterial thrombi and other observations in fatal acute myocardial infarction. A study of 107 necropsy patients. Am J Med **52**:425, 1972.

18. Paterson JC, Moffatt T, Mills J: Hemosiderin deposition in early atherosclerotic plaques. Arch Pathol **61**:496, 1956.

19. Schwartz CJ, Ardlie NG, Carter RF, Paterson JC: Gross aortic sudanophilia and hemosiderin deposition. A study on infants, children and young adults. Arch Pathol **83**:325, 1967.

20. Roberts WC, Jones AA: Quantification of coronary arterial narrowing at necropsy in acute transmural myocardial infarction: Analysis and comparison of findings in 27 patients and controls. Circulation **61**:786, 1980.

21. Roberts WC, Jones AA: Quantitation of coronary arterial narrowing at necropsy in sudden coronary death. Analysis of 31 patients and comparison with 25 control subjects. Am J Cardiol **44**:39, 1979.

22. Roberts WC, Virmani R: Quantification of coronary arterial narrowing in clinically-isolated unstable angina pectoris. An analysis of 22 necropsy patients. Am J Med **67**:792, 1979.

Thrombocytosis and Fatal Coronary Heart Disease

JEFFREY E. SAFFITZ, MD, PhD*
EDWIN R. PHILLIPS, MD, PhD
PETER N. TEMESY-ARMOS, MD
WILLIAM C. ROBERTS, MD

Although thrombocytosis may cause vascular thrombosis with resultant organ or tissue ischemia, the occurrence of coronary thrombosis and myocardial infarction (MI) in this circumstance is rare. To our knowledge, this association has been reported only once previously, in a 22-year-old man.[1] In this report, we describe another 22-year-old man with fatal congestive heart failure almost a year after a large MI associated with thrombocytosis.

A 22-year-old man developed intermittent hematuria at age 5 years and systemic hypertension and proteinuria at age 7 years. Although the hypertension and proteinuria persisted, extensive evaluation at age 19 years, including renal biopsy, disclosed no specific abnormalities. The platelet count at that time was 231,000/mm³. At age 21 years, sudden, severe precordial pain appeared and an acute anterior wall MI was documented. The platelet count ranged from 400,000 to 600,000/mm³. The MI was complicated by ventricular arrhythmias and thromboemboli, which required embolectomy in both legs. A month after onset of the acute MI, congestive heart failure (CHF) prompted catheterization, which disclosed total occlusion of the right and left anterior descending coronary arteries (R and LAD) and an apical left ventricular (LV) aneurysm. The total serum cholesterol level was 174 mg/dl. Sudden pain, cyanosis and coolness of the left index finger occurred 6 months after the acute MI. At that time, he underwent embolectomy of the left brachial and radial arteries and the LV aneurysm in the anterior wall was excised. The aneurysm contained thrombus. CHF persisted and he was hospitalized several times. The platelet counts

From the Pathology Branch, National Heart, Lung, and Blood Institute, Bethesda, Maryland, and the Department of Pathology, Medical College of Ohio, Toledo, Ohio. Dr. Saffitz's present address: Pathology Department, Washington University, 660 South Euclid Avenue, St. Louis, Missouri 63110. Manuscript received and accepted June 3, 1983.

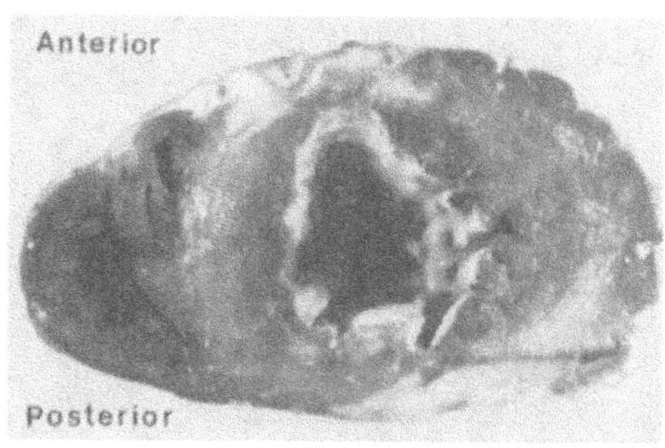

FIGURE 1. A transverse section of the heart at necropsy showing healed infarcts in the anterior and posterior left ventricular walls and fresh mural thrombus overlying dense white endocardial fibrous tissue.

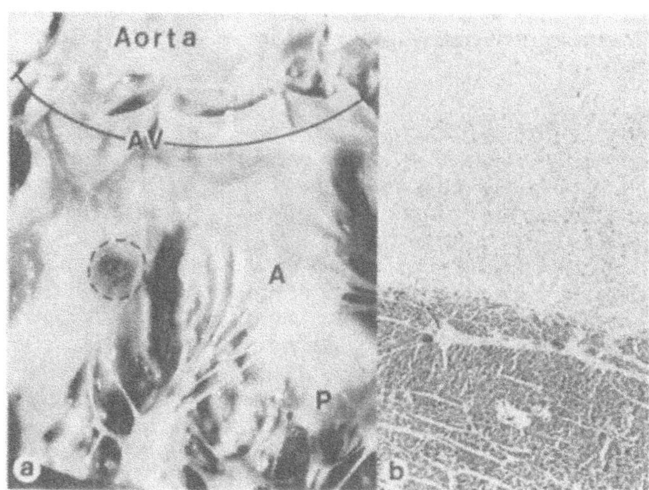

FIGURE 2. a, Opened left ventricle, aortic valve (AV) and aorta showing markedly thickened endocardial fibrous tissue overlying scarred myocardium. Enclosed in the dashed circle is a small thrombus. A and P = anterior and posterior mitral leaflets. **b,** Photomicrograph showing fibrous tissue overlying mural endocardium. The connective tissue is similar to that in the lumen of the occluded epicardial coronary arteries. Hematoxylin-eosin stain; magnification ×54, reduced 44%.

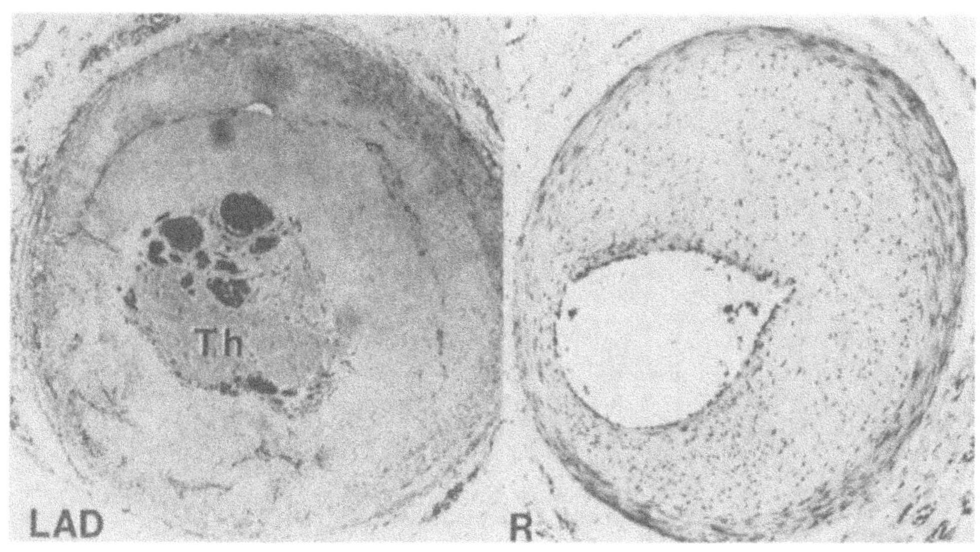

FIGURE 3. Photomicrographs of a cross section of the left anterior descending coronary artery (LAD) and a branch of the right coronary artery (R). The LAD is severely narrowed by fibrocellular tissue. Multiple channels and fresh platelet-fibrin thrombus (Th) are present. The branch of the right coronary artery is narrowed by connective tissue, similar to that shown in Figure 1. Neither vessel contains foam cells, cholesterol clefts, calcific deposits or pultaceous debris. Hematoxylin-eosin stains; magnification ×38 (LAD), ×107 (R); reduced 25%.

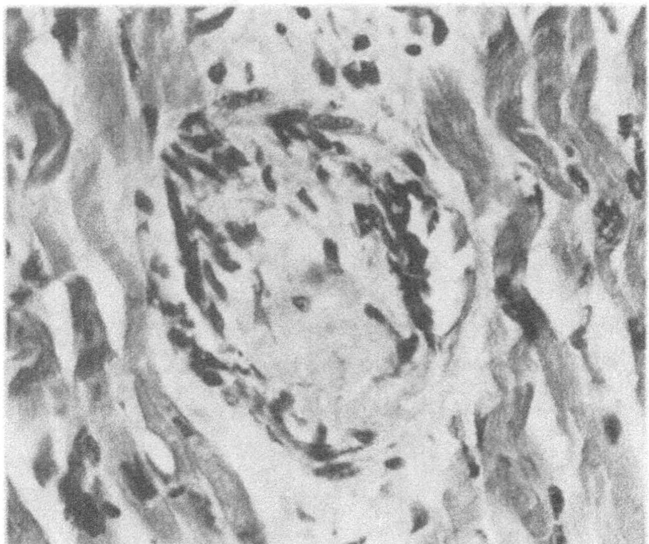

FIGURE 4. Photomicrograph of portion of left ventricular myocardium showing small intramural coronary artery containing platelet-fibrin thromboemboli. Hematoxylin-eosin stain; magnification ×430, reduced 13%.

ranged from 400,000 to 800,000/mm³. The final hospital admission at age 22 years was necessitated by severe CHF and ischemia of the distal left fourth finger. Cardiac output and blood pressure diminished progressively and the patient died 10.5 months after the acute MI.

At necropsy (Medical College of Ohio #A-82-2), the heart weighed 450 g. The apical half of the anterior LV free wall was replaced by dense scar at and adjacent to the LV aneurysectomy incision (Fig. 1). The posterior LV wall was also scarred. The LV apex contained mural thrombus adherent to underlying endocardial fibrous tissue. Fresh and organized mural thrombus also covered the LV outflow tract (Fig. 2). The R and LAD were totally occluded proximally; the length of the LAD occlusion was approximately 2 cm and that of the R 4 cm. The other portions of the LAD and R and the entire

left circumflex artery were normal. Branches of the major epicardial coronary contained discrete focal severe narrowings with normal intervening areas. Histologic examination of the narrowed coronary arterial segments showed fibrocellular intimal profileration without foam cells, cholesterol clefts, pultaceous debris or calcific deposits (Fig. 3). In some segments, the lumen contained several small channels, and a platelet-fibrin thrombus was present in the LAD (Fig. 3). The intima of the narrowed coronary arteries was similar histologically to the thickened fibrous tissue on the LV mural endocardium (Fig. 4). Histologic examination of LV myocardium disclosed necrosis adjacent to the healed MI and multiple small intramural coronary vessels with platelet-fibrin thromboemboli (Fig. 4). Both the spleen and lung contained discrete infarcts. The aorta was free of atherosclerotic plaques. The bone marrow, specifically the megakaryocytes, was normal. The kidneys contained focal hyaline sclerosis of glomerular capillary tufts consistent with organized microthrombi, but no other abnormalities to explain the hematuria and proteinuria throughout childhood. (Sections of kidney were examined by John M. Kissane, MD, a recognized renal expert, who agreed with our renal diagnosis.)

Thrombocytosis appears to be the only reasonable cause of the fatal coronary artery disease in the patient described here. The presence of thromboemboli in the intramural coronary arteries, in peripheral, splenic, pulmonary and renal arteries, the young age of the patient, the morphologic features of the luminal material that caused the multiple arterial narrowings (that is, its dissimilarity to atherosclerotic plaques) all strongly support the view that the arterial narrowings in this patient were the result of thrombocytosis.

Reference

1. Virmani R, Popvsky MA, Roberts WC. Thrombocytosis, coronary thrombosis and acute myocardial infarction. Am J Med 1979;67:498–506.

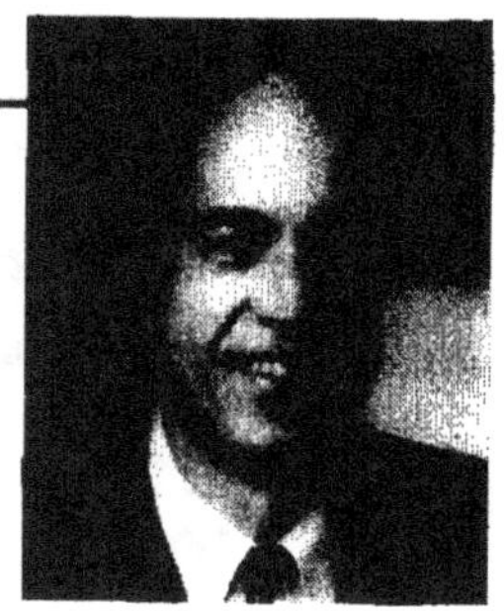

The "Blessing" Of Angina Pectoris

The use of the word "blessing" when speaking of angina pectoris needs considerable explanation because the patient who has angina clearly does not consider himself/herself "blessed." But when applied on a *relative* rather than on an *absolute* basis, there is justification for the use of this word. Over 95% of patients with atherosclerotic coronary heart disease (CAD) present clinically in 1 of 3 ways: acute myocardial infarction (AMI), cardiac arrest (sudden coronary death) or angina pectoris.

Although the amount of left ventricular myocardium lost is variable, AMI indicates permanent, irreplaceable loss of ventricular myocardium. The amount of myocardium lost is generally much less in the patients with so-called uncomplicated AMI compared to those in whom the acute event is complicated by cardiogenic shock or in whom chronic intractable congestive heart failure, with or without aneurysmal formation, is a late consequence. Irrespective of the size of the AMI, however, the patient whose initial manifestation of atherosclerotic CAD is AMI begins a symptomatic course with a partially but permanently damaged left ventricle, and therapy thereafter—either medical or surgical or both—is usually not as beneficial as in the patient with symptomatic CAD without permanent left ventricular damage.

The patient whose initial manifestation of atherosclerotic CAD is fatal cardiac arrest has no opportunity to receive long-term medical or surgical therapy irrespective of the presence or absence of underlying previous (clinically silent) myocardial damage. About 50% of successfully resuscitated survivors of cardiac arrest are left with no apparent permanent left ventricular damage.

Thus, relative to the initial clinical appearance of atherosclerotic CAD as manifested by AMI or fatal cardiac arrest, the patient whose initial clinical manifestation of CAD is angina pectoris (or nonfatal cardiac arrest) is "blessed." Angina, of course, in about 90% of the patients, indicates the presence of severe narrowing of ≥1 major epicardial coronary artery and is the result of *transient*, not permanent, myocardial ischemia. The left ventricular myocardium at the time of the initial appearance of angina is usually normal, or if a scar (indicative of a previously silent AMI which healed) is present, it is usually small and infrequently results in left ventricular dysfunc-

tion.[1] Thus, the patient with initial angina can undergo the definitive diagnostic study—selective coronary angiography—before the occurrence of permanent significant left ventricular damage. Of all patients with symptomatic CAD, those who deserve the most "aggressive" diagnostic and therapeutic approaches, unless contraindicated by extremely advanced age, presence of another more life-threatening condition or simply no desire on the part of the patient, are the patients whose only manifestation of atherosclerotic CAD is *unequivocal* angina pectoris. If I develop angina pectoris as the first manifestation of CAD, I want a coronary angiogram. Only 1 test during life can determine the presence or absence of significant coronary narrowing unequivocally and that is injection of contrast material into the coronary arteries. Angiography demonstrates the presence of normal (a 10% occurrence) or abnormal (a 90% occurrence) coronary arteries and if abnormal, the degree of, and the distribution of, the narrowings. In my view, most patients with significant (>50% diameter reduction) narrowing of ≥1 vital coronary arteries should be treated definitively at this juncture (before significant left ventricular damage has occurred from subsequent AMI or subsequent cardiac arrest). The most definitive therapy, of course, is dilatation of or bypass of the coronary narrowings.

In summary, *the initial appearance of angina pectoris is the time to do coronary angiography and if significant and appropriately located coronary narrowing is present, unless other factors preclude its performance, the time to dilate or to bypass the narrowing.* This aggressive approach initially almost certainly will delay for a reasonable period in most patients the occurrence of sudden coronary death (the most frequent cause of death in patients with angina) and permanent myocardial damage from AMI.

1. **Roberts WC.** The coronary arteries and left ventricle in clinically isolated angina pectoris. Circulation 1976;54:388–390.

William C. Roberts, MD
Editor-in-Chief

Fatal Cardiac Arrest during Cardiac Catheterization for Angina Pectoris*

A Marker of Quadruple Vessel Disease

Carole A. Warnes, M.B., B.S.; Joan C. Kishel, M.D.; and William C. Roberts, M.D., F.C.C.P.

Cardiac arrest during cardiac catheterization is uncommon, and fatal arrest is rare. In the coronary artery surgery study (CASS),[1] which includes 7,553 patients, the mortality rate of coronary arteriography was 0.2 percent. In the past 11 years, we have studied at necropsy 12 patients with severe angina pectoris who died during or shortly after coronary angiography. Ten of the 12 patients were described elsewhere[2] and in a recent one-month period, an additional two patients with unstable angina and fatal cardiac arrest during cardiac catheterization were studied at necropsy. Because the necropsy findings in patients with angina pectoris and fatal cardiac arrest in the peri-cardiac catheterization period are predictable, yet poorly recognized, a brief description of the latter two patients appears justified.

The patients, a 58-year-old woman (patient 1) and a 73-year-old woman (patient 2), had had stable angina for eight years, and unstable angina for three weeks (patient 1) and two weeks (patient 2), respectively. Neither had electrocardiographic or enzymatic evidence of myocardial necrosis immediately before catheterization. Both patients had a history of systemic hypertension, patient 2 had diabetes mellitus, and both had had acute myocardial infarcts three and six years, respectively, before death.

In each patient, cardiac catheterization was performed from the femoral artery by the Judkins technique. In patient 1, left ventricular angiography was performed first and then the Judkins catheter was placed directly into the left main (LM) coronary artery and 4 ml of contrast medium injected. Chest pain occurred immediately and the heart rate and systemic blood pressure fell. Despite endocardial pacing, electromechanical dissociation occurred and resuscitation was unsuccessful. In patient 2, contrast material was injected initially into the left sinus of Valsalva and then

into the LM and right coronary arteries. Severe narrowing of the lumens of the LM, left anterior descending, left circumflex and right coronary arteries was found. Left ventricular angiography was then performed. During these injections and for ten minutes thereafter, no problem occurred. Just before being transferred from the catheterization table to a stretcher, severe substernal chest pain developed followed quickly by cardiac arrest, electromechanical dissociation and unsuccessful resuscitation.

At necropsy, the heart of patient 1 weighed 400 g, and that of patient 2, 460 g. No foci of myocardial necrosis were evident; patient 1 had a transmural scar (anterior wall) and patient 2, a subendocardial scar (posterior wall). The four major (right, LM, left anterior descending, left circumflex) epicardial coronary arteries from each patient were excised, examined by x-ray, cut into 5-mm long segments, processed in alcohol and xylene, embedded in paraffin, stained by

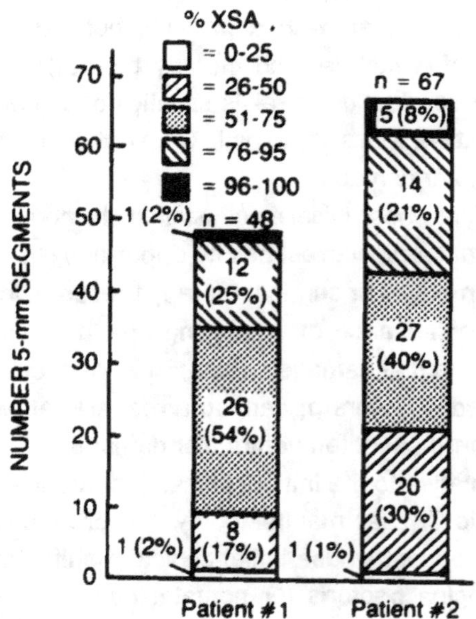

FIGURE 1. Bar graph showing the number and percentage of 5 mm segments of the four major epicardial coronary arteries narrowed to varying degrees by atherosclerotic plaque.

*From the Pathology Branch, National Heart, Lung, and Blood Institute, National Institutes of Health, Bethesda.
Reprint requests: Dr. Roberts, National Institutes of Health, Building 10, Room 3E30, Bethesda 20205

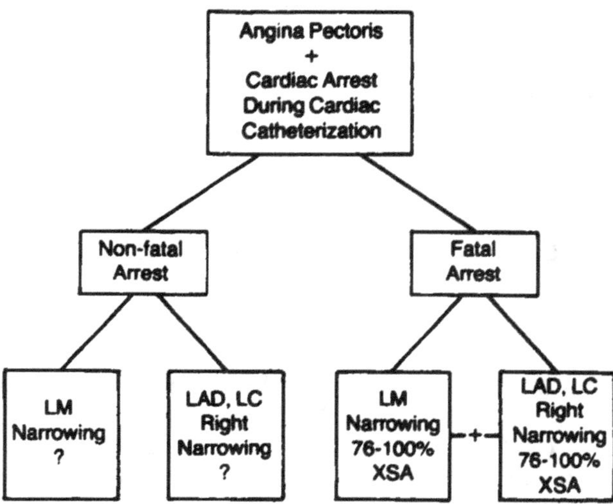

FIGURE 2. Status of the four major epicardial coronary arteries in patients with angina pectoris having fatal and non-fatal cardiac arrest during cardiac catheterization.

Movat technique, and examined histologically. The amount of luminal cross-sectional area (XSA) narrowing by atherosclerotic plaque of each 5 mm segment was determined (Fig 1): narrowing 76-100 percent in XSA was present in all four major epicardial coronary arteries in both patients. Of 48 segments in patient 1, 12 (25 percent) were narrowed 76-95 percent and one (2 percent), 96-100 percent; and of 67 segments in patient 2, 14 (21 percent) were narrowed 76-95 percent and five (8 percent), 96-100 percent. Extravasated erythrocytes were present in plaque in the LM coronary artery of patient 1, but the lumen of this artery did not appear to have been narrowed by this mechanism.

DISCUSSION

Several,[3] but not all,[4] investigators have suggested that patients with, compared with those without, severe narrowing of the LM coronary artery, are at greater risk of dying during cardiac catheterization. Many reports, however,[1,5] suggest that catheterization of patients with unstable angina pectoris is no more hazardous than in patients with stable symptoms. Both of our patients had unstable angina and neither had evidence of acute myocardial infarction immediately before catheterization.

Clinical and necropsy findings in our two patients confirm previous morphologic observation in patients having fatal cardiac arrest during or shortly after cardiac catheterization for angina.[2] Of our ten patients previously examined at necropsy, nine had narrowing of the LM>75 percent in XSA (by atherosclerotic

plaque in seven, and by thromboembolic material superimposed on plaque in two). In addition, at least three of four major epicardial coronary arteries were narrowed 76-100 percent in XSA in all ten patients. Severe narrowing of the LM coronary artery is often indicative of severe narrowing of the right, left anterior descending and left circumflex coronary arteries. Of 35 necropsy patients with fatal coronary heart disease and narrowing 76-100 percent in XSA of the LM coronary artery previously reported from our laboratory, 94 percent also had similar narrowing of the right, left anterior descending and left circumflex coronary arteries.[6]

In patients with angina pectoris suffering cardiac arrest during cardiac catheterization with successful resuscitation (Fig 2), the amount of narrowing of each of the four major coronary arteries has not been described. In contrast, of patients having cardiac arrest during cardiac catheterization and unsuccessful resuscitation, the previous study from this laboratory[2] and the present one, strongly suggest that the LM and all three other major coronary arteries will be narrowed 76-100 percent in XSA. Therefore, in patients with angina pectoris who cannot be resuscitated from cardiac arrest during cardiac catheterization, emergency aortocoronary bypass grafting, if performed, should include insertion of conduits to all three major coronary arterial systems because this event is usually a marker of severe quadruple vessel disease.

REFERENCES

1 Davis K, Ward Kennedy J, Kemp KG, Judkins MP, Gosselin AJ, Killip T. Complications of coronary arteriography from the collaborative study of coronary artery surgery (CASS). Circulation 1979; 59:1105-12

2 Cabin HS, Roberts WC. Fatal cardiac arrest during cardiac catheterization for angina pectoris: Analysis of 10 necropsy patients. Am J Cardiol 1981; 48:1-8

3 Bourassa MG, Noble J. Complication rate of coronary arteriography. A review of 5250 cases studied by a percutaneous femoral technique. Circulation 1976; 53:106-14

4 De Mots H, Bonchek LI, Rosch J, Anderson RP, Starr A, Rahimtoola SH. Left main coronary artery disease: risks of angiography, importance of coexisting disease of other coronary arteries and effects of revascularization. Am J Cardiol 1975; 36:136-41

5 Brooks N, Warnes CA, Cattell M, Balcan R, Honey M, Layton C, et al. Cardiac pain at rest. Management and follow-up of 100 consecutive cases. Br Heart J 1981; 45:35-41

6 Bulkley BH, Roberts WC. Atherosclerotic narrowing of the left main coronary artery: a necropsy analysis of 152 patients with fatal coronary heart disease and varying degrees of left main narrowing. Circulation 1976; 53:823-28

Amounts of Coronary Arterial Narrowing by Atherosclerotic Plaques in Clinically Isolated, Chronic, Pure Aortic Regurgitation: Analysis of 37 Necropsy Patients Older than 30 Years

PAUL J. DAY,* BRUCE M. McMANUS, MD, PhD, and WILLIAM C. ROBERTS, MD

The degree of cross-sectional area (XSA) narrowing by atherosclerotic plaque in each of the 4 major epicardial coronary arteries (right, left main, left anterior descending and left circumflex) was determined at necropsy in 37 patients (30 men and 7 women) aged 34 to 77 years (mean 54) with severe, isolated, chronic, pure aortic regurgitation (AR). In 7 patients (19%), ≥1 major coronary artery was narrowed 76 to 100% in XSA at some point. Of the 148 major coronary arteries examined in the 37 patients, 12 arteries (8%) were narrowed at some point 76 to 100% in XSA. Each of the 148 major coronary arteries were divided into 5-mm-long segments (average 53 per patient) and a histologic section from each segment was examined. Of the 1,977 segments, 1,087 were narrowed 0 to 25%, 669 (34%) 26 to 50%, 170 (9%) 51 to 75%, 48 (2%) 76 to 95% and 3 (0.001%) 96 to 100%. The average amount of XSA narrowing by atherosclerotic plaque per segment was about 28%. Of the 37 patients, 9 had had angina pectoris, 2 of whom had significant (>75% XSA reduction) coronary narrowing; 2 other patients had had acute myocardial infarction clinically, 1 of whom had significant coronary narrowing at necropsy. Thus, in general, the amount of coronary narrowing in our 37 adults with severe, pure, isolated, chronic AR was relatively mild. (Am J Cardiol 1984;53:173–177)

In recent years a number of articles have focused on the frequency and extent of coronary arterial narrowing and of angina pectoris in patients with aortic valve stenosis. Surprisingly, relatively little angiographic and no necropsy information about the frequency of and extent of coronary narrowing has been reported in patients with pure aortic regurgitation (AR). In this report we describe the amounts of narrowing by atherosclerotic plaques observed at necropsy in the 4 major epicardial coronary arteries in 37 patients >30 years with clinically isolated, pure, severe AR.

Patients

Certain clinical and morphologic findings in the 37 patients are summarized in Table I. For inclusion in this study the patients had to fulfill the following criteria: (1) age >30 years at death; (2) presence of AR by auscultation with the intensity of the basal diastolic blowing murmur grade ≥2 on a scale of 6; (3) absence of aortic valve stenosis as determined by left-sided cardiac catheterization (20 patients) and by morphologic examination of the aortic valve (at necropsy or the operatively excised valve) (all 37 patients); (4) absence of significant mitral valve dysfunction during life and presence of an anatomically normal mitral valve at necropsy; (5) presence of cardiomegaly at necropsy (heart weight >400 g); (6) absence of active infective endocarditis; (7) if aortic valve replacement had been performed (17 patients), the patient died within 60 days of the procedure; and (8) availability of the 4 major epicardial coronary arteries so that they could be examined in their entirety as discussed herein.

In the files of the Pathology Branch, National Heart, Lung, and Blood Institute, National Institutes of Health, 143 necropsy patients >20 years have been coded as having pure AR. Most of these cases were eliminated from the present study because of the presence of active infective endocarditis, the presence of only mild degrees of AR, age 30 years and younger or the unavailability of the heart specimen with intact epicardial coronary arteries.

In each of the 37 patients included in this study, the clinical records were examined, the heart was reexamined, and the 4 major (right, left main, left anterior descending and left cir-

From the Pathology Branch, National Heart, Lung, and Blood Institute, National Institutes of Health, Bethesda, Maryland. Manuscript received and accepted September 30, 1983.

* Student, Saint Mary's College, Saint Mary's City, Maryland 20686.

Address for reprints: William C. Roberts MD, Building 10A, Room 3E-30, National Institutes of Health, Bethesda, Maryland 20205.

TABLE I Clinical and Cardiac Morphologic Observations in the 37 Necropsy Patients with Severe Chronic Aortic Regurgitation

Pt	Cause of AR	Age (yr) & Sex	AP	Clinical AMI	Pressure (mm Hg) LV	SA*	AR by Cine (1+ = 4+)	AVR[†]	HW (g)	LV F	No. of 4 Major CAs >75%	No. of 5-mm Segs	No. of 5-mm Segs Narrowed 0–25%	26–50%	51–75%	76–95%	96–100%	Score[‡] Total	Mean
1	Syphilis	37M	+	0	152/50	152/55	4+	0	600	0	0	52	20	23	9	0	0	93	1.8
2	Syphilis	44M	0	0	160/5	160.85	3+	0	850	+	0	47	23	19	5	0	0	76	1.6
3	Syphilis	53M	+	0	150/20	150/40	4+	+	575	0	0	54	22	32	0	0	0	86	1.6
4	Syphilis	55M	0	0	138/37	160/51	4+	+	940	0	3	61	0	18	31	11	0	176	2.9
5	Syphilis	64M	0	0	⋯	145/55	⋯	0	540	0	0	55	22	32	1	0	0	89	1.6
6	Syphilis	64M	0	0	⋯	150/60	⋯	0	600	+	0	56	28	28	0	0	0	84	1.5
7	Syphilis	65F	0	0	170/8	184/50	4+	+	710	0	1	48	6	30	11	1	0	103	2.1
8	Syphilis	69M	+	0	⋯	170/50	⋯	0	640	0	0	61	51	10	0	0	0	71	1.2
9	Syphilis	69F	0	0	⋯	200/90	⋯	0	650	0	0	46	38	8	0	0	0	54	1.2
10	Syphilis	72F	0	0	⋯	155/95	⋯	0	500	0	0	70	41	27	2	0	0	101	1.4
11	Syphilis	75M	0	0	⋯	150/80	⋯	0	630	0	0	45	33	11	1	0	0	58	1.3
12	Syphilis	77M	0	0	⋯	200/100	⋯	0	620	0	1	64	25	26	11	2	0	118	1.8
13	IE	39M	0	0	140/20	140/38	4+	0	1010	0	0	72	45	16	11	0	0	110	1.5
14	IE	40M	0	0	⋯	120/40	⋯	0	600	0	0	54	54	0	0	0	0	54	1.0
15	IE	44M	0	0	⋯	130/40	⋯	0	610	0	0	54	50	4	0	0	0	58	1.1
16	IE	45M	0	0	120/50	120/50	⋯	+	610	0	0	36	20	16	0	0	0	52	1.4
17	IE	47M	0	0	⋯	135/45	⋯	0	590	0	0	69	44	25	0	0	0	94	1.4
18	IE	50M	0	+[§]	⋯	170/60	⋯	+	980	+[§]	0	54	54	0	0	0	0	54	1.0
19	IE	52F	0	0	130/44	150/40	4+	+	500	0	0	54	54	0	0	0	0	54	1.0
20	IE	53M	0	0	⋯	145/45	⋯	+	690	0	0	54	13	41	0	0	0	95	1.8
21	IE	55F	0	0	⋯	150/40	⋯	0	520	0	0	60	34	21	5	0	0	91	1.5
22	Anky S	34M	0	0	100/22	120/25	4+	+	700	0	0	54	50	4	0	0	0	58	1.1
23	Anky S	37M	+	0	⋯	230/125[‖]	⋯	0	765	+	2	34	1	5	15	11	2	108	3.2
24	Anky S	38M	0	0	170/16	175/50	4+	+	1100	0	0	60	53	7	0	0	0	67	1.1
25	Anky S	52M	+	0	160/18	168/30	4+	+	850	0	0	44	24	19	1	0	0	65	1.5
26	Anky S	55M	0	0	114/40	124/38	4+	0	680	0	0	54	7	31	16	0	0	117	2.2
27	Anky S	57M	+	0	⋯	170/60	⋯	0	500	0	0	52	43	8	1	0	0	62	1.2
28	Marfan	41M	0	0	100/30	100/40	3+	+	750	0	0	58	36	20	2	0	0	82	1.4
29	Marfan	48F	0	0	150/12	150/40	3+	+	520	0	0	32	16	16	0	0	0	48	1.5
30	Marfan	62M	0	0	105/32	105/50	4+	+	856	0	0	53	29	24	0	0	0	77	1.5
31	Marfan	69M	0	+	110/40	110/60	3+	+	650	+	2	43	12	16	9	6	0	95	2.2
32	Uncertain	34M	0	0	105/–	122/–	4+	+	460	0	1	56	4	18	20	14	0	156	2.8
33	Uncertain	41M	+	0	88/19	96/20	4+	+	920	0	0	54	41	12	1	0	0	68	1.3
34	Uncertain	58M	0	0	⋯	155.45	⋯	0	640	0	0	59	11	46	2	0	0	109	1.8
35	Trauma	71M	+	0	130/30	130/60	4+	0	470	+	2	50	0	31	15	3	1	123	2.5
36	SH	71M	0	0	160/30	160/80	3+	0	845	0	0	54	38	16	0	0	0	70	1.3
37	Congenital	51F	+	0	⋯	210/80	⋯	+	550	0	0	54	45	9	0	0	0	63	1.2

* When a left ventricular pressure is recorded, the SA pressure is direct; when not, it is indirect.

[†] Performed within 60 days of death.

[‡] The score is derived by assigning a number to each 5-mm segment according to its degree of luminal narrowing by atherosclerotic plaque: 1 = 0–25% cross- sectional area narrowing; 2 = 26–50%; 3 = 51–75%; and 4 = 76–100%. The *total score* was obtained for each patient by adding up the numbers for all 5-mm segments. The *mean score* was calculated by dividing the total score per patient by the number of 5-mm segments examined from that patient.

[§] Probably embolic in origin (during active infective endocarditis).

[‖] Recorded 5 years before death.

AMI = acute myocardial infarction; Anky S = ankylosing spondylitis; AP = angina pectoris; AR = aortic regurgitation; AVR = aortic valve replacement; CAs = coronary arteries; F = transmural fibrosis; HW = heart weight; IE = healed infective endocarditis; LV = left ventricle; SA = systemic artery; Segs = segments; SH = systemic hypertension.

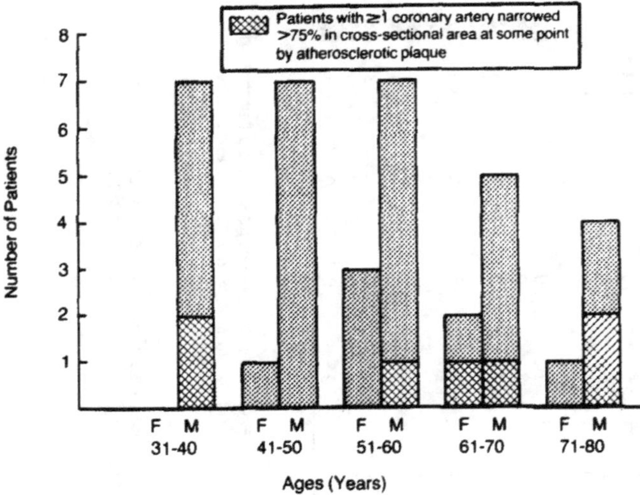

FIGURE 1. Number of necropsy patients by age decade and sex with severe pure aortic regurgitation in whom ≥ 1 major epicardial coronary artery (right, left main, left anterior descending and left circumflex) was narrowed 76 to 100% in cross-sectional area at some point by atherosclerotic plaques.

cumflex) epicardial coronary arteries were excised intact from the heart, decalcified if necessary, divided into 5-mm-long segments, cut transversely to the long axis of the artery, labeled sequentially from the origin of the artery from either the aorta or left main coronary artery, processed in alcohols and xylene, embedded in paraffin, cut 6 μ thick, and at least 1 histologic section from each 5-mm segment was stained by the Movat method[1] and examined. The degree of cross-sectional area (XSA) narrowing by atherosclerotic plaques was determined by examining the Movat-stained sections, which clearly delineate the internal elastic membrane. The amount of XSA luminal narrowing was determined by magnifying each cross section of coronary artery approximately 40 times via microscopy and estimating the degrees of luminal obliteration by dividing visually the XSA of the coronary artery into 4 quadrants, each comprising 25% of the total XSA luminal area. The degrees of XSA narrowing were categorized initially into 4 groups: 0 to 25, 26 to 50, 51 to 75 and 76 to 100%. Any section narrowed >75% was further classified into a group with narrowing 76 to 95% or into a group with narrowing 96 to 100%. Both the inter- and intraobserver error by this technique are <5%.[2]

Of the 37 patients, the cause of the AR was cardiovascular syphilis[3] in 12, infective endocarditis that healed[4] in 9, ankylosing spondylitis[5] in 6, the Marfan syndrome[6] (2 patients) or the Marfan cardiovascular disease without the skeletal features[7] (2 patients) in 4, undetermined in 3, and trauma,[3] systemic hypertension[8,9] and congenital (quadricuspid aortic valve) in 1 each, respectively. The 37 patients ranged in age from 34 to 77 years (mean 54) (Fig. 1); 30 (81%) were men and 7 (19%) were women. Ischemic-type chest pain occurred in 11 patients (30%): angina pectoris in 9 (24%) and clinical features diagnostic of acute myocardial infarction in 2 (5%). Of the 37 patients, 20 (54%) had left-sided cardiac catheterization, including aortic "root" angiography in 19 and selective coronary angiography in 5. The left ventricular (LV) peak systolic pressures ranged from 88 to 170 mm Hg (average 135) and the direct systemic arterial pressures from 96 to 184 mm Hg (average 140); the LV end-diastolic pressures ranged from 5 to 50 mm Hg (average 26) and the direct systemic arterial end-

diastolic pressures from 20 to 85 mm Hg (average 48). The degree of AR by cineangiography was graded 3+ or 4+ on a scale of 1 to 4+ in all 19 patients.

The cause of death in the 37 patients was variable: 17 (46%) died of complications of aortic valve replacement performed within 60 days of death; 13 (35%) died from chronic congestive heart failure secondary to the severe AR; 3 (8%) (Patients 11, 12 and 27) from cancer; 1 (3%) (Patient 9) from stroke; 1 (3%) (Patient 23) from associated severe coronary atherosclerosis; 1 (3%) (Patient 5) from chronic renal disease requiring chronic dialysis; and 1 (2%) (Patient 17) from an accident (kicked in the head by a horse). Thus, although all 37 patients had clinical evidence of severe AR, 30 (81%) died directly from consequences of the severe AR.

At necropsy, the hearts in the 30 men weighed 460 to 1100 g (mean 727) (normal ≤400 g); only 5 men (17%) had hearts that weighed <600 g. The hearts in the 7 women weighed 500 to 750 g (mean 564; normal weight ≤350 g); 5 of the 7 had hearts that weighed <600 g.

A grossly visible transmural LV scar (healed myocardial infarction) was found in 6 patients (16%), and none had scars limited to the LV subendocardium (inner half of the myocardial wall). Of the 6 patients, only 2 had a clinical event compatible with acute myocardial infarction, and in 1 of them (Patient 18) (Table I) the infarct occurred during active infective endocarditis and was most likely embolic in origin[10]; 2 others with LV scars had angina pectoris. Of the 6 patients with LV scars, 3 had significant and 3 had insignificant coronary narrowing at necropsy.

Results

Of the 37 patients, 7 (19%) had ≥1 of their 4 major epicardial coronary arteries narrowed >75% in XSA by atherosclerotic plaques (Fig. 1): in 3 patients, 1 of the 4 arteries was so narrowed; in 3 patients, 2 such arteries, and in 1 patient, 3 such arteries. In all 37 patients, the left main coronary artery was narrowed ≤50% in XSA. Of the 148 major epicardial coronary arteries examined in the 37 patients, 12 (8%) were narrowed at some point >75% in XSA by atherosclerotic plaque.

A total of 1,977 of the 5-mm segments of the 148 major coronary arteries were examined in the 37 patients. Of these, 1,087 segments (55%) were narrowed 0 to 25% in XSA by atherosclerotic plaque, 669 (34%) were narrowed 26 to 50%, 170 (9%) 51 to 75%; 48 (2%) 76 to 95%, and 3 (0.001%) 96 to 100%. The amount of narrowing by the patients' sex and age decade is summarized in Figure 2. Of the 7 patients in whom ≥1 major coronary artery was narrowed at some point >75% in XSA, 356 of the 5-mm segments of coronary artery were examined. Of these, 48 (13%) segments were narrowed 0 to 25%, 144 (41%) 26 to 50%, 113 (32%) 51 to 75%; 48 (13%) 76 to 95%, and 3 (1%) 96 to 100%. Of the 30 patients in whom none of the 4 major coronary arteries was narrowed >75%, 1,621 of the 5-mm segments were examined: 1,039 (64%) were narrowed 0 to 25%, 525 segments (32%) 26 to 50% and 57 (4%) 51 to 75%.

A scoring system was used to indicate the severity and extent of coronary arterial narrowing. Every 5-mm segment of coronary artery from each patient was assigned a score of 1 to 4, based on the amount of XSA narrowing by atherosclerotic plaque: 1 = 0 to 25% narrowing; 2 = 26 to 50%; 3 = 51 to 75%, and 4 = 76 to 100%. A total score was determined for each patient and the

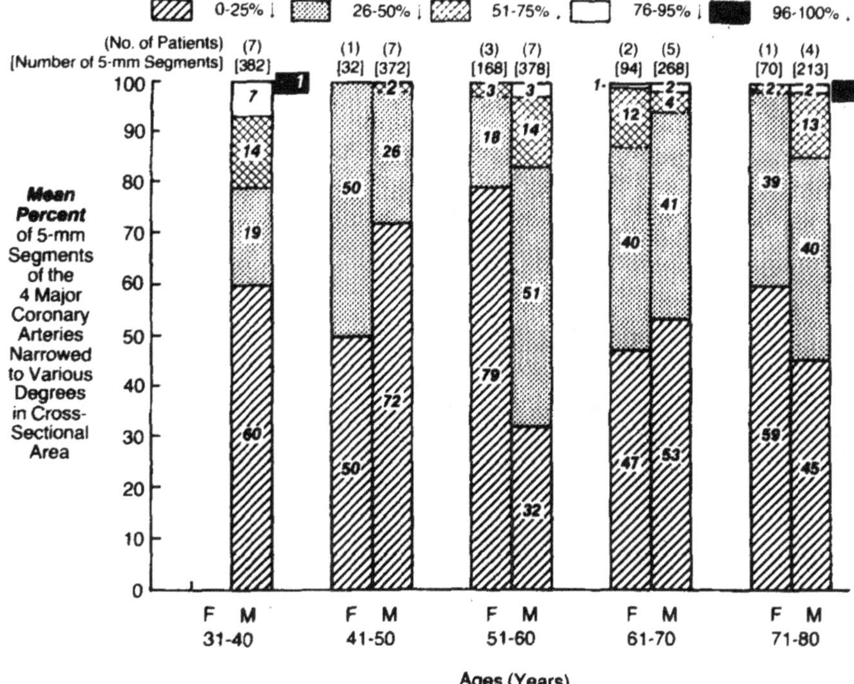

FIGURE 2. Number and percent of 1,977 five-millimeter segments of the 4 major epicardial coronary arteries narrowed to various degrees by atherosclerotic plaques in 37 patients (30 men, 7 women) aged 34 to 77 years with severe pure aortic regurgitation.

score per segment was then calculated by dividing the total score per patient by the number of segments examined from that patient. Of the 2,139 segments examined from the 37 patients, the total score was 3,352 and the mean score 1.6, indicating that the amount of XSA narrowing for each of the 2,139 segments was approximately 28%.

Of the 7 patients in whom ≥1 major coronary artery was narrowed 76 to 100% in XSA by atherosclerotic plaque, 2 had had angina pectoris, 1 had had a clinical event characteristic of acute myocardial infarction, and 3 had grossly visible LV scars, transmural in each; the mean score for the group of 7 patients was 2.1, indicating that each 5-mm segment from these patients was narrowed approximately 42%. In contrast, of the 30 patients with insignificant (≤75% reduction in XSA) coronary narrowing, 7 (23%) had had angina pectoris, 1 (3%) had had a clinical event diagnosed as acute myocardial infarction (probably embolic in origin), and 3 (10%) had grossly visible LV scars. The mean score for the 30 patients was 104, indicating that each 5-mm coronary segment in these patients was narrowed approximately 23%, or just over half that of the other group.

Thus, of the 9 patients considered to have angina pectoris, 2 had significant and 7 had insignificant coronary narrowing. Of the 2 patients with acute myocardial infarction clinically, 1 had significant coronary narrowing at necropsy and the other patient did not. The latter patient (Patient 18) had an acute myocardial infarction during active infective endocarditis, and therefore, the cause of the infarct likely was an embolus that subsequently lysed or organized, and at necropsy the narrowing was insignificant.[11]

Coronary angiography had been performed during life in 5 patients, 3 (Patients 7, 31 and 35) of whom had significant (>50% diameter reduction) and 2 (Patients 2 and 36) of whom had insignificant coronary narrowing.

Discussion

This study demonstrates that 7 (19%) of our 37 patients >30 years old with severe, chronic, pure isolated AR had narrowing >75% in XSA of ≥1 of the 4 major epicardial coronary arteries by atherosclerotic plaque. The extent of the severe (>75% XSA) coronary narrowing in these 7 patients, however, was relatively mild compared with the extent of severe narrowing observed in necropsy patients with fatal coronary heart disease unassociated with aortic valve dysfunction.[12–25] Of the 7 patients with AR and significant coronary narrowing, 14% of the 5-mm-long segments of the 4 major coronary arteries (average of 53 segments per patient) were narrowed >75%, whereas in patients with fatal symptomatic coronary heart disease unassociated with AR or aortic valve stenosis, an average of 33% of the coronary segments are narrowed >75%.[12–25]

The frequency of angina pectoris did not appear to be different in the 7 patients with compared to the 30 patients without significant coronary narrowing; angina was present in 2 of the 7 with and in 7 of the 30 without significant narrowing. Furthermore, the frequency of clinical acute myocardial infarction and LV scars was similar in the 7 patients with and in the 30 patients without significant coronary narrowing.

No previous study has examined the status of the epicardial coronary arteries in necropsy patients with pure AR, and indeed coronary angiographic data focusing exclusively on patients with pure AR is virtually nonexistent. Several reports,[26–33] however, have described coronary angiographic features of patients with aortic valve disease, and a number of them included findings in patients with severe AR. Of 20 patients (mean age 40 years, 10 with angina) with severe AR and peak gradients <30 mm Hg described by Basta et al,[26] 3 (10%) had significant (>50% diameter reduction) coronary narrowing (1 vessel in each) by angiography. Of 30 patients with "predominant" AR studied by Lacy et al,[27] 9 (30%) had significant coronary narrowing (1 vessel in 5) by angiography. Of 29 patients (mean age 49 years, 18 with angina) with severe AR (3+ or 4+/4+ AR by aortic angiography and <10 mm Hg peak pressure gradient) studied by Grayboys and Cohn,[28] 5 (17%) had significant coronary narrowing. Of 17 patients (mean age 42 years) with severe AR (peak pressure gradients <20 mm Hg) reported by Clark et al,[30] 3 (18%) had significant coronary narrowing (1 vessel in 1). Of 31 patients (mean age 55 years) with severe AR (pressure gradients <10 mm Hg) reported by Hakki et al,[31] 11 (35%) had significant coronary narrowing (1 vessel in 4). Of 17 patients with severe AR (pressure gradients <30 mm Hg) reported by Saltups,[32] 5 (29%) had significant coronary narrowing (1 vessel in 1). Of the 11 patients (mean age 48 years) with pure AR reported by Pichard and associates,[33] none had significant coronary narrowing by angiography.

References

1. **Movat HZ.** Demonstration of all connective tissue elements in a single section: pentachrome stains. Arch Pathol 1955;60:289–295.
2. **Isner JM, Wu M, Virmani R, Jones AA, Roberts WC.** Comparison of degrees of luminal narrowing determined by visual inspection of histologic sections under magnification among three independent observers and comparison to that obtained by video planimetry. An analysis of 559 five-millimeter segments of 61 coronary arteries from eleven patients. Lab Invest 1980;42:566–570.
3. **Roberts WC, Dangel JC, Bulkley BH.** Non-rheumatic valvular cardiac disease: a clinicopathologic survey of 27 different conditions causing valvular dysfunction. Cardiovasc Clinics 1973;5:333–446.
4. **Roberts WC, Buchbinder NA.** Healed left-sided infective endocarditis: a clinicopathologic study of 59 patients. Am J Cardiol 1977;40:876–888.
5. **Bulkley BH, Roberts WC.** Ankylosing spondylitis and aortic regurgitation. Description of the characteristic cardiovascular lesion from study of eight necropsy patients. Circulation 1973;48:1014–1027.
6. **Roberts WC, Honig HS.** The spectrum of cardiovascular disease in the Marfan syndrome: a clinico-morphologic study of 18 necropsy patients and comparison to 151 previously reported necropsy patients. Am Heart J 1982;104:115–135.
7. **Waller BF, Reis RL, McIntosh CL, Epstein SE, Roberts WC.** The Marfan cardiovascular disease without the Marfan syndrome. Chest 1980;77:533–540.
8. **Waller BF, Zoltick, JM, Rosen JH, Katz NM, Gomes MN, Fletcher RD, Wallace RB, Roberts WC.** Severe aortic regurgitation from systemic hypertension (without aortic dissection) requiring aortic valve replacement. Analysis of four patients. Am J Cardiol 1982;49:473–477.
9. **Waller BF, Roberts WC.** Severe aortic regurgitation secondary to systemic hypertension (without aortic dissection). Cardiovasc Rev Rep 1982;3:1504–1518.
10. **Roberts WC.** Coronary embolism: a review of causes, consequences, and diagnostic considerations. Cardiovasc Med 1978;3:699–710.
11. **Arnett EN, Roberts WC.** Acute myocardial infarction and angiographically normal coronary arteries. An unproven combination. Circulation 1976;53:395–400.
12. **Roberts WC, Jones AA.** Quantitation of coronary arterial narrowing at necropsy in sudden coronary death. Analysis of 31 patients and comparison with 25 control subjects. Am J Cardiol 1979;44:39–45.
13. **Roberts WC, Virmani R.** Quantification of coronary arterial narrowing in clinically-isolated unstable angina pectoris. An analysis of 22 necropsy patients. Am J Med 1979;67:792–799.
14. **Roberts WC, Jones AA.** Quantification of coronary arterial narrowing at necropsy in acute transmural myocardial infarction: analysis and comparison of findings in 27 patients and 22 controls. Circulation 1980;61:786–790.
15. **Virmani R, Roberts WC.** Quantification of coronary arterial narrowing and of left ventricular myocardial scarring in healed myocardial infarction with chronic eventually fatal, congestive cardiac failure. Am J Med 1980;68:831–838.
16. **Cabin HS, Roberts WC.** True left ventricular aneurysm and healed myocardial infarction. Clinical and necropsy observations including quantification of degrees of coronary arterial narrowing. Am J Cardiol 1980;46:754–763.
17. **Waller BF, Roberts WC.** Amount of narrowing by atherosclerotic plaque in 44 nonbypassed and 52 bypassed major epicardial coronary arteries in 32 necropsy patients who died within 1 month of aortocoronary bypass grafting. Am J Cardiol 1980;46:956–962.
18. **Virmani R, Roberts WC.** Non-fatal healed transmural myocardial infarction and fatal non-cardiac disease. Qualification and quantification of coronary arterial narrowing and of left ventricular scarring in 18 necropsy patients. Br Heart J 1981;45:434–441.
19. **Cabin HS, Roberts WC.** Fatal cardiac arrest during cardiac catheterization for angina pectoris: analysis of 10 necropsy patients. Am J Cardiol 1981;48:1–8.
20. **Brosius FC III, Roberts WC.** Comparison of degree and extent of coronary narrowing by atherosclerotic plaque in anterior and posterior transmural acute myocardial infarction. Circulation 1981;64:715–722.
21. **Cabin HS, Roberts WC.** Comparison of amount and extent of coronary narrowing by atherosclerotic plaque and of myocardial scarring at necropsy in anterior and posterior healed transmural myocardial infarction. Circulation 1982;66:93–99.
22. **Cabin HC, Roberts WC.** Relations of healed transmural myocardial infarct size to length of survival after acute myocardial infarction, age at death, and amount and extent of coronary arterial narrowing by atherosclerotic plaques: analysis of 70 necropsy patients. Am Heart J 1982;104:216–220.
23. **Cabin HS, Roberts WC.** Relation of serum cholesterol and triglyceride levels to the amount and extent of coronary arterial narrowing by atherosclerotic plaque in coronary heart disease. Quantification analysis of 2,037 five mm segments of 160 major epicardial coronary arteries in 40 necropsy patients. Am J Med 1982;73:227–234.
24. **Cabin HS, Roberts WC.** Quantitative comparison of extent of coronary narrowing and size of healed myocardial infarct in 33 necropsy patients with clinically recognized and in 28 with clinically unrecognized ("silent") previous acute myocardial infarction. Am J Cardiol 1982;50:677–681.
25. **Virmani R, Roberts WC.** Extravasated erythrocytes, iron, and fibrin in atherosclerotic plaques of coronary arteries in fatal coronary heart disease and their relation to luminal thrombus: frequency and significance in 57 necropsy patients and in 2958 five mm segments of 224 major epicardial coronary arteries. Am Heart J 1983;105:788–797.
26. **Basta LL, Raines D, Najjar S, Kioschos JM.** Clinical, haemodynamic, and coronary angiographic correlates of angina pectoris in patients with severe aortic valve disease. Br Heart J 1975;37:150–157.
27. **Lacy J, Goodin R, McMartin D, Masden R, Flowers N.** Coronary atherosclerosis in valvular heart disease. Annals Thorac Surg 1977;23:429–435.
28. **Graboys TB, Cohn PF.** The prevalence of angina pectoris and abnormal coronary arteriograms in severe aortic valvular disease. Am Heart J 1977;93:683–686.
29. **Storstein O, Enge I.** Angina pectoris in aortic valvular disease and its relation to coronary pathology. Acta Med Scand 1979;205:275–278.
30. **Clark DG, McAnulty JH, Rahimtoola SH.** Valve replacement in aortic insufficiency with left ventricular dysfunction. Circulation 1980;61:411–421.
31. **Hakki A-H, Kimbiris D, Iskandrian AS, Segal BL, Mintz GS, Bemis CE.** Angina pectoris and coronary artery disease in patients with severe aortic valvular disease. Am Heart J 1980;100:441–448.
32. **Saltups A.** Coronary arteriography in isolated aortic and mitral valve disease. Aust NZ J Med 1982;12:494–497.
33. **Pichard AD, Smith H, Holt J, Meller J, Gorlin R.** Coronary vascular reserve in left ventricular hypertrophy secondary to chronic aortic regurgitation. Am J Cardiol 1983;51:315–320.

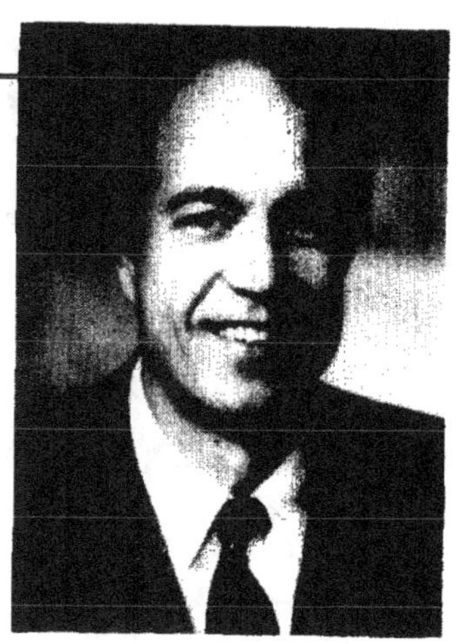

When I Have an Acute Myocardial Infarction Take Me to the Hospital That Has a Cardiac Catheterization Laboratory and Open Cardiac Surgical Facilities

When a sick person is taken to a hospital in an ambulance, the driver is required in most cities to transport this passenger to the nearest hospital irrespective of the diagnostic and therapeutic facilities present in that hospital. If available somewhere in the local community, when and if I develop an acute myocardial infarction (AMI), I want to be transported by ambulance *to the nearest hospital that has a cardiac catheterization laboratory and open cardiac surgical facilities.* If coronary flow is to be predictably reinstituted, appropriate therapy must be started within 6 hours after onset of the pain of AMI. If the passenger having an AMI is initially taken to a hospital where these facilities are unavailable, later transfer to a hospital equipped for invasive cardiologic procedures causes an additional delay that may prevent early reestablishment of coronary flow.

Another reason for wanting the patient with an AMI to be located in a hospital containing a cardiac catheterization laboratory is for definitive diagnostic procedures if certain complications arise. Additionally, cardiac angiographic and hemodynamic studies just before discharge from the hospital are important and useful in many patients with AMI, and some of these patients deserve coronary dilatation or bypass procedures during hospitalization for AMI.

I realize that it is impossible for all patients having an AMI in the USA to be treated in a hospital having a cardiac catheterization laboratory and open-cardiac surgical facilities; use of either or both during AMI has not been proved at this time to increase long-term survival after AMI. No data are available comparing mortality rates of patients with AMI treated in hospitals that have catheterization laboratories and cardiac operative facilities with those that do not. Nevertheless, in my view, in large metropolitan areas, patients with AMI ideally should be brought to hospitals with invasive cardiologic and cardiac surgical facilities. Without these invasive facilities, patients with AMI simply do not have access to today's presently available maximal care. With the introduction of coronary thrombolytic and dilating procedures, the traditionally diagnostic cardiac catheterization laboratory also is becoming a therapeutic laboratory, and committees determining certificates of need for various hospitals must recognize this fact.

Thus, for me, when and if I have an AMI, please, ambulance driver, *take me to the hospital that has a cardiac catheterization laboratory and a cardiac surgical unit even if that hospital is not the closest one.*

William C. Roberts, MD
Editor-in-Chief

Sudden Coronary Death: Relation of Amount and Distribution of Coronary Narrowing at Necropsy to Previous Symptoms of Myocardial Ischemia, Left Ventricular Scarring and Heart Weight

CAROLE A. WARNES, MB, BS, MRCP, and WILLIAM C. ROBERTS, MD

The amount and distribution of coronary arterial narrowing by atherosclerotic plaque at necropsy is described in 70 victims, aged 22 to 81 years (mean 50), of sudden coronary death. Of 3,484 five-millimeter segments examined (mean 50 per patient) from the 4 major (left main, left anterior descending, left circumflex and right) coronary arteries, 950 (27%) were narrowed 76 to 100% in cross-sectional area (XSA), 1,127 (32%), 51 to 75%; 689 (20%), 26 to 50%; and 718 (21%), 0 to 25%. More extensive severe narrowing occurred in the proximal than in the distal halves of the left anterior descending, left circumflex and right coronary arteries. Comparison between the 31 previously symptomatic victims (angina pectoris or a clinical acute myocardial infarction or both) with the 39 victims who had previously been asymptomatic disclosed a significantly higher mean percent of severely narrowed (76 to 100% XSA) 5-mm segments (30 vs 25%, p <0.005) and lower mean percent of minimally narrowed (0 to 25% XSA) segments in the symptomatic group (15 vs 25%, p <0.001). Comparison of the 31 patients who had a healed myocardial infarction at necropsy with the 39 patients who did not disclosed a higher mean percent of 5-mm segments narrowed 76 to 100% in XSA (33 vs 24%, p <0.001) and a lower mean percent of segments narrowed minimally in those with a left ventricular scar (13 vs 26%, p <0.001). Comparison between victims whose hearts weighed more than 450 g with those whose hearts weighed 450 g or less disclosed a higher mean percent of severely narrowed segments (19 vs 23%, p <0.01) and a lower mean percent of minimally narrowed segments (29 vs 24%, p <0.005) in the group with enlarged hearts.   (Am J Cardiol 1984;54:65–73)

It is well established that people who die suddenly from atherosclerotic coronary heart disease (CAD) have considerable narrowing of 1 or more major epicardial coronary arteries. We studied at necropsy 70 victims of sudden coronary death to determine the amount and distribution of cross-sectional area (XSA) luminal narrowing in each 5-mm segment of the 4 major coronary arteries, and compared the amount of narrowing both qualitatively and quantitatively in those with and without previous clinical evidence of myocardial ischemia, in those with and without left ventricular scars, and in those with and without cardiomegaly.

Methods

Patients: Only patients who fulfilled all the following criteria were included in this study: (1) Death was known to occur within less than 6 hours of the previously witnessed usual state of health. (2) Although the patient may have died in a hospital, he/she was not a patient in a hospital at the onset of symptoms suggestive of myocardial ischemia. (3) At necropsy, 1 or more of the 4 major coronary arteries (left main [LM], left anterior descending [LAD], left circumflex [LC] and right) was narrowed 76 to 100% in XSA. (4) Ventricular myocardial coagulation necrosis was absent at necropsy. (5) A cause of death, cardiac or noncardiac, other than CAD was absent. (6) Chronic congestive heart failure had never been present. (7) A cardiovascular operation had never been performed. Review of clinical and necropsy records in the Pathology Branch of the National Heart, Lung, and Blood Institute yielded 63 men and 7 women aged 22 to 81 years (mean 50) who fulfilled these criteria (Fig. 1). Of the 70 victims, 46 died outside the hospital; these hearts were obtained from the District of Columbia's Medical Examiner's Office. The other 24 had chest pain out-

From the Pathology Branch, National Heart, Lung, and Blood Institute, National Institutes of Health, Bethesda, Maryland. Manuscript received and accepted April 2, 1984.

Address for reprints: Carole A. Warnes, MB, BS, MRCP, Building 10A, Room 3E30, National Institutes of Health, Bethesda, Maryland 20205.

side the hospital and had fatal cardiac arrest soon after being brought to the hospital. These 24 patients underwent necropsy at 10 different hospitals. The intact, formalin-fixed heart in all 70 patients was submitted to us for detailed examination. The clinical information was obtained from the hospital where the patient had been hospitalized previously or from the patient's private physician; often, surviving family members were contacted for additional information.

The hearts were fixed for at least 24 hours in formalin. The 4 major coronary arteries were excised intact, x-rayed and, if necessary, decalcified. Each artery was then cut transversely into 5-mm segments and labeled sequentially, either from the aortic ostium or from its origin from the LM coronary artery. The segments were then dehydrated with alcohol and xylene, embedded in paraffin, and at least 2 histologic sections were cut from the paraffin block. Each histologic section was stained by the Movat technique.[1] The amount of luminal narrowing by atherosclerotic plaque was determined by visual inspection of these histologic sections when magnified 25 to 50 times. The percent XSA narrowing of each 5-mm segment was categorized into 5 groups: 0 to 25%, 26 to 50%, 51 to 75%, 76 to 95% and 96 to 100%. All sections were examined by 1 of us (CAW) and the accuracy of the assessment of luminal narrowing was spot-checked by videoplanimetry. The agreement between these 2 techniques is approximately 95%.[2] A total of 3,484 five-millimeter segments from the 70 victims were examined (mean of 50 segments per patient). In addition, at least 3 histologic sections extending from endocardium to epicardium were prepared from the wall of the left ventricle of each patient, and stained with hematoxylin-eosin. Absence of myocardial coagulation necrosis was confirmed by histologic examination.

Chi-square analysis was used to compare amounts of coronary narrowing by quantitative means.

Results

Qualitative studies: Of the 70 patients, 1 major coronary artery was narrowed 76 to 100% in XSA *at some point* in 11 patients (16%), 2 arteries in 19 (27%), 3 arteries in 33 (47%) and 4 arteries in 7 (10%). Of the 280 major epicardial coronary arteries in the 70 patients (4 per patient), 176 (63%) were narrowed at some point 76 to 100% in XSA, a mean of 2.5 of 4.0 major coronary arteries per patient. Excluding the LM coronary artery, 167 (80%) of the other 210 major coronary arteries were narrowed 76 to 100% in XSA, an average of 2.4 of 3.0 coronary arteries per patient. Of the individual major coronary arteries, the LM artery was severely narrowed (76 to 100% XSA) in 13% (9 of 70), the LAD in 86% (60 of 70), the LC in 74% (52 of 70) and the right in 79% (55 of 70).

Comparison of the number of coronary arteries narrowed 76 to 100% in XSA in the 39 previously *asymptomatic* patients with the 31 with *previous acute myocardial infarction (MI) or angina pectoris or both* disclosed the following (Fig. 2): 1 major artery so narrowed in 8 (21%) vs 3 (10%) (difference not significant [NS]); 2 arteries, 11 (28%) vs 8 (26%) (NS); 3 arteries, 18 (46%) vs 15 (48%) (NS); and 4 arteries, 2 (5%) vs 5 (16%) (NS).

Comparison of the number of arteries narrowed 76 to 100% in XSA in the 39 patients without to the 31 with *healed MI* revealed the following (Fig. 3): 1 major artery so narrowed in 9 (23%) vs 2 (7%) (NS); 2 arteries, 11 (28%) vs 8 (26%) (NS); 3 arteries, 13 (33%) vs 20 (64%) (p <0.02), and 4 arteries, 6 (15%) vs 1 (3%) (NS).

Comparison of the number of arteries narrowed 76 to 100% in XSA in the 35 patients in whom the *heart weight* was 450 g or less with the 35 patients in whom the heart weight was more than 450 g disclosed the following (Fig. 4): 1 major artery so narrowed in 6 (17%) vs 5 (14%) (NS); 2 arteries, 9 (26%) vs 10 (29%) (NS); 3 arteries, 17 (48%) vs 16 (46%) (NS); and 4 arteries, 3 (9%) vs 4 (11%) (NS).

Quantitative studies: Analysis of the 3,484 five-millimeter coronary segments showed that 950 (27%) were narrowed 76 to 100% in XSA, 1,127 (32%), 51 to 75%; 689 (20%), 26 to 50%; and 718 (21%), 0 to 25% (Fig. 5). The percent of segments severely narrowed per patient, however, varied enormously, from 2% (1 of 50) to 88% (86 of 98) (Table I). Sixteen patients had 10% or less of their 5-mm segments narrowed 76 to 100% in XSA;

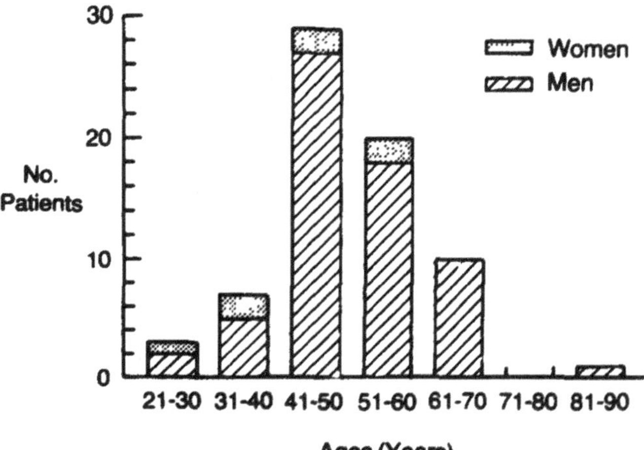

FIGURE 1. Age distribution in 70 patients with sudden coronary death.

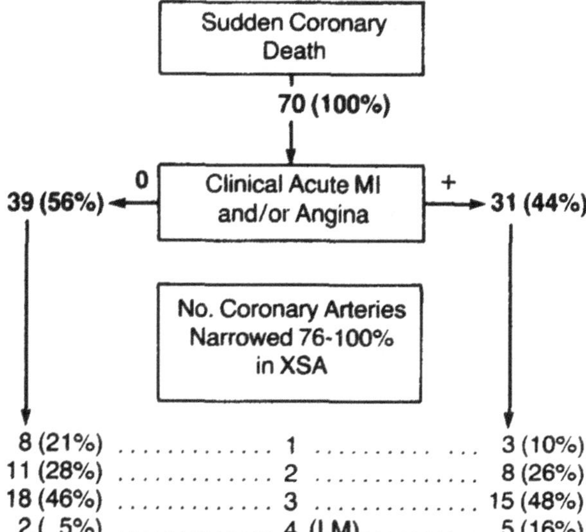

FIGURE 2. Qualitative comparison of the 39 previously asymptomatic patients with the 31 who had clinical acute myocardial infarction (MI) or angina pectoris or both before sudden coronary death. LM = left main coronary artery; XSA = cross-sectional area.

TABLE I Summary of Percentages of 5-mm Segments of the 4 Major Coronary Arteries Narrowed 76 to 100% in Cross-Sectional Area According to Age Group

Age Group (Yr)	No. of Pts	No. of Patients Listed According to Percent of 5-mm Segments of 4 Major Coronary Arteries Narrowed 76 to 100% in XSA								
		0–10	11–20	21–30	31–40	41–50	51–60	61–70	71–80	81–90
21–30	3	2	0	1	0	0	0	0	0	0
31–40	7	3	1	0	1	1	1	0	0	0
41–50	29	6	8	4	5	2	1	2	0	1
51–60	20	4	4	4	6	2	0	0	0	0
61–70	10	1	1	2	4	2	0	0	0	0
71–80	0	0	0	0	0	0	0	0	0	0
81–90	1	0	1	0	0	0	0	0	0	1
Totals	70	16 (23%)	15 (21%)	11 (16%)	16 (23%)	7 (10%)	2 (3%)	2 (3%)	0	1 (1%)

XSA = cross-sectional area.

15 patients had 11 to 20% of the segments so narrowed; 11 patients, 21 to 30% of the segments; 16 patients, 31 to 40% of the segments; 7 patients, 41 to 50% of the segments; 2 patients, 51 to 60% of the segments; 2 patients, 61 to 70% of the segments; and 1 patient had 81 to 90% of the segments so narrowed. The 5 categories of narrowing in each of the 4 major epicardial coronary arteries is also shown in Figure 5. Comparison of the mean percent of 5-mm segments narrowed 76 to 100% in XSA in the proximal and distal halves of the LAD, LC and right coronary arteries disclosed a significantly higher percent of severely narrowed segments proximally in the LAD and LC arteries (Fig. 6). A similar distribution of severe narrowing in the proximal and distal halves of these 3 arteries also was observed in the patients with and without previous symptoms of myocardial ischemia, in the patients with and without healed MI and in the patients without cardiomegaly (heart weight 450 g or less). In those patients with cardiomegaly (heart weight weighing more than 450 g), a higher mean percent of segments narrowed 76 to 100%

in XSA occurred in the proximal half than in the distal half of the LAD and LC arteries, but the reverse was true with the right coronary artery (37 vs 31% [NS]).

Of the 39 patients who had been asymptomatic, 502 (25%) of 1,991 five-millimeter segments were narrowed 76 to 100% in XSA, compared with 448 (30%) of 1,493 five-millimeter segments in the 31 patients who had had either a clinical acute MI or angina pectoris previously (Fig. 7) (p <0.005). Comparison of the mean percents of segments in all 5 categories of coronary narrowing in XSA between the previously asymptomatic and symptomatic groups disclosed significant differences in the category of minimal (0 to 25%) narrowing in XSA (25 vs 15%, p <0.001). Comparison of the amounts of narrowing in each of the 4 major coronary arteries disclosed a higher mean percent of 5-mm segments narrowed 76 to 100% in XSA in the symptomatic vs the asymptomatic victims in the LM, LAD and LC arteries, but not in the right coronary artery, and a lower mean percent of segments narrowed 0 to 25% in XSA in all 4 coronary arteries in the symptomatic group (Fig. 8).

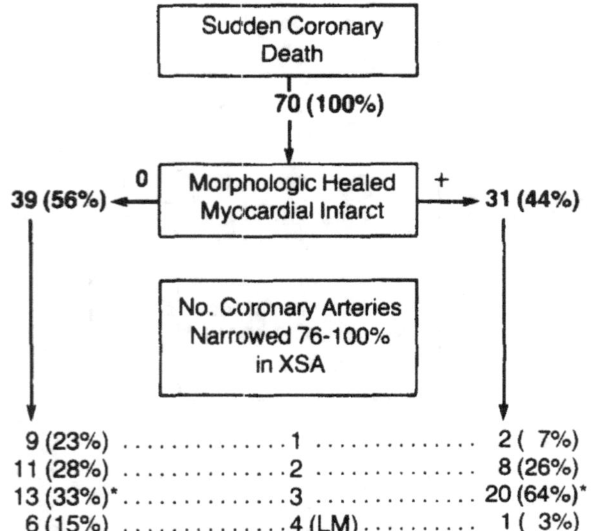

FIGURE 3. Qualitative comparison of the 39 patients who had no healed myocardial infarction at necropsy with the 31 who did have a left ventricular scar. LM = left main coronary artery; XSA = cross-sectional area. * p <0.02.

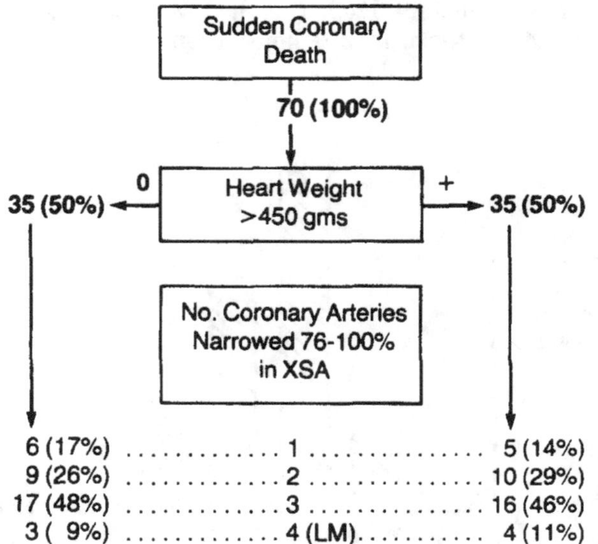

FIGURE 4. Qualitative comparison of the 35 patients who had hearts that weighed 450 g or less with the 35 who had hearts that weighed more than 450 g. LM = left main coronary artery; XSA = cross-sectional area.

Comparison of the mean percents of 5-mm segments in the 5 categories of narrowing between the 31 patients with and the 39 patients without *left ventricular scars* disclosed a higher mean percent of segments narrowed 76 to 100% in the healed MI group (33 vs 24%, p <0.001), and a lower mean percent of segments narrowed 0 to 25% (13 vs 26%, p <0.001) compared with those without healed MI (Fig. 9). When this comparison is made using the 4 individual coronary arteries, the same trends apply for each individual artery (Fig. 10). A higher mean percent of 5-mm segments were minimally narrowed in those with no healed MI, and a higher mean percent of segments were severely narrowed (76 to 100%) when a healed MI was present. Severe narrowing of the LM coronary artery, however, occurred more frequently in those without healed MI.

A similar comparison was made between the 35 patients who had hearts that weighed 450 g or less and those who had hearts that weighed more than 450 g (Fig. 11). A lower mean percent of segments narrowed 0 to 25% occurred in those with higher heart weights (19 vs 23%, p <0.01) and a higher mean percent of segments were narrowed 76 to 100% (29 vs 24%, p <0.005) in those with hearts that weighed more than 450 g. Comparison of the amounts of narrowing in each of the 4 major coronary arteries disclosed a higher mean percent of

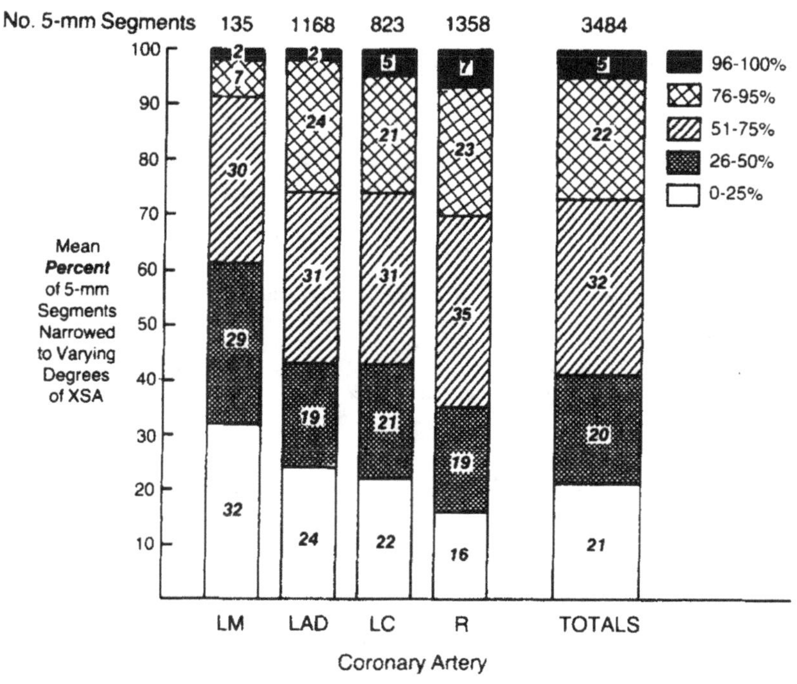

FIGURE 5. Mean percents of 5-mm segments of the 4 major coronary arteries narrowed to varying degrees in cross-sectional area (XSA) in 70 patients with sudden coronary death. LAD = left anterior descending; LC = left circumflex; LM = left main; R = right.

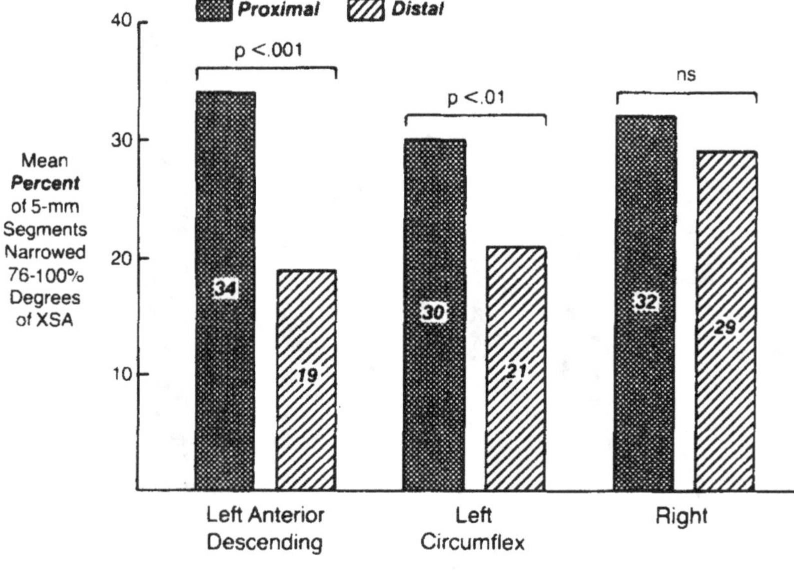

FIGURE 6. Comparison of the proximal and distal halves of mean percents of 5-mm segments of the 3 major coronary arteries narrowed 76 to 100% in cross-sectional area (XSA) in 70 patients with sudden coronary death.

5-mm segments narrowed 76 to 100% in XSA in those with higher heart weights in all coronary arteries except the LM (Fig. 12).

Figure 13 is a summary of the amounts of coronary narrowing quantitatively in the 70 patients after subdivision of heart weights in 100-g increments. The mean percent of 5-mm segments narrowed 76 to 100% in XSA did not increase with increasing heart weight.

Of the 70 patients, 13 were found at necropsy to have a thrombus in 1 coronary artery. In 6 patients, the thrombus consisted primarily of fibrin and erythrocytes, and in 7 patients, almost entirely of platelets. In all 13 patients, the thrombi were superimposed on atherosclerotic plaques that had already narrowed the lumina 26 to 50% (1 patient), 51 to 75% in XSA (4 patients) or 76 to 100% (8 patients).

Discussion

A major finding in our study was that victims of sudden death had severe and extensive narrowing of their 4 major (LM, LAD, LC and right) extramural coronary arteries by atherosclerotic plaque. Of the 70 patients, 59 (84%) had at least 2 major arteries narrowed 76 to 100% in XSA and 11 (16%) had only 1 artery so narrowed by atherosclerotic plaque. Of the 59 patients with multivessel CAD, 2 arteries were severely narrowed (76 to 100% XSA) in 19 patients (27%), 3 arteries in 33 (47%) and 4 arteries in 7 (10%). Of the 4 major coronary arteries per patient, 2.5 of 4 were severely narrowed. Of the 280 major coronary arteries in the 70 patients, 176 (63%) were severely narrowed and of them, the LAD artery was the most frequently narrowed (60 of 70, 86%). The 11 patients with 1-vessel CAD (1 artery narrowed 76 to 100% in XSA) were significantly younger than the 59 patients with multivessel CAD (mean age, 41 vs 51 years). The arteries severely narrowed in these 11 patients were the LAD in 5, the right in 4, the LC in 1 and the LM in 1.

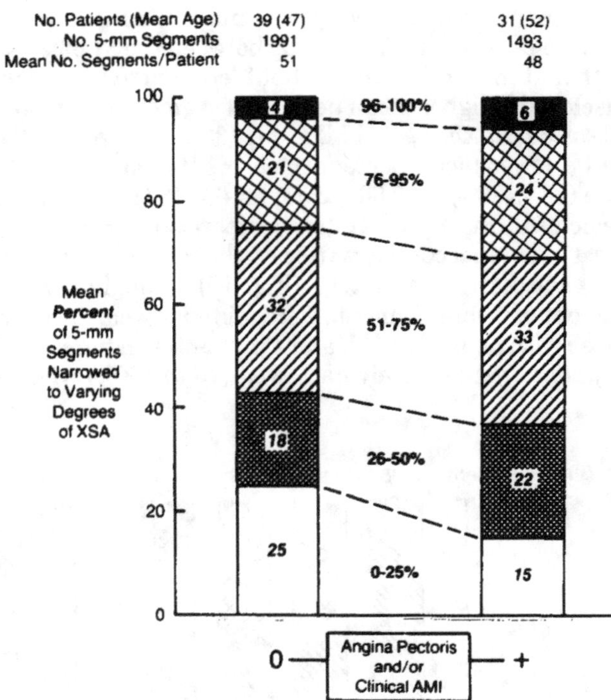

FIGURE 7. Mean percents of 5-mm segments of the sum of the 4 major coronary arteries narrowed to varying degrees in cross-sectional area (XSA) in 70 patients with sudden coronary death: comparison of 39 patients without and 31 patients with a clinical acute myocardial infarction (AMI) or angina or both.

Qualitative studies describing from gross inspection the number of 4 major coronary arteries severely narrowed in victims of nontraumatic sudden death have been performed by others.[3-7] Results of 5 such large necropsy studies are summarized in Table II. Of the 720 necropsy patients included in the 5 studies, 499 (69%) patients had 2 or more major coronary arteries narrowed

FIGURE 8. Comparison of mean percents of 5-mm segments of the 4 major coronary arteries narrowed to varying degrees in 70 patients with sudden coronary death: 39 patients without and 31 patients with a clinical acute myocardial infarction (AMI) or angina pectoris (AP) or both. XSA = cross-sectional area.

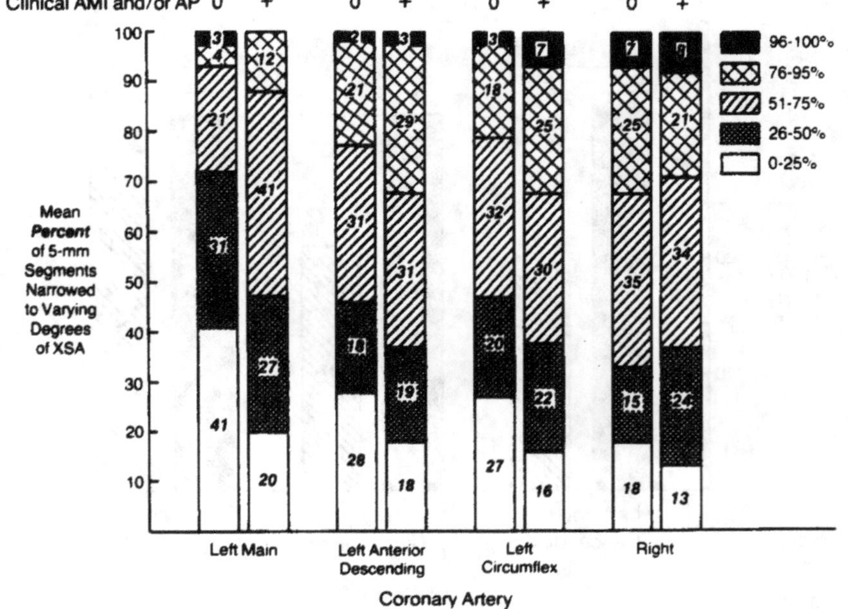

TABLE II Clinical and Cardiac Morphologic Observations in 5 Previously Reported Necropsy Studies on Sudden Death in Which the Number of Coronary Arteries Severely Narrowed was Described

Year of Study	First Author	No. of Pts	Ages (yr) (mean)	Sex M	Sex F	Definition of SD (Hours)	AP	Clinical Acute MI	Gross Exam of CA (Intervals in cm)	No. of Major CAs Narrowed >75% in XSA: 0	1	2	3	4	CA T	Acute MI	Healed MI	HW (g) (mean)
1972	Kuller	64	25–64(—)	—	—	<24	—	—	—	5 (8%)	16 (25%)	11 (17%)	22 (34%)	10 (16%)	12 (19%)	8 (13%)	—	*
1973	Friedman	59	----65(54)	53	6	<24	15	17	+(0.5)	4 (7%)	9 (15%)	11 (19%)	22 (37%)	13 (22%)	28 (47%)	7 (12%)	31 (53%)	310–585 (—) (448)
1974	Liberthson	220	—(59)	190	30	—	104[†] (47%)	57 (26%)	+(0.1)	13 (6%)	29 (13%)	53 (24%)	← 125 → (57%)		70 (32%)	59 (27%)	97 (44%)	
1975	Perper	169	25–64(—)	133	36	—	—[‡]	—[‡]	+(0.2)	16 (9%)	25 (15%)	25 (15%)	64 (38%)	39 (23%)	—	17/157 (11%)	68/157 (43%)	—
1979	Baroldi	208	<20–>70(—)	182	26	—	—[§]	—[§]	+(0.3) —	51 (24%)	53 (26%)	60 (29%)	← 44 → (21%)		54 (26%)	35 (17%)	170 (82%)	—‖

* Thirty-seven patients (58%) had hearts weighing more than 450 g.
[†] Chest pain. Possibly not angina in all.
[‡] History of "prior heart disease" in 51 (30%).
[§] History of "prior heart disease" in 102 (49%).
‖ Heart weight weighing more than 500 g in 87 (42%).
AP = angina pectoris; CA = coronary artery; HW = heart weight; MI = myocardial infarct; SD = sudden death; T = thrombus; XSA = cross-sectional area; — = unknown.

severely and 132 (18%) had only 1 coronary artery so narrowed. One difficulty in comparing any of these 5 previous necropsy studies with the present study is the varying criteria for inclusion of cases. To be included in our study, a patient had to have at least 1 of the 4 major coronary arteries narrowed 76 to 100% in XSA by atherosclerotic plaque. In the 5 previously reported studies, however, 89 of the 720 patients (12%) had none of the 4 coronary arteries narrowed to this extent; all apparently had at least 1 artery narrowed 51 to 75% in XSA. Another major problem in comparing our findings with those in previously reported studies concerns different temporal definitions of the term "sudden." We used a time period of 6 hours or less from the time of previously witnessed usual health to death, whereas the patients included in the studies both by Kuller et al[3] and by Friedman et al[4] used a time period of less than 24 hours. The time frame used in the other 3 studies[5–7] was not defined. Our study also included only patients without histologic evidence of left ventricular myocardial coagulation necrosis, whereas 126 of the 720 patients (18%) included in Table II had acute MI at necropsy.

Although 4 of the 5 previously reported studies (Table II) mentioned the number and percent of patients with previous clinical evidence of heart disease and with left ventricular scars (healed MI) at necropsy, none compared the amount of coronary narrowing in the group with to the group without clinical evidence of myocardial ischemia or the group with to the group without left ventricular scars. We found that the number of coronary arteries severely narrowed at some point (the qualitative

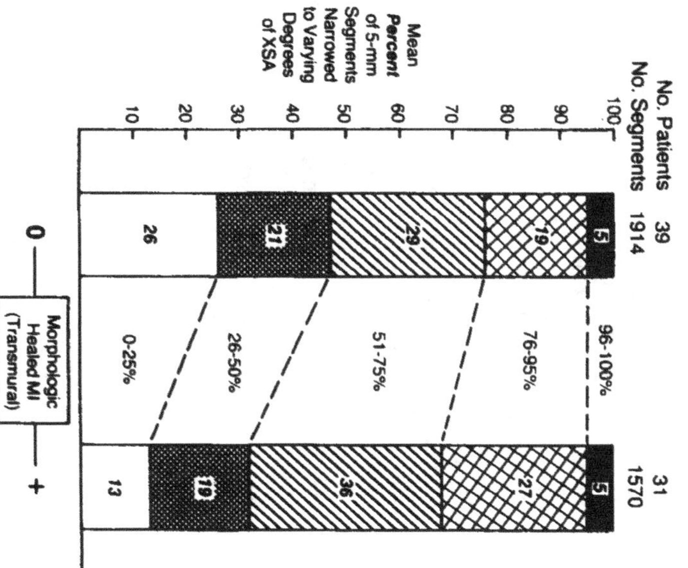

FIGURE 9. Mean percents of 5-mm segments of the sum of the 4 major coronary arteries narrowed to varying degrees in cross-sectional area (XSA) in 70 patients with sudden coronary death: comparison of 39 patients without to 31 with a morphologic healed myocardial infarct (MI).

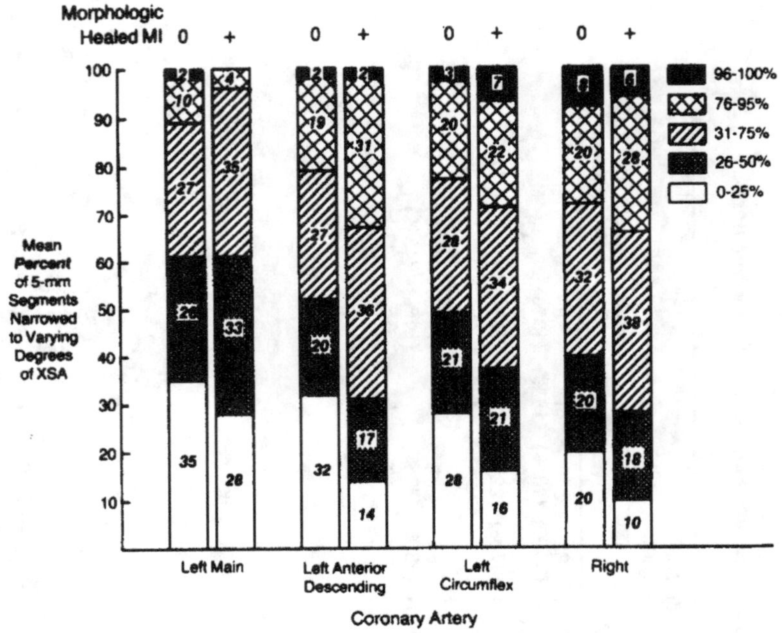

FIGURE 10. Mean percents of 5-mm segments of the individual 4 major coronary arteries narrowed to varying degrees in cross-sectional area (XSA) in 70 patients with sudden coronary death: comparison of 39 patients without to 31 with a morphologic healed myocardial infarct (MI).

approach) in the groups of patients with and without previous angina pectoris or acute MI or both, and the groups with and without grossly visible left ventricular scars at necropsy, were similar. Thirty-one of our 70 patients (44%) had had previous clinical acute MI (which healed) or angina or both, and 39 did not (Fig. 2). Comparison of those with to those without previous clinical evidence of myocardial ischemia disclosed similar percents of total coronary arteries (4 per patient) severely narrowed (84 of 124 [68%] vs 92 of 156 [59%] and roughly similar percents of 2 or more coronary arteries severely narrowed (28 of 31 [90%] vs 31 of 39 [79%]). Comparison of the 31 patients with to the 39 without left ventricular scars (Fig. 3) disclosed similar percents of total coronary arteries severely narrowed (82 of 124 [66%] vs 94 of 156 [60%]) and similar percents of 2 or more coronary arteries severely narrowed (29 of 31 [94%] vs 30 of 39 [77%]).

Cardiomegaly (heart weight more than 400 g) is frequently found at necropsy in patients who die suddenly from CAD. Of the 64 patients studied by Kuller et al,[3] 37 (58%) had hearts that weighed more than 450 g. Of the 208 victims studied by Baroldi et al,[7] 157 (75%) had hearts that weighed more than 400 g. In the 220 patients studied by Liberthson et al[5] the mean heart weight for 190 men was 460 g and that for the 30 women was 374 g. Only 1 of these previous necropsy studies[7] correlated the number of coronary arteries severely narrowed with heart weight. Comparison of our 35 patients with to the 35 patients without hearts that weighed more than 450 g (Fig. 4) disclosed similar percents of total coronary arteries severely narrowed (89 of 140 [64%] vs 87 of 140 [62%]) and similar percents of 2 or more coronary arteries severely narrowed (30 of 35 [86%] vs 29 of 35 [83%]).

None of the previously reported 5 necropsy studies[3–7] provided *quantitative* information on the amount and distribution of coronary narrowing in victims of sudden death. In our study, a total of 3,484 five-millimeter segments from the 70 patients were examined: 27% of the segments were narrowed 76 to 100% in XSA, including 5% narrowed 96 to 100%. The 96 to 100% narrowing in XSA is probably equivalent to angiographic total occlusion. Not a single 5-mm segment was entirely free of atherosclerotic plaque. A higher mean percent of segments was severely narrowed in the proximal compared with the distal halves of the 3 (LAD, LC and

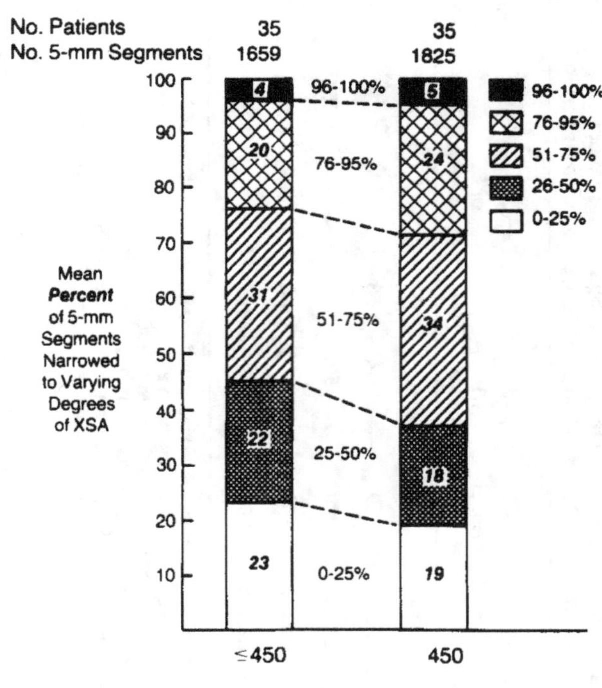

FIGURE 11. Mean percents of 5-mm segments of the sum of the 4 major coronary arteries narrowed to varying degrees in cross-sectional area (XSA) in 70 patients with sudden coronary death: comparison of 35 patients with hearts that weighed 450 g or less with 35 patients with hearts that weighed more than 450 g.

right) major coronary arteries. A previous report from this laboratory,[8] which included only 12 of the 70 patients included in the present study, also emphasized the diffuse extent of atherosclerosis in victims of sudden death. Although a control group was not examined in the present study, the previous study[8] from this laboratory included 25 control subjects (mean age 49 years), and in them, only 3% of the 5-mm segments of the 4 major coronary arteries were narrowed 76 to 100% in XSA by atherosclerotic plaque.

Of our 39 patients who previously had had no clinical evidence of myocardial ischemia (asymptomatic group), 25% of the 5-mm segments were narrowed 76 to 100% in XSA, compared with 30% in those who had had symptoms of ischemia (acute MI, which healed, or angina pectoris or both) (p <0.005). The asymptomatic groups also had a higher mean percent of segments minimally narrowed (25 vs 15%, p <0.001) (Fig. 7).

Similar differences were apparent in the quantitative comparisons between victims who had a healed MI at

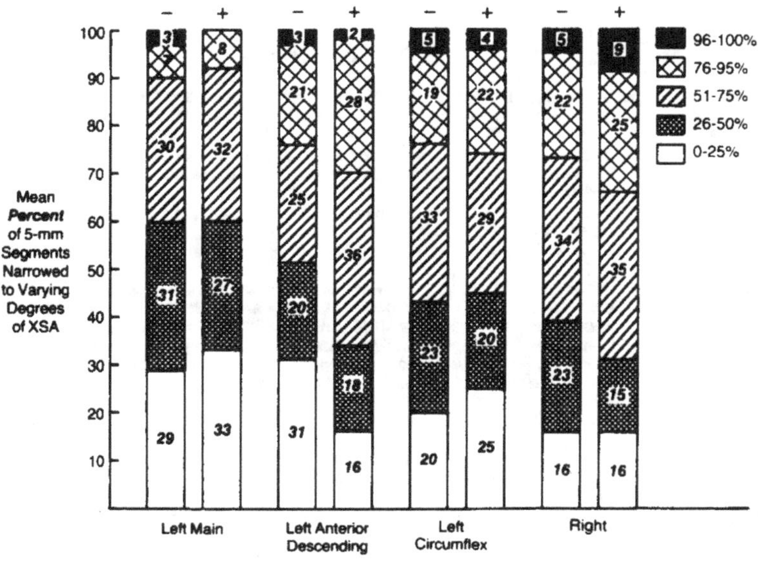

FIGURE 12. Mean percents of 5-mm segments of the individual 4 major coronary arteries narrowed to varying degrees in cross-sectional area (XSA) in 70 patients with sudden coronary death: comparison of 35 patients who had hearts that weighed 450 g or less (−) with 35 patients who had hearts that weighed more than 450 g (+).

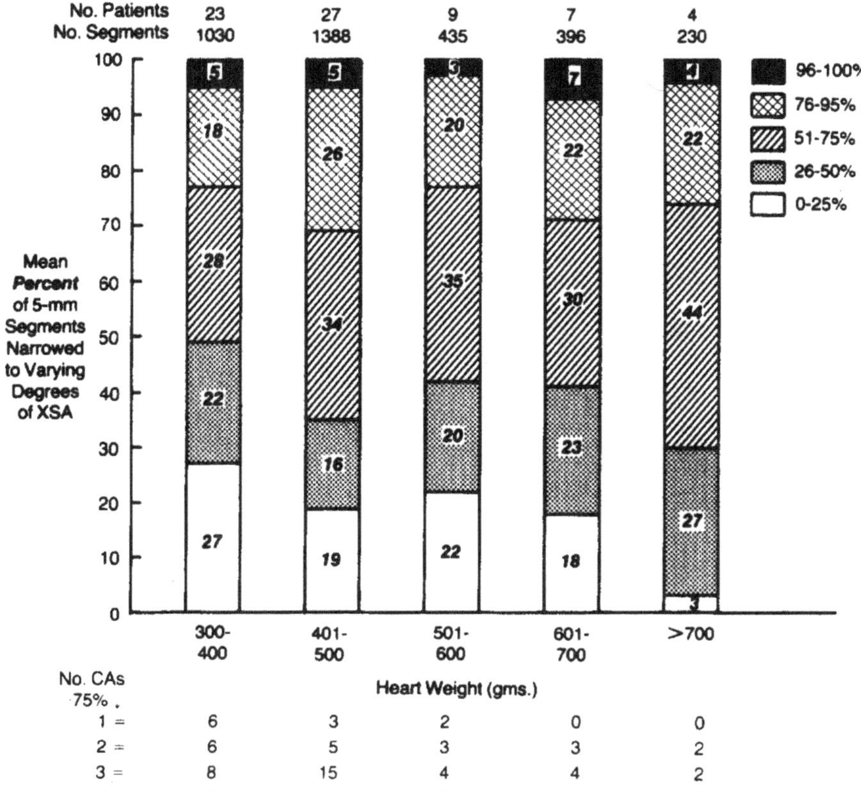

No. CAs 75%	300-400	401-500	501-600	601-700	>700
1 =	6	3	2	0	0
2 =	6	5	3	3	2
3 =	8	15	4	4	2
4 =	3	4	0	0	0

FIGURE 13. Relation of heart weight to the mean percent of 5-mm segments narrowed to varying degrees in 70 patients with sudden coronary death. CAs = coronary arteries; XSA = cross-sectional area.

necropsy and those who did not. More 5-mm segments were narrowed 76 to 100% in those with than in those without a left ventricular scar (33 vs 24%, p <0.001); fewer 5-mm segments were minimally narrowed in those with than in those without healed MI (13 vs 26%, p <0.001) (Fig. 9). Although a higher percentage of the 5-mm segments from the sum of all 4 major coronary arteries were severely narrowed in the patients with than in those without healed MI, analysis of the individual arteries disclosed that the LM coronary artery was different from the other 3 (Fig. 10). In the 31 patients with healed MI, only 4% of the 57 five-millimeter segments of the LM artery were severely narrowed; in contrast, in the 39 patients without healed MI, 12% of the 78 five-millimeter segments were severely narrowed. The more extensive severe narrowing in the LM coronary artery in the group without healed MI suggests that severe LM narrowing may prevent recovery from an acute MI and therefore the possibility of fatal cardiac arrest sometime later.

Comparison of patients with hearts that weighed 450 g or less to those with larger hearts disclosed a higher mean percent of segments narrowed 76 to 100% in those with cardiomegaly (29 vs 24%, p <0.005) and a lower mean percent of minimally narrowed segments (19 vs 23%, p <0.01) (Fig. 11). The cause of the cardiomegaly appears to have been systemic hypertension, which may have accelerated the atherosclerotic process.

Although our study patients as a group had severe and extensive coronary narrowing by atherosclerotic plaques, considerable variation in the percent of 5-mm segments narrowed severely was observed (Table I). The range was 2 to 86%: 16 patients (23%) had fewer than 10% of their coronary segments narrowed 76 to 100% in XSA and 12 patients (17%) had more than 40% of their 5-mm segments severely narrowed. Thus, the extent of the severe narrowing is difficult to predict in the individual patient put predictable in groups of patients dying suddenly from CAD. The previously symptomatic patients clearly had more severe narrowing and less minimal narrowing than the asymptomatic group, as did patients with a healed MI and those with cardiomegaly.

References

1. **Movat HZ.** Demonstration of all connective tissue elements in a single section. Pentachrome stains. Arch Pathol 1955;60:289–295.
2. **Isner JM, Wu M, Virmani R, Jones AA, Roberts WC.** Comparison of degrees of coronary arterial luminal narrowing determined by visual inspection of histologic sections under magnification among three independent observers and comparison to that obtained by videoplanimetry. An analysis of 559 five-millimeter segments of 61 coronary arteries from eleven patients. Lab Invest 1980;42:566–570.
3. **Kuller L, Cooper M, Perper J.** Epidemiology of sudden death. Arch Intern Med 1972;129:714–719.
4. **Friedman M, Manwaring JH, Rosenman RH, Donlon G, Ortega P, Grube SM.** Instantaneous and sudden deaths. Clinical and pathological differentiation in coronary artery disease. JAMA 1973;225:1319–1328.
5. **Liberthson RR, Nagel EL, Hirschman JC, Nussenfeld SR, Blackbourn BD, Davis JR.** Pathophysiologic observations in prehospital ventricular fibrillation and sudden cardiac death. Circulation 1974;49:790–798.
6. **Perper JA, Kuller LH, Cooper M.** Arteriosclerosis of coronary arteries in sudden, unexpected deaths. Circulation 1975;51,52:supplement III:III-27–III-33.
7. **Baroldi G, Falzi G, Mariani F.** Sudden coronary death. A postmortem study in 208 selected cases compared to 97 "control" subjects. Am Heart J 1979;98:20–31.
8. **Roberts WC, Jones AA.** Quantitation of coronary arterial narrowing at necropsy in sudden coronary death. Analysis of 31 patients and comparison with 25 control subjects. Am J Cardiol 1979;44:39–45.

The Coronary Artery Surgery Study (CASS): Do the Results Apply to Your Patient?

WILLIAM C. ROBERTS, MD, and DENNIS M. MANNING, MD

The Coronary Artery Surgery Study (CASS) appears to be having a major impact on the management of patients with coronary heart disease (CAD). CASS was initiated in 1973 by the National Heart, Lung, and Blood Institute as a prospective randomized study to determine the long-term benefit of coronary artery bypass grafting (CABG) in terms of survival and of prevention of nonfatal acute myocardial infarction (AMI) in patients with mild angina pectoris (with or without previous healed AMI) and in patients who were asymptomatic after healing of their last AMI (no angina). The findings of this study after an average follow-up of 5.5 years (range 3.8 to 7.7) were recently published.[1-4] No significant differences in survival rates or occurrence of nonfatal AMI were observed between the patients randomized to surgery and those to medicine. The quality of life (relief of chest pain, improvement in both subjective and objective measurements of functional status, and a diminished requirement for drug therapy), however, was better in the group randomized to surgery. These findings lead to the conclusion that patients similar to those enrolled in the CASS randomized trial can safely defer CABG (or maybe angioplasty) until symptoms worsen.

Crucial to understanding CASS is the realization that it consists of 2 major components: (1) the *registry* and (2) the *randomized study*. All patients having coronary angiograms for proved or suspected CAD at the 15 participating North American medical centers from August 1974 to May 1979 were asked to participate in

the registry; 94% agreed. Although the randomized study concerns patients with angiographically severe coronary narrowing (27%, however, had "single-vessel disease"), persons with angiographically normal or only minimally narrowed coronary arteries were included in the registry.

The patients included in the *randomized study* were a highly selected subset of patients included in the registry. Of the 24,959 patients included in the registry, 8,333 patients (33%) were excluded from the screening for randomization because they were studied in 4 medical centers that later did not participate in the randomized study or because they participated in a pilot study before the randomized trial began in August 1975. Thus, 16,626 (67%) of the initial 24,959 registry patients were screened to determine their eligibility for entry into the randomized trial. Of these 16,626 patients, 14,527 (87.3%) were not eligible for randomization because they had angiographically normal coronary arteries or minimal CAD (28.3%), or severely narrowed coronary arteries not suitable for bypass grafting (4.9%), or severe (class III or IV) angina pectoris (36.5%), or severe ($\geq$70% diameter reduction) narrowing of the left main coronary artery, or severe (New York Heart Association functional class III or IV) congestive heart failure, or excessive age (older than 65 years), or previous CABG (16.1%), or a combination of these. Thus, of the 16,626 patients screened for randomization, only 2,099 patients (12.7%) fulfilled the criteria that made them eligible for randomization. Of these 2,099 "randomizable" patients, however, 1,319 patients (63%) declined participation in the randomized study (often at the insistence of their referring physician). Consequently, 780 patients, or only 5% of the 16,626 patients screened for randomization, entered the trial. Of the 780 patients, 390 were assigned to the surgical group and 390 to the medical group.

From the Pathology Branch, National Heart, Lung, and Blood Institute, National Institutes of Health, Bethesda, Maryland. Dr. Manning's present address: Division of Cardiology (Fellow), Department of Medicine, The Mercy Hospital of Pittsburgh, Pittsburgh, Pennsylvania. Manuscript received May 15, 1984, accepted May 30, 1984.

Address for reprints: William C. Roberts, MD, Building 10A, Room 3E30, National Heart, Lung, and Blood Institute, National Institutes of Health, Bethesda, Maryland 20205.

A key to the understanding of CASS is an understanding of the types of coronary patients included in and excluded from the final randomized controlled clinical trial, and this understanding necessitates a familiarity with the definitions used to establish the criteria for either inclusion or exclusion. The patients included in the randomized study fulfilled the following criteria: (1) Age 65 years or younger at time of coronary angiography. (2) Performance of a technically satisfactory coronary angiogram. (3) Presence of *mild* (class I or II Canadian Cardiovascular Society (CCS) classification, to be defined later) angina pectoris and ejection fraction $\geq 35\%$ (with or without previous AMI which healed) or presence of AMI which healed and absence of angina pectoris after occurrence of the last AMI. (4) Presence of $\geq 70\%$ diameter narrowing of the proximal or middle portions of 1 or more major coronary arteries or of a major "bypassable" branch. The bypassable coronary artery should supply presumably viable left ventricular myocardium on basis of good contraction of ventricular segments and no evidence of Q waves in the area of myocardium in question.

The inclusion criteria can be further clarified by a description of criteria used for exclusion and they were: (1) Age older than 65 years at time of coronary angiography. (2) Absence of angina pectoris or of a clinical event diagnosed as AMI (with typical enzyme and/or electrocardiographic changes). (3) Presence of severe (classes III or IV Canadian Cardiovascular Society classification) angina pectoris, including unstable (or progressive) angina. (4) Presence of *normal* coronary arteries by angiogram with or without spasm. (5) Presence of *minimal* coronary narrowing by angiogram. (6) Presence of $\geq 70\%$ diameter reduction of the left main coronary artery. (7) Presence of $\geq 70\%$ diameter reduction in the distal portions of the right, left anterior descending and/or left circumflex coronary arteries. (8) Presence of chronic congestive heart failure (New York Heart Association functional class III or IV). (9) Presence of left ventricular aneurysm likely to require operative resection. (10) Presence of mitral regurgitation likely to necessitate mitral valve replacement. (11) Presence of left ventricular ejection fraction $<35\%$ in the patients with angina pectoris. (12) Presence of previous CABG. (Although not specifically stated, patients having had percutaneous transluminal coronary angioplasty were not included.)

Precise understanding of the including and excluding criteria requires knowledge of the definitions used for words or terms in the criteria.[5] The grading of the severity of angina pectoris was based on the 1972 classification of the CCS. Although this classification is probably unfamiliar to many American cardiologists, the CCS grading of effort angina is, as pointed out by Campeau,[6] really a modification of the New York Heart Association functional classification,[7] but it is quite different from the American Heart Association grading of the severity of chest pain.[8] The 4 grades of effort angina by the CCS are presented in Table I. The angina patients included in the CASS randomized study were patients limited to CCS grades I and II. In actuality, for purposes of the CASS study, *mild* angina was transient

TABLE I   Grading of Angina of Effort by the Canadian Cardiovascular Society*

I. "Ordinary physical activity does not cause . . . angina," such as walking and climbing stairs. Angina with strenuous or rapid or prolonged exertion at work or recreation.
II. "Slight limitation of ordinary activity." Walking or climbing stairs rapidly, walking uphill, walking or stair climbing after meals, or in cold, or in wind, or under emotional stress, or only during the few hours after awakening. Walking more than 2 blocks on the level and climbing more than one flight of ordinary stairs at a normal pace and in normal conditions.
III. "Marked limitation of ordinary physical activity." Walking one to two blocks on the level and climbing one flight of stairs in normal conditions and at normal pace.
IV. "Inability to carry on any physical activity without discomfort— anginal syndrome *may* be present at rest."

* Reproduced with permission from the American Heart Association.

chest pain which occurred only after walking more than 2 level blocks at a regular pace and/or after walking up more than 1 flight of stairs. The length of a block or the number of stairs in the flight was not defined. Thus, patients with effort angina when walking less than 2 level blocks or less than 1 flight of stairs were excluded from the CASS randomized study.

To understand the terms angiographically *normal* coronary arteries and *minimal* and *moderate* CAD, it is essential to be familiar with the Judkins angiographic terminology for coronary artery anatomy (Fig. 1).[5] The definitions of "normal," "minimal" and "moderate" used in CASS comprised 3 items: (1) the degree of internal diameter reduction of a coronary artery; (2) the distribution of the narrowings in the 27 angiographic coronary segments (Fig. 1); and (3) knowledge regarding coronary dominance (right, left, balanced or unknown). Angiographically "normal," for example, with a right-dominant, balanced or unknown dominant circulation required "0 stenosis" in 22 of the 27 coronary segments and with a left-dominant circulation, in 21 of the 27 coronary segments. "Minimal" CAD was defined as $<50\%$ diameter reduction of a major coronary segment or "$<70\%$ stenosis" of a minor segment or "$<30\%$ stenosis" of the left main coronary artery. "Moderate" CAD was defined as "50–69% stenosis" in 1 or more of 14 major coronary segments or "$>69\%$ stenosis" in segments 5 to 10 or 17 or a 30 to 49% narrowing in segment 11 for a right dominant, balanced or unknown dominant circulation; for a left dominant circulation, "50–69% stenosis" in 15 major segments or "$>69\%$ stenosis" in minor segment 17 or 30 to 49% narrowing in segment 11.[5]

Dominance of the coronary arteries was defined as follows: *right dominant* when the posterior descending artery arose from the right and at least 1 other branch of the right extended past the posterior descending artery into the atrioventricular groove giving off 1 or more posterolateral branches to the posterior left ventricular surface; *balanced* when the posterior descending artery arose from the right and was its terminal branch and no posterolateral branches to the posterior left ventricular surface were present; and *left dominant* when the posterior descending artery and all the posterolateral branches to the left ventricular posterior surface originated from the left circumflex artery.

The terms *proximal, middle* and *distal* for locations of coronary narrowings in the various major arteries were clearly defined only for the right and left circumflex coronary arteries. In fact, proximal, middle or distal makes no difference with the right coronary artery because its major function is to supply blood to the posterior left ventricular wall, a function not served until blood courses the entire length of the right coronary artery to enter the posterior descending branches. The proximal portion of the left circumflex coronary artery, which has no middle portion, extended from the bifurcation of the left main to and including the origin of the first obtuse marginal branch; the distal portion courses in the left atrioventricular sulcus distal to the origin of the first obtuse marginal branch. The proximal left anterior descending was that portion from the bifurcation of the left main to the origin of the first visible septal perforator; its middle and distal portions were not defined.

The term *bypassable artery* was not defined.

Left ventricular angiography was performed before coronary angiography. The volumes and ejection fractions were calculated using a single-plane adaption of the area-length method of Dodge and co-workers.[5]

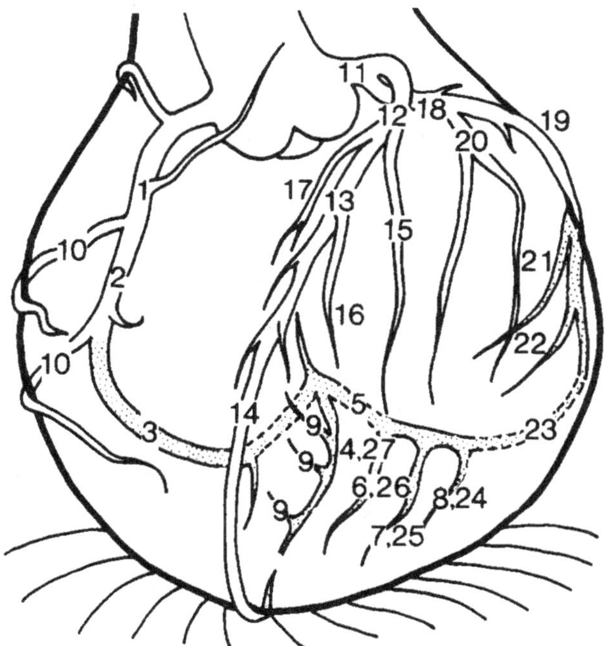

FIGURE 1. Judkins' angiographic terminology for coronary artery anatomy (reproduced with permission from the American Heart Association): (1) proximal right; (2) mid-right; (3) distal right; (4) right posterior descending; (5) right posterior lateral segment; (6) first right posterior lateral; (7) second right posterior lateral; (8) third right posterior lateral; (9) inferior septal; (10) acute marginal; (11) left main; (12) proximal left anterior descending; (13) mid-left anterior descending; (14) distal left anterior descending; (15) first diagonal; (16) second diagonal; (17) first septal; (18) proximal circumflex; (19) distal circumflex; (20) first obtuse marginal; (21) second obtuse marginal; (22) third obtuse marginal; (23) left atrioventricular; (24) first left posterior lateral; (25) second left posterior lateral; (26) third left posterior lateral; (27) left posterior descending.

The patients were analyzed according to the patient's original randomized group ("intention-to-treat" principle), irrespective of what type of treatment was given thereafter. Patients randomized to the surgical group but who did not have CABG were included in the "surgical group." Of the 390 patients assigned to the surgical group, 41 (11%) initially refused surgery, although 10 of them subsequently had CABG a mean of 2.5 years after randomization. Patients randomized to the "medical group" but who later had CABG were included in the "medical group." Of the 390 patients randomized to the medical group, 100 (26%) subsequently had CABG. Although the noncompliance to treatment assignment might appear to bias the results against CABG,[9] analysis of CASS mortality data by treatment received and by means of censoring at the time of crossover did not change the results.[3,10]

Thus, the patients included in the CASS randomized study had mild or absent symptoms of myocardial ischemia but severe ($\geq$70% diameter reduction) fixed narrowing of at least 1 major coronary artery. The degree of coronary narrowing of the right, left anterior descending or left circumflex coronary arteries for inclusion in the randomized study was severe ($\geq$70% diameter reduction), which corresponds roughly to a 91% cross-sectional area narrowing (Fig. 2). A 50% diameter reduction, which corresponds to a 75% cross-sectional area narrowing, was not sufficiently severe to warrant inclusion of the patient in the randomized study. Patients with narrowing of the left main coronary artery up to 69% in diameter were included in the randomized study. Of the many studies in the 1970s pointing out the danger of severe narrowing of the left main coronary artery, most defined "severe" as >50% diameter reduction.[11] It is remarkable how well the CASS patients randomized to medicine did in light of their severe degrees of coronary narrowing.

It might be useful to mention a few examples of patients to whom the CASS randomized data do not apply: (1) To the patient asymptomatic after healing of AMI who has never had a coronary angiogram. (2) To the patient with mild angina who has never had a coronary angiogram. (3) To the patient with mild stable angina or asymptomatic state after healing of AMI who is found to have >70% diameter reduction of the left main coronary artery by angiogram, or such extensive distal narrowing that insertion of grafts would not likely be successful. (4) To the patient admitted to the hospital (to rule out AMI) after his first episode of angina. Despite severe coronary narrowing by angiography, this patient would not be included in the CASS randomized study, which includes stable angina patients only. (5) To the asymptomatic patient who had never had chest pain but who has a positive exercise stress test, whether or not a coronary angiogram has been performed. (6) To the patient with severe coronary narrowing by angiogram but whose only clinical manifestation of CAD is an arrhythmia or congestive heart failure.

Although the CASS protocol specifically excludes patients with *unstable* angina, this exclusion has to do with how "unstable" is defined and at what time the

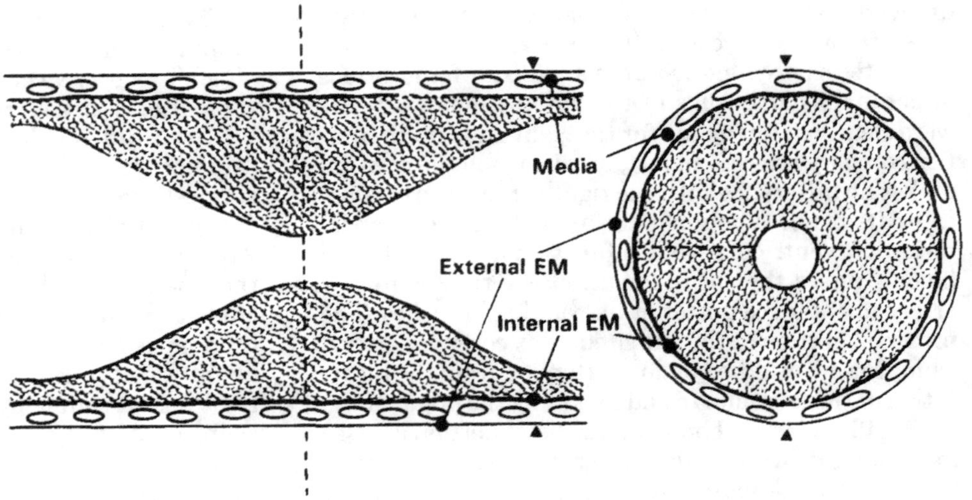

FIGURE 2. Diagrams showing a 70% diameter reduction (**left**), which corresponds to a 91% cross-sectional area narrowing (**right**).

instability occurred. If *initial* angina is included in the definition of unstable, then most of the CASS patients had unstable angina at some time. Furthermore, a patient with stable angina may have transient periods of unstable angina. If the later resolves either spontaneously or as a result of medical therapy and the patient has only mild stable angina 60 days before randomization, the patient would be eligible for randomization if the coronary and left ventricular angiographic requirements were fulfilled. Thus, it is the status of symptoms of myocardial ischemia 60 days before randomization (which virtually corresponds to the time of cardiac catheterization) that determined the patient's symptomatic status. (Incidentally, the fact that randomization was based on symptomatic status 60 days earlier was not mentioned in any of the CASS publications, only in the Manual of Operation.)

Despite the enormous amount of information thus far provided by the $24 million CASS, utilization of its results will not be easy. CASS implies that the patient who has mild angina pectoris or who is asymptomatic after healing of AMI does not need CABG (or possibly percutaneous transluminal coronary angioplasty), at least at the present time. Because coronary bypass or dilatation is unnecessary in this asymptomatic or mildly symptomatic state, justification for angiography to determine the status of the coronary arteries and left ventricle is lacking. But if angiography is not performed, the data acquired in CASS are really not applicable. If angiography is performed in the asymptomatic or mildly symptomatic patient, the finding of $\geq 70\%$ diameter reduction in 2 or more major (excluding left main) coronary arteries may result, in probably many medical centers, in the performance of coronary bypass or dilatation. The major worry in avoiding the performance of cardiac catheterization would be the missing of severe ($\geq 70\%$ diameter reduction) narrowing of the left main

coronary artery. But severe left main narrowing was found in only 4.3% of the more than 16,000 subjects screened for randomization. Therefore, it appears most reasonable, in light of CASS, *not* to perform coronary angiography in the patient who has mild angina (with or without previous AMI which healed) or is asymptomatic after healing of AMI. When symptoms of myocardial ischemia appear or worsen, coronary (and left ventricular) angiography can then be performed with coronary dilatation and/or bypass thereafter if appropriate. A major implication of CASS, therefore, is to avoid the performance of coronary (and left ventricular) angiography until symptoms of myocardial ischemia become moderate or severe (as opposed to absent or mild) despite medical therapy.

References

1. CASS Principal Investigators and their Associates. Coronary Artery Surgery Study (CASS): a randomized trial of coronary artery bypass surgery. Survival data. Circulation 1983;68:939–950.
2. CASS Principal Investigators and their Associates. Coronary Artery Surgery Study (CASS): a randomized trial of coronary artery bypass surgery. Quality of life in patients randomly assigned to treatment groups. Circulation 1983;68:951–960.
3. CASS Principal Investigators and their Associates. Coronary Artery Surgery Study: Myocardial infarction and mortality in the coronary artery surgery study (CASS) randomized trial. N Engl J Med 1984; 310:750–757.
4. CASS Principal Investigators and their Associates. Coronary Artery Surgery Study (CASS): a randomized trial of coronary bypass surgery. Comparability of entry characteristics and survival in randomized patients and nonrandomized patients meeting randomization criteria. J Am Coll Cardiol 1984;3:114–128.
5. Principal Investigators of CASS and their Associates. Killip T, (ed), Fisher LD, Mock MB (eds). The National Heart, Lung, and Blood Institute Coronary Artery Surgery Study (CASS). Circulation 1981;63:suppl I:I-1–I-81.
6. Campeau L. Grading of angina pectoris. Circulation 1976;54:522–523.
7. Nomenclature and Criteria for Diagnosis of Diseases of the Heart and Great Vessels, 7th ed. Boston: Little Brown & Co, 1973:1–347.
8. Council of Cardiovascular Surgery. American Heart Association: Coronary artery disease reporting systems. Circulation 1975;51:22.
9. Weinstein GS. Coronary-artery bypass grafting (letter to the editor). N Engl J Med 1984;310:1262.
10. Braunwald E. Coronary-artery bypass grafting (reply to letter to the editor). N Engl J Med 1984;310:1263.
11. Bulkley BH, Roberts WC. Atherosclerotic narrowing of the left main coronary artery. A necropsy analysis of 152 patients with fatal coronary heart disease and varying degrees of left main narrowing. Circulation 1976;53:823–828.

Comparison at necropsy by age group of amount and distribution of narrowing by atherosclerotic plaque in 2995 five-mm long segments of 240 major coronary arteries in 60 men aged 31 to 70 years with sudden coronary death

A comparison of the amount and distribution of coronary arterial narrowing by atherosclerotic plaque at necropsy is described in each of four decades (31 to 70 years) of 60 male victims of sudden coronary death (SCD). Of 2995 five-mm segments examined (mean 50 per patient) of the four major (left main [LM], left anterior descending [LAD], left circumflex [LC], and right) coronary arteries, no significant differences were observed in the mean percent of 5 mm long segments narrowed severely (76% to 100% in cross-sectional area [XSA]) in each decade: 33% in the five patients aged 31 to 40 years, 29% in the 27 patients aged 41 to 50 years, 26% in the 18 patients aged 51 to 60 years, and 30% in the 10 patients aged 61 to 70 years. The mean percent of 5 mm segments severely narrowed was significantly ($p < 0.05$) greater in the proximal halves than in the distal halves of the LAD, LC, and right coronary arteries in only the two older decades. The mean percent of 5 mm segments minimally (0% to 25%) narrowed, however, was significantly higher in the younger than in the older decades. Thus, as groups, both young and old victims of SCD have similar amounts of severe coronary narrowing, but the younger victims have a greater proportion of their major coronary arteries minimally narrowed. (Am Heart J 108:431, 1984.)

Carole A. Warnes, M.B., B.S., M.R.C.P., and William C. Roberts, M.D. *Bethesda, Md.*

Although it is recognized that patients who die suddenly from atherosclerotic coronary heart disease (CAD) have considerable narrowing of ≥ 1 major epicardial coronary arteries, no information is available on the amount and distribution of atherosclerotic plaques in different age groups of victims of sudden coronary death (SCD). To fill this void, the amount and distribution of cross-sectional area (XSA) luminal narrowing in each 5 mm segment of the four major coronary arteries was determined in 60 male victims of SCD.

From the Pathology Branch, National Heart, Lung, and Blood Institute, National Institutes of Health.

Received for publication Feb. 6, 1984; accepted March 1, 1984.

Reprint requests: Either Carole A. Warnes, M.B., B.S., M.R.C.P., or William C. Roberts, M.D., Bldg. 10A, Room 3E-30, NIH, Bethesda, MD 20205.

METHODS

Patients. Only men fulfilling all the following criteria were included in this study. (1) Death was known to occur within ≤ 6 *hours* of the previously witnessed usual state of health. (2) Although the patient may have died in a hospital, the individual was not a patient in a hospital at the onset of symptoms suggestive of myocardial ischemia. (3) At necropsy, ≥ 1 of the four major (left main [LM], left anterior descending [LAD], left circumflex [LC], and right) coronary arteries was narrowed 76% to 100% in XSA. (4) Ventricular myocardial coagulation necrosis was absent at necropsy. (5) A cause of death (cardiac or noncardiac) other than CAD was absent. (6) Chronic congestive heart failure had never been present. (7) A cardiovascular operation had never been performed. Review of clinical and necropsy records in the Pathology Branch, National Heart, Lung and Blood Institute, yielded 60 men, aged 32 to 67 years (mean 51), fulfilling these criteria (Fig. 1). Eleven of the 60 men were included in an earlier study from our laboratory.[1]

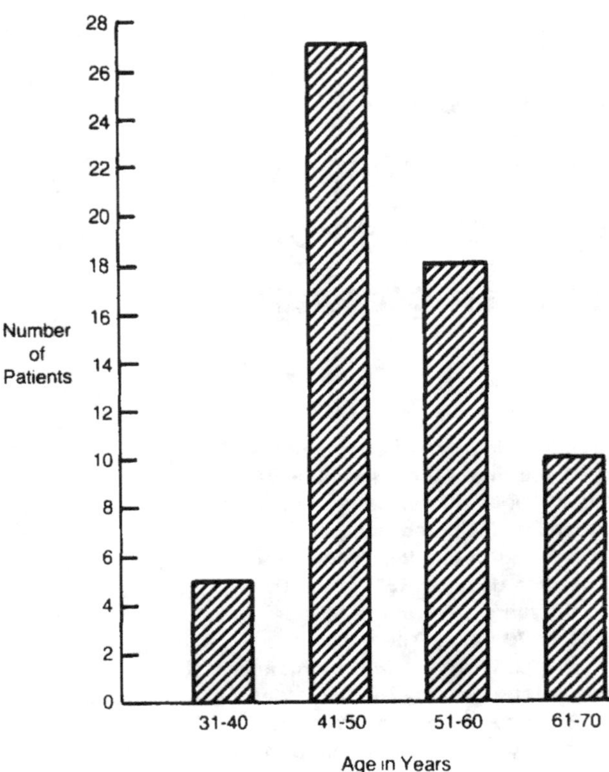

Fig. 1. Age distribution in the 60 men with sudden coronary death.

Of the 60 men, 37 died outside the hospital. The other 23 had onset of chest pain outside the hospital and had fatal cardiac arrest shortly after being brought to the hospital. In 31 of the 60 victims, SCD was the first manifestation of cardiac disease, and in the other 29, either a clinical acute myocardial infarction, which healed, and/or angina pectoris had occurred previously.

Necropsy. The hearts were fixed $\geq$ 24 hours in formalin. The four major coronary arteries were then excised intact, x-rayed, and decalcified if necessary. Each artery was then cut transversely into 5 mm segments and labelled sequentially, either from the aortic ostium, or from its origin from the LM coronary artery. The segments were then dehydrated with alcohol and xylene, embedded in paraffin, and at least two histologic sections were cut from the paraffin block. Each histologic section was stained by the Movat technique.[2] The amount of luminal narrowing by atherosclerotic plaque was determined by visual inspection of these histologic sections when magnified 25 to 50 times. The percent of XSA narrowing of each 5 mm segment was categorized into five groups: 0% to 25%, 26% to 50%, 51% to 75%, 76% to 95% and 96% to 100%. All sections were examined by one of us (C.W.), and the accuracy of the assessment of luminal narrowing was spot-checked by video-planimetry. The agreement between these two techniques is approximately 95%.[3] A total of 2995 five-mm segments from the 60 men were examined (mean number of segments per patient = 50). The absence of myocardial coagulation necrosis was confirmed by histologic examination. Chi square analysis was utilized for comparison of amounts of coronary narrowing by quantitative means.

RESULTS

Extent of stenoses. The mean percentages of 5 mm segments narrowed to varying degrees of XSA in the different age groups are shown in Fig. 2. No significant differences in the mean percent of segments narrowed 76% to 100% in XSA were observed in the four decades examined: 33% of segments in the 31 to 40 decade, 29% in the 41 to 50 decade, 26% in the 51 to 60 decade, and 30% in the 61 to 70 year decade. In each patient the number of the four major coronary arteries which had at least one 5 mm segment narrowed 76% to 100% in XSA is shown in Table I.

A scoring system was utilized to indicate numerically both the severity and extent of coronary narrowing. Every 5 mm segment of coronary artery from each patient was assigned a score from 1 to 5, based on the amount of XSA narrowing by plaque— i.e., 1 = 0% to 25% narrowing, 2 = 26% to 50%, 3 = 51% to 75%, 4 = 76% to 95%, and 5 = 96% to 100% narrowing. A total score was obtained for each patient, and the score per 5 mm segment was calculated by dividing the total score per patient by the number of 5 mm segments from that patient. Of the 2995 segments in the 60 patients, 156 segments (5%) were narrowed 96% to 100% in XSA (score = 780); 694 (23%) were narrowed 76% to 95% (score = 2,776); 995 (33%) were narrowed 51% to 75% (score = 2985); 604 (20%) were narrowed 26% to 50% (score = 1208); and 546 (18%) were narrowed 0% to 25% (score = 546). Thus, the *total score* for all 60 patients and the 2995 coronary 5 mm segments was 8295; the score per patient was 138, and the mean score per patient was 2.8, indicating that each of the 2995 segments was narrowed on an average between 26% to 75% in XSA. The mean coronary score per patient was 2.7 in the 31 to 40 decade, 2.7 in the 41 to 50 decade, 2.8 in the 51 to 60 decade, and 2.8 in the 61 to 70 decade, again demonstrating no increase in extent or severity of coronary narrowing with advancing age.

Proximal vs distal stenoses. In each age group, the sum of the mean percents of 5 mm segments narrowed 76% to 100% in XSA was higher in the proximal halves of the right, LAD, and LC arteries than the sum of the mean percents in the distal halves, but this difference was significant only in the 51 to 60 and 61 to 70 decades ($p < 0.0005$ and

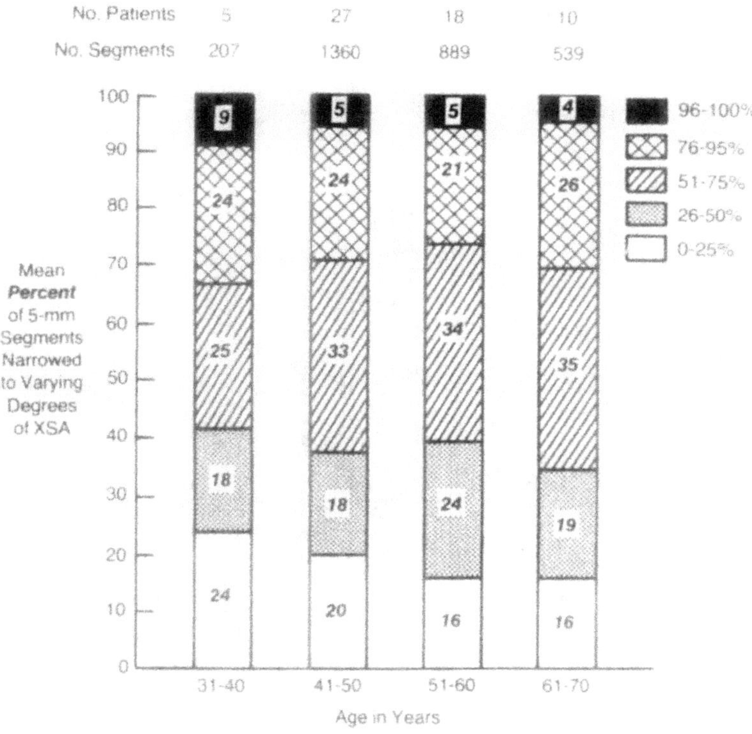

Fig. 2. Relation of age to the mean percent of 5 mm segments narrowed to varying degrees in 60 men with sudden coronary death.

Table I. Number of four major (left main, left anterior descending, left circumflex, and right) coronary arteries narrowed *at some point* 76% to 100% in cross-sectional area by atherosclerotic plaque in 60 men with sudden coronary death

Age (yr) decade	Number patients	Number of 4 coronary arteries per patient narrowed 76%-100% in XSA by plaque				
		4	3	2	1	(Mean)
31-40	5	0	3	0	2	(2.2)
41-50	27	5	11	6	5	(2.6)
51-60	18	1	9	8	0	(2.6)
61-70	10	1	7	1	1	(2.8)
Totals	60	7	30	15	8	(2.6)
		(12%)	(50%)	(25%)	(13%)	

XSA = cross-sectional area.

<0.005) (Fig. 3). In the distal halves of these three major coronary arteries the mean percent of segments narrowed 76% to 100% in XSA was similar in all four age decades and did not tend to increase with advancing age (correlation coefficient, $R = 0.06$). In the category of minimal XSA narrowing (0% to 25%), age-related differences were apparent. In the decade 31 to 40 years, a mean of 24% of 5 mm segments were narrowed 0% to 25%, and in the two older decades (51 to 60 and 61 to 70), only 16% of the segments had minimal (0% to 25%) luminal narrowing.

DISCUSSION

Stenoses related to age. Analysis of the amount and distribution of narrowing by atherosclerotic plaque in the four major coronary arteries in our 60 patients with SCD disclosed (1) similar degrees of severe (76% to 100% in XSA) narrowing by atherosclerotic plaque in all four decades studied (aged 41 to 70 years); (2) similar amounts of severe narrowing in the proximal halves of the right, LAD, and LC coronary arteries in all four decades and smaller but similar amounts of severe narrowing in the distal halves of these three arteries in each of the four

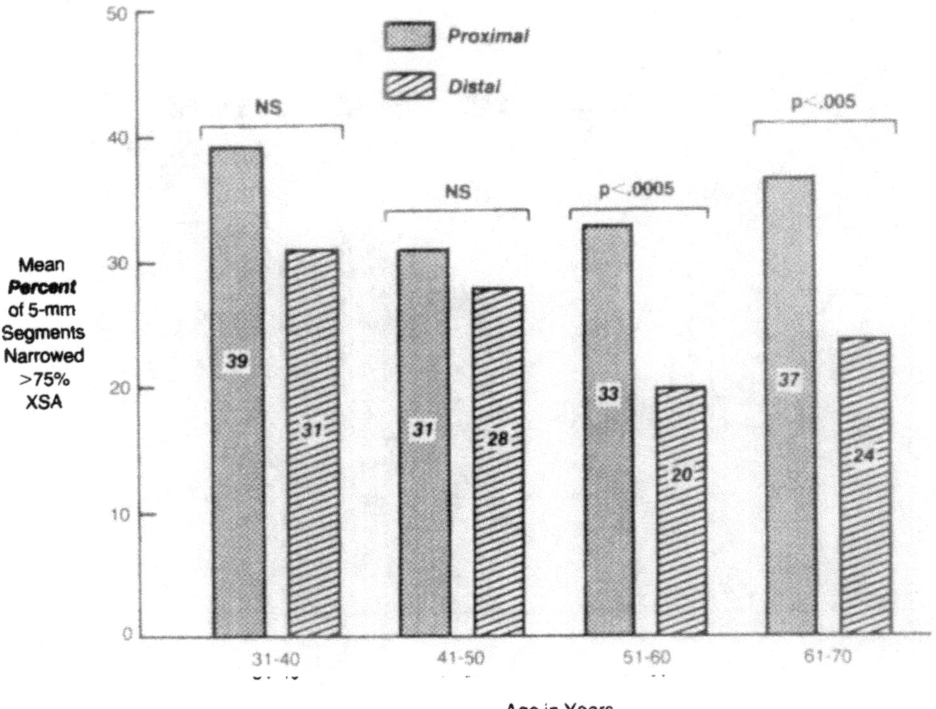

Fig. 3. Relation of age to the amount of 76% to 100% cross-sectional area *(XSA)* narrowing in the proximal and distal halves of the three major coronary arteries in 60 men with sudden coronary death.

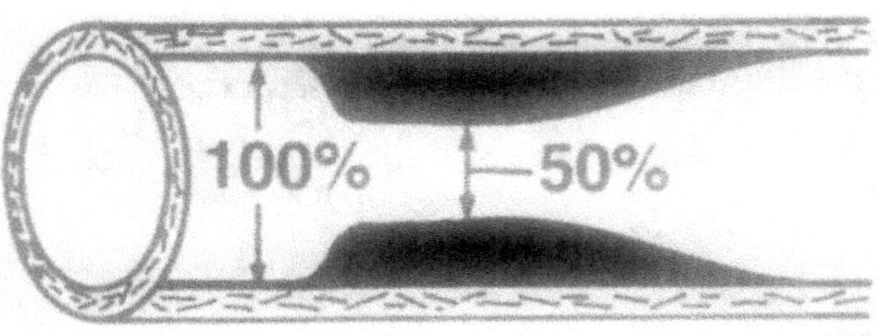

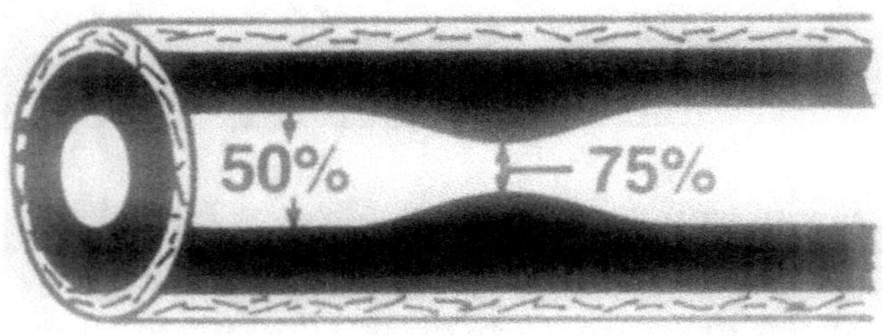

Fig. 4. Diagramatic representation of an angiographic view of two coronary arteries which have luminal plaque. Because the angiogram is a luminogram, and the width of the original arterial lumen is unknown, the least-narrowed segment is often presumed to be normal. Comparison of a narrowed segment to a near-normal segment *(upper)* is more likely to occur in the younger patients, whereas comparison of a severe narrowing to a less severe narrowing, which may be considered "normal" angiographically *(lower)*, is more likely in the older patients. This situation leads to an underestimation of the degree of stenosis in older patients.

decades; and (3) a higher proportion of near normal segments of the four major coronary arteries in the younger patients compared to the older ones.

Mean vs range of stenoses. Although the mean percent of 5 mm long segments narrowed 76% to 100% in XSA in all 60 patients in all four decades varied little (from 26% to 33%), the percent of segments severely narrowed per patient varied enormously, from 2% (1 of 50) to 88% (86 of 98). Twelve patients had ≤10% of their 5 mm segments narrowed 76% to 100% in XSA, 19 patients had 11% to 25% of segments so narrowed, 24 patients had 26% to 50% of the segments so narrowed, and only five patients had >50% of their segments so narrowed. Thus, the *extent* of severe coronary narrowing in SCD may be either minimal or spectacularly severe, and is unpredictable in the individual patient.

Distal segments. Because distal narrowing was no more severe in the older age groups, coronary arterial bypass grafting should be technically as feasible in the older as in the younger age groups, assuming similar left ventricular function. Although this study provides information about the amount and extent of narrowing in the distal portion of all three major arteries, conduits are rarely inserted into the LC coronary artery—the obtuse marginal branch is usually used—and conduits are often inserted into the posterior descending branch, rather than directly into the right coronary artery.

Normal segments. As might be anticipated, segments minimally narrowed (0% to 25% in XSA) were more frequent in the younger age groups. When extrapolated to angiographic assessment of coronary stenosis, this observation may have important implications. Such an assessment is usually made by visual comparison of the reduction in diameter of a portion of coronary artery (when filled with contrast medium) compared to an adjacent segment of coronary tree considered to be "normal." Even in patients 31 to 40 years old, however, a mean of 76% of the four major coronary arteries were narrowed >25% in XSA, and so not many truly "normal" segments would have been available for comparison to the more severely narrowed segments. In patients >50 years old, a mean of 84% of the four major coronary arteries were narrowed >25% in XSA, and so even fewer "normal" segments would have been available for comparison, and therefore the chance of underestimating a severe stenosis would have been greater in the older than in the younger age groups (Fig. 4).

Conclusions. This study emphasizes the diffuse nature of the atherosclerotic process in all age groups since, on average, 28% of the entire 25 cm length of the four major coronary arteries in each patient was narrowed 76% to 100% in XSA by atherosclerotic plaque. No previous studies have examined the extent of coronary luminal narrowing in relation to age.

REFERENCES

1. Roberts WC, Jones AA: Quantitation of coronary arterial narrowing at necropsy in sudden coronary death. Analysis of 31 patients and comparison with 25 control subjects. Am J Cardiol **44**:39, 1979.
2. Movat HZ: Demonstration of all connective tissue elements in a single section: Pentachrome stains. Arch Pathol **60**:289, 1955.
3. Isner JM, Wu M, Virmani R, Jones AA, Roberts WC: Comparison of degrees of coronary arterial luminal narrowing determined by visual inspection of histologic sections under magnification among three independent observers and comparison to that obtained by videoplanimetry. Lab Invest **42**:566, 1980.

Sudden Coronary Death: Comparison of Patients With to Those Without Coronary Thrombus at Necropsy

CAROLE A. WARNES, MB, BS, MRCP, and WILLIAM C. ROBERTS, MD

Among 70 victims of sudden coronary death (SCD), certain clinical and morphologic findings in the 13 with a coronary thrombus are compared with the findings in 57 victims without a coronary thrombus. The 13 with a thrombus were younger than those without (mean age 43 vs 51 years, p <0.02); had a lower mean percent of cross-sectional area (XSA) narrowing by plaque at the site of maximal coronary stenosis (89% vs 95%, p <0.01); and had a higher mean percent of 5-mm segments of the 4 major epicardial coronary arteries minimally narrowed (0 to 25% in XSA) by plaque (27% vs 19%, p <0.001). No differences occurred in the 2 groups with regard to sex, previous angina pectoris or clinical acute myocardial infarction, healed myocardial infarction at necropsy, mean heart weight, number of major coronary arteries narrowed 76 to 100% in XSA by atherosclerotic plaque, or the mean percent of 5-mm segments of the 4 major epicardial coronary arteries narrowed 76 to 100% in XSA by atherosclerotic plaque. Thus, coronary thrombi are infrequent in victims of SCD, and when observed, their significance is uncertain because victims of SCD without coronary thrombi have similar amounts of severe coronary narrowing.

(Am J Cardiol 1984;54:1206–1211)

Most necropsy studies of victims of sudden death resulting from atherosclerotic coronary heart disease (hereafter called "sudden coronary death" [SCD]) have disclosed a relatively low frequency of coronary thrombus (Table I). We recently reported necropsy findings in 70 victims of SCD, but the frequency and significance of coronary thrombus was not examined.[1] In this study of victims of SCD, we compare 13 patients with to 57 patients without coronary thrombus, a comparison not reported previously, and we describe the composition of the thrombi and their contribution to luminal narrowing.

Definitions

Sudden coronary death, for purposes of this study, was defined according to the following criteria: (1) Death known to occur within 6 hours of previously witnessed usual state of health. (2) Although the patient may have died in a hospital, he/she was not a patient in a hospital at the onset of symptoms suggestive of myocardial ischemia. (3) At necropsy, at least 1 of the 4 major (left main [LM], left anterior descending [LAD], left circumflex [LC] and right) epicardial coronary arteries was narrowed 76 to 100% in cross-sectional area (XSA) by atherosclerotic plaque. (4) Ventricular myocardial coagulation necrosis was absent at necropsy. (5) A cause of death, cardiac or noncardiac, other than coronary artery disease was absent. (6) Chronic congestive heart failure had never been present. (7) A cardiovascular operation had never been performed.

Thrombus was defined as a collection of fibrin or platelets or both, with or without associated erythrocytes and leukocytes, within the residual lumen, with the collection attached at some point to the luminal surface. An *occlusive thrombus* was defined as one that occupied the entire or nearly (>90% XSA) the entire lumen that was not occupied by atherosclerotic plaque, and a *nonocclusive (mural) thrombus* as one that occupied only a portion of the residual lumen.

Methods

In all 70 patients, the 4 major coronary arteries were excised intact, x-rayed and, if necessary, decalcified. Each artery was then cut transversely into 5-mm segments. The segments were dehydrated with alcohol and xylene, embedded in paraffin, and at least 1 histologic section was cut from the paraffin block and was stained by the Movat technique.[2] The amount of luminal narrowing by atherosclerotic plaque was determined by visual inspection of these histologic sections when magnified 25 to 50 times. The percent of XSA narrowing of each 5-mm segment was categorized into 5 groups: 0 to 25, 26 to 50, 51 to 75, 76 to 95 and 96 to 100. All sections were examined by 1 of us (CAW) and the accuracy of the assessment of luminal narrowing was spot-checked by videoplanimetry; the agreement between these 2 techniques is approximately 95%.[3] A total of 3,484 five-millimeter segments from the 70 victims were examined (mean 50 segments per patient). By video-

From the Pathology Branch, National Heart, Lung, and Blood Institute, National Institutes of Health, Bethesda, Maryland. Dr. Warnes' present address: National Heart Hospital, Westmoreland Street, London W1 England. Manuscript received and accepted August 3, 1984.

Address for reprints: William C. Roberts, MD, Chief, Pathology Branch, National Heart, Lung, and Blood Institute, National Institutes of Health, Building 10A, Room 3E30, Bethesda, Maryland 20205.

TABLE I Comparison of Clinical and Morphologic Observations Between 13 Victims of Sudden Coronary Death With a Coronary Thrombus at Necropsy and 57 Victims Without a Thrombus

Coronary Thrombus	+ 13 Pts.	0 57 Pts.	p Value
Mean age (years)	43	51	<0.02
Men:women	12:1	45:6	NS
Previous MI and/or AP	6(46%)	25(44%)	NS
Healed MI	4(31%)	27(47%)	NS
Mean heart weight (g)	430	483	NS
No. (%) CAs narrowed 76–100% in XSA by plaque			
1	4(31%)	7(12%)	NS
2	3(23%)	16(28%)	NS
3	3(23%)	30(53%)	NS
4	3(23%)	4(7%)	NS
No. (%) of 4 major CAs narrowed 76–100% in XSA by plaque/ total no. of 4 major CAs	31/52 (60%)	145/228 (64%)	NS
Mean percent of XSA narrowing by plaque at site of maximal stenosis	89%	95%	<0.01
Percent of 5-mm segments of 4 major CAs narrowed in XSA by plaque:			
0–25%	27%	19%	<0.001
76–100%	27%	27%	NS

AP = angina pectoris; CA = coronary artery; MI = myocardial infarction; NS = not significant; XSA = cross-sectional area; + = thrombus; 0 = thrombus absent.

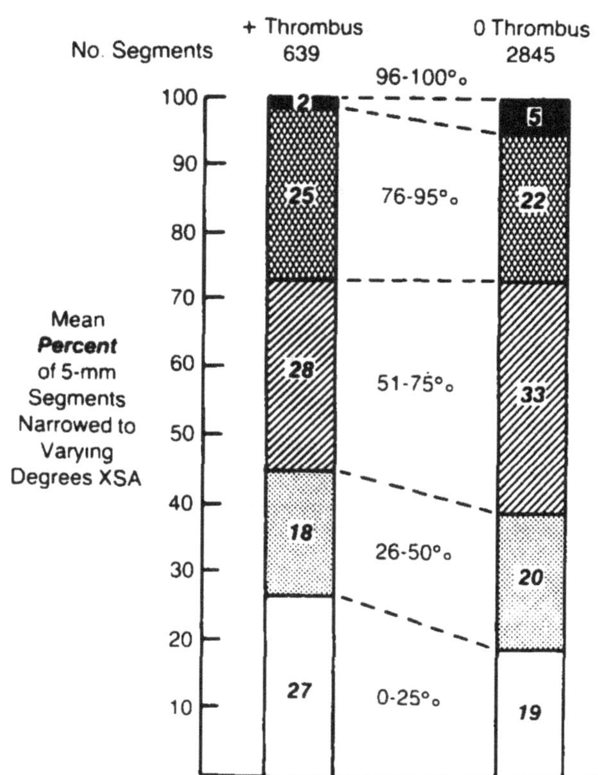

FIGURE 1. Mean percents of 5-mm segments of the 4 major coronary arteries narrowed to varying degrees in cross-sectional area (XSA) in the 13 patients with and in the 57 patients without coronary artery thrombus.

planimetry,[4] the amount of XSA narrowing by plaque was determined in the 5-mm segments containing the thrombus and in the 5-mm segment of any of the 4 major coronary arteries, which contained the most severe stenosis by plaque. In 12 of the 13 patients with coronary thrombus, each paraffin block that contained the 5-mm segment that contained thrombus was sectioned at 6-μ intervals, and every tenth section was stained by the Movat technique. In addition, 3 or more histologic sections extending from endocardium to epicardium were prepared from the wall of the left ventricle of each patient, and each section was stained with hematoxylin-eosin. Absence of myocardial coagulation necrosis in each patient was confirmed by histologic examination.

Statistics: Chi-square analysis was used to compare amounts of coronary narrowing in patients with and those without thrombi. A Student t test was used for all other comparisons between the patients with and those without coronary thrombi.

Results

Certain observations in the 70 patients—13 with and 57 patients without thrombus—are summarized in Table I.

Three significant differences in patients with and without thrombus: The mean ages, the mean percents of 5-mm segments narrowed 0 to 25% in XSA by atherosclerotic plaque, and the mean percents of XSA narrowing at sites of maximal stenosis by plaque were significantly (p <0.05) different between the 2 groups.

Quantitative comparison of amounts of XSA narrowing by plaque: Of the 639 five-millimeter segments from the 13 patients with thrombus, and of the 2,845 five-millimeter segments from the 57 patients without thrombus, similar mean percents of segments in each group were narrowed 76 to 100%, but a significantly higher mean percent of segments were minimally (0 to 25%) narrowed in the 13 patients with thrombi compared to the 57 patients without (Fig. 1).

Comparison of maximal XSA stenosis by plaque: The amount of XSA narrowing by plaque alone in the 5-mm segment that had the most severe stenosis of any of the 4 major coronary arteries in the 13 patients with coronary thrombus and in the 57 patients without thrombus is shown in Figure 2. Cross-sectional area narrowing of more than 85% by plaque occurred in 1 or more of the 4 major coronary arteries in 9 of the 13 patients (69%) with thrombus and in 53 of the 57 patients (93%) without thrombus. The maximal XSA narrowing by plaque was 98% or greater in only 1 of the 13 patients with thrombus and in 27 of the 57 patients (47%) without thrombus. The mean percent of XSA narrowing by plaque at the site of maximal stenosis was 89% (range 76 to 99) in the 13 patients with thrombus and 95% (range 79 to 100) in the 57 patients without (p <0.01) (Fig. 3).

General characteristics of the 13 patients with coronary thrombi: The general characteristics are summarized in Table II.

Number of coronary arteries containing thrombi and which artery involved: Thrombus (occlusive in 11, mural in 2) involved only 1 of the 4 major epicardial coronary arteries in all 13 patients: LAD in 6, LC in 5, LM in 1 and right in 1.

Location of thrombus within a coronary artery: In 12 of the 13 patients, the thrombus was located en-

TABLE II Clinical and Morphologic Observations in Sudden Coronary Death Victims in Whom a Coronary Thrombus Was Found at Necropsy

Pt	Age (yr) & Sex	Previous AMI and/or AP	Maximal Duration of Symptoms	No. 4 Major CAs Narrowed 76–100% in XSA	CA Containing Thrombus	Percent XSA Narrowing by Plaque at Site of Thrombus	Percent XSA Narrowing by Thrombus	Composition of Thrombus (0–3+)			
								P	F	E	L
1	22F	0	<1 hr	1	LM	79	21	+++	0	+	0
2	22M	0	<1 hr	1	LAD	70	30	+++	+	+	+
3	25M	0	<2 hr	3	LC	74	26	+++	0	+	0
4	32M	0	<2 hr	1	LAD	76	24	+++	+	++	0
5	44M	+	<6 hr	4	R	93	7	+	++	+++	0
6	45M	0	<4 hr	4	LC	80	20	+++	0	0	0
7	46M	0	<10 min	2	LC	95	5	+++	0	+	+
8	47M	+	<10 min	3	LAD	91	9	+	+++	+++	0
9	48M	0	<1 hr	1	LAD	75	25	+++	0	+	0
10	51M	+	<1 hr	2	LC	74	26	+	+++	++	0
11	56M	+	<1 hr	3	LC	62	12	0	+++	++	0
12	58M	+	<6 hr	2	LAD	95	5	0	+++	++	0
13	62M	+	<10 min	4	LAD	77	7	+	+++	+	0

AMI = acute myocardial infarction; AP = angina pectoris; CA = coronary artery; E = erythrocytes; F = fibrin; L = leukocytes; P = platelets; XSA = cross-sectional area; + = present; 0 = absent.

tirely in the proximal half of the coronary artery, including 8 in which the thrombus was located in the first 1-cm portion of the artery. In 1 patient thrombus was present only in the distal half of a coronary artery (the right).

Length of coronary thrombus: In 12 patients the thrombus was at least 5 mm long and in 1 patient, 6 to 10 mm long.

Amounts of luminal narrowing at site of thrombus: In all 13 patients, the thrombus occurred at a site already narrowed more than 50% in XSA by plaque: in 5 patients, 51 to 75%, and in 8 patients, 76 to 95%. The precise amount of XSA narrowing by atherosclerotic plaque at the site of thrombus in each of the 13 patients was determined by videoplanimetry and is shown in Table II. In the 11 patients with occlusive thrombi, the percent of XSA narrowing by plaque at the site of thrombus ranged from 70 to 95% (mean 82) and the percent of XSA narrowing by thrombus ranged from 5 to 30% (mean 18). In the 2 patients with nonocclusive thrombi (patients 11 and 13), the percent of XSA narrowing by plaque at the site of thrombus was 62% and 77%, respectively, and the percent of XSA narrowing by thrombus was 12% and 7%, respectively (mean 10) (Fig. 4).

Relation of coronary thrombus to site of maximal coronary narrowing by plaque alone: The thrombus occurred at the site of maximal narrowing by plaque (of any of the 4 major coronary arteries) in 5 patients. In the other 8 patients, the thrombus occurred at the site other than that which had the most severe stenosis by plaque: in 5, the site of maximal stenosis by plaque occurred in the same coronary artery, and in the remaining 3 patients the site of maximal stenosis by plaque occurred in a different artery.

Composition of coronary thrombus: In 12 patients with thrombi, the paraffin block containing the 5-mm segment with thrombus was serially sectioned and 9 to

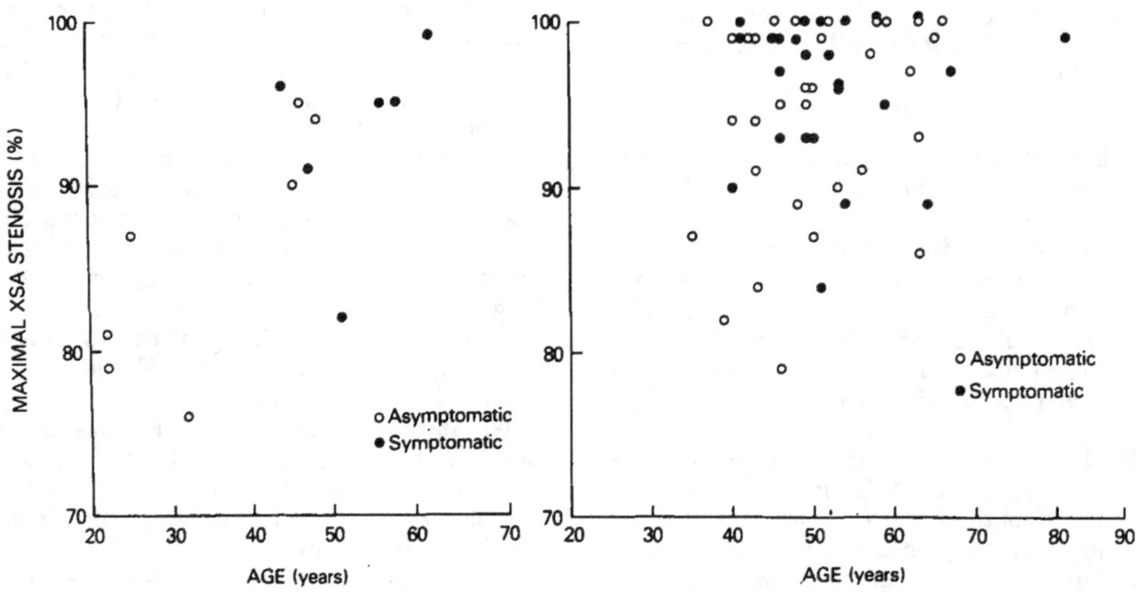

FIGURE 2. Relation of age to the maximal cross-sectional area (XSA) coronary artery narrowing by atherosclerotic plaque alone in the 13 patients with (**left**) and in the 57 patients without (**right**) coronary thrombus.

TABLE III   Frequency of Recent Coronary Thrombus in Sudden Coronary Death

First Author	Year of Publication	Interval Onset Symptoms to Death	Age range (years) (mean)	Interval of Cross Sectioning of CAs (mm)	Histology of CAs	No. of Pts.	Thrombus (%) in Extramural CA	Acute Myocardial Infarction (%)
Lie[5]	1975	<6 hr	(59)	3	+	120	17	33
Spain[6]	1970	<1 hr	—	3	+[a]	80	18	—
Friedman[7]	1973	<30 sec	<66	5	+[b]	25	4	0
		<24 hr				34	59	21
Baba[8]	1975	<24 hr	<65	1	+[c]	121	38	—
Liberthson[9]	1974	<30 min	—	1	+[d]	220	32	27
Baroldi[10]	1979	<3 hr	<20 to >70	3	+[e]	208	26	17
Haerem[11]	1974	<10 min	(64)	3	+	47	30	—
Scott[12]	1972	<1 hr	—	—[f]	—	183	45	47
Reichenbach[13]	1978	<12 hr	(63)	2[g]	+[h]	87	10	5
Rissanen[14]	1977	<24 hr	31–90	0[g]	0	141	32	26
Davies[15]	1984	<6 hr	<69	3[g]	+	100	74	—

[a] "Whenever required."
[b] With additional 200 micron step-sections.
[c] "Only if section grossly >75% narrowed."
[d] "Only if severe stenosis or acute lesions."
[e] "Sampled."
[f] Review of autopsy protocols and slides.
[g] Preceded by angiography.
[h] "From areas of interest."
CA = coronary artery; + = positive or present; 0 = negative or absent; — = no information available.

71 sections (mean 34) were stained and examined from each block. The thrombus was composed mainly of platelets in 7 patients and mainly of fibrin (with or without erythrocytes) in 6 patients. Compared to the 6 patients with predominantly fibrin thrombi, the 7 patients with predominantly platelet thrombi were younger (mean age 34 vs 53 years), and none had evidence of previous angina pectoris or acute myocardial infarction, whereas 6 of the other group did.

Composition of atherosclerotic plaque at the site of thrombus: In 9 patients the plaque consisted mainly of fibrocellular tissue, and 7 of them had disrupted fibrocellular caps at the site of thrombus. Of these 7 patients, erythrocytes were present under the surface of the plaque in 6. Small amounts of fibrin were present within the plaque in 8 patients. In 3 patients the plaque contained pultaceous debris, but in none was plaque hemorrhage observed within the pultaceous debris.

Discussion

This study discloses that the frequency of coronary arterial thrombus at necropsy in victims of SCD, in contrast to that observed in acute myocardial infarction, is low—19%. Other studies have reported higher or lower frequencies of coronary thrombi in SCD victims (Table III). Comparison of SCD studies is difficult because of differing criteria for inclusion, particularly differing definitions of *sudden* (minutes[9,11] to 24 hours[8,14]); inclusion[12] in some studies, and not in others, of patients with myocardial necrosis; differing methods of examining the coronary arteries; and differing or unstated definitions of coronary thrombus. Inclusion of patients with acute myocardial infarction, of course, among patients with SCD increases the frequency of coronary thrombus. Likewise, the longer the interval from onset of symptoms of myocardial ischemia to death, the higher the frequency of coronary thrombus.[6]

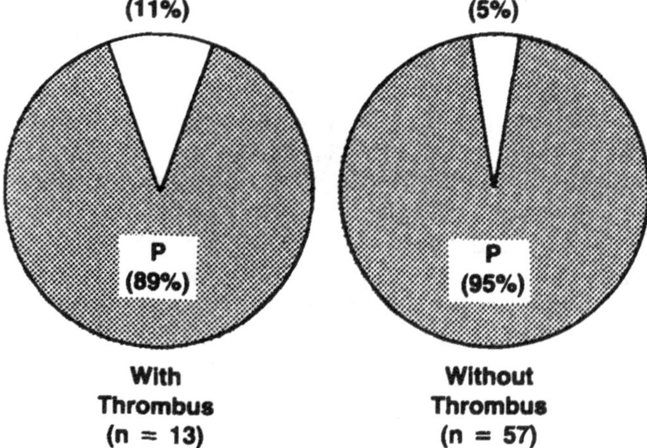

FIGURE 3. Mean amount of cross-sectional area coronary arterial narrowing at site of maximal narrowing by atherosclerotic plaque (P) alone in 70 victims of sudden coronary death, 13 with and 57 without coronary thrombus.

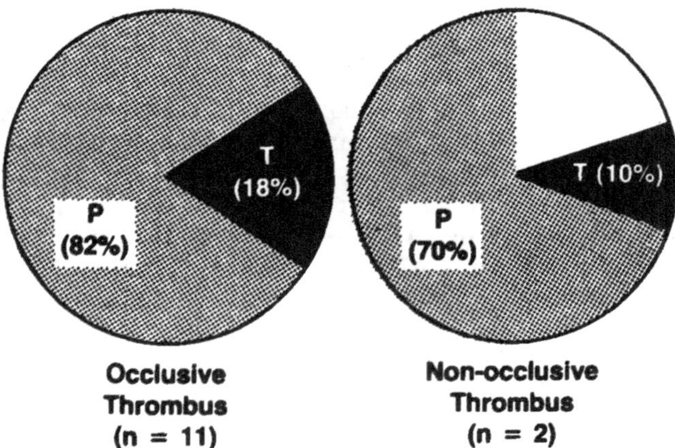

FIGURE 4. Mean amount of cross-sectional area coronary arterial luminal narrowing produced by thrombus (T) and mean amount produced by atherosclerotic plaque (P) at site of thrombus in 11 patients with occlusive thrombus and in 2 patients with nonocclusive thrombus.

Pathologists often disagree on what a thrombus is, and few studies actually provide definitions of coronary thrombus.

This study of victims of SCD is the first to compare in detail those with to those without coronary thrombus. Nine features in the 2 groups were compared: mean age; sex; presence of previous symptoms of myocardial ischemia; presence of a healed myocardial infarction at necropsy; heart weight; number of major coronary arteries narrowed 76 to 100% in XSA by atherosclerotic plaque per patient; total number of major coronary arteries (4 per patient) narrowed 76 to 100% in XSA by plaque; mean percent of XSA narrowing by plaque at the site of maximal coronary stenosis; and the mean percent of 5-mm segments of coronary artery narrowed to varying degrees.

The mean age of patients with a coronary thrombus was significantly less than that of those without (43 vs 51 years, p <0.02). A significantly greater mean percent of segments was minimally (0 to 25%) narrowed in the patients with thrombus compared to those without (27% vs 19%, p <0.001). This difference probably is the result of the younger mean age of the patients with thrombus. Our earlier study[16] had showed that younger victims of SCD, compared to older ones, had a higher mean percent of 5-mm coronary segments minimally narrowed by atherosclerotic plaque.

Although the mean percent of 5-mm segments narrowed severely (76 to 100%) in XSA by atherosclerotic plaque alone was identical in patients with and those without thrombi (27%), the mean percent of XSA narrowing by atherosclerotic plaque alone at the site of maximal coronary stenosis was smaller in those with compared to those without thrombus (89% vs 95%, p <0.01). Narrowing of more than 95% XSA by plaque was far less frequent in those with compared to those without thrombus (15% vs 60%, p <0.02). Narrowing of more than 95% XSA probably corresponds to total or near total occlusion at angiography; thus, 36 of the 70 patients (51%) probably would have had 1 or more major coronary arteries totally occluded, or nearly so, at angiography during life. Of the 13 patients with thrombus, 11 arteries containing the thrombus were totally occluded; of the 2 patients with nonocclusive thrombus, 1 had 99% XSA narrowing by plaque alone and 1 had 95% XSA narrowing by plaque alone in the same or in a different coronary artery. Thus, 12 of the 13 patients (92%) with a thrombus had near-total occlusion of 1 or more coronary arteries at some point by plaque alone, or plaque plus thrombus, compared to 34 of the 57 (60%) without thrombus.

The major coronary artery containing the thrombus also was determined. Of our 13 patients, the thrombus was located in the LAD in 6, in the LC in 5, the LM in 1 and the right coronary artery in 1. The artery containing the thrombus also was reported in 3 other studies.[7,8,15] Friedman et al[7] described coronary thrombus in 20 (of 34) victims of SCD; the thrombus was in the LAD in 10 (50%), in the LC in 2 (10%), LM in 1 (5%) and right coronary artery in 7 (35%). Baba et al[8] described "acute" coronary thrombus in 46 (of 121)

victims of SCD; the thrombus was in the LAD in 16 (35%), LC in 8 (17%), LM in 3 (7%), and right coronary artery in 19 (41%). Davies and Thomas[15] found coronary thrombus in 74 (of 100) victims of SCD; thrombus was in the LAD in 22 (30%), LC in 17 (23%), LM in none, and right coronary artery in 35 (47%).

The location of the thrombus in terms of proximal or distal halves in a single coronary artery was examined in our study, but not in the studies summarized in Table II. In our 13 patients, the thrombus was located in the proximal half of the LAD or LC coronary artery in 11; in the LM in 1; and in the distal half of the right coronary artery in 1.

The relation of coronary thrombus to the site of maximal coronary narrowing by atherosclerotic plaque alone also was examined. In 5 of our patients, the thrombus was located at the site of maximal narrowing by atherosclerotic plaque; in 5 others, the thrombus, although not located at the site of maximal narrowing by plaque, was nevertheless located in the coronary artery that contained the most severe degree of narrowing by plaque. Thus, in only 3 of the 13 patients was the thrombus located in the coronary artery that did not contain the site of most severe narrowing by plaque alone. In our study, the thrombi in all 13 patients occurred at a site already narrowed more than 50% in XSA by atherosclerotic plaque; 8 occurred at a site narrowed more than 75% in XSA, and only 1 thrombus (a nonocclusive thrombus) occurred at a site narrowed less than 70% in XSA. The amounts of luminal narrowing by plaque at the site of thrombus also was examined in 3 previous studies.[8,10,15] Baba et al[8] found 42 "acute" coronary thrombi (excluding 3 in the LM) among 121 victims of SCD and 41 (98%) were located at sites already obstructed at least 75% (presumably in XSA) by atherosclerotic plaque. Baroldi et al[10] found 54 "acute" coronary thrombi (32 occlusive, 22 "mural") in 208 SCD patients and 52 (96%) were located at a site with "lumen reduction" of at least 70%. Davies and Thomas[15] found at least 74 thrombi (in 100 victims of SCD) and 48 (65%) were located at sites already narrowed at least 75% by atherosclerotic plaque.

Although thrombi in SCD victims have previously been subdivided into "acute" and "organizing,"[8] the detailed composition of the "acute" thrombi has not been described. The coronary thrombus in our 13 patients consisted predominantly of platelets in 7 and of fibrin in 6. The mean age of the 7 patients with platelet thrombi was less than that of the 6 patients with fibrin-erythrocyte thrombi (34 vs 53 years, p <0.01). The maximal duration of acute terminal symptoms (chest pain, dyspnea or collapse), i.e., from time of onset (when the victim's usual state of health was interrupted) until death, was similar in the 7 patients with platelet thrombi and in the 6 with fibrin-erythrocyte thrombi. In 4 patients in both groups, the terminal event was within 1 hour of the onset of symptoms; the 2 patients (nos. 5 and 12) with the longest duration of terminal symptoms both had fibrin-erythrocyte thrombi. Only 1 of the 7 patients with predominantly platelet thrombi had a healed myocardial infarct at necropsy; 3 of 6 patients with predominantly fibrin-erythrocyte thrombi had a healed myocardial infarct. None of the 7 patients with predominantly platelet thrombi had had angina pectoris or a clinical event suggestive of acute myocardial infarction; in contrast, all 6 patients with predominantly fibrin-erythrocyte thrombi had had angina pectoris or a previous myocardial infarction that healed, or both. The explanation for this difference is unclear. The finding of large numbers of platelets in over half of the coronary thrombi suggests that antiplatelet agents may have been useful in them in preventing thrombus formation.

In our study, 4 features of the thrombus and adjacent atherosclerotic plaque were examined: presence of superficial plaque rupture; extravasation of erythrocytes into the underlying plaque, either into the adjacent fibrous capsule or into the deeper pultaceous debris; presence of lipid material or plaque debris within the luminal thrombus; and fibrin deposition in the underlying plaque. Of our 13 patients with thrombus, 7 had superficial plaque rupture and 6 had extravasation of erythrocytes under the superficial layer of the plaque. In only 3 patients did plaque at the site of thrombus contain pultaceous debris, but in none were extravasated erythrocytes present in the debris. In none of the 13 patients with thrombus was plaque debris found within the thrombus itself. Small amounts of fibrin were present within the atherosclerotic plaque at the site of thrombus in 8 patients. Friedman et al[7] found 20 acute thrombi (in 34 victims of SCD); 19 had plaque rupture and 18 had plaque hemorrhages. Debris fragments from the ruptured plaque were present in the overlying thrombus ". . . in the majority." Liberthson et al[9] found 70 acute thrombi (among 220 victims of SCD) and 28 (40%) had plaque rupture, but another 44 patients had plaque rupture without overlying thrombus. Among 115 instances of coronary thrombi, Davies and Thomas[15] found that 103 (90%) had coexistent "intraintimal" thrombus that resulted from plaque fissuring; of 26 cases without thrombus, however, 21 (81%) also had "intraintimal" thrombus, which in 19 cases was associated with plaque fissuring.

References

1. **Warnes CA, Roberts WC.** Sudden coronary death: Relation of amount and distribution of coronary narrowing at necropsy to previous symptoms of myocardial ischemia, left ventricular scarring and heart weight. Am J Cardiol 1984;54:65–73.
2. **Movat HZ.** Demonstration of all connective tissue elements in a single section. Pentachrome stains. Arch Pathol 1955;60:289–295.
3. **Isner JM, Wu M, Virmani R, Jones AA, Roberts WC.** Comparison of degrees of coronary arterial luminal narrowing determined by visual inspection of histologic sections under magnification among three independent observers and comparison to that obtained by videoplanimetry. An analysis of 559 five-millimeter segments of 61 coronary arteries from eleven patients. Lab Investigation 1980;42:566–570.
4. **Dvorak JA, Schuette WH, Whitehouse WC.** A simple video method for the quantification of microscopic objects. J of Microscopy 1974;102:71–78.
5. **Lie JT, Titus JL.** Pathology of the myocardium and the conduction system in sudden coronary death. Circulation 1975;52:suppl:III:III-41–III-52.
6. **Spain DM, Bradess VA.** Sudden death from coronary heart disease. Survival time, frequency of thrombi and cigarette smoking. Chest 1978;58:107–110.
7. **Friedman M, Manwaring JH, Rosenman RH, Donlon G, Ortega P, Grube SM.** Instantaneous and sudden death. Clinical and pathological differentiation in coronary artery disease. JAMA 1973;225:1319–1328.
8. **Baba N, Bashe WJ, Keller MD, Greer JC, Anthony JR.** Pathology of atherosclerotic heart disease in sudden death. I. Organizing thrombosis and acute coronary vessel lesions. Circulation 1975;52:suppl:III:III-53–III-59.
9. **Liberthson RR, Nagel EL, Hirschman JC, Nussenfeld SR, Blackbourne BD, Davis JR.** Pathophysiologic observations in prehospital ventricular fibrillation and sudden cardiac death. Circulation 1974;49:790–798.
10. **Baroldi G, Falzi G, Mariani F.** Sudden coronary death. A postmortem study in 208 selected cases compared to 97 "control" subjects. Am Heart J 1979;98:20–31.
11. **Haerem JW.** Mural platelet microthrombi and major acute lesions of main epicardial arteries in sudden coronary death. Atherosclerosis 1974;19:529–541.
12. **Scott RF, Briggs TS.** Pathologic findings in pre-hospital deaths due to coronary atherosclerosis. Am J Cardiol 1972;29:782–787.
13. **Reichenbach DD, Moss NS, Meyer E.** Pathology of the heart in sudden cardiac death. Am J Cardiol 1977;39:865–872.
14. **Rissanen V, Romo M, Siltanen P.** Prehospital sudden death from ischaemic heart disease. A postmortem study. Br Heart J 1978;40:1025–1033.
15. **Davies MJ, Thomas A.** Thrombosis and acute coronary-artery lesions in sudden cardiac ischemic death. N Engl J Med 1984;310:1137–1140.
16. **Warnes C, Roberts WC.** Comparison at necropsy by age group of amount and distribution of narrowing by atherosclerotic plaque in 2995 five-mm long segments of 240 major coronary arteries in 60 men aged 31–70 years with sudden coronary death. Am Heart J 1984;108:431–435.

Formation of New Coronary Arteries *Within* a Previously Obstructed Epicardial Coronary Artery (Intraarterial Arteries): A Mechanism for Occurrence of Angiographically Normal Coronary Arteries After Healing of Acute Myocardial Infarction

WILLIAM C. ROBERTS, MD
RENU VIRMANI, MD

Small vascular channels often develop within previously obstructed arteries, but usually such channels are small and the arterial lumen consequently remains narrowed. That large channels consisting of muscular arteries and capable of carrying large quantities of blood may develop in previously obstructed larger muscular arteries is not a well recognized observation. Such was the case, however, in 2 patients described herein.

Patient 1: A 26-year-old man was well until 36 months before death, when he had active infective endocarditis and he received antibiotic drugs. Five months later (31 months before death), he again had evidence of active infective endocarditis. He again received antibiotic drugs, but he had chronic congestive heart failure thereafter and evidence of severe aortic regurgitation. The electrocardiogram (Fig. 1) showed evidence of a healed anterior wall myocardial infarct. The aortic valve was replaced with a Teflon® leaflet valve 8 months before death. At operation, the aortic valve was congenitally bicuspid. Although the patient was asymptomatic thereafter, his blood pressure was 200/30 mm Hg 1 week before death. When severe aortic regurgitation was confirmed by angiography, he underwent replacement of the Teflon-leaflet aortic valve with a caged-ball prostheses. He died the next day. At necropsy (A63-170), an aneurysmal, large, anterior wall, healed transmural infarct was present. The left anterior descending coronary artery over a distance of approximately 4 cm was narrowed, primarily by fibrous tissue, in which numerous multiluminal channels were present (Fig. 2). Each channel was walled by a completely newly formed muscular artery (Fig. 3). The right, left main and left circumflex coronary arteries were normal.

Patient 2: A 25-year-old woman, who had always been healthy and asymptomatic, never awoke after going to sleep.

From the Pathology Branch, National Heart, Lung, and Blood Institute, National Institutes of Health, Bethesda, Maryland, and the Department of Cardiovascular Pathology, Armed Forces Institute of Pathology, Washington, D.C. Manuscript received and accepted July 23, 1984.

Necropsy (AFIP #1770851) disclosed a healed transmural infarct in the lateral wall of left ventricle. The ramus branch of the left main coronary artery was narrowed and histologic study of it disclosed numerous well formed, small channels in the narrowed portion (Fig. 4). The other major coronary arteries were normal.

Each patient described above had healed transmural left ventricular scars and severe narrowing of 1 major epicardial coronary artery without any narrowing of the other major arteries. Numerous small muscular arteries had formed in the narrowed lumens of a previously obstructed artery. Patient 1 had an embolus to the left anterior descending coronary artery during active infective endocarditis involving the aortic valve and the embolic material subsequently organized to form the new small muscular arteries within the larger muscular artery. Patient 2 presumably also had thrombus or embolus in the ramus branch of the left main coronary artery, but its source was not determined; it also subsequently organized, with development of multiple new muscular arteries within the obstructed artery. These 2 patients show that the human body is capable of forming normal coronary arteries *within* large epicardial coronary arteries.

Had coronary angiography been performed in each of these 2 patients after healing of the acute myocardial infarction, almost surely the artery containing the newly formed arteries within the previously obstructed artery would have appeared angiographically normal. Thus,

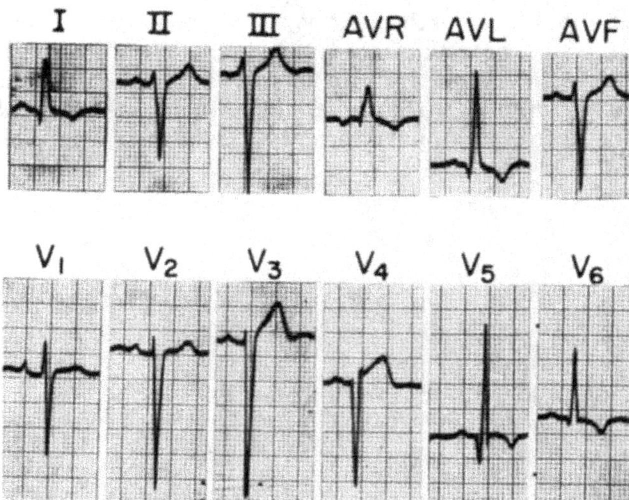

FIGURE 1. Patient 1—electrocardiogram recorded 3 days before the first aortic valve replacement, or 28 months after the first episode, and 23 months after the second episode of active infective endocarditis. The acute anterior wall myocardial infarct probably occurred during the second episode of infection. The infarct was large and aneurysmal at necropsy.

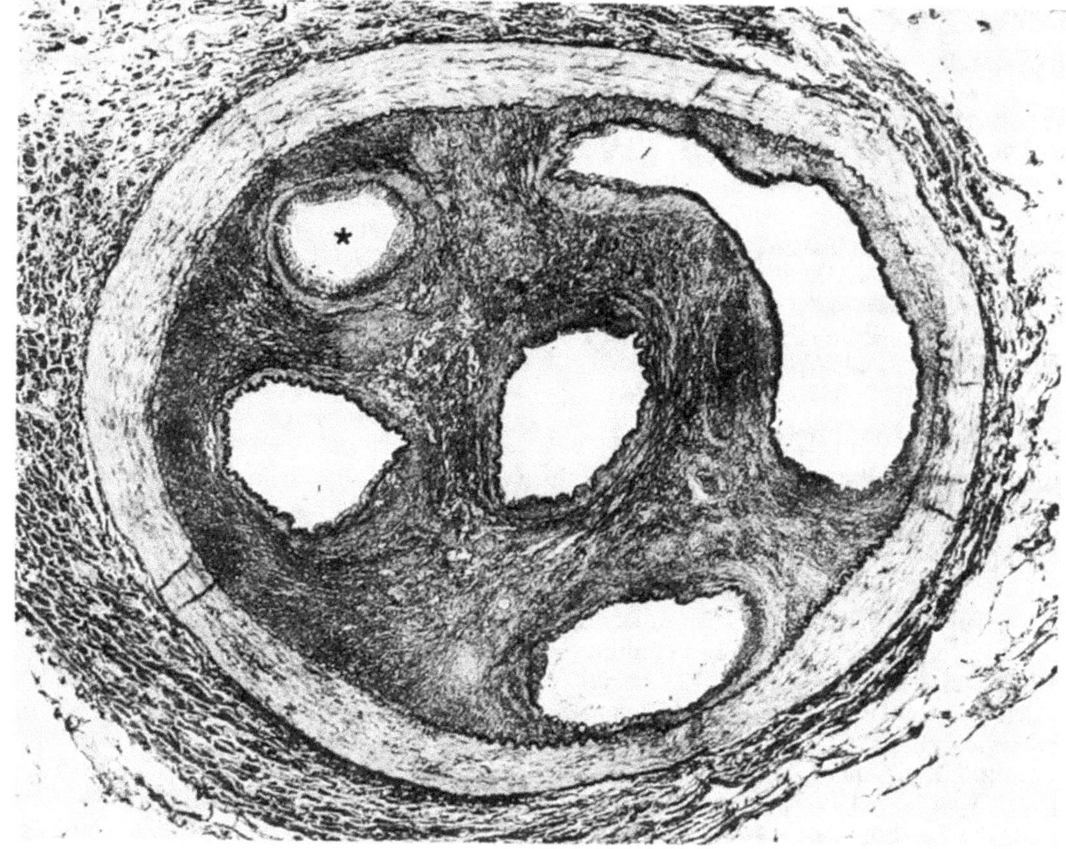

FIGURE 2. Patient 1—cross section of left anterior descending coronary artery showing 5 newly formed coronary arteries within the coronary artery. Each newly formed artery has an internal and external elastic membrane and a smooth-muscle media. Had angiography been performed, this artery probably would have appeared normal. A close-up of the small intraarterial artery marked with an asterisk is shown in Figure 3. Elastic tissue stain.

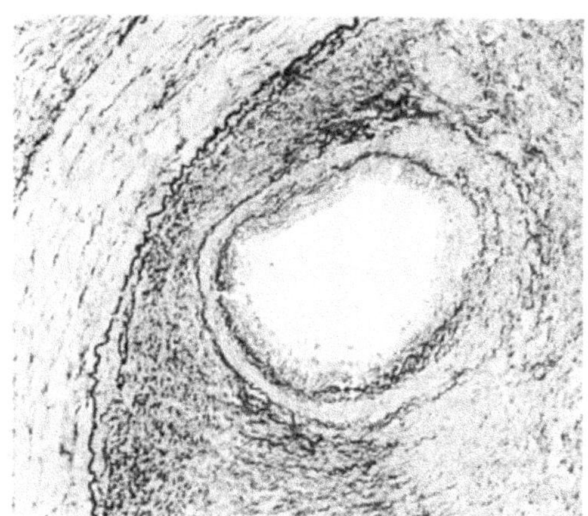

FIGURE 3. Patient 1—close-up of 1 intraarterial artery shown by asterisk in Figure 2. Elastic tissue stain; magnification ×160.

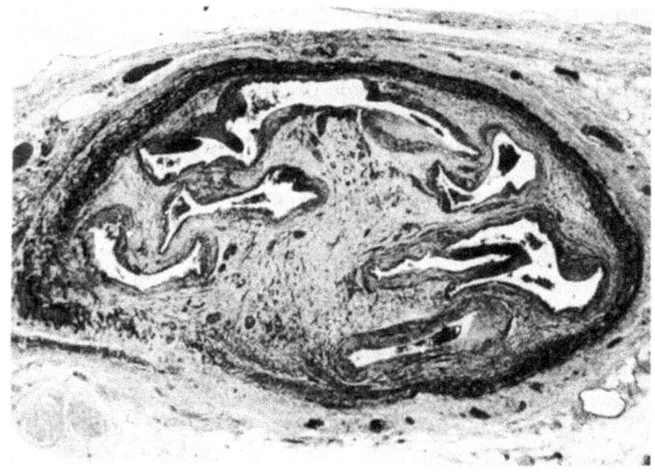

FIGURE 4. Patient 2—cross section of ramus branch of left main coronary artery demonstrating 6 newly formed coronary arteries within the previously obstructed major coronary artery. Movat stain; magnification ×25.

formation of multiple new small muscular arteries within previously obstructed large muscular coronary arteries is a mechanism of producing angiographically normal coronary arteries after healing of acute myocardial infarction.[1]

Reference

1. **Arnett EN, Roberts WC.** Acute myocardial infarction and angiographically normal arteries. An unproven combination. Circulation 1976;53:395–400.

Occluding Clot in the Left Main Coronary Artery with Survival Long Enough to Develop Massive Left Ventricular Wall Necrosis

ILDEFONSO J. MAS, MD
CHARLES W. BARTH, III, MD
PADMA K. SHUTLK, MD
MAZHAR U. SHEIKH, MD
WILLIAM C. ROBERTS, MD

Total occlusion of the left main (LM) coronary artery is rare in patients with acute myocardial infarction (AMI). We found published reports describing 5 patients with AMI who by angiography during the first day of presentation had total occlusion of the LM coronary artery.[1–3] All 5, each of whom had presented with cardiogenic shock, had early intracoronary thrombolytic therapy with opening of the lumen of the LM coronary artery and all survived. Additionally, another reported patient with AMI had total occlusion of the LM coronary artery by angiogram at day 15—but no coronary angiogram or thrombolytic therapy earlier—and this patient was alive 1 year later.[4] The present report was prompted by study at necropsy of a patient who survived 54 hours after onset of AMI and who had total occlusion of the LM coronary artery by clot superimposed on atherosclerotic plaque.

J.B., a 68-year-old previously healthy, active and asymptomatic man, while walking to a football game, felt nauseated, sat down on a curbstone and fainted. He was unconscious for about 45 seconds, during which time he did not urinate or defecate. Two hours later he arrived at the hospital emergency room. He appeared alert; he was still nauseated and he had mild, persistent pain in the left infrascapular region. The blood pressure was 120/80 mm Hg. (For several years he had taken a β-blocking drug for systemic hypertension.) Precordial examination disclosed no abnormalities except for softer heart sounds than expected. Bibasilar rales were present. The electrocardiogram shown in Figure 1 was recorded. Furosemide, nitrates, morphine, oxygen and lidocaine were administered. A repeat electro-

From the Division of Cardiology, Department of Medicine, Georgetown University Medical Division, District of Columbia General Hospital, Washington, D.C., and the Pathology Branch, National Heart, Lung, and Blood Institute, National Institutes of Health, Bethesda, Maryland 20205. Manuscript received December 17, 1984, accepted December 31, 1984.

cardiogram 6 hours after fainting revealed right bundle branch block and left-axis deviation, findings that had not been present in the earlier electrocardiogram. The pulmonary arterial wedge pressure 12 hours after fainting was 20 mm Hg and the pulmonary artery pressure was 50/18 mm Hg. Electrocardiogram recorded 12 hours after fainting is shown in Figure 1. On the echocardiogram (both M-mode and cross-sectional) recorded 13 hours after fainting, the left ventricular dimension at end-diastole was 50 mm and at peak systole, 42 mm; the walls of both ventricular septum and left ventricle contracted poorly. The heart size was normal on

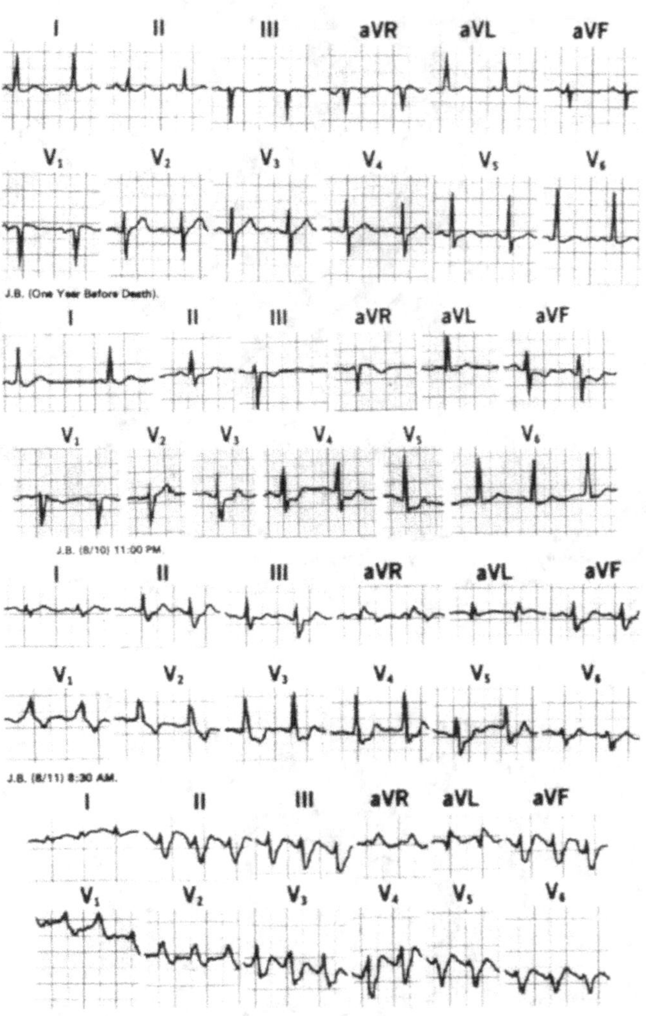

FIGURE 1. Electrocardiograms recorded 1 year before death (**first tracing**), at the time of presentation 2 hours after syncope (**second tracing**), 12 hours after syncope (**third tracing**), and 37 hours after syncope (**fourth tracing**).

chest radiograph. The serum total cholesterol level was 331 mg/dl. Other recorded electrocardiograms also are shown in Figure 1. The serum creatine kinase level rose to 2,490 MU/ml and the MB band was 11% at 22 hours after onset. During the 52 hours in the hospital, the systemic arterial pressure slowly fell, evidence of left-sided congestive heart failure gradually worsened despite vasopressors and endotracheal intubation, and fatal ventricular fibrillation occurred.

At necropsy, the heart weighed 450 g. Thromboembolic material protruded from the left coronary ostium into the aorta (Fig. 2). The LM coronary artery was totally occluded by a combination of thromboembolic material and underlying atherosclerotic plaque. The lumen of the LM just before its bifurcation was narrowed up to 88% by plaque and 12% by clot as determined by videoplanimetry; just after its origin from aorta, the lumen of the LM was narrowed 31% by plaque and 69% by clot. Thromboembolic material was found only in the LM coronary artery. Each of the 4 major coronary arteries was divided into 5-mm segments, each was prepared for histologic study, each was stained by the Movat method, and the degree of narrowing by plaque of each segment was determined (Fig. 3). The entire anterior and lateral left ventricular free walls and the anterior one-half of the ventricular septum were necrotic (Fig. 4).

It is unclear if the clot in the LM coronary artery in the patient was an embolus or a thrombus. That it

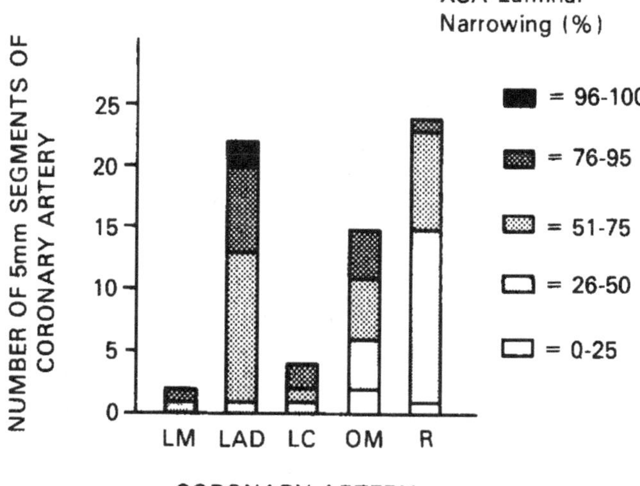

FIGURE 3. Bar graph showing number of 5-mm segments of the left main (LM), left anterior descending (LAD), left circumflex (LC), obtuse marginal (OM) and right (R) coronary arteries narrowed by atherosclerotic plaque only in 5 categories of cross-sectional area (XSA) narrowing. Of the 67 five-millimeter segments examined, 3% were narrowed 96 to 100% in XSA; 22%, 76 to 95%; 39%, 51 to 75%; 31%, 26 to 50%; and 5%, 0 to 25%. Each coronary artery was narrowed more than 75% in XSA by atherosclerotic plaque in 1 or more 5-mm segments.

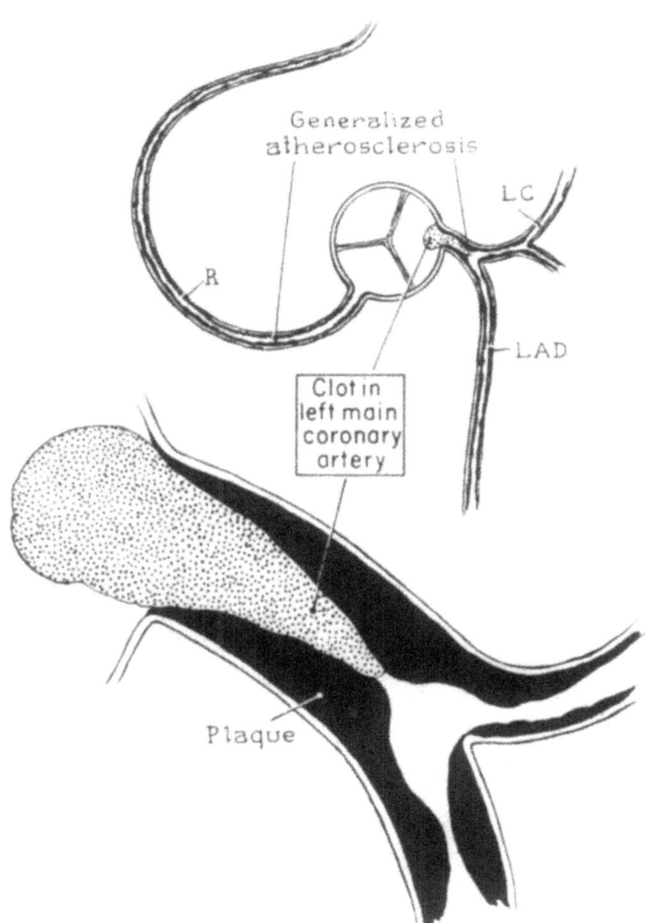

FIGURE 2. Diagram of clot and atherosclerotic plaque totally occluding the left main coronary artery with clot protruding from the left coronary ostium into the aorta. LAD = left anterior descending; LC = left circumflex; R = right coronary arteries.

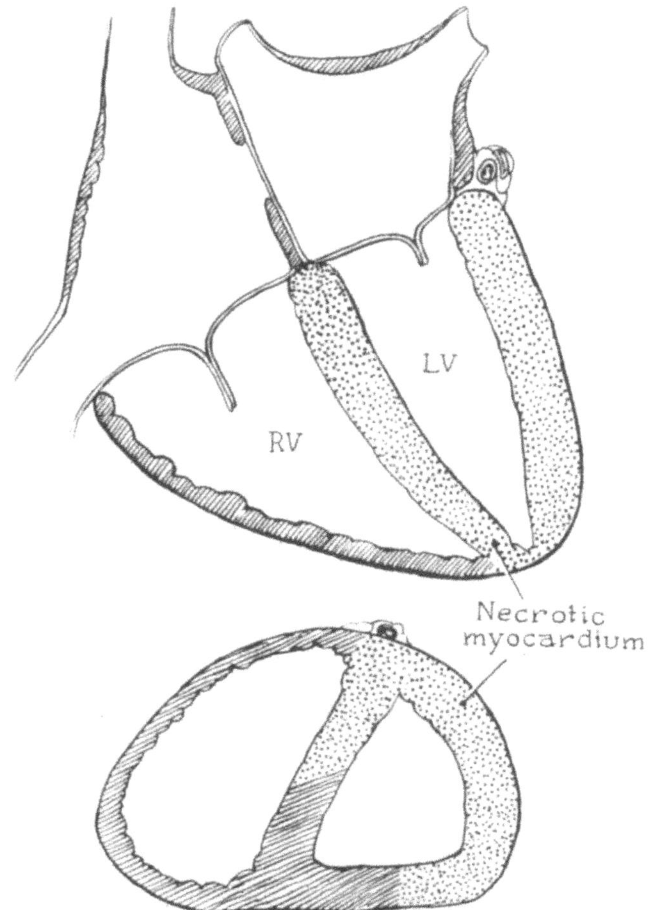

FIGURE 4. Diagram illustrating the extent of myocardial necrosis seen at necropsy. Only a portion of the posterior left ventricular free wall and posterior portion of ventricular septum were not necrotic. LV = left ventricular cavity; RV = right ventricular cavity.

protruded into the lumen of the aorta suggests that it may have been an embolus, but it is not known whether a thrombus located in the LM could protrude into the aorta. The lack of a source of embolism is against an embolus, but a source is not always recognized in patients with clear-cut embolism.[5] Emboli are difficult to recognize when superimposed on large atherosclerotic plaques, but clots in the LM coronary artery rarely are observed in patients with extensive atherosclerosis. In patients with fatal coronary heart disease studied at necropsy, thrombi are usually superimposed on atherosclerotic plaques that have already caused severe narrowing of the lumen of the coronary artery.[6] At the site of distal attachment of the clot in our patient, the lumen of the LM coronary artery was already narrowed 88% in cross-sectional area by atherosclerotic plaque.

It is also unclear why our patient with total occlusion of the LM coronary artery—in part by clot—survived long enough to allow the occurrence of massive left ventricular myocardial necrosis. Sudden occlusion of a previously normal LM coronary artery is incompatible with survival for more than a few minutes.[7] That our patient survived for 54 hours after onset of symptoms of myocardial ischemia likely resulted from the fact that the lumen of the LM coronary artery already was severely narrowed by atherosclerotic plaque, and therefore the clot occluded only 12% of the lumen of the LM artery. Additionally, the lumen of the right coronary artery in our patient was narrowed at one point 78% in cross-sectional area by plaque. Of course, collateral vessels probably were present between right and left coronary arteries before the final clot in the LM coronary artery appeared.

References

1. **Salvi A, Klugman S, Grazia ED, Maras P, Camerini F.** Myocardial reperfusion after acute occlusion of the left main coronary artery. Am J Cardiol 1983; 51:1791.
2. **de Feyter PJ, Serruys PW.** Thrombolysis of acute total occlusion of the left main coronary artery in evolving myocardial infarction. Am J Cardiol 1984;53:1727–1728.
3. **von Essen R, Lambertz H, Schmidt W, Rustige J, Uebis R, Effert S.** Successful recanalization of left main coronary artery occlusion. Am J Cardiol 1984;53:356–357.
4. **Flugelman MY, Shalit M, Shefer A, Yonathan H, Gotsman MS.** Survival after sudden obstruction of the left main coronary artery. Am J Cardiol 1983;51:900–901.
5. **Roberts WC.** Coronary embolism: a review of causes, consequences, and diagnostic considerations. Cardiovasc Med 1978;3:699–710.
6. **Brosius FC, Roberts WC.** Significance of coronary arterial thrombus in transmural acute myocardial infarction. A study of 54 necropsy patients. Circulation 1981;63:810–816.
7. **Waller BF, Dixon DS, Kim RW, Roberts WC.** Embolus to the left main coronary artery. Am J Cardiol 1982;50:658–660.

Right Ventricular Infarction with Electrocardiographic Anterior Left Ventricular Infarction and Thrombosis of the Left Anterior Descending Coronary Artery

DEBORAH J. BARBOUR, MD
PATRICK F. SAULINO, MD
WILLIAM C. ROBERTS, MD

At necropsy, right ventricular (RV) myocardial infarction secondary to coronary artery disease is observed only in patients with left ventricular (LV) infarction involving the LV posterior (inferior) wall.[1,2] The implication of this observation, of course, is that patients with electrocardiographic evidence of anterior wall LV infarction are spared from RV infarction. Although few reports describing patients with anatomically confirmed RV infarction have illustrated an electrocardiogram,[1–4] it is likely that more than 95% of patients with RV infarction have electrocardiographic evidence of posterior (inferior) LV infarction only. An occasional patient with electrocardiographic evidence of anterior wall myocardial infarction, however, has RV infarction. How can this be? The answer, demonstrated in the patient described herein, is: If the electrocardiogram indicates anterior wall LV infarction, but necropsy also shows RV infarction, the LV infarction in the basal third or so of the LV free wall is limited to the anterior LV free wall with or without involvement of the anterior portion of ventricular septum or lateral LV free wall or both; in the mid or apical third, or both, of the LV wall, however, the LV infarct is circumferential, or nearly so, such that the posterior (inferior) LV wall and posterior portion of ventricular septum indeed is infarcted. The RV infarct then represents an extension from the posterior portion of the ventricular septum.

B.S., a 67-year-old man with previous systemic hypertension and insulin-dependent diabetes mellitus, first had transient substernal chest pain 13 days before death. Six days before death, the pain recurred and persisted for 10 hours before his arrival at the hospital. The initial electrocardiogram (Fig. 1) showed marked ST-segment elevation in 10 of 12 leads (all except leads aVR and aVL, which showed depressed ST segments). (An electrocardiogram done 63 days earlier had disclosed Q waves in leads V_1 and V_2 [Fig. 1].) The chest pain, which lasted 14 hours, initially was relieved by nifedipine and nitrates. During his 6 days in the hospital, he had recurrent supraventricular tachycardia, which required cardioversion for correction. The creatine kinase level rose to 1,900 U/ml with 4% MB fraction. Chest pain recurred 2 days before death and evidence of congestive heart failure was apparent. On the day of death, the heart rate slowed and fatal asystole occurred.

At necropsy, the heart weighed 590 g. The cardiac cavities were of normal size. There were no myocardial scars; the

From the Pathology Branch, National Heart, Lung, and Blood Institute, National Institutes of Health, Bethesda, Maryland 20205, and Department of Medicine, Division of Cardiology, Washington Veterans Administration Hospital, Washington, D.C. Manuscript received and accepted December 31, 1984.

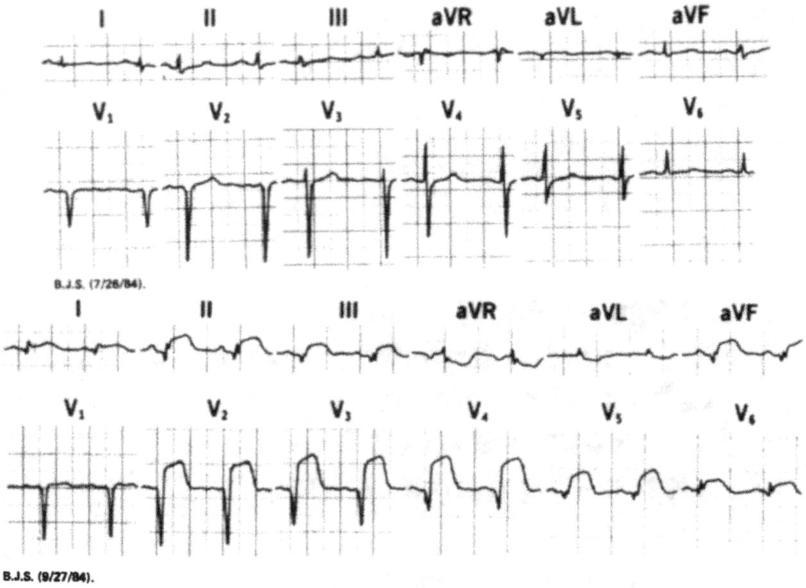

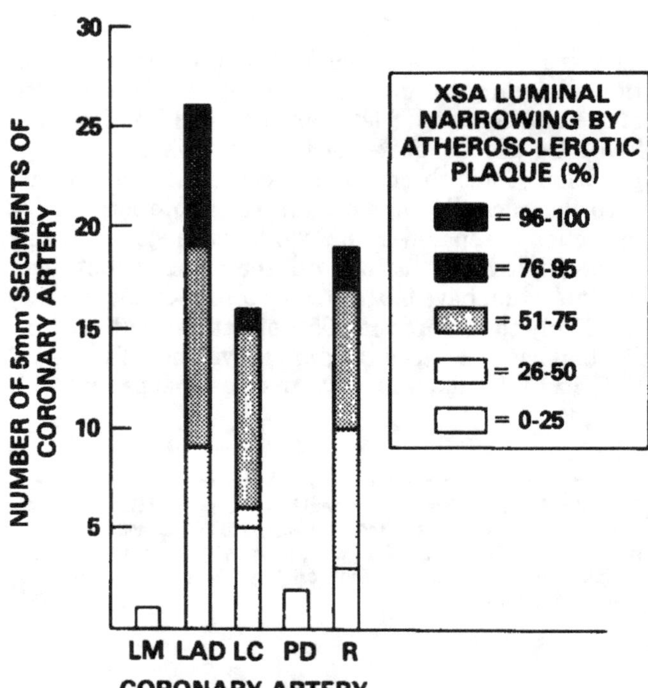

FIGURE 1. Electrocardiograms: **top,** recorded 70 days before death; **bottom,** 7 days before death. In the top tracing Q waves are present in leads aVR, aVL and V$_1$ and V$_2$; in the bottom tracing, Q waves are present in all leads except aVR and aVL.

anterior LV wall and ventricular septum at the base were necrotic; in the apical portion, the entire LV wall and septum were necrotic, as was the entire posterior and portions of the anterolateral RV wall. The right, left anterior descending and left circumflex (dominant) coronary arteries were all narrowed more than 75% in cross-sectional area at some point by atherosclerotic plaque. Each of these 3 arteries and the left main and posterior descending arteries were divided into 5-mm segments and 1 histologic section was prepared from each segment. The results of these examinations are summarized in Figure 2. An occluding thrombus was present in the proximal portion of the left anterior descending coronary artery; the distal portion of the left anterior descending coronary artery, however, was already totally occluded by atherosclerotic plaque.

The patient illustrates that RV infarction may indeed occur when there is electrocardiographic evidence of anterior wall LV infarction but that anatomically the LV infarction at least in the apical half does involve the posterior LV free wall and the posterior portion of ventricular septum. The RV infarct, therefore, represents extension of the posterior LV infarct across the posterior portion of ventricular septum to the posterior RV free wall. The RV anterior wall adjacent to ventricular septum was not involved by the myocardial infarct. Although our patient had clear electrocardiographic evidence of LV anterior wall infarction, the presence of Q waves in leads II, III and aVF indicated that the posterior (inferior) wall of LV wall also was infarcted.

FIGURE 2. Bar graph showing the number of 5-mm segments of the left main (LM), left anterior descending (LAD), left circumflex (LC), posterior descending (PD) and right (R) coronary arteries narrowed to various degrees in cross-sectional area (XSA) by atherosclerotic plaque. Of the total 62 five-millimeter segments examined, 2 (3%) were narrowed 96 to 100% in XSA; 10 (16%), 76 to 95%; and 26 (42%), 51 to 75%. There was total occlusion of the LAD by thrombus superimposed on the already severe luminal narrowing by atherosclerotic plaque.

References

1. **Isner JM, Roberts WC.** Right ventricular infarction complicating left ventricular infarction secondary to coronary heart disease. Am J Cardiol 1978;42:885–894.
2. **Ratliff NB, Hackel DB.** Combined right and left ventricular infarction: pathogenesis and clinicopathologic correlations. Am J Cardiol 1980;45:217–221.
3. **Wade WG.** The pathogenesis of infarction of the right ventricle. Br Heart J 1959;21:545–554.
4. **Cohn JN, Gulha NH, Broder MI, Limas CJ.** Right ventricular infarction. Clinical and hemodynamic features. Am J Cardiol 1974;33:209–214.

Severe Atherosclerotic Coronary Artery Disease, Healed Myocardial Infarction and Chronic Congestive Heart Failure: Analysis of 81 Patients Studied at Necropsy

ELIZABETH M. ROSS, MD, and WILLIAM C. ROBERTS, MD

Observations are described in 81 necropsy patients (aged 29 to 91 years [mean 62]; 77 [95%] men) with severe congestive heart failure (CHF) more than 3 months in duration, left ventricular (LV) transmural scar and >75% cross-sectional area narrowing by atherosclerotic plaque of 1 or more of the 4 major epicardial coronary arteries. The duration of symptoms from initial onset of acute myocardial infarction (59 patients) or CHF (18 patients) or angina pectoris (2 patients) to death ranged from 0.5 to 18 years (mean 7.1) (2 unknown). Angina pectoris occurred at some time, however, in 31 patients (38%). Cause of death was CHF in 48 patients (59%), sudden (arrhythmia) in 16 (20%), acute myocardial infarction in 11(14%), and emboli in 6 (7%). The heart weight ranged from 410 to 800 g (mean 585). Left or right ventricular thrombi or both occurred in 37 patients (46%), only 4 (10%) of whom had systemic emboli; of the 44 patients without intracardiac thrombi, none had any form of emboli. The severity of coronary narrowing was variable. In 24 patients (30%) only 1 artery was narrowed >75% in cross-sectional area; in 22 patients (27%), 2 arteries were so narrowed; in 32 patients (39%), 3 arteries; and in 3 patients (4%), 4 arteries. The size of the LV scar also varied. Of the 81 patients, 58 (72%) had large scars (involving >40% of the LV wall); 10 (12%) had moderate-sized scars (6 to 40% of the LV wall); and 13 (16%) had small scars (≤5% of the LV wall). Size of the LV scar correlated with a history of habitual alcoholism: of the 16 habitual alcoholics, 6 (38%) had small and 8 (50%) had large LV scars; of the 65 non-alcoholics, 7 (11%) had small and 50 (77%) had large LV scars (p <0.05). Chronic CHF in the 68 patients with either moderate or large-sized LV scars is readily attributed to the LV damage; in the 13 patients with small LV scars, however, chronic CHF more reasonably may be attributed to another factor, e.g., alcoholism, despite coronary artery narrowing similar in severity to that in the patients with large LV scars.

(Am J Cardiol 1986; 57: 44–50)

Chronic congestive heart failure (CHF) in patients with severe atherosclerotic coronary artery disease (CAD) and dilated cardiac ventricles usually is associated with considerable scarring of the left ventricular (LV) wall. This report describes clinical and necropsy findings in 81 necropsy patients with dilated cardiac ventricles, severe luminal narrowing by atherosclerotic plaques of 1 or more of the 4 major epicardial coronary arteries, and transmural LV scars.

Methods

Cardiac diagnoses were reviewed in the nearly 7,500 necropsy patients accessioned in the Pathology Branch of the National Heart, Lung, and Blood Institute. Records of all patients diagnosed as having CAD were reviewed. The present study was limited to patients who fulfilled the following criteria: (1) presence of at least 1 grossly visible healed, transmural (involvement of the entire inner one half and all or a portion of the outer one half of the wall) LV free wall scar; (2) presence of clinical evidence of left-sided CHF for longer than 3 months; (3) presence of dilated right and LV cavities by visual inspection at necropsy; (4) luminal narrowing by atherosclerotic plaque of 76 to 100% in cross-sectional area (XSA) of at least 1 major (right, left main, left anterior descending and left circumflex) epicardial coronary artery; (5) absence of LV free wall aneurysm; (6) heart weight >350 g in women and >400 g in men; (7) death resulting from or related to cardiac disease; (8) absence of primary anatomic cardiac valvular disease capable in itself of producing cardiac dysfunction; (9) absence of a pericardial condition sufficient to cause cardiac dysfunction; (10) absence of an

From the Pathology Branch of the National Heart Lung and Blood Institute, National Institutes of Health, Bethesda, Maryland. Manuscript received May 6, 1985, accepted June 21, 1985.

Dr. Ross' present address and address for reprints: Elizabeth M. Ross, MD, Washington Hospital Center, 110 Irving Street NW, Room 3B-44B, Washington, D.C. 20010.

infiltrative myocardial condition such as amyloid or sarcoid; and (11) absence of a cardiac operation at any time. Eighty-one patients fulfilled these criteria and form the basis of this report; 7 of the 81 patients had been included in an earlier report by Virmani and Roberts.[1]

In all 81 patients the hearts were examined at necropsy by one of us (WCR). The patients were separated into 3 groups based on gross estimation of the amount of LV or ventricular septal scar present relative to the total area of LV free wall and ventricular septum: small (≤5% of the LV free wall and wall of ventricular septum was scarred) moderate (involvement of 6 to 40% of the LV wall), and large (involvement of >40% of the LV wall). The coronary arteries were available for detailed quantitative examination in 56 of the 81 hearts. In them, the 4 major epicardial coronary arteries were removed from the heart intact, sectioned into 5-mm-long segments, decalcified, processed in alcohols and xylene, embedded in paraffin, cut into 6 μ-thick sections, placed on a glass slide, stained with Movat's trichrome method and examined by one of us (EMR) with a microscope at a magnification of 40 times. The XSA narrowing was graded in 5 categories: 0 to 25%, 26 to 50%, 51 to 75%, 76 to 95% and 96 to 100%. One to 6 (mean 3) hematoxylin-eosin–stained histologic sections of LV wall extending from endocardium to epicardium were examined from 70 of the 81 hearts.

The results were evaluated using a Student t test and chi-square test. A p value <0.05 was considered statistically significant.

Results

The 81 patients had died from 1967 through 1984. They were 29 to 91 years old (mean 62). Seventy-seven (95%) were men. Initial clinical evidence of myocardial ischemia, known in 79 patients, was acute myocardial infarction (AMI) in 59 (75%), CHF in 18 (23%) and angina pectoris in 2 (2%). At some time in their courses, 31 (38%) had angina pectoris, 65 (80%) had clinical events diagnosed as AMI, and all 81 (100%)

had evidence of chronic CHF. Duration of symptoms from initial clinical evidence of myocardial ischemia to death, known in 70 patients, ranged from 0.5 to 32 years (mean 7.2, median 3.0). The interval from first AMI to death, known in 55 patients, ranged from 0.5 to 32 years (mean 8.0, median 5.0) (Fig. 1). The interval from onset of CHF to death, known in 65 patients, ranged from 0.3 to 16 years (mean 3.4, median 2.0) (Fig. 1). Sixteen of the 81 patients (20%) were known to be habitual alcoholics, 22 (27%) were known to have diabetes mellitus (adult onset in each), and at least 34 (42%) by history had had systemic hypertension at some time. The systemic arterial pressures before AMI, however, were available in few patients. Ten patients had chronic obstructive pulmonary disease; 4 (5%) had a stroke at some time and 5 (6%) had symptomatic peripheral vascular disease.

Death was attributed to chronic CHF in 48 patients (59%), to cardiac arrest (arrhythmia) in 16 (20%), to AMI in 11 (14%) and to emboli in 6 (7%).

The heart weight ranged from 410 to 800 g (mean 585). Of the 324 major (right, left main, left anterior descending and left circumflex) epicardial coronary arteries in the 81 patients, 178 (55%) were narrowed at some point 76 to 100% in XSA by atherosclerotic plaque (right = 58, left main = 5, left anterior descending = 67 and left circumflex = 48). A mean of 2.2/4.0 coronary arteries per patient were narrowed 76 to 100% in XSA. Of the 81 patients, 24 (30%) had only 1 of the 4 major epicardial coronary arteries narrowed by atherosclerotic plaque 76 to 100%; 22 (27%) had 2 coronary arteries so narrowed; 32 (39%) had 3 coronary arteries so narrowed, and 3 (4%) had 4 coronary arteries so narrowed.

In 56 patients each 5-mm segment of the 4 major coronary arteries was examined histologically; 188

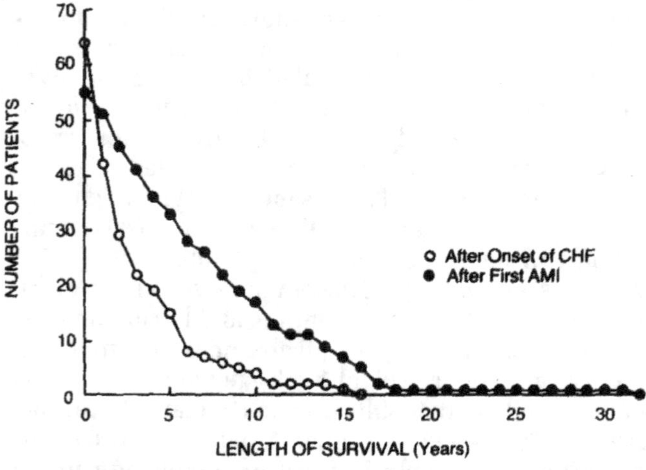

FIGURE 1. Length of survival after onset of either congestive heart failure (CHF) (65 patients) or acute myocardial infarction (AMI) (55 patients).

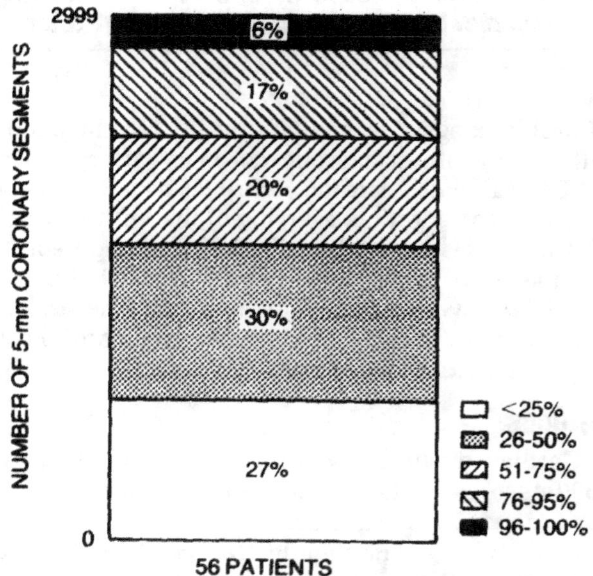

FIGURE 2. Number of 5-mm coronary segments and degree of cross-sectional area narrowing by atherosclerotic plaque in the 56 patients in whom every 5-mm segment of all 4 major (right, left main, left anterior descending and left circumflex) coronary arteries were examined.

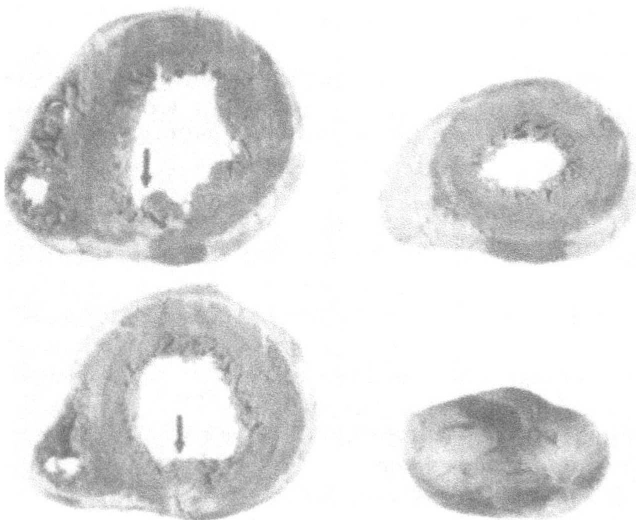

FIGURE 3. Transverse sections of the cardiac ventricles in a 54-year-old man (DCVAH #A80-108) with chronic congestive heart failure during the last 6 years of life. At necropsy, the heart weighed 625 g and only the right coronary artery was narrowed >75% in cross-sectional area. A small transmural scar (*arrows*) is in the posterior left ventricular wall.

segments (6%) were narrowed 96 to 100% in XSA by atherosclerotic plaque; 512 (17%), 76 to 95%; 584 (20%), 51 to 75%; 911 (30%), 26 to 50%; and 804 (27%), 0 to 25% (Fig. 2).

Although 23% of the 2,999 five-millimeter segments of coronary arteries in the 56 patients were narrowed >75% in XSA by atherosclerotic plaque, the percent of 5-mm segments narrowed to this extent per patient varied. Among the 56 patients, the number of 5-mm segments examined per patient ranged from 31 to 81 (mean 53) and the percent narrowed 76 to 100% in XSA by atherosclerotic plaque ranged from 1 to 80%: in 15 patients (27%), 1 to 5% of the coronary segments were narrowed to this extent; in 2 patients (4%), 6 to 10% of the 5-mm segments were so narrowed; in 13 patients (23%), 11 to 20% of the segments were so narrowed; in 19 patients (34%); 21 to 50% of the segments were so narrowed; and in 7 patients (13%), >50% of the segments were so narrowed.

The size of the LV scars was classified as small in 13 patients (16%) (Fig. 3), moderate in 10 (12%) (Fig. 4) and large in 58 (72%) (Fig. 5 and 6). Eleven of the 81 patients had AMI as a terminal event, but the amount of necrotic LV myocardium was not included in the percent of total LV wall involved by scar. The exact loca-

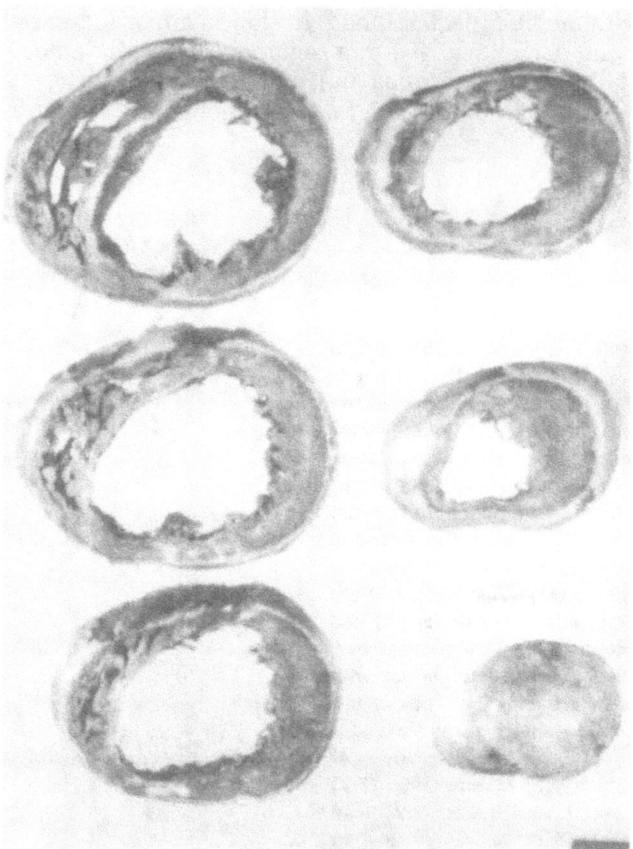

FIGURE 4. Transverse sections of the cardiac ventricles (*upper*) and of the basal portion of the heart (*lower*) in a 76-year-old man (DCVAH #A78-167) who had acute myocardial infarction 8 years before death and chronic congestive heart failure during his last 6 months of life. At necropsy, the heart weighed 460 g and 2 of the 4 major coronary arteries were narrowed >75% in cross-sectional area by atherosclerotic plaque. *Upper* and *lower*, the posteroseptal (P) left ventricular wall is thin and fibrotic and a mural thrombus (T) is attached to the mural endocardium of the anterior (A) wall, which is neither necrotic nor fibrotic.

FIGURE 5. Transverse sections of the cardiac ventricles in a 65-year-old man (SH #A79-88) who had acute myocardial infarction 18 months before death. Chronic severe congestive heart failure developed at the time of infarction and persisted thereafter. At necropsy, the heart weighed 580 g and 3 of the 4 major epicardial coronary arteries were narrowed >75% in cross-sectional area by atherosclerotic plaque. The entire ventricular septum and a portion of the posterior left ventricular free wall is thinned and scarred.

tion of the LV scars (known in 80 patients) was anterior wall only in 26 (32%), posterior (inferior) wall only in 36 (45%) and both anterior and posterior walls in 18 (22%). Thus, at least 18 of the 81 patients (22%) had 2 distinct healed myocardial infarcts. Among the 58 patients with large LV scars, 17 (29%) had 1-vessel CAD, 17 (29%) had 2-vessel CAD and 24 (42%) had 3-vessel CAD. Of the 13 patients with small LV scars, 4 (31%) had 1-vessel CAD, 1 (8%) had 2-vessel CAD, 5 (38%) had 3-vessel CAD and 3 (23%) had 4-vessel CAD. Additionally, examination of the 5-mm coronary segments in 38 patients with large LV scars disclosed that 22% were narrowed 76 to 100% in XSA by atherosclerotic plaque; in contrast, of 9 patients with small LV scars, 36% of the 5-mm coronary segments were so narrowed. The 22% and 36% values are not statistically significant.

Left or right ventricular thrombi, or both, occurred in 37 patients (46%), only 4 (10%) of whom had systemic emboli; of the 44 patients without intracardiac thrombi, none had emboli.

In the 81 patients, 8 factors were analyzed after the patients were classified into subgroups on the basis of presence or absence of angina pectoris, diabetes mellitus, systemic hypertension (by history), habitual alcoholism (by history), clinical evidence of AMI, and size of LV scar.

Compared to the 50 patients without, the 31 patients with angina pectoris had a significantly increased mean percentage of 5-mm segments of 4 major epicardial coronary arteries narrowed by atherosclerotic plaque 76 to 100% (31% vs 18%); there was no signifi-

cant difference in mean age (62 years vs 62 years), frequency of a history of systemic hypertension (29% vs 50%), diabetes mellitus (26% vs 28%), habitual alcoholism (13% vs 24%), mean duration of CHF (4.4 years vs 2.6 years), mean survival following clinically apparent AMI (9.4 years vs 6.6 years), or mean heart weight (604 g vs 571 g).

Compared to the 59 patients without, the 22 patients with a history of diabetes mellitus had a significantly longer mean duration of CHF (5.3 years vs 2.8 years); there was no significant difference in mean age (64 years vs 61 years), frequency of systemic hypertension (36% vs 44%), habitual alcoholism (27% vs 17%), mean survival after clinically apparent AMI (7.7 years vs 8.1 years), mean heart weight (575 g vs 588 g) and mean percent of 5-mm segments narrowed by atherosclerotic plaques 76 to 100% in XSA (27% vs 22%).

Compared to the 47 patients without, the 34 patients with a history of systemic hypertension had no significant difference in mean age (62 years vs 62 years), frequency of diabetes mellitus (24% vs 30%), habitual alcoholism (21% vs 19%), mean duration of CHF (3.9 years vs 3.0 years), mean survival after clinically apparent AMI (8.5 years vs 7.7 years), mean heart weight (585 g vs 585 g), and mean percent of 5-mm segments of 4 major epicardial coronary arteries narrowed by atherosclerotic plaque 76 to 100% (23% vs 23%).

Compared with the 65 patients without, the 16 patients with a history of habitual alcoholism had no significant difference in mean age (60 years vs 62 years), frequency of systemic hypertension (44% vs 42%), diabetes mellitus (38% vs 25%), mean duration

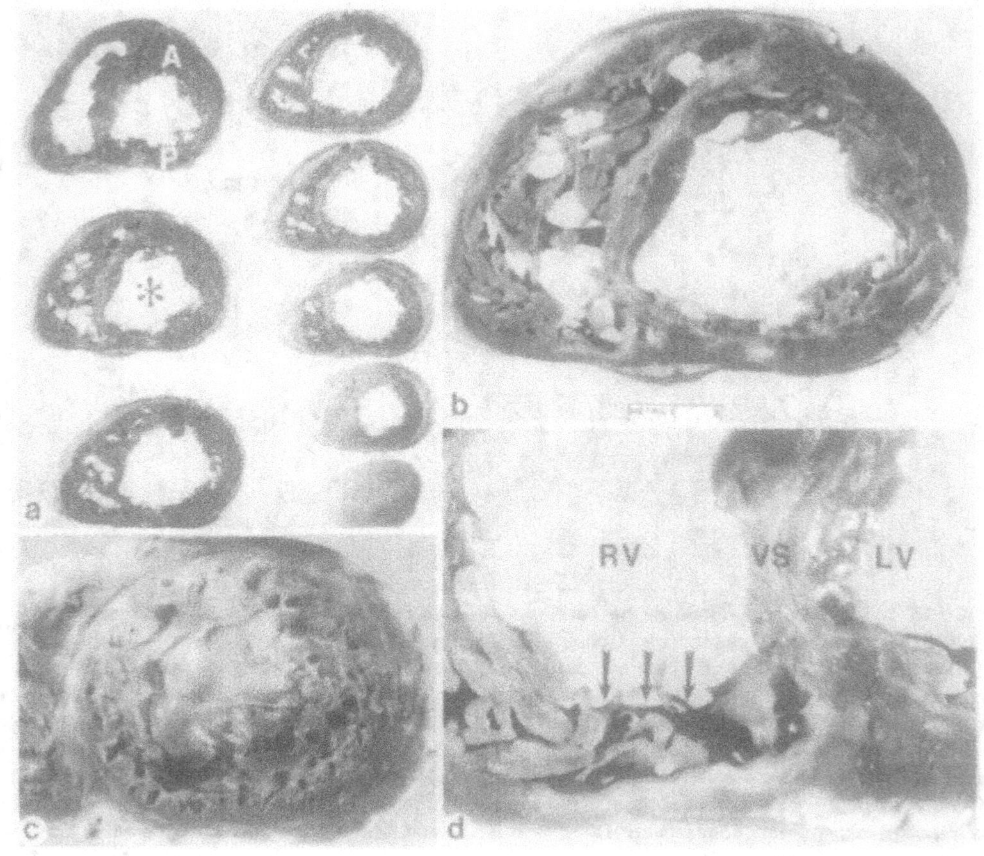

FIGURE 6. Cardic ventricles in a 56-year-old man (DCVAH #A83-47). At necropsy, the heart weighed 550 g and 3 of the 4 major epicardial coronary arteries were narrowed >75% in cross-sectional area by atherosclerotic plaque. a, transverse sections showing severe thinning and scarring of the ventricular septum and of adjacent anterior (A) and posterior (P) left ventricular free walls. b, transverse section with the asterisk in a. c, apex of left ventricle showing severe endocardial thickening. d, close-up of posterior right ventricular (RV) and left ventricular (LV) free walls and of ventricular septum (VS). Arrows point to severe scarring in the right ventricular wall.

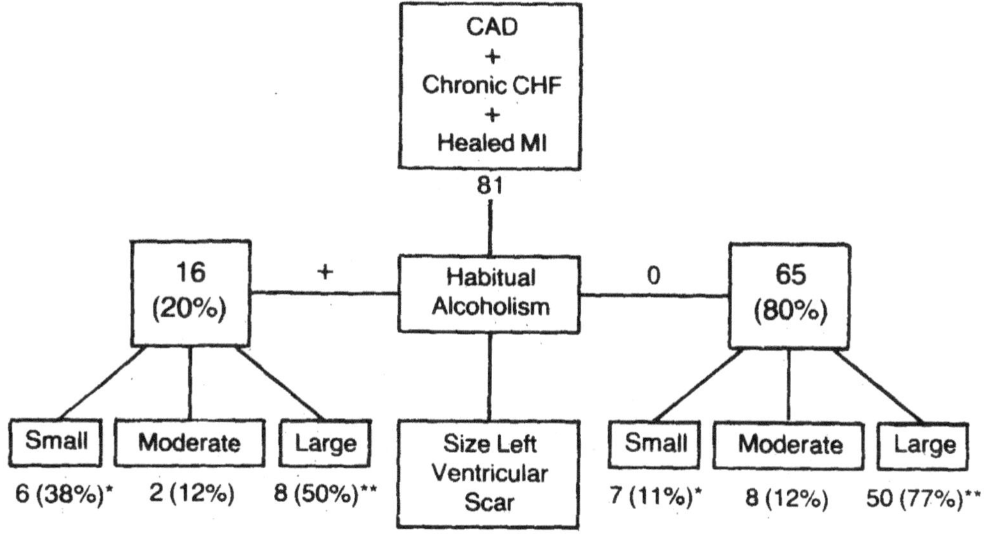

FIGURE 7. Comparison of myocardial infarct size in the 16 patients with a history of habitual alcoholism to the 65 patients without a history of habitual alcoholism. The percentage differences between the small (38% vs 11%) and between the large (50% vs 77%) infarcts in the 2 groups are significant (p <0.05). CAD = coronary artery disease; CHF = congestive heart failure; MI = myocardial infarction.

of CHF (3.5 years vs 3.4 years), mean survival after clinically apparent AMI (8.1 years vs 8.0 years), mean heart weight (600 g vs 580 g), and mean percent of 5-mm segments of the 4 major epicardial coronary arteries narrowed 76 to 100% in XSA by atherosclerotic plaque (28% vs 22%).

Compared to the 65 patients with, the 16 patients without a clinically apparent AMI had a significantly greater frequency of habitual alcoholism (44% vs 14%); there was no difference in frequency of systemic hypertension (56% vs 38%), mean age (60 years vs 62 years), diabetes mellitus (25% vs 28%), mean duration of CHF (4.1 years vs 3.3 years), mean heart weight (629 g vs 574 g), and mean percent of 5-mm segments of the 4 major epicardial coronary arteries narrowed 76 to 100% in XSA by atherosclerotic plaque (13% vs 25%). Of the 65 patients who had a clinically apparent AMI, 59 patients had AMI as their initial manifestation of CAD. Of the 65 patients with clinically apparent AMI, 19 (29%) lived 12 months or less after the onset of CHF; 12 (19%) lived 13 to 24 months after the onset of CHF; 23 (35%) lived longer than 24 months after the onset of CHF and 11 (17%) lived for an unknown number of months after the onset of CHF. Of the 16 patients without clinically apparent AMI, 4 (25%) lived for less than 12 months after the onset of CHF; 1 (6%) lived for less than 24 months after the onset of CHF; 6 (38%) lived longer than 24 months after the onset of CHF; and 5 (31%) lived for an unknown number of months.

After the initial manifestation of CAD, 11 patients (13.5%) survived 12 months or less; 8 patients (10%), 13 to 24 months; 51 patients (63%) lived longer than 24 months; and 11 (13.5%) for an unknown number of months. After clinically apparent AMI, 4 patients (6%) survived for 12 months or less; 6 patients (9%), 13 to 24 months; 44 patients (68%), longer than 24 months and 11 patients (17%), for an unknown number of months. After the onset of CHF 14 patients (17%) survived for 12 months or less; 22 patients (27%), 13 to 24 months; 29 patients (36%), longer than 24 months; and 16 (20%), for an unknown number of months.

Compared with the 58 patients with a large LV scar, the 13 patients with a small LV scar had a significantly increased frequency of habitual alcoholism (46% vs 14%) and increased heart weight (658 g vs 554 g); there was no significant difference in mean age (62 years vs 62 years), frequency of systemic hypertension (46% vs 43%), diabetes mellitus (38% vs 29%), mean duration of CHF (4.7 years vs 3.3 years), survival after clinically aparent AMI (6.2 years vs 8.2 years), and mean percent of 5-mm segments of 4 major epicardial coronary arteries narrowed 76 to 100% in XSA by atherosclerotic plaque (36% vs 22%).

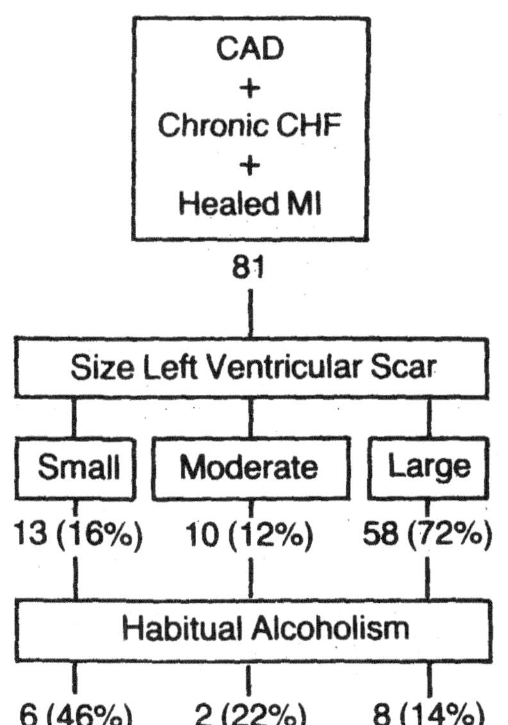

FIGURE 8. Relation of healed myocardial infarct size to frequency of a history of habitual alcoholism in the 81 patients. Patients with small left ventricular scars had a high frequency of alcoholism and those with large infarcts, a relatively low frequency. CAD = coronary artery disease; CHF = congestive heart failure; MI = myocardial infarction.

Discussion

Each of the 81 patients described herein had functional class III or IV (New York Heart Association classification) CHF for at least 3 months, each at necropsy had dilated right and left cardiac ventricles and hearts of increased weight (>400 g [mean 585]). Additional evidence of the severe degree of the CHF was the finding that 46% of the patients had intracardiac thrombi. Although the degree of CHF was similar, the duration of the CHF among the patients was variable (range 0.25 to 16 years, mean 3.4). In contrast to the similar degrees of CHF in all 81 patients, severity of the CAD and extent of LV scarring was variable. In all 81 patients at least 1 of the 4 major epicardial coronary arteries was narrowed 76 to 100% in XSA by atherosclerotic plaque: in 24 patients (30%) only 1 artery was so narrowed at some point (1 vessel CAD); in 22 patients (27%), 2 arteries were so narrowed; in 32 patients (39%), 3 arteries; and in only 3 patients (4%), 4 arteries (including the left main) were so narowed. The variability of the CAD was confirmed by examination of each 5-mm segment of the 4 major coronary arteries in 56 patients. Of 2,999 segments examined, 691 (23%) were narrowed 76 to 100% in XSA by atherosclerotic plaque, but the number of segments narrowed >75% in XSA in the 56 patients was variable (from 1 [1%] to 40 [80%]).

Size of LV scar also varied. Of the 81 patients, 58 (72%) had large scars, 10 (12%) had moderate-sized scars and 13 (16%) had small scars. The size of LV scar did not correlate with severity of the CAD.

Although it did not correlate with the severity of the coronary arterial narrowing, size of the LV scars did correlate with the presence of habitual alcoholism (Fig. 7 and 8). Of the 16 habitual alcoholics, 6 (38%) had small and 8 (50%) had large LV scars; in contrast, of the 65 non-alcoholics, 7 (11%) had small and 50 (77%) had large LV scars (p <0.05). Conversely, of the 13 patients with small LV scars, 6 (46%) were habitual alcoholics and 7 (54%) were not; in contrast, of the 58 patients with large LV scars, only 8 (14%) were habitual alcoholics and 50 (86%) were not (p <0.05) (Fig. 8).

Although mean severity of the coronary arterial narrowing in the 2 groups was similar, the explanation for chronic CHF may be different in patients with large and those with small LV scars. It is reasonable to attribute the chronic CHF in the patients with large LV scars to the presence of the LV scar. In contrast, it is not reasonable to attribute the chronic CHF in the patients with the small LV scars to ischemia-induced LV dysfunction. Because a large percentage of patients with small LV scars were habitual alcoholics (Fig. 8), it is likely that alcoholism contributed significantly to chronic CHF in them. By definition, however, one cannot diagnose idiopathic dilated cardiomyopathy (or alcoholic cardiomyopathy) in patients with severe coronary arterial narrowing. Nevertheless, these 2 conditions must coexist in an occasional patient.

Although all 81 patients at necropsy had healed myocardial infarcts, a clinical event diagnosed as AMI occurred in 65 patients (80%); in the other 16 patients (20%), the AMI had been clinically silent. The frequency of the small and large LV scars were different between the patients with clinically recognized and clinically unrecognized AMI (Fig. 9). Of the 65 patients with clinically recognized infarcts, 52 (80%) had large and 5 (8%) had small infarcts; in contrast, of the 16 patients with clinically unrecognized infarcts, 6 (38%) had large and 8 (50%) had small infarcts. Conversely, of the 58 patients with large LV scars, 52 (90%) had had clinically apparent acute myocardial infarcts, and of the 13 patients with small LV scars only 5 (38%) had had clinically apparent infarcts.

Although frequency of small and large LV scars was different between the patients with clinically recognized and those with unrecognized AMI, the severity of the CAD was similar in the 2 groups. The duration of chronic CHF was not significantly different between the patients with clinically recognized and those with clinically unrecognized AMI (3.3 years vs 4.1 years). The frequency of habitual alcoholism was different between the groups of patients with clinically recognized and clinically unrecognized AMI (14% vs 44%). Frequency of systemic hypertension and diabetes mellitus was similar between the 2 groups (38%

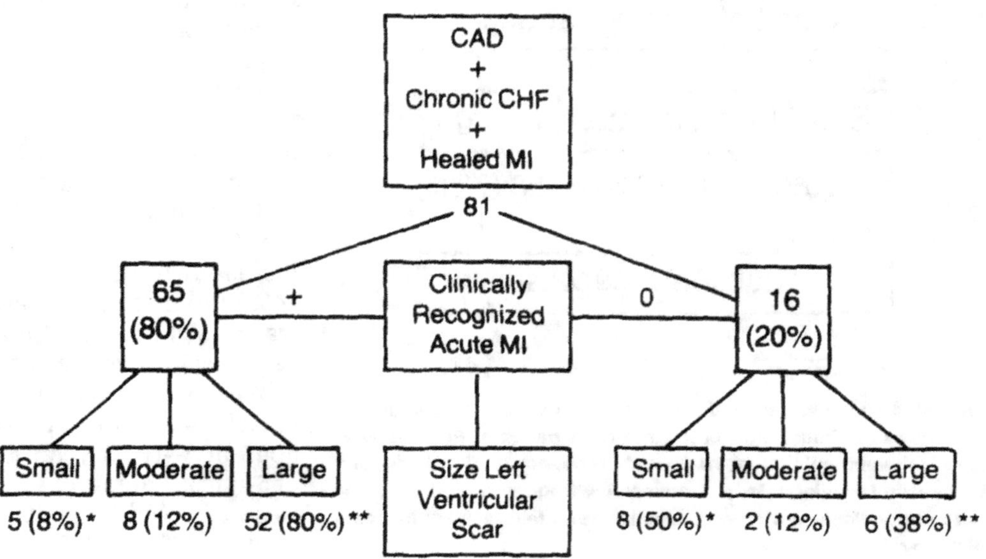

FIGURE 9. Comparison of the sizes of the left ventricular scars in the 65 patients with clinically recognized acute myocardial infarction (MI) to the 16 patients with a clinically inapparent acute MI. The percentage differences between the small (8% vs 50%) and large (80% vs 38%) sized left ventricular scars between the 2 groups are significant (p <0.05). CAD = coronary artery disease; CHF = congestive heart failure; MI = myocardial infarction.

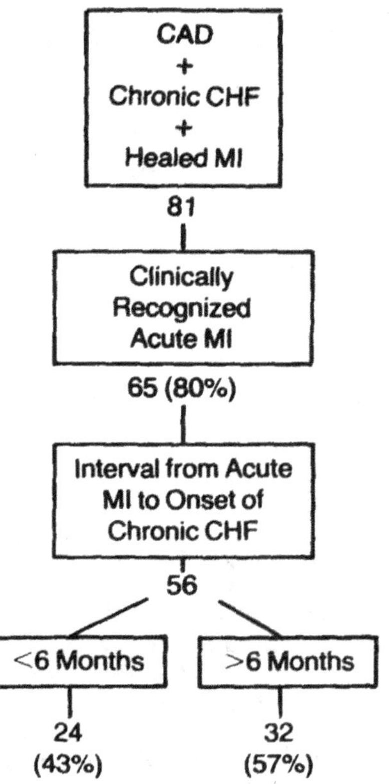

FIGURE 10. Frequency of an interval of less than or more than 6 months from clinically recognized acute myocardial infarction (MI) to onset of chronic congestive heart failure (CHF) in the 65 patients with clinically recognized acute MI. CAD = coronary artery disease.

vs 56% and 28% vs 25%, respectively). (Duration of symptoms of myocardial ischemia or of chronic CHF was determined from the onset of the initial AMI when more than 1 clinical infarct had occurred.)

Duration of survival from onset of clinical AMI to death in the 65 patients with clinically recognized AMI ranged from 5 to 384 months (mean 95). The duration of chronic CHF in these 65 patients ranged from 3 to 132 months (mean 39). This difference in duration of survival from onset of the first clinical AMI and onset of chronic CHF is explained by a delayed onset of CHF after AMI in many patients. Of the 65 with clinical evidence of AMI, time of onset of CHF after AMI was well established in 56 patients. This interval was ≤6 months in 24 (43%) and >6 months in 32 (57%) (Fig. 10). The explanation for this delay in onset of CHF after AMI is unclear. Mean duration of chronic CHF, however, was similar (p >0.05) in the 16 patients with clini-

cally unrecognized AMI and in the 65 with clinically recognized AMI (49 months vs 39 months).

Frequency distribution of mode of death in the 81 patients was a bit different from that of the usual group of patients with fatal CAD. Of the 81 patients, for example, only 16 (20%) died suddenly, whereas sudden death is the mode of death in about 50% of all patients with fatal CAD. Only 11 patients (14%) died of AMI. Progressive CHF was the major cause of death in 48 patients (59%). Six patients (7%) died of consequences of either systemic (2 patients) or pulmonary emboli (4 patients).

Few previous necropsy studies have been reported in patients with chronic CHF, severe CAD and LV transmural scars. Burch et al[2] described clinical and necropsy findings in 2 patients with "ischemic cardiomyopathy." Both had extensive LV scarring and CAD. Yatteau et al[3] described clinical features in 66 patients with severe CAD and LV ejection fractions ≤25%; 41 (62%) of them had functional class III or IV CHF (New York Heart Association classification). Of the 66 patients, 24 had died and necropsy was done in 5. All 5 had large LV scars and hearts of increased weight (mean 506 g), but all 5 had aortocoronary bypass grafting operations. Schuster and Bulkley[4] described necropsy findings in 14 patients who had chronic CHF, extensive CAD, dilated cardiac ventricles, hearts of increased weight (mean 600 g), and LV scars varying in size from small to large. These investigators, however, eliminated from the study patients with histories of systemic hypertension or habitual alcoholism. Thus, comparison of our data with those of others is not very useful.

Acknowledgment: We appreciate the technical assistance of Alvado Campbell, Filippina Giacometti and Barbara Winterrowd in preparation of the histology slides. The gross photographs were taken by Margaret Moore.

References

1. Virmani R, Roberts WC. *Quantification of coronary arterial narrowing and of left ventricular myocardial scarring in healed myocardial infarction with chronic, eventually fatal, congestive cardiac failure. Am J Med 1980; 68:831–838.*
2. Burch GE, Tsui CY, Harb JM. *Ischemic cardiomyopathy. Am Heart J 1972;83:340–350.*
3. Yatteau RF, Peter RH, Behar VS, Bartel AG, Rosati RA, Kong Y. *Ischemic cardiomyopathy: the myopathy of coronary artery disease. Natural history and results of medical versus surgical treatment. Am J Cardiol 1974; 34:520–525.*
4. Schuster EH, Bulkley BH. *Ischemic cardiomyopathy: clinicopathologic study of fourteen patients. Am Heart J 1980;100:506–512.*

Severe Atherosclerotic Coronary Arterial Narrowing and Chronic Congestive Heart Failure Without Myocardial Infarction: Analysis of 18 Patients Studied at Necropsy

ELIZABETH M. ROSS, MD, and WILLIAM C. ROBERTS, MD

Observations are reported on 18 patients (aged 38 to 73 years ([mean 58]; 16 [89%] men) studied at necropsy who had had chronic congestive heart failure (CHF) more than 3 months in duration, >75% cross-sectional area (XSA) narrowing of 1 or more of the 4 major epicardial coronary arteries, and no left ventricular fibrosis or necrosis. Duration of symptoms from onset of CHF to death ranged from 0.3 to 13 years (mean 5.7). Angina pectoris occurred in 2 patients (11%). The mode of death was CHF in 12 (67%), sudden (arrhythmia) in 5 (28%), and emboli in 1 (5%). Heart weight ranged from 410 to 890 g (mean 632). Of 72 major epicardial coronary arteries (right, left main, left anterior descending, left circumflex) in the 18 patients, 30 (42%) were narrowed 76 to 100% in XSA by atherosclerotic plaque (right = 10, left main = 0, left anterior descending = 9 and left circumflex = 11). A mean of 1.7 of 4 major epicardial coronary arteries per patient were narrowed 76 to 100% in XSA by atherosclerotic plaque. In 10 patients, each 5-mm segment of the 4 major coronary arteries was examined histologically (mean 53 per patient): 23 segments (3%) were narrowed 96 to 100% in XSA by atherosclerotic plaque; 58 (11%), 76 to 95; 93 (18%), 51 to 75%; 209 (40%), 26 to 50%, and 146 (28%), 0 to 25%. Left and right ventricular thrombi were found in 9 patients (50%); of the 9 patients, 1 had a systemic embolus; of the 9 patients without intraventricular thrombi, none had systemic emboli. Because grossly visible myocardial lesions were absent, the severe chronic CHF in these 18 patients cannot reasonably be attributed to coronary artery disease. It is most reasonable to believe that this group of patients had idiopathic dilated cardiomyopathy and the coronary artery disease was coincidental.

(Am J Cardiol 1986;57:51–56)

Chronic congestive heart failure (CHF) in patients with severe atherosclerotic coronary artery disease (CAD) and dilated cardiac ventricles usually is associated with considerable left ventricular (LV) wall scarring. Chronic CHF in patients without CAD, valvular, congenital, infiltrative or pericardial heart disease but with dilated LV cavities most commonly is a result of idiopathic dilated cardiomegaly. An occasional patient with severe CAD, however, may have chronic CHF and very dilated cardiac ventricular cavities but no ventricular wall scarring or necrosis. The explanation for the chronic CHF in this latter group of patients is unclear. This report describes clinical and necropsy findings in 18 patients with dilated cardiac ventricles and severe atherosclerotic coronary arterial narrowing but no LV scarring or necrosis.

From the Pathology Branch, National Heart, Lung, and Blood Institute, National Institutes of Health, Bethesda, Maryland. Manuscript received June 21, 1985, accepted June 24, 1985.

Dr. Ross's present address and address for reprints: Washington Hospital Center, 110 Irving Street, NW, Room 3B-44B, Washington, D.C. 20010.

Methods

The cardiac diagnoses were reviewed in the nearly 7,500 necropsy patients accessioned in the Pathology Branch of the National Heart, Lung, and Blood Institute. The records of all patients diagnosed as having CAD were reviewed. The criteria for inclusion in the study were: (1) narrowing >75% in cross-sectional area (XSA) by atherosclerotic plaque of at least 1 major epicardial coronary artery; (2) absence of LV or ventricular septal replacement fibrosis or necrosis; (3) dilatation, by visual inspection, of both right ventricular and LV cavities; (4) absence of infiltrative myocardial disease or of pericardial or cardiac valve disease sufficient to cause cardiac dysfunction; (5) absence of congenital anomalies of the heart or great vessels; (6) presence of left-sided CHF for more than 3 months; (7) death resulting from or related to cardiac disease; and (8) heart weight >350 g in a woman and >400 g in a man. Eighteen patients fulfilled these criteria and form the basis of this report. All 18 patients were studied from 1971 through 1984.

In the 10 hearts with intact epicardial coronary arteries, the 4 major epicardial coronary arteries were

TABLE I Clinical and Necropsy Findings in the 18 Patients

Pt	Age (yr)	Duration of CHF (yr)	Race	Sex	AP	A	DM	SH	Systemic BP (mm Hg)		Mode of Death	BBB	HW (g)	Thrombus				No. CA >75%	No.5-mm CA Segments	CA Segments Narrowed in XSA (%)				
									Systole	Diastole				RV	LV	RA	LA			0–25	26–50	51–75	76–95	96–100
1	38	4	B	M	0	+	0	0			CHF	U	660	+	+	0	0	3	53	9	7	9	21	7
2	43	4	W	M	0	0	0	0	110	70	CHF	0	700	0	0	0	0	2	42	2	32	4	1	3
3	50	2	W	M	0	0	0	0	85	60	S	0	555	+	+	0	0	3	39	0	6	10	11	12
4	50	4	W	M	0	0	+	0			CHF	0	790	0	0	+	+	1						
5	52	5	B	M	0	0	+	+	130	90	S	L	600	0	+	+	+	1						
6	53	*	W	F	0	0	+	+	150	100	CHF	0	550	+	+	0	0	2						
7	53	†	W	M	0	0	0	0			S	U	790	0	0	0	0	1	34	10	18	5	1	0
8	55	5	B	M	0	+	0	0			CHF	0	490	+	0	+	0	1						
9	57	4	B	M	0	+	+	+	150	80	PE	0	730	+	0	0	0	1	63	14	30	18	0	1
10	59	†	B	F	0	0	+	0			CHF	U	520	+	+	0	0	2						
11	60	6	W	M	0	+	0	0	120	70	CHF	0	440	0	0	0	0	1						
12	60	13	B	M	0	0	0	+	180	100	S	0	660	0	0	0	0	3	65	27	26	8	4	0
13	66	8	B	M	+	+	0	0	110	80	S	R	690	0	0	0	0	1	53	42	10	0	1	0
14	68	7	B	M	0	+	0	+	160	100	CHF	0	410	0	+	+	0	3	47	10	20	11	6	0
15	68	8	W	M	0	0	0	0			CHF	L	470	0	0	0	0	1						
16	70	10	W	M	0	0	0	+	150	100	CHF	L	810	0	+	0	0	1						
17	71	*	W	M	0	0	+	+			CHF	U	620	0	0	+	0	1	60	14	20	18	8	0
18	73	3	W	M	+	0	0	+	160	100	CHF	L	890	0	0	0	0	2	73	18	40	10	5	0

* = CHF for at least 3 months; † = CHF for at least 2 years.

A = history of habitual alcoholism; Age = age at death; AP = angina pectoris; B = black; BBB = bundle branch block; BP = blood pressure; CA = coronary artery; CHF = congestive heart failure; DM = diabetes mellitus; F = female; HW = heart weight; LA = left atrium; LV = left ventricle; M = male; PE = pulmonary embolus; R = right; RA = right atrium; RV = right ventricle; S = sudden; SE = systemic embolus; SH = history of systemic hypertension; U = unknown; W = white; XSA = cross-sectional area; + = present; 0 = absent.

removed from the heart intact, sectioned into 5-mm-long segments, decalcified, processed in alcohols and xylene, embedded in paraffin, cut into 6-μ-thick sections, placed on a glass slide, stained with Movat's trichrome method and examined by one of us (EMR) under the microscope at a magnification of 40 times. The XSA narrowing was graded in 5 categories: 0 to 25%, 26 to 50%, 51 to 75%, 76 to 95% and 96 to 100%. One to 4 (mean 3) histologic sections of LV free wall or ventricular septum extending from endocardium to epicardium and stained with hematoxalin-eosin were prepared and examined from 15 patients. The other 3 hearts were not available for reexamination.

Results were evaluated using Student t test and chi-square test. A p value of <0.05 was considered statistically significant.

Results

Certain observations in the 18 patients are provided in Table I. The 18 patients were 38 to 73 years old (mean 58); 16 (89%) were men. The duration of CHF from onset of symptoms to death ranged from 0.3 to 13 years (mean 5.7) (Fig. 1). Diabetes mellitus (adult-onset in all) was present in 6 patients (33%); a history of chronic alcohol abuse in 6 patients (33%); and a history of systemic hypertension in 8 patients (44%). Blood pressure recordings, available in 11 patients during the last year of life, ranged from 85/60 to 180/100 mm Hg (mean 137/86): the systolic pressure was >140 mm Hg in 6 and the diastolic pressure was >90 mm Hg in 5 patients. At least 2 patients had angina pectoris. Of 13 patients with available electrocardiograms recorded during the last 12 months of life, 1 had complete right and 4 had complete left bundle branch block. Two patients (nos. 13 and 17) had chronic obstructive pulmonary disease; 2 (nos. 3 and 9) had a stroke at some time and 2 (nos. 11 and 12) had symptomatic peripheral vascular disease. The mode of death was CHF in 12 patients (67%), sudden (arrhythmia) in 5 (28%) and embolus in 1 (5%).

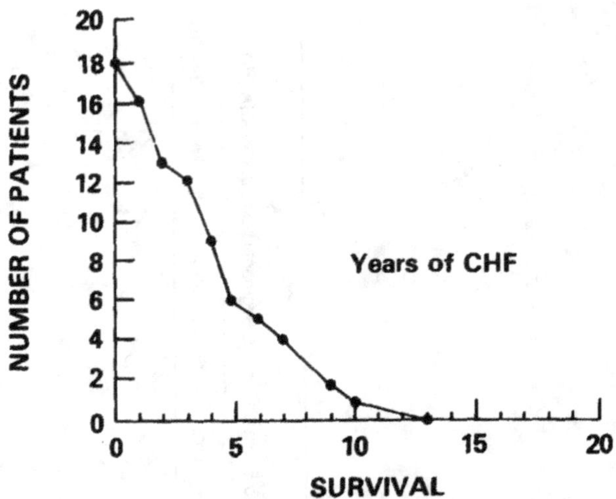

FIGURE 1. Length of survival (in years) after onset of congestive heart failure (CHF) in the 18 patients.

Heart weight ranged from 410 to 890 g (mean 632). Of 72 major coronary arteries examined in the 18 patients (4 per patient), 30 (42%) were narrowed 76 to 100% in XSA by atherosclerotic plaque at some point (right = 10; left main = 0; left anterior descending = 9; and left circumflex = 11). A mean of 1.7 of the 4 major coronary arteries per patient were narrowed 76 to 100% in XSA by plaque. Of the 18 patients, 10 (56%) had 1 of the 4 major coronary arteries narrowed 76 to 100% in XSA by plaque, 4 (22%) had 2 arteries so narrowed, and 4 (22%) had 3 arteries so narrowed. No patient had 4 arteries narrowed 75 to 100% in XSA.

In 10 patients, the entire lengths of each of the 4 major coronary arteries were divided into 5-mm-long segments and a histologic section was prepared from each 5-mm segment. The number of segments examined per patient ranged from 34 to 73 (mean 53). Of the 529 total segments examined (Fig. 2), 23 (3%) were narrowed 96 to 100% in XSA; 51 (11%), 76 to 95%; 93 (18%), 51 to 75%; 209 (40%), 26 to 50%; and 146 (28%), 0

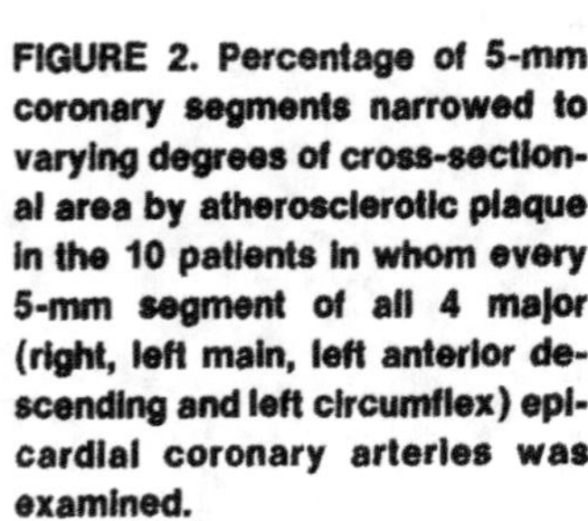

FIGURE 2. Percentage of 5-mm coronary segments narrowed to varying degrees of cross-sectional area by atherosclerotic plaque in the 10 patients in whom every 5-mm segment of all 4 major (right, left main, left anterior descending and left circumflex) epicardial coronary arteries was examined.

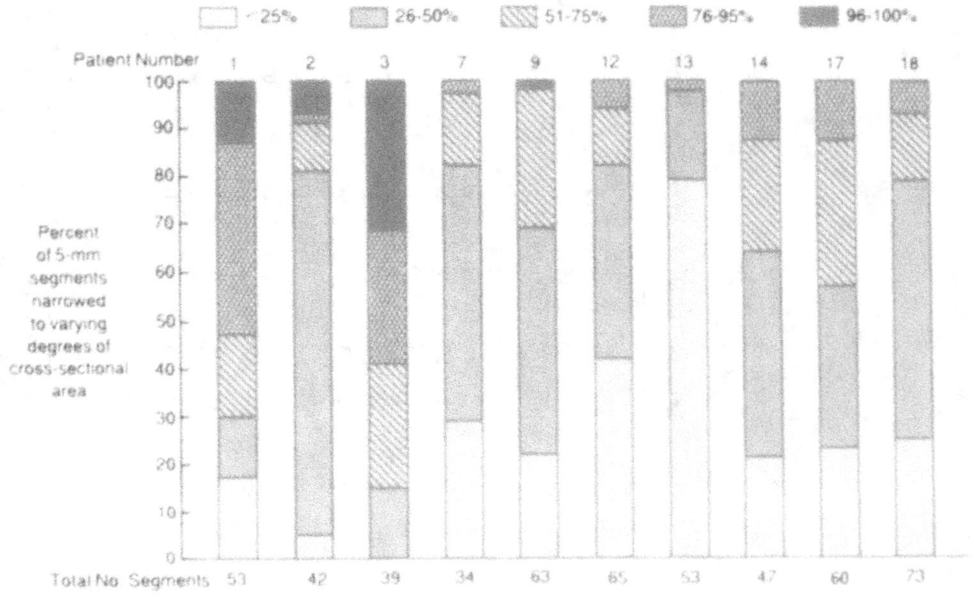

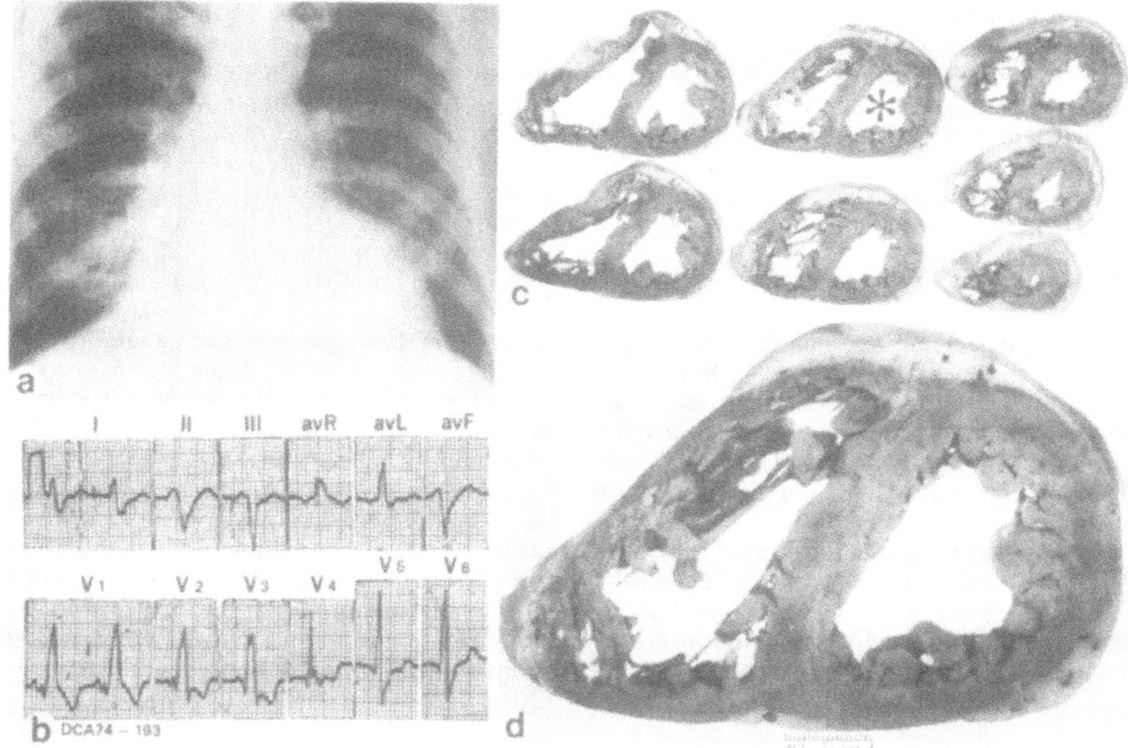

FIGURE 3. Patient 13 (Table I). *a*, chest radiograph showing an enlarged cardiac silhouette and pulmonary venous congestion. *b*, electrocardiogram showing left-axis deviation and right bundle branch block. *c*, transverse sections of the cardiac ventricles showing dilated cavities but no grossly visible myocardial lesions. *d*, close-up of section marked by *asterisk* in *c*.

to 25%. Histologic examination of the myocardial sections did not show significant abnormalities of the intramural coronary arteries with the exception of occasional intimal and medial thickening in the intramural coronary arteries of the LV papillary muscles. There

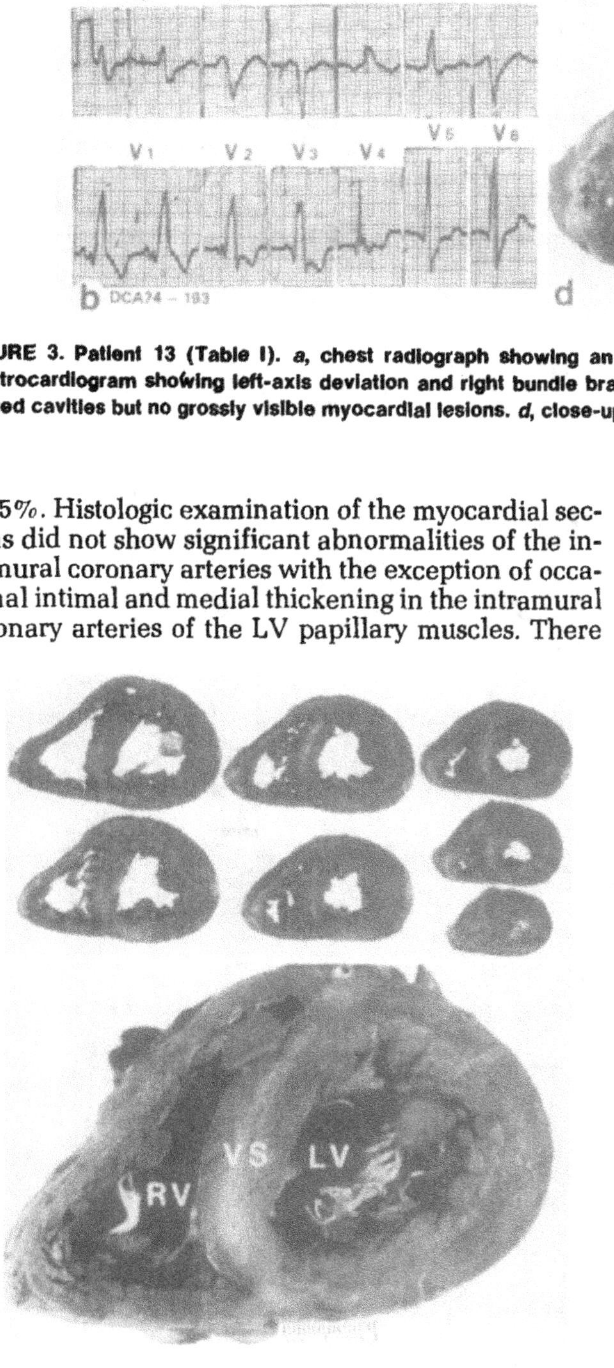

FIGURE 4. Patient 14 (Table I). Transverse sections of the cardiac ventricles (*upper*) and of the basal portion of the heart (*lower*) showing dilated right (RV) and left ventricles (LV) and no grossly visible myocardial lesions. VS = ventricular septum.

was no significant abnormalities of the intramural vessels of left or right ventricular free wall or ventricular septum.

Left or right ventricular thrombi, or both, were found in 9 patients (50%); 1 had a systemic embolus; of the 9 patients without intraventricular thrombi, none had systemic emboli (Fig. 3 to 5).

Seven factors were analyzed after the patients were divided into groups based on the presence or absence of diabetes mellitus, systemic hypertension (by history) and habitual alcoholism (by history).

Compared to the 10 patients without, the 8 patients with a history of systemic hypertension had an insignificant difference in mean age (63 years vs 54 years), frequency of diabetes mellitus (4 of 8 pateients vs 2 of 10 patients), habitual alcoholism (2 of 8 patients vs 4 of 10 patients), mean duration of CHF (7.0 years vs 5.1 years), mean heart weight (660 g vs 611 g) and mean percent of 5-mm segments of the 4 major epicardial coronary arteries narrowed 76 to 100% in XSA by atherosclerotic plaque (5% vs 26%).

Compared to the 12 patients without, the 6 patients with a history of diabetes mellitus had an insignificant difference in mean age (57 years vs 59 years), frequency of systemic hypertension (4 of 6 patients vs 4 of 12 patients), alcoholism (1 of 6 patients vs 5 of 12 patients), mean duration of CHF (4.3 years vs 6.4 years), mean heart weight (635 g vs 630 g), and mean percent of 5-mm segments of the 4 major epicardial coronary arteries narrowed 76 to 100% in XSA by atherosclerotic plaque (2% vs 17%).

Compared to the 12 patients without, the 6 patients with a history of habitual alcoholism had an insignificant difference in mean age (57 years vs 59 years), frequency of a history of systemic hypertension (2 of 6 patients vs 6 of 12 patients), history of diabetes mellitus (1 of 6 patients vs 5 of 12 patients), mean duration of CHF (5.7 years vs 6.1 years), mean heart weight (570 g vs 662 g), and mean percent of 5-mm segments of the 4 major epicardial coronary arteries narrowed 76 to 100% in XSA by atherosclerotic plaque (16% vs 11%).

Discussion

Each of the 18 patients described above had severe CHF for longer than 3 months, hearts of increased heart weight (mean 632 g) with dilated right and LV cavities and frequent (50%) ventricular thrombi. The severity of CAD, however, was less than is usually seen in patients with other types of fatal coronary events.[1-12] Ten patients (56%) had only 1 of the 4 major epicardial coronary arteries narrowed >75% in XSA by atherosclerotic plaque and for the entire group of 18 patients, a mean of only 1.7 of the 4 major epicardial coronary arteries were narrowed >75% in XSA by atherosclerotic plaque. Of the 529 five-millimeter segments of major coronary arteries examined micro-

scopically (10 patients), only 14% were narrowed >75% by atherosclerotic plaque and none had coronary arterial thrombi. In contrast, about 33% of the 5-mm segments from patients with fatal CAD who died suddenly or with acute myocardial infarction but without CHF were narrowed >75% in XSA by plaque.[1,3,8,11,12]

Only 2 patients (11%) had angina, 8 (44%) a history of systemic hypertension, 6 (33%) diabetes mellitus, and 6 (33%) habitual alcoholism. Insignificant differences occurred among the patients in frequency of a history of systemic hypertension, diabetes mellitus and habitual alcoholism; in mean age; mean duration of CHF; mean heart weight; and mean percent of 5-mm segments of the 4 major epicardial coronary arteries narrowed 76 to 100% in XSA.

If coronary arterial narrowing were not present, these 18 patients would have typical features of dilated cardiomegaly (increased heart weight, dilated right and LV cavities). Diagnosis of dilated cardiomegaly, however, is not proper when significant coronary arterial narrowing is present. Nevertheless, it is unreasonable to attribute the severe CHF in the 18 patients

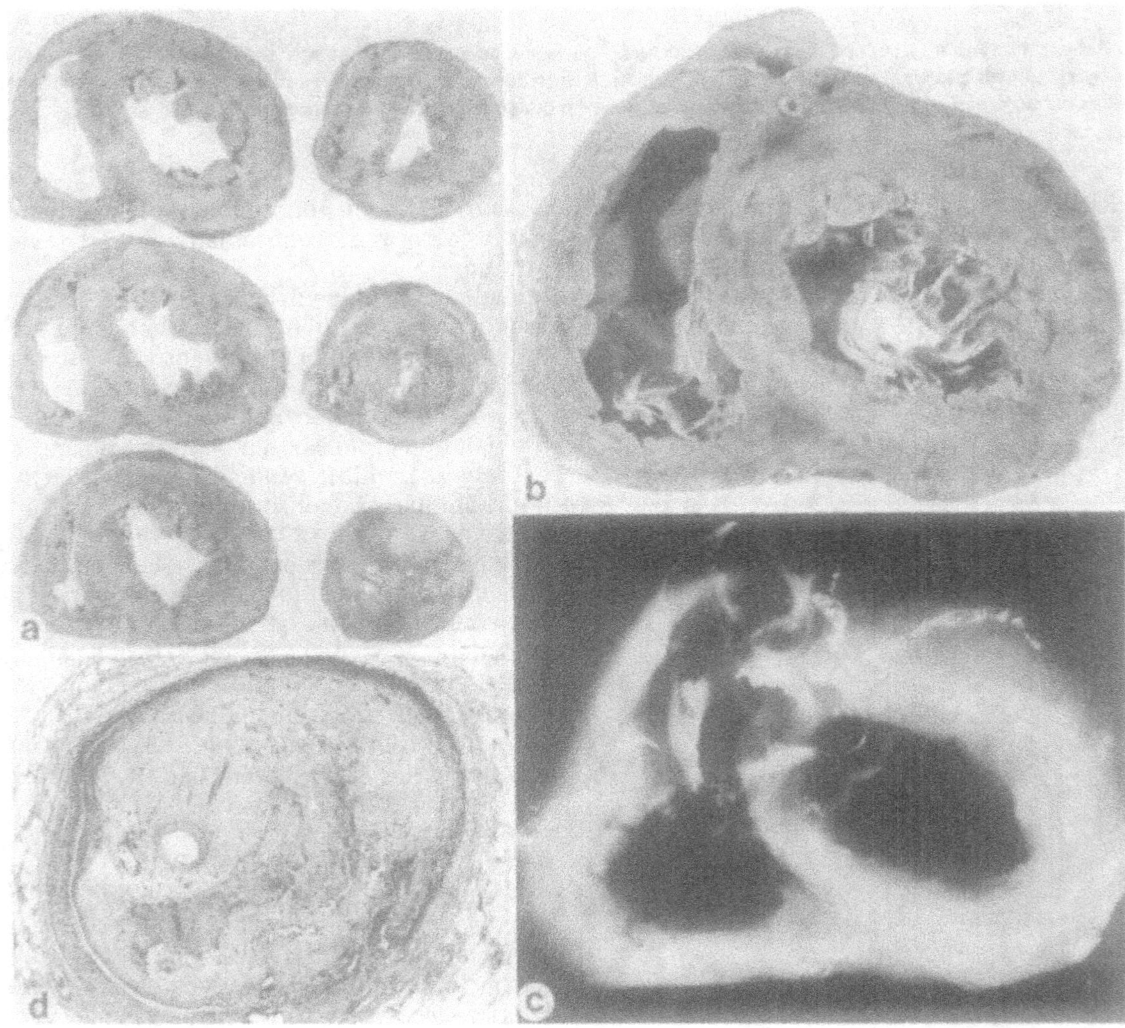

FIGURE 5. Patient 18 (Table I). *a* and *b*, transverse sections of the cardiac ventricles (*a*), basal portion of the heart (*b*), showing dilated right and left ventricular cavities and no grossly visible myocardial lesions. *c*, radiograph of postmortem specimen showing heavy calcific deposits of the epicardial coronary arteries. *d*, photomicrograph of a cross-section of right coronary artery showing severe luminal narrowing by atherosclerotic plaque. Movat trichrome stain; original magnification ×27.

solely to coronary narrowing in the absence of myocardial fibrosis or necrosis. Therefore, our 18 patients probably had dilated cardiomegaly and the CAD was coincidental.

Acknowledgment: We thank Filippina Giacometti, Barbara Winterrowd and Alvado Campbell for preparation of the histology slides, and Margaret Moore for taking the gross photographs.

References

1. Roberts WC, Jones AA. *Quantitation of coronary arterial narrowing at necropsy in sudden coronary death. Analysis of 31 patients and comparison with 25 control subjects. Am J Cardiol 1979;44:39–45.*

2. Roberts WC, Virmani R. *Quantification of coronary arterial narrowing in clinically-isolated unstable angina pectoris. An analysis of 22 necropsy patients. Am J Med 1979;67:792–799.*

3. Roberts WC, Jones AA. *Quantification of coronary arterial narrowing at necropsy in acute transmural myocardial infarction. Analysis and comparison of findings in 27 patients and 22 controls. Circulation 1980; 61:786–790.*

4. Virmani R, Roberts WC. *Quantification of coronary arterial narrowing and of left ventricular myocardial scarring in healed myocardial infarction with chronic, eventually fatal, congestive cardiac failure. Am J Med 1980;68:831–838.*

5. Cabin HS, Roberts WC. *True left ventricular aneurysm and healed myocardial infarction. Clinical and necropsy observations including quantification of degrees of coronary arterial narrowing. Am J Cardiol 1980;46:754–762.*

6. Cabin HS, Roberts WC. *Quantification of amounts of coronary arterial narrowing in patients with types II and IV hyperlipoproteinemia and in those with known normal lipoprotein patterns. Am Heart J 1981;101:52–58.*

7. Virmani R, Roberts WC. *Non-fatal healed transmural myocardial infarction and fatal non-cardiac disease. Qualification and quantification of coronary arterial narrowing and of left ventricular scarring in 18 necropsy patients. Br Heart J 1981;45:434–441.*

8. Brosius FC, Roberts WC. *Comparison of degree and extent of coronary narrowing by atherosclerotic plaque in anterior and posterior transmural myocardial infarction. Circulation 1981;64:715–722.*

9. Cabin HS, Roberts WC. *Comparison of amount and extent of coronary narrowing by atherosclerotic plaque and of myocardial scarring at necropsy in anterior and posterior healed transmural myocardial infarction. Circulation 1982;66:93–99.*

10. Cabin HS, Roberts WC. *Quantitative comparison of extent of coronary narrowing and size of healed myocardial infarct in 33 necropsy patients with clinically recognized and in 28 with clinically unrecognized ("silent") previous acute myocardial infarction. Am J Cardiol 1982;50:677–681.*

11. Warnes CA, Roberts WC. *Sudden coronary death: relation of amount and distribution of coronary narrowing at necropsy to previous symptoms of myocardial ischemia, left ventricular scarring and heart weight. Am J Cardiol 1984;54:65–73.*

12. Warnes CA, Roberts WC. *Comparison at necropsy by age group of amount and distribution of narrowing by atherosclerotic plaque in 2995 five-mm long segments of 240 major coronary arteries in 60 men aged 31 to 70 years with sudden coronary death. Am Heart J 1984;108:431–435.*

Intussusception of a Coronary Artery Associated with Sudden Death in a College Football Player

WILLIAM C. ROBERTS, MD
MARC A. SILVER, MD
JOSEPH C. SAPALA, MD

Sudden death in competitive athletes is usually the result of cardiac disease. In those younger than 35 years, the most common cause is hypertrophic cardiomyopathy[1] and in those older than 35 years, atherosclerotic coronary heart disease.[2] Among the younger age group, nonatherosclerotic but coronary causes of sudden death have included anomalies of origin, number and courses of these arteries and isolated dissection of 1 or more coronary arteries.[3–6] We recently

From the Pathology Branch, National Heart, Lung, and Blood Institute, National Institutes of Health, Bethesda, Maryland 20205, and the Department of Forensic Sciences, State of Alabama, Montgomery, Alabama. Manuscript received and accepted June 7, 1985.

encountered another nonatherosclerotic type of coronary abnormality associated with sudden death in a football player.

G.P., a 19-year-old black football fullback who weighed 235 pounds and was 68 inches tall, collapsed and died while running. He had been well except for heat stroke on 2 occasions 1 and 2 years earlier. Each episode was characterized by sudden collapse while exercising in hot weather. On the day he died, the first day of the season's football practice, he had a physical examination by the team's physician and no abnormalities were reported. During his final football practice, the temperature on the practice field was 118° F and the humidity nearly 100%. He completed three 440-yard sprints, collapsed during his fourth such sprint and could not be resuscitated.

At necropsy, all body organs except the heart were normal. The heart weighed 480 g and the ventricular septum and left ventricular free wall measured up to 1.9 cm in thickness. No foci of myocardial necrosis or fibrosis were present. All 4 cavities were of normal size, and the 4 valves and epicardium were normal. The right, left main, left anterior descending and left circumflex coronary arteries arose and coursed normally and their lumens were widely patent. The left circumflex artery, however, was hypoplastic. A large ramus intermedius coronary artery arose from the left main artery; at 1 cm from its origin the adventitia was darkened by blood and on sectioning the lumen appeared occluded (Fig. 1). The approximately 1.3-cm occluded segment of ramus intermedius was excised, processed for histologic study, and every twentieth section was stained by the Movat pentachrome method and examined (Fig. 2). Microscopic examination disclosed that the "occlusion" was the result of intussusception of a portion of media and intima.

Intussusception, an invagination or prolapse of a tubular wall into an adjacent protion, has been reported to involve the aorta, an elastic artery, in dissecting aneurysm[7] but not a coronary artery, and sudden death by this mechanism has not been reported previously.

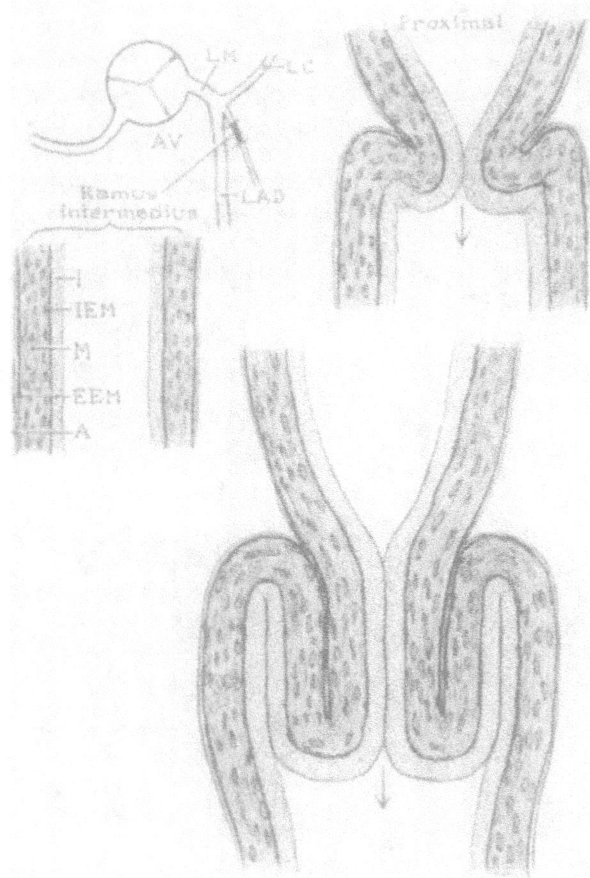

FIGURE 1. Location and appearance of the coronary arterial intussusception in the patient described. A = adventitia; AV = aortic valve; EEM = external elastic membrane; I = intima; IEM = internal elastic membrane; LAD = left anterior descending coronary artery; LC = left circumflex coronary artery; LM = left main coronary artery; M = media.

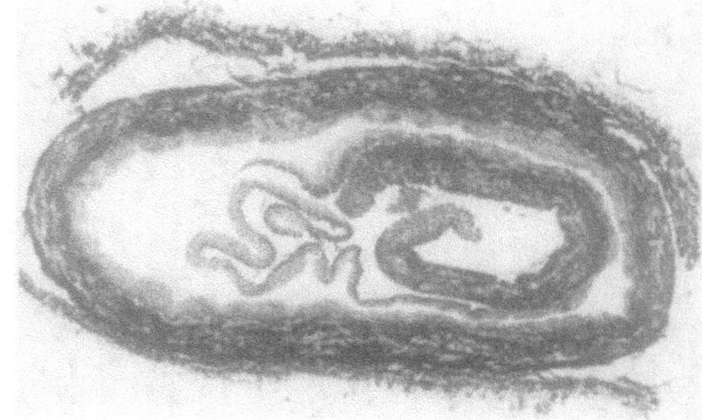

FIGURE 2. Photomicrograph of 1 of the many sections containing the intussusception in the ramus intermedius coronary artery. The intima of the intussusceptum is in apposition to the intima of the intussuscipiens. (Movat stain × 34, reduced 29%.)

References

1. Maron BJ, Roberts WC, McAllister HA, Rosing DR, Epstein SE. *Sudden death in young athletes. Circulation 1980;62:218-229.*

2. Waller BF, Roberts WC. *Sudden death while running in conditioned runners ages 40 years or over. Am J Cardiol 1980;45:1292-1300.*

3. Bulkley BH, Roberts WC. *Dissecting aneurysm (hematoma) limited to coronary artery. A clinicopathologic study of six patients. Am J Med 1973;55:747-756.*

4. Cheitlin MD, DeCastro CM, McCallister HA. *Sudden death as a complication of anomalous left coronary origin from the anterior sinus of Valsalva. A not so minor congenital anomaly. Circulation 1974;50:780-787.*

5. Roberts WC, Siegel RJ, Zipes DP. *Origin of the right coronary artery from the left sinus of Valsalva and its functional consequences: analysis of 10 necropsy patients. Am J Cardiol 1982;49:863-868.*

6. Topaz O, Edwards JE. *Pathologic features of sudden death in children, adolescents, and young adults. Chest 1985;87:476-482.*

7. Roberts WC. *Aortic dissection: anatomy, consequences, and causes. Am Heart J 1981;101:195-214.*

Amounts of Coronary Arterial Narrowing by Atherosclerotic Plaques in Clinically Isolated Mitral Valve Stenosis: Analysis of 76 Necropsy Patients Older Than 30 Years

RONALD N. REIS* and WILLIAM C. ROBERTS, MD

Although several studies have described the status of the coronary arteries by angiography in patients with mitral stenosis (MS), few necropsy studies of the coronary arteries in these patients are available. The present report describes in detail the amounts of narrowing by atherosclerotic plaque of the 4 major epicardial coronary arteries in 76 necropsy patients, aged 31 to 79 years (mean 53) with clinically isolated MS (with or without associated mitral regurgitation but without aortic valve dysfunction). Of the 76 patients, ≥ 1 major coronary artery was narrowed >75% in cross-sectional area (XSA) in 38 (50%) and in 10 of the 38 patients ≥ 1 major coronary artery was totally occluded or nearly so (>95% XSA narrowing). A higher percent of the 29 men had significant (>75% XSA) coronary narrowing than did the 47 women (62 vs 44%) and the men had more major coronary arteries significantly narrowed compared with the women (31 of 116 arteries [27%] vs 33 of 188 arteries [18%]).

The 4 major coronary arteries in the 76 patients were divided into 5-mm segments and examined histologically: of the 3,124 segments (41 per patient), 620 segments (20%) were narrowed 0 to 25% in XSA, 1,826 (58%) were narrowed 26 to 50%, 470 (15%) were narrowed 51 to 75%, 188 (6%) were narrowed 76 to 95%, and 20 segments (1%) were narrowed 96 to 100% in XSA. The percent of segments narrowed >75% in XSA was 9% in the men and 5% in the women. The percent of segments narrowed >75% in XSA was highly variable in the 38 patients with significant narrowing, ranging from 2 to 59% (mean 13%). Grossly visible left ventricular scars were present in 11 patients and in each they involved the posterior (inferior) wall; 8 of the 11 patients had significant coronary narrowing and 3 did not. Angina pectoris was present in 13 patients, 8 (62%) had significant coronary narrowing and 5 (38%) did not.

(Am J Cardiol 1986;57:1117–1123)

Although several reports have described coronary angiographic findings in patients with mitral stenosis (MS), few reports have described the frequency of and extent of coronary arterial narrowing at necropsy in patients with MS. In this report we describe the amounts of narrowing by atherosclerotic plaques observed at necropsy in the 4 major epicardial coronary arteries in 76 patients older than 30 years with clinically isolated MS with or without associated mitral regurgitation.

Methods

Patients classified as clinically isolated MS in the files of the Pathology Branch, National Heart, Lung, and Blood Institute (NHLBI), were reviewed and 76 patients fulfilled the following 4 criteria: (1) age >30 years at death; (2) presence of MS clinically and confirmation of MS at operation or at necropsy; (3) absence of clinical evidence of aortic valve dysfunction; (4) availability of the 4 major epicardial coronary arteries so that they could be examined in their entirety as discussed below. The hearts were received from 14 different medical centers: NHLBI = 39; Georgetown

*Sophomore Student, Albany Medical College, Albany, New York. From the Pathology Branch, National Heart, Lung, and Blood Institute, National Institutes of Health, Bethesda, Maryland. Manuscript received October 30, 1985, accepted December 6, 1985.

Address for reprints: William C. Roberts, MD, Building 10A, Room 3E-30, National Institutes of Health, Bethesda, Maryland 20205.

TABLE I Clinical and Cardiac Morphologic Observations in the 47 Women with Mitral Stenosis

| Pt | Age (yrs) | AP | AMI | Pressures (mm Hg) | | | LV Cine | Degree of MR (0–3+) | MVC | MVR | HW (g) | LA Clot | LV Scar | Major CAs >75% ↓ in XSA | 5-mm CA Segs | 5-mm Segments Narrowed in XSA (%) | | | | | Total | Mean |
				LA	LV	LA-LV mdg										0–25	26–50	51–75	76–95	96–100		
1	31	0	0	—*(w)	—	—*	0	—	+	0	450	0	0	1	53	12	39	1	1	0	97	1.8
2	31	0	0	—*	—	—*	+	0	+	0	540	0	0	0	42	11	31	0	0	0	73	1.7
3	31	0	0	—*	—	—*	0	—	0	84 mos	520	0	0	0	33	17	16	0	0	0	49	1.5
4	32	0	0	15	96/6	5	+	0	+	0	560	+	0	0	26	7	17	2	0	0	47	1.8
5	33	0	0	21	106/3	13	+	1+	+	0	550	+	0	1	44	2	38	3	1	0	91	2.1
6	35	0	0	—(w)*	—	—*	0	—	0	2 mos	780	0	0	0	40	25	15	0	0	0	55	1.4
7	39	0	0	—*	—	—*	0	—	+	12 mos	380	0	0	0	38	9	25	4	0	0	71	1.9
8	40	0	0	35(w)	120/30	28	+	0	0	12 days	440	0	0	0	43	9	27	7	0	0	84	2.0
9	41	0	0	24	110/13	10	+	0	+	0	360	0	+	3	35	9	6	4	14	2	97	2.8
10	41	0	0	19	108/7	10	+	0	+	5 days	370	0	+	1	27	4	10	12	0	1	64	2.4
11	41	0	0	—*(w)	—	—*	+	1+	+	0	450	+(LAA)	0	0	54	2	48	4	0	0	110	2.0
12	42	0	0	30(w)	125/10	24	+	3+	0	5 days	460	0	0	0	45	9	35	1	0	0	82	1.8
13	43	0	0	14(w)	150/12	5	+	3+	+	24 mos	540	0	0	0	43	33	10	0	0	0	53	1.2
14	44	0	0	20	95/6	20	+	3+	+	4 days	450	0	0	0	42	9	33	0	0	0	75	1.8
15	44	0	0	24(w)	95/20	14	0	—	+	1 day	480	0	0	1	45	6	10	24	5	0	118	2.6
16	47	+	0	—	—	—	0	—	0	0	430	0	0	1	42	2	25	8	7	0	104	2.5
17	47	0	0	18(w)	105/2	22	+	1+	0	22 days	380	0	0	0	35	3	27	5	0	0	72	2.1
18	48	0	+(po)	23	84/7	9	+	0	+	62 mos	510	0	0	0	38	14	24	0	0	0	62	1.6
19	48	+	0	—	—	—	0	—	0	0	370	0	0	0	43	23	12	8	0	0	71	1.7
20	49	+	0	—	—	—	0	—	+	0	525	0	0	3	36	0	17	11	8	0	99	2.8
21	50	+	0	18	112/7	12	+	0	+	0	465	+	0	0	38	3	33	2	0	0	75	2.0
22	52	0	0	30(w)	120/20	21	+	2+	0	0	645	+	+	2	50	16	17	11	6	0	107	2.1
23	54	+	0	19	136/10	12	+	3+	0	24 days	630	0	0	1	34	6	19	7	1	1	73	2.1
24	55	0	0	31(w)	137/12	26	+	2+	0	1 mo	420	0	0	1	37	2	30	4	1	0	78	2.1
25	56	+	0	14(w)	108/7	13	+	2+	+	OR	500	0	+	3	57	14	13	13	15	2	147	2.6
26	59	+	0	18(w)	130/16	7	+	3+	0	77 mos	540	0	0	0	47	15	28	4	0	0	83	1.8
27	59	+	0	20(w)	150/12	11	+	0	+	7 yrs	550	0	0	0	29	6	23	0	0	0	52	1.8
28	59	0	0	—*	—	10	+	1+	0	7 yrs	—	0	0	0	33	13	20	0	0	0	53	1.6
29	60	+	0	40(w)	160/15	22	+	1+	0	12 days	470	0	0	1	43	10	29	3	1	0	81	1.9
30	61	0	0	26(w)	105/8	18	+	2+	0	6 days	540	0	0	0	44	11	33	0	0	0	77	1.8
31	62	0	0	14(w)	120/8	11	0	—	0	5 mos	380	0	0	2	42	8	10	22	2	0	102	2.4
32	62	0	0	15(w)	120/5	16	+	1+	0	36 hrs	520	0	0	0	42	10	32	0	0	0	74	1.8
33	62	0	0	—*	140/6	6	+	3+	0	<1 day	660	0	0	1	25	12	7	5	1	0	45	1.3
34	62	0	0	13(w)	118/15	6	+	3+	0	3 hrs	500	0	0	0	46	21	23	2	0	0	73	1.6
35	64	0	0	25(w)	135/8	18	+	0	+	0	410	0	0	0	41	5	36	0	0	0	77	1.9
36	64	0	0	16(w)	—	10	+	0	+	0	420	0	0	2	37	3	20	7	7	0	92	2.5
37	65	0	0	—	—	—*	0	—	0	0	370	0	0	1	33	15	15	2	1	0	55	1.7
38	65	0	0	25	120/15	9	+	3+	0	6 days	640	0	0	0	38	20	18	0	0	0	56	1.5
39	65	0	0	—*	—	—*	0	—	0	OR	440	0	0	0	32	8	21	3	0	0	59	1.8
40	66	0	0	29(w)	110/16	13	+	3+	0	4 mos	560	0	0	1	48	7	32	7	2	0	100	2.1
41	68	0	0	—*	—	—*	0	—	0	13 yrs	545		0	3	52	3	20	17	11	1	142	2.7
42	69	0	0	30(w)	120/8	17	+	1+	+	0	380	+(LAA)	0	0	25	4	15	6	0	0	52	2.1
43	70	0	0	—	—	—	0	—	0	0	320	0	0	0	49	7	42	0	0	0	91	1.9
44	75	0	0	—	—	—	0	—	0	0	420	0	0	1	43	0	28	13	2	0	103	2.4
45	77	0	0	16(w)	100/14	12	+	0	0	2 mos	315	0	0	0	41	9	29	3	0	0	76	1.9
46	77	0	0	—*	—	—*	+	0	+	2 days	495	+	0	3	32	0	13	15	2	2	87	2.7
47	79	0	0	45(w)	155/15	20	+	0	+	0	625	+	0	0	42	10	24	8	0	0	82	2.0

* Known to be elevated but numbers not available. AMI = acute myocardial infarction; AP = angina pectoris; CA = coronary artery; HW = heart weight; LA = left atrium; LV = left ventricle; mdg = mean diastolic gradient; MR = mitral regurgitation; MVC = mitral valve commissurotomy; MVR = mitral valve replacement; OR = death in operating room; Segs = segments; w = pulmonary artery wedge pressure; XSA = cross-sectional area.

University Medical Center = 14; National Naval Medical Center = 8; District of Columbia Medical Examiners Office = 3; Suburban Hospital = 2; Franklin Square Hospital (Baltimore) = 2; and 1 came from each of 9 other medical centers. Of the 76 cases, in 3 (4%) necropsy had been performed in the 1950s, in 17 (22%) in the 1960s, in 21 (28%) in the 1970s, and in 35 (46%) in the 1980s.

In each of the 76 patients the clinical records were examined, the heart was reexamined, and the 4 major (right, left main, left anterior descending and left circumflex) epicardial coronary arteries were excised intact from the heart, decalcified if necessary, divided into 5-mm long segments, cut transversely to the long axis of the artery, labeled sequentially from the origin of the artery from either the aorta or left main coronary artery, processed in alcohols and xylene, embedded in paraffin, cut 6 μ thick, and at least 1 histologic section from each 5-mm segment was stained by the Movat method and examined.[1] The degree of cross-sectional area (XSA) narrowing by atherosclerotic plaques was determined by examining the Movat-stained sections, which clearly delineate the internal elastic membrane. The amount of XSA luminal narrowing was determined by magnifying each cross section of coronary artery 40 times via microscopy and estimating the degrees of luminal obliteration by visually dividing the XSA of the coronary artery into 4 quadrants, each comprising 25% of the total XSA luminal area. The degrees of XSA narrowing were categorized initially into 4 groups: 0 to 25, 26 to 50, 51 to 75 and 76 to 100%. All sections narrowed >75% were further classified into a group with narrowing 76 to 95% and into a group with narrowing 96 to 100% in XSA. Both the inter- and intraobserver error by this technique is <5%.[2]

The 76 patients ranged in age from 31 to 79 years (mean 53): 47 patients (62%) were women (mean age 54 years) (Table I) and 29 (38%) were men (mean age 51 years) (Table II). Ischemic-type chest pains occurred in 14 patients (18%): angina pectoris in 13 patients (17%) and clinical features diagnostic of acute myocardial infarction in 1 patient (1%). Of the 76 patients, left-sided cardiac catheterization was performed in 66 patients (87%); the catheterization data shown in Tables I and II are those recorded just before mitral valve replacement or if no valve replacement the data recorded at the last catheterization, usually many years after mitral commissurotomy if that procedure had been done. The mean diastolic gradient between left atrium or pulmonary arterial wedge position and left ventricle (52 patients) ranged from 5 to 28 mm Hg (average mean gradient 15 mm Hg). The degree of mitral regurgitation by left ventricular angiography (52 patients) was graded 0 (absent) (18 patients), 1+ (mild) (13 patients), 2+ (moderate) (8 patients) and 3+ (severe) (13 patients). Of the 76 patients, mitral valve commissurotomy had been performed in 32 patients (42%) and mitral valve replacement in 47. Of the 76 patients, 64 patients (84%) had either mitral valve commissurotomy (17 patients [27%]) or mitral valve replacement (32 patients [50%]) or both (15 patients [23%]). Of the 32 patients having commissurotomy, the commissurotomy had been performed >1 year before death in all

but 2 patients, who died just after the procedure. The replacement was performed within 30 days of death in 30 patients (64%), from 2 to 12 months of death in 6 patients (13%) and from 24 to 156 months (mean 95) before death in 11 patients (23%).

At necropsy, the hearts of the 47 women weighed 315 to 780 g (mean 485) (normal ≤350 g), and the hearts of the 29 men weighed 410 to 800 g (mean 559) (normal ≤400 g). Although functionally normal, each of the 3 aortic valve cusps were thickened in 17 patients: nos. 8, 11, 12, 26, 33, 38 and 46 in Table I and patients 1, 5 to 7, 11, 15, 20, 23, 25 and 27 in Table II.

A grossly visible left ventricular scar (healed myocardial infarction) was found at necropsy in 11 patients (14%): in 1 patient the scar was limited to the inner half of the left ventricular wall (endocardial) and in 10 patients the scar involved both inner and outer half of the left ventricular wall (transmural); in 9 patients the left ventricular scars were small and in 2 patients they were large (patients no. 9 and no. 17, Table II). The scars involved only the posterior (or inferior) left ventricular wall in 10 patients and both anterior and posterior walls in 1 patient (no. 17, Table II). Of the 11 patients with grossly visible left ventricular scars, 8 had narrowing by atherosclerotic plaque >75% in XSA of ≥1 of the 4 major epicardial coronary arteries and 3 did not.

Thrombi were present at operation or at necropsy in the left atrial cavity in 14 patients (18%). The thrombi were limited to the appendage in 3 patients and involved both left atrial appendage and body in 11 patients. Of the 14 patients with left atrial thrombi, 7 had narrowing >75% in XSA of ≥1 of the 4 major epicardial coronary arteries.

Only 2 patients (patient 25, Table I, and patient 4, Table II) had coronary artery bypass grafting. Both

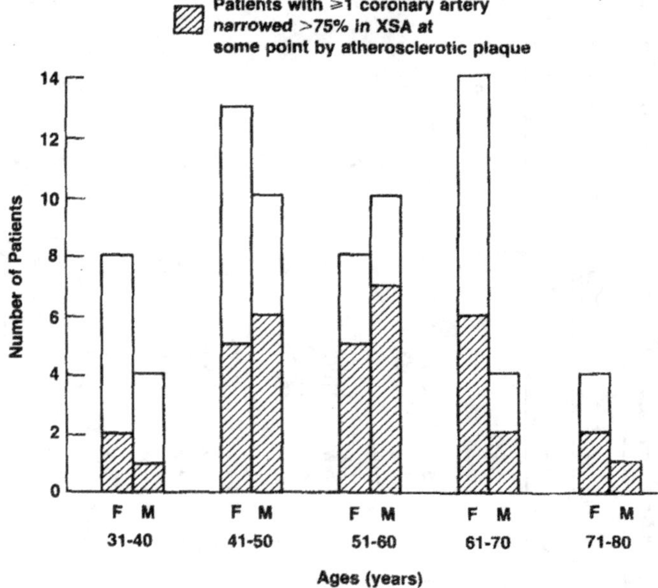

FIGURE 1. Number of necropsy patients by age decade and sex with clinically isolated mitral stenosis, with or without associated mitral regurgitation, in whom ≥1 major epicardial coronary artery was narrowed 76 to 100% in cross-sectional area at some point by atherosclerotic plaque.

TABLE II Clinical and Cardiac Morphologic Findings in the 29 Men with Mitral Stenosis

Pt	Age (yrs)	AP	AMI	LA	LV	LA-LV mdg	LV Cine	Degree of MR (0–3+)	MVC	MVR	HW (g)	LA Clot	LV Scar	No. of 4 Major CAs >75% ↓ in XSA	No. of 5-mm CA Segs	0–25	26–50	51–75	76–95	96–100	Total	Mean
				Pressures (mm Hg)												No. of 5-mm Segments Narrowed in XSA (%)						
1	31	0	0	16	93/6	12	+	2+	+	5d	570	+(po)	0	0	29	7	22	0	0	0	51	1.8
2	38	0	0	16	85/2	16	+	2+	0	2d	445	0	+	0	39	9	26	4	0	0	73	1.9
3	40	0	0	24	110/12	13	+	3+	0	2d	680	0	0	0	44	14	27	3	0	0	77	1.8
4	40	+	+po	26(w)	104/4	20	+	0	0	10h	495	0	0	1	27	0	25	1	1	0	57	2.1
5	42	0	0	27	100/9	19	0	—	+	0	480	0	0	2	43	0	18	20	5	0	116	2.7
6	42	0	0	17	135/2	20	+	0	+	0	470	0	0	0	19	0	16	3	0	0	41	2.2
7	44	0	0	34	129/10	21	0	—	0	6d	530	+	0	1	35	5	24	5	1	0	72	2.1
8	45	0	0	24	105/9	16	+	1+	0	4d	—	+	0	2	49	19	21	7	2	0	90	1.8
9	47	0	0	37(w)	100/21	17	+	2+	0	13d	570	+(po)	+	1	55	13	11	19	11	1	140	2.6
10	47	+	0	—	—	—	0	—	+	0	530	0	0	1	43	3	29	10	1	0	95	2.2
11	49	+	0	34	165/13	14	0	0	+	29d	665	0	+	3	39	1	10	19	9	0	114	2.9
12	49	0	0	32	86/7	17	0	—	0	0	410	0	0	1	38	0	27	10	1	0	88	2.3
13	49	0	0	30	105/5	17	+	3+	+	6h	800	0	0	0	31	1	28	2	0	0	63	2.0
14	50	0	0	25	110/11	15	+	2+	+	135m	600	0	0	0	50	9	41	0	0	0	91	2.8
15	51	0	0	41	—	—	0	—	0	0	480	+	0	0	49	0	48	1	0	0	99	2.0
16	52	0	0	—*	—	—*	+	1+	0	10y	490	0	0	0	53	19	31	3	0	0	90	1.7
17	53	0	+	—	—	—	0	—	0	0	445	0	+†	3	64	0	11	15	30	8	219	3.4
18	53	0	0	—	—	—	0	—	0	0	420	0	0	1	43	1	35	6	1	0	93	2.2
19	53	0	0	—*(w)	—	11	+	1+	0	11d	520	0	+	0	33	0	32	1	0	0	67	2.0
20	53	0	0	—*(w)	—	14	+	1+	0	0	470	0	0	3	49	4	29	8	7	1	118	2.4
21	54	0	0	22(w)	100/12	14	+	3+	+	87m	940	0	+	1	37	0	19	15	2	1	95	2.6
22	54	0	0	—*	—	—*	+	0	+	0	480	0	0	2	32	2	21	5	4	0	75	2.3
23	54	0	0	—*	—	—*	+	0	+	OR	420	+	0	1	43	1	20	20	2	0	109	2.5
24	56	0	0	—*(w)	—	25	0	—	0	17d	580	0	0	1	35	8	23	3	1	0	67	1.9
25	62	0	0*	25	155/17	7	+	3+	0	5d	720	0	0	3	88	0	49	27	12	0	227	2.6
26	65	0	0	28(w)	100/0	10	+	1+	+	11y	760	+	0	0	44	1	43	0	0	0	87	2.0
27	66	+	0	—*	—	—*	0	—	+	0	600	0	+	0	60	47	12	1	0	0	74	1.2
28	66	0	0	—*(w)	—	10	+	1+	0	9m	620	0	0	1	29	10	15	0	4	0	56	1.9
29	75	0	0	39(w)	—	—*	0	—	0	0	410	+(LAA)	0	3	40	2	18	14	6	0	104	2.6

* Numbers not available but known to be increased.
† Also healing anterior wall myocardial infarct.
Abbreviations as in Table I.

patients also had mitral valve replacement; 1 died in the operating room and the other within 10 hours after operation.

Results

Of the 76 necropsy patients, 38 (50%) had ≥1 of their 4 major epicardial coronary arteries narrowed >75% in XSA by atherosclerotic plaques (Fig. 1): in 22 patients (29%), 1 of the 4 arteries was so narrowed; in 6 patients (8%), 2 such arteries, and in 10 patients (13%) 3 such arteries. Thus, in the 38 patients, 64 major coronary arteries were narrowed >75% in XSA, an average of 1.7 coronary arteries per patient; of the entire 76 patients, an average of 0.8 coronary arteries were so narrowed.

Of the 47 women, 20 (44%) had ≥1 of the 4 major coronary arteries narrowed >75% in XSA by plaque and of the 29 men, 18 (62%) had ≥1 major coronary artery so narrowed. Not only did a higher percent of the men have narrowing ≥1 major coronary artery >75% in XSA by plaque, but a higher percent of their 4 major coronary arteries were so narrowed. Of the 188 major epicardial coronary arteries examined in the 47 women, 33 (18%) were narrowed at some point >75% in XSA by plaque; of the 116 major coronary arteries examined in the 29 men, 31 (27%) were narrowed >75% in XSA by plaque. Of the 304 major coronary arteries examined in the 76 patients, 64 (21%) were narrowed at some point >75% in XSA by plaque. Of the 64 coronary arteries narrowed >75% in XSA at some point, the right coronary artery was so narrowed in 26 patients (41%), the anterior descending in 22 (34%), the left circumflex in 16 (25%) and the left main in none. Of the 38 patients with ≥1 coronary artery narrowed >75% in XSA by plaque, 8 (21%) had a grossly visible left ventricular scar. The other 3 patients with grossly visible left ventricular scars had insignificant coronary arterial narrowing.

A total of 3,124 five-millimeter segments of the 304 major epicardial coronary arteries in the 76 patients were examined (Fig. 2): 620 segments (20%) were narrowed 0 to 25% in XSA by atherosclerotic plaque; 1,826 segments (58%) were narrowed 26 to 50%; 470 segments (15%) were narrowed 51 to 75%; 188 segments (6%) were narrowed 76 to 95% and 20 segments (1%) were narrowed 96 to 100% in XSA. The percent of 5-mm segments narrowed >75% in XSA was nearly 2 times higher in the men than in the women: of the 1,240 five-millimeter segments examined in the 29 men, 111 (9%) were narrowed >75% in XSA and of the 1,884 segments examined in the 47 women, 97 (5%) were narrowed >75% in XSA.

Among the 38 patients in whom narrowing >75% in XSA was present in ≥1 major coronary artery, the number and percent of 5-mm segments narrowed to this extent varied greatly. Among the 38 patients with significant (>75% in XSA) coronary arterial narrowing, 1,604 five-millimeter segments were examined and of them 208 segments (13%) were narrowed >75% in XSA: of the 815 segments examined in the 20 women, 97 (12%) were narrowed >75%. Of the 38 patients, however, with narrowing >75% of ≥1 coronary artery, 13 patients (34%) had only a single 5-mm segment narrowed to this degree, 6 (16%) others had only 2 segments so narrowed, and 6 (16%) others had 3 to 5 segments so narrowed. Thus, 25 (66%) of the 38 patients had ≤5 coronary segments narrowed >75% in XSA, and only 6 patients (16%) had >10 segments severely narrowed. The percent of 5-mm segments narrowed >75% in XSA in the 38 patients ranged from 2 to 59% (mean 13%).

The number and percent of 5-mm coronary segments totally occluded or nearly so (>95% in XSA) also varied greatly. Only 10 of the 76 patients had any coronary segment narrowed to this degree and all but 1 of them also had ≥1 coronary segment also narrowed

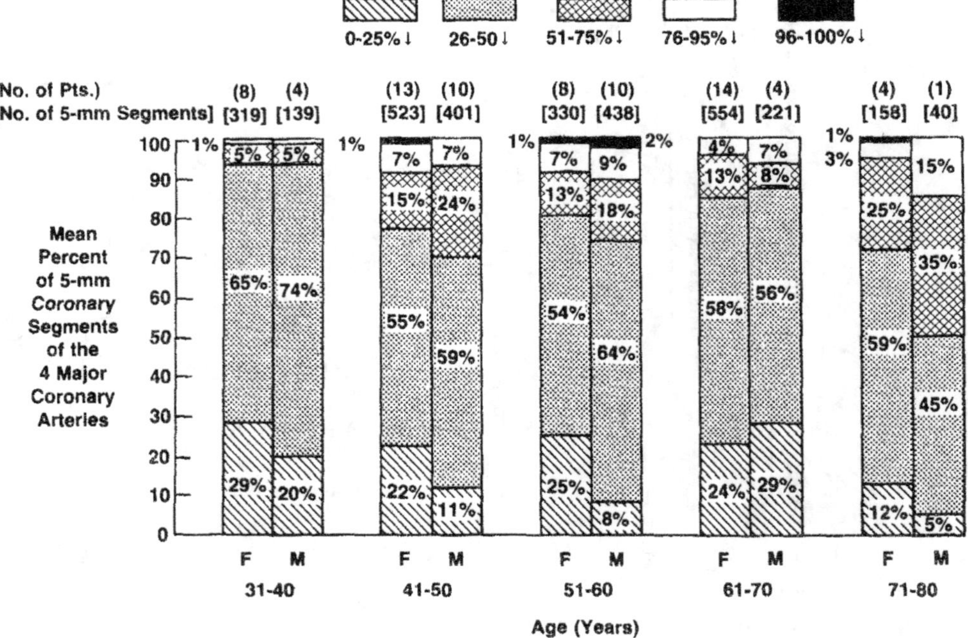

FIGURE 2. Number and percent of 3,124 five-millimeter segments of the 4 major epicardial coronary arteries narrowed to various degrees by atherosclerotic plaque in 76 patients (47 women, 29 men) aged 31 to 79 years with clinically isolated mitral stenosis with or without associated mitral regurgitation.

TABLE III Degrees of Coronary Arterial Narrowing By Angiogram During Life and at Necropsy in 13 Patients with Mitral Stenosis and Coronary Angiography

Table No.	Age (yr) & Sex	Maximal Narrowing by Angiogram (%DR)				Maximal Narrowing by Histology at Necropsy (%XSA)				AP	CABG
		R	LM	LAD	LC	R	LM	LAD	LC		
I	40F	0	0	0	0	51–75	51–75	51–75	26–50	0	0
I	54F	0	0	0	0	51–75	26–50	76–100	26–50	0	0
I	55F	25	0	25	0	51–75	26–50	76–100	26–50	0	0
I	56F	100	0	65	65	76–100	51–75	76–100	76–100	+	+
I	59F	0	0	0	0	51–75	0–25	26–50	26–50	0	+
I	62F	0	0	0	0	26–50	0–25	26–50	26–50	0	0
I	65F	0	0	0	0	26–50	26–50	26–50	26–50	0	0
I	69F	0	0	0	0	51–75	—	51–75	26–50	0	0
II	40M	0	0	50	95	51–75	—	26–50	76–100	+	+
II	52M	0	0	0	0	51–75	26–50	26–50	0–25	0	0
II	53M	0	0	0	0	26–50	26–50	26–50	51–75	0	0
II	54M	0	0	0	0	51–75	26–50	76–100	51–75	0	0
II	65M	0	0	0	0	26–50	26–50	26–50	26–50	0	0

AP = angina pectoris; CABG = coronary artery bypass grafting; DR = diameter reduction; LAD = left anterior descending coronary artery; LC = left circumflex coronary artery; LM = left main coronary artery; R = right coronary artery; XSA = cross-sectional area.

76 to 95% in XSA. Of these 10 patients, only 1 or 2 coronary segments were narrowed >95% in XSA in 9 patients; in the other patients, 8 of 38 segments (21%) were narrowed to this extent. Thus, of the 1,604 five-millimeter coronary segments narrowed >75% in XSA in the 38 patients, 20 segments (1%) were narrowed >95% in XSA.

A scoring system also was used to indicate the severity and extent of coronary arterial narrowing. Every 5-mm segment of coronary artery from each patient was assigned a score of 1 to 4 based on the amount of XSA narrowing by atherosclerotic plaque: 1 = 0 to 25% narrowing; 2 = 26 to 50%; 3 = 51 to 75% and 4 = 76 to 100%. A total score was determined for each patient and the mean score per segment was then calculated by dividing the total score per patient by the number of segments examined from that patient. The total score for the 3,124 five-millimeter coronary segments from the 76 patients was 6,514, indicating that the mean score for each 5-mm segment was 2.1. The latter number indicates that the amount of XSA narrowing for the 3,124 segments averaged about 40%.

Of the 10 patients with grossly visible left ventricular scars, 7 patients had ≥1 major coronary artery narrowed >75% and in 6 of the 7 patients ≥1 major coronary artery was narrowed >95% in XSA. Of the 496 five-millimeter coronary segments examined in these 10 patients, the total score was 1,197 for an average of 2.4 per segment, a number higher than that for the entire 76 patients.

Of the 13 patients with angina pectoris, 8 (62%) had narrowing >75% in XSA of ≥1 major epicardial coronary artery and 3 of the 13 patients (23%) also had grossly visible left ventricular scars. A total of 538 five-millimeter coronary segments were examined in these 13 patients and 46 (9%) of them were narrowed >75% in XSA. The total score in the 538 segments was 1,125, indicating a mean score of 2.1 per segment or approximately 40% XSA narrowing per segment.

Coronary angiography had been performed in life in 13 patients (Table III) and 2 patients (15%) had >50% diameter narrowing of ≥1 major epicardial coronary artery. At necropsy (within 2 months of angiography), 3 other patients—a total of 5—had narrowing >75% in XSA.

Discussion

This study demonstrates that 38 (50%) of our 76 necropsy patients over 30 years of age with clinically isolated MS (with or without associated mitral regurgitation but without aortic valve dysfunction) had narrowing of ≥1 major epicardial coronary artery between 76 and 95% in XSA by atherosclerotic plaque and that 10 of the 38 patients had XSA narrowing >95% in XSA by plaque. A higher percent of men than women had significant (>75% in XSA) narrowing of ≥1 major coronary artery (62% vs 44%). Moreover, the men had a higher number of major coronary arteries narrowed >75% in XSA than did the women (31 [27%] the 116 major coronary arteries in the 29 men vs 33 [18%] of the 188 major coronary arteries in the 47 women). Grossly visible left ventricular scars and/or angina pectoris were relatively infrequent in the patients with or without significant coronary narrowing. Of the 38 patients with narrowing >75% in XSA of ≥1 major coronary artery, only 8 (21%) had a grossly visible left ventricular scar and of the 38 without a major coronary artery narrowed >75% in XSA 3 (8%) had a grossly visible left ventricular scar. Of the 38 patients with significant coronary narrowing, 8 (21%) had angina pectoris and of the 38 patients in whom none of the major coronary arteries were narrowed >75% in XSA, 5 (13%) had had angina. Of the 64 coronary arteries narrowed >75% in XSA (average 1.7 per patient) in the 38 patients, the right one was narrowed most frequently (41% vs 34% for the left anterior descending and 25% for the left circumflex). The posterior (inferior) wall was the location of the grossly visible left ventricular scars in all 11 patients with scars.

Of the 3,124 five-millimeter segments of the 4 major epicardial coronary arteries examined in the 76 patients (mean 41 per patient), 188 segments (6%) were narrowed 76 to 95% in XSA and 20 segments (1%) were narrowed 96 to 100% in XSA. The percent of segments narrowed >75% in XSA was nearly twice as high in the men compared to the women. In the 38 patients in whom at least 1 segment was narrowed >75% in XSA, a total of 1,604 five-millimeter coronary segments were examined and 208 (13%) were narrowed >75% in XSA; the percent of segments narrowed >75% in XSA varied in these 38 patients from as few as 2% to as many as 59%. Of the 10 patients in whom at least 1 coronary segment was narrowed >95% in XSA, only 1 or 2 segments were narrowed to this degree in 9 patients.

Although one-half of the 76 patients had narrowing of >75% in XSA of at least 1 major coronary artery, the length of the narrowing, i.e., the number of 5-mm segments narrowed to this degree, was much less than in necropsy patients with fatal coronary heart disease studied in a similar fashion. Among 31 victims of sudden coronary death studied in this laboratory, 36% of the 5-mm segments of the 4 major coronary arteries were narrowed >75% in XSA by atherosclerotic plaque[3]; the percent in 27 victims of transmural acute myocardial infarction was 34%[4]; the percent in 22 patients with unstable angina pectoris was 48%,[5] and the percent in patients with healed myocardial infarction was 31%.[6-8]

The only other major necropsy study of the coronary arteries in patients with MS was by Tadavarthy et al.[9] These authors examined the major epicardial coronary arteries, primarily by gross inspection of cross sections of the arteries, of 60 patients, 47 women, aged "20s" to "70s" (mean "50s") with pure MS. Of the 60 patients, 21 (35%) had "significant" obstructive lesions in ≥1 major coronary artery: of the 47 women, 15 (32%) had ≥1 "severe" coronary narrowing and of the 13 men, 6 (46%) had ≥1 severe coronary narrowing. Of the 21 patients with significant coronary narrowing, 1 major artery was severely narrowed in 6 patients (29%), 2 arteries in 8 patients (38%), 3 arteries in 6 patients (14%) and 4 arteries in 1 patient (5%). As in the present study, the right coronary artery was more frequently severely narrowed than was the left anterior descending or the left circumflex.

Although morphologic studies of the coronary arteries in MS have been rare, several angiographic studies of the coronary arteries in patients with MS have been reported.[10-16] Befeler et al[10] performed coronary arteriography in 26 patients aged 32 to 69 years (mean 45) with isolated MS and found 5 patients (19%) to have >50% diameter reduction in ≥1 major coronary artery (complete obstruction in 4); 3 patients (12%) had clinical evidence of healed myocardial infarction, 2 with 100% obstruction and 1 with 50% obstruction of a coronary artery; and 3 (12%) patients had angina pectoris (1 also had a healed myocardial infarct) and all 3 had 100% obstruction of a coronary artery. Lacy et al[11] studied 67 patients (49 women) with "predominant" MS and by angiograms 13 (19%) had ≥1 coronary artery narrowed >50% in diameter: 3 arteries so narrowed in 1 patient, 2 arteries so narrowed in 6 patients,

and 1 artery so narrowed in 6 patients. Chun and associates[12] found angiographically significant (>50% diameter reduction) coronary narrowing in 16 (20%) of 82 patients (mean age 51 years, 47 women) with MS. Saltups[13] by angiography found ≥1 coronary arterial narrowing ≥50% in diameter in 7 (10%) of 68 patients with MS: angina was present in 4 and absent in 3 of the 7 patients with significant coronary narrowing; none of the 61 patients without significant coronary narrowing had angina. Ramsdale et al[14] found coronary arterial narrowing ≥50% diameter reduction in 24 (28%) of 86 patients with MS: of the 21 patients with angina pectoris, 13 had angiographically significant coronary narrowing and 8 did not. Czer and associates[15] found ≥50% diameter reduction of ≥1 major coronary artery by angiogram in 57 (29%) of 199 patients with MS in whom mitral valve replacement was performed. Mattina and colleagues[16] found ≥1 major coronary artery narrowed ≥70% in diameter in 27 (28%) of 96 patients aged 41 to 74 years (mean 60) (73 women) with severe MS; 21 (22%) of the 96 patients had angina pectoris and 10 of them had angiographically significant coronary narrowing and 11 did not.

References

1. Movat HZ. *Demonstration of all connective tissue elements in a single section: pentachrome stains. Arch Pathol* 1955;60:289–295.

2. Isner JM, Wu M, Renu V, Jones AA, Roberts WC. *Comparison of degrees of coronary arterial luminal narrowing determined by visual inspection of histologic sections under magnification among three independent observers and comparison to that obtained by video planimetry. An analysis of 559 five-millimeter segments of 61 coronary arteries from eleven patients. Lab Invest* 1980;42:566–570.

3. Roberts WC, Jones AA. *Quantitation of coronary arterial narrowing at necropsy in sudden coronary death. Analysis of 31 patients and comparison with 25 control subjects. Am J Cardiol* 1979;44:39–45.

4. Roberts WC, Jones AA. *Quantification of coronary arterial narrowing at necropsy in acute transmural myocardial infarction: analysis and comparison of findings in 27 patients and 22 controls. Circulation* 1980;61:786–790.

5. Roberts WC, Virmani R. *Quantification of coronary arterial narrowing in clinically-isolated unstable angina pectoris. An analysis of 22 necropsy patients. Am J Med* 1979;67:792–799.

6. Virmani R, Roberts WC. *Quantification of coronary arterial narrowing and of left ventricular myocardial scarring in healed myocardial infarction with chronic eventually fatal, congestive cardiac failure. Am J Med* 1980;68:831–838.

7. Cabin HS, Roberts WC. *True left ventricular aneurysm and healed myocardial infarction. Clinical and necropsy observations including quantification of degrees of coronary arterial narrowing. Am J Cardiol* 1980;46:754–763.

8. Virmani R, Roberts WC. *Non-fatal healed transmural myocardial infarction and fatal non-cardiac disease. Qualification and quantification of coronary arterial narrowing and of left ventricular scarring in 18 necropsy patients. Br Heart J* 1981;45:434–441.

9. Tadavarthy SM, Voldaver Z, Edwards JE. *Coronary atherosclerosis in subjects with mitral stenosis. Circulation* 1976;54:519–521.

10. Befeler B, Kamen AR, Macleod CA. *Coronary artery disease and left ventricular function in mitral stenosis. Chest* 1970;57:435–439.

11. Lacy J, Goodin R, McMartin D, Masden R, Flowers N. *Coronary atherosclerosis in valvular heart disease. Ann Thorac Surg* 1977;23:429–435.

12. Chun PKC, Gertz E, Davia JE, Cheitlin MD. *Coronary atherosclerosis in mitral stenosis. Chest* 1982;81:36–41.

13. Saltups A. *Coronary arteriography in isolated aortic and mitral valve disease. Aust NZ J Med* 1982;12:494–497.

14. Ramsdale DR, Bennett DH, Bray CL, Ward C, Beton DC, Faragher EB. *Angina, coronary risk factors and coronary artery disease in patients with valvular disease. A prospective study. European Heart J* 1984;5:716–726.

15. Czer LSC, Gray RJ, Derobertis MA, Bateman TM, Stewart ME, Chaux A, Matloff JM. *Mitral valve replacement: impact of coronary artery disease and determinants of prognosis after revascularization. Circulation* 1984;70:suppl I:I-198–I-207.

16. Mattina CJ, Green SJ, Tortolani AJ, Padmanabhan VT, Ong LY, Hall MH, Pizzarello RA. *Frequency of angiographically significant coronary artery disease in mitral stenosis. Am J Cardiol* 1986;57:802–805.

Relation of Size of Transmural Acute Myocardial Infarct to Mode of Death, Interval Between Infarction and Death and Frequency of Coronary Arterial Thrombus

JEFFREY E. SAFFITZ, MD, PhD, RURIK C. FREDRICKSON, and WILLIAM C. ROBERTS, MD

Seventy-eight necropsy patients with transmural acute myocardial infarction (AMI) were studied to correlate the mode of death, the interval between onset of AMI and death and the presence or absence of coronary thrombus with the extent of the infarct. Infarct size was assessed quantitatively as a percentage of total left ventricular (LV) mass. Death was caused by cardiogenic shock in 16 patients (21%), arrhythmia in 31 patients (40%) and cardiac rupture in 24 patients (31%). The mean interval between the onset of AMI and death was 12 ± 13 days. Infarct size averaged 23 ± 14% of LV mass. Patients who died in cardiogenic shock had the largest infarcts (37 ± 11%) and those who died of cardiac rupture had the smallest infarcts (15 ± 9%) and the shortest interval between onset of AMI and death (7 ± 8 days). Coronary thrombi were present in 58 patients (74%). When present, thrombus was observed in the coronary artery that had supplied the infarct area and was superimposed on advanced atherosclerotic plaque, but no relation was found between extent of luminal obstruction by thrombus and AMI size. The absence of coronary thrombus at necropsy was associated with either small infarcts or prolonged survival after AMI.

(Am J Cardiol 1986;57:1249–1254)

Prognosis after acute myocardial infarction (AMI) depends in part on the size of the myocardial infarct.[1] Although it has been demonstrated that patients in whom cardiogenic shock develops with AMI generally have large infarcts,[2–4] the relation of infarct size to other clinical and anatomic features of AMI has not been studied extensively. We quantified infarct size in 78 necropsy patients with fatal AMI and examined the relation of infarct size to mode of death, interval between the onset of symptoms of AMI and death and presence or absence of coronary arterial thrombus at necropsy.

Methods

Selection of necropsy patients: Cases from the files of the Pathology Branch of the National Heart, Lung,

From the Pathology Branch, National Heart, Lung, and Blood Institute, Bethesda, Maryland. Manuscript received December 17, 1985, accepted December 18, 1985.

Address for reprints: Jeffrey E. Saffitz, MD, PhD, Department of Pathology, Washington University School of Medicine, 660 South Euclid Avenue, St. Louis, Missouri 63110.

and Blood Institute were included in the study if the following criteria were met: (1) Death occurring from 1973 through 1983. (2) Presence of grossly discernible left ventricular (LV) necrosis involving, at some point, the entire inner one-half of the thickness of the LV wall and all or portions of the outer one-half of the wall (transmural). In most cases, necrosis extended to or near the LV epicardial surface. (3) Presence of the entire heart (except for small blocks removed for histologic examination) so that infarct size could be assessed. (4) Presence of all 4 major epicardial coronary arteries (right, left main, left anterior descending and left circumflex) for assessment of the presence or absence of coronary thrombus. (5) Presence of sufficient clinical information to determine accurately the interval between onset of symptoms of AMI and death, mode of death and whether congestive heart failure, systemic hypertension or angina pectoris had preceded the fatal AMI. Modes of death after AMI included cardiogenic shock, arrhythmia and cardiac rupture. Cardiogenic shock was considered to have caused death if the clinical course preceding death was characterized primarily by signs and symptoms of pump failure and low cardiac output. Patients in whom the course was characterized primarily by serious rhythm disturbances were considered to have died of arrhythmia, even though in some, low cardiac output states may have been present shortly before death. Patients with rupture of the LV free wall or ventricular septum were considered to have died of cardiac rupture, although some died hours to a few days after perforation of the ventricular septum. (6) Absence of coronary arterial or cardiac surgery, thrombolytic therapy, primary valvular heart disease, cardiomyopathy or congenital heart disease. (7) Presence of coagulation necrosis confirmed by histologic examination of the LV wall.

Measurement of infarct size: Hearts were cut transversely into slices approximately 1 cm thick from the apex to approximately 2 cm caudal to the posterior atrioventricular sulcus. The right ventricular free wall and all LV epicardial adipose tissue were removed (Fig. 1). The outlines of the epicardial and endocardial edges and the borders of the infarcted myocardium of each LV slice were traced onto transparent plastic sheets. Both cut surfaces of each slice were traced. The areas of infarcted and noninfarcted myocardium were measured to determine the percent of infarcted tissue per surface in every slice (Fig. 1). Weight of the infarcted myocardium (in grams) in each slice was calculated by multiplying the weight of the slice by the averaged percentage of surface area occupied by infarct and noninfarcted tissue in the 2 cut surfaces. Infarct size was expressed as a percentage of total LV mass. In most cases in which a healed infarct was present, the area occupied by scar was minimal and was ignored without significantly affecting the measurement of the size of the necrotic myocardium. In specimens containing more extensive healed infarcts, the scarred area was measured and calculations performed to determine the size of the healed infarct.

Evaluation of coronary thrombi: The 4 major epicardial coronary arteries were removed intact from the heart, decalcified if necessary and each was cut transversely to its longitudinal axis at 5-mm intervals. All segments were processed in alcohols and xylene, embedded in paraffin, cut with a microtome at 6-μm intervals and stained with hematoxylin-eosin and with Movat stains. Histologic criteria for the diagnosis of coronary thrombus included presence of fibrin plus erythrocytes or platelets and adhesion of the thrombus to the luminal surface at some point. Although most thrombi appeared to occlude the lumen either totally or almost totally, complete luminal occlusion was not required for the diagnosis of coronary thrombus. In each artery in which a thrombus was identified, the degree to which the lumen was obstructed by the thrombus and by atherosclerotic plaque was determined using methods developed and validated in this laboratory.[5]

Statistical analyses: Statistical comparisons of infarct size in selected subsets of the study population were performed using arcsin transformation to convert values of percent of LV mass to a normally distributed data set. Statistical significance (p $\leq$ 0.05) was determined with the t test or Fisher's exact test.

Results

Selected clinical and morphologic features in the 78 necropsy patients are listed in Table I. Compared with the 50 men, the 28 women were significantly older and

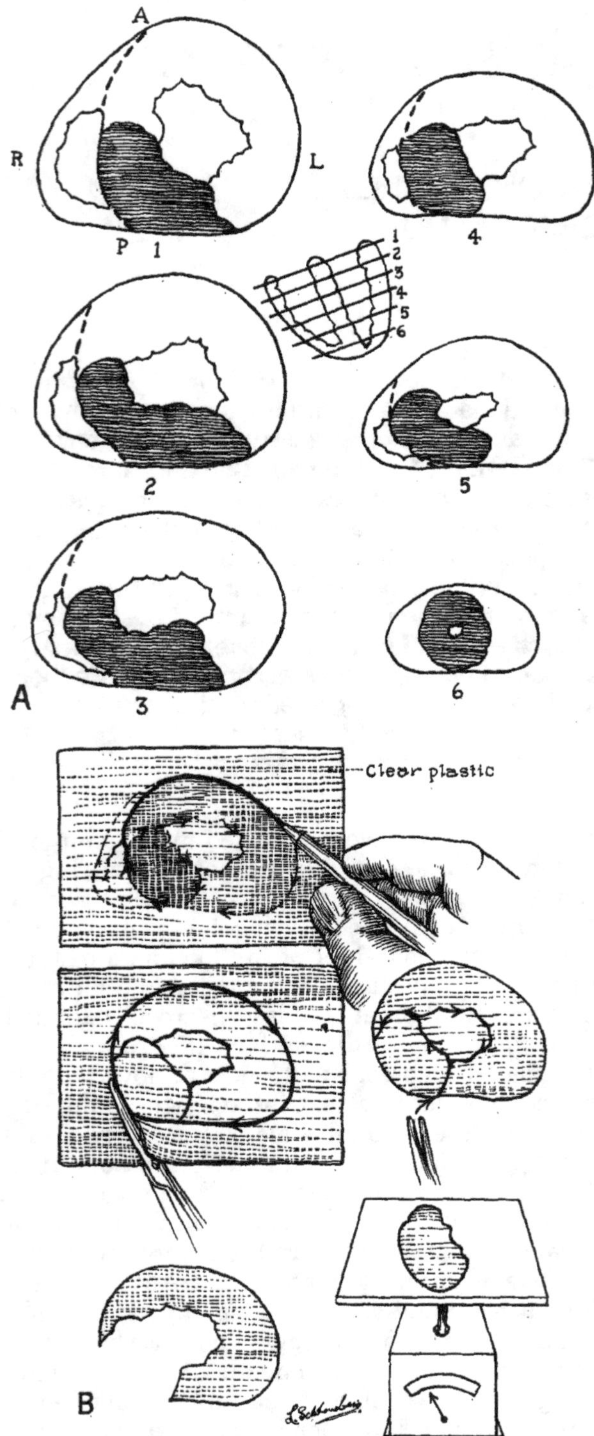

FIGURE 1. Method used to quantify myocardial infarct size. *A*, the cardiac ventricles were cut transversely from apex to base at 1-cm intervals parallel to the posterior atrioventricular sulcus. The right ventricular free wall and epicardial adipose tissue were removed. *B*, the slices were traced on transparent plastic and the areas occupied by infarcted and noninfarcted myocardium quantified by weighing the cut-out tracings.

TABLE I Clinical and Morphologic Features of 78 Necropsy Patients with Acute Myocardial Infarction (AMI)

	Totals	Men		Women
No. of pts	78	50 (64%)		28 (36%)
Mean age (yr)	67 ± 11	65 ± 10	‡	70 ± 12
Mean interval (days) from AMI to death	12 ± 13	14 ± 14		10 ± 9
Congestive heart failure*	9 (12%)	3 (6%)	‡	6 (21%)
Systemic hypertension*	48 (62%)	32 (64%)		16 (57%)
Angina pectoris*	26 (33%)	22 (44%)	§	4 (14%)
Mode of death				
Cardiogenic shock	16 (21%)	11 (22%)		5 (18%)
Arrhythmia	31 (40%)	19 (38%)		12 (43%)
Rupture	24 (31%)	15 (30%)		9 (32%)
LV free wall	17	10		7
Ventricular septum	7	5		2
Miscellaneous†	7 (9%)	5 (10%)		2 (7%)
Heart weight (g)	463 ± 97	484 ± 94	*	430 ± 93
Infarct size (% of LV mass)	23 ± 14	24 ± 14		21 ± 14
LV scar	22 (28%)	17 (34%)		5 (18%)
Coronary thrombus	58 (74%)	39 (78%)		19 (68%)

* Present before fatal AMI.

† Includes 1 each of: stroke, sepsis, diabetic ketoacidosis, pulmonary embolus, noncardiac postoperative complications, adenocarcinoma of the colon with volvulus and perforation of the colon.

‡ p <0.05; § p <0.01.

Mean values are ± standard deviation.

LV = left ventricular.

TABLE II Comparative Clinical and Morphologic Features in Patients with Different Modes of Death After Acute Myocardial Infarction (AMI)

Mode of Death	Cardiogenic Shock	Arrhythmia	Rupture
No. of pts	16	31	24
Mean age (yr)	69 ± 11	62 ± 11†	70 ± 8
Mean interval (days) from AMI to death	19 ± 18	13 ± 11	6 ± 4‡
Congestive heart failure*	5 (31%)‡	2 (6%)	0 (0%)
Systemic hypertension*	8 (50%)	21 (68%)	19 (79%)
Angina pectoris*	7 (44%)	10 (32%)	7 (29%)
Mean heart weight (g)	493 ± 98	476 ± 100	435 ± 91
Mean AMI size (% of LV mass)	37 ± 11‡	20 ± 12	14 ± 8‡
LV scar	5 (31%)	10 (32%)	4 (17%)

* Present before fatal AMI.

† p <0.05 compared with other groups; ‡ p <0.01 compared with other groups.

Mean values are ± standard deviation.

LV = left ventricular.

had smaller hearts, a higher frequency of congestive heart failure and a lower frequency of angina pectoris before the fatal AMI. The mean interval between the onset of symptoms of AMI and death was 12 ± 13 days. Death was attributed to cardiogenic shock in 16 patients (21%), arrhythmia in 31 patients (40%), cardiac rupture in 24 patients (31%) and other causes in 7 patients (8%). The mean size of the fatal AMI was similar in men and women (23 ± 14% of total LV mass). LV scar was present in 22 patients (28%), but in all cases it was patchy, confined to the subendocardium and amounted to <5% of LV mass. No transmural LV scar was seen. Coronary thrombi were observed in 58 of the 78 patients (74%).

Clinical and morphologic features of patients who died of cardiogenic shock, arrhythmia and cardiac rupture are compared in Table II. Patients who died of arrhythmia were younger than those who died of either cardiogenic shock or cardiac rupture. In patients who died of cardiogenic shock, a history of congestive heart failure before the fatal AMI was significantly more frequent than in patients who died from other causes. Patients who died of cardiogenic shock had the largest infarcts.

Of the 24 patients with cardiac rupture, none had had evidence of congestive heart failure before the fatal AMI. Infarct size was significantly smaller and the interval between AMI and death significantly shorter than in the patients who died from other causes.

The relation of mode of death to infarct size and interval between onset of symptoms and death is illustrated in Figures 2 and 3. Of the 24 patients who died of cardiac rupture, 14 (58%) had small infarcts (≤15% of LV mass); the 10 other patients with rupture had moderate-sized infarcts (16 to 30% of LV mass). The patients who died in cardiogenic shock had either large (>30% of LV mass) or moderate-sized infarcts, while the sizes of the infarcts in the patients who died of an arrhythmia varied broadly. Death occurred within the

TABLE III Comparative Clinical and Morphologic Features in Patients with Small, Moderate-Sized and Large Fatal Infarcts

Size of Myocardial Infarct (% LV mass)	Small (0 to 15%)	Moderate (16 to 30%)	Large (>30%)
No. of pts	28 (36%)	33 (42%)	17 (22%)
Mean interval (days) from AMI to death	6 ± 6[†]	16 ± 14	16 ± 14
Mean infarct size (% of LV mass)	9 ± 4	24 ± 4	43 ± 10
Congestive heart failure*	3 (11%)	4 (12%)	2 (12%)
Systemic hypertension*	17 (61%)	23 (70%)	8 (47%)
Angina pectoris*	8 (29%)	12 (36%)	6 (35%)
Mode of death			
Cardiogenic shock	0 (0%)	6 (18%)	11 (65%)
Arrhythmia	13 (46%)	12 (36%)	5 (29%)
Rupture	14 (50%)	10 (30%)	0 (0%)
Miscellaneous	1 (4%)	5 (15%)	1 (6%)
LV scar	8 (29%)	8 (24%)	6 (35%)
Coronary thrombus	21 (75%)	24 (73%)	13 (76%)

* Present before fatal AMI.

† p <0.01 compared with other groups.

Mean values are ± standard deviation.

AMI = acute myocardial infarction; LV = left ventricular.

first 10 days after the onset of symptoms of AMI in 22 of 24 patients who died of cardiac rupture, while in the patients who died from either arrhythmia or cardiogenic shock, the interval between AMI and death varied from 1 to 42 days.

In Table III and Figures 4 and 5, selected variables are compared in patients with small, moderate and large infarcts. Patients with small infarcts died earlier than those with moderate or large infarcts due to the high frequency of cardiac rupture in patients with small infarcts. The frequency of coronary thrombus was similar in patients with small, moderate and large infarcts.

In Table IV, clinical and morphologic features are compared in patients with and without coronary thrombi at necropsy. The 2 groups of patients were similar with respect to mode of death, interval between AMI and death and infarct size. When present, thrombus always occurred in the coronary artery responsible for supplying the infarcted area. Thrombi were always superimposed on atherosclerotic plaque. In Figure 6, the relation between AMI size and the extent of luminal obstruction caused by thrombus is examined. In 50 of 58 cases (86%), thrombus occupied ≤25% of the luminal cross-sectional area enclosed by the internal elastic membrane. Thus, thrombus was usually superimposed over areas of severe narrowing in which >75% of luminal cross-sectional area was occupied by plaque. There was, however, no clear relation between the degree of luminal obstruction caused by coronary thrombus and the size of the AMI.

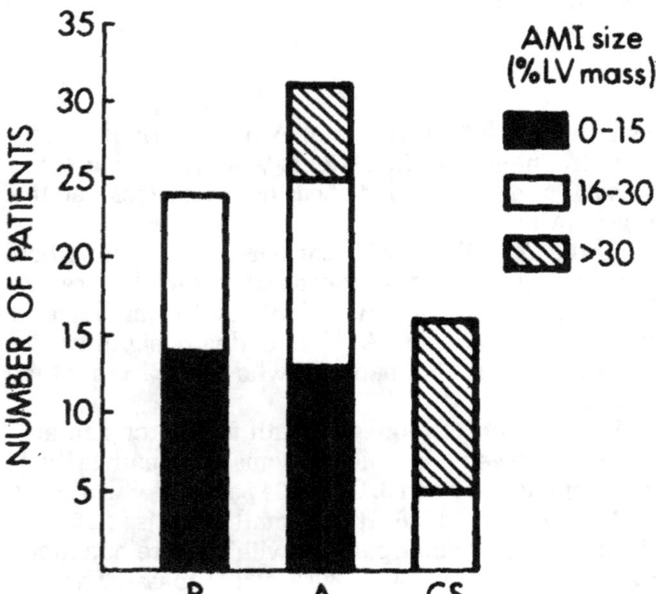

FIGURE 2. Relation of the mode of death to acute myocardial infarct (AMI) size. A = arrhythmia; CS = cardiogenic shock; LV = left ventricular; R = cardiac rupture.

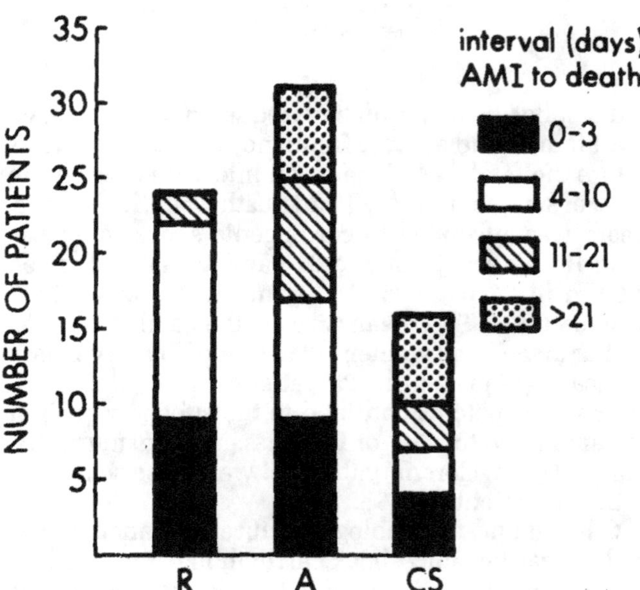

FIGURE 3. Relation of the mode of death to the interval between the onset of acute myocardial infarction (AMI) and death. Abbreviations as in Figure 2.

Coronary Thrombus	+	0
No. of pts	58	20
Mean age (yr)	66 ± 11	70 ± 11
Mode of death		
Cardiogenic shock	12/16 (75%)	4/16 (25%)
Arrhythmia	22/31 (71%)	9/31 (29%)
Rupture	21/24 (88%)	3/24 (12%)
Congestive heart failure*	5 (9%)	4 (20%)
Systemic hypertension*	34 (59%)	14 (70%)
Angina pectoris*	16 (28%)	10 (50%)
Mean interval (days) from AMI to death	11 ± 12	17 ± 16
Mean heart weight (g)	470 ± 95	448 ± 100
Mean infarct size (% of LV mass)	23 ± 13	21 ± 15

TABLE IV Comparative Clinical and Morphologic Features in Patients With and Without Coronary Thrombi at Necropsy

* Present before fatal AMI.

Mean values are ± standard deviation.

AMI = acute myocardial infarction; LV = left ventricular.

Thrombus occupying ≤5% of total luminal cross-sectional area, for example, was associated with a wide range of infarct sizes.

Although infarct size and survival interval were similar in all patients with and without coronary thrombi, the 20 patients without coronary thrombi could be separated into 3 groups on the basis of infarct size and interval between AMI and death (Table V). Group 1 patients had small infarcts (averaging 6 ± 4% of LV mass), and they died early after the onset of symptoms (5 ± 4 days). Group 2 patients died late (37 ± 13 days) after the onset of symptoms and they had large infarcts (32 ± 16% of LV mass). Group 3 patients had intermediate-sized infarcts (27 ± 8%) and intermediate intervals between onset of symptoms and death (8 ± 6 days); in 5 of the 6 patients in group 3, the infarct coronary artery was occluded either by pultaceous atheromatous debris or extensive plaque hemorrhage.

	Group I	Group II	Group III
No. of pts	7	7	6
Mean infarct size (% of LV mass)	6 ± 4*	32 ± 16	27 ± 8
Mean interval (days) from AMI to death	5 ± 4	37 ± 13*	8 ± 6

TABLE V Subgroups of Patients Without Coronary Thrombi Based on Infarct Size and Survival After Acute Myocardial Infarction (AMI)

* p <0.01 compared with other groups.

Mean values are ± standard deviation.

LV = left ventricular.

Discussion

In this study, the mode of death after AMI, the interval between AMI and death and the presence or absence of coronary arterial thrombus were examined in relation to the size of the AMI. Specimens were obtained from the files of the Pathology Branch of the National Heart, Lung, and Blood Institute and thus may not reflect general proportions of autopsy patients with fatal AMI. For example, the incidence of cardiac rupture of 31% in the present study is probably greater than the incidence in the general autopsy population.

Infarct size was measured by planimetry and expressed as a percentage of total LV mass, including the basal LV wall, in which extensive necrosis is uncommon. Two unavoidable types of error occur in quantification of infarct size by this technique. First, since

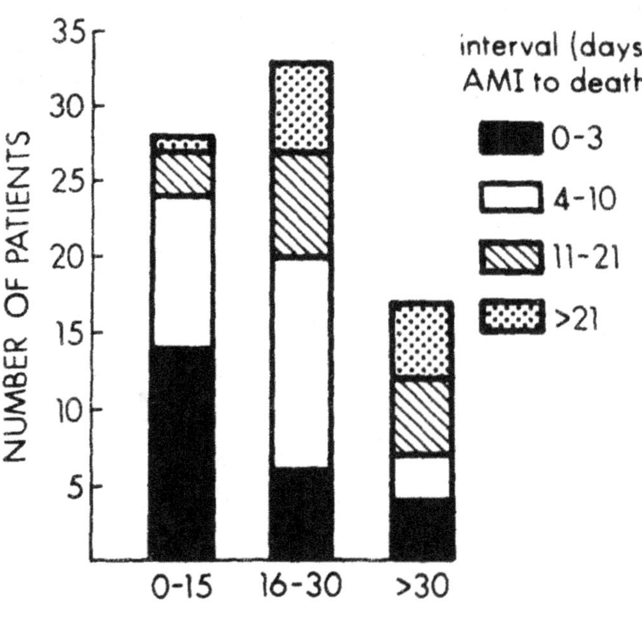

FIGURE 4. Relation of acute myocardial infarct (AMI) size and the interval between the onset of infarction and death.

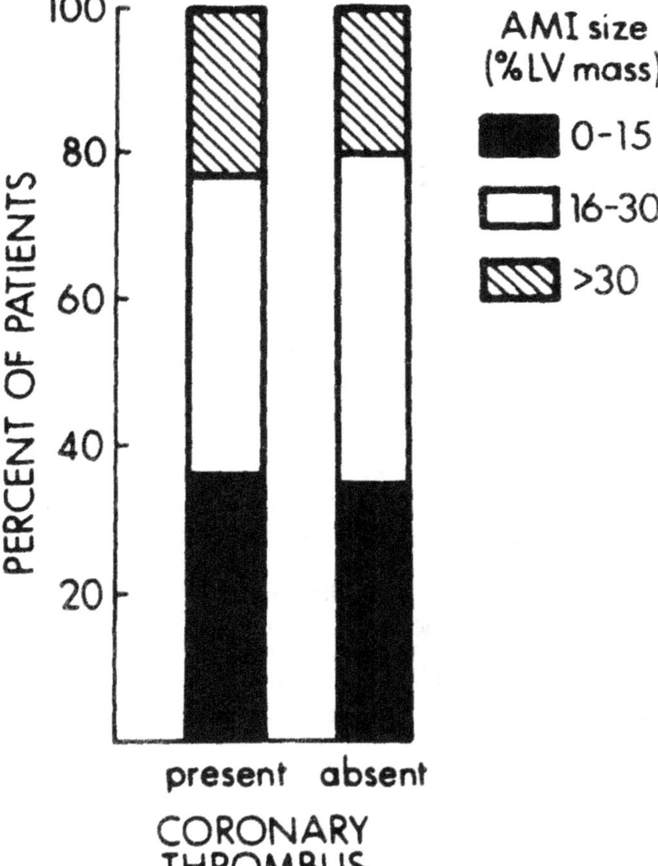

FIGURE 5. Relation of acute myocardial infarct (AMI) size and the presence or absence of coronary thrombus at necropsy.

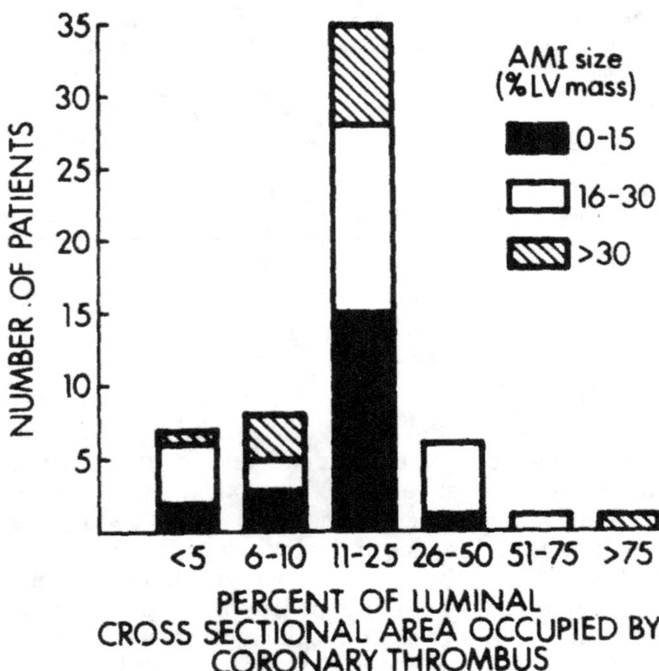

FIGURE 6. Relation of the extent of cross-sectional luminal area occupied by coronary thrombus and acute myocardial infarct (AMI) size. LV = left ventricular.

necrotic myocardium is resorbed during the healing of AMI, infarcts several weeks old would be underestimated. Second, the presence of a healed infarct diminishes total LV mass since the volume of the scar is considerably less than the previous volume of myocardium that the scar replaced. Thus, infarct size might be overestimated if a healed infarct is present. LV scar was observed in 22 of 73 cases (28%). However, in all cases it consisted of small patchy regions of subendocardial fibrosis rather than regional transmural scars. Although the patchy LV fibrosis was difficult to quantify precisely with the methods used for assessing acute infarct size, it amounted to <5% of LV mass in all cases.

Differences were observed in patients with large and small acute myocardial infarcts. In patients with *fatal* small acute infarcts (<15% of LV mass), death occurred early after AMI and was due to cardiac rupture or arrhythmia. Only 4 of 28 patients with small infarcts died more than 10 days after the onset of symptoms attributable to AMI. Thus, the risk of death after a small AMI was greater early and apparently decreased substantially with time.

Patients who died of cardiac rupture usually had small infarcts. Of the 24 patients who died of cardiac rupture, 14 (58%) had infarcts involving ≤15% of total LV mass and 10 had infarcts involving 16 to 30% of LV mass. No patient with a large infarct (>30% of LV mass) died of cardiac rupture.

Of the patients with large infarcts, most died in cardiogenic shock or from an arrhythmia. The length of survival after onset of symptoms of AMI in patients with large infarcts was variable. Our observation that patients who died in cardiogenic shock had large infarcts (averaging 37% of LV mass) is in general agreement with data of others[2-4] who reported infarct sizes of 40% or more in necropsy patients with AMI and cardiogenic shock. Six of our 16 patients who died in cardiogenic shock had infarcts involving only 25 to 35% of the total LV mass but some of these patients lived several weeks after the onset of AMI and infarct size in them may have been underestimated.

We examined the relation of coronary thrombus to infarct size and the interval between the onset of symptoms of AMI and death. Of the 78 patients, 58 (74%) had a coronary thrombus at necropsy. The 20 patients without a coronary thrombus at necropsy were subdivided into 3 groups determined by the infarct size and survival after AMI. In 7 (35%) of the 20 patients, a small infarct (averaging 6 ± 4% of total LV mass) was present. This group of patients had the smallest infarcts observed among the 78 patients and they died early (5 ± 4 days) after onset of symptoms. This observation suggests that very small transmural infarcts may develop in the absence of coronary thrombus. Another group without thrombi at necropsy survived many days (37 ± 13 days); they had much larger infarcts (32 ± 16%) compared with the first group. The prolonged survival may have allowed thrombi, if present earlier, to organize fully or to lyse. The third group included 6 patients without coronary thrombi at necropsy and intermediate-sized infarcts and survival periods; 5 of these 6 patients had coronary arterial lesions consisting of occlusive plugs of pultaceous atheromatous debris or extensive plaque hemorrhage, both of which may behave hemodynamically like occlusive thrombi. Thus, in patients who did not have coronary thrombus at necropsy after fatal AMI, either small infarcts were observed or survival was prolonged or both.

References

1. Sobel BE, Bresnahan GF, Shell WE, Yoder RD. *Estimation of infarct size in man and its relation to prognosis. Circulation 1972;46:640-648.*
2. Harnarayan C, Bennet MA, Pentecost BL, Brewer DB. *Quantitative study of infarcted myocardium in cardiogenic shock. Br Heart J 1970;32:728-732.*
3. Page DL, Caulfield JB, Kastor JA, DeSanctis RW, Sanders CA. *Myocardial changes associated with cardiogenic shock. N Engl J Med 1971;285:133-137.*
4. Alonso DR, Scheidt S, Post M, Killip T. *Pathophysiology of cardiogenic shock. Quantification of myocardial necrosis, clinical, pathological and electrocardiographic correlations. Circulation 1973;48:588-596.*
5. Isner JM, Wu M, Virmani R, Jones AA, Roberts WC. *Comparison of degrees of coronary arterial luminal narrowing determined by visual inspection of histological sections under magnification among three independent observers and comparison to that obtained by video planimetry. Lab Invest 1980;42:566-570.*

Sudden Cardiac Death: Definitions and Causes

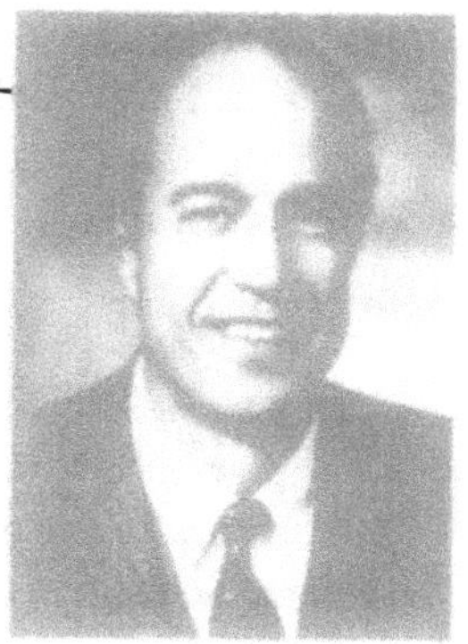

The phrase "sudden death" has been used by lay and medical persons for nearly 450 years. It has many definitions. "Sudden death" might be a game played to break a tie or the extra minutes of play added to a tied game, the winning team being the first team to score. In medicine "sudden death" generally denotes death which is *nonviolent* or nontraumatic, which is *unexpected*, which is *witnessed* and which is *instantaneous* or occurs within a few minutes of an abrupt change in previous clinical state. In heart disease the word "cardiac" is usually placed between the words "sudden" and "death," and the phrase "sudden cardiac death" usually is applied to persons who die suddenly from atherosclerotic coronary artery disease.[1] Necropsy studies of persons dying suddenly from cardiac disease, however, disclose many causes of "sudden cardiac death," and, therefore, greater specificity is required in terms to prevent confusion (Figure). Of persons dying suddenly from cardiovascular disease, the cause may be *cardiac* or *noncardiac*. The cardiac causes may be subdivided into *coronary* and *noncoronary*. Of the coronary causes, atherosclerosis is, of course, by far the most common, and the term *atherosclerotic sudden coronary death* may be applied to them.[2-18] In young persons particularly, several *nonatherosclerotic* coronary conditions, mainly coronary anomalies, cause sudden death.[19-28] Of the cardiac but noncoronary causes of sudden death, the most common are cardiomyopathy, particularly hypertrophic cardiomyopathy,[29-39] and valvular heart disease, most commonly the conditions causing left ventricular outflow obstruction,[40-50] sometimes associated with prosthetic or bioprosthetic heart valves.[51] Also, there are noncardiac but vascular causes of sudden death.[52-55] Some cardiac arrhythmic causes of sudden death not necessarily associated with morphologic abnormalities, e.g., prolonged QT interval syndrome, do not appear in the accompanying figure.[19,56-59]

Some examples of the many causes of sudden cardiac death:

(1) A 13-year-old athletic boy, the son of a former professional football player, collapsed while jogging and died. He had always been asymptomatic. His brother, a year older, had died a year earlier also while jogging. M.M.'s electrocardiogram 6 months earlier was considered "abnormal" but his left ventricular pressure was normal and there was no obstruction to left ventricular outflow.

(2) A 17-year-old girl, who ran 40 miles weekly, suddenly collapsed and died just after crossing the finish line of a 3-mile race. She had been "healthy" all of her life.

(3) A 19-year-old male midshipman was always asymptomatic until he suddenly collapsed and died while sitting on a bench immediately after running around the track several times. On admission examination a year earlier, electrocardiogram had shown ventricular premature complexes and left-axis deviation. The heart was of normal size by chest roentgenogram. The blood pressure was 135/80 mm Hg.

(4) A 28-year-old woman, well all her life, suddenly collapsed and died while running for a bus.

(5) A 28-year-old man died suddenly while pushing a brick-loaded wheelbarrow. He had been well until 2 days earlier when he complained of "pain in his neck," but this did not prevent him from performing his usual construction job activities.

(6) A 33-year-old woman, a domestic, collapsed while at work and died immediately. She had been healthy all her life.

(7) A 44-year-old woman, a secretary, collapsed while walking in her office and died. She had been asymptomatic all her life but on routine examination several years earlier was found to have precordial murmurs (each grade 2/6) consistent with "aortic stenosis and regurgitation." Chest radiograph had shown mild cardiomegaly and electrocardiogram had shown left ventricular hypertrophy.

(8) A 44-year-old male taxicab driver was well until about 1 hour before death when he became enraged because his taxicab was bombarded by snowballs thrown by 3 youths. One snowball entered an open window and hit him in the face, knocking off his glasses. He immediately radioed the police, who arrived several minutes later and apprehended the youths. The police described the taxicab driver as "livid with rage" over the incident and advised him to leave the scene. Thirty minutes later he radioed his dispatcher that he was having breathing difficulties. He arrived at the dispatcher's office a few minutes later, collapsed, and died.

(9) A 60-year-old male school teacher had been well all his life except for recognized systemic hypertension until a

few minutes before death, when he became enraged when trying to prevent 2 students in the school gymnasium from fighting. He finally broke up the fight and, while walking away from the event minutes later, collapsed and died.

(10) An 81-year-old woman, who had had a pacemaker inserted for complete heart block 23 months earlier, collapsed and died while climbing a flight of stairs in her home. During the preceding 2 days, she had noted excessive fatigue, nausea and vomiting.

The cause of death in each of the above 10 patients was different and had not a necropsy been performed, the cause of death could not have been accurately predicted. Patient 1 had *hypertrophic cardiomyopathy*. Patient 2 had *congenital hypoplasia of both right and left circumflex coronary arteries with inadequate perfusion of the posterior wall of the left ventricle*.[19] Patient 3 had *origin of the left main coronary artery from the right sinus of Valsalva with coursing of the left main between the pulmonary trunk and ascending aorta*.[23] Patient 4 had *isolated coronary arterial dissection* involving the left anterior descending and left circumflex coronary arteries.[28] Patient 5 had extensive *cardiac sarcoidosis*.[35] Patient 6 had a *ruptured sinus of Valsalva aneurysm* (into the pericardial sac rather than into the right side of the heart).[60] Patient 7 had *congenital origin of the left main coronary artery from the pulmonary trunk*.[24] Patient 8 had *atherosclerotic coronary artery disease* with severe narrowing of each of the 3 major coronary arteries. Patient 9 had a large heart (550 g [normal $\leq$ 400 g]) from *systemic hypertension* but no significant coronary arterial narrowing or other recognized cause of sudden death.[61] Patient 10 had severe *coronary arterial atherosclerosis* with *acute myocardial infarction* complicated by *rupture of the left ventricular free wall* and hemopericardium. Tests of the pacemaker after death disclosed that it had functioned normally.

In any study discussing sudden death from cardiovascular disease, the word *sudden* needs defining. The World Health Organization has used a 24-hour definition of sudden, meaning, of course, death occurring within 24 hours of an abrupt change in previous clinical status.[62] When this definition of sudden is used, many cases of acute myocardial infarction are intermixed with cases of sudden atherosclerotic coronary death unassociated with myocardial necrosis. Because it takes over 6 hours for histologic evidence of myocardial necrosis to be apparent and because most persons who die suddenly do so within an hour of change in previous clinical status, the 6-hour definition for "sudden" when applied to "atherosclerotic sudden coronary death" more clearly separates the infarct cases from the noninfarct ones.[2,4,16,17]

Although the term sudden implies *unexpected*, in only a quarter of victims of atherosclerotic coronary artery disease is sudden death the initial manifestation of coronary artery disease, and therefore, truly unexpected. Sudden death in patients with angina pectoris or healed myocardial infarction is really not so unexpected. Likewise, in persons with hypertrophic cardiomyopathy and certain forms of valvular heart disease, death suddenly is always a shock but, in actuality, not so unexpected.

Although sudden death is usually reserved for *nonviolent* or nontraumatic deaths, various mentally or even physically traumatic events can precipitate sudden death.[63,64]

The term "sudden death" is often used for persons in hospitals who are found dead, most often in their beds. I try to reserve the term "sudden death" for persons who have fatal or nonfatal cardiac arrest *outside* the hospital or at least

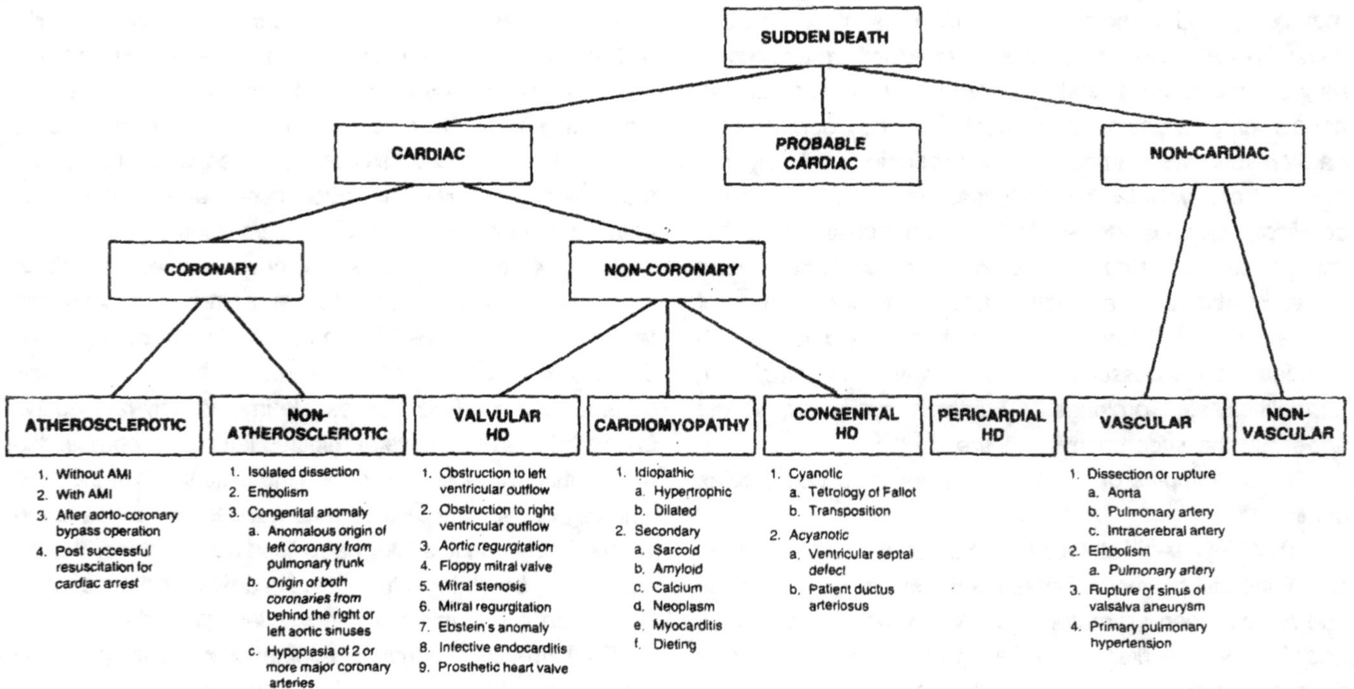

whose symptoms of cardiovascular dysfunction appear initially while outside a hospital. Some of these victims, of course, are rushed to hospitals, where fatal cardiac arrest occurs shortly after arrival.

I have examined many manuscripts that have used the phrase "sudden death" as a *cause* of death: "Patient so and so died of sudden death or patient so and so had sudden death but lived"! Obviously, the term "sudden death" should be used only as a *mode* of death or otherwise lawyers and editors will have a field day.

The use of the term "sudden death" in persons who are successfully resuscitated is not recommended. The use of the term *nonfatal cardiac arrest* (to contrast with *fatal cardiac arrest*) is preferable in this circumstance.

In summary, sudden cardiac death has many causes. Atherosclerotic coronary artery disease, obviously, is by far the most common cause of "sudden cardiac death," but the latter term is not synonmous with atherosclerotic coronary artery disease. "Sudden coronary death" is not ideal either because not all sudden coronary deaths are the result of atherosclerotic narrowing, but "sudden coronary death" is more precise than "sudden cardiac death." Sudden death is not always so *sudden*, or so *unexpected*, or *witnessed* and indeed it may be caused by or precipitated by mental or physical violence. Thus, greater precision is needed when discussing "sudden cardiac death."

William C. Roberts, MD
Editor in Chief

References

1. Eisenberg MS, Bergner L, Hallstrom AP, Cummins RO. Sudden cardiac death. Sci Am 1986(May);254:37–43.
2. Roberts WC, Buja LM. The frequency and significance of coronary arterial thrombi and other observations in fatal acute myocardial infarction. A study of 107 necropsy patients. Am J Med 1972;52:425–443.
3. Bulkley BH, Roberts WC. Atherosclerotic narrowing of the left main coronary artery. A necropsy analysis of 152 patients with fatal coronary heart disease and varying degrees of left main narrowing. Circulation 1976;53:823–828.
4. Roberts WC, Jones AA. Quantitation of coronary arterial narrowing at necropsy in sudden coronary death. Analysis of 31 patients and comparison with 25 control subjects. Am J Cardiol 1979;44:39–45.
5. Waller BF, Roberts WC. Sudden death while running in conditioned runners aged 40 years or over. Am J Cardiol 1980;45:1292–1300.
6. Brosius FC Jr, Blackbourne BD, Roberts WC. Death in the disco. Chest 1980;78:321–323.
7. Walker BF, Csere RS, Baker WP, Roberts WC. Running to death. Chest 1981;79:346–349.
8. Brosius FC III, Waller BF, Roberts WC. Radiation heart disease. Analysis of 16 young (aged 33 to 50 years) necropsy patients who received over 3,500 rads to the heart. Am J Med 1981;70:519–530.
9. Cabin HS, Roberts WC. Fatal cardiac arrest during cardiac catheterization for angina pectoris: analysis of 10 necropsy patients. Am J Cardiol 1981;48:1–8.
10. Roberts WC, Maron BJ. Sudden death while playing professional football. Am Heart J 1981;102:1061–1063.
11. McManus BM, Waller BF, Graboys TB, Mitchell JH, Siegel RJ, Miller HS Jr, Froelicher VF, Roberts WC. Exercise and sudden death. Part I. Current Prob Cardiol 1981;6(9):1–89.
12. McManus BM, Waller BF, Graboys TB, Mitchell JH, Siegel RJ, Miller HS Jr, Froelicher VF, Roberts WC. Exercise and sudden death. Part II. Current Prob Cardiol 1982;6(10):1–57.
13. Roberts WC, Curry RC Jr, Isner JM, Waller BF, McManus BM, Mariani-Constantini R, Ross AM. Sudden death in Prinzmetal's angina with coronary spasm documented by angiography. Analysis of three necropsy patients. Am J Cardiol 1982;50:203–210.
14. Warnes CA, Kishel JC, Roberts WC. Fatal cardiac arrest during cardiac catheterization for angina pectoris. A marker of quadruple vessel disease. Chest 1983;84:631–632.
15. Sprecher DL, Schaefer EJ, Kent KM, Gregg RE, Zech LA, Hoeg JM, McManus B, Roberts WC, Brewer HB Jr. Cardiovascular features of homozygous familial hypercholesterolemia: analysis of 16 patients. Am J Cardiol 1984;54:20–30.
16. Warnes CA, Roberts WC. Sudden coronary death: relation of amount and distribution of coronary narrowing at necropsy to previous symptoms of myocardial ischemia, left ventricular scarring and heart weight. Am J Cardiol 1984;54:65–73.
17. Warnes CA, Roberts WC. Comparison at necropsy by age group of amount and distribution of narrowing by atherosclerotic plaque in 2995 five-mm long segments of 240 major coronary arteries in 60 men aged 31 to 70 years with sudden coronary death. Am Heart J 1984;108:431–435.
18. Warnes CA, Roberts WC. Sudden coronary death: comparison of patients with to those without coronary thrombus at necropsy. Am J Cardiol 1984;54:1206–1211.
19. Maron BJ, Roberts WC, McAllister HA, Rosing DR, Epstein SE. Sudden death in young athletes. Circulation 1980;62:218–229.
20. Maron BJ, Epstein SE, Roberts WC. Causes of sudden death in competitive athletes. JACC 1986;7:204–214.
21. Roberts WC, Siegel RJ, Zipes DP. Origin of the right coronary artery from the left sinus of Valsalva and its functional consequences: analysis of 10 necropsy patients. Am J Cardiol 1982;49:863–868.
22. Roberts WC, Robinowitz M. Anomalous origin of the left anterior descending coronary artery from the pulmonary trunk with origin of the right and left circumflex coronary arteries from the aorta. Am J Cardiol 1984;54:1381–1383.
23. Barth CW III, Roberts WC. Left main coronary artery originating from the right sinus of Valsalva and coursing between the aorta and pulmonary trunk. JACC 1986;7:366–373.
24. Roberts WC. Major anomalies of coronary arterial origin seen in adulthood. Am Heart J 1986;111:in press.
25. Roberts WC, Silver MA, Sapala JC. Intussusception of a coronary artery associated with sudden death in a college football player. Am J Cardiol 1986;57:179–180.
26. Roberts WC. Coronary embolism: a review of causes, consequences, and diagnostic considerations. Cardiovasc Med 1978;3:699–710.
27. Waller BF, Dixon DS, Kim RW, Roberts WC. Embolus to the left main coronary artery. Am J Cardiol 1982;50:658–660.
28. Bulkley BH, Roberts WC. Dissecting aneurysm (hematoma) limited to coronary artery. A clinicopathologic study of six patients. Am J Med 1973;55:747–756.
29. Roberts WC, Ferrans VJ. Pathologic anatomy of the cardiomyopathies. Idiopathic dilated and hypertrophic types, infiltrative types and endomyocardial disease with and without eosinophilia. Hum Pathol 1975;6:287–342.
30. Maron BJ, Roberts WC, Edwards JE, McAllister HA, Foley DD, and Epstein SE. Sudden death in patients with hypertrophic cardiomyopathy: characterization of 26 patients without functional limitation. Am J Cardiol 1978;41:803–810.
31. Maron BJ, Lipson LC, Roberts WC, Savage DD, Epstein SE. "Malignant" hypertrophic cardiomyopathy: identification of a subgroup of families with unusually frequent premature death. Am J Cardiol 1978;41:1133–1140.
32. Maron BJ, Tajik AJ, Ruttenberg HD, Graham TP, Atwood GF, Victoria BE, Lie JT, Roberts WC. Hypertrophic cardiomyopathy in infants: clinical features and natural history. Circulation 1982;65:7–17.
33. Maron BJ, Roberts WC, Epstein SE. Sudden death in hypertrophic cardiomyopathy: a profile of 78 patients. Circulation 1982;65:1388–1394.
34. Maron BJ, Epstein SE, Roberts WC. Hypertrophic cardiomyopathy: a common cause of sudden death in the young competitive athlete. Eur Heart J 1983;4:suppl F:135–144.
35. Roberts WC, McAllister HA Jr, Ferrans VJ. Sarcoidosis of the heart. A clinicopathologic study of 35 necropsy patients (group I) and review of 78 previously described necropsy patients (group II). Am J Med 1977;63:86–108.
36. Virmani R, Bures JC, Roberts WC. Cardiac sarcoidosis: a major cause of sudden death in young individuals. Chest 1980;77:423–428.
37. Saffitz JE, Sazama K, Roberts WC. Amyloidosis limited to small arteries causing angina pectoris and sudden death. Am J Cardiol 1983;51:1234–1235.
38. Roberts WC, Waller BF. Cardiac amyloidosis causing cardiac dysfunction: analysis of 54 necropsy patients. Am J Cardiol 1983;52:137–146.
39. Saffitz JE, Ferrans VJ, Rodriquez ER, Lewis FR, Roberts WC. Histiocytoid cardiomyopathy: a cause of sudden death in apparently healthy infants. Am J Cardiol 1983;52:215–217.
40. Morrow AG, Fort L III, Roberts WC, Braunwald E. Discrete subaortic stenosis complicated by aortic valvular regurgitation. Clinical, hemodynamic, and pathologic studies and the results of operative treatment. Circulation 1965;31:163–171.
41. Roberts WC, Morrow AG. Aortico-left ventricular tunnel. A cause of massive aortic regurgitation and of intracardiac aneurysm. Am J Med

1965;39:662–667.

42. Roberts WC. *The structure of the aortic valve in clinically-isolated aortic stenosis. An autopsy study of 162 patients over 15 years of age.* Circulation 1970;42:91–97.

43. Roberts WC. *The congenitally bicuspid aortic valve. A study of 85 autopsy cases. Am J Cardiol* 1970;26:72–83.

44. Roberts WC. *Anatomically isolated aortic valvular disease. The case against its being of rheumatic etiology. Am J Med* 1970;49:151–159.

45. Roberts WC, Perloff JK, Constantino T. *Severe valvular aortic stenosis in patients over 65 years of age. A clinicopathologic study. Am J Cardiol* 1971;27:497–506.

46. Falcone MW, Roberts WC, Morrow AG, Perloff JK. *Congenital aortic stenosis resulting from unicommissural valve. Clinical and anatomic features in twenty-one adult patients.* Circulation 1971;44:272–280.

47. Roberts WC, Dangel JC, Bulkley BH. *Non-rheumatic valvular cardiac disease. A clinicopathologic survey of 27 different conditions causing valvular dysfunction.* Cardiovasc Clin 1973;5:333–446.

48. Maron BJ, Redwood DR, Roberts WC, Henry WL, Morrow AG, Epstein SE. *Tunnel subaortic stenosis. Left ventricular outflow tract obstruction produced by fibromuscular tubular narrowing.* Circulation 1976;54:404–416.

49. Roberts WC. *Morphologic features of the normal and abnormal mitral valve. Am J Cardiol* 1983;51:1005–1028.

50. Roberts WC. *The 2 most common congenital heart diseases. Am J Cardiol* 1984;53:1198.

51. Roberts WC. *The silver anniversary of cardiac valve replacement. Am J Cardiol* 1985;56:503–506.

52. Roberts WC. *The aorta: its acquired diseases and their consequences as viewed from a morphologic perspective.* In: Lindsay J Jr, Hurst JW, eds. The Aorta. New York: Grune & Stratton, 1979:51–117.

53. Roberts WC. *Aortic dissection: anatomy, consequences, and causes. Am Heart J* 1981;101:195–214.

54. Waller BF, Reis RL, McIntosh CL, Epstein SE, Roberts WC. *The Marfan cardiovascular disease without the Marfan syndrome.* Chest 1980;77:533–540.

55. Roberts WC, Honig HS. *The spectrum of cardiovascular disease in the Marfan syndrome: a clinico-morphologic study of 18 necropsy patients and comparison to 151 previously reported necropsy patients. Am Heart J* 1982;104:115–135.

56. Isner JM, Sours HE, Paris AL, Ferrans VJ, Roberts WC. *Sudden, unexpected death in avid dieters using the liquid-protein-modified-fast diet. Observations in 17 patients and the role of the prolonged QT interval.* Circulation 1979;60:1401–1412.

57. Siegel RJ, Cabeen WR Jr, Roberts WC. *Prolonged QT interval–ventricular tachycardia syndrome from massive rapid weight loss utilizing the liquid-protein-modified-fast diet: sudden death with sinus node ganglionitis and neuritis. Am Heart J* 1981;102:121–123.

58. Isner JM, Roberts WC, Heymsfield SB, Yager J. *Anorexia nervosa and sudden death.* Ann Intern Med 1985;102:49–52.

59. McManus BM, Fleury TA, Roberts WC. *Fatal catecholamine crisis in pheochromocytoma: curable cause of cardiac arrest. Am Heart J* 1981;102:930–932.

60. Roberts WC. *Congenital cardiovascular abnormalities usually "silent" until adulthood: morphologic features of the floppy mitral valve, valvular aortic stenosis, hypertrophic cardiomyopathy, sinus of Valsalva aneurysm, and the Marfan syndrome.* In: Roberts WC, ed. Congenital Heart Disease in Adults. Philadelphia: FA Davis, 1979:407–453 (Cardiovasc Clin 10;[1]:-574).

61. Roberts WC. *The hypertensive diseases. Evidence that systemic hypertension is greater risk factor to the development of other cardiovascular diseases than previously suspected. Am J Med* 1975;59:523–532.

62. *Classification of atherosclerotic lesions. Report of a study group.* WHO Techn Rep Ser 1958 (No. 143).

63. Engel GL. *Sudden and rapid death during psychological stress. Forklore or folk wisdom?* Ann Intern Med 1971;74:771–782.

64. Engel GL. *Psychologic stress, vasodepressor (vasovagal) syncope, and sudden death.* Ann Intern Med 1978;89:403–412.

Rupture of a Left Ventricular Papillary Muscle During Acute Myocardial Infarction: Analysis of 22 Necropsy Patients

DEBORAH J. BARBOUR, MD, WILLIAM C. ROBERTS, MD, FACC

Bethesda, Maryland

Certain clinical and cardiac morphologic findings are described in 22 patients, aged 45 to 80 years (mean 64) (15 men [68%]), in whom rupture of a papillary muscle occurred during acute myocardial infarction. In most, the acute infarction associated with papillary muscle rupture was a first coronary event (only 18% had a myocardial scar consistent with prior infarction and 29% had angina pectoris). The posteromedial papillary muscle, presumably because of its more tenuous blood supply, ruptured almost three times more frequently than the anterolateral one (73 and 27%, respectively).

Quantitative examination of the amounts of narrowing by atherosclerotic plaque in each of the four major epicardial coronary arteries (right, left main, left anterior descending and left circumflex) disclosed less narrowing in the patients with rupture than in the patients with fatal acute myocardial infarction unassociated with rupture. Of the 519 five mm sections of coronary artery examined (11 patients), only 68 sections (13%) were narrowed greater than 75% in cross-sectional area compared with 34% of 1,403 sections from 27 patients with fatal myocardial infarction without rupture.

(J Am Coll Cardiol 1986;8:558–65)

Although necrosis of one or both left ventricular papillary muscles during acute myocardial infarction is common, rupture of a papillary muscle during acute infarction is rare. Wei and associates (1,2) reported on 13 patients with papillary muscle rupture during acute myocardial infarction who were studied at necropsy at The Johns Hopkins Hospital in a 21 year period, and Nishimura et al. (3) reported on 11 such patients who were studied at necropsy at the Mayo Clinic in a 42 year period. During the past 14 years we have studied 22 patients at necropsy in whom one left ventricular papillary muscle ruptured during acute myocardial infarction. This report describes certain of their clinical and morphologic findings, with particular focus on the detailed evaluation of the amounts of narrowing in the major epicardial coronary arteries.

Results

Clinical Findings

Source of patients. The 22 patients had necropsy performed at 14 different institutions and the hearts were sub-

From the Pathology Branch, National Heart, Lung, and Blood Institute, National Institutes of Health, Bethesda, Maryland.

Manuscript received February 26, 1986; revised manuscript received April 8, 1986, accepted April 14, 1986.

Address for reprints: William C. Roberts, MD, Building 10A, Room 3E30, National Heart, Lung, and Blood Institute, National Institutes of Health, Bethesda, Maryland 20892.

sequently submitted to the Pathology Branch of the National Heart, Lung, and Blood Institute for examination (Table 1). Two patients (Cases 16 and 22) have been described previously (4,5). All hearts initially were examined by W.C.R.; 12 were reexamined by both authors. The medical records from each of the submitting hospitals were reviewed and the findings are tabulated in Table 1. Of the 22 patients, 20 died in a hopital and 2 patients (Cases 1 and 8) died at work or at home. The ages of the 22 patients ranged from 45 to 80 years (mean 64); 15 (68%) were men and 7 (32%) were women. Two patients (Cases 9 and 20) had had a myocardial infarct that healed before the fatal acute infarction associated with papillary muscle rupture.

Angina pectoris. This symptom had been present before the fatal acute infarction associated with papillary muscle rupture in 6 (27%) of the 22 patients. Two of these six patients had had an aortocoronary bypass operation because of angina; Patient 11 had the operation 3 months before death and Patient 13 had it 2 years before death.

Congestive heart failure. None of the 22 patients had evidence of congestive heart failure before the acute myocardial infarction associated with papillary muscle rupture.

Systemic hypertension and diabetes mellitus. Although the heart at necropsy was enlarged (heart weight > 350 g in women and > 400 g in men) in 17 (77%) of the 22 patients, a history of systemic hypertension had been recorded in only 8 patients (36%). Diabetes mellitus was known to be present in three patients (14%).

Table 1. Clinical and Morphologic Observations in 22 Patients With Acute Myocardial Infarction and Papillary Muscle Rupture

Case	Age (yr) & Sex	AP	SH	DM	AMI Diagnosed Clinically	Interval from AMI to Death (days)	Interval from AMI to Rupture (days)	Shock	CHF	Site of AMI By ECG	Site of AMI At N	Size of AMI	LV Scar	Papillary Muscle Ruptured	Type Rupture	HW (g)	No. of Four Major CA >75% in XSA
										A. Without mitral valve replacement							
1	50M	0	—	—	0	5	5	0	0	—	A	S	0	AL	I	470	1
2	51M	0	0	+	0	32	14	+	+	ND	P	L	0	PM	I	395	3
3	52M	+	+	0	+	5	2	+	+	P	P	S	0	PM	I	530	—
4	55M	0	0	0	+	6	3	+	+	ND	A	L	+	AL	C	380	—
5	59M	0	0	0	+	4	—	+	+	P	P	L	0	PM	C	550	2
6	61M	+	0	0	+	11	7	+	+	P	P	L	0	PM	C	510	—
7	66M	0	0	0	0	7	5	0	+	—	P	L	0	PM	C	550	—
8	66M	0	—	0	0	7	7	0	0	—	A	S	0	AL	C	500	2
9	67F	0	+	0	+	5	5	+	0	P	P	S	+	PM	I	395	2
10	67F	0	0	+	+	25	—	+	+	P	P	L	0	PM	I	645	2
11	72M	+	+	0	+	3	—	0	0	—	P	S	0	PM	I	530	3
12	76F	+	+	—	+	—	—	0	0	P	P	L	0	PM	I	450	3
13	76F	+	—	0	+	2	1	+	—	A	A	L	0	AL	I	550	3
14	77M	0	—	0	+	4	4	+	+	ND	A	L	0	AL	C	480	—
15	78F	—	0	—	+	—	—	—	—	—	P	L	0	PM	I	285	—
16	78F	0	+	+	+	1	1	0	+	ND	P	S	0	PM	I	360	1
17	80F	0	0	0	0	2	—	+	+	ND	P	L	+	PM	I	335	2
										B. With mitral valve replacement							
18	45M	0	+	0	+	4	3	+	0	P	P&A	L	0	AL	I	425	2
19	47M	0	+	0	+	6	1	0	+	ND	P	L	0	PM	I	450	1
20	63M	+	0	0	0	—	—	0	+	ND	P	S	+	PM	I	590	3
21	65M	0	0	0	+	7	5	+	+	P	P	L	0	PM	I	550	3
22	65M	0	+	0	+	84	6	0	+	P	P	—	+	PM	I	350	—

A = anterior; AL = anterolateral; AMI = acute myocardial infarction; AP = angina pectoris; C = complete; CA = coronary arteries; CHF = congestive heart failure; DM = diabetes mellitus; ECG = electrocardiogram; F = female; HW = heart weight; I = incomplete; L = large; LV = left ventricular; M = male; N = necropsy; ND = not diagnostic; P = posterior (inferior); PM = posteromedial; S = small; SH = systemic hypertension; XSA = cross-sectional area; + = present; 0 = absent; — = unknown.

Diagnosis of infarction. The acute myocardial infarction was diagnosed during life in 16 (73%) of the 22 patients by a typical pain pattern and diagnostic electrocardiographic or enzymatic changes, or both. Of the six patients in whom the diagnosis of acute infarction was not established during life, two (Cases 1 and 8) died suddenly outside the hospital; both had had intermittent chest pain for 5 to 7 days. Patient 2 died several days after a peripheral vascular operation; Patient 7 had Hodgkin's disease and his chest pain was attributed to the lymphoma rather than to acute myocardial infarction. Patient 17 was hospitalized for gastrointestinal bleeding and the electrocardiogram showed new left bundle branch block, and Patient 20 presented initially with severe congestive heart failure and mitral regurgitation without chest pain or electrocardiographic evidence of acute myocardial infarction.

Location of the acute myocardial infarct. The electrocardiographic findings during the acute myocardial infarction associated with papillary muscle rupture were available in 17 patients. The electrocardiogram was diagnostic of acute infarction in 10 patients: of the anterior left ventricular wall in 1 patient and the posterior (inferior) wall in 9. In the other seven patients, the findings were not diagnostic of acute myocardial infarction.

Time of papillary muscle rupture. The interval from onset of symptoms or signs compatible with acute myocardial infarction to death (19 patients) ranged from 1 to 84 days; in 15 patients (79%) the interval was 7 days or less. The interval from onset of symptoms or signs compatible with acute myocardial infarction to papillary muscle rupture as judged by clear-cut worsening of clinical status (14 patients) ranged from 1 to 14 days; in 13 patients (93%) this interval was 7 days or less. The interval from signs or symptoms, or both, considered indicative of papillary muscle rupture to death (14 patients) ranged from 0 to 78 days; this interval was 0 to 4 days (mean 1.8) in 5 patients with rupture of the entire papillary muscle trunk (complete rupture), and 0 to 78 days in 10 patients with incomplete rupture ($\leq$5 days in 8 of these 10 patients).

Consequences of papillary muscle rupture. At least 12 patients had hypotension or shock and at least 14 patients had evidence of congestive heart failure during the acute myocardial infarction associated with papillary muscle rupture.

Mitral valve replacement. Five of the 22 patients had mitral valve replacement because of severe mitral regurgitation associated with the papillary muscle rupture. A nontilting disc prosthesis was used in two patients, a tilting disc in two and a porcine bioprosthesis in one. Four patients died during operation and the fifth (Patient 20) lived less than 24 hours after operation.

Necropsy Findings

Heart weight. The 22 hearts ranged in weight from 285 to 645 g (mean 467). The heart weight in the 7 women ranged from 285 to 645 g (mean 431); the weight in the 15 men ranged from 350 to 590 g (mean 484).

Extent of acute infarct. The acute myocardial infarct (21 patients) involved more than 20% of the left ventricular and ventricular septal walls in 14 patients (66%) and 20% or less of these walls in 7 patients (33%).

Healed myocardial infarcts. Grossly visible left ventricular scar was present in five patients (Cases 4,9,17,20 and 22), and in each the scar was small but transmural (involving all the inner half and all or a portion of the outer half of the wall). Four of the patients (Cases 4,9,17 and 22), however, had a left ventricular scar (indicating previous myocardial infarction which, in three, was clinically silent) before the acute myocardial infarction associated with papillary muscle rupture. The infarction that was associated with papillary muscle rupture had healed in Patients 20 and 22.

Extent of papillary muscle rupture. The papillary muscle rupture, as assessed at either operation or necropsy, involved the entire papillary muscle trunk (complete rupture) in 6 patients (27%) and only a portion of the trunk, that is one or more heads (incomplete rupture), in 16 (73%) (Fig. 1). The anterolateral papillary muscle ruptured in 6 patients (27%) (Fig. 2) and the posteromedial muscle ruptured in 16 (73%) (Fig. 3 and 4).

Subepicardial fat. The amount of subepicardial adipose tissue present was recorded in 14 patients and graded on a scale of 1 + to 4 + . Four plus indicates that the subepicardial

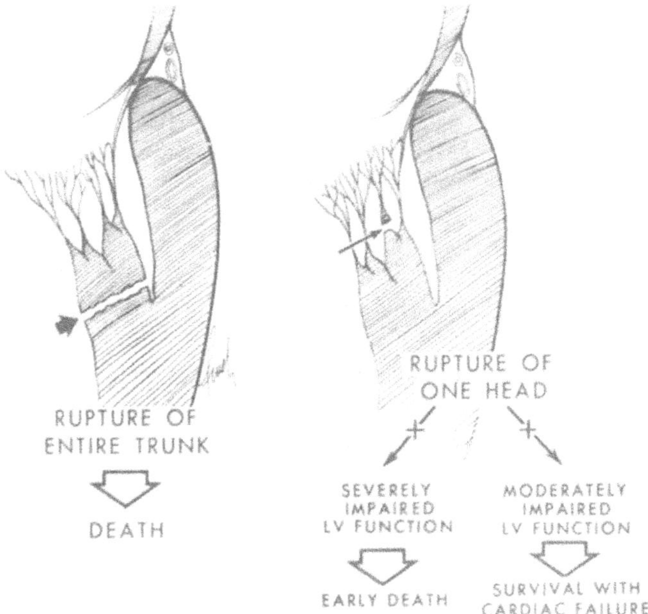

Figure 1. Forms of papillary muscle rupture: complete, involving the entire trunk (**left**) and incomplete, involving one or more heads of a trunk (**right**). LV = left ventricular. (Reprinted by permission of the American Heart Association, Inc. from Roberts WC, Cohen LS. Left ventricular papillary muscles. Description of the normal and a survey of conditions causing them to be abnormal. Circulation 1972;46:138–54.)

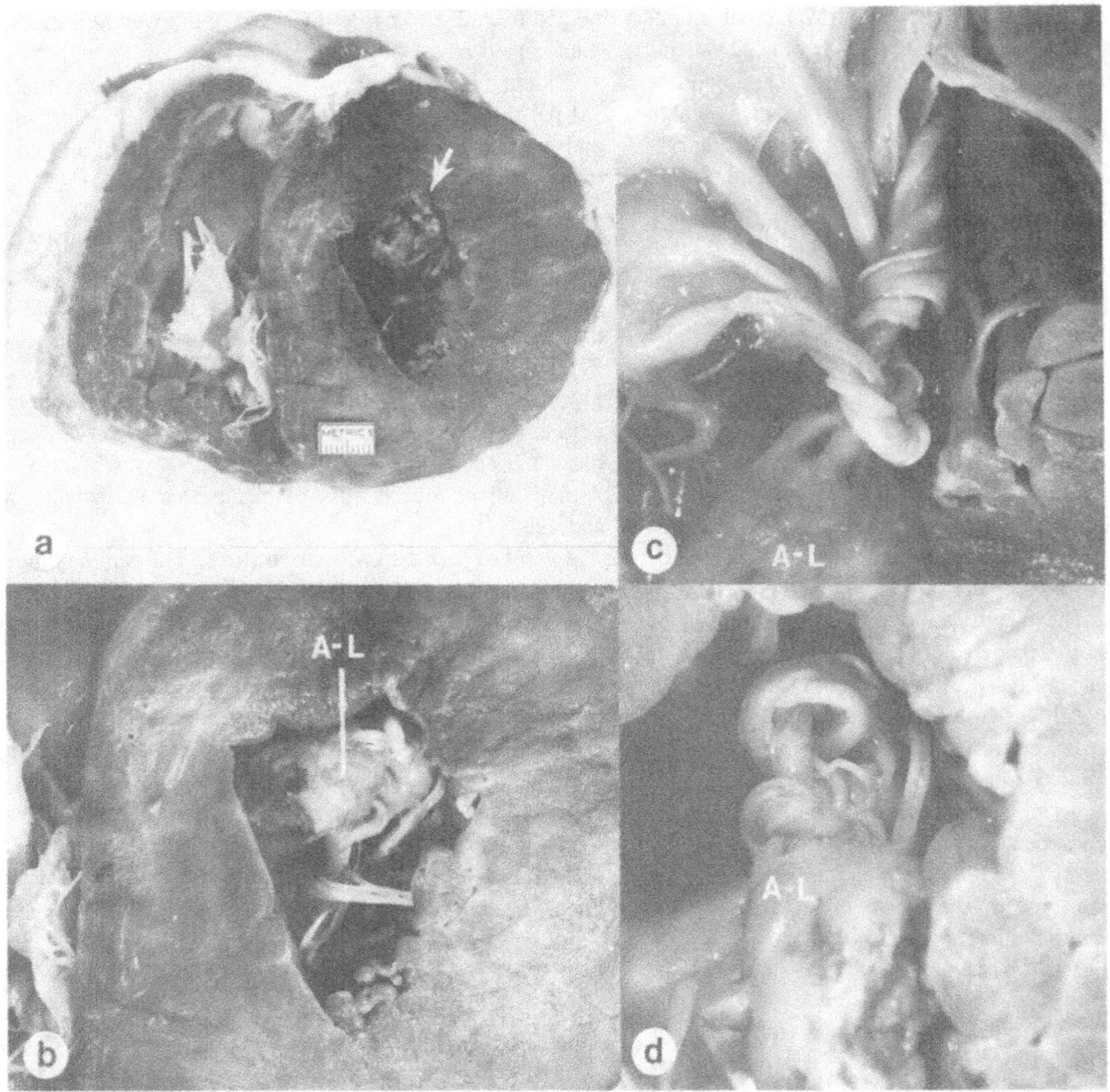

Figure 2. Patient 8. This 66 year old man collapsed and died while mowing his lawn. He was seen by his physician 7 days earlier for dyspnea and mild chest pain. **a** and **b**, Transverse sections of cardiac ventricles showing complete rupture (**arrow**) of the anterolateral (A-L) papillary muscle. **c** and **d**, Close-up of ruptured papillary muscle with attached tangled chordae tendineae.

fat was so extensive that the heart floated in water (6). The amount of subepicardial fat was grade 3 + in 9 of the 14 patients and grade 4 + in 5 patients (Fig. 2 to 4).

Extent of coronary artery narrowing: scoring system. In 15 patients, the number of the four major (right, left main, left anterior descending and left circumflex) coronary arteries narrowed more than 75% in cross-sectional area by atherosclerotic plaque was determined. In 6 patients 3 arteries were so narrowed; in 6 patients, 2 arteries; and in 3 patients, 1 major artery (mean, 2.2 coronary arteries per patient). Of these 15 patients, 7 had a thrombus in a coronary artery superimposed on atherosclerotic plaque.

In 11 patients, each of the four major epicardial coronary arteries was excised intact, decalcified if necessary and cut into 5 mm segments at right angles to the long axis of the artery. Each 5 mm segment was processed so that 6 μ thick histologic sections could be prepared from each. A total of 519 five mm segments (mean 47 per patient) were prepared and a Movat-stained section was examined under the microscope at 40 times magnification. The amount of cross-sectional area narrowing by atherosclerotic plaque was determined from each of the 519 five mm segments by estimating the amount of each of four quadrants of the lumen was obliterated by plaque. Lumen obliterated by thrombus was not included in the amount narrowed. The results of these examinations are summarized in Figure 5.

A scoring system was devised to numerically indicate

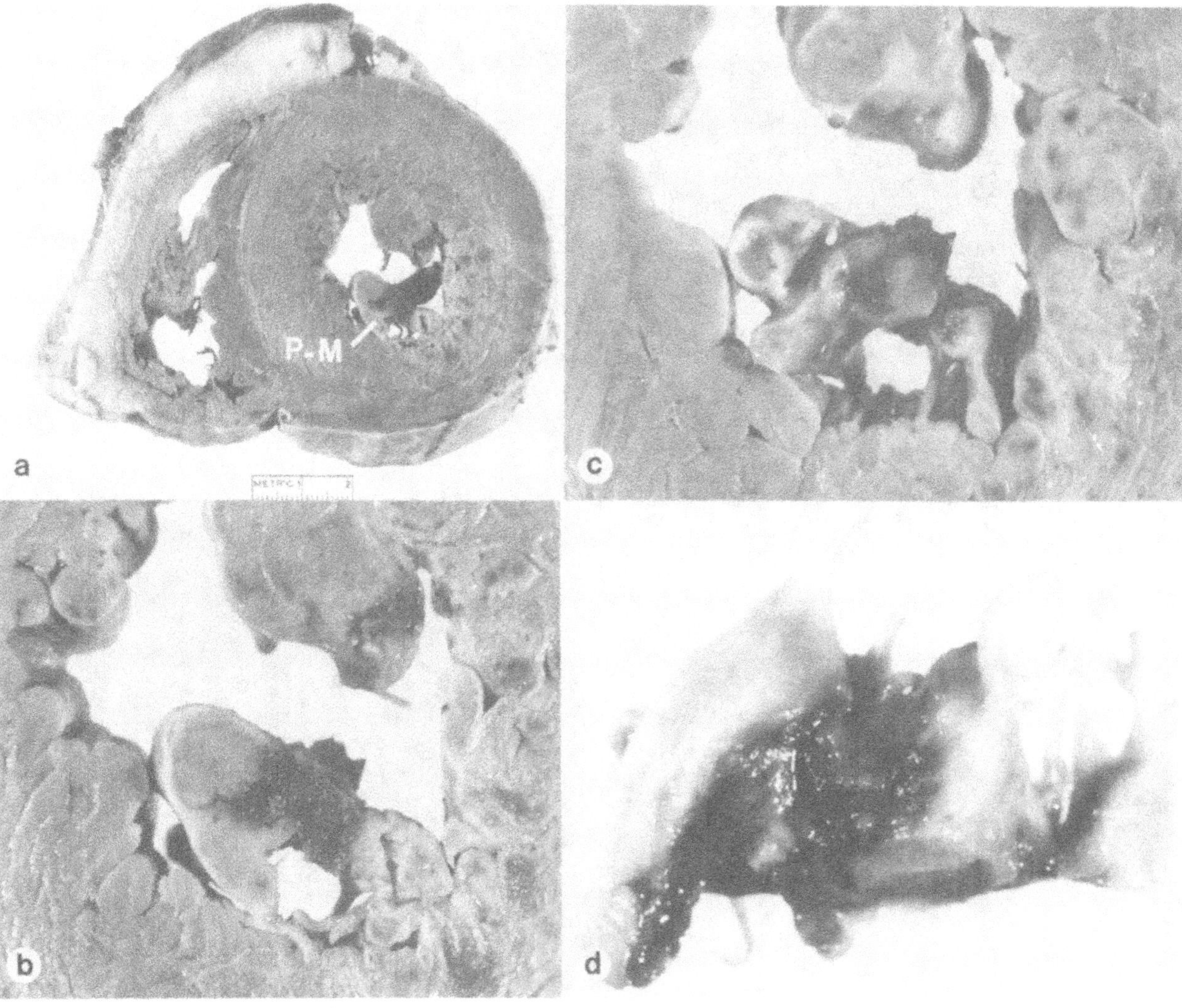

both the extent and the severity of coronary artery narrowing. Every 5 mm segment examined from each patient was assigned a score from 1 to 4, based on percent of cross-sectional area narrowing by plaque; that is, 1 = 0 to 25% narrowing, 2 = 26 to 50%, 3 = 51 to 75% and 4 = 76 to 100%. A total score was obtained for each patient and the mean score per 5 mm segment was derived by dividing the number of 5 mm segments from each patient into that patient's total score. Of the 519 segments examined from the 11 patients, 101 segments (20%) were narrowed 0 to 25% in cross-sectional area (score = 101), 158 segments (30%) were narrowed 26 to 50% (score = 316), 192 segments (37%) were narrowed 51 to 75% (score = 576) and 68 segments (13%) were narrowed 76 to 95% (score = 272). No segments were narrowed 96 to 100% in cross-sectional area. The total score, therefore, for all 11 patients and their 519 five mm coronary artery segments was 1,265, yielding a mean score of 115 per patient and a mean score per coronary artery segment of 2.4, indicating that each of the 519 segments, on average, was narrowed about 50% in cross-sectional area.

Figure 3. Patient 11. This 72 year old man had undergone aortocoronary bypass grafting to the left anterior descending, obtuse marginal and diagonal coronary arteries 3 months before having a nonfatal cardiac arrest en route to the hospital for recurrent chest pain. He died several days later from anoxic complications of his arrest. **a** to **c**, Transverse section of the cardiac ventricles showing acute infarction and incomplete rupture of the posteromedial (P-M) papillary muscle. **d**, The avulsed papillary muscle head with attached chordae tendineae.

Earlier aortocoronary bypass grafting. Patients 11 (Fig. 3) and 13 had undergone coronary artery saphenous vein bypass grafting 3 and 24 months, respectively, before death. Both grafts from Patient 11 were occluded by thrombus, and all three grafts from Patient 13 were occluded (two by fibrous tissue and one by thrombus).

Myocardial histologic studies. Sections of left ventricular wall extending from endocardium to epicardium were examined in 12 of the 20 patients with gross evidence of left ventricular wall necrosis, and in each, the presence of necrosis was confirmed histologically. In these 12 patients,

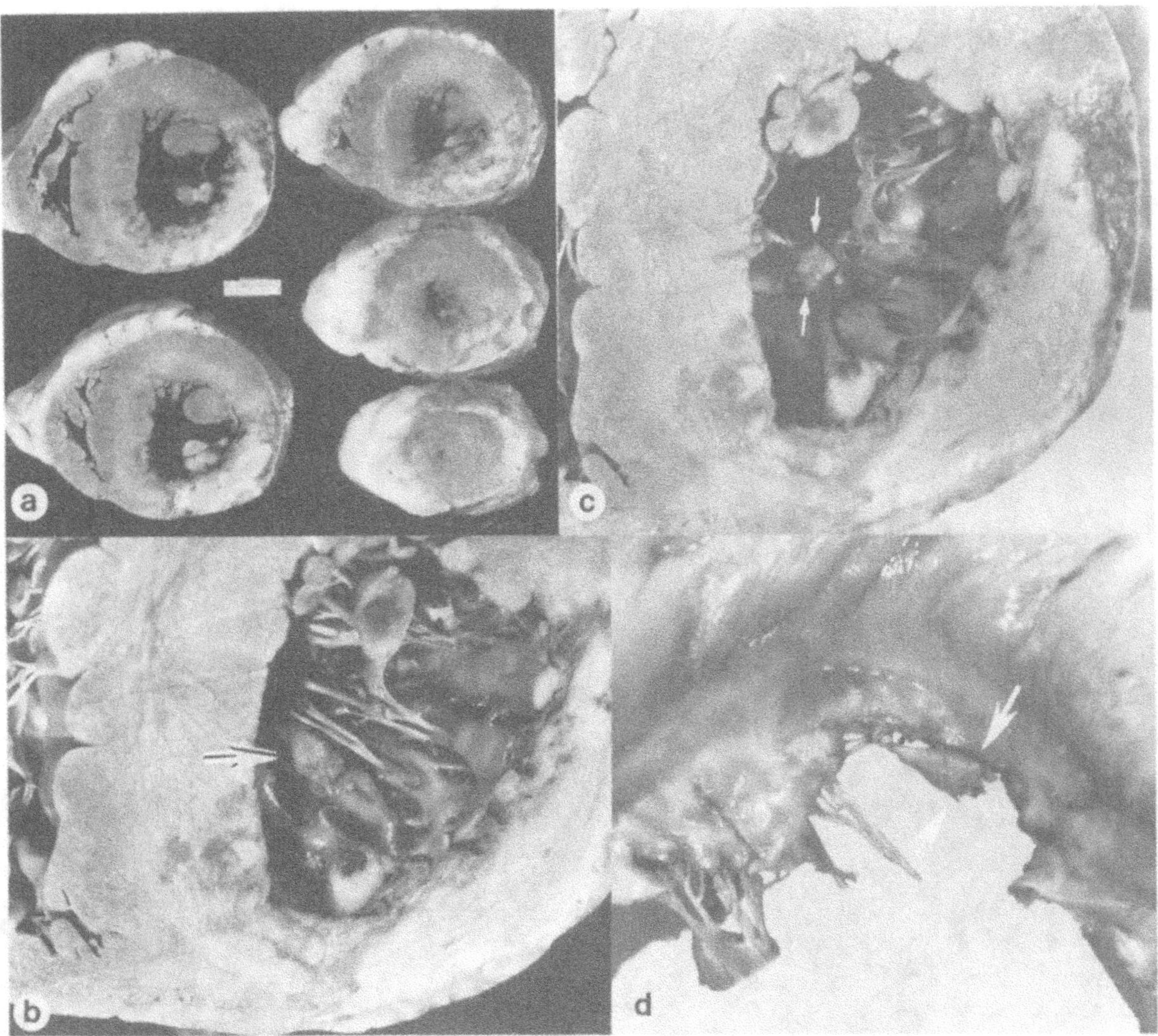

Figure 4. Patient 12. This 76 year old woman had a large posterior wall acute myocardial infarction with incomplete rupture of the posteromedial papillary muscle. **a,** Ventricular transverse slices from base (**top left**) to apex (**bottom right**) demonstrating the extent of the infarction. **b** and **c,** Close-up of the basal portion of the left ventricle showing a portion of the ruptured posteromedial papillary muscle (**arrows**). **d,** Opened mitral valve showing the ruptured papillary muscle head (**arrows**) and the tangled chordae tendineae.

2 to 12 sections (mean 5 each, total 55) of left ventricular wall were examined.

Discussion

Summary of findings. Analysis of our 22 patients with left ventricular papillary muscle rupture during acute myocardial infarction disclosed their mean age to be 64 years; 68% were men and most (81%) had shock or congestive heart failure or both, during the acute infarction. Most (73%) had posterior (inferior) wall infarction with rupture of the posteromedial papillary muscle and a few (18%) had had a previous myocardial infarction as indicated by the presence of a small left ventricular scar. The acute myocardial infarction associated with rupture was preceded by angina pectoris in only 29% of the patients; most (77%) had cardiomegaly at necropsy but few (36%) had had documented systemic hypertension. Most (79%) had rupture 7 days or less after onset of the acute myocardial infarction and all had large amounts of subepicardial adipose tissue. The amount of coronary narrowing by atherosclerotic plaque was less than that observed in groups of patients with myocardial infarction not associated with papillary muscle rupture (7–14).

Site of papillary muscle rupture. In 16 of our 22 patients, it was the posteromedial left ventricular papillary muscle that had ruptured. Other investigators have also observed rupture to involve more commonly the posteromedial than the anterolateral papillary muscle. Of 13 necropsy cases of papillary muscle rupture studied by Wei et al. (2) and 11 necropsy cases studied by Nishimura et al. (3), the posteromedial muscle was involved in 11 and 8, respectively;

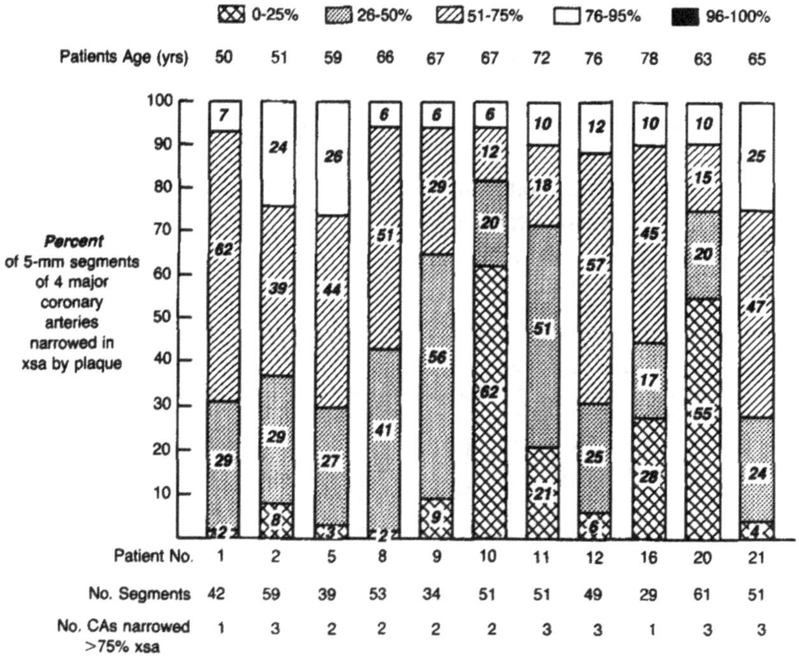

Figure 5. Bar graph showing numbers and percents of the 5 mm segments of the four major epicardial coronary arteries (CA) narrowed to various degrees in cross-sectional area (xsa) by atherosclerotic plaque in 11 of the 22 patients. Only 68 (13%) of the total 519 five mm segments were narrowed more than 75% and 259 segments (50%) were narrowed less than 50% in cross-sectional area.

of 14 operative cases studied by Clements et al. (15), the posteromedial muscle was involved in 12. Why the posteromedial muscle is more commonly involved than the anterolateral one is not clear; it appears that the posteromedial structure has a more tenuous blood supply (from a single coronary artery, that is, right or left circumflex, rather than from two arteries, that is, the left anterior descending and left circumflex) than does the anterolateral muscle (16). In contrast to papillary muscle rupture, rupture of either ventricular septum or left ventricular free wall is associated with equal frequency in anterior and posterior (inferior) wall infarction (17,18).

Papillary muscle rupture as the first coronary event. Rupture of a papillary muscle, like rupture of the left ventricular free wall or ventricular septum, secondary to coronary artery disease, is usually associated with a first acute myocardial infarction (19). Only 3 (14%) of our 22 patients had had a myocardial infarct before the one associated with the papillary muscle rupture, and in each the left ventricular scar was small. Wei et al. (2) found a left ventricular scar in 5 of their 13 necropsy cases but the size of the scar was not mentioned. Three of these five patients had clinically evident myocardial infarction that had healed. In the 11 necropsy cases of papillary muscle rupture described by Nishimura et al. (3), 3 patients had left ventricular scar but only 1 gave a history of prior myocardial infarction.

Size of left ventricular cavity. The left ventricular cavity of necropsy is usually of normal size in patients during or shortly after papillary muscle rupture. Thus, the left ventricular cavity is nearly always of normal size, or at least not dilated, at the time the papillary muscle ruptures. A corollary of this observation is that when patients with chronic congestive heart failure have an acute myocardial infarction,

rupture—be it of papillary muscle, left ventricular free wall or ventricular septum—virtually never occurs. In patients with chronic congestive heart failure secondary to coronary artery disease, the left ventricular cavity is dilated (20,21). The heart in the latter circumstance might be thought of as being "too weak" to rupture.

Amounts of coronary narrowing compared with other coronary events. A surprising finding in our study was the occurrence of less severe narrowing of the coronary arteries than in patients we studied who had fatal coronary artery disease unassociated with rupture. Of the 519 histologic sections examined from the four major epicardial coronary arteries in 11 of our 22 patients, only 68 (13%) were narrowed more than 75% in cross-sectional area by atherosclerotic plaque and none were narrowed more than 95%. In contrast, of 1,403 five mm histologic sections of the four major epicardial coronary arteries studied in 27 patients with fatal transmural acute myocardial infarction unassociated with rupture, 477 (34%) were narrowed more than 75% in cross-sectional area by plaque and 2% of them were narrowed more than 95% in cross-sectional area (7). Additionally, in victims of sudden coronary death (22), healed myocardial infarction (10,23,24) and unstable angina pectoris (25), the percent of 5 mm segments of the four major epicardial coronary arteries narrowed more than 75% by atherosclerotic plaque was 36, 31 and 47%, respectively. The explanation for the lesser degree of coronary narrowing in the patients with rupture is unclear. Detailed necropsy information on the major coronary arteries in patients with papillary muscle rupture has not been described by others.

Subepicardial adipose tissue increase. In each of our patients whose heart was available for reexamination, the amount of subepicardial adipose tissue was found to be excessive and it was so extensive in nearly half of them that the heart floated in water (6). The significance of the cardiac adiposity in fatal cases of papillary muscle rupture is unclear. We have also observed excessive subepicardial fat in virtually all cases of rupture of the left ventricular free wall and of the ventricular septum studied in our laboratory. The observation of excessive cardiac adiposity in these cases has not been described previously.

References

1. Wei JY, Hutchins GM. The pathogenesis of papillary muscle rupture complicating myocardial infarction. Hemorrhage accompanying contraction band necrosis. Lab Invest 1978;39:204–9.

2. Wei JY, Hutchins GM, Bulkley BH. Papillary muscle rupture in fatal acute myocardial infarction. A potentially treatable form of cardiogenic shock. Ann Intern Med 1979;90:149–53.

3. Nishimura RA, Schaff HV, Shub C, Gersh BJ, Edwards WD, Tajik AJ. Papillary muscle rupture complicating acute myocardial infarction: analysis of 17 patients. Am J Cardiol 1983;51:373–7.

4. Nagel MR, Ronan JA, Roberts WC. Left-to-right shunt at atrial level after rupture of papillary muscle from acute myocardial infarction. Am Heart J 1973;86:112–6.

5. Hammer WJ, Ferrans VJ, Roberts WC. Myocardial embolus to coronary artery. Result of rupture of papillary muscle during acute myocardial infarction. Chest 1975;68:843–4.

6. Roberts WC, Roberts JD. The floating heart or the heart too fat to sink: analysis of 55 necropsy patients. Am J Cardiol 1983;52:1286–9.

7. Roberts WC, Jones AA. Quantification of coronary arterial narrowing at necropsy in acute transmural myocardial infarction. Analysis and comparison of findings in 27 patients and 22 controls. Circulation 1980;61:786–90.

8. Brosius FC III, Roberts WC. Significance of coronary arterial thrombus in transmural acute myocardial infarction. A study of 54 necropsy patients. Circulation 1981;63:810–6.

9. Isner JM, Roberts WC. Right ventricular infarction complicating left ventricular infarction secondary to coronary heart disease. Frequency, location, associated findings and significance from analysis of 236 necropsy patients with acute or healed myocardial infarction. Am J Cardiol 1978;42:885–94.

10. Cabin HS, Roberts WC. True left ventricular aneurysm and healed myocardial infarction. Clinical and necropsy observations including quantification of degrees of coronary arterial narrowing. Am J Cardiol 1980;46:754–63.

11. Brosius FC III, Roberts WC. Comparison of degree and extent of coronary narrowing by atherosclerotic plaque in anterior and posterior transmural acute myocardial infarction. Circulation 1981;64:715–22.

12. Cabin HS, Roberts WC. Comparison of amount and extent of coronary narrowing by atherosclerotic plaque and of myocardial scarring at necropsy in anterior and posterior healed transmural myocardial infarction. Circulation 1982;66:93–9.

13. Cabin HS, Roberts WC. Relation of healed transmural myocardial infarct size to length of survival after acute myocardial infarction, age at death, and amount and extent of coronary arterial narrowing by atherosclerotic plaques: analysis of 70 necropsy patients. Am Heart J 1982;104:216–20.

14. Cabin HS, Roberts WC. Quantitative comparison of extent of coronary narrowing and size of healed myocardial infarct in 33 necropsy patients with clinically recognized and in 28 with clinically unrecognized (''silent'') previous acute myocardial infarction. Am J Cardiol 1982;50:677–81.

15. Clements SD Jr, Story WE, Hurst JW, Craver JM, Jones EL. Ruptured papillary muscle, a complication of myocardial infarction: clinical presentation, diagnosis, and treatment. Clin Cardiol 1985;8:93–103.

16. Estes EH, Dalton FM, Entman ML, Dixon HB II, Hackel DB. The anatomy and blood supply of the papillary msucles of the left ventricule. Am Heart J 1966;71:356–62.

17. Vlodaver Z, Edwards JE. Rupture of ventricular septum or papillary muscle complicating myocardial infarction. Circulation 1977;55:815–22.

18. Edwards BS, Edwards WD, Edwards JE. Ventricular septal rupture complicating acute myocardial infarction: identification of simple and complex types in 53 autopsied hearts. Am J Cardiol 1984;54:1201–5.

19. Roberts WC, Ronan JA, Harvey WP. Rupture of the left ventricular free wall (LVFW) or ventricular septum (VS) secondary to acute myocardial infarction (AMI): an occurrence virtually limited to the first transmural AMI in a hypertensive individual (abstr). Am J Cardiol 1975;35:166.

20. Ross EM, Roberts WC. Severe atherosclerotic coronary artery disease, healed myocardial infarction and chronic congestive heart failure: analysis of 81 patients studied at necropsy. Am J Cardiol 1986;57:44–50.

21. Ross EM, Roberts WC. Severe atherosclerotic coronary arterial narrowing and chronic congestive heart failure without myocardial infarction: analysis of 18 patients studied at necropsy. Am J Cardiol 1986;57:51–6.

22. Roberts WC, Jones AA. Quantitation of coronary arterial narrowing at necropsy in sudden coronary death. Analysis of 31 patients and comparison with 25 control subjects. Am J Cardiol 1979;44:39–45.

23. Virmani R, Roberts WC. Quantification of coronary arterial narrowing and of left ventricular myocardial scarring in healed myocardial infarction with chronic, eventually fatal, congestive cardiac failure. Am J Med 1980;68:831–8.

24. Virmani R, Roberts WC. Non-fatal healed transmural myocardial infarction and fatal non-cardiac disease. Qualification and quantification of coronary arterial narrowing and of left ventricular scarring in 18 necropsy patients. Br Heart J 1981;45:434–41.

25. Roberts WC, Virmani R. Quantification of coronary arterial narrowing in clinically-isolated unstable angina pectoris. An analysis of 22 necropsy patients. Am J Med 1979;67:792–9.

The Senile Cardiac Calcification Syndrome

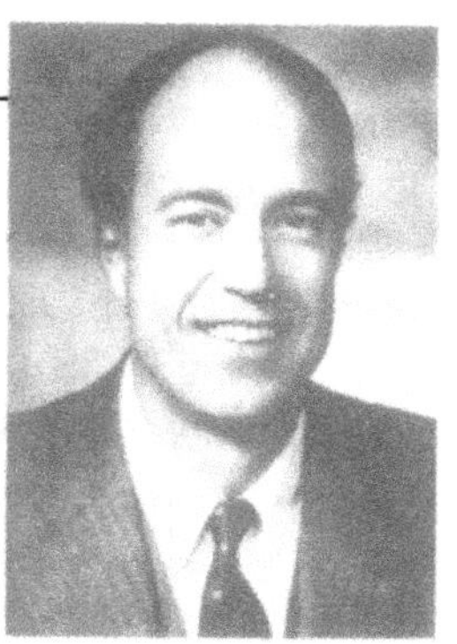

Calcific deposits in the heart are common in older individuals residing in areas where symptomatic atherosclerosis is common. The most common location of the calcific deposits is the *epicardial coronary arteries*. Calcific deposits in coronary arteries are located in intimal plaques, not in media, and therefore, their presence indicates the presence of atherosclerosis. In younger individuals, calcific deposits in epicardial coronary arteries not only indicate the presence of atherosclerotic plaques, but they nearly always indicate the presence of significant luminal narrowing of the arteries containing the calcified plaques. In persons >65 years of age, however, calcific deposits in epicardial coronary arteries do not necessarily indicate the existence of severe luminal narrowing.[1]

A second common site of cardiac calcific deposits is the *mitral anular area*. "Mitral anular calcium" (MAC) is really a misnomer because if calcific deposits were limited to the anulus they would not be visible grossly. The calcific deposits in actuality are located between the undersurface of the posterior mitral leaflet and the mural endocardium of left ventricular wall in apposition to posterior mitral leaflet.[2,3] These calcific deposits usually are located only behind the posterior mitral leaflet and because this leaflet has a C-shaped circumferential attachment to the anulus, the "anular" calcium, if extensive, has a C-shaped configuration. Rarely, the calcium also extends across anterior mitral leaflet to form an "O."[4] When these calcific deposits are small, no hemodynamic consequence results. If the calcific deposits are large, mild to moderate regurgitation may occur and, on rare occasion, actual "mitral" stenosis.[5] In older individuals with mitral "anular" calcium, the anular circumference is virtually never dilated, whereas in younger individuals, particularly those with mitral valve prolapse, the anulus may be dilated.[6-8] Mitral valve replacement in the setting of heavy mitral anular calcium can be hazardous.

The third common site of calcium in the heart in elderly individuals is the *aortic valve cusps*.[9] These calcific deposits are located nearly entirely on the aortic aspects of the cusps, and whether or not the valve is stenotic is determined by the quantity of calcium deposited. Large quantities of calcium impart an immobility to the cusps, which can prevent their opening adequately during ventricular systole. Calcific aortic valve disease in the elderly usually is not associated with commissural fusion and, therefore, the cusps coapt properly with each other during ventricular diastole and aortic regurgitation usually is absent or minimal.[9]

The fourth common location of calcific deposits in the elderly heart is the *left ventricular papillary muscles*, limited to their apical portions.[10] The papillary muscles are the last portions of the heart to be perfused with arterial blood, and, therefore, if any portion of the heart is likely to be short-changed of oxygenated blood, they are it, particularly the posteromedial papillary muscle, which has a single arterial supply, in contrast to the double coronary arterial supply of the anterolateral papillary muscle. Calcific deposits in the apices of the papillary muscles appear to have no functional consequence.

Calcific deposits in the coronary arteries are a manifestation of atherosclerosis, and thus the factors that predispose to noncalcific atherosclerosis also predispose to calcific atherosclerosis. the major predisposing factor, of course, is an elevated (>150 mg/dl) blood total cholesterol level. Because only 5% of Americans over 40 years of age have a total cholesterol level <150 mg/dl, 95% of the population >40 years of age are candidates for atherosclerosis extensive enough to produce luminal narrowing of 1 or more major coronary arteries.

It is my understanding that mitral anular calcium and aortic valve calcium are rare in elderly individuals residing in areas of the world where total blood cholesterol levels are <150 mg/dl. Because calcific deposits in the mitral anular area and in the aortic valve cusps are observed only in populations that develop significant coronary atherosclerosis, it is reasonable to suspect that the cause of the mitral anular calcium and the aortic valve cuspal calcium in the elderly is similar, namely, that the mitral anular and aortic cuspal calcium in the elderly is a form of atherosclerosis. Further support for this view is the frequent occurrence of calcific deposits in the coronary artery, mitral anular area and aortic valve in the same person (Fig. 1). In a study from my laboratory of necropsy persons age >65 years, 100% of those with mitral anular or aortic valve cuspal calcium also had calcific deposits in one or more coronary arteries.[3] Furthermore, of 100 persons >65 years of age with mitral anular calcium, 75 also had aortic cuspal calcium.[3]

The factors that predispose to atherosclerosis in the coronary arteries also predispose to calcific deposits in the mitral anular region and in the aortic valve cusps. Patients with extreme hypercholesterolemia (total cholesterol >500 mg/dl—type II homozygous hyperlipoproteinemia) develop severe coronary atherosclerosis by age 15 years and also calcific aortic valve stenosis in the teens.[11] Mitral anular calcium also occurs in these individuals in the teens.[11] Patients with systemic hypertension have a higher frequency of mitral anular and aortic valve calcific deposits than normotensive persons of similar age and sex.[3,12] Any condition causing hypercalcemia may lead to calcific deposits in the epicardial coronary arteries, mitral anular area, and aortic valve cusps.[13] Patients with diabetes mellitus have more coronary atherosclerosis and, specifically, more calcific deposits in these arteries than do nondiabetic persons of similar age and sex.[14–16] Diabetes mellitus patients also have more mitral anular and aortic cuspal calcific deposits than do nondiabetic persons of similar age and sex.[3]

Another factor suggesting that coronary atherosclerosis, mitral anular calcium and aortic valve calcium in the elderly have a similar etiology is a similar surface appearance of all 3 structures before the calcific deposits form. Specifically, during the teens, 20s and 30s, focal yellow deposits are observed on the endothelium of the epicardial coronary arteries, on the ventricular surfaces of the posterior mitral leaflet, and on the aortic aspects of each of the aortic valve cusps. These yellow deposits, of course, are foam cells. These collections of foam cells represent early or "young" atherosclerotic lesions. Experimentally induced systemic arterial atherosclerosis also is associated with deposition of fatty plaques on the aortic surfaces of the aortic valve cusps and on the ventricular surface of the posterior mitral leaflet.[17] As the fatty plaques get larger, their nutritional needs appear not be be fulfilled, and they degenerate into calcific deposits.

In persons under 65 years of age symptomatic coronary artery disease and clinical evidence of aortic valve stenosis is considerably more frequent in men than in women.[18–22] After age 65, however, the frequency of symptomatic coronary artery disease is nearly similar in men and women, and, likewise, after age 65 years, the frequency of aortic valve stenosis is similar in men and women.[9] After age 65, the frequency of mitral anular calcium is also similar in men and women, but of those persons with "massive" quantities of calcium in the mitral anular area, far more are women than men.[3]

Diagnosis of aortic valve stenosis in the elderly is more difficult than is this diagnosis in younger person.[2] The reason is not entirely certain, but the different configuration of the stenotic aortic valve in elderly compared to that in younger

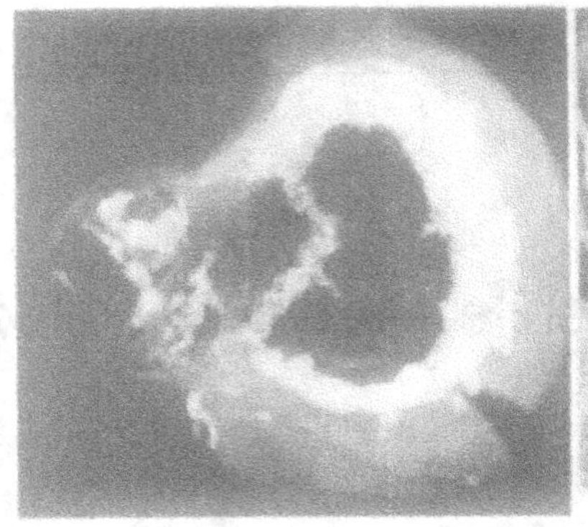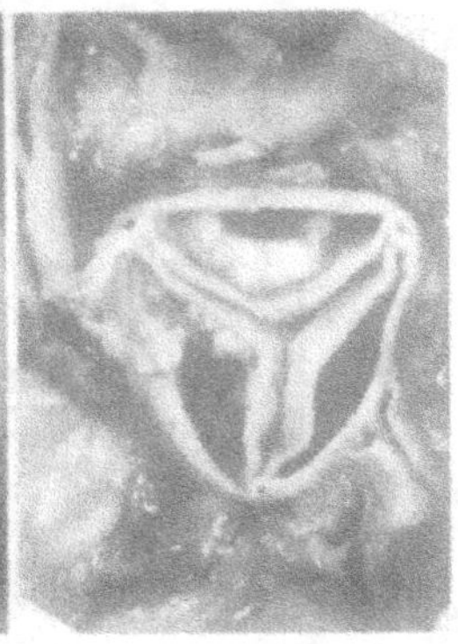

FIGURE 1. Radiograph of heart (*left*) and aortic valve (*right*) in an 82-year-old woman (NNMC #A70-200) who died of caecal volvulus. She never had symptoms of cardiac dysfunction, yet she has massive calcific deposits in the mitral "anular" region, across the anterior mitral leaflet, in the aortic valve cusps, and in the epicardial coronary arteries. The calcium in the aortic valve is located entirely on the aortic aspects of the cusps. None of the 3 commissures are fused, and therefore there was no aortic regurgitation. Reproduced with permission from Roberts and Perloff.[2]

individuals almost certainly is a factor. In the elderly, the aortic valve is usually (90%) 3-cuspid, the calcific deposits are limited to the aortic aspects of the cusps, the commissures are not fused, and aortic regurgitation is usually absent.[9] In the younger individuals, the stenotic aortic valve commonly is congenitally bicuspid and associated regurgitation as the rule rather than the exception.[21] Another factor is that most (75%) of the elderly individuals also have mitral anular calcium, which can also produce a precordial systolic murmur, and few younger persons with aortic valve stenosis have mitral anular calcium.[3] Third, the systemic systolic pressure is usually normal (<140 mm Hg) in younger individuals with aortic valve stenosis, but it often is >140 mm Hg in the older patients.[9] An older individual may have aortic valve stenosis despite the presence of systemic hypertension! And finally, the cardiac output generally is lower and the distance from precordium to heart is greater in older compared to young individuals and these 2 factors may decrease the intensity of the systolic precordial murmur.

Thus, cardiac calcium is not good. It may narrow the coronary arteries, mitral valve orifice and aortic valve orifice and it may prevent either or both of these valvular orifices from closing completely. It is reasonable to believe that both mitral anular and aortic cuspal calcific deposits in the elderly have the same etiology as the coronary atherosclerotic plaques because the 3 are commonly present in the same heart and the predisposing factors of all 3 are the same.

William C. Roberts, MD
Editor in Chief

References

1. Waller BF, Roberts WC. *Cardiovascular disease in the very elderly. Analysis of 40 necropsy patients aged 90 years or older. Am J Cardiol 1983;51:403-421.*

2. Roberts WC, Perloff JK. *Mitral valvular disease. A clinicopathologic survey of the conditions causing the mitral valve to function abnormally. Ann Intern Med 1972;77:939-975.*

3. Roberts WC. *Morphologic features of the normal and abnormal mitral valve. Am J Cardiol 1983;51:1005-1028.*

4. Roberts WC, Waller BF. *Mitral valve "annular" calcium forming a complete circle or "O" configuration: clinical and necropsy observations. Am Heart J 1981;101:619-621.*

5. Hammer WJ, Roberts WC, De Leon AC Jr. *"Mitral stenosis" secondary to combined "massive" mitral anular calcific deposits and small, hypertrophied left ventricles. Am J Med 1978;64:371-376.*

6. Roberts WC, Dangel JC, Bulkley BH. *Non-rheumatic valvular cardiac disease: a clinicopathologic survey of 27 different conditions causing valvular dysfunction. Cardiovasc Clin 1973;5:333-446.*

7. Roberts WC, Honing HS. *The spectrum of cardiovascular disease in the Marfan syndrome: a clinico-morphologic study of 18 necropsy patients and comparison to 151 previously reported necropsy patients. Am Heart J 1982;104:115-135.*

8. Waller BF, Morrow AG, Maron BJ, Del Negro AA, Kent KM, McGrath FJ, Wallace RB, McIntosh CL, Roberts WC. *Etiology of clinically isolated, severe, chronic, pure mitral regurgitation: analysis of 97 patients over 30 years of age having mitral valve replacement. Am Heart J 1982;104:276-288.*

9. Roberts WC, Perloff JK, Costantino T. *Severe valvular aortic stenosis in patients over 65 years of age. A clinicopathologic study. Am J Cardiol 1971;27:497-506.*

10. Roberts WC, Cohen LS. *Left ventricular papillary muscles. Description of the normal and a survey of conditions causing them to be abnormal. Circulation 1972;46:138-154.*

11. Sprecher DL, Schaefer EJ, Kent KM, Gregg RE, Zech LA, Hoeg JM, McManus B, Roberts WC, Brewer HB Jr. *Cardiovascular features of homozygous familial hypercholesterolemia: analysis of 16 patients. Am J Cardiol 1984;54:20-30.*

12. Roberts WC. *The hypertensive diseases. Evidence that systemic hypertension is a greater risk factor to the development of other cardiovascular diseases than previously suspected. Am J Med 1975;59:523-532.*

13. Roberts WC, Waller BF. *Effect of chronic hypercalcemia on the heart. An analysis of 18 necropsy patients. Am J Med 1981;71:371-384.*

14. Curry RC Jr, Roberts WC. *Status of the coronary arteries in the nephrotic syndrome. Analysis of 20 necropsy patients aged 15 to 35 years to determine if coronary atherosclerosis is accelerated. Am J Med 1977;63:183-192.*

15. Crall FV Jr, Roberts WC. *The extramural and intramural coronary arteries in juvenile diabetes mellitus. Analysis of nine necropsy patients aged 19 to 38 years with onset of diabetes before age 15 years. Am J Med 1978;64:221-230.*

16. Waller BF, Palumbo PJ, Lie JT, Roberts WC. *Status of the coronary arteries at necropsy in diabetes mellitus with onset after age 30 years. Analysis of 229 diabetic patients with and without clinical evidence of coronary heart disease and comparison to 183 control subjects. Am J Med 1980;69:498-506.*

17. Thubrikar MJ, Deck JD, Aouad J, Chen JM. *Intramural stress as a causative factor in atherosclerotic lesions of the aortic valve. Atherosclerosis 1985; 55:299-311.*

18. Roberts WC, Buja LM. *The frequency and significance of coronary arterial thrombi and other observations in fatal acute myocardial infarction. A study of 107 necropsy patients. Am J Med 1972;52:425-443.*

19. Roberts WC. *Anatomically isolated aortic valve disease. The case against its being of rheumatic etiology. Am J Med 1970;49:151-159.*

20. Roberts WC. *The structure of the aortic valve in clinically isolated aortic stenosis. An autopsy study of 162 patients over 15 years of age. Circulation 1970;42:91-97.*

21. Roberts WC. *The congenitally bicuspid aortic valve. A study of 85 autopsy cases. Am J Cardiol 1970;26:72-83.*

22. Falcone MW, Roberts WC, Morrow AG, Perloff JK. *Congenital aortic stenosis resulting from unicommissural valve. Clinical and anatomic features in twenty-one adult patients. Circulation 1971;44:272-280.*

Morphologic Findings in Sudden Coronary Death: A Comparison of Those With and Those Without Previous Symptoms of Myocardial Ischemia

Carole A. Warnes, M.D., and William C. Roberts, M.D.†*

Coronary atherosclerosis is a major cause of death in Western industrialized societies, and commonly, the mode of death is sudden and unexpected. It is well established that most victims of sudden coronary death have severe narrowing of one or more major epicardial coronary arteries, but little information is available regarding the amount of coronary artery narrowing in patients who have had previous symptoms of myocardial ischemia compared with those in whom sudden death was the first manifestation of coronary heart disease. We studied 70 victims of sudden coronary death at necropsy to determine the amount and distribution of cross-sectional area luminal narrowing in each 5-mm segment of the four major coronary arteries and compared the amount of narrowing both qualitatively and quantitatively in those with and without previous clinical evidence of myocardial ischemia.

PATIENTS STUDIED AND METHODS

Only patients fulfilling all of the following criteria were included in this study: (1) Death was known to occur within less than 6 hours of the previously witnessed usual state of health. (2) Although the patient may have died in a hospital, he or she was not a patient in a hospital at the onset of symptoms suggestive of myocardial ischemia. (3) At necropsy, one or more of the four major (left main, left anterior descending, left circumflex, and right) coronary arteries were narrowed 76 to 100 per cent in cross-sectional area. (4) Ventricular myocardial coagulation necrosis was absent at necropsy. (5) A cause of death, cardiac or noncardiac, other than coronary artery disease was absent. (6) Chronic congestive heart failure had never been present. (7) A cardiovascular operation had never been performed. Review of clinical and necropsy records in the Pathology Branch of the National Heart, Lung and Blood Institute yielded 63 men and 7 women, aged 22 to 81 years (mean age 50 years), who fulfilled these criteria (Fig. 1). Of the 70 victims, 46 died outside the hospital; these hearts were obtained from the District of Columbia's Medical Examiners Office. The other 24 victims had chest pain outside the hospital and had fatal cardiac arrest shortly after being brought to the hospital. The intact formalin-fixed hearts of all 70 patients were submitted to us for detailed examination. The clinical information was obtained from the patients' private physicians, and if there had been a previous hospitalization, a medical summary was obtained from the hos-

*Formerly Staff Associate, Pathology Branch, National Heart, Lung and Blood Institute, National Institutes of Health, Bethesda, Maryland; presently at National Heart Hospital, London, England

†Chief, Pathology Branch, National Heart, Lung and Blood Institute, National Institutes of Health, Bethesda, Maryland; Clinical Professor of Pathology and Medicine (Cardiology), Georgetown University School of Medicine, Washington, D.C.

Adapted from Warnes, C. A., and Roberts, W. C.: Sudden coronary death: Relation of amount and distribution of coronary narrowing at necropsy to previous symptoms of myocardial ischemia, left ventricular scarring, and heart weight. Am. J. Cardiol., 54:65–73, 1984.

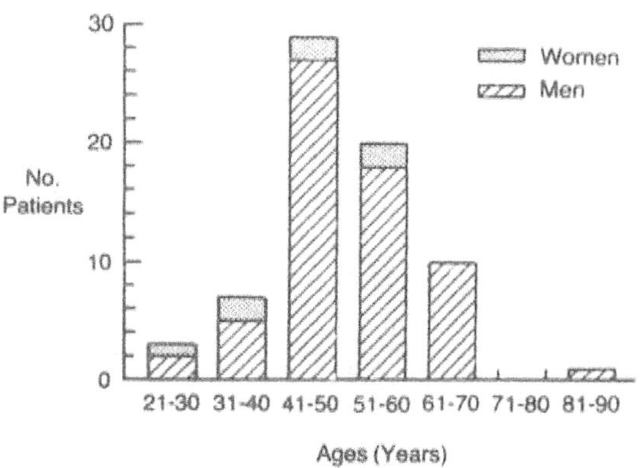

Figure 1. Age distribution in 70 patients with sudden coronary death. (*From* Warnes, C. A., and Roberts, W. C.: Sudden coronary death: Relation of amount and distribution of coronary narrowing at necropsy to previous symptoms of myocardial ischemia, left ventricular scarring, and heart weight. Am. J. Cardiol., 54:65–73, 1984, with permission.)

pital records. Surviving family members were contacted, when possible, for additional information.

The hearts were fixed in formalin for 24 hours or more. The four major coronary arteries were excised intact, radiographed, and decalcified, if necessary. Each artery was then cut transversely into 5-mm segments and labeled sequentially, either from the aortic ostium or from its origin from the left main coronary artery. The segments were then dehydrated with alcohol and xylene and embedded in paraffin, and at least two histologic sections were cut from the paraffin block. Each histologic section was stained by the Movat technique.[6] The amount of luminal narrowing by atherosclerotic plaque was determined by visual inspection of these histologic sections when magnified 25 to 50 times. The percentage of cross-sectional area narrowing of each 5-mm segment was categorized into five groups: 0 to 25, 26 to 50, 51 to 75, 76 to 95, and 96 to 100. All sections were examined by one of us (CAW), and the accuracy of the assessment of luminal narrowing was spot-checked by videoplanimetry. The agreement between these two techniques is approximately 95 percent.[3] A total of 3484 5-mm segments from the 70 victims were examined (mean number of segments per patient was 50). In addition, three or more histologic sections extending from endocardium to epicardium were prepared from the wall of the left ventricle of each patient and were stained with hematoxylin-eosin. Absence of myocardial coagulation necrosis was confirmed by histologic examination.

Chi square analysis was utilized for comparison of amounts of coronary narrowing by quantitative means.

RESULTS

Qualitative Analysis

Of the 70 patients , one major coronary artery was narrowed 76 to 100 per cent in cross-sectional area at some point in 11 patients (16 per cent), two arteries in 19 (27 per cent), three arteries in 33 (47 per cent), and four arteries in 7 (10 per cent). Of the 280 major epicardial coronary arteries in the 70 patients (4 per patient), 176 (63 per cent) were narrowed at some point 76 to 100 per cent in cross-sectional area, a mean of 2.5/4.0 major coronary arteries per patient. Excluding the left main coronary artery, 167 (80 per cent) of the other 210 major coronary arteries were narrowed 76 to 100 per cent in cross-sectional area, an average of 2.4/3.0 coronary arteries per patient. Of the individual major coronary arteries, the left main coronary artery was severely narrowed (76 to 100 per cent in cross-sectional area) in 13 per cent (9 out of 70), the left anterior descending coronary artery in 86 per cent (60 out of 70), the left circumflex coronary artery in 74 per cent (52 out of 70), and the right coronary artery in 79 per cent (55 out of 70).

Of the 70 patients, sudden coronary death was the first manifestation of cardiac disease in 39; the other 31 patients had had either a previous acute myocardial infarction that healed and/or angina pectoris. Comparison of the number of coronary arteries narrowed 76 to 100 per cent in cross-sectional area in the previously *asymptomatic* patients to the 31 with *previous acute myocardial infarction and/or angina pectoris* disclosed the following data (Fig. 2): one major artery so narrowed in 8 (21 per cent) versus 3 (10 per cent) (NS); two arteries so narrowed in 11 (28 per cent) versus 8 (26 per cent) (NS); three arteries so narrowed in 18 (46 per cent) versus 15 (48 per cent) (NS); and four arteries so narrowed in 2 (5 per cent) versus 5 (16 per cent) (NS).

Quantitative Analysis

Analysis of the 3484 5-mm coronary artery segments showed that 950 (27 per cent) were narrowed 76 to 100 per cent in cross-sectional area; 1127 (32 per cent) were narrowed 51 to

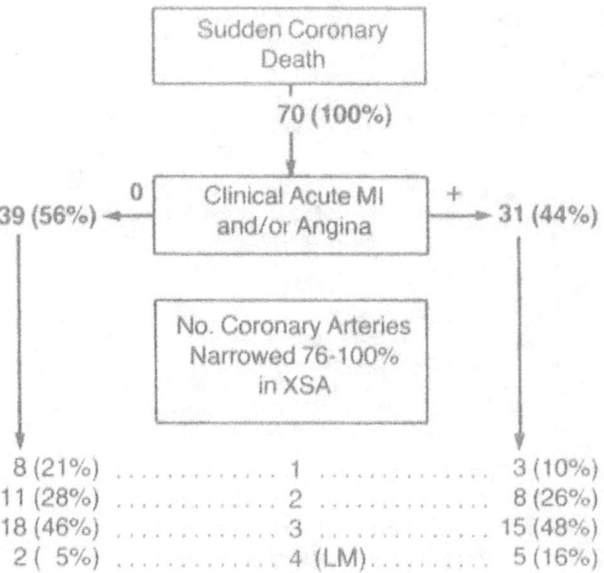

Figure 2. Qualitative comparison of the 39 previously asymptomatic patients with the 31 patients who experienced clinical acute myocardial infarction (MI) and/or angina pectoris before sudden coronary death. (LM = left main coronary artery; XSA = cross-sectional area.) (*From* Warnes, C. A., and Roberts, W. C.: Sudden coronary death: Relation of amount and distribution of coronary narrowing at necropsy to previous symptoms of myocardial ischemia, left ventricular scarring, and heart weight. Am. J. Cardiol., 54:65–73, 1984; with permission.)

75 per cent; 689 (20 per cent) were narrowed 26 to 50 per cent; and 718 (21 per cent) were narrowed 0 to 25 per cent (Fig. 3). The percentage of segments narrowed severely per patient, however, varied enormously, from 2 per cent (1 of 50) to 88 per cent (86 of 98) (Table 1). Sixteen patients had 10 per cent or less of their 5-mm segments narrowed 76 to 100 per cent in cross-sectional area; 15 patients had 11 to 20 per cent of the segments so narrowed; 11 patients had 21 to 30 per cent of the segments so narrowed; 16 patients had 31 to 40 per cent of the segments so narrowed; 7 patients had 41 to 50 per cent of the segments so narrowed; 2 patients had 51 to 60 per cent of the segments so narrowed; 2 patients had 61 to 70 per cent of the segments so narrowed; and 1 patient had 81 to 90 per cent of the segments so narrowed. The five categories of narrowing in each of the four major epicardial coronary arteries also are shown in Figure 3. Comparison of the mean percentage of 5-mm segments narrowed 76 to 100 per cent in cross-sectional area in the proximal and distal halves of the left anterior

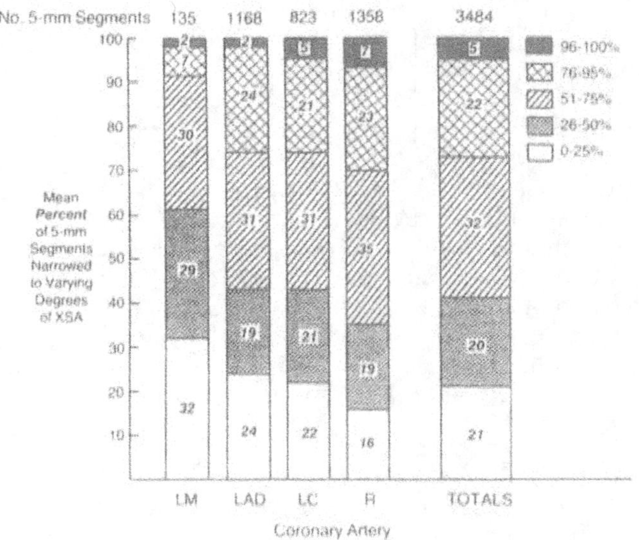

Figure 3. Mean percentages of 5-mm segments of the four major coronary arteries narrowed to varying degrees in cross-sectional area (XSA) in 70 patients with sudden coronary death. (LAD = left anterior descending; LC = left circumflex; LM = left main; R = right.) (*From* Warnes, C. A., and Roberts, W. C.: Sudden coronary death: Relation of amount and distribution of coronary narrowing at necropsy to previous symptoms of myocardial ischemia, left ventricular scarring, and heart weight. Am. J. Cardiol., 54:65–73, 1984; with permission.)

Table 1. *Summary of Percentages of 5-mm Segments of the Four Major Coronary Arteries Narrowed 76 to 100 Per Cent in Cross-Sectional Area According to Age Group*

AGE GROUP (YEARS)	NO. OF PATIENTS	NUMBER OF PATIENTS LISTED ACCORDING TO PERCENTAGE OF 5-MM SEGMENTS OF FOUR MAJOR CORONARY ARTERIES NARROWED 76 TO 100 PER CENT								
		0–10	11–20	21–30	31–40	41–50	51–60	61–70	71–80	81–90
21–30	3	2	0	1	0	0	0	0	0	0
31–40	7	3	1	0	1	1	1	0	0	0
41–50	29	6	8	4	5	2	1	2	0	1
51–60	20	4	4	4	6	2	0	0	0	0
61–70	10	1	1	2	4	2	0	0	0	0
71–80	0	0	0	0	0	0	0	0	0	0
81–90	1	0	1	0	0	0	0	0	0	0
Totals	70	16 (23%)	15 (21%)	11 (16%)	16 (23%)	7 (10%)	2 (3%)	2 (3%)	0	1 (1%)

descending, left circumflex, and right coronary arteries disclosed a significantly higher percentage of severely narrowed segments proximally in the left anterior descending and left circumflex coronary arteries (Fig. 4).

In contrast to the qualitative approach, significant differences were noted between the previously asymptomatic patients and the symptomatic patients when the quantitative analysis was utilized. Of the 39 patients who had been asymptomatic, 502 (25 per cent) of 1991 5-mm segments were narrowed 76 to 100 per cent in cross-sectional area compared with 448 (30 per cent) of 1493 5-mm segments in the 31 patients who had had either a clinical acute myocardial infarction and/or angina pectoris previously

(Fig. 5) (p < 0.005). Comparison of the mean percentages of segments in all five categories of cross-sectional area coronary narrowing between the previously asymptomatic and symptomatic groups disclosed significant differences in the category of minimal (0 to 25 per cent) cross-sectional area narrowing (25 per cent versus 15 per cent, p < 0.001). Comparison of the amounts of narrowing in each of the four major coronary arteries disclosed a higher mean percentage of 5-mm segments narrowed 76 to 100 percent in cross-sectional area in the symptomatic versus the asymptomatic victims in the left main, left anterior descending, and left circumflex coronary arteries but not in the right coronary artery, and a lower mean percentage

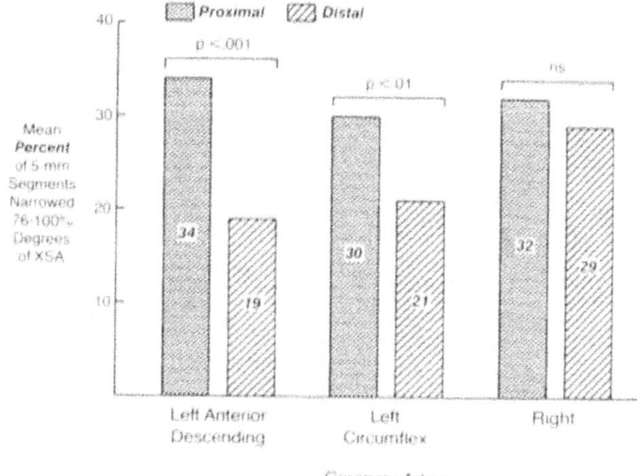

Figure 4. Comparison of the proximal and distal halves of mean percentages of 5-mm segments of the three major coronary arteries narrowed 76 to 100 per cent in cross-sectional area (XSA) in 70 patients with sudden coronary death. (*From* Warnes, C. A., and Roberts, W. C.: Sudden coronary death: Relation of amount and distribution of coronary narrowing at necropsy to previous symptoms of myocardial ischemia, left ventricular scarring, and heart weight. Am. J. Cardiol., 54:65–73, 1984; with permission.)

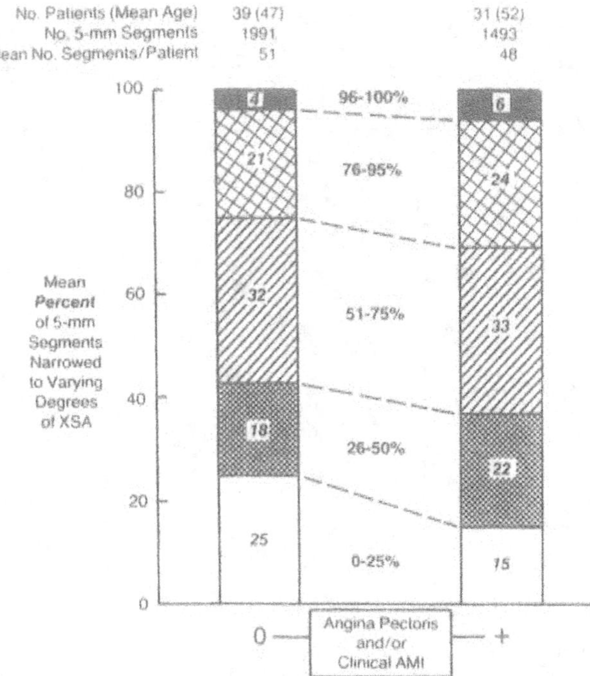

Figure 5. Mean percentages of 5-mm segments of the sum of the four major coronary arteries narrowed to varying degrees in cross-sectional area (XSA) in 70 patients with sudden coronary death: Comparison of 39 patients without and 31 patients with a clinical acute myocardial infarction (AMI) and/or angina pectoris. (*From* Warnes, C. A., and Roberts, W. C.: Sudden coronary death: Relation of amount and distribution of coronary narrowing at necropsy to previous symptoms of myocardial ischemia, left ventricular scarring, and heart weight. Am. J. Cardiol., *54:*65–73, 1984; with permission.)

of segments narrowed 0 to 25 per cent in cross-sectional area in all four coronary arteries in the symptomatic group (Fig. 6).

After it was established that the *extent* of severe narrowing was different in the previously asymptomatic and symptomatic patients, an analysis was made to determine whether the *distribution* of severe narrowing was different in the two groups. Comparison of the mean percentage of 5-mm segments narrowed severely in the proximal and distal halves of the left anterior descending, left circumflex, and right coronary arteries (Fig. 7) disclosed a significantly higher percentage of severely narrowed segments proximally in the left anterior descending coronary artery in both asymptomatic and symptomatic individuals. Proximal narrowing was also more extensive in the left circumflex coronary artery in both groups but did not achieve statistical significance in those who were symptomatic. No difference in the distribution of severe narowing occurred in the right coronary artery in either group. In other words, the distribution of severely narrowed

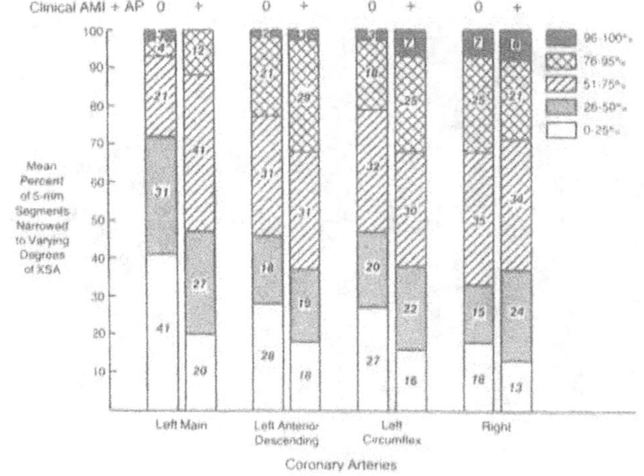

Figure 6. Comparison of mean percentages of 5-mm segments of the four major coronary arteries narrowed to varying degrees in 70 patients with sudden coronary death: Comparison of 39 patients without and 31 patients with a clinical acute myocardial infarction (AMI) and/or angina pectoris (AP). (XSA = cross-sectional area.) (*From* Warnes, C. A., and Roberts, W. C.: Sudden coronary death: Relation of amount and distribution of coronary narrowing at necropsy to previous symptoms of myocardial ischemia, left ventricular scarring, and heart weight. Am. J. Cardiol., *54:*65–73, 1984; with permission.)

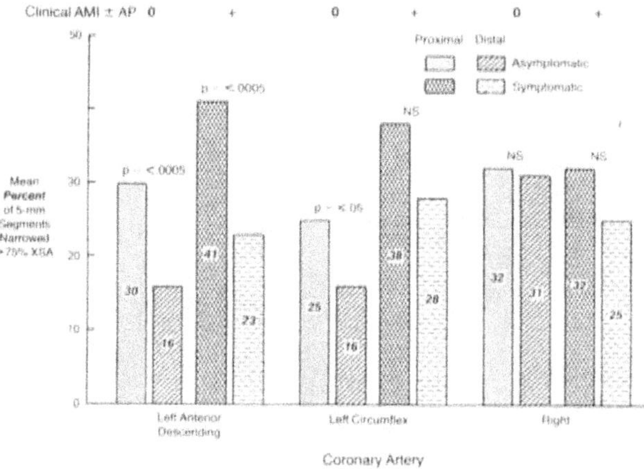

Figure 7. Mean percentages of 5-mm segments of the three major coronary arteries narrowed 76 to 100 per cent in cross-sectional area (XSA) proximally and distally in 70 patients with sudden coronary death. Comparison of 31 patients with and 39 patients without a clinical acute myocardial infarction (AMI) and/or angina pectoris (AP). (*From* Warnes, C. A., and Roberts, W. C.: Sudden coronary death: Relation of amount and distribution of coronary narrowing at necropsy to previous symptoms of myocardial ischemia, left ventricular scarring, and heart weight. Am. J. Cardiol., 54:65–73, 1984; with permission.)

segments was similar in asymptomatic and previously symptomatic patients.

Of the 70 patients, 13 were found at necropsy to have a thrombus in one coronary artery. In 6 patients, the thrombus consisted primarily of fibrin and erythrocytes, and in 7 patients, it consisted nearly entirely of platelets. None of the 7 patients with predominantly platelet thrombi had had angina pectoris or a clinical event suggestive of acute myocardial infarction previously; in contrast, all 6 patients with predominantly fibrin and erythrocyte thrombi had had angina pectoris or a previous myocardial infarction that healed, or both. In all 13 patients, the thrombi were superimposed on atherosclerotic plaques that had already narrowed the lumina 26 to 50 per cent in cross-sectional area (1 patient), 51 to 75 per cent in cross-sectional area (4 patients), or 76 to 100 per cent in cross-sectional area (8 patients).

DISCUSSION

A major finding in this study was that sudden death victims had severe and extensive narrowing of their four major (left main, left anterior descending, left circumflex, and right) extramural coronary arteries by atherosclerotic plaque. Of the 70 patients, 59 (84 per cent) had two or more major arteries narrowed 76 to 100 per cent in cross-sectional area, and 11 (16 per cent) had only one artery so narrowed by atherosclerotic plaque. Of the 59 patients with multivessel coronary artery disease, 19 (27 per cent) had two arteries severely narrowed (76 to 100 per cent in cross-sectional area), 33 (47 per cent) had three arteries so narrowed, and 7 (10 per cent) had four arteries so narrowed. Of the four major coronary arteries per patient, 2.5/4

were severely narrowed. Of the 280 major coronary arteries in the 70 patients, 176 (63 per cent) were narrowed severely, and of them, the left anterior descending coronary artery was the most commonly narrowed artery (60 of 70 = 86 per cent). The 11 patients with one-vessel coronary artery disease (one artery narrowed 76 to 100 per cent in cross-sectional area) were significantly younger than the 59 patients with multivessel coronary artery disease (mean age 41 years versus 51 years). The artery severely narrowed in these patients was the left anterior descending coronary artery in 5, the right coronary artery in 4, the left circumflex coronary artery in 1, and left main coronary artery in 1.

Qualitative studies describing from gross inspection the number of four major coronary arteries severely narrowed in nontraumatic death victims have been performed by others.[1, 2, 4, 5, 7] Results of five such large necropsy studies are summarized in Table 2. Of the 720 necropsy patients included in the five studies, 499 (69 per cent) had two or more major coronary arteries narrowed severely, and 132 (18 per cent) had only one coronary artery so narrowed. One difficulty in comparing any of these five previous necropsy studies with the present one is the varying criteria for inclusion of cases. To be included in our study, a patient had to have at least one of the four major coronary arteries narrowed 76 to 100 per cent in cross-sectional area by atherosclerotic plaque. In the five previously reported studies, however, 89 (12 per cent) of the 720 patients had none of the four coronary arteries narrowed to this extent; all apparently had at least one artery narrowed 51 to 75 per cent in cross-sectional area. Another major problem in comparing our findings with those in previously reported studies concerns different temporal definitions of the term "sud-

Table 2. *Clinical and Cardiac Morphologic Observations in Five Previously Reported Necropsy Studies on Sudden Death in Which the Number of Coronary Arteries Severely Narrowed Was Described*

YEAR OF STUDY	AUTHORS	NUMBER OF PATIENTS	AGES (YEARS) (MEAN)	M	F	DEFINITION OF SD (HOURS)	AP	CLINICAL ACUTE MI	GROSS EXAM OF CAs (INTERVALS IN CM)	NUMBER OF MAJOR CAs NARROWED >75% XSA					CA T	ACUTE MI	HEALED MI	HW (GM) (MEAN)
										0	1	2	3	4				
1972	Kuller et al.	64	25–64 (—)	—	—	<24	—	—	?	5 (8%)	16 (25%)	11 (17%)	22 (34%)	10 (16%)	12 (19%)	8 (13%)	—	—*
1973	Friedman et al.	59	–65 (54)	53	6	<24	15	17	+(0.5)	4 (7%)	9 (15%)	11 (19%)	22 (37%)	13 (22%)	28 (47%)	7 (12%)	31 (53%)	310–585 (—)
1974	Liberthson et al.	220	— (59)	190	30	—	104† (47%)	57 (26%)	+(0.1)	13 (6%)	29 (13%)	53 (24%)	125 (57%)		70 (32%)	59 (27%)	97 (44%)	(448)
1975	Perper et al.	168	25–64 (—)	133	36	—	—‡	—‡	+(0.2)	16 (9%)	25 (15%)	25 (15%)	64 (38%)	39 (23%)	—	17/157 (11%)	68/157 (43%)	—
1979	Baroldi et al.	208	<20–>70 (—)	182	28	—	—§	—§	+(0.3)	51 (24%)	53 (26%)	60 (29%)	44 (21%)		54 (26%)	35 (17%)	170 (82%)	—‖

*Thirty-seven patients (58 per cent) had hearts weighing more than 450 gm
†Chest pain; possibly not angina in all
‡History of "prior heart disease" in 51 (30 per cent)
§History of "prior heart disease" in 102 (49 per cent)
‖Heart weight greater than 500 gm in 87 (42 per cent)
AP = angina pectoris; CA = coronary artery; F = female; HW = heart weight; M = male; MI = myocardial infarction; SD = sudden death; T = thrombus; XSA = cross-sectional area

den." We used a time period of 6 hours or less from the time of previously witnessed usual health to death, whereas the patients included in the studies both by Kuller and associates[4] and by Friedman and colleagues[2] used a time period of less than 24 hours. The time frame utilized in the other three studies was not defined.[1, 5, 7] Our study also included only patients without histologic evidence of myocardial coagulation necrosis (infarction), whereas 126 (18 per cent) of the 720 patients included in Table 2 had acute myocardial infarction at necropsy.

Although the number and percentage of patients with previous clinical evidence of heart disease was mentioned in four of the five previously reported studies (see Table 2), in none of the studies was the amount of coronary artery narrowing in the group with clinical evidence of myocardial ischemia compared with that in the group without clinical evidence of myocardial ischemia. We found the number of coronary arteries to be severely narrowed at some point (the qualitative approach) in the groups of patients with and without previous angina pectoris and/or acute myocardial infarction to be roughly similar. As demonstrated in Figure 2, 31 (44 per cent) of our 70 patients had had previous clinical acute myocardial infarction (which healed) and/or angina, and 39 had not. Comparison of those with previous clinical evidence of myocardial ischemia with those without such evidence disclosed similar percentages of total coronary arteries (four per patient) severely narrowed (84 of 124 [68 per cent] versus 92 of 156 [59 per cent]) and roughly similar percentages of two or more coronary arteries severely narrowed (28 of 31 [90 per cent] versus 31 of 39 [79 per cent]).

None of the previously reported five necropsy studies provided *quantitative* information on the amount and distribution of coronary artery narrowing in sudden death victims. In our study, a total of 3484 5-mm segments were examined from the 70 patients: 27 per cent of the segments were narrowed 76 to 100 per cent in cross-sectional area, including 5 per cent narrowed 96 to 100 per cent. The 96 to 100 per cent cross-sectional area narrowing is probably equivalent to angiographic total occlusion. Not a single 5-mm segment was entirely free of atherosclerotic plaque. A higher mean percentage of segments was severely narrowed in the proximal compared with the distal halves of the three major coronary arteries (left anterior descending, left circumflex, and right). A previous

report from our laboratory[8] that included only 12 of the 70 patients included in the present study also emphasized the diffuse extent of atherosclerois in sudden death victims. Although a control group was not examined in the present study, the previous study[8] from our laboratory included 25 control subjects (mean age 49 years), and in these individuals, only 3 per cent of the 5-mm segments of the four major coronary arteries were narrowed 76 to 100 per cent by atherosclerotic plaque.

Of our 39 patients who previously had had no clinical evidence of myocardial ischemia (asymptomatic group), 25 per cent of the 5-mm segments were narrowed 76 to 100 per cent in cross-sectional area compared with 30 per cent in those who had had symptoms of ischemia (acute myocardial infarction that healed and/or angina pectoris) ($p < 0.005$). The asymptomatic group also had a higher mean percentage of segments minimally narrowed (25 per cent versus 15 per cent, $p < 0.001$) (see Fig. 5).

Although our study patients as a group had severe and extensive coronary artery narrowing by atherosclerotic plaque, considerable variation in the percentage of 5-mm segments narrowed severely was observed (see Table 1). The range was from 2 to 86 per cent: 16 patients had fewer than 10 per cent of their coronary artery segments narrowed 76 to 100 per cent in cross-sectional area, and 12 patients (17 per cent) had more than 40 per cent of their 5-mm segments severely narrowed. Thus, the extent of severe narrowing is difficult to predict in the individual patient but is predictable in groups of patients dying suddenly from coronary artery disease. The previously symptomatic patients clearly had more severe coronary artery narrowing and less minimal narrowing than the asymptomatic group.

REFERENCES

1. Baroldi, G., Falzi, G., and Mariani, F.: Sudden coronary death: A postmortem study in 208 selected cases compared to 97 "control" subjects. Am. Heart J., 98:20–31, 1979.
2. Friedman, M., Manwaring, J. H., Rosenman, R. H., et al.: Instantaneous and sudden deaths: Clinical and pathological differentiation in coronary artery disease. J.A.M.A., 225:1319–1328, 1973.
3. Isner, J. M., Wu, M., Virmani, R., et al.: Comparison of degrees of coronary arterial luminal narrowing determined by visual inspection of histologic sections under magnification among three independent observers and comparison to that obtained by videoplanimetry. An

analysis of 559 five-millimeter segments of 61 coronary arteries from 11 patients. Lab. Invest., 42:566–570, 1980.

4. Kuller, L., Cooper, M., and Perper, J.: Epidemiology of sudden death. Arch. Intern. Med., 129:714–719, 1972.

5. Liberthson, R. R., Nagel, E. L., Hirschman, J. C., et al.: Pathophysiologic observations in prehospital ventricular fibrillation and sudden cardiac death. Circulation, 49:790–798, 1974.

6. Movat, H. Z.: Demonstration of all connective tissue elements in a single section. Pentachrome stains. Arch. Pathol., 60:289–295, 1955.

7. Perper, J. A., Kuller, L. H., and Cooper, M.: Arterio-sclerosis of coronary arteries in sudden, unexpected deaths. Circulation, 51,52(Suppl. III):27–33, 1975.

8. Roberts, W. C., and Jones, A. A.: Quantitation of coronary arterial narrowing at necropsy in sudden coronary death. Analysis of 31 patients and comparison with 25 control subjects. Am. J. Cardiol., 44:39–45, 1979.

William C. Roberts, M.D.
The Pathology Branch
National Heart, Lung and Blood Institute
National Institutes of Health
Bethesda, Maryland 20205

Cardiac findings associated with sudden death secondary to atherosclerotic coronary artery disease: comparison of patients with and those without previous angina pectoris and/or healed myocardial infarction

DEBORAH J. BARBOUR, M.D., CAROLE A. WARNES, M.D., AND WILLIAM C. ROBERTS, M.D.

AMONG the many causes of sudden cardiac death, atherosclerotic coronary artery disease (CAD) is by far the most frequent. What is found at autopsy in victims of sudden death is to some extent dependent on how the term "sudden" is defined. Some studies define "sudden" as instantaneous death, others that within 1 hr, and others that up to 24 hr after onset the cardiac event. In our autopsy studies of victims of sudden coronary death we used the following definitions: (1) sudden death was that occurring within 6 hr of previously witnessed usual state of health. (2) Although death may have occurred in-hospital (usually in the emergency room), the victim was not a patient in a hospital at the onset of symptoms of myocardial ischemia. (3) At autopsy there was 76% to 100% narrowing by atherosclerotic plaque of cross-sectional area (XSA) of at least one of the four major (left main, left anterior descending, left circumflex, and right) epicardial coronary arteries. (4) Left ventricular myocardial coagulation necrosis was absent. (5) Another cause of death, either cardiac or noncardiac, was absent. (6) Chronic congestive heart failure had never been present. (7) No cardiovascular operation had ever been performed.

All four major epicardial coronary arteries were excised intact, decalcified, and cut into 5 mm sections; one histologic slide was prepared from each section. The slides were stained with Movat's stain and examined microscopically for the percentage of XSA narrowing caused by atherosclerotic plaque. The percentages of XSA narrowing were categorized into five groups: 0 to 25%, 26% to 50%, 51% to 75%, 76% to 95%, and 96% to 100%.

Many studies of victims of sudden coronary death have shown the amount of coronary artery narrowing by atherosclerotic plaque to be extensive. In a 1972

study of 24 victims of sudden death who were 28 to 85 years old (mean 54), Roberts and Buja[1] reported that 78% of the major coronary arteries examined (left main excluded) were narrowed more than 75% in XSA by atherosclerotic plaque, an average of 2.3/3.0 arteries per patient. Eleven patients (46%) had all three arteries so narrowed, 10 (42%) had two major arteries so narrowed, and only three (12%) had a single coronary artery narrowed more than 75% in XSA by atherosclerotic plaque. Fifteen of the 24 patients (62%) had evidence at autopsy of prior myocardial infarction that had healed.

Of 31 patients dying suddenly of atherosclerotic CAD studied by Roberts and Jones[2] in 1979, 29 (94%) had two or more of the four major epicardial coronary arteries narrowed more than 75% in XSA by atherosclerotic plaque. Of the 124 major epicardial coronary arteries examined in these 31 patients, 86 (67%) were more than 75% narrowed in XSA by plaque, an average of 2.8/4.0 coronary arteries per patient. Excluding the left main coronary artery, 83 (89%) of the other 93 major (left anterior descending, left circumflex, and right) coronary arteries were narrowed more than 75% in XSA by plaque, an average of 2.7/3.0 coronary arteries per patient. Of the 100 major coronary arteries in the 25 control subjects, 13 (13%) were narrowed more than 75% in XSA, an average of 0.5/4.0 coronary arteries per control subject.

More recently, Warnes and Roberts[3] studied patients with a history of angina pectoris and/or myocardial infarction and compared them with those in whom sudden death was the first manifestation of atherosclerotic CAD. This study is most relevant to the present discussion. The group of 70 patients examined at autopsy included seven women and 63 men 22 to 81 years old (mean 50). In a qualitative comparison of the 39 patients in whom sudden coronary death was the first manifestation of their CAD with the 31 patients with a history of prior myocardial infarction and/or angina pectoris, there was no significant difference in

From the Pathology Branch, National Heart, Lung, and Blood Institute, National Institutes of Health, Bethesda.

Address for correspondence: William C. Roberts, M.D., Pathology Branch, National Heart, Lung, and Blood Institute, National Institutes of Health, Building 10A, Room 3E30, Bethesda, MD 20892.

the number of major epicardial coronary arteries (of the four listed above) narrowed more than 75% in XSA (figure 1), no difference between the 31 patients with and 30 patients without myocardial scars (figure 2), and no difference between the 35 with and 35 without heart weights in excess of 450 g (figure 3).

Quantitative assessment of the 3484, 5 mm coronary artery segments from the four major coronary arteries in the 70 patients revealed that 950 (27%) were narrowed 76% to 100% in XSA and 718 (21%) were narrowed 0 to 25%. Comparison of the 39 previously asymptomatic patients with the 31 with previous myocardial ischemic symptoms revealed 76% to 100% XSA narrowing in 502 (25%) vs 488 (30%), respectively (p < .005). A similar comparison between these groups with respect to minimal (0 to 25% XSA) narrowing also disclosed significant differences (25% vs 15%, respectively; p < .001). When mean percent of coronary artery segments narrowed 76% to 100% in XSA in subjects with and those without myocardial scars was compared, a higher mean percent of segments were so narrowed in the group with scars (33% vs 24% p < .001). A surprising finding, however, was the more frequent occurrence of severe narrowing of the left main coronary artery in those without scar than in those with a healed myocardial infarct (12% vs 4%).

Similar comparisons made between those whose hearts weighed more than 450 g and those who had

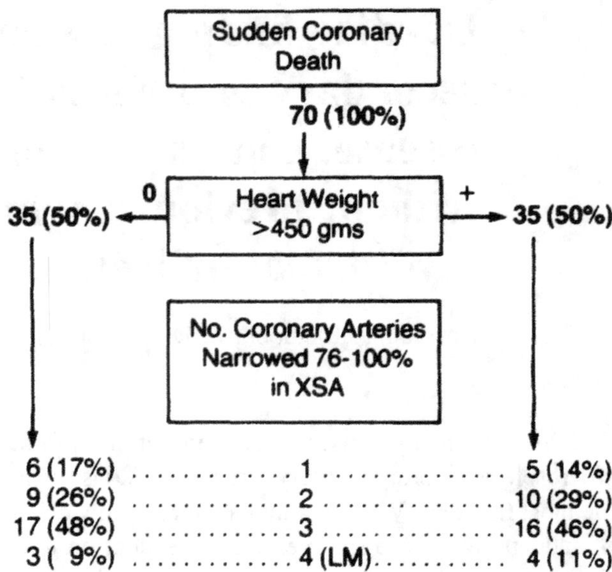

FIGURE 2. Qualitative comparison of the number of coronary arteries narrowed 76% to 100% in XSA by atherosclerotic plaque in 31 patients with morphologic evidence of healed myocardial infarction and that in 39 patients without such evidence revealed no differences between groups except for a significantly (p < .02) greater number with three-vessels so narrowed (*) among the 31 with prior myocardial infarction. Reproduced, with permission, from Warnes and Roberts.[3]

heart weights of 450 g or less revealed a lower mean percentage of segments narrowed 0 to 25% in XSA (19% vs 23%, p < .01) and a higher mean percentage of segments in all but the left main coronary artery narrowed 76% to 100% (29% vs 24%, p < .005) in those with the bigger hearts.

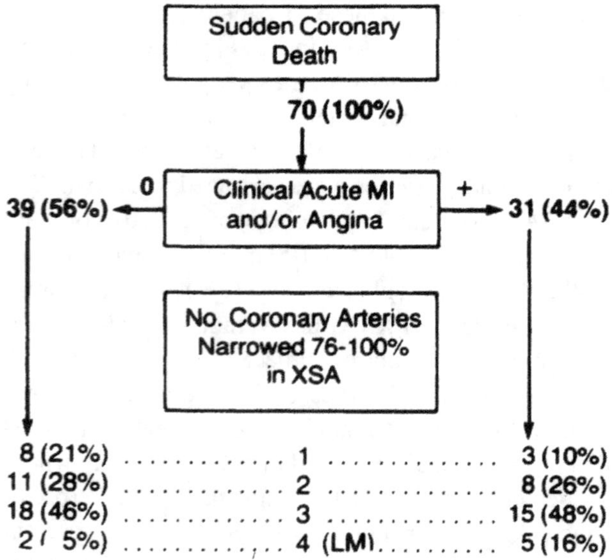

FIGURE 1. Qualitative analysis of data from 70 patients with sudden coronary death revealed no difference in the number of epicardial coronary arteries narrowed 76% to 100% in XSA by atherosclerotic plaque in those in whom sudden death was the first manifestation of their disease (n = 39) and the number in those in whom clinical myocardial infarction and/or angina pectoris had preexisted (n = 31). Reproduced, with permission, from Warnes and Roberts.[3]

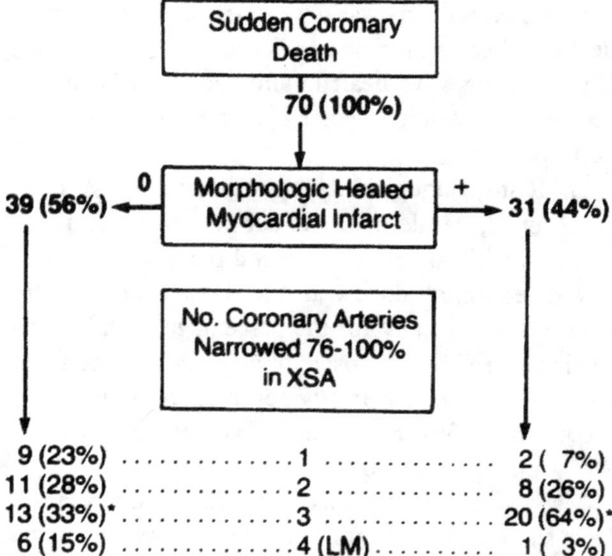

FIGURE 3. Qualitative comparison of 35 sudden coronary death patients whose hearts weighed more than 450 g with 35 whose hearts weighed 450 g or less. No difference in the numbers of coronary arteries narrowed 76% to 100% in XSA was found between the groups. Reproduced, with permission, from Warnes and Roberts.[3]

A comparison by age group of the amount and distribution of coronary artery narrowing in 60 men, 31 to 70 years old (mean 51), was made in a similar study by Warnes and Roberts.[4] In 31 of these 60 patients, sudden death was the first manifestation of their atherosclerotic CAD. The mean percentages of narrowing were compared for the four decades represented and no significant difference was found in the percent of segments narrowed 76% to 100% in XSA between groups: 33% of segments in the age group 31 to 40, 29% in the 41 to 50 year olds, 26% in the 51 to 60 year olds, and 30% in patients 61 to 70 years old. What was found was a higher proportion of minimally narrowed segments of the four major arteries in the younger patients, with fewer of the four major coronary arteries involved; i.e., 40% in the 31 to 40 year olds had one artery narrowed more than 75% in XSA compared with 10% of the 61 to 70 year olds. In their study of the 70 patients previously discussed, the same authors[3] noted that in the 11 patients who had only one artery narrowed more than 75% in XSA, the mean age was 41 years, in contrast to a mean age of 51 years in those patients with two or more arteries so involved. When the mean number of arteries narrowed more than 75% in XSA for each age group was examined, this differentiation was lost. There was no significant difference between age groups, i.e., 2.2/4 arteries were narrowed in the 31 to 40 year group, 2.6/4.0 were narrowed in the 41–50 year group, 2.6/4.0 were narrowed in the 51 to 60 year group, and 2.8/4.0 were narrowed in the 61 to 70 year group, for an overall average of 2.6/4.0 arteries narrowed more than 76% of XSA per patient in the 60 men having sudden coronary death in whom this comparison was made.

These investigations indicate that in patients dying suddenly from atherosclerotic CAD, coronary artery narrowing by atherosclerotic plaque is severe and extensive. The severity of narrowing is greater is those with prior myocardial ischemic symptoms, in those with healed myocardial infarcts, and in those with cardiomegaly than in individuals without these findings.

References

1. Roberts WC, Buja LM: The frequency and significance of coronary arterial thrombi and other observations in fatal acute myocardial infarction. A study of 107 necropsy patients. Am J Med **52:** 425, 1972
2. Roberts WC, Jones AA: Quantitation of coronary arterial narrowing at necropsy in sudden coronary death. Analysis of 31 patients and comparison with 25 control subjects. Am J Cardiol **44:** 39, 1979
3. Warnes CA, Roberts WC: Sudden coronary death: relation of amount and distribution of coronary narrowing at necropsy to previous symptoms of myocardial ischemia, left ventricular scarring and heart weight. Am J Cardiol **54:** 65, 1984
4. Warnes CA, Roberts WC: Comparison at necropsy by age group of amount and distribution of narrowing by atherosclerotic plaque in 2995 five-mm long segments of 240 major coronary arteries in 60 men aged 31 to 70 years with sudden coronary death. Am Heart J **108:** 431, 1984

Calcification of Healed Myocardial Infarcts

WILLIAM C. ROBERTS, MD, and REBECCA J. KAUFMAN*

Clinical and necropsy findings are described in 21 patients, aged 43 to 78 years (mean 63) (19 men [90%]), who had grossly visible calcified myocardial infarcts. The interval from the first clinically apparent acute myocardial infarct to death (20 patients) ranged from 2 to 26 years (mean 12). This interval was >5 years in 17 patients (85%) and >10 years in 11 patients (55%). The ages at the first clinically apparent acute myocardial infarct ranged from 36 to 72 years (mean 51). Of the 21 patients, 17 (81%) had clinical evidence of chronic congestive heart failure; 12 (57%) had left ventricular aneurysms; 8 (38%) had documented episodes of ventricular tachycardia; and 5 had angina pectoris. At necropsy, the heart weight was increased (>400 g) in all (mean 557 g), the left ventricular cavity was dilated in all, and at least 1 and usually 2 or 3 (86%) major epicardial coronary arteries were narrowed >75% in cross-sectional area by atherosclerotic plaque. Thus, patients with calcified myocardial infarcts are usually men, they usually have a myocardial infarct that calcifies at a relatively young age, the calcified wall is usually part of an aneurysmal wall, the left ventricular cavity is almost always dilated, heart weight is increased, and progressive congestive heart failure is the usual mode of death.

(Am J Cardiol 1987;60:28–32)

Calcific deposits are frequently observed in the human heart of persons residing in the Western world. Most commonly, the deposits are in atherosclerotic plaques in the epicardial coronary arteries, followed by mitral anular region, aortic valve cusps and apices of the left ventricular papillary muscles.[1] Calcific deposits are usually present in stenotic mitral[2,3] and aortic valves[4-6] in adults and occasionally in stenotic pulmonic valves in adults.[7] Calcification of individual myocardial fibers is common in hearts with generalized (noncoronary induced) myocardial ischemia, but the calcific deposits in this circumstance usually are not visible grossly.[8] During the past 15 years, one of us (WCR) has observed grossly at necropsy calcific deposits in the left ventricular wall at sites of healed myocardial infarcts in 21 patients. Search of *Index Medicus* on "calcification of myocardial infarcts" disclosed no reports on this subject since 1950. Because of the rarity of finding grossly visible calcific deposits in healed myocardial infarcts, we describe herein certain clinical and necropsy findings in our 21 patients.

From the Pathology Branch, National Heart, Lung, and Blood Institute, National Institutes of Health, Bethesda, Maryland. Manuscript received December 22, 1986, accepted February 5, 1987.

Address for reprints: William C. Roberts, MD, Building 10A, Room 3E-30, National Institutes of Health, Bethesda, Maryland 20892.

*High school student, Silver Spring, Maryland.

Patients

Sources of cases: The hearts of all 21 patients were examined originally by WCR and 16 were reexamined by both authors. The 21 cases were studied clinically at 10 different hospitals and the hearts were submitted to the Pathology Branch, National Heart, Lung, and Blood Institute, for study.

Ages, sexes and intervals: Clinical and morphologic findings in each of the 21 patients are tabulated in Table I and are illustrated in Figures 1 to 7. At death, the 21 patients were 43 to 78 years old (mean 63); 19 (90%) were men and 2 (10%) were women; 20 (95%) were white and 1 (5%) was black. In 20 of the 21 patients, 1 or more myocardial infarcts were clinically apparent. Of these 20 patients, 12 (60%) had a single clinically apparent infarct and 8 (40%) had more than 1 clinically apparent infarct. The interval from the first clinically apparent infarct to death in these 20 patients ranged from 2 to 26 years (mean 12); this interval was 2 to 5 years in 3 patients (15%), 6 to 10 years in 6 patients (30%) and >10 years in 11 patients (55%). The ages at the time of the first acute myocardial infarct in these 20 patients ranged from 36 to 72 years (mean 51). In the only patient (no. 10) in whom the acute infarct was clinically silent, an electrocardiogram at age 43 (19 years before death) was consistent with healed myocardial infarction.

Cardiac symptoms, arrhythmias, conduction disturbances: The most common manifestation of cardiac ischemia was chronic congestive cardiac failure, evi-

TABLE I   Clinical and Morphologic Findings in 21 Necropsy Patients with Calcified Myocardial Infarcts

Case	Age (yr) at Death	Race	Sex	Age First AMI (yr)	Interval First AMI Death (yr)	No. of AMIs	CHF	AP	VT	H SH	Mode of Death	HW (g)	A	P	Apical	Basal	LV Aneurysm	LV T	LAD	LC	R
1	43	W	M	37	6	1	+	0	0	0	CHF	610	+	0	+	+	+	0	+	+	+
2	50	W	M	36	14	1	+	+	+	0	AMI	480	+	0	+	+	+	0	+	0	0
3	52	W	M	50	2	1	0	0	0	0	Suicide	475	+	0	+	+	0	0	+	0	+
4	52	W	M	46	6	1	0	0	0	+	Sudden	510	+	0	+	+	0	+	+	0	+
5	54	W	M	44	10	3	+	0	0	0	CHF	730	+	0	+	+	0	+	+	+	+
6	57	W	M	45	12	2	+	0	0		Sudden	540	+	0[b]	+	+	0	0	+	0	+
7	57	W	M	43	14	1	0	0	+	+	HF	415	0	+	+	+	0	0	+	0	+
8	62	W	F	52	10	2	+	+	+	+	CHF	610	0	+	0	+	0	...	+[e]	+[e]	+
9	62	W	F	50	12	1	+	0	0	+	CHF	405	+	+	+	0	+[c]	+	+	0	0
10	62	W	M	...[a]	...	...	0	0	0	0	Cancer	500	0	+	+	+	+	0	+	+	+
11	63	W	M	38	25	4	+	+	0	0	CHF	470	+	+	+	0	+[c]	0	+	+	+
12	63	W	M	61	2	1	+	0	0	+	CHF	790	+	0	+	0	+	+	+	+	+
13	65	W	M	55	10	1	+	0	+	+	Sudden	570	+	0	+	0	+	+	+	+	0
14	65	W	M	50	15	2	+	0	0	0	CHF	610	+	0[b]	+	+	+[c,d]	0	+[e]	+	+
15	67	W	M	45	22	1	+	0	0	0	CHF	430	+	0	+	+	+[c]	0	+	+	0
16	68	W	M	52	16	1	+	0	0	0	CHF	480	+	0	+	+	0	0	+	+	+
17	69	B	M	56	13	4	+	0	+	+	CHF	470	+	0	+	0	+[c,d]	0	+	+	+[e]
18	74	W	F	62	12	1	+	+	+	+	AMI	...	+	0[b]	+	0	0	0	+	+	+
19	75	W	F	70	5	1	+	0	+	+	CHF	660	0	+	0	+	+	0	0	+	+
20	75	W	M	49	26	3	+	+	+	0	Hip Op	700	0	+	+	+	0	0	+	+	+
21	78	W	M	72	6	2	+	0	0	0	CHF	680	+	+	+	0	+[c]	+	+	0	0

a = electrocardiogram at age 43 was consistent with healed myocardial infarction; b = a second healed noncalcified infarct is located on this wall; c = also diagnosed clinically; d = aneurysm operatively excised 10 years before death; e = a bypass graft from aorta to this artery was implanted 10 years before death.

A = anterior; AMI = acute myocardial infarction; CA = coronary artery; CHF = chronic congestive heart failure; CSA = cross-sectional area; DM = diabetes mellitus; H = history of; HF = hepatic failure; HW = heart weight; LAD = left anterior descending; LC = left circumflex; LV = left ventricular; P = posterior; R = right; SH = systemic hypertension; T = thrombus; VT = ventricular tachycardia.

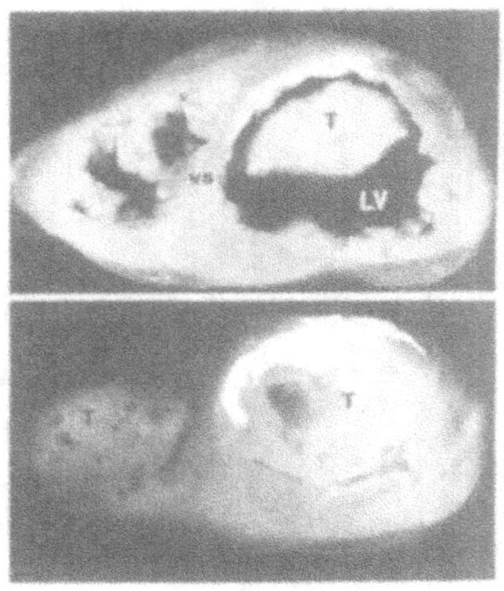
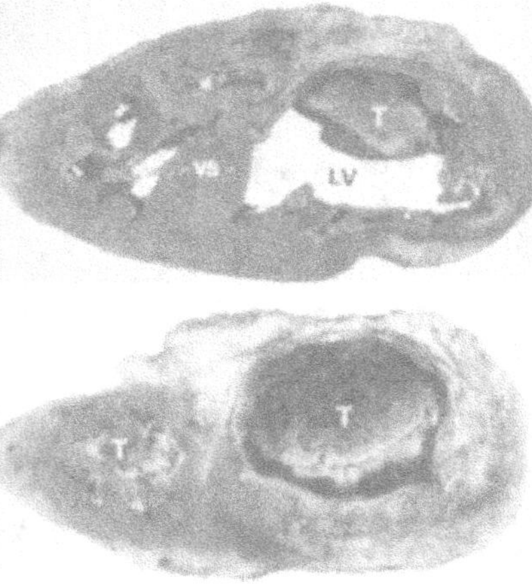

FIGURE 1. Patient 5 (Table I). Transverse slices of the cardiac ventricles in a 54-year-old man (NNMC #A84-142) who had his first acute myocardial infarct 10 years earlier and progressive and eventually fatal congestive cardiac failure thereafter. Large thrombi (T) were present in the cavities of both right and left ventricle (LV). Healed infarcts involved both anterior and posterior left ventricular walls, but calcific deposits were present only in the anterior wall. The radiographs of the 2 slices are shown at the *right*. VS = ventricular septum.

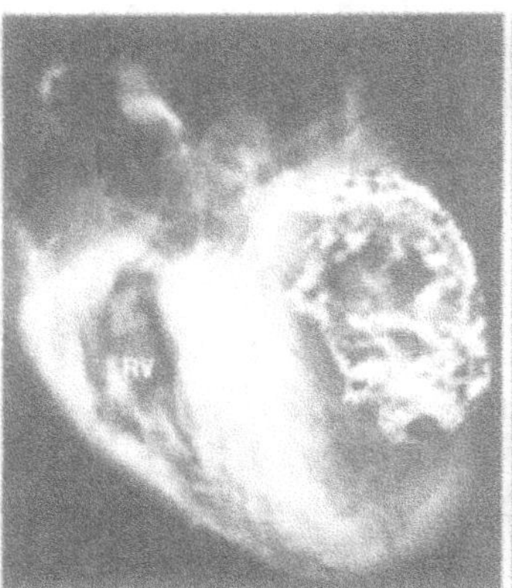
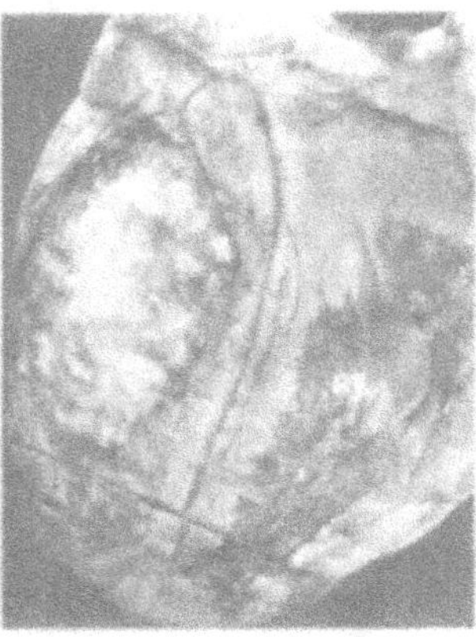

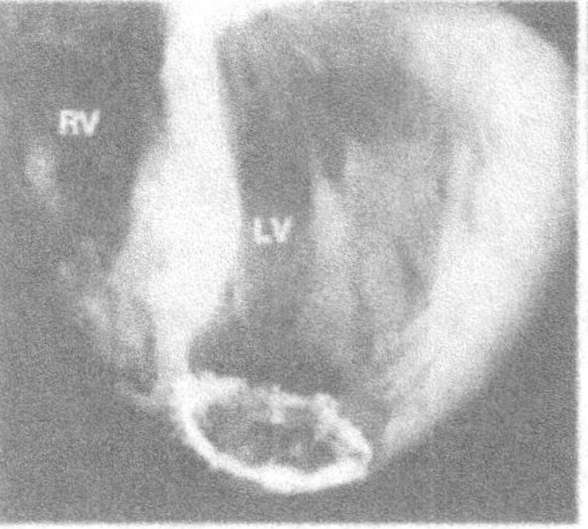
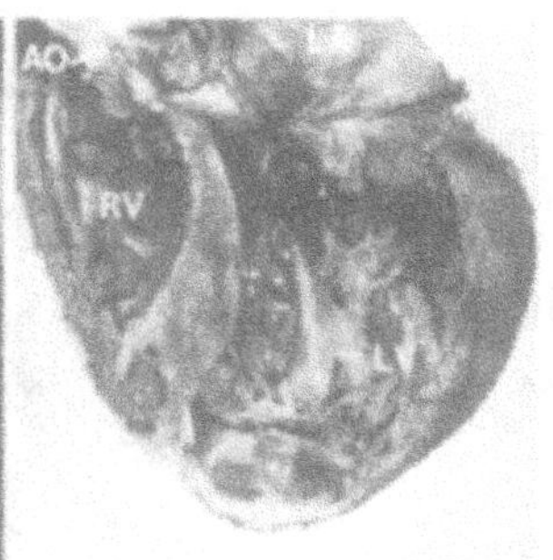

FIGURE 2. Patient 7 (Table I). Radiograph of heart (*left*) and view of posterior wall of the heart (*right*) in a 57-year-old man (NNMC #A86-75) who had an acute myocardial infarct 14 years earlier and episodic ventricular tachycardia subsequently. He never had congestive heart failure. This calcified infarct involved most of the posterior wall of the left ventricle (*right*). The calcified infarct was easily visible on chest radiograph during life. The calcific deposits were the largest of any of the 21 cases included in this study. RV = right ventricle.

FIGURE 3. Patient 11 (Table I). Calcified apical infarct in a 63-year-old man (GT# 71A-103) who had had an acute myocardial infarct 25 years earlier at age 38. *Left*, radiograph of heart specimen. *Right*, heart after removal of its anterior half. Both right (RV) and left (LV) ventricles are dilated. Ao = aorta; LA = left atrium.

dence of which was present in 17 patients (81%). Each of the 4 patients (nos. 3, 4, 7 and 10) without evidence of chronic congestive heart failure at necropsy had dilated left ventricular cavities and 1 had a true left ventricular aneurysm.[9,10] Five patients had angina pectoris at some time; in each it appears to have been infrequent or rare. At least 8 had documented episodes of recurrent ventricular tachycardia by electrocardiogram. Six patients had cardiac pacemakers in place at death; 2 (nos. 18 and 19) of them had complete heart block; the reason for the pacemaker insertion in the other 4 patients is unclear. Three patients (nos. 19 and 16) had complete left bundle branch block.

Diabetes mellitus: Three patients (nos. 11, 17 and 20) had diabetes mellitus; in all 3 it became apparent late in life.

Blood pressure: The level of the systemic arterial pressure before the first acute myocardial infarct was not known in any patient. At least 9 patients, however, were stated to have had "hypertension" at some time. Blood pressures during the last 3 months of life were available in 11 patients and in each it was <135/90 mm Hg.

Cardiac operation: Three patients (nos. 8, 14 and 17) had coronary artery bypass operations, each done 10 years before death, and in 2 of them (nos. 14 and 17), a left ventricular aneurysm also was resected.

Modes of death: Of the 21 patients, 12 (60%) died from progressive congestive heart failure; 3 (15%) died suddenly at home; 2 (10%) had a fatal acute myocardial infarction; and 4 (19%) died of noncardiovascular conditions (suicide in 1, cancer in 1, postoperative complications of hip replacement in 1 and hepatic failure in 1, possibly secondary to amiodarone therapy).

Necropsy findings: The heart weights ranged from 405 to 790 g (mean 565) (normal ≤400 g). The calcified left ventricular infarct involved the anterior wall only in 13 patients; the posterior wall only in 5 patients, and both anterior and posterior walls in 3 patients. The calcified infarct involved the left ventricle's apical half only in 7 patients; the basal half only in 2 patients; and portions of both apical and basal halves in 12 patients.

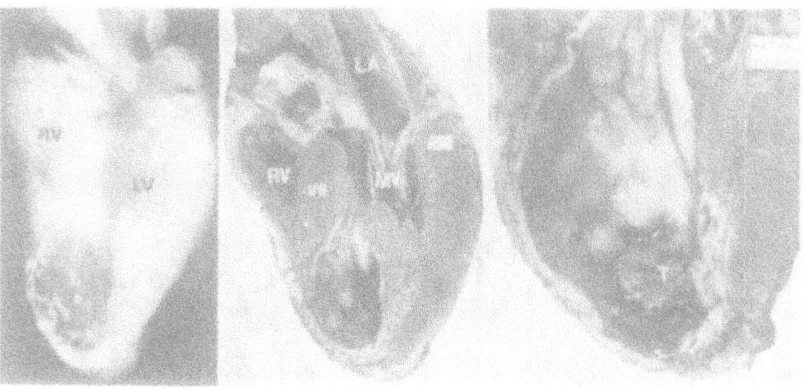

FIGURE 4. Patient 13 (Table I). Radiograph of heart specimen (*left*); interior of heart after longitudinal anterior-posterior cut (*center*) and close-up of the calcified apical aneurysm (*right*) in a 65-year-old man (GT #85A-74) who had an acute myocardial infarct 10 years earlier at age 55 and onset of congestive heart failure at age 64, about 1 year before death. Hypercalcemia developed, with serum calcium levels to 14 mg/dl (albumin 3.0 g/dl) from multiple myeloma. RV = right ventricle; LV = left ventricle; Ao = aorta; MV = mitral valve; LA = left atrium; T = thrombus; VS = ventricular septum.

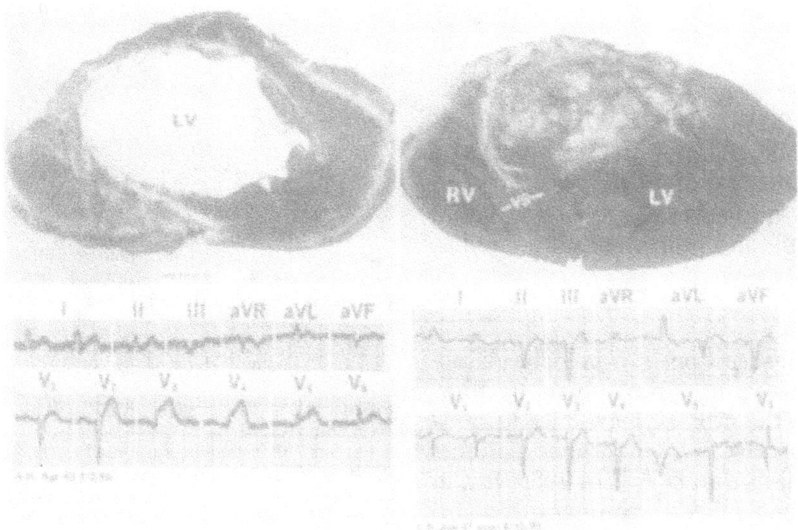

FIGURE 5. Patient 15 (Table I). Two slices of the cardiac ventricles (*upper*) showing a calcified anterior wall and most of the ventricular septum in a 67-year-old man (NNMC #A80-98) who had an acute myocardial infarct 22 years earlier at age 45. The electrocardiogram in the *lower left* was recorded during the acute myocardial infarct and the one on the lower right shortly before death 22 years later. LV = left ventricle; RV = right ventricle; VS = ventricular septum. Reproduced with permission from McManus BM, Roberts WC. Survival for 20 years or longer after transmural acute myocardial infarction: analysis of eight well documented necropsy cases. Am Heart J 1981;102:176–182.

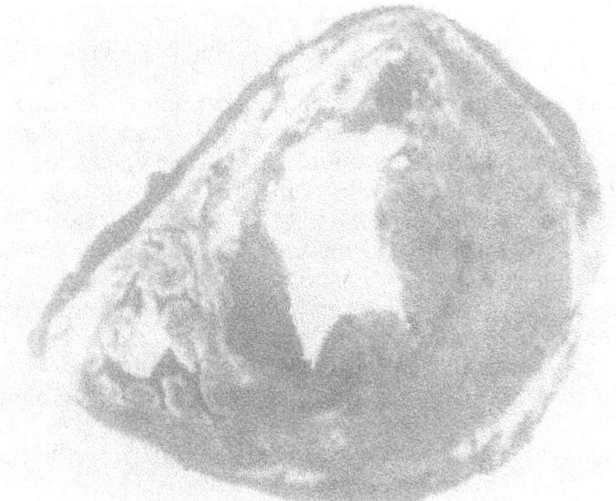

FIGURE 6. Patient 17 (Table I). Transverse section of cardiac ventricles showing a heavily calcified healed anterior wall myocardial infarct in a 69-year-old man (GT #82A-74) who had a portion of the left ventricular aneurysm operatively excised and 2 aortocoronary bypass conduits inserted 10 years earlier at age 59. It is not known whether the aneurysmally dilated infarct was calcified at the time of the cardiac operation.

The healed infarct that contained calcium was aneurysmally dilated in 12 patients (57%). In 2 (nos. 14 and 17) of the 12 patients the wall of the aneurysm had been operatively resected. Of the 12 patients with left ventricular aneurysms at operation (2 patients) or at necropsy (10 patients), the aneurysm had been diagnosed during life in 7. The aneurysm was "large" in 11 of the 12 patients. Of the 10 patients with left ventricular aneurysm at necropsy, 4 contained intraaneurysmal thrombus. Of the 9 patients without left ventricular aneurysms at necropsy, 2 had thrombi within the left ventricular cavity. The left ventricular cavity by gross inspection was dilated in all 21 patients at necropsy. Three patients (nos. 6, 8 and 18) had healed posterior wall right ventricular infarcts.

Of the 3 major (right, left anterior descending and left circumflex) epicardial coronary arteries, at least 1 was narrowed >75% in cross-sectional area by atherosclerotic plaque in all 21 patients: 1 artery only in 3 patients (15%); 2 arteries in 7 patients (33%), and all 3

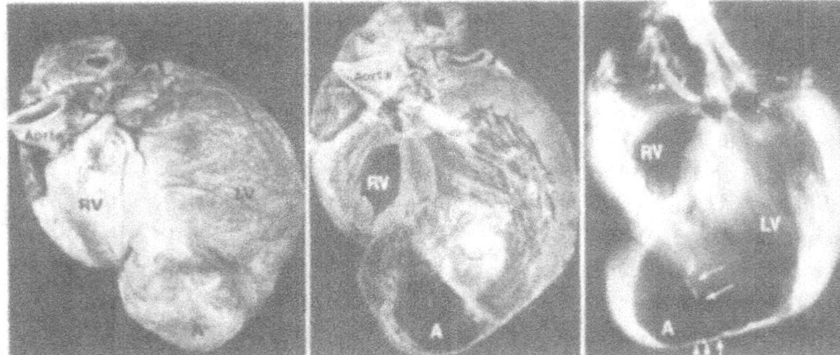

FIGURE 7. Patient 21 (Table I). Large apical, partially calcified left ventricular aneurysm with an intraneurysmal thrombus in a 78-year-old man (GT 76A-171) who had had an acute myocardial infarct 6 years earlier at age 72 and progressive congestive heart failure thereafter. *Left*, radiograph of heart specimen. *Center*, exterior view of heart showing the apical aneurysm (A). *Right*, view of heart after removing its anterior half. *Arrows* indicate the calcific deposits. This case contained the smallest deposits of calcium in the infarcted wall; LV = left ventricle; RV = right ventricle.

arteries in 11 patients (52%). Calcific deposits were present in atherosclerotic plaques in the epicardial arteries in 20 (95%) of the 21 patients. No patient had grossly visible calcific deposits in the aortic valve cusps; 1 patient (no. 9) had mitral anular calcific deposits.

Discussion

The first necropsy description of a grossly visible calcified myocardial infarct apparently was by Simmonds[12] in 1908. During the next 42 years, 15 additional reports appeared describing 23 necropsy patients with calcified myocardial infarcts.[13–27] In 1950, Brean and associates[27] described clinical, radiographic and necropsy findings in 9 patients with calcified myocardial infarcts, and since 1950, no reports have appeared describing clinical and necropsy findings in patients with calcified myocardial infarcts. All of the 24 necropsy patients reported previously with calcified myocardial infarcts were men.[12–27] Their ages ranged from 41 to 74 years (mean 62). Most (74%) had true left ventricular aneurysms and the aneurysmal wall was the portion of left ventricular wall that contained the calcific deposits. Other information in these 24 previously reported necropsy cases is scanny. The present study of 21 necropsy patients contains nearly as many cases as the total previously reported.

In all our 21 patients, the calcific deposits were located in the left ventricular wall, which was the site of the acute myocardial infarct that healed. Calcific deposits in healed infarcts must be distinguished from calcific deposits in left ventricular organized thrombi. The occurrence of calcific deposits in organized left ventricular thrombi appears to be more common than calcific deposits in healed myocardial infarcts.

The cause of calcification in some healed myocardial infarcts is unclear. The myocardial calcific deposits do not appear to be part of a generalized calcific process. Although all but 1 of our 21 patients had calcific deposits in atherosclerotic plaques in 1 or more epicardial coronary arteries, none had calcific deposits in the aortic valve cusps and only 1 had calcific deposits in the mitral anular area. Only 1 of our patients was known to have chronic hypercalcemia.

References

1. Roberts WC. *The senile cardiac calcification syndrome. Am J Cardiol 1986;58:572–574.*
2. Lachman AD, Roberts WC. *Calcific deposits in stenotic mitral valves. Extent and relation to age, sex, degree of stenosis, cardiac rhythm, previous commissurotomy and left atria body thrombus from study of 164 operatively-excised valves. Circulation 1978; 57:808–815.*
3. Roberts WC. *Morphologic features of the normal and abnormal mitral valve. Am J Cardiol 1983;51:1005–1028.*
4. Roberts WC. *The structure of the aortic valve in clinically-isolated aortic stenosis. An autopsy study of 162 patients over 15 years of age. Circulation 1970;42:91–97.*
5. Roberts WC. *The congenitally bicuspid aortic valve. A study of 85 autopsy cases. Am J Cardiol 1970;26:72–83.*
6. Roberts WC. *Anatomically isolated aortic valvular disease. The case against its being of rheumatic etiology. Am J Med 1970;49:151–159.*
7. Roberts WC. *Calcific pulmonic stenosis. Circulation 1968;86:77–80.*
8. Buja, LM, Levitsky S, Ferrans VJ, Souther SG, Roberts WC, Morrow AG. *Acute and chronic effects of normothermic anoxia on canine hearts. Light and electron microscopic evaluation. Circulation 1971;43,44:suppl I:I-44–I-50.*
9. Cabin HS, Roberts WC. *Left ventricular aneurysm, intraaneurysmal thrombus and systemic embolus in coronary heart disease. Chest 1980;77:586–590.*
10. Cabin HS, Roberts WC. *True left ventricular aneurysm and healed myocardial infarction. Clinical and necropsy observations including quantification of degrees of coronary arterial narrowing. Am J Cardiol 1980;46:754–763.*
11. Simmonds M. *Uber der Nachweis von Verkalkungen am Herzen durch das Rontgenverfahren. Fortschr a d Geb d Rontgenstrahlen 1908;12:371–374.*
12. Scholz T. *Calcification of the heart: its roentgenologic demonstration. Review of literature and theories on myocardial calcification. Arch Intern Med 1924;34:32–59.*
13. Davidson TW. *Two cases of cardiac infarction: one followed by calcification of the heart, the other by rupture. Br Med J 1928;1:212–213.*
14. Detterman A. *Beitrag zur Differentialdiagnose der Verschattungen in der Herzzilhouette. Fortschr Rontgenstrahlen 1932;46:137–142.*
15. Moore JJ. *Myocardial calcification. AJR 1934;31:766–769.*
16. Hirsehboek FJ. *Calcification of the myocardium following coronary occlusion: a case report. Am Heart J 1934;10:264–267.*
17. Redfearn JA. *Massive calcification of the myocardium: report of a case. Am Heart J 1936;12:365–367.*
18. Brenner F, Wachner G. *Uber einen ungewohnlichen Sitz cines Herzaneurysmas und seine Rontgendiagnostik. Fortschr Rontgenstrahlen 1936;54:243–248.*
19. Cohen JN, Levine HS. *Calcification of the myocardium with bone formation: report of a case. Arch Intern Med 1937;60:486–493.*
20. Schwedel JB, Gross H. *Ventricular aneurysm: roentgenographic and postmortem surveys. AJR 1939;41;32–36.*
21. Brown CE, Evans WD. *Primary, massive calcification of the myocardium. Am Heart J 1940;19:106–113.*
22. Peters JJ. *Aneurysm of the left ventricle. AJR 1941;45:371–378.*
23. Borman MC. *Calcification of left ventricular infarction recognized during life. Ann Intern Med 1943;18:857–865.*
24. McMillan RL, Rousseau JP. *Calcification of infarctions of the myocardium. Radiology 1945;44:181–183.*
25. Blackford LM. *Calcification of the myocardium. Ann Intern Med 1947;27:1036–1040.*
26. Brean HP, Marks JH, Sosman MC, Schlesinger MJ. *Massive calcification in infarcted myocardium. Radiology 1950;54:33–42.*

Rupture of the Ventricular Septum or Left Ventricular Free Wall from Acute Myocardial Infarction Early After Coronary Artery Bypass Grafting

JESSICA M. MANN, MD

JAY M. KALAN, MD

ROBERT B. WALLACE, MD

WILLIAM C. ROBERTS, MD

Rupture of the ventricular septum or of the left ventricular free wall from acute myocardial infarction (AMI) after coronary artery bypass grafting (CABG) is rare. Such was the case, however, in the 2 patients to be described below.

Case 1: *V.A., a 73-year-old man with diabetes mellitus, had been asymptomatic until 2 years earlier (age 71) when typical angina pectoris with exertion appeared. The angina was stable until age 73, when it became more frequent and appeared with less exertion. Exercise stress testing produced electrocardiographic ST depression and a decrease in systemic blood pressure. Coronary angiography disclosed up to 90% luminal diameter narrowing of the left anterior descending, and 51 to 75% diameter narrowing of the left circumflex and right coronary arteries. Left ven-*

From the Pathology Branch, National Heart, Lung, and Blood Institute, National Institutes of Health, Bethesda, Maryland, and the Department of Surgery, Georgetown University Medical Center, Washington, D.C. Manuscript received and accepted April 9, 1987.

tricular angiography disclosed a 73% ejection fraction and hypokinesia of the posterior wall. (There was never historical evidence of an AMI.) Seven days before death CABG was performed: 3 conduits were inserted with 3 aortic anastomotic sites and 1 each end-to-side anastomoses to the right, left anterior descending and left obtuse marginal coronary arteries. After discontinuing cardiopulmonary bypass, left ventricular contractions appeared good. During closure of the arterial cannulation site in the distal ascending aorta, the aorta tore with considerable bleeding. The arterial cannula was then placed in a femoral artery and a venous cannula in the right atrium. Cardiopulmonary bypass was reinstituted for 53 minutes, during which time the aortic tear was closed. After rewarming, cardiopulmonary bypass was discontinued and left ventricular contractions appeared good. The postoperative period was characterized by evidence of the low cardiac output syndrome. The electrocardiogram showed elevation of ST segments in leads V_2-V_5 and the serum creatine kinase level rose to 4,900 IU, with an 85% MB fraction. Seven days after operation the blood pressure became inadequate, ventricular fibrillation occurred and resuscitative efforts failed. At necropsy (85A-272), the heart weighed 375 g. Neither ventricular cavity was dilated. A small transmural scar was present in the posterior wall. A transmural acute myocardial infarct involved most of the ventricular septum, which had ruptured posteriorly and basally, and small portions of the anterior and posterior free walls (Fig. 1). The lumina of the left anterior descending and right coronary arteries were severely narrowed by atherosclerotic plaque. No coronary thrombi were found. All conduits were widely patent.

Case 2: *A.S., a 69-year-old man who had had mild stable angina pectoris for 7 years underwent cardiac catheterization because of a positive exercise stress*

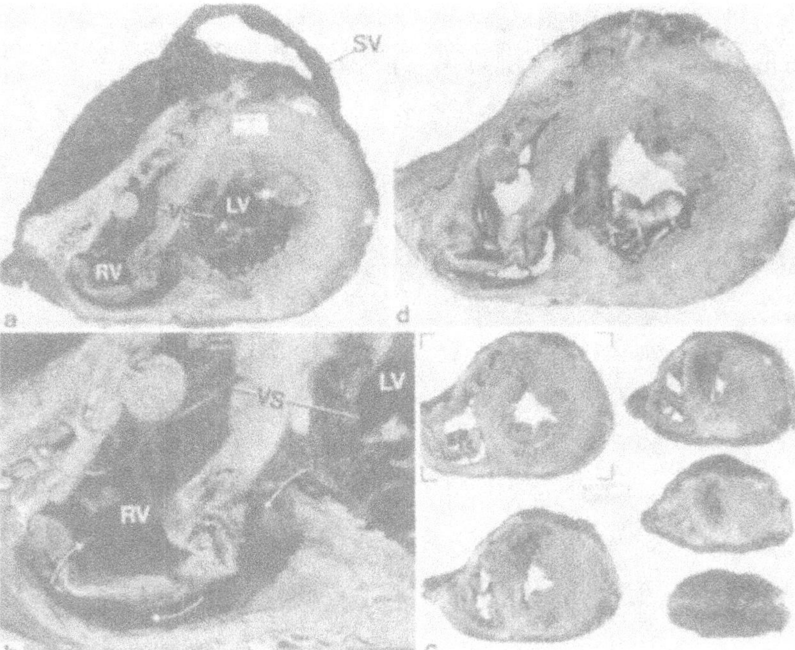

FIGURE 1. Case 1. Gross sections of the cardiac ventricles after multiple transverse cuts. *a*, most basal section showing the rupture site in the posterior portion of the ventricular septum (VS). LV = left ventricular cavity; RV = right ventricular cavity; SV = saphenous vein. *b*, close-up view of the rupture site (*arrows*) showing a dissection of the right ventricular wall. *c*, view of 5 cut surfaces showing the posterior wall healed myocardial infarct and the anterior wall acute myocardial infarct. *d*, view of the reverse side of the transverse slice enclosed by the brackets in *c*, again showing the septal rupture site.

test. *The lumina of the right, left anterior descending and left circumflex coronary arteries were severely narrowed. CABG was performed 26 days before death with aortocoronary saphenous vein grafts to the right, left anterior descending and left obtuse marginal coronary arteries. The early postoperative course was uneventful and he was discharged 7 days after CABG. At home, his recovery continued uneventful until 23 days after CABG or 3 days before death, when substernal chest pain recurred and he returned to the hospital. Electrocardiogram was diagnostic of anterior wall AMI. The initial serum creatine kinase level was 120, and it rose to 494 IU. Three days later, shortly after being transferred to the ward from the coronary care unit, fatal cardiac arrest occurred. At necropsy (A80-267), about 1,000 ml of blood were present in the pericardial sac. Transverse sections of the cardiac ventricles disclosed a large anterolateral acute myocardial infarct histologically compatible with 3 or 4 days duration. The rupture site was in the anterior left ventricular free wall. The distal portion of the conduit to the left anterior descending coronary artery was occluded by a thrombus and the native left anterior descending coronary artery just distal to the anastomotic site was severely narrowed by atherosclerotic plaque (Fig. 2). No thrombus was found in a native coronary artery.*

The 2 men described above had CABG because of angina pectoris. Neither had had a clinical event compatible with an AMI preoperatively. Patient 1 had an AMI within 3 days after CABG and the AMI was complicated by rupture of the ventricular septum. He died 7 days after CABG. Patient 2 had an AMI beginning 23 days after CABG and it was complicated by fatal rupture of the left ventricular free wall 3 days later or 26 days after CABG. Thus, both patients had AMI relatively early after CABG and the AMI in each was complicated by clinically undiagnosed cardiac rupture.

Rupture of the ventricular septum or left ventricular free wall complicating AMI shortly after CABG has been reported only once previously. Ibrahim and associates[1] described a 61-year-old woman who had a pos-

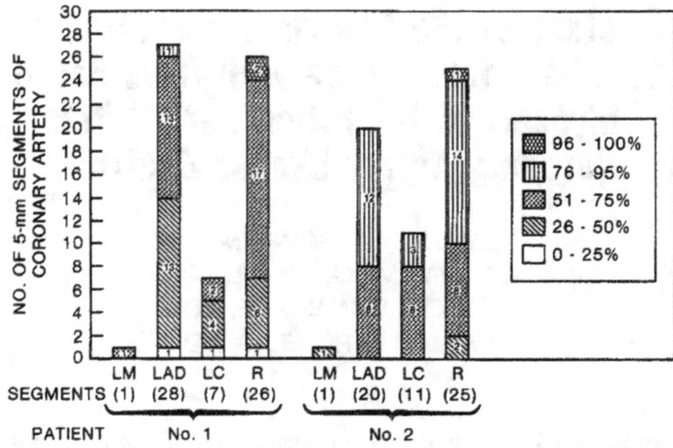

FIGURE 2. Bar graph showing the number of 5-mm-long coronary artery segments from the left main (LM), left anterior descending (LAD), left circumflex (LC) and right (R) epicardial coronary arteries in both patients and the number of segments narrowed to each of 5 categories of cross-sectional area narrowing by atherosclerotic plaque. The 4 major epicardial coronary arteries had been excised intact, decalcified if necessary, and each was divided into 5-mm-long segments cut at right angles to the longitudinal axis. Each section was processed in alcohols and xylene, dehydrated and a single section cut 6 μ thick was prepared from each 5-mm segment. The single section was stained by the Movat method. In patient 1, of 62 sections 1 was narrowed 76 to 95% (from the left anterior descending coronary artery) and 2 were narrowed 96 to 100% (from the right coronary artery). In patient 2, 29 of 57 sections were narrowed 76 to 95% (from the left anterior descending, left circumflex and right coronary arteries) and 1 section was narrowed 96 to 100% (from the right coronary artery).

terior wall AMI 3 days after CABG. Angiography disclosed the saphenous vein conduit to the distal right coronary artery to be totally occluded. Left ventricular angiography disclosed a perforation in the ventricular septum and a left ventricular-to-right ventricular shunt. The septal perforation was operatively closed 29 days after the CABG.

1. Ibrahim F, Kinard SA, Schwartz EL, Diethrich EB. *Transmyocardial left-to-right shunt complicating acute inferior wall myocardial infarction after aortocoronary bypass. Surgery 1975;75:285-290.*

Fatal Rupture of Both Left Ventricular Free Wall and Ventricular Septum (Double Rupture) During Acute Myocardial Infarction: Analysis of Seven Patients Studied at Necropsy

JESSICA M. MANN, MD
WILLIAM C. ROBERTS, MD

Rupture of the left ventricular (LV) free wall is a common complication of acute myocardial infarction (AMI). Rupture of either the ventricular septum (VS)

From the Pathology Branch, National Heart, Lung, and Blood Institute, National Institutes of Health, Bethesda, Maryland 20892. Manuscript received and accepted April 23, 1987.

or a LV papillary muscle during AMI is far less common.[1,2] Combined rupture of LV free wall and either VS or papillary muscle is rare and this possibility has received little attention.[3-5] In this report we describe certain clinical and necropsy findings in 7 patients who had combined rupture of both LV free wall and VS during AMI; in all of them the rupture was also associated with hemopericardium.

The ages of the 7 patients ranged from 57 to 81 years (mean 69 ± 9); 2 were women and 5 were men. Four had historical evidence of systemic hypertension before the fatal AMI and at least 2 of them had received antihypertensive treatment. Three had diabetes mellitus of late onset. Before the fatal AMI, 3 had had angina pectoris. None had had a previous clinical event compatible with AMI and none had had evidence of congestive heart failure. Thus, the fatal AMI with rupture was the first coronary event in 4 patients and angina pectoris was the first event in the other 3.

The interval from onset of chest pain (associated with the fatal AMI) to death ranged from 21 hours to 28 days (median 8 days). A "new murmur" appeared during the AMI in 5 patients; the interval from onset of chest pain associated with the fatal AMI to the appearance of a new precordial murmur compatible with rupture of the ventricular septum in them ranged from 15 hours to 6 days (mean 3 days, median 4 days). In patient 1, a murmur compatible with ventricular septal rupture was audible when the patient first entered the hospital; he died on the first hospital day. Two patients (nos. 3 and 7) did not have a precordial systolic murmur recorded during their hospital course for AMI. They were the only 2 patients in whom ventricular septal defect was not diagnosed or suspected during AMI. Rupture of the VS at necropsy in patient 7 was extremely small, the smallest by far of the 7 patients (Fig. 1). The location of the AMI by electrocardiography was posterior (inferior) wall in 6 patients and anterior wall in 1 patient (no. 1). Necropsy in the latter patient, however, disclosed that a portion of both the posterior and anterior LV walls was necrotic.

Of the 7 patients, 2 (nos. 1 and 6) had operative closure of the cardiac rupture sites (Fig. 2). At opera-

tion, both were found to have large quantities of blood in the pericardial sac. Patient 1 could not be weaned from cardiopulmonary bypass. Patient 6, who underwent surgery on day 1, died 28 days later. The septal defect reopened about day 2 as evidenced by the reappearance of a new murmur. The 5 patients who did not undergo cardiac operation died suddenly; necropsy disclosed large amounts of blood in the pericardial sac in each.

At necropsy, heart weights ranged from 350 to 590 g (mean 440 ± 102). The amount of subepicardial adi-

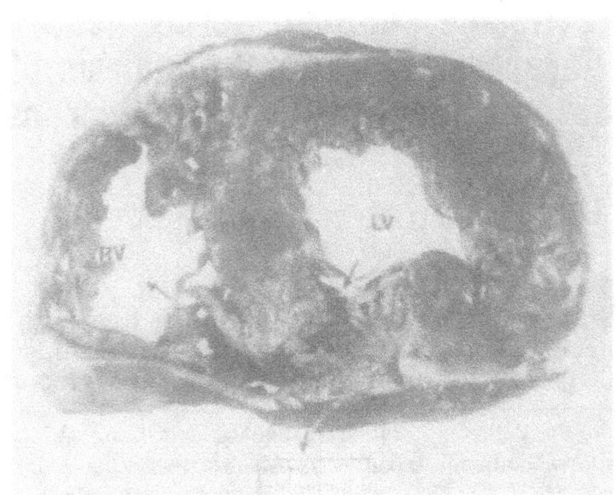

FIGURE 3. View of a transverse cut of the cardiac ventricles in still another patient showing a posterior acute myocardial infarct and the rupture site beginning at the posterior junction and dissecting through it into the right ventricular (RV) cavity and into the pericardial sac. Both ventricular cavities are dilated. LV = left ventricular cavity; VS = ventricular septum.

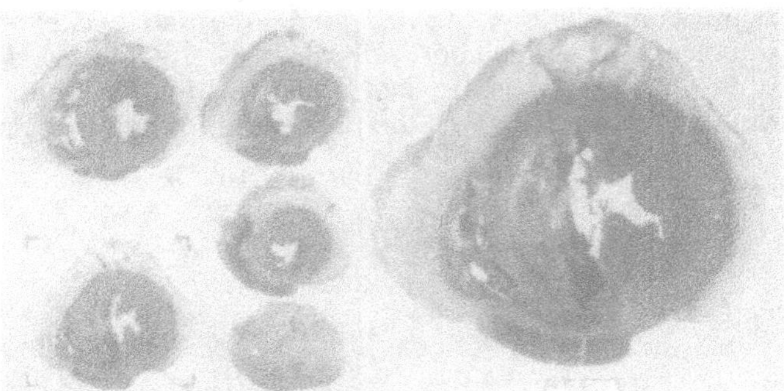

FIGURE 1. Gross sections of the cardiac ventricles after multiple transverse cuts in 1 patient. *Left*, view of 5 cut surfaces showing increased subepicardial fat, hemorrhagic on its posterior portion, and the posterior acute myocardial infarct. *Right*, view of the transverse slice (enclosed by the *brackets*) showing the small rupture site (*arrows*). LV = left ventricular cavity; RV = right ventricular cavity.

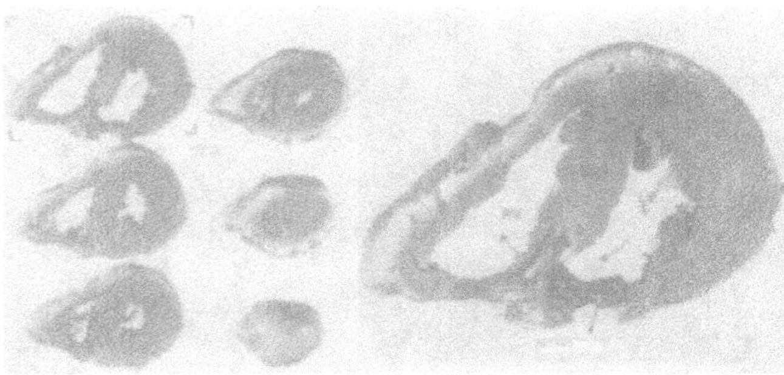

FIGURE 2. Gross sections of the cardiac ventricles after multiple transverse cuts in another patient. *Left*, view of 6 cut surfaces showing the surgical repair of the posterior double rupture. *Right*, close-up view of the transverse slice (enclosed by *brackets*) showing the thinned posterior ventricular septum (VS), a Dacron® patch on the left ventricular posterior wall and a posterior wall acute myocardial infarct. LV = left ventricular cavity; RV = right ventricular cavity.

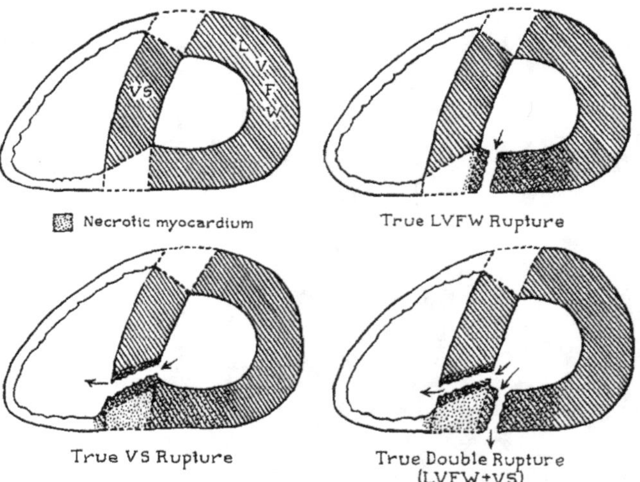

FIGURE 4. Types of "true" ventricular ruptures. *Top left*, portion of left ventricular free wall (LVFW) and ventricular septum (VS) that actually borders the LV cavity is in *hatched lines*. A true rupture occurs in a portion of wall actually bordering the LV cavity. *Top right*, an example of true LVFW rupture through an acute myocardial infarct (*dotted area*), allowing extravasation of blood into the pericardial space. *Bottom left*, example of true septal rupture, allowing free passage of blood from the left into the right ventricular cavity. *Bottom right*, example of a true double rupture of the ventricular septum and the LVFW.

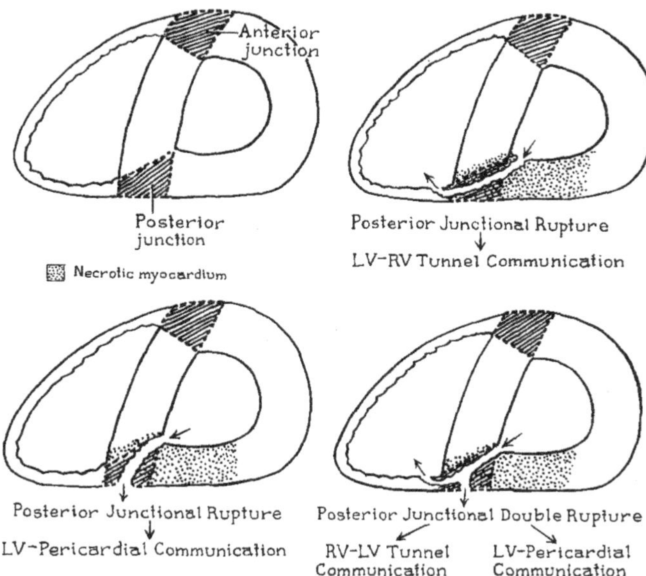

FIGURE 5. Types of "junctional" ventricular ruptures. *Top left,* junctional portions of the cardiac ventricle (*hatched lines*). A junctional rupture involves all or a portion of the junctional area. *Top right,* example of posterior junctional rupture through a posterior septal myocardial infarct (*dotted area*), with blood dissecting through the junction and producing a left ventricular (LV) to right ventricular (RV) tunnel communication. *Bottom left,* example of a posterior junctional rupture through a posterior myocardial infarct (*dotted area*) producing LV to pericardial communication. *Bottom right,* example of a posterior junctional double rupture, with passage of blood from the LV cavity into the right one and into the pericardial sac.

pose tissue was increased in all 7 patients, to a degree in 2 patients that the heart floated in water (Fig. 1). In no patient was the left main coronary artery significantly narrowed. Of the other 3 major (right, left anterior descending and left circumflex) epicardial coronary arteries, either 2 or 3 were narrowed >75% in cross-sectional area by atherosclerotic plaque. Only 1 patient (no. 2) had a left dominant coronary system. The cardiac ventricles were sectioned transversely. By visual inspection, both ventricular cavities were dilated in 2 patients (nos. 3 and 7) (Fig. 3). In the other 5 patients, neither ventricular cavity was dilated. In no patient was a scar present in the LV free wall or VS. The acute infarct involved the LV posterior free wall and the posterior portion of VS in all 7 patients and also the anterior LV free wall and anterior portion of VS in 1 patient (no. 1). Rupture of the LV free wall and VS was posteriorly located in 6 patients (nos. 2 through 7) (Fig. 1 to 3), and anteriorly located in 1 (no. 1).

At least 11 cases of double rupture studied at necropsy have been reported. Snyder[3] reported a 60-year-old man with posterior wall double rupture. Benrey and associates[4] reported a 45-year-old woman with posterior wall double rupture. Edwards et al[5] reported 9 cases of double rupture: The rupture sites were posterior in 7 and anterior in 2. Thus, of 11 reported double rupture necropsy cases, 9 had a posterior rupture site. The rupture site was the posterior wall in 6 of our 7 cases.

LV free wall or VS ruptures can be classified as "true" (Fig. 4) or "junctional" (Fig. 5) according to their location. The "junction" is the portion of myocardium located directly anterior and posterior to the ventricular septum, but does not contact either ventricular cavity. Junctional ruptures produce a left-to-right ventricular communication, a LV-to-pericardial communication, or both. "True rupture" of the ventricular septum and LV free wall involves the myocardial wall actually bordering the ventricular cavity, i.e., outside the junction area. In 5 of our 7 patients with double rupture, the type of rupture could be established: 4 were junctional double ruptures and only 1 was a true double rupture.

1. Lewis AJ, Burchell HB, Titus JL. *Clinical and pathologic features of postinfarction cardiac rupture. Am J Cardiol 1969;23:43–53.*
2. Bates RJ, Beutler S, Resnekov L, Anagnostopoulos CE. *Cardiac rupture challenge in diagnosis and management. Am J Cardiol 1977;40:429–437.*
3. Snyder GAC. *Spontaneous double rupture of the heart. Arch Pathol 1940;29:796–799.*
4. Benrey J, Krajcer Z, Hoeffler HB, Beard EF. *Myocardial infarction with cardiac rupture in isolated right coronary artery disease. Bull Texas Heart Inst 1976;4:294–302.*
5. Edwards BS, Edwards WL, Edwards JE. *Septal rupture complicating acute myocardial infarction: identification of simple and complex types in 53 autopsied hearts. Am J Cardiol 1984;54:1201–1205.*

Delayed Clinical Evidence of Coronary Arterial Disruption After Presumably Successful Percutaneous Transluminal Coronary Angioplasty for Angina Pectoris

BENJAMIN N. POTKIN, MD

RICHARD K. MYLER, MD

HAMID E. MOTAMED, MD

JESSICA M. MANN, MD

JEFFREY L. HENDEL, MD

DAVID C. SPERLING, MD

SIMON STERTZER, MD

WILLIAM C. ROBERTS, MD

Certain clinical and morphologic cardiac observations have been reported in at least 9 patients who died within 30 days of percutaneous transluminal coronary angioplasty (PTCA) for angina pectoris.[1-7] Of these 9 patients, 3 died of complications of PTCA either during the procedure or immediately after the balloon dilatation.[2,3,6] Of the remaining 6 patients, 4 had immediately recognizable complications of the PTCA procedure, and each of them either immediately[1,4] or the next day[1,7] had coronary artery bypass grafting. The remaining 2 reported patients who had PTCA for angina pectoris died 5 and 30 days, respectively, after the PTCA procedure, which was considered at the time uncomplicated, and the PTCA was followed by an asymptomatic period before sudden death.[5,7] The present report focuses on morphologic cardiac findings in another patient who had PTCA for angina pectoris and died suddenly the next day after a presumably uncomplicated and "successful" PTCA.

P.D., a 67-year-old man, had the onset of exertional angina pectoris 26 months before death. About 4 months before death, the frequency and intensity of the angina increased and 71 days before death the

From the Pathology Branch, National Heart, Lung, and Blood Institute, National Institutes of Health, Bethesda, Maryland; San Francisco Heart Institute of Seton Medical Center, Daly City, California; and the Department of Pathology, St. Francis Memorial Hospital, San Francisco, California. Manuscript received and accepted June 16, 1987.

patient underwent the first of a planned 2-stage PTCA for multivessel coronary artery disease. A totally occluded left anterior descending (LAD) coronary artery was crossed by a wire and then the balloon was inflated at several sites to 9 atm for up to 40 seconds with marked reduction in the mean gradient which was 60 mm Hg before the dilatation procedure. The LAD was widely patent at the end of the dilatation procedure. A ramus branch was severely narrowed (2 tandem narrowings) with a 60-mm Hg mean gradient across the narrowings. The balloon was inflated to 6 atm on several occasions for up to 40 seconds, resulting in a marked reduction in this mean gradient, a significant widening of the lumen and improved contrast flow of this branch as well. The moderately severe tandem stenoses in the right coronary artery were not dilated at that time.

There were no complications of this PTCA procedure. Shortly afterward, a thallium stress test showed persistent inferoapical ischemia of a mild to moderate degree and fixed perfusion defects of the inferior, apical and septal regions.

Seventy days later, a second PTCA procedure was performed because of recurrent angina. The previously dilated ramus branch was still widely patent. The LAD, however, was again severely narrowed at the site of the previous PTCA, with a measured 80-mm Hg gradient across the narrowing. The dilatation balloon was inflated on 4 occasions to 13 atm for 45 seconds, resulting in reduction of the gradient to <20 mm Hg. Shortly thereafter, however, the mean residual gradient across the proximal LAD rose to 60 mm Hg and for this reason, a fifth balloon dilatation to 14 atm for 60 seconds was applied with reduction of the gradient to <20 mm Hg. The angiogram thereafter showed insignificant LAD narrowing and the patient's condition was stable. After a suitable delay, the tandem narrowings in the mid-right coronary artery were dilated. A 60-mm Hg gradient was recorded across the narrowings. Seven atmospheres of balloon inflation pressure for 30 seconds was applied twice to the distal narrowing. The balloon was then withdrawn to the most proximal narrowing and inflated to 5 atm for 30 seconds. Repeat angiography then showed only minimal residual stenosis, an excellent flow of contrast material, and ablation of the pressure gradient.

In the next 24 hours, the patient was free of angina and had 3 normal electrocardiograms and 3 normal cardiac enzyme levels. He was then sent home. About 4 hours after leaving the hospital, while at a friend's

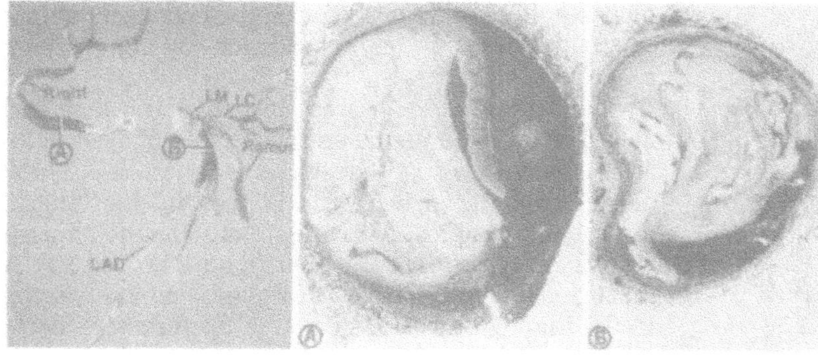

FIGURE 1. Epicardial coronary arteries in the patient described. *Left*, the coronary arteries were excised intact from the heart. In a portion of the right and left anterior descending (LAD) coronary arteries the outer wall of the artery is hemorrhagic. At the site labeled *A* in the right coronary artery, the cross section at this point is shown in *A*, and at the site shown in *B* of the LAD coronary artery, the cross section at this point is shown in *B*. Both *A* and *B* show tearing of the intimal plaque. In *A*, the media also is torn through and through creating a disruption at the former junction of media and adventitia. In *B*, the dissection occurs between intimal plaque and media. Movat stains: A × 20, B × 22.

apartment, chest pain developed that was unresponsive to sublingual nitroglycerin. An ambulance was called, shortly thereafter the paramedics arrived, ventricular fibrillation occurred and he was successfully defibrillated to sinus rhythm. He was taken to a nearby local hospital and the electrocardiogram showed marked ST-segment elevation in leads 2, 3 and aVF. About 2 hours after the onset of chest pain, complete atrioventricular block, widening of the QRS

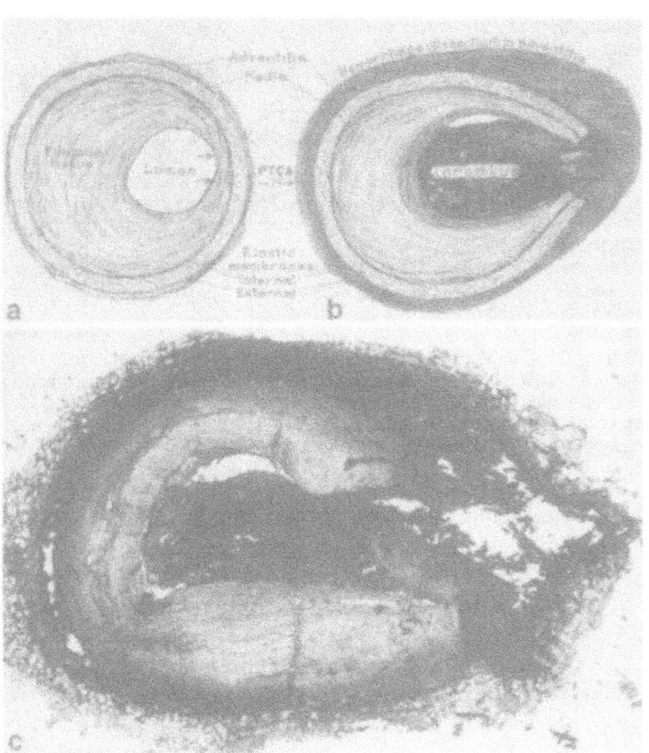

FIGURE 2. Another cross section of right coronary artery at the site of exterior wall hemorrhage shown in Figure 1. *a*, drawing of coronary artery as it probably appeared before balloon dilatation. The lumen is eccentric and the atherosclerotic plaque consists mainly of fibrous tissue. *b*, after the percutaneous transluminal coronary angioplasty (PTCA) procedure thrombus formed in the residual lumen and both intimal plaque and medial wall torn through and through to create a dissection at the previous junction of media and adventitia. *c*, photomicrograph of actual right coronary artery showing the thrombus in the lumen, through and through rupture of the plaque and medial walls, and extensive dissection at the former junction of media and adventitia. Movat stain, × 20.

complexes and then asystole developed. Resuscitation was unsuccessful.

At necropsy, both the LAD and right coronary arteries were focally disrupted (Fig. 1) and the dissection of the right coronary artery plus a luminal thrombus caused near-total occlusion of the residual eccentric lumen (Fig. 1 and 2). There was complete disruption of the medial wall and intimal plaque of the right coronary artery, allowing dissection between the media and adventitia. The extravasated blood compressed the residual coronary arterial lumen. Only the intimal plaque, not the media, of the LAD was disruptured. There was no hemopericardium and no extravasation of blood into the subepicardial adipose tissue. The heart weighted 485 g and there were no areas of myocardial necrosis. A small scar was present in the anterior wall of the left ventricle. The 2 coronary arteries that had been subjected to the second PTCA procedure were excised intact and cut into 5-mm-long segments transverse to the longitudinal axis of the artery. The 5-mm segments were processed in alcohols and xylene, embedded in paraffin and a 6-μ-thick section was prepared from each segment. Each section was stained by the Movat method. The degree of cross-sectional area narrowing of each section is shown in Figure 3.

In the present patient, no complications were recognized in the first 24 hours after clinically successful PTCA. Then chest pain appeared, followed by electrocardiographic changes, consistent with left ventricular posterior (inferior) wall myocardial injury and, subsequently, fatal cardiac arrest. Although necropsy disclosed disruption of both LAD and right coronary arteries at sites of the most recent PTCA, the residual lumen of the LAD did not appear to be compromised by the disruption, whereas the residual lumen of the right coronary artery was compressed to a point where it was nearly completely closed. The lumina at the sites of the disruption in both LAD and right coronary arteries were eccentrically located and the intimal plaque disrupture sites in both arteries were located at the junction between the "thin" outer border of the eccentric lumen and the "thick" underlying plaque beneath the lumen. The large atherosclerotic plaques between the eccentric lumina in both LAD and right coronary arteries contained calcific deposits, which may have

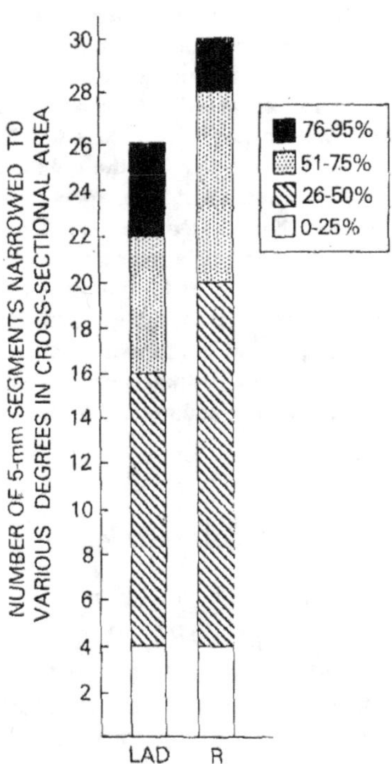

FIGURE 3. Bar graph showing the number of 5-mm segments of the left anterior descending (LAD) and right (R) coronary arteries narrowed to various degrees in cross-sectional area by atherosclerotic plaque alone. Of the 26 five-millimeter transverse sections of the LAD coronary artery, none was narrowed >95 % in cross-sectional area; 4 (15 %) were narrowed 76 to 95 %; 6 (23 %), 51 to 75 %; 12 (46 %), 26 to 50 %, and 4 (15 %), 0 to 25 % in cross-sectional area. Of the 30 five-millimeter segments of the right coronary artery, none was narrowed >95 % by plaque; 2 (7 %) were narrowed 76 to 95 %; 8 (27 %), 51 to 75 %; 16 (53 %), 26 to 50 %; and 4 (13 %) were narrowed 0 to 25 % in cross-sectional area. Of the 6 five-millimeter segments of both LAD and right coronary arteries narrowed 76 to 95 % in cross-sectional area by plaque, the lumina in all 6 were eccentrically located; of the 14 five-millimeter segments narrowed 51 to 75 %, the lumina were eccentrically located in 11(79 %); of the 28 five-millimeter segments narrowed 26 to 50 %, the lumina were eccentrically located in 12 (43 %), and of the 8 five-millimeter segments narrowed 0 to 25 %, the lumina were eccentrically located in none.

made the thick plaque beneath the eccentric lumina relatively resistant to compression by the balloon dilator.

The occurrence of dissection between intima and media or between media and adventitia of a coronary artery secondary to a tear at the junction of a "thin" outer border of an eccentric lumen and the "thick" underlying plaque also were found in photomicrographs of reports of at least 7 patients who had PTCA during acute myocardial infarction, but not during PTCA for angina pectoris only.[8-10] Furthermore, coronary dissection with luminal compression in our patient caused delayed (24 hours) clinical evidence of myocardial injury, without antecedent clinical, electrocardiographic or cardiac enzymatic warning, and this circumstance has not previously been reported, to our knowledge.

1. Block PC, Myler RK, Stertzer S, Fallon JT. *Morphology after transluminal angioplasty in human beings. N Engl J Med 1981;305:382–385.*
2. Saffitz JE, Rose TE, Oaks JB, Roberts WC. *Coronary arterial rupture during coronary angioplasty. Am J Cardiol 1983;51:902–904.*
3. Mizuno K, Kurita A, Imazeki N. *Pathological findings after percutaneous transluminal coronary angioplasty. Br Heart J 1984;52:588–590.*
4. Waller BF, Gorfinkel JH, Rogers FJ, Kent KM, Roberts WC. *Early and late morphologic changes in major epicardial coronary arteries after percutaneous transluminal angioplasty. Am J Cardiol 1984;53:42C–47C.*
5. Austin GE, Ratliff NB, Hollman J, Tabei S, Phillips DF. *Intimal proliferation of smooth muscle cells as an explanation for recurrent coronary artery stenosis after percutaneous transluminal coronary angioplasty. JACC 1985; 6:369–375.*
6. Soward AL, Essed CE, Serruys PW. *Coronary arterial findings after accidental death immediately after successful percutaneous transluminal coronary angioplasty. Am J Cardiol 1985;56:794–795.*
7. Schneider J, Grüntzig A. *Percutaneous transluminal coronary angioplasty: morphological findings in 3 patients. Path Res Pract 1985;180:348–352.*
8. Düber C, Junglbuth A, Rumpelt HJ, Erbel R, Meyer J, Thoenes W. *Morphology of the coronary arteries after combined thrombolysis and percutaneous transluminal coronary angioplasty for acute myocardial infarction. Am J Cardiol 1986;58:698–703.*
9. de Morais CF, Lopes EA, Checchi H, Arie S, Pileggi F. *Percutaneous transluminal coronary angioplasty—histopathological analysis of nine necropsy cases. Virchows Arch A 1986;410:195–202.*
10. Waller BF, Rothbaum DA, Pinkerton CA, Cowley MJ, Linnemeier TJ, Orr C, Irons M, Helmuth RA, Wills ER, Aust C. *Status of the myocardium and infarct-related coronary artery in 19 necropsy patients with acute recanalization using pharmacologic (streptokinase, r-tissue plasminogen activator), mechanical (percutaneous transluminal coronary angioplasty) or combined types of reperfusion therapy. JACC 1987;9:785–801.*

Cardiac Morphologic Observations After Operative Closure of Acquired Ventricular Septal Defect During Acute Myocardial Infarction: Analysis of 16 Necropsy Patients

JESSICA M. MANN, MD, and WILLIAM C. ROBERTS, MD

Certain cardiac morphologic findings are described in 16 necropsy patients having operative closure of an acquired ventricular septal defect (VSD) during acute myocardial infarction (AMI). Of the 16 patients, 6 were women (mean age 69 ± 7 years) and 10 were men (mean age 60 ± 11 years). The AMI associated with the VSD was the first coronary event in 13 patients (81%). At least 6 patients had a history of systemic hypertension. Conduction disturbances were diagnosed by electrocardiogram in 5 patients (31%). The median interval from the onset of the AMI to death was 11 days, and from the onset of the AMI to operative closure of the VSD, 4 days. Eight patients died in the operating room or within 2 hours of operation. Coronary artery bypass grafting was performed simultaneously with the VSD closure in 7 patients. Death was attributed to unsuccessful VSD closure in 5 patients, to inadequate left ventricular cavity after resection of necrotic myocardium in 5 patients and to inadequate viable left ventricular myocardium in 4 patients. Heart weights were increased in 14 patients (88%). The AMI associated with the VSD was anterior in 9 patients and posterior (inferior) in 7. Healed myocardial infarcts were present in 3 patients. All 16 patients had severe (>75% in cross-sectional area) narrowing of 1 or more of the 4 major epicardial coronary arteries. (Am J Cardiol 1987;60:981–987)

S everal studies have focused on morphologic findings at necropsy in patients with acquired ventricular septal defect (VSD) during acute myocardial infarction (AMI).[1-3] No studies, however, have focused on morphologic findings at necropsy in patients who had attempted operative closure of VSD secondary to AMI. The present report describes such observations in 16 necropsy patients.

Patients Studied

Clinical findings: Certain clinical and necropsy findings in the 16 patients are presented in Table I. Of the 16 patients, 6 were women (mean age 69 ± 7 years) and 10 were men (mean age 60 ± 11 years). The AMI associated with the acquired VSD was the first coro-

nary event in 13 patients (81%); 2 patients (nos. 2 and 10 [Table I]) had had angina pectoris and 1 patient (no. 5) had had a clinically apparent AMI that had healed. At least 6 patients had histories of systemic hypertension before the fatal AMI.

The AMI associated with the acquired VSD by electrocardiogram involved the anterior wall of left ventricle in 9 patients (56%) and the posterior wall in 6 (44%). In all 6 women, the AMI involved the anterior wall. Complete bundle branch block or second- or third-degree heart block was evident by electrocardiogram in 5 patients (31%). The interval from onset of AMI to death ranged from 2 to 115 days (median 11); the interval from onset of AMI to detection of a precordial systolic murmur consistent with VSD ranged from <1 to 8 days (median 2); the interval from onset of AMI to operative closure of the VSD ranged from 2 to 14 days (median 4); and the interval from "closure" of the VSD to death ranged from 0 to 113 days (median 14). Of the 16 patients, however, 8 (50%) died in the operating room (7 patients) or within 2 hours of completion of the operation (Table I).

From the Pathology Branch, National Institutes of Health, National Heart, Lung, and Blood Institute, Bethesda, Maryland. Manuscript received June 25, 1987, accepted July 14, 1987.

Address for reprints: William C. Roberts, MD, Building 10, Room 2N—258, National Institutes of Health, Bethesda, Maryland 20892.

TABLE I Clinical and Necropsy Findings in 16 Patients Having Operative "Closure" of Acquired Ventricular Septal Defect During Acute Myocardial Infarction

Case	Age (yr) & Sex	AP	SH	AMI Location by ECG	Conduction Disturbance During AMI	Int. (days) AMI to Death	Int. (days) Onset AMI to New Murmur	Int. (days) Onset to VSD "Closure"	Int. (days) VSD "Closure" to Death	Cause of Death	CABG	HW (g)	LV Scar	Location AMI	Site of VS Rupture	Incomplete VSD closure	No. CAs↓ >75% in CSA by Plaque	Thrombus CA
1	56M	0	+	P	0	4	–	4	OR	IM	0	↑	0	P	P	0	3	–
2	60M	+	+	P	+(2° AVB)	2	1	2	OR	IM	+	490	+*	P	P	+	3	+ (R)
3	65F	0	–	A	+(left BBB)	11	5	11	OR	IC	+	450	0	A	A	0	0	+ (LAD)
4	69F	0	0	A	0	4	2	4	OR	IC	0	290	0	A	A	0	1	0
5	76F	–	0	A	–	3	–	3	OR	IC	0	360	+	A	A	0	1	0
6	77M	0	0	P	–	14	3	14	OR	IC	0	560	0	P	P	0	3	0
7	79M	0	0	P	0	11	–	11	OR	IC	+	480	+*	P	P	0	3	+ (R)
8	43M	0	+	P	+(CHB)	4	2	4	<1	VSD	0	530	0	P	P	+	2	+ (R)
9	63F	0	0	A	0	9	6	7	2	Bleeding	0	405	0	A	A	0	1	0
10	79F	+	+	A	+(right BBB)	9	1	2	7	IM	+	600	0	A	A	0	2	0
11	51M	0	+	P	0	17	8	8	9	VSD	+	550	0	P	P	+	2	+ (R)
12	53M	0	+	A	0	21	6	7	14	WD	0	↑	0	A	A	0	2	0
13	63M	0	0	A	–	21	2	5	16	VSD	0	375	0	A	A	+	2	0
14	63F	0	0	A	0	18	<1	1	17	VSD	+	470	0	A	A	+	2	+ (LAD)
15	62M	0	0	P	0	47	–	5	42	VSD	0	650	0	P	P	+	2	0
16	56M	0	0	A	+(right BBB)	115	2	2	113	IM	+	615	0	A	A	+	1	0

*The AMI was clinically silent.

A = anterior; AMI = acute myocardial infarction; AP = angina pectoris; AVB = atrioventricular block; BBB = bundle branch block; CA = coronary artery; CABG = coronary artery bypass grafting; CHB = complete heart block; CSA = cross-sectional area; ECG = electrocardiogram; F = female; HW = heart weight; INT = interval; IC = inadequate left ventricular cavity; Int. = interval; IM = insufficient viable left ventricular myocardium; LAD = left anterior descending; LV = left ventricular; M = man; OR = operating room; P = posterior; R = right coronary artery; SH = history of systemic hypertension; VS = ventricular septum; VSD = ventricular septal defect; WD = wound dehiscence; + = present or positive; 0 = absent or negative; – = no information available; ↑ = increased.

Periods of operations, surgeons and institutions: Nine different surgeons performed the operations in the 16 patients to close the VSD during a 19-year period (1968 to 1987). The operations were performed at 6 different medical centers and the hearts in each patient were subsequently submitted to the Pathology Branch, National Heart, Lung, and Blood Institute. All hearts were initially examined by WCR and 10 were examined by JMM and reexamined by WCR. Operations to close the VSD were performed from 1968 through 1975 in 3 patients, from 1976 to 1980 in 5 patients, and from 1981 to 1987 in 8 patients. The operative approaches to close the VSD, of course, changed during the 19-year period.

Intervals from operation to death: Cardiac output in all 16 patients appeared to be inadequate immediately after closure of the VSD and after discontinuation of cardiopulmonary bypass. Of the 16 patients, 7 died in the operating room because of inability to be weaned from cardiopulmonary bypass (systemic arterial pressure always inadequate) and 1 patient died within 2 hours of leaving the operating room. The other 8 patients died 2 to 113 days after VSD closure. In 7 patients (44%) (nos. 2, 3, 7, 10, 11, 14 and 16) coronary artery bypass grafting was performed in addition to attempted closure of the VSD. One patient (no. 15, Table I) also had mitral valve replacement for mitral regurgitation 15 days after closure of the VSD, and he died 13 days after the second operation.

Causes of death: The immediate cause of death was attributed to incomplete closure of the VSD or reappearance of the VSD after initially successful closure in 5 patients (31%) (nos. 8, 11, 13, 14 and 15). Death in 5 patients (31%) (nos. 3 through 7) was attributed to inadequate left ventricular cavity after resection of necrotic ventricular septal and left ventricular free wall myocardium. None of these 5 patients could be separated from cardiopulmonary bypass. Death in 4 patients (25%) (nos. 1, 2, 10 and 16) was attributed to inadequate viable left ventricular myocardium because of extensive necrosis. Death in 1 patient (no. 9) was attributed to bleeding; she was returned to the operating room for tamponade on the first postoperative day and died the next day. Death in 1 patient (no. 12) was attributed to infection; the sternotomy incision could not be closed after VSD repair, the wound became infected and the patient died 14 days postoperatively.

Necropsy findings: Certain cardiac morphologic findings are illustrated in Figures 1 to 7. The hearts ranged in weight in the 6 women from 290 to 600 g (mean 430 ± 105) and the hearts in 8 men ranged from 375 to 650 g (mean 530 ± 85). The amount of subepicardial fat was increased in all 16 patients.[4] Three patients had small healed myocardial infarcts (scars) and all 3 involved the anterior wall. The acute myocardial infarcts associated with rupture of the ventricular septum involved the anterior wall in 9 patients and the posterior wall in 7 patients. The rupture site in the ventricular septum, accordingly, involved its anterior portion in 9 and the posterior portion in 7 patients. Neither ventricular cavity was dilated in the 7 patients

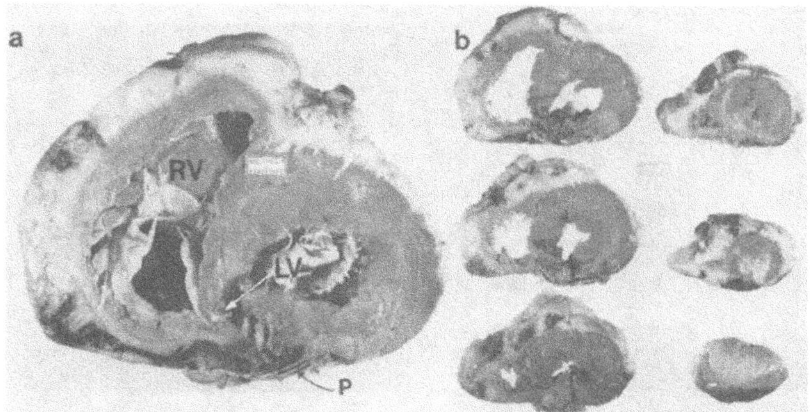

FIGURE 1. Case 2 (Table I). *a*, view of the most basal transverse cut of the cardiac ventricles showing the posterior wall acute myocardial infarct and ventricular septal defect (*arrow*) repaired with a patch (P). Neither right (RV) nor left (LV) ventricular cavities are dilated. *b*, sections of the cardiac ventricles after multiple transverse cuts showing the posterior wall necrosis.

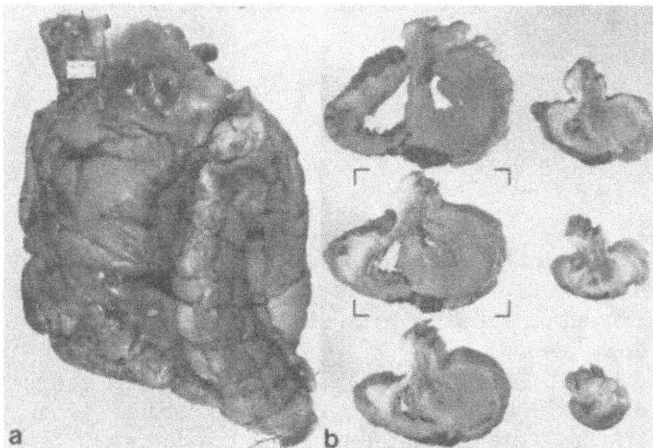

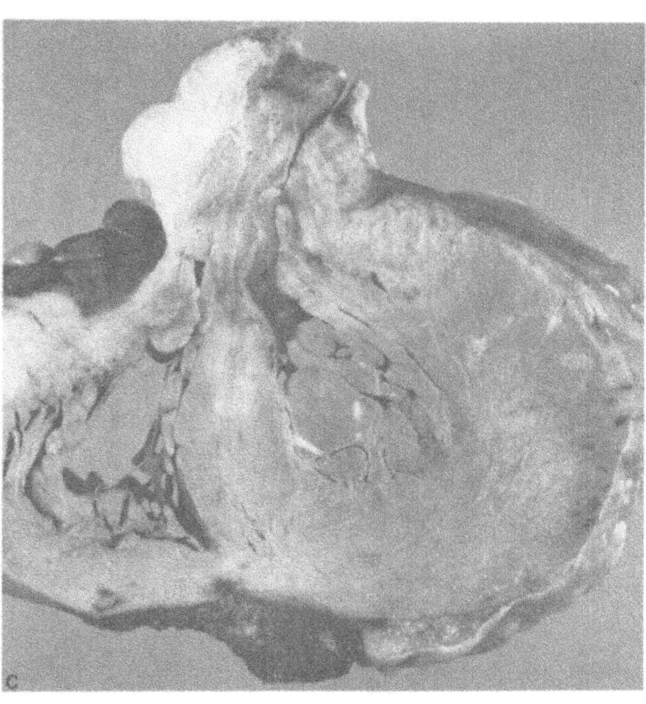

FIGURE 2. Case 3. *a*, external view of the heart showing a long ventriculotomy incision closed by sutures in cloth. *b*, sections of the cardiac ventricles after multiple transverse cuts showing the anterior acute myocardial infarct and the repair of the acquired anterior ventricular septal defect. The left ventricular cavity is minute. *c*, close-up view of the section in brackets in *b* showing the minute left ventricular cavity after operative closure of the ventricular septal defect. A small thrombus is present within the left ventricular cavity at the site of the left ventricular incision.

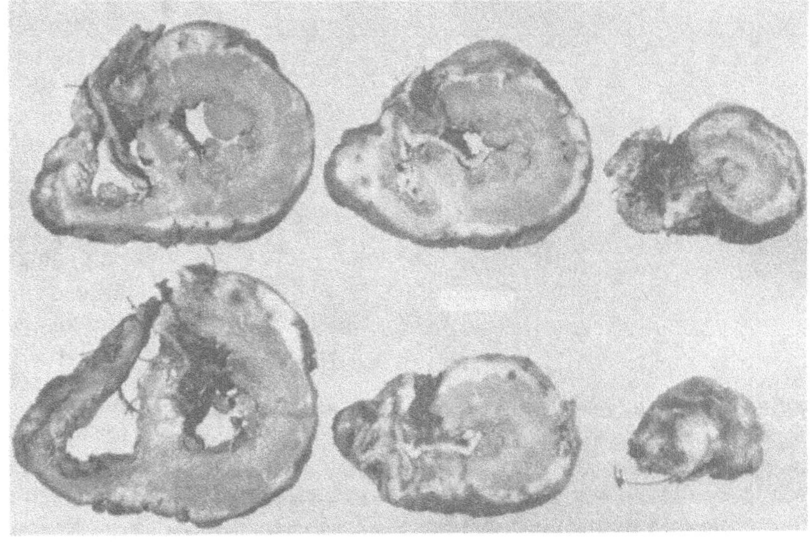

FIGURE 3. Case 4. Sections of the cardiac ventricles after transverse cuts showing an anterior wall acute myocardial infarct and the acquired ventricular septal defect repaired with a Dacron® patch. The left ventricular cavity is small.

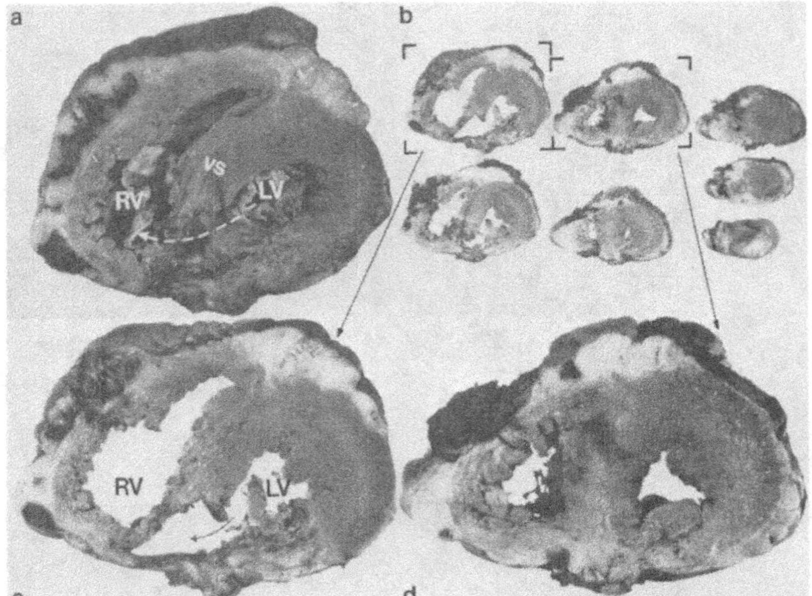

FIGURE 4. Case 6. *a*, view of the most basal transverse cut of the cardiac ventricles showing the posterior acute myocardial infarct and the acquired ventricular septal defect (*arrow*). The subepicardial fat over the right ventricle (RV) is focally hemorrhagic. LV = left ventricle; VS = ventricular septum. *b*, sections of the cardiac ventricles after multiple transverse cuts showing the posterior wall necrosis and ventricular septal defect in the most basal sections. *c*, close-up view of the section in brackets in *b*, showing the posterior wall necrosis and the thinning of the posterior portion of the ventricular septum. *d*, close-up view of the slice in brackets in *b*, showing the posterior wall necrosis.

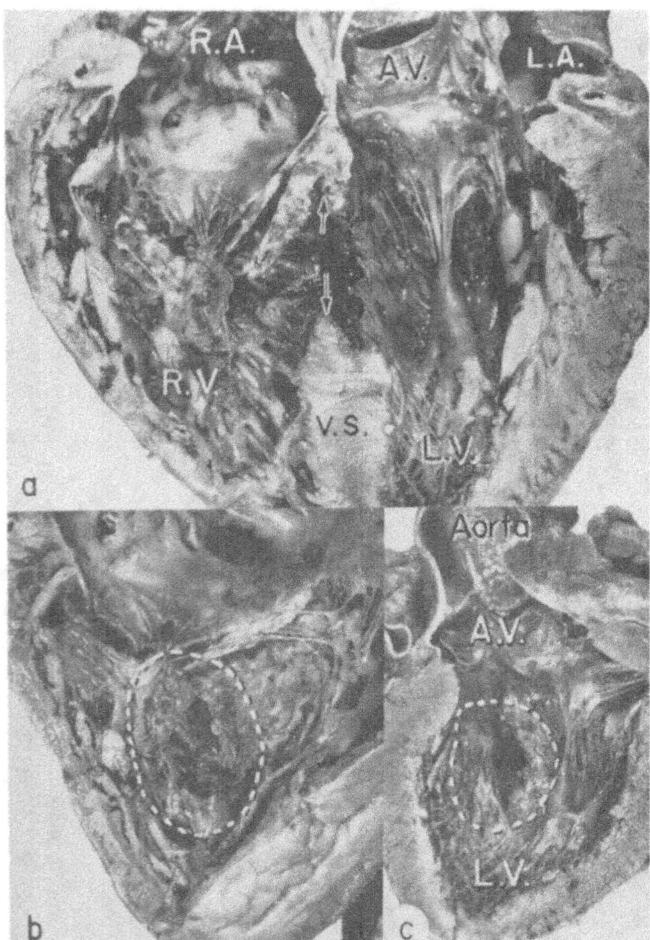

FIGURE 5. Case 8. *a*, view of the heart opened longitudinally showing the posterior and basal huge ventricular septal defect (*between arrows*). A.V. = aortic valve; L.A. = left atrium; L.V. = left ventricle; R.A. = right atrium; R.V. = right ventricle; V.S. = ventricular septum. *b*, close-up view of the defect (*dashed circle*) from the right ventricle. *c*, close-up view of the defect (*dashed circle*) from the left ventricle.

who could not be weaned from cardiopulmonary bypass. In contrast, both ventricular cavities by visual inspection appeared to be dilated in the 9 patients who died later.

In all 16 patients the 3 major (right, left anterior descending and left circumflex) epicardial coronary arteries were examined to assess the degree of cross-sectional area narrowing by atherosclerotic plaque. Of the 16 patients, none of the 3 epicardial coronary arteries was narrowed by plaque >75% in 1 patient (no. 3), but this patient did have a thrombus in the left anterior descending coronary artery and it plus the underlying plaque resulted in >75% luminal narrowing. A single coronary artery only was >75% narrowed by plaque in 4 patients; 2 arteries were so narrowed in 7 patients, and all 3 major coronary arteries were so narrowed in 4 patients.

In 10 patients, the 4 major (includes left main also) epicardial coronary arteries were excised intact, decalcified if necessary, and separated into 5-mm-long segments. A histologic section was then prepared from each segment and stained by the Movat method. A total of 384 five-mm-long coronary artery segments were examined: 16 from the left main, 127 from the left anterior descending, 80 from the left circumflex and 161 from the right coronary artery (Figure 8). The percentage of different degrees (0 to 25, 26 to 50, 51 to 75, 76 to 95 and 96 to 100) of cross-sectional narrowing by atherosclerotic plaque for each of the 4 coronary arteries in these 10 patients is shown in Figure 8 and for each patient in Figure 9. Of the 384 five-mm-long coronary artery segments, 32 (8%) were narrowed <25% by atherosclerotic plaque in cross-sectional area; 129 (34%) were narrowed 26 to 50%; 155 (40%), 51 to 75%, and 68 (18%), 76 to 95%. None of the 5-mm-long coronary artery segments in any of these 10 patients was narrowed by plaque as much as 96 to 100% in cross-sectional area. A thrombus was present in the infarct-related coronary artery in 6 patients (38%).

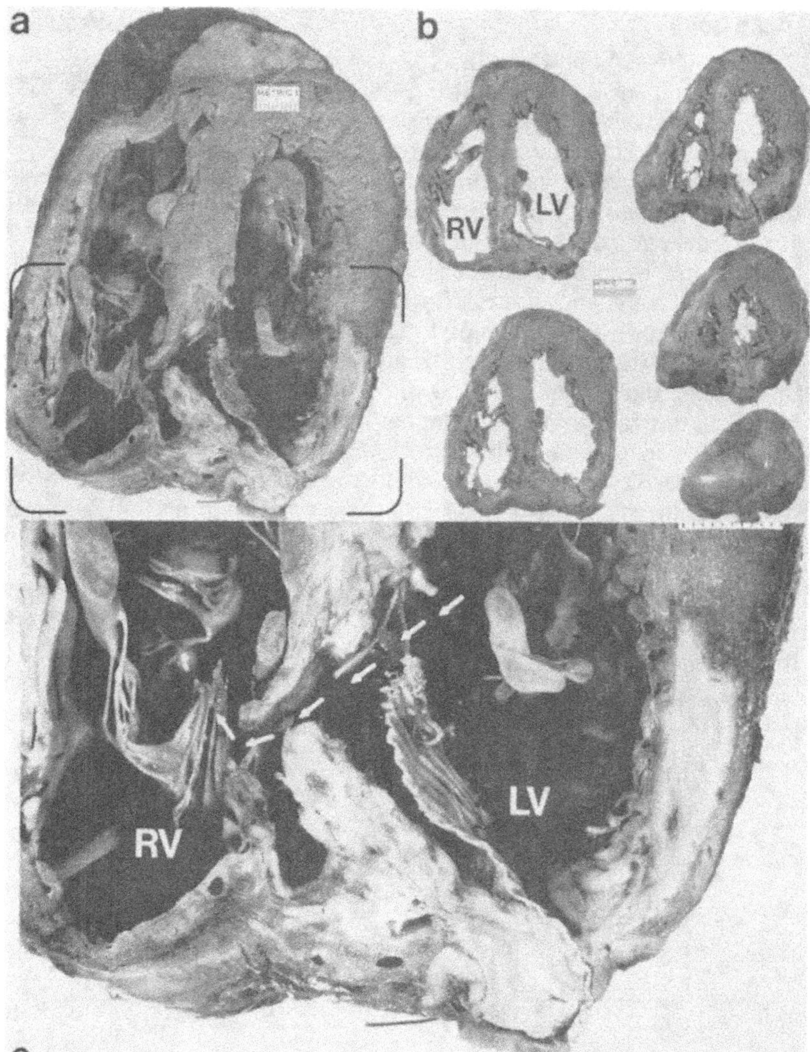

FIGURE 6. Case 11. *a*, view of the most basal transverse cut of the cardiac ventricles showing posterior wall necrosis and acquired ventricular septal defect repaired with a Dacron® patch. *b*, sections of the cardiac ventricles after multiple transverse cuts showing posterior wall necrosis and dilated right (RV) and left (LV) cavities. *c*, close-up view of the posterior wall necrosis and the ventricular septal defect (*arrows*).

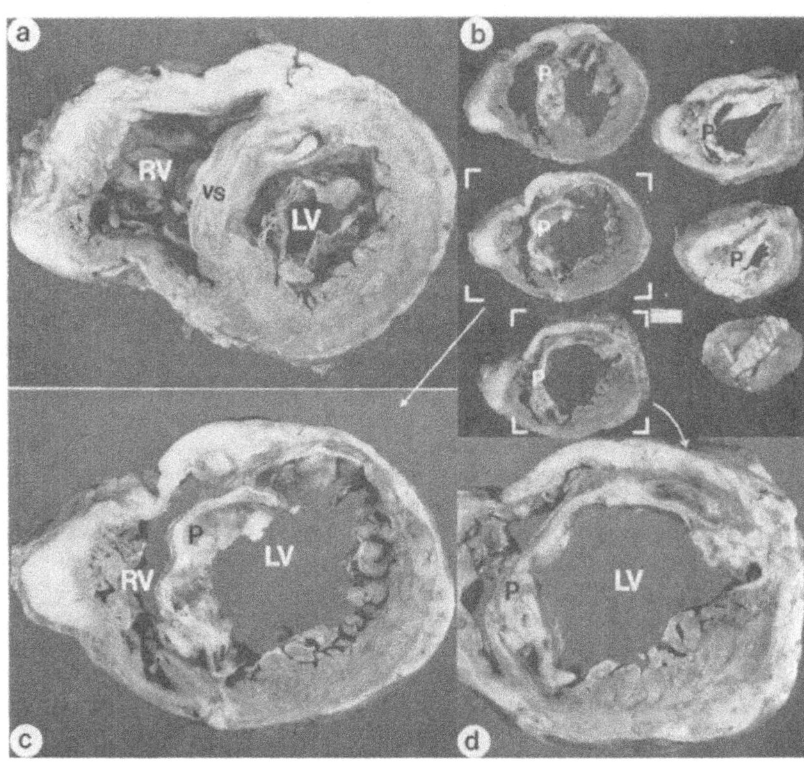

FIGURE 7. Case 16. *a*, view of the most basal transverse cut of the right (RV) and left (LV) ventricles showing a thinned and necrotic ventricular septum (VS). *b*, sections of the cardiac ventricles after multiple transverse cuts showing dilated cavities and a patch (P) comprising most of the ventricular septum. *c*, close-up view of the section in brackets in *b*. *d*, close-up view of the section in brackets in *b*. The patch extends into the anterior left ventricular wall. There is inadequate left ventricular myocardium.

Discussion

Each of the above-described 16 patients underwent operative closure of VSD during the first 2 weeks of AMI, which was the first coronary event in 13 (81%) of them. The AMI involved the anterior left ventricular wall and ventricular septum in 9 patients (56%) and the posterior wall in 7 patients (44%). Four (25%) of the 16 patients were older than 70 years. Of the 16 patients, 7 could not be separated from cardiopulmonary bypass, 1 patient died 2 hours after entering the "recovery room," and 4 patients lived longer than 2 weeks (up to 113 days) after cardiotomy. Death was attributed to incomplete closure of the VSD in 5 patients (31%), to inadequate sized left ventricular cavity after closure of the VSD and resection of necrotic myocardium in 5 patients (31%), to inadequate viable left ventricular myocardium in 4 patients (25%), to excessive bleeding in 1 patient (6%) and to infection in 1 patient (6%). Cardiac weight was increased (>350 g in women and >400 g in men) in 14 (88%) of the 16 patients. Only 3 patients (19%) had left ventricular scars, and in each they were small.

Closure of the VSD in all of our 16 patients was carried out during the first 2 weeks of the AMI. Several investigators have reported that the early mortality after closure of VSD secondary to AMI is much higher when operation is performed during the first 2 weeks of AMI than in later periods. Combining figures from 10 reports[5-14] showed the following: of 290 patients having VSD closure during AMI, 195 had the operation within 2 weeks of the onset of AMI and 95 (49%) of them died early; of 95 patients having closure at later times, 28 (29%) died in the early postoperative period.

The AMI associated with ventricular septal rupture involved the anterior left ventricular wall in 9 of our patients and the posterior (inferior) wall in the other 7. Other studies have shown that early operative mortality after closure of acquired VSD is higher when the AMI involves the posterior (inferior) wall compared to when it involves the anterior wall. Combining figures from 8 reports[5-7,9-12,14] showed the following: of 235 patients having operative closure of acquired VSD, the AMI involved the anterior wall in 139 patients (59%) and 38 (27%) of them died in the early postoperative period; of 95 patients (41%) having posterior wall infarcts, 56 (59%) died in the early postoperative period.

Of our 16 patients, 4 (25%) were older than 70 years at the time of VSD closure. Several studies show that the early mortality after closure of acquired VSD is higher in patients older than 70 years at the time of cardiotomy than in younger patients. Combining figures from 5 reports[5,7,10,12,13] showed the following: of 81 patients having operative closure of acquired VSD, 62 (76%) were younger than 70 years and 21 (34%) died in the early postoperative period; of 19 patients (24%) older than 70 years, 14 (74%) died in the early postoperative period.

Of our 16 patients, 7 (44%) had coronary artery bypass grafting at the time of operative closure of the VSD. Other reports indicate that performance of coronary artery bypass grafting at the time of VSD closure has nonpredictable effects on early operative mortali-

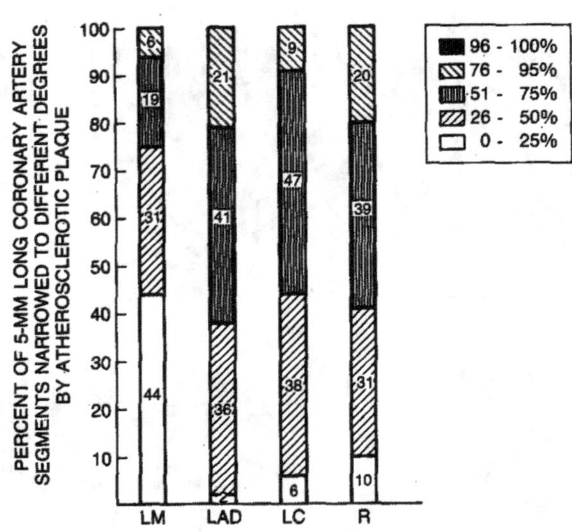

NO. CA SEGMENTS   16   127   80   161

FIGURE 8. Bar graph showing the amounts of cross-sectional area narrowing by atherosclerotic plaque alone in each of the 4 major (left main [LM], left anterior descending [LAD], left circumflex [LC] and right [R]) epicardial coronary arteries in 10 of the 16 necropsy patients with operative "closure" of an acquired ventricular septal defect during an acute myocardial infarction. Of the 16 segments of the left main, 44% were narrowed 0 to 25%; 31%, 26 to 50%; 19%, 51 to 75%; and 6%, 76 to 95%. Of the 127 segments of the left anterior descending, 2% were narrowed less than 25%; 36%, 26 to 50%; 41%, 51 to 75%; and 21%, 76 to 95%. Of the 80 segments of the left circumflex, 6% were narrowed less than 25%; 38%, 26 to 50%; 47%, 51 to 75%; and 9%, 76 to 95%. Of the 161 segments of the right, 10% were narrowed less than 25%; 31%, 26 to 50%; 39%, 51 to 75%; and 20%, 76 to 95%. None of the 5-mm-long coronary artery segments in any of the coronary arteries was narrowed 96 to 100%.

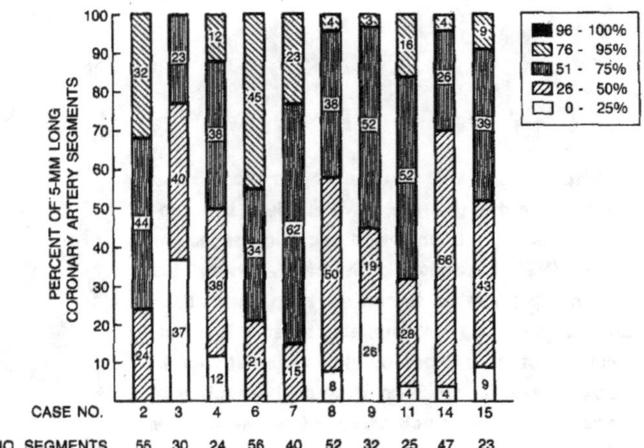

NO. SEGMENTS   55   30   24   56   40   52   32   25   47   23

FIGURE 9. Bar graph showing the amounts of cross-sectional area narrowing by atherosclerotic plaque of the 4 major (left main, left anterior descending, left circumflex and right) epicardial coronary arteries in each of the 10 necropsy patients having operative "closure" of an acquired ventricular septal defect during an acute myocardial infarction. None of the 5-mm-long coronary artery segments was narrowed 96 to 100%.

ty. Combining figures from 4 reports[7,8,10,11] showed the following: Of 77 patients having closure of acquired VSD, 18 (23%) had coronary artery bypass grafting performed simultaneously and 11 (61%) of them died in the early postoperative period; of 59 patients not having simultaneous coronary artery bypass grafting, 24 (41%) died in the early postoperative period. Additionally, Jones and associates[14] reported no differences in early operative mortality after VSD closure in patients having simultaneous coronary bypass compared to those not having coronary bypass, but numbers were not provided.

In 7 of our 16 patients (44%), the VSD was incompletely closed or it reopened in the early postoperative period. Other reports have described a much lower frequency of unsuccessful VSD closure. Combining figures from 7 studies[5-7,10-12,14] showed the following: of 180 patients having closure of acquired VSD, 14 (8%) had incomplete closure. In contrast to our patients, however, many of the 180 patients operated on by others had the procedure performed at later periods, including the period after healing of the AMI.

Modes or causes of death after operative closure of acquired VSD have received no attention previously from a morphologic aspect. Thus, our results cannot be compared with those of others. Nearly every report mentioning reasons for unsuccessful outcome after operative closure of acquired VSD has mentioned "inadequate cardiac output," "cardiogenic shock," "acute pulmonary edema," "renal failure," "respiratory failure," "sepsis," "stroke," and others, but the morphologic reasons for these clinical manifestations have essentially not been investigated.

References

1. Edmondson HA, Hoxie HJ. Hypertension and cardiac rupture: a clinical and pathologic study of seventy-two cases, in thirteen of which rupture of the interventricular septum occurred. Am Heart J 1942;24:719–733.
2. Roberts WC, Ronan JA Jr, Harvey WP. Rupture of the left ventricular free wall (LVFW) or ventricular septum (VS) secondary to acute myocardial infarction (AMI): an occurrence virtually limited to the first transmural AMI in a hypertensive individual (abstr). Am J Cardiol 1975;35:166.
3. Edwards BS, Edwards WD, Edwards JE. Ventricular septal rupture complicating acute myocardial infarction: identification of simple and complex types in 53 autopsied hearts. Am J Cardiol 1984;54:1201–1205.
4. Roberts WC, Roberts JD. The floating heart or the heart too fat to sink: analysis of 55 necropsy patients. Am J Cardiol 1983;52:1286–1289.
5. Donahoo JS, Brawley RK, Taylor D, Gott VL. Factors influencing survival following postinfarction ventricular septal defects. Ann Thorac Surg 1975;19:648–653.
6. Loisance DY, Cachera JP, Poulain H, Aubry P, Juvin AM, Galey JJ. Ventricular septal defect after acute myocardial infarction: early repair. J Thorac Cardiovasc Surg 1980;80:61–67.
7. Naifeh JG, Grehl TM, Hurley EJ. Surgical treatment of post-myocardial infarction ventricular septal defects. J Thorac Cardiovasc Surg 1980;79:483–488.
8. Matsui K, Kay JH, Mendez M, Zubiate P, Vanstrom N, Yokoyama T. Ventricular septal rupture secondary to myocardial infarction: clinical approach and surgical results. JAMA 1981;245:1537–1539.
9. Daggett WM, Buckley MJ, Akins CW, Leinbach RC, Gold HK, Block PC, Austen WG. Improved results of surgical management of postinfarction ventricular septal rupture. Ann Surg 1982;196:269–277.
10. Miyamoto AT, Lee ME, Kass RM, Chaux A, Sethna D, Gray R, Matloff JM. Post-myocardial infarction ventricular septal defect: improved outlook. J Thorac Cardiovasc Surg 1983;86:41–46.
11. Fananapazir L, Bray CL, Dark JF, Moussalli H, Deiraniya AK, Lawson RAM. Right ventricular dysfunction and surgical outcome in postinfarction ventricular septal defect. Eur Heart J 1983;4:155–167.
12. Scanlon PJ, Montoya A, Johnson SA, McKeever LS, Sullivan HJ, Bakhos M, Pifarre R. Urgent surgery for ventricular septal rupture complicating acute myocardial infarction. Circulation 1985;72:suppl II:185–190.
13. Kirklin JW, Barratt-Boyes BG. Postinfarction ventricular septal defect. In: Cardiac Surgery. New York, Wiley, 1986:301–310.
14. Jones MT, Schofield PM, Dark JF, Moussalli H, Deiraniya AK, Lawson RAM, Ward C, Bray CL. Surgical repair of acquired ventricular septal defect: determinants of early and late outcome. J Thorac Cardiovasc Surg 1987;93:680–686.

Aneurysmal Coronary Artery Disease in Cerebrotendinous Xanthomatosis

BENJAMIN N. POTKIN, MD

JEFFREY M. HOEG, MD

WILLIAM E. CONNOR, MD

GERALD SALEN, MD

ARSHED A. QUYYUMI, MD

JOHN E. BRUSH, Jr., MD

WILLIAM C. ROBERTS, MD

H. BRYAN BREWER, Jr., MD

Cerebrotendinous xanthomatosis (CTX), first described by van Bogaert et al in 1937,[1] is a rare (<100 cases reported), autosomal recessive disease characterized by accumulation of cholesterol and cholestanol

From the Molecular Disease, Cardiology and Pathology Branches, National Heart, Lung, and Blood Institute, National Institutes of Health, Bethesda, Maryland, the Oregon Health Sciences University, Portland, Oregon, and the University of Medicine and Dentistry of New Jersey, New Jersey Medical School, Newark, New Jersey. Manuscript received December 22, 1987; revised manuscript received and accepted January 19, 1988.

in tissues. Its clinical features can include tendon xanthomas, cataracts, neurologic dysfunction (dementia, ataxia, paresis and peripheral neuropathy) and accelerated arterial atherosclerosis. CTX results from a deficiency of a hepatic microsomal enzyme necessary for primary bile acid synthesis from cholesterol. Because bile acid synthesis is impaired, chenodeoxycholic acid in bile is reduced or absent, biliary cholesterol secretion is reduced, and, for reasons uncertain, the hepatic conversion of cholesterol to cholestanol is markedly increased and blood, biliary and tissue cholestanol levels are markedly elevated (Figure 1).[2,3] Cholestanol appears to be highly atherogenic and has been demonstrated in most tissues, including the coronary arteries.[3] Although accelerated coronary atherosclerosis is believed to be characteristic of this lipid disorder, coronary angiographic findings have not been reported in CTX. Herein, we describe such findings.

L.S., a 39-year-old black woman, born in Mississippi, developed xanthomas of the elbows at age 9 and tendon and tuberous xanthomas later, which became progressively enlarged. At age 35, systemic hypertension was noted and it was well controlled with prazosin (2 mg/day). She had always been asymptomatic and physically active. She never smoked cigarettes or had neurologic symptoms, cataracts or diabetes melli-

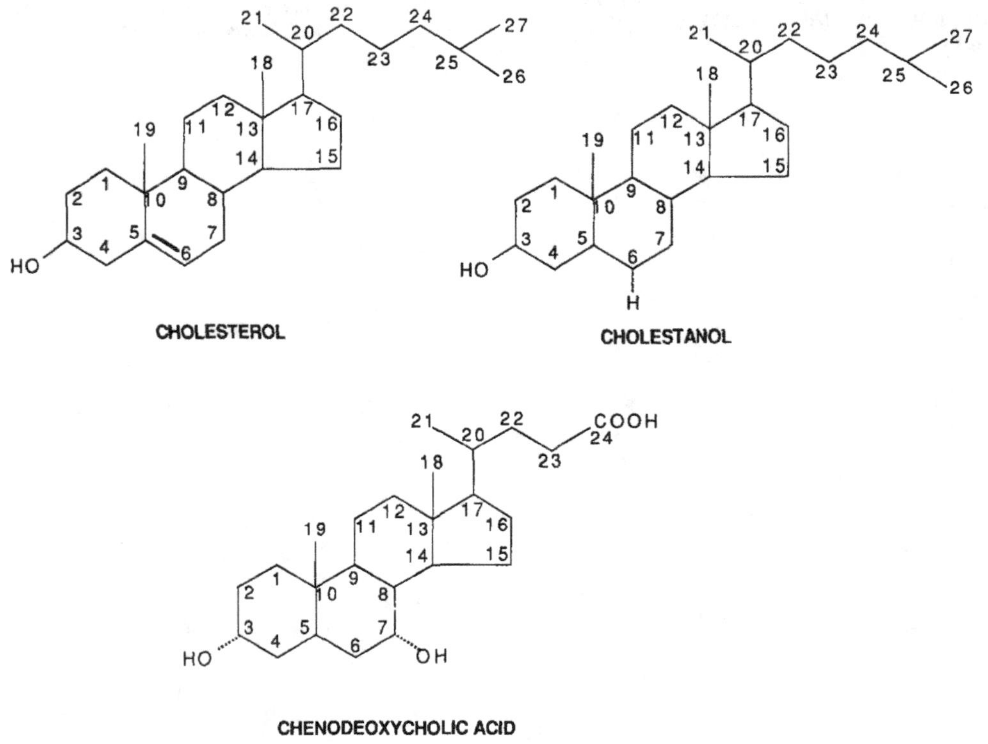

FIGURE 1. Chemical structure of cholesterol, cholestanol and chenodeoxycholic acid.

tus. Her intelligence was considered subnormal in that she was unable to perform simple mathematic computations. She had regular menstrual periods. None of her 11 siblings has symptoms of myocardial ischemia; 2 brothers, however, have tendon xanthomas. Both her mother and father died of a myocardial infarction at ages 62 and 82 years, respectively.

At age 39, she came to the National Institutes of Health. She had extensive tendon and tuberous xanthomas (Figure 2), arcus cornea and a bruit over the left carotid artery. Blood pressure was 140/80 mm Hg. Plasma lipid levels (in mg/dl) were as follows: total cholesterol = 266, high-density lipoprotein cholesterol = 72; low-density lipoprotein cholesterol = 177; very low-density lipoprotein cholesterol = 17 and triglycerides = 79. Serum bile acids were undetected. Endoscopic duodenal aspirate demonstrated virtually undetected amounts of chenodeoxycholic acid and 3 times normal cholestanol (normal biliary cholestanol <1% of biliary cholesterol). Total, free and esterified cholesterol and cholestanol in plasma and in a tendon xanthoma are shown in Table I. The resting electrocardiogram was normal. A treadmill stress test disclosed 1.5 mm of ST-segment depression in lead V_5 after 16 minutes of exercise using the combined NIH protocol (Figure 3). However, the patient remained asymptomatic, reached 92% of predicted heart rate and had a normal blood pressure increase with exercise. Resting ejection fraction by radionuclide angiogram was 50% and did not change at peak exercise (150 watts). Ambulatory electrocardiographic monitoring demonstrated 2 episodes of asymptomatic ST-segment depression lasting a total of 67 minutes. Coronary angiography demonstrated multiple aneurysms in the right, left anterior descending and left circumflex coronary arteries and narrowing (51 to 75% in diameter) of the posterior descending coronary artery (Figure 4). Left ventriculography disclosed mild anter-

oapical hypokinesis. Chenodeoxycholic acid (750 mg/day), diltiazem (90 mg/day) and aspirin (325 mg/day) were prescribed.[4]

This patient has a rare lipid disorder and silent myocardial ischemia in the setting of multiple aneu-

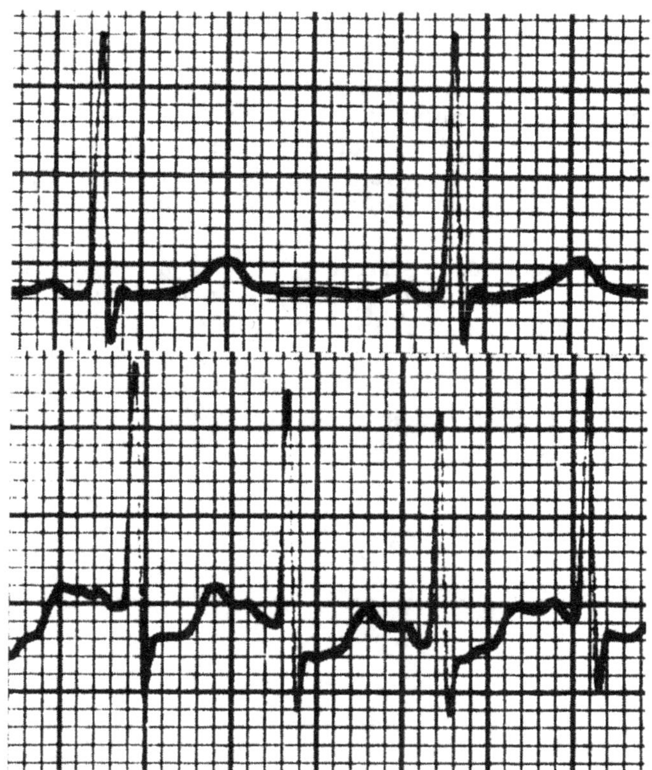

FIGURE 3. *Top*, normal rest electrocardiogram V_5 precordial lead, at a heart rate of 75 beats/min. *Bottom*, abnormal exercise electrocardiogram V_5 precordial lead, showing 1.5-mm ST-segment depression at a heart rate of 167 beats/min.

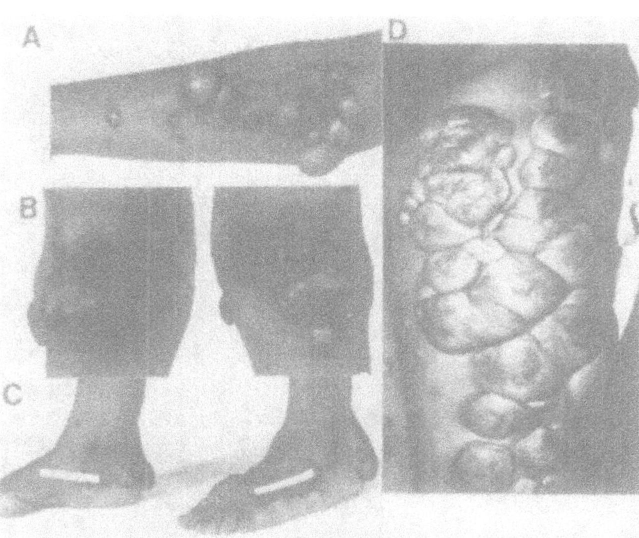

FIGURE 2. Photographs of extensive tendon xanthomas of elbow (*A*), knees (*B*) and achilles tendons (*C*), and tuberous xanthoma of posterior thigh (*D*).

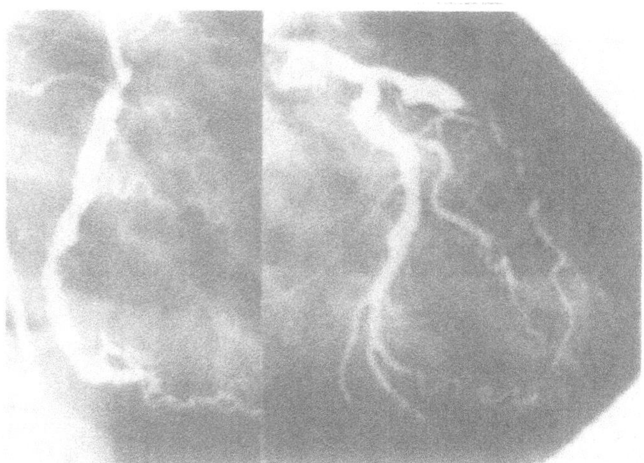

FIGURE 4. In the angiogram on the *left*, the right anterior oblique view of the right coronary artery shows a long coronary artery aneurysm with focal narrowing of the posterior descending coronary artery. The angiogram on the *right* encompasses a right anterior oblique view of the left main, left anterior descending and left circumflex coronary arteries showing aneurysmal dilation of most of the left circumflex and proximal left anterior descending coronary arteries.

TABLE I Patient's Plasma and Tendon Xanthoma Cholesterol and Cholestanol Measurements

	Cholesterol			Cholestanol		
	Total	Free	Esterified	Total	Free	Esterified
Plasma (mg/dl)	252	69	183	5.0*	0.7	4.3
Xanthoma (mg/g dried weight)	162	18	144	4.2	0.2	4.0

* Normal total plasma cholestanol level = 0.41 ± 0.17 mg/dl.

rysms of the major epicardial coronary arteries. It is likely that the multiple coronary arterial aneurysms are atherosclerotic in origin. Whether aneurysmal rather than obstructive disease of the coronary arteries is more characteristic of CTX is, of course, unknown.

The clue to the diagnosis of CTX in the present patient was the relatively low plasma total cholesterol level in the setting of extensive xanthomas. Determination of plasma cholestanol is an infrequently performed test and can be carried out in few laboratories. The findings of extensive xanthomas in the presence of a plasma total cholesterol <300 mg/dl, however, should suggest the possibility of a cholestanol lipid disorder like CTX and cardiac disease should be suspected even in the asymptomatic patient.

1. Van Bogaert L, Schere HJ, Epstein EE. *Une forme cérébrale de la cholestérinose généralisée. Paris: Masson, 1937;182.*

2. Salen G, Shefer S, Berginer VM. *Familial diseases with storage of sterols other than cholesterol: cerebrotendinous xanthomatosis and sitosterolemia with xanthomatosis. In: Stanbury JB, Wyngaarden JB, Frederickson DS, eds. The Metabolic Basis of Inherited Diseases. New York: McGraw-Hill, 1984: 713–730.*

3. Salen G. *Cholestanol deposition in cerebrotendinous xanthomatosis: a possible mechanism. Ann Intern Med 1971;75:843–851.*

4. Berginer VM, Salen G, Shefer S. *Long-term treatment of cerebrotendinous xanthomatosis with chenodeoxycholic acid. N Engl J Med 1984;311:1649–1652.*

Acquired Ventricular Septal Defect During Acute Myocardial Infarction: Analysis of 38 Unoperated Necropsy Patients and Comparison With 50 Unoperated Necropsy Patients Without Rupture

Jessica M. Mann, MD, and William C. Roberts, MD

Thirty-eight patients (24 men and 14 women) with an acquired ventricular septal defect during acute myocardial infarction (AMI) (rupture group) were studied and their clinical and necropsy findings were compared with 50 patients who died during their first AMI without rupture (nonrupture group). The frequency of systemic hypertension (54 vs 52%), angina pectoris (28 vs 22%) and congestive heart failure (5 vs 0%) before the fatal AMI was similar for both rupture and nonrupture groups. Mean heart weights for men (498 vs 526 g) and women (397 vs 432 g) with and without septal rupture also were insignificantly different. Whereas previous studies of fatal AMI cases have shown that 50% of cases of fatal AMI without rupture have left ventricular scars, only 4 (10%) of the rupture cases had a left ventricular scar before the infarct that ruptured. The rupture group had a significantly more frequent (p <0.01) posterior location of the infarcts (74 vs 40%) and, therefore, a higher frequency of associated right ventricular infarcts 50 vs 18%). The number of 3 major (right, left anterior descending and left circumflex) epicardial coronary arteries narrowed at some point >75% in cross-sectional area of atherosclerotic plaque was the same in both groups. The percent of these 3 arteries totally occluded or nearly so (>95% in cross-sectional area) by plaque was significantly less (p <0.001) in the rupture group compared with the nonrupture group (9 of 99 arteries [9%] vs 38 of 144 arteries [26%]). Analysis of each 5-mm long segment of these arteries in each group disclosed that the rupture group had significantly less narrowing than the nonrupture group. Of the 825 five-mm segments of artery examined in the rupture group (18 patients), only 101 (13%) were narrowed >75% in cross-sectional area by plaque; in contrast, of the 1,848 five-mm segments in the nonrupture group (38 patients), 508 (28%) were narrowed to this degree by plaque (p <0.01). Thus, rupture of the ventricular septum primarily is a complication of the first AMI. It is associated with less severe coronary arterial narrowing than observed in fatal AMI without rupture, and it is a more frequent complication of posterior (inferior) than anterior wall AMI.

(Am J Cardiol 1988;62:8–19)

Mortality rates due to complications of acute myocardial infarction (AMI) in the coronary care unit have been reduced in recent years, primarily because of the successful treatment of cardiac arrhythmias. Because of the decreased frequency of fatal cardiac arrhythmias during AMI, the frequency of cardiac rupture during AMI may be increasing. This study describes and illustrates cardiac findings in 38 necropsy patients who had rupture of the ventricular septum during AMI and who did not have a cardiac operation, and compares the findings with a group of 50 patients with their first AMI that was fatal but not associated with cardiac rupture or left ventricular scarring.

RUPTURE GROUP

Clinical findings: Certain clinical and necropsy findings in the 38 patients are presented in Table I. Of the 38 patients, 14 were women (mean age 73 ± 9 years) and 24 were men (mean age 65 ± 9 years). The AMI associated with the acquired ventricular septal defect (VSD) was the first coronary event in 32 patients (84%); 10 patients (nos. 5, 13, 17, 18, 21, 27, 28, 30, 37, 38 [Table I]) had had angina pectoris. At least 20 patients had histories of systemic hypertension before the fatal AMI, and 2 patients had symptoms of congestive heart failure. Of the 2 patients with congestive heart failure, 1 (no. 37 [Table I]) had had an AMI 7 months before death and the other 1 (no. 36 [Table I]), approximately 3 months before death. Of the 12 patients with an anterior AMI, 7 (58%) were women, whereas of the 26 patients with a posterior AMI, 6 (23%) were women. Conduction disturbances, ranging from increased PR interval (2 patients) to complete heart block (8 patients), were evident by electrocardiogram in 12 patients, of whom 11 had a posterior wall AMI. The interval from the onset of the AMI to death ranged from a few hours to 360 days (median 6 days) and the interval from the detection of a precordial systolic murmur consistent with VSD to death ranged from a few hours to 203 days (median 2 days). Of the 38 patients, 19 (50%) died <1 week after onset of the fatal AMI.

From the Pathology Branch, National Institutes of Health, National Heart, Lung, and Blood Institute, Bethesda, Maryland. Manuscript received February 22, 1988; revised manuscript received and accepted March 18, 1988.

Address for reprints: William C. Roberts, MD, Building 10, Room 2N258, Pathology Branch, National Heart, Lung, and Blood Institute, National Institutes of Health, Bethesda, Maryland 20892.

TABLE I Clinical and Necropsy Findings in 38 Patients with Rupture of the Ventricular Septum During Acute Myocardial Infarction and No Operative Therapy

Case	Age (yrs), Sex	History AP	SH	CHF	Location AMI by ECG	Conduction Disturbance During AMI	Interval AMI to Death (days)	Interval New Murmur to Death (days)	HW (g)	LV Scar Location	AMI Location	RV AMI	VSD Location	No CAs >75% ↓ by Plaque in CSA	CA Thrombus (CA)
1	68, F	—	0	0	P	0	<1	—	340	0	P	+	P	1	+ (R)
2	61, M	0	0	0	P	+ (CHB)	<1	—	405	0	P	+	P	3	0
3	68, M	0	+	0	P	0	<1	<1	450	0	P	+	P	3	+ (R)
4	77, M	0	0	0	P	+	<1	—	400	0	P	+	P	—	—
5	53, M	+	0	0	P	0	1	<1	335	0	P	0	P	2	+ (R)
6	74, F	0	0	0	A	+ (CHB)	2	2	370	0	A	0	A	2	0
7	76, F	0	+	0	P	+ (CHB)	2	1	410	0	P	+	P	1	0
8	55, M	0	+	0	P	0	2	2	450	0	P	0	P	—	—
9	79, F	0	0	0	P	+ (CHB)	3	<1	400	0	P	+	P	—	—
10	70, M	0	+	0	P	+ (CHB)	3	—	520	0	P	0	P	1	0
11	88, F	0	0	0	A	0	4	3	310	0	P	0	P	3	0
12	62, M	0	+	0	P	0	4	<1	510	0	P	+	P	2	0
13	84, M	+	—	0	P	0	4	—	—	0	P	0	P	—	—
14	58, M	0	+	0	P	+ (↑PR)	5	1	550	0	P	+	P	2	+ (R)
15	61, F	0	0	0	A	0	6	4	430	0	A	+	A	1	0
16	70, F	0	+	0	P	+ (CHB)	6	<1	450	0	P	+	P	2	0
17	77, F	+	+	0	A	0	6	5	450	0	A	0	A	3	0
18	64, M	+	0	0	P	+ (CHB)	6	—	465	0	P	+	P	3	0
19	77, M	0	+	0	P	+ (CHB)	6	<1	530	0	P	+	P	3	+ (R)
20	63, M	0	0	0	P	0	7	5	600	0	P	+	P	3	0
21	60, F	+	+	0	A	0	8	5	420	0	A	0	P	3	0
22	85, F	0	+	0	P	0	8	1	280	0	P	+	P	1	0
23	62, M	—	+	0	P	0	8	6	620	+ (P)	P	+	P	3	+ (R)
24	63, M	0	+	0	P	0	8	2	580	0	P	+	P	3	0
25	65, M	0	0	0	P	0	8	2	420	0	P	0	P	2	+ (R)
26	71, F	0	+	0	A	0	9	6	280	0	A	0	A	2	+ (LAD)
27	69, M	+	0	0	P	+ (RBBB)	10	6	440	0	P	0	P	0	+ (R)
28	60, M	+	0	0	P	0	13	—	700	0	P	0	P	3	0
29	53, M	0	0	0	P	0	14	—	500	0	P	+	P	3	0
30	83, M	+	+	0	P	+ (PR)	16	13	740	+ (P)	P	+	P	2	0
31	65, M	0	+	0	A	0	17	16	370	0	P	+	P	3	0
32	67, M	0	0	0	A	0	18	18	350	0	A	0	A	1	+ (LAD)
33	73, F	0	0	0	P	+ (2 AVB)	18	—	430	0	P	+	P	3	0
34	82, F	0	+	0	A	0	19	16	460	0	A	0	A	1	0
35	71, M	0	+	0	A	0	21	<2	420	+ (P)	A	0	A	3	0
36	54, M	0	0	+	A	0	76	7	620	+ (A)	A	0	A	1	0
37	60, F	+	+	+	A	0	210	203	530	+ (A)*	A	0	A	2	0
38	67, M	+†	+	0	P	0	360	—	480	+ (P)*	P	0	P	—	—

* Aneurysmal; † after healing of the AMI that ruptured.

A = anterior; AMI = acute myocardial infarction; AP = angina pectoris; AVB = atrioventricular block; CA = coronary artery; CHB = complete heart block; CHF = congestive heart failure; CSA = cross-sectional area; ECG = electrocardiogram; HW = heart weight; LAD = left anterior descending; LV = left ventricular; P = posterior; R = right coronary artery; RBBB = right bundle branch block; RV = right ventricular; SH = systemic hypertension; VSD = ventricular septal defect; ↑ = increased; ↓ = decreased; + = present; 0 = absent; — = no information available.

Necropsy findings: Certain cardiac morphologic findings are illustrated in Figures 1 to 16. The hearts ranged in weight in the 14 women from 280 to 530 g (mean 397 ± 73), and in 23 men from 335 to 740 g (mean 498 ± 108). The amount of subepicardial fat was increased in all 38 patients, and several hearts floated in water.[1] Six patients had healed myocardial infarcts (scars): 4 were small and were unassociated with the AMI that ruptured; the other 2 had large scars that were associated with the AMI that ruptured. Thus, only 4 (10%) of the 38 patients had had an AMI that healed unassociated with the infarct that ruptured. The AMI that ruptured involved anterior wall in 10 patients (26%), and posterior (inferior) wall in 28 (74%). Of the 38 patients, 19 (50%) also had a right ventricular AMI. By visual inspection at necropsy, 5 (13%) of the 38 pa-

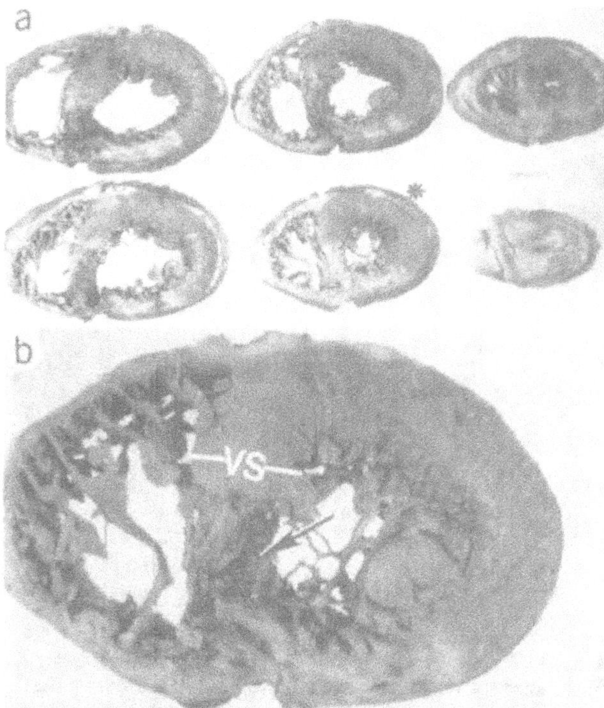

FIGURE 1. Case 3. *a,* sections of the cardiac ventricles after multiple transverse cuts showing the posterior acute myocardial infarct and the acquired ventricular septal defect in the posterior portion of the septum. *b,* close-up view of the underside of the slice designated by the *asterisk* in *a* showing the rupture site *(arrow).* VS = ventricular septum.

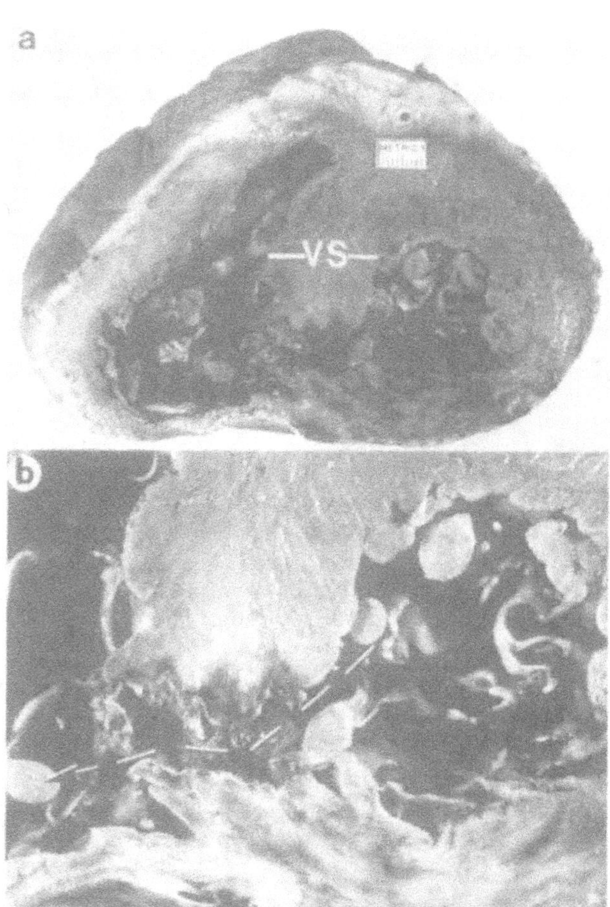

FIGURE 2. Case 7. *a,* view of the most basal transverse cut of the cardiac ventricles showing the posterior acute myocardial infarct and the posterior ventricular septal defect. The subepicardial adipose tissue is increased. Neither ventricle is dilated. VS = ventricular septum. *b,* close-up view of the rupture site *(arrow).*

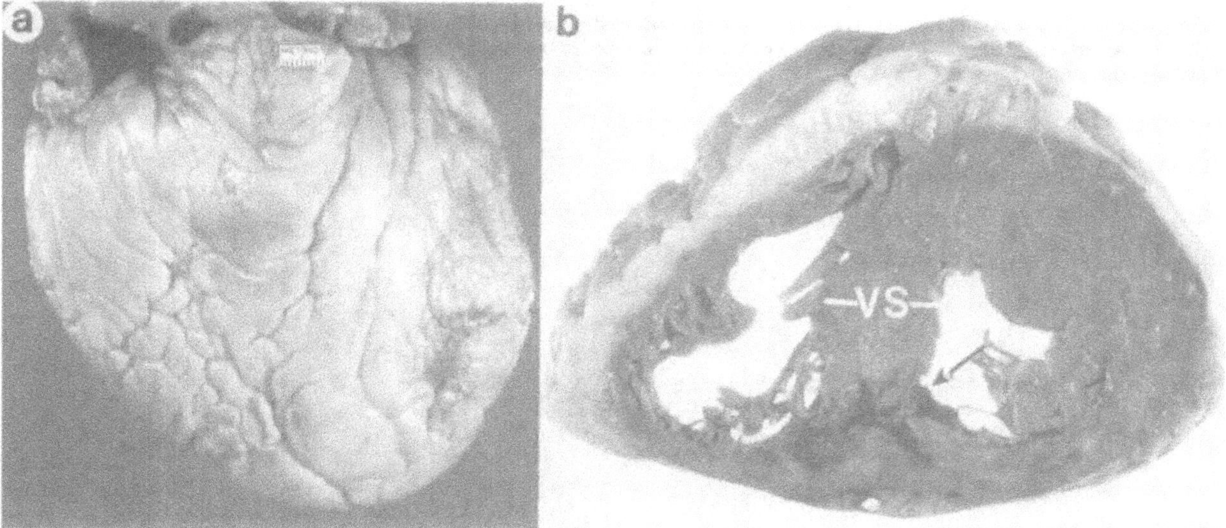

FIGURE 3. Case 10. *a,* external view of the heart showing a marked increased amount of subepicardial adipose tissue. *b,* view of a transverse section of the cardiac ventricles showing a posterior acute myocardial infarct and a posteriorly located ventricular septal defect *(arrow).* Neither ventricular cavity is dilated. VS = ventricular septum.

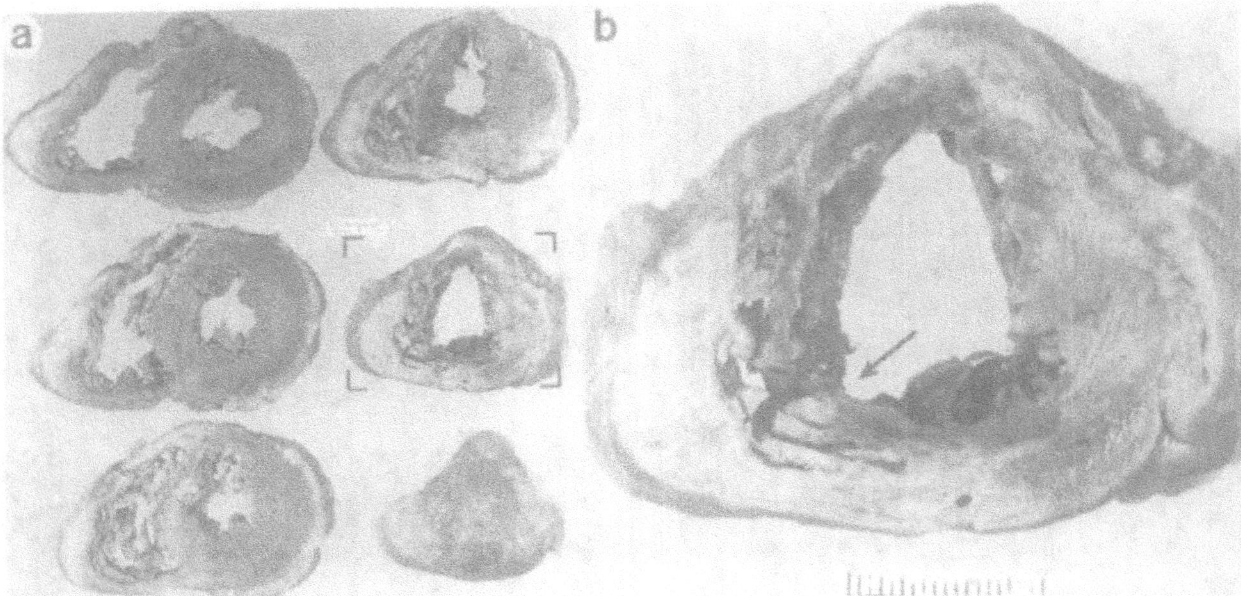

FIGURE 4. Case 11. *a*, sections of the cardiac ventricles after multiple transverse cuts showing an acute myocardial infarct, involving most of the ventricular septum apically and the free wall anteriorly. The ventricular septal defect involves the posterior portion of the ventricular septum. The right ventricle is mildly dilated. *b*, close-up view of the slice in brackets in *a* showing the acute myocardial infarct involving the entire ventricular septum, which is thinned. The *arrow* points toward the defect in the ventricular septum.

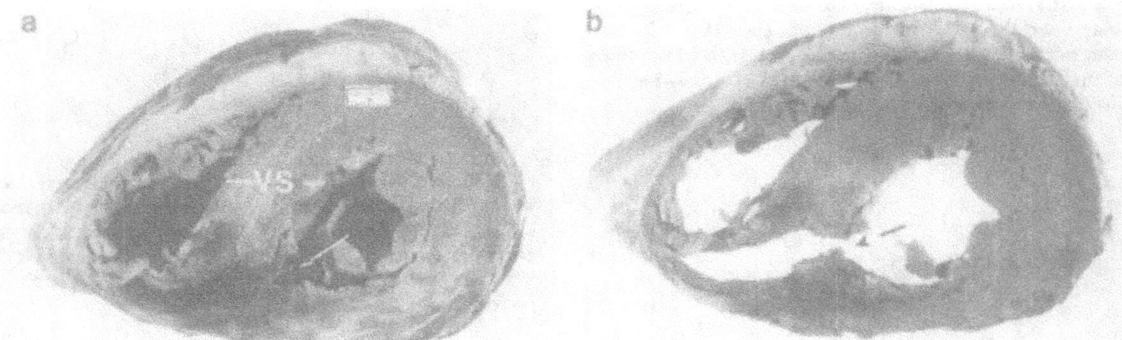

FIGURE 5. Case 12. *a*. view of the basal transverse section of the cardiac ventricles showing a posterior acute myocardial infarct and a posteriorly located ventricular septal defect (*arrow*). Neither ventricular cavity is dilated. VS = ventricular septum. *b*, view of the second most basal transverse section of the cardiac ventricles showing the defect (*arrow*), and a dissection of a portion of the right ventricular free wall.

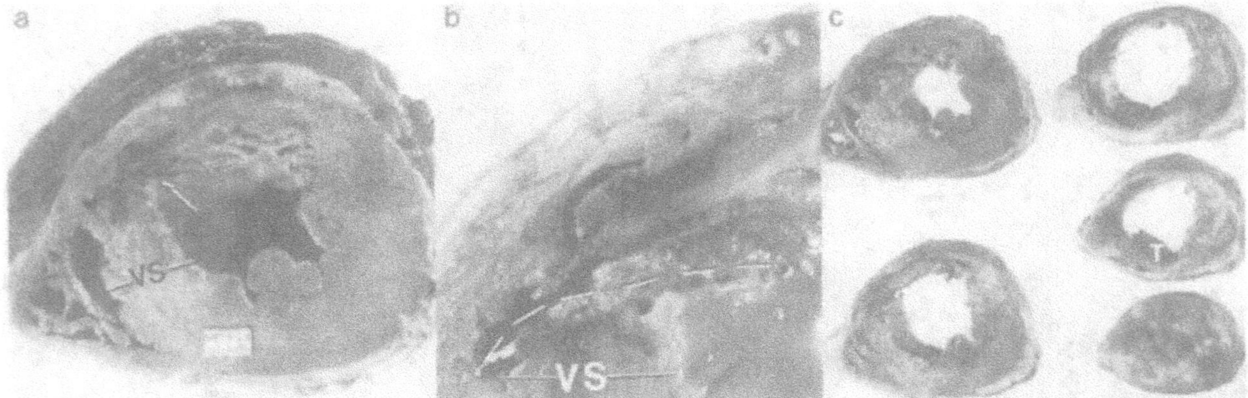

FIGURE 6. Case 15. *a*, view of the most basal transverse section of the cardiac ventricles showing an anterior acute myocardial infarct and an anteriorly located ventricular septal defect (*arrow*). VS = ventricular septum. *b*, close-up view of the rupture site (*arrow*). *c*, sections of the cardiac ventricles after multiple transverse cuts showing the anteriorly located acute myocardial infarct. The left ventricular cavity is dilated and its wall is thinned anteriorly. A thrombus (T) is present on the posterior left ventricular wall.

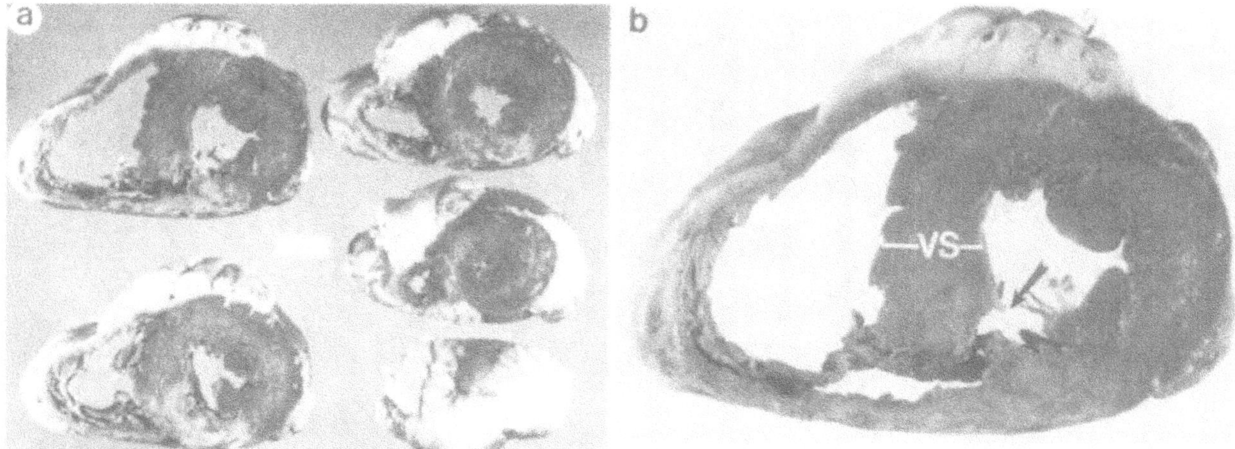

FIGURE 7. Case 16. *a*, sections of the cardiac ventricles after multiple transverse cuts showing a posterior wall acute myocardial infarct and ventricular septal defect. The subepicardial adipose tissue is increased. *b*, close-up view of the top left slice in *a* showing the site of rupture (*arrow*). A portion of right ventricular wall is dissected adjacent to the ruptured septum. The right ventricular cavity is dilated, whereas the left ventricular cavity is of normal size. VS = ventricular septum.

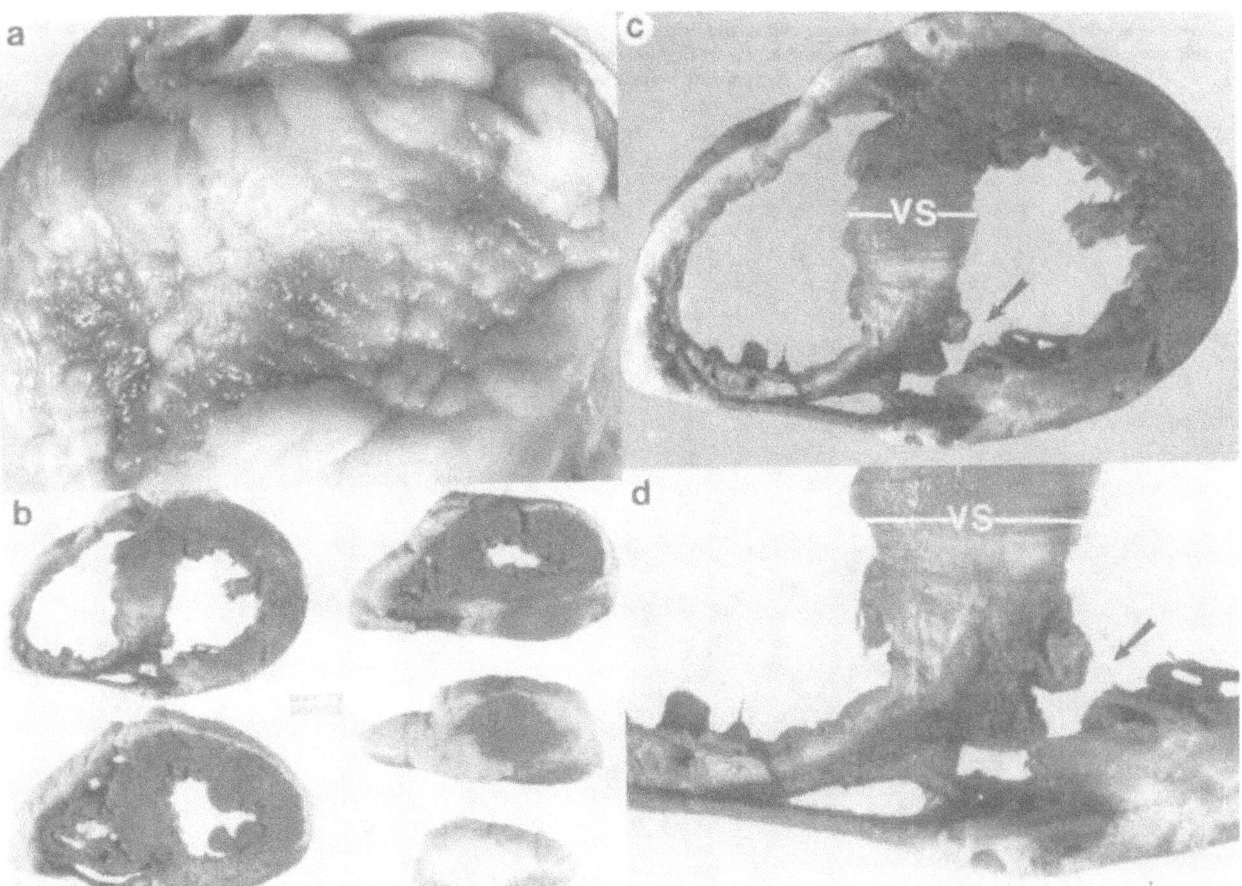

FIGURE 8. Case 18. *a*, external view of the right atrioventricular sulcus of the heart showing increased subepicardial adipose tissue. *b*, sections of the cardiac ventricles after multiple transverse cuts showing a posterior wall acute myocardial infarct and a posteriorly located ventricular septal defect. Both ventricular cavities are dilated. *c*, close-up view of the top left slice in *b* showing the rupture site (*arrow*). VS = ventricular septum. *d*, close-up view of the posterior ventricular septal defect seen in *c*. The right ventricular wall posteriorly is partially dissected.

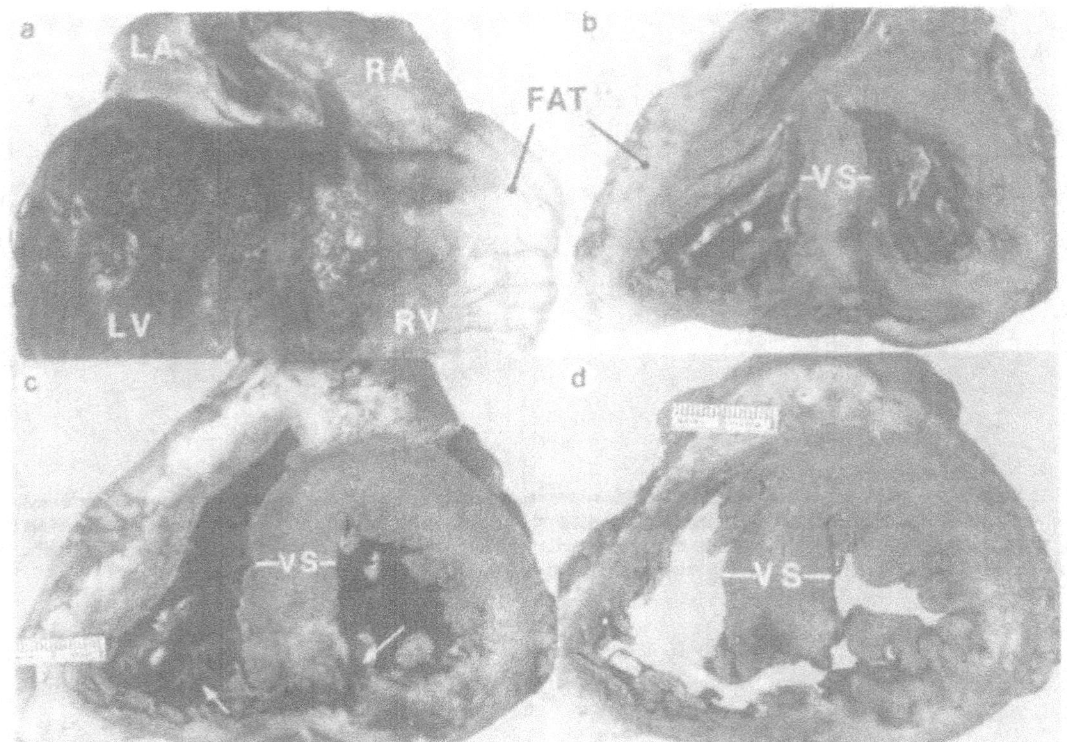

FIGURE 9. Case 19. *a*, view of the external aspect of the heart posteriorly showing increased subepicardial adipose tissue and hemorrhage into it. LA = left atrium; LV = left ventricle; RA = right atrium; RV = right ventricle. *b*, view of the most basal transverse section of the cardiac ventricles showing the posteriorly located myocardial infarct. VS = ventricular septum. Neither ventricular cavity is dilated. *c*, view of the most basal transverse section of the cardiac ventricles showing the site of rupture (*arrows*). *d*, view of a basal transverse section of the cardiac ventricles showing the infarct and the rupture site (*arrows*).

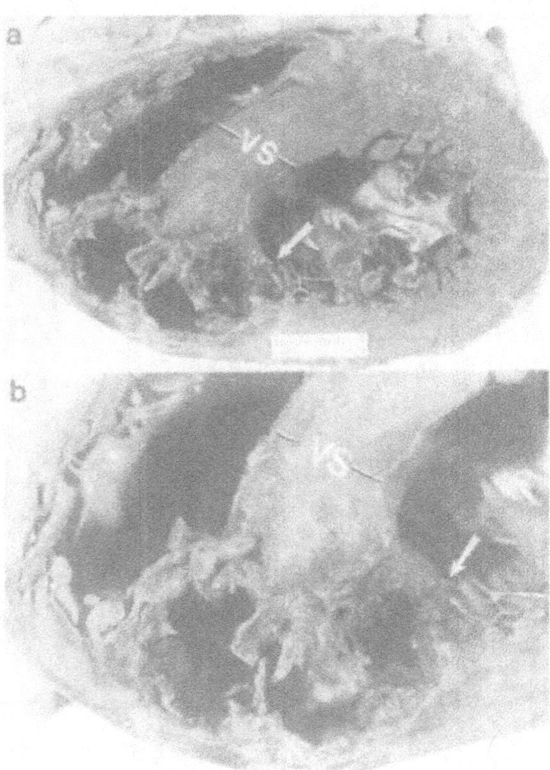

FIGURE 10. Case 20. *a*, view of the most basal transverse section of the cardiac ventricles showing the posterior acute myocardial infarct and the posterior ventricular septal defect (*arrow*). VS = ventricular septum. *b*, close-up view of the defect (*arrow*).

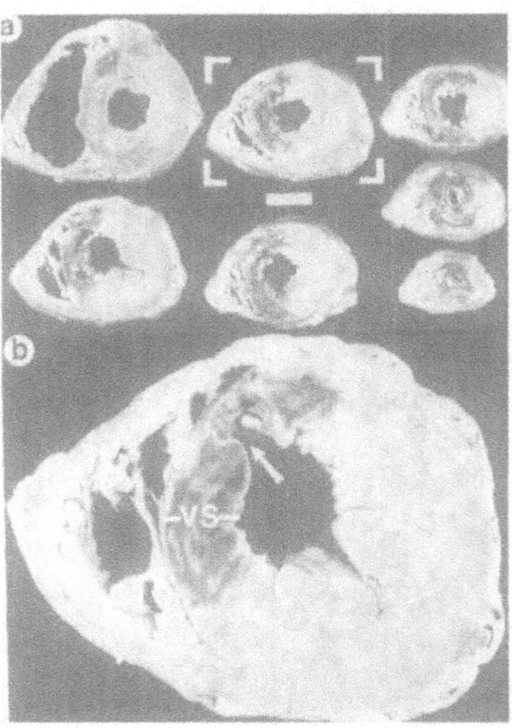

FIGURE 11. Case 26. *a*, sections of the cardiac ventricles after multiple transverse cuts showing the anterior acute myocardial infarct, which involves much of the ventricular septum (VS) and the anterior left ventricular free wall. The ventricular septal defect is anteriorly located. Neither ventricular cavity is dilated. *b*, close-up of the slice in *brackets* in *a* showing the acute myocardial infarct and defect (*arrow*).

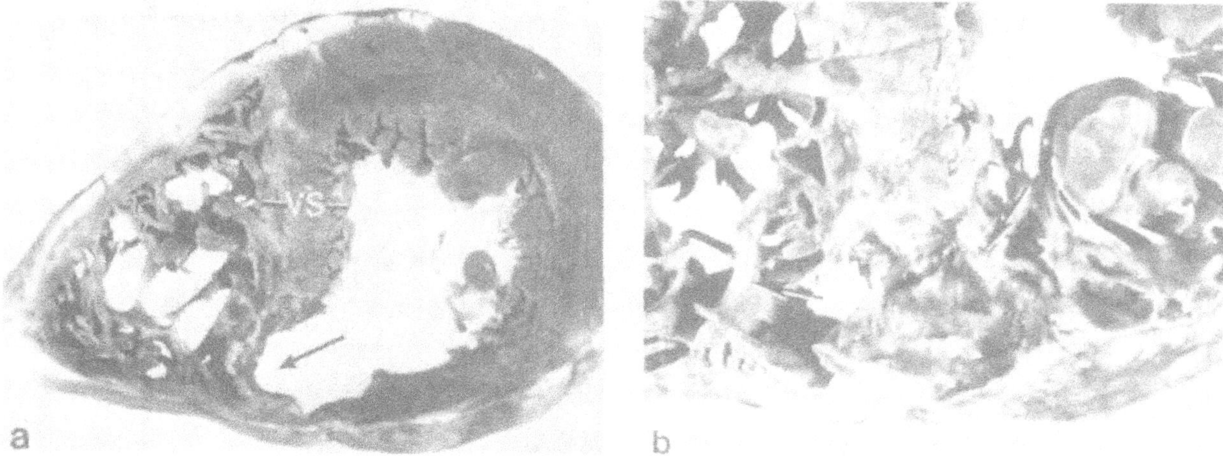

FIGURE 12. Case 30. *a,* transverse section of the cardiac ventricles showing a posterior acute myocardial infarct and a posteriorly located ventricular septal defect. Part of the posterior left ventricular wall and the ventricular septum (VS) is thinned. *b,* close-up view of the defect (*arrows*).

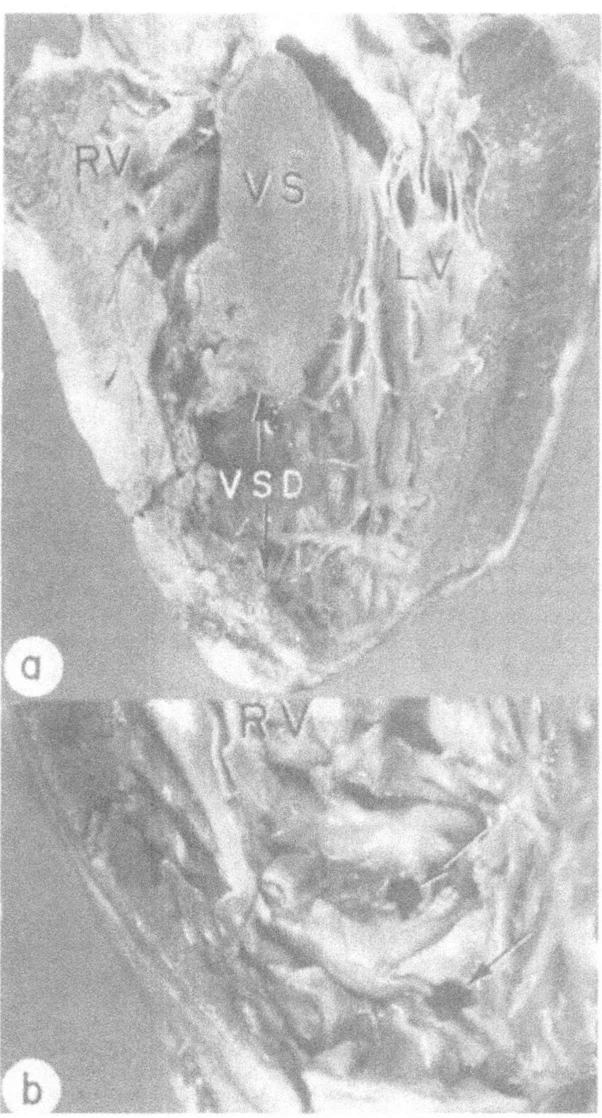

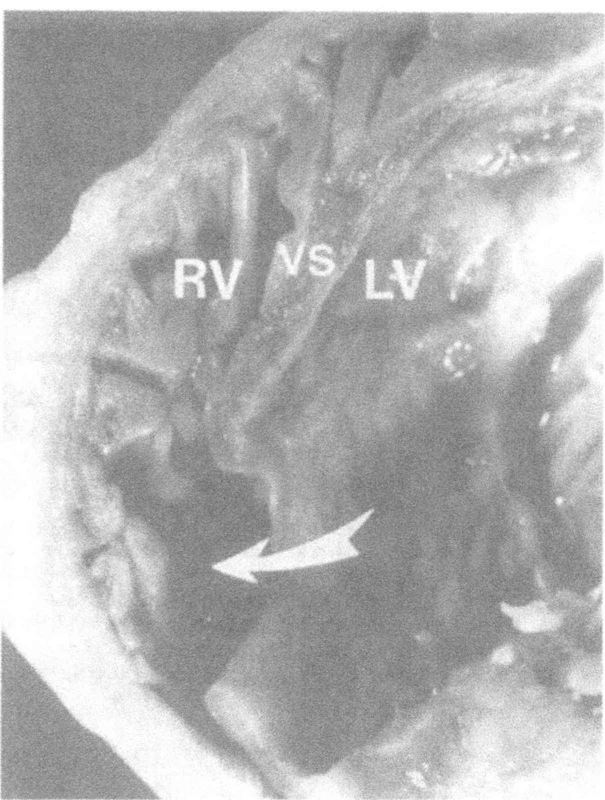

FIGURE 14. Case 34. View of a portion of a transverse slice of the cardiac ventricles showing a large ventricular septal defect (*arrow*) and a thin walled ventricular septum (VS). LV = left ventricle; RV = right ventricle.

FIGURE 13 (at *left*). **Case 31.** *a,* longitudinal cut of the cardiac ventricles showing an acute myocardial infarct and an apical ventricular septal defect (VSD), which is huge. LV = left ventricle; RV = right ventricle; VS = ventricular septum. *b,* close-up view of the 2 rupture sites (*arrows*) as seen from the right ventricular aspect.

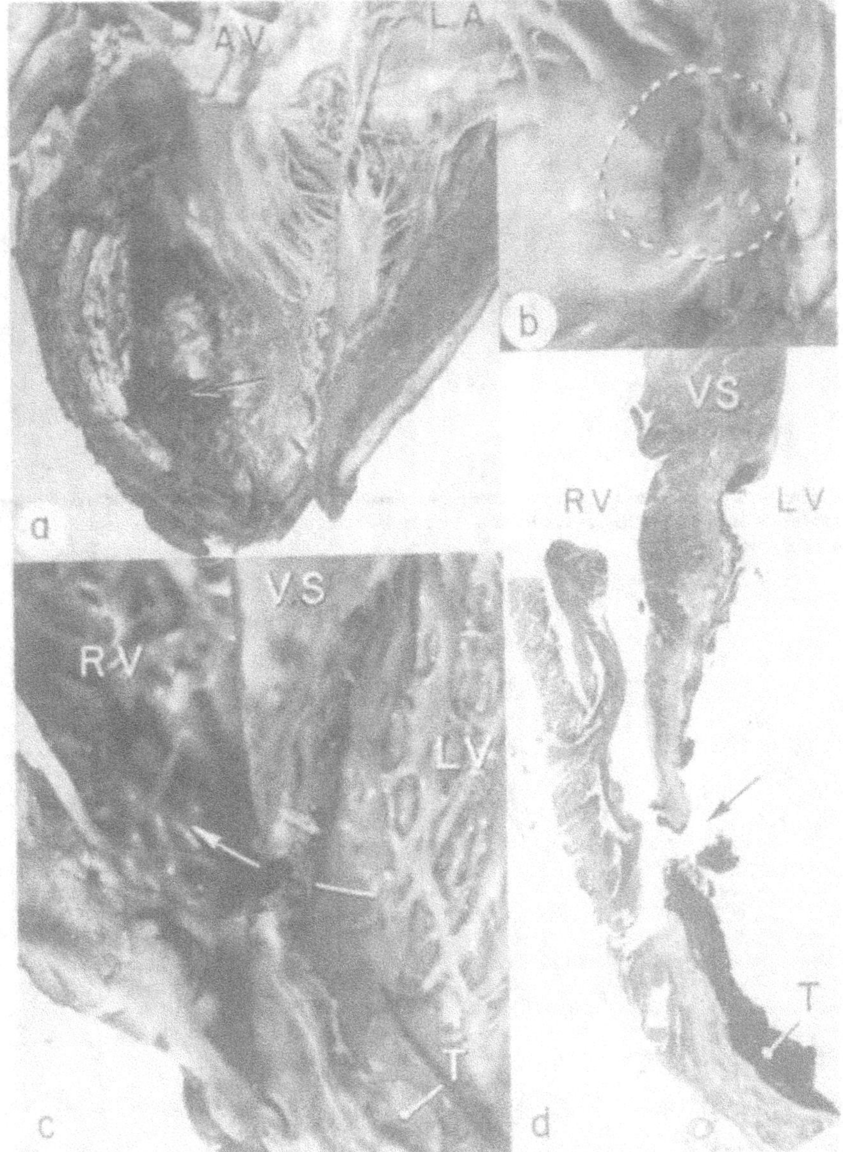

FIGURE 15. Case 36. *a*, longitudinal cut of the cardiac ventricles showing an anterior acute myocardial infarct and an antero-apical ventricular septal defect (*arrow*). AV = aortic valve; LA = left atrium. *b*, close-up view of the ventricular septal defect (*dotted circle*) from the right ventricular side. *c*, longitudinal cut of the cardiac ventricles showing the acute myocardial infarct and the small defect (*arrow*). The ventricular septum (VS) is thin, and a thrombus (T) overlies its most apical portion. LV = left ventricle; RV = right ventricle. *d*, histologic section of portions of the ventricular septum and the right ventricular walls showing the rupture site (*arrow*) and the thrombus. Hematoxylin and eosin stain, × 1.5.

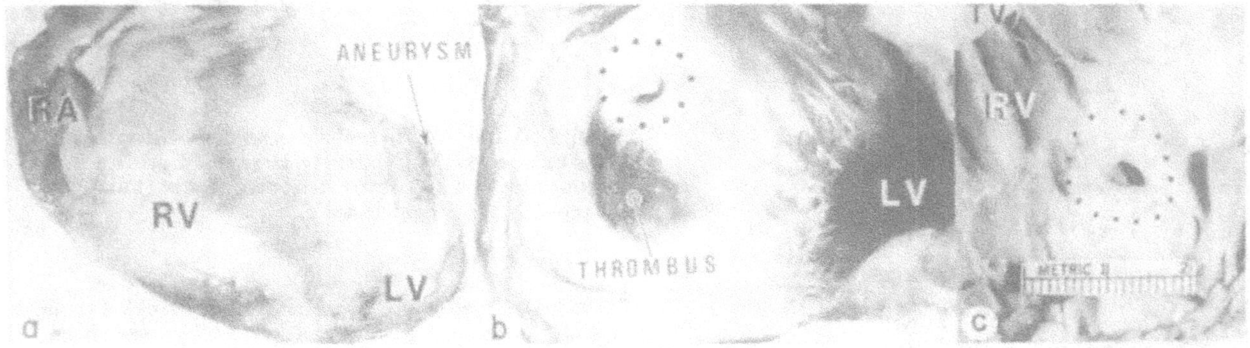

FIGURE 16. Case 37. *a*, external view of the heart showing a left ventricular (LV) aneurysm. RA = right atrium; RV = right ventricle. *b*, view of a "healed" ventricular septal defect (*dotted circle*) from the left ventricular side. A thrombus is seen. *c*, view of the healed ventricular septal defect (*dotted circle*) from the right ventricular side. TV = tricuspid valve.

tients had a dilated left ventricular cavity, 4 (10%) had a dilated right ventricular cavity and 11 (29%) had both ventricular cavities dilated. Patients 37 and 38 (Table I) had a healed left ventricular aneurysm.

In 33 of the 38 patients, the 3 major (right, left anterior descending and left circumflex) epicardial coronary arteries were examined in detail to assess their degree of cross-sectional area narrowing by atherosclerotic plaque: in 1 patient (no. 27) (3%) none of the 3 epicardial coronary arteries was narrowed >75% by plaque, but this patient had an occluding thrombus in the infarct-related coronary artery; in 8 patients (24%), 1 artery was narrowed >75% by plaque; in 9 patients (27%), 2 arteries were so narrowed, and in 15 patients (45%), all 3 major coronary arteries were so narrowed. Thus, of the 99 major epicardial coronary arteries examined in these 33 patients, 71 (72%) were narrowed >75% in cross-sectional area by plaque, an average of 2.2 of 3.0 major coronary arteries per patient. A thrombus was present in the infarct-related epicardial coronary artery in 10 (30%) of the 33 patients.

In 18 patients, the 4 major (including left main) epicardial coronary arteries were excised intact, decalcified if necessary and divided into 5 mm-long segments. A

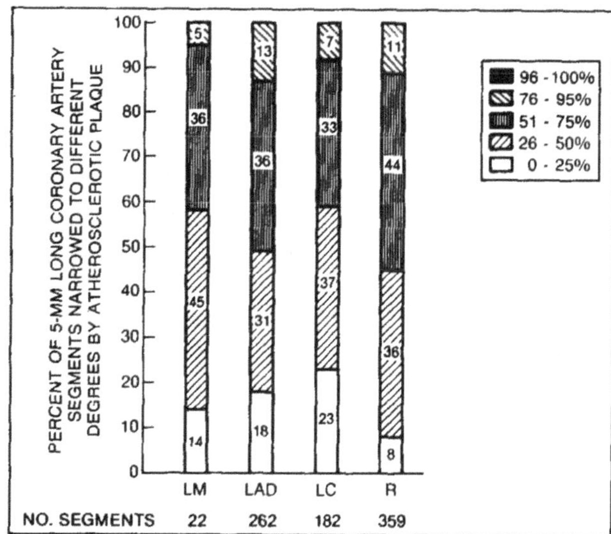

FIGURE 17. Bar graph showing the amounts of cross-sectional area narrowing by atherosclerotic plaque in each of the 4 major (left main [LM], left anterior descending [LAD], left circumflex [LC] and right [R]) epicardial coronary arteries in 18 of the 38 necropsy patients with an acquired ventricular septal defect during acute myocardial infarction.

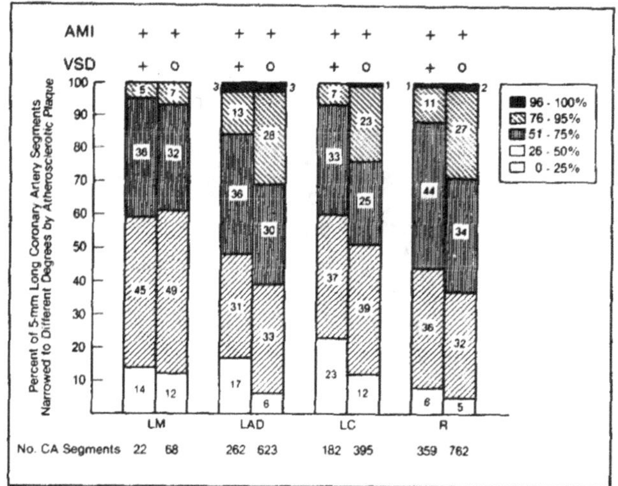

FIGURE 19. Bar graph showing the amounts of cross-sectional area narrowing by atherosclerotic plaque of the 4 major (left main [LM], left anterior descending [LAD], left circumflex [LC] and right [R]) epicardial coronary arteries in 18 of the 38 necropsy patients with an acquired ventricular septal defect (VSD) during acute myocardial infarction compared to 38 of the 50 patients with a fatal acute myocardial infarction (AMI) without rupture.

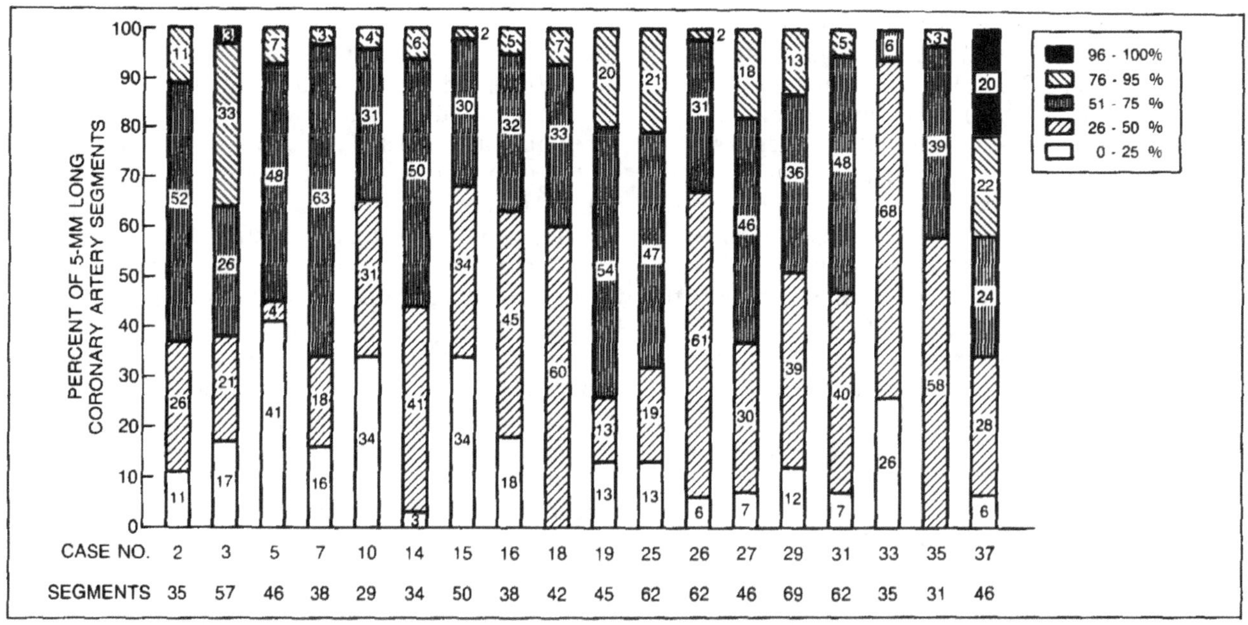

FIGURE 18. Bar graph showing the amounts of cross-sectional area narrowing by atherosclerotic plaque of the 4 major (left main, left anterior descending, left circumflex and right) epicardial coronary arteries in each of the 18 necropsy patients with an acquired ventricular septal defect during acute myocardial infarction.

TABLE II Clinical and Necropsy Findings in 32 Patients with an Acquired Ventricular Septal Defect (VSD) During Their First (*No Left Ventricular Scars*) Acute Myocardial Infarction (AMI) and in 50 Patients Without a VSD During Their First AMI (*No Left Ventricular Scars*)

	AMI With VSD	AMI Without VSD	p Value
Pts (n)	32	50	—
Mean ages (yrs)			
Men	65 ± 8	63 ± 11	NS
Women	74 ± 8	71 ± 16	NS
Men:Women	19 (59%):13 (41%)	32 (64%):18 (36%)	NS
Systemic hypertension*	15 (47%)	26 (52%)	NS
Angina pectoris*	7 (22%)	11 (22%)	NS
Congestive heart failure*	0	0	NS
Conduction disturbance[†]	11 (34)%	15 (30%)	NS
Interval (days) AMI → death	<1–360 (median 6)	<1–44 (median 10)	
Mean heart weight (g)			
Men	476 ± 95	526 ± 102	NS
Women	387 ± 65	432 ± 115	NS
Location LV AMI			
Anterior	7 (22%)	29 (58%)	<0.01
Posterior	25 (78%)	20 (40%)	<0.01
Lateral	0	1 (2%)	NS
Right ventricular AMI[‡]	17 (53%)	9 (18%)	<0.01
With anterior LV AMI	0/6	0/29	NS
With posterior LV AMI	18/26 (69%)	9/20 (45%)	NS
With lateral LV AMI	0	0/1	NS
Thrombus in infarct-related CA	9/28 (32%)	26/48 (52%)	NS
No. 3 major CAs > 75% ↓ in CSA by plaque			
0	1 (4%)	1 (2%)	NS
1	7 (25%)	7 (15%)	NS
2	7 (25%)	12 (25%)	NS
3	13 (46%)	28 (58%)	NS
No. of 5-mm segments examined	671	1,848	—
No. (%) of 5-mm CA segments narrowed:			
0 to 25 %	108 (16%)	132 (7%)	<0.01
26 to 50%	235 (35%)	632 (34%)	NS
51 to 75%	257 (38%)	576 (31%)	NS
76 to 95%	69 (10%)	472 (26%)	<0.01
96 to 100%	7 (<1%)	36 (2%)	<0.01

* Before the fatal AMI; [†] during the fatal AMI; [‡] all associated left ventricular infarcts involved its posterior (inferior wall).
CA = coronary artery; CSA = cross-sectional area; LV = left ventricular; NS = difference not significant.

histologic section was then prepared from each segment and stained by the Movat method. A total of 825 five-mm long coronary artery segments were examined: 22 from the left main, 262 from the left anterior descending, 182 from the left circumflex and 359 from the right coronary artery. The percent of different degrees (0 to 25, 26 to 50, 51 to 75, 76 to 95 and 96 to 100) of cross-sectional narrowing by atherosclerotic plaque for each of the 4 coronary arteries in all 18 patients is shown in Figure 17, and the amount of narrowing of all 5-mm segments of all 4 major coronary arteries in each of the 18 patients is shown in Figure 18. Of the 825 five-mm-long coronary artery segments, 118 (14%) were narrowed ≤25% by atherosclerotic plaque in cross-sectional area; 287 (35%) were narrowed 26 to 50%; 319 (39%), 51 to 75%; 89 (11%), 76 to 95%; and 12 (2%), 96 to 100%.

NONRUPTURE GROUP AND COMPARISON TO RUPTURE GROUP

The nonrupture group included 50 patients selected on the basis of a fatal transmural (involved all the endocardial one-half and all or a portion of the epicardial half of left ventricular wall) AMI unassociated with rupture of either the left ventricular free wall or ventricular septum or papillary muscle and on the basis of absence of a left ventricular scar. Certain clinical and necropsy findings in the nonrupture group are summarized in Table II and compared with those in the rupture group that had no left ventricular scars. Thus, only 32 of the rupture group patients were compared with the 50 nonrupture group patients. We excluded the 6 patients with healed myocardial infarct because none of the nonrupture group patients had left ventricular scars.

Of the 13 variables analyzed, 3 were significantly different between the rupture and nonrupture groups: (1) the extent of the coronary arterial narrowing by atherosclerotic plaque (Figure 19); (2) the frequency of associated right ventricular infarcts (53% in the rupture group vs 18% in the nonrupture group; however, among the patients with posterior (inferior) left ventricular infarcts, no significant differences were found between the rupture and nonrupture groups [Table II]); and (3) the location of the AMI (the posterior wall was the location of the AMI in 78% of the rupture group and in 40% of the nonrupture group). The number of coronary arteries narrowed >95% by atherosclerotic plaque was 9 of 99 (9%) in the rupture group and 38 of 144 (26%) in the

TABLE III Previously Published Necropsy Data on 78 Patients with Ventricular Septal Defect Secondary to Acute Myocardial Infarction and Comparison with 61 Necropsy Patients with an Acquired Ventricular Septal Defect during Acute Myocardial Infarction Described in the Present Report and in Two Previous Reports by the Present Authors

Authors (year)	Hutchins[2] (1979)	Edwards et al[3] (1984)	Cummings et al[4] (1988)	Total	Mann and Roberts (1987 and 1988)
Pts (n)	10	53	15	78	61[†]
Mean ages (yrs)	66	69	65	68	67
Men	—	67	—	—	64 ± 10
Women	—	73	—	—	72 ± 8
Men:Women	8:2	33:20	7:8	48 (62%):30 (38%)	40 (66%):21 (34%)
Systemic hypertension	5	—	9	14/25 (56%)	30 (49%)
Angina pectoris	—	—	3	—	15 (25%)
Congestive heart failure	—	—	0	—	2 (3%)
Conduction disturbance	4	6* (11%)	6	16 (21%)	19 (31%)
Interval (days) AMI → death	<1–100	—	—	—	<1–360 (median 8)
Mean heart weight (g)	537	482	477 ± 127	488	468
Men	—	514	—	—	502 ± 102
Women	—	430	—	—	403 ± 79
Location, LV AMI					
Anterior	4	24	8	36 (46%)	21 (34%)
Posterior	6	29	7	42 (54%)	40 (66%)
Right ventricular AMI	—	—	15	15/15	29 (47%)
LV infarct anterior	—	—	8/8	8/8	0
LV infarct posterior	—	—	7/7	7/7	29/40 (73%)
No. 3 major CAs >75% in CSA by plaque					
0	0	0	1 (7%)	1 (1%)	2 (4%)
1	0	0	3 (20%)	3 (4%)[‡]	12 (22%)[‡]
2	9	5 (9%)	3 (20%)	17 (22%)	18 (33%)
3	1	48 (91%)	8 (53%)	56 (73%)[‡]	23 (42%)[‡]
Thrombus in infarct-related CA	9	21	14	44 (57%)[‡]	17/55 (31%)[‡]
Healed myocardial infarct	0	—	0	0	9 (15)%

* Complete heart block in each; [†] this number includes the 38 patients described in the present article plus 16 previously described[5] patients with ventricular septal rupture secondary to AMI who underwent operative closure of the defect plus 7 previously described[6] patients who had rupture of the ventricular septum combined with rupture of the left ventricular free wall secondary to acute myocardial infarction. [‡] p <0.01.
AMI = acute myocardial infarct; CA = coronary artery; CSA = cross-sectional area; LV = left ventricular; — = no information available.

TABLE IV Reported Coronary Arterial Angiographic Findings in Patients with Ventricular Septal Defect Secondary to Acute Myocardial Infarction

First Author (year), Reference	Pts (n)	Mean Age of Pts (yrs)	Men (%)	CA Diameter Narrowing (%)	No. of Major (Right, LAD, LC) CAs Narrowed >50% or >70% in Diameter		
					1	2	3
Hill (1975)[7]	14	63	65	—	9	1	4
Miller (1978)[8]	26	—	63	>50	12	9	5
Killen (1981)[9]	29	69	61	>50	12	13	4
Radford (1981)[10]	25	63	61	—	6	12	7
Feneley (1983)[11]	13	65	58	—	6	5	2
Miyamoto (1983)[12]	8	64	63	>50	4	3	1
Fananapazir (1983)[13]	38	62	70	>70	28	9	0
Rebollar (1984)[14]	6	64	59	>50	2	3	1
Scanlon (1985)[15]	20	67	50	—	5	9	6
Jones (1987)[16]	54	62	68	>70	19	20	15
Total (%)	233				103 (44)	84 (36)	45 (19)

CA = coronary artery; LAD = left anterior descending; LC = left circumflex.

nonrupture group (p <0.001). A significantly lower percent of 5-mm coronary segments in the rupture group was narrowed 76 to 100% in cross-sectional area by plaque compared with the nonrupture group (76 of 671 [11%] vs 508 of 1,848 [28%]). Comparison of the rupture and nonrupture groups on the basis of men versus men, women versus women, anterior wall location versus anterior wall location, posterior wall location versus posterior wall location, heart weight ≤400 g versus heart weight ≤400 g and heart weight >400 g versus heart weight >400 g disclosed no significant differences between the 2 groups.

DISCUSSION

Comparison of certain findings in our patients with unoperated VSD secondary to AMI with those in patients with AMI without VSD disclosed 2 significant differences: (1) the patients with VSD had a higher frequency of posterior location of the left ventricular infarct (28 of 38 [74%] vs 20 of 50 [40%]), and (2) the patients with VSD had less severe narrowing of the major epicardial coronary arteries by atherosclerotic plaque. Other investigators have described necropsy findings in patients with VSD secondary to AMI, but none has compared findings to those in necropsy patients with AMI without VSD. Hutchins,[2] Edwards,[3] Cummings[4] and their co-workers did not find a higher frequency of posterior location of the left ventricular infarct in their patients and neither did they find a relatively low frequency of severe narrowing of the coronary arteries (Table III). Because each of the 3 previous necropsy studies[2-4] included both operative and nonoperative cases of VSD secondary to AMI, in Table III we combine findings in the present study with those of operative cases previously reported by us[5] and cases of double rupture[6] and compare our combined findings with those of the 3 previous necropsy reports. In our present study, we found a lower frequency of severe coronary atherosclerosis only because we examined each 5-mm long segment of the 4 major coronary arteries. None of the other 3 previously reported necropsy studies[2-4] of VSD secondary to AMI examined the coronary arteries in a quantitative fashion. Thus, our group of 38 unoperated patients with VSD secondary to AMI not only differed in 2 important respects from our control patients, but they also differed in these 2 respects compared with other reports focusing on necropsy findings in patients with VSD secondary to AMI.

Several studies[7-16] have described coronary angiographic findings in patients with VSD secondary to AMI and these findings are summarized in Table IV. Most of the studies showed a high percent of patients with single-vessel disease (44%) and a relatively small percent of patients with 3-vessel disease (19%). These findings support those of the present study.

The present study is the first necropsy study to describe quantitatively the amount of cross-sectional area narrowing by atherosclerotic plaque in patients with VSD secondary to AMI. The percent of 5-mm segments of the 4 major coronary arteries narrowed >75% by plaque was significantly less than in the patients without VSD (101 of 825 segments [13%] vs 508 of 1,848 segments [28%]). Comparison of our rupture cases with the nonrupture cases by the 1-, 2-, 3-vessel disease approach, however, did not show significant differences in the number of coronary arteries narrowed per patient at some point in the AMI patients with VSD compared with the AMI patients without VSD. The percent of 5-mm coronary segments narrowed minimally or not at all (0 to 25%) also differed in the rupture and nonrupture groups (118 of 825 segments [14%] vs 132 of 1,848 segments [7%]).

REFERENCES

1. Roberts WC, Roberts JD. *The floating heart or the heart too fat to sink: analysis of 55 necropsy patients. Am J Cardiol 1983;52:1286–1289.*
2. Hutchins GM. *Rupture of the interventricular septum complicating myocardial infarction: pathological analysis of 10 patients with clinically diagnosed perforations. Am Heart J 1979;97:165–173.*
3. Edwards BS, Edwards WD, Edward JE. *Ventricular septal rupture complicating acute myocardial infarction: identification of simple and complex types in 53 autopsied hearts. Am J Cardiol 1984;54:1201–1205.*
4. Cummings RG, Reimer KA, Califf R, Hackel D, Boswick J, Lowe JE. *Quantitative analysis of right and left ventricular infarction in the presence of postinfarction ventricular septal defect. Circulation 1988;77:33–42.*
5. Mann JM, Roberts WC. *Cardiac morphologic observations after operative closure of acquired ventricular septal defect during acute myocardial infarction: analysis of 16 necropsy patients. Am J Cardiol 1987;60:981–987.*
6. Mann JM, Roberts WC. *Fatal rupture of both left ventricular free wall and ventricular septum (double rupture) during acute myocardial infarction: analysis of seven patients studied at necropsy. Am J Cardiol 1987;60:722–724.*
7. Hill D, Lary D, Kerth W, Gerbode F. *Acquired ventricular septal defects. J Thorac Cardiovasc Surg 1975;70:440–444.*
8. Miller SW, Dinsmore RE, Greene RE, Daggett WM. *Coronary, ventricular and pulmonary abnormalities associated with rupture of the interventricular septum complicating myocardial infarction. AJR 1978;131:571–577.*
9. Killen DA, Reed WA, Wathanacharoen S, McCallister BD, Bell HH. *Postinfarctional rupture of the interventricular septum. J Cardiovasc Surg 1981; 22:113–126.*
10. Radford MJ, Johnson RA, Daggett WM Jr, Fallon JT, Buckley MJ, Gold HK, Leinbach RC. *Ventricular septal rupture: a review of clinical and physiologic features and an analysis of survival. Circulation 1981;64:545–553.*
11. Feneley M, Chang P, O'Rourke MF. *Myocardial rupture after acute myocardial infarction: ten year review. Br Heart J 1983;49:550–556.*
12. Miyamoto AT, Lee ME, Kass RM, Chaux A, Sethna D, Gray R, Matloff JM. *Post-myocardial infarction ventricular septal defect. J Thorac Cardiovasc Surg 1983;86:41–46.*
13. Fananapazir L, Bray CL, Dark JF, Moussalli H, Deiraniya AK, Lawson RAM. *Right ventricular dysfunction and surgical outcome in post-infarction ventricular septal defect. Eur Heart J 1983;4:155–167.*
14. Rebollar L, Jaramillo Uribe M, Gil M. *Ruptura del septum ventricular post infarto agudo del miocardio. Arch Inst Cardiol Mex 1984;54:267–281.*
15. Scanlon PJ, Montoya A, Johnson SA, McKeever LS, Sullivan HJ, Bakhos M, Pifarre R. *Urgent surgery for ventricular septal rupture complicating acute myocardial infarction. Circulation 1984;72(suppl II):185–190.*
16. Jones MT, Schofield PM, Dark JF, Moussalli H, Deiraniya AK, Lawson RAM, Ward C, Bray CL. *Surgical repair of acquired ventricular septal defect. Determinants of early and late outcome. J Thorac Cardiovasc Surg 1987;93:680–686.*

Location of an Acute Myocardial Infarct in Patients with a Healed Myocardial Infarct: Analysis of 129 Patients Studied at Necropsy

Benjamin N. Potkin, MD, and William C. Roberts, MD

To determine the relation of a single healed myocardial infarct to a fatal acute myocardial infarct, 129 patients with 1 grossly visible healed and 1 grossly visible acute infarct were studied at necropsy. It was determined whether the acute infarct was *opposite* to or *adjacent* to the healed infarct or if 1 infarct was so large that it was *both* opposite to and adjacent to the other infarct. In 74 (57%) of the 129 patients, the 2 infarcts were opposite one another, in 40 (31%) they were adjacent and in 15 (12%) they were both opposite and adjacent. The age, sex, mean size of the healed infarct and heart weight were similar among the 3 groups. Acute myocardial infarcts were larger in the group that had both opposite and adjacent infarcts than either of the other 2 groups (p <0.001). Information regarding whether the infarcts were clinically recognized or not was available in 108 patients: both infarcts were recognized in 41 (38%), neither infarct was recognized in 15 (14%) and 1 infarct was recognized and the other was not in 52 (48%). The number of the 4 major epicardial coronary arteries narrowed at some point >75% in cross-sectional area by atherosclerotic plaque was similar in patients with recognized and in those with unrecognized infarcts. Similar numbers of narrowed major epicardial coronary arteries also were found in each of the 3 infarct groups (opposite, adjacent or both).

(Am J Cardiol 1988;62:1017–1023)

From the Pathology Branch, National Heart, Lung, and Blood Institute, National Institutes of Health, Bethesda, Maryland. Manuscript received June 1, 1988; revised manuscript received and accepted July 11, 1988.

Dr. Potkin's present address: Division of Cardiology, Department of Medicine, Cedars-Sinai Medical Center, Los Angeles, California 90048.

Address for reprints: Pathology Branch, National Heart, Lung, and Blood Institute, National Institutes of Health, Building 10, Room 2N258, Bethesda, Maryland 20892.

Only 1 previous study has mentioned the location of an acute myocardial infarct in patients with a healed myocardial infarct. Macarie et al[1] described necropsy findings in 43 patients who had a healed myocardial infarct and an acute myocardial infarct: in 25 (58%), the new infarct was in a "different" territory than the initial infarct; in 6 (14%), the new infarct was in the "same" territory as the initial infarct and in 12 patients (28%), the new infarct was in both the "same" and in a "different" territory than the initial infarct. We studied 129 patients at necropsy with 1 grossly visible healed and 1 grossly visible acute myocardial infarct and determined whether the acute infarct was opposite to or adjacent to the healed infarct or if one infarct was so large that it was both opposite to and adjacent to the other infarct. The frequency of clinically recognized healed and acute infarcts was also determined and correlated with several clinical variables.

METHODS

Criteria for inclusion and exclusion: The cardiac diagnoses were reviewed in patients accessioned in the Pathology Branch, National Heart, Lung, and Blood Institute, from 1954 through 1987. A total of 271 patients were diagnosed at necropsy as having had both a healed myocardial infarct and an acute myocardial infarct. The records of the Pathology Branch in these 271 patients then were reviewed and patients having had cardiac surgery of any type (20 cases) and patients having significant valvular heart disease (11 cases) were excluded. Of the remaining 240 cases, an additional 111 were excluded for the following reasons: (1) the acute infarct was not grossly visible (32 cases); (2) the healed infarct was not grossly visible (1 case); (3) >1 healed infarct was present (36 cases); (4) neither the heart nor photographs of it was available (33 cases); (5) the healed infarct was neither transmural (scar involved more than inner one-half of the left ventricular wall) nor subendocardial (scar limited to inner one-half of the left ventricular wall) (5 cases); (6) a concomitant illness that could have caused death and the acute myocardial infarction may have been incidental (4 cases: fatal bronchospasm in 1, fatal gastrointestinal bleeding in 2 and suicide in 1). Thus, of the initial 271 cases reexamined, 142 were eliminated, thus leaving 129 cases to be included in this study. Of the 129 cases, all had 1 grossly visible healed subendocardial or transmural healed left ventricular infarct and all had 1 subendocardial or transmural grossly visible acute myocardial infarct that was fatal.

Definitions of anatomic locations of healed and acute myocardial infarcts (Figures 1 through 5): *Opposite:* the 2 infarcts were opposite one another and the intervening myocardial walls were normal, i.e., devoid of foci of fibrosis or necrosis. *Adjacent:* on 1 wall the 2 infarcts were contiguous with one another and on the opposite wall the myocardium was normal. *Both adjacent and opposite:* the 2 infarcts were opposite and adjacent when the necrotic and fibrotic walls of the 2 infarcts were contiguous with each other on one side and when 1 infarct was so extensive that a major portion of it was opposite to the other infarcted wall.

Characteristics of study patients (Table I): The 92 men ranged in age from 37 to 88 years (mean 64 ± 11) and the 37 women from 43 to 95 years (mean 70 ± 12). The heart weight in 81 men ranged from 330 to 685 g (mean 488 ± 84), and in 34 women from 270 to 555 g (mean 431 ± 79).

Statistical analysis: Analysis of variance was used to test for significant differences among sample means and variance; chi-square analysis for noncontinuous data. A probability value (p) <0.05 was considered significant.

RESULTS

Relation of healed to acute myocardial infarct (Table II): Of the 129 patients, 74 (57%) infarcts were op-

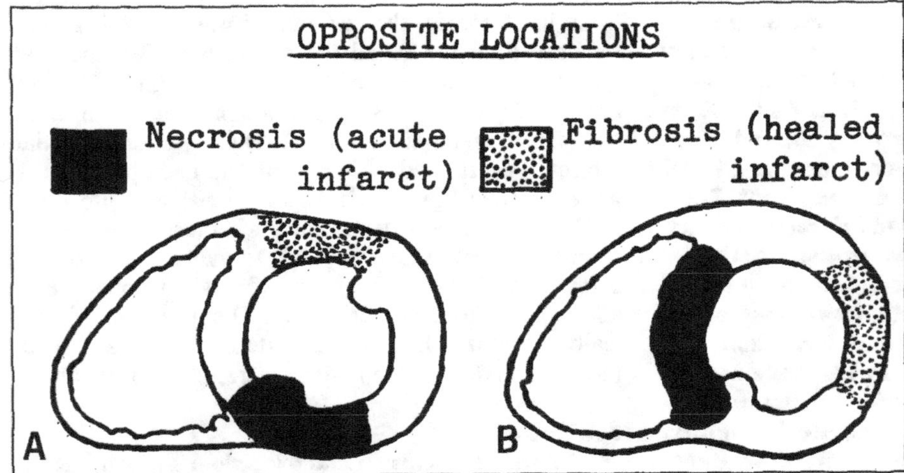

FIGURE 1. Diagrams of transverse sections of the cardiac ventricles illustrating the relation of an acute myocardial infarct being *opposite* to a healed myocardial infarct. *A*, 1 infarct is anterior and the other is posterior. *B*, 1 infarct is septal and the other is lateral.

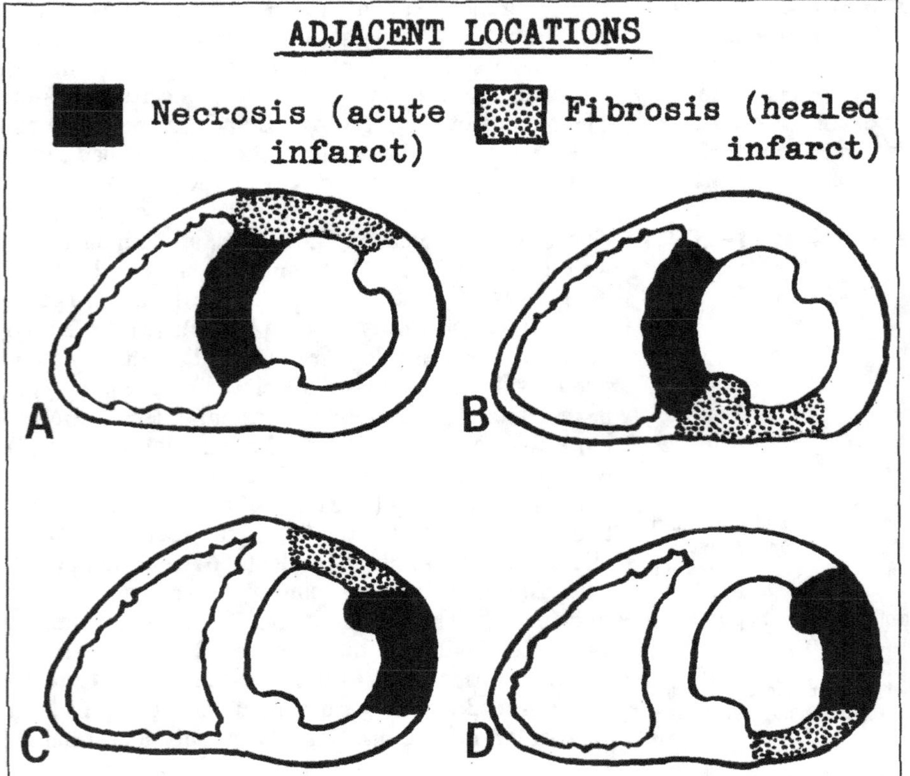

FIGURE 2. Diagrams of transverse sections of the cardiac ventricles illustrating the relation of an acute myocardial infarct being *adjacent* to a healed myocardial infarct. *A*, 1 infarct is septal and the other is anterior or posterior (*B*); *C*, 1 infarct is lateral and the other is anterior or posterior (*D*).

posite one another, 40 (31%) were adjacent and 15 (12%) were both opposite and adjacent. Of the 74 patients with the 2 infarcts located opposite to one another, the healed infarct involved the anterior wall in 21 (28%); the posterior wall in 47 (64%); the lateral wall in 5 (7%); and the ventricular septum in 1 (1%). Of the 40 patients in whom the 2 infarcts were located adjacent to one another, the healed infarct involved the anterior wall in 5 (13%); the posterior wall in 14 (35%); the lateral wall in 20 (50%); and the ventricular septum in 1 (2%). Of the 15 patients in whom the 2 infarcts were located both opposite to and adjacent to one another,

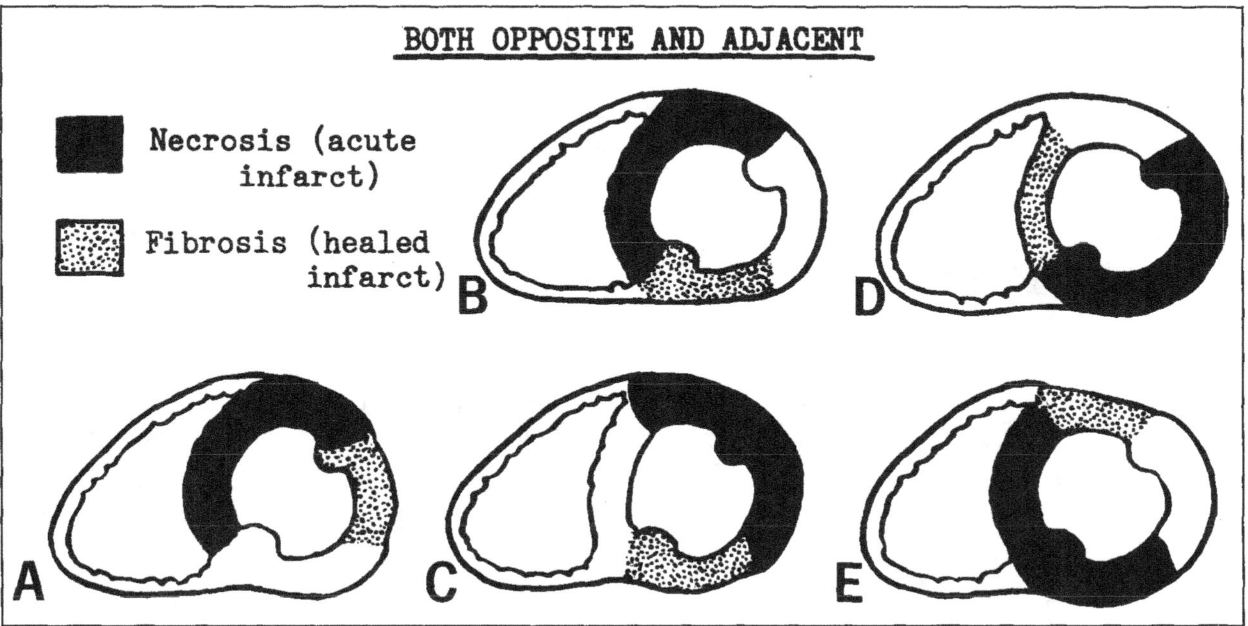

FIGURE 3. Diagram of transverse sections of the cardiac ventricles illustrating the relation of the acute myocardial infarct's being *both opposite and adjacent* to the healed myocardial infarct. *A*, the acute infarct is anteroseptal and the healed infarct is posterior. *B*, the acute infarct is anteroseptal and the healed infarct is posterior. *C*, the acute infarct is anterolateral and the healed infarct is posterior. *D*, the acute infarct is posterolateral and the healed infarct is septal. *E*, the acute infarct is posteroseptal and the healed infarct is anterior.

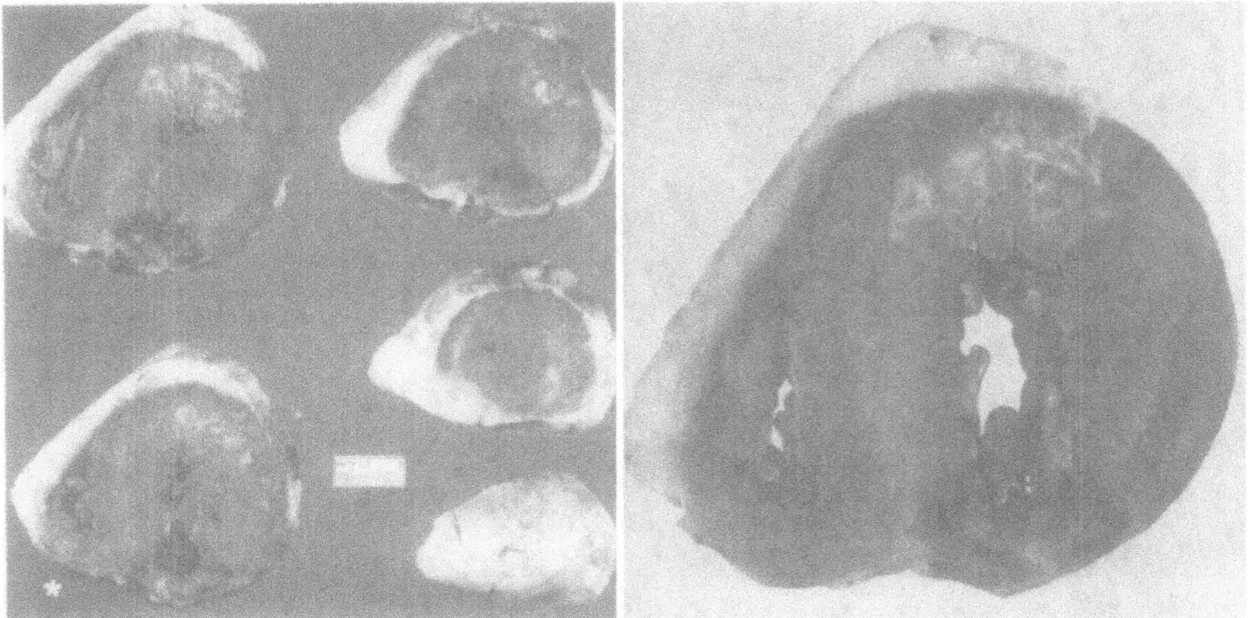

FIGURE 4. Transverse sections of cardiac ventricles from a 67-year-old man (N87-215) with a healed myocardial infarct and an acute myocardial infarct that ruptured. *Left,* transverse sections of the cardiac ventricles from base to apex showing a moderately sized transmural healed myocardial infarct involving the anterior wall and a moderately sized transmural acute infarct involving the posterior wall. *Right,* close-up view of the underside of the section marked with an *asterisk* on the *left.* The acute infarct is located opposite to the healed infarct.

TABLE I Ages, Sex and Heart Weights in 129 Patients Studied at Necropsy with an Acute and a Healed Myocardial Infarct

| | Total | Location of Myocardial Infarcts | | |
		Opposite	Adjacent	Both
No. of patients (%)	129 (100)	74 (57)	40 (31)	15 (12)
Men/women	92/37	54/20	28/12	10/5
Ages (yrs): mean (range)				
Men	64 ± 11 (37–88)	64 ± 10 (37–83)	64 ± 14 (39–88)	60 ± 8 (45–72)
Women	70 ± 12 (43–95)	70 ± 11 (44–89)	72 ± 13 (43–95)	63 ± 10 (48–73)
Men and women	66 ± 11 (37–95)	66 ± 10 (37–89)	67 ± 14 (39–95)	61 ± 9 (45–73)
Heart weight (g): mean (range)				
Men	488 ± 84 (330–685)	490 ± 87 (330–685)	476 ± 80 (360–620)	505 ± 89 (380–615)
Women	431 ± 79 (270–555)	451 ± 65 (330–555)	396 ± 92 (270–540)	421 ± 92 (320–530)
Men and women	471 ± 86 (270–685)	480 ± 83 (330–685)	452 ± 89 (270–620)	473 ± 96 (320–615)

TABLE II Relation of Healed to Acute Myocardial Infarcts in 129 Patients Studied at Necropsy

| Location of the Healed Infarct | Location of the Acute Infarct: Number (%) | | | |
	Opposite	Adjacent	Both	Totals
Anterior	21(72)	5(17)	3(10)	29(100)
Posterior	47 (66)	14(20)	10(14)	71(100)
Lateral	5(19)	20(77)	1(4)	26(100)
Septal	1(33)	1(33)	1(33)	3(100)
Total	74(57)	40(31)	15(12)	129(100)

the healed infarct involved the anterior wall in 3 (20%); the posterior wall in 10 (66%); the lateral wall in 1 (7%); and the ventricular septum in 1 (7%).

Of the 29 patients with a healed anterior wall myocardial infarct, the acute infarct was opposite in 21 (72%); adjacent in 5 (17%); and both opposite to and adjacent to the acute infarct in 3 (10%). Of the 71 patients with a healed posterior wall myocardial infarct, the acute infarct was opposite in 47 (66%); adjacent in 14 (20%); and both opposite to and adjacent to the acute infarct in 10 (14%). Of the 26 patients with a healed lateral wall myocardial infarct, the acute infarct was opposite in 5 (19%); adjacent in 20 (77%), and both opposite to and adjacent to the acute infarct in 1 (4%). Of the 3 patients with a healed ventricular septal infarct, the acute infarct was opposite in 1; adjacent in 1; and both opposite to and adjacent to the acute infarct in 1.

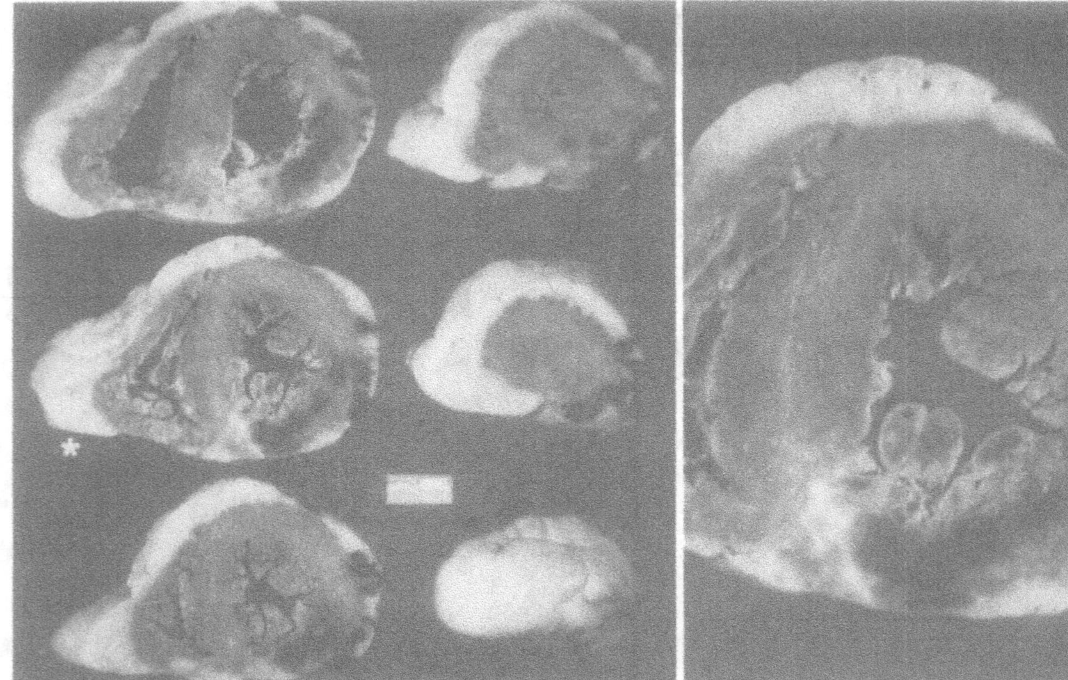

FIGURE 5. Transverse slices of the cardiac ventricles of a 73-year-old woman (A87-8) with a healed myocardial infarct and an acute myocardial infarct. *Left,* transverse sections of the cardiac ventricles from base to apex showing a small sized transmural healed myocardial infarct involving the posterior wall and a larger sized transmural acute infarct involving the lateral wall. *Right,* close-up view of the section marked with an *asterisk* on the *left*. The acute infarct is located adjacent to the healed infarct.

TABLE III Clinical and Morphologic Findings in Patients with a Healed and an Acute Myocardial Infarct: Analysis of Clinically Recognized and Unrecognized Infarcts

	Healed Myocardial Infarct		Acute Myocardial Infarct		Healed and Acute Myocardial Infarcts		
	Recognized	Unrecognized	Recognized	Unrecognized	Both Infarcts Recognized	Neither Infarct Recognized	One Infarct Recognized One Infarct Unrecognized
No. (%) of patients	57 (52%)	52 (48%)	89 (74%)	31 (26%)	41 (38%)	15 (14%)	52 (48%)
No. (%) men	41 (72%)	39 (75%)	65 (73%)	21 (68%)	31 (76%)	11 (73%)	37 (71%)
No. (%) women	16 (28%)	13 (25%)	24 (27%)	10 (32%)	10 (24%)	4 (27%)	15 (29%)
Age (yrs) mean (range)	65 ± 9 (44–85)	54 ± 13 (37–88)	65 ± 11 (37–95)	65 ± 12 (39–88)	64 ± 9 (44–81)	63 ± 14 (39–88)	65 ± 11 (37–87)
Location of healed MI							
Anterior	19 (33%)	7 (13%)	23 (26%)	4 (13%)	15 (37%)	1 (7%)	9 (17%)
Posterior	30 (53%)	30 (58%)	47 (53%)	20 (64%)	21 (51%)	10 (67%)	29 (56%)
Lateral	8 (14%)	13 (25%)	17 (19%)	7 (23%)	5 (12%)	4 (27%)	12 (23%)
Septal	0 (0%)	2 (4%)	2 (2%)	0 (0%)	0 (0%)	0 (0%)	2 (4%)
Location of acute MI							
Anterior	26 (46%)	25 (48%)	40 (45%)	16 (52%)	19 (46%)	8 (53%)	24 (46%)
Posterior	23 (40%)	16 (31%)	34 (38%)	8 (26%)	17 (41%)	3 (20%)	18 (35%)
Lateral	4 (7%)	7 (13%)	9 (10%)	5 (16%)	2 (5%)	3 (20%)	6 (12%)
Septal	4 (7%)	4 (8%)	6 (7%)	2 (6%)	3 (7%)	1 (7%)	4 (8%)
Relation of healed MI to acute MI							
Opposite	39 (68%)	26 (50%)	52 (58%)	17 (55%)	29 (71%)	7 (47%)	28 (54%)
Adjacent	12 (21%)	19 (37%)	26 (29%)	11 (35%)	7 (17%)	6 (40%)	18 (35%)
Both	6 (11%)	7 (13%)	11 (12%)	3 (10%)	5 (12%)	2 (13%)	6 (12%)
Size of healed/acute MI							
Small	22 (39%)/11 (20%)	21 (40%)/10 (19%)	40 (45%)/13 (15%)	11 (35%)/9 (29%)	18 (44%)/5 (12%)	6 (40%)/4 (27%)	19 (37%)/11 (21%)
Medium	23 (40%)/25 (43%)	24 (46%)/19 (37%)	37 (42%)/39 (44%)	13 (42%)/11 (35%)	15 (36%)/19 (46%)	6 (40%)/5 (33%)	25 (48%)/20 (38%)
Large	12 (21%)/21 (37%)	7 (13%)/23 (44%)	12 (13%)/37 (42%)	7 (23%)/11 (35%)	8 (20%)/17 (41%)	3 (20%)/6 (40%)	8 (15%)/21 (40%)
No. (%) with heart weight	47/53 (89%)	41/49 (84%)	69/82 (84%)	23/29 (79%)	34/38 (89%)	11/14 (79%)	42/49 (86%)
Heart weight (g) mean (range)							
Men	499 ± 77 (335–685)	490 ± 88 (330–660)	489 ± 80 (330–640)	497 ± 98 (350–685)	495 ± 75 (335–640)	490 ± 104 (350–660)	497 ± 84 (330–685)
Women	441 ± 83 (270–555)	431 ± 65 (320–530)	420 ± 67 (320–550)	464 ± 89 (270–555)	423 ± 63 (330–550)	450 ± 44 (420–500)	443 ± 88 (270–555)
Men and women	482 ± 83 (270–685)	475 ± 87 (320–660)	470 ± 82 (320–640)	487 ± 95 (270–685)	476 ± 78 (330–640)	481 ± 96 (350–660)	480 ± 88 (270–685)
No. (%) with AP	29/51 (57%)	20/49 (41%)	48/79 (61%)	4/27 (15%)	27/39 (69%)	2/15 (13%)	20/26 (77%)
No. (%) with SH	32/45 (71%)	18/42 (43%)	40/69 (58%)	14/23 (61%)	25/36 (69%)	7/14 (50%)	18/37 (49%)
No. (%) with DM	20/47 (43%)	14/44 (32%)	23/70 (33%)	13/25 (52%)	15/36 (42%)	8/14 (57%)	11/41 (27%)

AP = angina pectoris; DM = diabetes mellitus; MI = myocardial infarct; SH = systemic hypertension.

Age, sex and heart weight (Table I): The sex distribution, age and heart weight were similar among the 3 groups (*opposite, adjacent* and *both* opposite and adjacent). When the analyses were limited to only men or to only women, age and heart weight remained similar among the 3 groups; however, when comparing all the men with all the women, the women were older (p = 0.005) and had lighter heart weights than the men (p = 0.001).

Extent of coronary artery narrowing: All of the 129 patients had >75% narrowing in cross-sectional area by atherosclerotic plaque of at least 1 major (right, left main, left anterior descending, left circumflex) epicardial coronary artery. Of the 129 patients, 24 (19%) had severe narrowing of the left main (20 cases had left main plus all 3 other epicardial coronary arteries severely narrowed; 3 cases had left main plus 2 other epicardial arteries severely narrowed; and 1 case had left main plus 1 other epicardial coronary artery severely narrowed); 60 (47%) had severe narrowing of the left anterior descending, left circumflex and right coronary arteries; 25 (19%) had severe narrowing of 2 of the 3 major epicardial coronary arteries (excluding left main); 4 (3%) had severe narrowing of 1 of the 3 major epicardial coronary arteries (excluding left main); and 16 (12%) had severe narrowing of 1 or more major epicardial coronary arteries (exact number not known). The frequency of infarct location of opposite, adjacent or both was not related to the number of coronary arteries narrowed, and this finding remained when the 16 patients with the unknown exact number of coronary arteries severely narrowed were removed from the analysis. The heart weights and ages were similar when the patients were analyzed according to the number of major coronary arteries severely narrowed.

Infarct size: Of the 129 patients, the healed myocardial infarct was small in 54 (42%); moderate in 56 (43%) and large in 19 (15%). Of the 129 patients, the acute infarct was small in 24 (19%); moderate in 52 (40%); and large in 53 (41%). The size of the healed infarcts was similar among the 3 groups. The size of the acute infarct was larger in the group that had both opposite and adjacent infarcts than either the opposite (p = 0.0004) or adjacent groups (p = 0.001). The size of the acute infarct was similar in the adjacent and opposite groups. The acute infarcts were larger than the healed infarcts (p = 0.001). No relation between the size of the acute or healed infarcts and the number of severely narrowed epicardial coronary arteries was observed.

Infarct width: Of the 129 patients, the healed infarct was transmural in 122 (95%) and subendocardial in 7 (5%); the acute infarct was transmural in 121 (94%) and subendocardial in 8 (6%).

Frequency of clinical recognition of the healed and acute myocardial infarcts (Table III): Of the 129 patients with both a healed and an acute myocardial infarct, sufficient information regarding whether an acute infarct was clinically recognized or not was available in 109 (84%) patients with healed infarcts, in 120 (93%) patients with acute infarcts and in 108 (84%) patients with both healed and acute infarcts. Lateral wall healed infarcts were less frequently recognized than anterior but not posterior healed infarcts (62 vs 27%) (p = 0.05). The frequency of opposite, adjacent and both opposite and adjacent locations of both healed and acute infarcts was similar in the patients with recognized and unrecognized infarcts. The number of coronary arteries narrowed >75% in cross-sectional area by plaque was similar between patients with recognized and unrecognized infarcts. Patients with clinically recognized acute infarcts that healed (57 of 109 patients, 57%) had an increased frequency of systemic hypertension (32 of 45 [71%] vs 18 of 42 [43%]; p = 0.008). Patients with clinically recognized acute infarcts had an increased frequency of angina pectoris (48 of 79 [61%] vs 4 of 27 [15%]; p = 0.0001). Patients with one or both infarcts clinically recognized had an increased frequency of angina pectoris (27 of 39, 69% for both infarcts recognized; 20 of 26, 77% for 1 infarct recognized and 2 of 15, 13% for neither infarct recognized; p <0.001). Diabetes mellitus was present in similar percentages in patients with recognized and unrecognized infarcts.

DISCUSSION

In 129 patients with both a healed and an acute myocardial infarct, the acute infarct was opposite to the healed infarct in 74 patients (57%), adjacent in 40 (31%) and both opposite and adjacent in 15 (12%). In the 29 patients in whom the healed infarct involved the anterior wall, the fatal acute infarct was located on the opposite wall in 21 (72%), on the adjacent wall in 5 (all lateral) (17%) and on both the opposite and adjacent walls (all posteroseptal) in 3 (10%). In the 71 patients in whom the healed infarct involved the posterior wall, the fatal acute infarct was opposite in 47 (66%), adjacent (11 lateral and 3 septal) in 14 (20%) and on both opposite and adjacent walls (7 anteroseptal and 3 anterolateral) in 10 (14%). In the 26 patients in whom the healed infarct involved the lateral wall, the fatal acute infarct was opposite in 5 (19%), adjacent in 20 (77%) (17 posterior, 3 anterior) and both opposite and adjacent walls in 1 (4%).

Over 50% of the 2 infarcts in this study were related to one another in an opposite manner. A second myocardial infarct is more likely to be fatal when necrosis occurs opposite to a fibrotic myocardial wall rather than adjacent to it; possibly more left ventricular dysfunction occurs when 2 opposite walls, rather than 2 adjacent walls, even with similar infarcted areas, become infarcted.

Information regarding whether the infarcts were clinically recognized or not was available in 108 patients: both infarcts were recognized in 41 (38%), neither infarct was recognized in 15 (14%) and 1 infarct was recognized and the other was not in 52 (48%). The number of the 4 major epicardial coronary arteries narrowed >75% in cross-sectional area by plaque was similar between patients with recognized and unrecognized infarcts. Patients with 1 or both infarcts clinically recognized had an increased frequency of angina pectoris (69% for both infarcts recognized; 43% for 1 infarct recognized and 13% for neither infarct recognized; p = 0.001). The increased frequency of angina pectoris in patients with recognized myocardial infarcts also was observed in the Framingham Study.[2] In our study, patients with clinically recognized acute infarcts that healed (57 of 109 patients [57%]) as opposed to those in whom the healed infarct was unrecognized (52 of 109 patients [48%]) had an increased frequency of systemic hypertension (71 vs 43%; p = 0.008). Diabetes mellitus was present in a similar percentage between patients with recognized and unrecognized infarcts.

REFERENCES

1. Macarie C, Ionescu DD, Nicolescu M, Inoescu V, Dop R, Meclea G. [Repeat myocardial infarction and reinfarction. Clinical, developmental and peculiar anatomopathologic aspects]. *Rev Med Interna* [*Med Interna*] 1986;38:301–311.
2. Kannel WB, Abbott RD. Incidence and prognosis of unrecognized myocardial infarction. An update on the Framingham Study. *N Engl J Med* 1984;311:1144–1147.

Frequency of Acute and Healed Myocardial Infarcts in Fatal Cardiac Amyloidosis

Deborah J. Barbour, MD, and William C. Roberts, MD

Transmural (involvement of more than the inner one-half of the myocardial wall) left ventricular necrosis or fibrosis is most often secondary to severe (>75% cross-sectional area) narrowing by atherosclerotic plaques of 1 or more of the major epicardial coronary arteries. Myocardial infarction also may occur without significant narrowing of an epicardial coronary artery in several conditions, including hypertrophic cardiomyopathy,[1,2] dilated cardiomyopathy,[3] left or right ventricular outflow obstruction[4–10] and anomalies of coronary arterial origin or course.[11] Another condition associated with myocardial infarction without significant narrowing of 1 or more of the epicardial coronary arteries is cardiac amyloidosis.

From the Pathology Branch, National Heart, Lung, and Blood Institute, National Institutes of Health, Bethesda, Maryland 20892. Manuscript received June 9, 1988, and accepted July 13.

Our necropsy experience with myocardial infarction associated with cardiac amyloidosis is summarized here.

Of 61 necropsy patients aged 21 to 97 years (mean 64) with cardiac amyloidosis severe enough to cause cardiac dysfunction studied in this laboratory during the past 28 years,[12] 3 (5%) had transmural necrosis, 5 (8%) had transmural fibrosis of the left ventricular wall and 53 (87%) had neither necrosis nor fibrosis (Figure 1). One patient with necrosis, 3 with fibrosis and 9 with neither necrosis nor fibrosis had 1 or more epicardial coronary arteries severely narrowed by atherosclerotic plaque. Two patients with necrosis and 2 with fibrosis, plus 44 with neither, had no epicardial coronary artery narrowed >75% in cross-sectional area by atherosclerotic plaque.

In all 61 patients whose cardiac amyloid deposits were severe enough to cause dysfunction, amyloid depos-

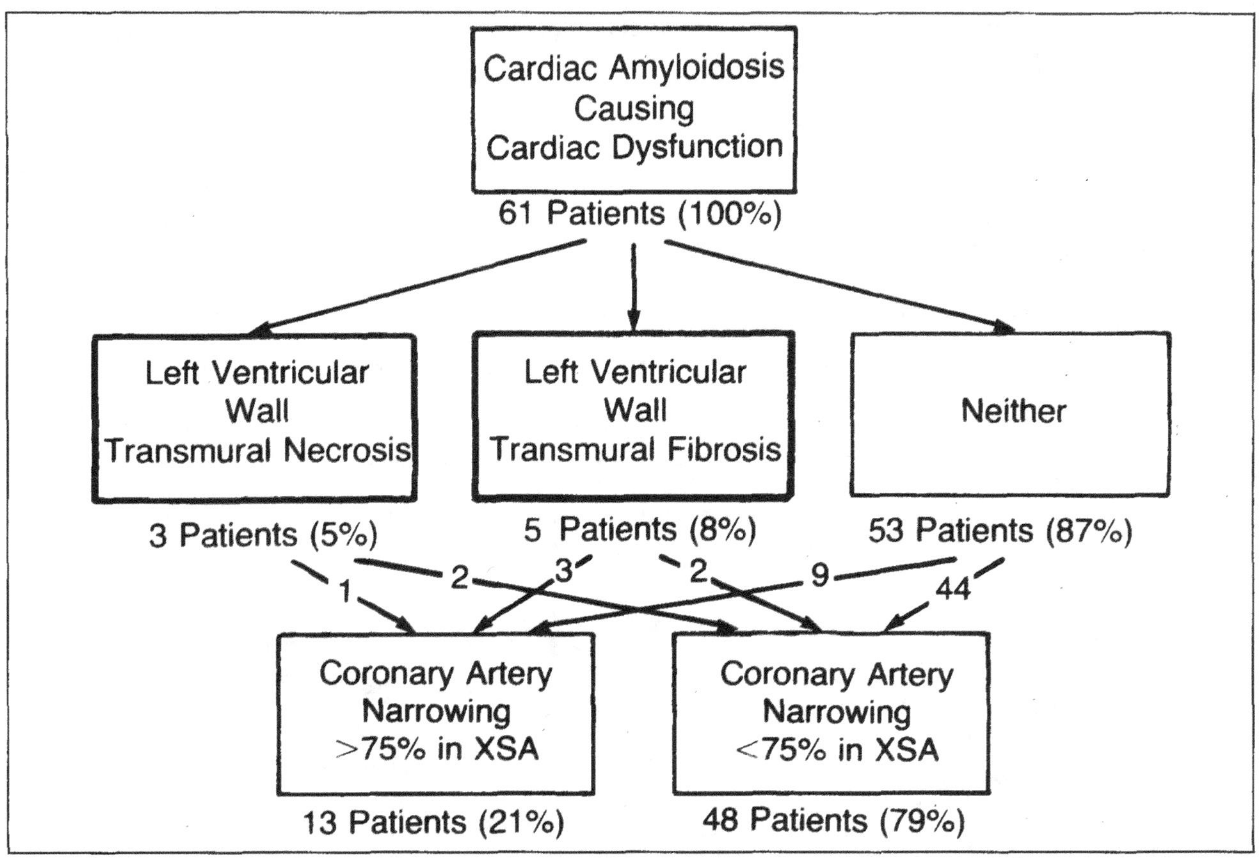

FIGURE 1. Diagram showing the frequency of left ventricular necrosis, the frequency of fibrosis and the frequency of coronary arterial narrowing in 61 necropsy patients with fatal cardiac amyloidosis. XSA = cross-sectional area.

its were present in the walls and lumens of the intramural coronary arteries, but the narrowing of the small coronary arteries by amyloid deposits did not appear to be greater in the patients with left ventricular necrosis and/or fibrosis than in those patients without myocardial lesions.

Of our 8 patients with transmural necrosis or fibrosis, none had clinical evidence of acute myocardial infarction. Of the 108 necropsy patients with cardiac amyloidosis reported by Smith and Hutchins[13], 5 (aged 54 to 89 years) had "severe . . . amyloid deposition" in the intramyocardial coronary arteries associated with myocardial necrosis or fibrosis. In all 5, the epicardial coronary arteries were free of atherosclerotic narrowing. No comment was made regarding the severity of intramural coronary artery amyloid deposits in those without myocardial necrosis or fibrosis or in those with concurrent atherosclerotic narrowing of the epicardial coronary arteries.

Jennette et al[14] reported a 70-year-old man with amyloidosis who had a clinically diagnosed fatal acute myocardial infarction. At necropsy, his epicardial coronary arteries were free of atherosclerotic narrowing; however, the lumens of the intramural coronary arteries were severely narrowed by amyloid deposits and the myocardium had multiple small areas of necrosis and fibrosis.

Thus, cardiac amyloidosis needs to be added to the list of conditions associated with transmural left ventricular necrosis or fibrosis unassociated with significant narrowing of 1 or more major epicardial coronary arteries.

1. McReynolds RA, Roberts WC. The intramural coronary arteries in hypertrophic cardiomyopathy (abstr). *Am J Cardiol 1975;35:120.*
2. Maron BJ, Wolfson JK, Epstein SE, Roberts WC. Intramural (small vessel) coronary artery disease in hypertrophic cardiomyopathy. *JACC 1986;8:545–557.*
3. Roberts WC, Siegel RJ, McManus BM. Idiopathic dilated cardiopathy: analysis of 152 necropsy patients. *Am J Cardiol 1987;60:1340–1355.*
4. Roberts WC. The structure of the aortic valve in clinically-isolated aortic stenosis. An autopsy study of 162 patients over 15 years of age. *Circulation 1970;42:91–97.*
5. Roberts WC. The congenitally bicuspid aortic valve. A study of 85 autopsy cases. *Am J Cardiol 1970;26:72–83.*
6. Roberts WC. Anatomically isolated aortic valvular disease. The case against its being of rheumatic etiology. *Am J Med 1970;49:151–159.*
7. Falcone MW, Roberts WC, Morrow AG, Perloff JK. Congenital aortic stenosis resulting from a unicommissural valve. Clinical and anatomic features in twenty-one adult patients. *Circulation 1971;44:272–280.*
8. Maron BJ, Redwood DR, Roberts WC, Henry WL, Morrow AG, Epstein SE. Tunnel subaortic stenosis. Left ventricular outflow tract obstruction produced by fibromuscular tubular narrowing. *Circulation 1976;54:406–416.*
9. Muna WFT, Ferrans VJ, Pierce JE, Roberts WC. Discrete subaortic stenosis in Newfoundland dogs: association of infective endocarditis. *Am J Cardiol 1978; 41:746–754.*
10. Roberts WC, Shemin RJ, Kent KM. Frequency and direction of interatrial shunting in valvular pulmonic stenosis with intact ventricular septum and without left ventricular inflow or outflow obstruction: An analysis of 127 patients treated by valvulotomy. *Am Heart J 1980;99:142–148.*
11. Roberts WC. Major anomalies of coronary arterial origin seen in adulthood. *Am Heart J 1986;111:941–963.*
12. Roberts WC, Waller BF. Cardiac amyloidosis causing cardiac dysfunction: analysis of 54 necropsy patients. *Am J Cardiol 1983;52:137–146.*
13. Smith RRL, Hutchins GM. Ischemic heart disease secondary to amyloidosis of intramyocardial arteries. *Am J Cardiol 1979;44:413–417.*
14. Jennette JC, Sheps DS, McNeill DD. Exclusively vascular systemic amyloidosis with visceral ischemia. *Arch Pathol Lab Med 1982;106:323–327.*

Morphologic Changes in Coronary Artery Seen Late After Endarterectomy

Amy H. Kragel, MD, Charles M. McIntosh, MD, PhD, and William C. Roberts, MD

Coronary endarterectomy occasionally is performed in conjunction with coronary artery bypass grafting. While information is available regarding the morphologic changes occurring late in the carotid artery after endarterectomy,[1-7] there is no information on histologic changes in coronary arteries late following endarterectomy. Herein we describe morphologic findings in a man who died 4.5 years after coronary endarterectomy.

W.N., a 77-year-old man, had his purely regurgitant mitral valve replaced and an endarterectomy of the right coronary artery followed by insertion of a saphenous vein conduit at age 73. Preoperatively, the left ventricular pressure was 144/14 mm Hg. Left ventricular angiography showed 4+/4+ mitral regurgitation. Coronary artery cineangiography before operation showed total occlusion of the right coronary artery distal to the second right ventricular branch. At operation, the mitral valve was typical of mitral valve prolapse. An endarterectomy was performed in the right coronary artery distal to the first right ventricular branch with removal of an 8-cm segment (Figure 1) of atheromatous plaque. A saphenous vein graft was inserted in the right coronary artery near the crux of the heart. He died

From the Pathology and Surgery Branches, National Heart, Lung, and Blood Institute, National Institutes of Health, Bethesda, Maryland 20892. Manuscript received November 18, 1988; revised manuscript received and accepted December 19, 1988.

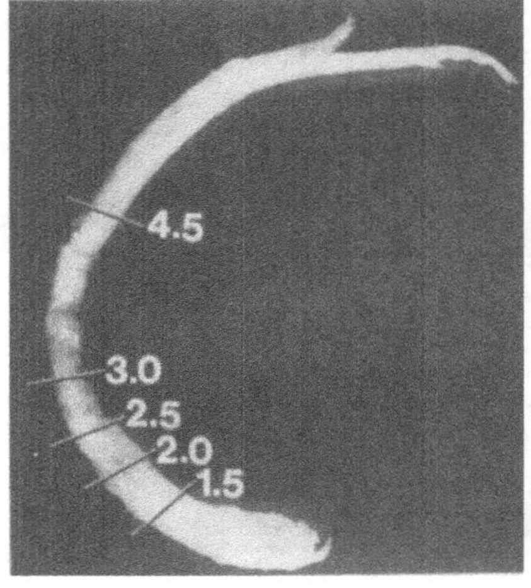

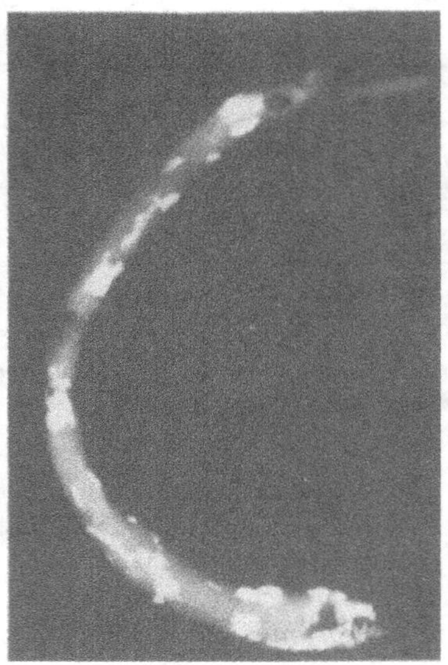

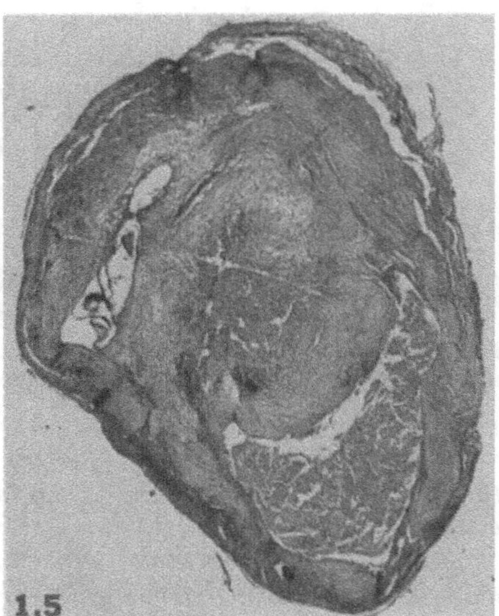

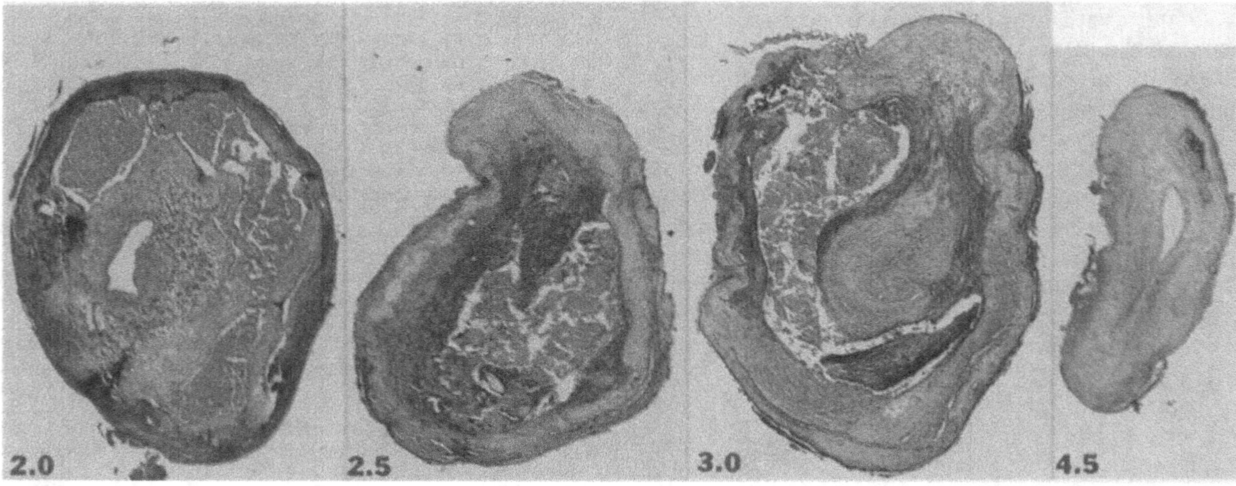

FIGURE 1. Gross photograph (original magnification × 2), radiograph (original magnification × 2) and Movat-stained sections (original magnification × 20) of the endarterectomy specimen. The approximate distance from the most proximal portion of the specimen (in cm) at which the histologic section was taken is noted on the gross photograph and in the corresponding panels. The specimen contains an atheromatous "core," which includes portions of internal elastic lamina and media (*arrow*). There is near total occlusion of the lumen by atherosclerotic plaque. The plaque contains large lipid "lakes" surrounded by fibrous tissue. In addition, foci of calcium, inflammatory infiltrates and small vascular channels are present.

suddenly at home 4.5 years after cardiac operation.

At necropsy, the heart weighed 970 g. A radiograph of the heart showed calcium in the mitral anulus and in the epicardial coronary arteries. There was no gross or histologic evidence of myocardial necrosis or fibrosis. The Hancock bioprosthesis in the mitral position appeared grossly free of any evidence of significant degeneration and no paravalvular communications were present.

The 4 major epicardial coronary arteries and the saphenous vein by-pass graft were excised, decalcified, sectioned at 5-mm intervals and examined histologically. The left anterior descending, left circumflex and right coronary arteries were all narrowed >75% in cross-sectional area by atherosclerotic plaque. Movat-stained sections of the native right coronary artery showed the proximal 3 cm (where endarterectomy presumably had not been performed) to be narrowed by calcified fibrous tissue containing scattered inflammatory infiltrates. The distal 8 cm (the presumed site of endarter-ectomy) was narrowed by a homogenous mixture of spindle cells and collagen. The internal elastic membrane could not be identified and the "media" were indistinguishable from intima (Figure 2). The saphenous vein graft was virtually occluded throughout its course by fibrous tissue containing small vascular channels (Figure 3).

Studies of the morphologic changes in surgical endarterectomy specimens removed for restenosis of the carotid artery have shown that restenosis occurring within 2 years of

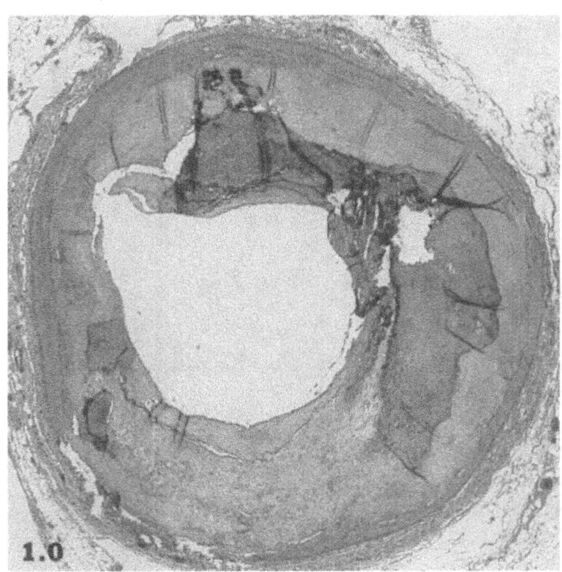
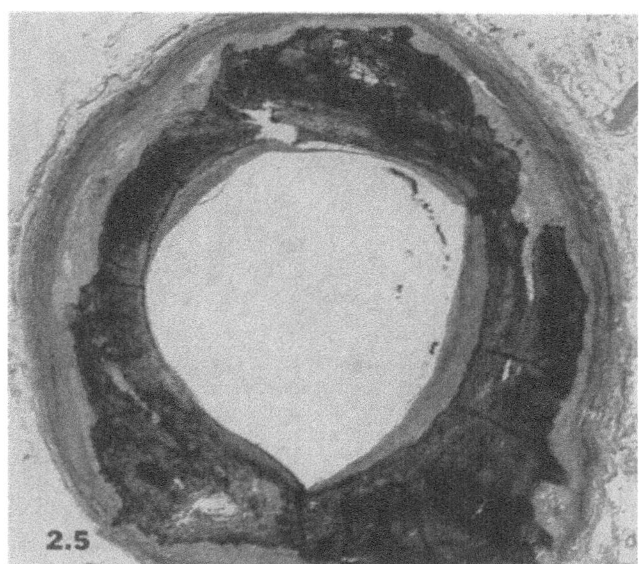
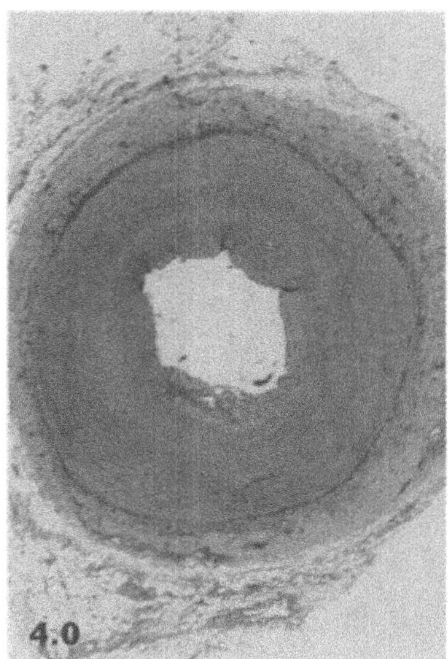
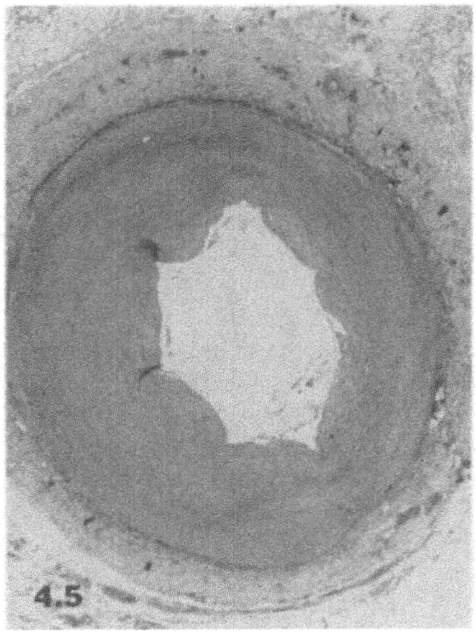
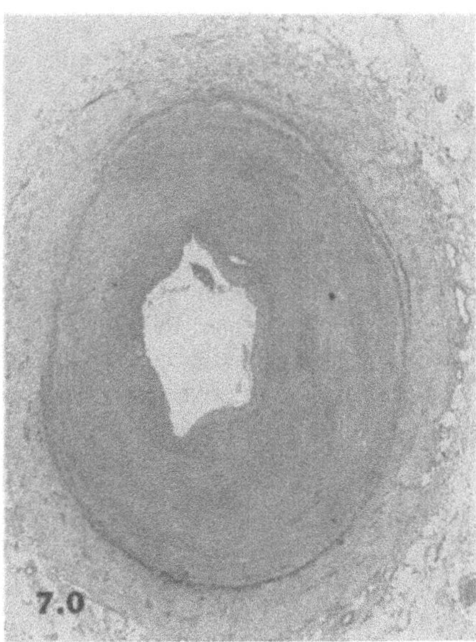

FIGURE 2. Movat-stained sections (each × 60) of the right coronary artery at necropsy. The distance (in cm) from the aortic ostium at which the section was taken is indicated on each section. Sections 1.0 and 2.5 were proximal to the endarterectomy site and they are composed of calcified fibrous tissue. Sections 4.0, 4.5 and 7.0 were taken from the site of endarterectomy and they are composed of a homogeneous mixture of spindle cells admixed with collagen. The internal elastic membrane cannot be identified in these distal sections.

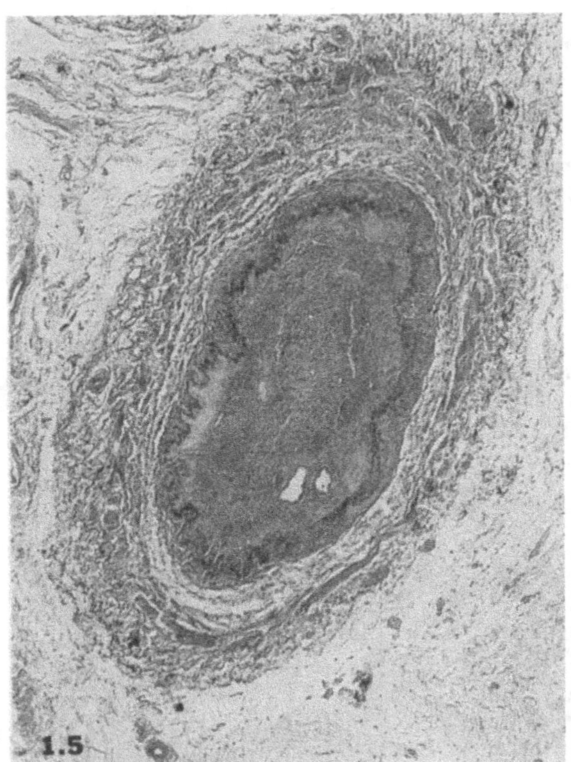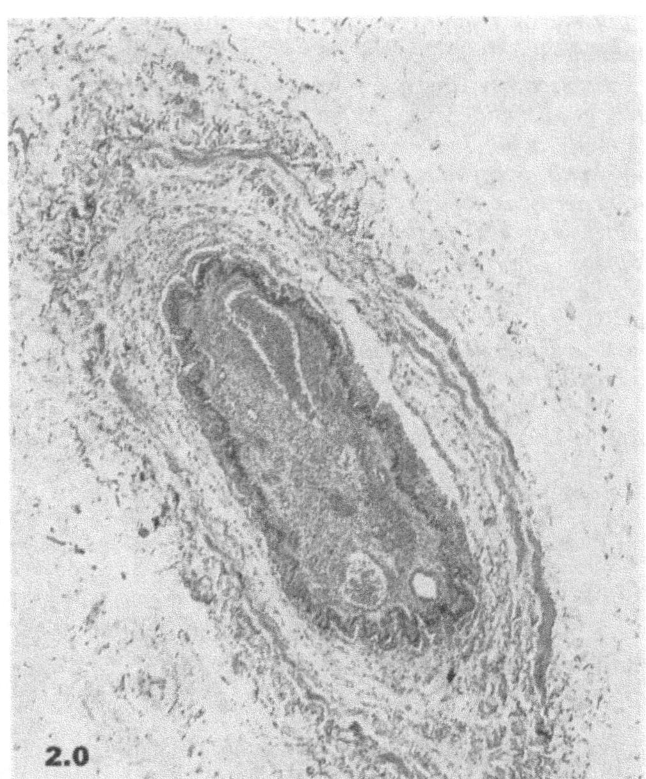

FIGURE 3. Movat-stained sections of the saphenous vein graft (× 60) taken at 1.5 cm and 2.0 cm from the proximal ostium showing near total obliteration of the lumen by fibrous tissue containing small vascular channels.

the initial surgical procedure is usually, but not always, due to a diffuse proliferation of spindle cells.[1,3,5] These cells, by electron microscopy, have features of both smooth muscle cells and fibroblasts.[2] Restenosis occurring late, i.e., >2 years after endarterectomy, is usually, but not always, due to "typical atherosclerotic plaque" containing various elements including fibrous tissue, hemosiderin and calcium.[1,3,5] Cases of early restenosis secondary to typical atherosclerotic plaque and late restenosis secondary to a proliferation of myofibroblasts have been described.[2,4,6,7]

In our patient, we studied plaque morphology of the native coronary artery at the site of endarterectomy and compared it to plaque morphology of the surgical endarterectomy specimen removed 4.5 years previously. The lumen of the endarterectomy specimen was narrowed by plaque composed of heavily calcified fibrous tissue containing pultaceous debris, inflammatory infiltrates and multiple small vascular channels. In contrast, the native coronary artery that had been the site of endarterectomy had no internal elastic membrane and its lumen was narrowed by nearly homogenous connective tissue containing spindle cells. While it is impossible to say when these changes occurred, they resemble those associated with early restenosis of the carotid artery. To our knowledge, this is the first description of coronary artery plaque morphology in a patient dying late after coronary endarterectomy.

1. Stoney RJ, String ST. Recurrent carotid stenosis. *Surgery 1976;80:705-710.*
2. French BN, Rewcastle NB. Recurrent carotid stenosis at the site of carotid endarterectomy. *Stroke 1977;8:597-605.*
3. Cossman D, Callow D, Stein A, Matsumoto G. Early restenosis after carotid endarterectomy. *Arch Surg 1978;113:275-278.*
4. Hertzer NR, Martinez BD, Beven EG. Recurrent stenosis after carotid endarterectomy. *Surg Gynecol Obstet 1979;149:360-364.*
5. Cantelmo NL, Cutler BS, Wheeler HB, Herrmann JB, Cardullo PA. Noninvasive detection of carotid stenosis following endarterectomy. *Arch Surg 1981;116:1005-1008.*
6. Das MB, Hertzer NR, Ratliff NB, O'Hara PJ, Bebin EG. Recurrent carotid stenosis: a five-year series of 65 reoperations. *Ann Surg 1985;202:28-35.*
7. Shumway SJ, Edwards WH, Jenkins JM, Mulherin JL Jr, Edwards WH Jr. Recurrent carotid stenosis: incidence and management. *Am Surg 1987; 53:61-65.*

Frequency of Rupture of the Left Ventricular Free Wall or Ventricular Septum Among Necropsy Cases of Fatal Acute Myocardial Infarction Since Introduction of Coronary Care Units

Shanthasundari G. Reddy, MD, and William C. Roberts, MD

Review of 18 published reports *before* the widespread use of cardiac care units disclosed that the frequency of rupture of the left ventricular free wall or ventricular septum among necropsy cases of acute myocardial infarction (AMI) ranged from 4 to 24% (mean 8%) (619 of 7,905 cases). The frequency of rupture of the left ventricular free wall or ventricular septum among necropsy patients with fatal AMI studied in this laboratory since 1968 was analyzed. Of 648 such patients, 204 (31%) had rupture of the left ventricular free wall or ventricular septum. Rupture occurred in 171 (40%) of 431 patients without healed myocardial infarcts (grossly visible left ventricular scars), and in 29 (13%) of 217 patients with a healed myocardial infarct (p <0.01). Thus, the frequency of rupture of the left ventricular free wall or ventricular septum during AMI appears to have increased substantially since the widespread use of coronary care units. Also, the frequency of rupture is nearly 3 times greater in those in whom rupture occurred during the first AMI compared to those with a previous infarct that healed.

(Am J Cardiol 1989;63:906–911)

From the Pathology Branch, National Heart, Lung, and Blood Institute, National Institutes of Health, Bethesda, Maryland. Manuscript received November 18, 1988; revised manuscript received and accepted January 26, 1989.

Address for reprints: William C. Roberts, MD, Pathology Branch, National Heart, Lung, and Blood Institute, Building 10, Room 2N258, National Institutes of Health, Bethesda, Maryland 20892.

In the period before the introduction of coronary care units, the reported frequency of cardiac rupture (left ventricular free wall or ventricular septum) among necropsy cases of fatal acute myocardial infarction (AMI) varied from 4 to 24% (mean 8%)[1-18] (Table I). Since the introduction of coronary care units, the reported frequency of rupture of the left ventricular free wall or ventricular septum among necropsy cases of fatal AMI has varied from 16 to 21% (mean 17%)[19-22] (Table II). We describe the frequency of rupture of the left ventricular free wall or ventricular septum in 648 patients with fatal AMI studied at necropsy.

METHODS

Inclusion and exclusion criteria: From January 1968 to March 1988 over 800 patients with AMI have been studied at necropsy in the Pathology Branch, National Heart, Lung, and Blood Institute. The present study was limited to patients with grossly visible AMI at necropsy associated with narrowing of 1 or more major (right, left anterior descending or left circumflex) epicardial coronary arteries >75% in cross-sectional area by atherosclerotic plaque with or without associated coronary arterial thrombus. Patients in whom the interval from onset of the AMI to death was >6 weeks were excluded. Patients with a major cardiac disease other than atherosclerotic coronary artery disease were excluded. Thus, patients with primary valvular heart disease including cases of mitral stenosis or pure mitral regurgitation (other than that caused by papillary muscle dysfunction), valvular aortic stenosis or pure aortic regurgitation, infective endocarditis and hypertrophic cardiomyopathy were excluded. With 1 exception, all patients who had had a cardiac operation were excluded. The exception was 21 patients who underwent coronary artery bypass grafting during the period of AMI; they were included. (Of these 21 patients, 2 had rupture: free wall in 1 and septum in 1.) Patients who had had coronary artery bypass grafting for myocardial ischemia (angina pectoris, congestive heart failure, positive exercise stress test) and had an AMI postoperatively were excluded. Also excluded were patients who had received long-term corticosteroid therapy, patients with

TABLE I Reported Frequency 1938–1968 of Rupture of the Left Ventricular Free Wall or Ventricular Septum 7905 Necropsy Patients with Fatal Acute Myocardial Infarction

Reference	Author (year)	No. of Patients With AMI	No. (%) with Rupture of LV or VS	Location of Rupture		Rupture Cases· M/F	Sex of Ages (yrs) of Rupture Cases Range (mean)
				LV	VS		
1	Bean (1938)	300	17 (6)	16	1	8/9	—
2	Edmonson & Hoxie (1942)	865	72 (8)	59	13	40/32	30–90 (—)
3	Friedman & White (1944)	105	10 (10)	10	0	7/3	51–80 (66)
4	Diaz-River & Miller (1948)	53	5 (9)	4	1	1/4	—
5	Wang et al (1948)	267	23 (9)	22	1	—	—
6	Selzer (1948)	95	8 (8)	7	1	—	—
7	Zinn & Cosby (1950)	430	34 (8)	34	0	12/22	54–82 (71)
8	Oblath et al (1952)	1,026	80 (9)	80	0	47/33	60–80 (—)
9	Wessler et al (1952)	124	20 (16)	15	5	—	—
10	Waldron et al (1954)	545	40 (8)	40	0	—	—
11	Goetz & Gropper (1954)	145	14 (10)	11	3	—	56–76 (—)
12	Maher et al (1956)	183	21 (12)	19	2	10/11	54–92 (69)
13	Griffith et al (1961)	1,212	52 (4)	44	8	—	—
14	Spiekerman et al (1962)	87	21 (24)	18	3	10/11	—
15	Ross & Young (1963)	606	43 (7)	43	0	27/16	35–90 (—)
16	London & London (1965)	1,001	47 (5)	42	5	27/20	— (69)
17	Sievers (1966)	811	104 (13)	104	0	52/52	— (69)
18	Sugiura et al (1968)	50	8 (16)	6	2	5/3	68–88 (77)
	Total	7,905	619 (8%)	574 (93%)	45 (7%)	246/216 (53%)/(47%)	30–92 (—)

AMI = acute myocardial infarction; LV = left ventricular free wall, VS = ventricular septum, — = no information available

TABLE II Reported Frequency 1970–1987 of Rupture of the Left Ventricular Free Wall or Ventricular Septum in 920 Necropsy Patients With Fatal Acute Myocardial Infarction

Reference	Author (year)	No. of Patients With Fatal AMI	No (%) with Rupture of LV or VS	Location of Rupture		Sex of Rupture Cases· M/F	Ages (yrs) of Rupture Cases Range (mean)
				LV	VS		
19	Hammer et al (1972)	47	10 (21)	7	3	6/4	55–80 (64)
20	Rasmussen et al (1979)	401	64 (16)	61	3	42/30	46–90 (—)
21	Dellborg et al (1985)	329	56 (17)	51	5	28/28	— (71)
22	Hiramori (1987)	143	26 (18)	20	6	—	23–92 (62)
	Total	920	156 (17)	139 (89%)	17 (11%)	76/98 (81%)/(18%)	23–92 (—)

Abbreviations as in Table I

a neoplasm involving the heart and patients with radiation heart disease.[23,24] After excluding patients with AMI associated with the aforementioned conditions, 648 patients remained and they form the basis of this study. Each heart had been examined initially by one of us (WCR). The grossly visible myocardial infarct was confirmed histologically in all cases.

Sources of cases: The 648 cases came from 81 different hospitals. Of the 648 cases, 552 (85%) came from 16 hospitals (Figure 1), and the remaining 96 cases came from 65 hospitals. Of these latter 96 cases, 58 were cases involved in multicenter studies where the Pathology Branch served as the central coordinating laboratory. Therefore, although 33 different hospitals submitted the 58 cases, in actuality the multicenter nature of the submitting protocol was as if only 2 hospitals provided the 58 cases. Thus, only 38 (6%) of the 648 cases came from hospitals that submitted only ≤3 cases; these 38 cases came from 32 different hospitals.

Statistical analysis: The analysis of variance both between and within groups was done by the chi-square and *t* test methods.

RESULTS

Frequency of cardiac rupture: Certain pertinent data in the 648 cases are summarized in Table III. Of the 648 cases, 204 (31%) had cardiac rupture and 444 (69%) did not (Figure 2). Of the 204 rupture cases, the site of rupture was *left ventricular free wall* in 137 (67%), *ventricular septum* in 55 (27%), *both* left ventricular free wall and ventricular septum in 7 (4%) and *both* left ventricular free wall and papillary muscle in 5 (2%).

Comparison of rupture to nonrupture cases: Comparison of the 204 rupture cases with the 444 nonrupture cases disclosed no significant differences in mean age (68 vs 64 years), frequency of a history of systemic hypertension (42 vs 50%) and mean heart

TABLE III Clinical and Necropsy Observations in Fatal Acute Myocardial Infarction (AMI) With and Without Rupture of the Left Ventricular Free Wall (LV) or Ventricular Septum (VS)

	AMI With Rupture of LV or VS (n = 204)	AMI Without Rupture of LV or VS (n = 444)	Total (n = 648)
Age range (yrs)	43–94 (68 ± 10)	35–95 (64 ± 12)	35–95 (65 ± 11)
Men	43–85 (63 ± 9)	35–93 (62 ± 11)	35–93 (63 ± 11)
Women	46–94 (73 ± 9)*	37–95 (69 ± 12)*	37–94 (71 ± 11)
Sex			
Men (%)	112 (55)*	311 (70)*	423 (65)
Women (%)	92 (45)*	133 (30)*	225 (35)
Systemic hypertension (%)	101 (50)	185 (42)	286 (44)
Diabetes mellitus (%)	28 (13)*	115 (27)*	143 (22)
Heart weight range (g)			
Men	320–810 (486 ± 96)	280–770 (496 ± 100)	280–810 (493 ± 99)
Women	275–645 (396 ± 79)	270–670 (426 ± 85)	270–670 (413 ± 83)
Left ventricular scar (%)	29 (13)*	188 (42)*	217 (33)

* p <0 01.
All ± values are mean ± standard deviation

weights in both men (486 vs 496 g) and women (396 vs 426 g). Significant (p <0.01) differences between the rupture and nonrupture groups were found in the frequency of men (55 vs 70%) and women (45 vs 30%), respectively, frequency of diabetes mellitus (adult onset in all) (13 vs 27%) and presence of left ventricular grossly visible scar (13 vs 42%).

Comparison of cardiac rupture frequency in patients with to those without a healed myocardial infarct: The patients with a grossly visible left ventricular scar (healed myocardial infarct) had a lower frequency of rupture than did the patients without an associated healed infarct (Figures 3 and 4). Of the 648 patients, 217 (33%) had a healed myocardial infarct and 29 (13%) of these had rupture of the left ventricular free wall or ventricular septum; of the 431 patients without a healed infarct, 171 (40%) had rupture at either of these 2 sites.

Frequency of cardiac rupture among the submitting hospitals: The frequency of rupture of the left ventricular free wall or ventricular septum among the 11 hospitals each submitting >15 cases was 25% (129 of 519); among the 5 hospitals each submitting 5 to 9 cases, 69% (22 of 32); among the 32 hospitals each submitting 3 or

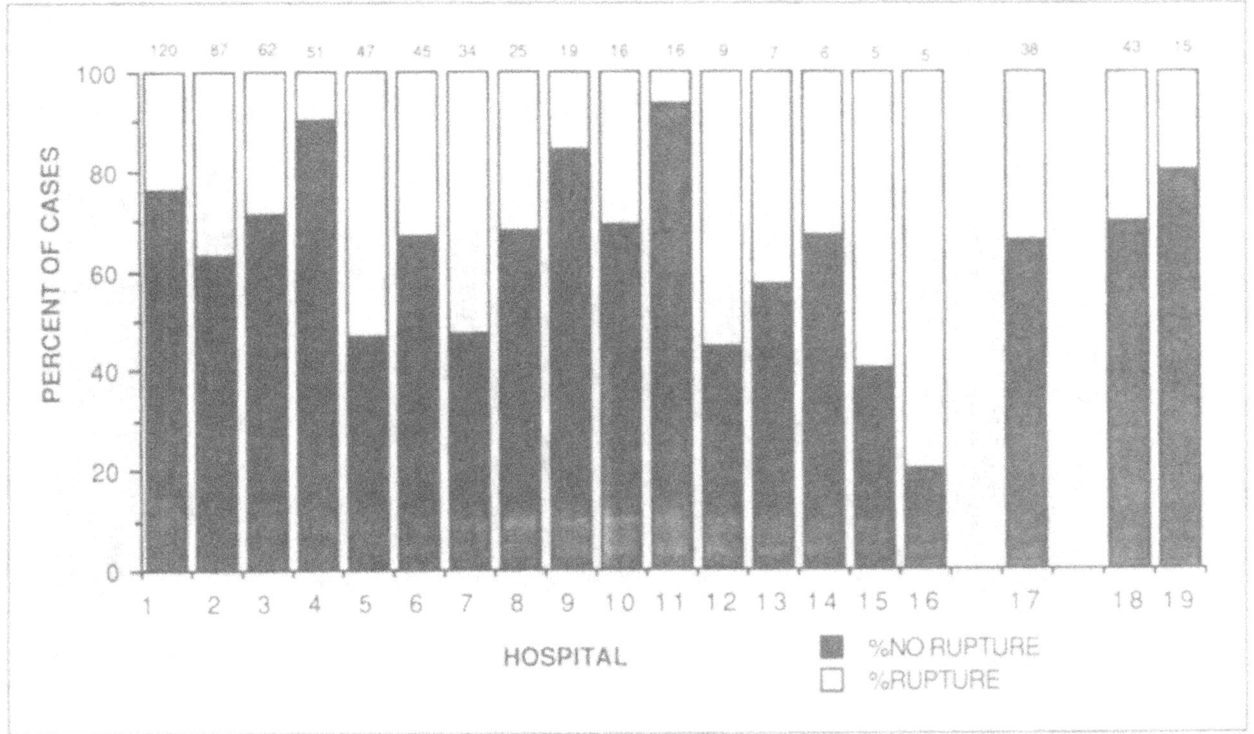

FIGURE 1. Percent of necropsy cases of acute myocardial infarction with and without rupture of the left ventricular free wall or ventricular septum from 16 hospitals (nos. 1 through 16) each submitting ≥5 cases, 32 hospitals (no. 17) each submitting ≤3 cases and from 2 multicenter studies (nos. 18 and 19) where the Pathology Branch served as the central receiving center. *Numbers* at the *top of the bars* are the number of cases.

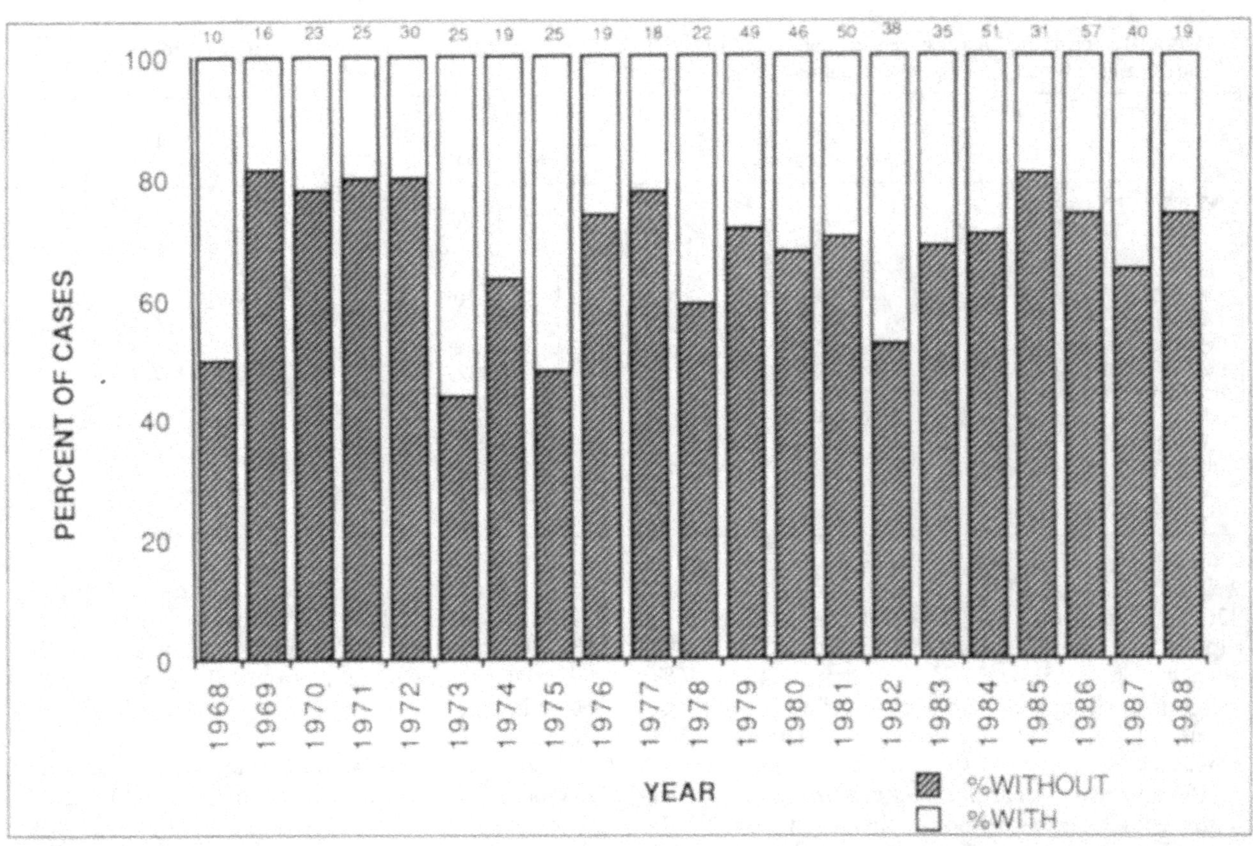

FIGURE 2. Comparison of percent of cases of fatal acute myocardial infarction studied each year at necropsy with and without rupture and including cases with a grossly visible left ventricular scar. *Numbers* at the *top of the bars* are the number of cases.

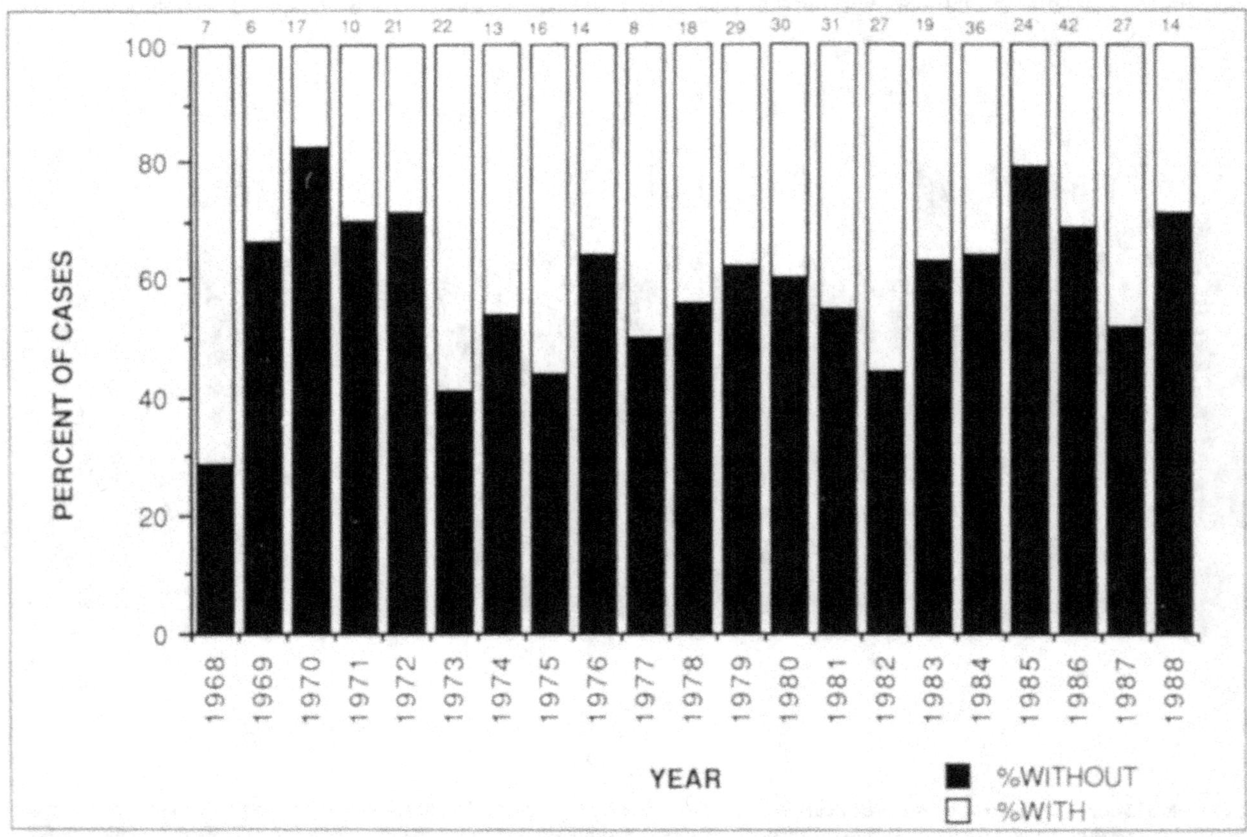

FIGURE 3. Comparison of percent of cases of acute myocardial infarction studied each year at necropsy with and without rupture in hearts without a grossly visible left ventricular scar. *Numbers* at the *top of the bars* are the number of cases.

fewer cases, 34% (13 of 38); and among the 33 submitting hospitals involved in multicenter studies, 28% (16 of 58).

DISCUSSION

The present study and the 4 previous ones[19–22] (Table II) since the introduction of coronary care units provide evidence that cardiac rupture during AMI has increased in frequency compared to the reported studies[1–18] before their introduction. Among our 648 patients with fatal AMI unassociated with other major cardiac conditions, rupture of the left ventricular free wall or ventricular septum was found at necropsy in 31%. The frequency of the 2 ruptures was much higher in the patients without a previous myocardial infarct compared to those with a left ventricular scar (healed infarct) (40 [171 of 431] vs 13% [29 of 217], p <0.01).

The reason the frequency of cardiac rupture during AMI appears to have increased since the widespread use of coronary care units is unclear. The most plausible explanation is that the frequency of fatal arrhythmias during AMI has significantly decreased. If the frequency of 1 cause of death, namely arrhythmias, has decreased, another cause of death must increase, and that other cause appears to be cardiac rupture. A much less likely explanation is the increased use of nonsteroidal antiinflammatory drugs in the last 2 decades. Anecdotal evidence has been presented by 1 center[25] but not by another[26] that patients with AMI receiving nonsteroidal

antiinflammatory agents for "pericarditis" have a higher frequency of cardiac rupture than do patients who do not receive these drugs during AMI. What percent of our patients were taking nonsteroidal antiinflammatory drugs during the period of AMI is uncertain. Corticosteroid therapy might also increase the frequency of cardiac rupture because these drugs delay the healing process.[27] Patients known to have taken corticosteroid therapy on a long-term basis, however, were excluded from the present study.

It has been suggested that rupture of the left ventricular free wall or ventricular septum occurs less frequently in patients with AMI treated immediately with β blockers, and that this accounts, in part, for the reduction in the very early mortality in such patients.[28] Although few of our 648 necropsy patients appeared to have received β blockers early after onset of AMI, the number of patients receiving such therapy is not known in either our rupture or nonrupture groups.

It also has been suggested that thrombolytic therapy might increase the frequency of rupture of the left ventricular free wall or ventricular septum during AMI and that this increase accounts for the higher mortality during the first 24 hours after onset of AMI compared to patients not treated with thrombolytic agents.[29] Among our 648 necropsy patients, 56 (9%) had received either streptokinase or recombinant tissue-type plasminogen activator during the first few hours after onset of infarction: 18 (32%) had rupture of the left ventricular free

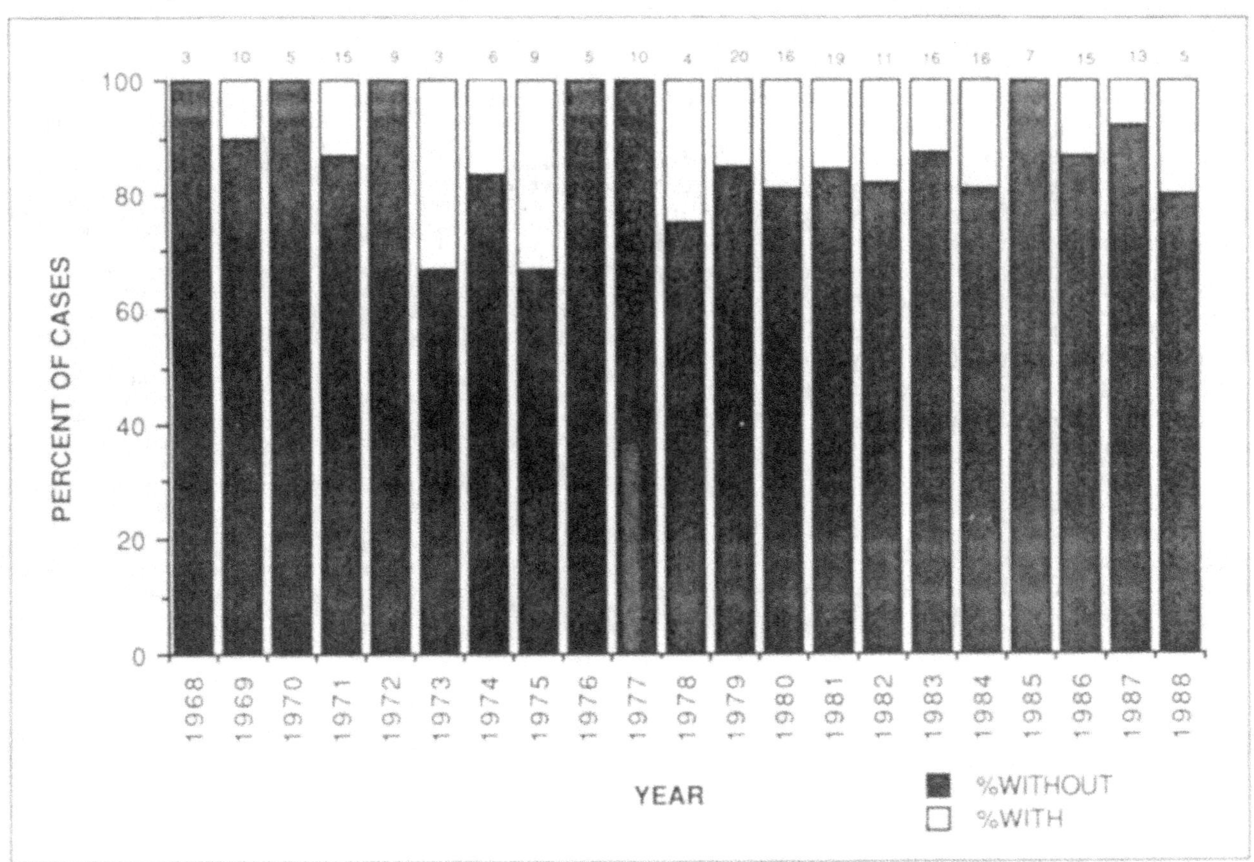

FIGURE 4. Comparison of percent of cases of fatal acute myocardial infarction studied each year at necropsy with and without rupture in hearts with a grossly visible left ventricular scar. *Numbers* at the *top of the bars* are the number of cases.

wall or ventricular septum, a percentage similar to that in the patients who had not received thrombolytic therapy (186 of 592 [31%]).

Patients with rupture of a left ventricular papillary muscle during AMI presented a problem for inclusion in this study. Among our 204 patients with rupture of the left ventricular free wall or ventricular septum, 5 (2%) also had rupture (partial or incomplete in all 5) of a left ventricular papillary muscle and they were included among the rupture cases. Among our 444 patients with fatal AMI without rupture of the left ventricular free wall or ventricular septum, 18 patients had rupture (partial in 14) of a left ventricular papillary muscle. We considered it preferable to include these 18 papillary muscle rupture cases with the 444 who did not have rupture of the left ventricular free wall or ventricular septum because none of the 18 reports,[1-18] which included 7,905 necropsy cases reported from 1938 to 1968, mentioned rupture of a left ventricular papillary muscle.

Finally, the question of biased case selection—accounting for the higher frequency of rupture in our patients compared to those reported before 1969—deserves comment. Figure 1 attempts to deal with this issue by showing the frequency of rupture of the left ventricular free wall or ventricular septum in the hearts studied from each of the submitting medical centers. It is clear that the frequency of rupture of either left ventricular free wall or ventricular septum varied considerably among the various submitting hospitals. It is our understanding that for many years our laboratory received all or nearly all of the "cardiac cases" from hospitals 1 to 5 (Figure 1), and the number of cases received from these 5 institutions, namely 367, accounts for 57% of the cases examined by us. Thus, although case selection is a potential bias in any clinical study and probably was a factor in the present study, it is unlikely in our view that case selection by itself could have produced such a high frequency of cardiac rupture in our cases compared to those reported before 1969. The reported frequency of left ventricular free wall or ventricular septal rupture during AMI after widespread use of coronary care units is also much higher than that in the period before coronary care units (17 [Table II] vs 8% [Table I]).

REFERENCES

1. Bean WB. Infarction of heart: III. Clinical course and morphological findings. *Ann Intern Med 1938;12:71–94.*

2. Edmonson HA, Hoxie HJ Hypertension and cardiac rupture. *Am Heart J 1942;24:719–733.*

3. Friedman S, White PD. Rupture of the heart in myocardial infarction. *Ann Intern Med 1944;21:778–782.*

4. Diaz-Rivera RS, Miller AJ. Rupture of heart following acute myocardial infarction: incidence in public hospital, with five illustrative cases including one of perforation of interventricular septum diagnosed ante mortem. *Am Heart J 1948;35:126–133.*

5. Wang CH, Bland EF, White PD. Note on coronary occlusion and myocardial infarction found post mortem at Massachusetts General Hospital during twenty year period from 1926 to 1945 inclusive *Ann Intern Med 1948;29:601–606.*

6. Selzer A. Immediate sequelae of myocardial infarction: their relation to prognosis. *Am J Med Sci 1948;216:172–178.*

7. Zinn WJ. Cosby RS. Myocardial infarction: statistical study of 679 autopsy proven cases. *Am J Med 1950;8:169–176.*

8. Oblath RW, Levinson DC, Griffith GC. Factors influencing rupture of the heart after myocardial infarction. *JAMA 1952;149:1276–1281.*

9. Wessler S, Zoll PM. Schlesinger MI. The pathogenesis of spontaneous cardiac rupture. *Circulation 1952;6:334–351.*

10. Waldron BR, Fennell RH, Castleman B, Bland EF. Myocardial rupture and hemopericardium associated with anticoagulant therapy. *N Engl J Med 1954; 251:892–894.*

11. Goetz AA, Gropper AN. Perforation of the interventricular septum. Report of three cases with ante-mortem diagnosis. *Am Heart J 1954;48:103–140.*

12. Maher JF. Mallory GK. Laurenz GA. Rupture of the heart after myocardial infarction. *N Engl J Med 1956;255:1–10.*

13. Griffith GC, Hedge B, Oblath RW. Factors in myocardial rupture. An analysis of 204 cases at Los Angeles County Hospital between 1924–1959. *Am J Cardiol 1961;8:792–798.*

14. Spiekerman RE, Brandenburg JT, Anchor RWP, Edwards JE. The spectrum of coronary heart disease in a community of 30,000. A clinicopathologic study. *Circulation 1962;35:57–65.*

15. Ross RM, Young JA. Clinical and necropsy findings in rupture of the myocardium. A review of 43 cases. *Scott Med J 1963;8:222–226.*

16. London RE, London SB Rupture of the heart. A critical analysis of 47 consecutive autopsy cases. *Circulation 1965;31:202–208.*

17. Sievers J. Cardiac rupture in acute myocardial infarction. *Geriatrics 1966;21:125–130.*

18. Sugiura M, Okada R, Morii T, Hiraoka K, Shimada H, Nakanishi A. A clinico pathological study on the cardiac rupture following myocardial infarction in the aged. *Jpn Heart J 1968;9:265–280.*

19. Hammer J, Fabian J, Pavlovic J, Smid J. Myocardial rupture in acute myocardial infarction. *Cor Vasa 1972;14:180–187.*

20. Rasmussen S, Leth A, Kjoller E, Pedersen A. Cardiac rupture in acute myocardial infarction. *Acta Med Scand 1979;205:11–16.*

21. Dellborg M, Held P, Swedberg K, Vedin A. Rupture of the myocardium. occurrence and risk factors. *Br Heart J 1985;54:11–16.*

22. Hiramori K. Major causes of death from acute myocardial infarction in a coronary care unit. *Jpn Circ J 1987;51:1041–1047.*

23. Brosius FC III, Roberts WC. Radiation heart disease. Analysis of 16 young (age 15 to 33 years) necropsy patients who received 3500 rads to the heart. *Am J Med 1981;70:519–530.*

24. Reynolds RA, Gold AL, Roberts WC. Coronary heart disease after mediastinal irradiation for Hodgkin's disease. *Am J Med 1976;60:39–45.*

25. Boden WE, Sadaniantz A. Ventricular septal rupture during ibuprofen therapy for pericarditis after acute myocardial infarction. *Am J Cardiol 1985;55:1631–1632.*

26. Spodick DH. Safety of ibuprofen for acute myocardial infarction pericarditis. *Am J Cardiol 1986;57:896–897.*

27. Bulkley BH, Roberts WC. Steroid therapy during acute myocardial infarction. A cause of delayed healing and of ventricular aneurysm *Am J Med 1974;56:244–250.*

28. ISIS-1 (First International Study of Infarct Survival) Collaborative Group. Randomised trial of intravenous atenolol among 16,027 cases of suspected acute myocardial infarction: ISIS-1. *Lancet 1986;2:57–65.*

29. ISIS-2 (Second International Study of Infarct Survival) Collaborative Group. Randomised trial of intravenous streptokinase, oral aspirin, both, or neither among 17,187 cases of suspected acute myocardial infarction: ISIS-2. *Lancet 1988;2:349–360.*

Qualitative and Quantitative Comparison of Amounts of Narrowing by Atherosclerotic Plaques in the Major Epicardial Coronary Arteries at Necropsy in Sudden Coronary Death, Transmural Acute Myocardial Infarction, Transmural Healed Myocardial Infarction and Unstable Angina Pectoris

William C. Roberts, MD

The amounts of narrowing of the 4 major (left main, left anterior descending, left circumflex and right) epicardial coronary arteries by atherosclerotic plaques were compared in 4 subsets of coronary patients. Of the 129 patients studied at necropsy, an average of 2.7 of the 4 arteries was narrowed >75% in cross-sectional area at some point (0.7/4 in controls), and the group with unstable angina pectoris (3.2/4) had more narrowing than did the groups with sudden coronary death (2.8/4), acute myocardial infarction (2.7/4) and healed myocardial infarction (2.3/4). Each of the 4 major epicardial coronary arteries was divided into 5-mm long segments and a histologic section was prepared and stained by the Movat method of each of the 6,461 segments in the 129 patients and in the 1,849 segments in the 40 control subjects. In the 129 patients, 35% of the 5-mm segments were narrowed 75 to 100% in cross-sectional area (3% in controls) and the group with unstable angina had the highest percent (48%) of segments severely narrowed compared to the groups with sudden coronary death (36%), acute myocardial infarction (34%) and healed myocardial infarction (31%). Thus, of the 4 subsets of patients with fatal coronary artery disease studied at necropsy, those with unstable angina pectoris had the most severe and extensive coronary artherosclerosis.

(Am J Cardiol 1989;64:324–328)

From the Pathology Branch, National Heart, Lung, and Blood Institute, Bethesda, Maryland. Manuscript received May 4, 1989, and accepted May 19.

Address for reprints: William C. Roberts, MD, Building 10, Room 2N258, National Institutes of Health, Bethesda, Maryland 20892.

Ten years ago my colleagues and I began examining at necropsy the 4 major epicardial coronary arteries in what we have called a *quantitative* manner. The left main, left anterior descending, left circumflex and right coronary arteries are excised from the heart intact and divided into 5-mm segments. A histologic section was then prepared from each segment. Using this approach, we have examined in the same manner and with similar control subjects the major epicardial coronary arteries in patients with sudden coronary death;[1] transmural acute myocardial infarction;[2] transmural healed myocardial infarction with noncardiac death,[3] with chronic and eventually fatal congestive heart failure without left ventricular aneurysm[4] and with left ventricular aneurysm;[5] and in patients with unstable angina pectoris dying at cardiac catheterization or shortly after coronary artery bypass grafting.[6] This article summarizes these previous studies and, in turn, compares the results of the previous separate studies in these various subsets of coronary patients.

METHODS

Patients: A total of 129 necropsy patients, each of whom had had a coronary event, were studied (Tables I and II). They included 27 patients with transmural (involving greater than the inner half of the left ventricular wall) acute myocardial infarction, which by history and by histologic examination was between 1 and 30 days old; 49 patients with transmural healed myocardial infarction with death either from progressive congestive heart failure ("ischemic cardiomyopathy") without left ventricular aneurysm (9 patients) or from a noncardiac condition (18 patients) or those with left ventricular aneurysm (22 patients); 22 patients with clinically isolated, unstable angina pectoris (without historical evidence at any time of acute myocardial infarction or congestive heart failure) and death within 7 days of an aortocoronary bypass operation or death during a cardiac catheterization procedure; and 31 patients who died suddenly, i.e., within 6 hours after onset of chest pain, which if

TABLE I Number of Major (Right, Left Main, Left Anterior Descending and Left Circumflex) Coronary Arteries Narrowed >75% in Cross-Sectional Area by Atherosclerotic Plaque in Fatal Coronary Artery Disease

Coronary Event	Pts (n)	Mean Age (yrs)	No. of Four Arteries/Pt >75% ↓ in CSA by Plaque				
			4	3	2	1	Mean
Sudden coronary death	31	47	3	20	6	2	2.8
Acute myocardial infarction	27	59	3	14	10	0	2.7
Healed myocardial infarction							
Asymptomatic	18	66	0	7	7	4	2.2
Chronic CHF without aneurysm	9	63	0	3	5	1	2.2
Left ventricular aneurysm	22	61	1	12	6	3	2.5
Angina pectoris/unstable	22	48	10	8	3	1	3.2
Total (%)	129	56	17 (13)	64 (50)	37 (29)	11 (8)	2.7
Controls (%)	40	52	0 (0)	5 (5)	12 (13)	21 (23)	0.7

CHF = congestive heart failure; CSA = cross-sectional area.

present, began outside the hospital, who never had evidence of congestive cardiac failure, and who at necropsy had >75% cross-sectional area narrowing of at least 1 of the 4 major coronary arteries and no ventricular wall myocardial coagulation necrosis. Patients with associated primary valvular, congenital or pericardial heart diseases, hypertrophic cardiomyopathy or other myocardial diseases not secondary to coronary artery disease (CAD) and patients who had had a cardiac operation (other than the unstable angina group) were excluded.

The coronary arteries in all 129 patients were studied in similar fashion. The hearts were fixed for at least 1 day in formalin. The 4 major epicardial coronary arteries were then excised intact, x-rayed and fixed for at least another day. Following decalcification (if necessary), each of the 4 major coronary arteries were cut transversely to their longitudinal axes into approximately 5-mm long segments and each segment was labeled sequentially from either its aortic ostium or from its origin from the left main. Of the coronary arteries, the average length (in cm) of the right was 11; left main, 1; left anterior descending, 10; and left circumflex, 6. The 5-mm segments were labeled, processed in alcohol and xylene, dehydrated and embedded in paraffin. Then 2 histologic sections were cut and stained from each paraffin block. The Movat stain was used on 1 histologic section, and all determinations of luminal narrowing were based on examination of the Movat-stained sections. The degrees of narrowing were based on histologic examination of each cross-section magnified 25 to 50 times. The judgment regarding the degree of luminal narrowing of each 5-mm segment was based on the degree of luminal obliteration within the luminal circle bordered by the internal elastic membrane. The circle was visually subdivided into 4 equally sized quadrants. The percent of narrowing in each 5-mm segment was determined as follows: 0 to 25, 26 to 50, 51 to 75 and 76 to 100%. The observations in the patients with CAD were compared to controls, all of whom died from noncardiac causes, mainly acute leukemia. None of the control subjects had evidence of cardiac dysfunction or myocardial ischemia during life, all had had normal

(<140/90 mm Hg) systemic arterial pressures and all had normal sized (<350 g in women and <400 g in men) hearts at necropsy.

RESULTS

Qualitative studies: Table I summarizes the number of major (right, left main, left anterior descending and left circumflex) epicardial coronary arteries narrowed >75% in cross-sectional area by atherosclerotic plaque alone in the patients with fatal CAD. Among the 129 patients, 516 major epicardial coronary arteries were examined and of them 345 (67%) were narrowed at some point 76 to 100% in cross-sectional area by atherosclerotic plaque. In contrast, of 40 control subjects, 160 major epicardial coronary arteries were examined and of them 60 (38%) were narrowed at some point >75% in cross-sectional area by plaque. Among the 129 coronary patients, only 11 (8%) had a single coronary artery severely (>75% in cross-sectional area) narrowed (controls = 23%); 37 (29%) had 2 arteries so narrowed (controls = 13%); 64 (50%) had 3 arteries severely narrowed (controls = 5%) and 17 patients (13%) had all 4 major arteries so narrowed (controls = 0). Thus, of the 4 major coronary arteries in the coronary patients an average of 2.7 were narrowed >75% in cross-sectional area by plaque and among the control subjects, 0.7 of 4.

The number of major coronary arteries severely narrowed by atherosclerotic plaque among the various subsets of coronary patients was relatively similar except for the unstable angina patients (Table I). Among the 31 *sudden coronary death* patients, an average of 2.8 of the 4 major arteries were narrowed severely; this is virtually identical to that of the 27 patients with *transmural acute myocardial infarction*, all of whom died in a coronary care unit. Only 2 of the 31 sudden death victims and none of the 27 acute myocardial infarction victims had only a single coronary artery ("1-vessel disease") severely narrowed.

The *healed myocardial infarction* group was divided into 3 subgroups. One consisted of patients who had had an acute myocardial infarct that healed; thereafter there was never clinical evidence of myocardial isch-

TABLE II Amounts of Cross-Sectional Area Narrowing of Each 5-mm Segment of the Four Major (Right, Left Main, Left Anterior Descending and Left Circumflex) Epicardial Coronary Arteries by Atherosclerotic Plaques in Subjects with Fatal Coronary Artery Disease

Subgroup	Pts (n)	Mean Age (yrs)	No. 5-mm Segments	Percent Segments Narrowed				Mean Score	Mean % Narrowing/ 5-mm Segments
				0–25%	26–50%	51–75%	76–100%		
Sudden coronary death	31	47	1,564	7	23	34	36	2.98	67
Acute myocardial infarction	27	59	1,403	5	23	38	34	3.01	68
Healed myocardial infarction									
Asymptomatic	18	66	924	11	23	35	31 ⎫	2.87	64
Chronic CHF							⎬ 31%		
without aneurysm	9	63	529	11	23	37	29	2.78	61
LV aneurysm	22	61	992	4	21	42	33 ⎭	3.03	68
Angina pectoris	22	48	1,049	11	12	29	48	3.12	70
Total	129	56	6,461	8	21	36	35	2.98	67
Controls	40	52	1,849	31	44	22	3	1.97	32

CHF = congestive heart failure; LV = left ventricular.

emia and they died from a noncardiac cause, usually cancer. Nevertheless, the average number of major coronary arteries severely narrowed at necropsy was 2.2 of 4. Another subgroup consisted of patients who had chronic congestive heart failure in the absence of left ventricular aneurysm after healing of an acute myocardial infarction. They might be called the *ischemic cardiomyopathy* group. Their average number of major coronary arteries severely narrowed also was 2.2 of 4. The other subgroup of healed myocardial infarction patients had a true left ventricular aneurysm. The average number of major coronary arteries severely narrowed in them was 2.5 of 4.

The final subgroup consisted of 22 patients with *unstable angina pectoris*. Nineteen of them had had coronary artery bypass grafting procedures within 7 days of death and the other 3 had cardiac arrest during cardiac catheterization. Preoperatively, all had normal left ventricular function and none had a clinically apparent acute myocardial infarct or congestive heart failure at any time. The average number of major coronary arteries severely narrowed by plaque was 3.2 of 4, and 10 of the 22 patients had severe narrowing of the left main coronary artery as well as severe narrowing of the other 3 major arteries ("4-vessel disease").

Quantitative studies: The results of the quantitative studies are summarized in Table II. A total of 6,461 five-mm segments were sectioned and examined histologically. The sections were stained by the Movat method to delineate the internal elastic membrane. The findings in the 129 coronary patients were compared to those in 1,849 five-mm segments from the 40 control subjects. In each coronary subgroup the 5-mm segments from each of the 4 major coronary arteries were pooled together; thus by this approach the amount of narrowing in an individual patient is not discernible. The percent of 5-mm segments narrowed 76 to 100% in cross-sectional area by atherosclerotic plaque was 35 for the coronary patients and 3 for the control subjects; the percent narrowed 51 to 75% was 36 for the coronary pa-

tients and 22 for the control subjects. Thus, 71% of the 5-mm segments in the coronary patients were narrowed >50% in cross-sectional area by atherosclerotic plaque. For the control subjects it was 25%. In contrast, only 29% of the 5-mm segments in the coronary patients were narrowed <50% and only 8% even approached normal, i.e., narrowed 25% or less in cross-sectional area. In contrast, 75% of the 5-mm segments in the control subjects were narrowed <50% and 31% of them were normal or nearly normal. Thus, in the coronary patients 92% of the 6,461 five-mm segments of the 4 major epicardial coronary arteries were narrowed >25% in cross-sectional area by atherosclerotic plaque.

Among the various subsets of coronary patients, those with *sudden coronary death* and *acute myocardial infarction* had similar percentages of 5-mm segments narrowed 76 to 100% in cross-sectional area by plaque (36 and 34%, respectively); patients with *healed myocardial infarction* as a group had the least severe narrowing (31% of segments narrowed >75%), and the patients with *unstable angina pectoris* had the most severe narrowing (48% of the 5-mm segments were narrowed >75% by plaque).

In an attempt to provide a single number for the amount of coronary arterial narrowing in each patient, a score system was used. A segment narrowed 0 to 25% in cross-sectional area was assigned a score of 1; a segment narrowed 26 to 50% = 2; a segment narrowed 51 to 75% = 3, and 1 narrowed 76 to 100% = 4. The mean score for all 129 patients or for each of the 6,461 five-mm coronary segments was 3.0 and that for the 40 control subjects or 1,849 five-mm segments, 2.0. Again, the unstable angina patients had the most extensive coronary narrowing by this approach.

In all of the aforementioned quantitative coronary arterial studies the amount of cross-sectional area luminal narrowing by atherosclerotic plaque in the right, left anterior descending and left circumflex coronary arteries was similar if the 5-mm segments in each of the 3 longest coronary arteries were pooled together from a number of patients. This statement might be best understood by examining a single subset of coronary patients with fatal CAD. Among the 27 patients with fatal transmural acute myocardial infarction, a total of 1,358 five-mm long segments were analyzed from the right, left anterior descending and left circumflex coronary arteries, and the percentage of segments narrowed 0 to 25, 26 to 50, 51 to 75 and 76 to 100% was similar at each of these 4 categories of cross-sectional area narrowing in each of these 3 major epicardial coronary arteries. The same findings were observed in the patients with sudden coronary death, healed myocardial infarction and unstable angina pectoris.

In a single patient, however, the percent of 5-mm long coronary segments severely (>75% in cross-sectional area) narrowed by atherosclerotic plaque in 1 major epicardial coronary artery may be greater or lesser than that of another major coronary artery. If the segments from 1 coronary artery (e.g., right), however, were pooled together from several patients with fatal CAD and compared to pooled 5-mm segments from another coronary artery (e.g., left anterior descending) from several patients with fatal CAD, the percentage of segments narrowed at each of the 4 categories of cross-sectional area narrowing in each artery was similar.

DISCUSSION

The information derived at necropsy quantitating the severity and extent of atherosclerosis in the 4 major epicardial coronary arteries in fatal CAD is potentially useful clinically in 2 areas: in interpreting degrees of coronary narrowing by angiography during life, and in deciding which of the major coronary arteries needs a conduit at the time of coronary artery bypass grafting.

Without coronary angiography neither coronary bypass nor angioplasty would be done. The only way during life to obtain information on the status of the epicardial coronary arteries is angiography, and, therefore, this procedure revolutionized diagnosis of CAD just as aortocoronary bypass grafting revolutionized therapy of CAD. But angiography—as good as it is—has certain deficiencies. Angiography is a luminogram and a narrowed segment is compared to a less narrowed segment, which is assumed to be normal. The angiogram does not delineate the internal elastic membrane of the artery, and, therefore, the artery's true lumen remains uncertain.

The aforementioned coronary quantitative studies[1-5] demonstrated that in fatal CAD 92% of the 5-mm long segments of the 4 major epicardial coronary arteries were narrowed >25% in cross-sectional area by atherosclerotic plaque. Thus, only 8% of the 5-mm segments even approached normal and virtually none was normal. Thus, at least in fatal CAD, and probably also in live patients with symptomatic myocardial ischemia, it is infrequent that an angiographically severely narrowed segment of a coronary artery can be compared to a segment of coronary artery that is actually normal. In patients with symptomatic myocardial ischemia, the coronary angiogram measures degrees of narrowing by comparing severely narrowed segments to segments that are simply less narrowed but by no means normal. Accordingly, coronary angiograms in patients with symptomatic myocardial ischemia usually underestimate the degrees of luminal narrowing.[7,8]

The unit of measuring degrees of narrowing by angiography is different than the unit of measurement at necropsy. In the anatomic quantitative studies presented herein, the unit was *cross-sectional area* narrowing. The unit of angiography is *diameter* narrowing. In general, a 75% cross-sectional area narrowing is equivalent to a 50% diameter reduction, and, therefore, a ≥50% diameter reduction during life has generally been considered the cutoff point between clinically significant and clinically insignificant coronary narrowing.

The second potential use of the information derived from these quantitative studies at necropsy is the appreciation that the atherosclerotic process in patients with symptomatic myocardial ischemia is usually diffuse and severe. Therefore, more rather than fewer aortocoronary conduits provide a higher frequency of relief or improvement in symptoms of myocardial ischemia, in improvement in results of exercise testing and in prolonging life. Among patients surviving ≤60 days or >60 days after aortocoronary bypass operations, the amount of severe narrowing in the *nonbypassed native* coronary arteries is usually similar to that in the *bypassed native* coronary arteries.[9] From study at necropsy of 102 patients dying either early (≤60 days) or late (2.5 to 108 months [mean 35]) after bypass operations, Waller and I[9] found that the bypassed and nonbypassed native coronary arteries had similar degrees of severe luminal narrowing by atherosclerotic plaques. Specifically, in 213 (94%) of the 226 bypassed native arteries and in 73 (91%) of 80 nonbypassed native arteries the lumens were narrowed >75% in cross-sectional area by atherosclerotic plaque. The reason the native arteries were not bypassed was not that they were too small or severely narrowed distally, but because by angiogram the lumens were judged not to be sufficiently narrowed to warrant the insertion of a conduit. Thus, if 2 of the major coronary arteries are severely narrowed by angiogram and the third major artery is "insignificantly" narrowed and if a bypass operation is to be done, the insertion of a conduit in all 3 major coronary arteries could be reasonably argued. There is, of course, potential danger in inserting a conduit in an artery insignificantly narrowed, but, nevertheless, it may be more advantageous to err on the side of too many conduits than too few. At necropsy, "3-vessel disease" is far more frequent than "2-vessel disease" and even when only 2 of the 3 major arteries at necropsy are narrowed >75% in cross-sectional area, the third one is usually narrowed 51 to 75% in cross-sectional area. Thus, an appreciation of the diffuse nature of coronary atherosclerosis in fatal CAD and probably also in symptomatic myocardial ischemia encourages the tilt toward more rather than fewer conduits at coronary bypass operations.

A possible criticism of the 5-mm segment approach to quantifying coronary arterial narrowing is that the epicardial coronary arteries were fixed in an unphysiologic pressure state, namely a zero pressure state, rather than at a systemic arterial diastolic pressure. In an attempt to take into account the unphysiologic fixation state, the degrees of narrowing were conservatively judged, that is, if a segment was more or less in between 2 quadrants (51 to 75% and 76 to 100%), the lesser degree of narrowing was always chosen. Second, in any segment in which a portion of wall was collapsed by the fixation process, the degree of narrowing was determined as if the segment was expanded. Most important, the segments narrowed the most, i.e., >75% in cross-sectional area, were affected the least by the fixation process. Irrespective of whether or not the histologic technique used in this study is perfect or imperfect, the same technique was used in all subsets of coronary patients and also in all control subjects, and, therefore, the comparison data are highly reliable. Irrespective of whether or not the degree of luminal narrowing should be slightly greater or slightly less than that determined by this technique, it is clear that the atherosclerotic process is a diffuse one in nearly all patients with fatal CAD. The accuracy of the technique determining degrees of cross-sectional area narrowing by estimating from stained histologic sections magnified about 40 times is similar ($\leq$5%) to that determined by planimetry.[10]

Another possible concern of the quantitative data is its applicability to living patients with symptomatic or other clinical evidence (e.g., positive exercise test) of myocardial ischemia. It is my view that the major difference in coronary arterial narrowing occurs at the stage of conversion from the asymptomatic to the symptomatic myocardial ischemia state and that there is relatively little difference in degrees of coronary narrowing between the symptomatic and the fatal states. Support for this view can be obtained by the presence of severe and extensive coronary narrowing on the angiogram during life, and by studying the coronary tree at necropsy in patients who had a coronary event and who died later from a noncardiac cause. Although data from the latter situation are minimal, the degrees of coronary narrowing at necropsy are similar to that in other patients with fatal symptomatic myocardial ischemia. Finally, among the subsets of coronary patients described herein, those with unstable angina pectoris had by far the worst degrees of coronary narrowing and the subjects in this group were the only ones in whom their natural course was interrupted by an iatrogenic event, namely coronary artery bypass grafting (within a week of death).

REFERENCES

1. Roberts WC, Jones AA. Quantitation of coronary arterial narrowing at necropsy in sudden coronary death. Analysis of 31 patients and comparison with 25 control subjects. *Am J Cardiol 1979;44:39–45.*

2. Roberts WC, Jones AA. Quantification of coronary arterial narrowing at necropsy in acute myocardial infarction: analysis and comparison of findings in 27 patients and 22 controls. *Circulation 1980;61:786–790.*

3. Virmani R, Roberts WC. Non-fatal healed transmural myocardial infarction and fatal non-cardiac disease. Qualification and quantification of coronary arterial narrowing and of left ventricular scarring in 18 necropsy patients. *Br Heart J 1981;45:434–441.*

4. Virmani R, Roberts WC. Quantification of coronary arterial narrowing and of left ventricular myocardial scarring in healed myocardial infarction with chronic, eventually fatal, congestive cardiac failure. *Am J Med 1980;68:831–838.*

5. Cabin HS, Roberts WC. True left ventricular aneurysm and healed myocardial infarction. Clinical and necropsy observations including quantification of degrees of coronary arterial narrowing. *Am J Cardiol 1980;46:754–763.*

6. Roberts WC, Virmani R. Quantification of coronary arterial narrowing in clinically-isolated unstable angina pectoris. An analysis of 22 necropsy patients. *Am J Med 1979;67:792–799.*

7. Arnett EN, Isner JM, Redwood DR, Kent KM, Baker WP, Ackerstein H, Roberts WC. Coronary artery narrowing in coronary heart disease: comparison of cineangiographic and necropsy findings. *Ann Intern Med 1979;91:350–356.*

8. Isner JM, Kishel J, Kent KM, Ronan JAJ, Ross AM, Roberts WC. Accuracy of angiographic determination of left main coronary arterial narrowing. Angiographic-histologic correlative analysis in 28 patients. *Circulation 1981;63:1056–1064.*

9. Waller BF, Roberts WC. Amount of narrowing by atherosclerotic plaque in 44 nonbypassed and 52 bypassed major epicardial coronary arteries in 32 necropsy patients who died within 1 month of aortocoronary bypass grafting. *Am J Cardiol 1980;46:956–962.*

10. Isner JM, Wu M, Virmani R, Jones AA, Roberts WC. Comparison of coronary arterial luminal narrowing determined by visual inspection of histologic sections under magnification among three independent observers and comparison to that obtained by video planimetry. An analysis of 559 five-millimeter segments of 61 coronary arteries from eleven patients. *Lab Invest 1980;42:566–570.*

Extensive Multifocal Myocardial Infarcts from Cloth Emboli After Replacement of Mitral and Aortic Valves with Cloth-Covered, Caged-Ball Prostheses

Allen L. Dollar, MD, Marie-Lydie Pierre-Louis, MD,
Charles L. McIntosh, MD, PhD, and William C. Roberts, MD

The early Starr-Edwards prosthetic heart valve models (series 1000, 1200 and 1260) contained no cloth on the inner aspects of the ring or on the struts. In an attempt to reduce the frequency of thrombus on the prostheses, a cloth covering was later added to cover the inside portion of the ring and the struts. Almost simultaneously, a stellite poppet was substituted for the silicone rubber poppet in many prostheses. Although these modifications did reduce the frequency of embolic events, a new problem was introduced, namely cloth wear. Cloth wear led in some patients to dysfunction of prostheses, hemolytic anemia and systemic emboli.[1-7] As the cloth on these prosthetic valves wore, cloth occasionally embolized to 1 or more systemic organs. Such resulting organ infarcts

From the Pathology and Surgery Branches, National Heart, Lung, and Blood Institute, National Institutes of Health, Bethesda, Maryland 20892, and the District of Columbia Medical Examiner's Office, District of Columbia, Washington, DC. Manuscript received April 19, 1989; revised manuscript received and accepted May 11, 1989.

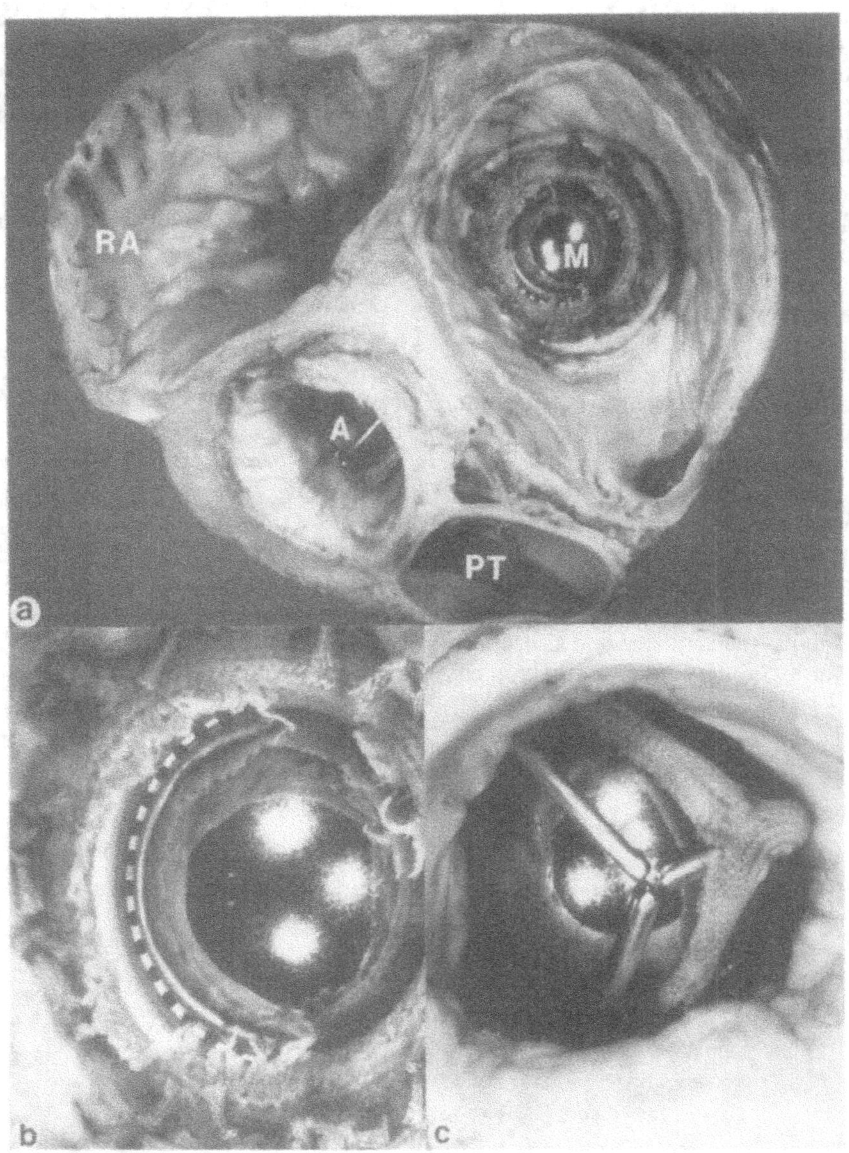

FIGURE 1. Photographs of the heart in the patient described. a, view of atria and great arteries from above showing the cloth-covered Starr-Edwards prostheses in the mitral (M) and aortic (A) valve positions. The cloth on the mitral prosthetic ring is frayed. PT = pulmonary trunk; RA = right atrium. b, close-up view of the mitral valve prosthesis from the left atrium with the torn cloth pulled away from the metallic ring. c, close-up view of the aortic valve prosthesis viewed from the aorta showing detachment of the cloth covering from each of the 3 struts due to wear of the cloth on the inside of the cage.

610

were usually not visible on gross inspection.

We recently studied a patient at necropsy who had multiple ventricular scars from cloth emboli from caged-ball prostheses. Such myocardial scars from this etiology have not been described previously.

A 58-year-old man underwent replacements of his stenotic mitral and aortic valves on January 23, 1970, and he died on November 1, 1988. Cloth-covered Starr-Edwards prostheses with metallic poppets, models 2310 and 6310, were implanted. Unilateral occlusion of a central retinal artery occurred at age 53 (13 years postoperatively); it re-solved spontaneously and sight returned. A ventricular demand pacemaker was implanted at age 54 because of symptomatic bradycardia. Cardiac catheterization at that time disclosed a 10 mm Hg mean diastolic gradient between the pulmonary artery wedge and left ventricle, and no peak systolic gradient between the left ventricle (140/11 mm Hg) and aorta (140/85 mm Hg). The coronary arteries were normal by angiogram. On echocardiogram, the diameter of the left ventricular cavity was 55 mm in end-diastole and 38 mm in peak systole. Left ventricular fractional shortening was 31%. On evaluation 8 months before death, he was asymptomatic. Death resulted from injuries sustained when, as a pedestrian, he was struck by a truck traveling at a high speed.

Thirteen electrocardiograms recorded from July 16, 1969, to March 16, 1988, were reviewed. Each of the 3 recorded before double valve replacement showed atrial fibrillation, Q waves in leads V_1 through V_3 and total 12-lead QRS amplitudes of 234, 240 and 216 mm (10 mm = 1 mV).[8] The first 8 electrocardiograms recorded from 5 days to 14 years after the double valve replacement also showed Q waves in leads V_1 through V_3 and total 12-lead QRS amplitudes ranging from 129

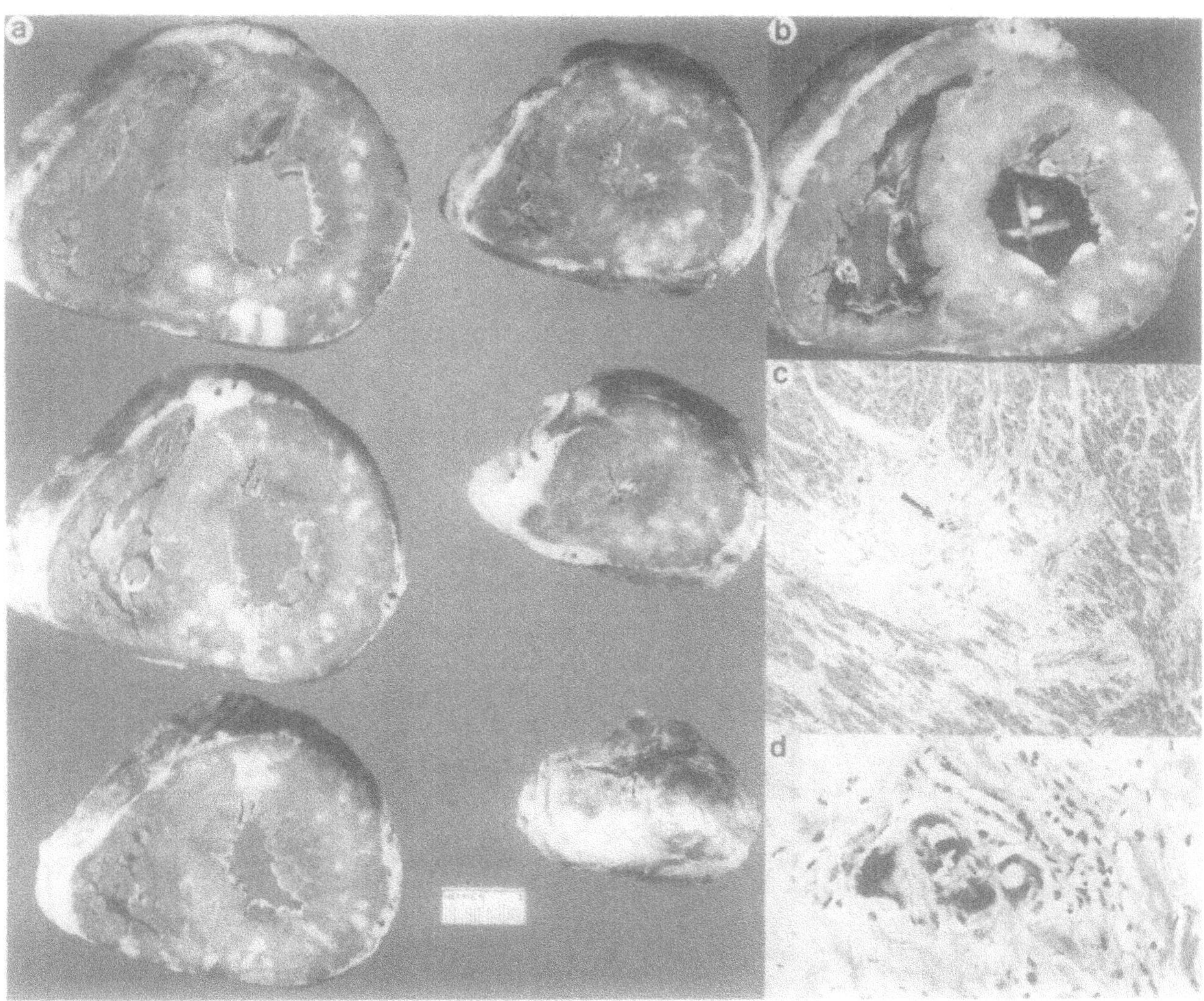

FIGURE 2. Ventricular myocardium in the patient described. *a,* views of the cardiac ventricles after transverse cutting showing numerous focal scars (*white*) in the walls of both ventricles. *b,* the most basal section showing the Starr-Edwards prosthetic valve in the mitral position. The cloth covering the struts of this valve is intact. *c,* photomicrograph of a portion of left ventricular myocardium showing a focal scar, in the center of which is basophilic staining, foreign body material (*arrow*) surrounded by multinucleated giant cells. *d,* higher power magnification of the embolized foreign-body material and associated giant cells seen in *c.* Hematoxylin and eosin stains, × 32 (*c*), × 250 (*d*).

to 179 mm (mean 164); atrial fibrillation was present in 5 and sinus rhythm in 3 of these 8 electrocardiograms. Two electrocardiograms recorded after the pacemaker was inserted showed total 12-lead QRS amplitudes of 199 and 213 mm, respectively.

At necropsy, the heart weighed 545 g. The epicardial coronary arteries were virtually devoid of atherosclerotic plaques. Cloth wear on both struts and rings was severe on both prostheses (Figure 1). There were numerous focal scars measuring 1 to 10 mm in the myocardial walls of both ventricles (Figure 2). Histologic examination revealed focal fibrosis and scattered basophilic staining, slightly refractile, foreign body material occluding small intramyocardial arteries, often surrounded by multinucleated giant cells (Figure 2). By polarized light this basophilic material was anisotropic and typical of cloth fragment. Histologic examination of the kidneys and brain disclosed similar foreign body material associated with multinucleated giant cells. The foreign body emboli in these organs was not associated with gross or microscopic scars. No foreign body material was found in lung, liver, spleen, pancreas or thyroid gland.

The extensive focal right and left ventricular wall scarring in this patient is presumed to have resulted from multiple cloth emboli dislodged from the cardiac valve prostheses. Despite these multiple emboli, there were no clinical or electrocardiographic consequences.

1. Niles NR, Sandilands JR. Pathology of heart valve replacement surgery: autopsies of 62 patients with Starr-Edwards prostheses. Dis Chest 1969;56: 373–382.

2. Niles NR. Teflon embolism from Starr-Edwards valves. J Thorac Cardiovasc Surg 1970;59:794–799.

3. Boruchow IB, Ramsey HW, Wheat MW Jr. Complications following destruction of the cloth covering of a Starr-Edwards aortic valve prosthesis. J Thorac Cardiovasc Surg 1971;62:290–293.

4. Thomas CS Jr, Killen DA, Alford WC Jr, Burrus GR, Stoney WS. Cloth disruption in the Starr-Edwards composite mitral valve prosthesis. Ann Thorac Surg 1973;15:434–438.

5. Crawford FA, Sethi GK, Scott SM, Takaro T. Systemic emboli due to cloth wear in a Starr-Edwards Model 2320 aortic prosthesis. Ann Thorac Surg 1973;16:614–619.

6. Shah A, Dolgin M, Tice DA, Trehan N. Complications due to cloth wear in cloth-covered Starr-Edwards aortic and mitral valve prostheses and their management. Am Heart J 1978;96:407–414.

7. Huber S, Burckhardt D, Raeder EA, Follath F, Hasse J, Gradel E. Complications in patients with cloth-covered Starr-Edwards prostheses. J Cardiovasc Surg 1980;21:19–24.

8. Siegel RJ, Roberts WC. Electrocardiographic observations in severe aortic valve stenosis: correlative necropsy study to clinical, hemodynamic, and ECG variables demonstrating relation of 12-lead QRS amplitude to peak systolic transaortic pressure gradient. Am Heart J 1982;103:210–221.

Morphometric Analysis of the Composition of Atherosclerotic Plaques in the Four Major Epicardial Coronary Arteries in Acute Myocardial Infarction and in Sudden Coronary Death

Amy H. Kragel, MD, Shanthasundari G. Reddy, MD, Janet T. Wittes, PhD, and William C. Roberts, MD

We studied at necropsy atherosclerotic plaque composition in the four major (right, left main, left anterior descending, and left circumflex) epicardial coronary arteries in 15 patients who died of consequences of an acute myocardial infarction (AMI) and in 12 patients with sudden coronary death (SCD) without AMI. The coronary epicardial arteries were sectioned at 5-mm intervals, and a Movat-stained section of each segment of artery was prepared and analyzed using a computerized morphometry system. Within the AMI group and within the SCD group, there were no differences in plaque composition among any of the four major epicardial coronary arteries. Within both groups, plaque morphology varied as a function of cross-sectional–area narrowing of the segments. In both groups, the amount of dense relatively acellular fibrous tissue, calcified tissue, and pultaceous debris (amorphous debris containing cholesterol clefts, presumably rich in extracellular lipid) increased in a linear fashion with increasing degrees of cross-sectional–area narrowing of the segments, and the amount of cellular fibrous tissue decreased linearly. In the AMI group, the percentage of plaque consisting of pultaceous debris and of cellular fibrous tissue separated significantly narrowed ($>75\%$ cross-sectional area) segments from less narrowed ($<75\%$) segments. A comparison of the AMI group to the SCD group showed significant differences. The percentage of plaque consisting of pultaceous debris (16% in the AMI group and 7% in the SCD group), of cellular fibrous tissue (11% vs. 18%), and of heavily calcified tissue (8% vs. 16%) were significantly different in the severely narrowed segments in the AMI and SCD groups. When all arteries containing thrombi were deleted from the analysis, there were no significant changes in the results. Occlusive coronary thrombi were present in 13 of the 15 AMI patients and in one of the 12 SCD patients. Thus, the frequency of coronary thrombi and plaque composition differ in patients with AMI and in those with SCD without AMI. (*Circulation* 1989;80:1747–1756)

several investigators have examined the degrees of cross-sectional–area luminal narrowing in the four major (left main, left anterior descending, left circumflex, and right) epicardial coronary arteries in patients with sudden coronary death (SCD)[1] and in those with acute myocardial infarction (AMI).[2-4] These studies have not been particularly useful in shedding light on why patients with severe coronary narrowing have different manifestations of myocardial ischemia. The present study examines in a quantitative fashion at necropsy the composition of coronary arterial plaques in patients with SCD and in those with AMI to determine whether the plaques are similar or different in these two subsets of patients and whether the differences offer potential explanations for the different outcomes in these two groups of patients, that is, thrombosis of a major epicardial coronary artery and left ventricular necrosis in the AMI group and sudden death in the absence of left ventricular necrosis in the SCD group.

From the Pathology Branch, National Heart, Lung, and Blood Institute, National Institutes of Health, Bethesda, Maryland.

Address for reprints: Amy H. Kragel, MD, Pathology Branch, National Heart, Lung, and Blood Institute, Building 10, Room 2N258, Bethesda, MD 20892.

Received March 22, 1989; revision accepted August 11, 1989.

Methods

Patients

The necropsy records of the Pathology Branch, National Heart, Lung, and Blood Institute, National Institutes of Health, were searched for patients coded as either AMI or SCD. Patients with AMI were selected in whom there was transmural (involvement of all the inner one half and all or a portion of the outer one half of the left ventricular freewall) left ventricular necrosis and in whom death was considered a direct consequence of that necrosis. Patients with SCD (death outside the hospital or shortly after admission to the hospital with an interval of less than 6 hours between onset of symptoms and death) were selected in whom there was greater than 75% cross-sectional–area narrowing of at least one of the four major epicardial coronary arteries, in whom there was no grossly visible myocardial necrosis, and in whom no other cause of death was identified at necropsy. To minimize other variables, the patients were selected such that all met the following criteria: 1) absence of left ventricular fibrosis, 2) absence of signs or symptoms of myocardial dysfunction or ischemia before the event leading to death, 3) absence of coronary angioplasty or bypass, 4) absence of thrombolytic or anticoagulant therapy, and 5) age 50–70 years, such that there was no significant difference in the mean ages between the two groups. Fifteen patients with AMI and 12 patients with SCD were selected for study.

Experimental Protocol

The coronary arteries from each patient were studied in a similar fashion. The hearts were fixed in formalin. The epicardial coronary arteries were excised intact, decalcified, and sectioned transversely at 5-mm intervals. The segments of each artery were labeled sequentially from their origin. In two patients the left main coronary artery was not available for examination. After transverse cutting of the coronary arteries, the 5-mm segments were decalcified again, if necessary, dehydrated (alcohols), cleared (xylene), embedded in paraffin, and cut. Two sections of each 5-mm segment were stained, one with hematoxylin and eosin and one by the Movat method.[5] Of 1,219 sections (620 from the AMI group and 599 from the SCD group) initially examined, 135 (65 from the AMI group and 70 from the SCD group) were excluded because the sections included branch points or sectioning artifacts, which left 1,084 sections (555 from the AMI group and 529 from the SCD group) for further examination.

Movat-stained sections were placed on the stage of a projection light microscope. The image was enlarged approximately 430 times, and a tracing of the artery was made on white opaque paper. The following areas were outlined: potential lumen (total area enclosed by the internal elastic membrane), residual lumen (potential lumen minus area of atherosclerotic plaque), and luminal thrombus (identified as aggregates of platelets, fibrin, and erythrocytes with sites of mural attachment). Components of the plaque outlined included dense fibrous tissue, loose fibrous tissue, cellular fibrous tissue, heavily calcified tissue, pultaceous debris (extracellular lipid), foam cells with and without lymphocytes, and inflammatory infiltrates without significant numbers of foam cells. Analyses of plaque components and luminal thrombus were performed in each of the four major epicardial coronary arteries in every patient.

The definitions and descriptions of potential and residual lumens, of luminal thrombus, and of components of plaques were finalized after approximately 60 sections had been reviewed (Figure 1). Dense fibrous tissue was defined as a relatively acellular area of dense collagen fibers. Loose fibrous tissue was a relatively acellular, more delicate arrangement of collagen fibers that stained pale blue with the Movat pentachrome stain. Cellular fibrous tissue consisted of spindle cells resembling myofibroblasts, smooth-muscle cells, or fibroblasts admixed with collagen or elastic fibers. Calcific deposits were detected by brown granular staining areas in Movat-stained sections and by blue-purple staining granules in hematoxylin and eosin–stained sections. Only solid areas and not isolated granules of calcium or faintly calcified tissue that can no longer be recognized because of the decalcification process were included in this analysis. The amount of calcium, therefore, does not represent the total amount of calcified tissue and should only be used in comparative analyses. Pultaceous debris (presumably rich in extracellular lipid) was indicated by pale staining areas composed of amorphous material with abundant cholesterol clefts with or without erythrocytes. This method does not analyze the total amount of intracellular or extracellular lipids but only pools of pultaceous debris admixed with large quantities of extracellular lipid. Foam cell aggregates were composed of plump, rounded, finely vacuolated cells. Foam cells and lymphocytes were areas containing round cells with finely granular or vaculated cytoplasm admixed with lymphocytes. Inflammatory infiltrates without foam cells were isolated aggregates of lymphocytes and other inflammatory cells that were almost always seen surrounding small vascular channels. The defined areas were recognized using the projection microscope and were confirmed by standard light microscopy using both the Movat- and hematoxylin and eosin–stained sections (Figure 2).

After a labeled drawing of each Movat-stained histologic section was made, each component was traced using a GTCO Micro Digi-Pad (GTCO Corp, Columbia, Maryland), and the area was calculated using Macmeasure,[6] which is a morphometric software package used in conjunction with a Macintosh SE computer. The area of each component of plaque was then converted to a percentage of the

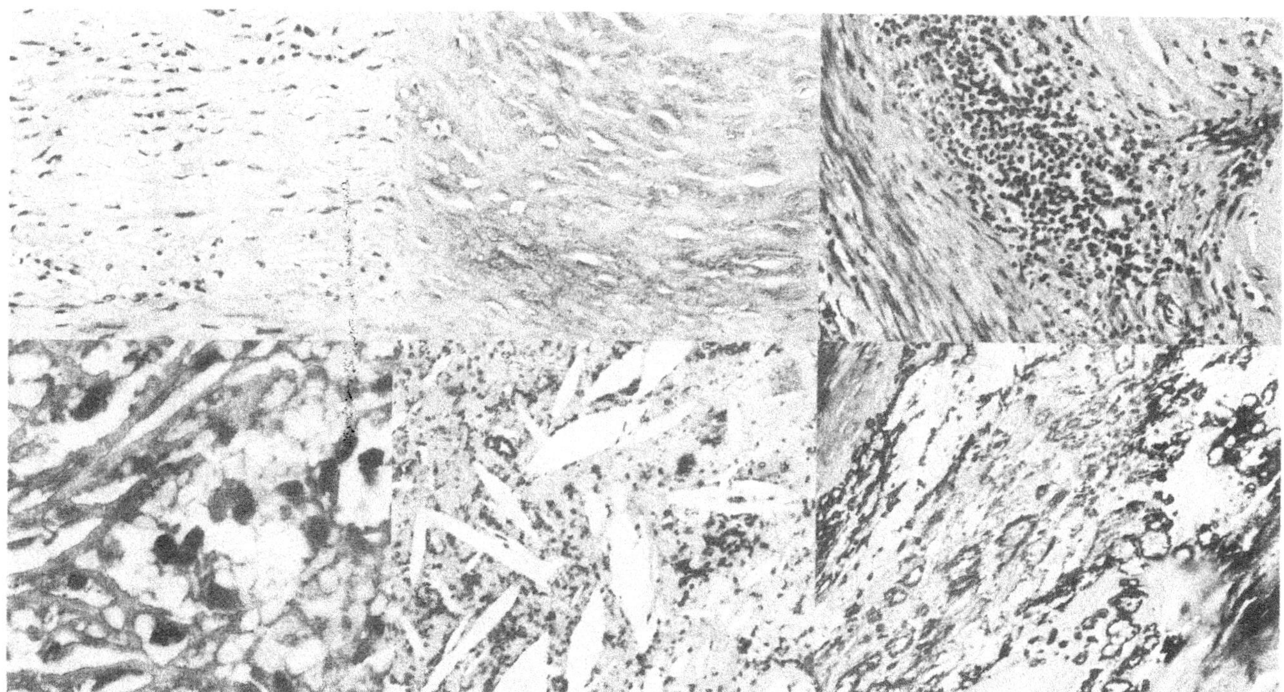

FIGURE 1. *Composite photograph of various components of coronary arterial plaque. From top left to bottom right: cellular fibrous tissue (×250), dense relatively acellular fibrous tissue (×250), lymphocytic inflammatory infiltrate (×250), foam cells (×1,350), pultaceous debris with abundant cholesterol clefts (×250), and heavily calcified tissue (×250). Movat stains on each.*

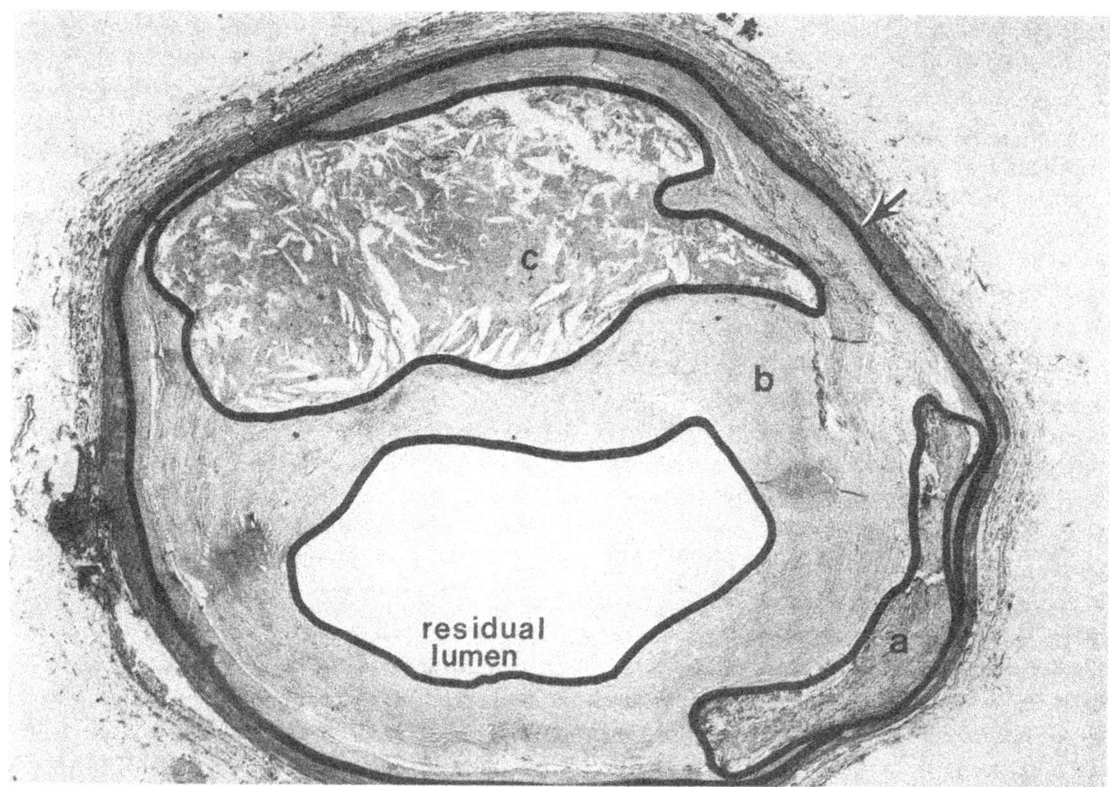

FIGURE 2. *Photograph of a Movat-stained section of coronary artery with the internal elastic membrane (arrow), the residual lumen, and the components of plaque outlined:* a, *heavily calcified tissue;* b, *dense fibrous tissue;* c, *pultaceous debris.*

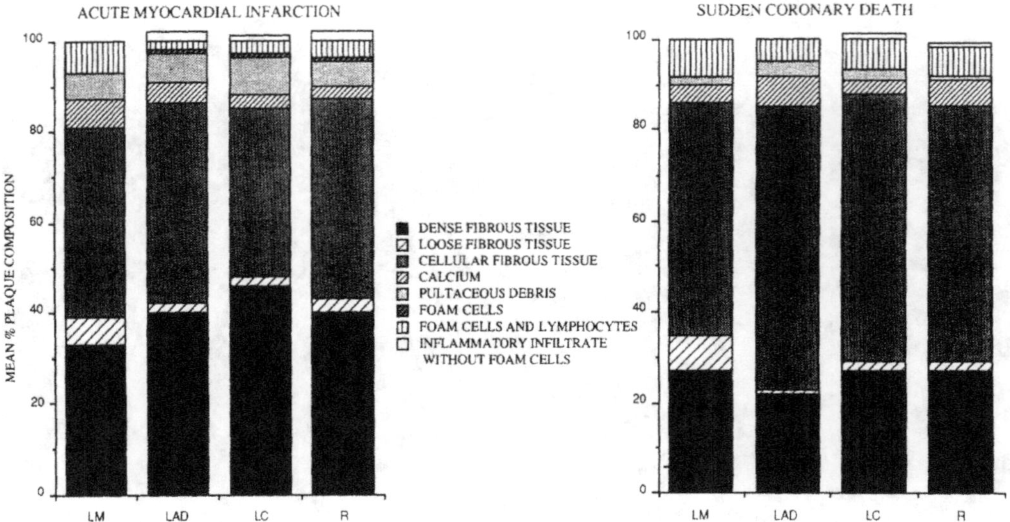

FIGURE 3. *Bar graph depicting mean coronary arterial plaque composition in the four major epicardial coronary arteries. LM, left main coronary artery; LAD, left anterior descending coronary artery; LC, left circumflex coronary artery; R, right coronary artery.*

total plaque area: the sum of dense fibrous, loose fibrous, cellular fibrous, pultaceous debris, foam cells, foam cells and lymphocytes, and inflammatory infiltrates without foam cells. Recent thrombus was not considered to be a component of plaque.

To assess interobserver and intra-observer variability, 20 segments from one patient were analyzed twice by one observer (with a 2-month interval between sets of observations), and 32 segments from another patient were analyzed once each by two observers. Pearson correlation coefficients were then calculated.

The percentage of cross-sectional–area narrowing was determined by using the measured values for residual luminal area and potential luminal area (percent cross-sectional–area narrowing $=[100-(\text{residual luminal area/potential luminal area})\times100]$). The degree of luminal narrowing was then categorized into four groups: 0–25%, 26–50%, 51–75%, and 76–100%. The results were verified by visual inspection of each segment. Discrepancies were said to occur when segments appeared to have been compressed during processing resulting in overestimation of the luminal narrowing by the above formula. For these segments, the value obtained by visual inspection alone was used.

The answers to the following questions were sought. 1) Is the distribution of each component of plaque among the four major epicardial coronary arteries different or similar between the two groups? 2) Is the distribution of each of the components of plaque over the four categories of cross-sectional–area narrowing different or similar between the two groups? 3) Are there differences in either the overall plaque composition, the composition of segments narrowed 0–25% in cross-sectional area or the composition of segments narrowed by more than 75% in cross-sectional area between the AMI and the SCD groups? 4) Does the presence of thrombus in the coronary arteries account for differences, if any, between the two groups?

Statistical Analysis

Analysis of plaque composition in each of the four major epicardial coronary arteries was performed by averaging the mean composition of all segments within a given artery in each patient adjusting for differing degrees of cross-sectional–area narrowing. Analysis of variance was used to assess the relation between the percentage of a given component of plaque and the specific epicardial coronary artery. The F tests comparing the composition by artery have (3, 99) degrees of freedom for the SCD group and (3, 129) degrees of freedom for the AMI group.

The plaque composition within the four categories of cross-sectional–area narrowing was analyzed by calculating the mean composition in each patient of all segments within each of the four groups of narrowing and averaging over the individuals using an analysis of variance model. A linear contrast model was used to assess whether a linear trend existed in the mean percentage of any component over the four categories of narrowing. F tests were used to compare the composition of plaque in sections narrowed 51–75% and those narrowed by more than 75%.

To assess whether there were differences in plaque composition, either overall, in segments narrowed 0–25% in cross-sectional area or in segments narrowed 76–100% in cross-sectional area between the two groups, the average of the mean composition for each patient of the appropriate segments was calculated. All t tests for these comparisons had at least 25 degrees of freedom.

TABLE 1. Clinical and Morphologic Features of the 27 Patients Studied

Feature	Acute myocardial infarction ($n=15$)	Sudden coronary death ($n=12$)
Age range (mean) (yr)	53–68 (61)	50–68 (57)
Men:women	11:4	12:0
Systemic hypertension	9 (60%)	5 (40%)
Diabetes mellitus	3 (20%)	0
Angina pectoris	0	0
Congestive heart failure	0	0
Thrombus in a major epicardial coronary artery	13 (87%)	1 (8%)
Left ventricular necrosis	15 (100%)	0
Left ventricular fibrosis	0	0
Approximate age of infarct,* range (mean) (day)	7–35 (11)	—

*Determined from a combination of clinical history and histologic evaluation of sections of left ventricular myocardium.

For all final statistical analyses, the individual patient was the unit of study. That is, a mean was calculated for each patient, and the number of units compared in each final analysis varied from 10 to 15, representing the number of patients within a given group rather than the number of sections or arteries studied.[7] PROC GLM of SAS[8] was used for the calculations. Because the number of sections per patient within a category varied markedly, an analysis of variance, weighted for the number of observations used to calculate each mean, was performed, and the relevant statistics were calculated. Because many highly correlated statistical tests of significance were performed, Bonferroni inequalities were used to ensure statistical rigor and to control the significance level.[9] Because the Bonferonni adjusted p values are more conservative than what is usually reported, F values are listed.

Results

Certain clinical and morphologic features of the patients studied are summarized in Table 1. No significant differences were found between the two groups in age, sex, history of systemic hypertension, or diabetes mellitus. Thirteen of the 15 patients in the AMI group and one of the 12 patients in the SCD group had thrombus in one of the four major epicardial coronary arteries. The approximate infarct age in the AMI group determined from a review of clinical data and histologic evaluation of left ventricular myocardium ranged from 4 to 35 days (mean, 10 days).

Pearson correlation coefficients, reflecting interobserver variability, were 0.83 for dense fibrous tissue, 0.72 for loose fibrous tissue, 0.95 for cellular fibrous tissue, 0.94 for calcium, and 0.90 for pultaceous debris. Pearson correlation coefficients, reflecting intraobserver variability, were 0.80 for dense fibrous tissue, 0.94 for cellular fibrous tissue, 0.92 for calcium, and 0.96 for pultaceous debris. Correlation coefficients for elements that represented small fractions of plaque composition, that is, less than 3–4% of the overall plaque composition, were either spuriously high because the frequency of the observations was small in the sections analyzed or were low. A comparison of the mean percentage of plaque occupied by these smaller components was quite good.

The degrees of cross-sectional–area narrowing in the four major epicardial coronary arteries in the two groups are summarized in Table 2. In the AMI group, the percentage of sections narrowed greater than 75% cross-sectional area varied from 6% in the left main to 32% in the left anterior descending coronary artery. In the SCD group, the percentage of sections narrowed greater than 75% in cross-sectional area varied from 18% in the left main to 33% in the right coronary artery. Overall, there was little difference in the degrees of cross-sectional–area narrowing between the two groups.

The results of the analysis of plaque composition in each of the four major epicardial coronary arteries in the AMI and SCD groups are summarized in Figure 3 and in Table 3. The results of this analysis and all subsequent analyses are listed as the mean composition for the subset of segments studied. Within both groups, no statistically significant differences were found in plaque composition among the four major epicardial coronary arteries. There was, however, a great deal of variability in plaque

TABLE 2. Number and Percentage of Coronary Arterial Sections Narrowed by a Given Degree of Cross-Sectional Area by Atherosclerotic Plaque

Coronary artery	Number and percent of 5-mm coronary segments narrowed to four categories of narrowing							
	Acute myocardial infarction				Sudden coronary death			
	0–25%	26–50%	51–75%	76–100%	0–25%	26–50%	51–75%	76–100%
LM	2 (11)	5 (28)	10 (55)	1 (6)	3 (13)	7 (32)	8 (36)	4 (18)
LAD	38 (23)	22 (13)	52 (32)	53 (32)	22 (11)	66 (32)	64 (31)	53 (26)
LCx	41 (34)	25 (20)	28 (23)	28 (23)	21 (16)	40 (30)	42 (31)	31 (23)
RCA	31 (12)	62 (25)	86 (34)	71 (29)	14 (8)	25 (15)	74 (44)	55 (33)
Total	112 (20)	114 (21)	176 (32)	153 (27)	60 (11)	138 (26)	188 (36)	143 (27)

LM, left main; LAD, left anterior descending; LCx, left circumflex; RCA, right coronary.
Numbers in parentheses are percentages.

TABLE 3. Mean Composition of Coronary Arterial Atherosclerotic Plaque in the Four Major Epicardial Coronary Arteries

| | Acute myocardial infarction | | | | | Sudden coronary death | | | | |
| | Mean percent (SEM) | | | | | Mean percent (SEM) | | | | |
Component of plaque	LM (n=13)†	LAD (n=15)	LCx (n=15)	Right (n=15)	F value*	LM (n=10)‡	LAD (n=12)	LCx (n=12)	Right (n=12)	F value*
Dense fibrous tissue	33 (7)	41 (3)	48 (3)	40 (2)	2.20	27 (6)	21 (2)	30 (3)	31 (2)	6.04
Loose fibrous tissue)	6 (2)	2 (1)	2 (1)	3 (1)	1.78	8 (2)	1 (1)	2 (1)	2 (1)	2.70
Cellular fibrous tissue)	42 (8)	44 (3)	37 (3)	46 (2)	2.04	51 (7)	64 (2)	58 (3)	55 (3)	2.98
Calcium)	6 (3)	5 (1)	3 (1)	3 (1)	1.03	4 (3)	6 (1)	2 (1)	6 (1)	1.93
Pultaceous debris)	6 (3)	6 (1)	8 (1)	5 (1)	1.20	3 (2)	3 (1)	2 (1)	1 (1)	0.90
Foam cells)	0 (1)	1 (0.3)	1 (0.3)	1 (0.3)	1.45	0 (0.1)	0 (0.1)	0 (0.1)	0 (0.1)	0.55
Foam cells and lymphocytes)	8 (2)	2 (1)	3 (1)	4 (1)	2.03	8 (4)	4 (1)	6 (2)	5 (2)	0.46
Inflammatory infiltrate without foam cells)	0 (1)	2 (0.4)	1 (0.4)	2 (0.3)	0.29	0 (1)	0 (0.2)	0 (0.2)	1 (0.2)	0.29

LAD, left anterior descending; LCx, left circumflex; LM, left main.
*No Bonferroni adjusted p value significant at $p=0.05$.
†In two cases, sections of left main coronary artery were not available.
‡In two cases, sections of left main coronary artery included artifacts.
Numbers in parentheses are percentages.

composition among individual 5-mm segments of artery within each subset.

The results of the analysis of plaque composition in the four categories of cross sectional–area narrowing are detailed in Table 4 and in Figure 4. In the AMI group, the amount of dense fibrous tissue, heavily calcified tissue, pultaceous debris, and foam cell aggregates increased in a linear fashion over the four categories of cross-sectional–area narrowing, whereas the amount of cellular fibrous tissue decreased in a linear fashion. The SCD group showed similar linear increases in the amount of dense fibrous tissue, heavily calcified tissue, and pultaceous debris, and inflammatory infiltrates without significant numbers of foam cells and a linear decrease in the amount of cellular fibrous tissue. The percentage of plaque occupied by foam cell aggregates was small in the SCD group in all four categories of narrowing and no statistically significant linear trend was seen.

A comparison of plaque composition in the AMI group of the critically narrowed sections (i.e., those narrowed by more than 75% in cross-sectional area) and those less critically narrowed (51–75% in cross-sectional area) showed a significant difference in the amount of pultaceous debris (16% in sections narrowed greater than 75% vs. 6% in sections narrowed 51–75%, $p<0.0001$) and cellular fibrous tissue (11% in sections narrowed by more than 75% vs. 22% in sections narrowed 51–75%, $p<0.05$). In the SCD group, no significant difference in the amount of pultaceous debris between sections narrowed 51–75% and those narrowed by more than 75% in cross-sectional area was seen. Significantly

TABLE 4. Mean Composition of Coronary Arterial Atherosclerotic Plaque at Varying Degrees of Cross-Sectional–Area Narrowing in the Four Major Epicardial Coronary Arteries

| | Acute myocardial infarction | | | | | | Sudden coronary death | | | | | |
| | Mean percent (SEM) | | | | F value for linear trend | F value for 51–75% vs. 76–100% | Mean percent (SEM) | | | | F value for linear trend | F value for 51–75% vs. 76–100% |
Component of plaque	0–25% (n=13)*	26–50% (n=15)	51–75% (n=15)	76–100% (n=15)			0–25% (n=12)	26–50% (n=12)	51–75% (n=12)	76–100% (n=12)		
Dense fibrous tissue	12 (4)	39 (3)	57 (2)	56 (3)	123.21†	0.25	12 (5)	15 (3)	34 (2)	46 (3)	55.53†	13.69†
Loose fibrous tissue	2 (2)	4 (1)	4 (1)	4 (1)	1.41	0.36	0 (1)	3 (1)	6 (1)	4 (1)	5.09	1.33
Cellular fibrous tissue	84 (5)	48 (3)	22 (3)	11 (3)	295.80†	7.45§	87 (5)	75 (3)	42 (3)	18 (3)	184.94†	36.17†
Calcium	1 (2)	2 (2)	6 (1)	8 (2)	20.10‡	0.74	0 (2)	2 (2)	6 (1)	16 (1)	54.75†	31.98†
Pultaceous debris	0 (2)	2 (1)	6 (1)	16 (1)	83.20†	41.70†	0 (2)	0 (1)	4 (1)	7 (1)	28.33†	7.07
Foam cells	0 (0)	1 (0.1)	1 (0.1)	1 (0.1)	11.40§	0.04	0 (0.1)	0 (0.1)	0 (0.1)	0 (0.1)	7.40	1.61
Foam cells and lymphocytes	1 (3)	6 (2)	4 (2)	5 (2)	4.67	0.18	1 (3)	5 (2)	9 (2)	7 (2)	3.77	0.99
Inflammatory infiltrate without foam cells	0 (0.4)	1 (0.2)	2 (0.2)	2 (0.3)	5.58	0.34	0 (0.4)	0 (0.2)	0 (0.2)	1 (0.3)	8.49§	17.31‡

*Two patients had no sections narrowed 0–25% cross-sectional area.
†Bonferroni adjusted p value <0.0001; ‡Bonferroni adjusted p value <0.001; §Bonferroni adjusted p value <0.05.
Numbers in parentheses are percentages.

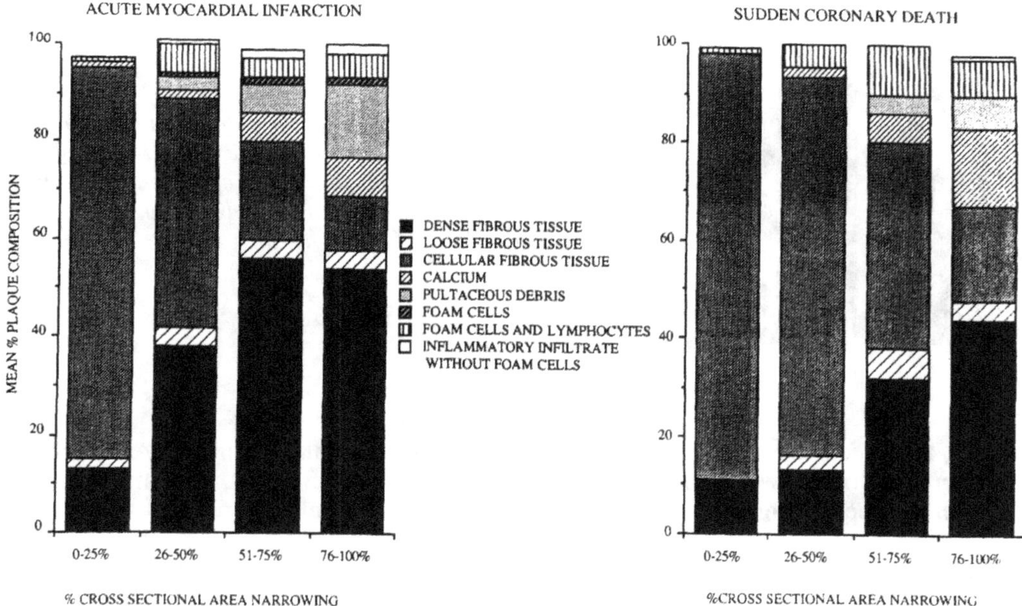

FIGURE 4. *Bar graphs depicting mean coronary arterial plaque composition of the four major epicardial coronary arteries analyzed according to degree of cross-sectional–area narrowing.*

TABLE 5. **Mean Composition of Coronary Arterial Atherosclerotic Plaque in the Four Major Epicardial Coronary Arteries**

	Mean percent (SEM) of plaque containing various components in the four major coronary arteries (1,084 segments)		
Component of plaque	Acute myocardial infarct ($n=15$)	Sudden coronary death ($n=12$)	F value
Dense fibrous tissue	46 (4)	29 (4)	10.3*
Loose fibrous tissue	3 (1)	3 (1)	0.22
Cellular fibrous tissue	32 (4)	50 (4)	11.1†
Calcium	4 (1)	8 (2)	3.8
Pultaceous debris	8 (1)	4 (1)	4.61
Foam cells	1 (0.5)	0 (0.5)	2.61
Foam cells and lymphocytes	4 (1)	6 (1)	2.32
Inflammatory infiltrates without significant numbers of foam cells	2 (0.4)	1 (0.4)	5.67

*Bonferroni adjusted p value <0.05.
†Bonferroni adjusted p value <0.01.
Numbers in parentheses are percentages.

more dense fibrous tissue (46% vs. 34%, $p<0.0001$), calcified tissue (16% vs. 6%, $p<0.0001$), and inflammatory infiltrates without foam cells (0% vs. 1%, $p<0.001$), and significantly less cellular fibrous tissue (18% vs. 42%, $p<0.0001$) were found in sections narrowed by more than 75% in cross-sectional area.

Comparison of the overall plaque composition between the AMI and SCD groups disclosed that the total percentage of fibrous tissue was similar (81% vs. 82%). Significantly more dense fibrous tissue (46% vs. 29%, $p<0.05$) and less cellular fibrous tissue (32% vs. 50%, $p<0.01$) were seen in

the AMI group (Table 5 and Figure 5). No significant differences were seen in plaque composition between the two groups in sections narrowed by less than 25% in cross-sectional area. In sections narrowed by more than 75% in cross-sectional area, the percentages of cellular fibrous tissue (18% vs. 11%, $p<0.05$) and calcified tissue (16% vs. 8%, $p<0.01$) were greater, and the percentage of pultaceous debris (7% vs. 16%, $p<0.01$) was less in the SCD group.

When all 5-mm segments from arteries containing thrombus were deleted (13 arteries from 13 patients in the AMI group and one artery from one patient in the SCD group), no significant differences were observed in the percentages of the various components of plaque in any of the various analyses.

Discussion

This study analyzed and compared plaque composition in two groups of patients with fatal coronary artery disease, one with AMI, and one with SCD. A Movat-stained histologic section of each 5-mm segment from the four major coronary arteries was examined using standard light microscopy in conjunction with a computerized morphometry system. To assure that artifacts associated with tissue handling and processing did not affect interpretation of the comparative results, all tissues were treated in an identical fashion.

Plaque composition of the four major epicardial coronary arteries was similar in each of the two groups, and no significant differences were seen among the arteries within each group. When all segments of each of the four major epicardial coronary arteries were analyzed, the percentages of fibrous tissue, pultaceous debris, calcium, foam

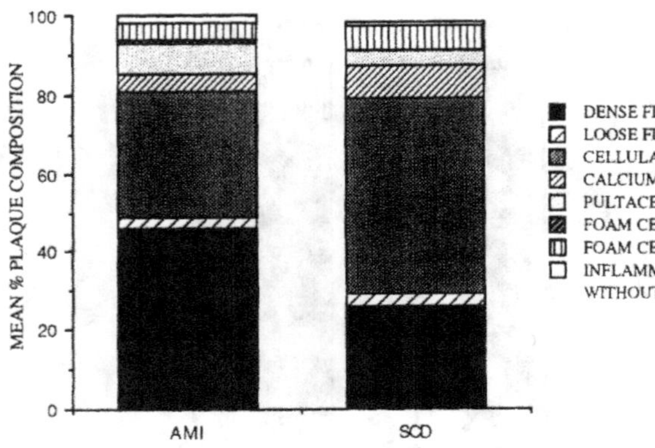

FIGURE 5. *Bar graph depicting mean coronary arterial plaque composition of all segments of the four major epicardial coronary arteries. AMI, acute myocardial infarction; SCD, sudden coronary death.*

cells, foam cells admixed with lymphocytes, and other inflammatory infiltrates were similar in the two groups. When the percentage of fibrous tissue (81–82%) was broken down into cellular and dense relatively acellular fibrous tissue, significantly more dense fibrous tissue (46% vs. 29%) and significantly less cellular fibrous tissue (32% vs. 50%) were found in the AMI group. When only sections with more than 75% cross-sectional–area narrowing were compared, significantly more pultaceous debris (16% vs. 7%), less calcium (8% vs. 16%), and less cellular fibrous tissue (11% vs. 18%) were found in the AMI group.

Analysis of plaque composition as a function of cross-sectional–area narrowing in the two groups disclosed several differences between the two groups. In both groups, the percentage of dense relatively acellular fibrous tissue, pultaceous debris, and calcium increased linearly across the four categories of narrowing, and the percentage of cellular fibrous tissue decreased. In the AMI group, the percentage of foam cells increased in linear fashion, and in the SCD group, the percentage of inflammatory infiltrates without foam cells and frequently associated with small vascular channels increased linearly across the four categories of narrowing.

Comparison of plaque composition between sections critically narrowed (>75% in cross-sectional area) and those less critically narrowed (51–75% in cross-sectional area) showed that in AMI patients the percentage of pultaceous debris was greater and that the percentage of cellular fibrous tissue was less in the critically narrowed sections. In the SCD group, these differences in the percentage of pultaceous debris were not seen. Significantly higher percentages of dense fibrous tissue, cellular fibrous tissue, calcium, and inflammatory infiltrates without foam cells were found in the more severely narrowed segments of artery.

Despite similar degrees of cross-sectional–area narrowing in the two groups of patients, several features serve to distinguish the AMI and SCD groups. First, the mean percentage of pultaceous debris was greater, and the mean percentage of cellular fibrous tissue and heavily calcified tissue was less in sections narrowed by more than 75% in cross-sectional area in the AMI group than in the SCD group. Second, the amounts of pultaceous debris and cellular fibrous tissue were the only components that distinguished between critically narrowed (>75% cross-sectional area) and less critically narrowed sections in the AMI group. Third, the frequency of intraluminal thrombi was much greater in the AMI group than in the SCD group (13 of 15 vs. one of 12).

It is recognized that intraluminal thrombi most commonly are seen at necropsy at sites where the underlying plaque contains a necrotic core (composed of pultaceous debris rich in cholesterol clefts).[10-14] Furthermore, intraluminal thrombi have been reported to occur primarily at sites where the underlying plaque has ruptured.[13,15] Falk,[13] in an analysis of 47 patients with fatal coronary artery disease, found that 82% of intraluminal thrombi were associated with plaque rupture. Similarly, Davies and Thomas,[15] in a study of 100 patients with fatal coronary artery disease, found 103 of 115 thrombi associated with sites of plaque rupture. The mean percentage of pultaceous debris, which is rich in thrombogenic substances, was more than two times greater in the AMI group than in the SCD group. It is not surprising, therefore, that the frequency of coronary thrombi in the AMI group was much higher than in the SCD group. The higher percentage of pultaceous debris in the AMI group appears to predispose to the formation of intraluminal thrombi.

If one assumes that differences in plaque composition are responsible for the differing frequencies of thrombi in patients with AMI and SCD, the fact that deletion of arteries containing thrombi did not significantly alter the composition of plaque in the AMI group suggests that all of the epicardial coronary arteries in a given patient in the AMI group are more at risk for development of thrombi than any artery in a patient in the SCD group.

Tracy et al[14] studied the morphology of 21 "thrombotic plaques" from 18 patients with SCD and compared it to that in 129 "nonthrombotic plaques" from the same 18 patients and to 94 plaques from 22 patients without coronary artery disease. Because the presence of a necrotic core was considered essential for development of a thrombus, the nonthrombotic plaques were all selected so that they also contained a central necrotic core. They used a scoring system and analyzed the presence or absence of hemorrhage, rupture, "deep cellularity," phagocytosis, "superficial cellularity," adventitial infiltrates, foam cells, medial erosion, and calcium. With the exception of calcium, which was decreased in thrombotic plaques, they found all of these components to occur with greater frequency in the thrombotic plaques when compared with nonthrombotic plaques in the same patients. In our study, we found little differences in mean plaque composition in the coronary arteries of patients with fatal AMI when arteries containing thrombus were deleted from the study. A comparison of severely narrowed "nonthrombotic" segments of coronary arteries (those narrowed >75% in cross-sectional area by atherosclerotic plaque in the SCD group) to severely narrowed segments in patients dying of consequences of coronary thrombosis, however, showed the thrombotic plaques to contain less calcium and cellular fibrous tissue and more pultaceous debris than did nonthrombotic segments of coronary artery.

Previously published semiquantitative or quantitative studies of plaque composition have been infrequent. Cliff et al[16] studied plaque composition at three sites of narrowing from each of 34 patients with coronary artery disease (25 patients with SCD and nine patients with AMI) and in 25 control patients. They used a scoring system to analyze the amounts of chronic inflammatory infiltrates, vascular channels, hemmorhage, and pultaceous debris in plaque. The major component of plaque, which from our study, appears to be a combination of cellular and dense fibrous tissue, was not analyzed in their study. They found a strong linear correlation between the average inflammation score and the degree of stenosis of the coronary segments studied. Yla-Herttuala et al[17] analyzed the biochemical composition of plaque and media in the left anterior descending, left circumflex, and right coronary arteries in 154 men who died accidentally. Because their analyses involved both media and atherosclerotic plaque and because their patient population differed dramatically from ours, the results cannot be compared.

The major limitations of this study are those imposed by the method of examination. Light microscopic examination was performed on partially decalcified formalin-fixed tissues, and as a consequence, the portion of plaque consisting of calcium was likely underestimated. Furthermore, it is possible that because some lipid deposits may be lost from the plaques during processing and because special stains for lipids were not performed, the total amount of lipid may be underestimated. In a comparative analysis such as this, however, the absolute amount of any given component is not critical because all segments of the coronary arteries were treated in a similar fashion. Likewise, any errors induced by the method of determination of the absolute degree of cross-sectional–area narrowing of a given segment is not critical because the determination is only used to compare relative degrees of stenosis within and between groups of patients.

To minimize variables, the AMI and SCD groups were selected such that they were of similar ages and that the final coronary event was the only manifestation of ischemic coronary artery disease. It is not known whether the findings in these two select groups are applicable to all patients with fatal AMI or SCD.

The differences in plaque composition observed in critically narrowed sections between two groups of patients suggest that plaque developed at either different rates or under different influences in the two subsets of patients. Why plaque in critically narrowed segments in patients with SCD had more cellular fibrous tissue and calcium and less pultaceous debris than in the AMI patients is not clear.

If plaque formation is viewed as the result of an intimal smooth muscle cell proliferation that then undergoes various degrees of secondary changes including scarring, deposition of calcium and necrosis, then the plaque in patients with SCD, because it is more cellular and contains less necrotic pultaceous debris, may be at an earlier stage of development when, perhaps, it has an adequate vascular supply. Alternatively, if pultaceous debris arises from breakdown of organizing thrombi, patients with AMI have more pultaceous debris and dense fibrous tissue because they develop more thrombi on a continual basis than do patients who die without left ventricular necrosis. Irrespective of their origin, real differences in plaque morphology between patients with AMI and SCD exist, and these differences may account for the higher incidence of coronary thrombi and left ventricular necrosis in the AMI group.

References

1. Roberts WC, Jones AA: Quantitation of coronary arterial narrowing at necropsy in sudden coronary death: Analysis of 31 patients and comparison with 25 control subjects. *Am J Cardiol* 1979;44:39–45
2. Virmani R, Roberts WC: Quantification of coronary arterial narrowing and of left ventricular myocardial scarring in healed myocardial infarction with chronic eventually fatal, congestive cardiac failure. *Am J Med* 1980;68:831–838
3. Roberts WC, Jones AA: Quantification of coronary arterial narrowing at necropsy in acute transmural myocardial infarction: Analysis and comparison of findings in 27 patients and 22 controls. *Circulation* 1980;61:786–790
4. Brosius FC III, Roberts WC: Comparison of degree and extent of coronary narrowing by atherosclerotic plaque in anterior and posterior transmural acute myocardial infarction. *Circulation* 1981;64:715–722
5. Movat HZ: Demonstration of all connective tissue elements in a single section. *Arch Pathol* 1955;60:289–295
6. Hook GR, Rasband W: Macmeasure: A low-cost, easy to operate quantitative morphometrics system for the Macintosh computer, in Bailey GW (ed): *Proceedings of the 45th Annual Meeting of the Electron Microscopy Society of*

America. San Francisco, Calif, San Francisco Press, Inc, 1987, pp 920–921

7. Armitage P: *Statistical Methods in Medical Research.* New York, Wiley, 1974, pp 253–259
8. SAS Institute Inc: *SAS User's Guide: Statistics*, ed 5. Cary, North Carolina, 1985
9. Miller RG: *Simultaneous Statistical Inference*, ed 2. Springer-Verlag, New York, 1981
10. Chapman I: Morphogenesis of occluding coronary artery thrombosis. *Arch Pathol* 1965;80:256–261
11. Constantinides P: Plaque fissures in human coronary thrombosis. *J Atheroscler Res* 1966;6:1–17
12. Friedman M: The coronary thrombus: Its origin and fate. *Human Pathol* 1971;2:81–128
13. Falk E: Plaque rupture with severe pre-existing stenosis precipitating coronary thrombosis: Characteristics of coronary atherosclerotic plaques underlying fatal occlusive thrombi. *Br Heart J* 1983;50:127–342
14. Tracy RE, Devaney K, Kissling G: Characteristics of the plaque under a coronary thrombus. *Virchows Arch* 1985;405:411–427
15. Davies MJ, Thomas A: Thrombosis and acute coronary-artery lesions in sudden cardiac ischemic death. *N Engl J Med* 1984;310:1137–1140
16. Cliff WJ, Heathcote CR, Moss NS, Reichenbach DD: The coronary arteries in cases of cardiac and noncardiac sudden death. *Am J Pathol* 1988;132:319–329
17. Yla-Herttuala S, Sumuvuori H, Karkola K, Mottonen M, Nikkari Tapio: Atherosclerosis and biochemical composition of coronary arteries in Finnish men: Comparison of two populations with different incidences of coronary heart disease. *Atherosclerosis* 1987;65:109–115

KEY WORDS • coronary heart disease • thrombosis • myocardial infarction • death, sudden

Mode of Death, Frequency of Healed and Acute Myocardial Infarction, Number of Major Epicardial Coronary Arteries Severely Narrowed by Atherosclerotic Plaque, and Heart Weight in Fatal Atherosclerotic Coronary Artery Disease: Analysis of 889 Patients Studied at Necropsy

WILLIAM C. ROBERTS, MD, FACC, BENJAMIN N. POTKIN, MD, DONALD E. SOLUS, BS, SHANTHASUNDARI G. REDDY, MD

Bethesda, Maryland

Mode of death, frequency of a healed or an acute myocardial infarct, or both, number of major epicardial coronary arteries severely narrowed by atherosclerotic plaque, and heart weight were studied at necropsy in 889 patients 30 years of age or older with fatal atherosclerotic coronary artery disease. No patient had had a coronary bypass operation or coronary angioplasty. The 889 patients were classified into four major groups and each major group was classified into two subgroups: 1) *acute myocardial infarct* without (306 patients) or with (119 patients) a healed myocardial infarct; 2) *sudden out of hospital death* without (121 patients) or with (118 patients) a healed myocardial infarct; 3) *chronic congestive heart failure with a healed myocardial infarct* without (137 patients) or with (33 patients) a left ventricular aneurysm; and 4) *sudden in-hospital death* without (20 patients) or with (35 patients) unstable angina pectoris.

The mean age of the 687 men (77%) was 60 ± 11 years, and of the 202 women (23%), 68 ± 13 years (p = 0.0001).

Although men included 77% of all patients, they made up approximately 90% of the out of hospital (nonangina) sudden death group. The frequency of systemic hypertension and angina pectoris was similar in each of the four major groups. The frequency of diabetes mellitus was least in the sudden out of hospital death group and similar in the other three major groups.

The mean heart weight and the percent of patients with a heart of increased weight were highest in the chronic congestive heart failure group; values were lower and similar in the other three major groups. All patients in the chronic congestive heart failure group (by definition) had a healed left ventricular infarct, which was similar in frequency in the other three major groups. The percent of patients in whom three or four of the four major coronary arteries were severely narrowed (>75% in cross-sectional area) by atherosclerotic plaque was highest in the unstable angina subgroup and similar in all other major groups.

(*J Am Coll Cardiol 1990;15:196–203*)

Atherosclerotic coronary artery disease usually manifests itself clinically by angina pectoris or acute myocardial infarction, and occasionally by evidence of congestive heart failure or arrhythmia without angina or myocardial infarction. The reason why one patient with coronary artery disease has angina and another has a myocardial infarct is not known. The mode of death in coronary artery disease and the frequency of the various morphologic consequences of severe coronary artery disease have not been examined in a large number of patients at necropsy in nearly 30 years. During the last 30 years, patients with atherosclerotic coronary artery disease have been categorized much differently than in earlier years. Unstable angina pectoris and ischemic cardiomyopathy are conditions not included in earlier studies of mode of death from coronary artery disease. In this report, we describe mode of death; frequency of a healed or an acute myocardial infarct, or both; number of major epicardial coronary arteries severely narrowed by atherosclerotic plaque; and heart weight in 889 patients >30 years of age studied at necropsy.

From the Pathology Branch, National Heart, Lung, and Blood Institute, National Institutes of Health, Bethesda, Maryland.

Manuscript received April 28, 1989; revised manuscript received July 19, 1989, accepted August 8, 1989.

Address for reprints: William C. Roberts, MD, Pathology Branch, Building 10, Room 2N258, National Institutes of Health, Bethesda, Maryland 20892.

Patients Studied and Methods

Study Patients

Exclusion and inclusion criteria. The accession files from 1961 until June 1, 1988 of the Pathology Branch, National Heart, Lung, and Blood Institute were examined for cases coded as "coronary artery disease." The records of the Pathology Branch for all such cases coded were then examined, and the following cases were excluded: 1) age at death <30 years; 2) coronary artery bypass grafting operation or any other type of cardiac operation at any time; 3) presence of a major associated cardiac condition, such as primary valvular heart disease (e.g., aortic stenosis, mitral regurgitation, aortic regurgitation), hypertrophic cardiomyopathy, infiltrative myocardial disease (e.g., amyloidosis, hemosiderosis, sarcoidosis, neoplasm) or major congenital cardiovascular anomaly (e.g., anomalous origin of one or more major epicardial arteries, ventricular septal defect). Also excluded were approximately 30 patients with severe atherosclerotic coronary artery disease with chronic congestive heart failure without a healed myocardial infarct (1). It is likely that these patients actually had "idiopathic dilated cardiomyopathy," a diagnosis not permitted in the presence of severe coronary artery disease; but nevertheless, most were habitual alcoholics. Patients with severe atherosclerotic coronary artery disease who died from a noncardiac cause were also excluded.

The present study was limited to patients aged >30 years of age whose cause of death was atherosclerotic coronary artery disease. A total of 889 patients fulfilled these criteria. All had one or more major (right, left main, left anterior descending and left circumflex) epicardial coronary arteries narrowed >75% in cross-sectional area by atherosclerotic plaque with or without associated coronary artery thrombus.

Source of cases. The necropsy in the 889 patients was performed at 110 different hospitals: 759 cases from 12 Washington, D.C. area hospitals; 45 cases from 13 nonlocal hospitals with each submitting ≥2 cases; and 85 cases from 85 different nonlocal hospitals, each submitting 1 case. All cases were initially examined by one of us (W.C.R.) who established the accessioning code for each case. Of the 889 cases included in this study, 63 were studied from 1961 to 1970, 346 from 1971 to 1980 and 480 from 1981 through June 1988.

Weighing the heart. The heart in cases included before 1971 was weighed on a Lipshaw scale, which is accurate to 10 g. The heart in cases included from 1971 onward was weighed on a Mettler P1210 scale, which is accurate to 0.1 g. Before the heart was weighed, it was "cleaned" of all extraneous material such as parietal pericardium and postmortem intracavitary clot. Before the heart was weighed, the pulmonary trunk and ascending aorta were excised about 2 cm cephalad to the sinotubular junction, i.e., an imaginary line corresponding to the most cephalad extension of the semilunar valve commissures, which also corresponds to the most cephalad portion of the semilunar valve sinuses. The weight of the heart was determined after fixation in formalin for 3 to 30 days.

Characteristics of patients studied (Table 1). The 889 patients were classified into four major groups and each major group was classified into two subgroups: 1) *acute myocardial infarct* without (306 patients) or with (119 patients) a healed myocardial infarct; 2) *sudden out of hospital death* (no myocardial necrosis) without (121 patients) or with (118 patients) a healed myocardial infarct; 3) *chronic congestive heart failure with a healed myocardial infarct* without (137 patients) or with (33 patients) a left ventricular aneurysm; and 4) *sudden in-hospital death* without (20 patients) or with (35 patients) unstable angina pectoris.

Definition of Terms

Acute myocardial infarct. All patients included in this group had histologically confirmed left ventricular wall coagulation necrosis. Of the 425 cases included in this group, over 400 had grossly visible foci of necrosis that, at some point, involved all of the inner one-half of the left ventricular wall and a portion of the outer one-half of the wall. In the few cases in which the necrosis had not been recorded as being grossly discernible, histologic sections disclosed the presence of coagulation necrosis.

Healed myocardial infarct. A healed infarct was a grossly visible scar in the left ventricular wall. A few scars involved only the inner one-half of the wall (subendocardial), but most (>90%) involved all of the inner half and a portion or all of the outer half.

Sudden out of hospital death. All 239 patients included in this group died suddenly, usually within 10 min—and always within 6 h—from the onset of a change in previous asymptomatic status (2). The onset of symptoms of myocardial ischemia occurred in all 239 patients while they were outside the hospital, usually at home. Death in 217 (91%) of the 239 patients occurred outside the hospital; in the other 22 patients (9%) it occurred shortly after arrival at the hospital, usually in the emergency room.

Chronic congestive heart failure. Evidence of chronic congestive heart failure was based on the clinical record. The 170 patients included in this group were stated by their physicians to have had evidence of chronic congestive heart failure. Nearly all had received drugs, usually digitalis and diuretics, for congestive heart failure. At necropsy, all had a dilated left ventricular cavity and a transmural left ventricular scar.

Left ventricular aneurysm. The cases included in this category had a true left ventricular aneurysm; i.e., the wall of the aneurysm originally had been a portion of the left ventricular wall (3,4). The aneurysmal wall consisted mainly of scar tissue. At necropsy, the bulge of the aneurysm

Table 1. Clinical and Morphologic Findings in 889 Necropsy Patients >30 Years of Age With Fatal Atherosclerotic Coronary Artery Disease

| | Acute Myocardial Infarct | | Sudden Out of Hospital Death | |
| | Healed Myocardial Infarct | | Healed Myocardial Infarct | |
Variable	Absent	Present	Absent	Present
No. of patients	306 (34%)	119 (13%)	121 (14%)	118 (13%)
Men/women	200 (65%)/106 (35%)	82 (69%)/37 (31%)	109 (90%)/12 (10%)	105 (89%)/13 (11%)
Age (yr) mean (range)				
Men	62 ± 11 (35 to 93)	63 ± 11 (37 to 88)	53 ± 11 (30 to 91)	57 ± 12 (30 to 90)
Women	72 ± 11 (37 to 94)	69 ± 12 (43 to 95)	60 ± 19 (31 to 85)	57 ± 11 (42 to 78)
Men and women	66 ± 12 (35 to 94)	65 ± 12 (37 to 95)	54 ± 12 (30 to 91)	56 ± 12 (30 to 90)
No. with SH	131/239 (55%)	50/89 (56%)	42/87 (48%)	33/66 (50%)
No. with AP	70/243 (29%)	48/99 (48%)	19/80 (24%)	34/71 (48%)
No. with DM	60/182 (33%)	35/92 (38%)	8/60 (13%)	16/60 (27%)
Heart weight (g) mean (range)				
Men	479 ± 94 (290 to 800)	490 ± 84 (330 to 685)	488 ± 123 (310 to 925)	517 ± 125 (315 to 915)
Women	407 ± 88 (219 to 670)	434 ± 77 (270 to 555)	418 ± 119 (290 to 650)	437 ± 107 (305 to 660)
Men and women	454 ± 98 (219 to 800)	472 ± 86 (270 to 685)	480 ± 124 (290 to 925)	508 ± 126 (305 to 915)
No. of men with HW ≤400 g	47/200 (24%)	14/82 (17%)	34/109 (31%)	20/105 (19%)
No. of women with HW ≤350 g	31/106 (29%)	7/37 (19%)	4/12 (33%)	3/13 (23%)
No. of men and women with normal HW	78/306 (25%)	21/119 (18%)	38/121 (31%)	23/118 (19%)
No. of major CAs >75% in CSA plaque				
1	51 (17%)	6 (5%)	24 (20%)	14 (12%)
2	62 (20%)	23 (19%)	39 (32%)	31 (26%)
3	135 (44%)	66 (55%)	48 (40%)	63 (53%)
4	14 (5%)	10 (9%)	4 (3%)	7 (6%)
≥1	44 (14%)	14 (12%)	6 (5%)	3 (3%)
Acute myocardial infarct	306 (100%)	119 (100%)	0	0
Healed myocardial infarct	0	119 (100%)	0	118 (100%)
Chronic CHF	0	20 (17%)	0	10 (8%)
Left ventricular aneurysm	0	4 (3%)	0	2 (2%)
Sudden death	0	0	121 (100%)	118 (100%)

AP = angina pectoris; CA = coronary artery; CHF = congestive heart failure; CSA = cross-sectional area; DM = diabetes mellitus; HW = heart weight; SH = systemic hypertension.

extended outward compared with the nonaneurysmal wall of the left ventricle. The mouth into the aneurysm was the largest diameter or equivalent to the largest diameter of the aneurysm. Most aneurysms contained intraaneurysmal thrombus.

Sudden in-hospital death. All 55 patients in this group died in the hospital. Of the 55 patients, 35 were hospitalized because of increasing frequency or intensity of angina pectoris; all 35 patients had cardiac arrest, usually several days after hospitalization. Nine of the 35 patients with unstable angina had cardiac arrest during cardiac catheterization, and died at the time or shortly after initially successful cardiac resuscitation (5); the other 26 patients had cardiac arrest outside the cardiac catheterization laboratory, but in the hospital. The initial cardiac arrest in 25 of the 26 patients was fatal; the remaining patient developed evidence of acute myocardial infarction after nonfatal arrest 36 h before the fatal arrest.

All 20 patients who died in the hospital without unstable angina had been admitted to the hospital for conditions other than myocardial ischemia. Four died suddenly during hemodialysis for chronic renal failure. Seven had cardiac arrest while being evaluated for a noncardiac problem. Nine died suddenly shortly after a noncardiac operation; seven after peripheral vascular surgery; one after eye surgery and one after spinal cord surgery; none had pulmonary emboli at necropsy.

Criteria for increased cardiac weight. A heart weighing >350 g in women and >400 g in men was considered increased in weight.

Table 1. Continued

| Chronic CHF and Healed Myocardial Infarct | | Sudden In-Hospital Death | | |
| Left Ventricular Aneurysm | | Unstable Angina Pectoris | | |
Absent	Present	Absent	Present	Totals
137 (15%)	33 (4%)	20 (2%)	35 (4%)	889 (100%)
118 (86%)/19 (14%)	28 (85%)/5 (15%)	19 (95%)/1 (5%)	26 (74%)/9 (26%)	687 (77%)/202 (23%)
63 ± 10 (38 to 86)	58 ± 11 (39 to 82)	67 ± 10 (48 to 81)	62 ± 11 (43 to 77)	60 ± 11 (30 to 93)
67 ± 14 (41 to 89)	61 ± 6 (55 to 71)	58	62 ± 11 (46 to 77)	68 ± 13 (31 to 95)
64 ± 10 (38 to 89)	59 ± 10 (39 to 82)	66 ± 8 (48 to 81)	62 ± 10 (43 to 77)	62 ± 12 (30 to 95)
46/92 (50%)	10/19 (53%)	15/19 (79%)	14/29 (43%)	341/640 (53%)
41/99 (41%)	7/20 (35%)	6/17 (35%)	35/35 (100%)	260/664 (39%)
37/78 (47%)	4/16 (25%)	8/18 (44%)	10/27 (37%)	178/533 (33%)
564 ± 109 (330 to 940)	553 ± 94 (350 to 790)	476 ± 73 (360 to 600)	475 ± 64 (390 to 560)	505 ± 110 (290 to 940)
511 ± 77 (340 to 650)	494 ± 115 (400 to 685)	405	405 ± 106 (260 to 620)	427 ± 94 (220 to 685)
557 ± 107 (330 to 940)	544 ± 101 (350 to 390)	472 ± 75 (360 to 600)	456 ± 82 (260 to 620)	488 ± 111 (220 to 940)
6/118 (5%)	1/28 (4%)	1/19 (5%)	6/26 (23%)	129/687 (19%)
1/19 (5%)	0/5	0/1	2/9 (22%)	48/202 (24%)
7/137 (5%)	1/33 (3%)	1/20 (5%)	8/35 (23%)	177/889 (20%)
22 (16%)	4 (12%)	5 (25%)	2 (6%)	128 (14%)
31 (23%)	11 (33%)	5 (25%)	5 (14%)	207 (23%)
56 (41%)	11 (33%)	9 (45%)	14 (40%)	402 (45%)
5 (4%)	2 (6%)	0	13 (37%)	55 (6%)
23 (17%)	5 (15%)	1 (5%)	1 (3%)	97 (11%)
0	0	0	0	425 (48%)
137 (100%)	33 (100%)	11 (55%)	19 (54%)	437 (49%)
137 (100%)	33 (100%)	3 (15%)	1 (3%)	204 (23%)
0	33 (100%)	0	0	39 (4%)
0	0	20 (100%)	35 (100%)	303 (34%)

Statistical analysis. In the analysis of variance, unpaired Student's *t* test was used to test for significant differences among and between sample means and variance; chi-square analysis was used for noncontinuous data. A probability value <0.05 was considered significant.

Results

Gender and age distribution. The 889 patients ranged in age from 30 to 95 years (mean 62 ± 12): the 687 (77%) men, from 30 to 93 years (mean 60 ± 11), and the 202 (23%) women, from 31 to 95 years (mean 68 ± 13) (p = 0.0001). The percent of men with an acute myocardial infarct was significantly less than that of the patients who died suddenly out of the hospital or those with chronic congestive heart failure with a healed myocardial infarct (p = 0.001). The mean age of the patients in the sudden out of hospital death group was younger than that in the other three major groups (p = 0.0001).

Frequency of systemic hypertension, angina pectoris and diabetes mellitus. *Clinical information concerning the presence or absence of systemic hypertension* was available in 640 (72%) of the 889 patients: 341 (53%) had systemic hypertension (229 by history alone; 56 by measured systolic and diastolic blood pressures [>140/90 mm Hg]; 56 by a history of antihypertensive drug treatment) and 229 (47%) did not. The frequency of systemic hypertension was similar among the four subgroups.

Clinical information concerning the presence or absence of angina pectoris was available in 664 patients (75%): 260 (39%) had angina and 404 (61%) did not. Patients with an acute myocardial infarct with a healed myocardial infarct had a higher frequency of angina than those with an acute myocardial infarct without a healed myocardial infarct (48

[48%] of 99 versus 70 [29%] of 243; p = 0.001). Among patients who died suddenly outside the hospital, those with a healed myocardial infarct had a higher frequency of angina pectoris than did those without a healed myocardial infarct (34 [48%] of 71 versus 19 [24%] of 80; p = 0.01).

Clinical information concerning the presence or absence of diabetes mellitus was available in 533 patients (60%): 178 (33%) had diabetes mellitus and 355 (67%) did not. The frequency of diabetes was lowest in the patients who died suddenly out of the hospital without a healed myocardial infarct (8 [13%] of 60) and highest in the patients with chronic congestive heart failure with a healed myocardial infarct without a left ventricular aneurysm (37 [47%] of 78; p = 0.001).

Coronary artery narrowing. In all 889 patients, at least one of the four major epicardial coronary arteries was narrowed >75% in cross-sectional area by atherosclerotic plaque. Of the 792 patients in whom all four major arteries were available for examination, only one artery was so narrowed by plaque in 128 patients (16%); two arteries were so narrowed in 207 patients (26%); three arteries were so narrowed in 402 patients (51%); and all four arteries were so narrowed in 55 patients (7%). Of the 3,168 major epicardial coronary arteries in these 792 patients, 1,968 arteries (62%) were narrowed >75% in cross-sectional area by atherosclerotic plaque, an average of 2.48 of 4 major arteries per patient. Thus, "multivessel" coronary artery disease was present in >80% of the patients, and none of the coronary arteries in any patient was devoid of atherosclerotic plaque.

Heart weight and mode of death. The heart weight in the 889 patients ranged from 220 to 940 g (mean 488 ± 111); the heart weight ranged from 290 to 940 g (mean 505 ± 110) in the 687 men and from 220 to 685 g (mean 427 ± 94) in the 202 women. The mean heart weight was greatest in the group with chronic congestive heart failure with a healed myocardial infarct; values were lower and similar among each of the other three groups. Of the 889 patients, 437 (49%) had a healed myocardial infarct, and they had a significantly heavier heart than those without a healed myocardial infarct (514 ± 109 versus 462 ± 108; p = 0.0001).

Of the 889 patients, 177 (20%) had a heart of normal weight. The percent of patients with normal heart weight was greatest for the group with sudden out of hospital death without a healed myocardial infarct (38 [31%] of 121) and least for the group with chronic congestive heart failure with a healed myocardial infarct (8 [5%] of 170) (p = 0.001). The percent of patients with a normal heart weight was greater for those without than for those with a healed myocardial infarct (118 [27%] of 437 versus 59 [13%] of 452; p = 0.001).

Heart weight and the number of coronary arteries severely narrowed. Of the 889 patients, 128 (14%) had >75% cross-sectional area narrowing by atherosclerotic plaque of only one major (right, left main, left anterior descending and left circumflex) epicardial coronary artery, and 100 (78%) of

them had increased heart weight; 207 (23%) had two major arteries so narrowed and 170 (82%) had increased heart weight; 402 (45%) had three major arteries so narrowed and 326 (81%) had increased heart weight; 55 (6%) had >75% narrowing of four arteries and 32 (58%) had increased heart weight; 97 (11%) patients had >75% narrowing of one or more major epicardial coronary arteries, but the exact number of arteries so narrowed was not known and 76 (78%) had increased heart weight. Therefore, the mean heart weight and the frequency of increased heart weight were similar among the patients with one, two, three and four or one or more coronary arteries narrowed >75% in cross-sectional area by plaque.

Analysis of Each Coronary Subgroup

Acute myocardial infarct. Of the 889 patients, the mode of death in 425 (48%) was acute myocardial infarction. Of these 425 patients, 119 (28%) had had a previous acute myocardial infarct that had healed, as indicated by the presence of a grossly visible scar in the left ventricular wall, and 326 (78%) had a heart of increased weight. Of these 425 patients, 282 (66%) were men and 143 (34%) were women; the mean age at death for the men was 62 years and for the women, 71 years. Systemic hypertension had been present (by history) in 55%, angina pectoris in 35%, diabetes mellitus in 35% and chronic congestive heart failure in 5%. Four of the 119 patients with a healed myocardial infarct had anatomically discernible left ventricular aneurysm.

Sudden out of hospital death. Of the 889 patients, the mode of death in 239 (27%) was cardiac arrest outside the hospital. Of these 239 patients, 118 (49%) had had an acute myocardial infarct that had healed, as indicated by the presence of a grossly visible scar in the left ventricular wall. Of these 239 patients, 214 (90%) were men and only 25 (10%) were women. The mean age at death in the men was 55 years and in the women, 58 years. Systemic hypertension had been present (by history) in 49%, angina pectoris in 35%, diabetes mellitus in 20% and chronic congestive heart failure in 4%. Only 2 of the 239 patients had a left ventricular aneurysm, and 178 (74%) had a heart of increased weight.

Chronic congestive heart failure with a healed myocardial infarct. Of the 889 patients, the mode of death in 170 (19%) was chronic congestive heart failure, and all of these patients had one or more healed left ventricular infarcts. (Patients with chronic congestive heart failure associated with coronary artery narrowing, but unassociated with left ventricular wall necrosis or fibrosis, were not included in this study.) Of the 170 patients, 146 (86%) were men and 24 (14%) were women; the mean age at death in the men was 62 years and in the women, 66 years. Systemic hypertension had been present (by history) in 50%, angina pectoris in 40%, diabetes mellitus in 44%, a heart of increased weight in 95% and a healed left ventricular aneurysm in 19%.

Sudden in-hospital death. Of the 889 patients, 55 (6%) died suddenly in the hospital without evidence of acute myocardial infarction either clinically or at necropsy. This group consisted of two distinct subgroups of patients. One subgroup consisted of 20 patients hospitalized for conditions not related to the heart, but each had cardiac arrest during evaluation of the noncardiac problem or during hemodialysis or early after a noncardiac operation. Eleven of the 20 patients had a previous acute myocardial infarction, as indicated by the presence of a left ventricular scar. Only 1 of the 20 patients was a woman (aged 58 years); the mean age of the men was 67 years.

The other subgroup consisted of 35 patients who were admitted because of unstable angina. All died suddenly, nine during diagnostic cardiac catheterization. Of these 35 patients, 26 (74%) were men and 9 (26%) were women; their mean age was 62 years. Of these 35 patients, systemic hypertension was present in 43%, diabetes mellitus in 37% and chronic congestive heart failure in 3%; at necropsy, 77% had a heart of increased weight and 54% had one or more healed myocardial infarcts.

Discussion

Clinicopathologic correlations. The present study presents data on mode of death in nearly 900 patients with fatal coronary artery disease studied at necropsy. All 889 patients died from consequences of atherosclerotic coronary artery disease, and the heart in all 889 was examined at necropsy by the same physician (W.C.R.). Of the 889 patients studied at necropsy, 425 (48%) had an acute myocardial infarct and 119 (28%) of them also had a grossly visible healed myocardial infarct; 239 patients (27%) died suddenly outside the hospital, and 118 (49%) of them had a healed myocardial infarct; 170 patients (19%) had chronic, intractable, eventually fatal congestive heart failure associated with one or more healed infarcts; 55 patients (6%) died suddenly in the hospital without an acute myocardial infarct, and 30 (55%) of these 55 had a healed myocardial infarct and 35 (64%) had unstable angina pectoris. None of the 889 patients had had coronary artery bypass grafting or coronary angioplasty. Thus, of the 889 patients, 437 (49%) had one or more grossly visible left ventricular scars.

Mode of death. Of the 437 patients (49%) with one or more grossly visible left ventricular scars, the fatal coronary event in 119 (27%) was an acute myocardial infarct; in 118 patients (27%) it was sudden out of hospital (or nearly so) cardiac arrest; in 170 patients (39%) it was chronic, intractable congestive heart failure; and in 30 patients (7%) it was sudden in-hospital death with or without preceding unstable angina pectoris. Of the 452 patients (51%) without a grossly visible left ventricular scar, the fatal coronary event in 306 (68%) was an acute myocardial infarct; in 121 patients (27%) it was sudden (or nearly so) out of hospital cardiac arrest,

and in 25 patients (5%) it was sudden in-hospital cardiac arrest with or without preceding unstable angina pectoris. Thus, the patients without a previous acute myocardial infarct were more likely (nearly 70%) to die from an acute myocardial infarct, and the fatal events in the patients with a previous acute myocardial infarct were more or less equally divided among the subgroups with fatal acute myocardial infarct, sudden (or nearly so) out of hospital cardiac arrest and chronic congestive heart failure.

Age at death. One of the major tragedies of coronary artery disease is the relatively young age of its victims. Among the 687 men in this study, the average age at death was 60 years; among the 202 women, the average age at death was 68 years, roughly 10 years less than the average life expectancy for men and women in the United States. Patients <30 years of age at death were excluded from the present study.

Comparison with previous studies. How representative of the modes of death from coronary artery disease are the patients in the present study? Most (73%) of the patients included in the present study died in a hospital, and this fact almost surely increases the percent of cases with a fatal acute myocardial infarct. Had more medical examiners' cases been included, the percent of patients who died suddenly outside the hospital almost surely would have been higher. Had only hospital deaths been included in the present study, the percent of sudden deaths would have been considerably less. Although the mode of death from coronary artery disease may or may not have been different from that in the present study had all victims of coronary artery disease in a single community been available for study at necropsy, the present study nevertheless provides opportunity to compare victims of one mode of death with victims of another mode of death when all cases had been studied and classified by the same physician (W.C.R.).

Although many reports (6–22) have described findings at necropsy in patients with coronary artery disease, it is surprisingly difficult and probably relatively meaningless to compare the present data with those reported in earlier decades by others. *There are several reasons why these comparisons are probably not useful, with one exception to be described subsequently.*

The use in older reports of cardiac terms that are no longer used and that were never defined or imprecisely defined. For example, are the terms "coronary thrombosis, sudden or acute coronary occlusion, acute coronary, acute coronary obstruction and myocardial accident," as used in older reports, synonyms for "acute myocardial infarction" used today, or are some of these terms synonyms for "sudden coronary death," (2) as used today? Are "coronary insufficiency" and "coronary failure," as used in the past, synonyms for "unstable angina" or "sudden death," as used today? The term unstable angina pectoris, introduced by Conti et al. (23), has been used for <2 decades. Are "myocardial insufficiency" or "myocardial failure" old terms for chronic congestive heart failure or "ischemic cardiomyopathy," as used today? "Sudden death" and "gradual death" in older reports were rarely defined.

The use of different inclusion and exclusion criteria. Some past studies included only young individuals, others only older individuals; some studies intermixed cases in which coronary artery disease caused death and in which death was not of coronary artery disease origin but coronary artery disease was present at necropsy or had produced symptoms of myocardial ischemia during life. Other studies included only patients who died in the hospital and others, only those who died outside the hospital; still other studies included only cases with a single coronary event—for example, acute myocardial infarction—and excluded those with sudden death, or vice versa.

The use of relatively few cases. Obviously, meaningful data on the frequency of the various modes of death from coronary artery disease cannot be obtained by studying relatively small numbers of patients, irrespective of how detailed those studies might be.

The use of data collected by numerous physicians with little expertise in cardiovascular disease versus that collected by a single individual or by relatively few individuals who specialize in cardiovascular disease. Nearly all publications focusing on the various modes of death from coronary artery disease or the cardiac findings in fatal coronary artery disease have been based on data recorded in autopsy protocols and collected by numerous physicians with little expertise in cardiovascular disease. In the present report, all hearts were examined by a single physician who has now specialized in cardiovascular diseases for 3 decades.

The treatment of patients in one time period is usually different from that of another, and the different treatments may alter frequency of the various modes of death and necropsy cardiac findings. Coronary care units were not widely employed until about 1970, and the mortality rate during acute myocardial infarction, and therefore, subsequent mortality, probably has been affected by their use. Pharmaceutical therapy for systemic hypertension was not used until about 1950, and in 1972 only 15% of patients in the United States with systemic hypertension were having their blood pressure adequately controlled by therapy; by 1987, this percent had climbed to nearly 60%. Thus, possibly, future studies of the heart at necropsy in fatal coronary artery disease will see a fall in the frequency of cardiomegaly and maybe other reflections of antihypertensive therapy on the heart. Future studies of modes of death from coronary artery disease may reflect the use or abuse of coronary angioplasty, coronary bypass grafting and various thrombolytic therapies.

The Rochester, Minnesota study. A superb study of the modes of death from coronary artery disease and cardiac findings at necropsy in its victims was reported by Spieker-

man and colleagues (20) in 1962. Their study analyzed deaths of residents in a single community (Rochester, Minnesota) during a 5 year period (1947 to 1952). During that period, 1,026 persons aged 20 years or older died (50% women, 50% men) and necropsy was performed in 691 (67%). Of the 1,026 patients, 563 (55%) died in the hospital and autopsy was done in 377 (67%), and 463 (45%) died outside the hospital and necropsy was done in 314 (68%). Of the 691 patients aged 20 years or over studied at necropsy, 221 (32%) died from coronary artery disease (40% of the men and 22% of the women). However, of the patients aged 30 to 64 years, 54% died from coronary artery disease and in the age group 65 years or older, 38% died from coronary artery disease.

In this Mayo Clinic study (20), the modes of death in the 221 patients with fatal coronary artery disease were as follows: 1) "acute coronary failure" (sudden death), 94 patients (43%); 2) acute myocardial infarction, 87 patients (39%); 3) congestive heart failure, 32 patients (14%); and 4) "thromboembolism," 8 patients (4%). A healed myocardial infarct was seen at necropsy in 115 (52%) of the 221 patients, a percent virtually identical to that of the present study. In their study, nine patients included in their sudden death group actually had an acute myocardial infarct. If these nine patients were transferred from the sudden death to the acute myocardial infarct group, the frequency of acute myocardial infarction as the mode of death would climb to 43%, and the frequency of sudden death would fall to 38%, percentages similar to those in the present study (48% and 34%).

Association between heart weight and coronary artery disease. Cardiomegaly (heart weight >400 g in men and >350 g in women) occurred in 80% of our 889 patients. The average heart weight in the men was 505 g and in the women, 427 g. Of the 170 patients with congestive heart failure, 162 (95%) had a heart of increased weight; in contrast, of the 239 patients who died suddenly outside the hospital, 178 (74%) had a heart of increased weight. Of all 889 patients, only 20% had a heart of normal weight.

Although several previous publications have described cardiac weight at necropsy in some subsets of coronary artery disease patients, the number of cases included in each study has been relatively small, and the heart weight was that mainly recorded in autopsy protocols where enormous variations occur, depending on the care of the prosector. The cardiac weights in our study were obtained in the same manner over nearly a 30 year period. Nevertheless, recordings by others are similar to ours. Romppanen et al. (24) described mean cardiac weight in 55 men and in 24 women with an acute or healed myocardial infarct, or both: the mean heart weight of 8 men and 4 women with an acute myocardial infarct was 487 ± 45 and 402 ± 73 g, respectively; of 22 men and 8 women with a healed myocardial infarct, 498 ± 122 and 412 ± 88 g, respectively; of 20 men and 11 women with both a healed and an acute myocardial infarct, 506 ± 54 and

403 ± 85 g, respectively; and of 5 men and 1 woman with left ventricular aneurysm, 599 ± 118 and 390 g, respectively.

The relation between heart weight and amount of coronary artery narrowing has been controversial. Romppanen et al. (24) found no correlation between heart weight and number of coronary arteries severely narrowed by atherosclerotic plaque in 79 patients studied at necropsy. We also found no significant difference in mean heart weight or the percent with normal or increased heart weight in patients with severe narrowing of one, two, three or four arteries in our 889 patients studied at necropsy. Dean and Gallagher (25) examined the relation between heart weight and number of coronary arteries narrowed in 34 patients at necropsy. They gave more significance to narrowing in the proximal portions of the major arteries and in the left main coronary artery, and they found a significant correlation between cardiac weight and the number of major coronary arteries severely narrowed. When we analyzed our data, as they did (giving significant left main coronary narrowing an equivalency of two major artery narrowing), we still found no significant association between heart weight and the number of major coronary arteries severely narrowed by atherosclerotic plaque.

References

1. Ross EM, Roberts WC. Severe atherosclerotic coronary arterial narrowing and chronic congestive heart failure without myocardial infarction: analysis of 18 patients studied at necropsy. Am J Cardiol 1986;57:51–6.

2. Roberts WC. Sudden cardiac death: definitions and causes. Am J Cardiol 1986;57:1410–3.

3. Cabin HS, Roberts WC. Left ventricular aneurysm, intra-aneurysmal thrombus and systemic embolus in coronary heart disease. Chest 1980;77:586–90.

4. Cabin HS, Roberts WC. True left ventricular aneurysm and healed myocardial infarction. Clinical and necropsy observations including quantification of degrees of coronary arterial narrowing. Am J Cardiol 1980;46:754–63.

5. Cabin HS, Roberts WC. Fatal cardiac arrest during cardiac catheterization for angina pectoris: analysis of 10 necropsy patients. Am J Cardiol 1981;48:1–8.

6. Levine SA, Brown CL. Coronary thrombosis: its various clinical features. Medicine 1929;8:245–418.

7. Barnes AR, Ball RG. The incidence and situation of myocardial infarction in one thousand consecutive postmortem examinations. Am J Med Sci 1932;183:215–25.

8. Willius FA, Smith HL, Sprague PH. A study of coronary and aortic sclerosis: incidence and degree in 5,060 consecutive postmortem examinations. Proc Mayo Clin 1933;8:140–4.

9. Levy RL, Bruenn HB, Kurtz D. Facts on disease of the coronary arteries, based on a survey of the clinical and pathologic records of 762 cases. Am J Med Sci 1934;187:376–90.

10. Saphir O, Priest WS, Hamburger WW, Katz LN. Coronary arteriosclerosis, coronary thrombosis, and the resulting myocardial changes. An evaluation of their respective clinical pictures including the electrocardiographic records, based on the anatomical findings. Am Heart J 1935;10:567–95, 762–92.

11. Hedley OF. A study of 450 fatal cases of heart disease occurring in Washington (D.C.) hospitals during 1932, with special reference to etiology, race, and sex. Public Health Rep 1935;50:1127–53.

12. Bruenn HG, Turner KB, Levy RL. Notes on cardiac pain and coronary disease: correlation of observations made during life with structural changes found at autopsy in 476 cases. Am Heart J 1936;11:34–40.

13. Gordon WH, Bland EF, White PD. Coronary artery disease analyzed postmortem with special reference to the influence of economic status and sex. Am Heart J 1939;17:10–4.

14. Hedley OF. Five years' experience (1933–1937) with mortality from acute coronary occlusion in Philadelphia. Ann Intern Med 1939;13:598–611.

15. Yater WM, Traum AH, Brown WG, Fitzgerald RP, Geisler MA, Wilcox BB. Coronary artery disease in men eighteen to thirty-nine years of age: report of eight hundred sixty-six cases, four hundred fifty with necropsy examination. Am Heart J 1948;36:334–72, 481–526, 683–722.

16. Harrison CV, Wood P. Hypertensive and ischemic heart disease: a comparative clinical and pathological study. Br Heart J 1949;11:205–29.

17. McCain FH, Kline EM, Gilson JS. A clinical study of 281 autopsy reports on patients with myocardial infarction. Am Heart J 1950;39:263–72.

18. Yater WM, Welsh PP, Stapleton JF, Clark ML. Comparison of clinical and pathologic aspects of coronary artery disease in men of various age groups: a study of 950 autopsied cases from the Armed Forces Institute of Pathology. Ann Intern Med 1951;34:352–92.

19. Branwood AW, Montgomery GL. Observations on the morbid anatomy of coronary artery disease. Scott Med J 1956;1:367–75.

20. Spiekerman RE, Brandenburg JT, Achor RWP, Edwards JE. The spectrum of coronary heart disease in a community of 30,000. A clinicopathologic study. Circulation 1962;25:57–65.

21. Roberts WC, Buja LM. The frequency and significance of coronary arterial thrombi and other observations in fatal acute myocardial infarction: a study of 107 necropsy patients. Am J Med 1972;52:425–43.

22. Kuller LH, Cooper M, Perper J, Fisher R. Myocardial infarction and sudden death in an urban community. Bull NY Acad Med 1973;49:532–43.

23. Conti CR, Brawley RK, Griffith LSC, et al. Unstable angina pectoris: morbidity and mortality in 57 consecutive patients evaluated angiographically. Am J Cardiol 1973;32:745–50.

24. Romppanen T, Seppa A, Roilas H. Ischemic heart disease and heart weight. Cardiology 1983;70:206–12.

25. Dean JH, Gallagher PJ. Cardiac ischemia and cardiac hypertrophy: an autopsy study. Arch Pathol Lab Med 1980;104:175–8.

Sudden Cardiac Death: A Diversity of Causes with Focus on Atherosclerotic Coronary Artery Disease

William C. Roberts, MD

There are many causes of sudden cardiac death, and the younger the patient the more diverse the cause. Among persons dying suddenly in the Western World atherosclerotic coronary artery disease is the most common. This group might best be called atherosclerotic sudden coronary death. This article summarizes a previously published necropsy study by Warnes and Roberts of 70 victims aged 22 to 81 years (mean 50) of sudden coronary death.

Of 3,484 five-mm coronary segments examined (mean 50 per patient) from the 4 major (left main, left anterior descending, left circumflex and right) coronary arteries, 950 (27%) were narrowed 76 to 100% in cross-sectional area by plaque; 1,127 (32%), 51 to 75%; 689 (20%), 26 to 50%, and 718 (21%), 0 to 25%. More extensive severe narrowing occurred in the proximal compared with the distal halves to the left anterior descending, left circumflex and right coronary arteries. Comparison between the 31 previously symptomatic victims (either angina pectoris and/or a clinical acute myocardial infarction) to the 39 victims who had previously been asymptomatic disclosed a significantly higher mean percent of severely (76 to 100% in cross-sectional area) narrowed 5-mm segments (30 vs 25% [p <0.0051]) and a lower mean percent of minimally (0 to 25%) narrowed segments in the symptomatic group (15 vs 25%, p <0.001). Thus, the major coronary arteries at necropsy in victims of sudden coronary death are diffusely involved by atherosclerotic plaque and in nearly one-third of the lengths of the major arteries the lumens are narrowed >75% in cross-sectional area by plaque. The average amount of severe (>75%) narrowing is similar in the age groups 31 to 40 years, 41 to 50, 51 to 60, and 61 to 70 years.

(Am J Cardiol 1990;65:13B–19B)

From the Pathology Branch, National Heart, Lung, and Blood Institute, National Institutes of Health, Bethesda, Maryland 20892.

Address for reprints: William C. Roberts, MD, Pathology Branch, Building 10, Room 2N258, National Heart, Lung, and Blood Institute, National Institutes of Health, Bethesda, Maryland 20892.

The phrase "sudden death" has been used by lay and medical persons for nearly 450 years. It has many definitions. Sudden death might be a game played to break a tie or the extra minutes of play added to a tied game, the winning team being the first team to score. In medicine, sudden death generally denotes death which is *nonviolent* or nontraumatic, which is *unexpected*, which is *witnessed* and which is *instantaneous* or occurs within a few minutes of an abrupt change in previous clinical state. In heart disease the word "cardiac" is usually placed between the words "sudden" and "death," and the phrase "sudden cardiac death" usually is applied to persons dying suddenly from atherosclerotic coronary artery disease.[1] Necropsy studies of persons dying suddenly from cardiac disease, however, disclose many causes of sudden cardiac death, and, therefore, greater specificity is required in terms to prevent confusion (Fig. 1). Of persons dying suddenly from cardiovascular disease, the cause may be *cardiac* or *noncardiac*. The cardiac causes can be subdivided into *coronary* and *noncoronary*. Of the coronary causes, atherosclerosis is, of course, by far the most common and the term *atherosclerotic sudden coronary death* may be applied to them.[2-10] In young persons particularly, several *nonatherosclerotic* coronary conditions, mainly coronary anomalies, cause sudden death.[11-13] Of the cardiac, but noncoronary, causes of sudden death, the most common are cardiomyopathy,[14,15] particularly hypertrophic cardiomyopathy,[16,17] and valvular heart disease, most often the conditions causing left ventricular outflow obstruction,[18-23] sometimes associated with prosthetic or bioprosthetic heart valves.[24] Also, there are noncardiac but vascular causes of sudden death.[25,26] Some cardiac arrhythmic causes of sudden death not necessarily associated with morphologic abnormalities, e.g., prolonged QT interval syndrome, do not appear in Figure 1.

Some examples of the many causes of sudden cardiac death:

1. M.M., a 13-year-old athletic boy, the son of a former professional football player, collapsed while jogging and died. He had always been asymptomatic. His brother, 1 year older, had died a year earlier also while jogging. M.M.'s electrocardiogram 6 months earlier was considered "abnormal" but his left ventricular pressure was normal and there was no obstruction to left ventricular outflow.

2. A 17-year-old girl, who ran 40 miles weekly, suddenly collapsed and died just after crossing the finish line of a 3-mile race. She had been "healthy" all her life.

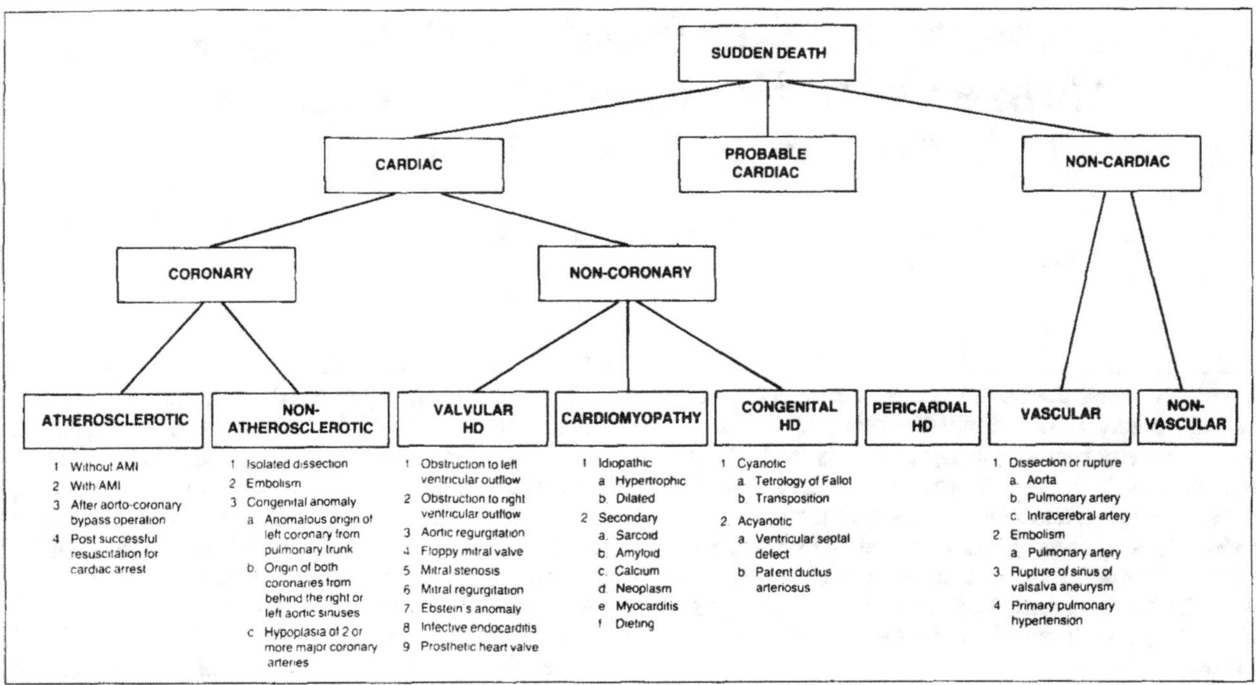

FIGURE 1. Various causes of sudden death. HD = heart disease. (Reproduced with permission from *Am J Cardiol*.[1])

3. A 19-year-old male midshipman was always asymptomatic until he suddenly collapsed and died while sitting on a bench immediately after running around the track several times. On admission examination 1 year earlier, electrocardiogram had shown ventricular premature complexes and left-axis deviation. The heart was of normal size by chest roentgenogram. The blood pressure was 135/80 mm Hg.

4. A 28-year-old woman, well all her life, suddenly collapsed and died while running for a bus.

5. A 28-year-old man died suddenly while pushing a brick-loaded wheelbarrow. He had been well until 2 days earlier when he complained of "pain in his neck," but this did not prevent him from performing his usual construction job activities.

6. A 33-year-old woman, a domestic, collapsed while at work and died immediately. She had been healthy all her life.

7. A 44-year-old woman, a secretary, collapsed while walking in her office and died. She had been asymptomatic all her life but on routine examination several years earlier was found to have precordial murmurs (each grade 2/6) consistent with "aortic stenosis and regurgitation." Chest radiograph had shown mild cardiomegaly and electrocardiogram had shown left ventricular hypertrophy.

8. A 44-year-old male taxicab driver was well until 1 hour before death when he became enraged because his taxicab was bombarded by snowballs thrown by 3 youths. One snowball entered an open window and hit him in the face, knocking off his glasses. He immediately radioed the police who arrived several minutes later and apprehended the youths. The police described the taxicab driver as "livid with rage" over the incident and advised him to leave the scene. Thirty minutes later he radioed his dispatcher that he was having breathing difficulties. He arrived at the dispatcher's office a few minutes later, collapsed and died.

9. A 60-year-old male school teacher had been well all his life except for recognized systemic hypertension until a few minutes before death when he became enraged when trying to prevent 2 students in the school gymnasium from fighting. He finally broke up the fight and, while walking away from the event minutes later, collapsed and died.

10. An 81-year-old woman, who had had a pacemaker inserted for complete heart block 23 months earlier, collapsed and died while climbing a flight of stairs in her home. During the preceeding 2 days, she had noted excessive fatigue, nausea and vomiting.

The cause of death in each of these 10 patients was different and had not a necropsy been performed the cause of death could not have been accurately predicted. Patient 1 had *hypertrophic cardiomyopathy*. Patient 2 had *congenital hypoplasia of both right and left circumflex coronary arteries with inadequate perfusion of the posterior wall of the left ventricle*.[27] Patient 3 had *origin of the left main coronary artery from the right sinus of Valsalva with coursing of the left main between the pulmonary trunk and ascending aorta*.[28] Patient 4 had *isolated coronary arterial dissection* involving the left anterior descending and left circumflex coronary arteries.[29] Patient 5 had extensive *cardiac sarcoidosis*.[15] Patient 6 had a *ruptured sinus of Valsalva aneurysm* (into the pericardial sac rather than into the right side of the heart).[30] Patient 7 had *congenital origin of the left main coronary artery from the pulmonary trunk*.[12] Patient 8 had *atherosclerotic coronary artery disease* with severe narrowing of each of the 3 major coronary arteries. Patient 9 had a large heart (550 g [normal ≤400 g]) from *systemic hypertension* but no significant coronary arterial narrowing or other recognized cause of sudden death.[31] Patient 10 had severe *coronary arterial atherosclerosis* with *acute myocardial infarction* complicated by *rupture of the left ventricular free wall* and hemopericardium.[32] Tests of the pacemaker after death disclosed that it had functioned normally.

In any study discussing sudden death from cardiovascular disease, the word *sudden* needs defining. The World Health Organization has used a 24-hour definition of sudden, meaning, of course, death occurring within 24 hours from an abrupt change in previous clinical status.[33] When this definition of sudden is used, many cases of acute myocardial infarction are intermixed with cases of sudden atherosclerotic coronary death unassociated with myocardial necrosis. Because it takes over 6 hours for histologic evidence of myocardial necrosis to be apparent and because most persons dying suddenly do so within an hour of change in previous clinical status, the 6-hour definition for sudden when applied to "atherosclerotic sudden coronary death" more clearly separates the infarct cases from the noninfarct ones.

Although the term sudden implies *unexpected*, in only one-quarter of victims of atherosclerotic coronary artery disease is sudden death the initial manifestation of coronary artery disease, and therefore, truly unexpected. Sudden death in patients with angina pectoris or healed myocardial infarction is really not so unexpected. Likewise, in persons with hypertrophic cardiomyopathy and certain forms of valvular heart disease, death suddenly is always a shock but, in actuality, not so unexpected.

Although sudden death is usually reserved for *nonviolent* or nontraumatic deaths, various mentally or even physically traumatic events can precipitate sudden death.[34-36]

The term "sudden death" is often used for persons in hospitals who are found dead, most often in their beds. I try to reserve the term "sudden death" for persons who have fatal or nonfatal cardiac arrest *outside* the hospital or at least whose symptoms of cardiovascular dysfunction appear initially while outside a hospital. Some of these victims, of course, are rushed to hospitals where fatal cardiac arrest occurs shortly after arrival.

I have examined many manuscripts which have used the phrase "sudden death" as a *cause* of death: "Patient so and so died of sudden death or patient so and so had sudden death but lived!" Obviously, the term "sudden death" should be used only as a *mode* of death or otherwise lawyers and editors will have a field day.

The use of the term "sudden death" in persons who are successfully resuscitated is not recommended. The use of the term *nonfatal cardiac arrest* (to contrast with *fatal cardiac arrest*) is preferable in this circumstance.

Thus, sudden cardiac death has many causes. Atherosclerotic coronary artery disease, obviously, is by far the most common cause of sudden cardiac death, but the latter term is not synonomous with atherosclerotic coro-

nary artery disease. The term "sudden coronary death" is not ideal either because not all sudden coronary deaths are the result of atherosclerotic narrowing, but "sudden coronary death" is more precise than "sudden cardiac death." Sudden death is not always so *sudden*, or so *unexpected* or *witnessed*, and indeed it may be caused by or precipitated by mental or physical violence. Thus, greater precision is needed when discussing sudden cardiac death.

ATHEROSCLEROTIC CORONARY ARTERY DISEASE

Warnes and I[8] studied at necropsy 70 victims of sudden coronary death to determine the amount and distribution of cross-sectional area luminal narrowing in each 5-mm segment of the 4 major coronary arteries, and compared the amount of narrowing both qualitatively and quantitatively in those with and without previous clinical evidence of myocardial ischemia.

All patients fulfilled the following criteria: (1) Death was known to occur within 6 hours of the previously witnessed usual state of health. (2) Although the patient may have died in a hospital, he/she was not a patient in a hospital at the onset of symptoms suggestive of myocardial ischemia. (3) At necropsy, ≥1 of the 4 major (left main, left anterior descending, left circumflex and right) coronary arteries was narrowed 76 to 100% cross-sectional area. (4) Ventricular myocardial coagulation necrosis was absent (histologic examination) at necropsy. (5) A cause of death, cardiac or noncardiac, other than coronary artery disease was absent. (6) Chronic congestive heart failure had never been present. (7) A cardiovascular operation had never been performed. Review of clinical and necropsy records in the Pathology Branch, National Heart, Lung, and Blood Institute, yielded 63 men and 7 women aged 22 to 81 years (mean 50) fulfilling these criteria. Of the 70 victims, 46 died outside the hospital. The other 24 had chest pain outside the hospital and had fatal cardiac arrest shortly after being brought to the hospital.

The hearts were fixed for ≥24 hours in formalin. The 4 major coronary arteries were excised intact, x-rayed and decalcified if necessary. Each artery was then cut transversely into 5-mm segments and labeled sequentially, either from the aortic ostium, or from its origin from the left main coronary artery. The segments were then dehydrated with alcohol and xylene, embedded in paraffin, and at least 2 histologic sections were cut from the paraffin block. Each histologic section was stained by the Movat technique. The amount of luminal narrowing by atherosclerotic plaque was determined by visual inspection of these histologic sections when magnified 25 to 50 times. The percent of cross-sectional area narrowing of each 5-mm segment was categorized into 5 groups: 0 to 25, 26 to 50, 51 to 75, 76 to 95 and 96 to 100. All sections were examined and the accuracy of the assessment of luminal narrowing was spot-checked by video planimetry. A total of 3,484 five-mm segments from the 70 victims were examined (mean number of segments per patient = 50).

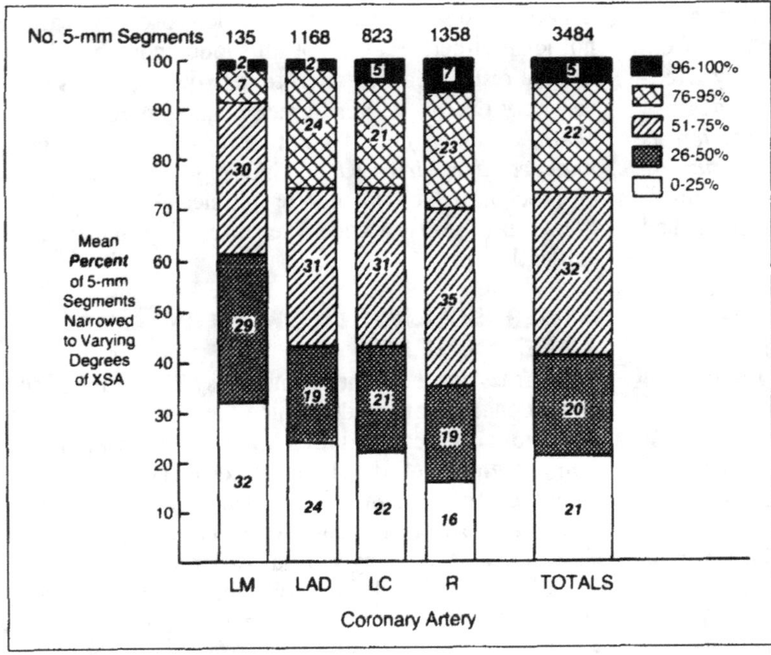

FIGURE 2. Mean percents of 5-mm segments of the 4 major coronary arteries narrowed to varying degrees in cross-sectional area (XSA) in 70 patients with sudden coronary death. LAD = left anterior descending; LC = left circumflex; LM = left main; R = right. (Reproduced with permission from *Am J Cardiol.*[9])

Qualitative studies: Of the 70 patients, 1 major coronary artery was narrowed 76 to 100% in cross-sectional area *at some point* in 11 patients (16%), 2 arteries in 19 (27%), 3 arteries in 33 (47%), and 4 arteries in 7 (10%). Of the 280 major epicardial coronary arteries in the 70 patients (4 per patient), 176 (63%) were narrowed at some point 76 to 100% in cross-sectional area, a mean of 2.5 of 4.0 major coronary arteries per patient. Excluding the left main coronary artery, 167 (80%) of the other 210 major coronary arteries were narrowed 76 to 100% in cross-sectional area, an average of 2.4 of 3.0 coronary arteries per patient. Of the individual major coronary arteries, the left main was severely (76 to 100% in cross-sectional area) narrowed in 13% (9 of 70), the left anterior descending in 86% (60 of 70), the left circumflex in 74% (52 of 70), and the right in 79% (55 of 70).

Comparison of the number of coronary arteries narrowed 76 to 100% in cross-sectional area in the 39 previously *asymptomatic* patients to the 31 with *previous acute myocardial infarction and/or angina pectoris* disclosed the following: 1 major artery so narrowed in 8 (21%) vs 3 (10%) (difference not significant [NS]); 2 arteries, 11 (28%) vs 8 (26%) (NS); 3 arteries, 18 (46%) vs 15 (48%) (NS), and 4 arteries, 2 (5%) vs 5 (16%) (NS).

Comparison of the number of arteries narrowed 76 to 100% in cross-sectional area in the 39 patients without to the 31 with a *healed myocardial infarct* revealed the following: 1 major artery so narrowed in 9 (23%) vs 2 (7%) (NS); 2 arteries, 11 (28%) vs 8 (26%) (NS); 3 arteries, 13 (33%) vs 20 (64%) (p <0.02), and 4 arteries, 6 (15%) vs 1 (3%) (NS).

Quantitative studies: Analysis of the 3,484 five-mm coronary segments showed that 950 (27%) were narrowed 76 to 100% in cross-sectional area; 1,127 (32%), 51 to 75%; 689 (20%), 26 to 50%, and 718 (21%), 0 to 25% (Fig. 2). The percent of segments severely narrowed per patient, however, varied enormously; from 2% (1 of 50) to 88% (86 of 98). Sixteen patients had ≤10% of their 5-mm segments narrowed 76 to 100% in cross-sectional area; 15 patients had 11 to 20% of the segments so narrowed; 11 patients, 21 to 30% of the segments; 16 patients, 31 to 40% of the segments; 7 patients, 41 to 50% of the segments; 2 patients, 51 to 60% of the segments; 2 patients,

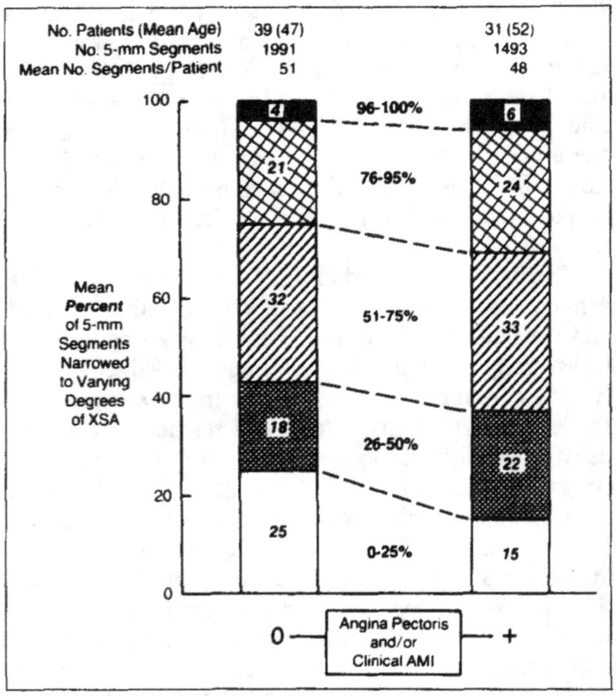

FIGURE 3. Mean percents of 5-mm segments of the sum of the 4 major coronary arteries narrowed to varying degrees in cross-sectional area (XSA) in 70 patients with sudden coronary death: comparison of 39 patients without and 31 patients with a clinical acute myocardial infarction (AMI) and/or angina. (Reproduced with permission from *Am J Cardiol.*[9])

61 to 70% of the segments, and 1 patient had 81 to 90% of the segments so narrowed. Comparison of the mean percent of 5-mm segments narrowed 76 to 100% in cross-sectional area in the arteries' proximal and distal halves disclosed a significantly higher percent of severely narrowed segments proximally in the left anterior descending and left circumflex coronary arteries than in the distal portion of these arteries, but a similar percent in the proximal and distal halves of the right coronary artery.

Of the 39 patients who had been asymptomatic, 502 (25%) of 1,991 five-mm segments were narrowed 76 to 100% in cross-sectional area compared with 448 (30%) of 1,493 five-mm segments in the 31 patients who had had either a clinical acute myocardial infarction and/or angina pectoris previously (p <0.005) (Fig. 3). Comparison of the mean percents of segments in all 5 categories of cross-sectional area coronary narrowing between the previously *asymptomatic* and *symptomatic* groups disclosed significant differences in the category of minimal (0 to 25%) cross-sectional area narrowing (25 vs 15%, p <0.001). Comparison of the amounts of narrowing in each of the 4 major coronary arteries disclosed a higher mean percent of 5-mm segments narrowed 76 to 100% in cross-sectional area in the symptomatic vs the asymptomatic victims in the left main, left anterior descending and left circumflex, but not in the right coronary arteries, and a lower mean percent of segments narrowed 0 to 25% in cross-sectional area in all 4 coronary arteries in the symptomatic group.

Comparison of the mean percents of 5-mm segments in the 5 categories of narrowing between the 31 patients with and the 39 patients without *left ventricular scars* disclosed a higher mean percent of segments narrowed 76 to 100% in the healed myocardial infarction group (33 vs 24%, p <0.001), and lower mean percent of segments narrowed 0 to 25% (13 vs 26%, p <0.001) compared to those without healed myocardial infarction (Fig. 4). A higher mean percent of 5-mm segments were minimally narrowed in those with no healed myocardial infarction, and a higher mean percent of segments were severely narrowed when a healed myocardial infarction was present. Severe narrowing of the left main coronary artery, however, occurred more frequently in those without healed myocardial infarction.

Of the 70 patients, 13 at necropsy had a thrombus in 1 coronary artery.[10] In 6 patients, the thrombus consisted primarily of fibrin and erythrocytes, and in 7 patients, nearly entirely of platelets. In all 13 patients, the thrombi were superimposed on atherosclerotic plaques which had already narrowed the lumina 26 to 50% (1 patient), 51 to 75% in cross-sectional area (4 patients) or 76 to 100% (8 patients).

DISCUSSION

A major finding in the aforementioned study was that the sudden death victims had severe and extensive narrowing of their 4 major extramural coronary arteries by atherosclerotic plaque. Of the 70 patients, 59 (84%) had ≥2 major arteries narrowed 76 to 100% in cross-sectional area and 11 (16%) had only 1 artery so narrowed by

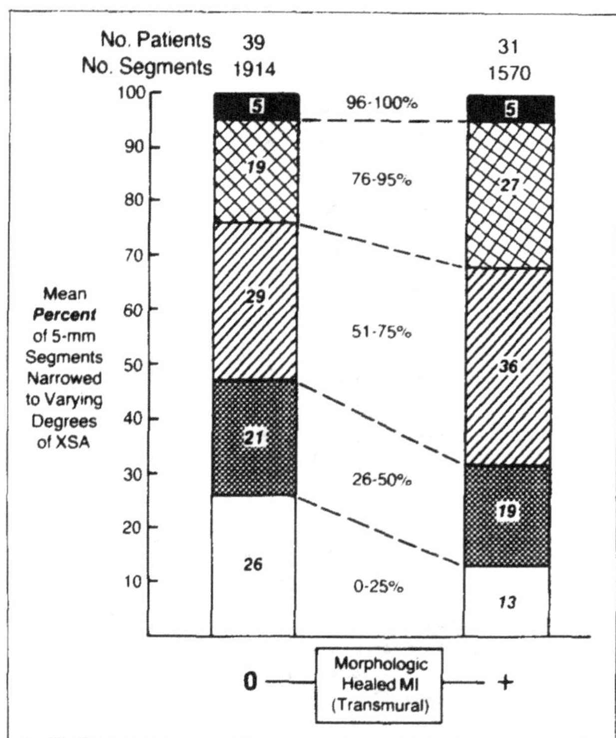

FIGURE 4. Mean percents of 5-mm segments of the sum of the 4 major coronary arteries narrowed to varying degrees in cross-sectional area (XSA) in 70 patients with sudden coronary death: comparison of 39 patients without and 31 patients with a morphologic healed myocardial infarction (MI). (Reproduced with permission from *Am J Cardiol.*[9])

atherosclerotic plaque. Of the 59 patients with multivessel coronary artery disease, 2 arteries were severely (76 to 100% in cross-sectional area) narrowed in 19 patients (27%), 3 arteries in 33 (47%) and 4 arteries in 7 (10%). Of the 4 major coronary arteries per patient, 2.5 of 4 were severely narrowed. Of the 280 major coronary arteries in the 70 patients, 176 (63%) were narrowed severely, and of them, the left anterior descending was the most frequently narrowed artery (60 of 70 = 86%). The 11 patients with 1-vessel coronary artery disease were significantly younger than the 59 patients with multivessel coronary artery disease (mean age 41 vs 51 years).

Warnes and I[8] found the number of coronary arteries to be severely narrowed at some point (the qualitative approach) in the groups of patients with and without previous angina pectoris and/or acute myocardial infarction, and the groups with and without grossly visible left ventricular scars at necropsy to be roughly similar. Of our 70 patients, 31 (44%) had had previous clinical acute myocardial infarction (which healed) and/or angina, and 39 did not. Comparison of those with previous clinical evidence of myocardial ischemia to those without disclosed similar percents of total coronary arteries (4 per patient) severely narrowed (84 of 124 [68%] vs 92 of 156 [59%]) and roughly similar percents of ≥2 coronary arteries severely narrowed (28 of 31 [90%] vs 31 of 39 [79%]). Comparison of the 31 patients with to the 39 without left ventricular scars disclosed similar percents of

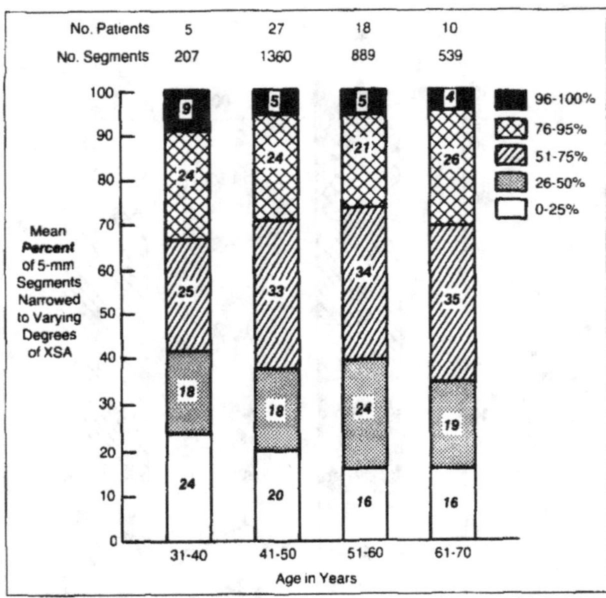

FIGURE 5. Relation of age to the mean percent of 5-mm coronary segments narrowed to varying degrees in 60 men with sudden coronary death. XSA = cross-sectional area. (Reproduced with permission from Am Heart J.[9])

total coronary arteries severely narrowed (82 of 124 [66%] vs 94 of 156 [60%]) and similar percents of ≥2 coronary arteries severely narrowed (29 of 31 [94%] vs 30 of 39 [77%]).

Of the 39 patients who previously had had no clinical evidence of myocardial ischemia (asymptomatic group), 25% of 5-mm segments were narrowed 76 to 100% in cross-sectional area compared with 30% in those who had had symptoms of ischemia (acute myocardial infarction which healed and/or angina pectoris) (p <0.05). The asymptomatic group also had a higher mean percent of segments minimally narrowed (25 vs 15%, p <0.001).

Similar differences were apparent in the quantitative comparisons between those victims who had a healed myocardial infarction at necropsy and those who did not. More 5-mm segments were narrowed 76 to 100% in those with than in those without a left ventricular scar (33 vs 24%, p <0.001); fewer 5-mm segments were minimally narrowed in those with compared to those without myocardial infarction (13 vs 26%, p <0.001). Although a higher percentage of the 5-mm segments from the sum of all 4 major coronary arteries were severely narrowed in the patients with compared to those without healed myocardial infarction, analysis of the individual arteries disclosed that the left main coronary artery was different from the other 3. In the 31 patients with healed myocardial infarction only 4% of the 57 five-mm segments of left main were severely narrowed; in contrast, in the 39 patients without healed myocardial infarction, 12% of the 78 five-mm segments were severely narrowed.

Although the study by Warnes and I[8] disclosed the patients as a group to have severe and extensive coronary narrowing by atherosclerotic plaque, considerable variation in the percent of 5-mm segments narrowed severely was observed. The range was from 2 to 86%: 16 patients

(23%) had <10% of their coronary segments narrowed 76 to 100% in cross-sectional area and 12 patients (17%) had >40% of their 5-mm segments severely narrowed. Thus, the extent of the severe narrowing is difficult to predict in the individual patient, but predictable in groups of patients dying suddenly from coronary artery disease. The previously symptomatic patients clearly had more severe narrowing and less minimal narrowing than the asymptomatic group, as did those patients with compared to those without a healed myocardial infarction.

The average amount of coronary narrowing in patients with atherosclerotic sudden coronary death was similar in both younger and older victims.[9] Among 60 men (all included in the aforementioned study) aged 31 to 70 years with atherosclerotic sudden coronary death, Warnes and I[9] found similar mean percents of 5-mm-long coronary segments narrowed severely (>75% in cross-sectional area) in each of 4 decades: 33% in the 5 patients aged 31 to 40 years, 29% in the 27 patients aged 41 to 50 years, 26% in the 18 patients aged 51 to 60 years, and 30% in the 10 patients aged 61 to 70 years (Fig. 5). The mean percent of 5-mm segments minimally narrowed (0 to 25%), however, was significantly higher in the younger than in the older decades. Thus, as groups, both young and old victims of sudden coronary death have similar amounts of severe coronary narrowing, but the younger victims have a greater proportion of their major coronary arteries minimally narrowed.

REFERENCES

1. Roberts WC. Sudden cardiac death: definitions and causes. *Am J Cardiol* 1986;57:1410–1413.
2. Roberts WC, Buja LM. The frequency and significance of coronary arterial thrombi and other observations in fatal acute myocardial infarction. A study of 107 necropsy patients. *Am J Med* 1972;52:426–443.
3. Roberts WC, Jones AA. Quantitation of coronary arterial narrowing at necropsy in sudden coronary death. Analysis of 31 patients and comparison with 25 control subjects. *Am J Cardiol* 1979;44:39–45.
4. Waller BF, Roberts WC. Sudden death while running in conditioned runners aged 40 or over. *Am J Cardiol* 1980;45:1292–1300.
5. McManus BM, Waller BF, Graboys TB, Mitchell JH, Siegel RJ, Miller HS Jr, Froelicher VF, Roberts WC. Exercise and sudden death. Part I. *Curr Probl Cardiol* 1982;6(9):1–89.
6. McManus BM, Waller BF, Graboys TB, Mitchell JH, Siegel RJ, Miller HS Jr, Froelicher BF, Roberts WC. Exercise and sudden death. Part II. *Curr Probl Cardiol* 1982;6(10):1–57.
7. Roberts WC, Curry RC Jr, Isner JM, Waller BF, McManus BM, Mariani-Constantini R, Ross AM. Sudden death in Prinzmetal's angina with coronary spasm documented by angiography. Analysis of three necropsy patients. *Am J Cardiol* 1982;50:203–210.
8. Warnes CA, Roberts WC. Sudden coronary death: relation of amount and distribution of coronary narrowing at necropsy to previous symptoms of myocardial ischemia, left ventricular scarring and heart weight. *Am J Cardiol* 1984;54:65–73.
9. Warnes CA, Roberts WC. Comparison at necropsy by age group of amount and distribution of narrowing by atherosclerotic plaque in 2995 five-mm long segments of 240 major coronary arteries in 60 men aged 31 to 70 years with sudden coronary death. *Am Heart J* 1984;108:431–435.
10. Warnes CA, Roberts WC. Sudden coronary death: comparison of patients with to those without coronary thrombus at necropsy. *Am J Cardiol* 1984;54:1206–1211.
11. Roberts WC, Robinowitz M. Anomalous origin of the left anterior descending coronary artery from the pulmonary trunk with origin of the right and left circumflex coronary arteries from the aorta. *Am J Cardiol* 1984;54:1381–1383.
12. Roberts WC. Major anomalies of coronary arterial origin seen in adulthood. *Am Heart J* 1986;111:941–963.
13. Kragel AH, Roberts WC. Anomalous origin of either the right or left main coronary artery from the aorta with subsequent coursing between aorta and pulmonary trunk: analysis of 32 necropsy cases. *Am J Cardiol* 1988;62:771–777.
14. Roberts WC, Siegel JM, McManus BM. Idiopathic dilated cardiomyopathy: analysis of 152 necropsy patients. *Am J Cardiol* 1987;60:1340–1355.

15. Roberts WC, McAllister HA Jr, Ferrans VJ. Sarcoidosis of the heart. A clinicopathologic study of 35 necropsy patients (Group I) and review of 78 previously described necropsy patients (Group II). *Am J Med 1977;63:86-108.*

16. Maron BJ, Roberts WC, Epstein SE. Sudden death in hypertrophic cardiomyopathy: a profile of 78 patients. *Circulation 1982;65:1388-1394.*

17. Roberts CS, Roberts WC. Morphologic features of hypertrophic cardiomyopathy. In: Zipes DP, Rowlans DJ, eds. Progress in Cardiology. *Philadelphia: Lea & Febiger, 1989;(2/2):3-32.*

18. Morrow AG, Fort L III, Roberts WC, Braunwald E. Discrete subaortic stenosis complicated by aortic valvular regurgitation. Clinical, hemodynamic, and pathologic studies and the results of operative treatment. *Circulation 1965; 31:163-171.*

19. Roberts WC. The structure of the aortic valve in clinically-isolated aortic stenosis. An autopys study of 162 patients over 15 years of age. *Circulation 1970;42:91-97.*

20. Roberts WC. The congenitally bicuspid aortic valve. A study of 85 autopsy cases. *Am J Cardiol 1970;26:72-83.*

21. Roberts WC. Anatomically isolated aortic valvular disease. The case against its being of rheumatic etiology. *Am J Med 1970;49:151-159.*

22. Roberts WC, Perloff JK, Costantino T. Severe valvular aortic stenosis in patients over 65 years of age. A clinicopathologic study. *Am J Cardiol 1971;27:497-506.*

23. Falcone MW, Roberts WC, Morrow AG, Perloff JK. Congenital aortic stenosis resulting from unicommissural valve. Clinical and anatomic features in twenty-one adult patients. *Circulation 1971;44:272-280.*

24. Roberts WC. The silver anniversary of cardiac valve replacement. *Am J Cardiol 1985;56:503-506.*

25. Roberts WC. The aorta: its acquired diseases and their consequences as viewed from a morphologic perspective. In: Lindsay J Jr, Hurst JW, eds. The Aorta. *New York: Grune & Stratton, 1979;51-117.*

26. Roberts WC. Aortic dissection: anatomy, consequences, and causes. *Am Heart J 1981;101:195-214.*

27. Maron BJ, Roberts WC, McAllister HA, Rosing DR, Epstein SE. Sudden death in young athletes. *Circulation 1980;62:218-229.*

28. Barth WC III, Roberts WC. Left main coronary artery originating from the right sinus of Valsalva and coursing between the aorta and pulmonary trunk. *JACC 1986;7:366-373.*

29. Bulkley BH, Roberts WC. Dissecting aneurysm (hematoma) limited to coronary artery. A clinicopathologic study of six patients. *Am J Med 1973; 55:747-756.*

30. Roberts WC. Congenital cardiovascular abnormalities usually silent until adulthood. In: Roberts WC, ed. Adult Congenital Heart Disease. *Philadelphia. FA Davis, 1987;631-691.*

31. Kragel AH, Roberts WC. Sudden death and cardiomegaly unassociated with coronary, valvular, congenital or specific myocardial disease. *Am J Cardiol 1988;61:659-660.*

32. Mann JM, Roberts WC. Rupture of the left ventricular free wall during acute myocardial infarction: analysis of 138 necropsy patients and comparison with 50 necropsy patients with acute myocardial infarction without rupture. *Am J Cardiol 1988;62:847-859.*

33. Classification of atherosclerotic lesions. Report of a study group. *WHO Techn Rep Ser 1958 (No. 143).*

34. Engel GL. Sudden and rapid death during psychological stress. Forklore or folk wisdom? *Ann Intern Med 1971;74:771-782.*

35. Engel GL. Psychologic stress, vasodepressor [vasovagal] syncope, and sudden death. *Ann Intern Med 1978;89:403-412.*

36. Roberts WC. The most powerful cause of sudden death. *Am J Cardiol 1986;57:190.*

Quantitative Analysis of Amounts of Coronary Arterial Narrowing in Cocaine Addicts

Frederick A. Dressler, MD, Sonya Malekzadeh, BA, and William C. Roberts, MD

From January 1979 to February 1989, 22 cocaine addicts were studied at necropsy. The 22 patients were divided into 2 groups: death associated with increased cocaine levels at necropsy (13 patients, aged 23 to 45 years [mean 32], and mean total blood cocaine level, 0.36 mg/dl) and noncocaine-related death (9 patients, aged 15 to 50 years [mean 32]). Of the 22 patients, 17 were men and 5 were women; 19 were black and 3 were white. Gross examination in the 22 patients disclosed that 8 patients (36%) had 1 or more of the 4 major (left main, left anterior descending, left circumflex, and right) coronary arteries narrowed at some point >75% in cross-sectional area by atherosclerotic plaque. In 17 cases, the 4 major epicardial coronary arteries were divided into 805 five-mm long segments and a histologic section was prepared from each segment: of the 12 patients with a cocaine-related death, 41 (8%) of 544 five-mm coronary segments were narrowed 76 to 100% and 106 segments (19%) were narrowed 51 to 75% in cross-sectional area by plaque. Of the 5 cocaine addicts who did not die from cocaine overdose, 8 (3%) of 261 five-mm coronary segments were narrowed 76 to 100% and 19 segments (7%) were narrowed 51 to 75% in cross-sectional area by plaque. The frequency of coronary artery disease was greater in patients dying with cocaine in their blood at necropsy compared to those whose death was not cocaine related. Also the frequency of severe coronary arterial narrowing is considerably greater than expected for the entire group of patients whose mean age was only 32 years. Thus, either of 2 possibilities, alone or in combination, may explain our findings: coronary atherosclerosis is accelerated by cocaine addiction for reasons as yet undetermined, or cocaine provides a fatal stress in patients with premature coronary atherosclerosis from other causes.

(Am J Cardiol 1990;65:303–308)

From the Pathology Branch, National Heart, Lung, and Blood Institute, National Institutes of Health, Bethesda, Maryland. Manuscript received August 22, 1989; revised manuscript received and accepted October 4, 1989.

Dr. Dressler's present address: Division of Cardiology, Department of Medicine, Saint Louis University School of Medicine, St. Louis, Missouri.

Ms. Malekzadeh's present address: George Washington University School of Medicine, Washington, DC.

Address for reprints: William C. Roberts, MD, Building 10, Room 2N258, National Institutes of Health, Bethesda, Maryland 20892.

Since the outbreak of epidemic drug abuse in the USA, several reports have described coronary (myocardial infarction, angina pectoris, arrhythmias and coronary arterial narrowing by angiogram) and noncoronary heart conditions (cardiomyopathy, myocarditis, contraction band necrosis and primary myocardial toxicity) in cocaine addicts.[1-19] Although several studies have mentioned coronary arterial findings at necropsy in cocaine addicts, no reports have provided results of detailed examination of these arteries at necropsy. The present report provides such findings.

METHODS

During the last 10 years we have studied at necropsy 22 known cocaine addicts, who also were known not to use opiates. The autopsies were performed at 5 different institutions and subsequently the heart and often portions of other organs were submitted for examination to the Pathology Branch, National Heart, Lung, and Blood Institute. Each heart was examined initially by one of us (WCR) and in 18 cases the heart was reexamined by 2 of us (FAD, SM). Of the 18 hearts that were reexamined, the coronary arteries were intact in 17, and in each of these 17 the 4 major (right, left main, left anterior descending, left circumflex) epicardial coronary arteries were studied in detail. Also examined in 20 patients were 1 to 11 histologic sections (mean 5) of left ventricular wall. These sections extended from endocardium to epicardium and measured at least 2 cm in longitudinal length.

The ages of the 22 patients ranged from 15 to 50 years (mean 32); 17 (77%) were men and 5 (23%) were women; 19 (86%) were black and 3 (14%) were white. The form and route of cocaine use was known in 9 patients: powder inhaled through the nose in 4; powder inhaled through the nose and slurry injected into a systemic vein in 2; smoke inhaled through the mouth in 2; smoke inhaled through the mouth and powder eaten in 1. Systemic hypertension was believed to be present in 5 patients (23%) and 3 (14%) were known to use alcohol to excess.

Of the 22 patients, the only symptom of cardiac dysfunction or myocardial ischemia before death was congestive heart failure in 4 (nos. 5, 11, 14 and 22, Table I). The onset of congestive heart failure in each was within 2 months of death; each had hearts weighing >400 g, and each had massively dilated ventricular cavities. A single coronary artery was narrowed >75% in cross-sectional area by plaque at some point in 2 of these 4 patients (nos. 11 and 22, Table I). Patient 14 had a large, posterior wall, transmural left ventricular scar without significant coronary narrowing, and he was awaiting cardiac transplantation when he died.

TABLE I Clinical and Morphologic Cardiac Findings in 22 Cocaine Addicts

Pt No.	Age (yrs), Race, Sex	Modes of Death	Death Outside Hospital	Total Blood Cocaine at Necropsy (mg/dl)	BW (lbs)	HW (g)	LM	LAD	LC	R	No. 5-mm Coronary Segments	0–25%	26–50%	51–75%	76–95%	96–100%	Mean Score	No. Sections LV + VS	Myocarditis (0 to 3+)	N	Fib
							\<— Narrowing >75% in CSA by Plaque —>					\<— No. of 5-mm Coronary Segments Narrowed in CSA by Plaque —>								\<— LV —>	
Group I: Cocaine-related death																					
1	23, B, M	Overdose	+	0.28	149	355	0	0	0	0	29	27	2	0	0	0	1.07	4	0	0	0
2	23, W, M	Overdose	+	0.10*	216	480	0	0	0	0	31	28	3	0	0	0	1.10	4	0	+ (Mi) (PM)	0
3	25, B, M	Overdose	+	0.60	—	380	0	+	+‡	0	48	14	13	16	5	0	2.25	7	0	+ (Mi)	0
4	30, B, M	Overdose	+	0.40	216	460	0	0	0	0	62	56	5	1	0	0	1.11	3	0	0	0
5	32, B, M	Overdose	+	0.22	164	880†	0	0	0	0	43	43	0	0	0	0	1.00	4	0	+ (Mi)§,||	0
6	32, W, M	Overdose	+	0.08*	174	450	0	+	0	0	50	6	11	30	2	1	2.60	5	0	0	0
7	32, B, F	Overdose	+	0.44	133	295	0	+	0	+	44	4	3	18	16	3	3.18	6	0	0	0
8	33, B, M	Overdose	+	0.30	330	990	0	0	+	0	42	14	12	14	2	0	2.10	11	0	0	0
9	36, B, M	Overdose	+	0.25	164	500	0	0	0	0	—	—	—	—	—	—	—	6	0	0	0
10	38, B, M	Overdose	+	0.72	134	325	0	0	0	0	49	39	8	2	0	0	1.24	9	+	0	0
11	41, B, M	Overdose	+	0.15	144	600†	0	+	0	0	61	51	7	2	1	0	1.23	3	0	0	0
12	45, B, M	Aortic dissection	+	0.90	206	500	0	+	+	+	55	13	8	23	11	0	2.58	7	0	0	0
13	—, B, F	Gunshot wound	+	0.25	158	330	0	0	0	0	30	30	0	0	0	0	1.00	4	0	0	0
Subtotal (mean) [%]			13	(0.36)	(182)	(503)	0	5	3	2	544 [100]	325 [60]	72 [13]	106 [19]	37 [7]	4 [1]	(1.71)	73 (6)	1	3	0
Group II: Death not due to cocaine																					
14	15, B, M	Chronic CHF	0¶	0	152	460	0	0	0	0	47	47	0	0	0	0	1.00	2	+++	0	+ (A)
15	26, B, F	Infective endocarditis	0¶	0	—	—	0	0	0	0	—	—	—	—	—	—	—	—	—	+ (SE)	0
16	27, B, M	Sudden (myocarditis)	0¶	0	161	—	0	0	0	0	—	—	—	—	—	—	—	3	+++	0	0
17	29, B, F	Sudden‡‡	0**	—††	—	300	0	0	0	0	49	49	0	0	0	0	1.00	6	0	+ (Mi)||	0
18	30, W, M	Sudden (CAD)	+	0	145	410	0	+	+	+	52	16	11	17	8	0	2.33	2	0	0	0
19	35, B, M	Chronic renal failure	0¶	0	121	380	0	0	0	0	—	—	—	—	—	—	—	3	0	+ (Mi)	0
20	39, B, M	Sudden‡‡	+	0	322	835	0	0	0	0	69	62	7	0	0	0	1.10	8	0	0	0
21	39, B, M	Sudden (bleeding varices)	+	0§§	185	500	0	0	0	0	44	41	1	2	0	0	1.11	1	0	0	0
22	50, B, F	CAD (chronic CHF)	0**	0	—	—	0	0	0	+	—	—	—	—	—	—	—	—	—	+(T)	0
Subtotal (mean) [%]			3		(181)	(481)	0	1	1	2	261[100]	215[82]	19[7]	19[7]	8[3]	0	(1.31)	25(4)	2	4	1

* excessive alcohol consumption also during the several hours before death; † idiopathic dilated cardiomyopathy; ‡ thrombus also present superimposed on plaque; § organized thrombus, left ventricular cavity; || dystrophic calcification; ¶ in hospital last 9 to 86 days of life; ** in hospital ≤24 hours; †† no cocaine measurements at time of death; ‡‡ etiology unknown; §§ although no cocaine was detected in blood, the urine-free cocaine was 0.0029 mg/dl, and the urine cocaine metabolite was 0.042 mg/dl.

BW = body weight; CAD = coronary artery disease; CHF = congestive heart failure; CSA = cross-sectional area; Fib = fibrosis; HW = heart weight; LAD = left anterior descending; LC = left circumflex; LM = left main; LV = left ventricular wall; Mi = microscopic only; N = necrosis; PM = papillary muscle; R = right; SE = subendocardial; T = transmural; VS = ventricular septum; — = not determined.

Mean score was determined by assigning a number to each 5-mm segment. A segment narrowed ≤25% in CSA has a score of 1; a segment narrowed 26 to 50%, 2; a segment narrowed 51 to 75%, 3; and a segment narrowed 76 to 100% a score of 4. The mean score is determined by dividing the sum of the scores of all 5-mm segments by the number of 5-mm segments examined.

The 22 patients were divided into 2 groups. The 13 group I patients all died suddenly outside the hospital and all had toxic levels of cocaine in their blood. Cocaine overdose was the mode of death in 11 of these 13 patients. Of the other 2 patients, 1 died of an aortic dissection and he had the highest blood cocaine levels of any of the 13 patients. It is believed that his cocaine intake raised the systemic blood pressure acutely and that the resulting hypertension led to the aortic dissection. This patient has been reported elsewhere.[21] The other patient, a middle-aged woman (no. 13, Table I), whose identity was never known, died of a gunshot wound but had toxic levels of cocaine in her blood at necropsy.

The 9 group II patients were known to be habitual users of cocaine. In contrast to the group I patients,

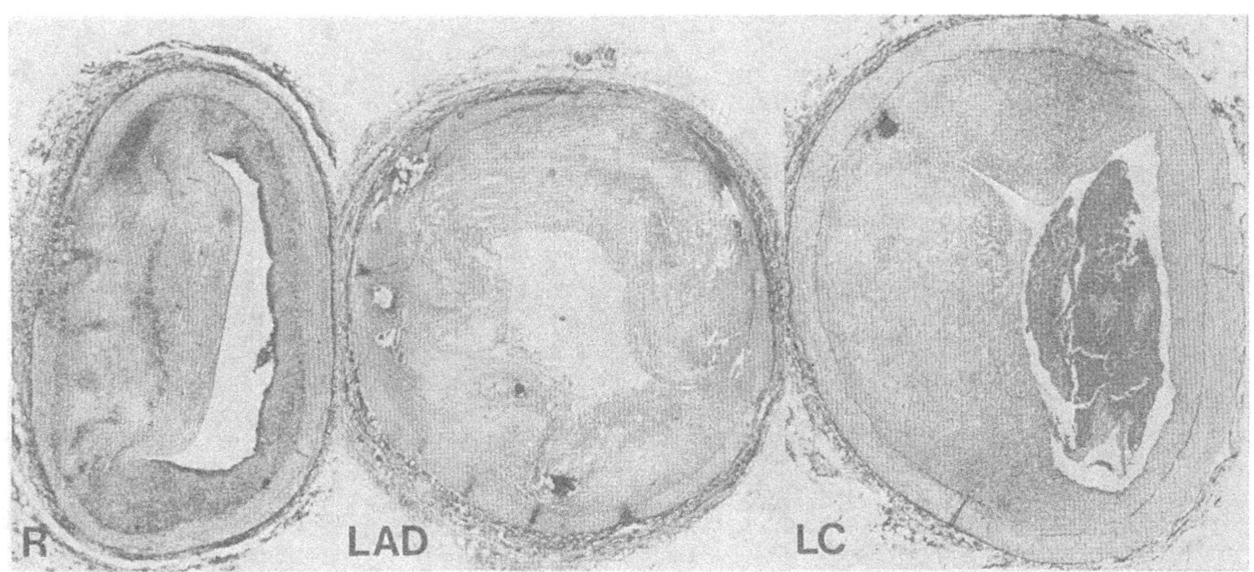

FIGURE 1. (Patient 3, Table I). Right (R), left anterior descending (LAD) and left circumflex (LC) coronary arteries at sites of maximal narrowing in a 25-year-old man (DCMEO #79-01-107) who suddenly developed chest pain shortly after a meal and died. The blood cocaine concentration at necropsy was 0.60 mg/dl. Considerable amounts of atherosclerotic plaque were present in 21 of the 48 five-mm segments of coronary artery. A thrombus also is present in the residual lumen of the left circumflex coronary artery. Movat stains, × 25 (R and LAD), × 40 (LC).

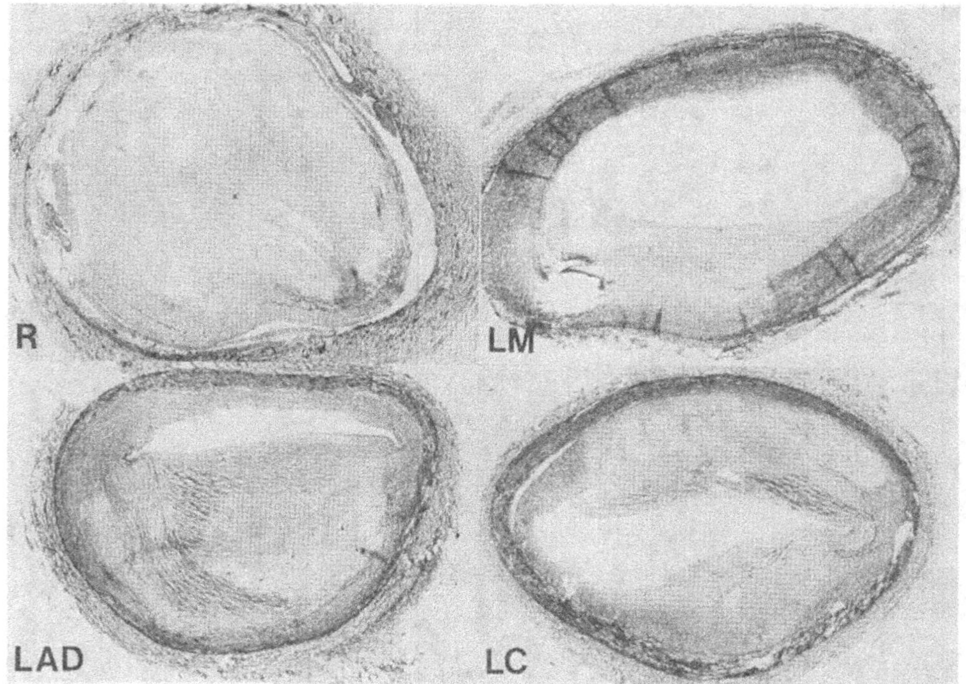

FIGURE 2. (Patient 7, Table I). Right (R), left main (LM), left anterior descending (LAD) and left circumflex (LC) coronary arteries at sites of maximal narrowing in a 32-year-old woman (DCMEO #88-04-450) who developed abdominal pain shortly after eating a sandwich and smoking cocaine. She died 2 hours later. The lumens of the right and left anterior descending coronary arteries are considerably narrowed by atherosclerotic plaque. Movat stains, × 32 (R, LAD and LC) × 40 (LM).

however, 6 of these 9 patients died in the hospital; 4 of them from 9 to 86 days after admission, and, therefore, cocaine would not have been expected in the blood; the other 2 patients died 10 and 24 hours, respectively, after admission and a toxicology screen was not performed in 1 and was negative in the other. The remaining 3 patients died suddenly outside the hospital: none had cocaine in the blood, but 1, who died from esophageal bleeding related to hepatic cirrhosis, had cocaine in the urine. Death in 1 patient was attributed to coronary artery disease, and the cause of the sudden death in the other patient was not determined.

RESULTS

In 8 of the 22 patients, 1 or more of the 4 major epicardial coronary arteries, by gross examination, was narrowed at some point >75% in cross-sectional area by atherosclerotic plaque: in 6 men aged 25 to 45 years (mean 34), and in 2 women, aged 32 and 50 (mean 41) (Figures 1 through 4). Of the 32 major epicardial coronary arteries in these 8 patients, 14 (44%) were so narrowed, a mean of 1.8/patient.

In 17 of the 22 cases, the 4 major epicardial coronary arteries were removed from the heart, cut into 5-mm segments, decalcified, processed in alcohols and xylene, sectioned 6 μ thick, stained by the Movat method and examined. Of the 805 five-mm coronary artery segments examined, 4 (<1%) were narrowed 96 to 100% in cross-sectional area by plaque; 45 (6%) were narrowed 76 to 95%; 125 (16%), 51 to 75%; 91 (11%), 26 to 50%; and 540 segments (67%) were narrowed 0 to 25%. A great variation in percents of 5-mm coronary segments severely narrowed occurred among the 17 patients (Table I).

The group I patients had more coronary arterial narrowing than did the group II patients. Six of the 13 group I patients and 2 of the 9 group II patients had 1 or more major coronary artery severely (>75% in cross-sectional area) narrowed by atherosclerotic plaque. Forty-one (8%) of the 544 five-mm segments of major coronary artery in the group I patients and 8 (3%) of the 261 five-mm segments in the group II patients were narrowed severely by plaque. The average amount of narrowing of each 5-mm coronary segment (determined by mean score [Table I]) also was greater in the group I compared to the group II patients.

Calcific deposits were present in atherosclerotic plaques in 1 or more of the 4 major epicardial coronary arteries in 5 of the 17 patients examined histologically. Of the 805 five-mm coronary segments examined 19 (2%) had calcium. *Multiluminal channels* were present within atherosclerotic plaques in only 1 (<1%) of the 805 five-mm segments. *Intraluminal thrombus* was observed in a coronary artery superimposed on atherosclerotic plaque in 1 patient.

Of the 22 patients, 7 (32%) had 1 or more foci of left ventricular wall necrosis. The foci of necrosis were visible on gross examination of the heart in 2 cases (nos. 15 and 22, Table I): in 1, the necrosis was limited to the inner half of the left ventricular wall (subendocardium), and in 1, the necrosis involved all of the inner half and portions of the outer half of the left ventricular wall (transmural). In the other 5 patients, the foci of necrosis were visible only on examination of the histologic sections of left ventricular wall. Only 2 of the 7 patients with left ventricular necrosis had severe narrowing of 1 or more major epicardial coronary artery.

DISCUSSION

Our findings indicate that a large percent of young cocaine addicts have significant coronary artery disease at necropsy. Of the 22 cocaine addicts studied, 8 (36%) had severe (>75% cross-sectional area) narrowing of 1 or more of the epicardial coronary arteries by atherosclerotic plaque, a percent much higher than expected in a group of persons whose mean age is only 32 years.

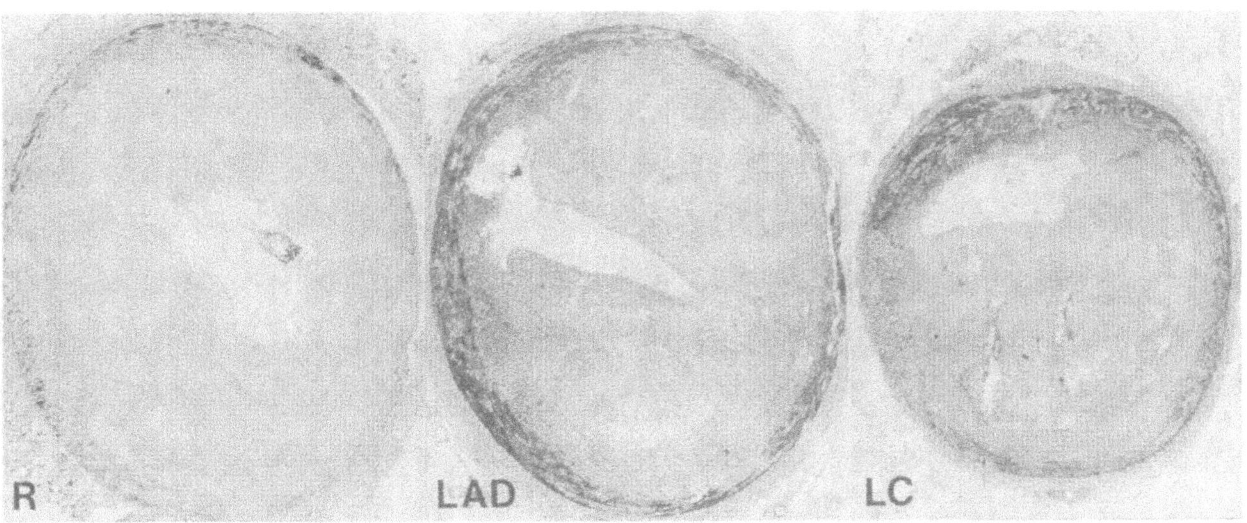

FIGURE 3. (Patient 12, Table I). Right (R), left anterior descending (LAD) and left circumflex (LC) coronary arteries at sites of maximal narrowing in a 45-year-old man (DCMEO #85-03-195) who suddenly collapsed and died after smoking "free-base" cocaine off and on for several hours. He died of an acute aortic dissection with through-and-through aortic rupture. At necropsy, however, the R, LAD and LC coronary arteries were each narrowed >75% in cross-sectional area of atherosclerotic plaque. Movat stains, × 32 (R and LC) and × 40 (LAD).

One (no. 3) of the 8 patients had an occluding thrombus superimposed on atherosclerotic plaque. Only 1 of 8 patients had a grossly visible acute myocardial infarct. (Of the other 14 patients without significant coronary artery disease, 1 [no. 15] had a grossly visible acute myocardial infarct, and 1 [no. 14] had a large healed myocardial infarct.)

At least 5 other reports have described young cocaine addicts at necropsy with "narrowing" in 1 or more epicardial coronary artery by atherosclerotic plaque with or without superimposed thrombus. Simpson and Edwards[22] described a 21-year-old male cocaine addict who died suddenly, and necropsy disclosed "chronic coronary obstruction . . . the result of a nonatherosclerotic intimal proliferation of smooth-muscle cells, with or without the deposition of collagen and elastin." The lumen of the left main was narrowed 65%, the left anterior descending 95%, the right 95%, and the left circumflex coronary artery, apparently up to 50% in cross-sectional area. Platelet thrombus also was present in 1 or more major coronary arteries. Isner et al[23] described a 37-year-old male addict who was found dead in bed and necropsy disclosed 90% cross-sectional narrowing by plaque of the left anterior descending coronary artery with superimposed obstructing thrombus, and up to 50% narrowing of the right coronary artery. The lumen of the left circumflex was narrowed up to 25% in cross-sectional area. Mittleman and Wetli[20] reported 24 cocaine addicts studied at necropsy and all had died suddenly. Death in 15 (aged 29 to 71 years [mean 47]) of the 24 patients was attributed to coronary atherosclerosis with ≥70% stenosis in 1 or more of the coronary arteries. This degree of luminal narrowing involved only 1 coronary artery in 8 patients and >1 in 7 patients.

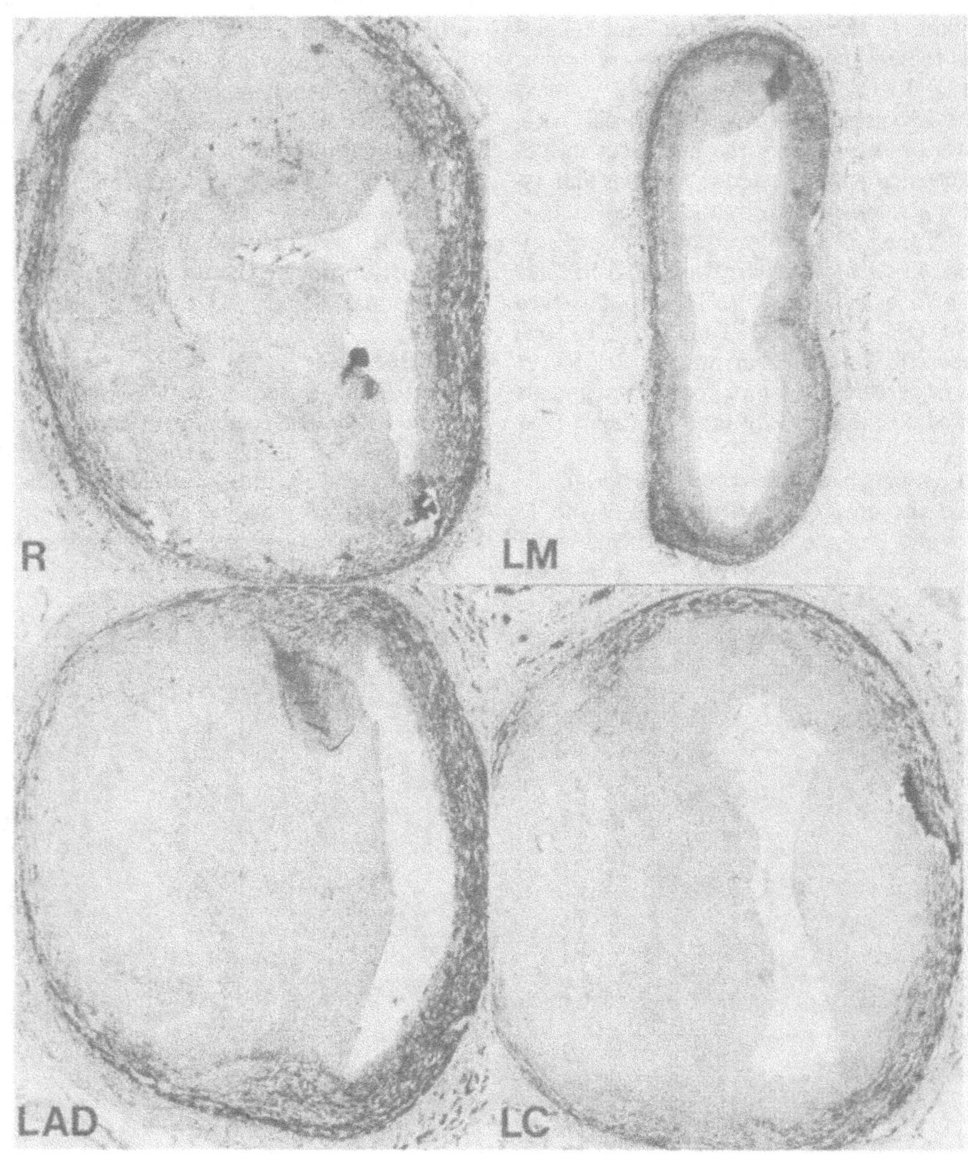

FIGURE 4. (Patient 18, Table I). Right (R), left main (LM), left anterior descending (LAD) and left circumflex (LC) coronary arteries at sites of maximal narrowing in a 30-year-old man (WCH #A85-28) who died suddenly at work while using a hydraulic lift. He had exertional chest pains periodically during the previous 1 year. Three of the 4 major coronary arteries contained considerable quantities of atherosclerotic plaque. Movat stains, × 32 (R), × 15 (LM), × 50 (LAD) and × 40 (LC).

Two patients had hemorrhage into an arteriosclerotic plaque, and 3 cases had complete thrombotic occlusion of the residual lumen. Virmani et al[24] described 2 cocaine addicts with "severe coronary atherosclerosis," and another, a 23-year-old woman, who had an occlusive platelet thrombus in the left anterior descending coronary artery superimposed on a plaque that had narrowed the lumen about 40% in cross-sectional area. Finally, Stenberg et al[25] described a 38-year-old male cocaine addict who died about 13 hours after onset of acute myocardial infarction. Necropsy disclosed occluding platelet thrombi in both the left anterior descending and right coronary arteries superimposed on plaque that had narrowed the lumen by 70 and 50%, respectively.

Our study is the first to describe in cocaine addicts the degree of cross-sectional area narrowing by atherosclerotic plaque in each 5-mm long segment of each of the 4 major epicardial coronary arteries. Of the 544 five-mm segments in the 12 patients who had documented toxic cocaine levels in their blood at necropsy (group I), 41 (8%) were narrowed >75% in cross-sectional by plaque alone, and 106 segments (19%) were narrowed 51 to 75% in cross-sectional area by plaque. Of the 261 five-mm segments in the 5 patients (group II) who did not have cocaine in their blood at necropsy but who were known to be habitual cocaine addicts, 8 segments (3%) were severely (>75% cross-sectional area) narrowed. Thus, it is apparent that severe coronary artery narrowing was strongly associated with death due to cocaine overdose in our patients.

The amount of severe coronary narrowing in our 2 groups of patients was higher than that expected for groups of persons whose average age is only 32 years. Of 40 patients whose epicardial coronary arteries were studied in similar fashion, who died mainly of leukemia, who never had evidence of cardiovascular disease, and whose average age was 52 years, only 3% of their 5-mm segments of the 4 major coronary arteries were narrowed >75% in cross-sectional area by plaque, and only 22% were narrowed 51 to 75% in cross-sectional area, and this group of "control subjects" was 20 years older on the average than were the cocaine addicts in the present study.[26]

In summary, this study suggests that cocaine addicts studied at necropsy have an increased amount of atherosclerotic plaque in their major epicardial coronary arteries. One explanation for the high frequency of premature coronary artery narrowing is that chronic cocaine use, by mechanisms not yet understood, accelerates coronary atherosclerosis. Another view is that of the large number of people, mostly young adults, who use cocaine, a small number have premature coronary atherosclerosis due to other causes. Cocaine may provide a fatal stress for this minority. Our study, like previous ones, focused on cocaine addicts who came to medical attention or died, and thus probably overestimates the frequency of coronary artery disease among all cocaine users.

REFERENCES

1. Young D, Glauber JJ. Electrocardiographic changes resulting from acute cocaine intoxication. *Am Heart J* 1946;34:272–279.

2. Coleman DL, Ross TF, Naughton JL. Myocardial ischemia and infarction related to recreational cocaine use. *West J Med* 1982;136:444–446.

3. Nanji AA, Filipenko JD. Asystole and ventricular fibrillation associated with cocaine intoxication. *Chest* 1984;85:132–133.

4. Schachne JS, Roberts BH, Thompson PD. Coronary-artery spasm and myocardial infarction associated with cocaine use. *N Engl J Med* 1984;310:1665–1666.

5. Kossowsky WA, Lyon AF. Cocaine and acute myocardial infarction. A probable connection. *Chest* 1984;86:729–731.

6. Boag F, Havard CWH. Cardiac arrhythmia and myocardial ischaemia related to cocaine and alcohol consumption. *Postgrad Med J* 1985;61:997–999.

7. Pasternack PF, Colvin SB, Baumann FG. Cocaine-induced angina pectoris and acute myocardial infarction in patients younger than 40 years. *Am J Cardiol* 1985;55:847.

8. Howard RE, Hueter DC, Davis GJ. Acute myocardial infarction following cocaine abuse in a young woman with normal coronary arteries. *JAMA* 1985;254:95–96.

9. Gould L, Gopalaswamy C, Patel C, Betzu R. Cocaine-induced myocardial infarction. *NY State J Med* 1985;85:660–661.

10. Wilkins CE, Mathur VS, Ty RC, Hall RJ. Myocardial infarction associated with cocaine abuse. *Texas Heart Inst J* 1985;12:385–387.

11. Weiss RJ. Recurrent myocardial infarction caused by cocaine abuse. *Am Heart J* 1986;111:793.

12. Rollingher IM, Belzberg AS, Macdonald IL. Cocaine-induced myocardial infarction. *Can Med Assoc J* 1986;135:45–46.

13. Mathias DW. Cocaine-associated myocardial ischemia. Review of clinical and angiographic findings. *Am J Med* 1986;81:675–678.

14. Wiener RS, Lockhart JT, Schwartz RG. Dilated cardiomyopathy and cocaine abuse. Report of two cases. *Am J Med* 1986;81:699–701.

15. Rod JL, Zucker RP. Acute myocardial infarction shortly after cocaine inhalation. *Am J Cardiol* 1987;59:161.

16. Tazelaar HD, Karch SB, Stephens BG, Billingham ME. Cocaine and the heart. *Hum Pathol* 1987;18:195–199.

17. Zimmerman FH, Gustafson GM, Kemp HG. Recurrent myocardial infarction associated with cocaine abuse in a young man with normal coronary arteries: evidence for coronary artery spasm culminating in thrombosis. *JACC* 1987;9:964–968.

18. Smith HWB, Liberman HA, Brody SL, Battey LL, Donohue BC, Morris DC. Acute myocardial infarction temporally related to cocaine use. *Ann Intern Med* 1987;107:13–18.

19. Peng S-K, French WJ, Pelikan PCD. Direct cocaine cardiotoxicity demonstrated by endomyocardial biopsy. *Arch Pathol Lab Med* 1989;113:842–845.

20. Mittleman RE, Wetli CV. Cocaine and sudden "natural" death. *J Forensic Sci* 1987;32:11–19.

21. Barth CW III, Bray M, Roberts WC. Rupture of the ascending aorta during cocaine intoxication. *Am J Cardiol* 1986;57:496.

22. Simpson RW, Edwards WD. Pathogenesis of cocaine-induced ischemic heart disease. Autopsy findings in a 21-year-old man. *Arch Pathol Lab Med* 1986;110:479–484.

23. Isner JM, Estes NAM III, Thompson PD, Costanzo-Nordin MR, Subramanian R, Miller G, Katsas G, Sweeney K, Sturner WQ. Acute cardiac events temporally related to cocaine abuse. *N Engl J Med* 1986;315:1438–1443.

24. Virmani R, Robinowitz M, Smialek JE, Smyth DF. Cardiovascular effects of cocaine: an autopsy study of 40 patients. *Am Heart J* 1988;115:1068–1076.

25. Stenberg RG, Winniford MD, Hillis LD, Dowling GP, Buja LM. Simultaneous acute thrombosis of two major coronary arteries following intravenous cocaine use. *Arch Pathol Lab Med* 1989;113:521–524.

26. Roberts WC. Qualitative and quantitative comparison of amounts of narrowing by atherosclerotic plaques in the major epicardial coronary arteries at necropsy in sudden coronary death, transmural acute myocardial infarction, transmural healed myocardial infarction and unstable angina pectoris. *Am J Cardiol* 1989;64:324–328.

Diffuse Extent of Coronary Atherosclerosis in Fatal Coronary Artery Disease*

William C. Roberts, MD

In 4 subsets of patients with coronary artery disease, the amounts of narrowing of the 4 major epicardial coronary arteries were compared (left main, left anterior descending, left circumflex and right) by atherosclerotic plaques. Among 129 patients studied at necropsy, an average of 2.7 of the 4 arteries were narrowed >75% in cross-sectional area at some point; in control subjects, narrowing was seen in an average of 0.7 arteries. Patients with unstable angina pectoris had a greater incidence of narrowing (3.2 arteries) than did patients with sudden coronary death (2.8), acute myocardial infarction (MI) (2.7) or healed MI (2.3). Each of the 4 major arteries was divided into segments 5 mm in length, and histologic sections were prepared and stained by the Movat method. A total of 6,461 segments were analyzed from the 129 patients and 1,849 from the 40 controls. In the 129 patients, 35% of the 5-mm segments were narrowed 75 to 100% in cross-sectional area (compared with 3% in control subjects). The group with unstable angina had the highest percentage (48%) of severely narrowed segments compared with the groups with sudden coronary death (36%), acute (34%) and healed MI (31%). Only 8% of the 6,461 segments were narrowed ≤25% in cross-sectional area, and virtually none of the 6,461 segments was normal; thus, 92% of the coronary segments were narrowed >25% in cross-sectional area by atherosclerotic plaque alone. Among patients with fatal coronary artery disease studied at necropsy, therefore, the atherosclerotic process is severe and diffuse in the major epicardial coronary arteries.

(Am J Cardiol 1990;65:2F–6F)

From the Pathology Branch, National Heart, Lung, and Blood Institute, National Institutes of Health, Bethesda, Maryland.

Address for reprints: William C. Roberts, MD, Pathology Branch, National Heart, Lung, and Blood Institute, Building 10, Room 2N258, National Institutes of Health, 9000 Rockville Pike, Bethesda, Maryland 20892.

*This article in nearly similar form appeared in the August 1, 1989, issue of *The American Journal of Cardiology*.

Atherosclerotic coronary artery disease (CAD) is the most common cause of death in the Western world. In the United States, 1 person dies every minute because of atherosclerotic CAD, and approximately 6 million persons have symptomatic myocardial ischemia due to this disease. Furthermore, approximately 250,000 coronary artery bypass grafting procedures and a similar number of coronary angioplasties were performed in the United States in 1988.

The evidence is now overwhelming that atherosclerosis is caused by elevated cholesterol levels; the higher the level of total blood cholesterol (specifically low-density lipoprotein cholesterol), the greater the risk of developing symptomatic CAD, the greater the chance of having fatal CAD, and the greater the extent of the atherosclerotic plaques. Conversely, lowering total blood cholesterol decreases the risk of symptomatic or fatal CAD and increases the likelihood that some atherosclerotic plaques will actually become smaller (i.e., regress). Although the coronary arteries have been examined by visual inspection at necropsy for more than 100 years, only recently has the extent of the atherosclerotic process in patients with symptomatic or fatal CAD become appreciated. This article reviews the status of the major epicardial coronary arteries in various subsets of patients with fatal atherosclerotic CAD. A similar review has appeared previously.[1]

NUMBER OF SEVERELY NARROWED MAJOR EPICARDIAL CORONARY ARTERIES

The most common method of describing the severity of CAD in patients with clinical evidence of myocardial ischemia is by the number of major epicardial coronary arteries narrowed >50% in luminal diameter, as determined on angiography. Thus, patients are categorized as having either 1-, 2-, or 3-vessel or "left main" CAD. Because a 50% diameter reduction is generally equivalent to a 75% cross-sectional area narrowing, the latter figure is used as the cut-off point for "significant" as opposed to "insignificant" luminal narrowing at necropsy. Physiologically, arterial flow is not obstructed until the lumen is narrowed >75% in cross-sectional area.

Table I summarizes the number of major (right, left main, left anterior descending and left circumflex) epicardial coronary arteries narrowed >75% in cross-sectional area by atherosclerotic plaque alone in a study of patients with fatal CAD.[1] Among 129 patients with fatal CAD studied at necropsy, 516 major epicardial coronary arteries were examined; of these, 345 arteries (67%) were narrowed 76 to 100% in cross-sectional area at some point by atherosclerotic plaque. Among 40 control subjects (mainly victims of acute leukemia who had no clinical evidence of myocardial ischemia during life), 160 major epicardial coronary arteries were examined; in contrast to the findings in the CAD patients, only 60 arteries (37%) were narrowed >75% in cross-sectional area at some point by plaque. Only 11 (8%) of CAD patients, vs 23% of controls, had a single coronary artery severely narrowed. Severe narrowing was present in 2 arteries in 37 patients (29%) vs 13% of controls, in 3 arteries in 64 patients (50%) vs 5% of controls, and in all 4 major arteries in 17 patients (13%) vs no controls. Overall, then, an average of 2.7 arteries in CAD patients, as opposed to 0.7 in controls, were narrowed >75% in cross-sectional area by plaque.

The numbers of severely narrowed arteries among the various subsets of patients with CAD were similar, with the exception of the group with unstable angina (Table I). Among 31 patients with sudden coronary death,[2] all of whom died outside the hospital (usually within a few minutes of onset of symptoms of myocardial ischemia), an average of 2.8 of the 4 major arteries were severely narrowed; this number was identical to that in 27 patients with transmural acute myocardial infarction (MI),[3] all of whom died in a coronary care unit. Only 2 of the 31 sudden death victims, and none of the 27 acute MI victims, had 1-vessel disease.

Patients with healed MI were separated into 3 subgroups. One subgroup consisted of those who had had an acute MI that had healed, with no subsequent clinical evidence of myocardial ischemia; these patients died from noncardiac causes (usually cancer).[4] Nevertheless, an average of 2.2 of the 4 major coronary arteries were severely narrowed at necropsy in these patients. A second subgroup consisted of patients who had chronic congestive heart failure after healing of an acute MI, but in the absence of a left ventricular aneurysm[5]; this group might be referred to as having "ischemic cardiomyopathy." An average of 2.2 major coronary arteries were severely narrowed in these patients. The other subgroup of patients with healed MI had true left ventricular aneurysms.[6] The average number of severely narrowed major coronary arteries in this group was 2.5.

The third subgroup consisted of 22 patients with unstable angina pectoris, all of whom had undergone coronary artery bypass grafting within 7 days of dying.[7] Preoperatively, all had normal left ventricular function and none had had a clinically apparent acute MI or congestive heart failure at any time. The average number of major coronary arteries severely narrowed by plaque was 3.2, and 10 of the 22 patients had severe narrowing of the left main coronary artery as well as the other 3 major coronary arteries (4-vessel disease). (Bulkley and I[8] found that severe narrowing of the left main coronary artery is usually an indicator that the other 3 major arteries also are severely narrowed.) The unstable angina group thus had the largest average number of severely narrowed major coronary arteries of any of the subgroups, but nevertheless had excellent left ventricular function.

AMOUNTS OF NARROWING IN SEGMENTS OF THE MAJOR CORONARY ARTERIES

Although the classifications of 1-, 2-, 3- and 4-vessel disease have been useful clinically, this type of analysis of severity might be thought of as a qualitative approach. Differences in degrees of coronary narrowing in various subsets of patients with CAD cannot usually be discerned by this approach. To obtain a better appreciation of the extent of the atherosclerotic process in patients with fatal CAD, my colleagues and I began examining 5-mm-long segments of each of the 4 major coronary arteries several years ago. In adults, the average length of the right coronary artery is 10 cm; the left main, 1 cm; the left anterior descending, 10 cm; and the left circumflex, 6 cm. Thus, 27 cm of major epicardial coronary artery are available for examination in each adult. Because each 1 cm is divided into 2 segments, each measuring 5 mm in length, an average of 54 such segments are available for examination in each heart. This approach allows one to ask not only how many of the 5-mm segments are narrowed 76 to 100% in cross-sectional area, but also how many are narrowed 51 to 75%, 26 to 50%, or 0 to 25%. This might be considered a quantitative approach.

The same patients previously described by the qualitative approach also were examined at necropsy by the quantitative approach; the findings are summarized in

TABLE II Amounts of Cross-Sectional Area Narrowing of Each 5-mm Segment of the Four Major (Right, Left Main, Left Anterior Descending and Left Circumflex) Epicardial Coronary Arteries by Atherosclerotic Plaques in Subjects with Fatal Coronary Artery Disease

Subgroup	Pts (n)	Mean Age (yrs)	No. 5-mm Segments	Percent Segments Narrowed				Mean Score	Mean % Narrowing/ 5-mm Segments
				0–25%	26–50%	51–75%	76–100%		
Sudden coronary death	31	47	1,564	7	23	34	36	2.98	67
Acute myocardial infarction	27	59	1,403	5	23	38	34	3.01	68
Healed myocardial infarction									
Asymptomatic	18	66	924	11	23	35	31 ⎫	2.87	64
Chronic CHF							⎬ 31%		
without aneurysm	9	63	529	11	23	37	29 ⎮	2.78	61
LV aneurysm	22	61	992	4	21	42	33 ⎭	3.03	68
Angina pectoris	22	48	1,049	11	12	29	48	3.12	70
Total	129	56	6,461	8	21	36	35	2.98	67
Controls	40	52	1,849	31	44	22	3	1.97	32

CHF = congestive heart failure; LV = left ventricular.
Reproduced with permission from *Am J Cardiol*.[1]

Table II. A total of 6,461 segments (each 5 mm in length) were sectioned and later examined histologically. The sections were stained by the Movat method to delineate the internal elastic membrane. The findings in the 129 patients with CAD were compared with those in 40 control subjects, from whom 1,849 segments were obtained. In each coronary subgroup, the 5-mm segments from each of the 4 major coronary arteries were pooled together. With this approach, the amount of narrowing in an individual patient was not discernible. Among the CAD patients, 35% of segments were narrowed 76 to 100% in cross-sectional area by atherosclerotic plaque; in contrast, only 3% were narrowed in controls. The segments narrowed 51 to 75% totaled 36 and 22%, respectively. Thus, 71% of the segments in the CAD patients, and 25% in controls, were narrowed >50% in cross-sectional area by atherosclerotic plaque. In contrast, only 29% of the segments in the CAD patients were narrowed <50% and only 8% even approached normal (i.e., narrowed ≤25% in cross-sectional area). In contrast, 75% of the segments in the control subjects were narrowed <50% and 31% of them were normal or nearly normal. Thus, in the CAD patients, 92% of the 6,461 segments of the 4 major epicardial coronary arteries were narrowed >25% in cross-sectional area by atherosclerotic plaque. Accordingly, the coronary atherosclerotic process is diffuse, rather than focal, in patients with fatal CAD.

Among the various subsets of CAD patients, those with sudden coronary death[2] and acute MI[3] had similar percentages of 5-mm segments narrowed 76 to 100% in cross-sectional area by plaque (36 and 34%, respectively); patients with healed MI[4-6] as a group had the least severe narrowing (31% of segments narrowed >75%), and those with unstable angina pectoris[7] had the most severe narrowing (48% of segments narrowed >75% by plaque).

In an effort to arrive at a single number for the amount of coronary arterial narrowing in each patient, a score system was utilized for each 5-mm segment. Nar-rowing of 0 to 25% was assigned a score of 1; 26 to 50%, 2; 51 to 75%, 3; and 76 to 100%, 4. The mean score for all 129 patients (or for the 6,461 coronary segments) was 3.0, and that for the 40 control subjects (or 1,849 segments) was 2.0. Using this scoring system, patients with unstable angina again had the most extensive coronary narrowing.

A possible criticism of the analysis of 5-mm segments to quantify coronary arterial narrowing is that the epicardial coronary arteries were fixed in an unphysiologic pressure state—namely, a zero-pressure state—rather than at a systemic arterial diastolic pressure. The degrees of narrowing were conservatively judged to take into account the unphysiologic fixed state. For example, if a segment was between 2 quadrants (51 to 75% and 76 to 100%), the lesser degree of narrowing was always chosen. Second, for any segment in which a portion of wall was collapsed by the fixation process, the degree of narrowing was determined as if the segment was expanded. Most important, the segments narrowed the most (>75% in cross-sectional area) were affected the least by the fixation process. Whether the histologic technique in this study is perfect or flawed, the same technique was in all subsets of coronary patients and all controls. The comparison data are, therefore, highly reliable. Also, regardless of whether the degrees of luminal narrowing are slightly greater or less than those determined by this technique, it is clear that the atherosclerotic process is a diffuse one in nearly all patients with fatal CAD. The accuracy of the technique of determining degrees of cross-sectional area narrowing by estimating from stained histologic sections magnified approximately 40 times is similar (≤5%) to that determined by planimetry.[9]

Another possible concern of the aforementioned quantitative data is its applicability to living patients with symptomatic or other clinical evidence (e.g., positive exercise test results) of myocardial ischemia. I believe that the major difference in coronary arterial narrowing occurs at the stage of conversion from the asymptomatic to the symptomatic myocardial ischemia state, and that there is relatively little difference in degrees of coronary narrowing between the symptomatic and the fatal states. Assessment of the presence of severe, extensive coronary narrowing on angiography during life, as well as by study of the coronary tree at necropsy in patients who had coronary events and later died from noncardiac causes, supports this view. Although only minimal data are available from the latter group, the degrees of coronary narrowing at necropsy are similar to those in other patients with symptomatic myocardial ischemia that proves fatal.[4] Also, of the subsets of CAD patients described, those with unstable angina pectoris had significantly greater degrees of coronary narrowing. Furthermore, these patients were the only subjects in whom the natural course was interrupted by an iatrogenic event, i.e., coronary artery bypass grafting within 7 days of death.

DISTRIBUTION OF SEVERE NARROWING IN THE THREE LONGEST EPICARDIAL CORONARY ARTERIES

In all the quantitative studies described herein, the amount of cross-sectional area luminal narrowing by atherosclerotic plaque in the right, left anterior descending and left circumflex coronary arteries was similar if the 5-mm segments in each of the 3 longest arteries were pooled together from a number of patients. Examination of a single subset of patients with fatal CAD may help to better understand this concept. Among the 27 patients with fatal transmural acute MI, a total of 1,358 segments were analyzed from the right, left anterior descending and left circumflex coronary arteries. The percentages of segments narrowed 0 to 25%, 26 to 50%, 51 to 75% and 76 to 100% were similar in each of these 4 categories in each of the 3 major epicardial coronary arteries. Analysis of the patients with sudden coronary death, healed MI and unstable angina pectoris yielded the same results.

In an individual patient, however, the percentage of 5-mm segments severely narrowed (>75% in cross-sectional area) by atherosclerotic plaque in 1 major epicardial coronary artery may be greater or less than that in another major coronary artery. Nonetheless, if the segments from 1 coronary artery (e.g., right) were pooled together from several patients with fatal CAD and compared with segments from another coronary artery (e.g., left anterior descending) pooled from several patients with fatal CAD, the percentages of segments narrowed in each of the 4 categories of cross-sectional area narrowing in each artery would be similar. The definition of "several" has not yet been established, but, with infrequent exceptions, this principle may apply to as few as 3 patients with pooled 5-mm segments from each of the 3 major coronary arteries. Thus, the quantity of atherosclerotic plaque is similar for similar lengths of the right, left anterior descending and left circumflex coronary arteries. Furthermore, because the amount of atherosclerotic plaque is similar, the amount of resulting luminal narrowing also is similar. The cholesterol thesis might not be tenable if the amount

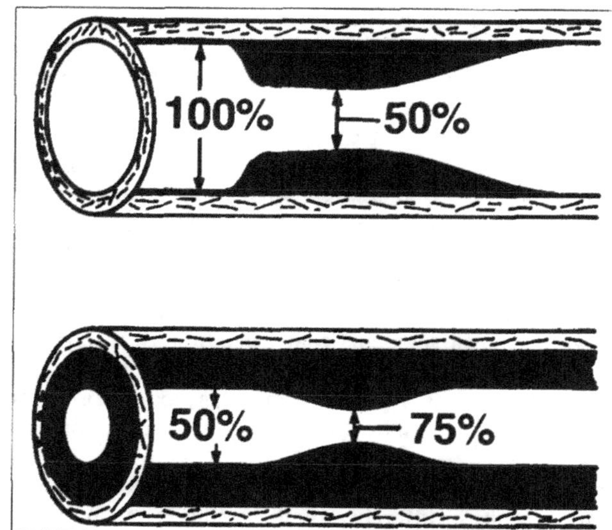

FIGURE 1. Representation of an angiographic view of 2 coronary arteries with luminal plaque. Because the angiogram is a luminogram, and the width of the original arterial lumen is unknown, the least narrowed segment is often presumed to be normal. Comparison of a narrowed segment to a near-normal segment (*upper panel*) provides an accurate measurement of the degree of narrowing, but normal or near-normal segments are infrequent in patients with symptomatic myocardial ischemia. More frequently, severely narrowed segments are simply compared with less severely narrowed segments, but none of the segments approach normal (*lower panel*). (Reproduced with permission from *Am Heart J*.[13])

of atherosclerotic plaque were highly different in the different major epicardial coronary arteries, because the same serum cholesterol level presumably is present in each major coronary artery.

CLINICAL USEFULNESS OF THE QUANTITATIVE APPROACH

The quantitative information derived at necropsy on the severity and extent of atherosclerosis in the 4 major epicardial coronary arteries in fatal CAD has possible clinical applications in (1) interpreting degrees of coronary narrowing by angiography during life and (2) deciding which of the major coronary arteries requires a conduit at the time of coronary artery bypass grafting.

Without coronary angiography, neither coronary bypass nor angioplasty would be performed. The only way to obtain information on the status of the epicardial coronary arteries during life is with angiography; consequently, this procedure revolutionized the diagnosis of CAD, just as aortocoronary bypass grafting revolutionized the therapy of CAD. However, despite the advantages of angiography, this technique has certain failings. For one, the angiogram is a luminogram, which compares a narrowed segment with a less narrowed segment that is assumed to be normal. The angiogram does not delineate the internal elastic membrane of the artery, and, therefore, the artery's true lumen remains uncertain.

The quantitative studies of fatal CAD mentioned herein demonstrated that 93% of the 5-mm long segments of the 4 major epicardial coronary arteries were narrowed >25% in cross-sectional area by atherosclerotic plaque. Thus, only 7% of the 5-mm segments even approached normal, and virtually none were normal. In fatal CAD, and probably also in live patients with symptomatic myocardial ischemia, therefore, only rarely can a coronary artery segment that is severely narrowed on angiography be compared with a segment of coronary artery that is normal. In other words, in patients with symptomatic myocardial ischemia, the coronary angiogram measures degrees of narrowing by comparing severely narrowed segments with segments that are simply less narrowed and by no means normal (Fig. 1). Thus, coronary angiograms in patients with symptomatic myocardial ischemia usually underestimate the degrees of luminal narrowing.[10,11]

The unit of measurement for degrees of narrowing on angiography is different from the unit of measurement at necropsy. In the aforementioned anatomic quantitative studies, the unit was cross-sectional area narrowing, whereas the unit used in angiography is diameter narrowing. In general, a 75% cross-sectional area narrowing is equivalent to a 50% diameter reduction, and, therefore, a 50% or more diameter reduction during life has generally been considered the cut-off point between clinically significant and clinically insignificant coronary narrowing.

The second potential clinical application of the information gleaned from the quantitative CAD studies at necropsy is the recognition that the atherosclerotic process in patients with symptomatic myocardial ischemia is usually diffuse and severe, and, therefore, more rather than fewer aortocoronary conduits provide a higher frequency of relief or improvement in symptoms of myocardial ischemia, improvement in results of exercise testing, and prolonged life. Among patients surviving <30 days or at later periods after aortocoronary bypass operations, the amount of severe narrowing in the nonbypassed native coronary arteries is usually similar to that in the bypassed native coronary arteries.[12] Waller and I[12] found from study at necropsy of 102 patients dying either early (≤60 days) or late (2.5 to 108 months, mean 35) after bypass operations that the bypassed and nonbypassed native coronary arteries had similar degrees of severe luminal narrowing by atherosclerotic plaques. In 213 of 226 bypassed native arteries (94%) and in 73 of 80 nonbypassed native arteries (91%), the lumens were narrowed >75% in cross-sectional area by atherosclerotic plaque. Bypass of the native arteries was not avoided because they were too small or severely narrowed distally, but, rather, because the lumens were judged to be insufficiently narrowed (on angiography) to warrant insertion of a conduit. Thus, if 2 of the major coronary arteries are found to be severely narrowed on angiography and the third major artery is "insignificantly" narrowed, and if bypass is to be performed, an argument could be made for insertion of a conduit in all 3 major coronary arteries. Of course, insertion of a conduit in an insignificantly narrowed artery is potentially dangerous. Nevertheless, it may be more prudent to have too many conduits rather than too few. Three-vessel disease is far more frequent than is 2-vessel disease at necropsy, and even when only 2 of the 3 major arteries are narrowed >75% in cross-sectional area, the third is usually narrowed 51 to 75%. Thus, an appreciation of the diffuse nature of coronary atherosclerosis in fatal CAD, and probably also in symptomatic myocardial ischemia, encourages the use of more, rather than fewer, conduits in coronary bypass operations.

REFERENCES

1. Roberts WC. Qualitative and quantitative comparison of amounts of narrowing by atherosclerotic plaques in the major epicardial coronary arteries at necropsy in sudden coronary death, transmural acute myocardial infarction, transmural healed myocardial infarction and unstable angina pectoris. *Am J Cardiol 1989;64:324–328.*

2. Robert WC, Jones AA. Quantitation of coronary arterial narrowing at necropsy in sudden coronary death. Analysis of 31 patients and comparison with 25 control subjects. *Am J Cardiol 1979;44:39.*

3. Roberts WC, Jones AA. Quantification of coronary arterial narrowing at necropsy in acute transmural myocardial infarction: analysis and comparison of findings in 27 patients and 22 controls. *Circulation 1980;61:786–790.*

4. Virmani R, Roberts WC. Non-fatal healed transmural myocardial infarction and fatal non-cardiac disease. Qualification and quantification of coronary arterial narrowing and of left ventricular scarring in 18 necropsy patients. *Br Heart J 1981;45:434–441.*

5. Virmani R, Roberts WC. Quantification of coronary arterial narrowing and of left ventricular myocardial scarring in healed myocardial infarction with chronic eventually fatal, congestive cardiac failure. *Am J Med 1980;68:831–838.*

6. Cabin HS, Roberts WC. True left ventricular aneurysm and healed myocardial infarction. Clinical and necropsy observations including quantification of degrees of coronary arterial narrowing. *Am J Cardiol 1980;46:754–763.*

7. Roberts WC, Virmani R. Quantification of coronary arterial narrowing in clinically-isolated unstable angina pectoris. An analysis of 22 necropsy patients. *Am J Med 1979;67:792–799.*

8. Bulkley BH, Roberts WC. Atherosclerotic narrowing of the left main coronary artery. A necropsy analysis of 152 patients with fatal coronary heart disease and varying degrees of left main narrowing. *Circulation 1976;53:823–828.*

9. Isner JM, Wu M, Virmani R, Jones AA, Roberts WC. Comparison of coronary arterial luminal narrowing determined by visual inspection of histologic sections under magnification among three independent observers and comparison to that obtained by video planimetry. An analysis of 559 five-millimeter segments of 61 coronary arteries from eleven patients. *Lab Invest 1980;42:566–570.*

10. Arnett EN, Isner JM, Redwood DR, Kent KM, Baker WP, Ackerstein H, Roberts WC. Coronary artery narrowing in coronary heart disease: comparison of cineangiographic and necropsy findings. *Ann Intern Med 1979;91:350–356.*

11. Isner JM, Kishel J, Kent KM, Ronan JAJ, Ross AM, Roberts WC. Accuracy of angiographic determination of left main coronary arterial narrowing. Angiographic-histologic correlative analysis in 28 patients. *Circulation 1981;63:1056–1064.*

12. Waller BF, Roberts WC. Amount of narrowing by atherosclerotic plaque in 44 nonbypassed and 52 bypassed major epicardial coronary arteries in 32 necropsy patients who died within 1 month of aortocoronary bypass grafting. *Am J Cardiol 1980;46:956–962.*

Coronary Arterial Morphology 10 Years After "Endarterectomy"

A. H. KRAGEL, M.D., C. L. MCINTOSH, M.D., Ph.D., W. C. ROBERTS, M.D.

Pathology and Cardiac Surgery Branches, National Heart, Lung, and Blood Institute, National Institutes of Health, Bethesda, Maryland, USA

Summary: Little information is available regarding coronary artery morphology after endarterectomy. In this report, we describe coronary artery morphology seen at necropsy 10 years after coronary artery endarterectomy and compare it with the morphology of the original endarterectomy specimen. Surprisingly, in some areas, all of the internal elastic membrane and most of the media were observed in the "endarterectomy" specimen.

Key words: coronary artery disease, coronary artery bypass surgery

Introduction

Coronary artery endarterectomy is performed on occasion as an adjunct to coronary artery bypass surgery. While there is extensive information regarding the morphology of changes in saphenous vein grafts and native coronary arteries following coronary artery bypass grafting, only two previous reports have described morphologic findings in the coronary arteries which have been sites of endarterectomy.[1,2] In this report we compare the histologic changes in the native coronary artery seen at necropsy 10 years after "endarterectomy" with those seen in the surgical "endarterectomy" specimen.

Address for reprints:

A. H. Kragel, M.D.
Pathology Branch
National Heart, Lung, and Blood Institute
Building 10, Room 2N258
Bethesda, MD 20892, USA

Received: November 7, 1989
Accepted: November 20, 1989

Case Report

G.O., a 62-year-old man with systemic hypertension, diabetes mellitus, and hypercholesterolemia, first developed angina pectoris at age 48. After a 4-year period of stable exertional angina, the angina worsened to functional class 4/4. Angiography disclosed 50–75% diameter narrowing of the left main and left obtuse marginal, 75–99% narrowing of the left circumflex, total occlusion of the right, and less than 50% narrowing of the left anterior descending coronary arteries. The left ventricular pressure was 145/10 mmHg. Saphenous vein grafts were placed to the left anterior descending, left obtuse marginal, and distal right coronary arteries, with endarterectomy of the distal right and proximal posterior descending coronary arteries (Fig. 1). Cardiac catheterization per-

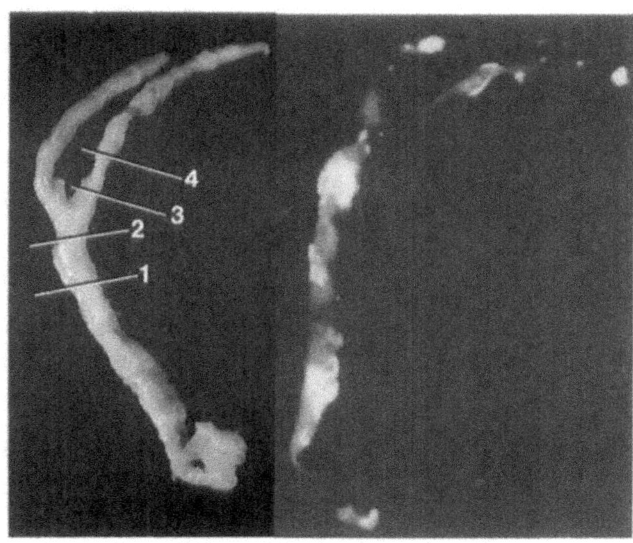

FIG. 1. Photograph (left) and radiograph (right) of the endarterectomy specimen removed 10 years before death from the distal right and proximal posterior descending coronary artery. The numbers approximate locations of the corresponding sections from the distal right (1 and 2), and proximal posterior descending (3 and 4), coronary arteries illustrated in Fig. 2.

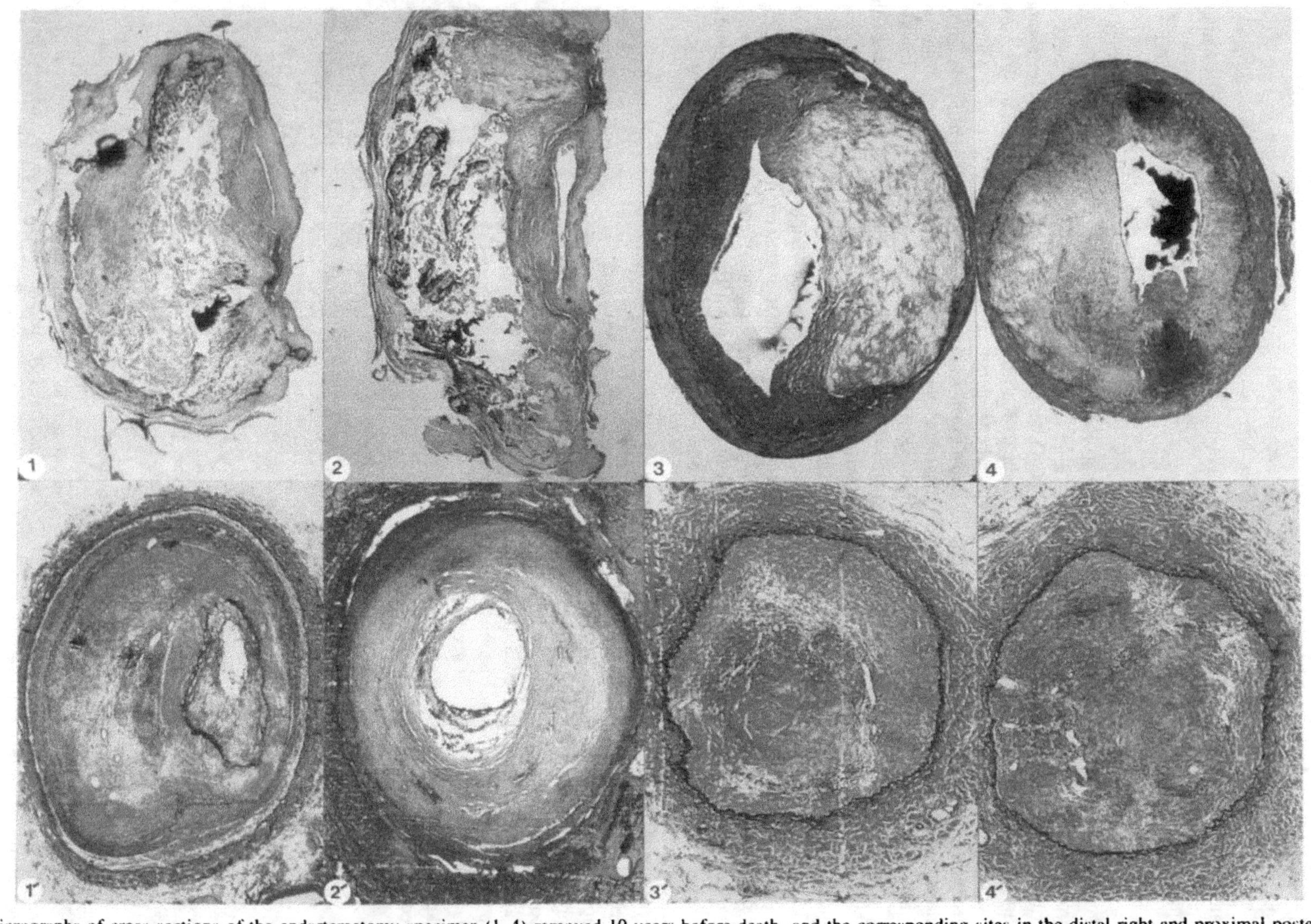

FIG. 2. Photomicrographs of cross-sections of the endarterectomy specimen (1–4) removed 10 years before death, and the corresponding sites in the distal right and proximal posterior descending coronary artery at necropsy (1'–4'). The lumen of the endarterectomy specimen is severely narrowed by focally calcified atherosclerotic plaque. The sections from the proximal posterior descending coronary artery portion (3 and 4) of the surgical specimen contain internal elastic membrane plus media. The lumen of the distal right coronary artery (1', 2') at necropsy also is severely narrowed by focally calcified plaque. Sections of proximal posterior descending coronary artery (3' and 4'), show that internal elastic membrane and media are absent, but there is severe luminal narrowing by a nearly homogeneous proliferation of spindle cells admixed with collagen and containing small vascular channels and scattered inflammatory cells. Movat stains; ×5.2[1], ×3.9[2], ×9.75[3], ×9.75[4], ×4.88[1'], ×6.5[2'], ×9.75[3'], ×9.75[4'].

formed 6 months postoperatively showed all three saphenous vein grafts to be patent. At age 58, the angina returned and by age 60 he was reclassified as functional class 3/4. Repeat catheterization disclosed the saphenous vein grafts to the left anterior descending and the right coronary arteries to be completely occluded. He continued to be severely limited by angina and underwent repeat coronary artery bypass surgery. Saphenous vein grafts were placed to the distal posterior descending, the second diagonal, and the first obtuse marginal coronary arteries, and a left internal mammary graft was placed in the distal left anterior descending coronary artery. The saphenous vein grafts placed 10 years previously were resected. He developed severe pump failure and sepsis and died 26 days after this second operation.

The "endarterectomy" specimen (Fig. 1) removed 10 years before death measured 7 cm in length and consisted of distal right coronary artery and two posterior descending branches. The native right and posterior descending coronary arteries were dissected from the epicardial surface of the heart and, using the bifurcation of the right coronary artery as a landmark, corresponding areas of the surgical and necropsy specimens were identified. Both specimens were decalcified, sectioned transversely at 5 mm intervals, processed in xylene, cleared in alcohol, and stained using the Movat method.

Sections from the proximal endarterectomy specimen (Fig. 2), corresponding to the distal portion of the right coronary artery, showed severe luminal narrowing by calcified atherosclerotic plaque. Small portions of internal elastic membrane and media also were present in these segments. Distal portions of the "endarterectomy" specimen, corresponding to the posterior descending coronary artery, not only showed severe luminal narrowing by calcified atherosclerotic plaque, but also contained large portions of internal elastic membrane and media.

Movat-stained sections of the native distal right coronary artery, examined 10 years after endarterectomy, showed severe luminal narrowing by atherosclerotic plaque composed of admixtures of focally calcified cellular and acellular connective tissue containing small vascular channels and chronic inflammatory cells. The internal elastic membrane and media were focally disrupted. Sections of the proximal posterior descending coronary artery showed near total occlusion of the lumen by cellular fibrous tissue composed of a homogeneous admixture of spindle cells and collagen which contained small vascular channels and chronic inflammatory cells. Both the internal elastic membrane and media were absent (Fig. 2).

Comment

Comparison of features of the native coronary artery and the "endarterectomy" specimen removed 10 years previously showed differences in plaque morphology between segments devoid of internal elastic membrane and media (which had been removed along with plaque) and those segments containing internal elastic membrane and media. In areas where the internal elastic membrane was largely intact, the plaque was pleomorphic, and consisted of cellular and acellular fibrous tissue and calcium. In contrast, where the internal elastic membrane and media had been excised at the time of "endarterectomy," the plaque was much more homogeneous in appearance, and consisted of an admixture of spindle cells and collagen containing only a few inflammatory cells and a few small vascular channels. This homogeneous proliferation of spindle cells admixed with collagen in the absence of the internal elastic membrane is similar to what we reported in a previous case in which death occurred 4.5 years after endarterectomy of the right coronary artery.[2] Byard and associates earlier had described similar changes in 6 of 9 patients who died 6 to 9 years after coronary endarerectomy.[1] Similar changes also have been described in operative specimens in association with early restenosis of the carotid artery after endarterectomy.[3-6] The spindle cells in these plaques have been shown by electron microscopy to have features of both smooth muscle cells and fibroblasts.[7]

References

1. Byard RW, Keon WJ, Walley VM: Coronary endarterectomy: The long-term local effects. *Am J Cardiovasc Pathol* 2, 31 (1988)

2. Kragel AH, McIntosh CL, Roberts WC: Morphologic changes in coronary artery seen late after endarterectomy. *Am J Cardiol* 63, 757 (1989)

3. Stoney RJ, String ST: Recurrent carotid stenosis. *Surgery* 80, 705 (1976)

4. Cossman D, Callow AD, Stein A, Matsumoto G: Early restenosis after carotid endarterectomy. *Arch Surg* 113, 275 (1978)

5. Cantelmo NL, Cutler BS, Wheeler HB, Herrmann JB, Cardullo PA: Noninvasive detection of carotid stenosis following endarterectomy. *Arch Surg* 116, 1005 (1981)

6. Palmaz JC, Hunter G, Carson SN, French SW: Postoperative carotid restenosis due to neointimal fibromuscular hyperplasia. Clinical, angiographic and pathologic findings. *Radiology* 148, 699 (1983)

7. Hertzer NR, Martinez BD, Beven EG: Recurrent stenosis after carotid endarterectomy. *Surg Gynecol Obstet* 149, 360 (1979)

Cardiac Morphologic Findings in Patients with Acute Myocardial Infarction Treated with Recombinant Tissue Plasminogen Activator

S. David Gertz, MD, PhD, Jay M. Kalan, MD, Amy H. Kragel, MD, William C. Roberts, MD, Eugene Braunwald, MD, and The TIMI Investigators

The hearts of 52 patients (aged 61 ± 11 years, 34 men) who participated in the Thrombolysis in Myocardial Infarction (TIMI) Study and died from 5 hours to 260 days (median 2.7 days) after onset of chest pain were studied. One heart became available at cardiac transplantation. Of the 52 patients, 38 received recombinant tissue plasminogen activator (rt-PA) not followed by percutaneous transluminal coronary angioplasty (PTCA) or coronary artery bypass grafting (CABG). Eight had PTCA, and 6 had CABG. The infarcts were hemorrhagic by gross inspection (with histologic confirmation) in 23 patients, nonhemorrhagic in 20, not visible grossly in 2 and, in 7, there was no myocardial necrosis by either gross or histologic examination. Comparisons between the 23 patients with hemorrhagic infarcts and the 20 patients with nonhemorrhagic infarcts showed: (1) similar frequencies of myocardial rupture (left ventricular free wall or ventricular septum) [6 (26%) of 23 vs 5 (25%) of 20], cardiogenic shock [10 (43%) of 23 vs 9 (47%) of 19], and fatal hemorrhage [2 (9%) of 23 vs 2 (10%) of 20]; (2) similar percents of necrotic portions of left ventricular wall among patients surviving >18 hours from onset of chest pain (26 ± 11 vs 23 ± 11%) with the hemorrhage confined to areas of necrotic myocardium in all cases; (3) similar frequencies of thrombi in the infarct-related arteries [7 (32%) vs 7 (37%)], but all thrombi in patients with hemorrhagic infarcts were nonocclusive, and all thrombi in those with nonhemorrhagic infarcts were occlusive (p = 0.0002); (4) similar degrees of luminal cross-sectional area narrowing over all 5-mm segments of the 4 major (left main, left anterior descending, left circumflex and right) epicardial coronary arteries in 27 patients receiving rt-PA alone between patients with hemorrhagic and nonhemorrhagic infarcts; (5) similar numbers of patients in whom the infarct-related artery was narrowed >75% in cross-sectional area at some point by plaque [21 (95%) of 22 vs 16 (84%) of 19], and similar mean percent reduction in cross-sectional area by plaque of the infarct-related arteries calculated by planimetry (67 ± 10 vs 68 ± 9%); (6) similar frequencies of plaque rupture [11 (55%) of 20 vs 12 (75%) of 16] and similar frequencies of hemorrhage into a plaque [13 (65%) of 20 vs 13 (81%) of 16] in patients without PTCA; (7) fewer right ventricular infarcts in patients with hemorrhagic infarcts (2 of 10 posterior hemorrhagic infarcts vs 6 of 9 posterior nonhemorrhagic infarcts); (8) similar percents of plaque with pultaceous debris (13 ± 11 vs 18 ± 9%), calcific deposits (14 ± 12 vs 20 ± 14%) and acellular fibrous tissue (49 ± 14 vs 53 ± 11%). Thus, hemorrhage occurs frequently in the infarcts of patients who receive rt-PA. Hemorrhage into an infarct does not appear to extend the infarct, and patients with hemorrhagic (vs nonhemorrhagic) infarcts have no greater frequency of myocardial rupture or cardiogenic shock, and no significant differences in coronary luminal narrowing, plaque rupture or plaque composition. However, those with hemorrhagic infarcts had only nonocclusive thrombi and fewer right ventricular infarcts.

(Am J Cardiol 1990;65:953–961)

Until thrombolytic and revascularization therapy of acute myocardial infarction (AMI) was introduced, virtually all AMIs observed at necropsy were nonhemorrhagic. Treatment with thrombolytic agents has been shown to restore the patency of occluded coronary arteries,[1-3] but this has been associated with an apparently marked, although heretofore undetermined, increase in the frequency of hemorrhagic infarcts. It has been suggested that myocardial hemorrhage after coronary reperfusion is confined to zones of the myocardium that were already necrotic, and that

From the Pathology Branch, National Heart, Lung, and Blood Institute, National Institutes of Health, Bethesda, Maryland; The Department of Anatomy and Embryology, The Hebrew University, Hadassah Medical School, Jerusalem, Israel; and the Department of Medicine, Brigham and Women's Hospital, Boston, Massachusetts. Manuscript received November 22, 1989; revised manuscript received December 19, 1989, and accepted December 21.

Address for reprints: S. David Gertz, MD, Pathology Branch, National Heart, Lung, and Blood Institute, National Institutes of Health, Building 10, Room 2N258, Bethesda, Maryland 20892.

the hemorrhage is probably a consequence of severe microvascular injury and not its cause.[4–6] However, concerns that myocardial hemorrhage after administration of recombinant tissue plasminogen activator (rt-PA) might increase the frequency of complications of infarction such as myocardial rupture or cardiogenic shock have not been resolved. Accordingly, during the last 3 years, we have studied at necropsy the hearts of 52 patients who received rt-PA during the course of AMI to compare clinical and cardiac morphologic findings in patients with hemorrhagic infarcts to those with non-hemorrhagic infarcts.

METHODS

The hearts of 52 patients who received rt-PA during evolving AMI were studied. All patients were part of the Thrombolysis in Myocardial Infarction (TIMI) study. Full details concerning criteria for inclusion into the TIMI studies have been previously reported.[1–3] The Pathology Branch, National Heart, Lung, and Blood Institute, served as the central pathology laboratory for the TIMI study. The hearts were submitted from 25 different centers participating in the TIMI trial (see Appendix). In 2 patients the coronary arteries were not available for examination. Of the 52 patients, 38 had been treated with rt-PA not followed by percutaneous transluminal angioplasty (PTCA) or coronary artery bypass grafting (CABG). In 8 patients, rt-PA was followed by PTCA after 2 hours (2 patients), 18 hours (5 patients) and 2 days (1 patient). In 6 patients, rt-PA was followed by CABG after 1 day (2 patients) and after 2, 10, 16 and 71 days (1 patient each). One of the 38 patients treated with rt-PA alone underwent cardiac transplantation 40 days after treatment and is still alive. Fourteen (27%) of the 52 had healed (previous) myocardial infarcts at necropsy.

The hearts were fixed in 10% buffered formaldehyde for at least 3 days. The epicardial coronary arteries were excised intact and decalcified by the formic acid-sodium citrate method[7] for approximately 12 hours. (Gross decalcification by this technique does not preclude the identification of calcific deposits in histologic sections stained by the Movat technique.) The arteries were sectioned transversely at 5-mm intervals and the segments were labeled sequentially. All specimens were then dehydrated in ethanol and xylene and embedded in paraffin. One section (5 μ thick) from each 5-mm segment was stained by the Movat method[8] and another section from each 5-mm segment was stained with hematoxylin and eosin. The hearts were then cut transversely into slices approximately 1 cm thick from the apex to approximately 2 cm caudal to the posterior atrioventricular sulcus for gross, histologic and morphometric examination of the myocardium.

Patients were compared with respect to age, sex, interval from chest pain to administration of rt-PA, peak creatine kinase, death, history of systemic hypertension, frequency of myocardial rupture, fatal cardiogenic shock, fatal arrhythmias, major or fatal bleeding, heart weight, postmortem location of the recent and previous infarcts, infarct size, presence of left ventricular dilatation and the status of the infarct-related coronary arter-

ies—including the presence of occlusive and nonocclusive thrombi, composition of thrombi, frequency of plaque rupture and its frequency of association with thrombus and pultaceous debris within the plaque, frequency of hemorrhage into a plaque and its frequency of association with thrombus, frequency of the presence of fibrin within the plaque, luminal narrowing, and composition of the atherosclerotic plaque.

All clinical parameters were verified with the records of the TIMI Data Coordinating Center.

Hemorrhagic infarcts were identified by grossly visible blood within the necrotic myocardium with confirmation of the presence and extent of the hemorrhage relative to the necrosis by histologic examination.

Infarct size was quantitated in 23 patients who survived at least 18 hours after the onset of chest pain. Each transverse ventricular slice was weighed and the percent of each slice that was necrotic or fibrotic was calculated by planimetric measurement.

The infarct-related coronary artery was identified as the left anterior descending artery for anterior wall infarcts and the dominant right or dominant left circumflex coronary artery for posterior (inferior) wall infarcts.

Plaque rupture was identified by a fissure within the atherosclerotic plaque that was associated with thrombus or hemorrhage into the plaque with the defect in the plaque being continuous with the arterial lumen.

The amounts of fibrin, platelets, erythrocytes and leukocytes in thrombi were estimated microscopically on a 0+ to 3+ scale.

Luminal narrowing of the 4 major (left main, left anterior descending, left circumflex and right) coronary arteries was estimated by examination of histologic sections of each 5-mm segment. With the internal elastic lamina as the perimeter of the luminal circle, the degree of luminal narrowing for each segment was assessed by visually subdividing the circle into 4 equal quadrants.[9] These quadrants corresponded to the 4 degrees of reduction of luminal cross-sectional area—0 to 25, 26 to 50, 51 to 75 and 76 to 100%, with the latter being subdivided further into 76 to 95 and 96 to 100%. In addition, a coronary score (of luminal narrowing) was calculated by assigning each of the 4 degrees of luminal narrowing a numerical value from 1 to 4. A 5-mm segment narrowed 0 to 25% in cross-sectional area had a score of 1, a segment narrowed 26 to 50% had a score of 2, and so forth. Each degree of narrowing was multiplied by the number of segments found to be narrowed by that degree. The sum for all 4 degrees of narrowing was then divided by the total number of segments studied for that artery, giving an overall coronary score from 0 to 4.

Plaque composition was assessed by planimetric measurement as follows. Movat-stained sections from each 5-mm coronary segment were projected onto white paper using a Bausch and Lomb Tri-simplex microprojector. The image was magnified $\times$ 40 (approximately) and the following areas were traced: external elastic lamina (corresponding to the outer border of the media), internal elastic lamina (potential lumen minus total area of atherosclerotic plaque), relatively acellular fibrous tissue (primarily collagenous and rich in mucopolysaccharides), cellular fibrous tissue (consisting primarily of smooth muscle cells and fibroblasts mingled with collagen and elastic fibers), calcific deposits (granular, brown-stained areas in Movat-stained sections) (single, isolated granules were not included in this quantification) and pultaceous debris (extracellular lipid represented by pale-staining areas consisting of amorphous material with numerous cholesterol clefts with a variable amount of inflammatory and foam-cell infiltrates). After tracing these components, the relative area occupied by each was determined by reoutlining these areas using a GTCO Micro Digi-pad and stylus (model 1212) in association with the Macmeasure morphometric software package adapted to a Macintosh SE computer.[10] Only those patients without PTCA or CABG were used for this quantitation of plaque composition to avoid misinterpretation of histopathologic findings.

Statistical comparisons of numerical data were performed by 2-tailed *t* tests (paired or unpaired as appropriate) without adjustment for multiple testing. Categorical data were compared by coded chi-square analysis. For these calculations the Stat View 512+ statistical package (Brain Power, Inc.) was used in association with a Macintosh SE computer.

RESULTS

Baseline characteristics: Of the 52 patients studied [age 61 ± 11 years, 34 (65%) men], 38 received rt-PA alone, 8 had rt-PA followed by PTCA and 6 had rt-PA followed by CABG. The interval from chest pain to death ranged from 5 hours to 260 days (mean 15 ± 40, median 2.7 days). The acute infarcts were hemorrhagic by gross inspection (with histologic confirmation) in 23 patients, nonhemorrhagic in 20, not visible grossly in 2 and in 7 there was no acute necrosis by either gross or histologic examination. Three patients enrolled in phase I and phase I pilot of the TIMI study received rt-PA within 7 hours of onset of chest pain, but all remaining patients were treated within 4 hours with similar intervals from onset of chest pain to treatment between patients with hemorrhagic and nonhemorrhagic infarcts (3.0 ± 1.0 vs 2.9 ± 1.3; p = 0.68). There was a history of systemic hypertension before admission in 27 patients (52%) with similar frequencies in patients with hemorrhagic and nonhemorrhagic infarcts [11 (48%) vs 11 (55%); p = 0.64]. The hearts weighed 471 ± 91 g in men and 404 ± 89 g in women with similar heart weights by sex between patients with hemorrhagic and nonhemorrhagic infarcts (men 447 ± 68 vs 487 ± 101 g, p = 0.28; and women 394 ± 72 vs 428 ± 132 g, p = 0.49). The percentage of women was greater [13 (57%) vs 5 (25%); p = 0.04], and the peak creatine kinase was higher (5,535 ± 6,219 vs 2,248 ± 1,472; p = 0.047) in patients with hemorrhagic compared to nonhemorrhagic infarcts.

Complications contributory to death: Myocardial rupture (left ventricular free wall or ventricular septum) occurred in 12 (23%) of the 52 patients, cardiogenic shock in 23 (45%) of 51, fatal arrhythmias in 19 (37%) of 51 and fatal bleeding in 5 (10%) of 52. Comparisons of the 23 patients with hemorrhagic infarcts with the 20 with nonhemorrhagic infarcts showed similar frequen-

cies of myocardial rupture [6 (25%) of 23 vs 5 (25%) of 20], cardiogenic shock [10 (43%) of 23 vs 9 (47%) of 19; p = 0.80], fatal arrhythmias [8 (35%) of 23 vs 6 (32%) of 19; p = 0.83] and fatal hemorrhage [2 (9%) of 23 vs 2 (10%) of 20; p = 0.70] (Table I).

Location and quantitation of infarct size: Of the 43 patients in whom myocardial necrosis was confirmed by gross and histologic examination, 22 (51%) had anterior wall infarcts, 19 (44%) had posterior wall infarcts, 1 had an infarct confined to the lateral wall and 1 to the ventricular septum. The frequency of anterior wall and posterior wall infarcts was similar in patients with hemorrhagic and in those with nonhemorrhagic infarcts [anterior 12 (52%) vs 10 (50%); posterior 10 (43%) vs 9 (45%)]. Histologic examination of the 23 patients with hemorrhagic infarcts showed the interstitial hemorrhage, in every case, to be confined to, and not extend beyond, the area of necrosis.

Right ventricular infarcts occurred in 8 (19%) of the 43 patients with infarcts confirmed at necropsy. All were associated with infarcts of the posterior wall of the left ventricle, but there were fewer in patients with hemorrhagic than nonhemorrhagic infarcts (2 of 10 hemorrhagic posterior infarcts vs 6 of 9 nonhemorrhagic posterior infarcts). Healed (previous) left ventricular infarcts were found in 14 (27%) of the 52 patients with 6 (26%) being among the 23 with hemorrhagic acute infarcts and 3 (15%) among the 20 with nonhemorrhagic infarcts (p = 0.37).

Of 23 patients who survived ≥18 hours from the onset of chest pain, and in whom AMI was confirmed both grossly and histologically, myocardial necrosis involved a mean of 25 ± 11% of the left ventricular wall with no significant difference between hemorrhagic and nonhemorrhagic infarcts (26 ± 11% vs 23 ± 11%; p = 0.42). There was no significant difference in percent of left ventricular wall that was necrotic between patients with previous (healed) infarcts (8 of 24) and those in which the recent (first) event was the fatal infarct (16 of 24) (23 ± 11 vs 26 ± 11%; p = 0.56). Furthermore, when restricting the analysis to patients with hemorrhagic infarcts, there was also no significant difference in size of the acute infarcts between those with and without healed infarcts (26 ± 12 vs 27 ± 11%; p = 0.96). The frequency of healed infarcts among the 23 (of 51) patients with cardiogenic shock was also not significantly different from that of patients without healed infarcts [7 (50%) vs 16 (43%); p = 0.67].

Coronary thrombus: Coronary thrombi were found in the infarct-related artery at necropsy in 16 (32%) of 50 patients. The frequency was similar in patients with hemorrhagic and nonhemorrhagic infarcts [7 (32%) of 22 vs 7 (37%) of 19; p = 0.74] (Table I). Of these 16 patients with thrombi at necropsy, 2 (13%) were among the 15 patients who died within 24 hours of the onset of chest pain, 7 were among the 14 (50%) patients who died between 24 and 72 hours and 7 were among the 21 (33%) who died >72 hours after the onset of chest pain. Similar frequencies of thrombi were also found within each of the 3 intervals from chest pain to death between patients with hemorrhagic and nonhemorrhagic infarcts [0 to 24 hours, 1 (17%) of 6 patients vs 0 of 3, p = 0.49;

TABLE I Comparisons of Selected Clinical and Morphologic Features Between Patients with Hemorrhagic and Nonhemorrhagic

Case	Age (yrs), Sex	CP to rt-PA (min)	CP to Death (days)	Dose rt-PA (mg)	Hours rt-PA to Peak CK	PTCA	CABG	Peak CK (IU)	SH	CS	A	H (0 to 2+)
Hemorrhagic infarcts												
1	36, F	160	0.2	90	—	0	0	—	+	0	+	0
2	72, F	138	0.3	100	—	0	0	—	0	0	+	0
3	61, M	140	0.3	117	—	0	0	—	0	0	0	0
4	75, F	150	0.4	100	4	0	0	2,328	0	0	+	0
5	70, M	195	0.5	100	—	0	0	—	0	0	0	0
6	74, F	230	0.5	100	8	0	0	1,688	0	+	0	++
7	37, M	150	0.5	100	4	0	0	6,780	+	0	+	0
8	62, F	390	1	150	24	0	0	4,065	+	+	+	+
9	66, F	185	1	150	16	0	0	2,140	+	0	0	0
10	68, F	123	1	100	8	0	0	4,908	+	0	0	++
11	42, M	210	2	80	16	0	0	4,536	0	+	0	0
12	59, M	180	2	100	4	0	0	5,000	0	+	0	0
13	68, F	105	3	100	48	0	0	30,200	0	+	0	+
14	67, F	233	4	100	4	+	+	3,824	+	+	+	0
15	73, F	205	4	100	12	0	0	2,582	0	+	0	0
16	40, M	233	8	150	8	+	0	4,290	+	0	0	0
17	72, F	150	10	100	8	0	0	3,795	+	0	+	0
18	67, F	72	12	100	8	0	0	3,800	0	+	0	+
19	72, M	150	14	100	8	0	0	2,141	+	+	+	0
20	65, M	180	15	100	12	0	+	3,620	+	0	0	0
21	67, F	146	33	100	12	0	+	4,110	+	0	0	+
22	73, M	234	41	80	4	0	0	7,950	0	0	0	0
23	61, M	182	108	80	12	0	+	7,400	0	+	0	0
Total or Mean ± SD	63 ± 12 13 F (57%)	180 ± 63	11 ± 24	104 ± 20	12 ± 10	2	4	5,535 ± 6,219	11 (48%)	10 (43%)	8 (35%)	6 (26%)
Nonhemorrhagic infarcts												
24	50, M	89	0.2	83	—	0	0	—	+	+	0	0
25	69, M	115	0.3	60	—	0	0	—	0	0	0	0
26	45, M	185	0.3	87	—	0	0	—	0	0	+	0
27	62, M	77	1	100	12	0	0	999	0	+	+	+
28	59, M	225	1	85	—	0	0	—	+	+	0	0
29	62, M	240	1	100	24	0	0	2,704	+	+	0	0
30	75, M	230	2	150	36	0	0	2,838	+	+	0	0
31	47, F	140	2	100	12	0	0	5,005	0	0	+	0
32	65, F	66	2	80	6	0	+	610	+	+	0	0
33	51, M	210	2	100	30	+	0	1,242	0	0	0	0
34	67, M	150	3	100	12	0	0	687	0	0	0	++
35	59, M	227	4	80	6	0	0	1,385	0	+	+	0
36	63, F	375	5	100	8	0	0	1,905	+	+	0	0
37	49, M	105	6	100	12	+	0	1,730	0	0	+	0
38	57, M	215	7	100	8	+	0	2,400	+	+	0	+
39	67, M	90	8	100	16	0	0	1,844	+	0	+	+
40	63, F	161	17	80	22	0	+	1,400	0	0	0	0
41	67, M	120	21	150	8	0	0	2,976	+	0	0	++
42	71, F	233	25	150	36	0	0	6,000	+	0	0	+
43	65, M	175	40‡	100	8	0	0	2,240	+	—	—	+
Total or Mean ± SD	61 ± 8 5 F (25%)	171 ± 75	7 ± 10	100 ± 24	16 ± 10	3	2	2,248 ± 1,472	11 (55%)	9 (47%)	6 (32%)	7 (35%)

* Right ventricular necrosis, also; † blood in scar as well as in small amount of residual necrosis; ‡ transplant 40 days after onset of symptoms: patient still alive: infarct looks hemorrhagic but blood is in dilated vessels only; § those with fibrosis.

A = arrhythmia; AMI = acute myocardial infarction; CA = coronary artery; CABG = coronary artery bypass grafting; CK = creatine kinase; CP = chest pain; CS = cardiogenic shock; D = dilatation; H = hemorrhage (+ = major bleeding, ++ = fatal bleeding); HW = heart weight; IRA = infarct-related artery; LAD = left anterior descending coronary artery; LC = left

24 to 72 hours, 3 (50%) of 5 vs 4 (50%) of 8, p = 1.0; >72 hours, 3 (30%) of 10 vs 3 (38%) of 8, p = 0.74].

All thrombi in patients with hemorrhagic infarcts were nonocclusive, and all thrombi in patients with nonhemorrhagic infarcts were totally occlusive (p = 0.0002). The amounts of platelets, fibrin and erythrocytes appeared similar in the hemorrhagic and nonhemorrhagic groups, but the amount of leukocytes in thrombi of patients with hemorrhagic infarcts was less.

Luminal narrowing: By examination of 5-mm segments of the 4 major epicardial coronary arteries, 49 (98%) of the 50 patients had at least 1 major epicardial artery narrowed >75% in luminal cross-sectional area by atherosclerotic plaque alone. Five patients (10%) had only 1 vessel narrowed >75% in cross-sectional area by plaque, 13 (26%) had 2-vessel disease and 31 (62%) had

Acute Myocardial Infarcts

Rupture LVFW	Rupture VS	Location AMI at Necropsy	Healed AMI (Location)	HW (g)	LV Weight (g)	Percent LV Wall N	Percent LV Wall F	LV D	CA T	No. major CAS >75% by P	IRA	Total 5-mm S of IRA	PR	H in P
0	0	P	0	535	—	—	—	+	0	3	LC	19	0	+
0	0	A	+ (P)	350	—	—	—	++	0	3	LAD	16	0	0
0	+	P	0	405	—	—	—	+	0	3	R	15	+	+
+	0	A	0	375	—	—	—	0	—	—	—	—	—	—
+	0	A	0	570	—	—	—	+	0	1	LAD	27	+	+
0	0	A	0	295	—	—	—	0	0	1	LAD	12	+	+
0	0	P	0	350	—	—	—	0	+	3	R	19	+	0
0	0	P, VS	0	350	138	37	0	+	+	3	R	18	+	+
0	0	L	0	325	132	24	0	0	0	3	R	29	+	+
0	0	P*	0	360	138	25	0	0	+	3	R	19	+	+
0	0	P*	0	370	139	33	0	+	+	4	R	31	+	+
0	0	A	+ (P)	450	199	24	5	0	0	3	LAD	18	0	0
0	0	P	0	320	97	15	0	+	0	3	LC	9	+	+
+	0	A	0	420	146	15	0	0	+	2	LAD	19	+	+
+	0	P	+ (P)	405	139	16	13	0	0	3	R	21	0	+
0	0	P	0	465	227	17	0	+	0	2	R	12	+	+
0	0	A	+ (P)	430	195	19	8	+	0	3	LAD	26	0	+
0	+	A	0	480	—	—	—	0	+	1	LAD	14	+	+
0	0	A	0	455	151	48	0	+	+	3	LAD	23	0	+
0	0	P	0	450	169	18	0	0	0	3	R	16	+	+
0	0	A	+ (P)	480	141	26	10	0	0	2	LAD	15	0	0
0	0	A	0	415	121	33	0	0	0	1	LAD	10	0	0
0	0	A	+ (AP)	535	164	46	13	+	0	1	LAD	6	0	0
4 (17)%	2 (9%)	12 A (52%)	6 (26%)	418 ± 74 M = 447 ± 68	153 ± 33	26 ± 11	3 ± 5 / 10 ± 3§	11 (48%)	7 (32%)	14, 3 or 4 (61%)		394 (18 ± 6)	13 (59%)	15 (68%)
0	0	A	0	440	—	—	—	+	0	3	LAD	17	0	0
+	0	P	0	555	—	—	—	0	0	3	R	28	+	+
0	0	A	+ (P)	615	—	—	—	+	0	2	LAD	20	0	0
0	0	P*	0	465	—	—	—	0	0	2	R	25	+	+
0	0	A	+ (A)	490	197	20	5	+	0	3	LAD	17	+	+
0	0	P*	0	615	—	—	—	0	+	3	R	22	+	+
0	0	P	0	620	—	—	—	+	+	3	R	18	+	+
0	0	P*	0	350	143	31	0	0	+	2	R	21	+	+
0	0	VS	0	630	—	—	—	0	0	2	LAD	27	+	+
+	0	P*	0	610	249	38	0	0	+	2	R	24	+	+
+	0	P	+ (A)	445	181	10	5	0	0	3	R	27	+	+
0	0	P*	0	435	—	—	—	+	0	3	R	17	+	+
0	+	A	0	405	—	—	—	0	0	2	LAD	9	0	+
0	0	A	0	420	—	—	—	0	0	3	LAD	23	+	0
0	0	A	0	355	167	10	0	0	0	3	LAD	22	+	0
0	0	A	0	505	—	—	—	0	—	—	—	—	—	—
0	+	A	0	470	—	—	—	+	+	2	LAD	11	0	0
0	0	A	0	455	186	22	0	+	+	3	LAD	23	+	+
0	0	P*	0	285	109	14	0	0	0	0	R	18	+	+
0	0	A	0	280	144	35	0	++	+	3	LAD	20	+	+
3 (15%)	2 (10%)	10 A (50%)	3 (15%)	472 ± 109 M = 487 ± 101	172 ± 42	23 ± 11	1 ± 2 / 5 ± 0§	8 (40%)	7 (37%)	11, 3 or 4 (58%)		389 (20 ± 5)	15 (79%)	14 (74%)

circumflex coronary artery; LV = left ventricle; LVFW = left ventricular free wall; M = mean; N = necrosis; P = plaque; PM = postmortem; PR = plaque rupture; PTCA = percutaneous transluminal coronary angioplasty; R = right coronary artery; rt-PA = recombinant tissue plasminogen activator; S = segments; SD = standard deviation; SH = history of systemic hypertension; T = thrombus; VS = ventricular septum; + = present; 0 = absent; — = no information or not applicable.

3- or 4-vessel disease. The infarct-related arteries were narrowed >75% by plaque at some point in 44 (88%) of 50 patients. Comparisons between patients with hemorrhagic infarcts and those with nonhemorrhagic infarcts showed similar numbers with at least 1 major coronary artery narrowed >75% [22 (100%) of 22 vs 18 (95%) of 19] and similar numbers with 3 or 4 arteries narrowed >75% [14 (64%) of 23 vs 11 (58%) of 19; p = 0.71].

The number of infarct-related arteries narrowed >75% by plaque at some point was also similar between groups [21 (95%) of 22 vs 16 (84%) of 19]. Analysis of the 27 patients who received rt-PA without PTCA or CABG, and in whom AMI was confirmed at necropsy, showed no significant differences in degrees of cross-sectional area narrowing by atherosclerotic plaque alone between patients with hemorrhagic and nonhemorrha-

TABLE II Quantitative Histopathologic Comparisons of Coronary Luminal Narrowing and Plaque Composition of Patients Treated With rt-PA Without PTCA or CABG

| | | Numbers (%) Narrowed in CSA by Plaque | | | | | | Quantitation of Plaque (%)* | | | | | | | | | |
| | | | | | | | Mean | Acellular FT | | Cellular FT | | Calcium Deposits | | Pultaceous Debris | | | No. 5-mm S with |
Case	No. 5-mm Coronary S	0–25%	26–50%	51–75%	76–95%	96–100%	Coronary Score	All	>75%	All	>75%	All	>75%	All	>75%	M%† CSA N	Plaque Quantitation
		Hemorrhagic infarcts															
1	60	6 (10)	12 (20)	26 (43)	13 (22)	3 (5)	2.87	57	51	12	8	14	11	14	22	70	13
2	50	7 (14)	10 (20)	21 (42)	10 (20)	2 (4)	2.76	67	48	11	13	16	21	5	16	61	17
3	38	3 (8)	5 (13)	20 (51)	10 (26)	0 (0)	2.91	49	59	22	18	16	12	9	8	78	12
5	59	15 (25)	25 (42)	15 (25)	4 (7)	0 (0)	2.12	64	48	8	14	20	13	8	23	60	20
6	37	5 (14)	17 (46)	13 (35)	2 (5)	0 (0)	2.31	47	34	5	4	20	20	27	41	70	11
9	47	10 (21)	6 (13)	18 (38)	13 (28)	0 (0)	2.73	74	50	18	30	5	9	1	3	72	16
11	41	4 (10)	10 (24)	14 (34)	13 (32)	0 (0)	2.88	49	61	41	25	0	0	9	13	68	20
12	66	4 (6)	26 (39)	22 (33)	14 (21)	0 (0)	2.67	59	62	20	17	14	11	5	5	74	28
13	49	0 (0)	2 (4)	19 (39)	26 (53)	2 (4)	3.53	72	69	11	17	10	12	4	5	83	17
16	48	3 (6)	25 (52)	14 (29)	6 (13)	0 (0)	2.49	57	51	19	18	6	4	3	8	70	21
18	57	15 (26)	9 (16)	15 (26)	16 (28)	2 (4)	2.64	78	56	10	13	5	12	5	18	49	19
19	37	23 (62)	10 (27)	4 (11)	0 (0)	0 (0)	1.49	33	21	39	15	16	0	4	10	47	13
20	54	0 (0)	17 (30)	13 (23)	21 (38)	3 (5)	3.01	73	53	11	15	13	26	1	3	68	23
23	32	17 (53)	8 (25)	6 (19)	1 (3)	0 (0)	1.72	33	27	30	23	35	45	2	5	72	10
Subtotal	675	112	182	220	149	12											240
M ± SD		18 ± 19%	27 ± 14%	32 ± 11%	21 ± 15%	2 ± 2%	2.6 ± 5	58 ± 14%	49 ± 14%	18 ± 11%	16 ± 7%	14 ± 9%	14 ± 12%	7 ± 7%	13 ± 11%	67 ± 10%	17 ± 5
		Nonhemorrhagic infarcts															
25	46	12 (26)	10 (22)	16 (35)	8 (17)	0 (0)	2.43	87	42	1	5	5	30	6	22	46	13
27	48	9 (19)	13 (27)	10 (21)	14 (29)	2 (4)	2.68	75	48	9	13	12	22	1	16	68	8
28	43	1 (2)	12 (28)	22 (51)	8 (19)	0 (0)	2.87	81	58	11	24	0	0	5	12	69	23
29	44	6 (14)	17 (39)	6 (14)	12 (27)	3 (7)	2.70	73	74	4	6	5	17	17	13	79	14
30	50	2 (4)	13 (26)	23 (46)	12 (24)	0 (0)	2.90	51	46	4	2	28	20	15	29	75	18
31	40	1 (3)	10 (25)	23 (58)	6 (15)	0 (0)	2.87	60	49	18	4	6	7	15	37	65	19
32	46	9 (20)	17 (37)	10 (22)	10 (22)	0 (0)	2.48	70	65	14	13	1	1	12	17	76	20
35	57	4 (7)	8 (14)	24 (42)	20 (35)	1 (2)	3.09	48	42	4	1	38	45	9	12	74	22
36	43	7 (16)	13 (30)	14 (33)	8 (19)	1 (2)	2.59	70	63	12	0	4	10	13	26	65	16
37	32	9 (28)	6 (19)	13 (40)	4 (13)	0 (0)	2.38	34	53	49	11	9	20	8	15	60	15
42	48	2 (4)	8 (16)	19 (37)	14 (27)	5 (10)	2.95	65	57	8	3	14	25	11	14	72	16
43	35	6 (17)	16 (46)	13 (37)	0 (0)	0 (0)	2.20	77	62	15	3	5	16	2	18	62	17
44	53	0 (0)	6 (11)	24 (45)	21 (40)	2 (4)	3.33	36	36	14	16	46	45	3	3	78	15
Subtotal	585	68	149	217	137	14											216
M ± SD		12 ± 10%	26 ± 10%	37 ± 12%	22 ± 10%	2 ± 3%	2.7 ± 0.3	64 ± 17%	53 ± 11%	13 ± 12%	8 ± 7%	13 ± 15%	20 ± 14%	9 ± 5%	18 ± 9%	68 ± 9%	17 ± 4
		No AMI grossly, AMI histologically															
45	54	1 (2)	4 (7)	23 (43)	24 (44)	2 (4)	3.37	57	52	30	32	3	1	9	12	74	22
		No AMI grossly or histologically															
47	49	4 (8)	26 (53)	16 (33)	3 (6)	0 (0)	2.37	59	—	22	—	7	—	1	—	61	12
48	32	8 (25)	5 (16)	9 (28)	9 (28)	1 (3)	2.65	50	36	12	10	11	21	26	33	67	10
49	44	0 (0)	18 (41)	21 (48)	5 (11)	0 (0)	2.70	72	50	15	19	10	24	3	6	70	15
50	43	10 (23)	4 (9)	21 (49)	8 (19)	0 (0)	2.64	73	53	2	0	19	43	6	4	63	9
53	43	9 (21)	18 (42)	14 (33)	2 (4)	0 (0)	2.20	51	64	3	0	39	36	8	0	63	8
Subtotal	211	31	71	81	27	1											54
M ± SD		15 ± 11%	32 ± 19%	38 ± 10%	14 ± 10%	1 ± 1%	2.5 ± 0.2	61 ± 11%	51 ± 12%	11 ± 8%	7 ± 9%	17 ± 13%	31 ± 10%	9 ± 10%	11 ± 15%	65 ± 4%	
Totals	1,573	212	406	541	337	29											532
M ± SD		15 ± 14%	27 ± 13%	35 ± 11%	21 ± 13%	2 ± 3%	2.7 ± 0.4	61 ± 15%	51 ± 12%	15 ± 12%	12 ± 9%	14 ± 12%	18 ± 14%	8 ± 7%	15 ± 10%	68 ± 9%	

* Each number represents the mean percent (± standard deviation) of plaque area occupied by the 4 plaque components listed calculated for all 5-mm segments or just those segments narrowed >75% in luminal cross sectional area by plaque; † mean % of all 5-mm segments. Luminal narrowing calculated by planimetry.
CSA = cross-sectional area; FT = fibrous tissue; N = narrowing; other abbreviations as in Table I.

gic infarcts (Table II). The overall coronary score of luminal narrowing was similar between the 2 groups (2.6 ± 0.5 vs 2.7 ± 0.3; p = 0.39). The mean percent reduction in luminal cross-sectional area of the infarct-related coronary arteries by planimetric measurement of all 5-mm segments was also similar between the 2 groups (67 ± 10 vs 68 ± 9%; p = 0.77).

Plaque rupture: Of the 42 patients without PTCA, rupture of an atherosclerotic plaque was present at some point in the infarct-related artery in 26 (62%). Of these 26 patients with plaque rupture, 8 were among 14 patients (57%) in whom the interval from chest pain to death was <24 hours, 12 were among 13 (92%) who died between 24 and 72 hours and 6 were found in the

15 patients (40%) in whom the interval was >72 hours. The plaque rupture occurred at sites of pultaceous debris in all 26 of these patients and at 11 (85%) of the 13 sites of thrombi in patients without PTCA; it was associated with hemorrhage into the plaque in all cases. The frequency of plaque rupture was similar between patients with hemorrhagic and nonhemorrhagic infarcts [11 (55%) of 20 vs 12 (75%) of 16; p = 0.21]. When patients with CABG were excluded in addition to those with PTCA, the frequency of plaque rupture in the 2 groups still was similar [9 (56%) of 16 vs 11 (79%) of 14; p = 0.20].

Plaque hemorrhage: Hemorrhage into the atherosclerotic plaque was present at some point in the infarct-related artery in 30 (71%) of 42 patients who did not have PTCA, and it occurred at 14 (88%) of the 16 sites of thrombus formation. The frequency of plaque hemorrhage was similar in patients with and without hemorrhagic infarcts [13 (65%) of 20 vs 11 (81%) of 16; p = 0.28] even when patients with CABG were excluded as well [11 (69%) of 16 vs 12 (86%) of 14; p = 0.27].

Plaque composition: By planimetric analysis of all 5-mm segments of the infarct-related arteries of the 33 patients receiving rt-PA without PTCA or CABG, the mean percent reduction in luminal cross-sectional area by atherosclerotic plaque was 68 ± 9%. By analysis of all segments irrespective of the degree of luminal narrowing, the plaques consisted of acellular fibrous tissue (61 ± 15%, cellular fibrous tissue (15 ± 12%), calcific deposits (14 ± 12%) and lipid-rich pultaceous debris (amorphous, pale staining areas with abundant cholesterol clefts with or without erythrocytes and inflammatory cells) (8 ± 7%). However, the percents of plaque occupied by calcific deposits and pultaceous debris were significantly greater in sections narrowed >75% in cross-sectional area by plaque than those narrowed <75% (calcific deposits, 18 ± 14 vs 11 ± 13%; p = 0.002; pultaceous debris, 15 ± 10 vs 5 ± 7%; p = 0.0001), and the amount of acellular fibrous tissue was less (51 ± 12 vs 64 ± 20%; p = 0.0003). However, analysis of all 5-mm sections narrowed >75% showed no significant differences in mean percents of these plaque components between patients with hemorrhagic and nonhemorrhagic infarcts (pultaceous debris, 13 ± 11 vs 18 ± 9%, p = 0.18; calcific deposits, 14 ± 12 vs 20 ± 14%, p = 0.25; acellular fibrous tissue, 49 ± 14 vs 53 ± 11%, p = 0.39).

DISCUSSION

We studied at necropsy the hearts of 52 patients treated for AMI with rt-PA who died from 5 hours to 260 days after onset of chest pain. All but 3 patients received rt-PA within 4 hours of the onset of chest pain. The acute infarcts were hemorrhagic by gross inspection (with histologic confirmation) in 23, nonhemorrhagic in 20, not visible grossly in 2 and, in 7, there was no acute necrosis by either gross or histologic examination of multiple sections of the myocardium. In 4 of these 7 patients without acute infarcts, the interval from chest pain to death was <10 hours, which is often too early to detect the presence of necrosis by histologic examination. In the remaining 3, only healed infarcts were

found, and the interval from chest pain to death was 37, 62 and 260 days, which is often (certainly so in the latter 2 cases) sufficient time for the infarct to heal. Of the 8 patients who had PTCA after rt-PA, the infarcts were hemorrhagic in 2, nonhemorrhagic in 3, visible only histologically in 1, and not visible either grossly or histologically in 2. Of the 6 patients who had CABG after rt-PA, the infarcts were hemorrhagic in 4 and nonhemorrhagic in 2.

The frequency of hemorrhagic infarcts in patients with fatal AMI without mechanical revascularization or thrombolytic therapy is rare. Mathey et al[11] found no hemorrhagic infarcts on review of 195 patients, Waller et al[12] found 3 (2%) of 119, and Fujiwara et al[6] reported 2 cases (3%) of hemorrhagic infarction in 60 patients with fatal AMI without thrombolytic therapy.

The frequency of hemorrhagic infarcts in patients with fatal AMI treated with thrombolytic therapy is not well established due to the paucity of necropsy studies on such patients in general and on patients treated with rt-PA alone in particular. Fujiwara et al[6] found hemorrhagic infarcts in 15 (83%) of 18 patients treated with intracoronary urokinase surviving 15 hours to 11 days from the onset of the AMI, including 3 (of the 15) patients who had hemorrhagic infarcts with no evidence of recanalization during intracoronary infusion. Mathey et al[11] found hemorrhagic infarcts in 4 of 6 patients whose infarct-related arteries were recanalized by intracoronary streptokinase, and nonhemorrhagic infarcts in all of 5 patients in whom streptokinase failed. Richardson et al[13] found hemorrhagic infarcts in 6 of 8 patients treated with intravenous streptokinase with the infarct-related artery said to be patent in 4 of these 6. Waller et al[14] found hemorrhagic infarcts in 14 (74%) of 19 patients who were successfully recanalized by either streptokinase alone (9 patients), streptokinase with PTCA or guidewire manipulation (4 patients) or rt-PA with PTCA (1 patient). There were no comparisons with patients in whom thrombolytic therapy or mechanical manipulation was unsuccessful. Previous studies have, therefore, not established the frequency of hemorrhagic infarction among patients treated with rt-PA. In the present study of 43 patients receiving intravenous rt-PA during AMI, 23 (53%) had hemorrhagic infarcts, 20 had nonhemorrhagic infarcts and 9 could not be classified. When considering only those patients who received intravenous rt-PA alone (without PTCA or CABG), the frequency of hemorrhagic infarcts was still 53% (17 of 32).

There were no significant differences between patients with hemorrhagic and nonhemorrhagic infarction with respect to mean age, frequency of history of systemic hypertension, heart weight (by sex), interval from chest pain to rt-PA infusion, interval from chest pain to peak creatine kinase, interval from chest pain to death, location of the myocardial necrosis, frequency of left ventricular dilatation, frequency of myocardial rupture (left ventricular free wall or ventricular septum) or frequencies of cardiogenic shock, fatal arrhythmias or fatal bleeding.

The percent of women was greater among patients with hemorrhagic infarcts (57 vs 25%, p = 0.04). Califf et al[15] found a greater blood loss among women with AMI treated intravenously with rt-PA compared to men. We found also that the peak creatine kinase level was higher among patients with hemorrhagic compared to nonhemorrhagic infarcts (p = 0.047), which may be a reflection of the increased frequency of reperfusion in patients with hemorrhagic infarcts.

Rupture of the left ventricular free wall or ventricular septum occurred in 12 (23%) of the 52 patients. This does not exceed the range derived from necropsy studies of the frequency of rupture of the left ventricular free wall or ventricular septum published before the widespread use of cardiac care units (4 to 24%).[16] The percent reported here is, in addition, lower than the overall frequency of rupture (31%) reported for 648 patients with fatal AMI studied in this laboratory since 1968.[16] The frequency of rupture reported here is also similar to that reported among patients who participated in the ISAM trial[17] [10 (20%) of 49 cardiac deaths in streptokinase-treated group and 13 (21%) of 62 cardiac deaths in the placebo group]. We found the infarcts to be hemorrhagic in 6 patients with myocardial rupture, nonhemorrhagic in 5, and in 1, no infarct was visible grossly or histologically; thus, no increase in frequency of myocardial rupture was found among patients with hemorrhagic compared to nonhemorrhagic infarcts.

Of 23 patients who survived ≥18 hours from the onset of chest pain, myocardial necrosis involved a mean of 25 ± 11% of the left ventricular wall. This percent is similar to the size of infarcts reported in patients with fatal AMI who did not receive thrombolytic therapy.[18] This is not surprising since the patients who formed the present studies are those who died despite thrombolytic therapy. We found similar infarct sizes between patients with hemorrhagic and nonhemorrhagic infarcts. Furthermore, the interstitial hemorrhage was always confined to, and did not extend beyond, areas of necrosis. These results, therefore, support the suggestions that hemorrhage does not expand the infarct area.[4–6,19,20] They also suggest that the interstitial hemorrhage itself after rt-PA therapy does not increase the frequency of myocardial rupture or cardiogenic shock.

We found significantly fewer right ventricular infarcts in patients with hemorrhagic compared to nonhemorrhagic posterior infarcts. Right ventricular infarcts are virtually always associated with infarcts of the posterior left ventricular wall and adjacent posterior portion of the ventricular septum.[21] Whether the increased frequency of right ventricular infarcts in patients with nonhemorrhagic infarcts is a reflection of the lower frequency of successful reperfusion suggested to occur in patients with posterior wall infarcts[1] is uncertain.

Thrombi were found in the infarct-related artery at necropsy in 16 (32%) of 50 patients treated with rt-PA. This is lower than the reported frequency of coronary thrombi at necropsy in patients with fatal AMI who did not receive thrombolytic therapy [(60%)[9], (74%)[18]]. In addition, of the 16 thrombi, only 2 were in patients who died <24 hours after the onset of chest pain, while 7 were in patients who died between 24 and 72 hours, and

7 thrombi were in patients dying >72 hours. It must be emphasized that the percentages of coronary thrombi found in the present study at necropsy include an uncertain number of thrombotic reocclusions in initially reperfused arteries. There was no significant difference in infarct size between patients in whom a thrombus was found at necropsy and those in whom thrombi were not found. This is consistent with previous observations in patients with fatal AMI without thrombolytic therapy.[18]

The frequencies of thrombi were similar in patients with hemorrhagic and nonhemorrhagic infarcts. However, all thrombi remaining at necropsy in patients with hemorrhagic infarcts were nonocclusive and all thrombi in patients with nonhemorrhagic infarcts were totally occlusive (p = 0.0002). This finding supports the suggestion that vascular patency had been restored before death among patients with hemorrhagic infarcts.

By examination of 5-mm segments of all 4 major epicardial coronary arteries, we found that 49 of the 50 patients had at least 1 major epicardial coronary artery narrowed >75% at some point in cross-sectional area by atherosclerotic plaque alone, and that most of these had 3- or 4-vessel disease. This extensive amount of coronary artery disease is consistent with previous studies of patients with first fatal AMI without thrombolytic therapy.[9] Comparisons between patients with and without hemorrhagic infarcts also showed no qualitative or quantitative differences in luminal narrowing of the 4 major epicardial arteries or of the infarct-related arteries when analyzed separately.

Plaque rupture was found at some point in the infarct-related artery in 26 (62%) of 42 patients who did not have PTCA. It always occurred at sites of pultaceous debris in these patients, was seen at most sites of thrombi and was usually associated with hemorrhage into the plaque. These findings are consistent with the previous reports of association between plaque rupture, hemorrhage into a plaque and AMI in patients without thrombolytic therapy.[22–26] The association of plaque rupture with sites of extensive pultaceous debris formation has been emphasized by others.[26–28] The frequencies of plaque rupture or hemorrhage into the plaque were similar in patients with hemorrhagic and nonhemorrhagic infarcts. In addition, as emphasized by Chesebro and Fuster,[29] even after successful thrombolysis, plaque rupture, with the exposed thrombogenic stimuli such as collagen fibrils and pultaceous debris, remains a predisposing factor for thrombotic reocclusion. Of the 26 patients with plaque rupture, the majority were among those who died within 72 hours of onset of chest pain. However, 6 died >72 hours after chest pain, suggesting that plaque rupture cannot be excluded as a threat for reocclusion after this interval.

By planimetric analysis of all 5-mm coronary segments narrowed >75%, the percents of plaque occupied by acellular fibrous tissue, cellular fibrous tissue, calcific deposits and pultaceous debris were found to be similar to those of coronary artery plaques in patients with fatal AMI not receiving thrombolytic therapy.[30] By analysis of all 5-mm coronary segments, we also found similar percents of these plaque components in the infarct-related arteries between patients with hemorrhagic and those with nonhemorrhagic infarcts.

The present study shows that, although the frequency of hemorrhagic infarction increases after thrombolytic therapy with intravenous rt-PA, the hemorrhage does not appear to extend the infarct, and patients with hemorrhagic infarcts (compared to patients with nonhemorrhagic infarcts) have no greater frequency of myocardial rupture, cardiogenic shock or fatal hemorrhage, no differences in luminal narrowing, no difference in frequency of coronary thrombi, plaque rupture or hemorrhage into the plaque and no differences overall in plaque components. However, patients with hemorrhagic infarcts had fewer right ventricular infarcts and had only nonocclusive thrombi.

Acknowledgment: The authors gratefully acknowledge the technical assistance of Alvado M. Campbell, Richard M. Frederickson, Filippina M. Giacometti, Eutha E. Harrigan, Glen R. Longenecker, and Michael W. Spencer.

REFERENCES

1. Chesebro JH, Knatterud G, Roberts R, Borer J, Cohen LS, Dalen J, Dodge HT, Francis CK, Hillis D, Ludbrook P, Markis JE, Mueller H, Passamani ER, Powers ER, Rao AK, Robertson T, Ross A, Ryan TJ, Sobel BE, Willerson J, Williams DO, Zaret BL, Braunwald E. Thrombolysis in myocardial infarction (TIMI) trial, phase I: a comparison between intravenous tissue plasminogen activator and intravenous streptokinase: clinical findings through hospital discharge. *Circulation 1987;76:142–154.*

2. The TIMI Research Group. Immediate vs delayed catheterization and angioplasty following thrombolytic therapy for acute myocardial infarction: TIMI II A results. *JAMA 1988;260:2849–2858.*

3. The TIMI Study Group. Comparison of invasive and conservative strategies after treatment with intravenous tissue plasminogen activator in acute myocardial infarction. Results of the thrombolysis in myocardial infarction (TIMI) phase II trial. *N Engl J Med 1989;320:618–627.*

4. Fishbein MC, Y-Rit J, Lando U, Kanmatsuse K, Mercier JC, Ganz W. The relationship of vascular injury and myocardial hemorrhage to necrosis after reperfusion. *Circulation 1980;62:1274–1279.*

5. Kloner RA, Ellis SG, Lange R, Braunwald E. Studies of experimental coronary artery reperfusion. Effects of infarct size, myocardial function, biochemistry, ultrastructure and microvascular damage. *Circulation 1983;68(suppl I):I-8-I-15.*

6. Fujiwara H, Onodera T, Tanaka M, Fujiwara T, Wu D-J, Kawai C, Hamashima Y. A clinicopathologic study of patients with hemorrhagic myocardial infarction treated with selective coronary thrombolysis with urokinase. *Circulation 1986;73:749–757.*

7. Luna LG. Manual of Histological Staining Methods of the Armed Forces Institute of Pathology. Third edition. *New York: McGraw-Hill, 1968:8.*

8. Movat H. Demonstration of all connective tissue elements in a single section. *Arch Pathol Lab Med 1955;60:289–295.*

9. Brosius FC, Roberts WC. Comparison of degree and extent of coronary narrowing by atherosclerotic plaque in anterior and posterior transmural acute myocardial infarction. *Circulation 1981;64:715–722.*

10. Hook GR, Rasband W. Macmeasure: a low-cost, easy-to-operate quantitative morphometrics system for the Macintosh computer. In: Bailey GW, ed. Proceedings of the 45th Annual Meeting of the Electron Microscopy Society of America. *San Francisco: San Francisco Press, Inc. 1987:920–921.*

11. Mathey DG, Schofer J, Kuck K-H, Beil U, Kloppel G. Transmural, haemorrhagic myocardial infarction after intracoronary streptokinase: Clinical, angiographic and necropsy findings. *Br Heart J 1982;48:546–551.*

12. Waller BF. Pathology of new interventions in the treatment of coronary heart disease. *Curr Probl Cardiol 1986;11:666–760.*

13. Richardson SG, Callen D, Morton P, Murtagh JG, Scott ME, O'Keeffe DB. Pathological changes after intravenous streptokinase treatment in eight patients with acute myocardial infarction. *Br Heart J 1989;61:390–395.*

14. Waller BF, Rothbaum DA, Pinkerton CA, Cowley MJ, Linnemeier TJ, Orr C, Irons M, Helmuth RA, Wills ER, Aust C. Status of the myocardium and infarct-related coronary artery in 19 necropsy patients with acute recanalization using pharmacologic (streptokinase, r-tissue plasminogen activator), mechanical (percutaneous transluminal coronary angioplasty) or combined types of reperfusion therapy. *JACC 1987;9:785–801.*

15. Califf RM, O'Neil W, Stack RS, Aronson L, Mark DB, Mantell S, George BS, Candela RJ, Kereiakes DJ, Abbottsmith C, Topol EJ. Failure of simple clinical measurements to predict perfusion status after intravenous thrombolysis. *Ann Intern Med 1988;108:658–662.*

16. Reddy SG, Roberts WC. Frequency of rupture of the left ventricular free wall or ventricular septum among necropsy cases of fatal acute myocardial infarction since introduction of coronary care units. *Am J Cardiol 1989;63:906–911.*

17. The ISAM Study Group. A prospective trial of intravenous streptokinase in acute myocardial infarction (ISAM): mortality, morbidity and infarct size at 21 days. *N Engl J Med 1986;314:1465–1471.*

18. Saffitz JE, Fredrickson RC, Roberts WC. Relation of size of transmural acute myocardial infarct to mode of death, interval between infarction and death and frequency of coronary arterial thrombus. *Am J Cardiol 1986;57:1249–1254.*

19. Kloner RA, Alker KJ. The effect of streptokinase on intramyocardial hemorrhage, infarct size, and the no-reflow phenomenon during coronary reperfusion. *Circulation 1984;70:513–521.*

20. Higginson LAJ, Sheldrick KR, Temple SV, Beanlands DS. Intracoronary streptokinase; effects on reperfusion hemorrhage and regional myocardial blood flow in the anesthetized dog. *J Cardiovasc Pharmacol 1987;9:509–514.*

21. Isner JM, Roberts WC. Right ventricular infarction complicating left ventricular infarction secondary to coronary heart disease: frequency, location, associated findings and significance from analysis of 236 necropsy patients with acute or healed myocardial infarction. *Am J Cardiol 1978;42:885–894.*

22. Chapman I. Morphogenesis of occluding artery thrombosis. *Arch Pathol Lab Med 1965;80:256–261.*

23. Friedman M, Van Den Bovenkamp GJ. The pathogenesis of a coronary thrombus. *Am J Pathol 1966;48:19–31.*

24. Ridolfi RL, Hutchins GM. The relationship between coronary artery lesions and myocardial infarcts: ulceration of atherosclerotic plaques precipitating coronary thrombosis. *Am Heart J 1977;93:468–486.*

25. Horie T, Sekiguchi M, Hirosawa K. Coronary thrombosis in pathogenesis of acute myocardial infarction: Histopathological study of coronary arteries in 108 necropsied cases using serial section. *Br Heart J 1978;40:153–161.*

26. Falk E. Plaque rupture with severe pre-existing stenosis precipitating coronary thrombosis: Characteristics of coronary atherosclerotic plaques underlying fatal occlusive thrombi. *Br Heart J 1983;50:127–134.*

27. Tracy RE, Devaney K, Kissling G. Characteristics of the plaque under a coronary thrombus. *Virchows Arch (Pathol Anat) 1985;405:411–427.*

28. Davies MJ, Thomas AC. Plaque fissuring—the cause of acute myocardial infarction, sudden ischaemic death, and crescendo angina. *Br Heart J 1985;53:363–373.*

29. Chesebro JH, Fuster V. Antithrombotic therapy for acute myocardial infarction: mechanisms and prevention of deep venous, left ventricular, and coronary artery thromboembolism. *Circulation 1986;74(suppl III):1–10.*

30. Kragel AH, Reddy SG, Wittes JT, Roberts WC. Morphometric analysis of the composition of atherosclerotic plaques in the 4 major epicardial coronary arteries in acute myocardial infarction and in sudden coronary death. *Circulation 1989;80:1747–1756.*

APPENDIX
Submitting Medical Centers:

Baylor College of Medicine, Houston, Texas: Ben Taub General Hospital, Methodist Hospital and Houston Veterans Administration Hospital;

Boston University, Boston, Massachusetts: Boston University Hospital, Boston City Hospital and Norwood Hospital;

Brown University, Providence, Rhode Island: Rhode Island Hospital;

Columbia University, New York, New York: Columbia Presbyterian Medical Center and Harlem Hospital;

Cornell Medical Center, New York: New York Hospital;

George Washington University Hospital, Washington, DC;

Harvard University, Beth Israel Hospital, Boston;

Mayo Clinic and Foundation, Rochester, Minnesota;

University of Massachusetts Medical Center, Worcester;

Baystate Medical Center, Springfield;

Bridgeport Hospital, Bridgeport, Connecticut;

Maine Medical Center, Portland, Maine;

New York Medical College, Valhalla: United Hospital;

Northwestern University, Chicago, Illinois: Evanston Hospital;

University of Alabama at Birmingham, Birmingham, Alabama: Carraway Methodist Medical Center; and

Yeshiva University, Albert Einstein College of Medicine, New York: Montefiore Hospital, North Central Bronx Hospital, Englewood Hospital, New Rochelle Hospital and Nyack Hospital.

Rupture of the Left Ventricular Free Wall During Acute Myocardial Infarction Without Hemopericardium

William C. Roberts, MD

Rupture of the left ventricular free wall is a major complication of acute myocardial infarction, and it usually leads to hemopericardium with tamponade. During the last 16 years, 138 patients with left ventricular free wall rupture during acute myocardial infarction have been studied at necropsy in this laboratory [1,2]: 131 (95%) had associated hemopericardium with probable or definite tamponade and 7 (5%) had no blood in the pericardial sac. This report describes certain clinical and morphologic findings in these 7 patients without hemopericardium.

The 7 patients ranged in age from 46 to 93 years (mean 67); 4 were women and 3 were men; 6 were white and 1 was black (Table I). Two (nos. 5 and 7) had had angina pectoris before the fatal acute myocardial in-

From the Pathology Branch, National Heart, Lung, and Blood Institute, National Institutes of Health, Bethesda, Maryland 20892. Manuscript received November 29, 1989; revised manuscript received December 14, 1989, and accepted December 15.

farct. None of the 7 had had a previous acute myocardial infarction by history, and at necropsy none had a grossly visible left ventricular scar. The interval from onset of chest pain typical of acute myocardial infarction to death was <1 day in 3 patients, 2 days in 1, 4 days in 2, and 31 days in 1 patient. Before the fatal cardiac arrest, 2 patients (nos. 3 and 5) had dyspnea (at rest) and hypotension for ≥1 hour; 1 patient (no. 6) had prolonged hypotension, and the other 4 patients had neither dyspnea nor hypotension before the sudden fatal cardiac arrest. None of the 7 patients ever had pericardiocentesis. If cardiac resuscitative efforts were carried out, they were apparently of short duration. No patient had fractured ribs at necropsy.

At necropsy, the pericardial sac was devoid of blood in all 7 patients. Five patients had small amounts (<30 ml) of serous fluid in the pericardial sac; 1 patient (no. 3) had diffuse fibrinous deposits on the visceral and parietal pericardia, and 1 patient (no. 7) had diffuse pericar-

TABLE I Clinical and Necropsy Findings in 7 Patients With Rupture of the Left Ventricular Free Wall During Acute Myocardial Infarction Without Hemopericardium

Pt No.	Age (yrs), Sex	SH	AMI By ECG (Location)	Conduction Disturbance During AMI	Interval (days) AMI to Death	HW (g)	Necropsy Site of LV Rupture	No. CAs >75% ↓ by Plaque	Coronary Thrombus (Artery)
1	71, F	+	+ (A)	0	<1	430	Anterior	1	+ (LAD)
2	78, F	+	+ (P)	+ (CHB)	<1	360	Posterior	1	+ (R)
3	93, F	+	0	0	<1	550	Posterior	2	0
4	59, M	0	+ (A)	0	2	450	Anterior	3	+ (LAD)
5	46, F	0	—	+ (LBBB)	4	600	Posterior	1	0
6	59, M	0	0	0	4	550	Posterior	2	+ (R)
7	61, M	0	+ (A)	+ (LBBB)	31	580	Anterior	—	—

AMI = acute myocardial infarction; CA = coronary artery; CHB = complete heart block; ECG = electrocardiogram; HW = heart weight; LAD = left anterior descending; LBBB = left bundle branch block; LV = left ventricular; P = posterior; R = right; SH = systemic hypertension (by history); + = present; 0 = absent; — = no information available.

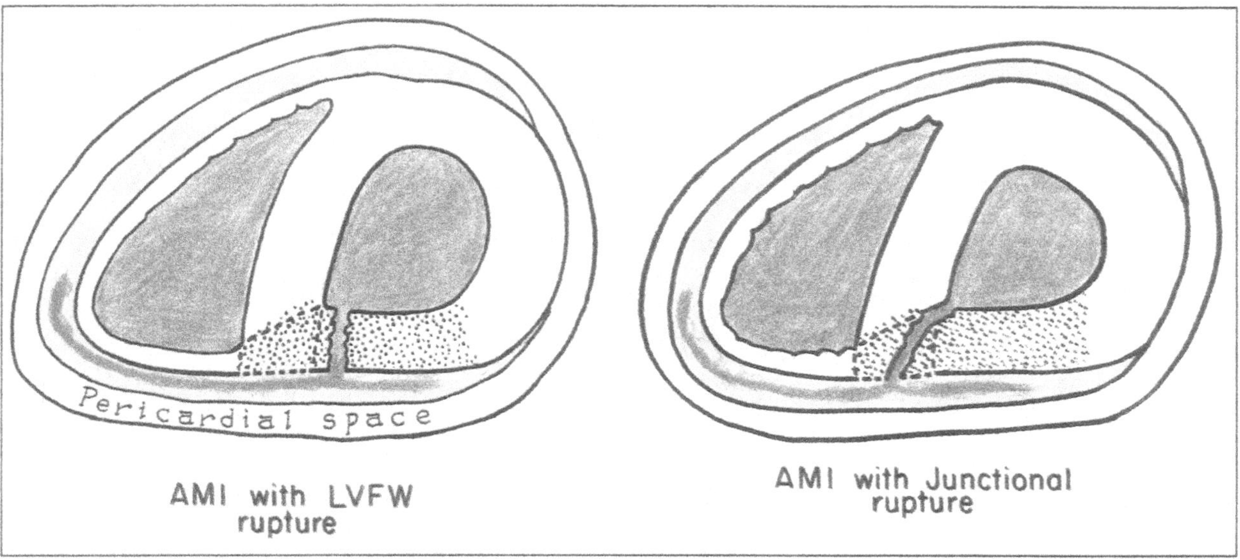

FIGURE 1. Diagram showing transverse sections of the cardiac ventricles with rupture of the left ventricular free wall (LVFW) (*left*) **or junctional portion of the ventricular septum** (*right*) **during acute myocardial infarction (AMI) into the epicardial adipose tissue without rupture into the pericardial sac.**

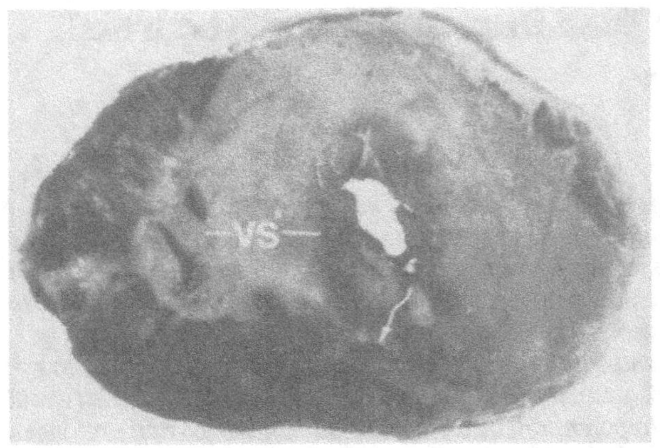

FIGURE 2. (Patient 3, Table I). Transverse section of cardiac ventricles showing a posterior wall acute myocardial infarct with rupture (*arrow*) into the epicardial adipose tissue but without rupture of the epicardium. VS = ventricular septum.

dial fibrous adhesions. The hearts in the 3 men weighed 527 ± 68 g, and in the 4 women, 485 ± 110 g. The left ventricular infarct involved the posterior wall in 4 patients and the anterior wall in 3. In all 7 patients the subepicardial adipose tissue was excessive (Figures 1 and 2). In all 7 patients blood had dissected into the subepicardial fat but no tears or rupture sites involving the epicardium were found. In addition to the left ventricular free wall rupture in all 7 patients, 2 patients (nos. 2 and 6) also had a partially ruptured posteromedial papillary muscle.

The 4 major epicardial coronary arteries were available for examination in 6 patients: a single artery was narrowed >75% in cross-sectional area by atherosclerotic plaque in 3 patients, 2 arteries were so narrowed in 2 patients, and 3 arteries in 1 patient. In 3 patients, each of the 4 major epicardial coronary arteries was divided into 5-mm segments and a histologic section was prepared and examined from each segment. Of the 113 segments studied, only 1 was narrowed >95% in cross-sectional area by plaque alone; 12 (11%) were narrowed 76 to 95%; 47 (42%) were narrowed 51 to 75%; 25 (22%), 26 to 50%, and 28 (25%), ≤25%. A thrombus was found in a major epicardial coronary artery in 4 patients.

The presence of fairly large deposits of blood (hematoma) in the subepicardial adipose tissue and a tear in the left ventricular myocardial wall in each of the aforementioned 7 patients indicate that a through-and-through rupture had occurred in the myocardial wall of the left ventricle. The absence of blood in the pericardial sac indicates that the epicardium had not ruptured. The result was a complete myocardial rupture and an incomplete epicardial rupture. In all 7 patients the amount of subepicardial adipose tissue was excessive. Had not a lot of fat covered portions of ventricular wall, the myocardial tear would likely have led to hemopericardium.

Despite the absence of hemopericardium, each of the 7 patients had clinical features consistent with a through-and-through rupture of both myocardium and epicardium with fatal hemopericardium and tamponade: 4 had sudden fatal cardiac arrest not preceded by shock or evidence of congestive heart failure and the other 3 had sudden cardiac arrest preceded by failure or hypotension.

To my knowledge, rupture through the entire thickness of the myocardial wall of left ventricle during acute myocardial infarction unassociated with either hemopericardium or false left ventricular aneurysm has been reported only once previously.[3] Edwards[3] described "subtotal" left ventricular free wall rupture in a 69-year-old woman who had severe valvular aortic stenosis and died 7 days after onset of acute myocardial infarction.

1. Mann JM, Roberts WC. Rupture of the left ventricular free wall during acute myocardial infarction: analysis of 138 necropsy patients and comparison with 50 necropsy patients with acute myocardial infarction without rupture. *Am J Cardiol* 1988;62:847–859.
2. Reddy SG, Roberts WC. Frequency of rupture of the left ventricular free wall or ventricular septum among necropsy cases of fatal acute myocardial infarction since introduction of coronary care units. *Am J Cardiol 1989;63:906–911.*
3. Edwards JE. An Atlas of Acquired Diseases of the Heart and Great Vessels. Volume II. Coronary Arterial Disease, Systemic Hypertension, Myocardiopathies, the Heart in Systemic Disease, and Cor Pulmonale, Acute and Chronic. *Philadelphia: WB Saunders, 1961:578.*

Coronary Artery Imaging With Intravascular High-Frequency Ultrasound

Benjamin N. Potkin, MD, Antonio L. Bartorelli, MD, James M. Gessert, BS,
Richard F. Neville, MD, Yaron Almagor, MD,
William C. Roberts, MD, and Martin B. Leon, MD

Safe and effective clinical application of new interventional therapies may require more precise imaging of atherosclerotic coronary arteries. To determine the reliability of catheter-based intravascular ultrasound as an imaging modality, a miniaturized prototype ultrasound system (1-mm transducer; center frequency, 25 MHz) was used to acquire two-dimensional, cross-sectional images in 21 human coronary arteries from 13 patients studied at necropsy who had moderate-to-severe atherosclerosis. Fifty-four atherosclerotic sites imaged by ultrasound were compared with formalin-fixed and fresh histological sections of the coronary arteries with a digital video planimetry system. Ultrasound and histological measurements correlated significantly (all $p<0.0001$) for coronary artery cross-sectional area ($r=0.94$), residual lumen cross-sectional area ($r=0.85$), percent cross-sectional area narrowing ($r=0.84$), and linear wall thickness (plaque and media) measured at 0°, 90°, 180°, and 270° ($r=0.92$). Moreover, ultrasound accurately predicted histological plaque composition in 96% of cases. Anatomic features of the coronary arteries that were easily discernible were the lumen-plaque and media-adventitia interfaces, very bright echoes casting acoustic shadows in calcified plaques, bright and homogeneous echoes in fibrous plaques, and relatively echo-lucent images in lipid-filled lesions. These data indicate that intravascular ultrasound provides accurate image characterization of the artery lumen and wall geometry as well as the presence, distribution, and histological type of atherosclerotic plaque. Thus, ultrasound imaging appears to have great potential application for enhanced diagnosis of coronary atherosclerosis and may serve to guide new catheter-based techniques in the treatment of coronary artery disease. (*Circulation* 1990;81:1575–1585)

Although coronary arteriography provides adequate imaging for routine diagnostic studies, more precise definition of lumen surface characteristics and identification of transmural components of atherosclerotic coronary arteries may be an important adjunct to standard angiography. Alternative imaging modalities may be especially useful for guidance during new experimental angioplasty procedures such as mechanical atherectomy, placement of expandable permanent stents, and laser angioplasty.

The potential value of ultrasound to characterize the morphological features of cardiovascular tissue has been extensively studied in recent years.[1-3] Ultrasound tissue characterization can detect the presence and severity of atherosclerotic lesions as well as differentiate normal from fatty, fibrous, and calcified regions within the vessel wall.[4-6] Transepicardial high-frequency ultrasound has been used intraoperatively to image coronary artery anatomic features.[7-9] In addition, recent studies suggest that catheter-based intraluminal ultrasound imaging provides similar high-resolution images of blood vessel wall architecture.[10-15] The present report is a feasibility and validation study comparing the capability of

See p 1715

quantitative histological findings with miniature intravascular high-frequency ultrasound to discern vessel wall geometry and structural composition of diseased necropsy coronary arteries.

Methods

Ultrasound Probe

Ultrasound images were obtained with a prototype intravascular imaging system (InterTherapy, Costa

From the Cardiology and Pathology Branches, National Heart, Lung, and Blood Institute, National Institutes of Health, Bethesda, Maryland.

Address for reprints: Martin B. Leon, MD, Cardiology Branch, National Heart, Lung, and Blood Institute, Building 10, Room 7B15, National Institutes of Health, Bethesda, MD 20892.

Received February 28, 1989; revision accepted January 17, 1990.

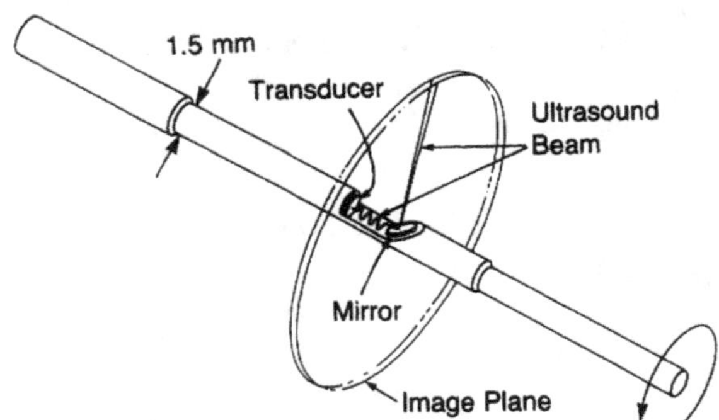

FIGURE 1. *Schematic diagram of the ultrasound probe. The 1-mm diameter transducer element (center frequency 25 MHz) is mounted in a rigid probe housing (outer diameter, 1.5 mm). The ultrasound beam is reflected perpendicular to the long axis of the probe by a mirror positioned at 45°. Two-dimensional, cross-sectional images of the coronary artery segments are created by manual rotation of the ultrasound probe inside the vessel lumen.*

Mesa, California). A 1-mm diameter transducer element (center frequency, 25 MHz), acting as transmitter and receiver, was mounted in a rigid probe (outer diameter, 1.5 mm) designed for in vitro imaging (Figure 1). With pulse-echo techniques, the ultrasound beam was reflected perpendicular to the long axis of the probe by a mirror, and planar two-dimensional images were formed in real time by manual circumferential rotation of the probe. The received A-mode echo signal was detected, sampled by an eight-bit analog-to-digital converter, converted by scan from a radial ultrasound data format to a rectangular format, and viewed as B-mode images on a 640×480–pixel grey scale video display. Image resolution was approximately 0.1 mm axially along the ultrasonic beam (i.e., perpendicular to the lumen long axis). The "slice thickness" and the lateral resolution of the ultrasound beam varied directly with distance from the probe and was approximately 0.4 mm for the 2–4-mm diameter vessels examined in this study. The image magnification factor could be selected in eight steps yielding image display scales from 3 to 32 mm in diameter. About 500 lines of echo data were used to form an ultrasound image.

Ultrasound and Histological Examination

A total of 32 coronary artery 1.5-cm segments were excised from 21 epicardial coronary arteries (three left main, eight left anterior descending, one left circumflex, seven right, one ramus intermedius, and one first diagonal) from 13 patients studied at necropsy (seven men and six women). The mean age at death was 64±17 years (range, 30–83 years). Five patients died from acute myocardial infarction, two from cardiogenic shock after coronary bypass graft surgery, and six from noncardiac causes (three sepsis, two neoplasia, and one stroke). Of the 32 coronary segments, 22 had been excised from heart specimens that were preserved in 10% formaldehyde, and the remaining 10 artery segments were excised from a fresh unfixed heart and later preserved with formaldehyde after the ultrasound scanning was performed.

Each of the 32 coronary artery segments was mounted vertically on a stage with cyanoacrylate ester glue applied to the distal end of the excised vessel. A 27-gauge stainless-steel needle was inserted transversely into the adventitia in 58 sites of the 32 mounted artery segments (Figure 2, bottom). The transverse needle served as a spatial marker to precisely identify the ultrasound imaging site that would later be examined by histological study. Each of the 32 mounted coronary segments was placed in a beaker of water (or 0.9% saline for the fresh unfixed specimens), and the ultrasound probe was advanced into the residual lumen with an X-Y-Z micropositioner (1.3 cm travel, 0.025 mm accuracy) until the needle marker was clearly imaged (Figure 2, top). Two potentiometers, placed around the probe, were used to define the position of the ultrasound transducer in relation to the artery segment. Manual rotation of the probe inside the artery resulted in a cross-sectional image of the artery wall at the needle marker site. The hard copy images were stored on a computer file for digital processing and subsequent analysis.

Of the 58 imaged sites, 14 (24%) were imaged before (fresh) and 5 days after fixation in 10% formaldehyde; the other 44 sites were imaged only in the formaldehyde-preserved state. After all the ultrasound images were obtained, each vessel segment with two needle markers ($n=26$) was cut transversely in two portions, 2–5 mm above and below the imaged site marked with the needle. Therefore, a total number of 58 coronary artery segments was obtained for histological processing. A 1.5-mm diameter stainless steel probe (the same size as the ultrasound probe and housing) was inserted into the residual lumen of any collapsed arteries to help maintain the geometric dimensions present when the vessel was imaged by the ultrasound probe. All 58 artery segments were then processed in alcohols and xylene; 24 segments had also required partial decalcification for 24 hours in a formic acid and sodium citrate solution to avoid crush artifacts during microtome sectioning. Care was used in preserving the spatial orientation of the vessel specimens when, before paraffin embedding, the needle marker was removed. Of the 58 artery segments, two had lost position markers in the tissue processing, and two were destroyed during the embedding process leaving 54 coronary segments for histological analysis. Each of the remaining 54 segments was serially sectioned (5 μm thick), and every 50th section was placed on a glass slide and stained with a Movat pentachrome stain to identify anatomic features of the intima, media, and adventitia.[16]

Quantitative Ultrasound and Histological Measurements

Ultrasound images and the corresponding histological sections were analyzed with a digital video analyzer (Magiscan, Nikon, Instrument Division,

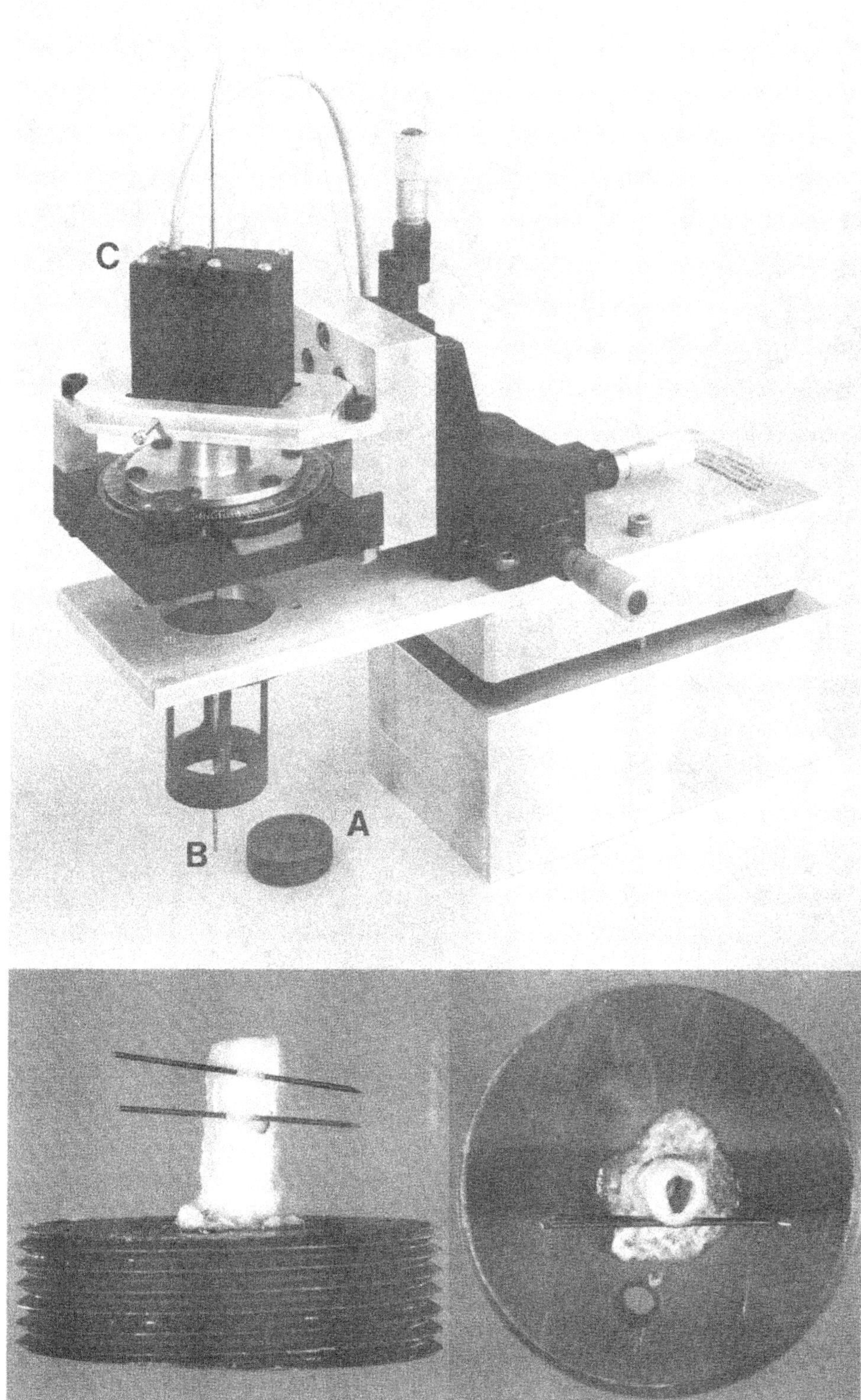

FIGURE 2. *Photograph of the apparatus for in vitro ultrasound imaging of the coronary arteries* (top panel). *The stage for mounting coronary segments (A), the ultrasound probe (B), and the positioning potentiometers (C) are shown. A proximal right coronary artery segment glued on the stage is shown in long axis (left) and short axis (right) view* (bottom panel). *Two 27-gauge needles were inserted as spatial markers, 0.75 cm apart from one another, within the adventitia.*

Garden City, New York). Each image was acquired by a television camera, linked to a light microscope (×10) for the histological specimen evaluation, and reproduced on the analyzer video screen where perimeters and linear dimensions were traced with a light pen. Areas (mm^2) and linear dimensions (mm)

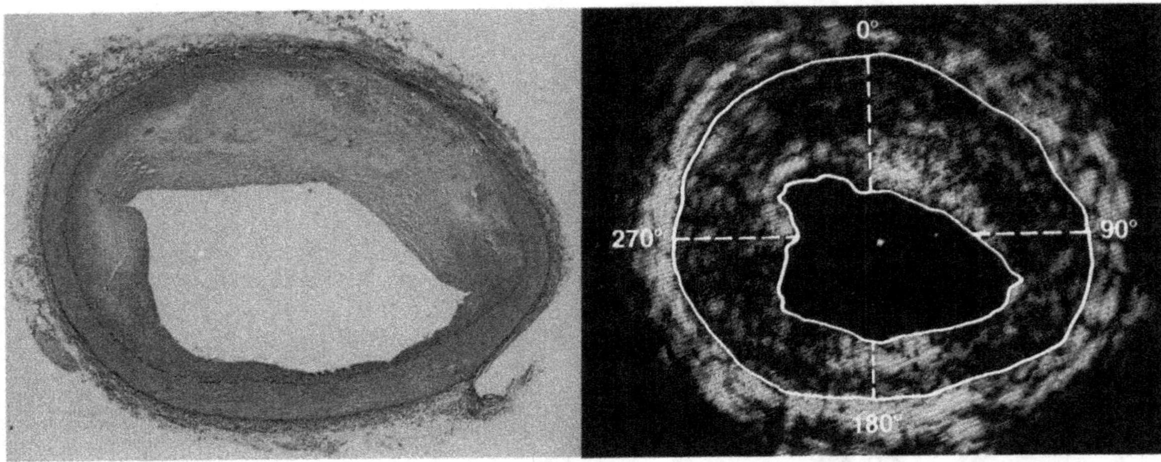

FIGURE 3. *Photomicrograph (×25) of histological section from the right coronary artery* (left panel) *and the corresponding ultrasound image* (right panel). *In the ultrasound image, the artery cross-sectional area is circumscribed by the outer circle, histologically corresponding to the external elastic membrane. The lumen cross-sectional area is enclosed by the inner circle. The four dashed radial lines define wall thickness (plaque and media) at 0°, 90°, 180°, and 270°.*

were then calculated by the computer from the tracings. Ultrasound cross-sectional area, which was representative of the coronary artery cross-sectional area (area confined within the external elastic membrane), and the residual lumen cross-sectional area were measured from the ultrasound images and compared with the corresponding histological areas (Figure 3). Linear dimensions of the wall (plaque and media) thickness at 0°, 90°, 180°, and 270° were also measured from the ultrasound images and histological sections (Figure 3). Percent cross-sectional area narrowing caused by atherosclerotic plaque was calculated from the equation: [(coronary artery CSA−residual lumen CSA)/coronary artery CSA]×100.

Tissue Characterization

Skills in interpretation of arterial wall structure and plaque composition were learned after repetitive comparisons between the first 54 ultrasound images and the corresponding histological specimens. Histological analysis of specimens indicated that all plaques contained variable amounts of fibrous tissue. Plaques with only fibrous constituents were classified as fibrous. Plaques with fibrous components and discrete areas of extracellular lipid material or calcific deposits were classified as lipid filled or calcified, respectively.

To test the predictive accuracy of ultrasound imaging for tissue characterization, 28 arterial segments excised from 12 additional coronary arteries (seven right coronary, two left anterior descending, one left circumflex, one patent ductus, and one left main) from four patients (two men and two women; mean age at death, 63±18 years) were studied. A total of 28 fresh coronary segments were imaged by ultrasound and then processed with the technique previously described. Plaque composition by ultrasound was determined by an investigator unaware of the histological classification in 112 quadrants obtained by

dividing each of the 28 ultrasound images into four equal quadrants. Ultrasound prediction was then compared with the histological analysis previously performed by a second investigator on the corresponding 112 histological quadrants.

Reproducibility

Intraobserver and interobserver variability of ultrasound and histological measurements was determined by remeasuring 26 of 54 coronary artery cross-sectional areas, lumen cross-sectional areas, and linear dimensions without knowledge of the original values. The second measurements were performed after 1 month by the original examiner and by a different observer.

Statistical Analysis

Correlations were determined by a linear regression analysis for two variables. The regression lines were compared with the line of identity (slope=1, y intercept=0) for each correlation to test the level of significance. Analysis of variance was used to test for significant differences among sample means and variances. A probability value less than 0.05 was considered significant.

Results

Arterial Wall Structure and Plaque Characterization

Ultrasound images of the coronary arteries were presented as a two-dimensional, 360° display of vessel cross-section perpendicular to the long axis of the probe. The typical image pattern consisted of three concentric layers around an echo-free lumen that could be clearly distinguished by sharp changes in ultrasound reflecting properties (Figures 4, 6, and 7). The ultrasound scanning provided an accurate description with high resolution of lumen structure and lumen-intima interface in all vessel specimens

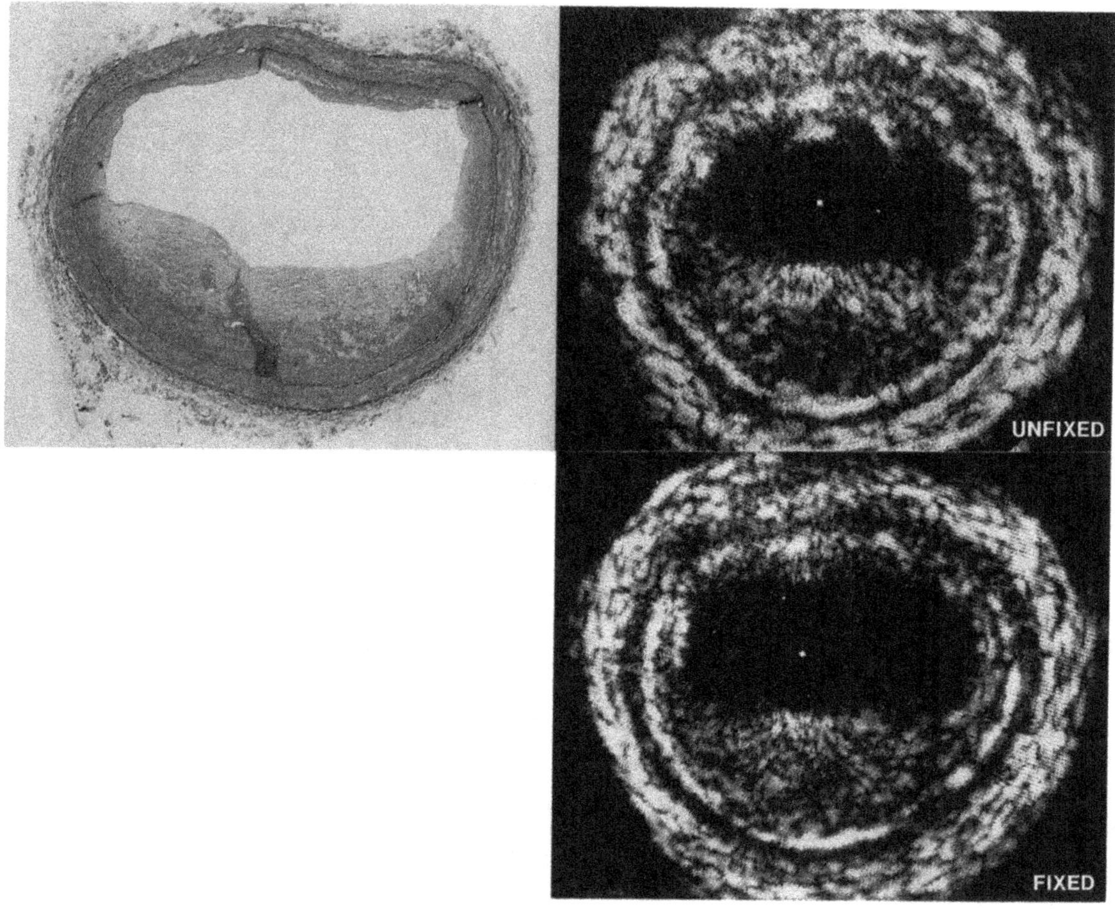

FIGURE 4. *Photomicrograph (×27) of a histological section from the right coronary artery* (left panel) *and the corresponding ultrasound images before* (center panel) *and 5 days after fixation with 10% formaldehyde* (right panel). *The ultrasound image shows a typical concentric three layer pattern consisting of plaque-intima, media, and adventitia. No significant qualitative or quantitative differences are discerned after tissue fixation.*

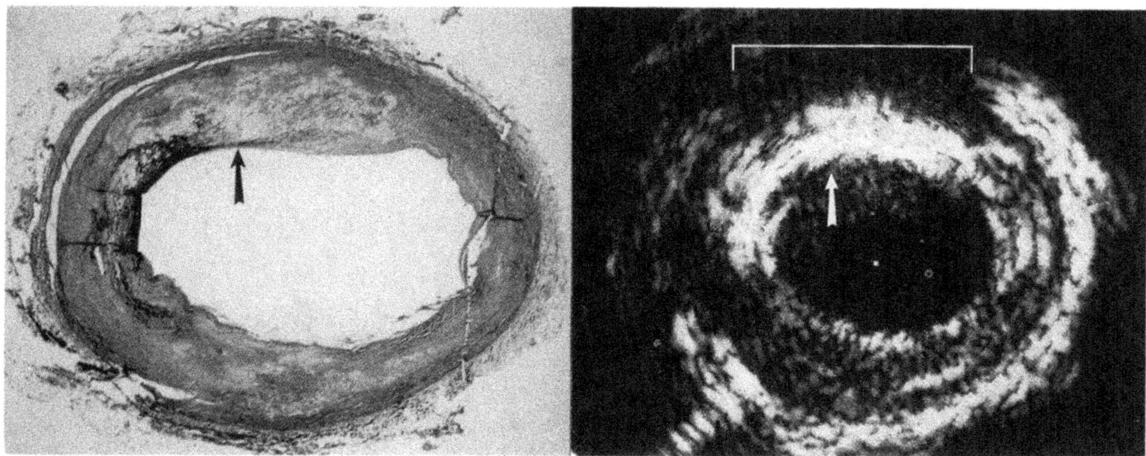

FIGURE 5. *Photomicrograph (×24) of a histological section from the left anterior descending coronary artery showing a calcified plaque (black arrow)* (left panel). *In the corresponding ultrasound image* (right panel), *the very bright echoes due to the calcium deposits (white arrow) and the acoustic shadow behind the calcium (bracket) are visible. Also shown in the ultrasound image are the echo reverberations from the needle marker inserted in the adventitia (at the seven o'clock position).*

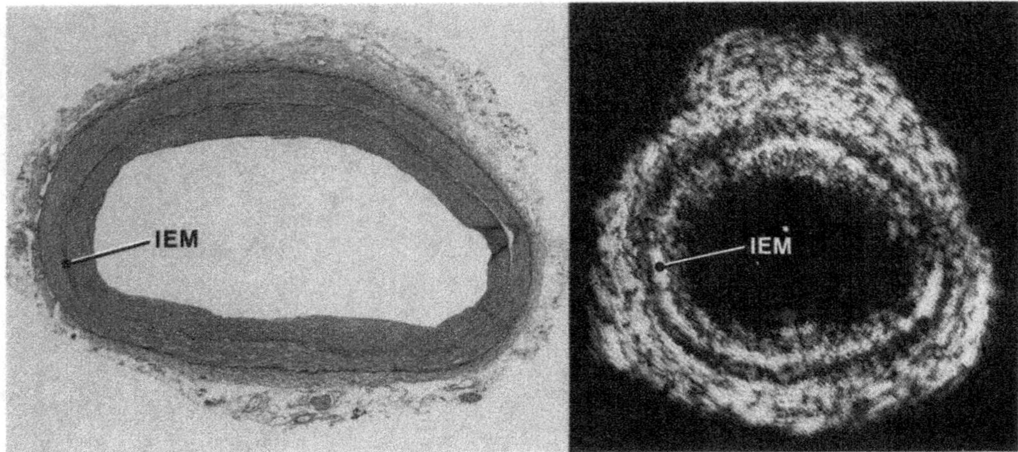

FIGURE 6. *Photomicrograph (×26) of a histological section from the left anterior descending coronary artery showing concentric mural thickening by a thin fibrous plaque* (left panel). *The bright and homogeneous echoes, characteristic of fibrous tissue, are shown in the corresponding ultrasound image* (right panel). *Also, the thin internal elastic membrane (IEM) is represented by a thicker echo-dense zone on the ultrasound image.*

(Figures 3–8). The tunica media was seen as an echo-lucent zone between the more intense echoes of the intima and adventitia laminae (Figures 4, 6, and 7). The junction between media and adventitia (external elastic membrane) could be identified in all 54 segments (Figures 3–8). However, the junction between intima and media (internal elastic membrane) could be clearly seen only in less-diseased coronary arteries that had minimal or moderate fibrous intimal thickening. In these arteries, the intima-media interface, corresponding histologically to the internal elastic membrane, appeared as a thin echo-dense layer (Figures 4, 6, and 7).

From comparative analyses between the first 54 ultrasound images and corresponding histological sections, plaque morphological subtypes were characterized. Plaques with calcific deposits were clearly identified by the presence of bright echoes casting echo-free shadows onto deeper tissue zones (Figure 5). Fibrous lesions yielded dense, homogeneous echo reflections without echo-free shadowing (Figures 4, 6, and 7), whereas extracellular lipid components were much less echogenic (Figure 8).

The histological analysis of the 112 quadrants obtained from the 28 additional arterial sections showed that 84 (75%) were composed of fibrous tissue, 19 (17%) were composed of calcific deposits, and nine (8%) were composed of lipid. Of the 84 fibrous plaque quadrants areas, 81 (96%) were correctly identified by ultrasound. In the three areas incorrectly diagnosed, the low echo density of the images, probably due to technical echo dropout, was erroneously interpreted as lipid deposits. Of the 19 calcific plaque quadrants areas, all were correctly identified by ultrasound. Of the nine lipid quadrants areas, seven (78%) were correctly identified by ultra-

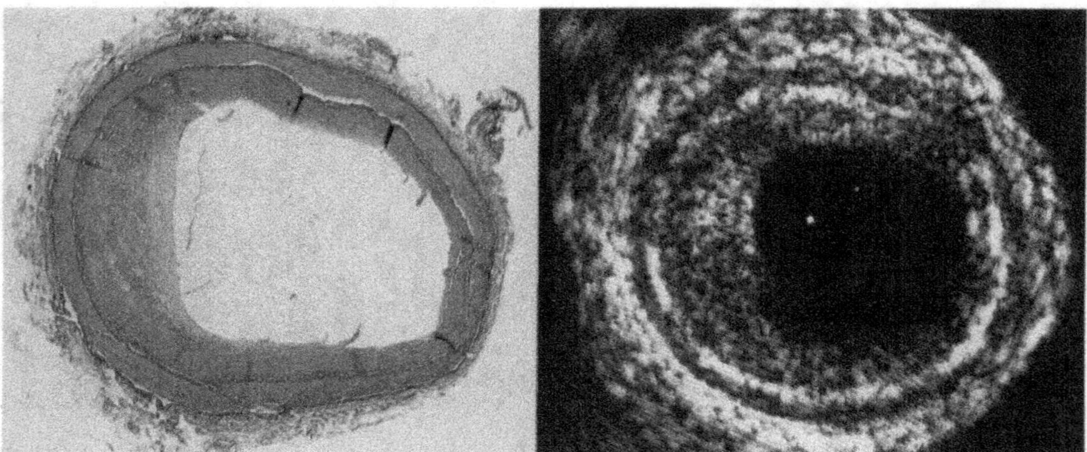

FIGURE 7. *Photomicrograph (×26) of a histological section from the right coronary artery showing an eccentric fibrous plaque* (left panel). *Bright and fairly homogeneous echoes are reflected by the fibrous tissue in the corresponding ultrasound image* (right panel).

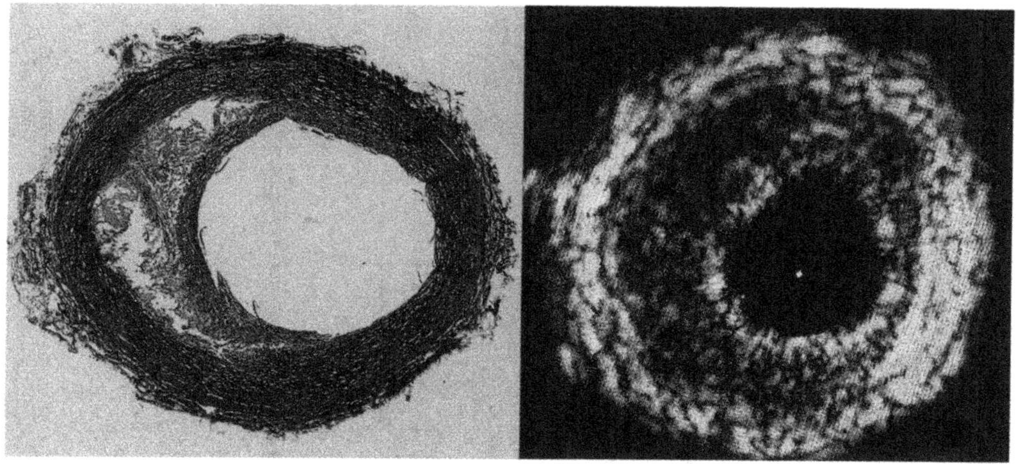

FIGURE 8. *Photomicrograph (×27) of a histological section from the right coronary artery showing a fatty plaque that is partially dissolved by tissue processing* (left panel). *The relative echo lucency of the lipid material is discernible in the corresponding ultrasound image* (right panel).

sound. The two (22%) areas incorrectly diagnosed were identified as fibrous plaque with echo dropout rather than lipid deposits. Thus, ultrasound accurately predicted histological plaque composition in 96% of quadrants analyzed.

Coronary Artery Cross-Sectional Area

The mean coronary artery cross-sectional area of the 54 coronary artery sites was 9.43 ± 3.70 mm^2 by ultrasound and 8.25 ± 3.18 mm^2 by histological analysis ($r=0.94$, $p=0.0001$) (Table 1, Figure 9A). The histological area was smaller than the corresponding ultrasound area in 43 of 54 segments (80%), and the average decrease was $10\pm13\%$.

Residual Lumen Cross-Sectional Area

The mean residual lumen cross-sectional area of the 54 coronary artery sites was 2.65 ± 1.19 mm^2 by ultrasound and 2.86 ± 0.90 mm^2 by histological analysis ($r=0.85$, $p=0.0001$) (Table 1, Figure 9B). The histological lumen area was equal to or larger than the corresponding ultrasound lumen area in 39 of 54 sites (72%), and the average increase was $18\pm36\%$.

Percent Narrowing of Cross-Sectional Area

The mean percent narrowing of cross-sectional area by plaque of the 54 coronary artery sites was $70\pm10\%$ by ultrasound and $63\pm11\%$ by histological analysis ($r=0.84$, $p=0.0001$) (Table 1, Figure 9C). The histological percent area narrowing was less than the corresponding ultrasound area narrowing in 48 of 54 sites (89%), and the average decrease was $11\pm9\%$.

Wall Thickness

The mean wall thickness (plaque and media) of the 54 coronary artery sites (216 measurements obtained at 0°, 90°, 180°, and 270°) was 0.75 ± 0.38 mm by ultrasound and 0.61 ± 0.36 mm by histological analysis ($r=0.92$, $p=0.0001$) (Table 2, Figure 9D). The histo-

logical wall thickness was less than the corresponding ultrasound wall thickness at 184 of 216 sites (85%), and the average decrease was $19\pm19\%$. An excellent correlation was also found when ultrasound and histological measurements performed at the four different locations were compared individually ($r=0.85$ at 0°, 0.91 at 90°, 0.94 at 180°, and 0.91 at 270°; $p=0.0001$ for each).

Intraobserver and Interobserver Variability

The mean percent difference between the initial and the second measurement by the same examiner for ultrasound images and histological sections, respectively, was $-0.5\pm5\%$ and $1\pm3\%$ for coronary artery cross-sectional area, $2\pm9\%$ and $2\pm2\%$ for residual lumen cross-sectional area, and $-3.6\pm18\%$ and $0.1\pm6\%$ for wall thickness. The mean percent difference between the two different observers for ultrasound images and histological sections, respectively, was $2.8\pm7\%$ and $0.2\pm1\%$ for coronary artery cross-sectional area, $1.8\pm15\%$ and $-2\pm9\%$ for residual lumen cross-sectional area, and $12\pm15\%$ and $-0.9\pm12\%$ for wall thickness.

Effect of Formaldehyde Fixation and Tissue Processing

In 14 arterial sites from 10 coronary segments, no significant qualitative or quantitative differences were noted when imaging of fresh specimens was repeated after 5 days of fixation with 10% formaldehyde (Figure 4). The mean percent difference between the fresh and fixed coronary artery measurements, respectively, was $4\pm6\%$ for coronary artery cross-sectional area, $2\pm10\%$ for residual lumen cross-sectional area, and $1\pm13\%$ for wall thickness.

On the other hand, analysis of the first 54 arterial sites indicated that tissue processing after fixation elicited important systematic changes in vessel wall dimensions. The histological cross-sectional area and

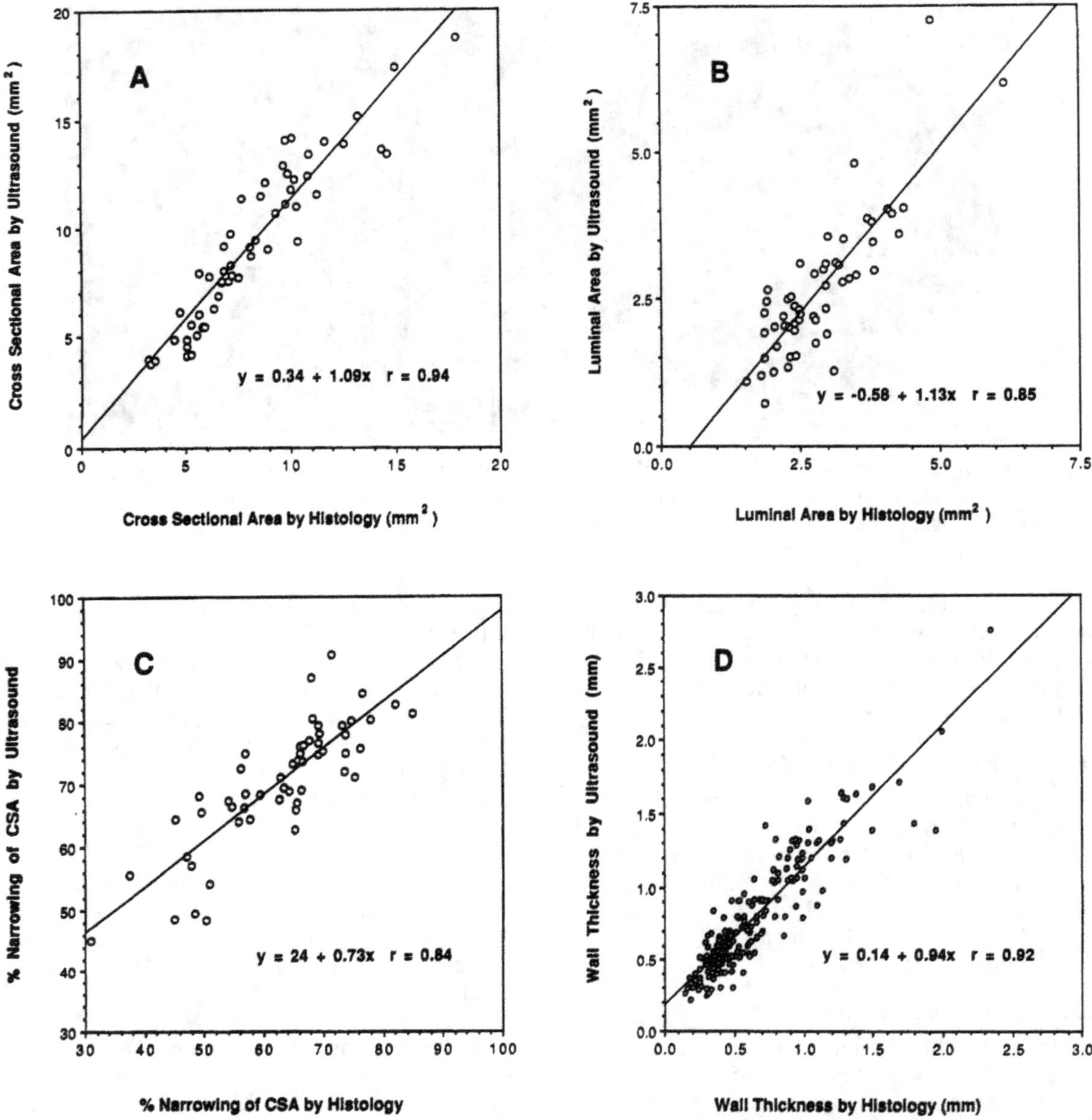

FIGURE 9. *Linear regression plots of the ultrasound and histological measurements of coronary artery cross-sectional area, luminal cross-sectional area, percent narrowing of cross-sectional area, and wall thickness. Correlation coefficients and regression lines are shown. CSA, cross-sectional area.*

wall thickness were reduced after tissue processing an average of 10% ($p<0.001$) and 19% ($p<0.001$), respectively, compared with the ultrasound images. In contrast, lumen cross-sectional area was 18% larger than the ultrasound areas ($p<0.05$).

Discussion

Contrast angiography of coronary arteries is currently the standard technique for in vivo quantification of the presence and severity of coronary atherosclerosis. However, several studies have provided anatomic and physiological evidence that angiography consistently underestimates the severity of coronary atherosclerosis.[17–19] These findings result from the inaccuracy of visual interpretation based on axial contrast angiograms. Angiography estimates coronary diameter narrowing as the difference between markedly narrowed and adjacent less narrowed sites without considering the absolute lumen size or the true cross-sectional area of the vessel. In addition, there is evidence that atherosclerosis is associated with vessel wall dilatation, and therefore, even in diffusely diseased arteries, the residual lumen diameter may appear angiographically normal.[20,21] These important limitations suggest that standard angiography does not provide a reliable quantitative assessment of coronary atherosclerosis and is grossly inadequate for evaluating vessel wall structure. Thus, new imaging modalities with the capacity for enhanced analysis of coronary atherosclerosis may provide valuable diagnostic and pathological insights and could be used for real-

TABLE 1. Coronary Artery Cross-Sectional Area, Residual Lumen Cross-Sectional Area, and Percent Cross-Sectional Area Narrowing by Ultrasound and Histological Analysis in 54 Coronary Artery Sites

	Cross-sectional area		
	Coronary	Lumen	% Narrowing
Ultrasound			
Mean	9.43±3.70	2.65±1.19	70±10
Range	3.77–18.71	0.71–7.24	45–91
Histological			
Mean	8.25±3.18	2.86±0.90	63±11
Range	3.20–17.95	1.53–6.17	31–85
Correlation (ultrasound vs. histological)			
r	0.94	0.85	0.84
p	0.0001	0.0001	0.0001
Histological<ultrasound (n, %)	43, 80	15, 28	48, 89
Histological≥ultrasound (n, %)	11, 20	39, 72	6, 11
% Difference*			
Mean	−10±13	18±36	−11±9
Range	−33 to +26	−33 to +161	−33 to +6

All areas are cross-sectional measured in millimeters squared.
*% Difference=[(histological−ultrasound)/ultrasound]×100.

time guidance of new catheter-based therapeutic intracoronary devices.

Ultrasound Plaque Geometrical and Morphological Features

In this in vitro study, a new intravascular ultrasound imaging system was used to create high-resolution, two-dimensional, cross-sectional images of human atherosclerotic coronary arteries that were quantitatively and qualitatively compared with corresponding histological specimens. Significant correlations were found between the ultrasound and histological paired measurements of coronary artery cross-sectional area, residual lumen cross-sectional area, percent cross-sectional area narrowing by atherosclerotic plaque and linear wall thickness dimensions (Figure 9). In addition to these significant morphometric correlations, ultrasound images accurately predicted the plaque distribution and its histological composition in most of the examined sites.

Heavily calcified lesions were characterized by bright echoes and a significant acoustic "shadow." Calcium salts, having the highest acoustic impedance among biological materials,[22,23] behave as total reflectors, and preclude ultrasound interrogation of deeper structures. This results in an echo-free space behind the calcified lesion. Thus, calcified coronary

TABLE 2. Wall Thickness (Intima and Media) at 0°, 90°, 180°, and 270° by Ultrasound and Histological Analysis in 54 Coronary Artery Sites

	0°	90°	180°	270°	Sum of all sites
Sites (n)	54	54	54	54	216
Ultrasound					
Mean	0.64±0.24	0.78±0.38	0.87±0.49	0.72±0.36	0.75±0.38
Range	0.24–1.33	0.29–1.71	0.26–2.76	0.21–1.60	0.21–2.76
Histological analysis					
Mean	0.49±0.21	0.68±0.40	0.71±0.45	0.57±0.31	0.61±0.36
Range	0.19–1.27	0.16–1.95	0.15–2.35	0.19–1.50	0.15±2.35
Correlation (ultrasound vs. histological)					
r	0.85	0.91	0.94	0.91	0.92
p	0.0001	0.0001	0.0001	0.0001	0.0001
Histological<ultrasound (n, %)	49, 91	49, 76	47, 87	47, 87	184, 85
Histological≥ultrasound (n, %)	5, 9	13, 24	7, 13	7, 13	32, 15
% Difference*					
Mean	−23±17	−15±21	−18±20	−20±18	−19±19
Range	−58 to +25	−51 to +40	−54 to +63	−53 to +33	−58 to +63

Plaque thickness measured in millimeters.
*% Difference=[(histological−ultrasound)/ultrasound]×100.

plaques, though easily identified by ultrasound, impair quantitative analysis of circumferential and linear dimensions of the vessel wall.

Bright and homogeneous ultrasound reflections were also seen in lesions characterized histologically by fibrous tissue accumulation. Experimental and clinical studies have demonstrated that ultrasound properties of fibrous tissue are related to a high concentration of collagen, which has been shown to possess high acoustic reflectivity.[24–27] However, because fibrous tissue has lower density than calcium deposits, and therefore less acoustic impedance, fibrous plaques do not manifest shadow artifacts and are less echo dense. Unlike calcified and fibrotic lesions, lipid deposition within the plaque was more difficult to identify by ultrasound techniques. Although lipid-filled areas have relatively less echo density than other plaque components, the ultrasound appearance of lipid lesions was variable depending largely on the presence and magnitude of surrounding fibrous tissue.

These findings are consistent with previous in vitro studies identifying the predominant constituents of atherosclerotic plaque, with quantitative ultrasound indexes based on attenuation or backscatter.[4,5] These studies also demonstrated a significant increase in integrated backscatter and attenuation in calcified and fibrotic regions of human aorta; in contrast, ultrasound interrogation of lipid deposits demonstrated a reduction in both these indexes.

A constant ultrasound feature in our images was the presence of prominent lumen-intima and media-adventitia interfaces that were separated by reduced echo signals from the media. These observations have been previously reported in vitro[28,29] and in vivo[30] in normal and diseased human arteries, and this distinctive pattern appears to be caused by relatively sharp changes in acoustic impedance at these interfaces. The increased echo density of adventitia, compared with the relatively silent acoustic behavior of media, may be related either to multiple impedance mismatches from inhomogeneous loose connective tissue or to the scattering effect of collagen whose content is increased in the adventitia. In vessels with mild-to-moderate atherosclerotic disease, there was also a thin echo-dense layer at the intima-media interface corresponding histologically to the internal elastic membrane. Previous reports, based on ultrasound imaging and backscatter,[11,28] have suggested that the thin elastic membranes, present within the media and oriented perpendicular to the ultrasound beam axis, result in multiple specular scattering and therefore, despite their thinness, are seen as bright reflecting structures. The external elastic membrane is less well seen as a discrete layer because of its proximity to more echo-dense adventitial structures.

Effect of Tissue Fixation and Processing

The influences of formaldehyde fixation on the ultrasound properties of coronary arteries were qualitatively and quantitatively minor, which is in agreement with the findings of other investigators examining fixation effects in vascular[22] and nonvascular tissues.[31]

Of importance, significant changes of vessel geometric features were seen after tissue processing. Tissue processing (dehydration with alcohols, cleaning with xylene, and embedding in paraffin) is known to cause significant shrinkage artifacts.[32,33] Siegel and colleagues[34] compared measurements in 61 human coronary artery segments before and after fixation and tissue processing. Although no significant changes were observed after fixation, tissue processing resulted in a 19% decrease in coronary artery cross-sectional area in 29 sites with less than 50% cross-sectional area narrowing and a 31% decrease in 32 sites with more than 50% cross-sectional area narrowing. Those findings are in agreement with the present study, in which histological cross-sectional area and wall thickness measurements of necropsy coronary arteries after tissue processing were reduced an average of 10% and 19%, respectively, compared with the ultrasound images. Plaque composition probably contributes greatly to the degree of shrinkage with tissue processing. In this study, although not statistically significant, the linear dimensions and vessel cross-sectional area of fibrous and fatty plaques manifested increased shrinkage after tissue processing compared with plaques containing large calcific deposits. These differences are probably due to variations in plaque water content that are directly proportional to the degree of tissue shrinkage during processing.

Unlike the coronary artery cross-sectional area and the wall thickness, the histological residual lumen cross-sectional areas of the 54 coronary sites were 18% larger than the corresponding ultrasound values. This may be explained by the much more pronounced shrinkage of the vascular tissue in the radial direction (18.7%) compared with that in the circumferential direction (0.9%), after fixation and processing, resulting in a larger residual lumen cross-sectional area of the histological sections. These anisotropic shrinkage changes had important artifactual effects on the calculated histological percent narrowing of cross-sectional area, which was 11% less than that determined from the corresponding ultrasound images. Thus, inhomogeneous tissue shrinkage during processing of diseased coronary arteries causes an unpredictable underestimation of percent narrowing of cross-sectional area measured from histological sections. Although additional corroborative studies are needed, our data suggest that quantitative ultrasound imaging of atherosclerotic coronaries may more accurately represent true vessel wall geometric features and disease severity than previous histological techniques.

Conclusion

This study demonstrates that intracoronary ultrasound imaging with a 25-MHz transducer of necropsy human coronary arteries can precisely determine coronary artery cross-sectional area, percent cross-sectional area narrowing by atherosclerotic plaque, and wall thickness. Ultrasound characterization of plaque composition is feasible and may provide important new perspectives on anatomic features of coronary artery disease.

Future studies are necessary to determine the feasibility and the clinical application of catheter-based intra-arterial ultrasound. Compared with an in vitro setting, where optimal coaxial position can be achieved by accurate probe manipulation, in vivo imaging inside a pulsatile artery presents new challenges. Technical improvements will be required to develop flexible and steerable miniature ultrasound probes capable of precise imaging within pulsatile tortuous coronary vessels overlying a beating heart.

Acknowledgments

We thank Richard Fredrickson for preparation of the artwork and Filippina Giacometti for histological processing. We deeply appreciated the cooperation and assistance from the dedicated scientists and engineers of InterTherapy, Inc, Costa Mesa, California.

References

1. Mimbs JW, Yuhas DE, Miller JG, Weiss AN, Sobel BE: Detection of myocardial infarction in vitro based on altered attenuation of ultrasound. *Circ Res* 1977;41:192–198

2. Mimbs JW, Bauwens D, Cohen RD, O'Donnell M, Miller JG, Sobel BE: Effect of myocardial ischemia on quantitative ultrasonic backscatter and identification of responsible determinants. *Circ Res* 1981;49:89–96

3. Mimbs JW, O'Donnell M, Miller JG, Sobel BE: Detection of cardiomyopathic changes induced by doxorubicin based on quantitative analysis of ultrasonic backscatter. *Am J Cardiol* 1981;47:1056–1060

4. Picano E, Landini L, Distante A, Sarnelli R, Benassi A, L'Abbate A: Different degrees of atherosclerosis detected by backscattered ultrasound: An in vitro study on fixed human aortic walls. *J Clin Ultrasound* 1983;11:375–379

5. Picano E, Landini L, Lattanzi F, Mazzarisi A, Sarnelli R, Distante A, Benassi A, L'Abbate A: The use of frequency histograms of ultrasonic backscatter for detection of atherosclerosis in vitro. *Circulation* 1986;74:1093–1098

6. Barzilai B, Saffitz JE, Miller JG, Sobel BE: Quantitative ultrasonic characterization of the nature of atherosclerotic plaques in human aorta. *Circ Res* 1987;60:459–463

7. Sahn DJ, Barratt-Boyes BG, Graham K, Kerr A, Roche A, Hill D, Brandt PWT, Copeland JG, Mammana R, Temkin LP, Glenn W: Ultrasonic imaging of the coronary arteries in open-chest humans: Evaluation of coronary atherosclerotic lesions during cardiac surgery. *Circulation* 1982;66:1034–1044

8. Sahn DJ, Copeland JG, Temkin LP, Wirt DP, Mammana R, Glenn W: Anatomic-ultrasound correlations for intraoperative open chest imaging of coronary artery atherosclerotic lesions in human beings. *J Am Coll Cardiol* 1984;3:1169–1177

9. McPherson DD, Hiratzka LF, Lamberth WC, Brandt B, Hunt M, Kieso RA, Marcus ML, Kerber RE: Delineation of the extent of coronary atherosclerosis by high-frequency epicardial echocardiography. *N Engl J Med* 1987;316:304–309

10. Pandian NG, Kreis A, Brockway B, Isner JM, Sacharoff A, Boleza E, Caro R, Muller D: Ultrasound angioscopy: Real-time, two-dimensional, intraluminal ultrasound imaging of blood vessels. *Am J Cardiol* 1988;62:493–494

11. Meyer CR, Chiang EH, Fechner KP, Fitting DW, Williams DM, Buda AJ: Feasibility of high-resolution, intravascular ultrasonic imaging catheters. *Radiology* 1988;168:113–116

12. Gussenhoven EJ, Essed CE, Lancee CT, Mastik F, Frietman P, Van Egmond FC, Reiber J, Bosch H, Van Hurk H, Roelandt J, Bom N: Arterial wall characteristics determined by intravascular ultrasound imaging: An in vitro study. *J Am Coll Cardiol* 1989;14:947–52

13. Mallery JA, Griffith J, Gessert J, Morcos NC, Tobis JM, Henry WL: Intravascular ultrasound imaging catheter assessment of normal and atherosclerotic arterial wall thickness (abstract). *J Am Coll Cardiol* 1988;2:22A

14. Yock PG, Linker DT, Thapliyal HV, Arenson JW, Samstad S, Saether O, Angelsen AJ: Real-time, two-dimensional catheter ultrasound: A new technique for high-resolution intravascular imaging (abstract). *Circulation* 1988;78(suppl II):II-21

15. Hodgson JM, Eberle MJ, Savakus AD: Validation of a new real time percutaneous intravascular imaging catheter (abstract). *Circulation* 1988;78(suppl II):II-21

16. Movat HZ: Demonstration of all connective tissue elements in a single section. *AMA Arch Path* 1955;60:289–295

17. Arnett EN, Isner JM, Redwood DR, Kent KM, Baker WP, Ackerstein H, Roberts WC: Coronary artery narrowing in coronary heart disease: Comparison of cineangiographic and necropsy findings. *Ann Intern Med* 1979;91:350–356

18. Schwartz JN, Kong Y, Hackel DB, Bartel AG: Comparison of angiographic and postmortem findings in patients with coronary artery disease. *Am J Cardiol* 1975;36:174–178

19. Grondin CM, Dyrda I, Pasternac A, Campeau L, Bourassa MC, Lesperance J: Discrepancies between cineangiographic and postmortem findings in patients with coronary artery disease and recent myocardial revascularization. *Circulation* 1974;49:703–708

20. Glagov S, Weisenberg E, Zarins CK, Stankunavicius R, Kolettis GJ: Compensatory enlargement of human atherosclerotic coronary arteries. *N Engl J Med* 1987;316:1371–1375

21. Zarins CK, Weisenberg E, Kolettis G, Stankunavicius R, Glagov S: Differential enlargement of artery segments in response to enlarging atherosclerotic plaques. *J Vasc Surg* 1988;7:386–392

22. Hartley CJ, Strandness DE: The effects of atherosclerosis on the transmission of ultrasound. *J Surg Res* 1969;9:575–582

23. Rogers EW, Feigenbaum H, Weyman AE, Godley RW, Johnston KW, Eggleton RC: Possible detection of atherosclerotic coronary calcification by two-dimensional echocardiography. *Circulation* 1980;62:1046–1053

24. Fields S, Dunn F: Correlation of echographic visualizability of tissue with biological composition and physiological state. *J Acoust Soc Am* 1973;54:809–812

25. Mimbs JW, O'Donnell M, Bauwens D, Miller JW, Sobel BE: The dependence of ultrasonic attenuation and backscatter on collagen content in dog and rabbit hearts. *Circ Res* 1980;47:49–58

26. Rasmussen S, Corya BC, Feigenbaum H, Knoebel SB: Detection of myocardial scar tissue by M-mode echocardiography. *Circulation* 1978;57:230–237

27. O'Donnell M, Mimbs JW, Miller JG: The relationship between collagen and ultrasonic attenuation in myocardial tissue. *J Acoust Soc Am* 1979;65:512–517

28. Picano E, Landini L, Lattanzi F, Salvadori M, Benassi A, L'Abbate A: Time domain echo pattern evaluations from normal and atherosclerotic arterial walls: A study in vitro. *Circulation* 1988;77:654–659

29. Pignoli P, Tremoli E, Poli A, Oreste P, Paoletti R: Intimal plus media thickness of the arterial wall: A direct measurement with ultrasound imaging. *Circulation* 1986;74:1399–1406

30. James EM, Earnest F IV, Forbes GS, Reese DF, Houser OW, Folger WN: High-resolution dynamic ultrasound imaging of the carotid bifurcation: A prospective evaluation. *Radiology* 1982;144:853–858

31. Bamber JC, Hill CR, King JA, Dunn F: Ultrasound propagation through fixed and unfixed tissues. *Ultrasound Med Biol* 1979;5:159–165

32. Stowell RE: Effect on tissue volume of various methods of fixation, dehydration, and embedding. *Stain Technology* 1941;16:67–83

33. Baker JR: The reactions of fixatives with tissue cells: Methods of research, in *Principles of Biological Microtechnique*. London, Methuen, 1958, pp 76–88

34. Siegel RJ, Swan K, Edwalds G, Fishbein MC: Limitations of postmortem assessment of human coronary artery size and luminal narrowing: Differential effects of tissue fixation and processing on vessels with different degrees of atherosclerosis. *J Am Coll Cardiol* 1985;5:342–346

KEY WORDS • coronary artery disease • ultrasound

Morphometric Analysis of the Composition of Coronary Arterial Plaques in Isolated Unstable Angina Pectoris with Pain at Rest

Amy H. Kragel, MD, Shanthasundari G. Reddy, MD, Janet T. Wittes, PhD, and William C. Roberts, MD

Coronary artery plaque morphology was studied in 354 five-mm segments of the 4 major (left main, left anterior descending, left circumflex and right) epicardial coronary arteries in 10 patients with isolated unstable angina pectoris with pain at rest. The 4 major coronary arteries were sectioned at 5-mm intervals and a drawing of each of the resulting 354 Movat-stained histologic sections was analyzed using a computerized morphometry system. The major component of plaque was a combination of dense acellular and cellular fibrous tissue with much smaller portions of plaque being composed of pultaceous debris, calcium, foam cells with and without inflammatory infiltrates and inflammatory infiltrates without foam cells. There were no differences in plaque composition among any of the 4 major epicardial coronary arteries. Plaque composition varied as a function of the degree of luminal narrowing. Linear increases were observed in the mean percent of dense fibrous tissue (from 5 to 50%), calcific deposits (from 1 to 10%), pultaceous debris (from 0 to 10%) and inflammatory infiltrates without significant numbers of foam cells (from 0 to 5%), and a linear decrease was observed in the mean percent of cellular fibrous tissue (from 94 to 22%) in sections narrowed up to 25% to more than 95% in cross-sectional area. Multiluminal channels were seen in all 10 patients (28 [19%] of the 146 sections narrowed >75% in cross-sectional area and in 36 [10%] of all 354 segments); occlusive thrombi in no patient; nonocclusive thrombi in 2 patients (1 section each of 2 arteries); plaque rupture in 2 patients (4 segments from 2 arteries); and plaque hemorrhages in 6 patients (11 sections from 10 arteries).

(Am J Cardiol 1990;66:562–567)

From the Pathology and Biostatistics Research Branches, National Heart, Lung, and Blood Institute, National Institutes of Health, Bethesda, Maryland 20892. Manuscript received February 28, 1990; revised manuscript received April 30, 1990, and accepted May 1.

Address for reprints: Pathology Branch, National Heart, Lung, and Blood Institute, Building 10, Room 2N258, Bethesda, Maryland 20892.

Since the early 1970s several angiographic and morphologic studies have described the degrees of luminal narrowing of the major epicardial coronary arteries, some acute lesions in the coronary arteries, and the status of the left ventricular myocardium in patients with unstable angina pectoris.[1-4] No previous studies, however, have described the composition of coronary arterial atherosclerotic plaques in patients with unstable angina pectoris shortly before death. Such was the purpose of the present study. The focus is on the composition of the plaques, not the types and frequency of acute lesions in the coronary arteries. We examined, in a quantitative fashion, the components of coronary arterial plaques in each of 354 five-mm segments of the 4 major (left main, left anterior descending, left circumflex and right) epicardial coronary arteries in 10 patients with isolated angina pectoris with pain at rest.

METHODS

The autopsy records of the Pathology Branch of the National Heart, Lung, and Blood Institute were searched for cases coded as unstable angina pectoris. Patients were selected with isolated unstable angina at rest. All patients had unstable angina pectoris as recently defined by Braunwald.[5] Cases were excluded in whom unstable angina developed in the presence of an aggravating extracardiac condition. Cases were excluded when death occurred during or immediately after cardiac catheterization or when coronary artery bypass surgery or percutaneous coronary angioplasty had been performed or thrombolytic therapy administered. Cases were selected in whom death occurred during or immediately after a hospital admission for evaluation of unstable angina and in whom there was no gross or microscopic evidence at necropsy of either transmural left ventricular necrosis or fibrosis.

The 4 major epicardial coronary arteries were excised intact from the heart, decalcified (if necessary), sectioned transversely at 5-mm intervals and labelled sequentially. The 5-mm segments then were decalcified again (if necessary), dehydrated in alcohols, cleared in xylene, embedded in paraffin and two 5-micron-thick sections were prepared from each segment. One section was stained by the Movat method,[6] and 1 by hematoxylin and eosin.

The Movat stained sections were placed on the stage of a projection microscope. Using a 40× objective, the image was enlarged and a tracing of the artery was made on opaque white paper. The following areas were outlined: potential lumen (total area outlined by the internal elastic membrane), residual lumen (potential lumen minus area of atherosclerotic plaque) and luminal thrombus (platelets, fibrin, erythrocytes and leukocytes). Components of plaque identified and outlined included dense fibrous tissue, loose fibrous tissue, cellular fibrous tissue, heavily calcified tissue, pultaceous debris, foam cells with and without lymphocytes, and inflammatory infiltrates without significant numbers of foam cells.

Definitions and descriptions of the various components of plaque were the following: *dense fibrous tissue* was an area of relatively acellular tissue composed primarily of dense collagen fibers; *loose fibrous tissue* was a relatively acellular, more delicate arrangement of collagen fibers; *cellular fibrous tissue* was composed of spindle cells resembling myofibroblasts, smooth muscle cells or fibroblasts admixed with collagen or elastic fibers, or a combination of these; *calcific deposits* were detected by red-brown granular staining areas (only solid heavily calcified areas were included in the analysis); *pultaceous debris* (presumably rich in extracellular lipid) were pale staining areas composed of amorphous material with abundant cholesterol clefts; *foam-cell aggregates* were composed of collections of plump, rounded, finely vacuolated cells; *foam cells and lymphocytes* were areas containing round, finely vacuolated or granular cells admixed with lymphocytes; *inflammatory in-filtrates* without foam cells were isolated aggregates of lymphocytes and other inflammatory cells that were almost always seen surrounding small vascular channels. All areas were initially recognized with the projection microscope and confirmed by standard light microscopy.

After a labeled drawing of each section was made, the area of potential and residual lumens and the area of each component was determined using a computerized morphometry system. The individual areas were traced using a GTCO Micro Digi-Pad® and the area calculated using Macmeasure,[7] a morphometric software package used in conjunction with a Macintosh SE® computer. The area of each component was then converted to a percentage of the total plaque area. Intraluminal thrombus was not considered to represent a component of plaque. Inter- and intraobserver variability using this method has been previously shown to be good.[8]

The percent luminal narrowing was determined by using the following formula: percent luminal narrowing = (1-residual lumen area/potential lumen area) × 100. The degrees of cross-sectional area luminal narrowing were then categorized into 5 groups: 0 to 25%, 26 to 50%, 51 to 75%, 76 to 95% and 96 to 100%. The results were verified by visual inspection of the section. If the outer circumference of the artery was not rounded and if the percent luminal narrowing appeared to have been

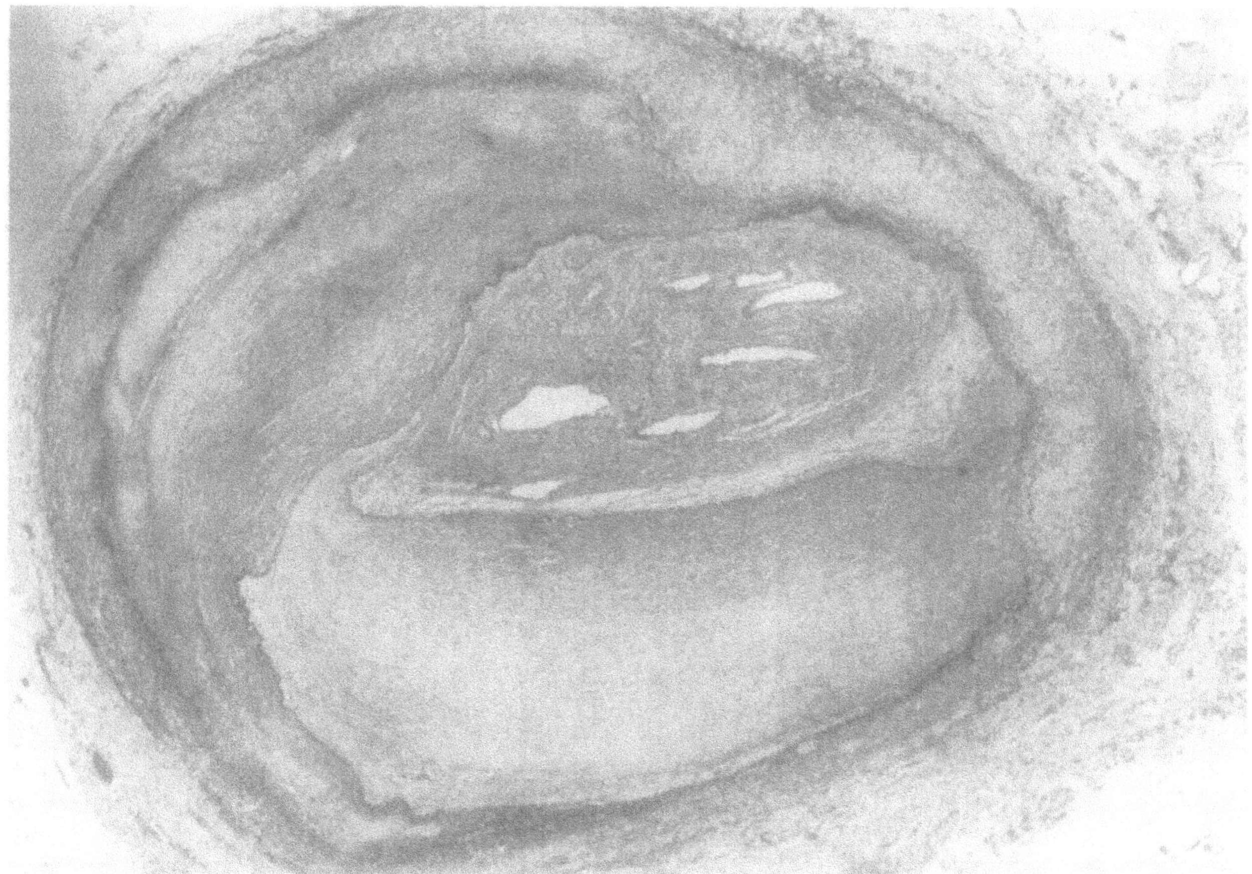

FIGURE 1. Photomicrograph of a Movat stained section of coronary artery that is severely narrowed by atherosclerotic plaque. The plaque is composed almost entirely of fibrous tissue and contains multiluminal channels. (Original magnification × 30.)

TABLE I Degrees of Luminal Narrowing in 10 Patients with Unstable Angina Pectoris

Case	Age (yrs)	Number (%) of Segments with a Given Degree of Cross-Sectional-Area Narrowing				
		0–25%	26–50%	51–75%	75–95%	96–100%
1	47	1 (3)	6(18)	10(29)	14(41)	3 (9)
2	48	2 (4)	10(20)	12(23)	23(45)	4 (8)
3	49	8(22)	13(35)	9(24)	4(11)	3 (8)
4	51	0 (0)	0 (0)	12(43)	16(57)	0 (0)
5	58	0 (0)	14(28)	18(36)	10(20)	8(16)
6	65	0 (0)	7(21)	16(49)	8(24)	2 (6)
7	68	4(10)	5(13)	18(46)	9(23)	3 (8)
8	68	3(10)	8(29)	7(25)	8(29)	2 (7)
9	68	0 (0)	1 (4)	6(21)	14(50)	7(25)
10	70	0 (0)	12(46)	6(23)	8(31)	0 (0)
Total		18 (5)	76(22)	114(32)	114(32)	32 (9)

overestimated by this formula then the estimate obtained by visual inspection alone was used. The presence or absence of plaque rupture (a tear extending from the plaque's luminal surface into its substance), plaque hemorrhage, centrally located multiluminal channels (Figure 1) and thrombus was noted in each 5-mm segment.

Statistical methods: The mean percent of each component of plaque in the 4 major epicardial coronary arteries was determined by calculating a mean for each patient and averaging over individual persons, and adjusting for different distributions of luminal narrowing. An analysis of variance was used to assess the association between the percent composition of a given component and the specific artery of origin. In each analysis, the individual patient was the unit of study[9]; all calculations were performed using SAS.[10]

The analysis of plaque composition within each of the 5 categories of narrowing was performed by determining the mean composition for each patient of all segments within each of the 5 categories and averaging over individuals using analysis of variance model. A linear contrast model was used to assess whether a linear trend existed in the mean percent of any of the components over the 5 categories of narrowing. To correct for the fact that 8 correlated significance tests were performed, Bonferroni adjustments were used.[11]

The analysis of plaque composition in segments of artery containing thrombus, hemorrhage, rupture or multiluminal channels was performed by calculating a mean for each component, averaging over individuals and adjusting for varying degrees in luminal narrowing. F tests were then used to compare the composition of segments with and without a given characteristic.

RESULTS

Clinical features: The 10 patients ranged in age from 47 to 70 years (mean 59). Only 1 patient (no. 8, Table I) was a woman. The duration of angina in the 9 patients in whom it was known ranged from 6 weeks to 19 years. All 10 patients had angina at rest during at least their last 48 hours of life and, additionally, the angina either had increased in frequency or the amount of stress required to elicit it had diminished during their last 2 months of life. Nine patients died during an admission to the hospital for the evaluation of angina, and the other patient died outside the hospital 9 days after hospitalization for unstable angina. At necropsy, none had gross or microscopic evidence of transmural (involvement of greater than the inner one half of the left ventricular wall) left ventricular necrosis. In 7 patients non-transmural left ventricular scars were present. The hearts ranged in weight from 330 to 540 g (mean 458).

Five-mm segments studied: Of 449 five-mm sections of coronary artery prepared, 95 were excluded from analysis because they contained either branch points or sectioning artifacts such that the entire cross-

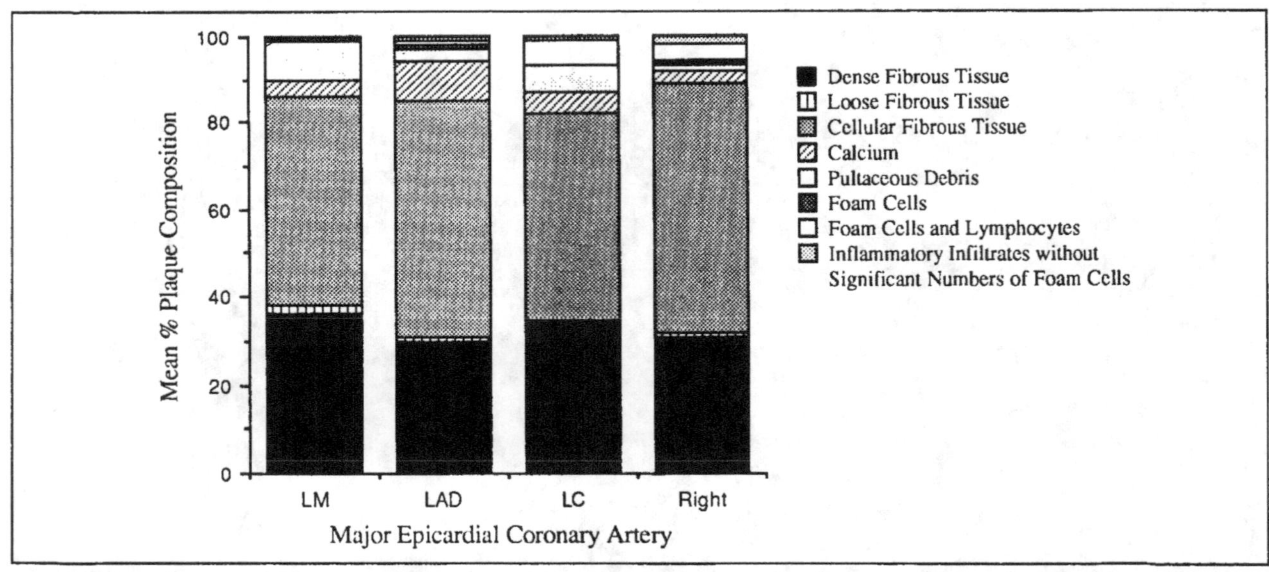

FIGURE 2. Mean percent plaque composition in each of the 4 major epicardial coronary arteries. LAD = left anterior descending; LC = left circumflex; LM = left main.

TABLE II Mean Percent of Various Components of Plaque in Each of the Five Categories of Narrowing

	0–25% mean (SE) (n = 5)	26–50% mean (SE) (n = 9)	51–75% mean (SE) (n = 10)	76–95% mean (SE) (n = 10)	96–100% mean (SE) (n = 8)	Normal p for Linear Trend
Dense fibrous tissue	5(5)	23(3)	39(3)	42(3)	50(3)	0.0001*
Loose fibrous tissue	0(1)	2(1)	2(1)	1(1)	1(2)	0.25
Cellular fibrous tissue	94(6)	66(4)	41(4)	30(4)	22(5)	0.0001*
Heavily calcified tissue	1(2)	0(2)	7(2)	9(2)	10(2)	0.0002†
Pultaceous debris	0(2)	0(2)	2(2)	8(2)	10(2)	0.0001*
Foam cells	0(1)	1(1)	1(1)	1(1)	1(1)	0.45
Foam cells and lymphocytes	0(3)	8(2)	7(2)	8(2)	2(2)	0.31
Inflammatory infiltrates without significant numbers of foam cells	0(2)	0(1)	1(1)	1(1)	4(1)	0.005‡

n = number of cases from which the mean was calculated (5 cases had no sections narrowed <25%, 1 had no sections narrowed 26–50% and 2 had no sections narrowed 96–100%).

* = Bonferroni p < 0.001; † = Bonferroni p < 0.01; ‡ = Bonferroni p < 0.05.

sectional area could not be studied. The remaining 354 sections (an average of 35/case) were studied in detail.

Amounts of coronary narrowing: The degrees of luminal narrowing in each case are listed in Table I. All cases had severe (>75% decrease in cross-sectional area) narrowing of ≥1 of the 4 major epicardial coronary arteries by plaque. Nine had >75% cross-sectional area narrowing of the left anterior descending, left circumflex and right coronary arteries by plaque, and 4 had this degree of narrowing of all 4 major epicardial coronary arteries. Segments narrowed >95% in cross-sectional area were present in 8 of the 10 patients. The percent or segments narrowed >75% cross-sectional area in each case ranged from 19 to 75% (mean 41%).

Atherosclerotic plaque composition: The mean compositions of plaque, corrected for varying degrees of luminal narrowing, of the 4 major epicardial coronary arteries are detailed in Figure 2. In each of the 4 arteries, the major component of plaque was a combination of dense and cellular fibrous tissue. Smaller amounts of loose fibrous tissue, pultaceous debris, calcium, foam cells with and without inflammatory infiltrates and in-

flammatory infiltrates without foam cells were present. The mean percent of any given component was similar in each of the 4 major coronary arteries.

The mean composition of plaque, analyzed in each of the 5 categories of luminal narrowing, is detailed in Table II and in Figure 3. Linear increases in the mean percent of dense fibrous tissue (from 5 to 50%, Bonferroni p <0.001), calcium (from 1 to 10%, Bonferroni p <0.01), pultaceous debris (from 0 to 10%, Bonferroni p <0.001), and lymphocytes without foam cells (from 0 to 5%, Bonferroni p <0.05) occurred across the 5 categories of narrowing. The mean percent of cellular fibrous tissue decreased across the 5 categories from 94 to 22% (Bonferroni p <0.001).

Intraluminal coronary thrombus: Minute intraluminal thrombi were seen in 2 sections, 1 from each of 2 patients. In both cases, the thrombus was nonocclusive and composed of platelets and fibrin. Both thrombi were located in segments narrowed >75% in cross-sectional area by plaque and neither was associated with underlying plaque hemorrhage or rupture. The mean percent of plaque occupied by foam cell aggregates was

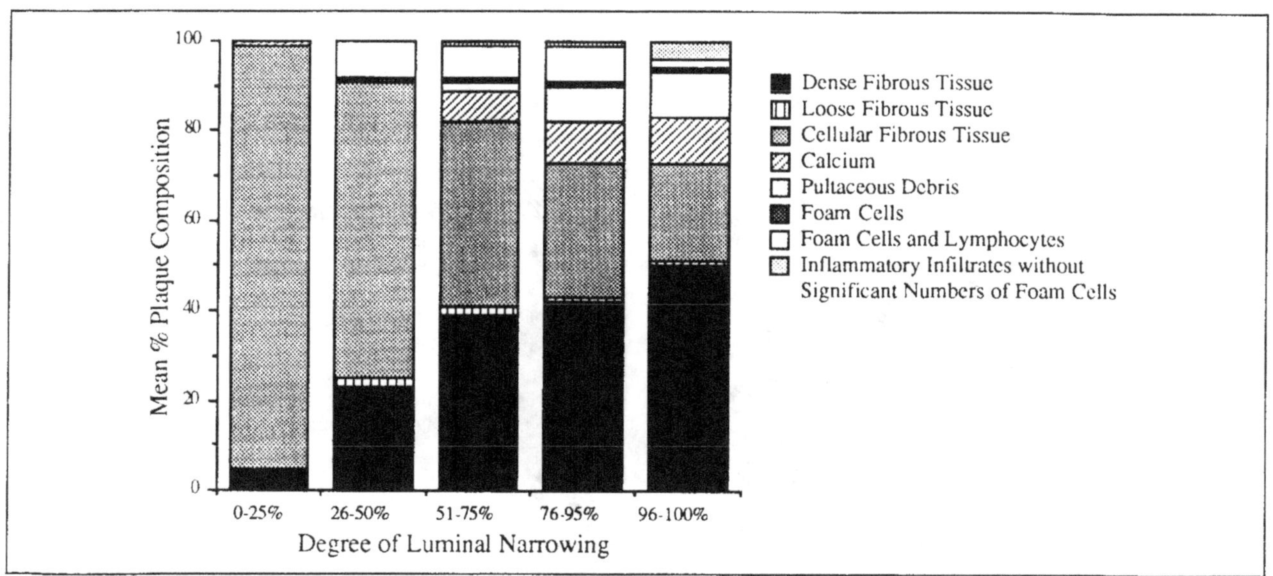

FIGURE 3. Mean percent plaque composition in each of the 5 categories of cross-sectional-area narrowing.

significantly greater (5 vs 1%, p = 0.04) in the 2 sections containing thrombus compared to the segments without thrombus.

Plaque rupture: This was seen in 4 sections from 2 patients. In each, both sections were from the same artery. In 1 case, both segments containing rupture were associated with hemorrhage into plaque. The composition of plaque in these sections was similar to that of sections without rupture.

Plaque hemorrhage: This was present in 11 sections from 10 arteries in 6 patients. The mean percents of pultaceous debris and loose fibrous tissue were greater (12 ± 3 vs 3 ± 2, p = 0.008 and 9 ± 3 vs 1 ± 1, p = 0.04, respectively) and the mean percent of dense fibrous tissue (21 ± 5 vs 32 ± 2, p = 0.04) was less in sections with hemorrhage than in those without.

Multiluminal channels: These were identified in all 10 patients, in 28 (19%) of 146 sections narrowed >75% in cross-sectional area and in 36 (10%) of all of the 354 5-mm segments. Of the 36 segments containing >1 channel, the lumen was narrowed >75% in cross-sectional area in 28; from 51 to 75% in 6 and from 26 to 50% in 2. Sections of artery containing multiluminal channels contained a higher percent of dense acellular fibrous tissue (41 ± 4 vs 32 ± 2%, p = 0.03) and less pultaceous debris (0.0 ± 1 vs 4 ± 1, p = 0.001) than did sections without multiluminal channels.

DISCUSSION

Plaque composition: The findings in this study indicate that the major component of atherosclerotic plaques in the 4 major epicardial coronary arteries in patients with isolated unstable angina pectoris at rest is a combination of cellular and dense acellular fibrous tissue (82 to 88%). Pultaceous debris, calcium, loose fibrous tissue, inflammatory infiltrates, and foam cell aggregations made up much smaller portions of the plaques. Plaque composition was similar in each of the 4 major coronary arteries. Plaque composition changed as a function of the degree of luminal narrowing. The mean percent of dense fibrous tissue, pultaceous debris, calcium and inflammatory infiltrates without foam cells increased and the amount of cellular fibrous tissue decreased in a linear fashion over the 5 categories of cross-sectional area narrowing.

While quantitative information on coronary arterial plaque composition is now available on other patients with fatal coronary artery disease—that is, acute myocardial infarction and sudden coronary death[8]—there is no previously published information on plaque composition in patients with clinically isolated unstable angina pectoris. The mean percent of the various components of plaque in 5-mm segments of coronary arteries narrowed >75% in cross-sectional area in these 3 groups of patients is shown in Figure 4. While the major component of plaque in all 3 groups is a combination of dense and cellular fibrous tissue, significant differences occur in the mean percent of plaque occupied by pultaceous debris. The mean percent of plaque occupied by pultaceous debris is about 8% in patients with angina pectoris at rest and sudden coronary death, conditions associated with a low frequency of occlusive intraluminal thrombi, and about 16% in patients with fatal acute myocardial infarction, a condition associated with a high frequency of intraluminal thrombi. Because occlusive thrombi usually overlie plaque rich in pultaceous debris,[8,12–16] the differences in the mean percent of pultaceous debris in these subsets of patients with coronary artery disease may explain the differences in the frequency of intraluminal thrombi.

Multiluminal channels within atherosclerotic plaques: These were seen in every patient, in 19% of segments narrowed >75% in cross-sectional area and in 10% of all coronary segments. The segments with multiluminal channels contained significantly more dense fibrous tissue than did the segments without multiluminal channels but with a similar degree of luminal narrowing. If thrombi are injected into the lumens of systemic veins, the clots migrate to the lungs, and they often organize into fibrous plaques containing multiluminal

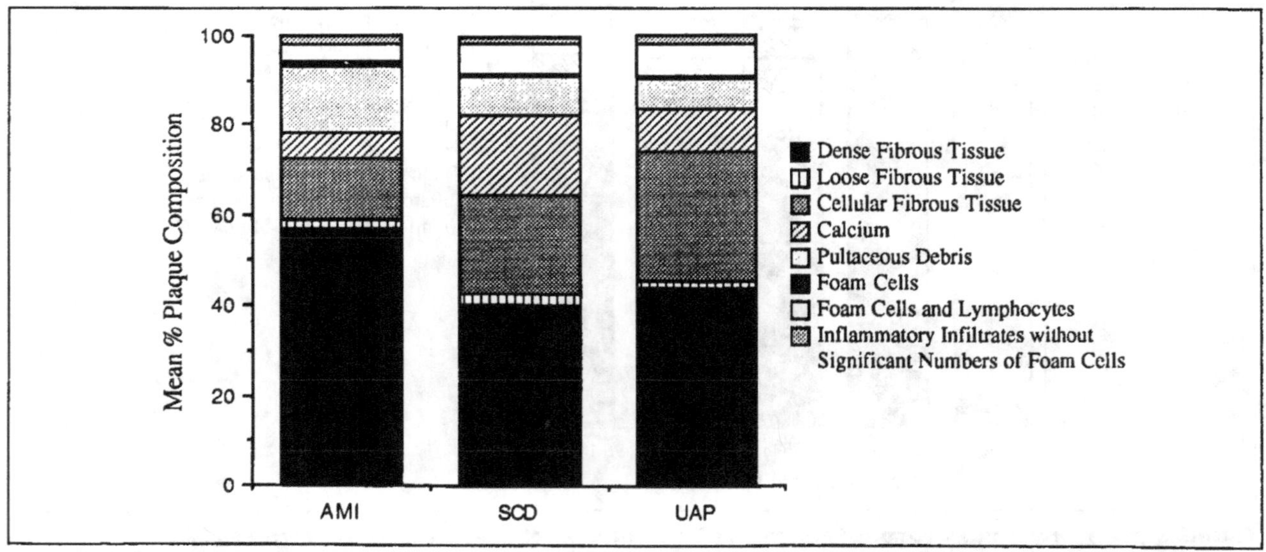

FIGURE 4. Mean percent plaque composition of sections of coronary artery narrowed >75% in cross-sectional area. AMI = acute myocardial infarction; SCD = sudden coronary death without left ventricular necrosis; UAP = unstable angina pectoris.

channels.[17] This fact suggests that arteries containing multiluminal channels are the result of organization of thrombi. It is therefore likely that a large portion of the plaque in the 19% of segments narrowed >75% in cross-sectional area is due to the organization of thrombi into fibrous plaques containing multiluminal channels.

The frequency of segments of coronary artery containing multiluminal channels in patients with isolated unstable angina pectoris has not been noted in other studies. Levin and Fallon[18] compared postmortem angiographic and histologic findings in patients with fatal coronary artery disease of various types. They demonstrated that angiographic narrowings with either irregular borders or intraluminal lucencies by histologic examination consisted of a variety of lesions including "recanalized thrombi," nonocclusive thrombi, plaque hemorrhage or plaque rupture. While narrowings containing recanalized thrombi were not illustrated, presumably they contained multiluminal channels. Narrowings with a similar angiographic appearance (eccentric lumens with irregular or overhanging borders) were observed by Ambrose et al[19] in 50 of 92 narrowings in 63 patients with unstable angina pectoris and in only 4 of 55 narrowings in 47 patients with stable angina pectoris. While histologic evaluation of these narrowings, which they believed were characteristic of patients with unstable angina, was not possible, they attributed the angiographic appearances to the presence of either plaque rupture or intraluminal thrombi. We found plaque rupture in only 2 of our 10 patients and nonocclusive intraluminal thrombi in only 2 of our 10 patients. In contrast, multiluminal channels were observed in all 10 patients. While coronary angiography of the epicardial coronary arteries was not available for comparison in the 10 patients we studied, it is likely that a great proportion of the narrowings would have been due to plaque containing multiluminal channels.

Limitations: Identification of calcium in formalin fixed partly decalcified tissue may result in an underestimation of the total mean percent of calcium. Likewise, processing of tissues in xylenes prevented us from using specific lipid stains and hence the total amount of lipid may be underestimated.

In summary, the major component of plaque in patients with unstable angina is fibrous tissue. Multiluminal channels, a finding suggesting the earlier presence of thrombus that organized, was present in all patients and in 10% of the segments studied. Plaque rupture was seen in 2 patients, nonocclusive thrombi were seen in 2 patients, and plaque hemorrhage in 6 of the 10 cases. The zero frequency of occlusive thrombi at necropsy might be explained in part by the low mean percent of pultaceous debris in the 4 major epicardial coronary arteries.

REFERENCES

1. Roberts WC. The coronary arteries and left ventricle in clinically isolated angina pectoris. A necropsy analysis. *Circulation* 1976;54:388–390.
2. Bodenheimer MM, Banka VS, Trout RG, Hermann GA, Pasdar H, Helfant RH. Pathophysiologic significance of S-T and T wave abnormalities in patients with the intermediate coronary syndrome. *Am J Cardiol* 1977;39:153–158.
3. Alison HW, Russell RO, Mantle JA, Kouchoukos NT, Moraski RE, Rackley CE. Coronary anatomy and arteriography in patients with unstable angina pectoris. *Am J Cardiol* 1978;41:204–209.
4. Roberts WC, Virmani R. Quantification of coronary arterial narrowing in clinically-isolated unstable angina pectoris. An analysis of 22 necropsy patients. *Am J Med* 1979;67:792–799.
5. Braunwald E. Unstable angina, a classification. *Circulation* 1989;80:410–414.
6. Movat HZ. Demonstration of all connective tissue elements in a single section. *Arch Pathol* 1955;60:289–295.
7. Hook GR, Rasband W. Macmeasure. A low-cost, easy to operate quantitative morphometrics system for the Macintosh computer. In: Barley GW, ed. Proceedings of the 45th Annual Meeting of the Electron Microscopy Society of America. *San Francisco:* 1987;920–921.
8. Kragel AH, Reddy SG, Wittes JT, Roberts WC. Morphometric analysis of the composition of atherosclerotic plaques in the four major epicardial coronary arteries in acute myocardial infarction and in sudden coronary death. *Circulation* 1989;80:1747–1756.
9. Armitage P. Statistical Methods in Medical Research. *New York: Wiley,* 1974;253–259.
10. SAS Institute Inc. SAS User's Guide: Statistics, Version 5th Edition. *Cary: SAS Institute, 1985.*
11. Miller RG. Simultaneous Statistical Inference, Second Edition. *New York: Springer-Verlag, 1981.*
12. Chapman I. Morphogenesis of occluding coronary artery thrombosis. *Arch Pathol* 1965;80:256–261.
13. Constantinides P. Plaque fissures in human coronary thrombosis. *J Atheroscler Res* 1966;6:1 17.
14. Friedman M. The coronary thrombus: its origin and fate. *Human Pathol* 1971;2:81–128.
15. Falk E. Plaque rupture with severe pre-existing stenosis precipitating coronary thrombosis. Characteristics of coronary atherosclerotic plaques underlying fatal occlusive thrombi. *Br Heart J* 1983;50:127–134.
16. Tracey RE, Devaney K, Kissling G. Characteristics of the plaque under a coronary thrombus. *Virchows Arch* 1985;405:411–427.
17. Hand RA, Chandler AB. Atherosclerotic metamorphosis of autologous pulmonary thromboemboli in the rabbit. *Am J Pathol* 1962;40:469–486.
18. Levin DC, Fallon JT. Significance of the angiographic morphology of localized coronary stenosis: histopathologic correlations. *Circulation* 1982;66:316–320.
19. Ambrose JA, Winters SL, Stern A, Eng A, Teichholz LE, Gorlin R, Fuster V. Angiographic morphology and the pathogenesis of unstable angina pectoris. *JACC* 1985;5:609–616.

Myocarditis or Acute Myocardial Infarction Associated With Interleukin-2 Therapy for Cancer

Amy H. Kragel, MD,* William D. Travis, MD,† Ronald G. Steis, MD,‡
Steven A. Rosenberg, MD,§ and William C. Roberts, MD*

The hearts of eight patients aged 22 to 67 years (mean, 41 years) who died during or within 4 days of interleukin-2 (IL-2) based immunotherapy for treatment of renal cell carcinoma or melanoma were studied at necropsy. Death resulted from combined cardiorespiratory failure in two patients, sepsis in four patients, acute myocardial infarction in one patient, and myocarditis in one patient. Transmural left ventricular necrosis was present in one of the two patients with significant atherosclerotic coronary artery narrowing. Noninfectious myocarditis was present in five patients: the inflammatory infiltrate was lymphocytic in four and composed of a mixture of eosinophils and lymphocytes in one. Although treatment-related deaths associated with high-dose IL-2 therapy are uncommon (1.5% in 652 consecutive patients), the potential for significant myocardial ischemia or myocarditis exists, and careful monitoring for arrhythmias or myocardial failure is warranted. *Cancer* 66:1513–1516, 1990.

NTERLEUKIN-2 (IL-2) BASED immunotherapy for the treatment of cancer has been associated with a variety of hemodynamic and cardiac alterations, including hypotension, tachycardia, decreased systemic vascular resistance, decreased ejection fraction, variable changes in pulmonary arterial wedge pressure, and peripheral edema.[1-3] In addition, atrial and ventricular arrhythmias, angina pectoris, myocarditis (noninfectious), and acute myocardial infarction have been reported.[4-8] Some of these abnormalities can be explained by the development of a "capillary leak syndrome" with profound hypotension. We studied the hearts at necropsy of eight patients who died during or within 4 days of cessation of IL-2-based immunotherapy to identify anatomic cardiac abnormalities associated with IL-2 administration.

Patients and Methods

The autopsy records of the Pathology Laboratory, National Cancer Institute, were searched for patients in whom IL-2-based immunotherapy had been administered and in whom death had occurred within 5 days of the cessation of therapy. Nine such patients were identified; in one patient, however, neither the heart nor histologic sections were available for review. The remaining eight cases are the subject of this report. In each case, the clinical records, necropsy report, heart specimen, and multiple hematoxylin and eosin stained sections of right and left ventricular myocardium were examined.

Results

The clinical and morphologic features of the five men and three women are summarized in Table 1. Certain features of patients 1, 2, 6, and 8 were reported previously.[8] Therapy was administered for the treatment of melanoma in six patients and for renal cell carcinoma in two. In

From the *Pathology Branch, National Heart, Lung, and Blood Institute, and the †Laboratory of Pathology, ‡Clinical Research Branch, Biological Response Modifiers Program, and §Surgery Branch, National Cancer Institute, National Institutes of Health, Bethesda, Maryland.

The authors thank all of the many people involved in the care of the patients included in this study, including Dr. Mario Sznol, Clinical Research Branch, National Cancer Institute, Frederick Memorial Hospital, and the physicians and nurses of the Clinical Center, National Institutes of Health, Bethesda, Maryland.

Address for reprints: Amy H. Kragel, MD, Pathology Branch, National Heart, Lung, and Blood Institute, Building 10, Room 2N258, Bethesda, MD 20892.

Accepted for publication February 22, 1990.

TABLE 1. Clinical and Cardiac Necropsy Findings in 8 Patients Receiving Interleukin-2-Based Immunotherapy

| Case no. | Age (yr) | Sex | Immunotherapy regimen | Interval treatment to death (days) | Mode of death | Evidence of toxicity while on therapy | | | | | HW (g) | Dilated cavity | | CA narrowing (% CSA) | Myocarditis |
						Hypotension*	Ischemia†	Atrial‡	Ventricular§		RV	LV		
1	22	F	IL2/LAK	0	CR Failure	4+	3+	4+	4+	295	+	0	0–25	+
2	24	M	IL2/LAK	4	Sepsis	4+	0	0	4+	355	+	0	0–25	+
3	30	M	IL2/TILs/C	4	Sepsis	−	−	−	−	440	+	0	0–25	+
4	34	M	IL2/TILs/C	4	Sepsis	−	−	−	−	430	0	0	0–25	0
5	50	F	IL2/LAK	1	CR Failure	0	0	0	0	330	+	0	0–25	+
6	51	M	IL2	4	Sepsis	2+	0	2+	1+	365	0	0	0–25	+
7	53	F	IL2	1	Sudden Death	1+	0	−	−	415	0	0	76–95	+
8	67	M	IL2	1	AMI	4+	4+	4+	4+	520	0	0	76–95	0

(0): negative; (−): information not available; AMI: acute myocardial infarction; C: cyclophosphamide; CA: coronary artery; CR: cardiorespiratory; CSA: cross-sectional area narrowing; HW: heart weight; IL2: interleukin 2; LAK: lymphokine-activated killer cells; LV: left ventricle, RV: right ventricle; TIL: tumor infiltrating lymphocytes.

* Hypotension: 1+ = hypotension not requiring therapy, 2+ = hypotension responding to fluid therapy, 3+ = hypotension requiring and responsive to pressors, 4+ = hypotension unresponsive to pressors.

† Ischemia: 2+ = nonspecific electrocardiographic changes, elevated CK, 3+ = angina, ischemic changes on electrocardiogram, elevated MB band, 4+ = AMI.

‡ Atrial arrhythmias: 1+ = sinus tachycardia > 110 beats/min, 2+ = premature atrial complexes, 3+ = atrial fibrillation or sinus tacchycardia > 150 beats/min, 4+ = atrial arrhythmia with hypotension.

§ Ventricular arrhythmias: 1+ = unifocal ventricular premature complexes, 2+ = multifocal ventricular premature complexes, bigeminy, trigeminy, 3+ = nonsustained ventricular tachycardia (VT), 4+ = sustained VT.

addition to IL-2, the immunotherapy regimens of three of the patients included lymphokine-activated killer (LAK) cells and two included tumor-infiltrating lymphocytes and cyclophosphamide.

The immediate cause of death varied. Severe combined cardiorespiratory failure immediately following an infusion of LAK cells occurred in two patients. Patient 1 (Table 1) had extensive plugging of pulmonary capillaries and widening of alveolar septae by lymphoid cells with early focal diffuse alveolar damage, and patient 5 (Table 1) had extensive intra-alveolar hemorrhage and early diffuse alveolar damage. Both patients also had a noninfectious myocarditis at necropsy. Patient 7 (Fig. 1) was found dead in bed following LAK therapy; the extent of metastatic disease was not considered sufficient to account for her death, but the left anterior descending coronary artery was narrowed greater than 75% in cross-sectional area by atherosclerotic plaque and a lymphocytic myocarditis also was present. Patient 8 had an acute myocardial infarction while on therapy. The remaining four patients died of consequences of bacterial sepsis, including one with severe renal failure (patient 4).

The heart weight was increased (> 350 g in women and > 400 g in men) in four patients. Two patients with cardiomegaly had coronary artery disease with more than 75% cross-sectional area narrowing by plaque of at least one of the four major epicardial coronary arteries. In one of these two (patient 8, Table 1), gross and microscopic examination of the heart showed transmural myocardial necrosis histologically compatible with a 24-hour-old infarct. Of the remaining seven patients, six had evidence of a diffuse, patchy myocarditis (Fig. 1). In four patients (1, 3, 6, and 7 [Table 1]), the inflammatory infiltrate was predominately lymphocytic; in one (patient 5), the infiltrate was composed of a mixture of eosinophils and lymphocytes; and in one (patient 2), it was composed of a mixture of polymorphonuclear leukocytes, lymphocytes, and eosinophils with microabscess formation. Only in this last patient was the etiology of the myocarditis believed to be infectious: colonies of organisms were identified within the abscesses. In all six of these patients, there was myofiber degeneration and scattered foci of myocyte necrosis. In the two patients dying with severe cardiorespiratory failure and in the one case of sudden death due to myocarditis, the myocarditis was of greater severity than in the other two cases of noninfectious myocarditis.

In no patient was there grossly visible right or left ventricular fibrosis. Microscopic examination of hematoxylin and eosin stained sections disclosed mild interstitial fibrosis in three cases (patients 2, 4, and 6). Foci of contraction-band necrosis were noted in several cases, including one (patient 2) in whom the final resuscitative measures were prolonged and had included open cardiac massage.

Discussion

While death associated with high-dose IL-2 therapy is rare (1.5% in 652 consecutive patients treated with high-dose IL-2-based immunotherapy),[6] we found cardiac morphologic abnormalities in seven of our eight patients who died within 4 days of therapy. These abnormalities

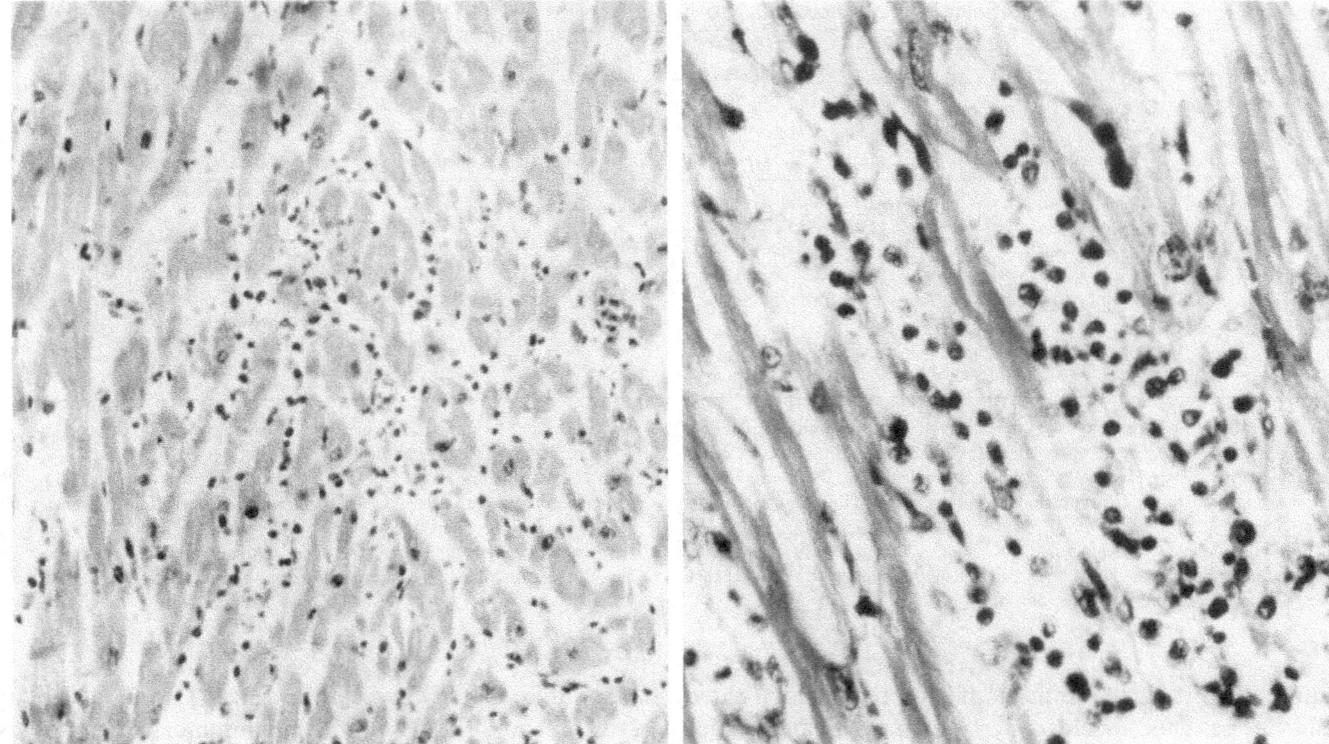

FIG. 1. Hematoxylin and eosin stained sections of left ventricular myocardium showing an interstitial lymphocytic infiltrate with degeneration and necrosis of myocytes. These sections were taken from patient 7, a 53-year-old woman who was found dead in bed, unexpectedly, 1 day after receiving her last dose of IL-2 (left, ×250; right, ×500).

included acute myocardial infarction associated with severe atherosclerotic coronary artery disease in one patient, noninfectious myocarditis in five patients, and bacterial myocarditis in one patient.

Clinical evidence of angina pectoris and acute myocardial infarction has been reported previously in patients receiving IL-2-based immunotherapy for cancer.[2,4–6] In addition to the patient described in this report in whom acute myocardial infarction was associated with severe atherosclerotic coronary artery disease and whose death occurred within 4 days of cessation of IL-2-based therapy, we have seen two additional cases at necropsy in which acute myocardial infarction occurred during therapy in the absence of atherosclerotic coronary artery disease but in whom death did not occur until later. The first patient[8] was a 53-year-old man who died 71 days after cessation of therapy, and necropsy disclosed cardiomegaly, biventricular dilatation, and a large transmural left ventricular circumferential infarct extending from apex to base. The second patient was a 20-year-old woman who died 21 days after therapy was stopped, and necropsy disclosed transmural left ventricular necrosis. In both of these cases, the epicardial coronary arteries were virtually devoid of atherosclerotic plaque. Thus, it appears that the profound

hypotension associated with IL-2 therapy can precipitate ischemic myocardial injury even in the absence of underlying atherosclerotic coronary artery disease.

Noninfectious myocarditis associated with IL-2-based immunotherapy has been described previously.[7,8] It is likely that myocarditis is responsible, at least in part, for the arrhythmias and decreased ejection fractions in patients receiving this therapy. The exact role that IL-2 plays in the development of myocarditis, however, is unknown.

The presence of a direct effect of IL-2 on myocardial function has not been identified in humans. Changes in myocyte contractility in response to IL-2, however, have been observed in rat myocyte cell cultures.[9] In addition, interleukin-1 and tumor necrosis factor, whose production may be stimulated by IL-2-based immunotherapy, decrease myocardial contractility in cell culture in response to β-adrenergic stimulation.[10]

We have not observed noninfectious myocarditis in other patients who died at intervals longer than 7 days after the cessation of therapy.[8] This observation suggests that it is either a transient phenomenon or that it occurs in patients who may have an increased susceptibility to IL-2 toxicity and subsequently die shortly after therapy. Because of the high frequency of myocarditis observed in our study and the potential for ischemic myocardial damage, patients receiving IL-2 should be monitored for the development of cardiac arrhythmias and cardiac failure during IL-2-based therapy.

REFERENCES

1. Gaynor ER, Vitek L, Sticklin L *et al.* The hemodynamic effects of treatment with interleukin-2 and lymphokine-activated killer cells. *Ann Intern Med* 1988; 109:953–958.

2. Nora R, Abrams JS, Tait NS, Hiponia DJ, Silverman HJ. Myocardial toxic effects during recombinant interleukin-2 therapy. *J Natl Cancer Inst* 1989; 81:59–63.

3. Lee RE, Lotze MT, Skibber JM *et al.* Cardiorespiratory effects of immunotherapy with interleukin-2. *J Clin Oncol* 1989; 7:7–20.

4. Rosenberg SA, Lotze MT, Muul LM *et al.* A progress report on the treatment of 157 patients with advanced cancer using lymphokine-activated killer cells and interleukin-2 or high dose interleukin-2 alone. *N Engl J Med* 1987; 316:889–897.

5. Fisher RI, Coltman CA, Doroshow JH *et al.* Metastatic renal cancer treated with interleukin-2 and lymphokine-activated killer cells. A phase II clinical trial. *Ann Intern Med* 1988; 108:518–523.

6. Rosenberg SA, Lotze MT, Yang JC *et al.* Experience with the use of high dose interleukin-2 in the treatment of 652 patients with cancer. *Ann Surg* 1989;210:474–485.

7. Samlowski WE, Ward JH, Craven CM, Freedman RA. Severe myocarditis following high dose interleukin-2 administration. *Arch Pathol Lab Med* 1989; 113:838–841.

8. Kragel AH, Travis WD, Feinberg L *et al.* Pathologic findings associated with interleukin-2 based immunotherapy for cancer: A postmortem study of 19 patients. *Hum Pathol* 1990;21:493–502.

9. Fink S, Finiasz M, Sterin-Borda L, Borda E, de Bracco MM. Interleukin 2 stimulates heart contractility in the presence of exogenous arachidonate or the calcium ionophore A 23187. *Immunol Lett* 1988; 17:183–188.

10. Gulick T, Chung MK, Pieper SJ, Lange LG, Schreiner GF. Interleukin 1 and tumor necrosis factor inhibit cardiac myocyte β-adrenergic responsiveness. *Proc Natl Acad Sci* 1989; 86:6753–6757.

Comparison of Coronary and Myocardial Morphologic Findings in Patients With and Without Thrombolytic Therapy During Fatal First Acute Myocardial Infarction

S. David Gertz, MD, PhD, Amy H. Kragel, MD, Jay M. Kalan, MD, Eugene Braunwald, MD, William C. Roberts, MD, and The TIMI Investigators

The hearts of 61 patients (39 men aged 64 ± 11 years) who died from 5 hours to 42 days (median 3 days) after a fatal first acute myocardial infarction without having undergone percutaneous transluminal coronary angioplasty or coronary bypass surgery were studied to compare clinical and cardiac morphologic features of patients receiving thrombolytic therapy with tissue-plasminogen activator (t-PA) to those not receiving thrombolytic therapy. Comparison of findings in the 23 patients who received t-PA intravenously 3 ± 1 hours after onset of symptoms, with the 38 patients who did not, showed similar baseline characteristics with respect to: age, gender, history of hypertension; location of the infarct; heart weight; severity and numbers of coronary arteries narrowed; and frequencies of plaque rupture, plaque hemorrhage and coronary thrombi. Among the patients receiving t-PA, however, there was a greater frequency of platelet-rich (fibrin-poor) thrombi in the infarct-related coronary arteries (6 of 11 vs 4 of 25 thrombi; p = 0.02), more nonocclusive than occlusive thrombi (6 of 11 vs 4 of 25 thrombi; p = 0.02), and a lower frequency of myocardial rupture (left ventricular free wall or ventricular septum) (5 of 23 [22%] vs 18 of 38 [46%]; p = 0.045).

(Am J Cardiol 1990;66:904–909)

From the Pathology Branch, National Heart, Lung, and Blood Institute, National Institutes of Health, Bethesda, Maryland; the Department of Anatomy and Embryology, The Hebrew University, Hadassah Medical School, Jerusalem, Israel; and the Department of Medicine, Brigham and Women's Hospital, Boston, Massachusetts. Manuscript received June 4, 1990, and accepted June 12.

Address for reprints: S. David Gertz, MD, Pathology Branch, National Heart, Lung, and Blood Institute, National Institutes of Health, Building 10, Room 2N258, Bethesda, Maryland 20892.

Administration of thrombolytic agents early in the course of acute myocardial infarction often restores the patency of occluded coronary arteries,[1] improves left ventricular function[2–4] and improves survival.[5] Early reperfusion frequently converts "ischemic" to hemorrhagic infarcts.[6] The frequencies of myocardial rupture and cardiogenic shock, degrees of coronary luminal narrowing and frequency of plaque rupture are similar between patients with hemorrhagic and nonhemorrhagic infarcts.[6] The present study of 61 patients after a fatal first acute myocardial infarction compares the clinical and cardiac morphologic features of patients who received thrombolytic therapy with recombinant tissue-plasminogen activator (t-PA) to those who did not.

METHODS

No patient had a healed (previous) myocardial infarct at necropsy, and none had undergone coronary artery bypass surgery or percutaneous transluminal coronary angioplasty. Of the 61 patients, 23 received thrombolytic therapy with t-PA during the acute myocardial infarction as participants in the Thrombolysis in Myocardial Infarction (TIMI) studies. (For full details concerning criteria for inclusion into the TIMI studies see references 1, 7 and 8). The Pathology Branch, National Heart, Lung, and Blood Institute, served as the central pathology laboratory for the TIMI study. The hearts of 23 patients were submitted from 16 different centers participating in the TIMI trial (see Appendix). One of these 23 patients underwent cardiac transplantation 40 days after treatment and is still alive. The remaining 38 patients did not receive thrombolytic therapy and thus were not participants in the TIMI studies. The hearts of these 38 patients were submitted to the Pathology Branch from 14 different centers (see Appendix) between 1960 and 1986. The criteria for selection of these hearts were the same as for those of the TIMI participants—no patient had a previous (healed) myocardial infarct, no patient had coronary artery bypass surgery and none had angioplasty.

The hearts were fixed in 10% buffered formaldehyde for at least 3 days. The epicardial coronary arteries were excised intact and lightly decalcified by the formic acid-sodium citrate method[9] for approximately 12 hours. The arteries were sectioned transversely at 5-mm intervals and the segments were labeled sequentially. All specimens were then dehydrated in ethanol and xylene and embedded in paraffin. One section (5 μ thick) from each 5-mm segment was stained by the Movat method[10] and another section from each 5-mm segment was stained with hematoxylin and eosin. The cardiac ventricles were cut transversely into slices approximately 1-cm thick from the apex to approximately 2-cm caudal to the posterior atrioventricular sulcus.

Luminal narrowing of the 4 major (left main, left anterior descending, left circumflex and the right) coronary arteries was determined by examination of histologic sections of each 5-mm segment. The degree of luminal narrowing for each segment was assessed by subdividing a circle, with the perimeter formed by the internal elastic lamina, into 4 equal quadrants.[11] These quadrants corresponded to the 4 degrees of reduction of luminal cross-sectional area—0 to 25, 26 to 50, 51 to 75 and 76 to 100%—with the latter being subdivided into 76 to 95 and 96 to 100%. In addition, a "coronary score" (of luminal narrowing) was calculated by assigning each of the 4 degrees of luminal narrowing a numerical value from 1 to 4. A 5-mm segment narrowed 0 to 25% in cross-sectional area had a score of 1, a segment narrowed 26 to 50%, a score of 2, and so forth. Each degree of narrowing was multiplied by the number of segments found to be narrowed by that degree. The sum for all 4 degrees of narrowing was then divided by the total number of segments studied for that artery, giving an overall coronary score from 0 to 4.

Plaque rupture was identified by a fissure within the atherosclerotic plaque that was associated with thrombus or hemorrhage into the plaque, with the defect in the plaque being continuous with the arterial lumen.

The amounts of fibrin, platelets and erythrocytes in thrombi were estimated microscopically on a 0 to 3+ scale (0 = none seen, 3+ = maximum seen). With observers not being aware of whether the patient received t-PA or did not, thrombi were estimated to be "platelet-rich" or "fibrin-rich" when the number of plusses scored for either component was greater than the number of plusses scored for the other.

Statistical comparisons of numerical data were performed by 2-tailed t tests (paired or unpaired as appropriate). Categorical data were compared by coded chisquare analysis. For these calculations the Stat View 512+ statistical package (Brain Power, Inc., Calabasas, California) was used in association with a Macintosh SE computer. All values reported are mean ± standard deviation.

RESULTS

Baseline characteristics: The 2 patient groups were quite similar; of the 61 patients with a fatal first acute myocardial infarct (39 men aged 64 ± 11 years), 23 received thrombolytic therapy with t-PA intravenously (doses as described previously[1,8,12]) within 3.1 ± 1.3 hours of onset of symptoms (Table I). Comparisons among patients receiving thrombolytic therapy with those who did not showed similar ages (62 ± 12 vs 65 ± 11 years; p = 0.22), gender (14 [61%] vs 25 [66%] men;

	TABLE I Baseline Clinical Characteristics in 61 Patients With First Fatal Acute Myocardial Infarction With and Without Thrombolytic Therapy		
	Thrombolytic Therapy		
	+ n = 23	0 n = 38	p Value
Age (years)	62 ± 12	65 ± 11	0.22
Men/women	14/9	25/13	0.70
Interval chest pain to			
rt-PA (hours)	3.1 ± 1.3	—	—
Death (days)	8 ± 12	8 ± 9	0.88
median	2.0	4.2	
History of hypertension	14	20 (n = 30)	0.66
Location of AMI [no. (%)]			
Anterior	9 (39)	16 (42)	0.82
Posterior	13 (57)	22 (58)	0.92
Lateral (only)	1 (4)	0	—
Right ventricle*	7 (30)	7 (18)	0.28
Heart weight (g)			
Men	460 ± 100	479 ± 117	0.60
Women	376 ± 84	408 ± 94	0.42
Dilated left ventricle [no. (%)]	11 (48)	15 (39)	0.52
Myocardial rupture [no. (%)]			
LVFW	2	11	
VS	3	7	
Total (%)	5 (22)	18 (47)	0.045

* Always associated with an infarct of the posterior wall of the left ventricle. Values are mean ± standard deviation.

AMI = acute myocardial infarction; LVFW = left ventricular free wall; VS = ventricular septum; + = yes, 0 = no.

p = 0.70), frequency of a history of systemic hypertension (14 of 23 [61%] vs 20 of 30 [67%]; p = 0.66), locations of the infarct (13 [57%] vs 22 [58%] posterior wall infarcts; p = 0.92), and heart weights by gender (men, 460 ± 100 g vs 479 ± 117 g, p = 0.60; women, 376 ± 84 g vs 408 ± 94 g, p = 0.42). The interval from chest pain to death for all 61 patients ranged from 5 hours to 42 days (mean 8 ± 11 days, median 3.2) with no significant difference between patients who received t-PA and those who did not (8 ± 12 days [median 2.0] vs 8 ± 9 days [median 4.2]; p = 0.88).

Myocardial rupture: The frequency of myocardial rupture was lower among patients who received thrombolytic therapy than those who did not (5 of 23 [22%] vs 18 of 38 [47%]; p = 0.045). The frequency of myocardial rupture among the subset of 29 patients who died within 72 hours of the onset of chest pain was also lower in patients who received thrombolytic therapy than in those who did not (3 of 15 [20%] vs 9 of 14 [64%]; p = 0.02).

Left ventricular dilatation: Left ventricular dilatation, judged by visual inspection at necropsy, occurred in 26 of 61 patients (43%), with similar frequencies between patients with and without thrombolytic therapy (11 [48%] vs 15 [39%]; p = 0.52) and between patients with and without myocardial rupture (8 [35%] vs 18 [47%]; p = 0.34).

Coronary arterial narrowing: Of the 61 patients, 60 had narrowing >75% of the luminal cross-sectional area by atherosclerotic plaque alone in at least 1 of the 4 major epicardial arteries: 8 patients (13%) had only 1 artery so narrowed; 9 patients (15%), 2 arteries; and 43 (70%), 3 or 4 arteries so narrowed. Nine patients (15%)

TABLE II Degrees of Luminal Cross-Sectional Narrowing by Atherosclerotic Plaque in Patients With and Without Thrombolytic Therapy for First Fatal Acute Myocardial Infarction

Thrombolytic Therapy (no.)	Mean % (± SD) 5-mm Coronary Segments Narrowed by Various Degrees in Cross-Sectional Area by Plaque					Coronary Score (mean ± SD)	No. (mean ± SD) of 5-mm Segments
	0–25%	26–50%	51–75%	76–95%	96–100%		
Four Major Epicardial Arteries							
+ (23)	13 ± 12	22 ± 12	34 ± 11	27 ± 14	2 ± 4	2.78 ± 0.49	1,025 (45 ± 9)
0 (38)	11 ± 12	20 ± 13	35 ± 12	31 ± 15	3 ± 4	2.90 ± 0.40	1,756 (46 ± 11)
p Value	0.55	0.68	0.92	0.36	0.88	0.32	
Infarct-Related Artery							
+	9 ± 17	18 ± 14	40 ± 18	32 ± 21	2 ± 4	2.97 ± 0.55	420 (18 ± 6)
0	9 ± 14	17 ± 14	33 ± 9	38 ± 22	2 ± 5	3.07 ± 0.51	647 (17 ± 8)
p Value	0.95	0.90	0.16	0.25	0.48	0.49	

SD = standard deviation; + = yes; 0 = no.

had severe narrowing of the left main coronary artery (>75%). The infarct-related arteries were narrowed >75% by plaque at some point in 59 of 61 patients (97%). Comparison between patients who received thrombolytic therapy and those who did not showed similar percentages with 3 or 4 arteries so narrowed (15 of 23 [65%] vs 28 of 38 [74%], p = 0.48) and similar percentages of patients with infarct-related arteries narrowed >75% by plaque at some point (21 of 23 [91%] vs 37 of 38 [97%], p = 0.99). Similar percentages of coronary segments narrowed to the 5 degrees (0 to 25, 26 to 50, 51 to 75, 76 to 95 and 96 to 100%) by atherosclerotic plaque were found in patients who had and who had not received thrombolytic therapy (Table II). The overall coronary score of luminal narrowing was similar between the 2 groups for all 4 major epicardial coronary arteries together (2.8 ± 0.5 vs 2.9 ± 0.4, p = 0.32) and for the infarct-related arteries analyzed independently (3.0 ± 0.6 vs 3.1 ± 0.5, p = 0.49).

Coronary thrombus: Coronary thrombi were found in the infarct-related artery at necropsy in 36 of the 61 patients (59%) (Figure 1). Of these 36 patients with thrombi at necropsy, 2 were among the 10 patients (20%) who died within 24 hours of the onset of chest pain, 13 were among the 19 (68%) patients who died between 24 and 72 hours, and 19 were among the 29 (66%) who died >72 hours after the onset of chest pain. The frequencies of thrombi among all patients who died within 72 hours compared with the frequencies in those who died >72 hours from onset of symptoms were similar between those who received thrombolytic therapy and those who did not. The frequencies of thrombi were similar between all patients who received thrombolytic therapy and those who did not (11 of 23 [48%] vs 25 of 38 [66%], p = 0.17) (Table III). However, the number of nonocclusive thrombi was greater in patients who had received thrombolytic therapy than in those who had not (nonocclusive thrombi: 6 of 11 [55%] vs 4 of 25 [16%] thrombi; p = 0.02).

A greater frequency of platelet-rich thrombi in the infarct-related coronary arteries was found in patients who received thrombolytic therapy than those who did not (6 of 11 [55%] vs 4 of 25 [16%]; p = 0.02), with a lower frequency of fibrin-rich thrombi in the group receiving thrombolytic therapy (3 of 11 [27%] vs 19 of 25 [76%], p = 0.006) (Table III).

Plaque rupture and plaque hemorrhage: Rupture of an atherosclerotic plaque was present in the infarct-related coronary artery in 37 of the 61 hearts (61%) (Table III), and an additional 3 patients (40 [66%]) had plaque rupture involving a non-infarct-related artery (Figure 1). The plaque rupture occurred at sites of pultaceous debris (pale-staining areas rich in extracellular lipid consisting of amorphous gruel with numerous cholesterol clefts and variable amounts of inflammatory and foam cell infiltrates) in all but 2 patients. Plaque rupture was found in 26 (72%) of the 36 sites of thrombi, and was associated with hemorrhage into the plaque in 34 (92%) of the 37 cases of plaque rupture. Hemorrhage into an atherosclerotic plaque was present at some point in the infarct-related artery in 45 (74%) of the 61 patients and in a non-infarct-related artery in an additional 4 patients (49 [80%]); it occurred at 27 (75%) of the 36 sites of thrombus formation.

The frequency of plaque rupture was similar between patients who received thrombolytic therapy and those who did not, whether the infarct-related arteries were considered independently (17 [74%] vs 20 [53%], p = 0.10) or all 4 major epicardial coronary arteries were considered together (17 [74%] vs 23 [61%], p = 0.29). The frequency of plaque hemorrhage was also similar between the 2 groups (the 4 major epicardial arteries, 19 [83%] vs 30 [79%], p = 0.73; the infarct-related arteries, 19 [83%] vs 26 [68%], p = 0.22).

Plaque rupture by itself resulted in total or near-total obstruction of the infarct-related artery in only 2 of the 23 patients who received thrombolytic therapy and in 2 of the 38 patients who did not receive t-PA. Of the

TABLE III Frequency of Luminal Thrombi, Plaque Rupture and Plaque Hemorrhage in the Infarct-Related Arteries of Patients With and Without Thrombolytic Therapy for First Fatal Acute Myocardial Infarction

| Thrombolytic Therapy (no.) | Coronary Thrombus | | | | Plaque Rupture (no. [%] pts.) | Hemorrhage into Plaque (no. [%] of pts.) |
| | Total No. (%) of Pts. | Occlusive No. (% of total) | Composition | | | |
			Platelet-Rich (no. [%])	Fibrin-Rich (no. [%])		
+ (23)	11 (48)	5 (45)	6 (55)	3 (27)	17 (74)	19 (83)
0 (38)	25 (66)	21 (84)	4 (16)	19 (76)	20 (53)	26 (68)
p Value	0.17	0.02	0.02	0.006	0.10	0.22

Abbreviations as in Table II.

TABLE IV Degrees of Luminal Cross-Sectional Area Narrowing at Sites of Plaque

| Thrombolytic Therapy | No. of S PR | No. (%) of S Narrowed in CSA by Plaque at Sites of PR | | | | |
		0–25%	25–50%	51–75%	76–95%	96–100%
+	42	0	1 (2)	10 (24)	29 (69)	2 (5)
0	59	0	2 (3)	17 (29)	37 (63)	3 (5)
Total	101	0	3 (3)	27 (27)	66 (65)	5 (5)

CSA = cross-sectional area; PR = plaque rupture; S = segments; + = yes; 0 = no.

total of 101 five-mm coronary segments with plaque rupture (from the 37 patients with plaque rupture), the lumen was narrowed 51 to 75% in cross-sectional area by plaque in 27 segments (27%); 76 to 95% in 66 segments (65%); and 96 to 100% in 5 segments (5%) (Figure 1). Similar degrees of narrowing at sites of plaque rupture were noted between patients who received thrombolytic therapy and those who did not (Table IV).

The mean percentages of all 5-mm segments of the 4 major coronary arteries with plaque rupture and plaque hemorrhage are listed in Table V. This analysis of the 46 ± 11 five-mm coronary segments from each of the 61 patients (total = 2,781 segments including 17 ± 8 segments from each infarct-related artery alone) disclosed similar frequencies of these structural features between patients who did and did not receive t-PA.

DISCUSSION

We studied the hearts of 61 patients who died shortly (mean 8 ± 11 days) after a first acute myocardial infarction: 23 of these had received intravenous thrombolytic therapy with t-PA an average of 3 ± 1 hours after the onset of chest pain, and 38 had not. Myocardial rupture (left ventricular free wall or ventricular septum) occurred in 38% of these 61 patients. An earlier study from this laboratory of patients dying during

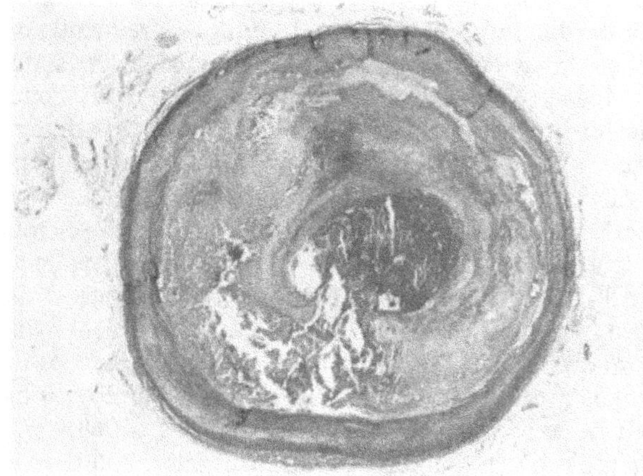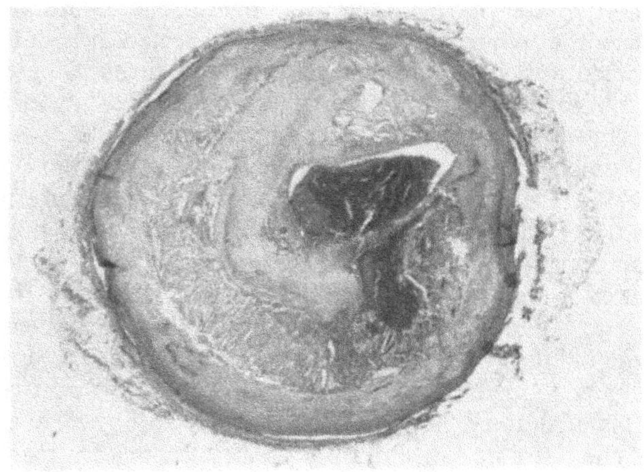

FIGURE 1. Rupture of atherosclerotic plaque in the infarct-related coronary artery of patients with first fatal acute myocardial infarction who did not receive thrombolytic therapy showing occlusion of the residual lumen by thrombus at sites of exposed pultaceous debris. By visual inspection, both lumens are narrowed 76 to 95% in cross-sectional area by atherosclerotic plaque alone. Right coronary artery *(left)* and left anterior descending coronary artery *(right)*. (Movat stains: × 15 *(left)*, × 20 *(right)*, reduced by 30%.)

TABLE V Mean Percent (± SD) of All 5-mm Segments with Plaque Rupture and Hemorrhage into a Plaque: Relation to Thrombolytic Therapy and to Interval from Chest Pain to Death

	IRA (no. of S = 1,067)		4 MEA (no. of S = 2,781)	
	PR	HIP	PR	HIP
Relation to Thrombolytic Therapy				
Thrombolytic therapy				
+	10 ± 9	17 ± 15	7 ± 7	9 ± 8
0	12 ± 16	15 ± 12	8 ± 10	7 ± 6
p Value	0.52	0.76	0.60	0.25
Relation to Interval from Chest Pain to Death				
>72 hours	14 ± 16	18 ± 23	8 ± 8	7 ± 6
<72 hours	9 ± 10	14 ± 15	7 ± 9	8 ± 7
p Value	0.20	0.43	0.55	0.50

HIP = hemorrhage into a plaque; IRA = infarct-related artery; MEA = major epicardial coronary arteries; SD = standard deviation. Other abbreviations as in Table IV.

acute myocardial infarction disclosed a higher frequency of myocardial rupture among those without a previous myocardial infarct (40%) compared to those with a previous (healed) infarct (13%),[13] and none of the patients included in the present study had a healed myocardial infarct. There has been concern that thrombolytic therapy might increase the frequency of rupture of the left ventricular free wall or ventricular septum during acute myocardial infarction. In the International Study of Infarct Survival-2 study, the frequency of myocardial rupture among all vascular deaths was apparently higher in patients treated with streptokinase within 24 hours of onset of chest pain than in those receiving placebo.[14] However, other studies have shown similar frequencies of cardiac rupture between patients who received thrombolytic therapy and control groups.[15,16]

The 61 patients comprising the present study died shortly after having their first myocardial infarction; thus, the frequency of rupture was expected to be, and indeed was, higher than in unselected patients dying of acute myocardial infarction. The frequency of myocardial rupture, however, was less in patients who received thrombolytic therapy (22%) than in those who did not (47%). This lower frequency of myocardial rupture in patients who received thrombolytic therapy was even more marked among those who died within 72 hours of onset of chest pain. One can argue that the higher frequency of myocardial rupture among our 38 patients who did not receive thrombolytic therapy might be due, in part, to selection bias from the 14 submitting centers. This laboratory, however, has received all or nearly all of the "cardiac cases" from 9 of these centers for many years accounting for 31, or 82%, of these cases. These results show that, even when considering the possibility of such bias, the previously feared increase in cardiac rupture in patients receiving thrombolytic therapy has not been confirmed.

The frequency at necropsy of thrombi in the infarct-related arteries of these patients with a fatal first acute myocardial infarction was not significantly lower in patients who received thrombolytic therapy than in those who did not. This finding does not imply that thrombolytic therapy fails to lyse coronary thrombi since our observations were limited to patients who died. Moreover, the frequency of occlusive thrombi was significantly lower in the t-PA–treated group, and this difference persisted when the analysis was restricted to patients who died within 72 hours of onset of chest pain. The greater frequency of platelet-rich, and lower frequency of fibrin-rich, thrombi in patients who had received t-PA supports suggestions that residual or recurrent thrombi in such patients are thrombolytic-resistant platelet-rich thrombi which might require treatment with an antiplatelet agent.[17]

Rupture of an atherosclerotic plaque was found at some point in the infarct-related artery in 61% of the total 61 patients and in 51% of patients who died >72 hours from the onset of chest pain. Similar frequencies of plaque rupture, and its usually associated hemorrhage, were found between patients who received thrombolytic therapy and those who did not. A number of angiographic and necropsy studies have suggested a direct pathogenetic relation between rupture of an atherosclerotic plaque, coronary thrombus formation and acute myocardial infarction.[18–24] In the present study, plaque rupture usually occurred at sites of pultaceous debris formation. The association of plaque rupture with sites of extensive lipid-rich pultaceous debris also has been emphasized by others.[25–28] Rupture of the atherosclerotic plaque, however, was found to be responsible itself for total or near-total obstruction of the infarct-related artery, resulting in 96 to 100% reduction in luminal cross-sectional area, in only 4 of the 37 patients with plaque rupture. In most patients with plaque rupture, it was the associated thrombus that appeared to account for the total, or almost total, luminal obstruction.

Recent angiographic studies have suggested that the degree of stenosis of infarct-related coronary arteries is not a reliable predictor of the time or location of future myocardial infarction, and that infarction frequently develops in association with infarct-related arteries that previously were not severely narrowed.[29,30] We found the lumen to be narrowed by <75% in cross-sectional area (<50% diameter reduction) in 30% of segments with plaque rupture—a finding that supports the concept that even moderately obstructing atherosclerotic plaques may rupture and be responsible for the patients' death, but this appears to be responsible in only a minority of such patients. In 65% of the segments with plaque rupture, the cross-sectional area narrowing ranged from 76 to 95%. Thrombolytic therapy would still be expected to be of value in most patients with plaque rupture (and nonresistant thrombi), and the fact that intravenous administration of t-PA is known to result in the restoration of vascular patency in approximately 75% of patients[1,7,8] does not exclude plaque rupture as an integral pathogenetic step in the evolution of acute myocardial infarction. However, even after successful thrombolysis, plaque rupture, with its associated exposed thrombogenic stimuli, remains a predisposing factor for thrombotic reocclusion, and this threat persists even after 72 hours.

The present study of hearts of patients dying a median of 2 to 4 days after their first myocardial infarction shows that those who received intraveous t-PA 3 ± 1 hours after onset of symptoms (compared to those with similar baseline characteristics who did not receive thrombolytic therapy) had greater frequencies of non-occlusive and platelet-rich (fibrin-poor) thrombi and a lower frequency of myocardial rupture.

Acknowledgment: We gratefully acknowledge the technical assistance of Leslie K. Berry, Alvado M. Campbell, Filippina M. Giacometti, Eutha E. Harrigan and Michael W. Spencer.

REFERENCES

1. Chesebro JH, Knatterud G, Roberts R, Borer J, Cohen LS, Dalen J, Dodge HT, Francis CK, Hillis D, Ludbrook P, Markis JE, Mueller H, Passamani ER, Powers ER, Rao AK, Robertson T, Ross A, Ryan TJ, Sobel BE, Willerson J, Williams DO, Zaret BL, Braunwald E. Thrombolysis in myocardial infarction (TIMI) trial, phase I: a comparison between intravenous tissue plasminogen activator and intravenous streptokinase: clinical findings through hospital discharge. *Circulation* 1987;76:142–154.
2. Serruys PW, Simoons ML, Suryapranata H, Vermeer F, Wijns W, van den Brand M, Bar F, Zwaan C, Hanno Krauss X, Remme WJ, Res J, Verheugt FWA, van Domburg R, Lubsen J, Hugenholtz PG. Preservation of global and regional left ventricular function after early thrombolysis in acute myocardial infarction. *J Am Coll Cardiol* 1986;7:729–742.
3. White HD, Norris RM, Brown MA, Takayama M, Maslowski A, Bass NM, Ormiston JA, Whitlock T. Effect of intravenous streptokinase on left ventricular function and early survival after acute myocardial infarction. *N Engl J Med* 1987;317:850–855.
4. O'Rourke M, Baron D, Keogh A, Kelly R, Nelson G, Barnes C, Raftos J, Graham K, Hillman K, Newman H, Healey J, Woolridge J, Rivers J, White H, Whitlock R, Norris R. Limitation of myocardial infarction by early infusion of recombinant tissue-type plasminogen activator. *Circulation* 1988;77:1311–1315.
5. Gruppo Italiano Per Lo Studio Della Streptochinasi Nell'infarto Miocardico (GISSI). Effectiveness of intravenous thrombolytic treatment in acute myocardial infarction. *Lancet* 1986;1:397–401.
6. Gertz SD, Kalan JM, Kragel AH, Roberts WC, Braunwald E, TIMI Investigators. Cardiac morphologic finding in patients with acute myocardial infarction treated with recombinant tissue plasminogen activator. *Am J Cardiol* 1990;65:953–961.
7. The TIMI Research Group. Immediate vs delayed catheterization and angioplasty following thrombolytic therapy for acute myocardial infarction: TIMI II A results. *JAMA* 1988;260:2849–2858.
8. The TIMI Study Group. Comparison of invasive and conservative strategies after treatment with intravenous tissue plasminogen activator in acute myocardial infarction. Results of the thrombolysis in myocardial infarction (TIMI) phase II trial. *N Engl J Med* 1989;320:618–627.
9. Luna LG. Manual of Histological Staining Methods of the Armed Forces Institute of Pathology. 3rd ed. New York, McGraw-Hill, 1968:8.
10. Movat H. Demonstration of all connective tissue elements in a single section. *Arch Pathol Lab Med* 1955;60:289–295.
11. Brosius FC, Roberts WC. Comparison of degree and extent of coronary narrowing by atherosclerotic plaque in anterior and posterior transmural acute myocardial infarction. *Circulation* 1981;64:715–722.
12. Mueller HS, Rao AK, Forman SA, The TIMI Investigators. Thrombolysis in myocardial infarction (TIMI): Comparative studies of coronary reperfusion and systemic fibrinolysis with two forms of recombinant tissue-type plasminogen activator. *J Am Coll Cardiol* 1987;10:479–490.
13. Reddy SG, Roberts WC. Frequency of rupture of the left ventricular free wall or ventricular septum among necropsy cases of fatal acute myocardial infarction since introduction of coronary care units. *Am J Cardiol* 1989;63:906–911.
14. ISIS-2 Collaborative Group. Randomised trial of intravenous streptokinase, oral aspirin, both, or neither among 17,187 cases of suspected acute myocardial infarction ISIS-2. *Lancet* 1988;2:349–360.
15. Yusuf S, Collins R, Peto R, Furberg C, Stampfer MJ, Goldhaber SZ, Hennekens CH. Intravenous and intracoronary fibrinolytic therapy in acute myocardial infarction: overview of results on mortality, reinfarction and side-effects from 33 randomized controlled trials. *Eur Heart J* 1985;6:556–585.
16. The ISAM Study Group. A prospective trial of intranveous streptokinase in acute myocardial infarction (ISAM): mortality, morbidity and infarct size at 21 days. *N Engl J Med* 1986;314:1465–1471.
17. Jang I-K, Gold HK, Ziskind AA, Fallon JT, Holt RE, Leinbach RC, May JW, Collen D. Differential sensitivity of erythrocyte-rich and platelet-rich arterial thrombi to lysis with recombinant tissue-type plasminogen activator. A possible explanation for resistance to coronary thrombolysis. *Circulation* 1989;79:920–928.
18. Friedman M, Van Den Bovenkamp GJ. The pathogenesis of a coronary thrombus. *Am J Pathol* 1966;48:19–31.
19. Ridolfi RL, Hutchins GM. The relationship between coronary artery lesions and myocardial infarcts: ulceration of atherosclerotic plaques precipitating coronary thrombosis. *Am Heart J* 1977;93:468–486.
20. Horie T, Sekiguchi M, Hirosawa K. Coronary thrombosis in pathogenesis of acute myocardial infarction: histopathological study of coroary arteries in 108 necropsied cases using serial section. *Br Heart J* 1978;40:153–161.
21. Ambrose JA, Winters SL, Stern A, Eng E, Teichholz LE, Gorlin R, Fuster V. Angiographic morphology and the pathogenesis of unstable angina pectoris. *J Am Coll Cardiol* 1985;5:609–616.
22. Falk E. Morphologic features of unstable atherothrombotic plaques underlying acute coronary syndromes. *Am J Cardiol* 1989;63:114E–120E.
23. Muller JE, Tofler GH, Stone PH. Circadian variation and triggers of onset of acute cardiovascular disease. *Circulation* 1989;79:733–743.
24. Alpert JS. The pathophysiology of acute myocardial infarction. *Cardiology* 1989;76:85–95.
25. Falk E. Plaque rupture with severe pre-existing stenosis precipitating coronary thrombosis: characteristics of coronary atherosclerotic plaques underlying fatal occlusive thrombi. *Br Heart J* 1983;50:127–134.
26. Tracy RE, Devaney K, Kissling G. Characteristics of the plaque under a coronary thrombus. *Virchows Arch (Pathol Anat)* 1985;405:411–427.
27. Davies MJ, Thomas AC. Plaque fissuring-the cause of acute myocardial infarction, sudden ischaemic death, and crescendo angina. *Br Heart J* 1985;53:363–373.
28. Richardson PD, Davies MJ, Born GVR. Influence of plaque configuration and stress distribution on fissuring of coronary atherosclerotic plaques. *Lancet* 1989;2:941–944.
29. Little WC, Constantinescu M, Applegate RJ, Kutcher MA, Burrows MT, Kahl FR, Santamore WP. Can angiography predict the site of a subsequent myocardial infarction in patients with mild-to-moderate coronary artery disease? *Circulation* 1988;78:1157–1166.
30. Ambrose JA, Tannenbaum MA, Alexopoulos D, Hjemdahl-monsen CE, Leavy J, Weiss M, Borrico S, Gorlin R, Fuster V. Angiographic progression of coronary artery disease and the development of myocardial infarction. *J Am Coll Cardiol* 1988;12:56–62.

APPENDIX

List of Submitting Medical Centers (TIMI Patients):

Baystate Medical Center, Springfield, MA; Baylor College of Medicine, Houston, TX (Ben Taub General Hospital and Methodist Hospital); Boston University, Boston, MA (Boston University Hospital and Boston City Hospital); Columbia University, New York, NY (Columbia Presbyterian Medical Center); Cornell Medical Center, New York, NY (New York Hospital); George Washington University Hospital, Washington, DC; Harvard University, Beth Israel Hospital, Boston, MA; Mayo Clinic and Foundation, Rochester, MN; New York Medical College, Valhalla, NY (United Hospital); Northwestern University, Chicago, IL (Evanston, Hospital); University of Alabama at Birmingham, Birmingham, AL (Carraway Methodist Medical Center); University of Massachusetts Medical Center, Worcester, MA; Yeshiva University, Albert Einstein College of Medicine, New York, NY (New Rochelle Hospital).

Non–TIMI Patients: National Institutes of Health, National Heart, Lung, and Blood Institute, Bethesda, MD; District of Columbia Medical Examiners Office, Washington, DC; District of Columbia Veterans Administration Hospital, Washington, DC; National Naval Medical Center, Bethesda, MD; George Washington University Medical Center, Washington, DC; Georgetown University Medical Center, Washington, DC; Suburban Hospital, Bethesda, MD; Emory University Hospital, Atlanta, GA; Washington Adventist Hospital, Takoma Park, MD; Franklin Square Hospital, Baltimore, MD; Mt. Sinai Medical Center, Miami Beach, FL; St. Vincent Health Center, Erie, PA; Hollywood Presbyterian Medical Center, Los Angeles, CA; Prince William Hospital, Manassas, VA.

Sudden Death Behind the Wheel from Natural Disease in Drivers of Four-Wheeled Motorized Vehicles

David H. Antecol, MD, and William C. Roberts, MD

The heart was studied in 30 persons who died suddenly from natural causes in the driver's seat of an automobile, truck or bus. Twenty had cardiac arrest while driving and the other 10 while sitting in the driver's seat of a parked vehicle. Of the 20 drivers, 16 died from atherosclerotic coronary artery disease (CAD): 12 (75%) had minor collisions and 4 did not. Of the 16 with fatal CAD, an average of 2.3 ± 0.8 of the 4 major coronary arteries were narrowed >75% in cross-sectional area (CSA) by plaque; of 668 five-mm segments of the 4 major (right, left main, left anterior descending, left circumflex) coronary arteries in 13 of these 16 cases, 27 (4%) were narrowed 96 to 100% and 127 (19%) were narrowed 76 to 95% in CSA by plaque. The remaining 4 drivers died from noncoronary conditions: aortic rupture associated with the Marfan syndrome in 1; cardiac sarcoidosis in 1; thoracic aortic dissection in 1; and severe mitral regurgitation from infective endocarditis, which had healed in 1. The other 10 persons were found dead in the driver's seat of a parked vehicle and 8 of them had fatal CAD. Of the 8 CAD victims, an average of 2.5 ± 1.2 of the 4 major coronary arteries was narrowed >75% by plaque; of the 283 five-mm segments of coronary arteries in 7 of the 8 cases, 44 (16%) were narrowed 96 to 100% and 69 (24%) were narrowed 76 to 95% in CSA by plaque.

Victims dying suddenly from CAD while driving are similar to other out-of-hospital sudden coronary death victims with respect to mean age, gender, heart weight, frequency of healed myocardial infarcts, number of major epicardial coronary arteries severely narrowed, and the percentage of 5-mm-long segments of the major arteries severely narrowed by atherosclerotic plaque. Most drivers stopped the vehicle without injury to themselves or to others.

(Am J Cardiol 1990;66:1329–1335)

From the Pathology Branch, National Heart, Lung, and Blood Institute, National Institutes of Health, Bethesda, Maryland. Manuscript received June 21, 1990; revised manuscript received July 19, 1990, and accepted July 20.

Dr. Antecol's present address is the Division of Cardiology, Department of Medicine, 2C2 Walter Mackenzie Health Sciences Center, University of Alberta, Edmonton, Alberta, Canada.

Address for reprints: William C. Roberts, MD, Pathology Branch, Building 10, Room 2N258, National Institutes of Health, Bethesda, Maryland 20892.

In the USA approximately 50,000 deaths occur each year from accidents involving 4-wheeled motorized vehicles, a death rate of 20/100,000 population.[1] Most deaths are the result of trauma incurred by the accident. Some deaths, however, occur in occupants of 4-wheeled motorized vehicles as a result of natural causes, and an accident may or may not result when the sudden illness affects the vehicle's driver. The most common cause of sudden death from natural disease in drivers is cardiovascular disease, and coronary artery disease (CAD) is by far the most common of them. Myerburg and Davis[2] in 1964 analyzed medical examiners' reports in 1,348 cases of natural death from CAD in their local medical examiner's office, and found that 71 (5%) occurred in drivers; 24 accidents (34%), all minor, resulted from these 71 deaths. Bowen[3] in 1973 analyzed medical examiner's reports in 9,330 cases of sudden death from CAD and found that 98 (1%) occurred in drivers: 46 accidents (47%), all minor, resulted from these 98 deaths. In the present report we examined the heart and major arteries and reports of other body organs in 30 persons who died behind the wheel from natural disease; 12 (40%) deaths resulted in accidents, all minor. The major focus of this report is on the extent of CAD present and on the frequency and types of myocardial lesions.

METHODS

Cases studied: Records from the Pathology Branch, National Heart, Lung, and Blood Institute, were searched for cases of sudden natural death that occurred in the driver's seat of automobiles, trucks, or buses. On the basis of findings at necropsy, the cases were divided into 3 groups: group I, fatal cardiac arrest from significant (>75% cross-sectional area [CSA] narrowing of 1 or more arteries) CAD while driving, 16 cases; group II, sudden natural death not due to CAD while driving, 4 cases; and group III, persons found dead in the driver's seat of a parked vehicle but who were not known to be driving at the onset of the terminal event, 10 cases. The autopsies in all 30 subjects were performed at 1 of 4 local institutions, and subsequently the hearts were submitted to the Pathology Branch for study. Available clinical records, autopsy records and police reports were examined in all 30 subjects.

Examination of heart: The hearts were fixed in 10% buffered formalin for at least 24 hours before weighing and examination. The major (left main, left anterior descending, left circumflex, and right) epicardial coronary arteries were excised intact after fixation. The arteries

TABLE I Clinical and Morphologic Observations of Drivers

Case	Cause of Death	Age (yrs) & Sex	AP	AMI	CHF	Duration of Symptoms of Heart Disease (yrs)	SH	DM	Blood Alcohol Present	HW (g)	N	F	RV	LV	No. of Major Coronary Arteries Narrowed >75% CSA	No. of 5-mm Segments Examined	0–25%	26–50%	51–75%	76–95%	96–100%	Coronary Thrombus
				History of							LV		Chamber Dilation				Percent of 5-mm Segments Narrowed in CSA					
16 Drivers with Cardiac Arrest Associated with Coronary Artery Disease While Driving and Without Significant Bodily Injury (Group I)																						
1	CAD	38M	0	0	0	—	—	—	0	480	0	0	+	0	3	47	6	9	40	32	13	0
2	CAD	38M	—	+	+	3	—	—	0	550	0	+(T)	+	+	2	37	22	24	35	19	0	0
3	CAD	51M	—	—	—	—	—	—	0	555	0	+(E)	+	+	1	63	41	30	25	3	0	0
4	CAD	52M	+	—	—	2	—	—	—	370	0	0	0	0	2	41	10	22	49	20	0	0
5	CAD	52M	+	+	—	10	+	—	—	370	+(T)	+(SE)	0	0	3	50	14	32	42	8	4	+(NO)
6	CAD	53M	—	—	—	—	—	—	0	415	0	0	0	0	3	52	10	21	42	27	0	+(O)
7	CAD	54M	+	+(a)	+	1.3	+	—	0	690	0	+(T)	0	+	3(a)	0	—	—	—	—	—	—
8	CAD	54M	—	—	—	—	+	+	0	550	0	+(T)	0	+	3	40	0	25	38	35	3	0
9	CAD	56M	—	—	—	—	—	—	0	490	0	+(T)	+	+	3	60	8	15	43	20	13	0
10	CAD	56M	—	+	+	—	+	—	0	550	0	+(E)	+	+	1	48(b)	60	27	8	4	0	0
11	CAD	57M	—	+	—	—	+	—	—	430	0	+(T)	0	+	2	43(b)	49	21	16	14	0	0
12(c)	CAD	60F	—	—	—	—	—	+	0	480	+(T)	0	0	0	1	66	86	9	2	3	0	+(NO)
13(c, d)	CAD	60M	—	+	+	4	—	—	—	—	+(T)	+(T)	0	0	≥1	0	—	—	—	—	—	—
14	CAD	63M	—	—	—	—	—	—	0	590	0	+(T)	0	0	2	0	—	—	—	—	—	—
15	CAD	63M	—	—	—	—	—	—	0	610	0	+(SE)	+	+	2	59	19	17	39	22	3	0
16	CAD	66M	—	—	—	—	—	—	0	705	0	+(T)	+	+	3	62	10	5	42	34	10	0
4 Drivers who Became Unconscious While Driving and Death was not from Coronary Artery Disease or Significant Bodily Injury (Group II)																						
17(e)	Aortic rupture	21M	0	0	0	—	0	0	—	460	0	0	+	+	0	54	96	4	0	0	0	0
18(f)	Cardiac sarcoidosis	35M	0	0	0	—	—	0	0	570	0	0	+	+	0	45	84	13	2	0	0	0
19(g)	Healed IE, MR	37M	—	—	+	3	—	—	0	800	0	0	+	+	0	64	98	2	0	0	0	0
20(h)	Aortic dissection	69F	—	—	—	—	—	—	—	400	0	0	0	0	2	31	16	13	48	19	3	0

(a), coronary bypass surgery and left ventricular aneurysm resection 9 months before death; one saphenous vein graft occluded at autopsy.
(b), left main coronary artery not available.
(c), severe anoxic brain injury with biologic death 2 weeks later.
(d), acute myocardial infarct 3 weeks before fatal cardiac arrest while driving.
(e), Marfan syndrome, aortic regurgitation, mitral valve prolapse.
(f), a passenger on the bus took over control and stopped the bus safely.
(g), backed into a fence then stopped and died a few minutes later in the vehicle.
(h), functionally normal bicuspid aortic valve.
(i), right coronary artery from the left sinus of Valsalva; right coronary artery courses between the aorta and pulmonary trunk; healed right ventricular infarct; left main and left anterior descending coronary arteries not available.
(j), left anterior descending artery tunneled for 3 cm.
(k), sexual activity inferred immediately before death.
(l), jogging inferred before death.
(m), left main, left anterior descending, and left circumflex coronary arteries not available.
AMI = acute myocardial infarct; AP = angina pectoris; CAD = coronary artery disease; CHF = congestive heart failure; CSA = cross-sectional area; DM = diabetes mellitus; E = subepicardial; F = fibrosis; HW = heart weight; IE = infective endocarditis; LV = left ventricle; MR = mitral regurgitation; N = necrosis; NO = nonocclusive; O = occlusive; RV = right ventricle; SAH = subarachnoid hemorrhage; SE = subendocardial; SH = history of systemic hypertension; T = transmural.

TABLE I Continued

10 Victims Found Dead in the Driver's Seat of a Parked Vehicle and who were not Known to be Driving at the Onset of the Terminal Event (Group III)

21	SAH	38M	—	—	—	—	+	—	—	380	0	0	0	0	0	55	100	0	0	0	0	0
22	CAD	41M	+	—	—	1.5	+	—	—	325	0	0	0	0	3	35	0	17	26	29	29	+(O)
23 (i)	CAD	49M	—	—	+	6	—	—	0	540	0	+(T)	0	+	1	29 (i)	72	7	18	3	0	—
24	CAD	50M	+	0	0	3.5	0	0	—	450	0	0	+	+	4	50	20	8	40	30	2	0
25	Unknown	51M	—	—	—	—	—	—	+	410	0	0	0	0	0	50	88	12	0	0	0	0
26 (j)	CAD	56M	0	0	0	—	0	0	—	565	0	0	0	0	1	0	—	—	—	—	—	—
27	CAD	56M	—	—	—	—	+	—	0	640	0	0	0	0	4	48	2	4	42	33	19	0
28 (k)	CAD	59M	—	+	—	>1	—	—	0	630	0	+(T)	0	+	3	65	3	15	28	25	29	0
29 (l)	CAD	59M	0	+	0	4	0	0	—	220	0	+(T)	0	+	2	41	32	29	17	17	5	0
30	CAD	62F	—	0	+	1	—	—	0	465	0	+(T)	+	+	2	15 (m)	7	13	33	27	20	—

(a), coronary bypass surgery and left ventricular aneurysm resection 9 months before death; one saphenous vein graft occluded at autopsy.
(b), left main coronary artery not available.
(c), severe anoxic brain injury with biologic death 2 weeks later.
(d), acute myocardial infarct 3 weeks before fatal cardiac arrest while driving.
(e), Marfan syndrome, aortic regurgitation, mitral valve prolapse.
(f), a passenger on the bus took over control and stopped the bus safely.
(g), backed into a fence then stopped and died a few minutes later in the vehicle.
(h), functionally normal bicuspid aortic valve.
(i), right coronary artery from the left sinus of Valsalva; right coronary artery courses between the aorta and pulmonary trunk; healed right ventricular infarct; left main and left anterior descending coronary arteries not available.
(j), left anterior descending artery tunneled for 3 cm.
(k), sexual activity inferred immediately before death.
(l), jogging inferred before death.
(m), left main, left anterior descending, and left circumflex coronary arteries not available.
AMI = acute myocardial infarct; AP = angina pectoris; CAD = coronary artery disease; CHF = congestive heart failure; CSA = cross-sectional area; DM = diabetes mellitus; E = subepicardial; F = fibrosis; HW = heart weight; IE = infective endocarditis; LV = left ventricle; MR = mitral regurgitation; N = necrosis; NO = nonocclusive; O = occlusive; RV = right ventricle; SAH = subarachnoid hemorrhage; SE = subendocardial; SH = history of systemic hypertension; T = transmural.

TABLE II Clinical and Cardiac Morphologic Observations in the 30 Drivers

	Group I Sudden Death While Driving Due to CAD (n = 16)	Group II Sudden Death While Driving Not Due to CAD (n = 4)	Group III Sudden Death Behind Wheel Vehicle Parked (n = 10)
Mean age ± SD (years)	55 ± 8	41 ± 20	52 ± 8
Men/women	15/1	3/1	9/1
Angina pectoris	3	0	2
Past acute myocardial infarction (history)	6	0	2
Congestive heart failure (history)	4	1	2
Systemic hypertension (history)	5	0	3
Diabetes mellitus (history)	2	0	0
Type of collision (no.):			
None	4	3	10
Parked vehicles only	4	0	—
Single-MVA, no parked vehicles	5	1	—
Multiple-MVA	3	0	—
Damage to driver's vehicle (no.):			
None	5	4	10
Minor	10	0	—
Major	1	0	—
Damage to other vehicles (no.):			
Minor	9	0	—
Major	1	0	—
Property damage (no.)	4	1	—
Blood alcohol present	0	0	1
Heart weight ±SD (g)	522 ± 103 (15)	558 ± 176	463 ± 135
HW >400 g (men); HW >350 g (women)	13/15	4	7
LV necrosis	3	0	0
LV fibrosis	12	0	4
RV dilation	7	3	2
LV dilation	9	3	5
No. of CAs narrowed >75% in CSA by plaque:			
0	0	3	2
1	3*	0	2
2	5*	1	2
3	7*	0	2
4	0*	0	2
Mean No. of CAs narrowed >75% in CSA by plaque ±SD	2.3 ± 0.8*	0.5 ± 1.0	2.0 ± 1.5
Nonocclusive coronary thrombus	2/13	0	0/7
Occlusive coronary thrombus	1/13	0	1/7

* One victim was not included here because although at least 1 coronary artery was severely narrowed, it was not known precisely how many were severely narrowed.
CA = coronary artery; MVA = motor vehicle accident; SD = standard deviation; other abbreviations as in Table I.

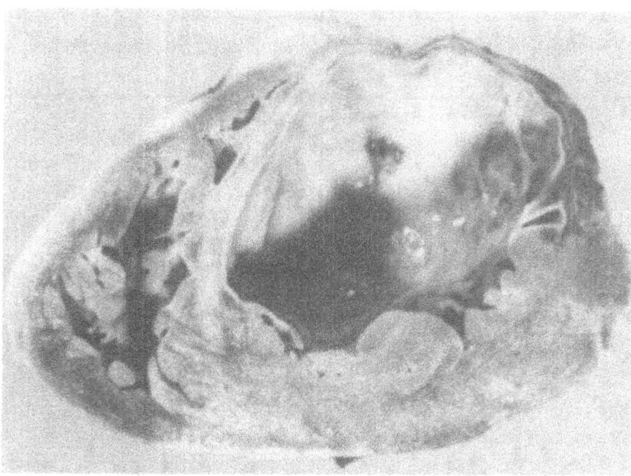

FIGURE 1. Case 2, Table I. Opened cardiac ventricles showing a healed large anterior wall infarct which is aneurysmal in a 38-year-old man (DCMEO #85-07-598). He had had evidence of congestive heart failure before his sudden death while driving.

then were decalcified if necessary with formic acid-sodium citrate for at least 24 hours. The coronary arteries then were cut transversely into 5-mm-long segments and labeled sequentially from origin to termination by a method described elsewhere.[4] The 5-mm segments were dehydrated in ethanol and xylene, and embedded in paraffin. At least one 6-μ-thick histologic section was cut from each 5-mm segment and stained by the Movat method. The percent CSA luminal narrowing by atherosclerotic plaque was determined by microscopic examination with approximately 40 times magnification. The percent luminal narrowing was graded into 1 of 5 CSA categories: 0 to 25, 26 to 50, 51 to 75, 76 to 95 and 95 to 100%. The accuracy of this technique of grading CSA narrowing has been validated to be >95%.[5] Histologic sections, at least 2 per heart, extending from

endocardium to epicardium of the left ventricle, were prepared. Foci of myocardial necrosis or fibrosis were confirmed histologically.

RESULTS

Clinical and terminal event features in each of the 30 subjects, divided by the 3 groups, are detailed in Table I, summarized in Table II, and some hearts are illustrated in Figures 1 to 7.

Etiology of deaths: All 20 subjects who died suddenly from natural causes while driving (groups I and II) died from cardiovascular disease: CAD in 16 (80%) and 1 each from rupture of the thoracic aorta in the Marfan syndrome; cardiac sarcoidosis; severe mitral regurgitation from infective endocarditis that had healed; and rupture of an aortic dissection. Of the 10 persons found dead in the driver's seat of a parked vehicle (group III), 8 died from CAD. Case 23 (Table I) had origin of the right coronary artery from the left sinus of Valsalva and it coursed between the aorta and pulmonary trunk.

Previous symptomatic myocardial ischemia: Angina pectoris or acute myocardial infarction that had healed and/or congestive heart failure was known to be present in 7 (44%) of the 16 group I subjects, in none of the 4 group II subjects, and in 6 of the 10 group III victims. A coronary bypass operation with simultaneous resection of a left ventricular aneurysm had been performed earlier in 1 subject (case 7).

Accidents: Among the 16 group I cases, 4 collisions occurred with parked vehicles only, 5 collisions involved property damage apart from other vehicles, 3 collisions were with other operating vehicles (1 head-on, 1 broadside, 1 rear-end), and no collision occurred in 4 cases. Therefore, an accident occurred in 12 (75%) group I subjects. These collisions resulted in minor damage to 10 drivers' vehicles and to 9 other vehicles, and major damage to 1 driver's vehicle and to 1 other vehicle. Only

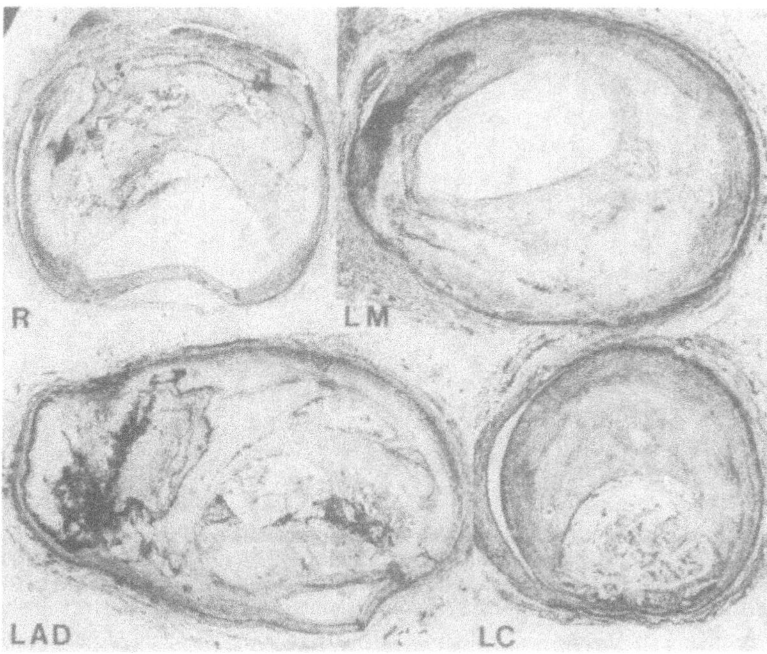

FIGURE 2. Case 5. Photomicrographs of sites of maximal narrowing of the right (R), left main (LM), left anterior descending (LAD) and left circumflex (LC) coronary arteries in a 52-year-old man (SH #A80-47) with previous angina pectoris. A large acute myocardial infarct was found at necropsy. (Movat stain, original magnification of each × 26, reduced 34%.)

1 collision occurred in the 4 group II subjects, and it involved non-vehicle property damage and no damage to the driver's vehicle. In case 18, an accident was prevented by a passenger on the bus who took over control when the driver collapsed. In the 16 group I subjects, 4 (25%) received minor body injuries. Only 1 driver in group I had passengers, and the 3 passengers in his taxi were not injured in the collision. No injuries and no fatalities occurred to passengers in the drivers' vehicles, to occupants of other vehicles or to pedestrians.

Blood alcohol levels: No blood alcohol or illicit mind-altering drugs were present in any of the drivers in whom this information was known (Table I). The cause of death was undetermined in the 1 subject with a positive blood alcohol level (case 25).

Myocardial damage: Left ventricular necrosis was present in 3 (19%) of the 16 drivers in group I; 2 of these drivers (cases 12 and 13) had been severely brain injured from anoxia during the cardiac arrest while driving and proceeded to biologic death 2 weeks later. In addition, case 13 had been hospitalized for an acute myocardial infarct 3 weeks before the cardiac arrest while driving. Left ventricular fibrosis was present in 12 (75%) of the 16 group I victims, and in 4 of the 10 group III victims.

Coronary arteries: In the 16 drivers who died suddenly from CAD, the mean number of coronary arteries narrowed >75% in CSA by atherosclerotic plaque was 2.3 (standard deviation 0.8): 3 (20%) had 1 artery so narrowed; 5 (33%) had 2 arteries, and 7 (47%) had 3 arteries so narrowed. One had >75% CSA narrowing of at least 1 coronary artery, but the exact number so narrowed is not known. None had a left main coronary artery narrowed >75% in CSA. In addition, the 1 subject with previous cardiac surgery (case 7) had total oc-

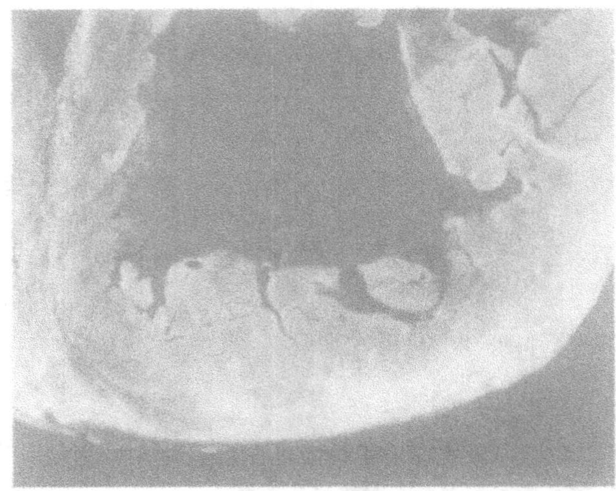

FIGURE 3. Case 10. Healed subepicardial infarct of the left ventricular free wall with left ventricular dilation in a 56-year-old man (DCMEO #88-01-68) with a previous clinical event compatible with acute myocardial infarction with evidence of congestive heart failure thereafter.

clusion of 1 of 2 saphenous vein bypass grafts. The coronary arteries were available for histologic review in 13 of 16 group I cases, and from them 668 five-mm-long segments were examined. The mean percents of 5-mm segments narrowed in CSA by 0 to 25, 26 to 50, 51 to 75, 76 to 95 and 96 to 100% were 26, 20, 33, 19 and 4%, respectively. In the 8 group III victims with CAD, the mean number of major epicardial coronary arteries narrowed >75% CSA was 2.5 (standard deviation 1.2): 2 had 1 artery so narrowed; 2 had 2 arteries so narrowed; 2 had 3 arteries so narrowed; and 2 had 4 arteries so narrowed. Of the 283 five-mm segments of coronary artery in 7 of these 8 victims, 44 (16%) were nar-

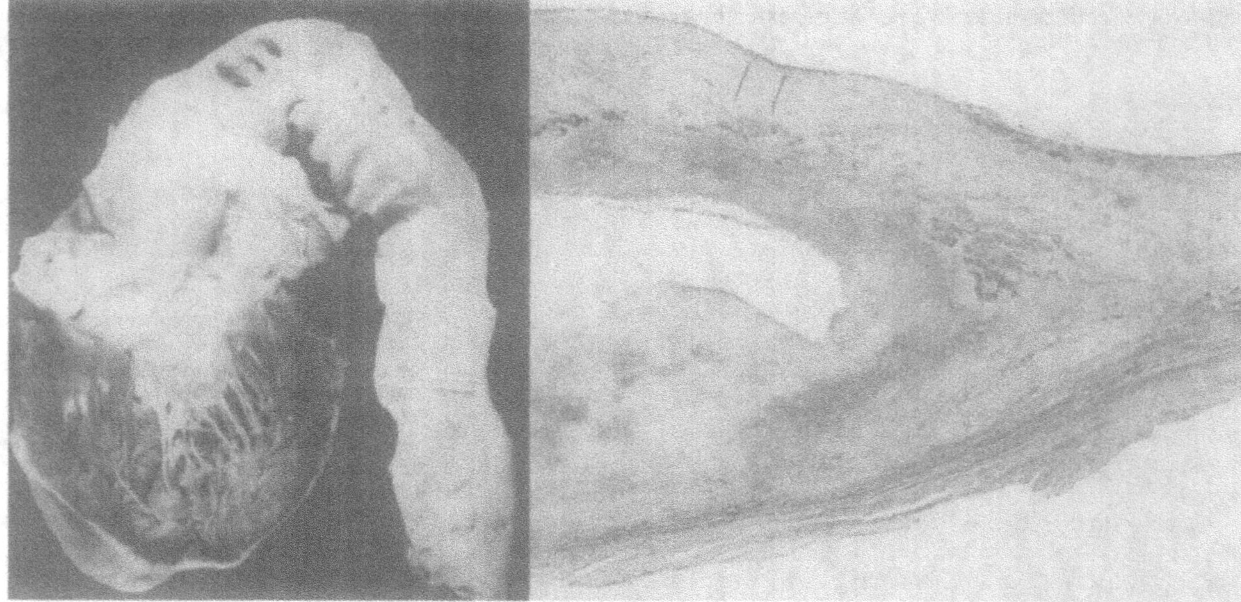

FIGURE 4. Case 17. Heart and aorta in a 21-year-old man (A67-120) with the Marfan syndrome who died suddenly from rupture of the thoracic aorta after parking his car in his garage. A tear is present in the ascending aorta, which is quite dilated. This patient was known to have had aortic regurgitation since childhood. A photomicrograph of a healed tear in ascending aorta is shown on the right. The media is virtually depleted of elastic fibers, the classic aortic lesion of the Marfan syndrome. (Elastic van Gieson stain, original magnification × 19, reduced 23%.)

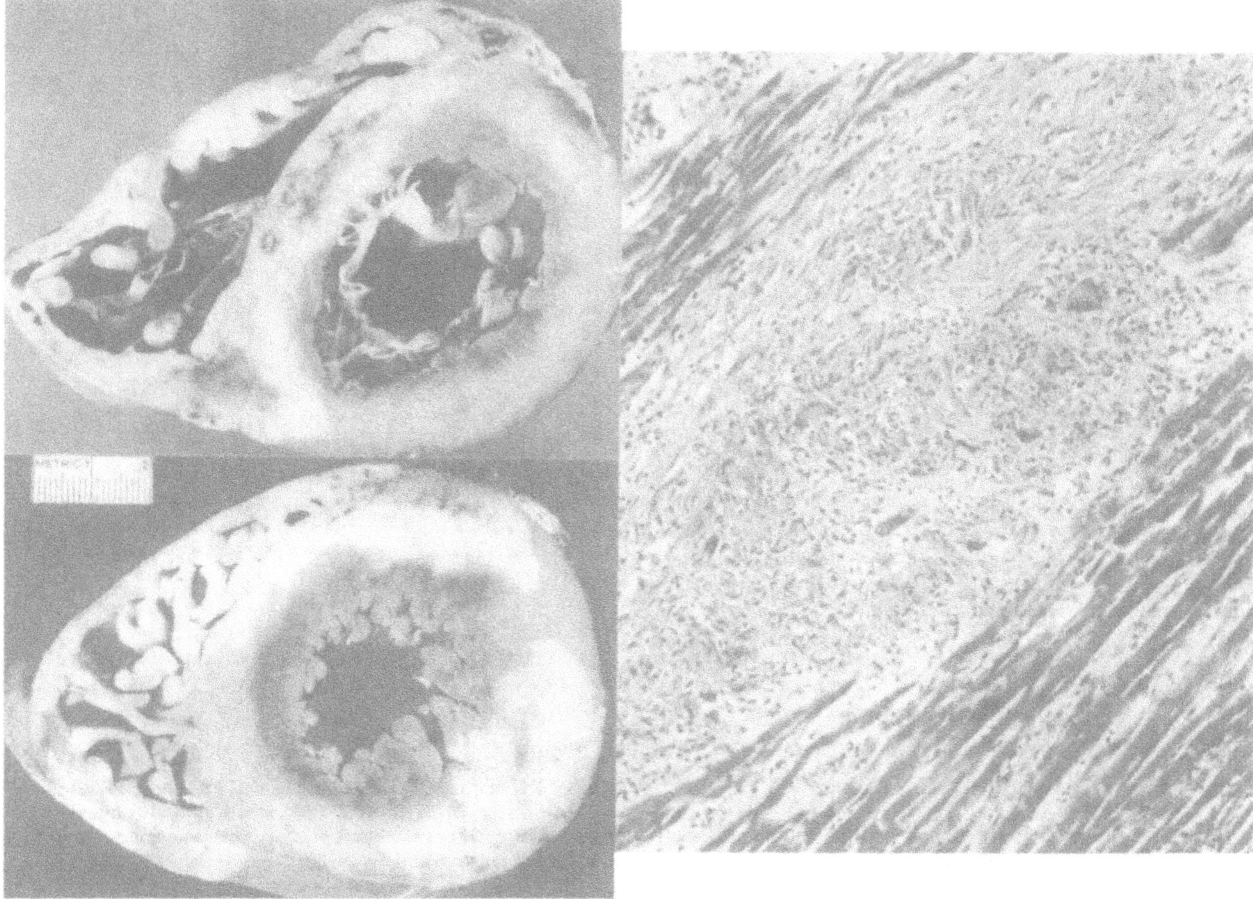

FIGURE 5. Case 18. Two views (left) of the cardiac ventricles showing extensive replacement of myocardium of the right ventricular wall, ventricular septum, and left ventricular wall in a 35-year-old man (DCMEO #88-01-140) who died suddenly from cardiac sarcoidosis while operating a bus. Photomicrograph (right) of portion of left ventricular wall. (Hematoxylin and eosin stain, original magnification × 300, reduced 25%.)

rowed 96 to 100% and 69 (24%) were narrowed 76 to 95% in CSA by plaque.

DISCUSSION

Death in 29 of the aforementioned 30 drivers was the result of a cardiovascular condition, CAD in 24 (80%). The mean age of the 24 CAD victims was 54 ± 7 years and most (92%) were men. This age is similar to that of out-of-hospital nondriving sudden coronary death victims.[3,6–9] The preponderance of men may be explained by 2 factors: (1) Men die suddenly from CAD more often than do women, and (2) men drive more than women.[10] Previous clinical evidence of heart disease is fairly common in persons dying from heart disease behind the wheel, occurring in 13 (43%) of our 30 victims, and in 17 to 67% of such previously reported victims.[2,3,8–10]

Among the 20 drivers dying suddenly from natural disease, a collision occurred in 12 cases, 4 drivers received injuries (all minor), and no other persons received injuries. This proportion of cases involving collisions is similar to previously published studies that have ranged from 26 to 67%.[2,3,8,9,11–13] Setting features such as the density of vehicles on the roads, road speed limits,

and the number of other persons at risk for injury are important when considering observations of collisions, property damage, and injury to others. Among the 16 drivers dying from CAD while driving, the vehicle was brought to a safe stop without collision in 4 (25%) cases. Kerwin[14] suggested that electrical disturbances in the heart "may take sufficient time to evolve that some cerebral circulation is maintained for a brief time. The driver therefore has a warning period during which a serious accident can be and nearly always is avoided."

Few previous studies of natural sudden death while driving or at the wheel have noted heart weights or the frequency of myocardial necrosis and healed infarcts. Cardiomegaly was present in 13 (87%) of 15 hearts in the drivers dying suddenly from CAD and in 6 (75%) of the 8 persons dying from CAD in the parked vehicle group; respective mean heart weights were 522 and 479 g. These heart weights and proportions of cardiomegaly are similar to those of out-of-hospital nondriving sudden coronary death victims.[7] Three victims who died from CAD had transmural necrosis. Previous reports of sudden coronary death while driving or behind the wheel have found the proportion with myocardial necrosis to be 2%,[3] 22%[9] and 39%.[8] Most drivers dying suddenly

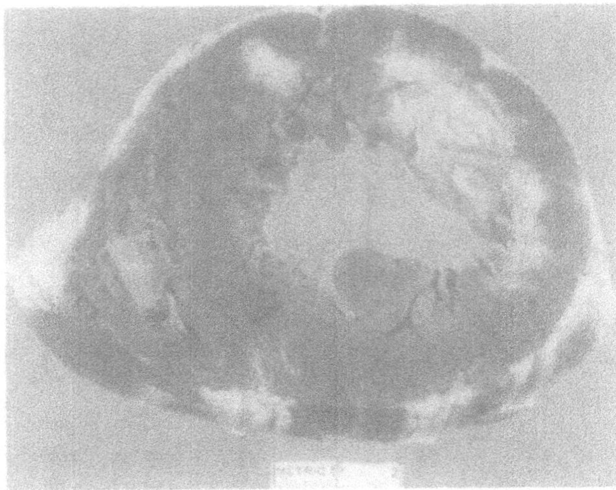

FIGURE 6. Case 29. A portion of the cardiac ventricles showing a healed infarct of the anterolateral left ventricular wall in a 59-year-old man (NNMC #A79-148) with a previous clinical event 4 years earlier compatible with acute myocardial infarction. He was found dead in his car. He had returned to his car shortly after jogging.

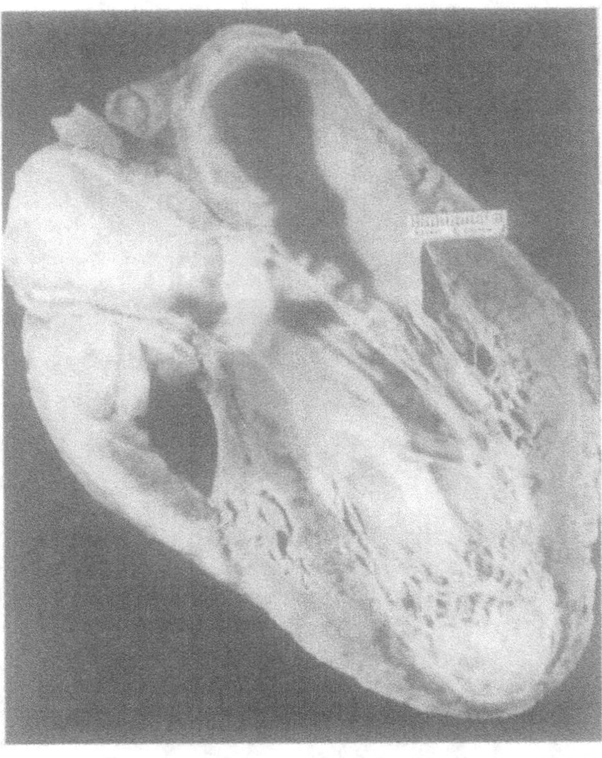

FIGURE 7. Case 30. Longitudinal view of the heart showing a dilated left ventricle with a large healed infarct in a 62-year-old woman (DCMEO #79-02-133) who had had congestive heart failure. She was found dead after a snowstorm in her car, which was parked on the street.

from CAD have healed myocardial infarcts: 67% in our 24 cases, and 56%[3,8] and 67%[9] in previously published reports.

One previous autopsy study of natural sudden deaths "in motor vehicles" (both drivers and nondrivers, both moving and parked vehicles) reported the extent of the coronary atherosclerosis. The study by Copeland[12] involved 133 autopsied cases of natural sudden death that occurred "in a motor vehicle," and in 106 of the 133 cases the coronary arteries were examined: in 70 (66%) victims 1 or more coronary arteries were narrowed 76 to 100% in CSA. In our study, the mean number of major epicardial coronary arteries narrowed >75% CSA was 2.3. In comparison, of 230 out-of-hospital and out-of-automobile sudden coronary death victims,[7] the mean number of major epicardial coronary arteries narrowed >75% CSA by plaque was 2.4.

REFERENCES

1. Hoffman MS, editor. The World Almanac and Book of Facts 1989. World Almanac, 1988:928.

2. Myerburg RJ, Davis JH. The medical ecology of public safety. I. Sudden death due to coronary heart disease. *Am Heart J* 1964;68:586–595.

3. Bowen DA. Deaths of drivers of automobiles due to trauma and ischaemic heart disease: a survey and assessment. *Forensic Sci* 1973;2:285–290.

4. Roberts WC, Jones AA. Quantitation of coronary arterial narrowing at necropsy in sudden coronary death: analysis of 31 patients and comparison with 25 control subjects. *Am J Cardiol* 1979;44:39–45.

5. Isner JM, Wu M, Virmani R, Jones AA, Roberts WC. Comparison of degrees of coronary arterial luminal narrowing determined by visual inspection of histologic sections under magnification among three independent observers and comparison to that obtained by video planimetry: an analysis of 559 five-millimeter segments of 61 coronary arteries from eleven patients. *Lab Invest* 1980;42:566–570.

6. Kannel WB, Doyle JT, McNamara PM, Quickenton P, Gordon T. Precursors of sudden coronary death. Factors related to the incidence of sudden death. *Circulation* 1975;51:606–613.

7. Roberts WC, Potkin BN, Solus DE, Reddy SG. Mode of death, frequency of healed and acute myocardial infarction, number of major epicardial coronary arteries severely narrowed by atherosclerotic plaque, and heart weight in fatal atherosclerotic coronary artery disease: analysis of 889 patients studied at necropsy. *J Am Coll Cardiol* 1990;15:196–203.

8. Ostrom M, Eriksson A. Natural death while driving. *J Forensic Sci* 1987;32:988–998.

9. Hossack DW. Death at the wheel. A consideration of cardiovascular disease as a contributory factor to road accidents. *Med J Aust* 1974;1:164–166.

10. West I, Nielsen GL, Gilmore AE, Ryan JR. Natural death at the wheel. *JAMA* 1968;205:266–271.

11. Peterson BJ, Petty CA. Sudden natural deaths among automobile drivers. *J Forensic Sci* 1962;7:274–285.

12. Copeland AR. Sudden natural death 'at the wheel'—revisited. *Med Sci Law* 1987;27:106–113.

13. Christian MS. Incidence and implications of natural deaths of road users. *Br Med J* 1988;297:1021–1024.

14. Kerwin AJ. Sudden death while driving. *Can Med Assoc J* 1984;131:312–314.

Hemodynamic Shear Force in Rupture of Coronary Arterial Atherosclerotic Plaques

S. David Gertz, MD, PhD, and William C. Roberts, MD

Angiographic and necropsy studies have suggested a direct pathogenetic relation among rupture of a coronary arterial atherosclerotic plaque, coronary thrombus formation, and acute myocardial infarction (AMI).[1-11] However, the local pathophysiologic factor or factors responsible for the initiation of plaque rupture have not been identified. Suggestions have included hemorrhage into a plaque after injury to vasa vasora; mechanical compression associated with coronary spasm; increased intraluminal arterial pressure; and circumferential tensile stress on the "fibrous cap" of the plaque. In this article we summarize the evidence for and against each of these theories and present the case for hemodynamic (rheologic) shear forces as a factor in the pathogenesis of plaque rupture.

Rupture of vasa vasora: Damage to small vascular channels within atherosclerotic plaques has been suggested by a number of investigators to be a source of plaque hemorrhage,[12-15] but none has shown how this might result in plaque rupture. Extravasation of erythrocytes from injury to intraplaque vascular channels is known to occur in large plaques, but this has been distinguished from hemorrhage associated with plaque rupture by the absence in the former of associated fibrin and platelets.[16] Moreover, Constantinides,[17] in an analysis of serial sections of 17 cases of fatal coronary thrombosis, showed that the associated plaque hemorrhage could always be traced to an entry of blood from the lumen through the same crack in the plaque. Thus, although intraplaque vascular channels are seen often, it is our experience that they are not seen within lipid-rich pultaceous debris, and there is no evidence that such channels are associated with plaque hemorrhage which accompanies rupture of a coronary atherosclerotic plaque.

Plaque compression by coronary vasospasm: Vasoconstriction or spasm has been proposed as a cause of rupture of an atherosclerotic plaque,[18-20] but can vasospasm occur in severely narrowed coronary arteries? The dominant histopathologic component of coronary atherosclerotic plaques is fibrous tissue, and, when the luminal narrowing is severe, the underlying media is often severely attenuated.[21,22] Nevertheless, angiographic

studies, particularly those involving provocative testing with ergonovine maleate, have identified spasm in coronary arteries at, and in close proximity to, sites of severe luminal narrowing.[23-27] Recent experimental studies have suggested that sites of atherosclerotic narrowing may be hypercontractile because of possible loss of endothelial-dependent arterial relaxation associated with structural or functional damage to these cells.[28,29] Joris and Majno[30] and Kurgan et al[31] reported endothelial desquamation after experimental vasospasm induced by periarterial application of L-epinephrine and calcium chloride. Thus, it appears that vasospasm may occur at sites of atherosclerotic stenosis and that vasospasm may be associated with damage to the arterial intima. However, that vasospasm may cause plaque rupture remains an important but still unanswered question.

Sudden increase in intraluminal arterial pressure: Constantinides reported that intravenous injection of various vasopressor amines, in combination with Russel viper venom, induced thrombus formation associated with plaque fissure and hemorrhage in arteries with advanced atherosclerosis.[32,33] It was hypothesized, therefore, that plaque fissures can be produced in mammalian atherosclerotic arteries by a sudden surge of intraluminal pressure in synergy with endothelial damage.[17] It can be questioned, however, whether this model provides a sufficiently convincing case for increased intraluminal pressure as a factor in the initiation of plaque rupture, and whether an agent such as Russel viper venom, which can cause endothelial damage, might not by itself contribute to plaque rupture.

Increased circumferential tensile stress: Richardson et al[34] recently suggested that the eccentric "pools" of extracellular lipid within the atherosclerotic plaque are associated with increased circumferential tensile stress on the thin residuum of fibrous tissue adjacent to the lumen, particularly during ventricular systole, and that variations in the mechanical strength of the plaque cap, such as that which may result from infiltration of foam cells, might further contribute to the likelihood of rupture at such sites. This hypothesis is based on a computerized reconstruction of the distribution of tensile stress within the arterial wall in response to theoretic elevation of intraluminal pressure. Values for tensile strengths of the various components of the atherosclerotic plaque were obtained from previous studies involving micromechanical testing of samples of intima and media obtained from the coronary arteries of human cadavers. Although the applicability of this model to the biophysical forces generated in vivo in the highly pulsatile coronary arterial system may be questioned, this study pro-

From the Pathology Branch, National Heart, Lung, and Blood Institute, National Institutes of Health, Bethesda, Maryland; and The Department of Anatomy and Embryology, The Hebrew University, Hadassah Medical School, Jerusalem, Israel. Manuscript received July 20, 1990, and accepted July 23.

Address for reprints: S. David Gertz, MD, Pathology Branch, National Heart, Lung, and Blood Institute, National Institutes of Health, Building 10, Room 2N258, Bethesda, Maryland 20892.

vides valuable information concerning the potential for components of the atherosclerotic plaque to yield in response to increased lateral pressure forces, which are well within the realm of physiologic possibility.

In the following discussion we present evidence supporting hemodynamic shear forces as a major factor in the initiation of plaque rupture.

Plaque rupture involves plaques heavily laden with extracellular lipid material (pultaceous debris) covered by a thin residuum of fibrous tissue (cap) adjacent to the lumen.[16,34–36] Morphometric analysis (performed by a computerized technique described elsewhere[22]) of Movat-stained sections of the infarct-related coronary arteries of patients who died after their first acute myocardial infarction showed the atherosclerotic plaques at sites of plaque rupture to consist of about 32% pultaceous debris, whereas plaques not associated with rupture contained approximately 5% pultaceous debris (Table I).

Although plaque rupture occurs at sites of luminal narrowing, the degree of narrowing is usually insufficient to reduce the rate of distal coronary blood flow. Histologic study of Movat-stained sections from 101 five-mm-long segments at sites of plaque rupture in the infarct-related arteries of 37 patients with first and fatal acute myocardial infarction showed the lumen to be narrowed by 51 to 75% in cross-sectional area by plaque in 27 (27%) segments; by 76 to 95% in 66 (65%) segments; and by 96 to 100% in 5 (5%) segments[37] (Figure 1). By planimetry, with the internal elastic lamina as the perimeter of the luminal circle, the mean percent reduction in luminal cross-sectional area by atherosclerotic plaque alone (of all 5-mm coronary segments) at sites of plaque rupture was 81 ± 9%. Although the latter is significantly greater than the mean percent cross-sectional narrowing of all segments of the infarct-relat-

| Segments with Plaque Rupture (no. of S) | Plaque Components (%) | | | | | |
| | Fibrous Tissue | | Calcific Deposits | | Pultaceous Debris | |
	All S	S >75%	All S	S >75%	All S	S >75%
+ (39)	63 ± 14*	63 ± 12	6 ± 9	5 ± 9	32 ± 14	32 ± 14
0 (229)	77 ± 13	69 ± 15	14 ± 13	15 ± 15	5 ± 5	12 ± 10
p Value	0.002	0.10	0.02	0.30	0.0001	0.02

TABLE I Planimetric Measurements of Components of Atherosclerotic Plaque for All Segments (5-mm Intervals) of the Infarct-Related Coronary Arteries of 17 Patients with Plaque Rupture

* Each number represents the mean percent (± standard deviation) of plaque area occupied by the 3 plaque components listed for all 5-mm coronary segments of each patient (all S) or just segments of each patient that were narrowed >75% in luminal cross-sectional area by plaque (S >75%). p values were calculated by paired 2-tailed *t* tests, no. of S = number of segments.

ed arteries that did not have plaque rupture (68 ± 9%, p = 0.002), this "severe" degree of cross-sectional narrowing corresponds, if considering a perfect circle, to approximately 56% reduction in transluminal diameter by plaque alone, which is insufficient, by itself, to reduce the rate of distal coronary flow substantially. This observation is supported by the necropsy studies of Falk,[5] which show that, of 103 sites of plaque rupture, the lumen was narrowed, in cross-sectional area, by <75% in 39 (38%), by 75 to 94% in 69 (67%), and >94% at only 12 (12%) sites of plaque rupture. From quantitative high-resolution angiographic studies, the "critical stenosis," beyond which coronary flow is sufficiently reduced to cause symptoms, has been determined to range between 70 and 80% reduction in luminal diameter, which corresponds to approximately 90 to 95% reduction in cross-sectional area.[38] Because angiographic images may underestimate the degree of diameter reduction, in that the most narrowed areas are compared to less narrowed and not necessarily normal areas,[39] the degree of actual diameter reduction necessary to result in critical reduction in flow might be even greater (Figure 2). In contrast, techniques of specimen preparation for histopathologic study, such as fixation

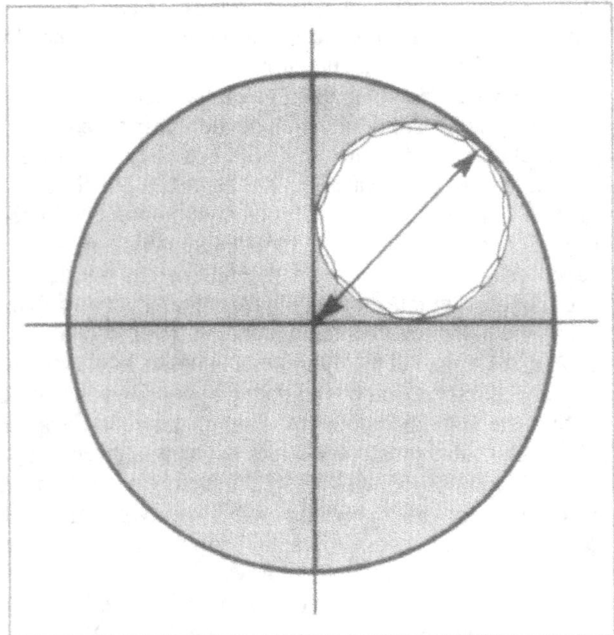

FIGURE 1. Seventy-five percent reduction in cross-sectional area corresponds to approximately 50% diameter reduction.

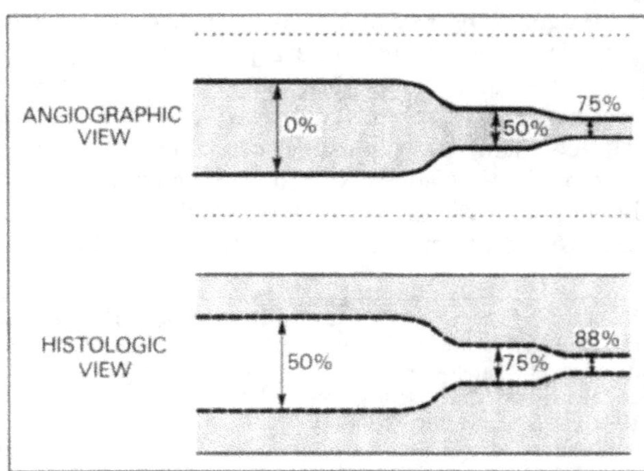

FIGURE 2. Comparison between angiographic and necropsy views of luminal narrowing.

and dehydration, may cause tissue shrinkage and, hence, slight overestimation of absolute values of luminal narrowing.[40]

Angiographic studies have suggested that the degree of stenosis of infarct-related coronary arteries is not a reliable predictor of the time or location of future myocardial infarcts, and that infarcts frequently develop in association with coronary arteries that previously were not severely narrowed.[41,42] It can be argued that the hypothesis—that coronary arteries subtending a myocardial infarct frequently are not critically narrowed—is not strongly supported by the latter studies, because they were based on angiograms performed weeks to years before the infarction, and these images may underestimate the degree of diameter reduction.[39] Nonetheless, we and others have found the lumen at sites of plaque rupture frequently to be narrowed by <75% in cross-sectional area (<50% diameter reduction)—a finding that supports the concept that even moderately narrowed atherosclerotic plaques may rupture.

Hemodynamic wall shear at sites of "subcritical" arterial narrowing has been calculated to be sufficiently strong to cause marked endothelial damage followed by platelet deposition and thrombus formation on exposed subendothelial tissues. Correlative scanning electron microscopic and blood flow studies of the coronary arteries of dogs and the common carotid artery of rabbits have shown that marked endothelial damage, with extensive platelet deposition and thrombus formation on exposed subendothelial tissues, may occur at the site of a partial arterial constriction (40 to 60% reduction in transluminal diameter) even, and perhaps particularly, when the reduction in luminal diameter is insufficient to alter substantially the rate of distal coronary blood flow.[30,43] This observation is supported by reports of functional and structural changes in the endothelial lining[44-48] associated with arterial curvatures and "flow dividers"[49] of branch orifices. These sites are normally subjected to increases in the magnitude of wall shear stress (force of the flowing blood, which is parallel to the luminal surface and independent of turbulence) or wide variations in the direction of these forces, or both. This observation is further supported by Fry,[50] in whose study a partially occlusive, intravascular grooved plug was used to narrow the arterial lumen acutely. He reported that when the shear forces of the blood approach 379 ± 85 dynes/cm^2, the "acute yield stress of the endothelial surface" in his model system, rapid cellular deterioration occurred, resulting in endothelial desquamation. That shear forces of this magnitude might be possible at sites of plaque rupture in humans can be estimated as follows: By applying Poiseuille's law, shear stress may be expressed as $\tau = 4Q\rho/\pi r^3$, where τ = shear force in dynes/cm^2, Q = coronary blood flow distal to the site of constriction in ml/s, ρ = viscosity of the blood in units of poise, and r = the luminal radius at the site of constriction in centimeters. Assuming the average luminal diameter of a "normal" coronary artery to be 3.0 mm, the luminal radius of such a coronary artery at the site of a 50% diameter reduction would be 0.075 cm. The average viscosity of the blood, assuming normal hematocrit, is approximately 0.047 poise, and coronary blood flow in, for example, the left anterior descending coronary artery distal to the site of a 50% subcritical stenosis, can be assumed to remain at 150 ml/min with maintenance of normal arterial pressure, although flow may increase more than 3-fold during exercise. The shear force under these conditions is calculated to be 353 dynes/cm^2, which is well within the range of shear forces hypothesized by Fry to be capable of inducing endothelial damage. These calculations assume steady, laminar flow. Accurate calculations of shear forces in pulsatile arterial systems like the coronary arteries are virtually impossible without knowing the precise velocity profile across the arterial lumen. The marked blunting of the velocity profile that occurs across the arterial lumen in circumstances of pulsatile flow results in a much greater velocity gradient at the arterial wall, especially at sites of arterial constriction, such that it would be reasonable to expect a 5-fold increase or more in shear stress in pulsatile flow over that for the same mean flow rate in steady flow.[51,52] The shear force might increase even further during exercise, but this increase may be offset at least partially by autoregulatory mechanisms.

It may be argued that just because shear forces cause marked endothelial damage does not prove that

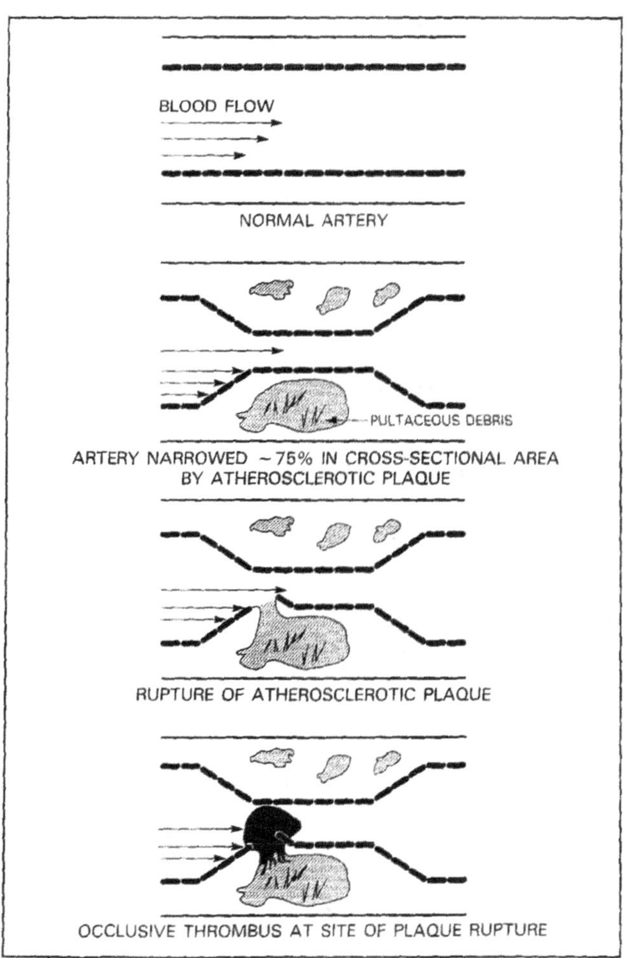

FIGURE 3. Hemodynamic shear force as a factor in rupture of atherosclerotic plaque.

they are capable of causing plaque rupture. Indeed, further multidisciplinary studies are necessary to confirm this hypothesis. Nonetheless, intimal damage thus produced, even if initially of minimal mural depth, may increase the likelihood of rupture at such sites, particularly when occurring in segments with extensive amounts of pultaceous debris and correspondingly thinner residuum of fibrous tissue between the pultaceous debris and the arterial lumen (Figure 3). Exposure of thrombogenic stimuli, such as collagen fibrils and pultaceous debris, followed by platelet adhesion and thrombus formation, may result in partial or total arterial occlusion at such sites by thrombus, with facilitation of such occlusion by superimposed spasm consequent to the release of vasoactive compounds from platelets at the sites of damaged or absent endothelium. Vasoconstriction at sites of endothelial desquamation also might increase the likelihood of plaque rupture, by the mechanical effects of the constriction itself on the arterial wall, or by further increasing the intensity of the hemodynamic shear on the already damaged intima, provided that the constriction remains below the "critical stenosis."

Intimal damage associated with hemodynamic shear might also be expected to facilitate the sequence proposed by Richardson et al,[34] by decreasing the circumferential tensile force necessary to rupture the plaque at sites of extensive pultaceous debris and an attenuated fibrous tissue residuum.

Thus, it appears likely that coronary atherosclerotic plaques may rupture even when, and perhaps particularly because, the reduction in luminal cross-sectional area is insufficient to reduce distal coronary flow. Increased shear force associated with the acutely narrowed arterial segments may, by itself, cause intimal damage sufficiently severe to cause plaque rupture, or it may participate with either or both intramural circumferential stress or mechanical forces associated with active vasoconstriction as a component of a multifactorial pathogenesis of plaque rupture.

REFERENCES

1. Chapman I. Morphogenesis of occluding artery thrombosis. *Arch Pathol Lab Med* 1965;80:256–261.

2. Friedman M, Van Den Bovenkamp GJ. The pathogenesis of a coronary thrombus. *Am J Pathol* 1966;48:19–31.

3. Ridolfi RL, Hutchins GM. The relationship between coronary artery lesions and myocardial infarcts: ulceration of atherosclerotic plaques precipitating coronary thrombosis. *Am Heart J* 1977;93:468–486.

4. Horie T, Sekiguchi M, Hirosawa K. Coronary thrombosis in pathogenesis of acute myocardial infarction: histopathological study of coronary arteries in 108 necropsied cases using serial section. *Br Heart J* 1978;40:153–161.

5. Falk E. Plaque rupture with severe pre-existing stenosis precipitating coronary thrombosis: characteristics of coronary atherosclerotic plaques underlying fatal occlusive thrombi. *Br Heart J* 1983;50:127–134.

6. Ambrose JA, Winters SL, Stern A, Eng A, Teichholz LE, Gorlin R, Fuster V. Angiographic morphology and the pathogenesis of unstable angina pectoris. *J Am Coll Cardiol* 1985;5:609–616.

7. Fuster V, Badimon L, Cohen M, Ambrose JA, Badimon JJ, Chesebro J. Insights into the pathogenesis of acute ischemic syndromes. *Circulation* 1988;77:1213–1220.

8. Davies MJ. Successful and unsuccessful coronary thrombolysis. *Br Heart J* 1989;61:381–384.

9. Falk E. Morphologic features of unstable atherothrombotic plaques underlying acute coronary syndromes. *Am J Cardiol* 1989;63:114E–120E.

10. Muller JE, Tofler GH, Stone PH. Circadian variation and triggers of onset of acute cardiovascular disease. *Circulation* 1989;79:733–743.

11. Alpert JS. The pathophysiology of acute myocardial infarction. *Cardiology* 1989;76:85–95.

12. Paterson JC. Vascularization and hemorrhage of the intima of arteriosclerotic coronary arteries. *Arch Pathol* 1936;22:313–324.

13. Paterson JC. Capillary rupture with intimal hemorrhage as a causative factor in coronary thrombosis. *Arch Pathol* 1938;25:474–487.

14. Barger AC, Beeuwkes R, Lainey LL, Silverman KJ. Hypothesis: vasa vasorum and neovascularization of human coronary arteries. A possible role in the pathophysiology of atherosclerosis. *New Engl J Med* 1984;310:175–177.

15. Baroldi G, Mariani F, Silver MD, Giuliano G. Correlation of morphologic variables in the coronary atherosclerotic plaque with clinical patterns of ischemic heart disease. *Am J Cardiovasc Pathol* 1988;2:159–172.

16. Davies MJ, Thomas AC. Plaque fissuring—the cause of acute myocardial infarction, sudden ischaemic death, and crescendo angina. *Br Heart J* 1985;53:363–373.

17. Constantinides P. Plaque fissures in human coronary thrombosis. *J Atheroscler Res* 1966;6:1–17.

18. Leary T. Coronary spasm as a possible factor in producing sudden death. *Am Heart J* 1934;10:338–344.

19. Hellstrom HR. Evidence in favor of the vasospastic cause of coronary artery thrombosis. *Am Heart J* 1979;97:449–452.

20. Alpert JS. Coronary vasomotion, coronary thrombosis, myocardial infarction and the camel's back. *J Am Coll Cardiol* 1985;5:617–618.

21. Kragel AH, Reddy SG, Wittes JT, Roberts WC. Morphometric analysis of the composition of atherosclerotic plaques in the 4 major epicardial coronary arteries in acute myocardial infarction and in sudden coronary death. *Circulation* 1989;80:1747–1756.

22. Gertz SD, Kalan JM, Kragel AH, Roberts WC, Braunwald E and TIMI investigators. Cardiac morphologic findings in patients with acute myocardial infarction treated with recombinant tissue plasminogen activator. *Am J Cardiol* 1990;65:953–961.

23. Maseri A, Pesola A, Marzilli M, Severi S, Parodi O, L'Abbate A, Ballestra AM, Maltinti G, De Nes DM, Biagini A. Coronary vasospasm in angina pectoris. *Lancet* 1977;1:713–717.

24. Chahine RA, Luchi RJ. Coronary arterial spasm: culprit or bystander? *Am J Cardiol* 1976;37:936–937.

25. Meller J, Pichard A, Dack S. Coronary arterial spasm in Prinzmetal's angina: a proved hypothesis. *Am J Cardiol* 1976;37:938–940.

26. Gensini GG. Coronary artery spasm and angina pectoris. *Chest* 1975;68:709–713.

27. Dalen JE, Ockene IS, Alpert JS. Coronary spasm, coronary thrombosis, and myocardial infarction: a hypothesis concerning the pathophysiology of acute myocardial infarction. *Am Heart J* 1982;104:1119–1124.

28. Ganz P, Alexander RW. New insights into the cellular mechanisms of vasospasm. *Am J Cardiol* 1985;56:11E–15E.

29. Hoak JC. The endothelium, platelets, and coronary vasospasm. *Adv Intern Med* 1989;34:353–375.

30. Joris I, Majno G. Endothelial changes induced by arterial spasm. *Am J Pathol* 1981;102:346–358.

31. Kurgan A, Gertz SD, Wajnberg RS. Intimal changes associated with arterial spasm following periarterial application of calcium chloride. *Exp Molec Pathol* 1983;39:176–193.

32. Constantinides P, Lawder J. Experimental thrombosis and hemorrhage in atherosclerotic arteries. *Fed Proc* 1963;22:251–259.

33. Constantinides P. Experimental Atherosclerosis. New York: Elsevier Publishing, 1965.

34. Richardson PD, Davies MJ, Born GVR. Influence of plaque configuration and stress distribution on fissuring of coronary atherosclerotic plaques. *Lancet* 1989;2:941–944.

35. Falk E. Plaque rupture with severe pre-existing stenosis precipitating coronary thrombosis: characteristics of coronary atherosclerotic plaques underlying fatal occlusive thrombi. *Br Heart J* 1983;50:127–134.

36. Tracy RE, Devaney K, Kissling G. Characteristics of the plaque under a coronary thrombus. *Virchows Arch (Pathol Anat)* 1985;405:411–427.

37. Gertz SD, Kragel AH, Kalan J, Braunwald E, Roberts WC, and the TIMI investigators. Comparison of coronary and myocardial morphologic findings in patients with and without thrombolytic therapy during fatal first acute myocardial infarction. *Am J Cardiol* 1990;66:904–909.

38. McMahon MM, Brown BG, Cukingnan R, Rolett EL, Bolson E, Frimer M, Dodge HT. Quantitative coronary angiography: measurement of the "critical" stenosis in patients with unstable angina and single-vessel disease without collaterals. *Circulation* 1979;60:106–113.

39. Arnett EN, Isner JM, Redwood DR, Kent KM, Baker WP, Ackerstein H, Roberts WC. Coronary artery narrowing in coronary heart disease: comparison of cineangiographic and necropsy findings. *Ann Intern Med* 1979;91:350–356.

40. Siegel RJ, Swan K, Edwalds G, Fishbein MC. Limitations of postmortem assessment of human coronary artery size and luminal narrowing: differential effects of tissue fixation and processing on vessels with different degrees of atherosclerosis. *J Am Coll Cardiol* 1985;5:342–346.

41. Little WC, Constantinescu M, Applegate RJ, Kutcher MA, Burrows MT, Kahl FR, Santamore WP. Can angiography predict the site of a subsequent myocardial infarction in patients with mild-to-moderate coronary artery disease? *Circulation* 1988;78:1157–1166.

42. Ambrose JA, Tannenbaum MA, Alexopoulos D, Hjemdahl-Monsen CE, Leavy J, Weiss M, Barrico S, Gorlin R, Fuster V. Angiographic progression of coronary artery disease and the development of myocardial infarction. *J Am Coll Cardiol* 1988;12:56–62.

43. Gertz SD, Uretzky G, Wajnberg RS, Navot N, Gotsman MS. Endothelial cell damage and thrombus formation after partial arterial constriction: relevance to the role of coronary artery spasm in the pathogenesis of myocardial infarction. *Circulation* 1981;63:476–486.

44. Nelson E, Gertz SD, Forbes MS, Rennels MI, Heald FP, Kahn MA, Farber TM, Miller E, Husain MM, Earl FL. Endothelial lesions in the aorta of egg yolk-fed miniature swine: a study by scanning and transmission electron microscopy. *Exp Mol Pathol* 1976;25:208–220.

45. Flaherty JT, Pierce JE, Ferrans VJ, Patel DJ, Tucker WK, Fry DL. Endothelial nuclear patterns in the canine arterial tree with particular reference to hemodynamic events. *Circ Res* 1972;30:23–33.

46. Wright HP. Endothelial turnover. In: Koller F, Brinkhous KM, Biggs R, Rodman NF, Hinnom S, eds. Vascular Factors and Thrombosis. Stuttgart: FK Schattauer Verlag, 1970:79–84.

47. Fry DL. Response of arterial wall to certain physical factors. In: Porter R, Knight J, eds. Atherogenesis: Initiating Factors. Ciba Foundation Symposium 12. Amsterdam: Ciba Foundation, 1973:93–125.

48. Fry DL. Hemodynamic forces in atherogenesis. In: Scheinberg P, ed. Cerebrovascular Diseases. New York: Raven Press, 1976:77–95.

49. Flaherty JT, Ferrans VJ, Pierce JE, Carew TE, Fry DL. Localizing factors in experimental atherosclerosis. In: Likoff W, Segal BL, Insull W, Moyer JH, eds. Atherosclerosis and Coronary Heart Disease. New York: Grune and Stratton, 1972:40–83.

50. Fry DL. Acute vascular endothelial changes associated with increased blood velocity gradients. *Circ Res* 1968;22:165–197.

51. Blaumanis OR, Grady PA, Nelson E. Hemodynamic and morphological aspects of cerebral vasospasm. In: Price TR, Nelson E, eds. Cerebrovascular Diseases. New York: Raven Press, 1979;283–294.

52. McDonald DA. Blood Flow in Arteries. Baltimore: Williams and Wilkins, 1974.

Ages at Death and Sex Distribution in Age Decade in Fatal Coronary Artery Disease

William C. Roberts, MD, Amy H. Kragel, MD, and Benjamin N. Potkin, MD

A prominent article in the lay press in 1989 stressed that coronary artery disease was an "old person's disease."[1] Apparently many physicians also consider coronary artery disease to be an "old person's disease." Recently, Roberts et al[2] reported a large series of necropsy patients with fatal coronary artery disease. Using data from the earlier study, these investigators examined the age of death in men and in women with fatal coronary artery disease, the ages at death in the various types of fatal coronary events, and the ages at death in 3 different decades.

This study analyzes 867 patients >30 years of age with fatal coronary artery disease, and each patient was studied at necropsy. None at any time had a coronary bypass operation or another type of cardiac operation, and none ever had coronary angioplasty or another type of therapeutic invasive coronary procedure. The hearts in all patients were examined by WCR and classified by him into 4 modes of death: acute myocardial infarction, sudden out-of-hospital death, chronic congestive heart failure after healing of acute myocardial infarction, and sudden in-hospital death with unstable angina pectoris. Further details on the patients included and the definitions used can be obtained from the earlier study.[2]

The results are displayed in Figures 1 through 4. The mean age of the 667 men was 60 years, and that of the 200 women, 68 years. Three hundred ninety-three (45%) of the 867 patients died from age 31 to 60 years (343

From the Pathology Branch, National Heart, Lung, and Blood Institute, National Institutes of Health, Bethesda, Maryland 20892. Manuscript received July 6, 1990; revised manuscript received July 19, 1990, and accepted July 20.

[87%] were men and 50 [13%] were women) (Figure 1). The percentage of women progressively increased in the 3 decades aged 61 to 70, 71 to 80 and 81 to 90 years. Of the 256 patients aged 61 to 70 years, 53 (21%) were women and 203 (79%) were men; of the 161 patients aged 71 to 80 years, 65 (40%) were women and 96 (60%) were men; and of the 51 patients aged 81 to 90 years, 28 (55%) were women and 23 (45%) were men. Of the entire group of 867 patients, 667 (77%) were men and 200 (23%) were women.

The mean ages of death in the men and women in each of the 4 modes of death are displayed in Figure 2. The group with sudden coronary death had a significantly (p <0.05) younger (55 years) mean age than the other 3 groups; the mean age of the acute myocardial infarction group was significantly (p <0.05) older (65 years) than that of the other 3 groups. The groups with chronic congestive heart failure and unstable angina pectoris had similar and intermediate mean ages (62 and 63 years). The sudden coronary death group and the chronic congestive heart failure group had the highest percentage of men (90 and 86%). In both the acute myocardial infarction and unstable angina pectoris groups the percentage of men was less (66 and 73%).

The ages at death in the men (Figure 3) and in the women (Figure 4) in each of 3 decades (1961 to 1990) according to the 4 modes of death are shown in Figures 3 and 4. No significant changes were noted in the 3 decades in either gender within each of the 4 groups.

These data from 867 patients with fatal coronary artery disease studied at necropsy indicate that the mean

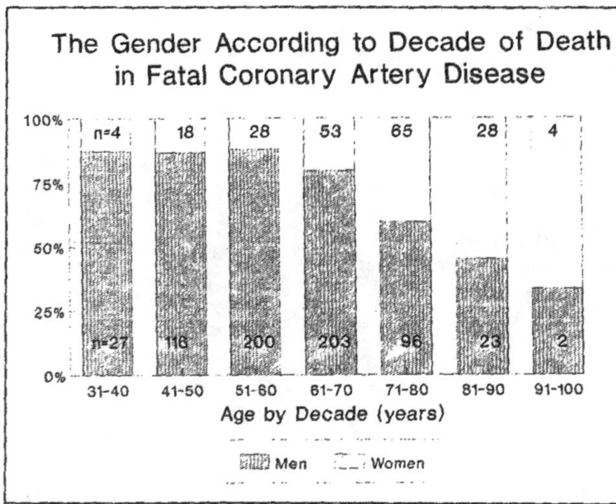

FIGURE 1. Numbers and percent of patients of each sex by age decade with fatal coronary artery disease.

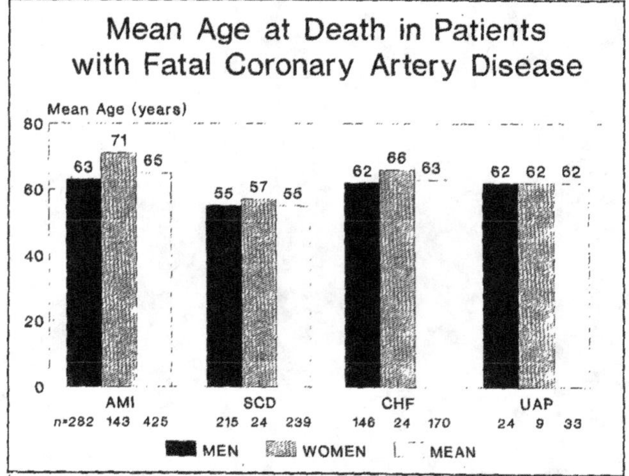

FIGURE 2. Mean age at death in men and women in each of 4 modes of death. AMI = acute myocardial infarction; CHF = chronic congestive heart failure after healing of acute myocardial infarction; SCD = sudden coronary death; UAP = unstable angina pectoris.

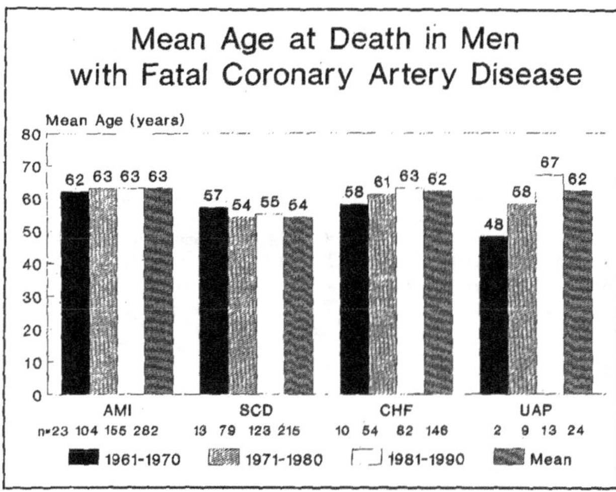

FIGURE 3. Mean age of death in men in the 4 modes of death in each of 3 decades. Abbreviations as in Figure 2.

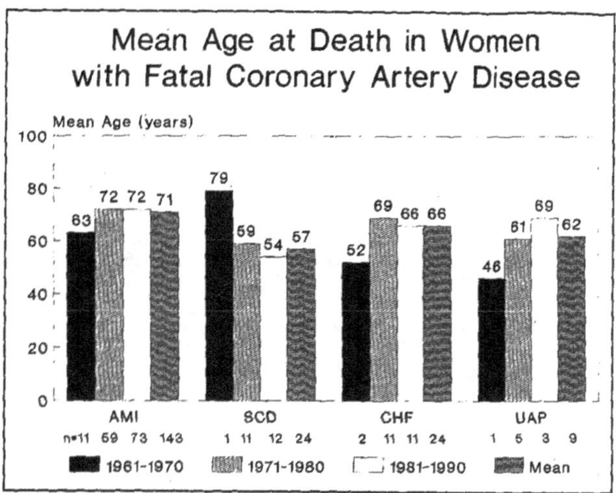

FIGURE 4. Mean age of death in women in the 4 modes of death in each of 3 decades. Abbreviations as in Figure 2.

age of death in the men, who comprised 77% of the patients, was 60 years, and that of the women, who comprised 23% of the patients, was 68 years. The age at death varied a bit depending on the mode of death. The mean age at death was youngest in the sudden coronary death group (55 years), oldest in the acute myocardial infarction group (65 years), and intermediate in the unstable angina pectoris and chronic congestive heart failure groups (62 years).

Although women comprised only 23% of the 867 patients, their percentage increased progressively after age 60 years. Of the 393 patients aged 31 to 60 years, only 50 (13%) were women; in the 61- to 70-year decade, 21% were women; in the 71- to 80-year decade, 40% were women, and in the 81- to 90-year decade, 55% were women. Thus, the gender distribution in any coronary study is in part dependent on the age group of the patients analyzed. A 1939 report by Gordon et al[3] on the frequency and extent of atherosclerotic plaques in coronary arteries of 3,400 cases studied at autopsy (data were based on information obtained from autopsy protocols) stated that "... no significant sex difference in the occurrence of coronary changes" was noted after age 70 years.

Some differences in gender also were observed in the various modes of death. Because the mean age of the sudden coronary death group was the youngest of the 4 groups, it might be expected that the frequency of men in this group would be the highest and indeed that was the case (215 of 239 [90%]). Likewise, because the mean age of the acute myocardial infarction group was the oldest, it might be expected that the percentage of men in this group would be the lowest and indeed that was the case (282 of 425 [66%]). In the unstable angina group, 72% were men and in the chronic congestive heart failure group, 86% were men. Thus, the gender distribution in any coronary study is in part dependent on the mode of death or type of coronary event present.

Because none of the 867 patients included had had coronary bypass or angioplasty or any type of cardiac operation or therapeutic invasive procedure, the present data may serve as baseline values for comparison to that acquired in patients undergoing "revascularization" procedures.

Comparison of the data on age and gender in the present study to that reported earlier by others is difficult for several reasons: (1) The numbers of patients in other studies were insufficient to provide meaningful mean age or gender data; (2) the study was limited to a single gender; (3) the study was limited to a specified age group; (4) the study was limited to a single subset of coronary patients, usually acute myocardial infarction or sudden coronary death; (5) the study did not separate patients with fatal coronary artery disease from those dying from noncoronary causes but in whom coronary atherosclerosis was present at necropsy; and (6) the study did not mention mean age or it was not possible to determine mean age because age was described only in terms of the numbers and percentages of patients in the various age decades. Five reported necropsy studies, all concerning patients with either acute myocardial infarction or sudden coronary death, provided data to which those in the present study can be compared. Bean[4] in 1938 examined autopsy protocols in 300 patients with fatal acute myocardial infarction: 209 (70%) were men (mean age 60 years) and 91 (30%) were women (mean age 62 years). McCain et al[5] in 1950 similarly analyzed 281 patients with acute myocardial infarction: 198 (70%) were men (mean age 61) and 83 (30%) were women (mean age 63). McQuay et al[6] in 1955 similarly analyzed 133 patients with acute myocardial infarction: 81 (61%) were men (mean age 63) and 52 (39%) were women (mean age 68). Silver et al[7] in 1980 analyzed 100 patients with acute myocardial infarction: 72 (72%) were men (mean age 61) and 28 (28%) were women (mean age 69). Titus et al[8] in 1973 analyzed 286 patients in whom sudden coronary death was the first manifestation of coronary artery disease: 213 (74%) were men (mean age 58) and 73 (26%) were women (mean age 62).

In summary, the mean age of men with fatal coronary artery disease is about 8 years younger than that of women. The gender distribution in any coronary study is in part dependent on the age group of the patients analyzed, and in part on the mode of death or type of coronary event present.

1. Moore TJ. The cholesterol myth. *The Atlantic* 1989;264:37–70.
2. Roberts WC, Potkin BN, Solu DE, Reddy SG. Mode of death, frequency of healed and acute myocardial infarction, number of major epicardial coronary arteries severely narrowed by atherosclerotic plaque, and heart weight in fatal atherosclerotic coronary artery disease: analysis of 889 patients studied at necropsy. *J Am Coll Cardiol* 1990;15:196–203.
3. Gordon WH, Bland EF, White PD. Coronary artery disease analyzed post mortem with special reference to the influence of economic status and sex. *Am Heart J* 1939;17:10–14.
4. Bean WB. Infarction of the heart. A morphologic and clinical appraisal of three hundred cases. Part 1. Predisposing and precipitating conditions. *Am Heart J* 1939;17:684–702.
5. McCain FH, Kline EM, Gibson JS. A clinical study of 281 autopsy reports on patients with myocardial infarction. *Am Heart J* 1950;39:263–272.
6. McQuay NW, Edwards JE, Burchell HB. Types of death in acute myocardial infarction. *Arch Intern Med* 1955;96:1–10.
7. Silver MD, Baroldi G, Mariani F. The relationship between acute occlusive coronary thrombi and myocardial infarction studied in 100 consecutive patients. *Circulation* 1980;61:219–227.
8. Titus JL, Oxman HA, Connolly DC, Nobrega FT. Sudden unexpected death as the initial manifestation of coronary heart disease: clinical and pathological observations. *Singapore Med J* 1973;14:291–293.

Composition of atherosclerotic plaques in the coronary arteries in homozygous familial hypercholesterolemia

Amy H. Kragel, MD, and William C. Roberts, MD.
Bethesda, Md.

Homozygous familial hypercholesterolemia (FH) is a rare disorder occurring in one of every one million persons. In the affected individuals the serum total cholesterol levels are >700 mg/dl and the low-density lipoprotein (LDL) levels are >500 mg/dl. In untreated affected individuals, death most commonly occurs in the second decade of life and is usually the consequence of severe atherosclerosis, affecting particularly the coronary arteries.[1] In young individuals with such elevated serum total and LDL-cholesterol levels, the atherosclerotic plaques might be expected to consist predominately of lipid material. This report describes quantitatively the composition of atherosclerotic plaques in each 5 mm-long segment of each of the four major epicardial coronary arteries in a young man with homozygous FH and fatal coronary artery disease.

LF, a 28-year-old white man, developed xanthomas at age 2 years and a diagnosis of homozygous FH was made.

From the Pathology Branch, National Heart, Lung, and Blood Institute, National Institutes of Health.

Reprint requests: Pathology Branch, NHLBI, NIH, Bldg. 10, Room 2N258, Bethesda, MD 20892.

4/4/25185

During his second decade his serum total cholesterol levels were usually >700 mg/dl. When first seen at the National Institutes of Health (NIH) at age 27, his serum total cholesterol was 588 mg/dl; LDL-cholesterol was 535 mg/dl; high-density lipoprotein cholesterol was 29 mg/dl; and very-low density lipoprotein was 24 mg/dl. His serum triglyceride level was 100 mg/dl. He first developed clinical evidence of myocardial ischemia at 17 years of age, with the appearance of typical anginal pectoris. At age 27, several months before coming to NIH, he had an acute myocardial infarct. On examination on admission to NIH, his blood pressure was 120/70 mm Hg. Bruits were audible over the carotid and femoral arteries. Xanthomas were present over tendons in the hands, elbows, and heels. Arcus was present. A grade 3/6 precordial systolic murmur, loudest just to the right of the sternum in the second left intercostal space, was present. During his last 4 years of life he was treated with a low cholesterol, low-fat diet plus cholestyramine, and when seen a few months before death his serum total cholesterol was 340 mg/dl. He died suddenly at home. At necropsy, each of the three cusps of the aortic valve were thickened by fibrous tissue and calcium and the aortic valve orifice was stenotic. A healed left ventricular infarct was present. Each of the four major (right, left main, left anterior descending, and left circumflex) coronary arteries were excised intact from the heart, decalcified, and sectioned into 5 mm-long segments. A Movat-stained section was prepared after the usual processing of each 5 mm segment. A total of 30 sections were analyzed.

Plaque composition was determined using methods that have been described previously.[2, 3] Briefly, a drawing of each section of coronary artery was made using a projection microscope. The internal elastic membrane, the residual lumen, and each component of plaque were traced manually and the actual area was calculated using a computerized morphometry system. Of the 30 sections, 14 (47%) were narrowed >95% in cross-sectional area, 14 (47%) were narrowed 76% to 95%, and two (6%) were narrowed 51% to 75%. The predominant component of plaque was dense acellular fibrous tissue (83 ± 22%, mean ± standard deviation) (Figs. 1 and 2). In 29 of the 30 segments >50% of the plaque was made up of dense fibrous tissue, and in 13 segments >90% of the plaque consisted of fibrous tissue. The remaining portions of the plaques consisted of cellular fibrous tissue, 7% ± 19%; heavily calcified tissue, 3% ± 7%; pultaceous debris, 5% ± 11%; and foam cell aggregates, 0.2% ± 0.9%.

The atherosclerotic plaques in each 5 mm segment of the four major epicardial coronary arteries in the aforementioned patient consisted primarily (83%) of dense acellular fibrous tissue; in contrast, lipid deposits, nearly entirely extracellular, made up only 5% of the plaques. Thus while atherosclerotic plaques in young persons without FH with and without fatal coronary artery disease are rich in cellular fibrous tissue and lipid-laden foam cells,[4, 5] the atherosclerotic plaques in the young man described here with homozygous FH were "hard," acellular, and calcified. In fact, of all of the 46 patients in whom plaque composition was quantitated in this laboratory,[2-4] the present patient had the highest mean percent of plaque composed of dense fi-

Fig. 1. Photomicrograph of a section of left anterior descending coronary artery in the patient described. The lumen is severely narrowed and the plaque consists primarily of dense fibrous tissue. (Movat stain; original magnification ×40.)

Fig. 2. Pie diagram showing the composition of the atherosclerotic plaques in each 5 mm segment of major coronary artery in the patient described.

brous tissue and yet the highest serum total—and LDL—cholesterol levels.

REFERENCES

1. Sprecher DL, Schaefer EJ, Kent KM, Gregg RE, Zech LA, Hoeg JM, McManus B, Roberts WC, Brewer HB Jr. Cardiovascular features of homozygous familial hypercholesterolemia: analysis of 16 patients. Am J Cardiol 1984;54:20-30.
2. Kragel AH, Reddy SG, Wittes JT, Roberts WC. Morphometric analysis of the composition of atherosclerotic plaques in the 4 major epicardial coronary arteries in acute myocardial infarction and sudden coronary death. Circulation 1989;80:1747-56.
3. Kragel AH, Reddy SG, Wittes JT, Roberts WC. Morphometric analysis of the composition of coronary arterial plaques in isolated unstable angina pectoris with pain at rest. Am J Cardiol 1990;66:562-7.
4. Dollar AL, Kragel AH, Fernicola DJ, Waclawiw MA, Roberts WC. Morphometric analysis of the composition of atherosclerotic plaques in the 4 major epicardial coronary arteries in women <40 years of age with fatal coronary artery disease. (Submitted for publication).
5. Stary HC. Changes in the cells of atherosclerotic lesions as advanced lesions evolve in coronary arteries of children and young adults. In: Glagov S, Newman WP III, Schaffer SA, eds. Pathobiology of the human atherosclerotic plaque, New York: Springer-Verlag, 1989:93-106.

To-and-fro left ventricular-to-right atrial shunting after valve replacement shown by transesophageal echocardiography

Edward S. Katz, MD, Paul A. Tunick, MD, and Itzhak Kronzon, MD. *New York, N.Y.*

Transesophageal echocardiography has a demonstrated utility in clearly defining atrial septal defects and ventricular septal defects, especially in the membranous region.[1] Isolated left ventricular-to-right atrial shunts are rare phenomena that are usually congenital.[2] These may be di-

From the Department of Medicine, New York University Medical Center.

Reprint requests: Paul A. Tunick, MD, 560 First Ave. New York, NY 10016.

4/4/25184

Composition of Atherosclerotic Plaques in Coronary Arteries in Women <40 Years of Age with Fatal Coronary Artery Disease and Implications for Plaque Reversibility

Allen L. Dollar, MD, Amy H. Kragel, MD, Daniel J. Fernicola, MD, Myron A. Waclawiw, PhD, and William C. Roberts, MD

This study analyzes the composition of atherosclerotic plaques in the 4 major epicardial coronary arteries in 8 women <40 years of age (mean 34) with fatal coronary artery disease (CAD) and compares these data to previous studies of 37 adults >45 years of age (mean 59) with fatal CAD. Histologic sections were taken at 5-mm intervals from the entire lengths of the right, left main, left anterior descending and left circumflex coronary arteries. With the use of a computerized morphometry system, analysis of the 4 major epicardial coronary arteries showed the major component of plaque to be a combination of cellular (mean percent total plaque area = 65%, standard error = 6%) and dense (19%, standard error = 6%) fibrous tissue. Arterial segments narrowed >75% in cross-sectional area from these young women were compared with similarly narrowed arteries from 37 older patients (32 men [86%]) with fatal CAD previously reported by this laboratory, and showed significantly more cellular fibrous tissue and lipid-rich foam cells, and lesser amounts of dense fibrous and heavily calcified tissue. The large amount of lipid-containing foam cells and relative lack of acellular scar tissue in coronary plaques in these young women suggests a greater potential for reversibility of these plaques in this subset of patients with CAD.

(Am J Cardiol 1991;67:1223–1227)

Death from coronary artery disease (CAD) in young women is uncommon. Most published information regarding characteristics of CAD in young persons is based on angiographic data.[1-10] No published studies have provided a quantitative analysis at necropsy of the degree of coronary arterial narrowing or of the composition of atherosclerotic plaques in such persons. This study describes quantitatively the degrees of coronary arterial narrowing and the composition of the atherosclerotic plaques at necropsy in 8 women <40 years of age with fatal CAD, and compares the results to similar studies of the coronary arteries in older persons with fatal CAD.

METHODS

Patients: The necropsy files of the Pathology Branch, National Heart, Lung, and Blood Institute, National Institutes of Health, were searched for women who were <40 years of age at death and who were coded as having fatal CAD. The coding of CAD was based on the presence of at least 1 major (right, left main, left anterior descending and left circumflex) epicardial coronary artery being narrowed >75% in cross-sectional area by plaque. Patients who had undergone coronary artery surgery or angioplasty were excluded. Patients having hemodialysis or radiation therapy were also excluded. Nine women met these criteria. In 1 woman, histologic examination of the narrowed artery showed that the lumen was narrowed entirely by thromboembolic material, without underlying atherosclerotic plaque, and, therefore, the clot was believed to be embolic in origin. This case was deleted from subsequent analysis. The remaining 8 women form the basis of this study.

Histologic techniques: The hearts studied were fixed in formalin. The 4 major epicardial coronary arteries were dissected off of the hearts intact, decalcified, and then sectioned transversely at 5-mm intervals. The segments were labeled sequentially from the origin of each artery. The 5-mm segments were dehydrated in alco-

From the Pathology and Biostatistics Branches, National Heart, Lung, and Blood Institute, National Institutes of Health, Bethesda, Maryland. Dr. Dollar's present address is: Division of Cardiology, Department of Medicine, The Washington Hospital Center, Washington, D.C. Manuscript received December 6, 1990; revised manuscript received and accepted February 5, 1991.

Address for reprints: William C. Roberts, MD, Pathology Branch, Building 10, Room 2N258, National Institutes of Health, Bethesda, Maryland 20892.

TABLE I Clinical and Morphologic Features in Eight Women Aged <40 Years with Fatal Coronary Artery Disease

						LV		Percent Segments Narrowed a Given Degree in CSA					Coronary Artery Narrowed >75% in CSA			
Pt.	Age (yr)	Mode of Death	DM	SH	HW (g)	N	F	0–25%	26–50%	51–75%	76–95%	96–100%	Right	LM	LAD	LC
1	31	Sudden	—	—	240	0	0	32	40	16	4	0	+	0	0	0
2	32	Sudden	0	0	390	0	0	12	26	40	23	0	+	0	+	0
3	32	Sudden*	0	0	300	0	+	5	24	14	19	38	+	+	0	+
4	33	Sudden†	0	+	385	0	0	27	57	11	5	0	0	0	0	+
5	39	Sudden	0	+	520	0	0	18	47	21	14	0	0	0	+	+
6	33	AMI	—	—	285	+	+	0	50	43	7	0	+	0	0	0
7	37	AMI	+	+	520	+	0	6	6	56	26	6	+	0	+	+
8	38	AMI	+	+	300	+	0	3	20	34	40	3	+	0	+	+
Mean	34				368			13	35	29	17	6				

* Unexpected intraoperative death during femoral artery embolectomy, the source of which was presumed to be the left ventricular cavity.
† Death in the hospital during admission for unstable angina pectoris and ventricular arrhythmias.
AMI = acute myocardial infarct; CSA = cross-sectional area; DM = diabetes mellitus; F = fibrosis; HW = heart weight; LAD = left anterior descending; LC = left circumflex; LV = transmural left ventricular; LM = left main; N = necrosis; SH = history of systemic hypertension; 0 = absent; + = present; — = no information available.

hols, cleared in xylene, and embedded in paraffin. Each 5-mm section of coronary artery was sectioned and stained both with hematoxylin and eosin and by the Movat method. Two hundred fifty-nine segments were analyzed.

Morphometric techniques: The morphometric techniques used in this study have been described in detail previously.[11] In brief, the individual sections of coronary artery were projected onto a sheet of paper using a projection microscope, and a tracing was made of the internal elastic membrane of the artery, the actual lumen of the artery (including any fresh intraluminal thrombus, if present), and the areas of the various components of the atherosclerotic plaque including dense, relatively acellular fibrous tissue, pultaceous debris (extracellular lipid), foam cells with and without lymphocytes, and inflammatory infiltrates without significant numbers of foam cells. The actual areas of each component of the artery and plaque outlined were measured using a digitalized computer morphometric system. The composition of atherosclerotic plaque in each histologic section from the 259 segments of coronary arteries in the young women (mean age 34 years) and in each of the sections prepared from the 1,533 segments in the 37 control subjects (mean age 59 years, 32 men [86%]) was determined by the same investigator (AHK).

The degree of cross-sectional area luminal narrowing (excluding fresh intraluminal thrombus) was determined by measuring the difference in the area bounded by internal elastic membrane and that occupied by plaque. Each segment of artery was then classified as belonging to 1 of 4 subgroups of cross-sectional area narrowing: 0 to 25%, 26 to 50%, 51 to 75% and 76 to 100%. The subgroup of cross-sectional narrowing in segments of artery that were significantly compressed during processing were determined visually because calculated areas in these cases may overestimate the degrees of luminal narrowing.

Statistical analysis: The mean plaque composition of each of the 4 major epicardial coronary arteries and in each of the 4 categories of cross-sectional area narrowing were calculated by determining first the mean for a given subset of sections in each patient and then calculating the mean for all 8 patients. Analyses of variance were then used to study the difference in plaque composition among the 4 arteries (correcting for differing degrees of luminal narrowing). A linear contrast model was used to study whether a linear trend existed in the mean percentage of any component over the 4 categories of luminal narrowing.

In all analyses, the individual patient was the unit of study rather than the number of sections or arteries studied.[12] General linear models procedure (PROC GLM) of SAS[13] was used for all analyses. The analyses were weighted for the numbers of observations used to calculate each mean to account for the differing number of sections in each subset of the analysis.

RESULTS

Clinical and morphologic findings in the 8 women are summarized in Table I. Three patients had only 1 of the 4 major epicardial coronary arteries narrowed >75% in cross-sectional area, 2 had 2 arteries so narrowed and 3 had 3 arteries so narrowed. Only 1 patient had significant narrowing of the left main coronary artery.

Plaque composition in the four major epicardial coronary arteries: The mean plaque composition of the 4 major coronary arteries is shown in Figure 1. The major component of plaque in all 4 arteries was a combination of cellular (mean percent total plaque area, 65%; standard error [SE] = 6%) and dense (19%, SE = 6%) fibrous tissue. Foam cells (9%, SE = 2%), pultaceous debris (3%, SE = 1%), heavily calcified tissue (2%, SE = 2%), loose fibrous tissue (1%, SE = 0.4%) and foam cells admixed with lymphocytes (0.6%, SE = 0.4%) accounted for small portions of the plaque. No significant difference in plaque composition was noted among the 4 major epicardial coronary arteries.

Plaque composition in the four categories of narrowing: When the segments of coronary artery in each patient were divided into 4 categories of narrowing, significant linear trends in the composition of plaque were observed (Figure 2). As the cross-sectional area narrowing increased, the mean percentage of most components of the plaque increased: As the narrowing increased from 0 to 25 to 76 to 100%, the mean proportion of plaque composed of dense fibrous tissue increased from 1 to 33% (p = 0.003); pultaceous debris, from 0 to 8% (p = 0.002); foam cell aggregates, from 1 to 20% (p = 0.01); and foam cells and lymphocytes, from 0 to 2% (p = 0.02). The only plaque component that had a linear decrease as the artery became more narrowed was cellular fibrous tissue, which decreased from 98 to 35% (p = 0.0001).

DISCUSSION

Recent reports from this laboratory have described the composition of atherosclerotic plaques, studied in a manner similar to that in the present study, in 37 older patients (32 men) with fatal CAD (acute myocardial infarction, sudden coronary death and unstable angina pectoris).[13,14] The composition of atherosclerotic plaque in severely narrowed segments of artery from these older patients (mean age 59 years) and the young women (mean age 34 years) in this study are summarized in Table II and in Figure 3. There were striking differences in the mean percentage of plaque occupied by dense and cellular fibrous tissue, heavily calcified tissue and foam cell aggregates. The dominant component of severely narrowed segments in the older patients with acute myocardial infarction, sudden coronary death and unstable angina pectoris was dense fibrous tissue (mean 40 to 53%) with a lesser amount of cellular fibrous tissue (12 to 29%). In the present study, the significantly narrowed plaques contained approximately equal amounts of dense and cellular fibrous tissue (33 and 34%, respectively). Foam cell aggregates, which

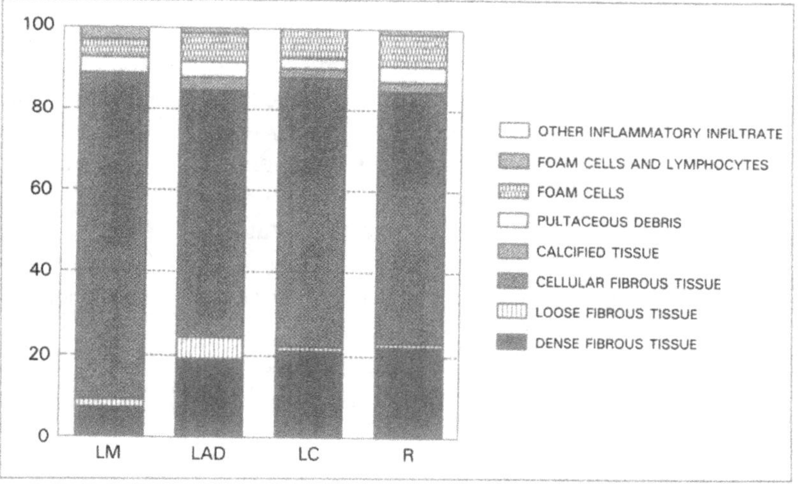

FIGURE 1. Graph showing the plaque composition (mean percentage) in each of the 4 major epicardial coronary arteries. LAD = left anterior descending coronary artery; LC = left circumflex coronary artery; LM = left main coronary artery; R = right coronary artery.

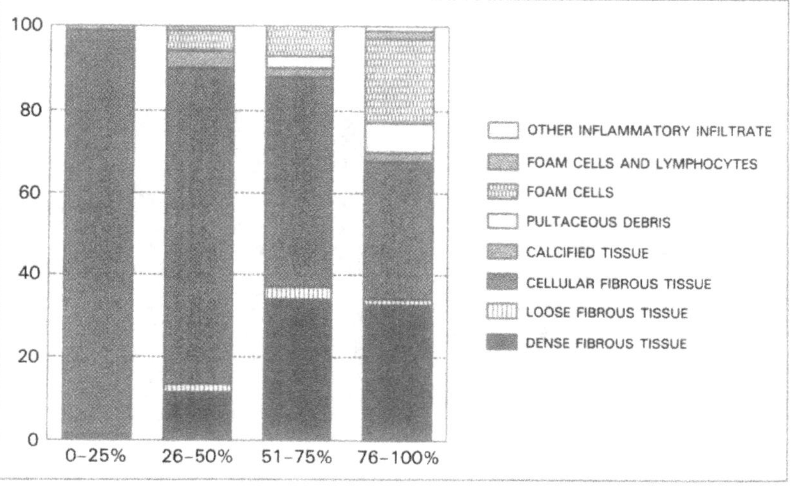

FIGURE 2. Graph showing the plaque composition (mean percentage) in each of the 4 categories of cross-sectional area narrowing.

TABLE II Comparison of Plaque Composition in Women <40 Years of Age with Fatal Coronary Artery Disease with That in Older Patients with Fatal Coronary Artery Disease

	Present Study	Combined Previous Studies	Subsets of Previous Studies			p Value*
			AMI	SCD	UAP	
No. of patients	8	37	15	12	10	—
No. of 5-mm coronary segments	259	1533	555	529	449	—
Age (yr) (mean)	31–39(34)	47–70(59)	53–68(61)	51–68(57)	47–70(59)	—
Dense fibrous tissue	33	46	53	40	44	0.0003
Loose fibrous tissue	1	2	3	2	2	0.2
Cellular fibrous tissue	34	20	12	22	29	0.003
Heavily calcified tissue	2	10	6	17	10	0.004
Pultaceous debris	8	12	19	8	7	0.2
Foam cells	19	1	2	0	1	0.0001
Foam cells and lymphocytes	2	5	4	7	6	0.9
Other inflammatory infiltrates	1	2	2	1	2	0.4

The header "Mean Percent Plaque Composition in Segments Narrowed >75% in Cross-Sectional Area" spans the Present Study, Combined Previous Studies, and Subsets of Previous Studies columns.

* p value is for comparison between the mean percent composition in the present study group and the combined previous studies.
AMI = first and only acute myocardial infarction; SCD = sudden death as first and only manifestation of coronary artery disease; UAP = unstable angina pectoris (pain at rest without acute myocardial infarction).

are rich in intracellular lipid, comprised a strikingly greater percentage of plaques in the young patients (19%) compared to that in the previous studies (0 to 2%). Plaques containing calcified deposits were present in only 2 of the 8 patients in the present study as opposed to being present in virtually every older patient.

Few other studies have described morphologic features of atherosclerotic plaques in young persons with CAD.[15,16] Strong et al[15] studied longitudinally opened coronary arteries in 74 men aged 24 to 44 years with fatal CAD. The percentage of intimal surface containing grossly visible fatty streaks (Sudan IV stain), fibrous plaques, complicated lesions and calcified lesions was determined: 59% of the intimal surface was covered by grossly visible atherosclerotic plaques, consisting of fibrous (49%), calcified (32%), fatty (12%) and "complicated" lesions (7%). Because the methods used

in their earlier study are very different from ours, meaningful comparison with our findings is not possible. Corrado et al[16] studied histologic sections of coronary arteries at sites of severe narrowing in 19 patients (17 men) aged 18 to 35 years with fatal CAD, and found the plaque in 16 cases to be "uncomplicated" and "mainly fibromatous."

The high percentage of cellular fibrous tissue and foam cells and the relative lack of calcium in severely narrowed segments of coronary artery in our young women, compared with our older patients, suggests that plaques in the younger group are either "younger" (i.e., have been present for a shorter period of time or developed more quickly), or developed under different influences or by different mechanisms, or both. Wissler[17] found that the plaques in hypercholesterolemic rabbits and fowl, whose atherosclerotic plaques developed

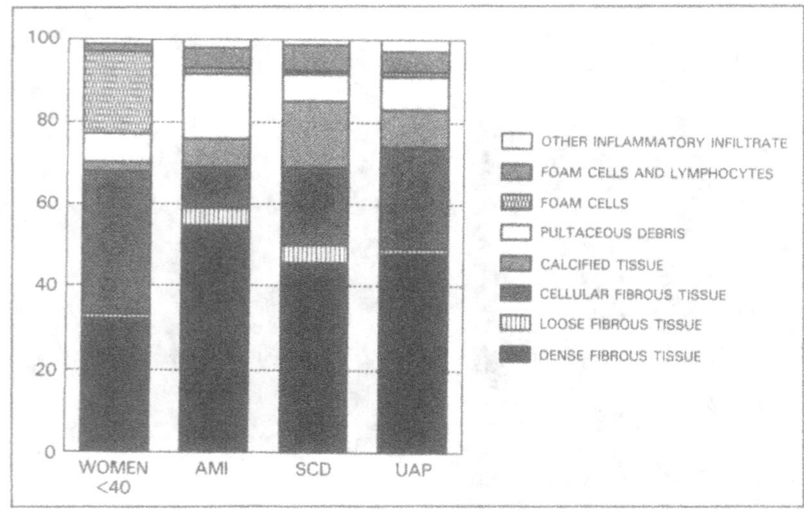

FIGURE 3. Graph comparing plaque composition (mean percentage) in sections narrowed >75% in cross-sectional area in the present study and in older patients with a fatal acute myocardial infarct (AMI), sudden coronary death (SCD) and unstable angina pectoris (UAP).

quickly, were composed predominantly of foam cells, whereas the plaques in swine and monkeys that developed atherosclerosis more slowly were composed mainly of spindle cells (cellular fibrous tissue). Wilson et al[18] studied coronary atherosclerotic plaques at various periods up to 5 years in rabbits fed butterfat, and found a decrease in the lipid content of the plaques, a decrease in "normal" smooth muscle (cellular fibrous tissue), and an increase in the amount of fibrosis (dense fibrous tissue) and calcium over time. Both the observations of Wissler and Wilson et al suggest that young atherosclerotic plaques that develop rapidly are characterized by a rich foam-cell content, by the presence of large amounts of cellular fibrous tissue and by a lack of calcific deposits. Our observations suggest that this pattern is also found in young women.

The large amount of foam cells and the relative lack of acellular scar tissue (dense fibrous tissue) and calcium in these young women may have important clinical implications. Armstrong and Megan[19,20] showed that during regression of atherosclerotic plaques in nonhuman animals, there may be a preferential loss of lipid and "young" collagen rather than "older" heavily cross-linked collagen fibers. The lipid-rich, cellular plaques in young patients may have a higher degree of reversibility compared with the densely fibrotic and calcified plaques in older patients.

REFERENCES

1. Wolfe MW, Vacek JL. Myocardial infarction in the young: angiographic features and risk factor analysis of patients with myocardial infarction at or before the age of 35 years. *Chest* 1988;94:926–930.
2. Klein LW, Agarwal JB, Herlich MB, Leary TM, Helfant RH. Prognosis of symptomatic coronary artery disease in young adults aged 40 years or less. *Am J Cardiol* 1987;60:1269–1272.
3. Weinberger I, Rotenberg Z, Fuchs J, Sagy A, Friedmann J, Agmon J. Myocardial infarction in young adults under 30 years: risk factors and clinical course. *Clin Cardiol* 1987;10:9–15.
4. Davia JE, Hallal FJ, Cheitlin MD, Gregoratos G, McCarty R, Foote W. Coronary artery disease in young patients: arteriographic and clinical review of 40 cases aged 35 and under. *Am Heart J* 1974;87:689–696.
5. Underwood DA, Proudfit WL, Lim J, MacMillan JP. Symptomatic coronary artery disease in patients aged 21 to 30 years. *Am J Cardiol* 1985;55:631–634.
6. Uhl GS, Farrell PW. Myocardial infarction in young adults: risk factors and natural history. *Am Heart J* 1983;105:548–553.
7. Wei JY, Bulkley BH. Myocardial infarction before age 36 years in women: predominance of apparent nonatherosclerotic events. *Am Heart J* 1982;104:561–566.
8. Glover MU, Kuber MT, Warren SE, Vieweg WVR. Myocardial infarction before age 36: risk factor and arteriographic analysis. *Am J Cardiol* 1982;49:1600–1603.
9. Morris DC, Hurst JW, Logue RB. Myocardial infarction in young women. *Am J Cardiol* 1976;38:299–304.
10. Roth O, Berki A, Wolff A. Long range observations in fifty-three young patients with myocardial infarction. *Am J Cardiol* 1967;19:331–338.
11. Kragel AH, Reddy SG, Wittes JT, Roberts WC. Morphometric analysis of the composition of atherosclerotic plaques in the four major epicardial coronary arteries in acute myocardial infarction and in sudden coronary death. *Circulation* 1989;80:1747–1756.
12. Armitage P. Statistical Methods in Medical Research. New York: Wiley, 1974:253–259.
13. SAS Institute, Inc. SAS User's Guide: Statistics, Version 5 ed. Cary: SAS Institute, 1985.
14. Kragel AH, Reddy SG, Wittes JT, Roberts WC. Morphometric analysis of the composition of coronary arterial plaques in isolated unstable angina pectoris with pain at rest. *Am J Cardiol* 1990;66:562–567.
15. Strong JP, Oalmann MC, Newman WP III, Tracey RE, Malcom GT, Johnson WD, McMahan LH, Rock WA Jr, Guzman MA. Coronary heart disease in young black and white males in New Orleans: community pathology study. *Am Heart J* 1984;108:747–759.
16. Corrado D, Thiene G, Pennelli N. Sudden death as the first manifestation of coronary artery disease in young people (≤35). *Eur Heart J* 1988;9:139–144.
17. Wissler RW. Atherosclerosis—its pathogenesis in perspective. *Adv Cardiol* 1974;13:10–31.
18. Wilson RB, Miller RA, Middleton CC, Kinden D. Atherosclerosis in rabbits fed a low cholesterol diet for five years. *Arteriosclerosis* 1982;2:228–240.
19. Armstrong ML, Megan MB. Lipid depletion in atheromatous coronary arteries in rhesus monkeys after regression diets. *Circ Res* 1972;30:675–680.
20. Armstrong ML, Megan MB. Arterial fibrous proteins in cynomolgus monkeys after atherogenic and regression diets. *Circ Res* 1975;36:256–261.

Composition of Atherosclerotic Plaques in the Four Major Epicardial Coronary Arteries in Patients ≥90 Years of Age

S. David Gertz, MD, PhD, Sonya Malekzadeh, BA, Allen L. Dollar, MD,
Amy H. Kragel, MD, and William C. Roberts, MD

The composition of atherosclerotic plaques in 733 five-mm segments of the 4 major (left main, left anterior descending, left circumflex and right) epicardial coronary arteries of 18 patients ≥90 years of age was determined by computerized planimetric analysis. By analysis of all coronary segments of all patients >90, the plaques consisted primarily of fibrous tissue (87 ± 8%) with calcific deposits (7 ± 6%), pultaceous debris (5 ± 4%) and foam cells (1 ± 1%) occupying a much smaller percentage of plaque area. Analysis of composition according to the 4 degrees of luminal cross-sectional area narrowing revealed marked step-wise increases in pultaceous debris (from 0 ± 0% at 0 to 25% narrowing to 18 ± 22% at 76 to 100% narrowing, p = 0.0001) and calcific deposits (from 0 ± 0 to 10 ± 15%, p = 0.002), and decreases in fibrous tissue (from 99 ± 3 to 71 ± 23%, p = 0.0001) and area occupied by the media (from 35 ± 8 to 16 ± 8%, p = 0.0001). When the analysis was restricted to sections narrowed >75%, no significant differences were found in plaque components or medial area between patients with (11 patients) and without (7 patients) myocardial infarcts at necropsy.

(Am J Cardiol 1991;67:1228–1233)

From the Pathology Branch, National Heart, Lung, and Blood Institute, National Institutes of Health, Bethesda, Maryland, and the Department of Anatomy and Embryology, The Hebrew University, Hadassah Medical School, Jerusalem, Israel. Manuscript received December 6, 1990; revised manuscript received and accepted February 20, 1991.

Address for reprints: S. David Gertz, MD, Pathology Branch, National Heart, Lung, and Blood Institute, National Institutes of Health, Building 10, Room 2N258, Bethesda, Maryland 20892.

The percentage of people surviving ≥90 years has continued to increase, and coronary artery disease is still the most frequent cause of death in the elderly population.[1-4] The frequency of myocardial infarcts at necropsy in patients dying at ages ≥90 years has been reported to be lower than in younger populations.[5-7] The few reported necropsy studies of patients aged ≥90 years suggest that the severity of coronary atherosclerosis in the subset with symptomatic myocardial ischemia is similar to[4,7,8] or less than[5,9,10] that of younger patients with symptomatic myocardial ischemia, but that the severity of coronary artery disease in unselected or asymptomatic patients >90 years old is similar to[8] or more than[7,9,10] that of younger unselected or asymptomatic patients. The present study examines the composition of atherosclerotic plaques in the coronary arteries of patients ≥90 years old.

METHODS

The hearts of 18 patients ≥90 years of age at death were studied. The hearts were selected from the necropsy files of the Pathology Branch of the National Heart, Lung, and Blood Institute. The patients in this study were included in a previous study from this laboratory of clinical and cardiac morphologic features of 40 patients ≥90 years of age.[9] Patients who had undergone coronary artery bypass surgery or percutaneous transluminal coronary angioplasty were excluded. Eleven patients had myocardial infarcts (acute, healed, or both) at necropsy, and 7 patients died from noncardiac causes and had no infarcts at necropsy. Certain characteristics of each patient are listed in Table I.

The hearts were fixed in 10% buffered formaldehyde for ≥3 days. The 4 major epicardial coronary arteries (left main, left anterior descending, left circumflex and right) were excised intact and decalcified by the formic acid-sodium citrate method[11] for approximately 12 hours. (The gross decalcification by this technique does not preclude the identification of calcific deposits in histologic sections stained by the Movat or the hematoxylin and eosin techniques.) The arteries were sectioned transversely at 5-mm intervals and the segments were labeled sequentially. All specimens were then dehydrated in ethanol and xylene, and embedded

Case No.	Age (yrs)	Sex	SH	DM	HW (g)	Mean HW by Sex	LV N	LV F'	Location AMI	Location OMI	No. of Major CAs Narrowed >75% by P	No. 5-mm Coronary S All
TABLE I Pertinent Characteristics in the 18 Patients ≥90 Years Old												
AMI, OMI, or Both												
1	90	M	+	0	465		++	0	A	0	3	43
2	90	F	+	+	400		++	0	A	0	2	22
3	91	M	+	0	390		0	++	0	P	3	50
4	91	F	0	0	560		++	++	C	P	3	45
5	92	F	0	0	280		++	0	L	0	3	31
6	93	M	+	0	470		+	0	A	0	3	44
7	93	F	+	+	450		+	0	A	0	3	41
8	93	F	+	0	560		+	+	P	P	2	32
9	93	F	+	0	500		0	+	0	P	1	46
10	95	F	0	0	440		0	+	0	P	2	47
11	100	M	0	—	335		0	+	0	P	2	42
Subtotal n = 11	93 ± 3	4M 7F	7	2	441 ± 86	M415 ± 65 F456 ± 98					2.5 ± 0.7	443
No AMI or OMI												
12	90	F	+	0	235		0	0	0	0	2	36
13	91	M	+	0	490		0	0	0	0	0	39
14	95	M	+	0	580		0	0	0	0	1	51
15	95	M	0	0	385		0	0	0	0	3	46
16	97	F	0	0	320		0	0	0	0	2	38
17	97	F	0	0	360		0	0	0	0	2	44
18	103	F	—	0	320		0	0	0	0	1	36
Subtotal n = 7	95 ± 4	3M 4F	3	0	384 ±116	M485 ± 98 F309 ± 53					1.6 ± 1.0 0.04	290 0.82*
	P = 0.14	0.78	0.59	0.21	0.25	M0.3 F0.02					2.1 ± 0.9	733
Totals (Mean ± SD)	94 ± 4	7M 11F	10	2	419 ± 100	M445 ± 82 F402 ± 110						

* Calculated from means.

All = all segments of the 4 major epicardial coronary arteries; AMI = acute (recent) myocardial infarct; CA = coronary artery; CD = calcific deposits; CSA = cross-sectional area; DM = diabetes mellitus; F = female; F' = fibrosis; FO = foam cells; FT = fibrous tissue; HW = heart weight; M = male; n = number of patients; N = necrosis; LV = left ventricular; OMI = old (healed) myocardial infarct; P = plaque; PD = pultaceous debris; S = segments; SD = standard deviation; SH = systemic hypertension.

in paraffin. One section (5-μm thick) from each 5-mm segment was stained by the Movat method,[12] and another section from each 5-mm segment was stained with hematoxylin and eosin. Seven hundred thirty-three coronary segments were examined in detail. The hearts were cut transversely into slices approximately 1.0-cm thick from the ventricular apex to approximately 2.0 cm caudal to the posterior atrioventricular sulcus.

Plaque composition and luminal narrowing were assessed by planimetry as follows: Movat-stained sections from each 5-mm coronary segment were projected onto white paper using a Bausch & Lomb Tri-simplex microprojector. The image was magnified approximately 40 times and the following areas were traced: external elastic lamina (corresponding to the outer border of the media); internal elastic lamina (potential lumen); residual lumen; fibrous tissue (cellular and acellular, primarily collagenous with some elastic fibers intermingled with smooth muscle cells and fibroblasts with a variable amount of mucopolysaccarides); pultaceous debris (extracellular lipid represented by pale-staining areas consisting of amorphous material with numerous cholesterol clefts and a variable amount of inflammatory infiltrates); calcific deposits (granular, brownstained areas in Movat-stained sections) (single, isolated granules were not included in this quantification); and foam cells.

After tracing the aforementioned components, the relative area occupied by each component was determined by re-outlining these areas with a GTCO "Micro Digi-pad" and stylus (model 1212) in association with the "Macmeasure" morphometric software package adapted to a MacIntosh SE computer.[13]

Luminal narrowing was determined by the difference between the area bounded by the internal elastic lamina and that occupied by plaque (percent cross-sectional area narrowing = [100 − (area of residual lumen/area bounded by internal elastic lamina) × 100]). The percent reduction in cross-sectional area by atherosclerotic plaque alone thus obtained was expressed as an absolute number and as belonging to 1 of 4 degrees of cross-sectional area narrowing—0 to 25%, 26 to 50%, 51 to 75% and 76 to 100%.

Plaque composition was analyzed for each of the 4 major epicardial coronary arteries by averaging the means for each component of all segments for each artery in each patient. For all final statistical analyses, the individual patient was the unit of study[14] unless

TABLE I CONTINUED

| Case No. | All | | | | | Mean % of Plaque Area for All 5-mm S | | | | | | | |
| | No. (%) S Narrowed in CSA by Plaque | | | | | FT | | FO | | PD | | CD | |
	0–25%	26–50%	51–75%	76–95%	96–100%	All	>75%	All	>75%	All	>75%	All	>75%
						AMI, OMI, or Both							
1	0 (0)	12 (28)	18 (42)	13 (30)	0 (0)	80 ± 22	62 ± 24	0	0	11 ± 19	24 ± 27	9 ± 15	14 ± 19
2	0 (0)	9 (41)	10 (45)	3 (14)	0 (0)	89 ± 18	65 ± 29	0 ± 1	1 ± 2	2 ± 5	9 ± 12	9 ± 14	23 ± 15
3	4 (8)	8 (16)	27 (54)	8 (16)	3 (6)	84 ± 20	71 ± 27	1 ± 4	1 ± 2	10 ± 14	17 ± 16	6 ± 14	11 ± 19
4	0 (0)	7 (16)	27 (60)	10 (22)	1 (2)	88 ± 17	73 ± 26	1 ± 2	2 ± 4	7 ± 13	20 ± 20	5 ± 9	6 ± 10
5	0 (0)	14 (45)	12 (39)	4 (13)	1 (3)	82 ± 24	43 ± 19	0 ± 1	0	14 ± 23	57 ± 19	5 ± 12	0
6	0 (0)	3 (7)	33 (75)	6 (14)	2 (5)	93 ± 11	95 ± 7	1 ± 2	2 ± 4	1 ± 2	0	6 ± 11	3 ± 7
7	0 (0)	1 (2)	25 (61)	11 (27)	4 (10)	83 ± 19	74 ± 21	1 ± 2	2 ± 3	9 ± 15	17 ± 21	7 ± 13	6 ± 11
8	3 (9)	4 (12)	14 (44)	9 (28)	2 (6)	78 ± 22	66 ± 18	0	0	4 ± 6	5 ± 6	18 ± 22	28 ± 19
9	2 (4)	31 (63)	11 (22)	2 (4)	0 (0)	66 ± 25	61 ± 4	0 ± 1	0	7 ± 12	12 ± 7	27 ± 25	28 ± 3
10	0 (0)	18 (38)	27 (57)	2 (4)	0 (0)	94 ± 11	91 ± 5	1 ± 2	1 ± 2	3 ± 7	6 ± 7	3 ± 6	2 ± 3
11	1 (2)	7 (17)	31 (74)	3 (7)	0 (0)	94 ± 11	84 ± 23	4 ± 10	16 ± 23	1 ± 5	0	1 ± 3	0
12	10 (2)	114 (26)	235 (53)	71 (16)	13 (3)	85 ± 8	71 ± 15	1 ± 1	2 ± 5	6 ± 4	15 ± 16	9 ± 7	11 ± 11
						No AMI or OMI							
13	7 (19)	11 (31)	12 (33)	5 (14)	1 (3)	78 ± 25	59 ± 28	0	0	13 ± 21	39 ± 27	8 ± 18	2 ± 5
14	5 (13)	32 (82)	0 (0)	0 (0)	2 (5)	98 ± 5	0	0 ± 2	0	0 ± 0	0	1 ± 5	0
15	1 (2)	24 (47)	22 (43)	1 (2)	3 (6)	86 ± 17	47 ± 0	1 ± 3	4 ± 0	6 ± 9	49 ± 0	7 ± 15	0 ± 0
16	0 (0)	14 (30)	26 (57)	5 (11)	1 (2)	91 ± 17	81 ± 7	0 ± 3	4 ± 9	1 ± 4	7 ± 11	8 ± 16	8 ± 9
17	2 (5)	19 (50)	12 (32)	2 (5)	3 (8)	88 ± 19	75 ± 12	1 ± 3	0	4 ± 8	15 ± 10	8 ± 17	10 ± 2
18	0 (0)	17 (39)	23 (52)	2 (5)	2 (5)	95 ± 11	89 ± 16	0 ± 1	0	1 ± 3	11 ± 16	4 ± 10	0
19	0 (0)	18 (50)	15 (42)	1 (3)	2 (6)	97 ± 8	65 ± 0	0 ± 1	0	2 ± 7	35 ± 0	0 ± 3	0
20	15 (5)	135 (47)	110 (38)	16 (6)	14 (5)	90 ± 7	59 ± 30	0	1 ± 2	4 ± 5	22 ± 19	5 ± 3	3 ± 4
21	0.21*	0.03	0.08	0.01	0.19	0.15	0.27	0.27	0.55	0.28	0.4	0.26	0.08
	25 (3)	249 (34)	345 (47)	87 (12)	27 (4)	87 ± 8	67 ± 22	1 ± 1	2 ± 4	5 ± 4	18 ± 17	7 ± 6	8 ± 10

otherwise specified. Comparisons of plaque composition were made between the various degrees of luminal narrowing, between infarct-related and non-infarct-related arteries, between patients with infarcts at necropsy and those without, and between patients ≥90 years of age with infarcts at necropsy and patients 53 to 68 years of age[14,15] and patients <40 years of age with infarcts at necropsy[16] studied previously.

The infarct-related coronary artery was the left anterior descending artery for anterior wall infarcts and the dominant right or dominant left circumflex coronary artery for posterior (inferior) wall infarcts.

Statistical comparisons of numerical data were performed by 2-tailed *t* tests (paired or unpaired as appropriate). Categorical data were compared by coded chi-square analysis. For these calculations, the Stat View

TABLE II Comparison of Plaque Composition of the Four Major Epicardial Coronary Arteries in Patients ≥90 Years Old With and Without Myocardial Infarcts at Necropsy

| CA | Plaque Components | | | | Media[†] | M%[‡] CSAN |
	FT	PC	PD	CD		
LM + (8)[16]	80 ± 17*	0	7 ± 7	13 ± 17	23 ± 9	55 ± 12
0(6)[8]	87 ± 13	2 ± 3	8 ± 9	3 ± 5	15 ± 10	59 ± 18
p Value	0.47	0.10	0.75	0.18	0.12	0.61
LAD + (11)[157]	82 ± 13	1 ± 1	5 ± 4	12 ± 12	23 ± 6	61 ± 10
0(7)[103]	90 ± 11	0	3 ± 5	6 ± 7	26 ± 7	49 ± 9
p Value	0.18	0.24	0.32	0.29	0.35	0.01
LC + (10)[98]	84 ± 14	0	9 ± 13	7 ± 6	25 ± 7	57 ± 14
0(7)[68]	88 ± 11	1 ± 1	7 ± 11	5 ± 5	26 ± 6	50 ± 13
p Value	0.55	0.17	0.65	0.56	0.75	0.31
R + (10)[172]	85 ± 8	1 ± 2	6 ± 4	7 ± 8	22 ± 8	62 ± 10
0(7)[111]	94 ± 7	0 ± 1	2 ± 3	4 ± 5	26 ± 8	47 ± 10
p Value	0.03	0.52	0.03	0.33	0.36	0.01

* Each number represents the mean percentage (± standard deviation) of plaque area occupied by each component listed for all 5-mm segments of each of the 4 major epicardial coronary arteries of each patient with (+) or without (0) myocardial infarcts (acute or healed, or both) at necropsy.
[†] Mean percentage (± standard deviation) of the area encircled by the external elastic lamina that is media.
[‡] Mean percent reduction (± standard deviation) in luminal cross-sectional area calculated by planimetry.
CSAN = cross-sectional area narrowing; LAD = left anterior descending; LC = left circumflex; LM = left main; M = mean; R = right; S = segments; other abbreviations as in Table I.

512+ statistical package (Brain Power, Inc., Calabasas, California) was used in association with a MacIntosh SE computer.

RESULTS

Baseline characteristics: Of the 18 patients ≥90 years of age (mean age ± standard deviation 94 ± 4, 11 women), 11 had myocardial necrosis or fibrosis, or both, and 7, who died of noncardiac causes, had no gross or histologic evidence of myocardial necrosis or fibrosis. Comparisons between patients with and without infarcts at necropsy revealed similar ages (93 ± 3 vs 95 ± 4 years, p = 0.14), gender (7 [64%] vs 4 [57%] women, p = 0.78), frequency of a history of systemic hypertension (7 [64%] vs 3 [50%], p = 0.59) and frequency of a history of diabetes mellitus (2 [20%] vs 0, p = 0.21). The mean heart weight of the women who died from coronary artery disease was significantly higher than those who died of noncardiac causes (456 ± 98 vs 309 ± 53 g, p = 0.02), but this difference was not found between the small number of men in each group (415 ± 65 vs 485 ± 98 g, p = 0.30).

Coronary arterial narrowing: Of the 18 patients ≥90 years of age at death, all (100%) had narrowing >75% of the luminal cross-sectional area by atherosclerotic plaque alone of ≥1 of the 4 major epicardial coronary arteries: 7 patients (39%) had 3 arteries so narrowed and 2 had a left main artery narrowed to this extent. Patients with infarcts at necropsy had a greater mean number of coronary arteries narrowed >75% by plaque than patients without infarcts (2.5 ± 0.7 vs 1.6 ± 1.0, p = 0.04), higher percentages of 5-mm coronary segments narrowed 76 to 95% in cross-sectional area by plaque (p = 0.01) and a correspondingly lower percentage of segments narrowed 26 to 50% (p = 0.03) (Table I). The mean percent reduction in luminal cross-sectional area by plaque for all 5-mm segments of all 4 major epicardial arteries was significantly greater in nonagenarians with, than in those without, infarcts (60 ± 7 vs 49 ± 8%, p = 0.007). Among the 11 patients

with infarcts at necropsy, the mean percent reduction in luminal cross-sectional area for all segments of the infarct-related arteries was significantly greater than that for all non-infarct-related arteries of each patient (66 ± 11 vs 57 ± 9%, p = 0.03).

Plaque composition: By planimetric analysis of all 733 five-mm segments of all 4 major epicardial coronary arteries of patients aged ≥90 years (by patient), irrespective of the degree of luminal narrowing, the plaques consisted of fibrous tissue (87 ± 8%), foam cells (1 ± 1%), lipid-rich pultaceous debris (pale-staining areas with abundant cholesterol clefts with or without erythrocytes and inflammatory cells) (5 ± 4%) and calcific deposits (7 ± 6%) (Table I). The mean percentage (for all segments, by patient) of the area bounded by the external elastic lamina that is media was 24 ± 6%.

Analysis of each of the 4 major coronary arteries individually revealed similar plaque composition between the 4 arteries (Table II).

Analysis of plaque composition of all segments according to the 4 degrees of luminal narrowing revealed marked step-wise increases in pultaceous debris (from 0

TABLE III Comparison of Plaque Composition in 18 Patients ≥90 Years of Age According to the Four Degrees of Luminal Cross-Sectional Area Narrowing

| | Degrees of CSAN by Atherosclerotic Plaque | | | | |
Component	0–25% [25]	26–50% [249]	51–75% [345]	76–100% [94][†]	p Value[‡]
FT	99 ± 3*	95 ± 14	85 ± 19	71 ± 23	0.0001
FC	1 ± 3	0 ± 2	1 ± 4	1 ± 4	0.28
PD	0	1 ± 6	5 ± 10	18 ± 22	0.0001
CD	0	4 ± 12	9 ± 17	10 ± 15	0.002
Media	35 ± 8	30 ± 11	21 ± 8	16 ± 8	0.0001

* Each number represents the mean percentage ± standard deviation of plaque area occupied by each component for all 5-mm segments of all 4 major epicardial coronary arteries in each of the 4 degrees of luminal cross-sectional narrowing.
[†] Excludes 20 unpaired segments.
[‡] p values for paired comparisons between components of segments narrowed 0 to 25% and those narrowed 76 to 100%.
Numbers in brackets are numbers of segments of each degree of narrowing.
Abbreviations as in Table I.

TABLE IV Comparison of Plaque Composition of Segments Narrowed <75% to Those Narrowed >75% in Cross-Sectional Area in Patients ≥90 Years Old With and Without Myocardial Infarct at Necropsy

| | Myocardial Infarct | | | | | | | | | |
| | +(11) | | | | | 0(7) | | | | |
CSAN	FT	FC	PD	CD	Media	FT	FC	PD	CD	Media
>75%	71 ± 15*	2 ± 5	15 ± 16 [84]	11 ± 11	18 ± 7[†]	59 ± 30	1 ± 2	22 ± 19 [30]	3 ± 4	16 ± 9
<75%	88 ± 8	0 ± 1	4 ± 3 [359]	8 ± 7	25 ± 6	92 ± 6	0	3 ± 3 [260]	5 ± 3	26 ± 6
p Value	0.003	0.15	0.03	0.19	0.004	0.04	0.27	0.02	0.15	0.08

* Each number represents the mean percentage ± standard deviation of plaque area occupied by each of the 4 plaque components for all 5-mm segments narrowed greater than or <75% in cross-sectional area in all 4 major epicardial coronary arteries of patients with or without a myocardial infarct (acute or healed, or both) at necropsy.
[†] See Table II.
Numbers in parentheses = numbers of patients; numbers in brackets = numbers of segments.
Abbreviations as in Table I.

TABLE V Comparison of Plaque Composition of the Infarct-Related to Non-Infarct-Related Arteries of Patients ≥90 Years Old with Myocardial Infarct at Necropsy

Infarct-Related Artery	Plaque Components				M%[†]
	FT	FC	PD	CD	CSAN
+ All S [169]	81 ± 12*	1 ± 2	9 ± 12	9 ± 8	66 ± 11
S >75% [41]	72 ± 25	2 ± 5	15 ± 22	11 ± 17	
0 All S [274]	84 ± 9	0	6 ± 5	10 ± 8	57 ± 9
S >75% [38]	69 ± 23	1 ± 3	19 ± 21	11 ± 15	
p Value	0.4	0.13	0.53	0.75	0.03
	0.49	0.67	0.38	0.96	

* Each number represents the mean percentage ± standard deviation of plaque area occupied by each component listed for all 5-mm segments of the infarct-related artery (or segments narrowed >75%) compared (by paired t tests) with segments of all non-infarct-related arteries of each patient.
[†] Mean percent reduction in luminal cross-sectional area by planimetry.
Numbers in brackets = numbers of 5-mm coronary segments.
Abbreviations as in Table I.

± 0% at 0 to 25% narrowing to 18 ± 22% at 76 to 100% narrowing, p = 0.0001) and calcific deposits (from 0 ± 0 to 10 ± 15%, p = 0.002), and concomitant decreases in fibrous tissue (from 99 ± 3 to 71 ± 23%, p = 0.0001) and area occupied by the media (from 35 ± 8 to 16 ± 8%, p = 0.0001) (Table III). The mean percentage of plaque occupied by pultaceous debris was significantly greater in sections narrowed >75% in cross-sectional area by plaque than in those narrowed <75% (18 ± 17 vs 3 ± 3%, p = 0.001), and the amount of fibrous tissue was correspondingly less (67 ± 22 vs 89 ± 7%, p = 0.0007). The mean percent area occupied by the media was also significantly less in sections narrowed >75% than in those <75% (17 ± 8 vs 25 ± 6%, p = 0.002). These differences in plaque composition and medial thickness (by area) between sections narrowed more and those <75% were also apparent when patients with and without infarcts were analyzed separately (Table IV). However, when restricting the analysis to sections narrowed >75%, no significant differences were found in plaque components or media between patients with and without infarcts at necropsy (Table I).

In patients with infarcts, comparisons between the infarct-related artery and the noninfarct arteries also revealed no significant differences in plaque composition whether considering all segments together or restricting the analysis to sections narrowed >75% (Table V).

DISCUSSION

By computerized planimetric analysis of all 5-mm segments of all 4 major epicardial coronary arteries, we have shown that the predominant component of atherosclerotic plaques in patients ≥90 years of age at necropsy is fibrous tissue. Analysis of the composition according to the 4 degrees of luminal narrowing (0 to 25%, 26 to 50%, 51 to 75%, 76 to 100%) revealed a marked step-wise increase in pultaceous debris and calcific deposits with increased luminal narrowing, and a corresponding decrease in the percentage of plaque occupied by fibrous tissue and in the area occupied by the media (Table III). With correction for degrees of narrowing, no differences were found between the composition of plaques or thickness of the media in the arteries of the elderly patients with and without infarcts.

Comparisons between the composition of plaques in the elderly patients with infarcts at necropsy with that of 2 populations of younger patients with infarcts at necropsy from this laboratory, calculated by the same planimetric technique, are presented in Table VI: Fibrous tissue was the dominant component in all 3 patient populations, with insignificant differences between the 3 whether restricting the analysis to sections narrowed >75% or to sections narrowed <75%. The per-

TABLE VI Comparison of Plaque Composition of Patients 90 to 100 Years Old with Those 53 to 68 and 33 to 38 Years Old with Myocardial Infarcts at Necropsy

Component	33–38+ (4) [39/108] (Dollar et al[16])	53–68 (15) [153/402] (Kragel et al[15])	90–100 (11) [84/359]	p1[†]	p2
FT >75%	62 ± 11*	68 ± 12	71 ± 15	0.53	0.25
<75%	88 ± 13	88 ± 6	88 ± 8	0.83	0.97
FC >75%	25 ± 23	5 ± 5	2 ± 5	0.12	0.006
<75%	5 ± 5	5 ± 4	0 ± 1	0.003	0.007
PD >75%	10 ± 13	19 ± 12	15 ± 16	0.51	0.57
<75%	3 ± 3	3 ± 3	4 ± 3	0.58	0.55
CD >75%	4 ± 7	6 ± 6	11 ± 11	0.15	0.22
<75%	4 ± 8	3 ± 4	8 ± 7	0.04	0.37

* Each number represents the mean percentage ± standard deviation of plaque area occupied by each component for all 5-mm segments narrowed greater than or <75% in cross-sectional area by plaque.
[†] p1 = p values for comparisons between components of patients >90 with those aged 53 to 68 years; p2 = values for comparisons between patients >90 with those <40 years.
Numbers in parentheses = numbers of patients; numbers in brackets = numbers of segments [>75%/<75%].
Abbreviations as in Table I.

centage of plaque occupied by foam cell aggregates rich in intracellular lipid, however, was significantly higher in patients aged 33 to 38 years with infarcts at necropsy than in patients ≥90 years old in sections narrowed >75% and in sections narrowed <75%, and was significantly higher in patients aged 53 to 68 years in sections narrowed <75%. There were insignificant differences in the amounts of lipid-rich pultaceous debris between the 3 groups for both categories of narrowing.

It has been suggested[4,9,10,17] that the increase in calcific deposits in the coronary arteries of elderly patients does not correlate with increased luminal narrowing. We found that the percentage of plaque occupied by calcific deposits does, in fact, increase with increasing degrees of luminal narrowing in patients ≥90 years old (Table III), but that the amount of calcium in sections narrowed <75% is greater than that found in the lesser narrowed sections of the younger patients (Table VI).

Acknowledgment: We gratefully acknowledge the technical assistance of Leslie K. Berry, Alvado M. Campbell, Filippina M. Giacometti, and Michael W. Spencer.

REFERENCES

1. Siegel JS. Recent and prospective demographic trends for the elderly population and some implications for health care. In: Haynes SG, Feinleib M, eds. Second Conference of the Epidemiology of Aging. NIH Publication No. 80-969. Washington, D.C.: U.S. Department of Health and Human Services, 1980: 289–314.

2. Wei JY. Heart disease in the elderly. *Cardiovasc Med* 1984;9:971–982.

3. Wenger NK, Furberg CD, Pitt E. Coronary Heart Disease in the Elderly. New York: Elsevier Publishing, 1986.

4. Lie JT, Hammond PI. Pathology of the senescent heart: anatomic observations on 237 autopsy studies of patients 90 to 105 years old. *Mayo Clin Proc* 1988;63:552–564.

5. Pomerance A. Pathology of the heart in the tenth decade. *J Clin Pathol* 1968;21:317–321.

6. Puxty JAH, Horan MA, Fox RA. Necropsies in the elderly. *Lancet* 1983;2:1262–1264.

7. Jónsson A, Agnarsson BA, Hallgrímsson J. Coronary atherosclerosis and myocardial infarction in nonagenarians: a retrospective autopsy study. *Age Aging* 1985;14:109–112.

8. Weber G, Bianciardi G, Bussani R, Gentilini R, Giarelli L, Novelli MT, Resi L, Salvi M, Silvestri F, Tanganelli P. Atherosclerosis and aging. A morphometric study on arterial lesions of elderly and very elderly necropsy subjects. *Arch Pathol Lab Med* 1988;112:1066–1070.

9. Waller BF, Roberts WC. Cardiovascular disease in the very elderly. Analysis of 40 necropsy patients aged 90 years or over. *Am J Cardiol* 1983;51:403–421.

10. Waller BF, Morgan R. The very elderly heart. In: Waller BF, Brest AN, eds. Contemporary Issues in Cardiovascular Pathology. Philadelphia: FA Davis, 1987:361–410.

11. Luna LG. Manual of Histological Staining Methods of the Armed Forces Institute of Pathology. 3 ed. New York: McGraw-Hill, 1968:8.

12. Movat H. Demonstration of all connective tissue elements in a single section. *Arch Pathol Lab Med* 1955;60:289–295.

13. Hook GR, Rasband W. Macmeasure: a low-cost, easy-to-operate quantitative morphometrics system for the MacIntosh computer. In: Bailey GW, ed. Proceedings of the 45th Annual Meeting of the Electron Microscopy Society of America. San Francisco: San Francisco Press, 1987:920–921.

14. Kragel AH, Reddy SG, Wittes JT, Roberts WC. Morphometric analysis of the composition of atherosclerotic plaques in the four major epicardial coronary arteries in acute myocardial infarction and in sudden coronary death. *Circulation* 1989;80:1747–1756.

15. Kragel AH, Reddy SG, Wittes JT, Roberts WC. Morphometric analysis of the composition of coronary arterial plaques in isolated unstable angina pectoris with pain at rest. *Am J Cardiol* 1990;66:893–895.

16. Dollar AL, Kragel AH, Fernicola DJ, Waclawiw MA, Roberts WC. Composition of atherosclerotic plaques in coronary arteries in women <40 years of age with fatal coronary artery disease and implications for plaque reversibility. *Am J Cardiol* 1990;67:1227–1231.

17. Eggen DA, Strong JP, McGill HC Jr. Coronary calcification, relationship to clinically significant coronary lesions and race, sex, and topographic distribution. *Circulation* 1965;32:948–955.

Morphologic Comparison of Frequency and Types of Acute Lesions in The Major Epicardial Coronary Arteries in Unstable Angina Pectoris, Sudden Coronary Death and Acute Myocardial Infarction

AMY H. KRAGEL, MD,* S. DAVID GERTZ, MD, PhD, WILLIAM C. ROBERTS, MD

Bethesda, Maryland

The frequency and type of acute lesions in the four major (right, left main, left anterior descending, left circumflex) epicardial coronary arteries were examined at necropsy in 14 patients with unstable angina pectoris, 21 patients with sudden coronary death and 32 patients with a fatal first acute myocardial infarction. None of the 67 patients had a grossly visible left ventricular scar (healed myocardial infarct) and only the group with acute myocardial infarction had left ventricular myocardial necrosis.

Although the frequency of *intraluminal thrombus* was similar in patients with unstable angina (29%) and sudden death (29%) and significantly lower than in those with acute infarction (69%) (p = 0.02), the thrombus in the patients with unstable angina and sudden death consisted almost entirely of platelets and was nonocclusive, whereas the thrombus in the group with acute infarction consisted almost entirely of fibrin and was occlusive. The frequency of *plaque rupture* was insignificantly different in the groups with unstable angina (36%) and sudden death (19%), and was significantly lower than in the group with acute infarction (75%) (p = 0.02).

The frequency of *plaque hemorrhage* was insignificantly dif-

ferent in the groups with unstable angina (64%) and sudden death (38%) and was significantly lower than in the group with acute infarction (90%) (p = 0.04). The frequency of atherosclerotic plaques containing *multiluminal channels* was similar in patients with unstable angina, sudden death and acute infarction (100%, 81% and 90%, respectively), but the percent of 5-mm long segments of the four major coronary arteries containing multiluminal channels (probably the result of organization of thrombus) was greatest in the unstable angina pectoris group (12% vs. 7% vs. 1%, respectively; p = 0.04).

Thus, the frequency of thrombus, plaque rupture and plaque hemorrhage in the coronary arteries among patients with unstable angina pectoris and sudden coronary death was similar and significantly less than in the patients with acute myocardial infarction. The type of thrombus and the amount of lumen obstructed by thrombus were similar in the groups with unstable angina pectoris and sudden coronary death and quite different from those in the group with acute myocardial infarct group.

(J Am Coll Cardiol 1991;18:801–8)

In recent years, considerable effort has been directed toward understanding the acute coronary events that may be responsible for the development of unstable angina pectoris, sudden coronary death and acute myocardial infarction. From angiographic, angioscopic and necropsy studies (1–14), it has been speculated that plaque rupture and hemorrhage with overlying intraluminal thrombus, which are the acute coronary lesions usually responsible for acute myocardial infarction, are also responsible for unstable angina pectoris. Although necropsy studies in patients with unstable angina have demonstrated plaque rupture or intraluminal thrombus, or both, all reported studies have included patients who also had acute myocardial infarction or sudden coronary death, or both. Thus, it is possible that patients with unstable angina complicated by acute myocardial infarction have acute coronary lesions similar to those in patients with acute infarction not preceded by unstable angina.

Because of the intermixing of unstable angina pectoris, sudden coronary death and acute myocardial infarction in previously reported studies, we examined in detail the major epicardial coronary arteries in patients whose only manifestation of myocardial ischemia was unstable angina not complicated by acute infarction and compared the frequency and type of acute coronary lesions in these patients with those in patients with a fatal first acute myocardial infarction and victims of sudden coronary death in whom myocardial necrosis was absent.

Methods

Cases studied and selection criteria. The autopsy records of the Pathology Branch, National Heart, Lung, and Blood Institute were searched and all cases coded as fatal coronary artery disease were reviewed. Patients who had one or more

From the Pathology Branch, National Heart, Lung, and Blood Institute, National Institutes of Health, Bethesda, Maryland.

Manuscript received November 19, 1990; revised manuscript received February 7, 1991, accepted April 3, 1991.

*Present address: Department of Pathology, St. Luke's Hospital, 44th and Wornall, Kansas City, Missouri 66103.

Address for reprints: William C. Roberts, MD, Pathology Branch, National Heart, Lung, and Blood Institute, Building 10, Room 2N258, 9000 Rockville Pike, Bethesda, Maryland 20892.

left ventricular scars (healed myocardial infarct), had undergone coronary angioplasty or coronary bypass surgery, had received thrombolytic therapy or were ≤40 years of age were excluded.

The patients with unstable angina pectoris included those who died in the hospital (13 patients) or shortly (<1 day) after hospital discharge (1 patient); none had gross or microscopic evidence of left ventricular necrosis at necropsy. In all 14 patients, there was electrocardiographic (ECG) evidence of ischemia during the final hospital admission or chest pain at rest within 24 h of death, or both. These 14 cases included all patients studied in the Pathology Branch with unstable angina pectoris in whom coronary angioplasty or bypass surgery or thrombolytic therapy had not been performed or administered, in whom no left ventricular scars were present and in whom the 5-mm coronary sections were available for examination.

All 32 patients with acute myocardial infarction were studied from 1970 to 1980 and all had transmural necrosis (involvement of all the inner half of the left ventricular wall and all or a portion of the outer half of the wall).

All 21 victims of sudden coronary death died suddenly outside the hospital usually within 15 min of onset of chest discomfort and all within 3 h of symptom onset. All 21 patients were studied at necropsy from 1978 to 1988; 10 of the 21 had been included in a previous study (15). All 21 were randomly selected from the files of the Pathology Branch. To be included, all had had histologic sections prepared from each 5-mm long segment of the four major coronary arteries. None had gross or histologic evidence of transmural left ventricular necrosis or fibrosis.

The only manifestation of myocardial ischemia in any of the 67 study patients was that which caused death. No patient with fatal acute myocardial infarction, for example, had angina pectoris; no patient with unstable angina had acute infarction and no victim of sudden coronary death had unstable or stable angina or acute infarction at any time. No patient had necropsy evidence of valvular, congenital or other specific cardiac disease. All patients with unstable angina and acute infarction were diagnosed as such by the physicians providing their clinical care.

Coronary artery preparation and examination. In each case, the four major (right, left main, left anterior descending, left circumflex) epicardial coronary arteries were dissected from the surface of the heart and processed in an identical fashion. The arteries were decalcified, sectioned gently with minimal pressure transversely at 5-mm intervals with a sharp knife blade, decalcified again if necessary, dehydrated in ethanol, cleared in xylene and embedded in paraffin. Both a Movat-stained and a hematoxylin-eosin-stained section of each 5-mm segment were prepared.

All sections containing intraluminal thrombus, plaque rupture, plaque hemorrhage and multiluminal channels were examined by all three authors and agreed on by each. In every section, the degree of cross-sectional area narrowing was estimated by examination of histologic sections magni-fied 40 times (occasionally 20 times) and the narrowing categorized into five groups: 0% to 25%, 26% to 50%, 51% to 75%, 76% to 95% or 96% to 100%. The presence or absence of thrombus, plaque rupture, plaque hemorrhage and multiluminal channels was noted in each section and confirmed by all three authors (Fig. 1 and 2).

Definitions of acute coronary lesions. *Thrombus* was defined as an occlusive or nonocclusive intraluminal aggregate of platelets or fibrin, or both, with or without associated erythrocytes and leukocytes with definite mural attachment. *Plaque rupture* was defined as a defect observed on histologic sections of coronary artery cross sections extending from the luminal surface of the plaque or with thrombus over the defect. Minor surface erosions were not considered plaque rupture. *Plaque hemorrhage* was defined as extravasation of erythrocytes into the plaque. *Multiluminal channels* were defined as multiple vascular channels present in the inner (luminal) half of the plaque.

Statistics. Statistical analysis compared the frequency of each lesion in each of the three patient groups by using either a chi-square analysis or a two-tailed Fisher's exact test.

Results

Number of patients, coronary arteries and 5-mm coronary segments studied. A total of 67 patients, 268 major epicardial arteries and 3,101 5-mm segments of the major arteries were studied: 14 patients (56 arteries and 592 5-mm segments) with unstable angina pectoris; 32 patients (128 arteries and 1,530 5-mm segments) with first fatal acute myocardial infarction and 21 patients (84 arteries and 999 5-mm segments) with sudden coronary death. Certain clinical and morphologic features in these patients are summarized in Tables 1 to 3. The age of the 67 patients ranged from 41 to 82 years (mean 61); the mean age was 61 years (11 men) in the 14 patients with unstable angina pectoris, 55 years (all men) in the 21 patients with sudden coronary death and 66 years (22 men) in the 32 patients with acute myocardial infarction. Of the 67 patients, 54 (81%) were men.

Degrees of luminal narrowing. Of the 268 major coronary arteries examined, 192 (72%) were narrowed >75% in cross-sectional area by atherosclerotic plaque, including 37 arteries (14%) narrowed >95% in cross-sectional area. The percent of arteries narrowed >75% in the unstable angina, sudden coronary death and acute myocardial infarction groups was insignificantly different (80% [45 of 56] vs. 67% [56 of 84] [p = 0.07] vs. 71% [91 of 128] [p = 0.02]), but the percent of arteries narrowed >95% was significantly higher in the unstable angina than the sudden death group (25% [14 of 56] vs. 5% [4 of 84]; p = 0.001), but not significantly different from that in the acute infarction group (15% [19 of 128]; p = 0.1).

Intraluminal thrombus. The frequency of intraluminal thrombus was similar in the unstable angina pectoris and sudden coronary death groups (29% [4 of 14] and 29% [6 of

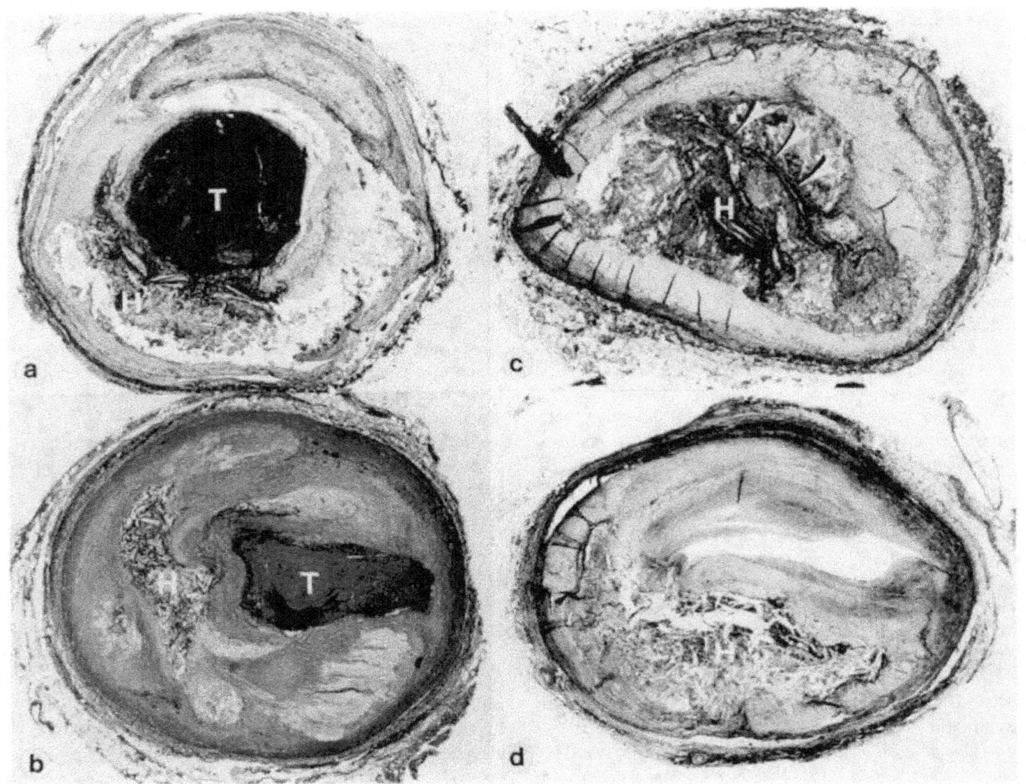

21]) and significantly lower than that in the acute myocardial infarction group (69% [22 of 32]). The thrombus was nonocclusive in all 4 patients with unstable angina, in 5 of the 6 patients with sudden death and in only 4 of the 22 patients with acute infarction. The composition of the nonocclusive and occlusive thrombi also was different: the nonocclusive thrombus consisted mainly of platelets and the occlusive thrombus mainly of fibrin. Of the 32 patients with thrombus, plaque rupture was found in association with the thrombus in 17 patients (53%): in none of the 4 patients with unstable angina, in 2 of the 6 patients with sudden death and in 15 (83%) of the 22 patients with acute infarction. In the 15 patients with thrombus unassociated with plaque rupture, hemorrhage into the plaque at the site of thrombus was found in 7; in 3 of the 4 patients with unstable angina, in 2 of the 6 patients with sudden death and in 2 of the 32 patients with acute myocardial infarction.

Plaque rupture. Plaque rupture was found in 33 (49%) of the 67 patients. Its frequency was insignificantly different in the groups with unstable angina pectoris (36% [5 of 14]) and sudden coronary death (19% [4 of 21]): in both groups, the

Figure 1. Photomicrographs of transverse sections of epicardial coronary artery in patients with fatal coronary artery disease. a. Section of the right coronary artery from a patient with fatal acute myocardial infarction and total occlusion of the lumen by thrombus (T). There is rupture of the underlying plaque with hemorrhage (H) into the plaque that is rich in pultaceous debris and contains numerous cholesterol clefts (Movat stain ×20, reduced by 15%). b. Section of the left circumflex coronary artery with total occlusion of the lumen by thrombus (T). Although hemorrhage (H) is present in the underlying plaque, no site of plaque rupture was identified (hematoxylin-eosin stain ×20, reduced by 15%). c. Section of the left circumflex coronary artery in a patient dying with unstable angina pectoris without left ventricular necrosis. The lumen (arrowheads) is compressed by plaque into which there has been extensive hemorrhage (H). A site of plaque rupture was identified in an adjacent section (Movat stain ×34, reduced by 15%). d. Section of the left anterior descending coronary artery in a patient with unstable angina pectoris with hemorrhage (H) into a lipid-rich plaque. Plaque rupture was not identified (Movat stain ×16, reduced by 15%).

frequency was significantly less than in the group with acute myocardial infarction (75% [24 of 32]; p < 0.02).

Plaque hemorrhage. This was observed in 27 (40%) of the 67 patients and its frequency was significantly lower in the

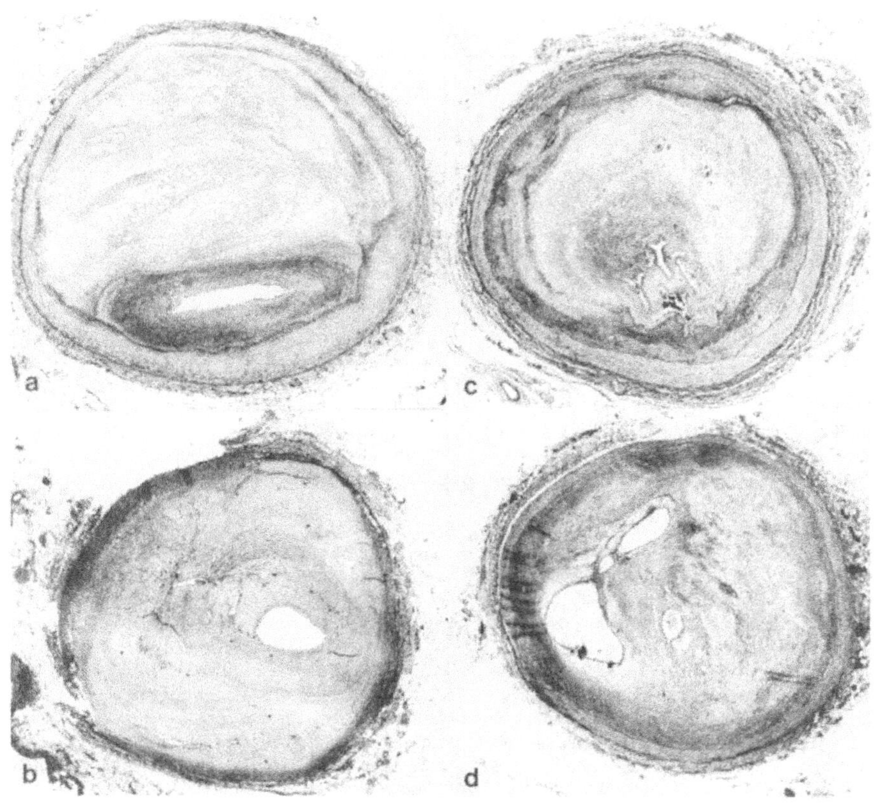

Figure 2. Photomicrographs of Movat-stained sections of an epicardial coronary artery in patients who died with unstable angina pectoris without evidence of left ventricular necrosis. **a** and **b**, Segments of a coronary artery severely narrowed by plaque composed almost entirely of fibrous tissue (Movat stain, ×27, ×26, both reduced by 15%). **c** and **d**, Segments of an artery narrowed by fibrous plaque with multiple small vascular channels (Movat stains, both ×27, both reduced by 15%).

groups with unstable angina pectoris (21% [3 of 14]) and sudden coronary death (19% [4 of 21]) compared with that in the group with acute myocardial infarction (63% [20 of 32]). Plaque hemorrhage was associated with plaque rupture or intraluminal thrombus in 20 (74%) of the 27 patients with plaque hemorrhage: in 4 of the 14 patients with unstable angina, in 4 of 21 with sudden death and in 12 of the 32 with acute infarction.

Multiluminal channels. Multiple small vascular channels were present in 60 (90%) of the 67 patients and with an insignificantly different frequency in each of the three patient groups (Table 1). The frequency of multiluminal channels in each 5-mm long segment of coronary artery was significantly

higher in the group with unstable angina pectoris (12% [66 of 572]) than in either the sudden coronary death group (7% [72 of 999]) or acute myocardial infarction group (7% [107 of 1,530]) (Table 3).

Discussion

Major morphologic complications. Comparison of findings from examination of a histologic section from each of 3,101 5-mm segments of 268 major epicardial coronary arteries from 67 patients with fatal coronary artery disease disclosed that the frequency of three acute coronary lesions (namely, intraluminal thrombus, plaque rupture and plaque hemorrhage) was similar in patients with unstable angina pectoris and sudden coronary death and that the frequency of each of these acute lesions was significantly higher in patients with fatal first transmural acute myocardial infarction. Furthermore, although multiluminal channels (not acute lesions) within plaques were frequent in all three patient groups, these lesions were found significantly more often in 5-mm segments of coronary arteries in the group

Table 1. Frequency of Acute Coronary Lesions and Multiluminal Channels at Necropsy in Patients With Unstable Angina Pectoris, Sudden Coronary Death and Acute Myocardial Infarction

Coronary Subset	No. of Patients	Coronary Arteries			
		Thrombus	Plaque Rupture	Plaque Hemorrhage	Multiluminal Channels
Unstable angina pectoris	14	4 (29%)*	5 (36%)*	3 (21%)*	14 (100%)
Sudden coronary death	21	6 (29%)*	4 (19%)*	4 (19%)*	17 (81%)
Acute myocardial infarction	32	22 (69%)†	24 (75%)†	20 (63%)†	29 (91%)
Total	67	32 (48%)	33 (49%)	27 (40%)	59 (90%)

* versus † in same vertical column = p < 0.02.

with unstable angina than in the groups with sudden death and acute infarction (where their frequency was similar).

Unstable Angina Pectoris

Previous studies. Several angiographic studies (1–5) have identified either intraluminal filling defects consistent with thrombus or specific morphologic lesions (eccentric narrowings with irregular borders) in patients with unstable angina pectoris, and these defects have been used to distinguish such patients from those with stable angina (1–3). Comparison of postmortem angiographic and histologic findings (6), however, in patients with coronary artery disease (not necessarily unstable angina pectoris) has shown that these irregular eccentric lesions may represent not only sites of intraluminal thrombus, but also plaque rupture, plaque hemorrhage or organized thrombus. In addition, three angioscopic studies (7–9) have identified intraluminal thrombus and ulceration or rupture of plaque in patients with unstable angina. On the basis of these studies, it has been widely speculated that the lesion responsible for the development of unstable angina pectoris is an ulcerated plaque over which nonocclusive intraluminal thrombus develops.

Limitations of previous studies. Before accepting that this hypothesis is indeed true for all or most patients with unstable angina pectoris, the limitations of the previous studies (1–9) need to be considered. Interpretation of the significance of the eccentric irregular lesions seen angiographically in patients with unstable angina is based largely on the work of Levin and Fallon (6), who compared postmortem coronary arteriograms and histologic sections of coronary artery narrowings in 39 patients who died either after coronary artery bypass surgery or of consequences of acute myocardial infarction. (Because the trauma of bypass surgery may be associated with plaque rupture or plaque hemorrhage, or both, patients who had undergone this procedure were excluded from our study.) They identified 38 narrowings that had irregular borders or intraluminal lucencies by angiography. Of these, 8 (21%) were acute or organizing nonocclusive thrombi overlying atherosclerotic plaque, 6 (16%) were nonocclusive thrombi overlying sites of plaque rupture or hemorrhage, 10 (26%) were sites of plaque hemorrhage or rupture without thrombus, 6 (16%) contained recanalized thrombus (presumably multiluminal channels) and 21% showed narrowing of the segment by plaque without any complicating acute lesion. More than a third of the irregular eccentric lesions studied, therefore, showed no acute lesion that would account for the abrupt change in symptoms in the setting of unstable angina. In our study, plaques containing multiluminal channels, although common to all three groups of patients, were seen with greatest frequency in the group with unstable angina.

When interpreting reports of angiographic or angioscopic studies in patients with unstable angina pectoris, it is assumed that the patients did not have left ventricular necrosis (acute myocardial infarction) at the time of study, an assumption that may or may not be true. Guthrie et al. (10) studied 12 patients with unstable angina who died shortly after coronary artery bypass surgery. At autopsy, 4 of the 12 patients had acute myocardial infarction that histologically appeared to have occurred before the operation and acute myocardial infarction was not suspected clinically in any of

Table 2. Frequency of Acute Lesions and Multiluminal Channels at Necropsy in the Four Major Epicardial Coronary Arteries in Unstable Angina Pectoris, Sudden Coronary Death and Acute Myocardial Infarction

Coronary Subset	No. of Coronary Arteries	Coronary Arteries			
		Thrombus	Plaque Rupture	Plaque Hemorrhage	Multiluminal Channels
Unstable angina pectoris	56	4 (7%)	9 (16%)	15 (27%)	32 (57%)
Sudden coronary death	84	6 (7%)	4 (5%)	10 (12%)	32 (38%)
Acute myocardial infarction	128	22 (17%)	27 (21%)	47 (37%)	69 (50%)
Total	268	32 (12%)	40 (15%)	72 (27%)	133 (50%)

Table 2. Frequency of Acute Coronary Lesions and Multiluminal Channels at Necropsy in 5-mm Long Segments of the Four Major Epicardial Coronary Arteries in Unstable Angina Pectoris, Sudden Coronary Death and Acute Myocardial Infarction

	No. of 5-mm Coronary Segments	Coronary Arteries			
Coronary Subset		Thrombus	Plaque Rupture	Plaque Hemorrhage	Multiluminal Channels
Unstable angina pectoris	572	11 (2%)	7 (1%)	24 (4%)	66 (12%)*
Sudden coronary death	999	6 (0.6%)	5 (0.5%)	19 (2%)	72 (7%)†
Acute myocardial infarction	1,530	105 (7%)	59 (4%)	117 (8%)	107 (7%)†
Total	3,101	122 (4%)	71 (2%)	160 (5%)	245 (8%)

* versus † in same vertical column = p < 0.004.

the 4 patients. Therefore, when studying living patients, it may be difficult to determine whether the patients have pure unstable angina pectoris or have combined unstable angina pectoris and acute myocardial infarction.

Information regarding coronary artery morphology in patients with unstable angina pectoris is scant, difficult to obtain and difficult to interpret for several reasons. Unstable angina pectoris is rarely fatal and those patients who do die during the period of unstable angina usually have had a coronary angioplasty or bypass procedure performed or have experienced an acute myocardial infarction shortly before death. In patients with acute infarction preceded by unstable angina pectoris, intracoronary lesions may not be representative of those occurring in patients with unstable angina not complicated by acute infarction.

Information regarding the acute coronary lesions in patients who died shortly after coronary artery bypass surgery has been provided in several studies. Guthrie et al. (10) described 12 patients and Roberts and Virmani (11) described 19 patients with unstable angina pectoris who died shortly after coronary bypass surgery. In both studies, the frequency of intraluminal thrombus was low (8% and 12%, respectively) when patients with acute myocardial infarction were excluded. In a separate report, Virmani and Roberts (12) described the frequency of extravasated erythrocytes and fibrin in the plaque of 17 of the 22 patients with unstable angina. Plaque hemorrhage (erythrocytes with or without fibrin) was identified in 94% of their patients. It is likely that surgical manipulation of the epicardial coronary arteries was responsible for the plaque hemorrhage in many of these cases.

In a study of unstable angina with fatal outcome, Falk (13) provided information regarding the frequency of acute lesions in the epicardial coronary arteries of patients with sudden coronary death, unstable angina pectoris and acute myocardial infarction. He described necropsy findings in ". . . 25 patients, all of whom died of acute coronary thrombosis within 24 hours after the onset of acute symptoms." Of the 24 patients for whom clinical information was available, 15 clearly had, 2 had an equivocal history of and 7 did not have unstable angina pectoris. Of these 25 patients, 15 had coagulative necrosis (acute myocardial infarction), that, as

determined histologically, was compatible with an age of <24 h. In these patients, he described lamellar thrombi (21 of 25 patients, including 14 of 15 with unstable angina pectoris) 81% of which were associated with plaque rupture and hemorrhage. Neither the frequency of plaque rupture nor the number of thrombotic episodes differed between the patients with and without unstable angina. Because all of these patients died suddenly (some with unstable angina and some with unstable angina complicated by acute infarction), the three ischemic syndromes cannot be analyzed individually.

Sudden Coronary Death With or Without Unstable Angina

Davies et al. (14) studied 90 patients who died suddenly outside the hospital within 6 h of the onset of pain "or other symptoms." The data were presented in a report entitled "Intramyocardial platelet aggregation in patients with unstable angina suffering sudden ischemic cardiac death." Of their 90 patients, 36 (40%) had chest or arm pain at some time in the 2 weeks preceding death. The history of chest pain was obtained by a coroner's police officer from the next of kin who had been living with the patient. Thus, the history was not obtained from the patient or a physician. None of the 90 patients had been admitted to a hospital with increasing chest pain. There was no information on any patient regarding the presence or absence of chest pain at rest. Thus, in none of the 90 patients was the type, location or severity of the pain known. Nevertheless, these patients were considered to have unstable angina pectoris. Necropsy in the 90 patients disclosed the following: 31 (30%) had nonocclusive intracoronary thrombus, 22 (24%) had sudden coronary death associated with "regional coagulative necrosis" (acute myocardial infarction) and 23 (25%) had nontransmural necrosis. Of the 36 patients with chest or arm pain at some time in the 2 weeks before death, 35 had plaque rupture identified in one of the major epicardial coronary arteries. Of the 54 without chest pain in the 2 weeks before death, 51 had plaque rupture. Thus, whether the patients in that study had unstable angina pectoris is unknown. Some probably did have unstable angina pectoris, but some clearly had acute myocardial infarction and the majority would

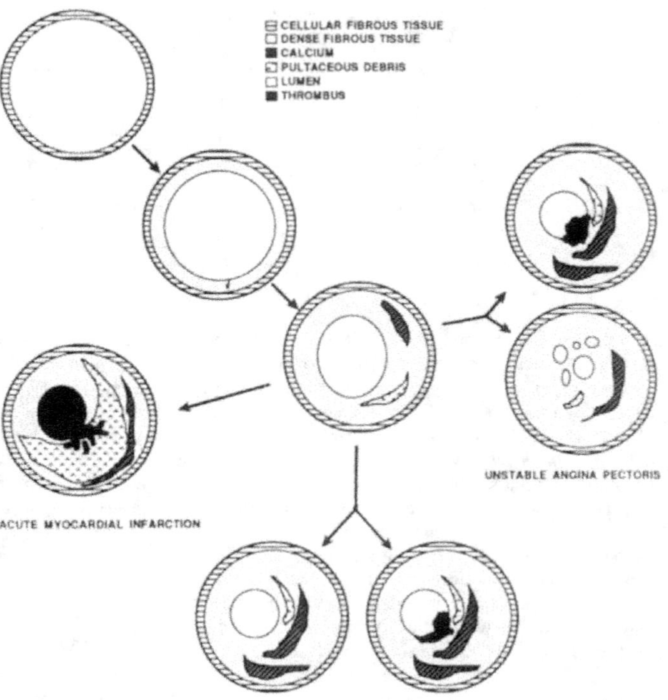

Figure 3. Diagram of coronary artery plaque morphology in patients with fatal coronary artery disease due to acute myocardial infarction, sudden coronary death without transmural left ventricular necrosis or unstable angina pectoris without transmural left ventricular necrosis. In all three groups, the mean percent of cellular fibrous tissue decreases with increasing degrees of luminal narrowing and the mean percent of dense fibrous tissue, calcific deposits and pultaceous debris rich in extracellular lipid increases. Severely narrowed segments in the group with acute myocardial infarction contain more pultaceous debris and are characterized by plaque rupture with associated hemorrhage and occlusive intraluminal thrombus. Severely narrowed segments in the group with unstable angina pectoris are characterized by the presence of multiluminal channels. Nonocclusive thrombus and plaque hemorrhage with or without plaque rupture can be seen in all three groups.

fulfill most investigators' definition of sudden coronary death. Diagnosing unstable angina pectoris in persons not admitted to the hospital whose history was obtained by a nonphysician is difficult to say the least.

Centrally placed multiluminal vascular channels. These vascular channels were present in 90% of our 67 patients. Most likely they represented organized thrombus (the consequence of a previous thrombotic event) and were usually at a site where the lumen was severely narrowed by plaque. Multiluminal channels were observed in a significantly higher percent of the 5-mm coronary segments in our patients with unstable angina pectoris compared with those with either sudden coronary death or acute myocardial infarction. Data on the frequency of multiluminal channels in coronary plaque in patients with unstable angina, sudden death and acute infarction have been reported in only one previous study (12).

Plaque rupture and hemorrhage. It is possible that small sites of plaque rupture were not detected by examining the epicardial coronary arteries at 5-mm intervals in our study. It is likely, however, that associated plaque hemorrhage would have been detected. Although hemorrhage into plaque theoretically may be derived from sources other than intimal plaque rupture, the percent of cases that actually had plaque rupture (detected or not in this study) should be equal to or

less than the percent of cases containing plaque hemorrhage. If this is the case, then the maximal percent of the unstable angina pectoris group that could have had plaque rupture is 64% of the acute myocardial infarction group, 90% and of the sudden coronary death group, 38%. Even under these circumstances, plaque rupture would be much more common in acute infarction than in unstable angina or sudden death. Small nonocclusive thrombus or intraluminal platelet aggregates might also have been missed. Because all cases were handled in an identical fashion, it is likely that they would have been missed in all three groups with equal frequency.

Unstable angina and sudden coronary death versus acute myocardial infarction (Fig. 3). The lower frequency of plaque rupture and occlusive thrombus in the groups with unstable angina pectoris and sudden coronary death compared with that in the group with acute myocardial infarction may be a reflection of differences in plaque composition between these groups (16). Likewise, the similarity in the frequency of these acute coronary lesions in patients with unstable angina and sudden death may be a reflection of the similarity in plaque composition in these two groups (15). It has been shown (15,16) that in all three types of patients, the mean percent of dense fibrous tissue, calcific deposits and pultaceous debris increases with increasing degrees of luminal narrowing and the mean percent of cellular fibrous tissue decreases (Fig. 3). Severely narrowed segments in the acute myocardial infarction group (those narrowed >75% in cross-sectional area) contain significantly more pultaceous debris and significantly less calcium and cellular fibrous tissue than do similarly narrowed segments in the unstable angina pectoris and sudden coronary death groups. Because occlusive thrombus is almost exclusively seen in association with rupture of a lipid-rich plaque, the greater the amount of pultaceous debris, the greater is the frequency of plaque rupture and occlusive thrombus in these patients (16).

The characteristic lesion in patients with a fatal first acute myocardial infarction, then, is an occlusive thrombus overlying a ruptured plaque rich in pultaceous debris (Fig. 3); in patients with unstable angina pectoris, it is a severely narrowed segment frequently containing multiluminal channels with or without a small nonocclusive thrombus (Fig. 3); in patients with sudden coronary death without left ventricular necrosis, it is a segment of coronary artery with significant luminal narrowing by atherosclerotic plaque with or without platelet-rich nonocclusive thrombus (Fig. 3). Thus, the frequency of acute coronary lesions (intraluminal thrombus, plaque rupture and plaque hemorrhage) in patients with unstable angina (not complicated by acute myocardial infarction) and sudden death (not complicated by acute infarction) is similar and the frequency of these lesions is significantly lower than that observed in patients with acute infarction.

References

1. Cowley MJ, DiSciasco G, Rehr RB, Vetrovec GW. Angiographic observations and clinical relevance of coronary thrombus in unstable angina pectoris. Am J Cardiol 1989;63:108E–13E.
2. Gotoh K, Minamino T, Katoh O, et al. The role of intracoronary thrombus in unstable angina: angiographic assessment and thrombolytic therapy during ongoing anginal attacks. Circulation 1988;77:526–34.
3. Ambrose JA, Winters SL, Stern A, et al. Angiographic morphology and the pathogenesis of unstable angina pectoris. J Am Coll Cardiol 1985;5:609–16.
4. Vetrovec GW, Leinbach RC, Gold HK, Cowley MJ. Intracoronary thrombolysis in syndromes of unstable ischemia: angiographic and clinical results. Am Heart J 1982;104:946–52.
5. Holmes DR, Hartzler GO, Smith HC, Fuster V. Coronary artery thrombosis in patients with unstable angina. Br Heart J 1981;45:411–6.
6. Levin DC, Fallon JT. Significance of the angiographic morphology of localized coronary stenoses: histopathologic correlations. Circulation 1982;66:316–20.
7. Hombach V, Hoher M, Kochs M, et al. Pathophysiology of unstable angina pectoris: correlations with angioscopic imaging. Eur Heart J 1988;9(suppl N):40–5.
8. Forrester JS, Litvack F, Grundfest W. A perspective of coronary disease seen through the arteries of living man. Circulation 1987;75:505–13.
9. Sherman CT, Litvack F, Grundfest W, et al. Coronary angioscopy in patients with unstable angina pectoris. N Engl J Med 1986;315:913–9.
10. Guthrie RB, Vlodaver Z, Nicoloff DM, Edwards JE. Pathology of stable and unstable angina pectoris. Circulation 1975;51:1059–63.
11. Roberts WC, Virmani R. Quantification of coronary arterial narrowing in clinically-isolated unstable angina pectoris: an analysis of 22 necropsy patients. Am J Med 1979;67:792–9.
12. Virmani R, Roberts WC. Extravasated erythrocytes, iron, and fibrin in atherosclerotic plaques of coronary arteries in fatal coronary heart disease and their relation to intraluminal thrombus: frequency and significance in 57 necropsy patients and in 2958 five-mm segments of 224 major epicardial coronary arteries. Am Heart J 1983;105:788–97.
13. Falk E. Unstable angina with fatal outcome: dynamic coronary thrombosis leading to infarction and/or sudden death. Circulation 1985;71:699–708.
14. Davies MJ, Thomas AC, Knapman PA, Hangartner JR. Intramyocardial platelet aggregation in patients with unstable angina suffering sudden ischemic cardiac death. Circulation 1986;73:418–27.
15. Kragel AH, Reddy SG, Wittes JT, Roberts WC. Morphometric analysis of the composition of coronary arterial plaques in isolated unstable angina pectoris with pain at rest. Am J Cardiol 1990;66:562–7.
16. Kragel AH, Reddy SG, Wittes JT, Roberts WC. Morphometric analysis of the composition of atherosclerotic plaques in the four major epicardial coronary arteries in acute myocardial infarction and sudden coronary death. Circulation 1989;80:1747–56.

The Heart in Fatal Unstable Angina Pectoris

William C. Roberts, MD, Amy H. Kragel, MD, S. David Gertz, MD, PhD
Charles S. Roberts, MD, Jay M. Kalan, MD

Compared to patients with sudden coronary death and acute myocardial infarction, relatively little morphologic data has been reported in patients with unstable angina pectoris. This article reviews necropsy data collected from one laboratory on unstable angina pectoris. From these data, several observations are appropriate: (1) Patients with unstable angina as a group have more coronary narrowing by atherosclerotic plaque than do patients with sudden coronary death or acute or healed myocardial infarction. (2) Patients with unstable angina have a much higher frequency of severe narrowing of the left main coronary artery than do patients in other coronary subsets. (3) The coronary atherosclerotic plaques in unstable angina consist primarily of fibrous tissue, and they are more similar to those found in patients with sudden coronary death than in patients with acute myocardial infarction. (4) The frequency of acute coronary lesions (thrombi, plaque rupture, and plaque hemorrhage) is similar to that observed in patients with sudden coronary death and significantly less than that observed in acute myocardial infarction. (5) The frequency of multiluminal channels throughout the major coronary arteries is significantly higher in unstable angina compared to sudden coronary death or acute myocardial infarction. (6) The major epicardial arteries and the heart are smaller in patients with unstable angina than in patients with sudden coronary death or acute myocardial infarction. (7) The left ventricular cavity is usually of normal size in patients with unstable angina and therefore left ventricular function is usually normal.

(Am J Cardiol 1991;68:22B–27B)

Most patients with severe atherosclerotic coronary artery disease die suddenly (sudden coronary death[1]) from a ventricular arrhythmia or from an acute myocardial infarction. As a consequence a great deal of information is available on necropsy cardiac findings in patients with sudden coronary death or with acute myocardial infarction. Although angina pectoris is the most common symptom of severe atherosclerotic coronary artery disease, angina pectoris is rarely fatal. When a person with stable angina dies during an anginal attack, death is usually attributed to the sudden development of a ventricular arrhythmia (sudden coronary death) and not to angina pectoris. Likewise, death during unstable angina pectoris is uncommon, and then usually when acute myocardial infarction supervenes or an unsuccessful invasive procedure (coronary bypass or angioplasty) is performed. If acute infarction occurs, the patient is placed in the acute myocardial infarction category at necropsy; if death occurs after an invasive procedure, death is usually attributed to one or more complications of the procedure rather than to unstable angina per se. As a consequence, the amount of information available at necropsy on patients with isolated stable angina is minimal.[2] More information, although still limited, is available on necropsy findings in patients with unstable angina pectoris shortly before death. The data accumulated in the last 25 years at the Pathology Branch, National Heart, Lung and Blood Institute, on patients with unstable angina will be summarized in this article.

AMOUNTS OF CORONARY ARTERIAL LUMINAL NARROWING IN UNSTABLE ANGINA

In 1979 Roberts and Virmani[3] reported necropsy findings in the 4 major (right, left main, left anterior descending, and left circumflex) epicardial coronary arteries in 22 patients with clinically-isolated unstable angina pectoris. "Clinically-

From the Pathology Branch, National Heart, Lung, and Blood Institute, National Institutes of Health, Bethesda, Maryland.

Dr. Kragel's present address is Department of Pathology, St. Luke's Hospital, Kansas City, Missouri. Dr. Gertz's present address is Department of Anatomy, The Hebrew University, Hadassah Medical School, Jerusalem, Israel. Dr. Kalan's present address is Section of Cardiology, University of Virginia Medical Center, Charlottesville, Virginia. Dr. C.S. Robert's present address is Department of Surgery, Medical University of South Carolina, Charleston, South Carolina.

Address for reprints: William C. Roberts, MD, Building 10, Room 2N-258, National Institutes of Health, 9000 Rockville Pike, Bethesda, Maryland 20892.

isolated" was defined as absence of clinical evidence at any time of acute myocardial infarction or of congestive cardiac failure. No patient had associated valvular, congenital, primary myocardial, or pericardial heart disease. "Unstable angina" was defined as anterior thoracic pain of recent (<1 month) onset or a recent change in the pattern of the pain in terms of frequency, severity, intensity, and ease of provocation. Nocturnal or rest angina or prolonged angina within 3 months of death was considered unstable. All 22 patients had an aorto-coronary bypass operation and each died within 7 days of the procedure. The 22 patients ranged in age from 37 to 59 years (mean 48); 13 were men and 9 were women. The angina had been present periodically from 2 to 120 months (mean 18). Ten had had systemic hypertension (blood pressure $>140/90$ mm Hg).

Among the 22 patients, 85 major epicardial coronary arteries were examined: 71 (81%) were narrowed by atherosclerotic plaque occupying $>75\%$ of the luminal cross-sectional area in an average of 3.2/4.0 coronary arteries per patient. If the left main coronary artery was excluded, 61 (93%) of the other 66 major coronary arteries were narrowed $>75\%$ in cross-sectional area by plaque, an average of 2.8/3.0 coronary arteries per patient. Of the 22 patients, 21 (95%) had 76–100% cross-sectional area narrowing by plaque of 2 or more major epicardial coronary arteries, including 10 patients (45%) who had this degree of narrowing in all 4 major epicardial arteries. Only 1 patient (5%) had this degree of narrowing involving just 1 artery. Comparison of these findings to other subsets of coronary patients is summarized in Table I.[4,5]

To determine the extent of the atherosclerotic process in the coronary arteries, the epicardial arteries in each of the 22 patients were divided into 5-mm segments and a histologic section stained by the Movat method was prepared from each segment. A total of 1,049 segments 5-mm in length were prepared from the 85 epicardial coronary arteries in the 22 patients. Of them, 497 segments (47%) were narrowed 76–100% in cross-sectional area by atherosclerotic plaque; 304 segments (29%) were narrowed 51–75%; 129 were narrowed 26–50%; and 119 segments (11%) were narrowed 0–25%. The mean percentage of 5-mm segments narrowed 76–100% in cross-sectional area in the proximal halves of the left anterior descending and right coronary arteries was greater than the mean percentage of 5-mm segments similarly narrowed in the distal halves of these 2 arteries. The 7 patients aged ≤ 45 years had a higher percentage of 5-mm segments severely ($>75\%$) narrowed than did the 15 patients aged 46–65 years (63 ± 6% vs 41 ± 6%; p <0.05). Sex, heart weight, and the presence or absence of a healed left ventricular infarct (clinically silent) did not alter the percentage of segments severely narrowed. Compared with other subsets of coronary patients, unstable angina patients have by far the severest degree of coronary narrowing by atherosclerotic plaque (Table II).[4,5]

In 1990 Kragel and associates[6] reported necropsy findings in 10 patients with isolated unstable pectoris with pain at rest. In contrast to the 1979 study by Roberts and Virmani,[3] the 1990 study excluded patients whose death occurred during or immediately after cardiac catheterization or coronary bypass or angioplasty. All 10 patients died during or immediately after a hospital admission for evaluation of unstable angina and none had gross or microscopic evidence at necropsy of either transmural left ventricular necrosis or fibrosis. The 10 patients ranged in age from 47 to 70 years (mean 59); 9 were men. The duration of angina ranged from 6 weeks to 19 years. Of the 10 patients, 9 had

TABLE I Number of Major (Right, Left Main, Left Anterior Descending and Left Circumflex) Coronary Arteries Narrowed $>75\%$ in Cross-Sectional Area by Atherosclerotic Plaque in Fatal Coronary Artery Disease

Coronary Event	Pts (n)	Mean Age (yrs)	Number of Patients with CSA Narrowing $>75\%$ by Plaque in 1–4 Arteries				
			4	3	2	1	Mean
Sudden coronary death	31	47	3	20	6	2	2.8
Acute myocardial infarction	27	59	3	14	10	0	2.7
Healed myocardial infarction							
Asymptomatic	18	66	0	7	7	4	2.2
Chronic CHF without aneurysm	9	63	0	3	5	1	2.2
Left ventricular aneurysm	22	61	1	12	6	3	2.5
Angina pectoris/unstable	22	48	10	8	3	1	3.2
Total (%)	129	56	17 (13)	64 (50)	37 (29)	11 (8)	2.7
Controls (%)	40	52	0 (0)	5 (5)	12 (13)	21 (23)	0.7

CHF = congestive heart failure; CSA = cross-sectional area.

TABLE II Amounts of Cross-Sectional Area Narrowing of Each 5-mm Segment of the Four Major (Right, Left Main, Left Anterior Descending and Left Circumflex) Epicardial Coronary Arteries by Atherosclerotic Plaque in Subjects with Fatal Coronary Artery Disease

Subgroup	Pts (n)	Mean Age (yrs)	No. 5-mm Segments	Percentage of Segments per Occlusion Quartile				Mean Score	Mean % Narrowing/ 5-mm Segments
				0–25%	25–50%	51–75%	76–100%		
Sudden coronary death	31	47	1,564	7	23	34	36	2.98	67
Acute myocardial infarction	27	59	1,403	5	23	38	34	3.01	68
Healed myocardial infarction									
Asymptomatic	18	66	924	11	23	35	31	2.87	64
Chronic CHF								31%	
without aneurysm	9	63	529	11	23	37	29	2.78	61
LV aneurysm	22	61	992	4	21	42	33	3.03	68
Angina pectoris	22	48	1,049	11	12	29	48	3.12	70
Total	129	56	6,461	8	21	36	35	2.98	67
Controls	40	52	1,849	31	44	22	3	1.97	32

CHF = congestive heart failure; LV = left ventricular

> 75% cross-sectional area narrowing by plaque of the left anterior descending, left circumflex, and right coronary arteries, and 4 patients had this degree of narrowing of all 4 major coronary arteries. Eight of the 10 patients had at least 1 major coronary artery narrowed > 95% in cross-sectional area by plaque.

A total of 354 of these 5-mm segments from the 40 major epicardial coronary arteries were examined in the 10 patients: 32 segments (9%) were narrowed 96–100% in cross-sectional area by plaque; 114 segments (32%) were narrowed 75–95%; 114 segments (32%) were narrowed 51–75%; 76 segments (22%), 26–50%, and 18 segments (5%) were narrowed 0–25% by plaque alone. Among the 10 patients, considerable range of severity of narrowing by plaque was observed. Although 41% of all 354 of the 5-mm segments were narrowed 76–100% by plaque, the percentage of segments severely narrowed per patient varied from 18% to 75%.

COMPOSITION OF ATHEROSCLEROTIC PLAQUES IN THE EPICARDIAL CORONARY ARTERIES IN UNSTABLE ANGINA

In 1990 Kragel and associates[6] reported for the first time the composition of coronary atherosclertic plaques in a group of patients with unstable angina. Using the same 10 patients heretofore described, plaque composition in each of the 354 Movat-stained histologic sections of coronary artery was analyzed using a computerized morphometry system. The major component of plaque was a combination of dense acellular and cellular fibrous tissue with much smaller portions of plaque being composed of pultaceous debris, calcium deposits, and foam cells. No differences in plaque composition were observed in specimens taken from any of the 4 major epicardial coronary arteries. Plaque composition varied as a function of the degree of luminal narrowing. Linear *increases* were observed in the mean percentage of dense fibrous tissue (from 5% to 50%), calcific deposits (from 1% to 10%), pultaceous debris (from 0% to 10%), and inflammatory infiltrates without significant numbers of foam cells (from 0% to 5%), and a linear *decrease* was observed in the mean percentage of cellular fibrous tissue (from 94% to 22%) in sections narrowed 25% to > 95% in cross-sectional area. Comparison of plaque composition in the large coronary plaques (those causing > 75% luminal narrowing) in the unstable angina patients with other subsets of coronary patients is summarized in Figure 1.[6,7]

FREQUENCY AND TYPES OF ACUTE LESIONS IN THE EPICARDIAL CORONARY ARTERIES IN UNSTABLE ANGINA

In 1991, Kragel and associates[8] reported the frequency and type of acute lesions in the 4 major epicardial coronary arteries in 3 subsets of coronary patients, including 14 patients with unstable angina. Ten of the 14 patients had been included in the 1990 study by Kragel and associates.[7] Of the 14 patients, 13 died in the hospital and 1 died within 24 hours of hospital discharge. None had gross or microscopic evidence of left ventricular necrosis or fibrosis. In all 14 patients there was electrocardiographic evidence of myocardial ischemia during the final hospital admission or chest pain at rest within 24 hours of death, or both. None had had coronary bypass, angioplasty, or thrombolytic therapy, and none had left ventricular scars by gross examination of the heart.

Intraluminal thrombus occurred in 4 (29%) of the 14 patients, in 4 (7%) of the 56 epicardial

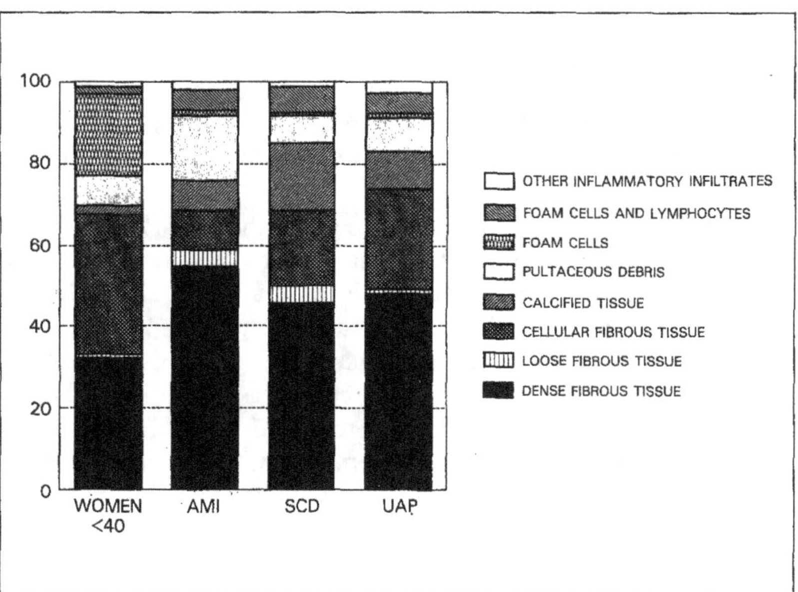

FIGURE 1. Graph comparing plaque composition (mean percentage) in specimens causing > 75% cross-sectional area luminal narrowing in the patients with unstable angina pectoris (UAP) to those in patients whose coronary event was sudden coronary death (SCD) and acute myocardial infarction (AMI). All patients with UAP, SCD, or AMI were > 40 years of age (mean 59 years). The findings in the older patients are compared with those of 8 women aged 31–39 years (mean 34) with fatal coronary events. In all subgroups, fibrous tissue was the dominant component of the large coronary plaques. (Reproduced with permission from Dollar AL, Kragel AH, Fernicola DJ, Waclawiw MA, and Roberts WC. Composition of atherosclerotic plaques in coronary arteries in women < 40 years of age with fatal coronary artery disease and implications for plaque reversibility. *Am J Cardiol* 1991;67:1223–1227.)

coronary arteries in the 14 patients, and in 11 of 572 (2%) 5-mm segments of the 56 arteries. The thrombi were small, nonocclusive, and consisted mainly of platelets. *Plaque rupture* was found in 5 (36%) of the 14 patients, including only 1 of the 4 patients with nonocclusive thrombi, in 9 (16%) of the 56 coronary arteries, and in 7 of the 572 (1%) 5-mm coronary segments. *Plaque hemorrhage* was found in 3 (21%) of the 14 patients, each of whom also had plaque rupture; in 15 (27%) of the 56 coronary arteries; and in 24 (4%) of the 572 coronary segments. Intraluminal thrombus and/or plaque rupture and/or plaque hemorrhage were found in 9 (64%) of the 14 patients. Thus, 5 (36%) of the 14 patients had no acute lesions. The frequency of thrombi, plaque rupture, and plaque hemorrhage was similar to that found in patients with sudden coronary death and significantly less than in acute myocardial infarction patients.[8]

Multiluminal channels within coronary atherosclerotic plaques were seen in all 14 patients, in 32 (57%) of the 56 coronary arteries in the 14 patients, and in 66 of the 572 (12%) 5-mm segments of the 56 coronary arteries (Figure 2). These channels are more frequent in unstable angina compared with patients with sudden coronary death or acute myocardial infarction.[8]

SIZES OF THE EPICARDIAL CORONARY ARTERIES IN UNSTABLE ANGINA

In 1980, Roberts and Roberts[9] reported cross-sectional area of the most proximal portions of the right, left anterior descending, and left circumflex coronary arteries in necropsy patients with fatal coronary artery disease, including 20 patients with clinically isolated angina pectoris who died shortly

after an aorto-coronary bypass operation. The cross-sectional area of the most proximal 5-mm segment of each of the 3 major coronary arteries (excludes left main) was determined by planimetry. A histologic section (Movat staining method) was prepared from each of the three 5-mm segments from each of the 3 coronary arteries from each patient. Each histologic section was positioned on the stage of a projection-light microscope that magnified the image 650 times. The circumference of the internal elastic membrane was then traced on paper. Each tracing was placed under a focused camera, passed through an electronic integrator, and displayed on a television monitor. The analog

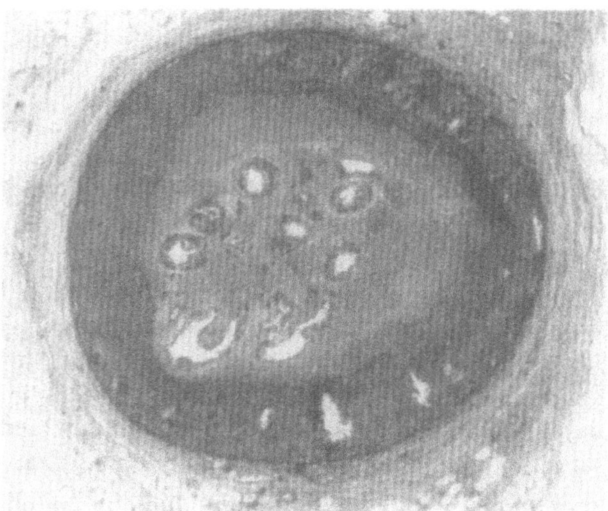

FIGURE 2. Photomicrograph of section of left circumflex coronary artery in a patient with unstable angina pectoris showing multiluminal channels within the fibrous plaque. These multiluminal channels are significantly more frequent in the sections of 5-mm segments of the major epicardial coronary arteries compared to patients with fatal acute myocardial infarction or sudden coronary death. Movat stain, ×30.

output voltages of the video planimeters, calibrated on a grid system, provided on-line measurements of the cross-sectional area. The area of each artery enclosed by the internal elastic membrane provided by the videoplanimetry was converted to the actual area.

The mean cross-sectional area of each of the 60 arteries in the 20 patients with angina pectoris was 6.2 mm^2. These were the smallest arteries of any of the coronary subsets studied. In contrast, the mean cross-sectional area of each of the 3 arteries in 23 patients with acute myocardial infarction was 7.6 mm^2; in 19 patients with sudden coronary death, 7.7 mm^2; and in 18 patients with ischemic cardiomyopathy (chronic congestive heart failure with healed myocardial infarction), 8.6 mm^2. The mean size in 31 cancer control subjects was 5.0 mm^2 and in 15 patients with aortic valve disease, 9.6 mm^2.

The differences in cross-sectional area of the coronary arteries among the coronary subsets and between and among the control subjects was due primarily to differences in heart weight. The angina pectoris group had the smallest hearts (mean 386 g) and the ischemic cardiomyopathy subgroup had the largest hearts (mean 588 g). The acute myocardial infarction and sudden coronary death subgroups were intermediate. The cancer control subjects had the smallest coronary arteries and the smallest hearts (mean 309 g) and the aortic valve control subjects had the largest coronary arteries and the largest hearts (mean 703 g). When the heart weights in the coronary subgroups and in the 2 control groups were equalized by using the same regression coefficient, no significant differences were present among the mean values of cross-sectional area of the coronary arteries.

SIGNIFICANCE OF CARDIAC WEIGHT IN PATIENTS HAVING CORONARY ARTERY BYPASS GRAFTING FOR ANGINA PECTORIS

Kalan and Roberts[10] in 1988 reported cardiac weight at necropsy in 211 patients who had isolated coronary artery bypass grafting (coronary bypass) for angina pectoris. They sought the relation of heart weight to early (<60 days) and late (>60 days) death after coronary bypass. Cases selected for study included only patients who had coronary bypass because of angina pectoris. Patients having coronary bypass within 2 months of acute myocardial infarction were excluded. The 121 patients dying early had a lower mean heart weight than did the 90 patients dying late (444 ± 94 vs 498 ± 107 g; p <0.001). The mean heart weight of the 85 men dying early was less than that of the 75 men dying late (472 vs 506 g; p <0.05), and the mean heart weight of the 36 women dying early was less than that of the 15 women dying late (377 vs 459 g; p <0.005). Most patients with hearts of normal weight were in the early death group: of the 17 women with hearts of normal weight (≤350 g), 16 (94%) died early (p <0.01), and of the 34 men with hearts of normal weight (≤400 g), 21 (62%) died early (difference not significant). Conversely, most patients in the late death group had hearts of increased weight: of the 15 women dying late, 14 (93%) had hearts of increased weight, and of the 75 men dying late, 62 (83%) had hearts of increased weight. The mean cardiac weight of the 125 patients with left ventricular scars was larger than that of the 86 patients without scars (492 vs 432 g; p <0.01), and these differences were observed within each sex and in both early (463 vs 425 g) and late (520 vs 448 g) death groups. This study suggests that patients with normal or near normal sized hearts have a higher early mortality after coronary bypass than do persons with hearts of increased weight.

THE LEFT VENTRICLE IN UNSTABLE ANGINA

Roberts[11] in 1976 described morphologic features of the left ventricle in 22 patients with unstable and in 5 patients with stable angina. These 27 patients included 3 patients who had fatal cardiac arrest during cardiac catheterization and 24 patients who had an operative procedure to relieve myocardial ischemia (coronary bypass = 21 patients; carotid–sinus stimulator = 2 patients; and Vineburg procedure = 1 patient). Patients who had had clinical evidence of acute myocardial infarction, congestive heart failure, or nonfatal cardiac arrest before cardiac catheterization or surgery were excluded. The 27 patients ranged in age from 39 to 67 years (mean 50). Eleven patients (41%) had had systemic hypertension. The cardiac silhouette by chest radiograph was within normal limits in all 27 patients, and none had electrocardiographic criteria compatible with left ventricular hypertrophy.

The hearts ranged in weight from 320 to 520 g (mean 407); for the 6 women, 320–480 g (mean 375) and for the 21 men, 330–520 g (mean 417). The weight of the heart was normal (≤350 g in women; ≤400 g in men) in 15 patients (56%) and increased in 12 patients (44%). The average increase above the upper limit of normal for the latter 12 patients was 19%. The hearts of the 5 men with stable angina weighed 350–475 g (mean 393) and those of the 16 men with unstable angina, 350–520 g (mean 424).

The left ventricular cavity was of normal size in 26 (96%) of the 27 patients. Grossly visible left ventricular wall scars (excluding those limited to papillary muscle) were present in 14 patients (52%), 4 of the 5 with stable, and 10 of the 22 patients with unstable angina. In only 4 of the 14 patients was the scarring transmural, i.e., involving all of the inner one half of the wall and all or a portion of the outer one half of the wall. The scars in all 14 patients were small, involving <20% of the circumference of a transverse section of left ventricle, and none extended >2 cm in length on the apical–basal longitudinal dimension. In none of the 14 patients did the scarring appear to result in thinning of the myocardial wall.

Foci of myocardial necrosis were present in the left ventricular wall or ventricular septum in 4 (15%) of the 27 patients. The foci were visible grossly (and confirmed histologically) in 3 patients and visible by histologic study only in the fourth patient. The acute infarcts were transmural in 2 patients and entirely subendocardial (limited to the inner one half of wall) in 2 patients. Each of the 4 patients with myocardial necrosis died from 18 to 48 hours from the start of an aorto-coronary bypass operation. The histologic age of the myocardial necrosis corresponded in each of the 4 patients to the postoperative time interval, indicating that the necrosis was almost certainly operatively induced and not present before the operation.

REFERENCES

1. Roberts WC. Sudden cardiac death: definitions and causes. *Am J Cardiol* 1986;57:1410–1413.
2. Virmani R, Roberts WC. Disappearance of symptomatic coronary heart disease and death from a noncardiac condition. *Chest* 1980;77:91–93.
3. Roberts WC, Virmani R. Quantification of coronary arterial narrowing in clinically-isolated unstable angina pectoris. An analysis of 22 necropsy patients. *Am J Med* 1979;67:792–799.
4. Roberts WC. Qualitative and quantitative comparison of amounts of narrowing by atherosclerotic plaques in the major epicardial coronary arteries at necropsy in sudden coronary death, transmural acute myocardial infarction, transmural healed myocardial infarction and unstable angina pectoris. *Am J Cardiol* 1989;64:324–328.
5. Roberts WC. Diffuse extent of coronary atherosclerosis in fatal coronary artery disease. *Am J Cardiol* 1990;65:2F–6F.
6. Kragel AH, Reddy SG, Wittes JT, Roberts WC. Morphometric analysis of the composition of coronary arterial plaques in isolated unstable angina pectoris with pain at rest. *Am J Cardiol* 1990;66:562–567.
7. Kragel AH, Reddy SG, Wittes JT, Roberts WC. Morphometric analysis of the composition of atherosclerotic plaques in the four major epicardial coronary arteries in acute myocardial infarction and in sudden coronary death. *Circulation* 1989;80:1747–1756.
8. Kragel AH, Gertz SD, Roberts WC. Morphologic comparison of frequency and types of acute lesions in the major epicardial coronary arteries in unstable angina pectoris, sudden coronary death and acute myocardial infarction. *J Am Coll Cardiol* 1991;18.
9. Roberts CS, Roberts WC. Cross-sectional area of the proximal portions of the three major epicardial coronary arteries in 98 necropsy patients with different coronary events. Relationship to heart weight, age and sex. *Circulation* 1980;62:953–959.
10. Kalan JM, Roberts WC. Significance of cardiac weight in patients having coronary artery bypass grafting for angina pectoris. *Am J Cardiol* 1988;62:36–40.
11. Roberts WC. The coronary arteries and left ventricle in clinically isolated angina pectoris. A necropsy analysis. *Circulation* 1976;54:388–390.

Reported Frequency of Coronary Arterial Narrowing by Angiogram in Patients with Valvular Aortic Stenosis

Gisela C. Mautner, MD, and William C. Roberts, MD

During the past 25 years most patients aged >40 years of age having aortic valve replacement have had coronary angiography preoperatively. At least 33 studies have reported the frequency of significant (>50% diameter reduction) coronary arterial narrowing in patients with valvular aortic stenosis, and most of these reported studies included only patients who had the stenotic valve replaced with a prosthesis or bioprosthesis[1-33] (Table I). Patients with mitral valve dysfunction usually were excluded. Analysis of the studies, which unfortunately also included a small percentage of patients <40 years of age, disclosed that 37% of the patients (1,302 of 3,509) had significant narrowing by angiogram of 1 or more major epicardial coronary arteries.

1. Linhart JW, de la Torre A, Ramsey HW, Wheat MW. The significance of coronary artery disease in aortic valve replacement. *J Thorac Cardiovasc Surg* 1968;55:811–819.

2. Harris CN, Kaplan MA, Parker DP, Dunne EF, Cowell HS, Ellestad MH. Aortic stenosis, angina, and coronary artery disease. Interrelations. *Br Heart J* 1975;37:656–661.

From the Pathology Branch, National Heart, Lung, and Blood Institute, National Institutes of Health, Bethesda, Maryland 20892. Manuscript received March 4, 1992, and accepted March 24.

3. Basta LL, Raines D, Najjar S, Kioschos JM. Clinical, haemodynamic, and coronary angiographic correlates of angina pectoris in patients with severe aortic valve disease. *Br Heart J* 1975;37:150–157.

4. Gross B, Mason DT, Amsterdam EA. Angina pectoris in aortic stenosis: clinical, hemodynamic and coronary angiographic correlates (abstr). *Circulation* 1975;51,52(suppl II):II-192.

5. Moraski RE, Russell RO, Mantle JA, Rackley CE. Aortic stenosis, angina pectoris, coronary artery disease. *Cathet Cardiovasc Diagn* 1976;2:157–164.

6. Mandal AB, Gray IR. Significance of angina pectoris in aortic valve stenosis. *Br Heart J* 1976;38:811–815.

7. Paquay PA, Anderson G, Diefenthal H, Nordstrom L, Richman HG, Gobel FL. Chest pain as a predictor of coronary artery disease in patients with obstructive aortic valve disease. *Am J Cardiol* 1976;38:863–869.

8. Hancock EW. Aortic stenosis, angina pectoris, and coronary artery disease. *Am Heart J* 1977;93:382–393.

9. Lacy J, Goodin R, McMartin D, Masden R, Flowers N. Coronary atherosclerosis in valvular heart disease. *Ann Thoracic Surg* 1977;23:429–435.

10. Graboys TB, Cohn PF. The prevalence of angina pectoris and abnormal coronary arteriograms in severe aortic valvular disease. *Am Heart J* 1977;93:683–686.

11. Swanton RH, Brooksby IAB, Jenkins BS, Coltart DJ, Webb-Peploe MM, Williams BT, Braimbridge MV. Determinants of angina in aortic stenosis and the importance of coronary arteriography. *Br Heart J* 1977;39:1347–1352.

12. Thompson RH, Ahmed MS, Mitchell AG, Towers MK, Yacoub MH. Angina, aortic stenosis and coronary heart disease. *Clin Cardiol* 1979;2:26–32.

13. Storstein O, Enge I. Angina pectoris in aortic valvular disease and its relation to coronary pathology. *Acta Med Scand* 1979;205:275–278.

14. Hakki AH, Kimbiris D, Iskandrian AS, Segal BL, Mintz GS, Bemis CE. Angina pectoris and coronary artery disease in patients with severe aortic valvular disease. *Am Heart J* 1980;100:441–449.

15. Bonow RO, Kent KM, Rosing DR, Lipson LC, Borer JS, McIntosh CL, Morrow AG, Epstein SE. Aortic valve replacement without myocardial revascularization in patients with combined aortic valvular and coronary artery disease. *Circulation* 1981;63:243–251.

16. Bermudez GA, Abdelnur R, Midell A, DeMeester T. Coronary artery disease in aortic stenosis: importance of coronary arteriography and surgical implications. *Angiology* 1983;34:591–596.

17. Crochet D, Petitier H, de Laguerenne J, Wanlin P, Chiffoleau S, Grossète R, Godin JF. Adult aortic stenosis: value of catheterization for the study of associated lesions: a series of 137 cases. *Arch Mal Coeur* 1983;76:1057–1064.

18. Exadactylos N, Sugrue DD, Oakley CM. Prevalence of coronary artery disease in patients with isolated aortic valve stenosis. *Br Heart J* 1984;51:121–124.

19. Monsuez JJ, Drobinski G, Verdière C, Chollet D, Grosgogeat Y. Étude prospective de la fréquence de l' atteinte coronarienne en cas de rétrécissement aortique pur. *Ann Cardiol Angeiol (Paris)* 1985;34:65–69.

20. Abdulali SA, Baliga BG, Clayden AD, Smith DR. Coronary artery luminal diameter in aortic stenosis. *Am J Cardiol* 1985;55:450–453.

21. Green SJ, Pizzarello RA, Padmanabhan VT, Ong LY, Hall MH, Tortolani AJ. Relation of angina pectoris to coronary artery disease in aortic valve stenosis. *Am J Cardiol* 1985;55:1063–1065.

22. Turina J, Goebel N, Hess O, Krayenbühl HP. Indications for coronary arteriography in aortic valve disease. *Z Kardiol* 1986;75(suppl 2):68–72.

23. Sechtem U, Müller-Haake RC. Coronary artery disease in aortic stenosis. *Z Kardiol* 1986;75(suppl 2):86–89.

24. Lombard JT, Selzer A. Valvular aortic stenosis. A clinical and hemodynamic profile of patients. *Ann Intern Med* 1987;106:292–298.

25. Safford RE, Bove AA. Prediction of coronary artery disease by left ventricular regional wall motion abnormalities in patients with stenosis of the aortic valve. *Br Heart J* 1987;57:237–241.

26. Vandeplas A, Willems JL, Piessens J, de Geest H. Frequency of angina pectoris and coronary artery disease in severe isolated valvular aortic stenosis. *Am J Cardiol* 1988;62:117–120.

27. Bessone LN, Pupello DF, Hiro SP, Lopez-Cuenca E, Glatterer MS, Ebra G. Surgical management of aortic valve disease in the elderly: a longitudinal analysis. *Ann Thorac Surg* 1988;46:264–269.

28. Kishore AGR, Gupta SK, Reddy KN, Murthy JSN, Prasad SV, Abraham KA. Coronary artery disease in patients with isolated aortic valve stenosis. *Indian Heart J* 1988;40:481–484.

29. Chobadi R, Wurzel M, Teplitsky I, Menkes H, Tamari I. Coronary artery disease in patients 35 years of age or older with valvular aortic stenosis. *Am J Cardiol* 1989;64:811–812.

30. Vekshtein VI, Alexander RW, Yeung AC, Plappert T, St John Sutton MG, Ganz P, Selwyn AP, Bittl JA. Coronary atherosclerosis is associated with left ventricular dysfunction and dilatation in aortic stenosis. *Circulation* 1990;82:2068–2074.

31. Lund O, Nielsen TT, Pilegaard HK, Magnussen K, Knudsen MA. The influence of coronary artery disease and bypass grafting on early and late survival after valve replacement for aortic stenosis. *J Thorac Cardiovasc Surg* 1990;100:327–337.

32. Danielsen R, Nordrehaug JE, Vik-Mo H. Clinical and haemodynamic features in relation to severity of aortic stenosis in adults. *Eur Heart J* 1991;12:791–795.

33. Mautner GC, Cannon RO III, Mautner SL, Hunsberger SA, Roberts WC. Clinical factors useful in predicting aortic valve structure in patients >40 years of age with isolated valvular aortic stenosis. Submitted to *Am J Cardiol* 1992; in press.

TABLE I Published Reports on the Frequency of Significant (≥ 50% diameter narrowing) Coronary Arterial Narrowing on Angiogram in Patients with Valvular Aortic Stenosis

First Author	Year of Publication	No. of Pts.	Age (years) Range (mean)	Men	Women	Mitral Valve Dysfunction	AVR	CA ↓ ≥50% in Diameter	CABG
1. Linhart	1968	52	19–68 (51)	41	11	0	33 (63%)	33/52 (63%)	—
2. Harris	1975	69	38–77 (58)	58	11	+	—	16*/69 (23%)	—
3. Basta	1975	68	34–77 (56)	50	18	—	68 (100%)	10/41 (24%)	—
4. Gross	1975	48	— (61)	—	—	—	—	16*/48 (33%)	—
5. Moraski	1976	88	31–81 (59)	67	21	—	81 (92%)	41/88 (47%)	19 (22%)
6. Mandal	1976	28	45–66 (58)	20	8	0	20 (71%)	14†/28 (50%)	8 (29%)
7. Paquay	1976	48	39–84 (60)	48	0	—	—	21*/48 (44%)	—
8. Hancock	1977	173	40–83 —	—	—	0	156 (90%)	97/173 (56%)	—
9. Lacy	1977	56	18–74 —	39	17	—	—	12/56 (21%)	—
10. Graboys	1977	19	47–76 (62)	12	7	0	19 (100%)	4*/19 (21%)	—
11. Swanton	1977	140	18–75 (60)	90	50	12	122 (87%)	32/140 (23%)	6 (4%)
12. Thompson	1979	139	30–79 —	—	—	—	127 (91%)	45‡/139 (32%)	36 (26%)
13. Storstein	1979	44	— —	—	—	—	—	13*/44 (30%)	—
14. Hakki	1980	39	43–79 (65)	26	13	0	—	18/39 (46%)	—
15. Bonow	1981	78	— (58)	—	—	0	78 (100%)	26/78 (33%)	0
16. Bermudez	1983	64	40–71 (55)	38	26	—	64 (100%)	32*/64 (50%)	—
17. Crochet	1983	137	— (63)	93	44	14	—	34/110 (31%)	—
18. Exadactylos	1984	88	38–77 (58)	64	24	0	88 (100%)	22/64 (34%)	—
19. Monsuez	1984	148	20–81 (62)	89	59	0	—	27/148 (18%)	—
20. Abdulali	1985	32	— (55)	26	6	—	—	11‡/32 (34%)	—
21. Green	1985	103	44–87 (66)	68	35	0	—	46‡/103 (45%)	—
22. Turina	1986	300	— (54)	—	—	—	300 (100%)	54/300 (18%)	—
23. Sechtem	1986	75	25–75 (59)	35	40	—	—	17/75 (23%)	12 (16%)
24. Lombard	1987	397	15–>80 (61)	276	121	0	—	135/234 (58%)	—
25. Safford	1987	83	33–85 (66)	65	18	—	—	55/83 (66%)	—
26. Vandeplas	1988	192	28–82 (59)	121	71	0	—	47/192 (24%)	—
27. Bessone	1988	219	70–88 (75)	132	87	+	219 (100%)	112‡/219 (51%)	107 (49%)
28. Kishore	1988	106	40–63 (48)	100	6	0	—	6/106 (6%)	—
29. Chobadi	1989	146	38–80 (63)	88	58	0	—	54/146 (37%)	—
30. Vekshtein	1990	78	— (74)	32	46	0	—	35/78 (45%)	—
31. Lund	1990	205	— —	—	—	—	205 (100%)	83/205 (40%)	55 (27%)
32. Danielsen	1991	100	41–79 (65)	64	36	3	—	54/100 (54%)	—
33. Mautner	1992	188	42–81 (61)	139	49	0	188 (100%)	80/188 (43%)	43 (23%)
Totals		3,750	15–88 (61)	1,881/ 2,763 (68%)	882/ 2,763 (32%)	29/ 2,500 (1%)	1,768/ 1,849 (96%)	1,302/ 3,509 (37%)	286/ 1,040 (28%)

*Coronary diameter narrowing > 75%.
†Coronary diameter narrowing > 60%.
‡Coronary diameter narrowing > 70%.
AVR = aortic valve replacement; CA ↓ = coronary artery narrowing; CABG = coronary artery bypass grafting.

The Heart in Tangier Disease

Severe Coronary Atherosclerosis with Near Absence of High-Density Lipoprotein Cholesterol

SUSANNE L. MAUTNER, M.D., JULIAN A. SANCHEZ, M.D., DANIEL J. RADER, M.D.,
GISELA C. MAUTNER, M.D., VICTOR J. FERRANS, M.D., PH.D.,
DONALD S. FREDRICKSON, M.D., H. BRYAN BREWER, JR., M.D.,
AND WILLIAM C. ROBERTS, M.D.

Cardiac necropsy findings are described in a 72-year-old man with Tangier disease whose plasma total cholesterol levels averaged 70 mg/dL, low-density lipoprotein cholesterol level was 45 mg/dL, and high-density lipoprotein cholesterol level was 1.4 mg/dL, and who had coronary artery bypass grafting for severe atherosclerotic coronary artery disease. At necropsy, 24 of the 72 (33%) 5-mm segments of the 4 major (right, left main, left anterior descending, and left circumflex) native coronary arteries and 4 of the 27 (15%) 5-mm segments of the saphenous vein aortocoronary bypass conduits were narrowed by more than 75% in cross-sectional area by atherosclerotic plaques. The plaques were composed primarily (91% to 97%) of fibrous tissue. Oil red O staining, polarized light microscopy, and electron microscopy revealed cholesterol deposits in the plaques and in the walls of coronary arteries, saphenous vein grafts, and aorta. Such deposits also were found in foam cells of histiocytic origin, fibroblasts in all four cardiac valves, and in Schwann cells of cardiac nerves. (Key words: Tangier disease; Atherosclerosis; High-density lipoprotein; Low-density lipoprotein; Coronary artery disease; Coronary artery bypass surgery) Am J Clin Pathol 1992; 98: 191–198

Tangier disease, a rare disorder of lipoprotein metabolism, is characterized by extremely low plasma levels of high-density lipoprotein (HDL) cholesterol and low levels of total and low-density lipoprotein cholesterol. The low levels of HDL are due to rapid catabolism of HDL rather than to defective biosynthesis of HDL.[1] Patients with Tangier disease have accumulation of cholesteryl esters in various tissues, including tonsils, lymph nodes, thymus, bone marrow, intestinal mucosa, liver, spleen, skin, and cornea. The disease is manifested by enlarged orange-yellow tonsils, splenomegaly, and peripheral neuropathy and is transmitted in an autosomal co-dominant mode. Little information is available on clinical and morphologic aspects of coronary artery disease in patients with genetic syndromes characterized by HDL deficiency, and no reports are available describing cardiovascular findings at necropsy in patients with Tangier disease. Such is the purpose of this report.

REPORT OF A PATIENT

A 72-year-old white man, who had been an oil-refinery worker, had a tonsillectomy at age 14 years because of markedly enlarged tonsils. He remained well until age 42 years, when he noted excessive fatigue. At age 43 years (in 1962), he was found to have malabsorption, thrombocytopenia, and splenomegaly that resulted in splenec-

From the Pathology and Molecular Disease Branches, National Heart, Lung, and Blood Institute, National Institutes of Health, Bethesda, Maryland.

Received August 28, 1991; received revised manuscript and accepted for publication February 28, 1992.

Address reprint requests to Dr. Mautner: Pathology Branch, National Heart, Lung, and Blood Institute, National Institutes of Health, Building 10, Room 2N-258, Bethesda, Maryland 20892.

"""

tomy. At age 44 years, he was referred to the National Institutes of Health, where the diagnosis of Tangier disease was made on the basis of clinical and biochemical studies. Some of these studies have been subjects of previous publications.[2-4] Morphologic examination of various tissues from this patient constituted part of the original description of the pathologic features of Tangier disease (including the presence of lipid deposits in lymph nodes, spleen, bone marrow, liver, rectal mucosa, skin, and small nerves). At age 45 years, gynecomastia and an omental mass developed. At age 48 years, peripheral neuropathy was evident. At age 50 years, bilateral neural hearing loss developed and 4 years later glucose intolerance and corneal opacities were discovered.

Angina pectoris developed at age 59 years. Angiography at that time disclosed severe coronary arterial narrowing with total occlusion of the left circumflex and 75% and 50% diameter narrowing of the left anterior descending and right coronary arteries, respectively. He smoked fewer than 10 cigarettes a month, was slightly overweight (weight, 88 kg; height, 179 cm), and had no history of systemic hypertension. Eighteen indirect systemic arterial pressure measurements were recorded from age 44 (in 1963) until age 72 years (in 1990): the systolic pressures averaged 120 mmHg and the diastolic averaged 77 mmHg. In May 1979 (at age 60 years), the patient underwent coronary artery bypass grafting with insertion of saphenous venous grafts from the aorta to the left anterior descending, first diagonal, and right coronary arteries. Repeated angiography in 1986 and 1989 revealed narrowing of the grafts and total occlusion of the right coronary artery, 75% diameter narrowing of the left main and left anterior descending coronary arteries, and total occlusion of the saphenous vein graft to the right coronary artery. At age 64 years, dementia was first observed and it progressed thereafter. A progressive wasting illness developed, the origin of which was never determined, and he died of bronchopneumonia at age 72 years.

During a 17-year period (1973 to 1990), multiple determinations of plasma lipoproteins were made: total cholesterol ranged from 43 to 101 mg/dL (mean, 70 mg/dL); HDL cholesterol ranged from 0 to 7 mg/dL (mean, 1.4 mg/dL); low-density lipoprotein cholesterol ranged from 26 to 65 mg/dL (mean, 45 mg/dL); and triglyceride levels ranged from 113 to 396 mg/dL (mean, 203 mg/dL) (Table 1).

TABLE 1. LIPID CUMULATIVE FLOW SHEET (MG/DL)

Date	Total Cholesterol	Triglycerides	HDL Cholesterol	LDL Cholesterol
10/01/73	101	362	0	65
10/03/73	71	396	0	48
10/05/73	78	212	0	46
10/07/73	81	263	0	42
10/09/73	66	238	0	32
06/17/74	91	172	0	56
06/19/74	76	175	0	55
11/07/75	75	137	2	59
06/21/78	74	207	2	47
09/30/78	85	251	6	43
04/23/79	77	214	0	55
05/21/79	75	245	0	40
06/17/79	83	256	0	52
06/20/79	78	251	0	48
06/25/79	66	183	0	46
07/02/79	43	160	0	26
07/09/79	53	153	0	41
12/03/79	61	164	0	44
12/07/79	74	174	2	51
09/08/80	72	185	7	39
01/23/81	60	188	5	32
01/30/81	58	139	4	38
07/06/82	69	216	1	46
07/13/82	62	219	1	39
09/21/82	65	227	0	47
04/14/83	79	213	1	57
03/05/84	64	113	1	39
06/25/84	61	116	1	45
10/10/84	59	143	4	39
02/20/90	52	113	4	36
Average	70	203	1.4	45

His father had hearing loss and died at age 75 years of an acute myocardial infarct; his mother died at age 84 years of natural causes. One sister had systemic hypertension and died of an acute myocardial infarct, as did the patient's brother, who was homozygous for Tangier disease and who developed angina at age 42 years. He died suddenly at age 48 years and autopsy was not performed. Two younger siblings died in infancy of "diphtheria." The son of the patient, who is obligate heterozygous for Tangier disease, had a tonsillectomy at age 7 years but is otherwise asymptomatic. The father and mother were distant cousins with no known relationship to the Chesapeake Bay Tangier kindred (Fig. 1).[4]

Gross Findings

Autopsy was performed at the Chief Medical Examiner's Office in Louisville, Kentucky. The heart and other tissues were submitted to the National Institutes of Health for examination. Necropsy confirmed the presence of extensive acute bronchopneumonia. Foamy macrophages were found in lymph nodes. The liver weighed 1,200 g; most portal areas were fibrotic and foamy macrophages were located in the periportal and pericentral vein areas. In the omentum, a firm, yellow mass was present and consisted of dense fibrosis with cholesterol clefts and calcific deposits. No sections of skeletal muscle were available for examination. The heart weighed 310 g. There were no gross foci of fibrosis or necrosis in the left ventricular myocardium. Calcific deposits were present in the mitral anulus (2+/4+) and in the bases of the aortic valve cusps (1+/4+). Atherosclerotic plaques were present in the descending thoracic and abdominal aorta.

Microscopic Findings

Tissue samples from left ventricular myocardium, ventricular septum, all 4 cardiac valves, coronary arteries, saphenous venous grafts, coronary sinus, and thoracic aorta were fixed in buffered formalin, embedded in paraffin, sectioned, and stained with hematoxylin and eosin. Frozen sections of formalin-fixed tissues from these sites were stained with oil red O. Unstained and oil red O-stained sections from these blocks were examined by polarized light microscopy to detect birefringent materials. These sections also were examined using Nomarski differential interference contrast microscopy to obtain further details of tissue morphology. The Schultz reaction,[5] specific for cholesterol, was performed in sections of aortic valve leaflet, aorta, coronary arteries, and saphenous vein grafts. Additional pieces of tissue that had been fixed in

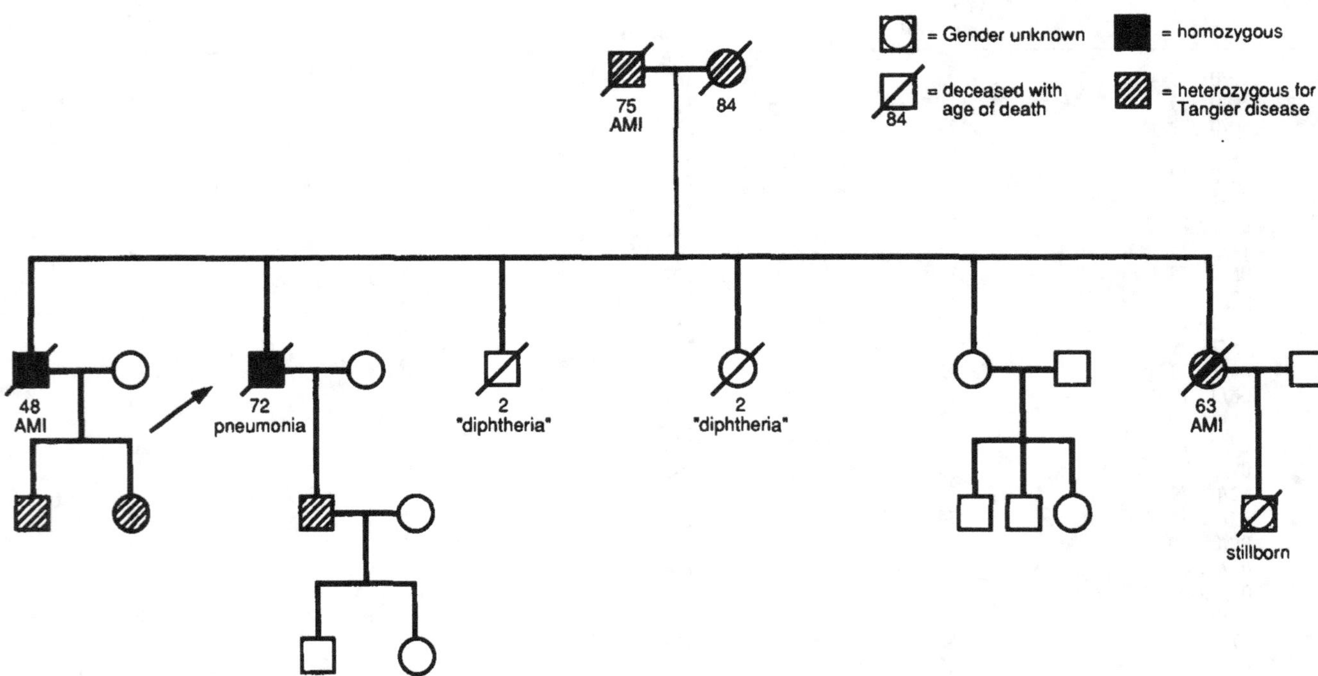

FIG. 1. Genealogical tree of affected family. It represents an update of the pedigree illustrated in 1965 by Hoffman and Fredrickson.[4] The propositus (arrow) was homozygous for Tangier disease, had coronary bypass surgery at age 60 years, and died of pneumonia at age 72 years. His brother, who also was homozygous for Tangier disease, died at age 48 years of an acute myocardial infarct, as did one heterozygous sister. Two siblings died at age 2 years of presumed "diphtheria." The obligate heterozygous children of the brother and the son of the propositus are in good health. The latter had tonsillectomy at age 7 years. The parents of the propositus were both heterozygotes; the father had hearing loss and died of a myocardial infarct at age 75 years, and the mother died of natural causes at an advanced age.

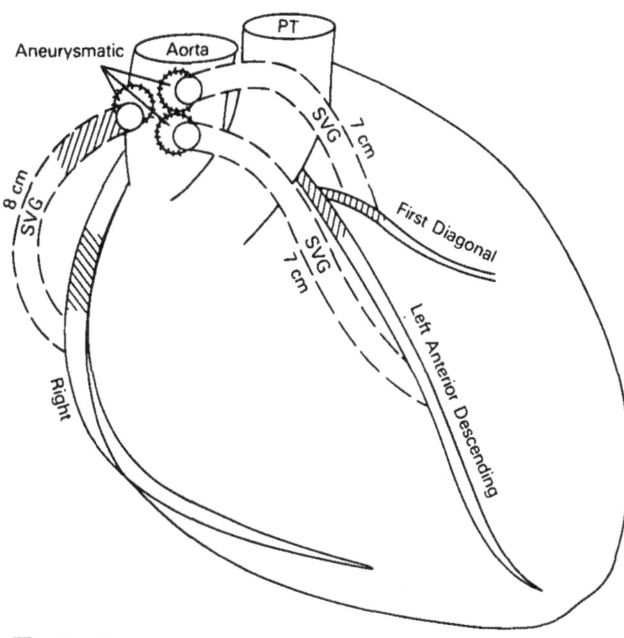

FIG. 2. Diagram of the heart showing distribution and extent of areas of severe narrowing of the coronary arteries and saphenous venous bypass grafts (SVG). PT = Pulmonary trunk.

formalin were refixed in glutaraldehyde and prepared for electron microscopic examination.

For quantitative assessment of the degree of narrowing and evaluation of plaque composition in the coronary arteries and in saphenous venous grafts, the vessels were dissected from the heart, decalcified, and sectioned transversely at 5-mm intervals. They were dehydrated, cleared, embedded in paraffin, cut, and stained by the Movat method. Seventy-two segments of the major epicardial coronary arteries and 27 segments of the saphenous venous grafts were taken. Evaluation was done by planimetry,[6] outlining the internal elastic membrane, residual lumen, and components of the plaque, such as fibrous tissue, calcified tissue, pultaceous debris, and foam cells. The area of each component of plaque was then converted to a percentage of the total plaque area. The degree of cross-sectional luminal narrowing was categorized into 5 groups: 0 to 25%, 26% to 50%, 51% to 75%, 76% to 95%, and 96% to 100%.

The myocardium revealed normal myocytes but the amount of interstitial myocardial fibrous tissue was increased. The location of the stenoses in the coronary arteries and histologic examples are shown in Figures 2 and 3. Thirty-three percent of the 72 5-mm segments of the

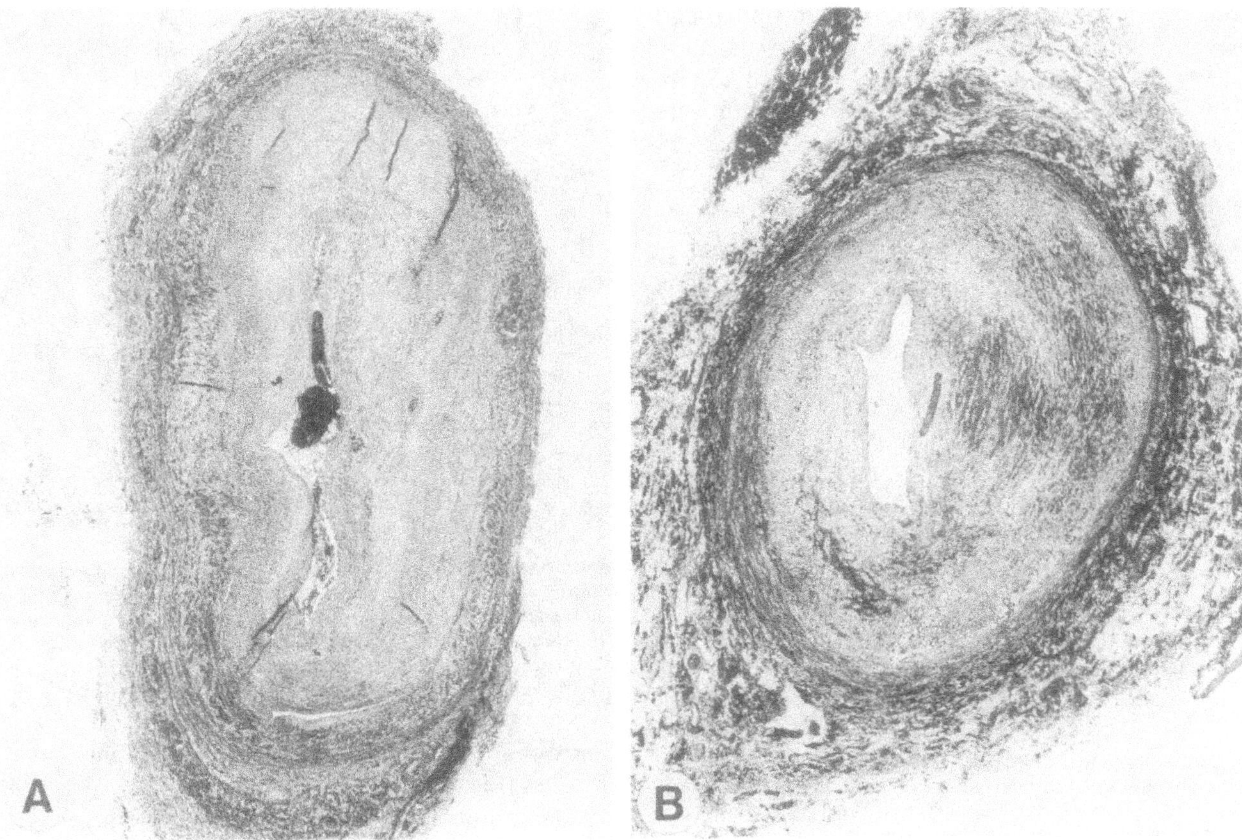

FIGS. 3A and B. Histologic section of a saphenous vein graft to the right artery (A) and of a left circumflex coronary artery (B). The plaques consist mainly of fibrous tissue (Movat stains; A, ×27; B, ×39).

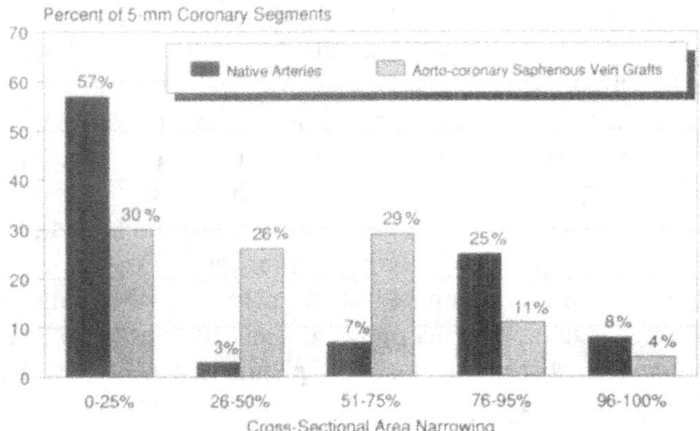

FIG. 4. Histogram demonstrating the percentage of cross-sectional area narrowing of 5-mm segments of the four major epicardial coronary arteries (n = 72) and saphenous vein grafts (n = 27). In the native coronary arteries, 57% of all segments were narrowed less than 25% and 33% had plaques with narrowing of the lumen of more than 75% in cross-sectional area. The saphenous vein grafts showed a more homogeneous distribution of atherosclerotic plaques with less segments in the first category but also less in the category of narrowing more than 75% in cross-sectional area.

4 major (right, left main, left anterior descending, and left circumflex) coronary arteries were narrowed more than 75% in cross-sectional area by plaque and 15% of the 27 5-mm segments of the saphenous vein grafts were

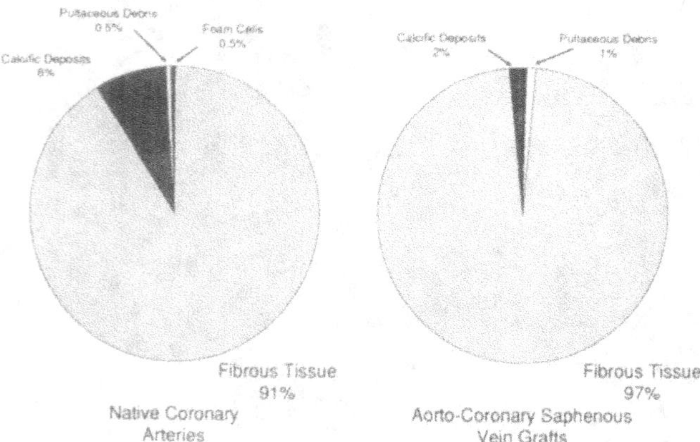

FIG. 5. Composition of atherosclerotic plaques in all 5-mm segments of the four major epicardial coronary arteries (n = 72) and saphenous vein grafts (n = 27). The plaques of the saphenous veins grafts consisted to a higher percentage of fibrous tissue (97%) compared to native coronary arteries (91%). The latter contained more calcific deposits (8% *versus* 2%) and foam cells.

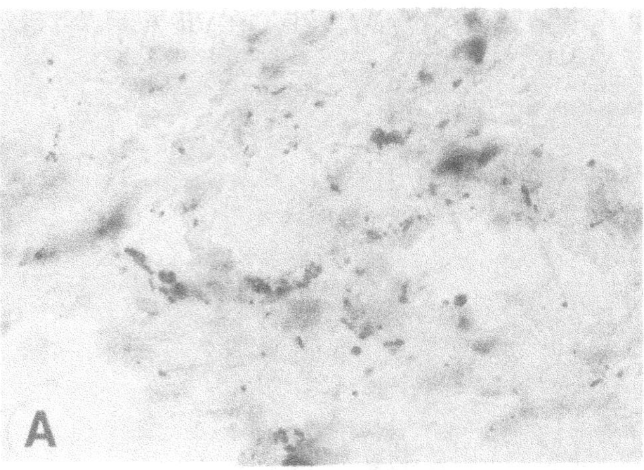

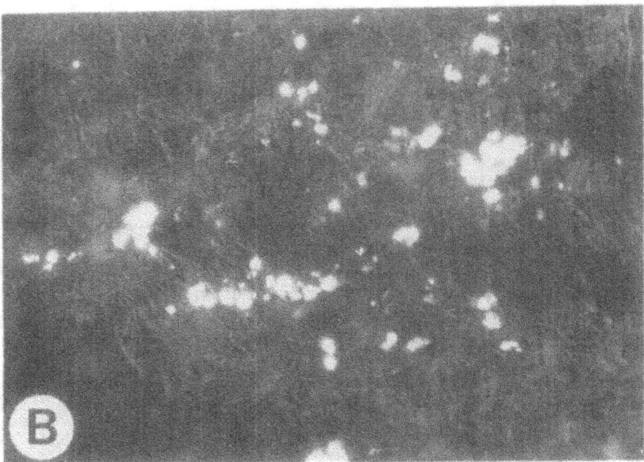

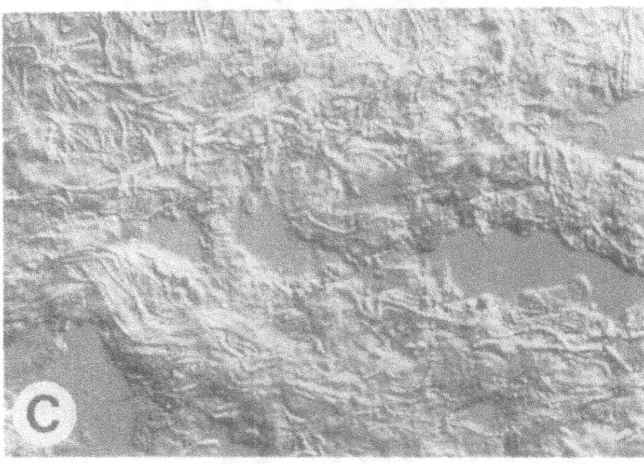

FIGS. 6A–C. Photomicrographs of lipid deposits in frozen sections of the mitral valve, using different techniques (A) showing positive oil red 0 staining; (B) same area examined with polarized light microscope and (C) using Nomarski interference contrast optics to demonstrate details of tissue morphology in an area surrounding lipid-containing fibroblasts (×400, A, B, C).

narrowed more than 75% in cross-sectional area by plaques (Fig. 4).

The plaques in both native coronary arteries and in the saphenous vein grafts consisted almost entirely of fibrous tissue (91% and 97%, respectively); the native coronary

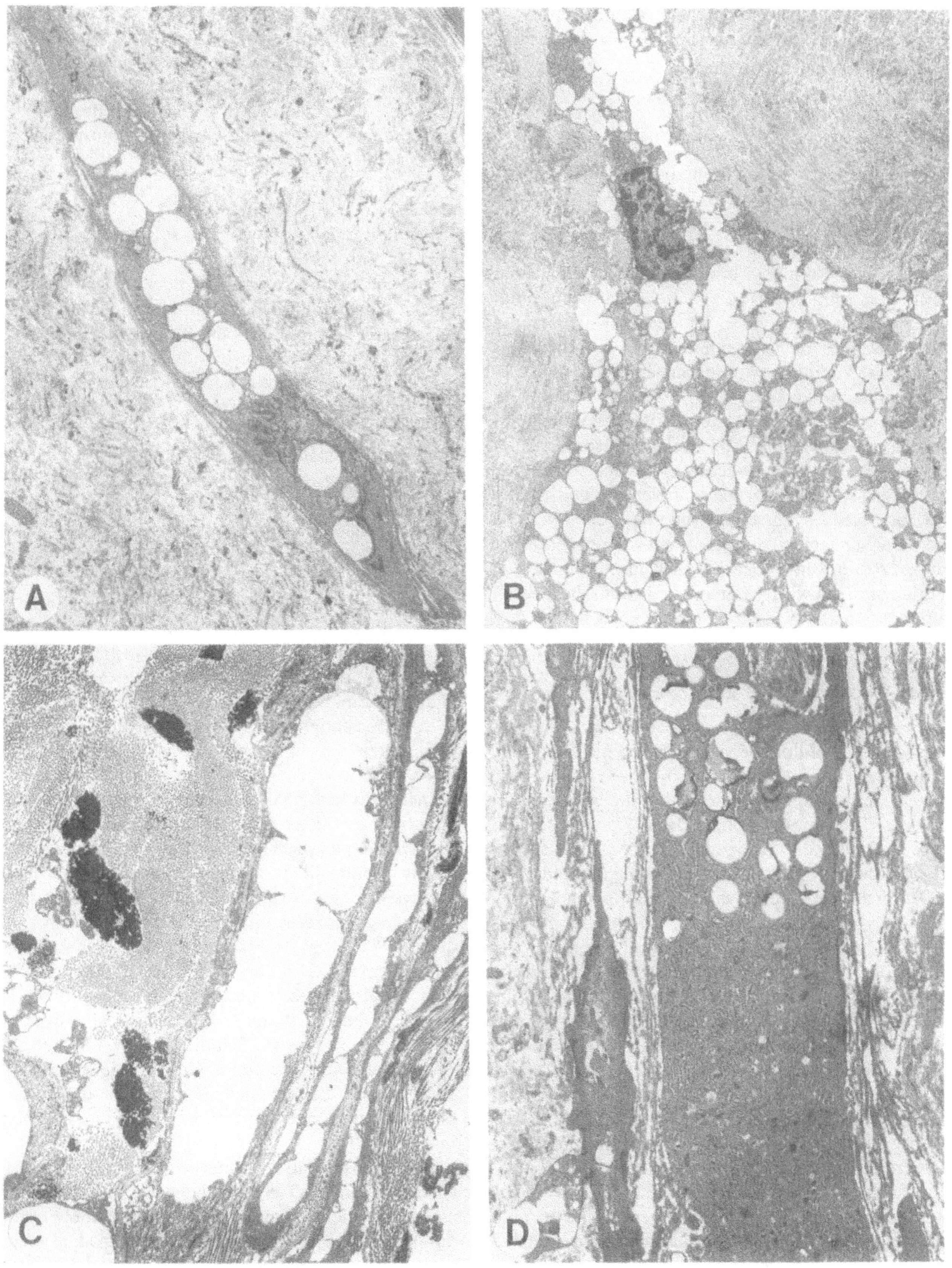

FIGS. 7A–D. Ultrastructure of four different types of lipid-containing cells. *A.* Smooth muscle cell in the left anterior descending coronary artery. The cell has basement membrane, many actin-type filaments, and peripherally located myofilament insertion sites. It contains prominent lipid deposits, which correspond to those shown in other smooth muscle cells by polarized light microscopy (×4,000). *B.* Foam cells, probably of histiocytic origin, located in the adventitia of a coronary artery. It lacks a basement membrane and it contains many lipid droplets (×4,000). *C.* Smooth muscle cell in a saphenous venous bypass graft demonstrates ultrastructural characteristics similar to those of the smooth muscle cell in the coronary artery shown in (*A*). The lipid deposits in these cells tend to be more extensive and confluent (×6,000). *D.* Cell containing large amounts of endoplasmic reticulum and abundant lipid droplets was present in connective tissue of the mitral valve and was considered to represent a valvular fibroblast (×5,000).

artery plaques had a higher content of calcium (8% *versus* 2%), and intra- and extracellular lipid deposits were minimal (Fig. 5).

Oil Red O stain, Polarized Light Microscopy and Schultz Reaction

Cardiac myocytes did not contain birefringent lipids. The four cardiac valves showed diffuse oil red O-positive reaction (Fig. 6*A*), which corresponded to areas of birefringence suggesting cholesterol deposits (Fig. 6*B*). Examination with Nomarski optics showed that the lipid deposits were intracellular (Fig. 6*C*). The distribution of oil red O-positive material in the coronary arteries and saphenous venous grafts was inhomogeneous and variable in location and amount, with this material present in media, adventitia, and plaque.

Sections of left main and left anterior descending coronary arteries showed birefringence only in some atherosclerotic plaques. The left circumflex coronary artery revealed extensive birefringence in adventitia and in atherosclerotic plaques (corresponding to oil red O-positive areas). The saphenous vein grafts showed extensive birefringence in adventitia, media, and in plaques. In the sections examined with the Schultz reaction, the areas of birefringence partially corresponded to areas stained positive for cholesterol.

Electron Microscopy

The endothelial cells of the coronary arteries and capillaries were free of lipid deposits. The oil red O-positive lipid deposits observed by light microscopy in the coronary arteries were located in both smooth muscle cells and in foam cells. The number of lipid droplets in the smooth muscle cells varied considerably. These droplets were electronlucent and were not limited by membranes (Fig. 7*A*). The foam cells were oval or round in shape. They were usually larger in size than the smooth muscle cells (Fig. 7*B*). They did not have basement membranes, and their cytoplasm was completely filled by small lipid droplets, which at times tended to become confluent. In the saphenous vein grafts, no foam cells were observed and lipid deposits were present only in smooth muscle cells (Fig. 7*C*). On the basis of electron microscopic observations, it was not possible to distinguish extracellular lipid deposits in the atherosclerotic plaques specifically related to Tangier disease, that is, those containing masses of cholesterol, from those occurring as nonspecific components of ordinary atherosclerotic plaques.

In cardiac valves, lipid deposits were found in both foam cells and in fibroblasts. The latter cells were identified by their content of cisterns of rough-surfaced endoplasmic reticulum, elongated shape, and lack of basement membranes. Foam cells were larger in size and resembled those in coronary arteries (Fig. 7*D*). The changes in the thoracic aorta were similar to those in the coronary arteries and saphenous vein grafts. Lipid deposits also were present in epicardial nerves and consisted of small droplets in the cytoplasm of Schwann cells enveloping unmyelinated axons, and within the axons.

DISCUSSION

The only previously reported information on cardiovascular morphologic findings in Tangier disease was the description of coronary intimal thickening and the presence of patchy lipid deposits in the mitral and tricuspid valves in a 5-year-old boy[7] and the presence of focal lipid deposits in the wall of the pulmonary artery in a 10-year-old girl.[2] The present study documents the occurrence of severe atherosclerosis in a patient with Tangier disease. Quantitative analysis revealed narrowing of more than 75% in cross-sectional area in 33% and 15% of all 5-mm segments of the native coronary arteries and saphenous vein grafts, respectively. Analysis of the plaque composition revealed that fibrous tissue was the major component, a finding similar to those reported in patients without Tangier disease having fatal atherosclerotic coronary artery disease.[6,8-11] This is especially interesting in light of the fact that Tangier disease results in the abnormal accumulation of cholesteryl ester in the histiocytes of many organs, and therefore may have been expected to result in an abnormal form of atherosclerosis as well.[2]

In both plaques and in the walls of the vessels, cholesterol was present in smooth muscle cells. Accumulation of cholesterol often was not suspected in preparations stained with hematoxylin and eosin and was recognized only by the positive reaction with oil red O stain, birefringence in polarized light microscopy, Schultz reaction, and by the ultrastructural appearance. Cholesterol deposits also were present in cardiac valves and cardiac nerves, resembling those described in several patients with Tangier disease.[2,7,12] It was demonstrated in previous studies that the lipid deposits in various organs of patients affected with Tangier disease were histochemically similar. They were birefringent, stainable by lipid-soluable dyes, such as oil red O, and by the Schultz reaction for cholesterol. These results are concordant with the extensive chemical data showing that an increased content of cholesteryl esters in those lipid droplets was the consistent abnormality.[1,2,13-16]

Epidemiologically, plasma concentrations of HDL cholesterol are inversely associated with risk of premature atherosclerotic cardiovascular disease.[17] Apolipoprotein (apo) A–I is the primary protein in HDL and serves a variety of structural and functional roles in HDL metabolism.[18] Genetic defects that result in the inability to synthesize apoA–I result in very low plasma concentrations of HDL cholesterol and premature coronary artery disease.[18-21] Conversely, in Tangier disease, plasma levels of HDL cholesterol and apoA–I are very low as a result of exceptionally rapid catabolism.[22-24] Are the very low HDL cholesterol and apoA–I concentrations in Tangier disease a risk factor for premature atherosclerotic cardiovascular disease? In a review of the clinical features of Tangier disease,[3,25] five of eight homozygous patients older than 40 years had definite clinical evidence of atherosclerotic cardiovascular disease, with four having onset of symptoms before age 60 years. Obligate heterozygotes for Tangier disease have HDL cholesterol levels approximately one half of normal.[3,25] Of 14 heterozygous patients older than 40 years, 7 had clinical evidence of atherosclerotic cardiovascular disease, with 5 having onset of symptoms before age 60 years. However, no homozygous or heterozygous patient developed symptoms of atherosclerotic cardiovascular disease before the age of 40 years. The conclusion is that patients with Tangier disease are at some increased risk for premature vascular disease, but not to the degree expected from the extremely low plasma HDL cholesterol levels. Two factors may potentially offset this enhanced risk. First, Tangier disease patients almost always have significantly lower plasma low-density lipoprotein cholesterol levels than the normal population,[3,25] and thus may be partially protected from the usual atherogenic process. Second, the mechanism of the low HDL cholesterol, specifically normal synthesis with markedly accelerated catabolism of HDL, allows a high "flux" of HDL and may permit some HDL-mediated removal of excess cholesterol from tissues (reverse cholesterol transport), despite the very low steady-state plasma levels of HDL.

In summary, we describe in this report the first cardiac necropsy findings in an adult patient with Tangier disease. This patient had clinical symptoms of coronary artery disease by age 59 years and was found at necropsy to have severe atherosclerotic disease that did not differ histologically from atherosclerosis occurring in patients without Tangier disease. However, cholesterol deposits in cardiac valves and cardiac nerves found in our patient were considered to be more specific features of Tangier disease.

REFERENCES

1. Assmann G, Schmitz G, Brewer HB Jr. Familial high density lipoprotein deficiency: Tangier disease. In: Scriver CR, Beaudet AL, Sly WS, Valle D, eds. Stanbury JB, Wyngaarden JB, Fredrickson DS, consulting eds. The Metabolic Basis of Inherited Disease. I. Sixth Edition. New York: McGraw-Hill, 1989, pp 1267–1282.
2. Ferrans VJ, Fredrickson DS. The pathology of Tangier disease. A light and electron microscopic study. Am J Pathol 1975;78:101–158.
3. Schaefer EJ, Zech LA, Schwartz DE, Brewer HB Jr. Coronary heart disease prevalence and other clinical features in familial high-density lipoprotein deficiency (Tangier disease). Ann Intern Med 1980;93:261–266.
4. Hoffman HN II, Fredrickson DS. Tangier disease (familial high density lipoprotein deficiency). Clinical and genetic features in two adults. Am J Med 1965;39:582–593.
5. Luna LG. Manual of Histologic Staining Methods of the Armed Forces Institute of Pathology, Third Edition. New York: McGraw-Hill, 1968, p 140.
6. Kragel AH, Shanthasundari GR, Wittes JT, Roberts WC. Morphometric analysis of the composition of atherosclerotic plaques in the four major epicardial coronary arteries in acute myocardial infarction and in sudden coronary death. Circulation 1989;80:1747–1756.
7. Bale PM, Clifton-Bligh P, Benjamin BN, Whyte HM. Pathology of Tangier disease. J Clin Pathol 1971;24:609–616.
8. Kragel AH, Reddy SG, Wittes JT, Roberts WC. Morphometric analysis of the composition of coronary arterial plaques in isolated unstable angina pectoris with pain at rest. Am J Cardiol 1990;66:562–567.
9. Kragel AH, Roberts WC. Composition of atherosclerotic plaques in the coronary arteries in homozygous familial hypercholesterolemia. Am Heart J 1991;121:210–211.
10. Dollar AL, Kragel AH, Fernicola DJ, et al. Composition of atherosclerotic plaques in coronary arteries in women < 40 years of age with fatal coronary artery disease and implications for plaque reversibility. Am J Cardiol 1991;67:1223–1227.
11. Gertz SD, Malekzadeh S, Dollar AL, et al. Composition of atherosclerotic plaques in the four major epicardial coronary arteries in patients ≥ 90 years of age. Am J Cardiol 1991;67:1228–1233.
12. Schmalbruch H, Stender S, Boysen G. Abnormalities in spinal neurons and dorsal root ganglion cells in Tangier disease presenting with a syringomyelia-like syndrome. J Neuropathol Exp Neurol 1987;46(5):533–543.
13. Herbert PN, Forte T, Heinen RJ, Fredrickson DS. Tangier disease. One explanation of lipid storage. N Engl J Med 1978;299(10):519–521.
14. Schmitz G, Bruening T, Williamson E, Nowicka G. The role of HDL in reverse cholesterol transport and its disturbances in Tangier disease and HDL deficiency with xanthomas. Eur Heart J 1990;11(Suppl E):197–211.
15. Katz SS, Small DM, Brook JG, Lees RS. The storage lipids in Tangier disease. A physical chemical study. J Clin Invest 1977;59:1045–1054.
16. Assmann G, Schaefer HE. High density lipoprotein deficiency and lipid deposition in Tangier disease. In: Carlson LA, Paoletti R, Sirtori CR, Weber G, eds. International Conference on Atherosclerosis. New York: Raven Press, 1978, pp 97–101.
17. Gordon DJ, Rifkind BM. High-density lipoprotein-the clinical implications of recent studies. N Engl J Med 1989;321:1311–1316.
18. Brewer HB Jr, Gregg RE, Hoeg JM, Fojo SS. Apolipoproteins and lipoproteins in human plasma: An overview. Clin Chem 1988;34:4–8.
19. Norum RA, Lakier JB, Goldstein S, et al. Familial deficiency of apolipoproteins A-I and C-III and precocious coronary-artery disease. N Engl J Med 1982;306:1513–1519.
20. Schaefer EJ, Ordovas JM, Law SW, et al. Familial apolipoprotein A-I and C-III deficiency, variant II. J Lipid Res 1985;26:1089–1101.
21. Matsunaga T, Hiasa Y, Yanagi H, et al. Apolipoprotein A-I deficiency due to a codon 84 nonsense mutation of the apolipoprotein A-I gene. Proc Natl Acad Sci USA 1991;88:2793–2797.
22. Schaefer EJ, Blum CB, Levy RI, et al. Metabolism of high-density lipoprotein apolipoproteins in Tangier disease. N Engl J Med 1978;299:905–910.
23. Schaefer EJ, Anderson DW, Zech LA, et al. Metabolism of high density lipoprotein subfractions and constituents in Tangier disease following the infusion of high density lipoproteins. J Lipid Res 1981;22:217–228.
24. Bojanovski D, Gregg RE, Zech LA, et al. In vivo metabolism of proapolipoprotein A-I in Tangier disease. J Clin Invest 1987;80:1742–1747.
25. Schaefer EJ. Clinical, biochemical, and genetic features in familial disorders of high density lipoprotein deficiency. Arteriosclerosis 1984;4:303–322.

Degrees of Coronary Arterial Narrowing at Necropsy in Men with Large Fusiform Abdominal Aortic Aneurysm

Gisela C. Mautner, MD, Katherine Berezowski, MD,
Susanne L. Mautner, MD, and William C. Roberts, MD

In 27 patients (mean age at death 72 ± 9 years) with abdominal aortic aneurysm (AAA) ≥5.0 cm in its widest transverse diameter, the amounts of narrowing at necropsy in the 4 major (left main, left anterior descending, left circumflex, and right) epicardial coronary arteries were determined. During life, 12 of the 27 patients (44%) had symptoms of myocardial ischemia: angina pectoris alone in 2, acute myocardial infarction alone in 3, angina pectoris and acute myocardial infarction in 5, and sudden coronary death in 2. Ten of the 27 patients (37%) died from consequences of myocardial ischemia. Six (22%) died from rupture of the AAA. Grossly visible left ventricular necrosis or fibrosis, or both, was present in 15 patients (56%). Of the 27 patients, 23 (85%) had narrowing 76 to 100% in cross-sectional area of 1 or more major coronary arteries by atherosclerotic plaque. The mean number of coronary arteries per patient severely (>75%) narrowed was 2.0 ± 1.3/4.0. Of the 108 major coronary arteries in the 27 patients, 55 (51%) were narrowed >75% in cross-sectional area by plaque. The 4 major coronary arteries in the 27 patients were divided into 5-mm segments and a histologic section, stained by the Movat method, was prepared from each segment. The mean percentages of the resulting 1,475 five-mm segments narrowed in cross-sectional area 0 to 25%, 26 to 50%, 51 to 75%, 76 to 95% and 96 to 100% were 17, 37, 28, 15 and 3%, respectively. The percentages of 5-mm coronary segments narrowed >75% in cross-sectional area were similar in the right, left anterior descending, and left circumflex coronary arteries. Thus, patients with AAA nearly always have diffuse and severe coronary atherosclerosis.

(Am J Cardiol 1992;70:1143–1146)

From the Pathology Branch, National Heart, Lung, and Blood Institute, National Institutes of Health, Bethesda, Maryland. Manuscript received June 4, 1992, and accepted June 29.

Address for reprints: Gisela C. Mautner, MD, Pathology Branch, National Heart, Lung, and Blood Institute, National Institutes of Health, Building 10, Room 2N258, 9000 Rockville Pike, Bethesda, Maryland 20892.

It is well known that patients with abdominal aortic aneurysm (AAA) often have symptoms of myocardial ischemia and that complications of atherosclerotic coronary artery disease are a common cause of death in persons with AAA. Although some reports have described degrees of coronary narrowing by angiogram during life in patients with AAA, no studies have described *at necropsy* the amounts of coronary narrowing in persons with AAA. Such is the purpose of this report.

METHODS

Sources of patients and general characteristics: Records from the Pathology Branch of the National Heart, Lung, and Blood Institute of the National Institutes of Health were searched for patients with AAA from the years 1968 to 1991. Only patients fulfilling the following criteria were included in this study: (1) men >50 years of age; (2) infrarenal AAA, fusiform, ≥5.0 cm in its largest transverse diameter at necropsy; (3) absence of syphilis, the Marfan syndrome and aortic dissection; (4) absence of surgery on the abdominal aorta; and (5) the presence of both, the epicardial coronary arteries and the abdominal aorta, for reexamination. Twenty-seven patients fulfilled these criteria, and their pertinent clinical and necropsy observations are detailed in Table I.

Examination of abdominal aortic aneurysm: After the abdominal aorta of each patient had been fixed in formalin for ≥24 hours, it was measured in its widest diameter and length. The mean of the largest diameter of the AAA in the 27 patients was 6.8 ± 1.8 cm (Figure 1). Six (22%) aneurysms ruptured and each was fatal. Three patients (11%) had an additional aneurysm of the descending thoracic aorta. During life, 12 of the 27 patients (44%) had symptoms of myocardial ischemia: angina pectoris alone in 2, acute myocardial infarction alone in 3, angina pectoris and acute myocardial infarction in 5, and sudden coronary death[1] in 2. Ten of the 27 patients (37%) died from consequences of myocardial ischemia.

Examination of the heart: The hearts were fixed for at least 1 day in formalin. The 4 major epicardial coronary arteries then were excised intact and fixed for at least another day. After decalcification (if necessary), each of the 4 major coronary arteries was cut transversely to its longitudinal axis into 5-mm-long segments, and each segment was labeled sequentially from either its aortic ostium or from its origin from the left main coronary artery. The 5-mm segments were labeled, de-

TABLE I Clinical and Morphologic Findings in the 27 Men with Large Abdominal Aortic Aneurysms

Case No.	Age at Death (yr)	Race	Maximal Diameter AAA (cm)	History of						
				AP	AMI	SCD	SH	DM	CS	S
1	57	W	5	0	0	+	0	0	0	0
2	57	W	10	0	0	0	0	0	+	0
3	59	W	5.5*	0	0	0	0	0	+	0
4	63	B	8	0	0	0	+	0	+	0
5	64	W	6	+	+	0	+	0	+	+
6	64	W	6	0	0	0	0	0	0	0
7	65	B	9.5*	+	0	0	+	0	0	+
8	66	W	6*	0	0	0	+	0	+	0
9	67	B	5	−	+	0	0	0	−	0
10	68	B	5	+	0	+	+	+	+	+
11	68	W	8.5	+	+	0	+	0	0	0
12	70	W	8	+	+	0	+	0	0	0
13	72	W	12*	−	0	0	−	−	−	−
14	72	W	7.5	+	+	0	−	0	−	0
15	73	W	6	0	0	0	+	0	0	+
16	73	B	8	0	0	0	+	0	+	0
17	73	B	7*	0	0	0	+	0	+	0
18	73	B	5	0	0	0	0	0	+	0
19	74	W	8	+	+	0	+	0	0	+
20	75	W	5	0	0	0	0	0	+	0
21	76	−	5	0	0	0	+	+	0	0
22	78	W	7	0	0	0	+	+	+	0
23	82	W	6*	+	0	0	+	0	0	0
24	82	W	5	0	+	0	0	0	+	+
25	85	W	5.5	0	0	0	0	0	0	0
26	87	W	7	0	+	0	0	0	0	+
27	90	W	6	0	0	0	0	0	0	0
Mean or totals	72		6.8	8	8	2	14	3	12	7

hydrated (alcohol and xylene) and embedded in paraffin, and 2 histologic sections were cut and stained from each paraffin block. The Movat stained section was used in this study for determining degrees of narrowing.[2] The degree of narrowing was determined after histologic examination of each cross section magnified 25 to 50 times. The judgment regarding the degree of luminal narrowing of each 5-mm segment was based on the degree of luminal obliteration within the luminal circle bordered by the internal elastic membrane. The circle was visually subdivided into 4 equal-sized quadrants and the percentage of cross-sectional area luminal narrowing in each 5-mm segment was classified as follows: 0 to 25%, 26 to 50%, 51 to 75%, 76 to 95% and 96 to 100%. The accuracy of this technique of grading cross-sectional area narrowing has been validated to be ≥95%.[3] In addition to sectioning the major epicardial coronary arteries, ≥2 histologic sections extending from endocardium into epicardium and for ≥2.0 cm in circumferential dimension were prepared from left ventricular myocardium from each patient and stained by hematoxylin and eosin. Foci of myocardial necrosis or fibrosis, or both, were confirmed histologically.

RESULTS

Grossly visible left ventricular wall necrosis or fibrosis, or both: Of the 27 patients, 1 (4%) had left ventricular foci of necrosis alone, 10 (37%) had foci of fibrosis alone, and 4 (15%) had foci of both necrosis and fibrosis.

Coronary arteries: In the 27 patients, the mean number of coronary arteries per patient narrowed >75% in cross-sectional area by atherosclerotic plaque was 2.0 ± 1.3: 4 patients (15%) had no arteries narrowed to this degree, 7 patients (26%) had 1 artery so narrowed; 2 (7%) had 2 arteries so narrowed; 12 (45%) had 3 arteries so narrowed; and 2 patients (7%) had 4 arteries so narrowed. Of the 23 patients with >75% narrowing of 1 or more major coronary arteries, the number/patient narrowed >75% was 2.4 ± 1.0. Of the 108 major epicardial coronary arteries in the 27 patients (4 per patient), 55 (51%) were narrowed by plaque at some point 76 to 100% in cross-sectional area. Of the individual major coronary arteries, the left main coronary artery was severely narrowed (76 to 100% in cross-sectional area) in 3 patients (11%), the left anterior descending coronary artery in 17 patients (63%), the left circumflex coronary artery in 17 patients (63%), and the right coronary artery in 18 patients (67%). Of the 1,475 five-mm-long coronary artery segments from the 108 major coronary arteries, the mean percentages narrowed in cross-sectional area 0 to 25%, 26 to 50%, 51 to 75%, 76 to 95% and 96 to 100% were 17, 37, 28, 15 and 3%, respectively.

DISCUSSION

Summary of major findings in the present study: Of the 27 men, 23 (85%) had 1 or more coronary arteries narrowed >75% in cross-sectional area by plaque, an average of 2.4 ± 1.0 for each of the 23 patients. The left

TABLE I (continued)

Case No.	HW (g)	LV N	LV F	Number of CAs ↓ >75%	Number of 5-mm CA Segments	Number (%) of Coronary Segments Narrowed by Plaque 0–25%	26–50%	51–75%	76–95%	96–100%
1	450	0	0	3	38	6 (16)	5 (13)	15 (39)	12 (32)	0
2	340	0	0	4	49	9 (19)	11 (22)	16 (33)	11 (22)	2 (4)
3	340	0	0	1	49	19 (39)	21 (43)	8 (16)	1 (2)	0
4	680	0	+	1	41	18 (44)	9 (22)	13 (32)	1 (2)	0
5	510	+	+	3	52	5 (10)	12 (23)	19 (36)	16 (31)	0
6	470	0	0	0	46	18 (39)	17 (37)	11 (24)	0	0
7	500	0	+	2	58	5 (8)	22 (38)	26 (45)	5 (9)	0
8	330	0	+	3	58	3 (5)	16 (28)	20 (34)	15 (26)	4 (7)
9	550	0	+	3	49	5 (10)	9 (18)	12 (25)	22 (45)	1 (2)
10	540	0	0	4	38	0	5 (13)	15 (39)	15 (40)	3 (8)
11	510	+	0	3	74	5 (7)	29 (39)	13 (18)	26 (35)	1 (1)
12	435	0	+	3	61	10 (16)	14 (23)	9 (15)	14 (23)	14 (23)
13	590	0	0	1	67	21 (31)	37 (55)	8 (12)	1 (2)	0
14	460	+	+	3	79	6 (8)	27 (34)	31 (39)	11 (14)	4 (5)
15	505	0	+	3	56	3 (5)	8 (15)	32 (57)	12 (21)	1 (2)
16	325	0	0	1	73	14 (19)	39 (54)	19 (26)	1 (1)	0
17	690	0	0	0	58	19 (33)	39 (67)	0	0	0
18	390	0	+	2	43	3 (7)	20 (46)	18 (42)	2 (5)	0
19	440	+	+	3	55	4 (7)	16 (29)	17 (31)	15 (28)	3 (5)
20	360	0	+	0	46	25 (54)	13 (28)	8 (18)	0	0
21	740	0	0	0	59	10 (17)	40 (68)	9 (15)	0	0
22	505	0	0	1	60	12 (20)	23 (38)	23 (38)	2 (4)	0
23	410	0	+	3	55	2 (4)	20 (36)	21 (38)	6 (11)	6 (11)
24	300	0	+	3	44	4 (9)	7 (16)	19 (43)	11 (25)	3 (7)
25	480	0	0	1	59	23 (39)	32 (54)	3 (5)	1 (2)	0
26	430	+	+	3	39	1 (3)	4 (10)	17 (43)	16 (41)	1 (3)
27	445	0	0	1	69	4 (6)	49 (71)	15 (22)	1 (1)	0
Mean or totals	471	5	14	2.0	1,475 (55)	254 (17%)	544 (37%)	417 (28%)	217 (15%)	43 (3%)

*Rupture of the AAA occurred and in each it was fatal.

AAA = abdominal aortic aneurysm; AMI = acute myocardial infarction; AP = angina pectoris; CA = coronary artery; CS = cigarette smoker; DM = diabetes mellitus (adult onset); F = fibrosis; HW = heart weight; LV = left ventricular; N = necrosis; S = stroke; SCD = sudden coronary death; SH = systemic hypertension.

anterior descending, left circumflex and right coronary arteries had similar amounts of severe coronary narrowing (31, 31 and 33%, respectively). Of a total of 1,475 five-mm segments of the 4 major coronary arteries, 18% were narrowed 76 to 100% in cross-sectional area. The numbers of coronary arteries narrowed >75% in cross-sectional area by plaque were significantly different in the 12 patients *with* compared to the 15 patients *without* clinical evidence of myocardial ischemia (angina pectoris or acute myocardial infarction or sudden coronary death, or a combination) (3.0 ± 0.4 vs 1.3 ± 1.2, p = 0.0001), and the percentage of 5-mm coronary segments narrowed >75% was also significantly greater in patients *with* than *without* clinical evidence of myocar-

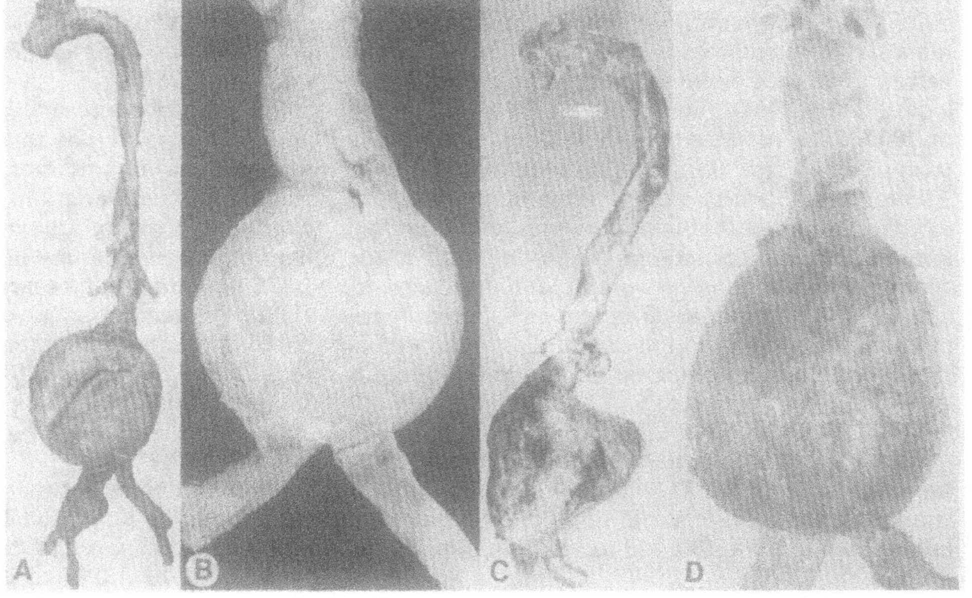

FIGURE 1. Abdominal aortic aneurysms in patients 2 *(A)*, 6 *(B)*, 13 *(C)* and 26 *(D)* (Table I). All 4 aneurysms contain large quantities of thrombus.

dial ischemia (32 vs 7%, p = 0.0001). Fifteen of the 27 patients at necropsy had acute and/or healed myocardial infarcts. The 15 patients *with* myocardial infarcts had significantly more coronary narrowing by plaque than did the 12 patients *without* (mean numbers of coronary arteries narrowed >75% = 2.5 ± 0.9 vs 1.4 ± 1.4, p = 0.02; 5-mm segments narrowed >75% = 26 vs 8%, p <0.05).

Previously reported necropsy studies on the coronary arteries in patients with abdominal aortic aneurysm: No previously reported study has examined at necropsy the amounts of coronary narrowing in patients having AAA.

Previously reported coronary angiographic studies in patients with abdominal aortic aneurysm: Although a number have described the frequency of clinical evidence of myocardial ischemia in patients with AAA,[4-13] few previously published studies have reported the amounts of coronary narrowing by angiogram in patients with AAA. Tomatis et al[14] in 1972 performed coronary angiography in 28 patients (aged 57 to 81 years [mean 67]) with AAA: 21 patients (75%) had narrowing 76 to 100% in diameter of 1 or more coronary arteries; 2 patients (7%) had narrowing 51 to 75%; and the remaining 5 patients (18%) had insignificant (≤50% diameter reduction) coronary narrowing. Hertzer et al[15] in 1984 described coronary angiographic findings in 263 patients with AAA and Young et al[16] in 1986 described 302 patients with AAA. Both studies were performed at the Cleveland Clinic and represent largely the same patient group. The 302 patients included in the study of Young et al[16] consisted of 289 patients with infrarenal AAA and 13 patients with thoracoabdominal aneurysms (aged 47 to 94 years [mean 68]): 199 (66%) had narrowing >70% in diameter of 1 or more coronary arteries; another 85 patients (28%) had 1 or more narrowings between "measurable" to 70% diameter reduction, and the remaining 18 patients (6%) had "angiographically normal" arteries.

Although the present study in many ways is quite different from the one reported by Young et al,[16] comparison of our study to theirs is nevertheless appropriate in some areas: *frequency of the presence of 1 or more major coronary arteries significantly (>75% in cross-sectional area narrowing at necropsy and >50% in diameter at angiography) narrowed* (23 of 27 patients [85%] vs 284 of 302 [94%]); *frequency of single, double and triple (or quadruple) coronary arterial narrowing* (26, 7 and 52% vs 26, 21 and 22%, respectively); *frequency of significant narrowing of the left main, left anterior descending, left circumflex, and right coronary arteries* (5, 31, 31 and 33% vs 6, 39, 39 and 50%, respectively); and *frequency of clinical evidence of myocardial ischemia* (44 vs 52%).

Acknowledgment: We appreciate the technical assistance of Michael W. Spencer, Filippina Giacometti and Leslie Berry, and thank Vivian Norman for the preparation of the manuscript.

REFERENCES

1. Roberts WC. Sudden cardiac death: a diversity of causes with focus on atherosclerotic coronary artery disease. *Am J Cardiol* 1990;65:13B–19B.

2. Roberts WC. Qualitative and quantitative comparison of amounts of narrowing by atherosclerotic plaques in the major epicardial coronary arteries at necropsy in sudden coronary death, transmural acute myocardial infarction, transmural healed myocardial infarction and unstable angina pectoris. *Am J Cardiol* 1989;64:324–328.

3. Isner JM, Wu M, Virmani R, Jones AA, Roberts WC. Comparison of degrees of coronary arterial luminal narrowing determined by visual inspection of histologic sections under magnification among three independent observers and comparison to that obtained by video planimetry: an analysis of 559 five-millimeter segments of 61 coronary arteries from eleven patients. *Lab Invest* 1980;42:566–570.

4. DeBakey ME, Crawford ES, Cooley DA, Morris Jr GC, Royster TS, Abbott WP. Aneurysm of abdominal aorta: analysis of results of graft replacement therapy one to eleven years after operation. *Ann Surg* 1964;160:622–639.

5. Hollier LH, Plate G, O'Brien PC, Kazmier FJ, Gloviczki P, Pairolero PC, Cherry KJ. Late survival after abdominal aortic aneurysm repair: influence of coronary artery disease. *J Vasc Surg* 1984;1:290–299.

6. Ruby ST, Whittemore AD, Couch NP, Collins JJ, Cohn L, Shemin R, Mannick JA. Coronary artery disease in patients requiring abdominal aortic aneurysm repair. Selective use of a combined operation. *Ann Surg* 1985;201:758–764.

7. Thurmond AS, Semler HJ. Abdominal aortic aneurysm: incidence in a population at risk. *J Cardiovasc Surg* 1986;27:457–460.

8. Graor RA. Preoperative evaluation and management of coronary and carotid artery occlusive disease in patients with abdominal aortic aneurysms. *Surg Clin North Am* 1989;69:737–743.

9. Roger VL, Ballard DJ, Hallett Jr JW, Osmundson PJ, Puetz PA, Gersh BJ. Influence of coronary artery disease on morbidity and mortality after abdominal aortic aneurysmectomy: a population-based study, 1971–1987. *J Am Coll Cardiol* 1989;14:1245–1252.

10. Freeman WK, Gibbons RJ, Shub C. Preoperative assessment of cardiac patients undergoing noncardiac surgical procedures. *Mayo Clin Proc* 1989;64:1105–1117.

11. Freeman WK, Gersh BJ, Gloviczki P. Abdominal aortic aneurysm and coronary artery disease: frequent companions, but an uneasy relationship. *J Vasc Surg* 1990;12:73–77.

12. Hinkamp TJ, Pifarre R, Bakhos M, Blakeman B. Combined myocardial revascularization and abdominal aortic aneurysm repair. *Ann Thorac Surg* 1991;51:470–472.

13. Abraham SA, Coles NA, Coley CM, Strauss HW, Boucher CA, Eagle KA. Coronary risk of noncardiac surgery. *Prog Cardiovasc Dis* 1991;34:205–234.

14. Tomatis LA, Fierens EE, Verbrugge GP. Evaluation of surgical risk in peripheral vascular disease by coronary arteriography: a series of 100 cases. *Surgery* 1972;71:429–435.

15. Hertzer NR, Beven EG, Young JR, O'Hara PJ, Ruschhaupt III WF, Graor RA, DeWolfe VG, Maljovec LC. Coronary artery disease in peripheral vascular patients: a classification of 1000 coronary angiograms and results of surgical management. *Ann Surg* 1984;199:223–233.

16. Young JR, Hertzer NR, Beven EG, Ruschhaupt III WF, Graor RA, O'Hara PJ, DeWolfe VG, Kramer JR, Simpfendorfer CC. Coronary artery disease in patients with aortic aneurysm: a classification of 302 coronary angiograms and results of surgical management. *Ann Vasc Surg* 1986;1:36–42.

Amounts of Coronary Arterial Narrowing by Atherosclerotic Plaque at Necropsy in Patients with Lower Extremity Amputation

Gisela C. Mautner, MD, Susanne L. Mautner, MD, and William C. Roberts, MD

In 26 patients (mean age at death 68 ± 9 years) who had undergone amputation (at mean age 63 ± 12 years) of 1 or both lower extremities due to severe peripheral arterial atherosclerosis, the amounts of narrowing at necropsy in the 4 major (left main, left anterior descending, left circumflex, and right) epicardial coronary arteries were determined. During life, 15 of the 26 patients (58%) had symptoms of myocardial ischemia: angina pectoris alone in 1, acute myocardial infarction alone in 5, and angina and/or infarction plus congestive heart failure or sudden coronary death in 9. Twelve of the 26 patients (42%) died from consequences of myocardial ischemia: acute myocardial infarction in 5, sudden coronary death in 3, chronic congestive heart failure in 3, and shortly after coronary bypass surgery in 1. Grossly visible left ventricular necrosis or fibrosis, or both, was present in 21 patients (81%). Of the 26 patients, 24 (92%) had narrowing 76 to 100% in cross-sectional area of 1 or more major coronary arteries by atherosclerotic plaque. The mean number of coronary arteries per patient severely (>75%) narrowed was 2.3 ± 1.0/4.0. Of the 104 major coronary arteries in the 26 patients, 60 (58%) were narrowed >75% in cross-sectional area by plaque. The 4 major coronary arteries in the 26 patients were divided into 5-mm segments and a histologic section, stained by the Movat method, was prepared from each segment. The mean percentages of the resulting 1,322 five-mm segments narrowed in cross-sectional area 0 to 25%, 26 to 50%, 51 to 75%, 76 to 95% and 96 to 100% were 17, 20, 35, 19 and 9%, respectively. The percentages of 5-mm coronary segments narrowed >75% in cross-sectional area were similar in the left anterior descending, left circumflex and right coronary arteries. Thus, patients with peripheral arterial atherosclerosis severe enough to warrant amputation nearly always have diffuse and severe coronary atherosclerosis at the time of necropsy.

(Am J Cardiol 1992;70:1147–1151)

From the Pathology Branch, National Heart, Lung, and Blood Institute, National Institutes of Health, Bethesda, Maryland. Manuscript received May 28, 1992; revised manuscript received and accepted June 30, 1992.

Address for reprints: Gisela C. Mautner, MD, Pathology Branch, National Heart, Lung, and Blood Institute, National Institutes of Health, Building 10, Room 2N-258, Bethesda, Maryland 20892.

It is well known that persons with atherosclerotic involvement of 1 arterial system frequently also have atherosclerotic involvement of 1 or more other arterial systems. Persons, for example, with peripheral arterial disease often have evidence of myocardial ischemia and vice versa. Indeed, coronary artery disease is a major cause of death in patients with known abdominal aortic aneurysm or vascular disease peripheral to the aorta. Despite the common occurrence of significant amounts of atherosclerosis in more than 1 vascular system, relatively little information is available on the actual amounts of atherosclerotic involvement in a vascular system other than the one actually causing symptoms of organ ischemia. In the present study we examined in detail the amounts of coronary arterial narrowing by atherosclerotic plaque in patients who had peripheral arterial disease by atherosclerosis severe enough to warrant amputation of 1 or both lower limbs. Such a study has not been reported previously.

METHODS

Sources of patients and general characteristics: Records from the Pathology Branch, National Heart, Lung, and Blood Institute, were searched for cases of amputation of the lower extremity due to severe peripheral arterial atherosclerotic disease. A total of 30 cases of lower extremity amputation were retrieved. Two cases were eliminated because the patients were <50 years of age at necropsy. Two other patients were eliminated because the hearts were not available for reexamination and the coronary arteries had never been sectioned in their entirety by the method to be described subsequently. The remaining 26 cases, all of whom were aged ≥50 years, formed the basis of this study. The autopsies were performed at 8 different local institutions and subsequently the hearts were submitted to this Branch for detailed study. The clinical and autopsy records and police reports were examined in all 26 patients. Pertinent clinical and necropsy findings in each of the 26 patients are listed in Table I. Of the 26 patients, 24 were men and 2 (cases 12 and 22, Table I) were women.

A total of 31 lower limb amputations were performed in the 26 patients: in 21 patients a single leg was amputated and in 5 patients both lower limbs were amputated. Seven (27%) patients had undergone either femoral-popliteal, femoral-femoral, axillofemoral or aortofemoral bypass operation. Another 2 patients had peripheral angioplasty.

During life, 15 of the 26 patients (58%) had symptoms of myocardial ischemia (cases 12 to 26 [Table I]): angina pectoris alone in 1, acute myocardial infarction

TABLE I Clinical and Morphologic Findings in the 26 Lower Limb Amputees

Case No.	Age at Death (yr)	Age at amputation (yr)	Interval Amputation to Death (mo)	Race	Leg Amputated		Location of Amputation/ Incision	AP	AMI	SCD	CHF	CS	DM
					Right	Left							
1	58	53	60	B	+	+	AK	0	0	0	0	−	0
2	59	53	72	B	+	0	BK	0	0	0	0	+	+
3	61	61	2 days	W	+	+	BK	0	0	0	0	−	0
4	64	64	19 days	W	+	+	AK	0	0	0	0	−	0
5	64	63	12	B	0	+	BK	0	0	0	0	−	+
6	69	69	24 days	B	0	+	BK	0	0	0	0	+	0
7	75	—	—	B	+	0	BK	0	0	0	0	+	0
8	79	—	—	W	+	0	AK	0	0	0	0	−	0
9	81	81	9 days	W	0	+	BK	0	0	0	0	−	+
10	82	—	—	W	0	+	BK	0	0	0	0	−	0
11	88	84	48	W	+	0	AK	0	0	0	0	0	0
12	50	45	60	B	+	+	BK	+	0	0	+	−	0
13	61	46	180	W	0	+	BK	0	+	0	+	−	+
14	61	61	11 days	W	0	+	AK	0	+	0	0	+	0
15	62	57	60	B	+	0	BK	+	0	0	+	+	0
16	63	53	120	B	+	+	BK/AK	0	+	0	0	−	0
17	63	—	—	B	0	+	BK	+	+	0	0	−	+
18	63	56	84	W	0	+	BK	+	+	0	0	−	0
19	66	—	—	B	+	0	BK	0	+	0	0	+	+
20	67	—	—	B	0	+	AK	0	+	+	0	−	0
21	67	67	19 days	W	0	+	BK	+	+	0	+	+	0
22	67	67	14 days	B	+	0	AK	0	+	0	0	−	−
23	69	54	180	B	+	0	BK	+	0	0	0	+	+
24	75	75	1	W	+	0	BK	−	+	+	0	+	0
25	77	—	—	B	0	+	BK	0	+	0	+	−	+
26	84	81	36	W	0	+	AK	0	+	0	0	−	0
Totals or mean	68 ± 9	63 ± 12	76 (14 days)		14	17		6	12	2	5	9	8

alone in 5, and angina and/or infarction plus congestive heart failure or sudden coronary death[1] in 9. Patients 1 to 11 never had symptoms of myocardial ischemia during life.

Twelve of the 26 patients (46%), including 2 (cases 5 and 9, [Table I]) who never had symptoms of myocardial ischemia during life, died from consequences of myocardial ischemia: acute myocardial infarction in 5, chronic congestive heart failure in 3, sudden coronary death in 3, and immediately after coronary bypass surgery in 1.

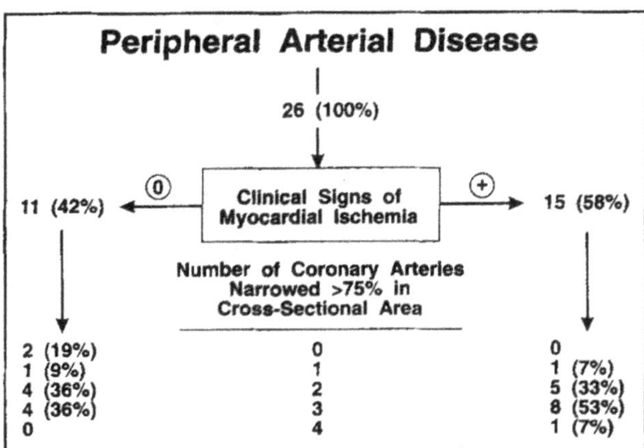

FIGURE 1. Qualitative comparison of the 11 patients *without* clinical evidence of myocardial ischemia (cases 1 to 11, Table I) with the 15 patients *with* clinical evidence of myocardial ischemia (cases 12 to 26, Table I).

Examination of the heart: The hearts were fixed in 10% buffered formalin for ≥24 hours before weighing and examination. The major (left main, left anterior descending, left circumflex, and right) epicardial coronary arteries were excised intact after fixation. The arteries then were decalcified, if necessary, with formic acid–sodium citrate for ≥24 hours. The coronary arteries then were cut transversely into 5-mm-long segments and labeled sequentially from origin to termination by a method described elsewhere.[2] The 5-mm segments were dehydrated in ethanol and xylene, and embedded in paraffin. At least 6 μm thick histologic sections were cut from each 5-mm segment and stained by the Movat method. The percent cross-sectional area luminal narrowing by atherosclerotic plaque was determined by microscopic examination with approximately 40 times magnification. The percent luminal narrowing was graded into 1 of 5 cross-sectional area categories: 0 to 25, 26 to 50, 51 to 75, 76 to 95 and 96 to 100%. The accuracy of this technique of grading cross-sectional area narrowing has been validated to be >95%.[3] Histologic sections, ≥2 per heart, extending from endocardium to epicardium of the left ventricular wall, were prepared. Foci of myocardial necrosis or fibrosis, or both, were confirmed histologically.

RESULTS

Grossly visible left ventricular wall necrosis or fibrosis, or both: Two patients (8%) had left ventricular foci of necrosis alone, 15 (58%) had foci of fibrosis

TABLE I (continued)

Case No.	S	SH	HW (g)	LV Wall N	LV Wall F	Number of CAs ↓ >75%	No. of 5-mm CA Segments	Number (%) of Coronary Segments Narrowed by Plaque 0–25%	26–50%	51–75%	76–95%	96–100%
1	0	+	770	0	+	3	65	2 (3)	24 (37)	35 (54)	4 (6)	0
2	0	0	370	0	+	3	48	2 (4)	3 (6)	21 (44)	20 (42)	2 (4)
3	0	+	600	0	0	2	41	8 (19)	4 (10)	14 (34)	6 (15)	9 (22)
4	0	−	490	0	+	2	53	18 (34)	10 (19)	19 (36)	6 (11)	0
5	0	+	660	+	+	3	37	11 (30)	4 (11)	10 (27)	10 (27)	2 (5)
6	0	+	380	0	+	2	59	25 (43)	6 (10)	22 (37)	6 (10)	0
7	+	+	405	0	+	3	49	4 (9)	11 (22)	23 (47)	11 (22)	0
8	+	+	490	0	0	1	39	2 (5)	19 (49)	17 (44)	1 (2)	0
9	0	0	560	+	+	2	53	10 (19)	12 (23)	15 (28)	15 (28)	1 (2)
10	+	0	495	0	0	0	50	40 (80)	6 (12)	4 (8)	0	0
11	0	+	350	0	0	0	53	16 (30)	22 (42)	15 (28)	0	0
12	0	+	650	0	+	3	52	6 (11)	3 (6)	12 (23)	17 (33)	14 (27)
13	0	0	410	0	+	2	65	4 (6)	13 (20)	30 (46)	8 (12)	10 (16)
14	+	0	405	+	0	4	59	8 (13)	9 (15)	21 (36)	11 (19)	10 (17)
15	0	+	645	0	0	1	38	25 (66)	8 (21)	4 (10)	1 (3)	0
16	0	+	430	0	+	3	42	13 (31)	1 (2)	11 (26)	10 (24)	7 (17)
17	0	+	450	+	+	3	65	0	18 (28)	16 (24)	20 (31)	11 (17)
18	0	+	480	0	+	3	47	0	9 (19)	14 (30)	20 (43)	4 (8)
19	+	+	475	0	+	2	47	1 (2)	9 (19)	24 (51)	8 (17)	5 (11)
20	−	−	350	0	+	3	56	7 (13)	5 (9)	14 (25)	12 (21)	18 (32)
21	0	+	595	0	+	3	47	3 (6)	11 (23)	20 (43)	12 (26)	1 (2)
22	−	−	510	+	0	2	43	2 (5)	4 (9)	31 (72)	6 (14)	0
23	0	0	450	0	+	3	61	3 (5)	14 (23)	13 (21)	19 (31)	12 (20)
24	+	0	430	0	+	3	45	12 (27)	1 (2)	18 (40)	12 (27)	2 (4)
25	0	+	595	+	+	2	56	0	14 (25)	25 (45)	14 (25)	3 (5)
26	−	0	330	0	+	2	52	11 (21)	24 (46)	10 (19)	1 (2)	6 (12)
Totals or mean	6	15	491 ± 113	6	19	2.3 ± 1.0	1,322 (51)	233 (17%)	264 (20%)	458 (35%)	250 (19%)	117 (9%)

AK = above knee; AMI = acute myocardial infarction; AP = angina pectoris; B = black; BK = below knee; CA = coronary artery; CHF = congestive heart failure; CS = cigarette smoker; DM = diabetes mellitus (adult onset); F = fibrosis; HW = heart weight; LV = left ventricular; N = necrosis; S = stroke; SCD = sudden coronary death; SH = systemic hypertension; W = white.

alone, and 4 patients (15%) had foci of both necrosis and fibrosis.

Coronary arteries: In the 26 patients, the mean number of coronary arteries per patient narrowed >75% in cross-sectional area by atherosclerotic plaque was 2.3 ± 1.0: 2 patients (8%) had no arteries narrowed to this degree, 2 patients (8%) had 1 artery so narrowed, 9 (34%) had 2 arteries so narrowed, 12 (46%) had 3 arteries so narrowed, and 1 patient (4%) had 4 arteries so narrowed (Figure 1). Of the 24 patients with >75% narrowing of 1 or more major coronary arteries, the number/patient narrowed >75% was 2.5 ± 0.7. Of the 104 major epicardial coronary arteries in the 26 patients (4 per patient), 60 (58%) were narrowed by plaque at some point 76 to 100% in cross-sectional area. Of the individual major coronary arteries, the left main coronary artery was severely narrowed (76 to 100% in cross-sectional area) in 1 patient (4%), the left anterior descending coronary artery in 21 patients (81%), the left circumflex coronary artery in 17 patients (65%), and the right coronary artery in 21 patients (81%). Of the 1,322 five-mm-long coronary segments from the 104 major coronary arteries, the mean percentages narrowed in cross-sectional area 0 to 25%, 26 to 50%, 51 to 75%, 76 to 95% and 96 to 100% were 17, 20, 35, 19 and 9%, respectively. The amount of narrowing in all 5-mm segments and in each major coronary artery in the pa-

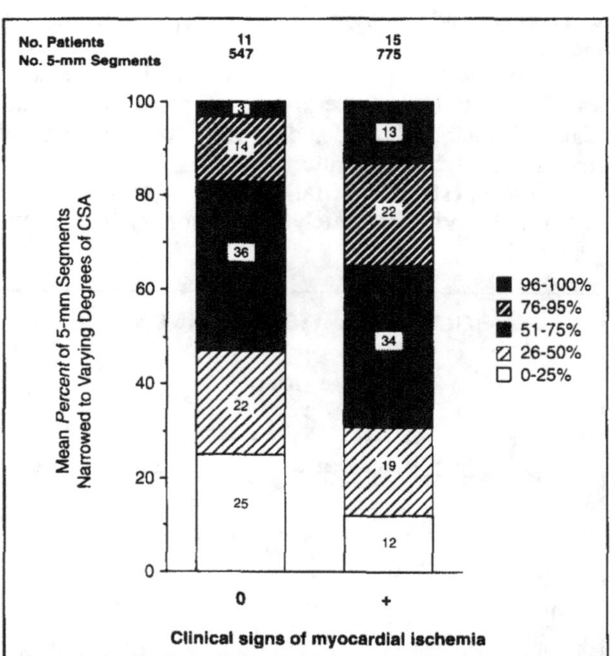

FIGURE 2. Mean percentages of 5-mm segments of the sum of the 4 major coronary arteries narrowed to varying degrees in cross-sectional area (CSA) in 26 amputees: comparison of 11 patients *without* (cases 1 to 11, Table I) with 15 patients *with* (cases 12 to 26, Table I) clinical evidence of myocardial ischemia.

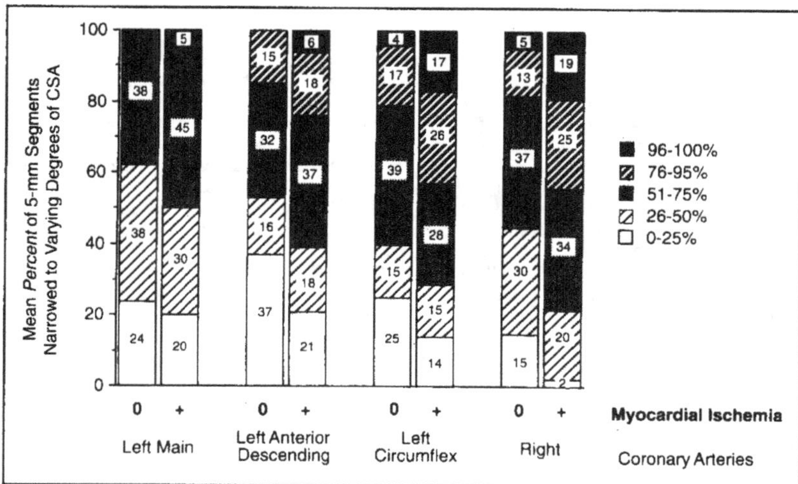

FIGURE 3. Comparison of mean percentages of 5-mm segments of the 4 major coronary arteries narrowed to varying degrees in cross-sectional area (CSA) in 26 amputees: comparison of 11 patients *without* (cases 1 to 11, Table I) and 15 patients *with* (cases 12 to 26, Table I) clinical evidence of myocardial ischemia.

tients with and without clinical evidence of myocardial ischemia is summarized in Figures 2 and 3.

DISCUSSION

Summary of major findings in the present study: Of the 26 amputees, 24 (92%) had 1 or more coronary arteries narrowed >75% in cross-sectional area by plaque, an average of 2.5 ± 0.7 for each of the 24 patients. The left anterior descending, left circumflex, and right coronary artery had similar amounts of severe coronary narrowing (35, 28 and 35%, respectively). Of a total of 1,322 five-mm segments of the 4 major coronary arteries, 28% were narrowed 76 to 100% in cross-sectional area. Although the numbers of coronary arteries narrowed >75% in cross-sectional area by plaque were not significantly different in the 15 patients *with* compared to the 11 patients *without* clinical evidence of myocardial ischemia (2.6 ± 0.7 vs 1.9 ± 1.1, p = 0.07), the percentage of 5-mm coronary segments narrowed >75% was significantly greater in patients *with* compared to those *without* clinical evidence of myocardial ischemia (35 vs 17%, p = 0.02). Twenty-one of the 26 patients at necropsy had acute and/or healed myocardial infarcts. The 21 patients *with* myocardial infarcts had more coronary narrowing by plaque than did the 5 patients *without* (mean numbers of coronary arteries narrowed >75% = 2.7 ± 0.6 vs 0.8 ± 0.8, p = 0.0001; 5-mm segments narrowed >75% = 32 vs 8%, p = 0.006).

Previously reported necropsy studies on the coronary arteries in patients with peripheral vascular disease with and without amputation: No previously reported study has examined at necropsy the amounts of coronary narrowing in patients having previous lower limb amputation.

Previously reported coronary angiographic studies in patients with symptomatic peripheral arterial atherosclerotic disease: Although a number have described the frequency of clinical evidence of myocardial ischemia in patients with peripheral arterial disease,[4-14] few previously published studies have reported the amounts of coronary narrowing by angiogram in patients with intermittent claudication or lower limb tissue necrosis, or both. Schoop et al[15] in 1966 performed cor-

onary angiography in 28 men (aged 26 to 70 years [mean 56]) with symptomatic peripheral arterial disease: only 3 patients (11%) had coronary narrowing >50% in diameter. Tomatis et al[16] in 1972 reported findings on coronary angiograms in 72 patients (aged 39 to 76 years [mean 58]) with symptomatic peripheral vascular disease: 34 patients (47%) had narrowing 76 to 100% in diameter of 1 or more major coronary arteries, 7 patients (10%) had narrowing 51 to 75%, and the remaining 31 patients (43%) had insignificant (≤50% diameter reduction) coronary narrowing. Hertzer et al[17] in 1984 described coronary angiographic findings in 381 patients (aged 29 to 90 years [mean 62]) with peripheral vascular disease: 218 (57%) had narrowing >70% in diameter of 1 or more major coronary arteries, another 125 patients (33%) had 1 or more narrowings between "measurable" to 70% diameter reduction, and the remaining 38 patients (10%) had "angiographically normal" arteries.

Although the present study in many ways is quite different from the one reported by Hertzer et al,[17] comparison of our study to theirs is nevertheless appropriate in some areas: *frequency of the presence of 1 or more major coronary arteries significantly* (>75% cross-sectional area narrowing at necropsy and >50% in diameter at angiography) *narrowed* (24 of 26 patients [92%] vs 343 of 381 patients [90%]); *frequency of single, double and triple (or quadruple) coronary arterial narrowing* (8, 34 and 50% vs 21, 20 and 18%, respectively); *frequency of significant narrowing of the left main, left anterior descending, left circumflex and right coronary arteries* (2, 35, 28 and 35% vs 4, 30, 35 and 46%, respectively); and *frequency of clinical evidence of myocardial ischemia* (58 vs 56%).

Acknowledgment: We appreciate the excellent secretarial assistance of Vivian Norman, and the technical assistance of Filippina Giacometti and Leslie Berry.

REFERENCES

1. Roberts WC. Sudden cardiac death: a diversity of causes with focus on atherosclerotic coronary artery disease. *Am J Cardiol* 1990;65:13B–19B.
2. Roberts WC. Qualitative and quantitative comparison of amounts of narrowing by atherosclerotic plaques in the major epicardial coronary arteries at necrop-

sy in sudden coronary death, transmural acute myocardial infarction, transmural healed myocardial infarction and unstable angina pectoris. *Am J Cardiol* 1989;64:324–328.

3. Isner JM, Wu M, Virmani R, Jones AA, Roberts WC. Comparison of degrees of coronary arterial luminal narrowing determined by visual inspection of histologic sections under magnification among three independent observers and comparison to that obtained by video planimetry: an analysis of 559 five-millimeter segments of 61 coronary arteries from eleven patients. *Lab Invest* 1980;42:566–570.

4. McDonald L. Ischaemic heart disease and peripheral occlusive arterial disease. *Br Heart J* 1953;15:101–107.

5. Richards RL. Prognosis of intermittent claudication. *Br Med J* 1957;2:1091–1093.

6. Juergens JL, Barker NW, Hines EA Jr. Arteriosclerosis obliterans: review of 520 cases with special reference to pathogenic and prognostic factors. *Circulation* 1960;21:188–195.

7. Tillgren C. Obliterative arterial disease of the lower limbs. III. Prognostic influence of concomitant coronary heart disease. *Acta Med Scand* 1965;178:121–128.

8. Cooperman M, Pflug B, Martin EW, Evans WE. Cardiovascular risk factors in patients with peripheral vascular disease. *Surgery* 1978;84:505–509.

9. DeBakey ME, Lawrie GM. Combined coronary artery and peripheral vascular disease: recognition and treatment. *J Vasc Surg* 1984;1:605–607.

10. Kannel WB, McGee DL. Update on some epidemiologic features of intermittent claudication: the Framingham study. *J Am Geriat Soc* 1985;33:13–18.

11. Lassila R, Lepäntalo M, Lindfors O. Peripheral arterial disease-natural outcome. *Acta Med Scand* 1986;220:295–301.

12. Hertzer NR. Basic data concerning associated coronary disease in peripheral vascular patients. *Ann Vasc Surg* 1987;1:616–620.

13. Ledingham JGG. Peripheral vascular disease as a risk factor for ischaemic heart disease. *Eur Heart J* 1988;9(suppl G):65–68.

14. Gersh BJ, Rihal CS, Rooke TW, Ballard DJ. Evaluation and management of patients with both peripheral vascular and coronary artery disease. *J Am Coll Cardiol* 1991;18:203–214.

15. Schoop W, Kiefer H, Blümchen G. Koronarangiographische Befunde bei Kranken mit obliterierenden Veränderungen in den Extremitätenarterien und normalem Ruhe-EKG. *Z Kreislauf Forsch* 1966;55:884–890.

16. Tomatis LA, Fierens EE, Verbrugge GP. Evaluation of surgical risk in peripheral vascular disease by coronary arteriography: a series of 100 cases. *Surgery* 1972;71:429–435.

17. Hertzer NR, Beven EG, Young JR, O'Hara PJ, Ruschhaupt III WF, Graor RA, DeWolfe VG, Maljovec LC. Coronary artery disease in peripheral vascular patients: a classification of 1000 coronary angiograms and results of surgical management. *Ann Surg* 1984;199:223–233.

Composition of Atherosclerotic Plaques in the Epicardial Coronary Arteries in Juvenile (Type I) Diabetes Mellitus

Susanne L. Mautner, MD, Fengru Lin, MD, and William C. Roberts, MD

The composition of atherosclerotic plaques in 331 five-mm segments of the 4 major (left main, left anterior descending, left circumflex, and right) epicardial coronary arteries of 8 patients with juvenile (mean age at onset, 9 years; mean age at death, 29 years) diabetes mellitus was determined by computerized planimetric analysis. Analysis of all coronary segments disclosed that the plaques consisted primarily of dense (53%) and cellular (38%) fibrous tissue. Pultaceous debris (7%), foam cells (1.2%) and calcific deposits (0.7%) occupied a small percentage of the plaques. Thus, 91% of the coronary plaques in these young diabetic patients consisted of fibrous tissue and nearly all of the remaining 9% consisted of lipid deposits. Analysis of composition according to degrees of cross-sectional luminal narrowing revealed marked increases in dense fibrous tissue (from 31 to 74%), pultaceous debris (from 3 to 12%), and calcific deposits (from 0% to 3%) as the cross-sectional area narrowing increased from $\leq 25\%$ to $>75\%$. Compared with older patients with fatal coronary artery disease, the patients with juvenile diabetes had more dense fibrous tissue and pultaceous debris and less calcific deposits.

(Am J Cardiol 1992;70:1264–1268)

From the Pathology Branch, National Heart, Lung, and Blood Institute, National Institutes of Health, Bethesda, Maryland. Manuscript received April 24, 1992; revised manuscript received and accepted July 6, 1992.

Address for reprints: Susanne L. Mautner, MD, National Heart, Lung, and Blood Institute, National Institutes of Health, Building 10, Room 2N258, 9000 Rockville Pike, Bethesda, Maryland 20892.

It is well recognized that patients with diabetes mellitus have an increased risk of significant atherosclerosis compared with similar aged nondiabetic patients. Despite this fact, the composition of the atherosclerotic plaques in such patients has not been reported. Accordingly, we examined quantitatively the composition of atherosclerotic plaques in the 4 major epicardial coronary arteries in 8 patients with juvenile diabetes mellitus.

METHODS

Clinical features: Certain observations in the 8 patients are summarized in Table I. The patients ranged in age from 19 to 38 years (mean 29) at death, and at ages 2 to 13 (average 9) the onset of symptoms or signs of diabetes appeared. The duration of insulin therapy in the 8 patients averaged 20 years. The serum total cholesterol was >240 mg/dl in 5 of 6 patients. Three of the 8 patients had indirect systemic systolic arterial pressures >160 or diastolic pressures >100 mm Hg, or both, on multiple occasions. Although no patient had a clinical event recognized as acute myocardial infarction, 2 patients (cases 7 and 8, Table I) had transmural acute myocardial infarcts at necropsy, and death in each of them was attributed to the infarct.

Methods of examining the coronary arteries at necropsy: All 4 major epicardial coronary arteries were dissected from the heart intact, decalcified, and sectioned transversely at 5-mm intervals. They were dehydrated, cleared, embedded in paraffin, cut and stained by the Movat method. A total of 331 five-mm segments were examined. Evaluation was done by planimetry (described in detail in a previous publication[1]), outlining the internal elastic membrane, residual lumen, and components of the plaque, such as dense fibrous tissue, cellular fibrous tissue, calcific deposits, pultaceous debris, foam cells, foam cells with lymphocytes, and inflammatory cells without foam cells (Figure 1). The area of each component of plaque was then converted to a percentage of the total plaque area. For each patient the mean plaque composition was determined by calculating the mean of all 5-mm segments of the 4 coronary arteries of each patient. The total mean for the 8 patients was calculated as the mean of all 331 segments (Table II, Figures 2 and 3). For comparison with previous studies the total mean was calculated in the same fashion used in those studies, i.e., the total mean was based on the mean of each patient rather than on all segments (Figure 4). The degree of cross-sectional luminal narrowing was categorized into 5 groups: 0 to 25%, 26 to 50%, 51 to 75%, 76 to 95%, and 96 to 100%.

RESULTS

Cross-sectional area narrowing: The results are summarized in Table II and in Figures 2 and 3. In 6 of the 8 patients, 1 or more epicardial coronary arteries were narrowed by atherosclerotic plaque >75% in cross-sectional area. Of the 331 five-mm coronary segments examined, 68 (21%) were narrowed >75% in cross-sectional area by plaque.

Plaque composition: Plaque composition in all 331 five-mm segments in each of the 8 patients is summarized in Table II. *Fibrous tissue* was the domi-

	Age (years) at Death	Sex	Age (years) at Onset DM	Duration of DM (years)	NS	TC* (mg/dl)	BUN† mg/dl	BP† (mmHg) (s/d)	CHF	Cause of Death
TABLE I Clinical Observations in the Eight Patients with Juvenile Diabetes Mellitus										
Case										
1	19	F	10	9	0	174	10	100/80	0	Infection
2	20	M	11	9	0	244	20	130/80	0	Hodgkin's
3	25	F	9	16	+	254	60	120/70	0	Renal
4	26	M	2	25	+	240	60	240/140	+	Renal
5	28	M	9	19	+	365	60	270/150	0	Renal
6	35	M	9	26	+	249	50	240/140	+	CNS bleed
7	37	M	9	28	—	—	—	130/70	+	AMI
8	38	F	13	25	0	—	30	130/80	0	AMI
Total or Mean	29	3F:5M	9	20	4	254	41	170/101	3	

*Highest value recorded.
†Usual value one to six months before death.
AMI = acute myocardial infarction; BP = blood pressure; BUN = blood urea nitrogen; CHF = congestive heart failure; CNS = central nervous system; DM = diabetes mellitus; NS = nephrotic syndrome; s/d = peak systole/end diastole; TC = serum total cholesterol.

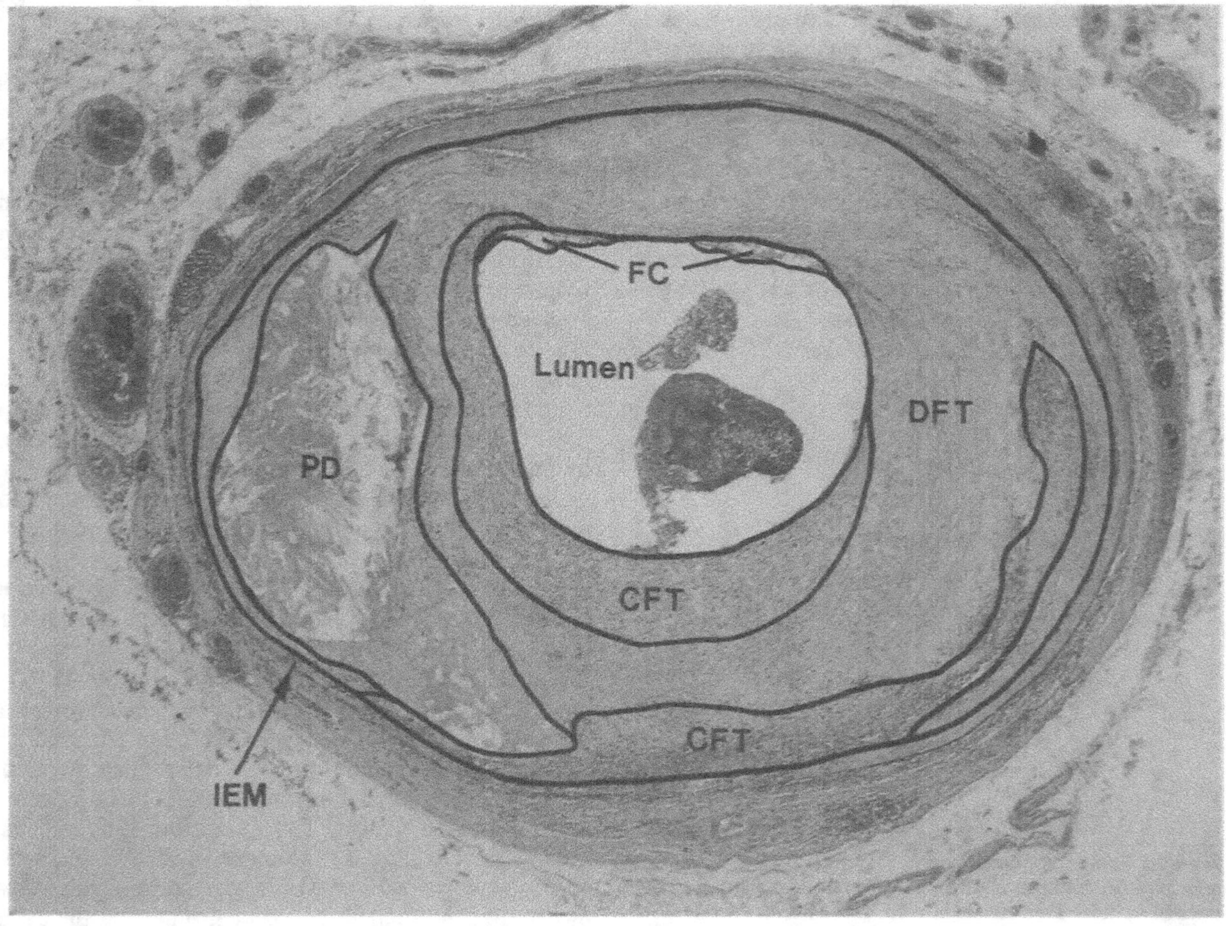

FIGURE 1. Photograph of a coronary artery in cross section with the internal elastic membrane (IEM), residual lumen, and the components of plaque outlined: cellular (CFT) and dense fibrous tissue (DFT) as predominant contributors to the narrowing of the lumen, foam cells (FC) located on the luminal surface, and an area of pultaceous debris (PD) located deeper in the plaque. In the lumen is some postmortem thrombotic material. The patient died at age 37 of an acute myocardial infarct. (Movat stain × 37, reduced by 32%).

nant component, comprising an average of 91% of the plaques: *dense* fibrous tissue made up 53% and *cellular* fibrous tissue 38%. *Pultaceous debris*, which is primarily extracellular lipid, comprised an average of 7% of the plaques. Intracellular lipid in the form of *foam cell aggregates* comprised an average of 1% of the plaques. Plaque composition was similar in each of the 4 major coronary arteries (Figure 2) and varied according to degrees of cross-sectional area narrowing (Figure 3): *Dense fibrous tissue* increased from 31% in the 0 to 25% narrowing category to 74% in the combined 76 to 100% narrowing category; *pultaceous debris* and *calcific deposits* increased from 3 and 0%, respectively, in the

TABLE II Necropsy Findings in the Eight Patients with Juvenile Diabetes Mellitus

Case	HW(g)	Gross LV N	Gross LV F	Number of 5 mm Segments	0–25%	26–50%	51–75%	76–95%	96–100%	DFT	CFT	CD	PD	FC	FC+L	ICWFC
					Number of Percent of 5 mm Segments Narrowed to 5 Categories of CSA by Plaque					Percent of Coronary Plaques Consisting of:						
1	160	0	0	47	24 (51)	14 (30)	7 (15)	2 (4)	0 (0)	39.8	43.3	0.0	14.4	2.4	0.0	0.0
2	310	0	0	36	32 (89)	4 (11)	0 (0)	0 (0)	0 (0)	64.1	23.9	0.0	5.8	6.2	0.0	0.0
3	300	0	0	29	18 (62)	9 (32)	1 (3)	1 (3)	0 (0)	2.6	91.7	0.0	4.1	1.6	0.0	0.0
4	340	0	0	37	36 (97)	1 (3)	0 (0)	0 (0)	0 (0)	4.1	95.9	0.0	0.0	0.0	0.0	0.0
5	430	0	0	43	7 (16)	7 (16)	15 (35)	12 (28)	2 (5)	62.8	32.0	0.0	4.8	0.2	0.0	0.2
6	450	+	+	48	1 (2)	17 (35)	20 (42)	9 (19)	1 (2)	84.8	7.2	0.0	7.2	0.4	0.0	0.1
7	450	+	+	55	1 (2)	4 (7)	21 (38)	26 (47)	3 (6)	76.5	14.0	4.2	4.3	0.1	0.2	0.2
8	340	+	0	36	11 (31)	6 (17)	7 (19)	12 (33)	0 (0)	61.5	23.0	0.0	14.9	0.2	0.0	0.1
Total or Mean	348	3	2	331 (100%)	130 (43%)	62 (19%)	71 (19%)	62 (17%)	6 (2%)	53.3%	37.9%	0.7%	6.7%	1.2%	0.1%	0.1%

CFT = cellular fibrous tissue; CD = calcific deposits; CSA = cross-sectional area; DFT = dense fibrous tissue; F = fibrosis; FC = foam cells; FC+L = foam cells plus lymphocytes; HW = heart weight; ICWFC = inflammatory cells without foam cells; LV = left ventricular; N = necrosis; PD = pultaceous debris.

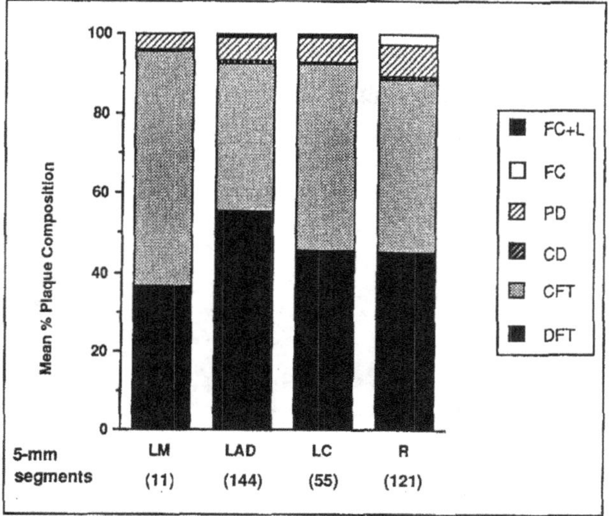

FIGURE 2. Graph showing mean coronary arterial plaque composition in the 4 major epicardial coronary arteries. The number of total 5-mm segments for each coronary artery is shown in parentheses. CD = calcific deposits; CFT = cellular fibrous tissue; DFT = dense fibrous tissue; FC = foam cells; FC + L = foam cells plus lymphocytes; LAD = left anterior descending coronary artery; LC = left circumflex; LM = left main; PD = pultaceous debris; R = right coronary artery.

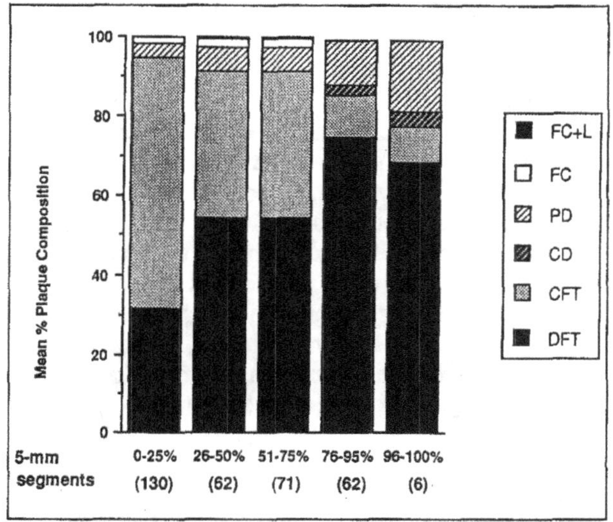

FIGURE 3. Graph showing mean coronary arterial plaque composition in each of the 5 categories of cross-sectional area narrowing. The number of total 5-mm segments for each coronary artery is shown in parentheses. Abbreviations as in Figure 2.

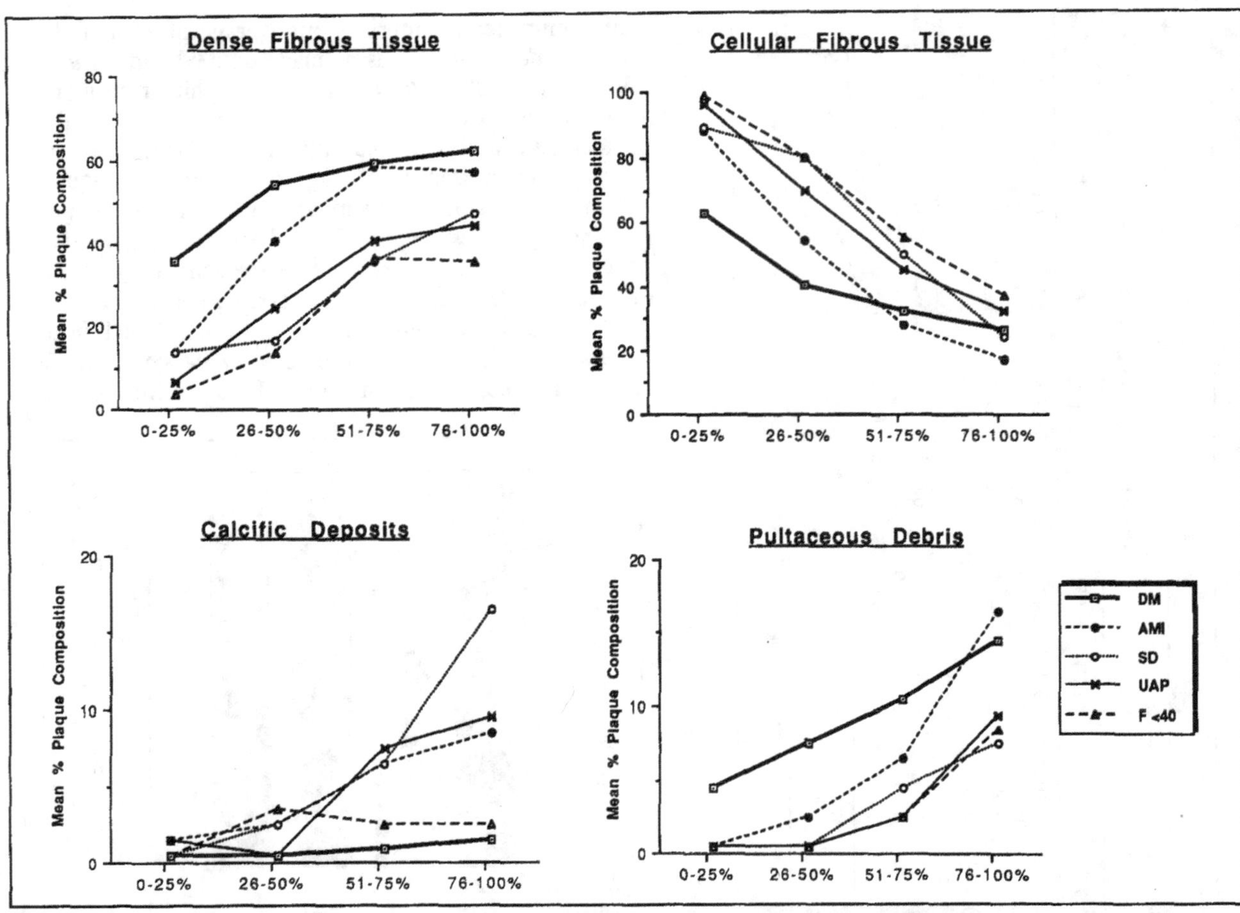

FIGURE 4. Graph comparing mean coronary arterial plaque composition in each of the 4 categories of cross-sectional narrowing in the present study of patients with juvenile diabetes mellitus (DM) and in previously reported patients with fatal acute myocardial infarct (AMI), sudden coronary death (SD), unstable angina pectoris (UAP), and women <40 years of age (F <40).

0 to 25% narrowing category and to 12 and 3%, respectively, in the combined 76 to 100% narrowing category. *Cellular fibrous tissue* and *foam cells* decreased with increasing degrees of cross-sectional area narrowing: from 63 and 2%, respectively, in the 0 to 25% narrowing category, and to 11 and 0%, respectively, in the 76 to 100% narrowing category.

DISCUSSION

As is well appreciated, patients with juvenile diabetes mellitus at necropsy generally have rather severe degrees of narrowing of the major epicardial coronary arteries by atherosclerotic plaque.[2] In 6 of the 8 patients, 1 or more major epicardial coronary arteries was severely (>75%) narrowed by plaque, and 21% of all 5-mm segments of the major coronary arteries were narrowed >75% in cross-sectional area. The dominant component (91%) of the plaques was *fibrous tissue*. In each of the 4 major coronary arteries, plaque composition was similar.

Comparing our findings in the 8 patients with juvenile diabetes to older patients (mean age 59 years) with fatal coronary artery disease (acute myocardial infarction,[1] sudden death,[1] unstable angina pectoris[3]), and to young nondiabetic women (mean age 34 years) with fatal coronary disease[4] disclosed similarities and dissimilarities in plaque composition (Figure 4): *dense fibrous tissue*, *pultaceous debris* and *calcific deposits* increased in all 5 patient groups with increasing degrees of cross-sectional area luminal narrowing. In contrast, *cellular fibrous tissue* decreased in all 5 patient groups as the luminal area decreased (or as plaque size increased). The patients with juvenile diabetes had the highest percentage of *dense fibrous tissue* in all categories of narrowing. They also had the smallest percentage of *calcific deposits* in nearly every category of cross-sectional area narrowing.

Although only 8% of the 331 five-mm sections of coronary plaque in the 8 patients with juvenile diabetes consisted of lipid (intracellular or extracellular), a wide variation was observed in individual patients. Patient 4 (Table II), for example, had no lipid in any of his plaques (37 five-mm coronary sections); in patient 1, in contrast, nearly 17% of her plaques (47 five-mm coronary sections) consisted of lipid. Because lipid deposits can regress with lowering of serum total cholesterol levels,[5] the potential for plaque reversibility or shrinkage is much greater in patient 1 than in patient 4. If cellular fibrous tissue is reversible as well, and there is some experimental evidence that that might be the case,[6] then the potential for plaque reversibility was present in all 8 patients.

Acknowledgment: We gratefully acknowledge the technical assistance of Filippina M. Giacometti, Leslie

K. Berry, Alvado M. Campbell, Michael W. Spencer
and Vivian E. Norman.

REFERENCES

1. Kragel AH, Reddy SG, Wittes JT, Roberts WC. Morphometric analysis of the composition of atherosclerotic plaques in the four major epicardial coronary arteries in acute myocardial infarction and in sudden coronary death. *Circulation* 1989;80:1747–1756.

2. Crall FV, Roberts WC. The extramural and intramural coronary arteries in juvenile diabetes mellitus. *Am J Med* 1978;64:221–230.

3. Kragel AH, Reddy SG, Wittes JT, Roberts WC. Morphometric analysis of the composition of coronary arterial plaques in isolated unstable angina pectoris with pain at rest. *Am J Cardiol* 1990;66:562–567.

4. Dollar AL, Kragel AH, Fernicola DJ, Waclawiw MA, Roberts WC. Composition of atherosclerotic plaques in coronary arteries in women <40 years of age with fatal coronary artery disease and implication for plaque reversibility. *Am J Cardiol* 1991;67:1223–1227.

5. Stary HC. Progression and regression of experimental atherosclerosis in rhesus monkeys. In: Goldsmith EI, Moor-Jankowski J, ed. Medical Primatology. Basel: S. Karger, 1972:356–367.

6. Armstrong ML, Megan MB. Arterial fibrous proteins in cynomolgus monkeys after atherogenic and regression diets. *Circ Res* 1975;36:256–261.

Scarring of the Left Ventricular Papillary Muscles in Sickle-Cell Disease

Katherine Berezowski, MD, Gisela C. Mautner, MD, and William C. Roberts, MD

A number of publications have described various findings in the heart in patients with sickle-cell disease.[1,2] In general, both ventricular cavities are dilated, cardiac mass is increased, and the epicardial coronary arteries are dilated. Although the cardiac valve leaflets are usually normal anatomically, precordial systolic murmurs are common in these patients.[2,3] Although infarcts are common at necropsy in the lungs, spleen, liver, kidneys and even brain in sickle-cell disease, grossly visible myocardial infarcts are rare in these patients.[4,5] Because patients with sickle-cell disease usually have severe and chronic

anemia, and because the papillary muscles are believed to be the last portion of the heart to be perfused by blood through the coronary system, we systematically examined the left ventricular papillary muscles at necropsy in a group of patients with sickle-cell anemia for foci of necrosis or fibrosis, findings indicative of inadequate myocardial perfusion.

The files of the Pathology Branch were searched for cases classified as "sickle-cell disease" or "anemia." In all, 20 cases were retrieved. On reexamination of clinical records, however, 2 cases were excluded because patients were toddlers (aged 2 and 3 years). Five other cases were eliminated because the hearts or histologic slides of papillary muscles were not available for reexamination. Thus, this study was limited to 13 cases of classic sickle-cell disease (diagnosed by electrophoresis). The perti-

From the Pathology Branch, National Heart, Lung, and Blood Institute, National Institutes of Health, Bethesda, Maryland 20892. Manuscript received March 6, 1992; revised manuscript received and accepted June 10, 1992.

TABLE I Clinical and Necropsy Findings in 13 Black Patients with Sickle-Cell Disease

Case	Age (yr) & Sex	Chronic CHF	SD	PE	HW (g)	Fibrosis LV PM	Major CA ↓ >75% CSA by Plaque	LVFW or VS Scarring	Myocardial Iron (0–3+)	Intra-cardiac Thrombi
1	13F	+	0	0	360	+	0	0	0	0
2	16F	0	0	+	380	+	0	0	0	0
3	27M	0	+	+	405	0	0	0	+	+
4	28F	−	0	0	305	0	0	0	+	0
5	28M	+	0	+	770	+	0	0	0	+
6	29M	0	0	0	485	+	0	0	0	0
7	32M	+	0	+	480	0	0	0	0	0
8	37M	+	0	0	715	+	0	0	0	0
9	40F	+	0	+	450	+	0	0	+	0
10	41F	+	0	0	345	+	0	0	+++	0
11	41M	0	+	0	480	+	+	+	+	0
12	45M	+	0	0	620	0	0	0	0	0
13	45F	+	+	0	500	+	0	0	+++	0

CA = coronary artery; CHF = congestive heart failure; CSA = cross-sectional area; HW = heart weight; LV = left ventricle; LVFW = left ventricular free wall; PE = pulmonary emboli; PM = papillary muscle; SD = sudden death; VS = ventricular septum.

nent clinical and morphologic findings are tabulated in Table I. All patients had severe chronic anemia (blood hematocrit <30%). Detailed information on the precordial examination was available in only 5 patients, and each had grade 2/6 systolic apical and basal murmurs. The heart in each patient was examined initially by WCR and reexamined by each investigator. Sections were prepared for histologic study from each left ventricular papillary muscle. Each section was stained by both hematoxylin and eosin, and for iron (Prussian blue).

At least 1 left ventricular papillary muscle was scarred in 9 patients (Figures 1 and 2). Additionally, a right ventricular papillary muscle was examined histologically in 12 patients, and this structure was scarred in 2. One patient (case 11; Table I) had a large, healed, left ventricular posterior wall infarct and severe narrowing of the lumen of the right coronary artery by atherosclerotic plaque. No patient had myocardial necrosis. Both ventricular cavities were dilated in all 13 patients. Six patients (46%) had iron in the myocardium, presumably the result of numerous blood transfusions in the past.

This study indicates that ischemic change (namely fibrosis) occurs frequently in 1 or both left ventricular

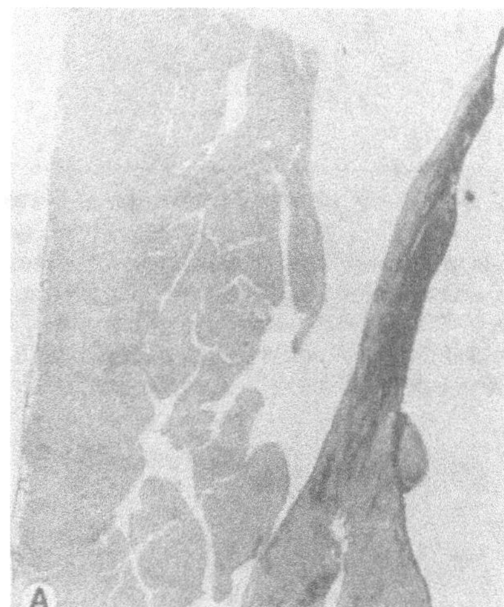

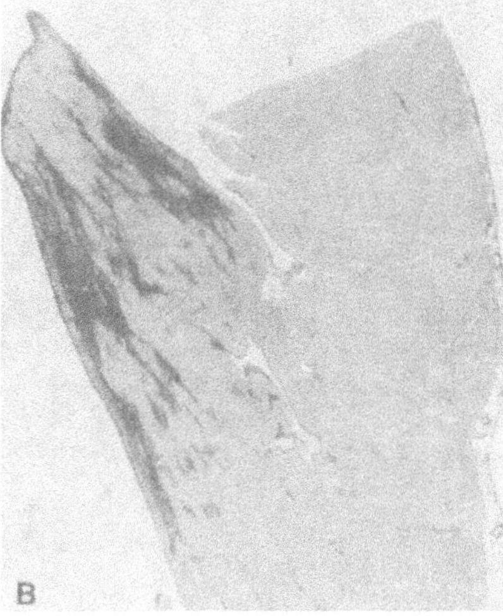

FIGURE 2. Case 1 (Table I). *Photomicrographs* of histologic sections of papillary muscles. *A*, fibrosis of right ventricular papillary muscle. *B*, focal areas of fibrosis in the left ventricular papillary muscle. Elastic van Gieson stains (original magnification ×5; reduced by 41%).

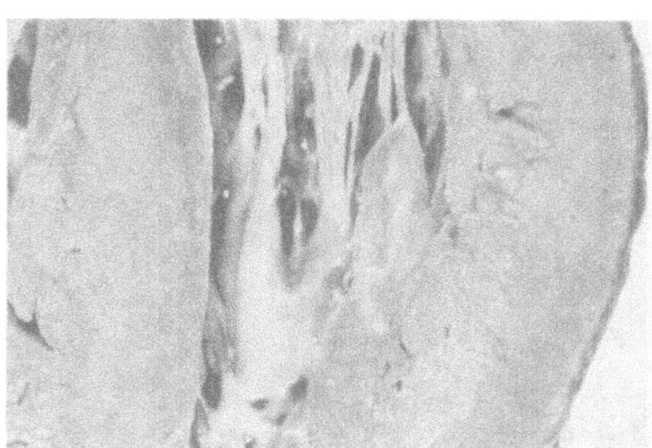

FIGURE 1. Case 8 (Table I). Close-up view of scarred left ventricular papillary muscle.

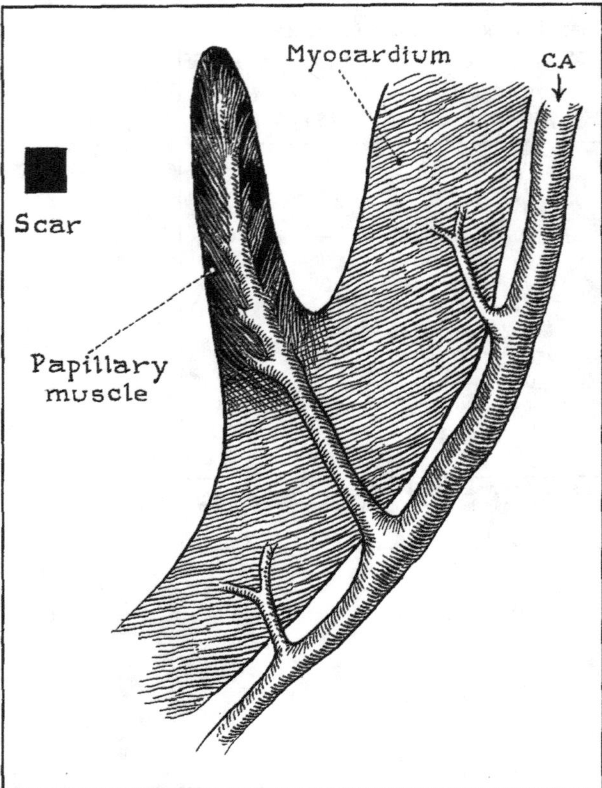

FIGURE 3. *Schematic view* of distribution of fibrosed areas in papillary muscle. The left ventricular papillary muscles are the last portions of the heart to be perfused with coronary arterial blood. To perfuse the apices of the papillary muscles, the coronary artery (CA) must extend through the entire thickness of the myocardial free wall, turn uphill, and ascend a distance of at least 1 and often 2 thicknesses of the free wall.

papillary muscles in patients with sickle-cell disease. The left ventricular papillary muscles appear to be the last cardiac structure to be perfused by arterial blood,[6] and therefore, if any cardiac structure is inadequately perfused it would logically be these structures (Figure 3). Although the epicardial coronary arteries are dilated in these chronically and severely anemic patients, this dilatation and resulting increased capacity for coronary blood flow is usually not a completely adequate, compensatory mechanism to prevent inadequate perfusion of the left ventricular papillary muscles. It is also possible that a sharp reduction in the usually chronically low blood hematocrit (as may occur in a sequestration, aplastic or hemolytic crisis) plays a role in the development of papillary muscle lesions.[7] Thus, these structures can be viewed as sensitive indicators of inadequate myocardial perfusion.

1. Gerry LJ Jr, Bulkley BH, Hutchins GM. Clinicopathologic analysis of cardiac dysfunction in 52 patients with sickle cell anemia. *Am J Cardiol* 1978;42: 211–216.
2. Falk RH, Hood WB Jr. The heart in sickle cell anemia. *Arch Intern Med* 1982;142:1680–1684.
3. Simmons BE, Santhanam V, Castaner A, Rao KRP, Sachdev N, Cooper R. Sickle cell heart disease. Two-dimensional echo and Doppler ultrasonographic findings in the hearts of adult patients with sickle cell anemia. *Arch Intern Med* 1988;148:1526–1528.
4. McCormick WF. Massive nonatherosclerotic myocardial infarction in sickle cell anemia. *Am J Forensic Med Pathol* 1988;9:151–154.
5. Martin CR, Cobb C, Tatter D, Johnson C, Haywood LJ. Acute myocardial infarction in sickle cell anemia. *Arch Intern Med* 1983;143:830–831.
6. Roberts WC, Cohen LS. Left ventricular papillary muscles. Description of the normal and a survey of conditions causing them to be abnormal. *Circulation* 1972;46:138–154.
7. Weatherall DJ, Clegg JB, Higgs DR, Wood WG. The hemoglobinopathies. In: Scriver CR, Beaudet AL, Sly WS, Valle D, eds. The Metabolic Basis of Inherited Disease. New York: McGraw-Hill, 1989:2293–2301.

Comparison of Composition of Atherosclerotic Plaques in Saphenous Veins Used as Aortocoronary Bypass Conduits with Plaques in Native Coronary Arteries in the Same Men

Susanne L. Mautner, MD, Gisela C. Mautner, MD,
Sally A. Hunsberger, PhD, and William C. Roberts, MD

This study describes quantitatively the components of atherosclerotic plaques in saphenous vein grafts used for aortocoronary bypass and compares the findings with the plaques in the native coronary arteries in the same men. A total of 607 five-mm segments of saphenous veins and 797 five-mm segments of native coronary arteries were examined by computerized planimetric technique in 19 men, aged 39 to 82 years (mean 61), who had survived bypass operation for >1 year. Comparison of the mean percentages of the plaque components in saphenous vein grafts in place for 14 to 26 months with those of the native coronary arteries revealed significant differences: *cellular* fibrous tissue, 86 vs 7%; *dense* fibrous tissue, 13 vs 82%; p <0.05. As survival time after the bypass operation increased, composition of the plaques in the saphenous veins changed so that by approximately 80 months the amounts of cellular and dense fibrous tissue in both saphenous vein grafts and native coronary arteries were similar: 10 vs 16%, and 75 vs 71%; p = not significant. Thus, by about 7 years after a coronary bypass operation the composition of plaques in saphenous vein grafts is similar to that in the native coronary arteries of the same patients.

(Am J Cardiol 1992;70:1380–1387)

From the Pathology and Biostatistics Research Branches, National Heart, Lung, and Blood Institute, National Institutes of Health, Bethesda, Maryland. Manuscript received June 16, 1992; revised manuscript received and accepted July 15, 1992.

Address for reprints: Susanne L. Mautner, MD, National Heart, Lung, and Blood Institute, National Institutes of Health, Building 10, Room 2N258, 9000 Rockville Pike, Bethesda, Maryland 20892.

Morphologic changes in saphenous veins that had been inserted into the aortocoronary position as bypass conduits have been described previously.[1-11] No studies, however, have examined the composition of the developing atherosclerotic plaques of saphenous vein bypass grafts in a detailed quantitative fashion including a comparison with the atherosclerotic plaques of the native coronary arteries of the same patients. Such is the purpose of this report.

METHODS

Patients: Cases selected were limited to men in whom the heart, the native coronary arteries, and the saphenous venous bypass grafts were available for study, and in whom the saphenous veins had been in the aortocoronary position for >1 year.[12]

Patient characteristics: Clinical features of the 19 men are listed in Table I. Their ages at death ranged from 39 to 82 years (mean 61). The interval from the coronary artery bypass grafting to death ranged from 14 to 185 months (mean 69). The 19 men had a total of 41 saphenous venous grafts; the number of grafts per patient ranged from 1 to 4 (mean 2.2). A saphenous vein having 1 aortic anastomosis and either 1 or >1 coronary arterial anastomosis was considered a single conduit.

Death was due to a cardiac cause in 9 patients (47%): sudden cardiac arrest in 4 patients without myocardial necrosis, chronic congestive heart failure in 3, and acute myocardial infarction in 2. Death was attributed to a noncardiac cause in 10 patients (53%): a vascular condition in 2 patients, cancer in 4, and miscellaneous conditions in 4 (Parkinson's disease, chronic obstructive lung disease, pancreatitis and infection).

Method of examination of saphenous vein grafts and native coronary arteries: The saphenous vein grafts and native coronary arteries were studied in a similar fashion. The hearts were fixed in formalin. The saphenous vein bypass grafts and the 4 major epicardial coronary arteries (left main, left anterior descending, left circumflex, and right) were removed from the heart intact and cut transversely into 5-mm-long intervals. (In 3 patients the left main coronary artery was not available for examination.) The segments were labeled sequentially from their origin. Each segment was processed in alcohol and xylene, embedded in paraffin, cut into 6 μm thick sections and stained by the Movat method.[13] Of 1,470 sections initially examined, 66 were excluded be-

TABLE I Clinical and Necropsy Findings in 19 Men Surviving More Than One Year After Coronary Bypass Grafting

Case	Age (years) at Death	Interval CABG–Death (months)	SH	DM	After CABG			Mode of Death	HW (g)	Dilated LV	LV Necrosis	LV Fibrosis
					AP	AMI	CHF					
1	59	14	0	0	0	0	0	Infection*	710	0	0	+
2	54	19	+	+	0	0	+	CHF	510	+	0	+
3	60	24	0	0	0	0	+	CHF	540	+	0	+
4	66	26	0	0	0	0	0	Sudden	460	0	0	+
5	62	27	+	0	0	0	0	Cancer	450	0	0	0
6	47	32	0	+	+	0	0	AMI	390	0	+	0
7	69	34	0	0	+	+	0	Sudden	550	+	0	+
8	49	39	0	0	0	0	0	Sudden	370	0	0	0
9	76	48	0	0	0	0	0	Cancer	395	0	0	+
10	58	52	+	+	+	0	0	Pancreatitis	340	0	0	0
11	73	60	+	0	0	0	0	COPD	540	0	0	+
12	69	82	0	0	0	0	0	Cancer	440	0	0	0
13	39	84	0	0	+	+	0	AMI	400	0	+	+
14	57	84	+	+	+	0	0	Sudden	515	0	0	+
15	49	96	0	0	+	0	+	CHF	520	+	0	+
16	54	120	+	0	+	0	0	Carotid operation	560	0	0	+
17	82	132	+	0	0	0	0	Stroke	485	+†	0	0
18	63	144	0	0	0	0	0	Cancer	310	0	0	+
19	63	185	0	0	+	0	0	Parkinsonism	345	0	0	0
Total or mean	61	69	7	4	8	2	3		465	5	2	12

*Multiple complications after CABG—never left hospital.
†Result of mitral regurgitation.
AMI = acute myocardial infarction; AP = angina pectoris; CABG = coronary artery bypass grafting; CHF = chronic congestive heart failure; COPD = chronic obstructive pulmonary disease; DM = diabetes mellitus; HW = heart weight; LV = left ventricle (ventricular); SH = systemic hypertension by history.

cause of sectioning artifacts. Thus, a total of 607 segments of saphenous vein grafts (mean 32/patient) and 797 five-mm segments of native coronary arteries (mean 42/patient) were studied. Evaluation of plaque composition was performed by planimetry: Movat-stained sections were placed on the stage of a projection light microscope enlarging the image approximately 150 times. A tracing of the artery was made using a GTCO micro Digi-Pad (GTCO Corp, Columbia, Maryland); the area was calculated using MacMeasure,[14] which is a morphometric software package used in conjunction with a Macintosh SE computer. The following areas were outlined: potential lumen (total area enclosed by the internal elastic membrane), residual lumen (potential lumen minus area of atherosclerotic plaque), and the components of the plaque separated into dense fibrous tissue, cellular fibrous tissue, calcific deposits, pultaceous debris (extracellular lipid), foam cells (intracellular lipid) with and without lymphocytes, and inflammatory infiltrates without significant numbers of foam cells. Analysis of components was performed in each of the 4 major epicardial coronary arteries and saphenous venous bypass grafts in every patient.

Dense fibrous tissue consisted of nearly acellular relatively homogeneous fibrous tissue staining yellow or yellow-brown by the Movat stain. *Cellular fibrous tissue* contained numerous spindle cells resembling myofibroblasts, smooth muscle cells, or fibroblasts admixed with fibrous tissue and often elastic fibers. *Calcific deposits* were detected by blackish, brownish or purple collections of granular staining areas in Movat-stained sections. *Pultaceous debris* (presumably rich in extracellular lipid) consisted of collections of amorphous pale-staining material with abundant cholesterol clefts.

Foam cell aggregates were composed of plump, rounded, finely vacuolated cells. *Foam cells and lymphocytes* were areas containing round cells with finely granular or vacuolated cytoplasm admixed with lymphocytes. *Inflammatory infiltrates without foams cells* were isolated aggregates of lymphocytes and other inflammatory cells that were almost always seen surrounding small vascular channels. The defined areas were recognized using the projection microscope and were confirmed by standard light microscopy. The area of each component of plaque was then converted to a percentage of the total plaque area. For each patient a mean percentage of each plaque component was determined by calculating the mean of all 5-mm segments of the grafts of each patient and the native coronary arteries, respectively. The total mean was calculated based on the means of the 19 men (Tables II and III).

The presence of *intraluminal thrombus, intraplaque hemorrhage, and intraplaque multiluminal channels* also was recorded in each 5-mm segment. Since intraplaque hemorrhage occupies part of the plaque area it was outlined in the same fashion as previously described and substracted from the total plaque area. The extent of hemorrhagic areas was highly variable, from <1% to as much as 37% in 1 patient. The lumina of the multiluminal channels also were outlined, added up and subtracted from the total plaque area. They were not added to the total luminal area and were usually <1% of the total plaque area. The total mean percentages of plaque components for each patient in Tables II and III therefore do not add up to 100% in patients in whom intraplaque hemorrhage or multiluminal channels were present. Intraluminal thrombus, intraplaque hemorrhage and multiluminal channels were listed based on their

TABLE II Degree of Narrowing and Composition of Atherosclerotic Plaques in the Saphenous Vein Grafts

Case	No. of 5-mm Segments	No. and Percent of 5-mm Segments Narrowed to 5 Categories of CSA by Plaque					Percent of Plaques Consisting of*						
		0–25%	26–50%	51–75%	76–95%	96–100%	DFT	CFT	CD	PD	FC	FC + L	ICWFC
1	53	52 (98)	1 (2)	0 (0)	0 (0)	0 (0)	0.6	99.4	0.0	0.0	0.0	0.0	0.0
2	42	8 (19)	15 (36)	10 (24)	9 (21)	0 (0)	1.3	98.5	0.0	0.0	0.1	0.0	0.0
3	48	0 (0)	39 (81)	1 (2)	2 (4)	6 (13)	30.8	67.8	0.0	0.0	0.0	0.0	0.0
4	51	27 (53)	23 (45)	1 (2)	0 (0)	0 (0)	21.1	78.0	0.0	0.0	0.9	0.0	0.0
5	30	13 (43)	16 (53)	1 (3)	0 (0)	0 (0)	94.9	3.5	0.0	0.8	0.5	0.3	0.0
6	9	2 (22)	4 (44)	2 (22)	1 (11)	0 (0)	50.4	0.0	0.0	13.5	10.1	0.0	0.0
7	45	8 (18)	8 (18)	7 (16)	14 (31)	8 (18)	81.7	6.3	1.3	8.5	0.8	1.2	0.2
8	27	0 (0)	4 (15)	8 (30)	15 (56)	0 (0)	79.6	2.4	0.3	9.3	1.8	1.0	0.3
9	62	36 (58)	23 (37)	3 (5)	0 (0)	0 (0)	0.0	100.0	0.0	0.0	0.0	0.0	0.0
10	32	9 (28)	13 (41)	4 (13)	3 (9)	3 (9)	78.6	15.7	1.8	3.0	0.1	0.03	0.8
11	38	29 (76)	9 (24)	0 (0)	0 (0)	0 (0)	69.0	30.9	0.1	0.1	0.04	0.0	0.0
12	55	3 (5)	22 (40)	22 (40)	8 (15)	0 (0)	96.9	3.1	0.0	0.0	0.0	0.0	0.0
13	10	0 (0)	3 (30)	2 (20)	5 (50)	0 (0)	48.3	0.5	1.2	10.8	0.5	1.0	0.3
14	30	13 (43)	11 (37)	3 (10)	1 (3)	2 (7)	94.2	4.6	0.0	0.5	0.6	0.0	0.0
15	19	0 (0)	2 (11)	1 (5)	5 (26)	11 (58)	29.9	61.3	5.6	2.5	0.1	0.02	0.6
16	21	13 (62)	0 (0)	0 (0)	1 (5)	7 (33)	98.8	0.0	0.7	0.4	0.0	0.0	0.01
17	12	8 (67)	3 (25)	0 (0)	1 (8)	0 (0)	93.4	1.5	0.3	3.9	0.4	0.5	0.1
18	15	0 (0)	0 (0)	0 (0)	1 (7)	14 (93)	49.9	7.2	0.1	20.0	0.0	0.0	0.7
19	8	2 (25)	6 (75)	0 (0)	0 (0)	0 (0)	91.3	0.0	3.4	1.3	1.6	2.4	0.0
Total	607	223 (37)	202 (33)	65 (11)	66 (11)	51 (8)	58.4	30.6	0.8	3.9	0.9	0.3	0.2

*Intraplaque hemorrhage and multiluminal channels are not listed; therefore numbers may not add up to 100% in each patient.
CD = calcific deposits; CFT = cellular fibrous tissue; CSA = cross-sectional area; DFT = dense fibrous tissue; FC = foam cells; FC + L = foam cells plus lymphocytes; ICWFC = inflammatory cells without foam cells; PD = pultaceous debris.

TABLE III Degree of Narrowing and Composition of Atherosclerotic Plaques in the (native) Coronary Arteries

Case	No. of 5-mm Segments	No. and Percent of 5-mm Segments Narrowed to 5 Categories of CSA by Plaque					Percent of Plaques Consisting of*						
		0–25%	26–50%	51–75%	76–95%	96–100%	DFT	CFT	CD	PD	FC	FC + L	ICWFC
1	51	5 (10)	6 (12)	9 (18)	21 (41)	10 (20)	60.1	17.9	19.5	1.5	0.01	0.03	0.2
2	37	0 (0)	19 (51)	10 (27)	2 (5)	6 (16)	81.3	4.3	2.2	10.7	1.2	0.2	0.3
3	45	13 (29)	8 (18)	13 (29)	11 (24)	0 (0)	93.5	0.0	3.5	1.7	0.2	0.2	0.0
4	40	10 (25)	7 (18)	11 (28)	11 (28)	1 (3)	93.7	4.5	1.8	0.0	0.0	0.0	0.1
5	39	9 (23)	7 (18)	5 (13)	12 (31)	6 (15)	86.5	0.6	11.0	1.7	0.0	0.2	0.0
6	30	16 (53)	8 (27)	0 (0)	5 (17)	1 (3)	96.6	1.4	1.4	0.0	0.5	0.0	0.1
7	49	5 (10)	5 (10)	2 (4)	24 (49)	13 (27)	69.5	15.8	13.4	0.2	0.01	0.0	0.04
8	47	2 (4)	5 (11)	12 (26)	17 (36)	11 (23)	89.1	0.5	4.9	4.6	0.2	0.2	0.5
9	48	0 (0)	1 (2)	6 (13)	34 (71)	7 (15)	78.1	6.5	12.0	3.1	0.0	0.0	0.01
10	25	1 (4)	2 (8)	5 (20)	14 (56)	3 (12)	78.1	12.8	3.5	4.8	0.1	0.1	0.04
11	29	2 (7)	5 (17)	9 (31)	8 (28)	5 (17)	61.6	12.7	18.1	5.5	0.04	0.0	0.01
12	56	0 (0)	5 (9)	5 (9)	20 (36)	26 (46)	92.9	2.0	4.1	0.5	0.1	0.0	0.01
13	55	6 (11)	3 (5)	9 (16)	27 (49)	10 (18)	33.9	58.0	2.5	5.2	0.02	0.2	0.2
14	44	0 (0)	2 (5)	6 (14)	26 (59)	10 (23)	90.9	1.9	4.0	2.5	0.3	0.1	0.2
15	47	7 (15)	6 (13)	4 (9)	8 (17)	22 (47)	44.2	41.7	10.5	3.1	0.0	0.0	0.1
16	44	6 (14)	1 (2)	5 (11)	20 (45)	12 (27)	87.3	0.0	4.0	8.0	0.1	0.0	0.6
17	37	9 (24)	5 (14)	11 (30)	12 (32)	0 (0)	76.8	0.0	21.8	0.7	0.2	0.1	0.0
18	40	10 (25)	4 (10)	2 (5)	10 (25)	14 (35)	60.9	26.5	8.9	1.5	0.0	0.0	0.2
19	34	3 (9)	1 (3)	4 (12)	24 (71)	2 (6)	84.8	0.0	14.8	0.4	0.1	0.0	0.0
Total	797	104 (13)	100 (13)	128 (16)	306 (38)	159 (20)	76.8	10.9	8.5	2.9	0.2	0.1	0.1

*Intraplaque hemorrhage and multiluminal channels are not listed; therefore numbers may not add up to 100% in each patient.
Abbreviations as in Table II.

TABLE IV Frequency of Coronary Intraluminal Thrombus, Intraplaque Hemorrhage, and Intraplaque Multiluminal Channels at Necropsy in the 19 Men Surviving Coronary Bypass More than One Year

	Saphenous Vein Grafts			Native Coronary Arteries		
	Thrombus	Plaque Hemorrhage	Multiluminal Channels	Thrombus	Plaque Hemorrhage	Multiluminal Channels
Patients	6/19 (32%)	5/19 (26%)	6/19 (32%)*	7/19 (37%)	9/19 (47%)	14/19 (74%)*
Vessels	6/41 (15%)	7/41 (17%)	7/41 (17%)	8/73 (11%)	15/73 (21%)	23/73 (32%)
Five-mm segments	40/607 (7%)†	34/607 (6%)‡	25/607 (4%)§	12/797 (2%)†	21/797 (3%)‡	72/797 (9%)§

*p <0.05; †p <0.001; ‡p <0.05; §p <0.001.

frequency in patients, vessels and 5-mm segments (Table IV).

Luminal narrowing, measured as a decrease in the cross-sectional area enclosed by the border of the internal elastic membrane, was graded by visual inspection of the histologic sections at a magnification of ×40. The amount of narrowing of each 5-mm segment was categorized into 5 groups: 0 to 25, 26 to 50, 51 to 75, 76 to 95 and 96 to 100%.

Statistical analysis: To analyze the plaque components a linear regression model was used. First, a test was performed on whether the slopes of the different plaque components in the saphenous vein grafts and native coronary arteries were the same, i.e., whether the components increased, decreased or remained constant over time. If the slopes were the same, a further examination was conducted to determine if the amount of each component differed in the veins compared with the native coronary arteries and whether there was a change over time. If the slopes for the saphenous vein grafts and native coronary arteries were not the same, then the components of the saphenous vein grafts and native coronary arteries only were compared at specific times. Because the measurements are percentages the values were transformed using a logit transformation, $\log[\%/(100 - \%)]$. As some percentages were 0, a constant (0.1667) was added so that the logit transformation could be applied. It was assumed that the components of the saphenous vein grafts are uncorrelated with those of the native coronary arteries. This assumption was examined and found to be valid. Figure 1 shows the regression curves plotted for cellular and dense fibrous tissue based on the actual data using the linear regression model.

Statistical comparisons of the frequencies of intraluminal thrombi, hemorrhage into plaques, and multiluminal channels in the vein grafts and the native coronary arteries were performed by chi-square tests. A p value <0.05 was considered significant (Table IV).

RESULTS

Cross-sectional area narrowing: The results are summarized in Tables II and III. Thirteen of the 19 men had 1 or more saphenous vein conduits narrowed by atherosclerotic plaque >75% in cross-sectional area. Of the 607 five-mm saphenous vein segments examined, 117 (19%) were narrowed >75% in cross-sectional area by plaque (Table II). In all 19 men, 1 or more epicardial coronary arteries were narrowed by atherosclerotic plaque >75% in cross-sectional area. Of the 797 five-mm native coronary segments examined, 465 (58%) were narrowed >75% in cross-sectional area by plaque (Table III). In the saphenous vein grafts and native coronary arteries in all 5 categories of cross-sectional area narrowing there was no significant change noted across time, i.e., from bypass operation to death. Comparing patients *with* symptoms of myocardial ischemia such as angina pectoris or acute myocardial infarct late (>1 year) after bypass operation to those patients *without* symptoms disclosed no difference in the number of 5-mm segments narrowed significantly, i.e., >75% narrowing of cross-sectional area, in the saphenous veins

(35 vs 13%; p = not significant) and native coronary arteries (67 vs 52%; p = not significant).

Plaque composition: The results are summarized in Tables II and III, and in Figure 2.

FIBROUS TISSUE: The mean percentage of fibrous tissue in all plaques of the saphenous vein grafts and native coronary arteries was 89 and 88%, respectively. Fibrous tissue decreased as the degree of cross-sectional area narrowing increased, both in the saphenous vein grafts and in the native coronary arteries, which mainly

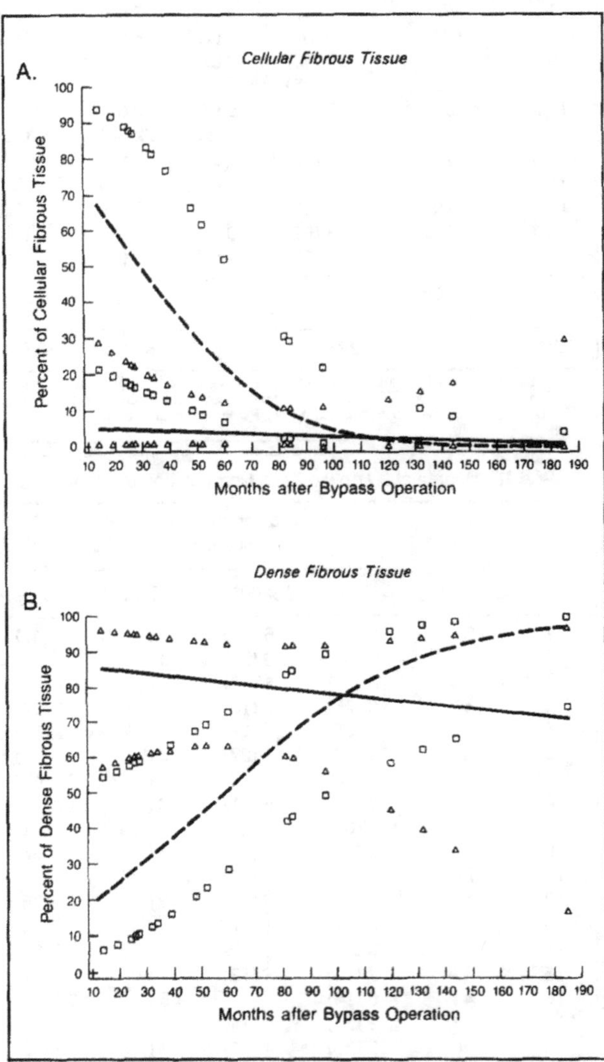

FIGURE 1. Graph showing development of fibrous tissue in plaques over time. As the time interval from bypass operation was short, the mean percentage of cellular (A) and dense (B) fibrous tissue in the plaques of the saphenous vein grafts was significantly different compared with that of the native coronary arteries. As the time interval increased, the mean percentage of cellular fibrous tissue decreased and that of dense fibrous tissue increased and at ≥82 months reached the 95% confidence interval of that of the native coronary arteries. The mean percentage of cellular and dense fibrous tissue in the native coronary arteries remained constant over time. Thus after 82 months plaque composition of the plaques in the saphenous vein grafts and native coronary arteries have become similar. *Broken line*, regression curve for the plaques of the saphenous vein grafts; *solid line*, regression curve for the plaques of the native coronary arteries; *boxes*, 95% pointwise confidence interval of the regression curve of the saphenous vein grafts; *triangles*, 95% pointwise confidence interval of the regression curve of the native coronary arteries.

was due to a decrease in *cellular* fibrous tissue (Figure 2).

CALCIFIC DEPOSITS: The mean percentage of calcific deposits in all plaques of the saphenous veins was <1%, and in the native coronary arteries, 8.5%. The mean percentage of calcific deposits in both increased as the degree of cross-sectional area narrowing increased.

PULTACEOUS DEBRIS (EXTRACELLULAR LIPID): In the saphenous vein grafts pultaceous debris was found in the plaques in 13 of the 19 men. In these 13 men, the mean percentage of pultaceous debris in all plaques of the saphenous vein grafts was 6%. Extracellular lipid was not found in a saphenous vein graft in any of the 4 patients in whom the graft had been in place for ≤26 months. In the coronary arteries pultaceous debris was present in the plaques in 17 of the 19 patients. In these 17 patients, the mean percentage of pultaceous debris in all plaques of the coronary arteries was 3%. The mean percentage of pultaceous debris increased as the degree of cross-sectional area narrowing increased.

FOAM CELLS (INTRACELLULAR LIPID), FOAM CELLS WITH LYMPHOCYTES AND INFLAMMATORY INFILTRATES WITHOUT FOAM CELLS: The mean percentage of foam cells in all plaques of the saphenous vein grafts and native coronary arteries was 0.9 and 0.2%, respectively. Usually they were located on or near the borders of the lumen. The mean percentage of foam cells with lymphocytes was 0.3% in all plaques of the saphenous vein grafts and 0.1% in those of the native coronary arteries; the mean percentage of pure inflammatory cells was 0.2% in all plaques of the grafts and 0.1% in those of the native coronary arteries.

Development of plaque composition over time: The results are summarized in Table IV, and in Figures 1 to 3. The plots in Figure 1 give the predicted mean response for cellular and dense fibrous tissue at specified times after bypass operation along with the pointwise 95% confidence intervals. One year after bypass operation cellular fibrous tissue comprised a higher percentage of the plaques in the saphenous vein grafts compared with the plaques in the native coronary arteries (p <0.05); dense fibrous tissue comprised a lower percentage of the plaques in the saphenous vein grafts compared with the plaques in the native coronary arteries (p <0.05). With time, the mean percentage of cellular fibrous tissue in the grafts decreased, and that of dense fibrous tissue increased. At 82 months (about 7 years) after the bypass operation, the mean percentage of cellular and dense fibrous tissue in the plaques of the saphenous vein grafts was within the confidence interval of the mean percentage of the native coronary arteries (p = not significant). The mean percentage of cellular and dense fibrous tissue in the plaques of the native coronary arteries remained constant over the time interval from bypass operation to death. If divided into groups according to the time of survival after the bypass operation (Figure 3), in patients surviving 14 to 26 months, the mean percentage of cellular fibrous tissue in all venous plaques was 86% and that of dense fibrous tissue, 13%; in contrast, in patients surviving 82 to 185 months the mean percentage of cellular fibrous tissue in all venous plaques was 10% and that of dense fibrous tissue 75%. In the native coronary arteries the mean percentage of cellular fibrous tissue in all plaques in patients surviving 14 to 26 months was 7% and that of dense fibrous tissue 82%; in patients surviving 82 to 185 months the mean percentage of cellular fibrous tissue in all native coronary artery plaques was 16% and that of

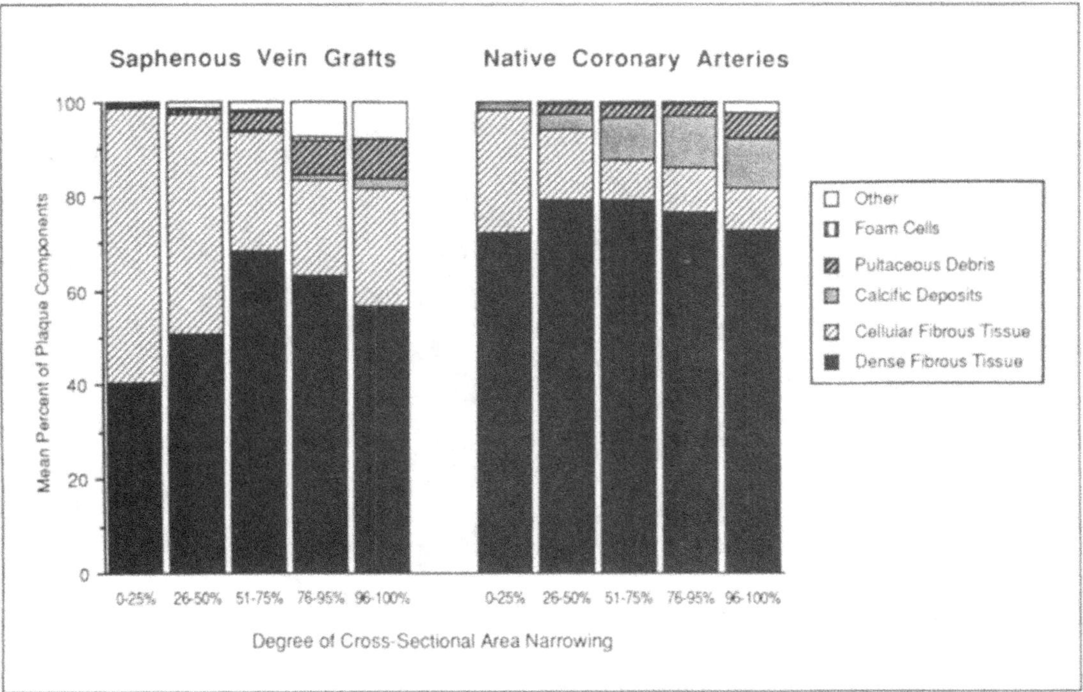

FIGURE 2. Graph showing the relation of plaque composition in the saphenous vein grafts and native coronary arteries according to the degrees of cross-sectional area narrowing. The mean percentage of fibrous tissue decreased, and that of calcific deposits and pultaceous debris increased as luminal narrowing increased both in the plaques of the saphenous vein grafts and of the native coronary arteries. The category "Other" includes foam cells plus lymphocytes and pure inflammatory infiltration.

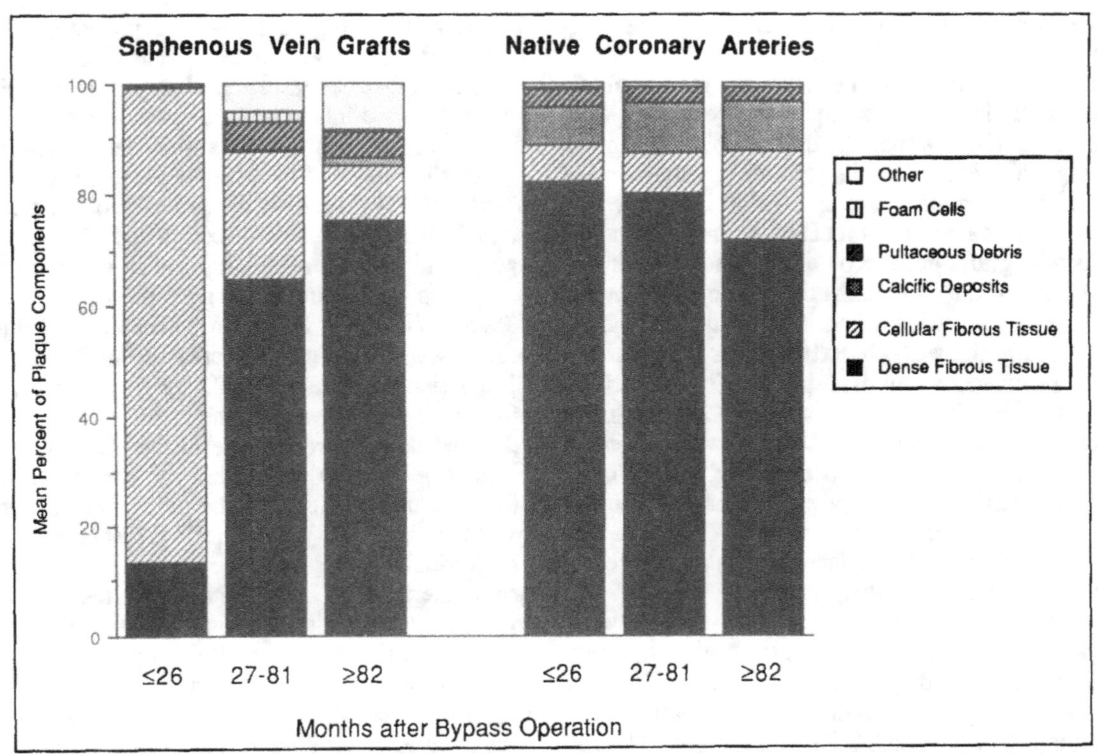

FIGURE 3. Graph showing the relation of plaque composition in saphenous vein grafts and in the native epicardial coronary arteries according to the time interval from bypass operation to death. In patients surviving ≤26 months cellular fibrous tissue was the dominant component in the plaques of the saphenous vein grafts. After ≥82 months the plaques of the saphenous vein grafts consisted predominantly of dense fibrous tissue, similar to the plaque composition in the native coronary arteries. The composition of the plaques in the native coronary arteries remained constant after bypass operation. The category "Other" includes foam cells plus lymphocytes and pure inflammatory infiltration.

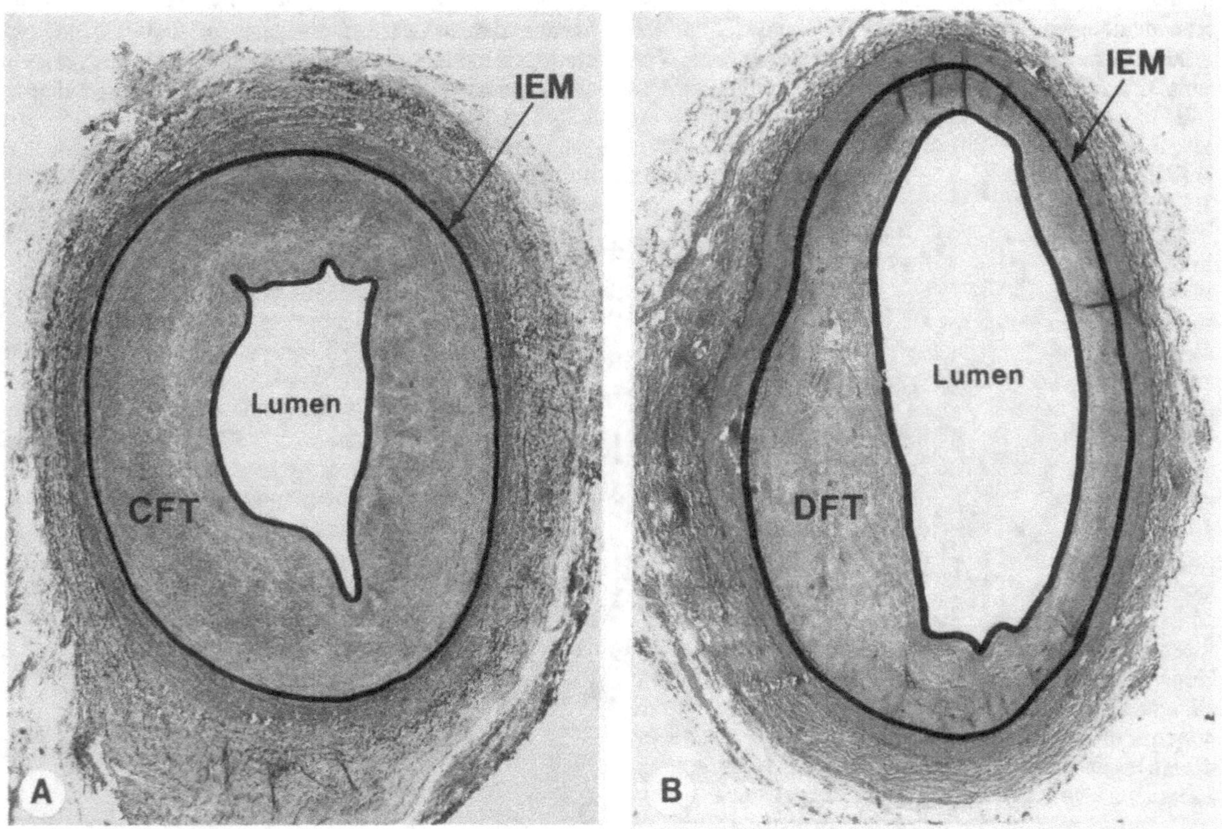

FIGURE 4. Patient 2, Table I. *A*, example of a saphenous vein graft (to the left anterior descending coronary artery), and *B*, a native coronary artery (left circumflex) of a patient surviving 19 months after coronary bypass surgery. The saphenous vein graft consists primarily of cellular fibrous tissue (CFT), whereas the dominant component in the native coronary artery is dense fibrous tissue (DFT). IEM = internal elastic membrane *(arrow)*. (Movat stains: *A*, ×25; and *B*, ×34).

dense fibrous tissue 71%, demonstrating no change of those plaque components in the native coronary arteries after bypass operation.

The mean percentage of calcific deposits was significantly higher in the native coronary arteries than in the vein grafts. This relation did not change over time. The mean percentages of pultaceous debris and foam cells remained constant in the grafts and in the native coronary arteries from the time of bypass operation to death and did not appear to be significantly different in the venous grafts compared with the coronary arteries.

Intraluminal thrombus, intraplaque hemorrhage, and intraplaque multiluminal channels: The frequency of these 3 lesions in patients, in vessels (both saphenous vein grafts and native coronary arteries) and in 5-mm segments of both saphenous vein grafts and native coronary arteries is summarized in Table IV. The frequency of intraluminal thrombus and of intraplaque hemorrhage was similar in both saphenous vein grafts and in native coronary arteries when analyzed from the standpoint of both patients and vessels, but was significantly different when examined from the standpoint of 5-mm segments. Thrombus was present, for example, in 7% (40 of 607) of all venous segments and in 2% (12 of 797) of all native coronary artery segments (p <0.001); intraplaque hemorrhage was present in 6% (34 of 607) of venous segments and in 3% (21 of 797) of native coronary artery segments (p <0.05). Intraplaque multiluminal channels were significantly less frequent in saphenous vein grafts than in native coronary arteries when examined from the standpoints of both patients and 5-mm segments but not from the standpoint of vessels alone. Intraplaque multiluminal channels were present in 32% (6 of 19) of grafts in patients and in 74% (14 of 19) of native arteries in patients (p <0.05); they were present in 4% (25 of 607) of all venous segments and in 9% (72 of 797) of all native coronary artery segments (p <0.001).

Although comparisons of intraluminal thrombus, intraplaque hemorrhage, and intraplaque multiluminal channels between saphenous venous grafts and native coronary arteries from the standpoints of patients, vessels, and 5-mm segments did show some significant differences (in 4 of 9 possible comparisons, Table IV), all differences were produced because of the virtual absence of the 3 lesions in the patients surviving 14 to 26 months compared with those surviving 27 to 185 months. For example, none of the 4 patients surviving 14 to 26 months had intracoronary thrombi or multiluminal channels and only 1 of these 4 patients had intraplaque hemorrhage (in 1 of 12 saphenous vein grafts and in 3 of 194 five-mm segments of saphenous vein). Indeed, comparison of intraluminal thrombus, intraplaque hemorrhage, and intraplaque multiluminal channels among patients, saphenous vein grafts and 5-mm segments of saphenous vein grafts disclosed significant differences in all 9 comparative areas when comparing patients surviving 14 to 26 months versus those surviving 27 to 185 months. In the native coronary arteries no differences in frequency of these 3 lesions were found irrespective of which time period was analyzed.

DISCUSSION

Composition of atherosclerotic plaques in the saphenous vein grafts of 19 men who underwent coronary bypass operation and survived >1 year was examined and compared with that in the native coronary arteries in the same patients. The data indicate that virtually all saphenous veins in place as aortocoronary conduits for >1 year develop atherosclerotic plaques in each 5-mm segment of their entire lengths. Furthermore, the degree of narrowing in the saphenous veins of our 19 men was striking: of the 607 five-mm segments of the 41 veins examined, 117 (19%) had luminal narrowing >75% in cross-sectional area by plaque alone. No differences in the amounts of significant (>75%) narrowing in the saphenous veins or in the native coronary arteries were observed in patients *with* compared to those *without* symptoms of myocardial ischemia (either angina pectoris or acute myocardial infarction) postoperatively.

The length of time that the saphenous vein grafts had been in place in the aortocoronary position influenced the composition of the atherosclerotic plaques in these venous conduits. The younger plaques in the veins consisted predominantly of cellular fibrous tissue, whereas the older plaques in the veins consisted predominantly of dense fibrous tissue. In the native coronary arteries the plaques consisted mainly of dense fibrous tissue and remained constant throughout the time periods studied (Figure 4). Thus, the plaques in the saphenous vein grafts became similar to those of the native coronary arteries over time. Intra- and extracellular lipids were infrequent in the plaques in both saphenous veins and native coronary arteries and their mean percentages did not change as the time interval from bypass operation to death increased. Calcific deposits were found at least 10 times less frequently in the plaques of the saphenous vein grafts than in those of the native coronary arteries. Intraluminal thrombus, intraplaque hemorrhage, and intraplaque multiluminal channels were found mainly in patients who had survived >26 months after bypass operation.

In summary, the amount of cross-sectional area narrowing did not change significantly after the saphenous vein grafts had been in place for >1 year. Therefore, it appears that the development of atherosclerotic plaques was a relatively fast process that within 1 year resulted in extensive luminal narrowing. Thereafter, the plaques did not increase significantly in size, but their structure changed, from predominantly *cellular* fibrous tissue to predominantly *dense* fibrous tissue. Because cellular fibrous tissue has some reversible characteristics, as opposed to dense fibrous tissue,[15] plaques in vein grafts may have the potential for reversal during the first 7 years after bypass surgery.

Acknowledgment: We thank Vivian E. Norman for her secretarial assistance, and Ricardo V. Dreyfuss and Christopher R. Dame for their photographic expertise.

REFERENCES

1. Vlodaver Z, Edwards JE. Pathologic changes in aortic coronary arterial saphenous vein grafts. *Circulation* 1971;64:719-728.

2. Barboriak JJ, Pintar K, Korns ME. Atherosclerosis in aortocoronary vein grafts. *Lancet* 1974;2:621–624.

3. Spray TL, Roberts WC. Changes in saphenous veins used as aortocoronary bypass grafts. *Am Heart J* 1977;94:500–516.

4. Smith SH, Geer JC. Morphology of saphenous vein-coronary artery bypass grafts. Seven to 116 months after surgery. *Arch Pathol Lab Med* 1983;107:13–18.

5. Atkinson JB, Forman MB, Vaughan WK, Robinowitz M, McAllister HA, Virmani R. Morphologic changes in long-term saphenous vein bypass grafts. *Chest* 1985;88:341–348.

6. Kern WH, Wells WJ, Meyer BW. The pathology of surgically excised aortocoronary saphenous vein bypass grafts. *Am J Surg Pathol* 1981;5:491–496.

7. Neitzel GF, Barboriak JJ, Pintar K, Qureshi I. Atherosclerosis in aortocoronary bypass grafts. Morphologic study and risk factor analysis 6 to 12 years after surgery. *Arteriosclerosis* 1986;6:594–600.

8. Ratliff NB, Myles JL. Rapidly progressive atherosclerosis in aortocoronary saphenous vein grafts. Possible immune-mediated disease. *Arch Pathol Lab Med* 1989;113:772–776.

9. Campeau L, Lespérance J, Corbara F, Hermann J, Grondin CM, Bourassa MG. Aortocoronary saphenous vein bypass graft changes 5 to 7 years after surgery. *Circulation* 1978;58(suppl I):I-170–I-175.

10. Walts AE, Fishbein MC, Matloff JM. Thrombosed, ruptured atheromatous plaques in saphenous vein coronary artery bypass grafts. Ten years experience. *Am Heart J* 1987;114:718–723.

11. Solymoss BC, Nadeau P, Millette D, Campeau L. Late thrombosis of saphenous vein coronary bypass grafts related to risk factors. *Circulation* 1988;78(suppl I):I-140–I-143.

12. Kalan JM, Roberts WC. Morphologic findings in saphenous veins used as coronary arterial bypass conduits for longer than 1 year: necropsy analysis of 53 patients, 123 saphenous veins and 1865 five-millimeter segments of veins. *Am Heart J* 1990;119:1164–1184.

13. Movat HZ. Demonstration of all connective tissue elements in a single section. *Arch Pathol* 1955;60:289–295.

14. Hook GR, Rasband W. Macmeasure: a low-cost, easy to operate quantitative morphometrics system for the Macintosh computer. In: Baily GW, ed. Proceedings of the 45th Annual Meeting of the Electron Microscopy Society of America. San Francisco, CA: San Francisco Press, 1987:920–921.

15. Armstrong ML, Megan MB. Lipid depletion in atheromatous coronary arteries in rhesus monkeys after regression diets. *Circ Res* 1972;30:675–680.

Amounts of Coronary Arterial Luminal Narrowing and Composition of the Material Causing the Narrowing in Buerger's Disease

Gisela C. Mautner, MD, Susanne L. Mautner, MD, Fengru Lin, MD, Gary M. Roggin, MD, and William C. Roberts, MD

Relatively little information is available on the status of the coronary arteries in patients with Buerger's disease (thromboangiitis obliterans). No detailed analyses of the coronary arteries have been reported at necropsy in patients with Buerger's disease. Such is the purpose of this report.

From the Pathology Branch, National Heart, Lung, and Blood Institute, National Institutes of Health, and the Department of Medicine, Suburban Hospital, Bethesda, Maryland. Manuscript received June 30, 1992, and accepted July 30.

M.C., a 37-year-old white man, was in good health until age 32 when he suddenly developed pain, pallor, and coldness of his right leg, and angiography disclosed severe luminal narrowing of the right femoral artery. Angioplasty was unsuccessful, and, as a consequence, an arterial bypass operation was performed. This too was unsuccessful and an above-the-knee amputation was performed at age 33 years. Shortly thereafter his left extremity was affected in a similar fashion and an above-the-knee am-

putation of the left leg also was performed. At age 34 he had an episode of prolonged chest pain. Electrocardiogram revealed sinus rhythm, and T-wave inversion in leads I, aVL, and V_4 to V_6. He was given intravenous streptokinase (250,000 U). Creatine phosphokinase increased to 599 IU/liter. A precordial murmur was absent. Angiography revealed no significant narrowing of the left anterior descending or right coronary arteries, but up to 75% diameter reduction of the proximal portion of the left circumflex coronary artery. Additionally, the left circumflex coronary artery arose from the right sinus of Valsalva and coursed in a retroaortic position to reach the left atrioventricular sulcus. (This finding was confirmed at necropsy.) The serum total, high-density lipoprotein, and

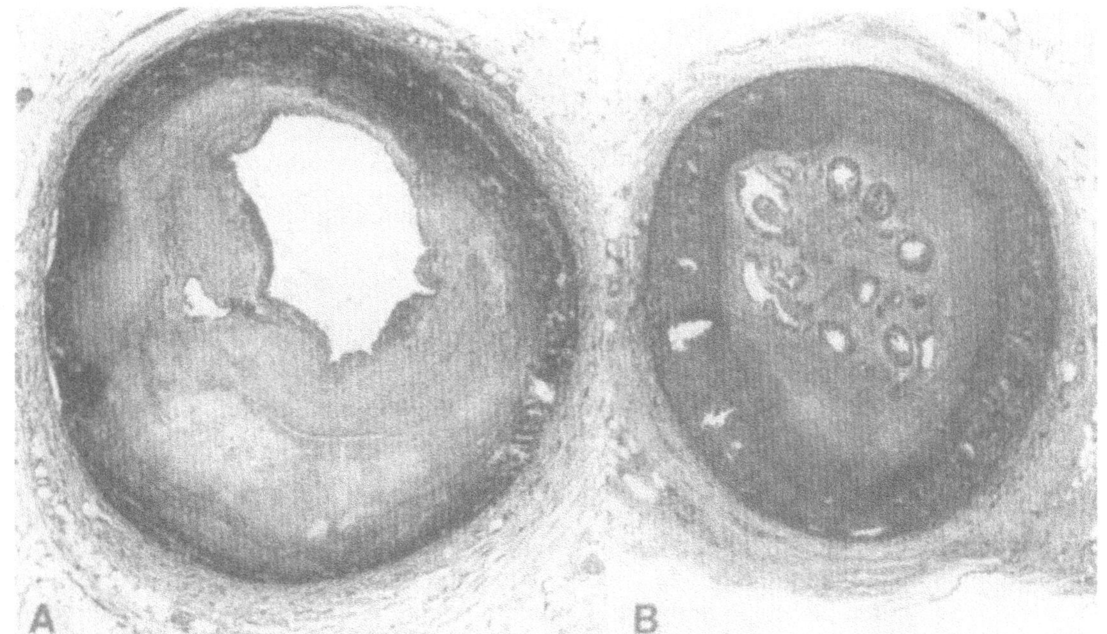

FIGURE 1. Photomicrographs of coronary arteries. *A*, right and *B*, left circumflex arteries showing multiluminal channels. Movat stains, each magnified ×27.

low-density lipoprotein cholesterol were 159, 35 and 91 mg/dl, respectively, and the triglycerides 113 mg/dl.

One year after coronary angiography (age 35 years) he developed abdominal pain and nausea. He subsequently had an arteriogram which disclosed significant narrowing of the first jejunal branches of the superior mesenteric artery and distal branches of the ileocolic artery. An anomalous origin of the right hepatic artery from the superior mesenteric artery was noted. The patient had no history of rash, fever, myalgia, arthralgia, Raynaud's syndrome, or upper extremity symptoms of ischemia. The ocular fundi were normal. Tests for rheumatoid factor, antinuclear antibody and serum cryoglobulins were negative. Total complement, C3 and C4, were normal. Hepatitis antigen was negative. He had smoked a pack of cigarettes daily for up to 15 years. His highest systemic blood pressure was 140/80 mm Hg, he was not obese, and he had no evidence of diabetes mellitus. Coagulation tests were normal: platelet count was 193,000 cu mm; prothrombin time 11.9 seconds, and partial thromboplastin time 30 seconds. He was treated with prednisone (10 mg/day). At his final hospitalization, he presented with severe abdominal pain. Angiography showed occlusion of the superior mesenteric artery. Necrotic small bowel was resected. He had a complicated postoperative course with a second laparotomy, but his condition deteriorated and he died.

The coronary arteries were excised intact from the heart, and sectioned into 5-mm segments. A Movat-stained section was prepared, after the usual processing, from each 5-mm segment. A total of 53 sections were analyzed. Plaque composition was determined using methods that have been described

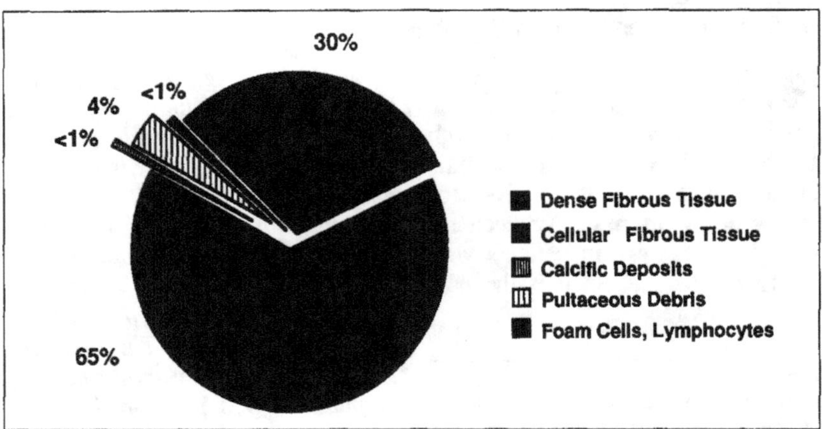

FIGURE 2. Diagram summarizing the components of the atherosclerotic plaques in the 53 five-mm segments of coronary artery in our patient.

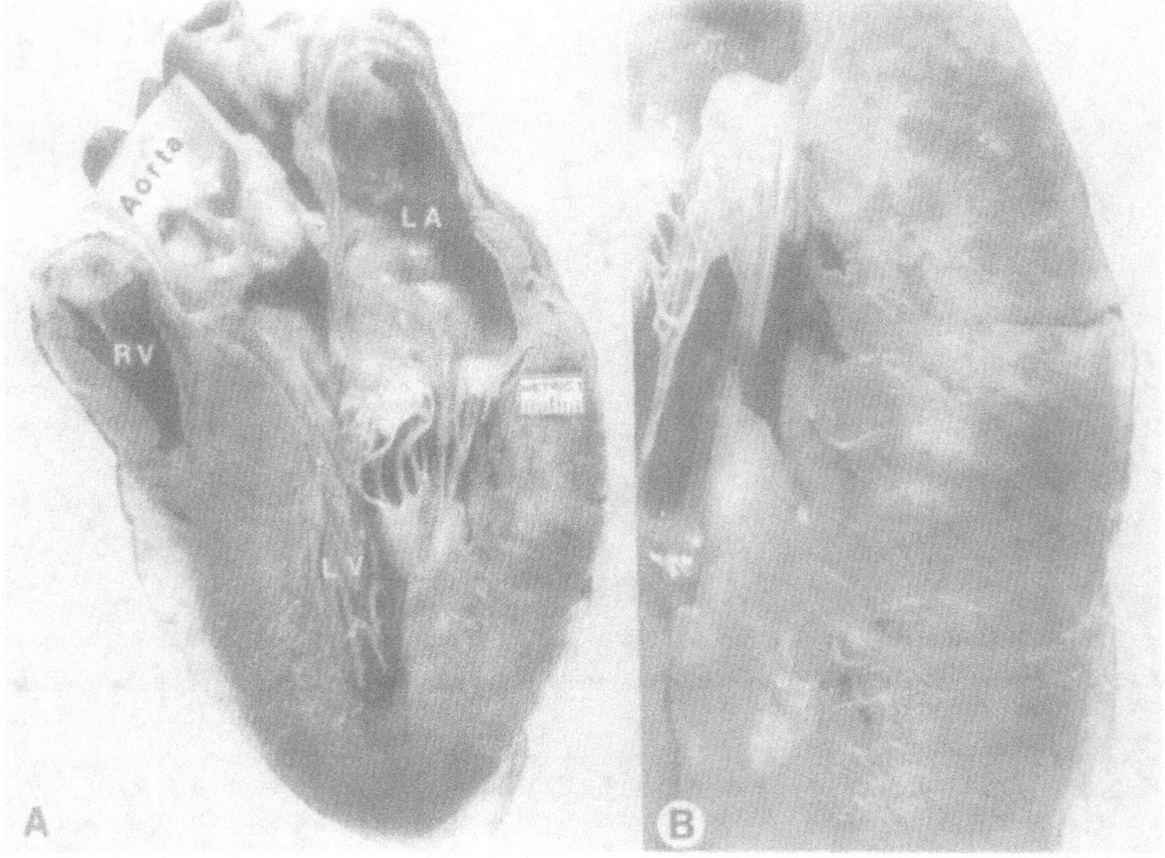

FIGURE 3. Heart. *A,* longitudinal section; *B,* close-up of the basal portion of the posterior left ventricular wall. This area shows transmural scarring (healed myocardial infarct). LA = left atrium; LV = left ventricle; RV = right ventricle.

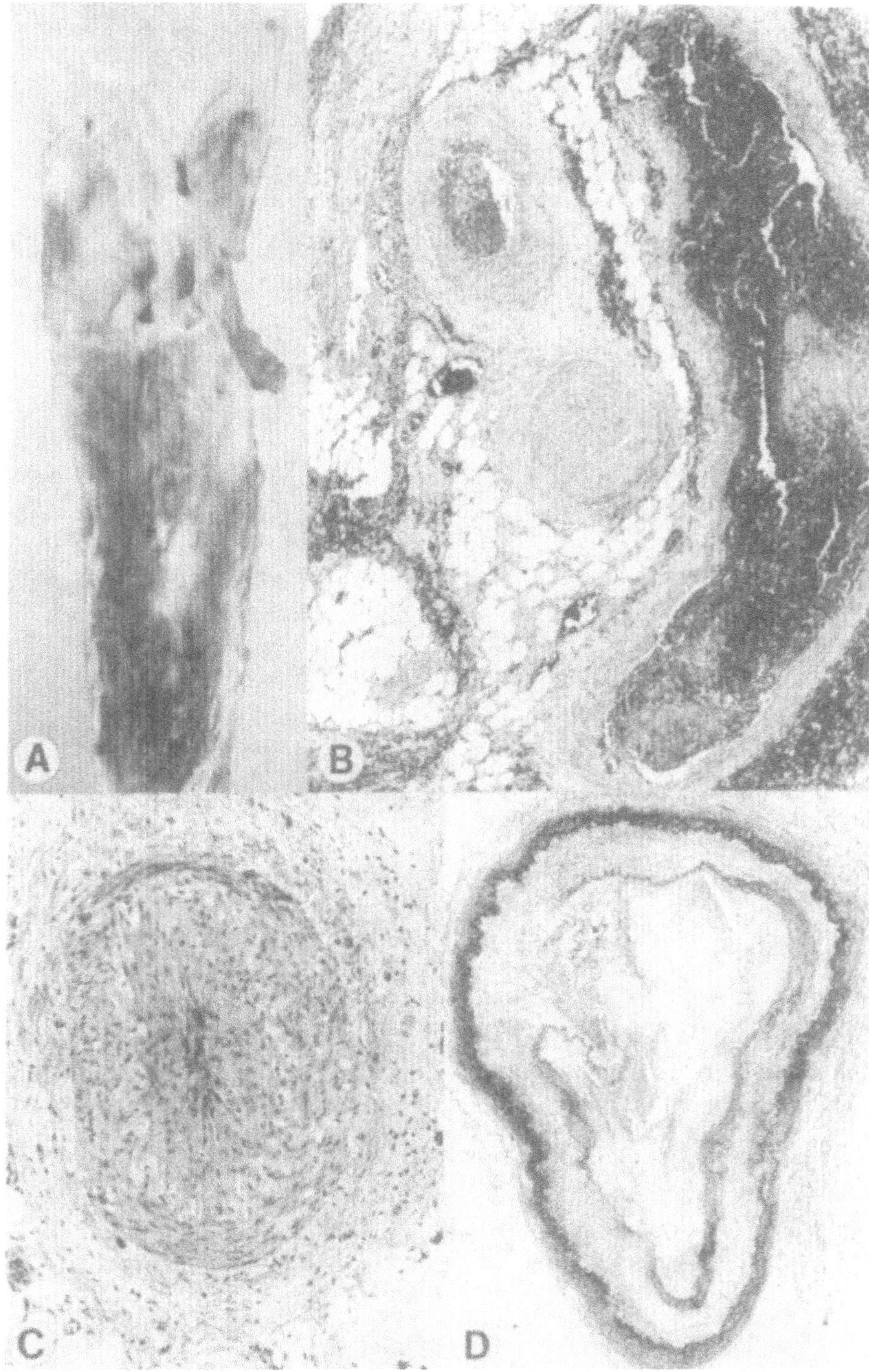

FIGURE 4. Abdominal aorta *(A)*, and photomicrographs *(B, C, D)* of intraabdominal arteries in the patient described. The aorta contains thrombus with underlying atherosclerotic plaque. *B*, sections of mesenteric artery which is occluded in portions by plaque and by thrombus in other portions. *C*, branch of mesenteric artery containing inflammatory cells. *D*, unspecified retroperitoneal artery occluded by fibrous tissue. Hematoxylin and eosin stains *(B and C)*, ×54 *(B)*, ×130 *(C)*; Movat stain *(D)*, ×14.

previously.[1,2] *Briefly, a drawing of each section of coronary artery was made using a projection microscope. The internal elastic membrane, the residual lumen, and each component of plaque were traced manually and the actual area was calculated using a computerized morphometry system. Of the 53 sections, 6 (11%) were narrowed 0 to 25% in cross-sectional area, 5 (9%) were narrowed 26 to 50%, 30 (57%) were narrowed 51 to 75%,* 11 (21%) were narrowed 76 to 95%, and 1 (2%) was narrowed 96 to 100% in cross-sectional area. Multiluminal channels were found in 3 (6%) of the 53 sections (Figure 1). The predominant component of the plaques was cellular (65%) and dense (30%) fibrous tissue (Figure 2). In all segments, >50% of the plaques was made up of fibrous tissue and in 44 (83%) of the 53 segments >90% of the plaques consisted of fibrous tissue. The remaining portions of the plaque consisted of pultaceous debris (extracellular lipid) (4%), foam cells (intracellular lipid) (<1%), and calcified tissue (<1%). Only 3 five-mm segments contained calcific deposits.

The heart weighed 350 g and a transmural basal scar was present in the posterior wall (Figure 3). The abdominal portion of the aorta had severe intimal involvement by atherosclerotic plaques and overlying thrombus (Figure 4). Histologic sections of the mesenteric and other retroperitoneal arteries showed typical atherosclerotic plaques with and without superimposed thrombi and occasionally slight inflammatory cell infiltrates (Figure 4).

The heretofore described patient had classic Buerger's disease, and, additionally, severe narrowing of each of the 3 major epicardial coronary arteries by atherosclerotic plaque. Of the 53 five-mm segments of the 4 major coronary arteries examined, 12 (23%) were narrowed >75% in cross-sectional area by plaque and 42 (79%) of the 53 segments were narrowed >50% by plaque. Thus, in this 37-year-old man with Buerger's disease, the coronary atherosclerotic process was diffuse and severe. The dominant component of the plaques in the coronary arteries was fibrous tissue, making up 95% of the plaques observed in the 53 segments of coronary artery studied.

The present patient is not the first with Buerger's disease to have the status of the coronary arteries described at necropsy. Leo Buerger (1879–1943) described many of the clinical and morphologic features of the disease, which he called thromboangiitis obliterans in 1908.[3] He also was the first to describe the status of the coronary arteries in the disease.[4] Table I lists previously reported necropsy cases of Buerger's disease in which the coronary arteries were studied histologically.[4–13] Several cases stated to have coronary artery disease in Buerger's disease were excluded from our analysis because of the lack of histologic study of the coronary arteries or because the patients were >50 years of age.[14–19] Analysis of the 12 cases, limited to patients <50 years of age at death, indicates that significant coronary arterial narrowing is common in this condition (10 of 11 cases where the information was available), and that the major reason for the coronary narrowing is "atherosclerosis" as was present in our patient. Three of the previously reported 12 patients, however, had histologic findings in the coronary arteries consistent with thromboangiitis obliterans. "Old thrombi" in 1 or more coronary arteries were described in 7 of the 12 previously

TABLE I Published Reports on 12 Men <50 Years of Age with Buerger's Disease and Histologic Examination of the Coronary Arteries

Case No.	First Author	Author's Case No.	Year of Publication	Age at Death (year)	Duration of Symptoms of BD (year)	Leg Amputation (+ = 1)(+ + = 2)	Habitual Smoker	Clinical AP	Clinical AMI	Clinical SD	LV F	LV N	No. of Major CAs Severely Narrowed (coronary artery)	Thrombus (fibrin)	"Atherosclerosis" G	"Atherosclerosis" M	TAO (M)	MLC
1	Buerger	1	1924	28	5	++	—	0	0	+	+	0	1 (LAD)	0	+	+	0	+
2	Goecke	—	1928	35	12	+	—	0	0	0	0	0	0	0	0	+	0	0
3	Dürck	—	1931	38	2	+	+	+	+	+	—	—	1 (R)	0	+	+	0	0
4	Jäger	1	1932	48	11	++	+	+	0	+	+	0	2 (LAD, R)	0	+	0	0	+
5	Averbuck	2	1934	45	14	+	+	0	0	0	+	0	– (–)	0	+	+	0	0
6	Averbuck	20	1934	42	13	++	+	0	0	0	0	0	1 (LAD)	0	+	+	0	+
7	Averbuck	46	1934	48	13	++	+	0	0	0	?+	?+	1 (LAD)	+	+	+	0	+
8	De Blasi	—	1934	31	10	++	—	0	0	0	+	—	1 (LAD)	0	+	+	0	0
9	Van Dooren	—	1934	38	7	++	+	+	0	0	+	+	2 (LAD, R)	+	+	+	0	+
10	Saphir	—	1936	35	6	0	—	0	0	+	+	0	1 (? > 1) (LAD)	+	+	+	+	0
11	Adler	—	1970	29	0.67	0	+	+	+	0	+	+	1 (? > 1) (R)	+	0	0	+	+
12	Nagalotimath	—	1986	30	0.17	0	+	+	+	0	0	+	1 (LAD)	+	0	0	+	+

AMI = acute myocardial infarction; AP = angina pectoris; BD = Buerger's disease; CA = coronary artery; F = fibrosis; G = gross; LAD = left anterior descending; LV = left ventricular; M = microscopic; MLC = multiluminal channels; N = necrosis; R = right; SD = sudden death; TAO = thromboangiitis obliterans; + = present or positive; 0 = absent or negative; — = no information.

reported patients and we believe that the "old thrombi" actually represent what we have called "multiluminal channels" such as occurred in our patient (Figure 1). Five (42%) of the 12 previously reported patients also had recent thrombi in 1 or more epicardial coronary arteries. Nine of the 12 patients had acute or healed left ventricular myocardial infarcts, as occurred also in our patient.

Coronary angiography, as was performed in our patient, also has been reported in at least 2 other patients with Buerger's disease. Ohno and associates[20] described a 32-year-old man who had an acute myocardial infarction in the anterior wall. Admission coronary angiogram showed 70% diameter narrowing of both the right and left anterior descending coronary arteries, and repeat angiogram 4 weeks later showed both of these coronary arteries to be normal. Kim and colleagues[21] described a 29-year-old man with acute myocardial infarction of the anterior wall, and 2 weeks later coronary angiogram disclosed "partial segmental occlusion" of the left anterior descending, "complete occlusion" of the first diagonal, and "irregular and tort-[u]ous contour" of the right coronary artery.

In summary, severe coronary artery disease may occur in patients with Buerger's disease, and at least at necropsy, the intimal material most often is typical atherosclerotic plaque rather than material resembling thromboangiitis obliterans.

REFERENCES

1. Kragel AH, Reddy SG, Wittes JT, Roberts WC. Morphometric analysis of the composition of atherosclerotic plaques in the four major epicardial coronary arteries in acute myocardial infarction and in sudden coronary death. *Circulation* 1989;80:1747–1756.

2. Kragel AH, Reddy SG, Wittes JT, Roberts WC. Morphometric analysis of the composition of coronary arterial plaques in isolated unstable angina pectoris with pain at rest. *Am J Cardiol* 1990;66:562–567.

3. Buerger L. Thrombo-angiitis obliterans: a study of the vascular lesions leading to presenile spontaneous gangrene. *Am J Med Sci* 1908;136:567–580.

4. Buerger L. The Circulatory Disturbances of the Extremities. Philadelphia and London: WB Saunders, 1924:628.

5. Goecke H. Zur Enstehung der Endarteriitis obliterans. *Virchows Arch Pathol Anat Physiol Klin Med* 1928;266:609–629.

6. Dürck H. Ueber pathologisch-anatomische Grundlagen plötzlicher Todesfälle. *Münch Med Wochenschr* 1931;78:627–632.

7. Jäger E. Zur pathologischen Anatomie der Thromboangiitis obliterans bei juveniler Extremitätengangrän. *Virchows Arch Pathol Anat Physiol Klin Med* 1932; 284:526–583.

8. Averbuck SH, Silbert S. Thrombo-angiitis obliterans: IX. The cause of death. *Virchows Arch Pathol Anat Physiol Klin Med* 1934;54:436–465.

9. De Blasi A. I reperti di autopsia nel morbo di Buerger. *Pathologica* 1934;26:258–274.

10. Van Dooren F. Maladie de Buerger avec atteinte des coronaires. Rélation du deuxième cas connu. Commentaires. *Brux Med* 1934;15:104–114.

11. Saphir O. Thromboangiitis obliterans of the coronary arteries and its relation to arteriosclerosis. *Am Heart J* 1936;12:521–535.

12. Adler CP, Stefani FH. Thrombangitis obliterans mit Beteiligung der Koronargefäßostien. *Med Welt* 1970;21:2095–2101.

13. Nagalotimath SJ, Chandargi SL, Pai N. Thrombo-angitis obliterance of coronary artery leading to myocardial infarction. *Indian Heart J* 1986; 38:483–485.

14. Perla D. An analysis of forty-one cases of thrombo-angiitis obliterans: with a report of a case involving the coronaries and the aorta. *Surg Gynecol Obstet* 1925;41:21–30.

15. Cserna S. Arteriitis obliterans mit analogen Veränderungen in den Venen. *Wien Arch Innere Med* 1926;12:213–226.

16. Lemann II. Coronary occlusion in Buerger's disease (thromboangiitis obliterans). *Am J Med Sci* 1928; 176:807–812.

17. Birnbaum W, Prinzmetal M, Connor CL. Generalized thrombo-angiitis obliterans: report of a case with involvement of retinal vessels and suprarenal infarction. *Arch Intern Med* 1934;53:410–422.

18. Telford ED, Stopford JSB. Thrombo-angiitis obliterans: with special reference to its pathology and the results of sympathectomy. *Br Med J* 1935; 1:863–866.

19. Korsgaard N, Johansen A, Baandrup U. A case of thromboangiitis obliterans affecting coronary, pulmonary, and splenic vessels. Is thromboangiitis obliterans a generalized vascular disease? *Am J Cardiovasc Pathol* 1988;2:263–267.

20. Ohno H, Matsuda Y, Takashiba K, Hamada Y, Ebihara H, Hyakuna E. Acute myocardial infarction in Buerger's disease. *Am J Cardiol* 1986;57:690–691.

21. Kim KS, Kim YN, Kim KB, Park SK. Acute myocardial infarction in a patient with Buerger's disease. A case report and a review of the literature. *Korean J Intern Med* 1987;2:278–281.

Comparison in Women Versus Men of Composition of Atherosclerotic Plaques in Native Coronary Arteries and in Saphenous Veins Used as Aortocoronary Conduits

SUSANNE L. MAUTNER, MD, FENGRU LIN, MD, GISELA C. MAUTNER, MD,
WILLIAM C. ROBERTS, MD, FACC

Bethesda, Maryland

Objectives. This study quantifies and compares the components of atherosclerotic plaques in native coronary arteries and in saphenous vein grafts used for aortocoronary bypass surgery in women versus those in men.

Background. Plaque composition has been described in various manifestations of fatal coronary artery disease and after the bypass operation, but no reports have investigated this composition according to gender.

Methods. A total of 979 5-mm segments of native coronary arteries and 842 5-mm segments of saphenous vein grafts were examined by computerized planimetric technique in 11 women and 11 men who were matched for survival time after the bypass operation.

Results. Comparison of the plaque components revealed that atherosclerotic plaques in women, compared with those in men, contained significantly more cellular fibrous tissue, both in native coronary arteries (mean 38% vs. 4%, p < 0.001) and in saphenous vein grafts (mean 70% vs. 36%, p < 0.05). In contrast, the proportion of dense fibrous tissue was significantly less in the atherosclerotic plaques of women than in those of men, both in native coronary arteries (mean 50% vs. 85%, p < 0.001) and in saphenous vein grafts (mean 25% vs. 57%, p < 0.05).

Conclusions. Cellular fibrous tissue is often found at an early stage of plaque development, whereas dense fibrous tissue is a major component in later stages. Thus, the plaque composition of the native coronary arteries and saphenous venous conduits differed in men and women, with the plaques of the women appearing younger than those of the men.

(J Am Coll Cardiol 1993;21:1312–8)

Although several studies have described the composition of atherosclerotic plaques in patients with various manifestations of coronary artery disease (1–5) and in patients who underwent aortocoronary bypass surgery (6–12), none have compared the composition of atherosclerotic plaques in women and men.

Accordingly, we examined in detail plaque composition in 11 women and 11 men, matched for survival time after an aortocoronary bypass operation performed >1 year earlier. Both the native coronary arteries and the saphenous veins used as aortocoronary conduits were studied.

Methods

Study patients. We limited our study to women and men in whom the heart, the native coronary arteries and the saphenous vein bypass grafts were available for examination and whose saphenous veins had been in the aortocoronary

From the Pathology Branch, National Heart, Lung, and Blood Institute, National Institutes of Health, Bethesda, Maryland.

Manuscript received July 8, 1992; revised manuscript received October 23, 1992, accepted October 28, 1992.

Address for correspondence: Susanne L. Mautner, MD, NHLBI-NIH, Building 10, Room 2N258, 9000 Rockville Pike, Bethesda, Maryland 20892.

position for >1 year. Because a previous study (13) had shown that the duration of saphenous vein placement in the aortocoronary position was the most important determinant of plaque composition, we selected pairs of women and men with a similar time interval from bypass operation to death. Of 19 women and 53 men who met the aforementioned criteria, 11 pairs were matched according to survival time after an aortocoronary bypass operation. In all three tables in this study, patients are listed by survival time (from the shortest to the longest); Patient 1 of the women matches to Patient 1 of the men, and so forth. The interval from the bypass operation to death ranged from 22 to 120 months (mean 45) in the 11 women and from 19 to 120 months (mean 46) in the 11 men. The age of the women ranged from 44 to 78 years (mean 63), that of the men ranged from 47 to 76 years (mean 62). The women had a total of 35 saphenous vein conduits, the men had 25; the number of grafts per patient ranged from one to four (mean 3.2 in women and 2.3 in men). A saphenous vein having one aortic anastomosis and one or more coronary artery anastomoses was considered a single conduit. Clinical features of the 22 patients are shown in Table 1. Death had a *cardiac cause* in seven women (64%) and six men (55%): sudden cardiac arrest without myocardial necrosis in four women and three men, chronic congestive heart failure in three women and two men

Table 1. Clinical and Necropsy Findings in 11 Women and 11 Men Surviving 1 Year After Coronary Artery Bypass Grafting

Case No.	Age at Death (yr)	Interval From CABG to Death (mo)	Htn	DM	AP	AMI	CHF	Mode of Death	Heart Weight (g)	Dilated LV	LV Necrosis	LV Fibrosis
A. Women												
1	65	22	+	+	0	+	0	Sudden	565	+	+	+
2	64	24	+	+	+	0	+	CHF	490	+	0	+
3	70	24	0	0	0	0	+	CHF	500	+	0	+
4	44	26	+	0	0	0	+	Sudden	600	+	0	+
5	68	30	−	+	+	0	+	Sudden	550	+	0	0
6	61	31	+	+	0	0	0	GI bleeding	440	+	0	+
7	78	37	+	0	0	0	0	Cancer	355	0	0	+
8	44	43	0	+	+	+	+	CHF	498	+	0	+
9	68	70	+	+	0	0	+	Sudden	550	+	0	+
10	59	72	0	0	0	0	0	Cancer	480	0	0	0
11	74	120	0	0	0	0	0	Trauma	466	0	0	0
Total* or mean	63	45	7*	6*	3*	2*	6*		499	8*	1*	8*
B. Men												
1	54	19	+	+	0	0	+	CHF	510	+	0	+
2	60	24	0	0	0	0	+	CHF	540	+	0	+
3	66	26	0	0	0	0	0	Sudden	460	0	0	+
4	62	27	+	0	0	0	0	Cancer	450	0	0	0
5	47	32	0	+	+	0	0	AMI	390	0	+	0
6	69	34	0	0	+	+	0	Sudden	550	+	0	+
7	49	39	0	0	0	0	0	Sudden	370	0	0	0
8	76	48	0	0	0	0	0	Cancer	395	0	0	+
9	73	60	+	0	0	0	0	COPD	540	0	0	+
10	69	82	0	0	0	0	0	Cancer	440	0	0	0
11	54	120	+	0	+	0	0	Carotid operation	560	0	0	+
Total* or mean	62	46	4*	2*	3*	1*	2*		473	3*	1*	7*

AMI = acute myocardial infarction; AP = angina pectoris; CABG = coronary artery bypass grafting; CHF = chronic congestive heart failure; COPD = chronic obstructive pulmonary disease; DM = diabetes mellitus; GI = gastrointestinal; Htn = systemic hypertension by history; LV = left ventricle (ventricular); + = present; 0 = absent.

and acute myocardial infarction in one man. Death was attributed to a *non-cardiac cause* in four women (36%) and five men (45%): cancer in two women and three men and miscellaneous conditions in the other patients (gastrointestinal bleeding, trauma, chronic obstructive pulmonary disease and carotid operation).

Method of examination of native coronary arteries and saphenous vein grafts. The native coronary arteries and saphenous vein grafts were studied in a similar fashion. The hearts were fixed in formalin. The four major epicardial coronary arteries (left main, left anterior descending, left circumflex and right) and the saphenous vein bypass grafts were removed from the heart intact and cut transversely at 5-mm intervals. In one woman and one man the left main coronary artery was not available for examination. Except for the segments adjacent to anastomoses, the entire lengths of the native coronary arteries and vein conduits were available for examination. The segments were labeled sequentially from their origin. Each segment was processed in alcohol and xylene, embedded in paraffin, cut into sections 6 μm thick and stained by the Movat method (14). Of 1,918 sections initially examined, 97 were excluded because of sectioning artifacts. Thus, a total of 979 5-mm segments of native coronary arteries (mean 45/patient) and 842 segments of saphenous vein grafts (mean 38/patient) were studied. Plaque composition was assessed by planimetry: Movat-stained sections were placed on the stage of a projection light microscope, enlarging the image approximately 150 times. A tracing of the artery was made using a GTCO micro Digi-Pad. The area was calculated using Macmeasure (15), a morphometric software package used in conjunction with a Macintosh computer. The following areas were outlined: potential lumen (total area enclosed by the internal elastic membrane); residual lumen (potential lumen minus area of atherosclerotic plaque), and the components of the plaque separated into dense fibrous tissue, cellular fibrous tissue, calcific deposits, pultaceous debris (extracellular lipid), foam cells (intracellular lipid) with and without lymphocytes and inflammatory infiltrates without significant numbers of foam cells. Analysis of components was performed in all 5-mm segments in each of the four major epicardial coronary arteries and all saphenous venous bypass grafts in every patient.

Dense fibrous tissue consisted of nearly acellular, relatively homogeneous fibrous tissue staining yellow or yellow-brown by the Movat stain. *Cellular fibrous tissue* contained numerous spindle cells resembling myofibroblasts, smooth muscle cells or fibroblasts admixed with fibrous tissue and often elastic fibers. *Calcific deposits* were detected by blackish, brownish or purple collections of granular staining areas in Movat-stained sections. *Pultaceous debris* (presumably rich in extracellular lipid) consisted of collections of amorphous pale-staining material with abundant cholesterol clefts. *Foam cell aggregates* were composed of plump, rounded, finely vacuolated cells. *Foam cells and lymphocytes* were areas containing round cells with finely granular or vacuolated cytoplasm admixed with lymphocytes. *Inflammatory infiltrates without foams cells* were isolated aggregates of lymphocytes and other inflammatory cells that were almost always seen surrounding small vascular channels. The defined areas were recognized using the projection microscope and were confirmed by standard light microscopy.

After outlining and measuring the area of the plaque components, the area of each plaque component was converted to a percentage of the total plaque area. Other findings, such as hemorrhage into plaques and multilumen channels, were recorded but were not part of the analysis because they were considered to be a result of complications such as rupture of a plaque or total occlusion of the lumen by plaque.

Lumen narrowing, measured as a decrease in the cross-sectional area enclosed by the border of the internal elastic membrane, was graded by visual inspection of the histologic sections at a magnification of ×40. The amount of narrowing of each 5-mm segment was categorized into five groups: 0% to 25%, 26% to 50%, 51% to 75%, 76% to 95% and 96% to 100%.

Statistical analysis. For each patient a mean percentage of segments narrowed in each category of cross-sectional area narrowing was determined. Based on the mean for each patient, the total mean $\pm$ SD for the women and men was calculated for each category of narrowing.

The area of each plaque component was converted to a percentage of the total plaque area. For each patient the average plaque composition in the native coronary arteries was determined by calculating the mean of all 5-mm segments of the four coronary arteries of each individual patient. On the basis of the mean value for each patient, the

Table 2. Degree of Narrowing and Composition of Atherosclerotic Plaques in the Native Coronary Arteries in Women Compared With Men

Case No.	5-mm Segments (no.)	5-mm Segments With CSA Plaque Narrowing (no. [%])					Plaque Composition*						
		0% to 25%	26% to 50%	51% to 75%	76% to 95%	96% to 100%	DFT (%)	CFT (%)	CD (%)	PD (%)	FC (%)	FC+L (%)	ICWFC (%)
A. Women													
1	64	34 [53]	15 [23]	10 [16]	4 [6]	1 [2]	34.1	58.7	0.8	5.9	0.1	0.2	0.1
2	50	4 [8]	4 [8]	11 [22]	22 [44]	9 [18]	61.9	14.5	21.1	0.7	0.1	0.4	0.2
3	42	15 [36]	4 [10]	10 [24]	13 [31]	0 [0]	52.9	38.6	7.9	0.5	0.1	0.0	0.1
4	46	7 [15]	4 [9]	7 [15]	20 [43]	8 [17]	49.4	39.4	6.1	2.4	1.8	0.1	0.2
5	35	1 [3]	3 [9]	11 [31]	16 [46]	4 [11]	84.5	8.9	3.2	3.0	0.1	0.0	0.0
6	49	4 [8]	5 [10]	29 [59]	11 [22]	0 [0]	26.9	63.9	6.9	1.1	0.6	0.5	0.1
7	51	12 [24]	15 [29]	15 [29]	7 [14]	2 [4]	30.2	61.4	5.0	2.9	0.2	0.3	0.0
8	48	3 [6]	6 [13]	11 [23]	16 [32]	12 [25]	51.6	26.8	19.8	1.4	0.0	0.1	0.4
9	36	4 [11]	2 [6]	11 [31]	16 [44]	3 [8]	69.6	21.3	0.0	7.9	0.1	0.0	1.1
10	40	8 [20]	7 [18]	12 [30]	10 [25]	3 [8]	20.7	62.0	17.2	0.1	0.0	0.0	0.0
11	54	12 [22]	10 [19]	11 [20]	10 [19]	11 [20]	63.3	24.4	7.6	3.9	0.0	0.0	0.0
Mean	47	9 [19]	7 [15]	13 [28]	13 [28]	5 [10]	49.6	38.2	8.7	2.7	0.3	0.1	0.2
B. Men													
1	37	0 [0]	19 [51]	10 [27]	2 [5]	6 [16]	81.3	4.3	2.2	10.7	1.2	0.2	0.3
2	45	13 [29]	8 [18]	13 [29]	11 [24]	0 [0]	93.5	0.0	3.5	1.7	0.2	0.2	0.0
3	40	10 [25]	7 [18]	11 [28]	11 [28]	1 [3]	93.7	4.5	1.8	0.0	0 0	0.0	0.1
4	39	9 [23]	7 [18]	5 [13]	12 [31]	6 [15]	86.5	0.6	11.0	1.7	0.0	0.2	0.0
5	30	16 [53]	8 [27]	0 [0]	5 [17]	1 [3]	96.6	1.4	1.4	0.0	0.5	0.0	0.1
6	49	5 [10]	5 [10]	2 [4]	24 [49]	13 [27]	69.5	15.8	13.4	0.2	0.0	0.0	0.0
7	47	2 [4]	5 [11]	12 [26]	17 [36]	11 [23]	89.1	0.5	4.9	4.6	0.2	0.2	0.5
8	48	0 [0]	1 [2]	6 [13]	34 [71]	7 [15]	78.1	6.5	12.0	3.1	0.0	0.0	0.0
9	29	2 [7]	5 [17]	9 [31]	8 [28]	5 [17]	61.6	12.7	18.1	5.5	0.0	0.0	0.0
10	56	0 [0]	5 [9]	5 [9]	20 [36]	26 [46]	92.9	2.0	4.1	0.5	0.1	0.0	0.0
11	44	6 [14]	1 [2]	5 [11]	20 [45]	12 [27]	87.3	0.0	4.0	8.0	0.1	0.0	0.6
Mean	42	6 [14]	6 [14]	7 [17]	15 [36]	8 [19]	84.5	4.4	6.9	3.3	0.2	0.1	0.1

*Hemorrhage into plaques or multilumen channels are not listed; therefore, numbers do not add up to 100% in each patient. CD = calcific deposits; CFT = cellular fibrous tissue; CSA = cross-sectional area; DFT = dense fibrous tissue; FC = foam cells; FC+L = foam cells plus lymphocytes; ICWFC = inflammatory cells without foam cells; PD = pultaceous debris.

Table 3. Degree of Narrowing and Composition of Atherosclerotic Plaques in the Saphenous Vein Grafts in Women Compared With Men

Case No.	5-mm Segments (no.)	5-mm Segments With CSA Plaque Narrowing (no. [%])					Plaque Composition*						
		0% to 25%	26% to 50%	51% to 75%	76% to 95%	96% to 100%	DFT (%)	CFT (%)	CD (%)	PD (%)	FC (%)	FC+L (%)	ICWFC (%)
A. Women													
1	15	0 [0]	0 [0]	0 [0]	1 [7]	14 [93]	1.1	87.0	0.0	0.0	0.0	0.0	0.0
2	58	24 [41]	31 [53]	3 [5]	0 [0]	0 [0]	2.7	95.0	0.0	0.0	0.0	0.0	0.0
3	54	8 [15]	37 [69]	9 [17]	0 [0]	0 [0]	0.9	99.0	0.1	0.0	0.0	0.0	0.0
4	33	1 [3]	7 [21]	7 [21]	4 [12]	14 [42]	37.6	59.2	0.0	0.0	0.0	0.0	0.0
5	34	6 [18]	28 [82]	0 [0]	0 [0]	0 [0]	0.0	99.8	0.0	0.0	0.2	0.0	0.0
6	46	0 [0]	0 [0]	0 [0]	19 [41]	27 [59]	3.5	96.2	0.2	0.0	0.0	0.0	0.0
7	31	5 [16]	13 [42]	11 [35]	2 [6]	0 [0]	10.0	86.7	0.0	0.3	0.1	0.1	0.0
8	41	0 [0]	7 [17]	17 [41]	15 [37]	2 [5]	56.6	31.2	0.0	5.6	0.6	0.1	0.3
9	25	1 [4]	9 [36]	2 [8]	7 [28]	6 [24]	28.7	49.9	0.0	19.4	0.7	0.2	0.1
10	26	6 [23]	20 [77]	0 [0]	0 [0]	0 [0]	42.8	56.7	0.3	0.0	0.2	0.0	0.0
11	51	25 [49]	24 [47]	2 [4]	0 [0]	0 [0]	89.7	9.1	0.0	0.9	0.1	0.04	0.1
Mean	38	7 [18]	16 [42]	5 [13]	4 [11]	6 [16]	24.9	70.0	0.1	2.4	0.2	0.04	0.04
B. Men													
1	42	8 [19]	15 [36]	10 [24]	9 [21]	0 [0]	1.3	98.5	0.0	0.0	0.1	0.0	0.0
2	48	0 [0]	39 [81]	1 [2]	2 [4]	6 [13]	30.8	67.8	0.0	0.0	0.0	0.0	0.0
3	51	27 [53]	23 [45]	1 [2]	0 [0]	0 [0]	21.1	78.0	0.0	0.0	0.9	0.0	0.0
4	30	13 [43]	16 [53]	1 [3]	0 [0]	0 [0]	94.9	3.5	0.0	0.8	0.5	0.3	0.0
5	9	2 [22]	4 [44]	2 [22]	1 [11]	0 [0]	55.4	0.0	0.0	13.5	10.1	0.0	0.0
6	45	8 [18]	8 [18]	7 [16]	14 [31]	8 [18]	81.7	6.3	1.3	8.5	0.8	1.2	0.2
7	27	0 [0]	4 [15]	8 [30]	15 [56]	0 [0]	79.6	2.4	0.3	9.3	1.8	1.0	0.3
8	62	36 [58]	23 [37]	3 [5]	0 [0]	0 [0]	0.0	100.0	0.0	0.0	0.0	0.0	0.0
9	38	29 [76]	9 [24]	0 [0]	0 [0]	0 [0]	69.0	30.9	0.1	0.1	0.04	0.0	0.0
10	55	3 [5]	22 [40]	22 [40]	8 [15]	0 [0]	96.9	3.1	0.0	0.0	0.0	0.0	0.0
11	21	13 [62]	0 [0]	0 [0]	1 [5]	7 [33]	98.8	0.0	0.7	0.4	0.0	0.0	0.01
Mean	39	13 [33]	15 [38]	5 [13]	5 [13]	2 [5]	57.2	35.5	0.2	3.0	1.3	0.2	0.04

*Hemorrhage into plaques or multilumen channels are not listed; therefore, numbers do not add up to 100% in each patient. Abbreviations as in Table 2.

total mean value ± SD for the women and men was calculated for the native coronary arteries. In the same fashion, the total plaque composition of the saphenous vein grafts was determined.

For statistical evaluation, the mean percentages for each patient were used. The unit of comparison was the pairs of women and men matched by survival time after bypass operation. A paired t test was performed with a probability of < 0.05 (two-tailed) considered to be significant.

Results

Cross-sectional area narrowing. The results are summarized in Tables 2 and 3. In all 22 patients, one or more epicardial coronary arteries were narrowed significantly (>75% in cross-sectional area) by atherosclerotic plaque; an average of 38 ± 19% of coronary artery segments in the women and 55 ± 25% of segments in the men were narrowed to this degree. Six of the 11 women and 7 of the 11 men had one or more saphenous vein conduits narrowed by atherosclerotic plaque >75% in cross-sectional area; an average of 27 ± 40% of saphenous vein segments in the women and 18 ± 20% in the men were narrowed to this degree. Statistical comparison based on the pairs of women and men matched according to time interval from bypass operation to death did not reveal any difference between women and men with respect to narrowing in cross-sectional area in the native coronary arteries and in the saphenous vein grafts.

Plaque composition. The results are summarized in Tables 2 and 3 and Figures 1 and 2.

Fibrous tissue. The mean percentage of fibrous tissue in all plaques of the native coronary arteries was 88 ± 6% in women and 89 ± 7% in men; in the saphenous vein grafts it was 95 ± 7% and 93 ± 14%, respectively (paired t test: p = NS).

Analysis of the subtypes of fibrous tissue revealed that the mean percentage of *cellular* fibrous tissue in the plaques of the native coronary arteries was 38 ± 21% in women and 4 ± 5% in men (p < 0.001); in the plaques of the saphenous vein grafts it was 70 ± 31% and 36 ± 42%, respectively (p < 0.05). The mean percentage of *dense* fibrous tissue in the plaques of the native coronary arteries was 50 ± 20% in women and 85 ± 11% in men (p < 0.001); in the plaques of the saphenous vein grafts it was 25 ± 29% and 57 ± 38%, respectively (p < 0.05).

Calcific deposits. Calcific deposits were present in the plaques of the native coronary arteries in all patients except one woman. The mean percentage was 9 ± 7% in women and

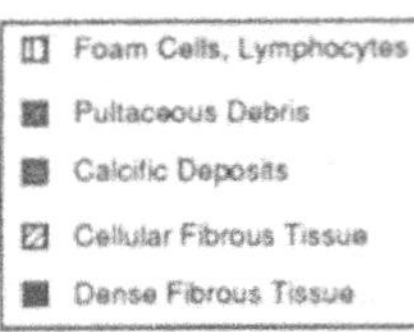
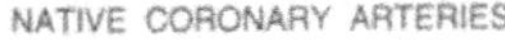
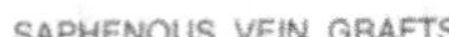
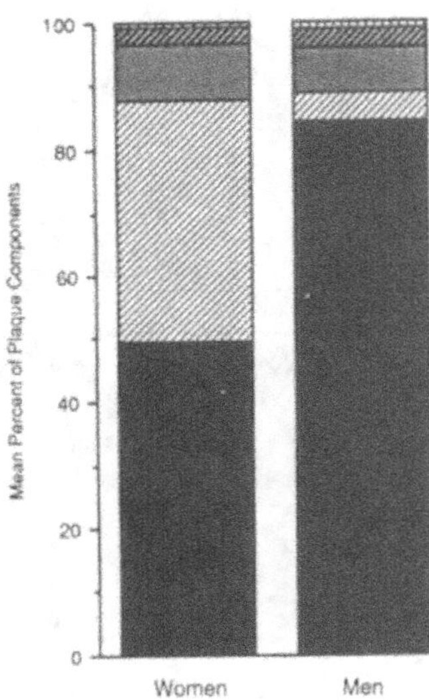
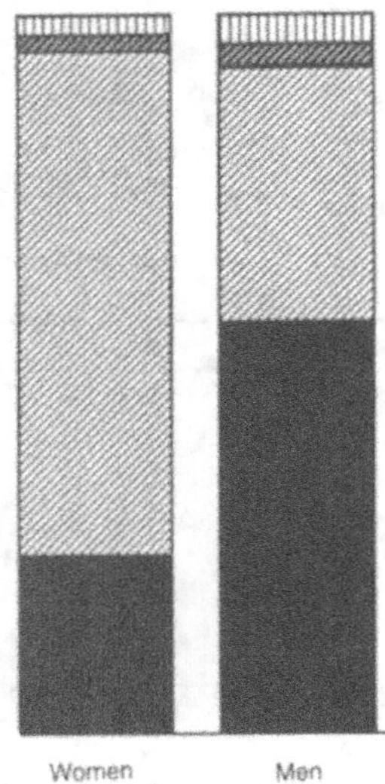

Figure 1. Graph comparing the mean composition of the plaques in the native coronary arteries and saphenous vein grafts of women and men. The plaques in women had a higher percentage of cellular fibrous tissue than did those in men. This difference was observed in the saphenous vein grafts and was even more pronounced in the native coronary arteries. In both men and women, calcific deposits were found mainly in native coronary arteries.

7 ± 6% in men. In the saphenous veins, calcific deposits were present in the plaques of three women and four men. The mean percentage was <1% in both groups. Statistically, the percentage of calcific deposits in the plaques did not differ between women and men in either the native coronary arteries or the vein grafts (p = NS).

Pultaceous debris (extracellular lipid). In the native coronary arteries, pultaceous debris was present in the plaques in 20 of the 22 patients. The mean percentage of pultaceous debris in all plaques of the coronary arteries was 2.7 ± 2.4% in women and 3.3 ± 3.6% in men (p = NS). In the saphenous vein grafts, pultaceous debris was found in the plaques in 4 of the 11 women and 6 of the 11 men. The mean percentage of pultaceous debris in all plaques of the saphenous vein grafts was 2.4 ± 5.9% in women and 3.0 ± 5.0% in men (p = NS).

Foam cells (intracellular lipid), foam cells with lymphocytes and inflammatory infiltrates without foam cells. The mean percentage of foam cells in all plaques of the native coronary arteries was 0.3 ± 0.5% in women and 0.2 ± 0.3% in men, and in the saphenous vein grafts it was 0.2 ± 0.2% in women and 1.3 ± 3.0% in men. Usually these cells were located on or near the borders of the lumen. The mean percentage of foam cells with lymphocytes and pure inflammatory cells was <1% in all plaques of both the native

coronary arteries and the saphenous vein grafts in women as well as in men. Statistically, the percentage of foam cells, foam cells with lymphocytes, and inflammatory infiltrates without foam cells in the plaques did not differ between women and men in the native coronary arteries or the saphenous vein grafts (p = NS for all comparisons).

Figure 2 (opposite page). Photomicrographs of sections of native coronary arteries and saphenous vein grafts. **Left panels (A to D),** From a woman who survived 26 months after a coronary bypass operation (Case 4, Table 1A). **Right panels (E to H),** From a man who survived 27 months after a coronary bypass operation (Case 4, Table 1B). **A,** Section of a native coronary artery from a woman (Case 4). **B,** Higher magnification of the section in A. The plaque consists of 68% dense and 32% cellular fibrous tissue. **C and D,** The saphenous vein graft in this patient consists mostly of cellular fibrous tissue (90%). **E, F,** Example of a native coronary artery of a man (Case 4, Table 1B), revealing as main plaque component dense fibrous tissue (95%). A small area of calcific deposit is also present. **G, H,** In the plaque of the saphenous vein graft in this patient, dense fibrous tissue (89%) is the predominant component, whereas only a small amount (11%) of cellular fibrous tissue is present. CA = native coronary artery; SVG = saphenous vein graft; B, D, F, H are each higher magnifications of the area indicated by the rectangle in the section above. Movat stains: A ×34; C ×16; E ×34; G ×22; B, D, F, H ×200, all reduced by 22%.

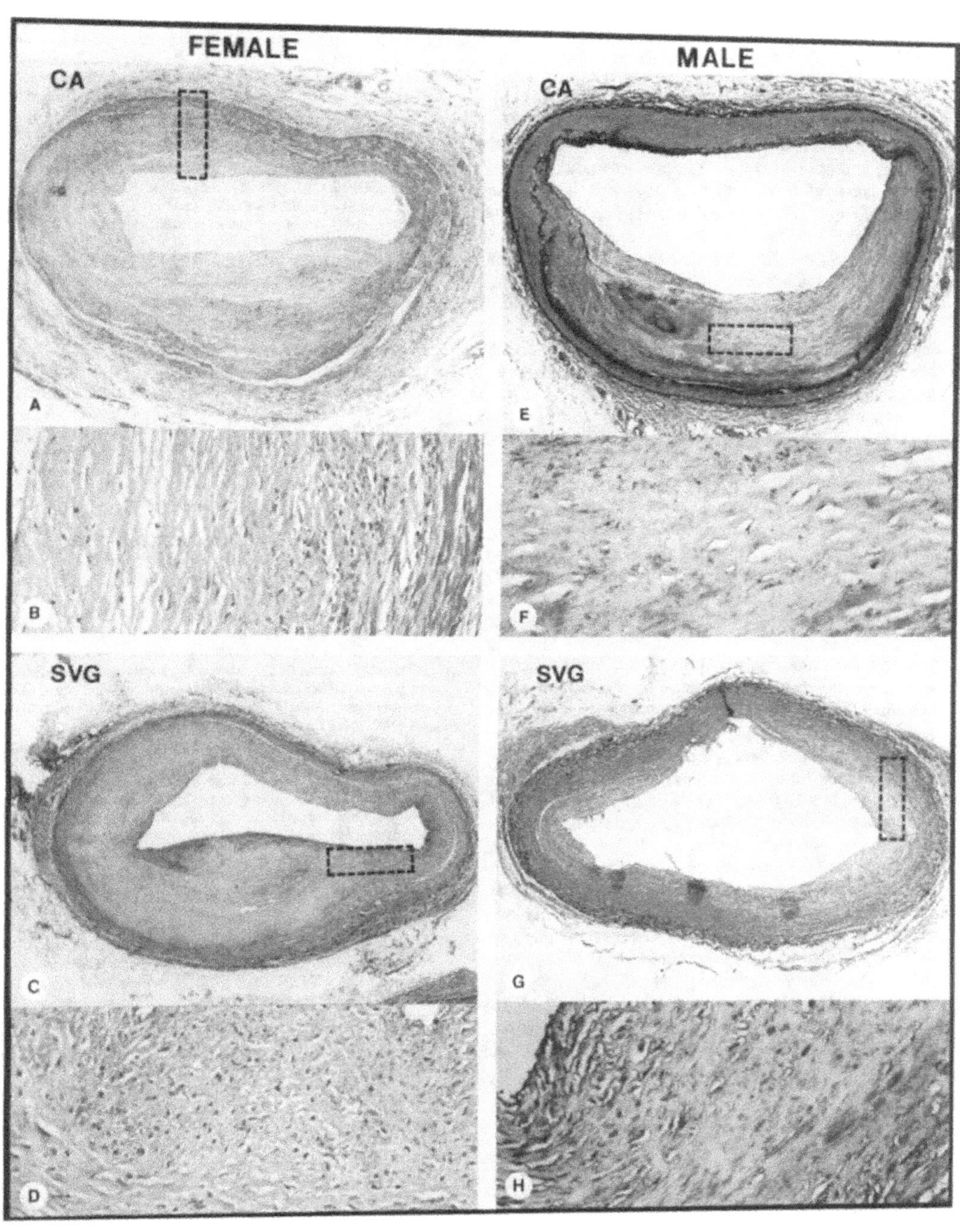

FEMALE
MALE
CA
CA
A
E
B
F
SVG
SVG
C
G
D
H

Discussion

Although several studies have compared clinical features of myocardial ischemia and results after coronary angioplasty and after bypass surgery in women versus men (16–23), no study has compared the composition of atherosclerotic plaques in the coronary arteries or in other vascular systems in those two groups. The present study compared plaque composition according to gender in both native epicardial coronary arteries and in saphenous veins used as aortocoronary conduits. The 11 women and 11 men studied were matched for the length of time that the saphenous vein aortocoronary conduits had been in place. The native coronary arteries and the saphenous vein grafts of each patient were studied by dividing their entire lengths into 5-mm segments, which then were examined histologically. In all, nearly 2,000 sections were examined by a computerized morphometric technique.

Comparison of all categories of degree of lumen narrowing of the native coronary arteries and the saphenous vein grafts revealed no difference between findings in women versus those in men.

In contrast, analysis of plaque composition disclosed that the plaques in both the native coronary arteries and saphenous vein grafts differed in women and men: in the native coronary arteries, the mean percentage of dense, acellular fibrous tissue in the plaques was much lower in women than in men (mean 50% vs. 85%), and the mean percentage of cellular fibrous tissue in the plaques was much higher in women than in men (mean 38% vs. 4%). Similar findings were present in the saphenous veins used as aortocoronary conduits: dense, acellular fibrous tissue in the plaques of the saphenous vein grafts comprised a significantly smaller percentage in women than in men (mean 25% vs. 57%) and cellular fibrous tissue constituted a higher percentage in women than in men (mean 70% vs. 36%).

It was established previously (2,4,5,13) that cellular fibrous tissue, which was present in a higher amount in the plaques of the 11 women studied, is often found at an early stage of plaque development, whereas dense fibrous tissue, the dominant component in the plaques of the 11 men studied, is seen in later stages. These differences in plaque composition, that is, the younger appearance of plaques in the native coronary arteries and saphenous venous conduit in women and the older appearance in men, might be due to differences in duration or speed of the atherosclerotic process or to different mechanisms or influences in women and men, which will require further investigation.

We thank Michael A. Proschan, PhD for statistical advice and Ricardo V. Dreyfuss and Christopher R. Dame for photographic expertise.

References

1. Roberts CS, Roberts WC. Cross-sectional area of the proximal portions of the three major epicardial coronary arteries in 98 necropsy patients with different coronary events: relationship to heart weight, age, and sex. Circulation 1980;62:953–9.

2. Dollar AL, Kragel AH, Fernicola DJ, Waclawiw MA, Roberts WC. Composition of atherosclerotic plaques in coronary arteries in women <40 years of age with fatal coronary artery disease and implication for plaque reversibility. Am J Cardiol 1991;67:1223–7.

3. Gertz SD, Malekzadeh S, Dollar AL, Kragel AH, Roberts WC. Composition of atherosclerotic plaques in the four major epicardial coronary arteries in patients ≥90 years of age. Am J Cardiol 1991;67:1228–33.

4. Kragel AH, Reddy SG, Wittes JT, Roberts WC. Morphometric analysis of the composition of atherosclerotic plaques in the four major epicardial coronary arteries in acute myocardial infarction and in sudden coronary death. Circulation 1989;80:1747–56.

5. Kragel AH, Reddy SG, Wittes JT, Roberts WC. Morphometric analysis of the composition of coronary arterial plaques in isolated unstable angina pectoris with pain at rest. Am J Cardiol 1990;66:562–7.

6. Vlodaver Z, Edwards JE. Pathologic changes in aortic coronary arterial saphenous vein grafts. Circulation 1971;64:719–28.

7. Barboriak JJ, Pintar K, Korns ME. Atherosclerosis in aortocoronary vein grafts. Lancet 1974;2:621–4.

8. Spray TL, Roberts WC. Changes in saphenous veins used as aortocoronary bypass grafts. Am Heart J 1977;94:500–16.

9. Smith SH, Geer JC. Morphology of saphenous vein-coronary artery bypass grafts. Seven to 116 months after surgery. Arch Pathol Lab Med 1983;107:13–8.

10. Atkinson JB, Forman MB, Vaughan WK, Robinowitz M, McAllister HA, Virmani R. Morphologic changes in long-term saphenous vein bypass grafts. Chest 1985;88:341–8.

11. Campeau L, Lesperance J, Corbara F, Hermann J, Grondin CM, Bourassa MG. Aortocoronary saphenous vein bypass graft changes 5 to 7 years after surgery. Circulation 1978;58(suppl I):I-170–5.

12. Kalan JM, Roberts WC. Morphologic findings in saphenous veins used as coronary arterial bypass conduits for longer than 1 year: necropsy analysis of 53 patients, 123 saphenous veins and 1865 five-millimeter segments of veins. Am Heart J 1990;119:1164–84.

13. Mautner SL, Mautner GC, Hunsberger SA, Roberts WC. Comparison of composition of atherosclerotic plaques in saphenous veins used as aortocoronary bypass conduits with plaques in native coronary arteries in the same men. Am J Cardiol 1992;70:1380–7.

14. Movat HZ. Demonstration of all connective tissue elements in a single section. Arch Pathol 1955;60:289–95.

15. Hook GR, Rasband W. Macmeasure: a low-cost, easy to operate quantitative morphometrics system for the Macintosh computer. In: Bailey GW, ed: Proceedings of the 45th Annual Meeting of the Electron Microscopy Society of America. San Francisco: San Francisco Press, 1987:920–1.

16. Johansson S, Bergstrand R, Schlossman D, Selin K, Vedin A, Wilhelmsson C. Sex differences in cardioangiographic findings after myocardial infarction. Eur Heart J 1984;5:374–81.

17. Loop FD, Golding LR, MacMillan JP, Cosgrove DM, Lytle BW, Sheldon WC. Coronary artery surgery in women compared with men: analyses of risks and long-term results. J Am Coll Cardiol 1983;1:383–90.

18. Fisher LD, Kennedy JW, Davis KB, et al. Association of sex, physical size, and operative mortality after coronary artery bypass in the Coronary Artery Surgery Study (CASS). J Thorac Cardiovasc Surg 1982;84:334–41.

19. Bolooki H, Vargas A, Green R, Kaiser GA, Ghahramani A. Results of direct coronary artery surgery in women. J Thorac Cardiovasc Surg 1975;69:271–7.

20. Tyras DH, Barner HB, Kaiser GC, Codd JE, Laks H, Willman VL. Myocardial revascularization in women. Ann Thorac Surg 1978;25:449–53.

21. Golding LR, Groves LK. Results of coronary artery surgery in women. Cleve Clin Q 1976;43:113–5.

22. Killen DA, Reed WA, Arnold M, McCallister BD, Bell HH. Coronary artery bypass in women. Long-term survival. Ann Thorac Surg 1982;34:559–63.

23. Douglas JS Jr, King SB III, Jones EL, Craver JM, Bradford JM, Hatcher CR Jr. Reduced efficacy of coronary bypass surgery in women. Circulation 1981;64(suppl II):II-11–6.

Subepicardial myocardial lesions

Subepicardial myocardial lesions are rarely seen at necropsy, and a description of them and their causes has not been reported. Over the last 13 years we have studied 22 patients with subepicardial myocardial lesions. They ranged in age from 14 to 73 years (mean 47), and 20 were men. The lesions were associated with atherosclerotic coronary artery disease in six patients, sarcoidosis in five, idiopathic dilated cardiomyopathy in four, lymphocytic myocarditis in two, and hypoplastic right and left circumflex coronary arteries in one. In four patients the cause was unclear. In the patients with atherosclerotic coronary artery disease, the subepicardial myocardial lesions were small, few in number, and located in the left ventricular posterior wall. In patients with sarcoidosis or myocarditis, the subepicardial lesions were extensive and commonly associated with transmural left and right ventricular lesions. The right ventricular half of the ventricular septum also was frequently affected. In the remaining nine patients, the subepicardial lesions were small and unassociated with transmural left ventricular lesions. Thus subepicardial myocardial lesions occur in a variety of cardiac diseases. (AM HEART J 1993;125:1346.)

Jamshid Shirani, MD, and William C. Roberts, MD* *Bethesda, Md.*

Necrotic, fibrotic, or other types of lesions in the left ventricular free wall have most commonly been categorized as subendocardial (limited to the inner half of the myocardial wall) or transmural (involving more than the inner half of the myocardial wall) (Fig. 1). Because most subendocardial lesions resulting from myocardial ischemia involve only the inner 33% of the myocardial wall and most transmural lesions resulting from myocardial ischemia involve more than the inner 67% of the myocardial wall, the 50% demarcation point has served well in separating the subendocardial from the transmural foci of fibrosis or necrosis. Another location for left ventricular lesions is the subepicardial half of the wall. Myocardial lesions rarely are limited to this portion of the left ventricular wall, and no study has focused on causes of lesions in such locations. This report describes subepicardial left ventricular lesions observed at necropsy in a variety of cardiac conditions.

METHODS

Patients studied. Cases recorded in the Pathology Branch of the National Heart, Lung, and Blood Institute

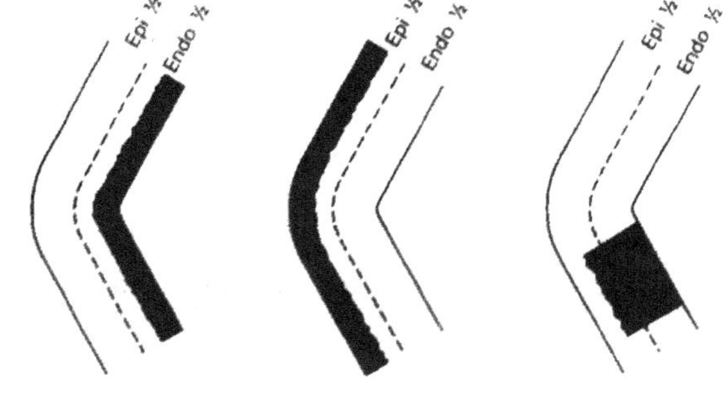

Fig. 1. Diagram showing terms used to describe left ventricular myocardial lesions according to percentage of wall thickness involved. *Broken line* represents 50% demarcation point, which separates subendocardial *(Endo ½)* from subepicardial *(Epi ½)* portion. *Transmural* refers to involvement of more than half the thickness of the wall.

as having "subepicardial scar(s)" were retrieved. The files from 1954 through August 1992 were searched. A total of 22 cases were located, and they constitute the subject of this report. The first case coded as "subepicardial scar" was seen in February 1979. Since then approximately 5500 hearts have been added to the records accessioned in the Pathology Branch. The hearts of all 22 cases were originally examined and coded by one of us (W. C. R.) and subsequently examined by another (J. S.). The hearts of the 22 cases were submitted by five different medical centers including 13 cases from the District of Columbia Medical Examiner's Office (DCMEO), six from the District of Columbia Veterans Administration Hospital (DCVAH), and one each from three other (two local and one nonlocal) medical centers.

Definition of subepicardial lesion. In this report the

From the Pathology Branch, National Heart, Lung, and Blood Institute, National Institutes of Health.

Received for publication Oct. 2, 1992; accepted Nov. 6, 1992.

Reprint requests: Pathology Branch, National Heart, Lung, and Blood Institute, National Institutes of Health, Building 10, Room 2N258, Bethesda, MD 20892.

*Present address: Baylor Cardiovascular Institute, Baylor University Medical Center, PO Box E010, Dallas, TX 75246.

4/1/44701

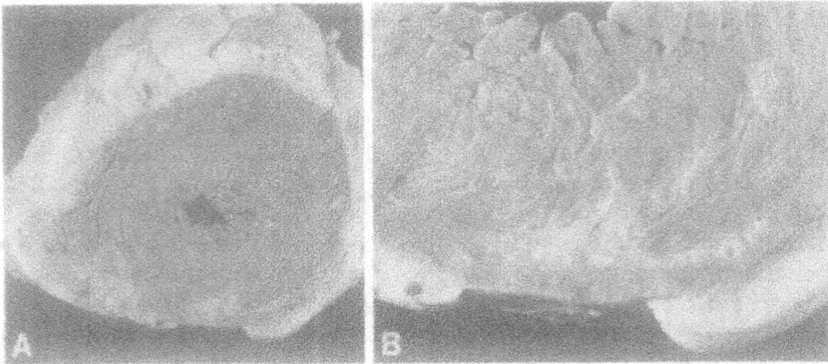

Fig. 2. A, Transverse section of apical portion of left ventricle (DCVAH# 92A-11; patient 5) showing small subepicardial scar in posterior wall. **B,** Close-up view of scar.

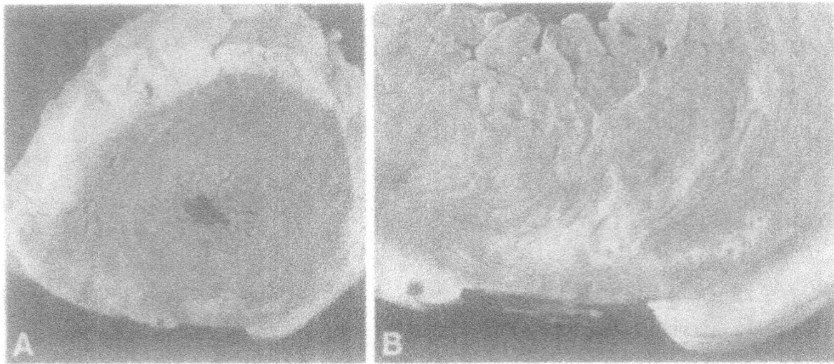

Fig. 3. A, Transverse section of cardiac ventricles (DCVAH# 91A-58; patient 6) showing small scar in posterior left ventricular wall. **B,** Close-up view.

subepicardial lesion is defined as a lesion limited to no more than the outer half of the left ventricular wall (Fig. 1). Although an argument can be made to consider any lesion that spares the innermost (subendocardial) portion of the left ventricular wall as "subepicardial," even if it involves more than 50% of the wall, we did not include such cases in this study. The right ventricular half of the ventricular septum was also considered as being equivalent to the "subepicardial region" of the left ventricular free wall. Thus the left ventricle was divided into four anatomic regions (anterior, lateral, posterior, and septal), and the presence of myocardial lesions was assessed morphologically in each segment (Fig. 1).

RESULTS

Certain clinical and cardiac morphologic findings in the 22 patients are summarized in Table I. Their ages ranged from 14 to 73 years (mean 47); 20 (91%) were men, and 17 (77%) were black. Sudden death occurred in 16 (73%); three patients died of cerebrovascular accidents and one each from acute myo-

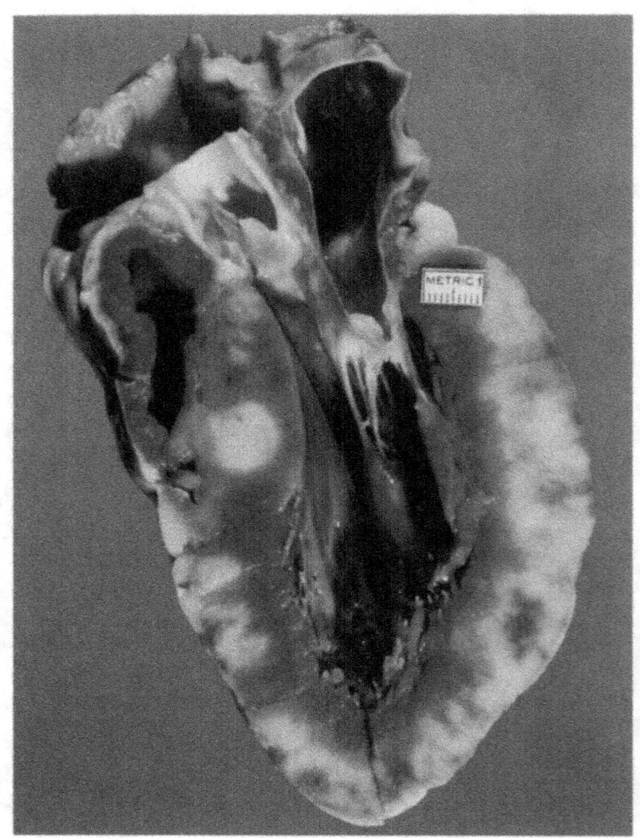

Fig. 4. Longitudinal view of heart (DCMEO #83-10-670; patient 8) showing extensive primarily subepicardial myocardial lesions that were sarcoid granulomas histologically.

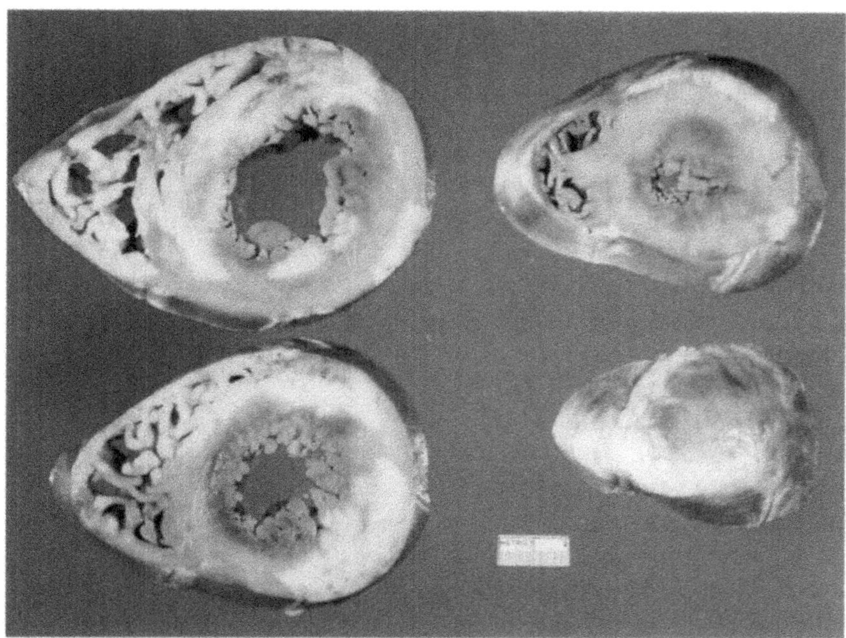

Fig. 5. Multiple transverse slices of cardiac ventricles (DCMEO #88-01-140; patient 10) showing extensive involvement of right and left ventricular myocardium by sarcoid granulomas. *Upper right* view shows subepicardial myocardial lesions; all of these lesions are sarcoid granulomas.

Table I. Clinical and morphologic findings in 22 patients with subepicardial myocardial lesions

Patient No.	Age (yr)	Sex	Race	Mode of death	Death in hospital	Morphologic diagnosis
1	51	M	B	Sudden	0	Atherosclerotic CAD
2	55	M	W	AMI	+	Atherosclerotic CAD
3	62	M	B	Stroke	+	Atherosclerotic CAD
4	65	M	B	Renal failure	+	Atherosclerotic CAD
5	67	M	B	Cancer	+	Atherosclerotic CAD
6	73	M	W	Stroke	+	Atherosclerotic CAD
7	25	M	B	Sudden	0	Sarcoidosis
8	27	F	B	Sudden	0	Sarcoidosis
9	34	M	W	Sudden	0	Sarcoidosis
10	35	M	B	Sudden	0	Sarcoidosis
11	37	M	B	Sudden	+	Sarcoidosis
12	32	M	B	Sudden	0	IDC
13	46	M	W	Sudden	+	IDC
14	52	M	B	Sudden	0	IDC
15	68	M	B	Sudden	0	IDC
16	29	M	B	Sudden	0	Cardiomegaly*
17	30	M	B	Sudden	0	Cardiomegaly*
18	35	M	W	Sudden	0	Cardiomegaly*
19	56	M	B	Sudden	0	Cardiomegaly*
20	14	M	B	Sudden	0	Myocarditis†
21	28	F	B	Sudden	0	Myocarditis†
22	62	M	B	Stroke	+	Hypoplastic RCA and LCCA
Totals (mean or %)	14-73 (47)	20 M (91%)	17 B (77%)	16 SD (73%)	8 (36%)	

AMI, Acute myocardial infarction; *B*, black; *CAD*, coronary artery disease; *CSA*, cross-sectional area; *IDC*, idiopathic dilated cardiomyopathy; *LCCA*, left circumflex coronary artery; *LV*, left ventricular; *RCA*, right coronary artery; *RV*, right ventricular; *SD*, sudden death; *T*, transmural; *VS*, ventricular septal; *W*, white.

*Undetermined cause.

†Lymphocytic myocarditis.

cardial infarction, renal failure, and lung cancer. The heart weights ranged from 275 to 940 gm (mean 565), and the weight was increased (>350 gm in women and >400 gm in men) in 21 (95%) patients. The frequency of left ventricular subepicardial lesions at different locations as follows: posterior wall, 19 of 22 (86%); lateral wall, 11 of 22 (50%); and anterior wall, 6 of 22 (27%). In addition, 11 patients (50%) had myocardial lesions in the right ventricular half of the ventricular septum. In eight patients (36%) left ventricular transmural lesions also were present: two had atherosclerotic coronary artery disease, four had sarcoidosis, and one each had idiopathic dilated cardiomyopathy or lymphocytic myocarditis. Myocardial lesions were present in the right ventricular wall in 10 (45%) patients. The intramural coronary arteries were normal in all 22 patients. In two patients (Nos. 1 and 17) the subepicardial myocardium was replaced by adipose tissue intermixed with fibrous tissue.

Atherosclerotic coronary artery disease (Figs. 2 and 3). In six patients the lumen of at least one of the four ma-

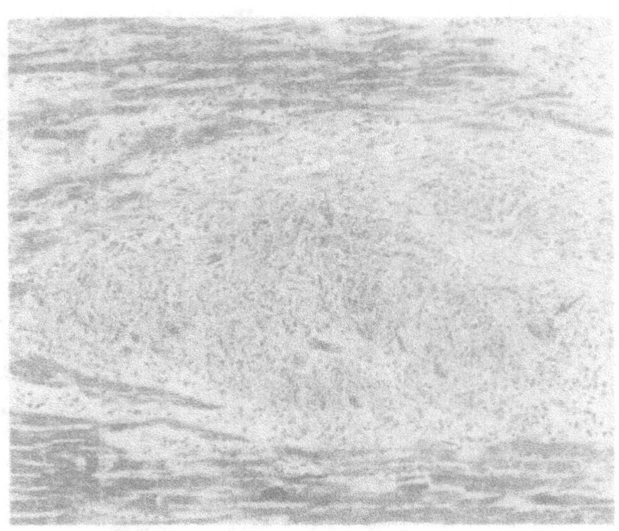

Fig. 6. Histologic section of left ventricular myocardium in patient whose heart is shown in Fig. 5 showing noncaseating sarcoid granulomas. *Arrows* point out some multinucleated giant cells. (Hematoxylin & eosin stain; original magnification ×200.)

Heart weight (gm)	Distribution of subepicardial LV lesions			Lesions			No. of major coronary arteries ↓ >75% in CSA by plaque
	Posterior	Lateral	Anterior	VS (RV½)	RV T	LV T	
555	+	+	0	0	0	0	1
530	+	+	0	0	0	+	4
790	+	0	0	+	0	+	1
490	+	0	0	0	0	0	2
420	+	0	0	0	0	0	1
475	+	0	0	0	+	0	2
430	0	+	0	+	+	+	0
405	+	+	+	+	+	+	0
460	+	+	0	0	0	0	0
570	+	+	+	+	+	+	0
700	+	+	+	+	+	+	0
930	+	0	0	0	0	+	0
940	0	0	+	+	0	0	0
710	0	+	0	0	0	0	0
780	+	0	0	0	0	0	0
520	+	+	0	0	0	0	0
490	+	0	0	+	+	0	0
475	+	0	0	0	+	0	0
550	+	+	0	+	+	0	0
275	+	+	+	+	+	0	0
340	+	0	+	+	+	+	0
540	+	0	0	+	0	0	0
275-940 (565)	19 (86%)	11 (50%)	6 (27%)	11 (50%)	10 (45%)	8 (36%)	

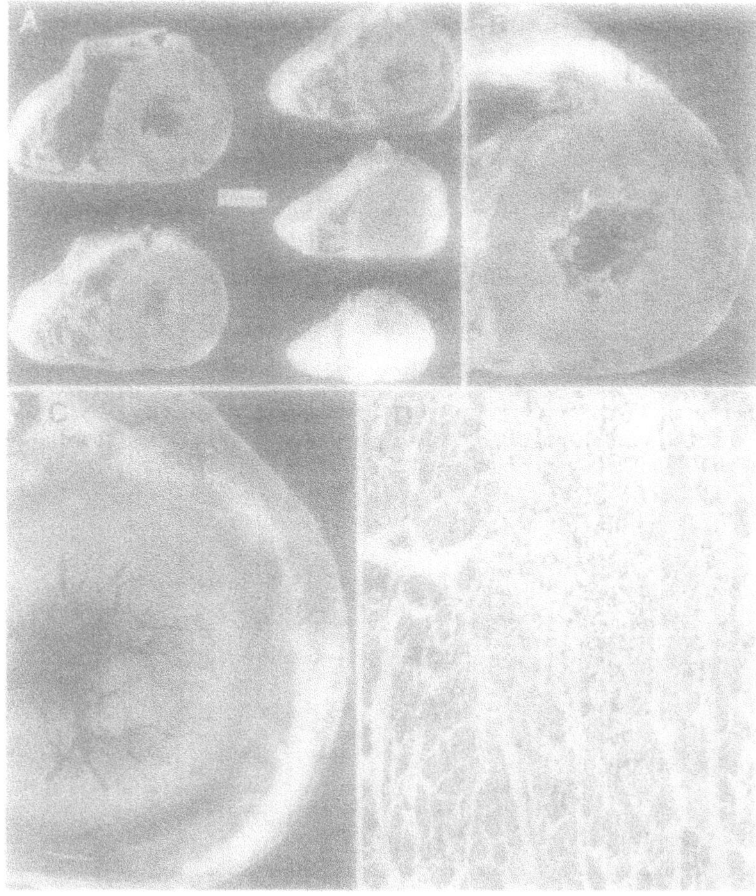

Fig. 7. Multiple transverse slices **(A)** and close-up view of basal portion **(B** and **C)** of cardiac ventricles (DCMEO# 92-04-402; patient 20) showing extensive subepicardial myocardial necrosis in 14-year-old boy with lymphocytic myocarditis **(D).** (Hematoxylin & eosin stain; original magnification ×200.)

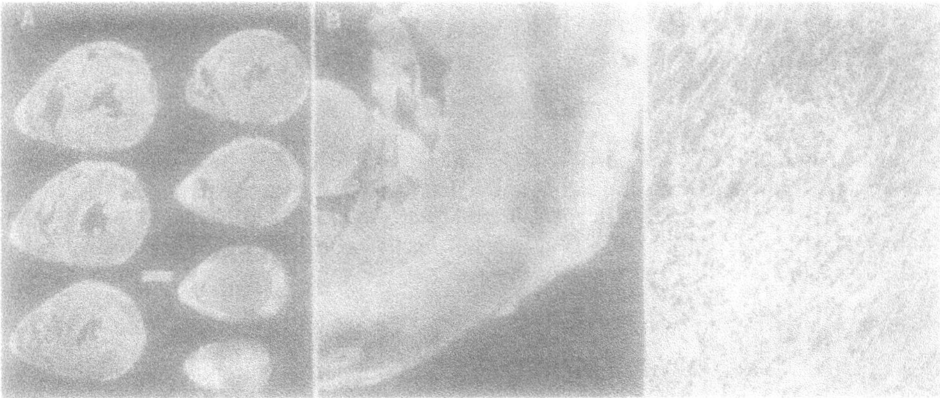

Fig. 8. Multiple transverse sections of cardiac ventricles **(A)** and close-up view **(B)** in 28-year-old woman (DCMEO# 91-07-735; patient 21) with lymphocytic myocarditis **(C).** (Hematoxylin & eosin stain; original magnification ×200.)

jor (left main, left anterior descending, left circumflex, and right) epicardial coronary arteries was narrowed >75% in cross-sectional area by atherosclerotic plaque.

Cardiac sarcoidosis (Figs. 4 to 6) **or lymphocytic my-ocarditis** (Figs. 7 and 8). All seven patients died suddenly. The subepicardial myocardial lesions were extensive and in five patients were associated with transmural lesions. The right ventricular myocardium was involved in six of the

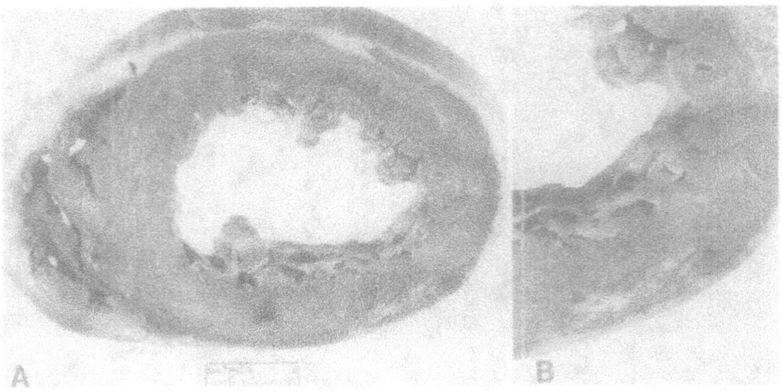

Fig. 9. Transverse section **(A)** and close-up view **(B)** of cardiac ventricles of 32-year-old man (DCMEO #84-1-12; patient 12) with idiopathic dilated cardiomyopathy showing subepicardial scar involving posterior and lateral segments of left ventricular wall.

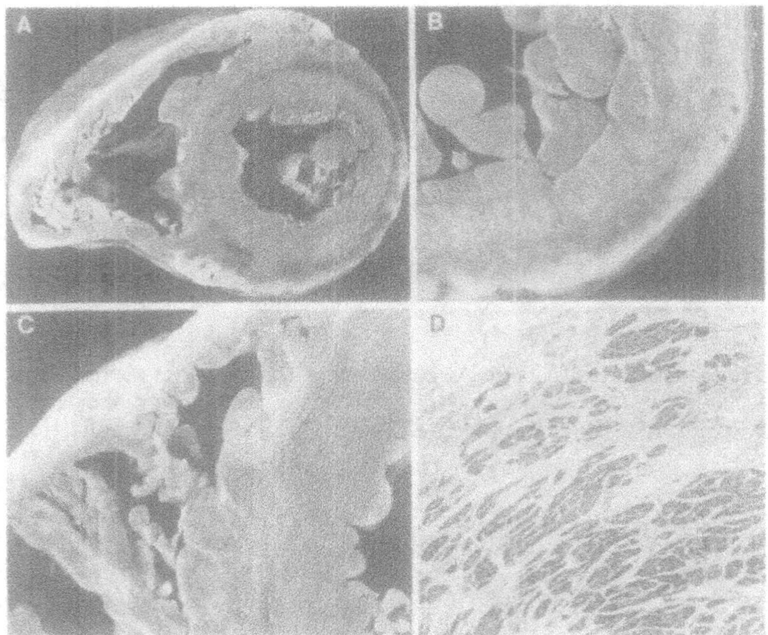

Fig. 10. Transverse section of basal portion **(A)** of cardiac ventricles and close-up views of left ventricular free wall **(B)** and ventricular septum and right ventricular wall **(C)** in 30-year-old man (DCMEO# 91-5-476; patient 17) showing extensive scarring in subepicardial portion of left ventricular wall **(A and B)** and right ventricular half of ventricular septum **(C)**. Histologically lesions consisted of adipose and fibrous tissues **(D)**. (Hematoxylin & eosin stain; original magnification ×50.)

seven patients. In six patients the right ventricular half of the ventricular septum also was involved.

Idiopathic dilated cardiomyopathy (Fig. 9), **cardiomegaly of undetermined cause** (Figs. 10 and 11), **and hypoplastic right and left circumflex coronary arteries** (Fig. 12). In these nine patients the subepicardial lesions were small and consisted of areas of fibrosis and except for two patients were unassociated with a transmural scar.

DISCUSSION

This report indicates that subepicardial myocardial lesions occur in a variety of cardiac diseases.

Previous reports have described isolated cases of sarcoidosis[1] or idiopathic dilated cardiomyopathy[2] with subepicardial myocardial lesions. The occurrence of myocardial lesions at this location of the left ventricular wall has not been seen in other cardiac diseases. Myocardial lesions in the subepicardial area are rare in patients with atherosclerotic coronary artery disease. The portion of the myocardium most vulnerable to the effect of ischemia is of course the subendocardial area. The subepicardial area is relatively protected from the effect of ischemia and is

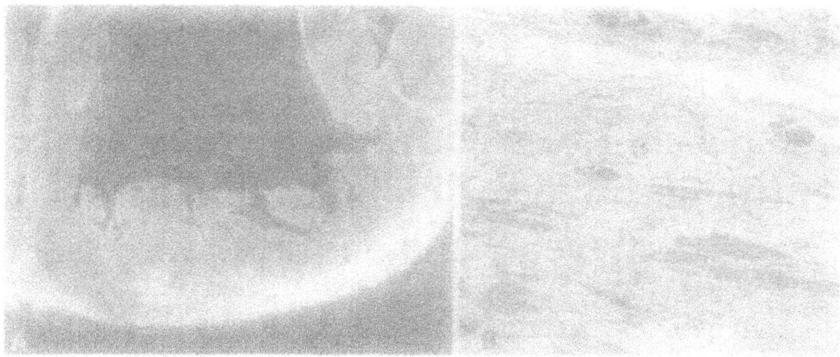

Fig. 11. Transverse section of mainly posterior wall of left ventricle **(A)** showing extensive subepicardial scarring in 56-year-old man (DCMEO# 88-01-68; patient 19) with cardiomegaly of unclear cause. Histologically subepicardial lesion consisted of adipose and fibrous tissues **(B)**. *(Hematoxylin & eosin stain; original magnification ×50.)*

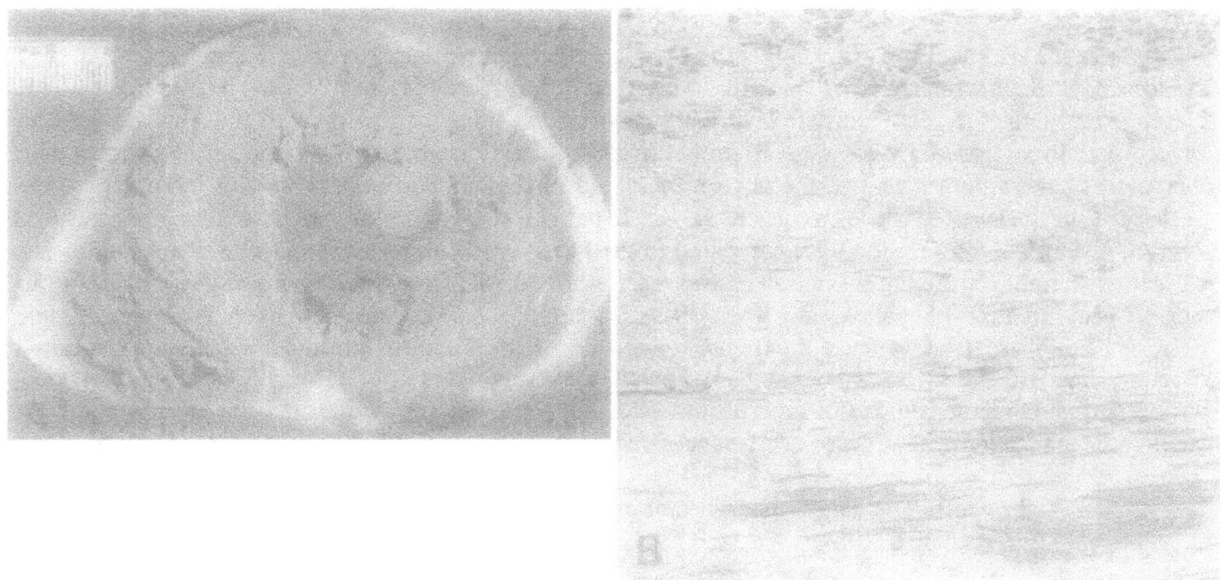

Fig. 12. Transverse section of cardiac ventricles showing subepicardial scarring in posterior segment of left ventricle **(A)** in 62-year-old man (DCVAH# 87A-54; patient 22) with hypoplastic right and left circumflex coronary arteries. Histologically lesion consists of fibrous tissue **(B)**. *(Hematoxylin & eosin stain; original magnification ×50.)*

spared in most patients with acute myocardial infarcts unless the subendocardial portion is also affected.[3]

REFERENCES

1. Roberts WC, McAllister HA, Ferrans VJ. Sarcoidosis of the heart: a clinicopathologic study of 35 necropsy patients (group I) and review of 78 previously described necropsy patients (group II). Am J Med 1977;63:86-108.
2. Roberts WC, Siegel RJ, McManus BM. Idiopathic dilated cardiomyopathy: analysis of 152 necropsy patients. Am J Cardiol 1987;60:1340-55.
3. Lee JT, Ideker RE, Reimer KA. Myocardial infarct size and location in relation to the coronary vascular bed at risk in man. Circulation 1981;64:526-34.

Effects of tissue plasminogen activator therapy on the frequency of acute right ventricular myocardial infarction associated with acute left ventricular infarction

Jay M. Kalan[a], S. David Gertz[b], Amy H. Kragel[a], Peter B. Berger[c], William C. Roberts[a] and Thomas J. Ryan[c]

[a]Pathology Branch, National Heart, Lung and Blood Institute, National Institutes of Health, Bethesda, Maryland 20892, USA, [b]Department of Anatomy and Embryology, The Hebrew University, Hadassah Medical School, Jerusalem, Israel and [c]Section of Cardiology, University Hospital, Boston University Medical Center, Boston, Massachusetts 02118, USA.

(Received 18 February 1992; revision accepted 18 September 1992)

To assess the effects of reperfusion therapy on acute right ventricular myocardial infarction, we studied at necropsy the hearts from 51 patients who died after receiving intravenous recombinant tissue plasminogen activator for acute left ventricular myocardial infarction as part of the Thrombolysis in Myocardial Infarction (TIMI) study. Right ventricular infarction occurred in none of 29 patients with infarction of the anterior wall of the left ventricle and in 8 of 22 patients (36%) with infarction of the posterior (inferior) wall of the left ventricle. Of the 22 patients with posterior wall infarction, the 8 patients with right ventricular infarction were compared to the 14 patients without right ventricular infarction. The patients with right ventricular infarction had a longer mean interval from tissue plasminogen activator infusion to peak creatine phosphokinase level (19 vs. 11 h, $P < 0.03$), a lower frequency of hemorrhagic necrosis (2 of 8 vs. 10 of 14, $P < 0.04$) and higher frequency of luminal thrombus in the infarct-related coronary artery (6 of 8 vs. 3 of 14, $P = 0.054$). Each of these findings is associated with the absence of coronary reperfusion. Thus, successful reperfusion following acute left ventricular myocardial infarction appears to be associated with a decreased frequency of concomitant right ventricular myocardial infarction.

Key words: Right ventricular infarction; Thrombolysis; Reperfusion; Coronary artery disease

---

Introduction

Necropsy studies in the pre-thrombolytic era demonstrated that acute myocardial infarction in-

Correspondence to: William C. Roberts, M.D., Chief, Pathology Branch, National Heart, Lung and Blood Institute, Building 10, Room 2N258, National Institutes of Health, Bethesda, Maryland 20892, USA.
From the Thrombolysis in Myocardial Infarction (TIMI) Trial.

volves the right ventricle in about 25% of patients having an acute left ventricular infarct [1–4]. Right ventricular infarction is nearly always limited to patients with infarction involving the posterior (inferior) left ventricular wall [3–5]. Little is known about the effect of reperfusion therapy on the morphologic characteristics of right ventricular infarction and no data are available on whether successful reperfusion alters the frequency of right ventricular infarction. To evaluate the influence of thrombolytic therapy on right ventricular infarction, we studied, at necropsy, 51 patients who died after receiving recombinant tissue plasminogen activator therapy for acute left ventricular myocardial infarction.

Materials and Methods

The patients studied all received intravenous recombinant tissue plasminogen activator after being enrolled in either the Thrombolysis in Myocardial Infarction (TIMI) I or II trial [6–7]. The 51 hearts came from 24 separate hospitals, with the largest number from any 1 hospital being 7. These represent all hearts undergoing autopsy study at the TIMI Core Pathology Laboratory at the Pathology Branch, National Heart, Lung and Blood Institute, National Institutes of Health. Clinical data were received from each submitting hospital and from the TIMI data coordinating center. The hearts were fixed in 10% formaldehyde, sectioned and examined for the presence of myocardial necrosis and fibrosis, cavity dilatation, ventricular hypertrophy and valvular abnormality. The coronary arteries were removed, decalcified and cut into 5-mm long segments. Histologic sections from each segment were stained by the Movat pentachrome technique [8]. A narrowing of greater than 75% in cross-sectional area was considered hemodynamically significant.

Of the 51 patients receiving tissue plasminogen activator for acute myocardial infarction, 29 had necrosis involving the anterior left ventricular wall and 22, the inferior (posterior) wall. Right ventricular infarction was defined as necrosis, observed grossly and confirmed histologically, of any part of the free wall of the right ventricle. None of the 29 patients with anterior wall left ventricular infarction had necrosis involving the right ventricular wall. Of the 22 patients with inferior wall left ventricular infarcts, 8 (36%) also had necrosis of a portion of the right ventricular free wall. The dominant right coronary artery was the infarct-related artery in all 8 patients with right ventricular infarcts. The 22 patients with inferior wall myocardial infarction were divided into 2 groups: 8 patients with right ventricular infarction and 14 patients without. These 22 patients comprise our study group.

A peak creatine kinase level was definable in 16 patients by measuring a post-peak value. Creatine kinase levels were obtained every 4 h for the first 24 h following enrollment in the trial and then every 6 h for the subsequent 24 h.

Composition of the atherosclerotic plaque in the infarct-related coronary artery was determined in 13 patients, who did not have angioplasty or bypass surgery, by computerized histomorphometry as described previously [9]. The percentage of the plaque consisting of cellular and acellular fibrous tissue, calcific deposits and lipid (pultaceous debris) was determined.

TABLE 1

Clinical characteristics of 22 patients dying after receiving intravenous tissue plasminogen activator therapy for inferior wall myocardial infarction as part of the Thrombolysis in Myocardial Infarction Study.

	RVMI		$P =$
	Present ($n = 8$)	Absent ($n = 14$)	
Men (%)	5 (63)	8 (57)	N.S.
Mean age (y)	58	61	N.S.
Systemic hypertension (%)	3 (38)	8 (57)	N.S.
Mean interval:			
Chest pain to death (d)	5 (mode = 2)	6 (mode = 2)	N.S.
rt-PA infusion to peak CK (h)	11	19	0.03
Mean peak CK (IU)	2933	2787	N.S.
Frequency of complete heart block	5 (63)	3 (21)	0.054
Mode of death:			
Cardiogenic shock	3	5	N.S.
Ventricular arrhythmia	2	3	N.S.
Myocardial rupture	1	4	N.S.
Bleed	1	0	N.S.
Other	1	2	N.S.

CK, creatine kinase; d, days; h, hours; IU, international units; RVMI, right ventricular myocardial infarction; y, years; N.S., not significant. Statistical significance $P < 0.05$.

Sixteen patients survived greater than 18 h after the onset of infarction (at which time necrosis can be fully defined by gross inspection). In these patients, the size of the infarct was determined by planimetry of 1-cm thick transverse slices of left ventricular wall and was expressed as the percent of total left ventricular mass that was necrotic.

Statistical analyses were performed using the Statview 512 statistical package. Analysis of noncontinuous data was performed by the χ^2, test. Continuous data were analyzed by Students t-test and coronary artery morphology data by analysis of variance where appropriate.

Results

Patients with and without right ventricular myocardial infarction had similar clinical characteristics and modes of death (Table 1). Differences were suggested in the frequency of complete heart block and in the interval from the start of the tissue plasminogen activator infusion to the peak level of serum creatine kinase. Complete heart block occurred in 5 of 8 patients with and in 3 of 14 patients without right ventricular infarcts ($P = 0.054$). The mean interval from tissue plasminogen activator infusion to peak creatine kinase level was 19 h in patients with, and 11 h in those without, right ventricular infarcts ($P = 0.03$) (Fig. 1). The mean value of the peak creatine kinase was similar in the 2 groups (2933 IU vs. 2787 IU).

No differences were observed in the mean heart weight, presence of left ventricular dilatation, presence of scar, or the size of the infarct as determined by planimetry (Table 2) (Fig. 2). Hemorrhage into necrotic myocardium (hemorrhagic infarct) occurred in 2 of 8 patients with, compared to 10 of 14 patients without, right ventricular infarcts ($P = 0.035$). Right ventricular cavity dilatation occurred in 5 of 8 patients with, compared to 2 of 14 patients without, right ventricular infarcts ($P < 0.02$). Hypertrophy of the right ventricular wall was not noted in any heart.

The number of major epicardial coronary arteries narrowed >75% in cross-sectional area at some point by atherosclerotic plaque was similar in the

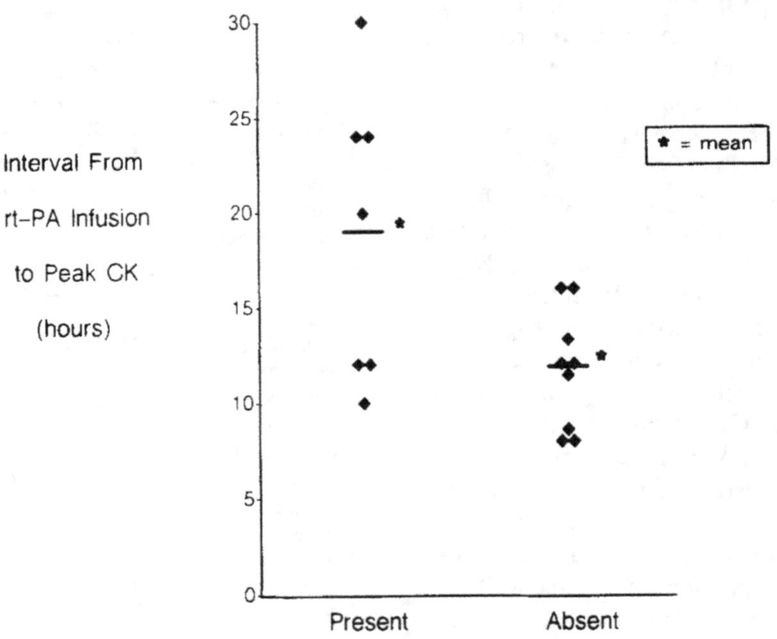

Fig. 1. Interval from intravenous infusion of tissue plasminogen activator (rt-PA) to peak creatine kinase (CK) level in 7 patients with and in 9 patients without, right ventricular myocardial infarction.

TABLE 2

Morphologic characteristics at necropsy of 22 patients dying after receiving intravenous tissue plasminogen activator therapy for inferior left ventricular wall myocardial infarction as part of the Thrombolysis in Myocardial Infarction Study

	RVMI		$P =$
	Present $(n = 8)$	Absent $(n = 14)$	
Mean heart weight (g)	438	458	N.S.
Dilated LV (%)	1 (13)	5 (36)	N.S.
Dilated RV (%)	5 (63)	2 (14)	0.02
Hemorrhagic necrosis (%)	2 (25)	10 (71)	0.035
Planimetered infarct size (% of LV weight)	26 $(n = 6)$	20 $(n = 10)$	N.S.
Myocardial fibrosis (%)	2 (25)	6 (43)	N.S.
Luminal thrombus in the IRA (%)	5 (63)	3 (21)	0.054
Mean no. CAs narrowed >75% CSA	2.1	2.9	N.S.
Mean no. (%) 5-mm segments of CA narrowed >75% CSA	10.6 (20)	15.0 (32)	0.018
Mean no (%) 5-mm segments of IRA narrowed >75% CSA	4.5 (20)	6.1 (33)	0.064

CA, coronary artery; CSA, cross-sectional area; g, grams; IRA, infarct related artery; LV, left ventricle; RV, right ventricle; RVMI, right ventricular myocardial infarction; N.S., not significant.

2 groups (mean = 2.1/4 vs. 2.9/4). Quantitative analysis of 1078 5-mm segments of coronary artery showed a mean of 11 segments per patient (20% of all segments of the 4 major epicardial arteries) narrowed >75% in cross-sectional area in the 8 patients with right ventricular infarcts compared to an average of 15 segments per patient (32%) in 14 patients without right ventricular infarcts $(P = 0.02)$ (Fig. 3). However, analysis of segments of the infarct-related artery of all patients with posterior wall left ventricular infarcts showed similar degrees of luminal narrowing between those with and those without right ventricular infarcts. The stenosis was found primarily within the proximal half of the dominant right coronary artery (20 patients) in both groups.

Thrombus in the lumen of the infarct-related coronary artery was present in 5 of 8 patients with and in 3 of 14 patients without right ventricular infarcts. The thrombi were totally occlusive in 3 of the 5 with, and in 1 of the 14 without right ventricular infarcts.

Histomorphometric analysis of the infarct-related artery by light microscopy showed no significant differences in plaque components between the two groups (Table 3) (Fig. 4). Comparisons restricted to segments narrowed >75% in cross-sectional area showed a slightly higher percentage of acellular fibrous tissue in the plaques of patients with compared to those without right ventricular infarcts (60% vs. 50%), but the amounts of the other components of the plaque were similar.

Discussion

Of the 51 patients studied, 8 (16%) had right ventricular myocardial infarcts and all were among the 22 patients with posterior (inferior) wall left ventricular infarcts. Thus, 36% of our 22 patients with inferior wall left ventricular infarcts had concomitant right ventricular infarcts. This frequency of right ventricular infarcts is comparable to that found in 3 previously reported autopsy series of patients with acute left ventricular myocardial infarcts performed before the use of thrombolytic therapy [2–4]. Thus, therapy with intravenous tissue plasminogen activator did not appear to change the frequency of right ventricular infarcts seen at autopsy.

Three observations suggest that the frequency of right ventricular infarcts is decreased in patients with morphologic and enzymologic findings suggestive of successful reperfusion. Firstly, a shortened interval from myocardial infarction to peak creatine kinase level has been shown to be a marker for reperfusion [10–12]. In this study, a longer mean interval from the time of infusion of tissue plasminogen activator to peak creatine kinase level was found in patients with posterior

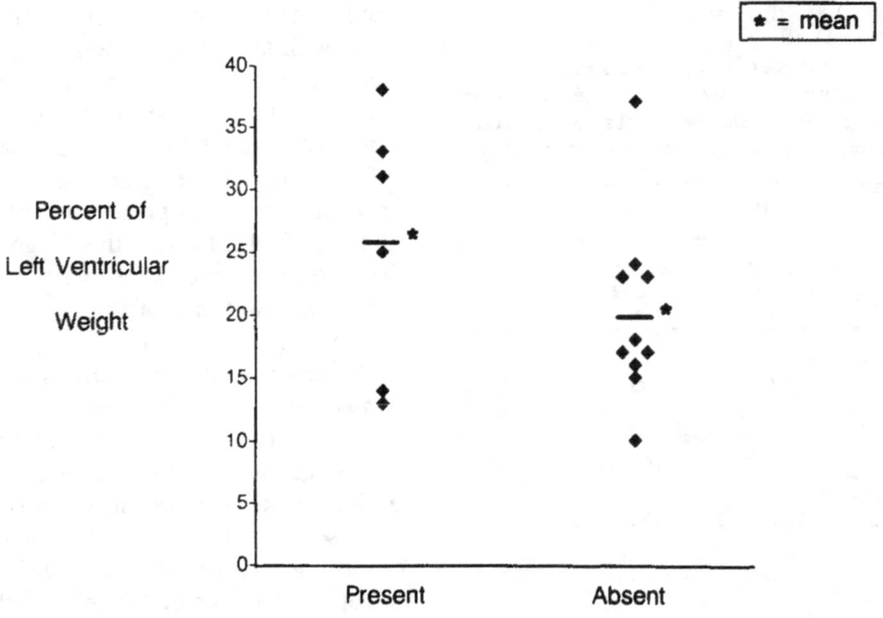

Fig. 2.   Left ventricular infarct size by planimetry in 6 patients with and in 10 patients without right ventricular myocardial infarcts.

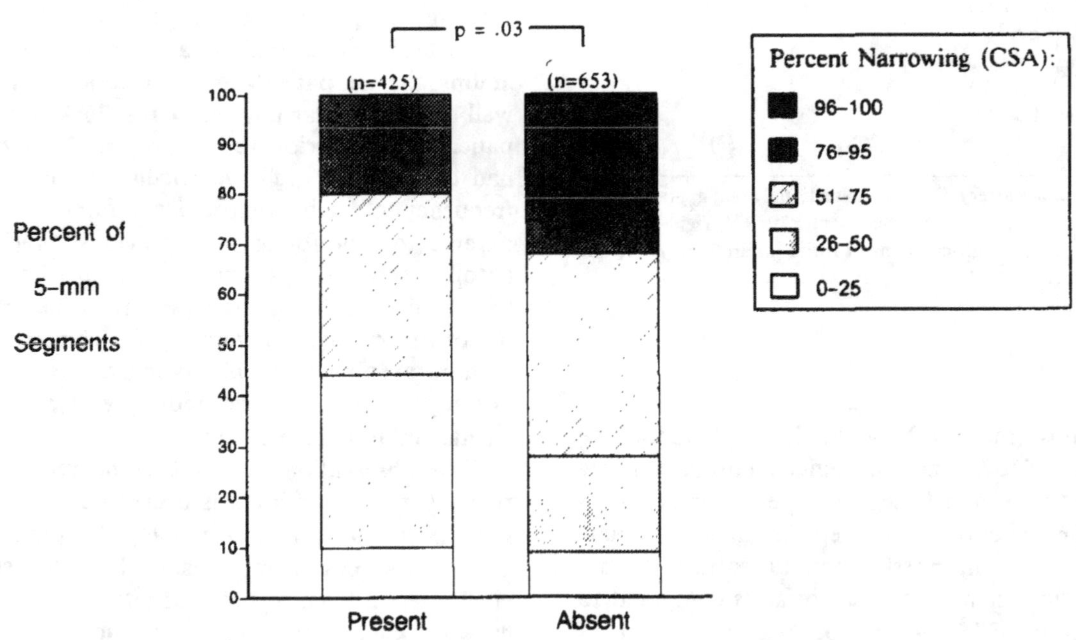

Fig. 3.   Percent of 5-mm segments of coronary artery narrowed to various degrees in a cross-sectional area (CSA) by atherosclerotic plaque in 8 patients with and in 14 patients without right ventricular myocardial infarcts.

TABLE 3

Composition of atherosclerotic plaque in the infarct related coronary artery in 7 patients with and 6 patients without right ventricular myocardial infarcts.

| | Right ventricular myocardial infarction | | | | | |
| | All Segments | | | Only segments narrowed >75% CSA | | |
	Present ($n = 154$)	Absent ($n = 118$)	$P =$	Present ($n = 36$)	Absent ($n = 34$)	$P =$
Acellular fibrous tissue	0.65	0.58	N.S.	0.60	0.50	0.02
Cellular fibrous tissue	0.17	0.16	N.S.	0.12	0.13	N.S.
Calcium deposits	0.07	0.14	N.S.	0.08	0.15	N.S.
Pultaceous debris (lipid)	0.08	0.09	N.S.	0.17	0.15	N.S.

CSA, cross-sectional area; N.S., not significant. Statistical significance defined as $P < 0.05$.

wall left ventricular infarcts associated with right ventricular infarcts than those with posterior wall infarcts alone (19 h vs. 11 h, $P < 0.03$). Although peak creatine kinase level was available in only 16 of the 22 patients, this sample was sufficient to identify statistically significant differences between these groups. Three patients with right ventricular infarcts had intervals to peak creatine kinase which were shorter than the mean. While the possibility of partial or total reperfusion cannot be

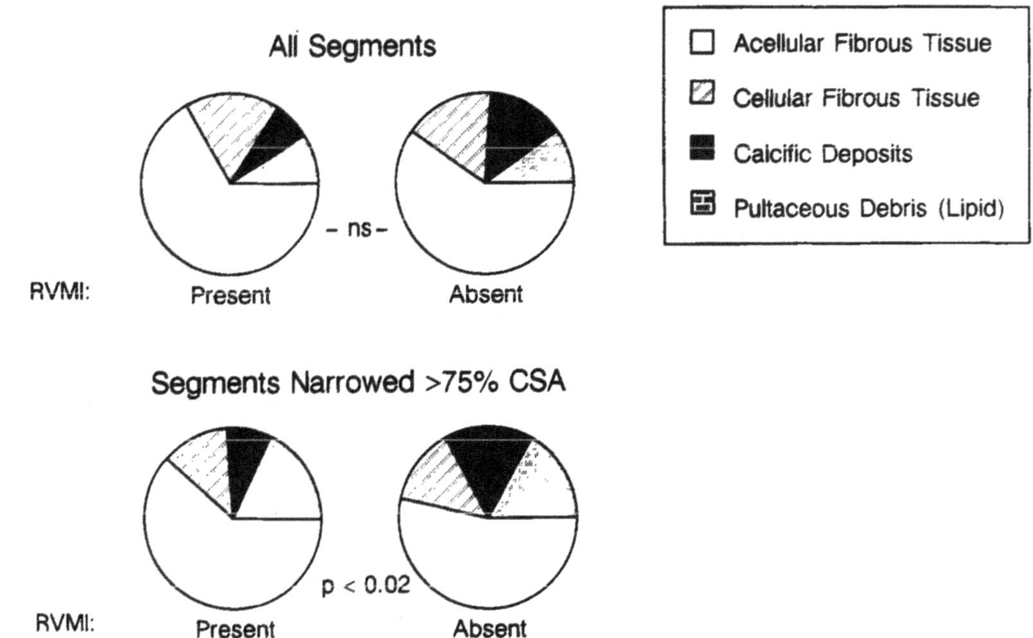

Fig. 4. Composition of atherosclerotic plaque in the infarct-related coronary artery from 7 patients with and from 6 patients without right ventricular myocardial infarction.

excluded, it is likely that this is a reflection of smaller infarct size as depicted in Fig. 2. Secondly, hemorrhagic infarction [13,14], which is thought to be a manifestation of myocardial reperfusion following a period of ischemic injury to the myocardial capillaries, was less common (than non-hemorrhagic infarcts) in patients with right ventricular infarcts than in patients with infarcts of the posterior wall of the left ventricle (not associated with the right ventricular infarction) (2 of 8 [25%] vs. 10 of 14 [71%], $P = 0.035$). Lastly, the frequency of luminal thrombi at necropsy in the infarct-related coronary artery appeared greater in patients with right ventricular infarction than those without (5 of 8 [63%] vs. 3 of 14 [21%], $P = 0.054$).

A lower frequency of right ventricular myocardial infarction after successful reperfusion is supported by angiographic data from the TIMI II trial. Berger et al. reported on 524 patients randomly assigned to cardiac catheterization 18–48 h following infarction [15]. Patients with right ventricular infarction, as diagnosed by right ventricular wall motion abnormalities on radionuclide angiogram, had a higher frequency of persistent occlusion of the infarct-related artery, defined as TIMI grade 0 or 1 flow, than did patients without right ventricular infarction. Of 31 patients with right ventricular infarction, 15 (48%) had persistent occlusion, compared to 67 of 493 patients (14%) without right ventricular infarction ($P < 0.001$).

No significant differences were found in the degrees of luminal narrowing of the infarct-related artery of patients with, and those without, right ventricular infarction. In fact, the number of coronary arteries per patient which were severely narrowed (>75% luminal cross-sectional area narrowing at some point) was similar between those with and those without right ventricular infarction and the percent of 5-mm long segments of all 4 major coronary arteries narrowed >75% in cross-sectional area was actually somewhat lower in the patients with right ventricular infarction ($P = 0.03$). Very proximal location of stenosis within the dominant right coronary artery has been reported to be associated with right ventricular myocardial infarction [16], but this finding

was noted equally in both of our groups. No difference was found in the presence or extent of stenosis in the left anterior descending coronary artery. The presence of left anterior descending stenosis has been reported to be more common in patients with inferior wall left ventricular infarction complicated by right ventricular infarction than in those without right ventricular infarction [17]. Finally, the morphology of the atherosclerotic plaque of the infarct-related coronary artery was not significantly different in patients with and without right ventricular infarction.

Although treatment with intravenous recombinant tissue plasminogen activator does not appear to influence the frequency of right ventricular infarction as seen at autopsy, keeping in mind the limitations of not having confirmatory angiographic data, this study reports a decrease in the frequency of right ventricular infarction in patients with morphologic and biochemical evidence of successful reperfusion. Since patients with inferior wall left ventricular infarction complicated by right ventricular infarction are believed to be at increased risk [18], these findings may explain, at least in part, the improved prognosis of patients with inferior wall infarction treated with thrombolytic therapy.

References

1 Wartman WB, Hellerstein HK. The incidence of heart disease in 2,000 consecutive autopsies. Annals Intern Med 1948;28:41–65.

2 Erhardt LR. Clinical and pathological observations in different types of acute myocardial infarction. A study of 84 patients deceased after treatment in a coronary care unit. Acta Med Scand 1974;560(Suppl 560):7–78.

3 Isner JM, Roberts WC. Right ventricular infarction complicating left ventricular infarction secondary to coronary heart disease. Frequency, location, associated findings and significance, from analysis of 236 necropsy patients with acute or healed myocardial infarction. Am J Cardiol 1978;42:885–894.

4 Ratliff NB, Hackel DB. Combined right and left ventricular infarction. Pathogenesis and clinicopathologic correlations. Am J Cardiol 1980;45:217–221.

5 Cabin HS, Clubb KS, Wackers FJT, Zaret BL. Right ventricular myocardial infarction with anterior wall left ventricular infarction. An autopsy study. Am Heart J 1987;113:16–22.

6 The TIMI Study Group. Comparison of invasive and conservative strategies after treatment with intravenous tissue

plasminogen activator in acute myocardial infarctions. Results of the Thrombolysis in Myocardial Infarction (TIMI) Phase II Trial. New Engl J Med 1989;320:618–627.

7 The TIMI Research Group. Immediate vs. delayed catheterization and angioplasty following thrombolytic therapy for acute myocardial infarction. TIMI 11A Results. J Am Med Assoc 1988;260:2849–2858.

8 Movat MZ. Demonstration of all connective tissue elements in a single section. Arch Pathol 1985;60:289–295.

9 Kragel AH, Reddy SG, Wittes JT, Roberts WC. Morphometric analysis of the composition of atherosclerotic plaques of the 4 major epicardial coronary arteries in acute myocardial infarction and in sudden coronary death. Circulation 1989;80:1747–1756.

10 Vatner SF, Baig H, Manders WT, Maroko PR. Effects of coronary artery reperfusion on myocardial infarct size calculated from creatine kinase. J Clin Invest 1978;61:1048–1056.

11 Mathey DG, Kuck K, Tilsner V, Krebber H, Bleifeld W. Nonsurgical coronary artery recanalization in acute transmural myocardial infarction. Circulation 1981;63:489–497.

12 Gore JM, Roberts R, Ball SP, Montero A, Goldberg RJ, Dalen JE. Peak creatine kinase as a measure of effectiveness of thrombolytic therapy in acute myocardial infarction. Am J Cardiol 1987;59:1234–1238.

13 Higginson LAJ, White F, Heggtveit HA, Sanders TM, Bloor CM, Covell JW. Determinants of myocardial hemorrhage after coronary reperfusion in the anesthetized dog. Circulation 1982;65:62–69.

14 Gertz S.D., Kalan JM, Kragel AH, Roberts WC, Braunwald E and the TIMI Investigators. Cardiac morphologic findings in patients with acute myocardial infarction treated with recombinant tissue plasminogen activator. Am J Cardiol 1990;65:953–961.

15 Berger PB, Ruocco NA Jr, Timm TC, Zaret BL, Wackers FJT, Ryan TJ. The impact of thrombolytic therapy on right ventricular infarction complicating inferior myocardial infarction. Results from TIMI II. Circulation;80(Suppl II):II-313.

16 Anderson HR, Falk E, Nielson D. Right ventricular infarction. Frequency, size and topography in coronary artery disease. A prospective study comprising 107 consecutive autopsies from a coronary care unit. J Am Coll Cardiol 1987;10:1223–1232.

17 Haupt HM, Hutchins GM, Moore GW. Right ventricular infarction. Role of the moderator band in determining infarct size. Circulation 1983;67:1268–1272.

18 Berger PB, Ryan TJ. Inferior myocardial infarction. High-risk subgroups. Circulation 1990;81:401–411.

Out-of-Hospital Sudden Death from Left Ventricular Free Wall Rupture During Acute Myocardial Infarction as the First and Only Manifestation of Atherosclerotic Coronary Artery Disease

Jamshid Shirani, MD,* Katherine Berezowski, MD,† and William C. Roberts, MD‡

From the Pathology Branch, National Heart, Lung, and Blood Institute, National Institutes of Health, Bethesda, Maryland 20892. Manuscript received May 4, 1993, and accepted June 12.

*Present address: Department of Medicine, Division of Cardiology, Medical College of Virginia, Box 128, MCV Station, Richmond, Virginia, 23298-0128.

†Present address: Department of Pathology, Medical College of Virginia, MCV Station, Richmond, Virginia 23298-0128.

‡Present address: Baylor Cardiovascular Institute, Baylor University Medical Center, 3500 Gaston Avenue, Dallas, Texas 75246.

Rupture of the left ventricular (LV) free wall is a frequent complication of acute myocardial infarction (AMI). It most often occurs 4 to 7 days after hospitalization in patients with their first AMI. Sudden out-of-hospital death from LV free wall rupture during AMI in patients with no apparent previous symptoms of myocardial ischemia is unusual. We describe certain clinical and cardiac morphologic findings in 12 such patients, and compare findings in them with those in 226 patients with in-hospital fatal cardiac rupture during AMI.

Of 226 patients with a fatal cardiac rupture during AMI studied at the Pathology Branch, National Heart, Lung, and Blood Institute from January 1968 to February 1993, 137 (61%) had isolated LV free wall rupture (Table I), and 12 of them are the subjects of this report. All 12 patients died suddenly outside a hospital, and in

TABLE I Ages, Sexes, and Sites of Cardiac Rupture During Acute Myocardial Infarction (AMI) in 226 Patients

	Number of Patients	Age (years)	Men (%): Women (%)	Location of AMI		
				Anterior	Posterior	Lateral
Rupture of the:						
Left ventricular free wall	137	46–94 (66)	62 (45%):75 (55%)	62 (45%)	51 (37%)	24 (18%)
Ventricular septum	52	43–90 (66)	32 (62%):20 (38%)	20 (38%)	29 (56%)	3 (6)
Papillary muscle	27	45–80 (63)	17 (63%):10 (37%)	5 (19%)	18 (67%)	4 (14%)
Double rupture*	8	58–75 (67)	5 (63%):3 (37)	1 (12%)	7 (88%)	0
Triple rupture*	1	81	1	0	1	0
Right ventricular free wall	1	89	0	0	1	0
Total	226	43–94 (mean 66)	117 (52%):108 (48%)	88 (39%)	107 (47%)	31 (14%)

*Simultaneous rupture of the left ventricular free wall and ventricular septum (double rupture) and right ventricular free wall (triple rupture).

TABLE II Clinical and Cardiac Morphologic Findings in 12 Patients Who Died or Collapsed Suddenly Outside the Hospital

Patient	Age (years)	Race	Sex	SH	DM	Place of Death	HW (g)	Heart Floated in Water	A	P	L	Number of CAs >75% ↓ in CSA by Plaque	LM	LAD	LC	R	Infarct Size (1–3+)
1	50	W	M	0	0	Work	470	—	0	0	+	2	0	0	+	+	+
2	64	B	M	+	0	Work	500	0	0	0	+	3	0	+	+	+	+
3	66	B	M	0	0	Street	510	—	+	0	0	2	0	+	0	+	+++
4	70	W	M	0	0	Home	390	0	0	0	+	3	0	+	+	+	+
5	73	W	M	0	0	Garage	340	0	0	0	+	3	0	+	+	+	+
Subtotal	(65)			1	0		(440)	—	1	1	3	(2.6)	0	4	4	5	(1.4+)
6	58	W	F	0	+	Home	400	0	0	0	+	3	0	+	+	+	+
7	61	W	F	0	0	ER*	345	+	+	0	0	1	0	0	+	0	+
8	64	W	F	+	+	Street	520	+	0	0	+	1	0	+	0	0	+
9	68	B	F	+	0	Home	330	—	+	0	0	1	0	+	0	0	+
10	69	W	F	+	+	Home	345	+	0	0	+	1	0	0	+	+	+
11	74	W	F	0	0	Home	310	+	0	0	+	2	0	0	+	0	+
12	79	W	F	+	0	Home	475	0	+	0	0	1	0	0	+	0	+++
Subtotal	(68)			4	3		(390)	4	3	0	4	(1.4)	0	3	5	2	(1.3+)
Total	(66)			5	3		(410)	4/8	4	1	7	(1.9)	0	7	9	7	(1.3+)

*Collapsed at home and was brought to emergency room (ER) where she died <90 minutes after arrival. AMI was not considered during life.
A = anterior; AMI = acute myocardial infarct; B = black; CA = coronary artery; CSA = cross-sectional area; DM = diabetes mellitus; F = female; HW = heart weight; L = lateral; LAD = left anterior descending; LC = left circumflex; LM = left main; M = male; P = posterior; R = right; SH = systemic hypertension; W = white; 0 = absent or negative; + = present or positive; — = no information available.

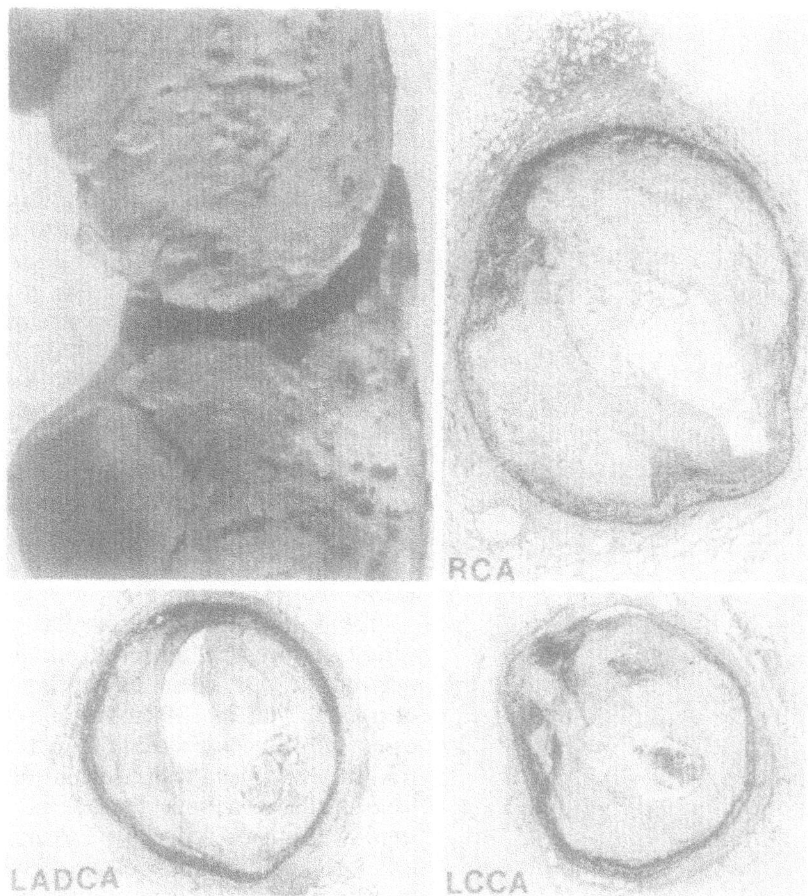

FIGURE 1. Heart of a 64-year-old black man (patient 2, DCMEO#80-8-683) who was found dead in the storage room of the building in which he worked. The left ventricular free wall had ruptured at the site of a small lateral wall myocardial infarct *(top left)*. The right (RCA), left anterior descending (LADCA) and left circumflex (LCCA) coronary arteries each show significant reduction in cross-sectional area by atherosclerotic plaque at the sites of maximal luminal narrowing. Thrombus is present inside the lumen of the left circumflex coronary artery (i.e., infarct-related coronary artery). (Movat stain ×15; reduced by 28%.)

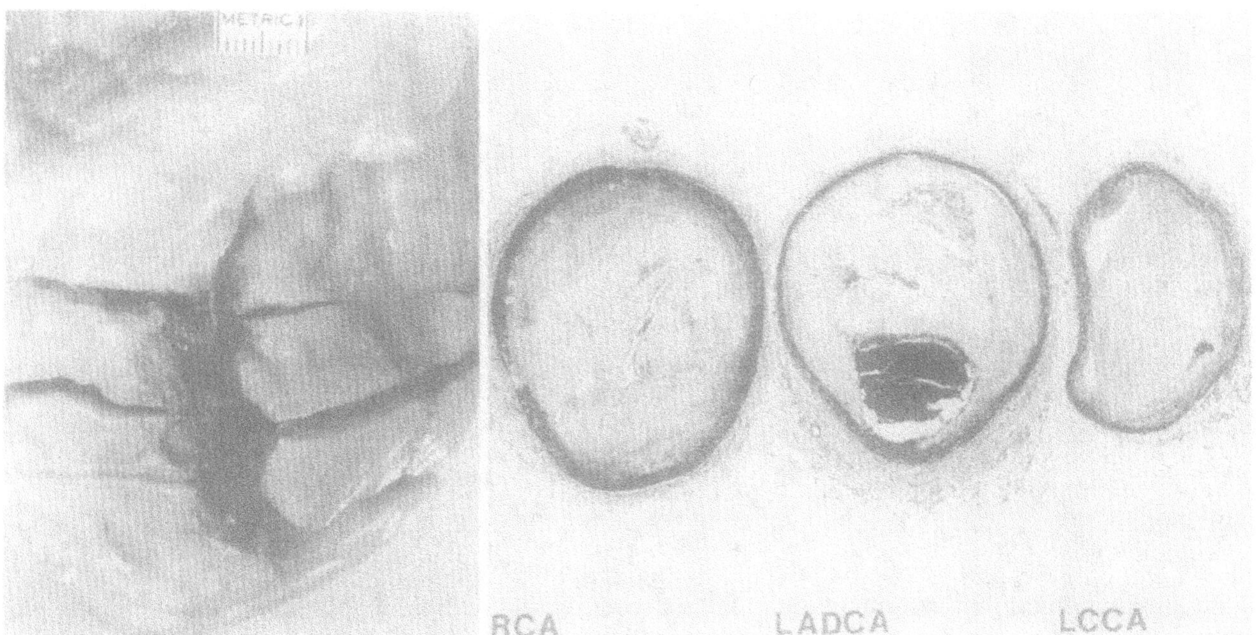

FIGURE 2. Heart of a 66-year-old white man (patient 3, CMH#A84-5) who died suddenly on the street without any premonitory symptoms. Rupture of the free wall occurred through the left ventricular anterior wall *(left)*. The amount of epicardial adipose tissue is increased. The lumens of the right (RCA) and left anterior descending (LADCA) coronary arteries are narrowed >75% in cross-sectional area, and that of the left circumflex coronary artery (LCCA) is narrowed 51 to 75% at the site of maximal obstruction. An adherent thrombus is seen in the lumen of the left anterior descending coronary artery (i.e., infarct-related artery). (Movat stain ×16; reduced by 24%.)

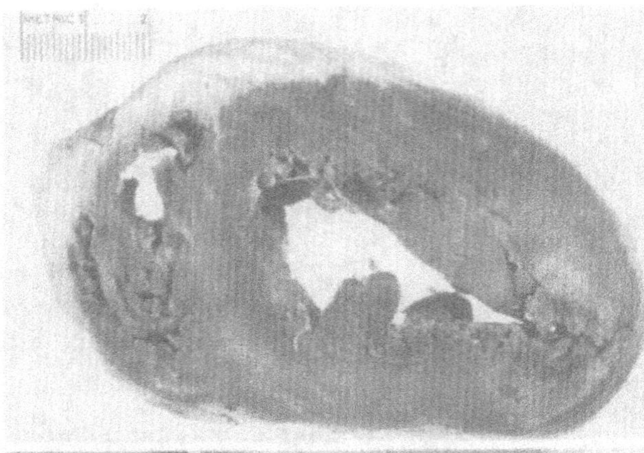

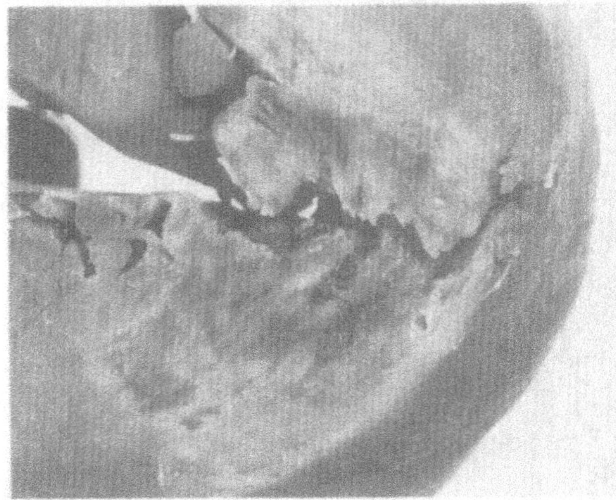

FIGURE 3. Heart of a 73-year-old white man (patient 5, DCMEO#88-6-575) who died suddenly while wiping the windshield of his car outside a shopping center. Transmural left ventricular free wall rupture occurred through a small lateral wall infarct *(top)*, a close-up of which is shown at the *bottom.*

them, rupture was the first and only manifestation of atherosclerotic coronary artery disease. Certain clinical and cardiac morphologic findings in these 12 patients are listed in Table II and shown in Figures 1 to 6. The LV free wall had ruptured into the pericardial cavity in all patients, and hemopericardium was present in each case. A mean 1.9 major epicardial (left main, left anterior descending, left circumflex and right) coronary arteries were narrowed >75% in cross-sectional area by atherosclerotic plaque. Men had a higher number of significantly narrowed coronary arteries than did women (mean 2.6 vs 1.4; p <0.05). In 8 patients, the 4 major epicardial coronary arteries were excised and cut in 5 mm segments, and 1 Movat-stained section of each segment was then examined (Table III). Of the total of 433 five mm segments of the coronary arteries examined, 63 (15%) showed cross-sectional area narrowing >75% by atherosclerotic plaque. Three patients (numbers 3, 7 and 11) had a thrombus in the infarct-related artery.

The number of major epicardial coronary arteries severely narrowed by atherosclerotic plaque (by gross or microscopic visualization) differs among various subsets of patients with fatal atherosclerotic coronary artery disease.[1] Of patients who die of AMI, those with rupture (LV free wall, ventricular septum or papillary muscle) have smaller mean infarct sizes[2] and a lower number of significantly narrowed major epicardial coronary arteries[3–5] than do a nonrupture subset. Whereas a mean 2.5 major epicardial coronary arteries were narrowed in 50 patients who died of AMI without rupture (Table IV; group III), in the 137 who died of AMI with rupture (Table IV; groups I and II), only a mean 1.9 major epicardial coronary arteries were significantly narrowed (p <0.05). Comparison of the 2 groups with rupture (Table

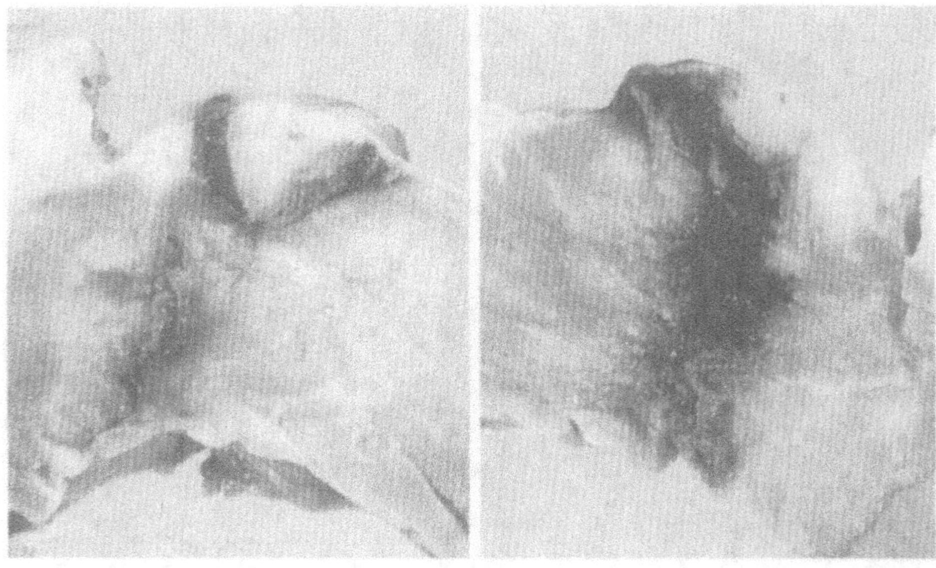

FIGURE 4. Heart of a 61-year-old white woman (patient 7, MVH#12-92A) who collapsed at home, was transferred to emergency room in shock and died <90 minutes later. At necropsy, the myocardial infarct was small and confined to the most basal portion of the anterior wall of the left ventricle. Photograph of 2 adjacent (1 cm apart) transverse sections of the left ventricular anterior wall showing the site of rupture.

IV; groups I and II) showed that patients who died suddenly outside a hospital and in whom no apparent previous symptoms or signs of myocardial ischemia were known often had small lateral wall infarcts (7 of 12). There was no other significant difference between the 2 groups.

1. Roberts WC, Potkin BN, Solus DE, Reddy SG. Mode of death, frequency of healed and acute myocardial infarction, number of major epicardial coronary arteries severely narrowed by atherosclerotic plaque, and heart weight in fatal atherosclerotic coronary artery disease: analysis of 889 patients studied at necropsy. *J Am Coll Cardiol* 1990;15:196–203.
2. Saffitz JE, Fredrickson RC, Roberts WC. Relation of size of transmural myocardial infarct to mode of death, interval between infarction and death and frequency of coronary arterial thrombus. *Am J Cardiol* 1986;57:1249–1254.

TABLE III Quantitative Morphologic Analysis of the Four Major Epicardial Coronary Arteries in Eight Patients Who Died Suddenly of Left Ventricular Free Wall Rupture as the First Manifestation of Atherosclerotic Coronary Artery Disease

	Number of 5 mm Segments					% CSA Narrowing by Plaque					Number (%) of 5 mm Segments >75% ↓ in CSA	CA Thrombus	CAs >75% ↓ in CSA by Plaque				Number of CAs >75% ↓ in CSA by Plaque
Patient	Total	LM	LAD	LC	R	0–25	26–50	51–75	76–95	96–100			LM	LA	LC	R	
1	48	3	16	7	22	2	29	12	3	2	5 (10%)	0	0	0	+	+	2
2	74	2	31	18	23	2	15	45	11	1	12 (16%)	0	0	+	+	+	3
3	69	2	29	18	20	7	6	30	23	3	26 (38%)	+	0	+	0	+	2
5	44	1	11	9	23	6	4	25	8	1	9 (20%)	0	0	+	+	+	3
7	43	1	13	11	18	14	10	14	5	0	5 (12%)	+	0	0	+	0	1
8	55	2	18	8	27	22	18	14	1	0	1 (2%)	0	0	+	0	0	1
11	40	—	11	8	21	18	6	12	3	1	4 (10%)	+	0	0	+	+	2
12	60	—	13	14	33	10	23	26	1	0	1 (2%)	0	0	0	+	0	1
Total	433	11	142	93	187	81 (19%)	111 (25%)	178 (41%)	55 (13%)	8 (2%)	63 (15%)	3	0	5	6	4	(1.9)

Abbreviations as in Table II.

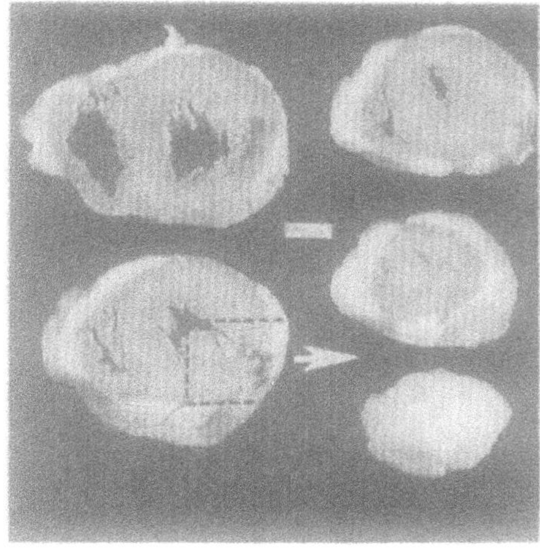
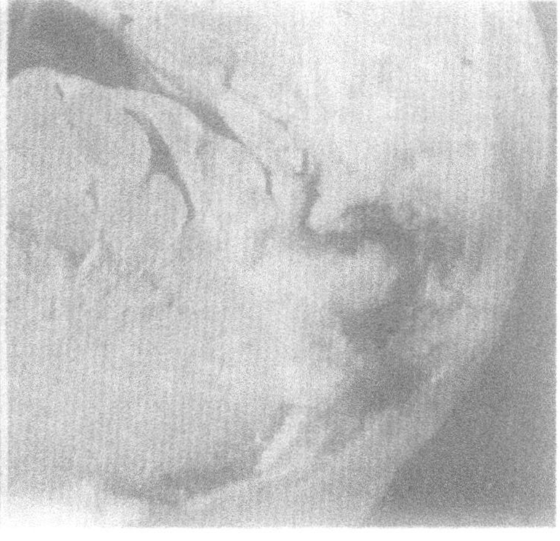

FIGURE 5. Heart of a 64-year-old white woman (patient 8, DCMEO#92-2-184) who was found dead on the sidewalk of a street. *Left,* transverse sections through the ventricular cavities showing excess epicardial fat and rupture through a small lateral wall infarct. *Right,* close-up view of the infarct area shown on the left (broken lines).

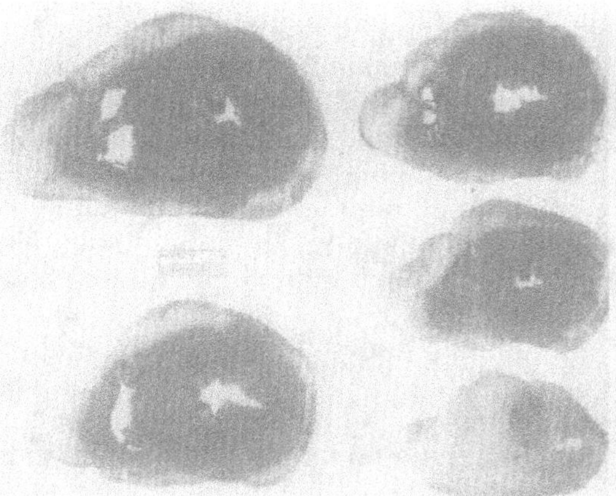
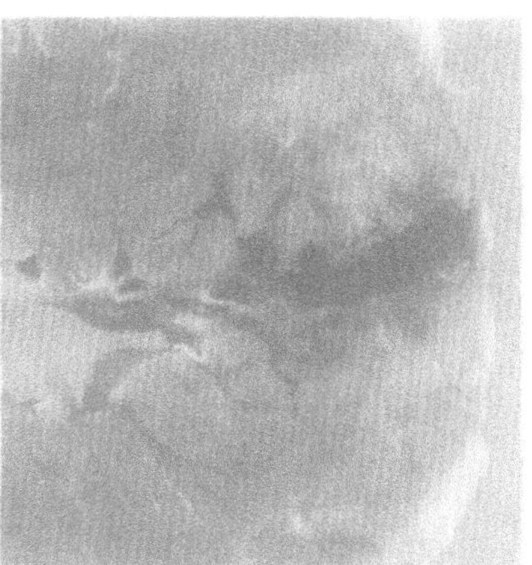

FIGURE 6. Heart of a 69-year-old woman (patient 10, SH A82-20) who collapsed and died at home. Transverse sections of cardiac ventricles showing excess epicardial fat *(left),* and close-up view of the site of rupture through the lateral left ventricular wall *(right).*

TABLE IV Comparison of the Clinical and Cardiac Morphologic Findings in Patients with Acute Myocardial Infarction, and With and Without Left Ventricular Free Wall Rupture

| | AMI With Rupture | | AMI Without Rupture[3,4] |
Group	I	II	III
Number of patients	12	125	50
Mean age (years)			
Men	65 ± 6	61 ± 8	63 ± 11
Women	68 ± 7	70 ± 9	71 ± 16
Men:women	5 (42%):7 (58%)	60 (48%):65 (52%)	32 (64%):18 (36%)
Systemic hypertension	5 (42%)	70 (56%)	26 (52%)
Angina pectoris	0	17 (14%)	11 (22%)
Mean heart weight (g)			
Men	440 ± 46*	475 ± 82	526 ± 102
Women	390 ± 35	404 ± 75	432 ± 115
Location of LV AMI			
Anterior	4 (33%)	58 (46%)	29 (58%)
Posterior	1 (9%)	50 (40%)	20 (40%)
Lateral	7 (58%)	17 (14%)	1 (26%)
Number of major epicardial CAs ↓ >75% by plaque			
0	0	4 (3%)	1 (2%)
1	5 (42%)	53 (42%)	7 (14%)
2	3 (25%)	26 (21%)	12 (24%)
3	4 (33%)	33 (26%)	28 (56%)
4	0	9 (8%)	2 (4%)
Mean number of CAs ↓ >75% by plaque	1.9*	1.9*	2.5

*p <0.05 compared with group III.
AMI = acute myocardial infarction; CAs = coronary arteries; LV = left ventricular.

3. Mann JM, Roberts WC. Rupture of left ventricular free wall during acute myocardial infarction: analysis of 138 necropsy patients and comparison with 50 necropsy patients with acute myocardial infarction without rupture. *Am J Cardiol* 1988;62:847–859.

4. Mann JM, Roberts WC. Acquired ventricular septal defect during acute myocardial infarction: analysis of 38 unoperated necropsy patients and comparison with 50 unoperated necropsy patients without rupture. *Am J Cardiol* 1988;62:8–19.

5. Barbour DJ, Roberts WC. Rupture of a left ventricular papillary muscle during acute myocardial infarction: analysis of 22 necropsy cases. *J Am Coll Cardiol* 1986;8:558–565.

Status of the Major Epicardial Coronary Arteries at Necropsy in Paraplegia and Quadriplegia

Jamshid Shirani, MD,* and William C. Roberts, MD†

To study the possible effects of physical inactivity on the extent of coronary artery atherosclerosis, we examined at necropsy the hearts of 10 patients with paraplegia or quadriplegia. Such a study has not been reported previously.

From March 1979 to August 1991, the hearts of 13 patients with paraplegia (n = 11) or quadriplegia (n = 2 patients) were submitted to the Pathology Branch of the National Heart, Lung, and Blood Institute. Three of 11 patients with paraplegia were excluded because either paralysis occurred gradually rather than suddenly (n = 2) or symptomatic myocardial ischemia was present before the onset of paralysis (n = 1). The remaining 10 patients are the subjects of this study; cer-

tain clinicopathologic findings in them are listed in Table I. The paralysis was caused by gunshot wounds to the spinal cord in 7 of 10 patients, by spinal cord injury in an automobile accident in 1, and by fall in another. The remaining patient had an embolus to a spinal cord artery during mitral valve replacement for rheumatic mitral stenosis. The duration of paralysis ranged from 6 months to 47 years (mean 17 years). Systemic hypertension was present in 2 patients; none had diabetes mellitus. Only 1 patient (number 8) died of a cardiac cause; this man, 58 years old at time of death, had congestive heart failure after a silent myocardial infarct 1 year before death. Two patients died of stroke: 1 (number 7) had systemic hypertension, and the other (number 6) had mitral valve replacement, 14 years before death, for mitral stenosis. The other 7 patients died of noncardiovascular causes. None of the 10 patients was known to be a "wheelchair athlete."

Heart weight ranged from 300 to 770 g (mean 515) in men and from 215 to 565 g (mean 335) in women, and was increased in 3 of 10 patients (>350 g in women, and >400 g in men). Healed myocardial infarcts were present in 2 patients (numbers 2 and 7), and

From the Pathology Branch, National Heart, Lung, and Blood Institute, National Institutes of Health, Bethesda, Maryland 20892. Manuscript received May 4, 1993, and accepted June 12.

*Present address: Division of Cardiology, Medical College of Virginia, Box 128, MCV Station, Richmond, Virginia 23298-0128.

†Present address: Baylor Cardiovascular Institute, Baylor University Medical Center, 3500 Gaston Avenue, Dallas, Texas 75246.

TABLE I Clinical and Cardiac Morphologic Findings in 10 Patients with Paraplegia or Quadriplegia

Patient	Age (years)	Race	Sex	Type and Duration (years) of Paralysis	Clinical AP	AMI	CHF	SH	DM	Arrhythmia*	Cause of Death	HW (g)	LV Fi	N
1	22	B	M	P 0.5	0	0	0	0	0	0	PE	390	0	0
2	31	B	M	P 8	0	0	0	0	0	0	Opiate overdose	300	+	0
3	37	B	F	P 7	0	0	0	0	0	0	Infection	305	0	0
4	42	B	M	P 20	0	0	0	0	0	0	Alcoholism	360	0	0
5	47	B	F	Q 0.9	0	0	0	0	0	0	Cancer	325	0	0
6	54	W	F	P 14	0	0	+	0	0	+	Stroke	565	0	0
7	58	W	M	P 36	0	0	0	+	0	+	Stroke	760	0	0
8	58	B	M	P 38	0	+	+	+	0	+	CHF	770	+	0
9	61	B	F	P 47	0	0	0	0	0	0	Cancer	215	0	0
10	73	W	F	Q 1.3	0	0	0	0	0	0	Infection	265	0	0
Totals or (mean)	(48)	7B	5M	(17.3)	0	1	2	2	0	3		(men 515) vs (women 335)	2	0

TABLE I (continued)

Patient	Dilated (0–3+) RV	LV	MAC	Number of Major Epicardial CAs >75% ↓ in CSA by Plaque	CA <75% ↓ in CSA by Plaque LM	LAD	LC	R	Total	Number of 5 mm Segments of Epicardial CAs by % CSA Narrowing 0–25	26–50	51–75	76–95	96–100
1	++	+	0	0	0	0	0	0	51	49	2	0	0	0
2	+	+	0	1	0	+	0	0	54	34	11	6	3	0
3	0	0	0	0	0	0	0	0	42	42	0	0	0	0
4	+	++	0	0	0	0	+	0	43	36	7	0	0	0
5	+	0	0	1	0	0	0	+	56	55	1	0	0	0
6	0	0	0	1	0	0	0	+	43	35	4	2	2	0
7	++	++	0	0	0	0	0	0	83	46	27	10	0	0
8	++	+++	+	3	0	+	+	+	65	2	24	35	4	0
9	0	0	0	0	0	0	0	0	51	44	7	0	0	0
10	0	0	0	0	0	0	0	0	32	31	1	0	0	0
Totals or (mean)	6	5	1	(0.5)	0	2	1	2	520	374 (72%)	84 (16%)	53 (10%)	9 (2%)	0

*Atrial arrhythmias only; no patient had ventricular arrhythmias.
AMI = acute myocardial infarct; AP = angina pectoris; B = black; CA = coronary artery; CHF = congestive heart failure; CSA = cross-sectional area; DM = diabetes mellitus; F = female; Fi = fibrosis; HW = heart weight; LAD = left anterior descending; LC = left circumflex; LM = left main; LV = left ventricle; M = male; MAC = mitral annular calcium; N = necrosis; P = paraplegia; PE = pulmonary embolism; Q = quadriplegia; R = right; RV = right ventricle; SH = systemic hypertension; W = white.

none had acute myocardial infarcts at necropsy. One patient (number 7) had mitral annular calcium. The 4 major epicardial (left main, left anterior descending, left circumflex and right) coronary arteries were excised, cut transversely at approximately 5 mm intervals, stained with Movat, and studied microscopically to determine the degree of luminal narrowing by atherosclerotic plaque. Of the resulting 520 five mm segments, none were narrowed 96 to 100%, 9 (2%) were narrowed 76 to 95%, 53 (10%) were narrowed 51 to 75%, 84 (16%) were narrowed 26 to 50%, and 374 (72%) were narrowed ≤25% in cross-sectional area.

If physical activity alone is an important factor in prevention of coronary atherosclerosis, considerable coronary artery narrowing might be expected in patients with paraplegia or quadriplegia over many years. This was not the case in the patients discussed herein. Even in 1 patient (number 9) with paraplegia for 47 years, none of the 51 five mm segments of the major epicardial coronary arteries were narrowed >50%.

In summary, adults with paraplegia or quadriplegia for many years may have minimal degrees of coronary arterial luminal narrowing by atherosclerotic plaques.

Coronary arteries in unstable angina pectoris, acute myocardial infarction, and sudden coronary death

William C. Roberts, MD, Amy H. Kragel, MD, S. David Gertz, MD, PhD, and Charles S. Roberts, MD *Bethesda, Md., and Dallas, Texas*

This article reviews and compares coronary arterial findings in patients with fatal unstable angina pectoris (UAP), acute myocardial infarction (AMI), and sudden coronary death (SCD).

AMOUNTS OF CORONARY ARTERIAL LUMINAL NARROWING IN THE THREE CORONARY SUBSETS

The amount of coronary arterial narrowing observed at autopsy in patients with UAP, AMI, and SCD is generally enormous.[1] As shown in Table I, from a study of 80 patients at autopsy with these three coronary events (SCD in 31, AMI in 27, and UAP in 22), an average of 2.9 of the four major (right, left main, left anterior descending, and left circumflex) coronary arteries were severely (>75% decrease in cross-sectional area) narrowed at some points, and no significant differences were observed among the three coronary subsets.[1] Patients with UAP had a much higher frequency of severe narrowing of the left main coronary artery (10 of 22 patients [45%]) compared with those with AMI (3 of 27 patients [11%]) and SCD (3 of 31 patients [10%]).

A more sophisticated approach to determining degrees of luminal narrowing is to examine the entire lengths of the four major epicardial coronary arteries. One technique involves incising each of the four major coronary arteries transversely at 5 mm intervals and then preparing a histologic section from each 5

mm segment. Normally the total length of the four major arteries is approximately 27 cm (right = 10 mm, left main = 1 mm, left anterior descending = 10 mm, and left circumflex = 6 mm), and thus approximately 55 five-mm long segments are available for examination from each heart. Results of studies that used this approach in patients with UAP, AMI, and SCD are summarized in Table II.[1] Of the 4016 five-mm segments studied in the 80 patients, 38% were narrowed 76% to 100% in cross-sectional area by plaque alone (control 3%), 34% were narrowed 51% to 75% (control 3%), 34% were narrowed 51% to 75% (control 22%), 20% were narrowed 26% to 50% (control 44%), and only 7% were narrowed 25% or less (control 31%). Similar degrees of narrowing by plaque alone in all four categories of narrowing were observed in the groups with AMI and SCD; patients with UAP had significantly more severe coronary narrowing than the other two groups.

Thus, in general, patients with fatal UAP have more extensive severe narrowing by plaque alone of the four major epicardial coronary arteries than patients with either AMI or SCD, and patients with UAP compared with the other two groups have a significantly higher frequency of severe narrowing of the left main coronary artery.

COMPOSITION OF CORONARY ATHEROSCLEROTIC PLAQUES IN THE THREE CORONARY SUBSETS

Until recently[2, 3] no detailed information was available concerning the composition of atherosclerotic plaques in the epicardial coronary arteries of patients with fatal coronary events. Kragel et al.,[2, 3] with the use of a computerized morphometry system, traced the various components of atherosclerotic plaques in histologic sections prepared from 1438 five-mm segments of the four major epicardial coronary arteries in 37 patients with fatal coronary artery disease

From the Pathology Branch, National Heart, Lung, and Blood Institute, National Institutes of Health; and the Baylor Cardiovascular Institute, Baylor University Medical Center.

Received for publication Sept. 16, 1993; accepted Nov. 1, 1993.

Reprint requests: William C. Roberts, MD, Baylor Cardiovascular Institute, Baylor University Medical Center, 3500 Gaston Ave., Dallas, TX 75246.

AM HEART J 1994;127:1588-93.

Table I. Number of major (right, left main, left anterior descending, and left circumflex) coronary arteries narrowed >75% in cross-sectional area by atherosclerotic plaques in fatal coronary artery disease

Coronary event	Patients (n)	Mean age (yr)	Number of 4 arteries/patient >75% narrowed in CSA by plaque				
			4	3	2	1	Mean
Sudden coronary death	31	47	3	20	6	2	2.8
Acute myocardial infarction	27	59	3	14	10	0	2.7
Unstable angina pectoris	22	48	10	8	3	1	3.2
TOTAL	80	51	16 (20%)	42 (52%)	19 (24%)	3 (4%)	2.9
Control	40	52	0 (0)	5 (5%)	12 (13%)	21 (23%)	0.7

CSA, Cross-sectional area.

Table II. Amount of cross-sectional area narrowing in each 5 mm segment of the four major (right, left main, left anterior descending, and left circumflex) epicardial coronary arteries by atherosclerotic plaques in subjects with fatal coronary artery disease

Subgroup	Patients (n)	Mean age (yr)	Number of 5 mm segments	Percentage of segments narrowed				
				0%-25%	25%-50%	51%-75%	76%-100%	Mean score
Sudden coronary death	31	47	1564	7%	23%	34%	36%	2.98
Acute myocardial infarction	27	59	1403	5%	23%	38%	34%	3.01
Unstable angina pectoris	22	48	1049	11%	12%	29%	48%	3.12
TOTAL	80	51	4016	7%	20%	34%	38%	3.02
Control	40	52	1849	31%	44%	22%	3%	1.97

Table III. Mean composition of coronary arterial atherosclerotic plaques in the four major epicardial coronary arteries

Components of plaque	Mean percentage of plaques containing various components in the major coronary arteries (1438 segments)		
	Unstable angina pectoris (n = 10)	Acute myocardial infarction (n = 15)	Sudden coronary death (n = 12)
Dense fibrous tissue	35	46	29
Loose fibrous tissue	1	3	3
Cellular fibrous tissue	52	32	50
Calcium	4	4	8
Pultaceous debris	4	8	4
Foam cells	0	1	0
Foam cells and lymphocytes	3	4	6
Inflammatory infiltrates without significant number of foam cells	1	2	1

(UAP in 10, AMI in 15, and SCD in 12 patients). The results are summarized in Table III. The dominant component of the coronary atherosclerotic plaques in all three subsets of patients was fibrous tissue, comprising about 80% of the plaques in each subset; extracellular lipid (pultaceous debris) and calcium each made up approximately 5% of the plaques, and several miscellaneous components comprised the remainder of the plaques. The cellular component of the fibrous tissue occupied a larger portion of plaque in the patients with UAP and SCD, and the acellular (dense) component of fibrous tissue occupied a larger portion of the plaque in the group with AMI. In all three subsets the amount of dense fibrous tissue in-

Table IV. Frequency of acute coronary lesions and multiluminal channels at autopsy in patients with unstable angina pectoris, sudden coronary death, and acute myocardial infarction

		Coronary arteries			
Coronary subset	*Number of patients*	Thrombus	Plaque rupture	Plaque hemorrhage	Multiluminal channels
Unstable angina pectoris	14	4 (29%)*	5 (36%)*	3 (21%)*	14 (100%)
Sudden coronary death	21	6 (29%)*	4 (19%)*	4 (19%)*	17 (81%)
Acute mycardial infarction	32	22 (69%)†	24 (75%)†	20 (63%)†	29 (90%)
Total	67	32 (48%)	33 (49%)	27 (40%)	60 (90%)

*Versus † in same verticle column = $p < 0.02$.

creased as plaque size increased (or a lumen size decreased), and the amount of cellular fibrous tissue decreased as plaque size increased.

FREQUENCY AND TYPES OF ACUTE LESIONS IN THE MAJOR CORONARY ARTERIES IN THE THREE CORONARY SUBSETS

In recent years considerable effort has been directed toward understanding the acute coronary events that may be responsible for the development of UAP, AMI, and SCD. From angiographic, angioscopic, and autopsy studies it has been speculated that plaque rupture and hemorrhage with overlying intraluminal thrombus, which are the acute lesions usually responsible for AMI, are also responsible for UAP and possibly SCD. Kragel et al.[4] examined 3101 five-mm segments of 268 epicardial coronary arteries from 67 patients with fatal coronary events (UAP in 14, AMI in 31, and SCD in 21 patients). The results of these detailed studies are summarized in Table IV. The frequency of *intraluminal thrombus* was similar in the groups with UAP and SCD (29% in each) and significantly lower than that in the group with AMI (69%). The thrombus was nonocclusive in all patients with UAP and in five of six patients with SCD but was nonocclusive in only 4 of 22 patients with AMI. The composition of the nonocclusive and occlusive thrombi also was different—that is, the nonocclusive thrombus consisted mainly of platelets and the occlusive thrombus mainly of fibrin. Of the 32 patients with thrombus, plaque rupture was found in association with thrombus in 17 (53%): in none of the four with UAP, in two of six with SCD, and in 15 (83%) of 22 with AMI. Among the 15 patients with thrombus unassociated with plaque rupture, hemorrhage into the plaque at the site of thrombus was found in seven: in three of four patients with UAP, in two of six with SCD, and in 2 of 32 with AMI.

Plaque rupture was found in 33 (49%) of 67 patients. Its frequency was insignificantly different in the groups with UAP (36% [5 of 14] and SCD (19%

[4 of 21]): in both groups the frequency was significantly lower than in the group with AMI (75% [24 of 32]).

Plaque hemorrhage was observed in 27 (40%) of 67 patients, and its frequency was significantly lower in the groups with UAP (21% [3 of 14]) and SCD (19% [4 of 21]) compared with that in the group with AMI (63% [20 of 32]). Plaque hemorrhage was associated with plaque rupture or intraluminal thrombus in 20 (74%) of 27 patients with plaque hemorrhage: in 4 of 14 with unstable angina, in 4 of 21 with sudden death, and in 13 of 32 with acute infarction.

Multiple small vascular channels were present in 60 (90%) of 67 patients and with an insignificantly different frequency in each of the three groups of patients (Table I). The frequency of multiluminal channels in each 5 mm long segment of coronary artery was significantly higher in the group with UAP (12% [66 of 572]) than in either the SCD (7% [72 of 999]) or the AMI group (7% [107 of 1530]).

Thus comparison of findings from examination of a histologic section from each of 3101 five-mm segments of 268 major epicardial coronary arteries from 67 patients with fatal coronary artery disease disclosed that the frequency of three acute coronary lesions (intraluminal thrombus, plaque rupture, and plaque hemorrhage) was similar in patients with UAP and SCD and that the frequency of each of these acute lesions was significantly higher in patients with a fatal first transmural AMI. Furthermore, although multiluminal channels (not acute lesions) within plaques were frequent in all three groups of patients, these lesions were found significantly more often in 5 mm segments of coronary arteries in the group with UAP than in the groups with SCD and AMI where the frequency was similar.

Several angiographic studies[5-9] have identified either intraluminal filling defects consistent with thrombus or specific morphologic lesions (eccentric narrowings with irregular borders) in patients with UAP, and these defects have been used to distinguish such patients from those with stable angina. Comparison of postmortem angiographic and histologic findings,[10] however, in patients with coronary artery disease (not necessarily UAP) has shown that these irregular eccentric lesions may represent not only sites of intraluminal thrombus but also plaque rupture, plaque hemorrhage, or organized thrombus. In addition, three angioscopic studies[11-13] have identified intraluminal thrombus and ulceration or rupture of plaque in patients with UAP. On the basis of these studies, it has been widely speculated that the lesion responsible for the development of UAP is an ulcerated plaque over which nonocclusive intraluminal thrombus develops.

Before accepting that this hypothesis is indeed true for all or most patients with UAP, the limitations of the previous studies[5-13] need to be considered. Interpretation of the significance of the eccentric irregular lesions seen angiographically in patients with UAP is based largely on the work of Levin and Fallon,[10] who compared postmortem coronary anteriograms and histologic sections of coronary artery narrowings in 39 patients who died either after coronary artery bypass surgery or of consequences of AMI. (Because the trauma of bypass surgery may be associated with plaque rupture or plaque hemorrhage or both, patients who had undergone this procedure were excluded from the study of Kragel et al.[4] Levin and Fallon[10] identified 38 narrowings that had irregular borders or intraluminal lucencies by angiography. Of these, eight (21%) were acute or organizing nonocclusive thrombi overlying atherosclerotic plaque, six (16%) were nonocclusive thrombi overlying sites of plaque rupture or hemorrhage, 10 (26%) were sites of plaque hemorrhage or rupture without thrombus, six (16%) contained recanalized thrombus (presumably multiluminal channels), and 21% showed narrowing of the segment by plaque without any complicating acute lesion. More than a third of the irregular eccentric lesions studied, therefore, showed no acute lesion that would account for the abrupt change in symptoms in the setting of UAP. In the study by Kragel et al.,[4] plaques containing multiluminal channels, although common to all three groups of patients, were seen with the greatest frequency in the group with UAP.

When interpreting results of angiographic or angioscopic studies in patients with UAP, it is assumed that these patients did not have left ventricular necrosis (AMI) at the time of study, an assumption that may or may not be true. Guthrie et al.[14] studied 12 patients with UAP who died shortly after coronary artery bypass surgery. At autopsy 4 of the 12 patients had AMI that histologically appeared to have oc-

curred before the operation, and AMI was not suspected clinically in any of the four patients. Therefore when studying living patients it may be difficult to determine whether the patients have pure UAP or a combination of UAP and AMI.

Information regarding coronary artery morphology in patients with UAP is scant, difficult to obtain, and difficult to interpret for several reasons. UAP is rarely fatal, and those patients who do die during the period of UAP usually have had coronary angioplasty or a bypass procedure performed or have had an AMI shortly before death. In patients with AMI preceded by UAP, intracoronary lesions may not be representative of those occurring in patients with UAP not complicated by AMI.

Information regarding acute coronary lesions in patients who died shortly after coronary artery bypass surgery has been provided in several studies. Guthrie et al.[14] described 12 patients and Roberts and Virmani[15] described 19 patients with UAP who died shortly after coronary bypass surgery. In both studies the frequency of intraluminal thrombus was low (8% and 12%, respectively) when patients with AMI were excluded. In a separate report Virmani and Roberts[16] described the frequency of extravasated erythrocytes and fibrin in the plaque of 17 of 22 patients with UAP. Plaque hemorrhage (erythrocytes with or without fibrin) was identified in 94% of their patients. It is likely that surgical manipulation of the epicardial coronary arteries was responsible for the plaque hemorrhage in many of these patients.

In a study of UAP with fatal outcome, Falk[17] provided information regarding the frequency of acute lesions in the epicardial coronary arteries of patients with SCD, UAP, and AMI. He described autopsy findings in "… 25 patients, all of whom died of acute coronary thrombosis within 24 hours after the onset of acute symptoms." Of the 24 patients for whom clinical information was available, 15 clearly had UAP, two had an equivocal history of UAP, and seven did not have UAP. Of these 25 patients, 15 had coagulative necrosis (AMI), which as determined histologically was compatible with an age of less than 24 hours. In these patients he described lamellar thrombi (21 of 25 patients, including 14 of 15 with UAP), 81% of which were associated with plaque rupture and hemorrhage. Neither the frequency of plaque rupture nor the number of thrombotic episodes differed between patients with and without UAP. Because all of these patients died suddenly (some with UAP and some with UAP complicated by AMI), the three ischemic syndromes cannot be analyzed individually.

Davies et al.[18] studied 90 patients who died suddenly outside the hospital within 6 hours of the on-

Table V. Mean cross-sectional area of the right, left anterior descending, and left circumflex coronary arteries and heart weight, age, and sex in three coronary subsets and in two groups of control subjects

Coronary subsets and control subjects	No. of patients	Male Female	Age (yr)	Heart weight (gm)	Mean cross-sectional area (mm^2) of right, LAD, and LC coronary arteries
Range (mean)	Range (mean)	Range (mean)			
Unstable angina pectoris	20	12	37-59	240-520	2.7-13.1
		8	(49)	(386)	(6.0)
Acute myocardial infarction	23	17	33-82	310-720	3.6-11.9
		6	(58)	(482)	(7.6)
Sudden coronary death	19	17	28-85	300-670	5.2-14.9
		2	(54)	(459)	(7.7)
Cancer	31	17	26-74	135-470	2.0-9.1
		14	(51)	(309)	(5.0)
Aortic valve disease	15	13	34-81	550-1050	7.1-14.9
		2	(56)	(730)	(906)

LAD, Left anterior descending; *LC*, left circumflex.

set of pain "or other symptoms." The data were presented in a report entitled, "Intramyocardial platelet aggregation in patients with unstable angina suffering sudden ischemic cardiac death." Of their 90 patients, 36 (40%) had chest or arm pain at some time in the 2 weeks preceding death. The history of chest pain was obtained by a coroner's police officer from the next of kin who had been living with the patient. Thus the history was not obtained from the patient or by a physician. None of the 90 patients had been admitted to a hospital with increasing chest pain. There was no information on any patient regarding the presence or absence of chest pain at rest. Thus in none of the 90 patients was the type, location, or severity of the pain known. Nevertheless, these patients were considered to have had UAP. Autopsies in the 90 patients disclosed the following: 31 (30%) had nonocclusive intracoronary thrombus, 22 (24%) had SCD associated with "regional coagulative necrosis" (AMI), and 23 (25%) had nontransmural necrosis. Of the 36 patients with chest or arm pain at some time in the 2 weeks before death, 35 had plaque rupture identified in one of the major epicardial coronary arteries. Of the 54 patients without chest pain in the 2 weeks before death, 51 had plaque rupture. Thus whether the patients in that study had UAP is unknown. Some probably did have UAP, but some clearly had AMI and most would have fulfilled most investigators' definitions of SCD. Diagnosing UAP in persons not admitted to the hospital, whose history was obtained by a nonphysician, is difficult to say the least.

Multiluminal vascular channels were present in 90% of the 67 patients studied by Kragel et al.[4] Most likely they represented organized thrombus (the consequence of a previous nonfatal thrombotic event) and were usually at a site where the lumen was severely narrowed by plaque. Multiluminal channels were observed in a significantly higher percentage of the 5 mm coronary segments in the patients with UAP compared with those with either SCD or AMI.

The lower frequency of plaque rupture and occlusive thrombus in the groups with UAP and SCD compared with the frequency in the group with AMI may be a reflection of differences in plaque composition among these groups. Likewise the similarity in the frequency of these acute coronary lesions in patients with UAP and SCD may be a reflection of the similarity in plaque composition in these two groups. As described earlier, in all three types of patients the mean percentage of dense fibrous tissue, calcific deposits, and pultaceous debris increased with increasing degrees of luminal narrowing, and the mean percentage of cellular fibrous tissue decreased. Severely narrowed segments in the group with AMI (those narrowed >75% in cross-sectional area) contained significantly more pultaceous debris and significantly less calcium and cellular fibrous tissue than similarly narrowed segments in the groups with UAP and SCD. Because occlusive thrombus is seen almost exclusively in association with rupture of a lipid-rich plaque, the greater the amount of pultaceous debris, the greater the frequency of plaque rupture and occlusive thrombus.

The characteristic lesion in patients with a fatal first AMI, then, is an occlusive thrombus overlying a ruptured plaque rich in pultaceous debris; in patients with UAP it is a severely narrowed segment frequently containing multiluminal channels with or without a small nonocclusive thrombus; in patients with SCD without left ventricular necrosis it is a segment of coronary artery with significant luminal narrowing by atherosclerotic plaque with or without platelet-rich nonocclusive thrombus. Thus the frequency of acute coronary lesions (intraluminal thrombus, plaque rupture, and plaque hemorrhage) in patients with UAP (not complicated by AMI) and SCD (not complicated by AMI) is similar, and the frequency of these lesions is significantly lower than that observed in patients with AMI.

SIZES OF THE CORONARY ARTERIES IN THE THREE CORONARY SUBSETS

The amount of blood that can flow down an artery is dependent on many factors including the degree of cross-sectional area narrowing and the size of the artery. A large artery and a small artery can be similarly narrowed in cross-sectional area, and yet the area through which blood can flow in the large artery obviously is greater than the area through which blood can flow in the smaller artery. At autopsy Roberts and Roberts[19] measured by videoplanimetry the area enclosed by internal elastic membrane in the proximal 1 cm of the right, left anterior descending, and left circumflex coronary arteries in 20 patients with UAP, 23 with AMI, and 19 with SCD. The results are summarized in Table V. The patients with UAP had the smallest coronary arteries (mean cross-sectional area of each of the 60 arteries 6.0 mm^2) and the smallest hearts (mean weight 386 gm). The patients with AMI and SCD had similar-sized coronary arteries (mean area 7.6 mm^2) and similar-sized hearts (mean weight 471 gm). The 31 control subjects with fatal cancer and normal or nearly normal-sized hearts (mean weight 309 gm) had the smallest coronary arteries (mean area 5.0 mm^2). The 16 control subjects with aortic valve disease had the largest hearts (mean weight 730 gm) and the largest coronary arteries (mean area 9.6 mm^2).

Thus significant ($p < 0.001$) differences are observed in the mean cross-sectional areas of the three major epicardial coronary arteries between patients with UAP and patients with either AMI or SCD. These differences result primarily from differences in heart weight. The anatomic determinant of myocardial oxygenation, therefore, is cross-sectional area narrowing, because the size of the epicardial coronary arteries is proportional to heart weight.

REFERENCES

1. Roberts WC. Qualitative and quantitative comparison of amounts of narrowing by atherosclerotic plaques in the major epicardial coronary arteries at necropsy in sudden death, transmural acute myocardial infarction, transmural healed myocardial infarction and unstable angina pectoris. Am J Cardiol 1989;64:324-8.
2. Kragel AH, Reddy SG, Wittes JT, Roberts WC. Morphometric analysis of the composition of atherosclerotic plaques in the four major epicardial coronary arteries in acute myocardial infarction and in sudden coronary death. Circulation 1989;80:1747-56.
3. Kragel AH, Reddy SG, Wittes JT, Roberts WC. Morphometric analysis of the composition of coronary arterial plaques in isolated unstable angina pectoris with pain at rest. Am J Cardiol 1990;66:562-7.
4. Kragel AH, Gertz SD, Roberts WC. Morphologic comparison of frequency and types of acute lesions in the major epicardial coronary arteries in unstable angina pectoris, sudden coronary death and acute myocardial infarction. J Am Coll Cardiol 1991;18:801-8.
5. Cowley JM, DiSciasco G, Rehr RB, Vetrovec GW. Angiographic observations and clinical relevance of coronary thrombus in unstable angina pectoris. Am J Cardiol 1989;63:108E-13E.
6. Gotoh K, Minamino T, Katoh O, Hamano Y, Fukui S, Hori M, Kusuoka H, Mishima M, Inoue M, Kamada T. The role of intracoronary thrombus in unstable angina: angiographic assessment and thrombolytic therapy during ongoing anginal attacks. Circulation 1988;77:526-34.
7. Ambrose JA, Winters SL, Stern A, Eng A, Teichholz LE, Gorlin R, Fuster V. Angiographic morphology and the pathogenesis of unstable angina pectoris. J Am Coll Cardiol 1985;5:609-16.
8. Vetrovec GW, Leinbach RC, Gold HK, Cowley MD. Intracoronary thrombolysis in syndromes of unstable ischemia: angiographic and clinical results. AM HEART J 1982;104:946-52.
9. Holmes DR, Hartzler GO, Smith HC, Fuster V. Coronary artery thrombosis in patients with unstable angina. Br Heart J 1981;45:411-6.
10. Levin DC, Fallon JT. Significance of the angiographic morphology of localized coronary stenoses: histopathologic correlations. Circulation 1982;66:316-20.
11. Hombach V, Hoher M, Kochs M, Eggeling T, Schmidt A, Hopp HW, Hilger HH. Pathophysiology of unstable angina pectoris: correlations with angioscopic imaging. Eur Heart J 1988;9(suppl N):40-5.
12. Forrester JS, Litvack F, Grundfest W. A perspective of coronary disease seen through the arteries of living man. Circulation 1987;75:505-13.
13. Sherman CT, Litvack F, Grundfest W, Lee M, Hickey A, Chaux A, Kass R, Blanche C, Matloff J, Morgenstern L, Ganz W, Swan HJC, Forrester J. Coronary angioscopy in patients with unstable angina pectoris. N Engl J Med 1986;315:913-9.
14. Guthrie RB, Vlodaver Z, Nicoloff DM, Edwards JE. Pathology of stable and unstable angina pectoris. Circulation 1975;51:1059-63.
15. Roberts WC, Virmani R. Quantification of coronary arterial narrowing in clinically isolated unstable angina pectoris: an analysis of 22 necropsy patients. Am J Med 1979;67:792-9.
16. Virmani R, Roberts WC. Extravasated erythrocytes, iron, and fibrin in atherosclerotic plaques in coronary arteries in fatal coronary heart disease and their relation to intraluminal thrombus: frequency and significance in 57 necropsy patients and in 2958 five-mm segments of 224 major epicardial coronary arteries. AM HEART J 1983;105:788-97.
17. Falk E. Unstable angina with fatal outcome: dynamic coronary thrombosis leading to infarction and/or sudden death. Circulation 1985;71:699-708.
18. Davies MJ, Thomas AC, Knapman PA, Hangartner JR. Intramyocardial platelet aggregation in patients with unstable angina suffering sudden ischemic cardiac death. Circulation 1986;73:418-27.
19. Roberts CS, Roberts WC. Cross-sectional area of the maximal portions of the three major epicardial coronary arteries in 98 necropsy patients with different coronary events. Relationship to heart weight, age and sex. Circulation 1980;62:953-9.

Radiation-induced cardiovascular disease including stenosis of coronary ostium, coronary and carotid arteries, and aortic valve

Leigh Anne C. Harvey, MD, *Pathology Resident*; Samuel J. DeMaio, MD, *Cardiology Division*; and William C. Roberts, MD, *Baylor Cardiovascular Institute*

Clinical and necropsy findings are described in a 42-year-old man who received mediastinal irradiation (about 40 Gy) for Hodgkin's disease when he was 24 years old. He subsequently developed virtually every cardiovascular manifestation of radiation heart disease, including constrictive pericardial disease, complete occlusion of the ostium of a coronary artery, severe narrowing of the right coronary artery and of both carotid arteries, complete heart block (infranodal), hemodynamically confirmed aortic valve stenosis, and transmural right ventricular infarction.

Before the 1940s, the heart was considered a "radio-resistant" organ. With the introduction of megavoltage radiotherapy for treatment of neoplasms, it became apparent that the heart could indeed be damaged by high-dose radiation, and numerous reports have documented such damage. The portion of the heart most frequently affected is the pericardium, the visceral and parietal aspects of which may eventually become thickened and adherent and cause myocardial constriction (1–4). The coronary arteries reside in the subepicardial adipose tissue; their lumens may be narrowed by atherosclerotic plaques, the development of which is greatly accelerated by irradiation. The myocardial wall frequently contains an increased amount of fibrous tissue, but usually no grossly visible myocardial lesions are seen in patients with radiation heart disease. Mural and valvular endocardium typically is focally thickened by fibrous tissue (4). Because the thickening is focal, the valvular involvement generally does not cause valvular dysfunction; if dysfunction does occur, it usually is pure regurgitation. Recently, we studied a man at necropsy who had received large-dose mediastinal irradiation 18 years earlier and 17 years later had hemodynamically demonstrated aortic valve stenosis, complete occlusion of a coronary ostium, coronary and carotid arterial stenosis, and other evidences of radiation-induced damage to vascular structures. A description of the extensive damage in this patient is the purpose of this report.

CASE DESCRIPTION

W.P., a 42-year-old white man who died on May 17, 1993, was well until age 24 years (1975) when he was found to have Hodgkin's disease, stage IA, with large supraclavicular and mediastinal lymph nodes. Following splenectomy he received approximately 40 Gy of irradiation to the upper mediastinum, lower neck, and axillary areas ("upper mantle"). At age 29 (1980), he developed clinical evidence of constrictive pericardial disease and underwent "total" pericardiectomy. The symptoms of cardiac dysfunction were relieved by this procedure.

He was then well until age 40 (April 1991, 25 months before death) when he developed respiratory symptoms, and pulmonary function tests disclosed evidence of both restrictive and obstructive pulmonary disease. During the next 2 years, he also had recurring acute pulmonary infections (cytomegalovirus, *Pseudomonas*) and pleural effusions. In April 1992, he had the first of several episodes of syncope. Examination in August 1992 disclosed a grade 3/6 harsh systolic murmur and a grade 2/6 blowing diastolic murmur over the precordium, loudest in the basal area. Echocardiogram disclosed thickening of the cusps of both mitral and aortic valves with poor mobility of the aortic valve cusps. Electrocardiogram showed sinus rhythm and complete right bundle branch block and later, complete heart block.

Cardiac catheterization on September 30, 1992, disclosed the following pressures in mm Hg: pulmonary artery, 19/10; right ventricle, 23/3; right atrium, mean 9; pulmonary arterial wedge, mean 6; left ventricle, 124/13; and aorta, 87/52, yielding on pullback of the catheter a peak systolic pressure gradient of 37 mm Hg between the left ventricle and aorta. The calculated aortic valve area was 1.2 cm^2 and the valve index, 0.59 cm^2/m^2. By left ventriculogram, the ejection fraction was 64%. Injection of contrast material into the left main coronary artery disclosed no narrowing of this artery or of the left anterior descending or left circumflex arteries The ostium of the right coronary artery could not be cannulated.

On October 1, 1992, an electrophysiologic study disclosed atrioventricular nodal block distal to the atrioventricular bundle. Wenckebach block occurred at atrial pacing with a cycle length of 490 milliseconds, and 2:1 block occurred at a cycle length of 470 milliseconds. Extra stimuli in the right ventricular outflow tract readily induced sustained monomorphic ventricular tachycardia that was easily terminated by burst pacing. An automatic pacer cardioverter-defibrillator was implanted.

The patient returned home and was treated daily with furosemide and enalapril. He remained in satisfactory condition until early May 1993, when a pacemaker lead was noted to have fractured. Following insertion of a new lead 7 days before death, he developed recurrent and progressive pulmonary insufficiency, his heart rate slowed, and he was found unresponsive in electromechanical dissociation.

Between September 28 and November 3, 1992, the serum total cholesterol was measured on at least 6 different occasions and ranged from 66 to 164 mg/dL (mean 121, median 129).

MORPHOLOGIC FINDINGS

At necropsy, the pleural spaces contained large, loculated effusions; the lungs were focally but extensively fibrotic; and histologic sections were compatible with chronic radiation pneumonitis. The epicardium was adherent by fibrous tissue to the surrounding structures. The heart weighed 420 g. Both atria were moderately dilated, and both ventricles were mildly dilated. The leaflets of all 4 cardiac valves were thickened by fibrous tissue, the mitral and aortic valves far more than the right-sided valves, and both left-sided valves also contained calcific deposits. The aortic valve cusps contained heavy calcific deposits on their aortic aspects; 1 cusp was made totally immobile by the deposits and was fixed in a ventricular diastolic position, and the mobility of the other 2 cusps also was limited (*Figure 1*). The adventitia of the sinus and proximal tubular portions of ascending aorta was severely thickened by dense, fibrous tissue, as was the adventitia about the arteries arising from the aortic arch (*Figure 2*). The

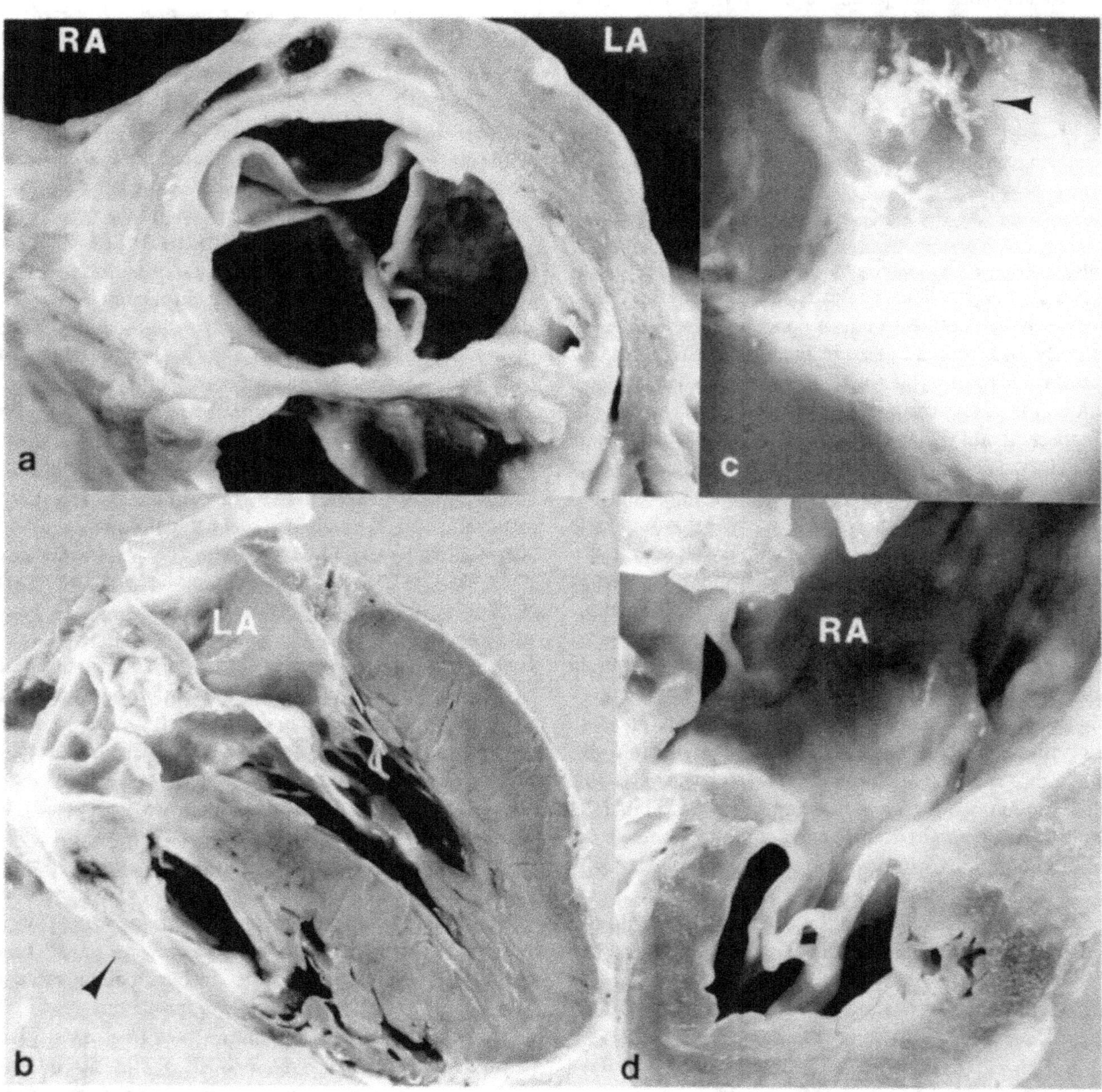

Figure 1. Photographs of the heart in the patient described. (**a**) Aortic valve from above. The cusps are thickened by fibrous tissue, and calcific deposits are present on the aortic aspects. LA = left atrial cavity, RA = right atrial cavity. (**b**) Long axis view showing the calcific deposits in the aortic valve. The arrow points to the right ventricular wall in the outflow tract, which is essentially replaced by fibrous tissue. (**c**) Radiograph of the heart showing heavy calcific deposits in the aortic valve cusps and also calcium at the posteromedial commissure area of the mitral valve. (**d**) Thickened tricuspid valve cusps and thickened mural endocardium of both right ventricle and right atrium.

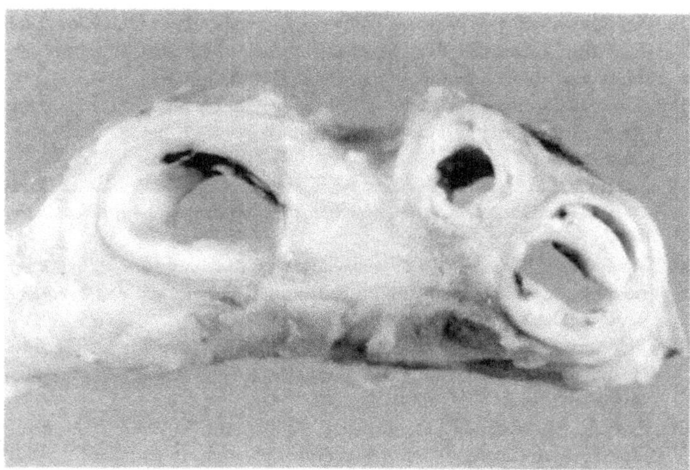

Figure 2. Great arteries arising from the aortic arch. The innominate artery is on the left and the left subclavian is on the right. All 3 contain atherosclerotic plaque. Doppler echocardiogram had shown considerable narrowing of both carotid arteries.

ostium of the right coronary artery was totally occluded by plaque. Small calcific deposits were present locally in all major epicardial coronary arteries. The lumen of the right coronary artery proximally was virtually totally occluded by plaque, and the left anterior descending coronary artery was narrowed up to 75% in cross-sectional area by plaque. Histologically, the adventitia of the major epicardial coronary arteries was thickened severely by dense fibrous tissue. No grossly visible foci of fibrosis or necrosis were noted in the left ventricular free wall or ventricular septum; in contrast, portions of the right ventricular wall, in its outflow tract, were completely replaced by fibrous tissue (*Figure 1*).

DISCUSSION

The heretofore described patient had evidence of radiation-induced heart disease. He had Hodgkin's disease at age 24 and received high doses of radiation to the mediastinum, including the heart. Five years later, he developed constrictive pericardial disease, and 17 years later, he developed a severe degree of heart block and hemodynamically confirmed aortic valve stenosis. At necropsy, he had typical morphologic features of radiation heart disease, including obliterative fibrous pericardial disease; fibrous replacement of the right ventricular wall (in its outflow tract) without grossly visible fibrosis of the left ventricular wall; obliteration of the aortic ostium of the right coronary artery; severe narrowing by plaque of the right coronary artery, with severe and extensive adventitial fibrosis (not a feature of atherosclerotic coronary artery disease) of all epicardial coronary arteries and thoracic aorta; focal fibrous thickening of the mural endocardium of the right atrium and right ventricle; and thickening of the valve cusps, particularly those of the aortic and mitral valves.

Hancock and associates (5) recently analyzed 2232 patients treated for Hodgkin's disease at Stanford University Medical Center, 2001 (90%) of whom had received mediastinal irradiation and 79% of whom had received doses of 40 Gy or more to the mediastinum. Of the 2232 patients, 88 (4%) died of heart disease: mode of death was acute myocardial infarction in 42 (48%), sudden coronary death (outside the hospital) in 13 (15%), ischemic cardiomyopathy in 11 (12%), radiation-induced pericardial disease in 14 (16%), valvular heart disease in 7 (8%), and doxorubicin-induced cardiomyopathy in 1 patient (1%). Of the 7 patients with valvular heart disease, 2 had infective endocarditis, 1 had a congenital valve abnormality, and 3 had aortic valve replacement. None of the 7 patients with valvular heart disease had a necropsy; or if so, the findings were not described, and therefore it is unclear if the valvular involvement was related to irradiation. The average interval between treatment for Hodgkin's disease and death from acute myocardial infarction or sudden unexpected cardiac arrest was 10.3 years (at an average age of 49 years), and from other types of cardiac disease, 11.3 years (at an average age of 51 years). The younger the patient at the time of radiation treatment, the greater was the risk of developing cardiac disease.

A number of case reports have described valvular abnormalities detected clinically many years after mediastinal irradiation, usually for Hodgkin's disease. In the 1991 publication by Carlson and associates (6), 35 previously reported cases (7–19) with valvular abnormalities were tabulated, and 3 additional patients were described (6). Subsequently, Suzuki and colleagues (20) reported an additional case. Of the total of 39 patients, 11 patients had echocardiographic evidence of thickening of the mitral (7 patients) or aortic valve (3 patients), or both (1 patient), without apparent valvular dysfunction; 6 patients had evidence of mitral regurgitation, 4 of aortic regurgitation, and 4 of both; 11 patients had evidence of aortic valve stenosis, including 5 with associated mitral regurgitation; 2 patients had pulmonic valve stenosis; and 1 had subpulmonic stenosis. None of the 39 patients had clinical evidence of mitral stenosis, and only 1 was reported to have associated tricuspid regurgitation. Seven of the 39 patients had attempted or actual replacement of the mitral (1 patient) or aortic (5 patients) valves, or both (1 patient), and 6 of these 7 patients had some degree of aortic valve stenosis (6, 11, 15, 17, 18).

Although narrowing of the major epicardial coronary arteries is a well-recognized complication of mediastinal irradiation, severe stenosis or total occlusion of a coronary ostium by this process, as occurred in our patient, is less recognized. Pilliere and colleagues (21) tabulated 11 reported patients with single coronary ostial stenosis following mediastinal radiotherapy, and at least 2 such patients with bilateral coronary ostial stenosis have been reported (22, 23). Orzan and associates (24) performed coronary angiography late after mediastinal irradiation in 15 patients, and 10 had evidence of coronary ostial stenosis, 9 of whom also had extensive involvement of other cardiac structures. Only 8 of the 15 patients had clinical evidence of myocardial ischemia.

Although myocardial lesions, usually interstitial myocardial fibrosis, are a recognized consequence of high-dose mediastinal irradiation, transmural right ventricular replacement fibrosis (right ventricular infarction), as occurred in our patient, has not been described previously as a consequence of this process.

High degrees of atrioventricular block, as occurred in our patient, are uncommon consequences of mediastinal irradiation. Orzan and associates (25) described 4 patients aged 31 to 46 years who developed complete heart block 13 to 20 years after therapeutic mediastinal irradiation for Hodgkin's disease. They also tabulated 18 previously reported patients with complete heart block from the same mechanism. Of these 18 patients, 11 were under 50 years of age when the complete heart block appeared, as occurred in our patient. The level of the atrioventricular block was infranodal in all but 2 patients with complete heart block. All patients with atrioventricular block of a high degree had other recognized consequences of radiation heart disease.

References

1. Cohn KE, Stewart JR, Fajardo LF, Hancock EW: Heart disease following radiation. *Medicine* 1967;46:281–298.
2. Fajardo LF, Stewart JR, Cohn KE: Morphology of radiation-induced heart disease. *Arch Pathol* 1968;86:512–519.
3. Ruckdeschel JC, Chang P, Martin RG, Byhardt RW, O'Connell MJ, Sutherland JC, Wiernik PH: Radiation-related pericardial effusions in patients with Hodgkin's disease. *Medicine* 1975;54:245–259.
4. Brosius FC III, Waller BF, Roberts WC: Radiation heart disease: analysis of 16 young (aged 15 to 33 years) necropsy patients who received over 3500 rads to the heart. *Am J Med* 1981;70:519–530.
5. Hancock SL, Tucker MA, Hoppe RT: Factors affecting late mortality from heart disease after treatment of Hodgkin's disease. *JAMA* 1993;270:1949–1955.
6. Carlson RG, Mayfield WR, Normann S, Alexander JA. Radiation-associated valvular disease. *Chest* 1991;99:538–545.
7. Stewart JR, Cohn KE, Fajardo LF, Hancock EW, Kaplan HS: Radiation-induced heart disease: a study of 25 patients. *Radiology* 1967;89:302–310.
8. Steinberg I: Effusive-constrictive radiation pericarditis: two cases illustrating value of angiocardiography in diagnosis. *Am J Cardiol* 1967;19:434–439.
9. Morton DL, Glancy DL, Joseph WL, Adkins PC: Management of patients with radiation-induced pericarditis with effusion: a note on the development of aortic regurgitation in two of them. *Chest* 1973;64:291–297.
10. Fouchard J, Joly J, Rousseau J, Herreman F: Pericardite constrictive et myocardite post-radiotherapique avec: insuffisance mitrale. *Semaine des Hopitaux* 1978;54:1283–1287.
11. Warda M, Khan A, Massumi A, Mathur V, Klima T, Hall RJ: Radiation-induced valvular dysfunction. *J Am Coll Cardiol* 1983;2:180–185.
12. Detrano RC, Yiannikas J, Salcedo EE: Two-dimensional echocardiographic assessment of radiation-induced valvular heart disease. *Am Heart J* 1984;107:584–585.
13. Perrault DJ, Levy M, Herman JD, Burns BJ, Bar Schlomo BZ, Drunk MN, Wu WQ, McLaughlin PR, Gilbert BW: Echocardiographic abnormalities following cardiac radiation. *J Clin Oncol* 1985;3:546–551.
14. Pohjola-Sintonen S, Totterman K-J, Salmo M, Siltanen P: Late cardiac effects of mediastinal radiotherapy in patients with Hodgkin's disease. *Cancer* 1987;60:31–37.
15. Lederman GS, Sheldon TA, Chaffey JT, Herman TS, Gelman RS, Coleman CN: Cardiac disease after mediastinal irradiation for seminoma. *Cancer* 1987;60:772–776.
16. Moncure AC, Mark EJ: A 38-year-old woman with a history of radiation treatment for a malignant tumor in the right hemithorax and persistent chest pain and pleural abnormality. *N Engl J Med* 1987;316:1075–1083.
17. McEniery PT, Dorosti K, Schiavone WA, Pedrick TJ, Sheldon WC: Clinical and angiographic features of coronary artery disease after chest irradiation. *Am J Cardiol* 1987;60:1020–1024.
18. Hancock SL, Hoppe RT, Horning SJ, Rosenberg SA: Intercurrent death after Hodgkin disease therapy in radiotherapy and adjuvant MOPP trials. *Ann Intern Med* 1988;109:183–189.
19. Mauch P, Tarbell N, Weinstein H, Silver B, Goffman T, Osteen R, Zajac A, Coleman CN, Canellos G, Rosenthal D: Stage IA and IIA supradiaphragmatic Hodgkin's disease: prognostic factors in surgically staged patients treated with mantle and paraaortic irradiation. *J Clin Oncol* 1988;6:1576–1583.
20. Suzuki M, Hamada M, Matsumoto Y, Hiwada K, Osuka Y. Aortic valvular disease and right coronary artery stenosis induced by mediastinal irradiation: report of a case. *Japanese Circ J* 1993;57:467–471.
21. Pilliére R, Luquel L, Brun D, Jault F, Gandjbakhch I, Bourdarias JP: Ostial stenosis of the left main coronary artery after mediastinal radiotherapy: a case report. *Arch Mal Coeur Vaiss* 1991;84:869–872.
22. Deloche A, Bellin J, Hennetier J, Carpentier A: Post-irradiation coronary ostial stenosis treated by bilateral ostial endarterectomy. *Presse Med* 1987;16:780–781.
23. Stegaru-Hellring B, Keller H, Bode G, Usadel KM, Wallwork J: Ostium stenosis of both coronary arteries and latent hypothyroidism as sequelae of radiotherapy in Hodgkin disease. *Z Kardiol* 1985;74:458–488.
24. Orzan F, Brusca A, Conte MR, Presbitero P, Figliomeni MC: Severe coronary artery disease after radiation therapy of the chest and mediastinum: clinical presentation and treatment. *Br Heart J* 1993;69:496–500.
25. Orzan F, Brusca A, Gaita F, Giustetto C, Figliomeni MC, Libero L: Associated cardiac lesions in patients with radiation-induced complete heart block. *Int J Cardiol* 1993;39:151–156.

Gisela C. Mautner, MD • Susanne L. Mautner, MD • Juergen Froehlich, MD • Irwin M. Feuerstein, MD
Michael A. Proschan, PhD • William C. Roberts, MD • John L. Doppman, MD

Coronary Artery Calcification: Assessment with Electron Beam CT and Histomorphometric Correlation[1]

PURPOSE: **To assess the reliability of electron beam computed tomography (CT) in the detection of calcific deposits in coronary arteries.**

MATERIALS AND METHODS: **The authors quantitatively evaluated a total of 4,298 segments of coronary arteries with electron beam CT and histomorphometry.**

RESULTS: **Regression analysis of the electron beam CT calcium score versus histomorphometric calcium area produced an r^2 value of .92 ($r = .96$; $P < .0001$). Ninety-three percent (78 of 84) of all coronary arteries with stenosis of 76%-100% contained calcific deposits, and 20% (17 of 83) of all coronary arteries with stenosis of 0%-50% contained calcific deposits.**

CONCLUSION: **The amount of calcific deposits detected with electron beam CT correlates highly with histomorphometric measurements. Also, the amount of calcific deposits correlates well with the degree of coronary artery stenosis. Electron beam CT, therefore, is a promising noninvasive technique that can help depict the presence and extent of atherosclerotic plaques.**

Index terms: Coronary vessels, calcification, 54.81 • Coronary vessels, CT, 54.12119, 54.76 • Coronary vessels, stenosis or obstruction, 54.76

Radiology 1994; 192:619–623

---

[1] From the Department of Diagnostic Radiology, Clinical Center (G.C.M., S.L.M., J.F., I.M.F., J.L.D.), the Biostatistics Research Branch (M.A.P.), and the Pathology Branch (W.C.R.), National Heart, Lung, and Blood Institute, National Institutes of Health, Bldg 10, Rm 1C 660, Bethesda, MD 20892. Received November 24, 1993; revision requested January 24, 1994; revision received April 11; accepted April 25. Supported in part by a research grant from the Henry M. Jackson Foundation. **Address reprint requests to** G.C.M.
· RSNA, 1994

See also the articles by Bielak et al (pp 631–636), Mautner et al (pp 625–630), and McCollough (pp 637–643), and the editorial by Baron (pp 613–614) in this issue.

CALCIFIC deposits in the coronary arteries occur almost only in atherosclerotic plaques and, therefore, are indicative of coronary artery disease (1–5). Unfortunately, methods such as radiography, fluoroscopy, and conventional computed tomography (CT) are not always accurate in the depiction of calcific deposits as a result of superimposition and motion artifacts.

In recent years, a new generation of CT scanners has been developed, namely electron beam CT. Due to its rapid image acquisition, electron beam CT eliminates motion artifacts from the heart and, to a lesser degree, from the respiratory system. As a result, it is hoped that it could be used to detect calcific deposits in the coronary arteries more reliably than any previously performed noninvasive method (6–10).

In this study, we correlated the calcific deposits depicted with electron beam CT with the "actual" amount of calcific deposits in coronary arteries as assessed with histomorphometric methods. We also examined how well the amount of calcific deposits as assessed with electron beam CT correlates with the degree of stenosis in coronary arteries. Finally, we studied the topographic distribution of calcific deposits in the coronary artery system.

MATERIALS AND METHODS

Heart specimens obtained at recent autopsies at different local institutions were submitted to the Pathology Department of the National Heart, Lung, and Blood Institute, Bethesda, Md. Fifty heart specimens were obtained from men aged 30–69 years with known cause of death. These specimens were consecutively selected with the addition of a few others aged 30–49 years. The cause of death was based on the pathologic findings at autopsy. Individuals who had congenital heart disease (except for mitral valve prolapse), coronary anomalies, cardiomyopathy (except for ischemic cardiomyopathy), interventions or manipulations to the heart (eg, left ventricular assisting device, percutaneous transluminal coronary angioplasty, or coronary artery bypass grafting), and severe states of tumor cachexia or emaciation were excluded. The four major epicardial coronary arteries (right coronary artery [RCA], left circumflex artery [LCA], left anterior descending artery [LADA], and left main artery [LMA]) were excised intact from the heart in their full length (G.C.M., S.L.M.).

The electron beam CT studies were performed with an electron beam scanner (Imatron C-100; San Francisco, Calif). The scanner permits high-resolution, thin-section tomographic images to be acquired in 50–100 msec. Details of the electron beam CT technology have been reported elsewhere (11–14). Images were acquired in the 100-msec single-section mode with the coronary arteries stretched out and arranged parallel to each other. The coronary arteries were scanned in their full length from the proximal to the distal end transversely to their longitudinal axis in contiguous, 3-mm-thick sections, with no intersection gaps. We obtained 40–65 sections per heart specimen, depending on the length of the examined coronary arteries. For each 3-mm-thick section of each of the four coronary arteries taken from each heart specimen, both a calcium area and a score were computed. Image analysis and quantification were performed without knowledge of the clinical data and histologic measurements of the heart specimens. All studies were performed in the same manner.

To compute the calcific deposit area and score, the electron beam CT images were inspected visually for areas of calcium. A calcific deposit was considered to be present if contiguous pixels with a CT number above 130 HU composed an area more than 1 mm². Since some tissue was present around the coronary arteries, areas of high attenuation occurred in the periphery of this tissue, mostly at sharp cutting edges, which were not evaluated. Regions of in-

---

Abbreviations: LADA = left anterior descending artery, LCA = left circumflex artery, LMA = left main artery, RCA = right coronary artery.

terest were placed around every lesion, and automated measurements of the lesion area (in square millimeters) and the peak CT number (in Hounsfield units) were computed and recorded. The calcium score for each lesion (hereafter called the electron beam CT calcium score) was calculated by multiplying the area of the lesion by an attenuation factor. The attenuation factor was determined on the basis of the peak electron beam CT number for that lesion: attenuation factor of 1 for lesions with CT number greater than 130–199 HU, 2 for 200–299 HU, 3 for 300–399 HU, and 4 for 400 HU and above (8).

The coronary arteries were prepared for histomorphometry by being cut transversely to their longitudinal axis into segments with the same section thickness as the electron beam CT images (3 mm thick). Each segment was labeled sequentially from the proximal portion of the coronary artery to its distal end. A total of 4,325 segments were prepared. There were 27 segments (0.6%) that could not be evaluated due to histologic artifacts. The electron beam CT images that corresponded to these segments were also not evaluated. On the average, 86 segments ± 16 (standard deviation) per specimen were evaluated. The segments were dehydrated in ethanol and xylene and embedded in paraffin. Histologic sections which were at least 6 μm thick, were cut from each segment and stained with use of the method of Movat (15). The Movat stain allows distinction of a variety of different components of the coronary artery wall and atherosclerotic plaque, among other calcific deposits. To assess the reliability of the Movat stain in its ability to stain calcific deposits, we also stained 500 segments with von Kossa stain, which is a specific stain for calcium. The Movat stain showed a high degree of accuracy in the identification of calcific areas compared with sections stained with von Kossa stain.

The degree of stenosis, which is defined as the degree of cross-sectional luminal obliteration within the luminal circle bordered by the internal elastic membrane, was assessed at histologic examination of each segment magnified 10 times. The degree of cross-sectional-area luminal stenosis in each segment was judged at visual inspection and was classified into one of four groups: 0%–25% stenosis, 26%–50%, 51%–75%, and 76%–100%. The accuracy of this technique of grading cross-sectional-area stenosis has been shown to be greater than 95% (16).

Quantitative morphometric analysis of the calcific deposits was then performed (17). Each section was placed on the stage of a projection light microscope. The image was enlarged and the artery was traced (Micro Digi-Pad; GTCO, Columbia, Md). The areas traced were potential lumen (total area enclosed by the internal elastic membrane), residual lumen (potential lumen minus area of atherosclerotic plaque), and calcified tissue (granular, brown-stained areas in Movat-stained sections). The area of calcific deposits, which will be referred to hereafter as the histolo-

morphometric calcium area, was calculated with use of a morphometric software package. The investigators were blinded to the measurements made with electron beam CT and to the clinical data of the specimens.

Regression methods and analysis of covariance were used to assess whether the amount of calcium present in coronary arteries can be accurately determined with electron beam CT. An average electron beam CT calcium score and an average histolomorphometric calcium area, respectively, were computed for all 3-mm-thick segments of each heart specimen. Averages were also computed separately for each of the four major epicardial coronary arteries. A univariate regression model was employed with the electron beam CT calcium score, as a function of the histolomorphometric calcium area. Square roots of the electron beam CT calcium scores and histolomorphometric calcium areas were used in the analysis to stabilize the variance and reduce skewness (18). Inverse regression (19) was applied to place bounds on the degree of error when using electron beam CT to predict the amount of calcium present. To investigate whether the amount of calcific deposit correlates with the degree of stenosis, we computed the correlation between the histomorphometric calcium area and the degree of stenosis between all segments of each specimen individually. The average correlation over all specimens was then computed, and a *t* test was performed to determine if the mean correlation was 0.

RESULTS

The four major epicardial coronary arteries of each of the 50 heart specimens were examined with electron beam CT and histologic morphometry (ie, 198 coronary arteries [in two patients the LMA was too short to be investigated]). We examined a total of 4,298 paired electron beam CT scans and histomorphometrically examined segments. The RCA comprised 1,611 segments; the LCA, 921; the LADA, 1,647; and the LMA, 119.

Of 198 coronary arteries examined with electron beam CT, there were 127 that showed at least one area of calcific deposit: 31 (62%) of the 50 segments in the RCA, 30 (60%) of the 50 segments in the LCA, 43 (86%) of the 50 segments in the LADA, and 23 (48%) of the 48 segments in the LMA. Of the 4,298 segments, 1,000 (23%) showed at least one area of calcific deposit: 395 (25%) of the 1,611 segments in the RCA, 226 (25%) of the 921 segments in the LCA, 340 (21%) of the 1,647 segments in the LADA, and 39 (33%) of the 119 segments in the LMA.

Of 198 coronary arteries examined with histomorphometry, there were

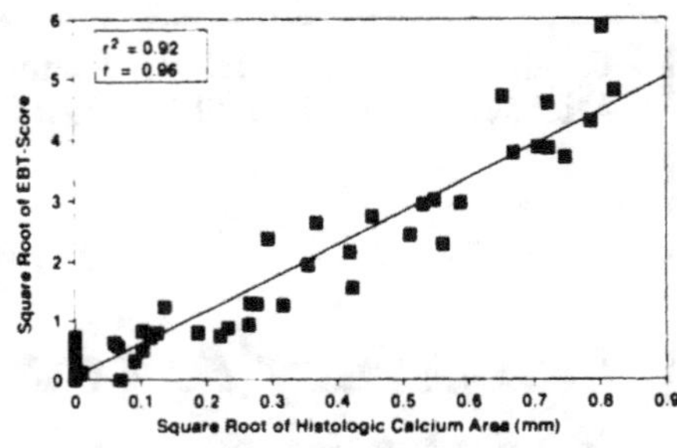

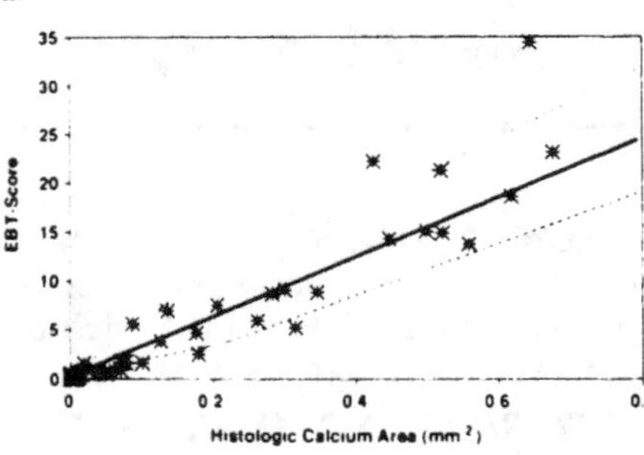

Figure 1. Correlation of the electron beam CT calcium score and the calcium area measured at histolomorphometric examination. **(a)** Plot of univariate regression analysis by use of square root transformation of the electron beam CT (*EBT*) calcium score versus histomorphometric assessment of the calcium area for the 50 heart specimens. There is an apparent high-positive correlation between the electron beam CT calcium score and histomorphometric calcium area ($r^2 = .92$; $r = .96$; $P < .0001$). **(b)** Plot of the inverse regression analysis of the actual data (not square root transformed), which allows prediction of the amount of calcium actually present on the basis of the electron beam CT calcium score. The lower and upper 80% fiducial limits (analogous to confidence intervals) are shown, which demonstrate the degree of error when the attempt is made to predict the amount of calcium actually present.

114 that showed at least one area of calcific deposit: 28 (56%) of the 50 segments in the RCA, 28 (56%) of the 50 segments in the LCA, 35 (70%) of the 50 segments in the LADA, and 23 (48%) of the 48 segments in the LMA. Of 4,298 segments, 980 (23%) showed at least one area of calcific deposit: 394 (24%) of the 1,611 segments in the RCA, 203 (22%) of the 921 segments in the LCA, 344 (21%) of the 1,647 segments in the LADA, and 39 (33%) of the 119 segments in the LMA.

Figure 1a is a plot of the square root–transformed electron beam CT calcium score versus histomorphometric calcium area for the 50 heart specimens. Univariate regression of √(electron beam CT calcium score) and √(histomorphometric calcium area) produced an r^2 value of .92 ($r = .96$; $P < .0001$), signifying that 92% of the variability in √(electron beam CT calcium score) is explained

Degree of Stenosis in the Four Major Epicardial Coronary Arteries

Coronary Artery	No. of Segments in the Four Categories of Stenosis*				
	0%–25%	26%–50%	51%–75%	76%–100%	Total
RCA	640 (40)	429 (27)	234 (15)	308 (19)	1,611 (100)
LCA	411 (45)	230 (25)	128 (14)	152 (17)	921 (100)
LADA	778 (47)	410 (25)	245 (15)	214 (13)	1,647 (100)
LMA	48 (40)	48 (40)	13 (11)	10 (8)	119 (100)
Total	1,877 (44)	1,117 (26)	620 (14)	684 (16)	4,298 (100)

Note.—Numbers in parentheses are percentages. (Some totals do not add to 100% because of rounding.)

* The degree of stenosis is defined as the degree of cross-sectional luminal obliteration within the luminal circle bordered by the internal elastic membrane.

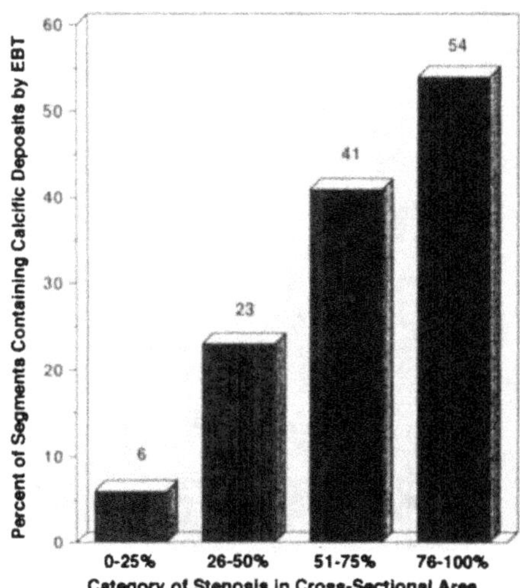

Figure 2. Relation of the degree of stenosis to the amount of calcific deposits. Histogram demonstrates that in the categories with a higher degree of stenosis, the percentage of segments that contained calcific deposits demonstrated at electron beam CT (*EBT*) increased from 6% (category with 0%–25% stenosis) to 54% (category with 76%–100% stenosis).

by the linear relationship with (histomorphometric calcium area). To predict how much calcium is present for a given electron beam CT calcium score, an inverse regression was performed. Lower and upper 80% fiducial limits (analogous to confidence intervals) were determined to assess the degree of error present when the attempt was made to predict the amount of calcium present in the arteries (19). Figure 1b is a plot of the actual data (not square roots) and the 80% fiducial limits. The squared correlation between the square root of the histomorphometric calcium area and the square root of the electron beam CT calcium *score* for each of the separate arteries was r^2 of .90 for the RCA, .88 for the LCA, .90 for the LADA, and .83 for the LMA. With the same analysis, an average of the electron beam CT calcium *area* for every heart specimen yielded an r^2 of .91, and for each

of the separate arteries of .90 for the RCA, .84 for the LCA, .89 for the LADA, and .82 for the LMA.

The percentage of stenosis in cross-sectional area in each segment was categorized into four groups: 0%–25% stenosis, 26%–50%, 51%–75%, and 76%–100%. Of 4,298 segments, 1,877 (44%) showed stenosis of 0%–25%; 1,117 (26%), of 26%–50%; 620 (14%), of 51%–75%; and 684 (16%), of 76%–100% in cross-sectional area as determined at histologic evaluation. The breakdown of the numbers in each of the individual epicardial coronary arteries showed a nearly equal distribution of stenoses (Table).

Of 4,298 segments evaluated with electron beam CT, 1,000 (23%) showed at least one area of calcific deposit. Calcific deposits were contained in 115 (6%) of the 1,877 segments that showed stenosis of 0%–25%, in 261 (23%) of the 1,117 segments that showed stenosis of 26%–50%, in 256 (41%) of the 620 segments that showed stenosis of 51%–75%, and in 368 (54%) of the 684 segments that showed stenosis of 76%–100% (Fig 2). Of 4,298 segments analyzed with histomorphometry, 980 (23%) showed at least one area of calcific deposit. Calcific deposits were contained in 26 (1%) of the 1,877 segments that showed stenosis of 0%–25%, in 201 (18%) of the 1,117 segments that showed stenosis of 26%–50%, in 311 (50%) of the 620 segments that showed stenosis of 51%–75%, and in 442 (65%) of the 684 segments that showed stenosis of 76%–100%. There were 84 coronary arteries that had at least one stenosis of more than 75% in cross-sectional area and 78 (93%) of these contained calcific deposits. Of 83 coronary arteries with no stenosis above 50% in cross-sectional area, 17 (20%) contained calcific deposits, and of 26 coronary arteries with no stenosis above 25% in cross-sectional area, one (4%) contained calcific deposits.

In assessing the correlation between percentage stenosis and calcium area determined at histomorphometry, the average correlation was 0.437 ± 0.215. A t test of whether the mean correlation was 0 was highly significant ($P < .0001$). Data from 13 heart specimens were not included because the variance of either the percentage stenosis or the histomorphometric calcium area was 0, making the correlation undefined. Figure 3 demonstrates the histomorphometric calcium area for every single segment, as well as the average histomorphometric calcium area of all segments for each category of stenosis. The greater the degree of stenosis, the greater was the average histomorphometric area of calcific deposits for that category of stenosis.

As seen in Figure 4, the calcific deposits measured at histomorphometry varied in their location and amount in the epicardial coronary arteries. The coronary arteries had most calcific deposits in the proximal portions. In the RCA, the majority of calcific deposits were present up to 5 cm past the aortic ostium, and in the LCA and LADA, calcific deposits were found up to 3 cm past the point where they branched from the LMA.

All heart specimens with calcific deposits in the RCA (31 specimens) had calcific deposits in the LADA or LCA as well. Of the 43 specimens with calcific deposits in the LADA, 37 (86%) also had calcific deposits in the RCA or LCA. Of the 23 specimens with calcific deposits in the LMA, all but two (91%) had at least two other coronary arteries with calcific deposits and 17 (74%) of the 23 specimens had calcific deposits in all four major coronary arteries. Six heart specimens had only one coronary artery with calcific deposits. This coronary artery was always the LADA.

DISCUSSION

Coronary artery disease is one of the major health care problems of the Western Hemisphere. Calcific deposits in plaques of coronary arteries have been shown to be an indicator of coronary artery disease (20–25). The techniques currently available to assess calcific deposits, however, are unsatisfactory in several aspects. Electron beam CT is a newly developed diagnostic tool with the ability to detect calcific deposits in coronary arteries. Of critical importance to the usefulness of electron beam CT is whether the calcific deposits measured with electron beam CT accurately reflect the amount of calcific deposits actually present in coronary arteries. To assess this accuracy, histopathologic examination was considered the most useful technique. We therefore compared quantitatively the data of calcific deposits as measured with electron beam CT with the actual amount of calcific deposit present as confirmed with histomorphometric techniques. To our knowledge, this is the only study in which this approach has been performed. The main goals of this study were (*a*) to investigate whether calcific deposits can be measured with electron beam CT and to determine how reliable these measurements were, (*b*) to determine whether the calcific deposits measured correlate with the degree of coronary artery stenosis present, and (*c*) to assess the topographic distribution of calcific deposits in the coronary artery system.

Results in our study showed that of 4,298 segments analyzed, 23% contained calcific deposits as measured with electron beam CT and histomorphometry. Regression analysis used to evaluate the data generated by these two techniques revealed a high correlation between the calcific deposits assessed with electron beam CT calcium *score* (area of calcific deposits × attenuation factor) and the calcific deposits assessed with histomorphometry ($r^2 = .92$, $r = .96$; $P < .0001$). A similar high correlation was found by analyzing the *area* of calcific deposits assessed with electron beam CT instead of the electron beam CT calcium score ($r^2 = .91$, $r = .95$; $P < .0001$). Thus, it appears that the amount of calcific deposits measured with electron beam CT (assessed with either area or score) closely represents the actual amount of calcific deposits present in atherosclerotic plaques. In another study that compared electron beam CT measurements with histologic evaluation, calcific deposits assessed with electron beam CT as number of voxels registering at greater than 130 HU were compared with the whole histologic plaque area (not the calcium area itself) (26). A good correlation was demonstrated (RCA, $r = .57$; LCA, $r = .69$; LADA, $r = .76$; $P < .001$). The results of our study also confirmed the results of another study in which measurements with electron beam CT were compared with pathologic data from the International Atherosclerosis Project. These researchers found that there is a close correlation in the data obtained at electron beam CT and pathologic evaluation (27).

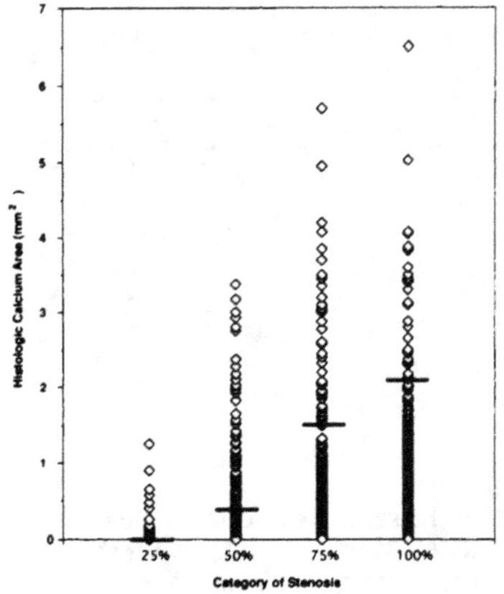

Figure 3. Histologic calcium area in relation to the degree of stenosis. Graph demonstrates the histomorphometric area of calcific deposits for every segment in each category of stenosis. Horizontal bars indicate the average histomorphometric area of calcific deposits for each category of stenosis. The greater the category of stenosis the greater the average histomorphometric area of calcific deposits.

Our results show that the higher the degree of stenosis in the coronary arteries, the more likely these arteries are to contain calcific deposits in their plaques. Ninety-three percent of all coronary arteries that had marked stenoses (ie, > 75% stenosis in cross-sectional area) contained calcific deposits, whereas only 20% of all coronary arteries with less than 51% stenosis in cross-sectional area contained calcific deposits. Analysis per segment revealed that of all segments with marked stenosis, 65% contained calcific deposits, and of all segments with minimal stenosis (< 25% stenosis in cross-sectional area), only 1% contained calcific deposits. A similar relationship between coronary artery disease and calcific deposits has been demonstrated in other pathologic, fluoroscopic, and electron beam CT studies (3,4,10,26,28–31). Hamby et al (32) examined 250 patients older than 30 years and found that of 550 coronary arteries with more than 50% stenosis, 47% contained calcific deposits, whereas in 200 coronary arteries with less than 50% stenosis, only 16% contained calcific deposits ($P < .01$). In a study that used conventional CT, it was found that of 46 coronary arteries with calcific deposits, 72% demonstrated more than 50% stenosis at angiography (30). In a study of Bartel et al (33), the stenoses demonstrated angiographically were located at the same site of the calcific deposits that were observed fluoroscopically in

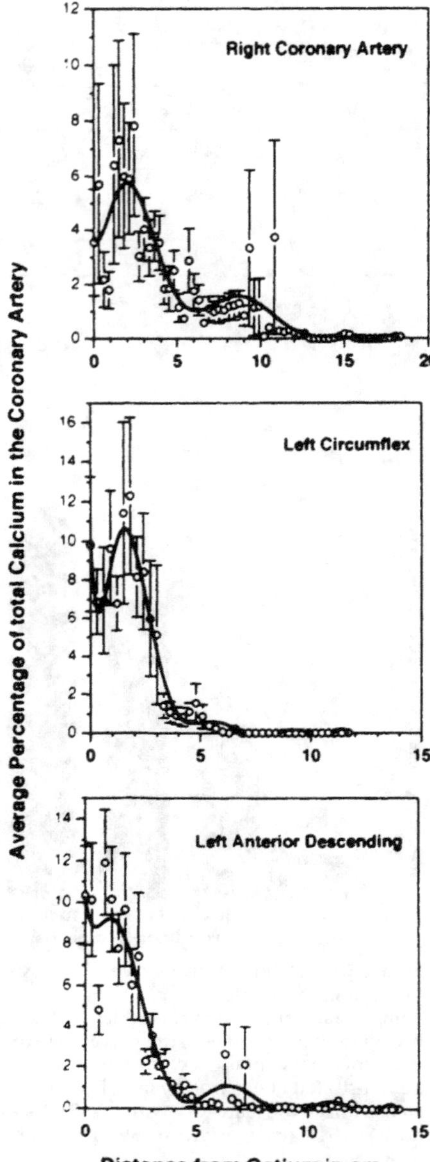

Figure 4. Topographic distribution of calcific deposits. In all investigated epicardial coronary arteries, the majority of calcific deposits were in the proximal portion, as assessed at histomorphometric examination. The RCA had the majority of calcific deposits up to 5 cm past the ostial orifice, and the LCA and LADA had calcific deposits up to 3 cm past their branching from the LMA (*Ostium*).

91% of the LADAs, in 93% of the LCAs, in 83% of the RCAs, and in 80% of the LMAs. Only 10% of the 66 calcified coronary arteries studied had no marked stenoses as demonstrated angiographically at the site of calcific deposits. Crawford et al (34) found calcific deposits more frequently in arteries that had been recently occluded or were the site of severe stenosis than in arteries in which stenosis was less severe. Most of the data are consistent with the conclusion that the amount of coronary calcium increases as the extent of atherosclerosis in coronary arteries increases (ie, the amount of calcific deposits reflects the degree of coronary artery disease). The results of this study cannot be transferred in their full extent to living patients, due to the in vitro approach in which the heart was removed from its thoracic position and the coronary arteries were dissected from the heart and scanned in a stretched position. Nevertheless, the in vitro data suggest that electron beam CT should be of value in the clinical assessment of the severity of atherosclerosis, both for individual cases and for epidemiologic investigations.

Our results showed that most of the calcific deposits were located in the proximal portions (up to 5 cm) of the coronary arteries. This was true for the RCA, LCA, and LADA. These results were shown earlier in other studies, which found that calcific deposits were most frequently observed in the proximal part of the coronary arteries (1,3,4,25). Agatston et al (8) reported that they had performed electron beam CT of the coronary arteries in their full length in 58 patients. Of the 26 patients in whom calcific deposits were detected, only one had calcific deposits exclusively in the distal portion of the coronary arteries, four had proximal and distal calcific deposits, and 21 had proximal calcific deposits only.

The topographic distribution of calcified lesions observed in our study agreed well with the distribution of markedly stenosed or occlusive lesions reported in other studies (1,4,34,35). Rodriguez et al (36) and Pitt et al (37) reported series in which 66% and 70%, respectively, of all occlusions in coronary arteries were within 4 cm of the ostia. Thus, to a large extent, calcified lesions are distributed among the three epicardial coronary arteries (RCA, LCA, and LADA) in about the same manner as are the stenoses present in the coronary arteries. Therefore, calcific deposits seem to be an indicator of the location of atherosclerotic plaques.

In conclusion, calcific deposits measured with electron beam CT correlate highly with actual calcific deposits measured with histomorphometry. The amount of calcific deposit also correlates well with the degree of coronary artery stenosis. Electron beam CT is, therefore, a promising noninvasive technique with which to diagnose the presence and extent of atherosclerotic plaques. ■

Acknowledgments: We thank Leslie K. Berry and Filippina M. Giacometti for their technical assistance.

References

1. Blankenhorn DH, Stern D. Calcification of the coronary arteries. AJR 1959; 81:772–777.
2. Frink RJ, Achor RWP, Brown AL Jr, Kincaid OW, Brandenburg RO. Significance of calcification of the coronary arteries. Am J Cardiol 1970; 26:241–247.
3. Oliver MF, Samuel E, Morley P, Young GB, Kapur PL. Detection of coronary artery calcification during life. Lancet 1964; 1:891–895.
4. Eggen DA, Strong JP, McGill HC Jr. Coronary calcification: relationship to clinically significant coronary lesions and race, sex, and topographic distribution. Circulation 1965; 32:948–955.
5. Pyke D, Symons C. Calcification of the aortic valve and of the coronary arteries. Br Heart J 1951; 13:355–363.
6. Hamada S, Takamiya M, Saito H. Evaluation of coronary artery calcification by ultrafast CT. Nippon Igaku Hoshasen Gakkai Zasshi 1991; 51:1299–1305. [Japanese]
7. Lipton MJ, Holt WW. Computed tomography for patient management in coronary artery disease. Circulation 1991; 84 (suppl 1): i72–i80.
8. Agatston AS, Janowitz WR, Hildner FJ, Zusmer NR, Viamonte M Jr, Detrano R. Quantification of coronary artery calcium using ultrafast computed tomography. J Am Coll Cardiol 1990; 15:827–832.
9. Georgiou D, Brundage BH. Conventional and ultrafast cine-computed tomography in cardiac imaging. Curr Opin Cardiol 1990; 5:817–824.
10. Tanenbaum SR, Kondos GT, Veselik KE, Prendergast MR, Brundage BH, Chomka EV. Detection of calcific deposits in coronary arteries by ultrafast computed tomography and correlation with angiography. Am J Cardiol 1989; 63:870–872.
11. Boyd DP, Couch JL, Napel SA, Peschmann KR, Rand RE. Ultra cine-CT for cardiac imaging: where have we been? what lies ahead? Am J Cardiac Imaging 1987; 1:175–185.
12. Lipton MJ, Holt WW. Value of ultrafast CT scanning in cardiology. Br Med Bull 1989; 45: 991–1010.
13. Flicker S, Naidech HJ, Altin RS, Eldredge J, Carr KF. Ultrafast computed tomography techniques in cardiac disease. J Thorac Imaging 1989; 4:42–49.
14. Boyd DP, Gould RG, Quinn JR, Sparks R, Stanley JH, Herrmannsfeldt WB. A proposed dynamic cardiac 3-D densitometer for early detection and evaluation of heart disease. IEEE Trans Nucl Sci 1979; 26:2724–2727.
15. Movat HZ. Demonstration of all connective tissue elements in a single section. Arch Pathol Lab Med 1955; 60:289–295.
16. Isner JM, Wu M, Virmani R, Jones AA, Roberts WC. Comparison of degrees of coronary arterial luminal narrowing determined by visual inspection of histologic sections under magnification among three independent observers and comparison to that obtained by video planimetry: an analysis of 559 five-millimeter segments of 61 coronary arteries from eleven patients. Lab Invest 1980; 42:566–570.
17. Kragel AH, Reddy SG, Wittes JT, Roberts WC. Morphometric analysis of the composition of atherosclerotic plaques in the four major epicardial coronary arteries in acute myocardial infarction and in sudden coronary death. Circulation 1989; 80:1747–1756.
18. Snedecor GW, Cochran WG. Statistical methods. 7th ed. Iowa City, Ia: Iowa State University Press, 1980; 287–292.
19. Draper N, Smith H. Applied regression analysis. 2nd ed. New York, NY: Wiley, 1981; 47–51.
20. Rienmueller R, Lipton MJ. Detection of coronary artery calcification by computed tomography. Dynamic Cardiovasc Imaging 1987; 1:139–145.
21. Habbe JE, Wright HH. Roentgenographic detection of coronary arteriosclerosis. AJR 1950; 63:50–62.
22. Lieber A, Jorgens J. Cinefluorography of coronary artery calcification: correlation with clinical arteriosclerotic heart disease and autopsy findings. AJR 1961; 86:1063–1072.
23. McGuire J, Schneider HJ, Chou TC. Clinical significance of coronary artery calcification seen fluoroscopically with the image intensifier. Circulation 1968; 37:82–87.
24. Tampas JP, Soule AB. Coronary artery calcification: its incidence and significance in patients over forty years of age. AJR 1966; 97:369–376.
25. Jorgens J, Blank N, Wilcox WA. The cinefluorographic detection and recording of calcifications within the heart: results of 803 examinations. Radiology 1960; 74:550–554.
26. Simons DB, Schwartz RS, Edwards WD, Sheedy PF, Breen JF, Rumberger JA. Noninvasive definition of anatomic coronary artery disease by ultrafast computed tomographic scanning: a quantitative pathologic comparison study. J Am Coll Cardiol 1992; 20:1118–1126.
27. Janowitz WR, Agatston AS, Kaplan G, Viamonte M Jr. Differences in prevalence and extent of coronary artery calcium detected by ultrafast computed tomography in asymptomatic men and women. Am J Cardiol 1993; 72: 247–254.
28. Breen JF, Sheedy PF II, Schwartz RS, et al. Coronary artery calcification detected with ultrafast CT as an indication of coronary artery disease. Radiology 1992; 185:435–439.
29. Rifkin RD, Parisi AF, Folland E. Coronary calcification in the diagnosis of coronary artery disease. Am J Cardiol 1979; 44:141–147.
30. Schultz KW, Thorsen K, Gurney JW, et al. Comparison of fluoroscopy, angiography and CT in coronary artery calcification. Appl Radiol 1989; 18:38–42.
31. Stanford W, Thompson BH, Weiss RM. Coronary artery calcification: clinical significance and current methods of detection. AJR 1994; 161:1139–1146.
32. Hamby RI, Tabrah F, Wisoff BG, Hartstein ML. Coronary artery calcification: clinical implications and angiographic correlates. Am Heart J 1974; 87:565–570.
33. Bartel AG, Chen JT, Peter RH, Behar VS, Kong Y, Lester RG. The significance of coronary calcification detected by fluoroscopy: a report of 360 patients. Radiology 1974; 49:1247–1253.
34. Crawford T, Dexter D, Teare RD. Coronary artery pathology in sudden death from myocardial ischaemia. Lancet 1961; 1:181–185.
35. Young W, Gofman JW, Tandy R, Malamud N, Waters ESG. The quantitation of atherosclerosis. I. Relationship to artery size. Am J Cardiol 1960; 6:288–293.
36. Rodriguez F, Robbins S, Banasiewicz M. Incidence and topography of coronary occlusions: relation to coronary anatomic pattern (abstr). Circulation 1963; 28:670.
37. Pitt B, Zoll PM, Blumgart HL, Freiman DG. Location of coronary arterial occlusions and their relation to the arterial pattern (abstr). Circulation 1963; 28:35.

Major Cardiac Findings at Necropsy in 366 American Octogenarians

Jamshid Shirani, MD,* Jamal Yousefi,† and William C. Roberts, MD‡

We examined the hearts of 366 octogenarians (184 women [50%], 264 white [72%], mean age 84 ± 4 years). The cause of death was cardiac in 195 (53%), noncardiac but vascular in 47 (13%), and noncardiac and nonvascular in 124 patients (34%). Of the 195 patients with fatal cardiac disease, atherosclerotic coronary artery disease was the cause of death in 127 (65%): acute myocardial infarction in 87 (69%), sudden cardiac arrest outside the hospital in 19 (15%), chronic congestive heart failure with healed myocardial infarction in 15 (12%), and complications of coronary bypass surgery in 6 (4%). At least 1 of the 4 major (left main, left anterior descending, left circumflex, and right) epicardial coronary arteries was narrowed >75% in cross-sectional area by atherosclerotic plaque in 218 patients (60%). The mean number of significantly narrowed major epicardial coronary arteries was 1.7, 1.3, and 0.7 in those who died of cardiac, peripheral vascular, or noncardiovascular causes, respectively. Among the 87 patients (33 men and 54 women) with fatal acute myocardial infarction, the women more often had ruptured ventricles (21 of 54 [39%] vs 3 of 33 [9%]), and fewer women had healed myocardial infarcts (11 of 54 [20%] vs 24 of 33 [73%], p <0.05). Calcific deposits were present in the epicardial coronary arteries in 285 patients (78%), in the mitral annulus in 140 (38%), and in aortic valve cusps in 153 (42%). Most octogenarian women with fatal acute myocardial infarction had no previous nonfatal infarcts, but had a high frequency of cardiac rupture; in contrast, most men with a fatal acute myocardial infarction had had a nonfatal infarct and a low frequency of cardiac rupture. Sudden death was uncommon in both sexes in this age group.

(Am J Cardiol 1995;75:151–156)

Octogenarians (aged 80 to 89 years) are the most rapidly growing segment of the population in the Western world.[1] A previous study from this laboratory summarized findings at necropsy in 93 patients aged ≥90 years.[2] The present study focuses on clinical and necropsy findings in 366 patients aged 80 to 89 years. Such a study has not been previously reported.

METHODS

Patients: The files of the Pathology Branch, National Heart, Lung, and Blood Institute, National Institutes of Health, were searched for all accessioned cases of patients aged 80 to 89 years at death. From 1966 to July 1, 1992, 379 cases were found: 13 (5 men aged 82 to 89 years) were excluded because of inadequate clinical (n = 11) or cardiac morphologic (n = 2) information. In the remaining 366 patients, the subjects of this study, records of clinical and pathologic findings, photographs and postmortem radiographs of the heart, histologic slides, and descriptions of the cardiac morphologic abnormalities were reviewed. All hearts were originally examined by WCR, who recorded the gross morphologic abnormalities in each case, and some were reexamined by JS.

Sources of patients: The necropsy was performed at the National Institutes of Health in 11 patients (3%), at 11 other hospitals in the Washington, D.C., area in 308 patients (84%), and at 36 hospitals and medical centers in nonlocal areas of Washington, D.C., in 47 patients (13%). Of the 366 hearts, 25 (7%) were studied from 1966 to 1970, 129 (35%) from 1971 to 1980, 191 (52%) from 1981 to 1990, and 21 (6%) from 1991 through June 1992.

Clinical information: Patient's age, race, sex, symptoms or signs of cardiac dysfunction or myocardial ischemia, diabetes mellitus, systemic hypertension, and cause of death were obtained from the patient's medical record supplied by the submitting hospital. *Sudden coronary death* was defined as death within 6 hours from the onset of new symptoms of myocardial ischemia in the presence of morphologic evidence of significant atherosclerotic coronary artery disease (≥1 major epicardial coronary artery narrowed >75% in cross-sectional area by atherosclerotic plaque). Most patients who died suddenly did so outside a hospital; a few, however, died shortly after admission to an emergency room. Sudden out-of-hospital death also occurred in some patients with cardiac diseases other than atherosclerotic coronary artery disease. In each case, an underlying cardiac disease generally accepted to cause sudden death was present at necropsy. *Acute myocardial infarction* was defined as a grossly visible left ventricular wall lesion confirmed histologically to represent coagulation-type myocardial necrosis. *Ischemic cardiomyopathy* was defined as chronic congestive heart failure associated with a transmural healed myocardial infarct and a dilated left ventricular cavity.

Cardiac morphologic data: Hearts were fixed in 10% phosphate-buffered formalin for 3 to 15 days before examination. They were then "cleaned" of parietal pericardium and postmortem intracavitary clot, and the pulmonary trunk and ascending aorta were incised approximately 2 cm cephalad to the sinotubular junction. *Heart weight* was then measured on accurate scales (Lipsaw scale before 1971, accurate to 10 g, and Mettler P1210

From the Pathology Branch, National Heart, Lung, and Blood Institute, National Institutes of Health, Bethesda, Maryland. Manuscript received August 18, 1994; revised manuscript received and accepted September 25, 1994.

*Present address: Albert Einstein College of Medicine of Yeshiva University, Department of Medicine/Division of Cardiology, 1300 Morris Park Avenue, Bronx, New York 10461.

†Medical student volunteer, Medical College of Virginia, Richmond, Virginia.

‡Present address: Baylor Cardiovascular Institute, Baylor University Medical Center, 3500 Gaston Avenue, Dallas, Texas 75246.

TABLE I Certain Clinicopathologic Findings in 366 Patients Aged 80 to 89 Years

	Men (n = 182)	Women (n = 184)	Total (n = 366)
1. Mean age (years)	83 ± 4	84 ± 3	84 ± 4
2. White:black	124:58	140:44	264 (72%):102 (28%)
3. Angina pectoris	69 (38%)	67 (36%)	136 (37%)
4. Acute myocardial infarction	51 (28%)*	24 (13%)*	75 (20%)
5. Chronic congestive heart failure	74 (41%)	61 (33%)	135 (37%)
6. Systemic hypertension	86 (47%)	73 (40%)	159 (43%)
7. Diabetes mellitus	25 (14%)	28 (15%)	53 (14%)
8. Heart weight (g):	230–830:	185–900:	185–900:
range (mean)	(495 ± 135)*	(410 ± 95)*	(450 ± 155)
9. Left ventricular			
Necrosis only	10 (5%)*	43 (23%)*	53 (14%)
Fibrosis only	57 (31%)	39 (21%)	96 (26%)
Both necrosis and fibrosis	24 (13%)	11 (6%)	35 (10%)
10. Dilated ventricle			
Right	67 (37%)*	47 (26%)*	114 (31%)
Left	69 (38%)*	47 (26%)*	116 (32%)
11. Calcific deposits			
Mitral annulus	49 (27%)*	90 (49%)*	139 (38%)
1+	31	38	69
2+	6	15	21
3+	12	37	49
Aortic valve	60 (33%)	92 (50%)	152 (42%)
1+	39	56	95
2+	7	10	17
3+	14	26	40
Coronary arteries	140 (77%)	145 (79%)	285 (78%)
Papillary muscle	22 (12%)	11 (6%)	33 (9%)
12. Valvular aortic stenosis	33 (18%)	33 (18%)	66 (18%)
Severity			
Mild	14	11	25
Moderate	5	3	8
Severe	14	19	33
Number of cusps			
2	8	5	13
3	25	5	13
Fused commissures	7	3	10
13. Mitral valve prolapse	6 (3%)	6 (3%)	12 (3%)
14. Number of major coronary arteries narrowed >75% by plaque			
0	71 (39%)	77 (42%)	148 (40%)
1	30 (16%)	35 (19%)	65 (18%)
2	32 (18%)	35 (19%)	67 (18%)
3	37 (20%)	31 (17%)	68 (19%)
4	12 (7%)	6 (3%)	18 (5%)
(mean)	(1.4)	(1.2)	(1.3)
15. Major coronary artery narrowed >75% in cross-sectional area by plaque			
Left main	16 (9%)	12 (7%)	28 (8%)
Left anterior descending	91 (50%)	85 (46%)	174 (48%)
Left circumflex	64 (35%)	52 (28%)	116 (32%)
Right	82 (45%)	73 (40%)	155 (42%)
16. Causes of death			
Cardiac	89 (49%)	106 (58%)	195 (53%)
Vascular	28 (15%)	19 (10%)	47 (13%)
Noncardiovascular	65 (36%)	59 (32%)	124 (34%)

*p <0.05.

TABLE II Causes of Death in Patients Aged 80 to 89 Years

I. Cardiac (n = 195)		
A. Coronary artery disease	127	(65%)
1. Acute myocardial infarction	87	
2. Ischemic cardiomyopathy	15	
3. Sudden	19	
4. Aorto-coronary bypass	6	
B. Vascular heart disease	40	(21%)
1. Aortic stenosis	32	
2. Aortic regurgitation	2	
3. Mitral regurgitation	1	
4. Mitral stenosis	1	
5. Mitral valve prolapse	4	
C. Primary cardiomyopathy	7	(4%)
1. Hypertrophic	4	
2. Idiopathic dilated	3	
D. Secondary cardiomyopathy	16	(8%)
1. Amyloidosis	14	
2. Transfusion hemochromatosis	1	
3. Eosinophilic myocarditis	1	
E. Cor pulmonale	2	(1%)
F. Pericardial heart disease	3	(2%)
II. Vascular (n = 47)		
A. Cerebrovascular accident	15	(32%)
B. Abdominal aortic aneurysm	14	(30%)
1. Rupture = 10		
C. Peripheral arterial disease	10	(21%)
D. Aortic dissection	3	(6%)
E. Pulmonary embolism	5	(11%)
III. Noncardiovascular (n = 124)		
A. Cancer	47	(38%)
B. Infection	30	(24%)
C. Fall complications	10	(8%)
D. Others	37	(30%)

teriorly. In each heart, the visually estimated sizes of cardiac ventricular cavities, presence of left ventricular fibrosis (healed myocardial infarct) or necrosis (acute myocardial infarct), status of the 4 cardiac valves, and the maximal degree of cross-sectional luminal narrowing in each of the 4 major epicardial (left main, left anterior descending, left circumflex, and right) coronary arteries were recorded.

Statistics: For each variable, number and mean value ± SD or percentage are reported. Student's t test was used to assess the significance of differences between continuous variables and chi-square analysis was used when data were noncontinuous. A probability value <0.05 was considered significant.

RESULTS

Certain clinicopathologic findings in the 366 patients (184 women [50%], 264 white [72%]) are listed in Table I. By history, diabetes mellitus was present in 53 (14%), acute myocardial infarction in 75 (20%), chronic congestive heart failure in 135 (37%), and systemic hypertension in 159 (43%) patients. Except for the number and percentage of patients with a history of acute myocardial infarction (51 men [28%] vs 24 women [13%], p <0.05), no significant differences in clinical data were present between men and women. More men also had

scale after 1971, accurate to 0.1 g). Heart weight was considered increased if it was >350 g in women and >400 g in men. Radiographs of the hearts were then taken to assess the presence of and extent of *calcific deposits* using a Hewlett-Packard 43805N x-ray system. In each location, the extent of calcific deposits was graded as none (0), mild (1+), moderate (2+), or severe (3+).

Most hearts were studied by cutting the ventricles transversely at approximately 1 cm thick intervals from apex to base parallel to the atrioventricular groove pos-

morphologic evidence of a healed myocardial infarct (81 [45%] vs 50 [27%], p <0.05) and dilated ventricular cavities (69 [38%] vs 47 [26%], p <0.05). Fewer men had morphologic evidence of acute myocardial infarction (34 [19%] vs 54 [29%], p <0.05) and calcific deposits in the mitral annulus (49 [27%] vs 90 [49%], p <0.05).

Causes of death: The causes of death are listed in Table II. Death was due to cardiac causes in 195 patients (53%), noncardiac but vascular causes in 47 (13%), and noncardiovascular causes in 124 patients (34%). Other cardiac findings according to cause of death are listed in Table III. No significant differences were found between men and women in the number of patients dying of each of the 3 causes.

Number of major epicardial coronary arteries severely narrowed by atherosclerotic plaque: At least 1 of the 4 major epicardial coronary arteries was narrowed >75% in cross-sectional area by atherosclerotic plaque in 218 of the 366 patients (60%). The mean number of major coronary arteries so narrowed was 1.3 and was not significantly different in men than in women (1.4 vs 1.2 major coronary arteries). Almost an equal number of patients had 1 (65 of 366 [18%]), 2 (67 of 366 [18%]), or 3 (68 of 366 [19%]) of their major epicardial coronary arteries significantly narrowed by atherosclerotic plaque. All 4 major epicardial coronary arteries were significantly narrowed by atherosclerotic plaque in 18 patients (5%). The left anterior descending coronary artery was the most frequently significantly narrowed artery (176 of 366 [48%]) followed by the right (155 [42%]), left circumflex (116 [32%]), and left main (28 [8%]). The mean number of major epicardial coronary arteries significantly narrowed by atherosclerotic plaque differed among patients who died of cardiac, vascular, and noncardiovascular causes (1.7, 1.3, and 0.7 coronary arteries, respectively).

Frequency of healed and acute myocardial infarcts: Of the 366 patients, 131 (36%) had healed myocardial infarcts (81 of 182 men [45%] and 50 of 184 women [27%]). Most (94 of 131 of those with healed myocardial infarcts [72%]) died of cardiac (75 of 131 [57%]) or vascular (19 of 131 [15%]) causes. An acute myocardial infarct was present at necropsy in 87 of the 366 patients (24%) (33 of 182 men [19%] and 54 of 184 women [29%]) (Table IV). In 1 of the 87 patients with acute myocardial infarction, death occurred due to cerebrovascular accident and myocardial necrosis was believed to be a secondary and terminal event and not directly the cause of the patient's death. Of the 87 patients with acute myocardial infarcts, 35 (40%) also had healed myocardial infarcts (24 of 33 men [72%] vs 11 of 54 women [20%], p <0.05).

Fatal complications of acute myocardial infarction: Acute myocardial infarction was the cause of death in 87 patients (54 women [62%]) (Table IV). Heart weight ranged from 280 to 750 g and was increased in 60 patients (69%). Only 11 of 54 women (20%) who died of acute myocardial infarction had morphologic evidence of a healed myocardial infarct compared with 24 of 33 men (73%). Cardiac rupture occurred 4.4 times more frequently in women (21 of 54 [39%]) than in men (3 of 33 [9%]). Rupture involved the left ventricular free wall in 17 patients (71%), the ventricular septum in 4 patients (17%), and a papillary muscle 1 patient (4%). In 2 patients (8%), rupture involved both the left ventricular free wall and the ventricular septum. Of the 24 patients with

TABLE III	Certain Clinicopathologic Findings in 195 Patients Aged 80 to 89 Years Dying of Cardiac Causes		
	Cardiac (n = 195)	Vascular (n = 47)	No CV (n = 124)
1. Mean age (years)	84 ± 4	84 ± 4	83 ± 4
2. White:	143 (73%):	30 (64%):	91 (73%):
black	52 (27%)	17 (36%)	33 (27%)
3. Angina pectoris	97 (50%)	8 (17%)	31 (25%)
4. Acute myocardial infarction	61 (31%)	5 (11%)	9 (7%)
5. Chronic congestive heart failure	104 (53%)	8 (17%)	23 (19%)
6. Systemic hypertension	96 (49%)	27 (57%)	36 (29%)
7. Diabetes mellitus	30 (15%)	8 (17%)	15 (12%)
8. Heart weight (g):	210–900:	285–555:	185–775:
range (mean)	(475 ± 140)	(430 ± 135)	(425 ± 135)
9. Left ventricular			
Necrosis only	52 (27%)	1 (2%)	0
Fibrosis only	40 (21%)	19 (40%)	37 (30%)
Both necrosis and fibrosis	35 (18%)	0	0
10. Calcific deposits			
Mitral annulus	77 (39%)	15 (32%)	48 (39%)
1+	44	7	18
2+	10	2	9
3+	23	5	21
Aortic valve	58 (30%)	12 (26%)	49 (40%)
1+	24	9	32
2+	5	2	7
3+	29	1	10
Coronary arteries	165 (85%)	36 (77%)	84 (68%)
11. Valvular aortic stenosis	48 (25%)	4 (9%)	14 (11%)
Severity			
Mild	24	4	8
Moderate	5	0	3
Severe	29	0	3
Number of cusps			
2	12	0	1
3	36	4	13
12. Mitral valve prolapse	5 (3%)	1 (2%)	6 (5%)
13. Major coronary artery narrowed >75% in cross-sectional area by plaque			
Left main	20 (10%)	2 (4%)	6 (5%)
Left anterior descending	120 (62%)	24 (51%)	32 (26%)
Left circumflex	86 (44%)	12 (26%)	18 (15%)
Right	102 (52%)	22 (47%)	31 (25%)
14. Number of major coronary arteries narrowed >75% in cross-sectional area by plaque			
0	53 (27%)	18 (38%)	77 (62%)
1	37 (19%)	10 (21%)	18 (15%)
2	38 (19%)	9 (19%)	20 (16%)
3	53 (27%)	8 (17%)	7 (6%)
4	14 (7%)	2 (5%)	2 (1%)
(mean)	(1.7)	(1.3)	(0.7)

CV = cardiovascular.

TABLE IV Certain Clinicopathologic Findings in 87 Patients Aged 80 to 89 Years with Fatal Acute Myocardial Infarction

	Men (n = 33)	Women (n = 54)	Total (n = 87)
1. Mean age (years)	83 ± 4	84 ± 4	84 ± 4
2. White:black	22:11*	45:9*	67 (77%):20 (23%)
3. Angina pectoris	23 (70%)	36 (67%)	59 (68%)
4. Acute myocardial infarction	16 (48%)	9 (17%)	25 (29%)
5. Chronic congestive heart failure	13 (39%)	17 (31%)	30 (34%)
6. Systemic hypertension	21 (64%)	27 (50%)	48 (55%)
7. Diabetes mellitus	5 (15%)	11 (20%)	16 (18%)
8. Heart weight (g): range (mean)	330–750: (535 ± 110)*	280–650: (415 ± 95)*	280–750: (460 ± 125)
9. Left ventricular			
Necrosis only	9 (27%)*	43 (80%)*	52 (60%)
Fibrosis only	0	0	0
Both necrosis and fibrosis	24 (73%)*	11 (20%)*	35 (40%)*
10. Location of myocardial infarction			
Healed	n = 24	n = 11	n = 35
Anterior	8 (33%)	3 (27%)	11 (31%)
Posterior	11 (46%)	5 (46%)	16 (46%)
Lateral	5 (21%)	3 (27%)	8 (23%)
Acute	n = 33	n = 54	n = 87
Anterior	15 (45%)	31 (57%)	46 (53%)
Posterior	15 (45%)	22 (41%)	37 (43%)
Lateral	3 (9%)	1 (2%)	4 (5%)
11. Cardiac rupture	3 (9%)	21 (39%)	24 (28%)
Left ventricular free wall	1	16	17
Ventricular septum	1	3	4
Left ventricular free wall and ventricular septum	1	1	3
Papillary muscle	0	1	1
12. Calcific deposits			
Mitral annulus	4 (12%)*		
1+	4	11	15
2+	0	3	3
3+	0	5	5
Aortic valve	10 (30%)	22 (41%)	31 (36%)
1+	6	22	18
2+	1	3	4
3+	3	6	9
Coronary arteries	25 (76%)	50 (93%)	75 (86%)
13. Valvular aortic stenosis	7 (21%)	6 (11%)	13 (15%)
14. Number of major coronary arteries narrowed >75% in cross-sectional area by plaque			
0	0	0	0
1	7 (21%)	26 (48%)	23 (26%)
2	7 (21%)	17 (31%)	24 (28%)
3	14 (42%)	18 (33%)	32 (37%)
4	5 (15%)	3 (6%)	8 (9%)
(mean)	(2.5)	(2.1)	(2.3)

*p <0.05.

cardiac rupture during acute infarction, the infarct involved the anterior wall in 16 patients (67%), the posterior wall in 7 (29%), and the lateral wall in 1 patient (4%). The location of the acute myocardial infarct was similar in the 24 patients with and the 63 patients without cardiac rupture.

The duration of survival from the onset of symptoms of acute myocardial infarction ranged from 0 to 26 days (mean 5), and was not significantly different in the groups with rupture (mean 4 days) and no rupture (mean 6 days). Necrosis of the right ventricular free wall was seen at necropsy in 8 patients. Intracavitary thrombi were found in the left ventricle in 9 patients, right ventricle in 3 patients, and left and right atria in 1 patient each. Only 2 of the 24 patients admitted after January 1985 received thrombolytic therapy, and none before that date.

Sudden coronary death: Of the 366 patients, 19 (5%) died suddenly outside of the hospital (n = 17) or within 6 hours of admission to an emergency room (n = 2). A history of myocardial ischemia was present in 8 (42%). Death most often occurred at home (12 of 19 [63%]); 5 deaths occurred on the street, of which 1 occurred while the person was driving her car. Heart weight was increased in 14 patients (74%). Six patients had healed myocardial infarcts. A mean of 2 major epicardial coronary arteries were narrowed >75% in cross-sectional area by atherosclerotic plaque in the 19 patients. The mean number of significantly narrowed major epicardial coronary arteries was lower in women than in men (1.4 vs 2.5), and fewer had healed myocardial infarcts (1 of 9 women vs 5 of 10 men). The mean number of significantly narrowed major coronary arteries in the 10 men who died suddenly was comparable to that of the 33 men who died of acute myocardial infarction. The mean number of major epicardial coronary arteries significantly narrowed by atherosclerotic plaque was lower in the 9 women who died suddenly compared with the 54 women who died of acute myocardial infarction (1.4 vs 2.1).

Valvular aortic stenosis: Some degree of valvular aortic stenosis was present at necropsy in 66 of the 366 patients (18%), and all had either 3+/4+ or 4+/4+ calcified deposits on the aortic aspects of the cusps (Table I). These included 25 patients with mild, 8 with moderate, and 33 with severe degrees of stenosis. Thirteen patients, including 10 of the 33 patients considered to have severe aortic stenosis, had a congenitally bicuspid aortic valve. Among the 33 patients with severe aortic stenosis, 3 died of noncardiac causes, 23 died of progressive congestive heart failure, 1 died suddenly outside the hospital, and 6 died during or immediately after cardiac catheterization (n = 2), percutaneous aortic balloon valvuloplasty (n = 2), or aortic valve replacement (n = 2).

Mitral valve prolapse: Twelve patients (6 men, mean age 83 years) had mitral valve prolapse. In 4 (1 man and 3 women) of the 12 patients, death appeared to be related to mitral valve prolapse. Clinical and cardiac morphologic findings in these 12 patients are described elsewhere.[3]

Other fatal valvular heart diseases: *Aortic regurgitation* was reported to have been present in 4 men and was either fatal or contributed significantly to death in 2 of them. The aortic valve cusps and ascending aorta, however, were normal except for the expected aging changes. *Rheumatic mitral stenosis* was the cause of death in an 87-year-old woman who died of pulmonary edema. One man died of left ventricular failure secondary to severe acute mitral regurgitation. His heart weighed 400 g; there was necrosis with rupture of the anterolateral papillary muscle, but the major epicardial coronary arteries were devoid of significant luminal narrowing.

Primary myocardial diseases: Four patients died of *hypertrophic cardiomyopathy* (3 women). Their heart weights ranged from 310 to 550 g (mean 455). Asymmetric ventricular septal hypertrophy was seen grossly, and severe disorganization of myofibers in the ventricular septum was observed histologically in each case. Two died suddenly outside the hospital, and in both hypertrophic cardiomyopathy was not diagnosed before death: one had a left ventricular apical transmural scar and aneurysm in the absence of significant atherosclerotic coronary artery disease; the other died of progressive congestive heart failure years after ventricular septal myotomy and myectomy. The last of these 4 patients, an 84-year-old man, died during cardiopulmonary bypass of suspected "constrictive pericarditis." At necropsy, no pericardial abnormality was found; he also had a small healed transmural myocardial infarct and significant coronary narrowing.

Idiopathic dilated cardiomyopathy caused death in 3 patients. All 3 died of progressive left ventricular failure. The heart weights ranged from 360 to 700 g (mean 545).

Secondary cardiomyopathy: Grossly visible *amyloid*, confirmed histologically, was observed in the hearts of 19 patients (12 men) and was severe and fatal in 14 patients (9 men). The remaining 5 patients died of acute myocardial infarction (n = 3), pancreatic cancer (n = 1), and cerebrovascular accident (n = 1). The presence of amyloid deposits in the heart was not routinely studied, however, and was only pursued if clinical or gross morphologic findings (e.g., left atrial endocardial granular deposits) indicated the possibility of its presence.

One patient with fatal chronic congestive heart failure had massive *cardiac hemosiderosis*. *Eosinophilic myocarditis* was the cause of death in a woman who died of congestive heart failure.

Calcific deposits in the heart: The most frequent location for calcific deposits in the heart was the major *epicardial coronary arteries.* Some degree of calcific deposits was seen in at least 1 of the 4 major epicardial coronary arteries in 285 of the 366 patients (78%) and were more frequently seen in those who died of cardiac (165 of 195 [85%]) causes than in those who died of vascular (36 of 47 [77%]) or noncardiovascular (84 of 127 [66%]) causes. The mean number of major epicardial coronary arteries narrowed >75% by atherosclerotic plaque was significantly higher in patients with than without calcific deposits (1.4 vs 0.9 major coronary artery, p <0.05). In only 17 patients were calcific deposits seen in the mitral annulus or aortic cusps in the absence of radiographically detectable calcific deposits in the major epicardial coronary arteries. In all 17 cases, the calcium deposits were small.

Mitral annular calcium was present in 139 patients (38%). It was seen more frequently in women than men (49% vs 27%, p <0.05). In no patient with mitral annular calcific deposits did the mitral orifice appear to have been made stenotic by the deposits.

TABLE V Comparison of Certain Clinicopathologic Findings in 366 Octogenarians with Findings in 93 Previously Reported[2] Patients Aged ≥90 Years at Death Examined in Our Laboratory

		Patient Age Group (years)	
		80–89 (n = 366)	90–103 (n = 93)
1.	Age, years (mean)	80–89 (84)	90–103 (93)
2.	Men:women	182 (50%):184 (50%)	51 (55%):42 (45%)
3.	Black:white	102 (28%):264 (72%)	33 (35%):59 (63%)
4.	Systemic hypertension	159 (43%)	50 (54%)
5.	Diabetes mellitus	53 (14%)	8 (9%)
6.	Angina pectoris	136 (37%)	4 (4%)
7.	Acute myocardial infarction	75 (20%)	17 (18%)
8.	Chronic congestive heart failure	135 (37%)	21 (23%)
9.	Cause of death		
	Cardiac	195 (53%)	29 (31%)
	Vascular	47 (13%)	17 (18%)
	Noncardiovascular	124 (34%)	47 (51%)
10.	Heart weight, g (mean)		
	Men	230–830 (495)	220–660 (436)
	Women	185–900 (410)	220–630 (397)
11.	≥1 Major coronary artery narrowed >75% in CSA by plaque	218 (60%)	59 (63%)
	Men	111/182 (61%)	33 (65%)
	Women	107/184 (58%)	26 (62%)
12.	Number of 4 major coronary arteries narrowed >75% in CSA by plaque	475/1,464 (32%)	107/372 (29%)
	Men	253/287 (35%)	57/204 (28%)
	Women	222/736 (30%)	60/168 (36%)
13.	Myocardial infarction	184 (50%)	35 (38%)
	Acute only	53	10
	Healed only	96	21
	Both	35	4
14.	Calcium in		
	Coronary arteries	285 (78%)	88 (95%)
	Mitral valve annulus	139 (38%)	39 (42%)
	1+	69 (50%)	20 (51%)
	2+	21 (15%)	8 (21%)
	3+	49 (35%)	11 (28%)
	Aortic valve cusps	152 (42%)	59 (63%)
	1+	95 (63%)	43 (73%)
	2+	17 (11%)	10 (17%)
	3+	40 (26%)	6 (10%)
15.	Dilated cardiac ventricles		
	Right	114 (31%)	20 (22%)
	Left	116 (32%)	18 (19%)
16.	Cardiac amyloidosis	19 (5%)	16 (17%)

CSA = cross-sectional area.

Calcific deposits were seen in the *aortic valve* cusps in 152 of the 366 patients (42%).

DISCUSSION

Summary of cardiac morphologic findings in octogenarians: Among the 366 hearts examined, at least 1 morphologic abnormality was found in 309 (84%). Only 27 hearts (19 women and 8 men) could be considered normal for the age. Of the latter 27 patients, 22 (81%) died of noncardiovascular and the remaining 5 died of vascular causes. Atherosclerotic coronary artery disease ($\geq$1 major epicardial coronary artery narrowed >75% in cross-sectional area by atherosclerotic plaque) was the most common abnormality (218 patients [60%]). Coronary artery disease was the most common single cause of death (127 of 366 patients [35%]), and its most common manifestation was acute myocardial infarction (87 of 127 [69%]). Sudden coronary death occurred in only 19 patients. Hypertrophic cardiomyopathy, cardiac amyloidosis, and mitral valve prolapse were present in a few patients; these cardiac diseases often manifested themselves for the first time in this age group, and the diagnosis was usually not made until necropsy.

Comparison of cardiac morphologic abnormalities in octogenarian men and women: Significant differences existed in the clinical presentation and fatal complications of acute myocardial infarction among the men and women. A history of myocardial ischemia, including prior myocardial infarction, and death from left ventricular systolic dysfunction ("pump failure") were more often present in men. Women, however, more often died of mechanical complications of acute myocardial infarction (left ventricular free wall and ventricular septal or papillary muscle rupture) and in them prior evidence for myocardial infarction was usually lacking. In the absence of healed myocardial infarcts, the difference in frequency of cardiac rupture between sexes was less (3 of 9 men vs 21 of 43 women).

Comparison of the cardiac morphologic abnormalities in octogenarians with those of other age groups: Some cardiac anatomic changes are considered to be the consequence of aging.[1–14] The heart of the very elderly, for example, typically has small ventricular cavities, relatively large atria, tortuous epicardial coronary arteries, and increased epicardial adipose tissue.[2,7,9] Ventricular septal thicknesses and valvular circumferences also increase with age in both sexes.[10] Information about cardiac morphologic abnormalities in specific age groups among the elderly (i.e., age >65 years) is sparse. In a 1965 necropsy study of 370 patients aged $\geq$75 years at death,[4] the frequency of "ischemic heart disease"—calcific deposits in mitral annulus and aortic valve cusps and calcific aortic stenosis—in octogenarians was found to be similar to that of patients aged 75 to 79 years at death. The frequency of these morphologic abnormalities, however, was higher in octogenarians than in those

$\geq$90 years of age at death. In this earlier study,[4] no information was given regarding the causes and modes of death or the number of significantly narrowed epicardial coronary arteries present.

Two recent studies[2,11] described cardiac morphologic findings in 330 patients aged $\geq$90 years. Compared with patients aged $\geq$90 years at death, our octogenarians had higher frequencies of significant atherosclerotic coronary artery disease (1.3 vs 0.9 of the 4 major epicardial coronary arteries significantly narrowed by atherosclerotic plaque) and acute (88 [24%] vs 51 [14%]) and healed (131 [36%] vs 61 [17%]) myocardial infarcts, and more often died of cardiovascular causes. Cardiac rupture after acute myocardial infarction also occurred more often in octogenarians than in the older age group. Comparison of the 80- to 89- and 90- to 103-year-old age groups is shown in Table V.

Study limitations: The patients presented in this study may not be representative of the general population of octogenarians today. Although all hearts were examined by the same physician, the observations were made over a span of almost 27 years. The hearts were studied from several different medical centers. Our laboratory is involved primarily in the study of cardiac diseases and consequently a selection bias toward abnormal and complex cardiac morphology may have taken place. Nevertheless, these data represent the largest necropsy study in octogenarians and delineates the differences between the manifestations of various cardiac diseases between men and women in this age group.

1. Coni N, Davison W, Webster S. Ageing, the Facts. Oxford, England: Oxford University Press, 1992:1–11.

2. Roberts WC. Ninety-three hearts $\geq$90 years of age. *Am J Cardiol* 1993;71:599–602.

3. Shirani J, Roberts WC. The clinical and morphologic features of mitral valve prolapse in octogenarians. *Am J Cardiol* 1993;73:1316–1319.

4. Pomerance A. Pathology of the heart with and without cardiac failure in the aged. *Br Heart J* 1965;27:697–710.

5. Roberts WC, Perloff JK, Costantino T. Severe valvular aortic stenosis in patients over 65 years of age. A clinicopathologic study. *Am J Cardiol* 1971;27:497–506.

6. Gerstenblith G, Frederiksen J, Yin FCP, Fortuin NJ, Lakatta EG, Weisfeldt ML. Echocardiographic assessment of a normal adult aging population. *Circulation* 1977;56:273–278.

7. Waller BF, Roberts WC. Cardiovascular disease in the very elderly. Analysis of 40 necropsy patients aged 90 years or older. *Am J Cardiol* 1983;51:403–421.

8. Fleg JL. Alterations in cardiovascular structure and function with advancing age. *Am J Cardiol* 1986;57:33C–44C.

9. Roberts WC. The aging heart. *Mayo Clinic Proc* 1988;63:205–206.

10. Kitzman DW, Scholz DG, Hagen PT, Ilstrup DM, Edwards WD. Age-related changes in normal human hearts during the first 10 decades of life. Part II (maturity): a quantitative anatomic study of 765 specimens from subjects 20 to 99 years old. *Mayo Clinic Proc* 1988;63:137–146.

11. Lie JT, Hammond PI. Pathology of the senescent heart: anatomic observations on 237 autopsy studies of patients 90 to 105 years old. *Mayo Clinic Proc* 1988;63: 552–564.

12. Morley JE, Reese SS. Clinical implications of the aging heart. *Am J Med* 1989; 86:77–86.

13. Kowalchuk GL, Siu SC, Lewis SM. Coronary artery disease in the octogenarian: angiographic spectrum and suitability for revascularization. *Am J Cardiol* 1990; 66:1319–1323.

14. Gertz SD, Malekzadeh S, Dollar AL, Kragel AH, Roberts WC. Composition of atherosclerotic plaques in the four major epicardial coronary arteries in patients $\geq$90 years of age. *Am J Cardiol* 1991;67:1228–1233.

Factors Involved in the Development of Symptom-Producing Atherosclerotic Plaques

William C. Roberts, MD

Symptom-producing atherosclerosis is rare in individuals whose serum total cholesterol is about 150 mg/dL (3.9 mmol/L), low-density lipoprotein cholesterol <100 mg/dL (2.6 mmol/L), and high-density lipoprotein cholesterol >35 mg/dL (1 mmol/L). Furthermore, lipid lowering therapy has been unequivocally demonstrated to prevent or delay atherosclerotic events in individuals without previous events and, when elevated cholesterol levels are considerably lowered, to prevent or delay subsequent events in individuals who have had previous atherosclerotic events. The role of thrombus in precipitating coronary atherosclerotic events has received considerable attention in recent years. The role of thrombus, however, in causing the atherosclerotic plaque has received much less attention in recent years. This symposium, underwritten by DuPont Pharma, attempts to provide evidence implicating both lipids and thrombus in plaque formation, and it also examines the role of the arterial wall itself. We are pleased with the results of this symposium and hope that you find it useful.

I would like to summarize the editorial published in December 1973 on the role of thrombus in the development of the atherosclerotic plaque.[1] There is morphologic evidence that thrombus plays a role in the development of the atherosclerotic plaque. Rokitansky, nearly 150 years ago, first proposed that atherosclerotic plaques resulted from the organization of thrombi.[2] Several observations suggest that atherosclerotic plaques result, at least in part, from the organization of thrombi:

1. *The presence of known components of thrombi—namely, fibrin and platelets—within atherosclerotic plaques, and commonly, particularly in the aorta, overlying atherosclerotic plaques.*

2. *The occurrence of known components of atherosclerotic plaques—namely, foam cells, cholesterol clefts, pultaceous debris, calcium—in organized hematomas or known thrombi wherever they might occur in the body.* An example is the left atrial thrombus in the patient with mitral stenosis. Organization of this thrombus may produce typical complicated atherosclerotic plaques in the left atrial wall.

3. *The presence of multiple channels in lumens—a* recognized consequence of organization of pulmonary arterial thromboemboli. Multiluminal

From the Baylor Cardiovascular Institute, Baylor University Medical Center, Dallas, Texas.

Address for reprints: William C. Roberts, M.D., Baylor Cardiovascular Institute, Baylor University Medical Center, 3600 Gaston Avenue, Dallas, Texas 75246.

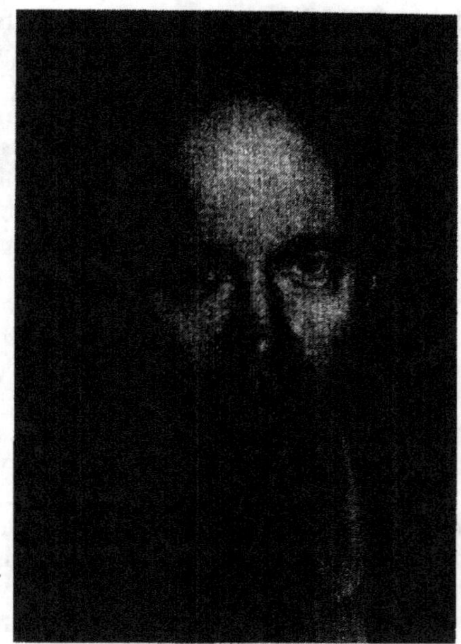

William C. Roberts, MD

channels are found in approximately 7% of severely atherosclerotic coronary arteries.[3] This observation suggests that thrombi or emboli were at one time present and that they organized. The tissue present between the multiluminal channels is similar to that found in arteries with only one channel. Because the artery with multiple channels has been recognized as the hallmark of an organized thrombus and because the tissue in both multi- and unichanneled arteries is similar, Duguid reasoned that the causative process also was similar.[4]

4. *The major component of coronary plaques in patients with fatal coronary artery disease is fibrous tissue.* Fibrous tissue makes up approximately 75% of coronary atherosclerotic plaques in patients with fatal coronary artery disease from any of the major subsets of coronary patients.[5] Even in patients with extreme hyperlipidemia, namely those with homozygous familial hypercholesterolemia, the major component of coronary plaques in these patients with fatal coronary artery disease is fibrous tissue.[6] Foam cells actually are infrequently observed in the coronary arteries in patients with fatal coronary artery disease. Often the "density" of the fibrous tissue plugging the coronary artery is different in different portions of the plaques. These subunits may be demarcated by distinct elastic lamellae. These subunits suggest that thrombus is deposited at different times. Possibly, the "density" of the resulting fibrous tissue may be determined by the composition of the initial thrombus, i.e., whether platelets or fibrin predominated.

5. *Experimentally induced thrombi under proper conditions may be transformed into atherosclerotic plaques closely resembling those observed in human coronary arteries.*

These factors obviously do not prove that thrombosis causes atherosclerotic plaques, but together they strongly suggest that organization of thrombi plays a major role in the development of the complicated atherosclerotic plaque. Indeed, most serious students of the morphology of the arterial plaque have supported, at least in part, the thrombogenic origin of atherosclerosis. Because the clotting factors in the blood appear to be similar in all population groups and because symptomatic atherosclerosis develops only in those populations with elevated blood lipids, the latter of course play the major and determining role in the development of plaques. Lipids may exert their effect both by their ability to alter the clotting mechanism as well as by their ability to infiltrate the arterial wall.

REFERENCES

1. Roberts WC. Does thrombosis play a major role in the development of symptom-producing atherosclerotic plaques? *Circulation* 1973;48:1161–1166.

2. Rokitansky CA. Manual of Pathological Anatomy, Vol. 4, translated by Day GE. London: Syndenham Society 1852:261–272.

3. Virmani R, Roberts WC. Extravasated erythrocytes, iron, and fibrin in atherosclerotic plaques of coronary arteries in fatal coronary heart disease and their relation to luminal thrombus: frequency and significance in 57 necropsy patients and in 2958 five-minute segments of 224 major epicardial coronary arteries. *Am Heart J* 1983;105:788–797.

4. Duguid JB. Thrombosis as a factor in the pathogenesis of coronary atherosclerosis. *J Pathol Bacteriol* 1946;58:207–215.

5. Roberts WC, Kragel AH, Gertz SD, Roberts CS. Coronary arteries in unstable angina pectoris, acute myocardial infarction, and sudden coronary death. *Am Heart J* 1994;127:1588–1593.

6. Kragel AH, Roberts WC. Composition of atherosclerotic plaques in the coronary arteries in homozygous familial hypercholesterolemia. *Am Heart J* 1991;121:210–211.

Clinical features and pathogenesis of intracerebral hemorrhage after rt-PA and heparin therapy for acute myocardial infarction:
The Thrombolysis in Myocardial Infarction (TIMI) II Pilot and Randomized Clinical Trial combined experience

M.A. Sloan, MD; T.R. Price, MD; C.K. Petito, MD; A.M.Y. Randall, BA; R.E. Solomon, MHS; M.L. Terrin, MD, MPH; J. Gore, MD; D. Collen, MD, PhD; N. Kleiman, MD; F. Feit, MD; J. Babb, MD; M. Herman, MD; W.C. Roberts, MD; G. Sopko, MD, MPH; E. Bovill, MD; S. Forman, MA; and G.L. Knatterud, PhD; for the TIMI Investigators

Article abstract—Parenchymatous intracerebral hemorrhage (ICH) is a serious, infrequent complication of thrombolytic therapy for acute myocardial infarction. We studied the clinical and radiologic features, manner of presentation, associated factors, and temporal course in 23 patients with ICH associated with 150 mg or 100 mg recombinant tissue-type plasminogen activator (rt-PA) and heparin therapy for acute myocardial infarction in the Thrombolysis in Myocardial Infarction (TIMI) II Pilot and Randomized Clinical Trial. In TIMI II, 13 of the 23 ICH patients developed or maintained systolic blood pressure ≥160 mm Hg or diastolic blood pressure ≥90 mm Hg during the rt-PA infusion and before the onset of neurologic symptoms. Six patients (26%) had life-threatening ventricular arrhythmias, five before onset of neurologic symptoms. A decreased level of consciousness was the earliest neurologic abnormality in 15 (65%) and the most common initial physical finding (in 19, or 82%). Onset was usually gradual (70%), but time to maximal deficit was frequently (61%) within 6 hours of onset. The locations of the primary ICH sites were lobar in 16 (70%), thalamic in four (17%), and brainstem-cerebellum in three (13%), but the putamen was never the primary site. Multiple lobar hemorrhages occurred in six cases (26%). The timing and size of ICH was similar among patients treated with 150 mg rt-PA and 100 mg rt-PA. Brain CT demonstrated an arteriovenous malformation in one case. Four patients had hypofibrinogenemia, which was profound in three patients. Pathologic findings were available for five patients. Of these, three patients had cerebral amyloid angiopathy, and one had hemorrhagic transformation of an ischemic cerebral infarction found at autopsy. We conclude that ICH following rt-PA and heparin therapy for acute myocardial infarction presents as a distinctive clinical syndrome. Intracerebral bleeding after combined thrombolytic and antithrombotic therapy may be associated with cerebral amyloid angiopathy and other vascular lesions. Acute or persistent hypertension before or during rt-PA infusion, life-threatening ventricular arrhythmias, and hypofibrinogenemia, either alone or in combination, may play roles in some cases. Care should be exercised when considering thrombolytic therapy for patients with risk factors for ICH.

NEUROLOGY 1995;45:649-658

Intracranial hemorrhage is an infrequent though severe complication of thrombolytic therapy for acute myocardial infarction. The reported frequencies of intracranial hemorrhage in previous studies are 0.1% to 0.8% for streptokinase,[1-12] 0.3% to 0.9% for recombinant tissue-type plasminogen activator (rt-PA),[6-10,12-18] and 0.8% for anisoylated plasminogen-streptokinase activator complex.[9] The Global

From the Maryland Medical Research Institute (Drs. Sloan, Price, Terrin, and Knatterud; Ms. Randall and Ms. Forman), Baltimore, MD; Department of Neurology (Drs. Sloan and Price), University of Maryland School of Medicine, Baltimore, MD; Department of Pathology (Dr. Petito), University of Miami School of Medicine, Miami, FL; Office of Program Planning and Evaluation (Ms. Solomon), National Heart, Lung, and Blood Institute, Bethesda, MD; Department of Medicine (Dr. Gore), University of Massachusetts School of Medicine, Worcester, MA; Department of Biochemistry (Dr. Collen), University of Vermont College of Medicine, Burlington, VT; Department of Medicine (Dr. Kleiman), Baylor College of Medicine, Houston, TX; Department of Medicine (Dr. Feit), New York University School of Medicine, New York, NY; Section of Cardiology (Dr. Babb), Bridgeport Hospital, Bridgeport, CT; Department of Medicine (Dr. Herman), New York Medical College, Valhalla, NY; Baylor Cardiovascular Institute (Dr. Roberts), Baylor University Medical Center, Dallas, TX; Division of Heart and Vascular Diseases (Dr. Sopko), National Heart, Lung, and Blood Institute, Bethesda, MD; and Department of Pathology (Dr. Bovill), University of Vermont School of Medicine, Burlington, VT.

Supported by National Heart, Lung, and Blood Institute research contracts and grants.

Received January 11, 1994. Accepted in final form September 19, 1994.

Address correspondence and reprint requests to Dr. Michael A. Sloan, Department of Neurology, University of Maryland Hospital, 22 South Greene Street, Baltimore, MD 21201.

Utilization of Streptokinase and rt-PA for Occluded Coronary Arteries (GUSTO) Trial reported[12] that intracranial hemorrhage occurred in 0.9% of patients treated with combined streptokinase plus accelerated rt-PA. Since these trials did not employ routine screening with brain CT following thrombolytic therapy, the frequency of occult or undiagnosed intracranial hemorrhages is unknown.

The Thrombolysis in Myocardial Infarction (TIMI) Phase II Pilot Study and Clinical Trial assessed the effects on mortality, re-infarction, other morbidity, and left ventricular function of an invasive treatment strategy (cardiac catheterization and, if angiographic findings demonstrated appropriate anatomy, percutaneous transluminal coronary angioplasty [PTCA] or coronary artery bypass grafting if coronary anatomy was too complex or hazardous for PTCA) versus a conservative strategy following intravenous rt-PA and heparin therapy for acute myocardial infarction.[19-21] As previously reported in TIMI II,[16] 23 of 56 cerebrovascular complications were primary parenchymatous intracerebral hemorrhages (ICHs), with a higher rate in patients treated with 150 mg rt-PA (1.3%) than in patients treated with 100 mg rt-PA (0.4%). Primary ICH was associated with increasing age but not female gender. In this report, we delineate the clinical and radiologic features, manner of presentation, and temporal course of primary ICH as well as limited hematologic and pathologic findings.

Methods. *TIMI II protocol.* Detailed descriptions of the TIMI II methods, cardiovascular and hemostatic findings, and overall results have been previously reported.[16,20,21] Patients presenting within the first 4 hours of acute MI with ST segment elevation received rt-PA, heparin, and aspirin. An initial 5,000-IU bolus of IV heparin was given at the start of rt-PA infusion; continuous infusion began within 1 hour at a rate of 1,000 IU/hr, and the dose was then adjusted to maintain the activated partial thromboplastin time (aPTT) between 1.5 and 2.0 times that of control. An unexpected number of intracranial hemorrhages occurred when patients were treated with 150 mg of rt-PA in the early part of TIMI II.[22,23] Protocol changes were made, and the dose of rt-PA was reduced to 100 mg for the remaining 3,016 patients (60 mg in the first hour, including a 6-mg bolus; 20 mg in the second hour; and 5 mg in each of the next 4 hours).[16,23,24] Aspirin (80 mg/d) on the same day as thrombolytic therapy was part of the study regimen in the first 627 patients in the TIMI II pilot and clinical trial. For the remaining 3,297 patients, initiation of aspirin was postponed to the next day and then increased to 325 mg/d on day 6, when IV heparin was replaced with subcutaneous heparin.

Clinical evaluation. Detailed information regarding circumstances surrounding the onset of the hemorrhage was recorded, including the date and time of onset of neurologic symptoms and signs. The earliest possible time was defined as the time of onset of first symptoms or signs compatible with CNS dysfunction. This could be a headache, with or without a focal deficit. When a patient was asleep or unconscious and responded or awoke with obvious signs of a focal deficit, the earliest possible time was defined as the time of loss of consciousness or going to sleep. The latest possible time was defined as the time when unequivocal evidence of CNS dysfunction was present.

Neurologic data were recorded by a neurologist or other responsible physician and abstracted by study staff on special data collection forms. Particular attention was paid to the mode of onset (rapid, gradual, or stepwise), time interval to maximal deficit, level of consciousness, and nature and distribution of presenting neurologic symptoms and signs. Diagnostic evaluation consisted of CT. CTs for 22 of 23 patients (96%) were reviewed centrally by two of the investigators (M.A.S. and T.R.P.). One patient with ICH whose CT could not be obtained for review was evaluated on the basis of a local CT report and a neurosurgeon's operative note.

Neuroradiology. A focal neurologic deficit associated with a focal collection of blood in the brain seen on CT without evidence of preceding ischemic infarction was classified as an ICH. The primary site was defined as the lesion most likely to be responsible for each patient's presenting symptoms and signs. A primary site was considered multilobar if multiple cerebral lobes were involved through contiguous spread. The presence of hemorrhage extending to other parenchymal sites, ventricles, subarachnoid space, or combination of sites was noted, as were multiple, distinct lesions.

The size of the ICH at the primary site was estimated by a modification of the methods of Hier et al[25] and Kase et al.[26] The volume of the hematoma was estimated by multiplying the maximum length and width (cross-sectional area) by the height of the high absorption lesion on the CT. This number was then divided by two in an attempt to correct for the deviation of the lesion from cuboid shape.[25,26]

Neuropathology. Postmortem records were available for five of the 11 fatal cases (45%). A limited number of hematoxylin-eosin–stained glass slides and paraffin blocks of the brain from four patients and slides stained with Luxol fast blue-periodic acid Schiff (LFB-PAS) from one were available for review by one of the authors (C.K.P.). Immunohistochemistry to detect amyloid β protein (ABP) was performed on all five cases using unstained glass slides of cerebral cortex in four and decolorized LFB-PAS–stained slides in the fifth. The slides were exposed to 88% formic acid for 5 minutes,[27] exposed to hydrogen peroxide (H_2O_2) for 20 minutes, and incubated with normal goat serum for 30 minutes. They were then incubated with rabbit polyclonal anti-ABP (gift of Dr. Samuel Gandy, Rockefeller University) diluted 1:500 in phosphate-buffered saline with 1% bovine serum albumin at 4 °C overnight. Following this, the slides were incubated with biotinylated secondary antibody at 27 °C for 30 minutes and the avidin-biotin complex[28] (Vector Labs, Carpenteria, CA) for 50 minutes. They were incubated with 3,3-diaminobenzidine and H_2O_2 for 5 minutes and lightly counterstained with hematoxylin. Phosphate-buffered saline with bovine serum albumin was substituted for the primary antibody as a negative control and a previously diagnosed case of cerebral amyloid angiopathy (CAA) was used as a positive control. Congo red stain and the modified Bielschowsky silver stain were performed on two to three sections of cerebral cortex from the four patients whose paraffin blocks were available for resectioning. The frequency of diffuse and neuritic plaques was evaluated according to the criteria of Khachaturian[29] and Mirra et al.[30]

Table 1. Clinical presentation, course, and outcome of intracerebral hemorrhage following rt-PA and heparin therapy

Pt no.	Age	WT	T_{i-o} (hr)	T_{o-c} (hr)	1° Site	Size (cc)	HA	Vomit	Sz	Focal deficit	$\downarrow$LOC	Coma	T_{o-m} (days)	ECI	Death	T_{o-f}	Deficit
					150 mg rt-PA												
1	55	54.1	2.4	0.50	Midbrain	6			+		+	+	Rapid	—	+	8	
2	60	57.7	74.3	14.50	R thalamus	4	?			+	+		Short	—	+	66	
3	62	81.8	8.6	1.00	R frontal	150		+		+	+		Rapid	—	+	11	
4	42	100.0	2.7	1.92	R fronto-parietal	40				+			Rapid	—	+	3.5	
5	60	?	5.7	2.50-26.50	Midbrain	1					+		Medium	Yes	+	53	
6	67	?	11.8	2.00	R parieto-occipital	116				+	+		Rapid	—	+	21	
7	58	80.0	7.4	3.00	L fronto-temporal	23	+						Rapid	—	+	4	
8	70	79.3	13.9	15.50	Cerebellum	14		+			+		Short	—		1490	Minor
9	61	78.6	17.3	<15.00	R thalamus	20				+			Rapid	—	+	26	
10	67	86.0	26.1	1.00	L occipital	3			+		+		Long	Yes	+	10	
11	66	76.3	19.6	?	L frontal	26		+	+		+		Rapid	—		1464	Major
12	64	64.0	1.3	8.00	L fronto-parietal	24					+		Medium	—		1101	Major
					100 mg rt-PA												
13	75	72.7	25.3	18.00	R frontal	3				+			Rapid	—		836	Minor
14	52	62.7	1.8	0.25	L thalamus	80				+	+	+	Rapid	—	+	2	
15	67	100.0	7.5	1.50-25.50	R parieto-occipital	30			+	+	+		Medium	Yes	+	3	
16	70	80.9	5.2	3.50	L temporo-parietal	166		+			+		Rapid	—	+	1	
17	72	67.0	1.8	1.50	R thalamus	2							Rapid	Yes		885	Minor
18	67	58.2	7.5	7.08	L temporo-parietal	23		+					Short	—		793	Major
19	61	70.0	12.6	7.50	L parietal	13							Rapid	Yes	+	227	
20	57	65.8	4.0	42.25	R frontal	27	+	+			+		Long	—		1096	Minor
21	68	68.0	9.5	6.02	L frontal	25					+		Rapid	—	+	2	
22	75	58.0	209.0	0.50	L fronto-parietal	1	?		+	?	+		Rapid	Yes		771	Full
23	60	93.6	3.5	11.33	L temporal	26	+						Short	—		1132	Full

WT — Weight (kg) at study entry.
T_{i-o} — Time from treatment initiation to symptom onset.
T_{o-c} — Time from earliest possible time of neurologic symptom onset to performance of first CT.
1° Site — Primary site.
cc — Cubic centimeters.
HA — Headache.
Sz — Seizure.
$\downarrow$LOC — Decreased level of consciousness.

T_{o-m} — Time from symptom onset to maximal deficit. Rapid = <6 hours; short = 6 to 12 hours; medium = >12 hours but <24 hours; and long = 24 to 48 hours.
ECI — Early clinical improvement within 24 hours of neurologic symptom onset.
T_{o-f} — Time from study entry to last follow-up or death.
? — Not available.
R — Right.
L — Left.

Results. Data from this study are presented in tabular form as follows. Table 1 contains each patient's age, weight, time interval between treatment initiation and neurologic symptom onset, time interval between neurologic symptom onset and performance of CT, site and size of primary ICH, earliest clinical abnormalities, time interval from neurologic symptom onset to maximal deficit, mortality, neurologic follow-up time, and residual deficit. Table 2 contains information on medical history (hypertension, atrial fibrillation, and prior cerebrovascular disease), ventricular arrhythmias, blood pressures, fibrinogen and aPTT (when available), presence of multiple hemorrhages, and underlying pathologic lesion (if known). Table 3 summarizes the neuropathologic data from the five autopsied patients.

Baseline characteristics. Of the 23 patients in this series, 14 (61%) were men and nine (39%) women. Twenty patients (87%) were white. The age range was 42 to 75 years, with a mean age of 63.3 years; 57% of the patients were in the seventh decade and 22% were in the eighth decade. Weight at study entry was available in 21 patients (91%); low body weight (<70 kg) was known to be present in three of 10 patients (30%) in the 150-mg rt-PA group and six of 11 patients (54%) in the 100-mg rt-PA group (table 1). Fourteen patients (61%) had histories of hypertension. Five patients had evidence of prior cerebrovascular disease: three with stroke, one with transient ischemic attacks, and one with transient ischemic attacks and stroke. No information is available about the type or location of stroke. The ECG location of myocardial infarction was anterior in 15 patients (65%).

At the time of study entry, 10 patients (43%) had systolic blood pressures greater than 140 mm Hg, and 10 patients (43%) had diastolic blood pressures greater than 90 mm Hg (table 2). Thirteen patients (56.5%) developed or maintained a blood pressure ≥160 mm Hg systolic or ≥90 mm Hg diastolic during the rt-PA infusion. Ten patients (43%) had systolic blood pressures ≥160 mm Hg during the rt-PA infusion; two of these were normotensive at study entry. Thirteen patients had diastolic blood pressures ≥90 mm Hg (five were ≥100 mm Hg) during

Table 2. Contributing factors and cerebrovascular lesions in ICH associated with thrombolytic therapy

Pt no.	HTN	AF	History of CD	VA	BP at entry	↑BP infusion	↑BP onset	FIB	↑aPTT (sec)	Mult ICH	Lesion
1	+				150/100	146/92 Pre					
2		+	Stroke		148/111	119/84 Pre					(late) HI
3	+				160/110	150/96 Pre					
4	+				140/105	167/110 During	167/110		150		?
5					120/90	167/94 Pre		15	150	+	
6	+		TIA, stroke	+	140/80	120/70 Pre		15		+	CAA
7					130/80	120/80 Pre		32	70		
8	+				110/60	204/80 Pre			150	+	
9	+		Stroke		130/100	182/122 Pre					
10	+		Stroke		160/100	190/100 Pre			(?150)		
11				+	138/66	126/82 Pre			(?100)		
12				+	130/86	100/72 Post	100/72		100		
13	+				92/60	120/86 Pre	130/70		>100		
14		+		+	150/90	190/110 Post	150/100				
15			TIA		130/82	160/92 Pre		85		+	CAA
16	+				160/75	176/99 Pre	200/—	107	82		
17					165/75	170 Pre/92 Post	150/70	181			
18	+			+	170/100	120/90 Pre		205	(?62)		AVM
19	+			+	174/114	120/88 Pre	160/110	232			
20					110/70	126/70 Pre		280	100	+	
21	+				84/58	102/60 Pre			89	+	CAA
22	+				126/92	150/92 Pre		245			
23	+				148/98	180/110 Pre	180/110	125	100		

HTN	History of hypertension.	
AF	Atrial fibrillation.	
CD	Cerebrovascular disease.	
VA	Ventricular arrhythmias.	
BP	Blood pressure.	
↑BP infusion	Highest blood pressure, systolic and diastolic, during the first 3 hours of rt-PA infusion.	
↑BP onset	Highest blood pressure, systolic and diastolic, nearest to time of symptom onset.	
FIB	Fibrinogen level 8 hours after initiation of rt-PA infusion (mg/dl).	
↑aPTT	Recorded activated partial thromboplastin time closest in time to onset of symptoms.	
Mult ICH	Multiple intracerebral hemorrhages.	
+	Present.	
—	Absent.	
TIA	Transient ischemic attack.	
Pre	Before symptom onset.	
Post	After symptom onset.	
HI	Hemorrhagic infarction.	
CAA	Cerebral amyloid angiopathy.	
AVM	Arteriovenous malformation.	

the rt-PA infusion; one had been normotensive at study entry. One of these patients had an ongoing hypertensive crisis that was difficult to control (patient 9). Of the eight patients with blood pressures recorded at or near the time of symptom onset, five had systolic blood pressures ≥160 mm Hg and/or diastolic blood pressures ≥100 mm Hg. In comparison, of the 3,901 patients who did not have ICH, 1,024 (26.2%) had a blood pressure ≥160 mm Hg systolic and/or ≥90 mm Hg diastolic during the first 3 hours of the rt-PA infusion.

Six of 23 patients (26%) had life-threatening cardiac arrhythmias (table 2). Ventricular fibrillation occurred in five and ventricular tachycardia occurred in one. The time of occurrence of ventricular fibrillation was before the rt-PA infusion in three, during the rt-PA infusion in one, and after termination of the rt-PA infusion but before onset of neurologic symptoms in one. The one instance of ventricular tachycardia occurred after termination of the rt-PA infusion and after onset of neurologic symptoms. Ventricular fibrillation occurred before or during the rt-PA infusion in four of 23 patients (17.4%) with ICH and 181 of 3,901 patients (4.6%) without ICH. Atrial fibrillation occurred in only two of the 23 patients (9%). In one of these (patient 2), symptoms occurred after cardioversion of rapid atrial fibrillation in the setting of acute anterior-wall myocardial infarction and a history of prior stroke.

Timing, clinical features, and temporal course. The earliest possible times of onset for 19 of the 23 hemorrhages (83%) were within the first 24 hours after initiation of treatment. Nine (39%) occurred during the 6-hour study drug infusion; six (26%) between 6 and 12 hours after initiation of the infusion; and four (17%) between 12 and 24 hours after initiation of the infusion. The times of occurrence of symptoms among the six patients with multiple hemorrhages were 4.0 hours, 5.7 hours, 7.5 hours, 9.5 hours, 11.8 hours, and 13.9 hours after initiation of treatment.

The most frequent earliest documented neurologic symptom and sign in the 23 patients studied was a decreased level of consciousness, observed in 15 patients (65%); two patients (9%) were in coma. Eight patients (35%) had focal neurologic deficits. Other presenting complaints included vomiting in six patients (26%), seizures in five (22%), and headache in three (13%). Headache was noted in

Table 3. Neuropathologic findings in five patients with fatal ICH following rt-PA and heparin therapy for acute myocardial infarction

Pt no.	Hematoma location	Amyloid β-protein	CNS, other	Probable etiology of ICH
2	Intraventricular	Negative	Lacunes, basal ganglia	Hemorrhagic transformation of infarct, periventricular centrum semiovale
4	Subcortical white matter	Negative	Slight vascular thickening	Undetermined
6	Subcortical	Blood vessels, neuritic plaques	Microhematomas of cortex, old; cortical neuritic plaques, frequent	CAA
15	Subcortical, multiple; intraventricular	Rare blood vessel, neuritic plaques	Cortical neuritic plaques, frequent; infarct, periventricular centrum semiovale	Possible CAA
21	Subcortical, multiple	Blood vessels, neuritic plaques	Microhematomas of cortex, old; cortical diffuse plaques, frequent; cortical neuritic plaques, few	CAA

ICH   Intracerebral hemorrhage.
rt-PA Recombinant tissue plasminogen activator.
CAA Cerebral amyloid angiopathy.

two patients with lobar hematomas and the one patient with multiple cerebellar hematomas. Eleven patients (48%) had more than one neurologic abnormality at symptom onset (table 1). In addition, documented symptoms and signs of neurologic deterioration at the time of examination in the 23 patients with ICH included decreased level of consciousness (lethargy or stupor) in 82%, coma in 30%, hemiparesis in 62%, disordered oculomotor function in 48%, nausea/vomiting in 39%, and disorientation in 30%. Of the five patients with seizures, four had lobar hemorrhages (25% of the 16 lobar cases), and one had a midbrain hemorrhage with extension to the subarachnoid space.

The onset of symptoms was rapid (less than 10 minutes) in seven (30%) and gradual in 16 (70%) patients. The time to maximal deficit was less than 6 hours in 14 (61%), 6 to 12 hours in four (17%), 12 to 24 hours in three (13%), and 24 to 48 hours in two (9%) patients. There was possible clinical improvement within 24 hours of onset in six patients (nos. 5, 10, 15, 17, 19, and 22). In patients 10 and 17, this may have represented recovery from a postictal state. In patient 15, the sedative effect of diazepam may have been resolving.

For 19 of 23 patients (83%), the time interval between the earliest possible time of neurologic symptom onset and performance of the first CT was known. The time interval was less than 2 hours in eight, 2 to 6 hours in two, 6 to 12 hours in five, 12 to 24 hours in three, and more than 24 hours in one. For four patients (nos. 5, 9, 11, and 15), the exact time interval could not be determined (table 1). For the patients with known time intervals between neurologic symptom onset and performance of CT, the time interval ranges were 0.50 to 7.50 hours (mean, 2.63 hours) for the four patients with clinical improvement within 24 hours of ICH onset, and 0.25 to 42.25 hours (mean, 8.52 hours) for the 16 patients without clinical improvement within 24 hours of ICH onset.

Hemostatic measurements. In the 17 patients with available platelet counts, thrombocytopenia (platelet count <150,000/mm^3) was not present at the onset of symptoms. The aPTT was greater than 65 seconds in close temporal relation to symptom onset in 12 of the 23 patients (52%). Three patients in the 150-mg rt-PA group had profound hypofibrinogenemia (15 mg/dl, 15 mg/dl, and 32 mg/dl) at or near the time of symptom onset; only one patient in the 100-mg rt-PA group had a fibrinogen level as low as 85 mg/dl (table 2). Three of the six patients with multiple hemorrhages had fibrinogen levels measured at or near the time of symptom onset; 15 mg/dl each in two patients (nos. 5 and 6) and 85 mg/dl in one (no. 15). There was no obvious relation between degree of hypofibrinogenemia and size of ICH.

Site and size of intracerebral hemorrhages. The sites of the primary hemorrhage for the 23 cases were lobar in 16 (70%), thalamic in four (17%), and brainstem-cerebellum in three (13%) (table 1). Specific primary lobar sites included frontal (5), parietal (1), temporal (1), occipital (1), and multiple contiguous sites (8). Multilobar sites were frontoparietal (3), parieto-occipital (2), temporoparietal (2), and frontotemporal (1). Extension of the ICH to other sites occurred in five patients (22%). Specific primary sites in the posterior fossa were midbrain (2) and cerebellum (1). Extension of the hemorrhage to the ventricular system occurred in 13 cases (57%) and to the subarachnoid space in nine cases (39%). In one patient (no. 18), a left temporoparietal ICH was associated with a serpentine structure coursing medially and inferiorly, suggestive of an arteriovenous malformation. Multiple distinct hemorrhages occurred in six of 23 patients (26%; nos. 5, 6, 8, 15, 20, and 21), three in the 150-mg rt-PA group and three in the 100-mg rt-PA group. Five of the six patients had multiple cerebral lobar hemorrhages and one had multiple cerebellar hemorrhages. Only one (no. 21) had more than five sites involved.

The size of the primary hematomas ranged from 1 cc to 166 cc, with a mean size of 35.8 cc (table 1). There were three distinct size groups: seven (30%) small-volume hemorrhages (1 to 9 cc), 12 (52%) moderate-volume hemorrhages (10 to 49 cc), and four (17%) large-volume hemorrhages (≥50 cc). Within 12 hours of initiation of rt-PA therapy, four of four large, eight of 12 medium, and three of seven small hemorrhages occurred. There were no important differences in the sizes of the hemorrhages associated with the 150-mg and 100-mg rt-PA regimens.

Neuropathologic findings. Table 3 summarizes the clinical and neuropathologic findings of the five patients with fatal ICH who had autopsy examinations. Four of these patients developed neurologic symptoms and signs within 12 hours of study entry, two of five patients (nos. 6 and 21) had ventricular arrhythmias, and none had uncontrolled hypertension.

Three patients had CAA associated with multiple subcortical hemorrhages. The arteries and arterioles of the cerebral leptomeninges and cortex were dilated, and the walls were thickened and replaced by amorphous pink material that was strongly immunoreactive to ABP. The vascular changes were extensive in two of the three patients but were only mild in the third. Congo red stains performed in two of the three patients (nos. 6 and 21) were positive and showed characteristic yellow-green dichroism when viewed under polarized light. In addition, frequent cortical neuritic plaques (>15 per 200× field) were present in two of these patients, and frequent diffuse plaques and a few neuritic plaques were found in the third. The etiology of the multiple subcortical hemorrhages in patient 4 was not identified. The cortical blood vessels were only slightly thickened, amyloid was not identified with either Congo red stain or immunohistochemistry, and neither thromboemboli nor infarcts were observed.

The massive intraventricular hemorrhage in one patient (no. 2) was anatomically contiguous with a hemorrhagic infarction in the periventricular white matter. The age of the infarct was consistent with the 3-month interval between the hemorrhagic complication and death. In retrospect, the diagnosis of hemorrhagic infarction may have been suspected in view of four distinctive clinical features: history of prior stroke, acute anterior-wall myocardial infarction, cardioversion for rapid atrial fibrillation, and late occurrence of neurologic symptoms (74 hours after initiation of thrombolytic therapy). In this patient, the time interval between neurologic symptom onset and performance of the CT was 18 hours.

Management and outcome. Eighteen of the 23 patients with ICH were treated medically with discontinuation of heparin (17), administration of protamine (5) and ε-aminocaproic acid (1), and infusion of fresh frozen plasma (4) and cryoprecipitate (4). One patient (no. 22) was not receiving anticoagulants at the time of onset of neurologic symptoms. Steroids or mannitol were given to six patients. Five had discontinuation of heparin and surgical evacuation of the hematoma, and two received ventriculostomies for hydrocephalus. Three of the five patients who underwent craniotomy died.

The overall case fatality rate within 1 month was 11 of 23 patients (48%): seven of 12 patients (58%) in the 150-mg rt-PA group and four of 11 patients (36%) in the 100-mg rt-PA group (table 2). Fatal hemorrhages occurred in five of nine patients (56%) with onset of symptoms within less than 6 hours after initiation of study drug infusion and five of six (83%) within 6 to 12 hours. In eight of these 10 fatal cases (80%), patients were comatose when initially examined. One patient succumbed due to underlying cardiac disease, possible mesenteric ischemia, and sepsis (no. 10), and another had a massive pulmonary embolus (no. 15).

Discussion. In TIMI II, 23 patients (0.58%) met previously defined criteria[16] for primary ICH associated with rt-PA and heparin therapy for acute myocardial infarction. Most of the hemorrhages (83%) occurred within 24 hours (with 15, or 65%, within 12 hours) of initiation of rt-PA infusion. This is similar to findings in other studies[1-5,13,15,31-41] and suggests a temporal relationship between rt-PA administration and ICH, with occurrence and enlargement of the hemorrhage during the period of active fibrinolysis.[42,43] This bleeding may be potentiated by concomitant administration of antithrombotic therapy[1,2,16,19,31,33,37,38,42,44] and other factors. An arteriovenous malformation was observed on CT in one patient. Pathologic examination in five ICH patients revealed important clues to pathogenesis in four patients: CAA in three and hemorrhagic transformation of cerebral infarction in one.

Clinical factors contributing to ICH occurrence. Fourteen patients (61%) had histories of hypertension, and 13 (57%) developed or maintained elevated blood pressure (≥160/90 mm Hg) during rt-PA infusion. In reported series of ICH occurring secondary to chronic hypertension, hemorrhages tended to be found most often in the basal ganglia. The predominance of lobar hemorrhages (70%) in TIMI II is unusual for hypertensive ICH.[45-47] The distribution of the primary hemorrhage sites in this series is similar to the distribution of ICH associated with long-term oral anticoagulant therapy,[48-50] although the cerebellum[48] was not a frequent site of bleeding.

These findings suggest that in TIMI II, chronic hypertension may not be the preeminent cause of ICHs associated with thrombolytic therapy.[26,45-47] Uncontrolled hypertension was a reason for exclusion of patients from enrollment in TIMI II. However, after enrollment, acute hypertension, ie, ≥160 mm Hg systolic or ≥100 mm Hg diastolic, arising during infusion of fibrinolytic agents may have contributed to the occurrence of ICH in 10 patients (43%).[14,51] Although elevated blood pressure was noted more frequently in the patients with ICH, this may reflect either different intensity of patient observation between the groups or a cardiovascular response to the ICH.

Life-threatening ventricular arrhythmias occurred in six patients (26%), with five of six (83%) cases occurring before onset of neurologic symptoms. Prolonged cardiopulmonary resuscitation (CPR) may lead to global hypoxic-ischemic encephalopathy. Several authorities recommend that CPR for less than 10 minutes should not be a contraindication to thrombolytic therapy.[52,53] Whether CPR is brief or prolonged, marked fluctuations in blood pressure due to pharmacologic therapy and electrical cardioversion are associated with hemodynamic instability that may lead to dramatic changes in cerebral perfusion. If cerebral vessels are structurally weakened, then the combined effect of thrombolytic therapy and blood pressure fluctuations may promote the occurrence of intracranial bleeding. While ventricular fibrillation before or during the rt-PA infusion was noted more frequently in the patients with ICH, this may reflect either a different level of patient observation between the groups or an association not previously reported that requires further study.

Underlying cerebrovascular pathology. The reported frequency of multiple sites of ICH in patients treated with thrombolytic agents is 15 to 38%.[13,15,42] The 26% frequency of multiple ICHs in TIMI II confirms these findings. Limited data in the literature[54-56] suggest that CT-detectable multiple hemorrhages may occur in 2%[55] to 11%[54] of spontaneous ICH cases. They occur most frequently in patients with leukemia and other blood dyscrasias, coagulopathies, neoplasms (primary and metastatic), vasculitis, venous sinus thrombosis, and CAA[57-60] but rarely with chronic hypertension.[54,55]

Structural lesions in the brain may predispose to ICH. Hemorrhage might occur by induction of de novo bleeding from a previously unruptured lesion or rebleeding from a vessel that had bled previously. In the setting of thrombolytic therapy for acute myocardial infarction, arteriovenous malformations[16,39] and CAA[40-42,61] are the only structural lesions that have been reported in patients with ICH.

CAA is due to the infiltration of cerebrum-specific amyloid into the media and adventitia of small to medium cerebral or cerebellar arteries, arterioles, and veins.[57-60] The affected vessels are structurally brittle and unable to withstand trauma or blood pressure changes.[57,59] The suspicion that CAA contributes to ICH in patients treated with thrombolytic agents is based on the cerebral or cerebellar lobar location, multiplicity, increasing frequency in older patients,[6-8,13-16,42,62,63] and the growing number of reports demonstrating the association in surgical[42,61] and autopsy[40,41] specimens. In the present study, four of five patients whose brains were examined at autopsy had subcortical lobar hemorrhages characteristic of CAA. In three of these four patients, we found multiple hemorrhages and immunohistochemical evidence of CAA. Four of the six multiple ICHs were fatal; three of these patients had CAA. In addition, two of these three patients had numerous neuritic plaques in the cerebral cortex; these plaque frequencies would have been consistent with the diagnosis of Alzheimer's disease had the patients been demented.[29,30] However, not all patients with CAA-related ICH after thrombolysis have microscopic Alzheimer's disease.[41,61]

Recent data support the possibility of a connection between increasing age, ICH, and CAA. The GUSTO Trial reported a three- or fourfold increase in the risk of hemorrhagic stroke in patients >75 years old treated with streptokinase or accelerated rt-PA compared with patients ≤75 years old.[12] In future studies, it would be interesting to briefly assess cognitive function in patients, particularly those over age 75, before thrombolytic treatment is given.

One of the five patients (no. 2) had pathologic evidence for a confluent hemorrhagic infarction that extended to the ventricular system. No other patient in this series had the combination of clinical features suggestive of preceding ischemic cerebral infarction that were present in this patient (no. 2). In the other patient with atrial fibrillation (no. 14), the timing of the ICH after thrombolytic treatment and the typical pattern of extension of the massive thalamic ICH make hemorrhagic transformation of a cerebral infarction less likely.

Even with stringent clinical and radiologic criteria, it may be extremely difficult to distinguish a primary ICH from a confluent hemorrhagic infarction.[62-66] Mutlu et al[65] observed that four cases of fatal lobar or white matter hemorrhages were actually "catabolic rupture hemorrhages" associated with thrombotic occlusion. Bogousslavsky et al[66] demonstrated that confluent hemorrhagic transformation of a cerebral infarction may occur within 16 ± 3 hours of stroke onset, particularly in patients with potential cardiac sources of embolism, prior TIAs, and previously undiagnosed stroke on CT. In one case in that study,[66] autopsy failed to demonstrate histologic evidence of an underlying ischemic cerebral infarction.

Some studies[67,68] suggest that hemorrhagic infarction following cardioembolic stroke generally occurs within 4 days of onset, rarely on the first day or as late as 11 days after onset. In TIMI II, there was a shorter mean time interval between ICH onset and performance of CT in patients with clinical improvement within 24 hours of ICH onset than in those who did not improve within 24 hours. The longer time to CT performance in patients who did not improve makes it less likely that confluent hemorrhagic infarctions occurred in patients who did improve and were not detected due to a delay in performance of CT.

Of the 29 ischemic cerebral infarctions in TIMI II,[64] eight (28%) had hemorrhagic infarctions. It is not known how often this event occurred in other studies.[1-10,13,14,31-38,62,69] It is presently unknown what proportion of "ICH" diagnosed on clinical grounds or with neuroimaging techniques would be classified pathologically as confluent hemorrhagic infarctions. In the GUSTO trial,[12] hemorrhagic transformation of ischemic cerebral infarction occurred in a small proportion of patients who had ischemic strokes. We therefore believe that the one misclassified patient (no. 2) in our series represents a small minority of patients who have hemorrhagic infarctions misclassified as ICHs.

Hemostatic measurements. In nine cases in the literature[15,36,44,70-72] and in three of our patients, ICH occurred in association with documented severe hypofibrinogenemia. In TIMI II,[73] patients with or without ICH who received 150 mg rt-PA had higher plasma rt-PA levels, higher fibrinogen degradation product levels, and lower plasminogen levels, and were more likely to have lower fibrinogen levels, than patients receiving 100 mg rt-PA. However, as previously reported,[16] there were no large differences in fibrinogen, fibrinogen degradation products, rt-PA antigen level, plasminogen levels, and aPTT among the 23 patients with ICH, the 29 patients with cerebral infarction, and all other patients who did not have cerebrovascular events. The small number of observations precludes firm conclusions regarding the relation between the existence of a systemic lytic state and CNS bleeding.

Role of multiple factors. A number of investigators have identified factors that may increase the risk of intracranial hemorrhage following thrombolytic therapy for acute myocardial infarction.[10,74] In a multiple logistic regression analysis of data on intracranial hemorrhage patients from a number of clinical trials, including the present study, Simoons et al[74] suggested that four variables known at hospital admission appeared to be related to intracranial hemorrhage: elderly age (>65 years), low body weight (<70 kg), hypertension upon admission (systolic blood pressure ≥170 mm Hg and/or diastolic blood pressure ≥95 mm Hg), and alteplase (rt-PA) regimen. In patients receiving alteplase, the odds ratios were 3.2 (95% CI = 1.8-5.6) for elderly age, 2.5 (95% CI = 1.4-4.4) for low body weight, and 2.0 (95% CI = 1.0-3.9) for hypertension on admission. Assuming an overall intracranial hemorrhage risk of 0.75%, the risk estimate varied from 0.26% for a patient without intracranial hemorrhage risk factors who received streptokinase to 5.0% for an elderly hypertensive patient with low body weight treated with alteplase.[74]

In TIMI II, prior cerebrovascular disease, wide fluctuations in blood pressure due to the occurrence and treatment of ventricular arrhythmias, marked hypofibrinogenemia, and prolonged aPTT after rt-PA and heparin therapy may have enhanced bleeding from weakened amyloid-infiltrated vessels and led to the multiple ICHs in one patient (no. 6). Ventricular arrhythmias in the setting of a prolonged aPTT may lead to ICH (patient 12). Persistent or acute hypertension (either systolic or diastolic)[14,44,51] in the presence of a prolonged aPTT may lead to single (patients 4, 8, 10, 16, and 23) or multiple (patient 15) ICH. In other ICH cases, presently unknown factors, other than the effects of combined thrombolytic/anticoagulant therapy, may be responsible for ICH.

Clinical features. The finding of a decreased level of consciousness at presentation in 15 of 23 (65%) and on initial examination in 20 of 23 patients (87%) is striking. Our patients frequently had a rapid onset and progression of symptoms and signs; 61% reached their maximal deficit within 6 hours (78% within 12 hours) of symptom onset. This temporal course is more characteristic of "hypertensive" hemorrhage[75] than of ICH related to long-term anticoagulant therapy.[48] Our findings differ from those of Wijdicks and Jack,[42] who found focal neurologic deficits at onset followed by a rapid decrease in level of consciousness in all eight of their patients. The variations in clinical presentation may be due to the site or size of ICH, rapidity of onset and progression before clinical recognition, and other factors. The occurrence of decreasing alertness, decreased level of consciousness, or focal neurologic deficits, especially if rapid in onset and progression, within 24 hours of rt-PA infusion for acute myocardial infarction should be interpreted as suggesting ICH, and this diagnosis must be excluded as soon as possible.

The reported observation of possible improvement within 24 hours of onset in six of the 23 cases (26%) is unusual for parenchymatous ICH.[75] In our study, two patients had motor seizures at presentation, and improvement in these cases may have reflected resolution of the postictal state. Improvement in the other four cases may have reflected the resolution of more clinically subtle complex partial seizures, toxic-metabolic disturbances, sedation, or improved cardiac function. There is no direct evidence to support or refute the hypothesis that these four patients had confluent hemorrhagic transformation of a preceding ischemic cerebral infarction.

Prognosis of intracerebral hemorrhage. Previous studies[76-78] have shown that decreased level of consciousness is associated with a poor prognosis in patients with ICH. In this study, 13 of the 20 patients (65%) with decreased level of consciousness at initial examination died (table 1). There was a high case fatality rate (10/15, or 67%) for patients with ICH within 12 hours of initiation of treatment. These findings are similar to those of Wijdicks and Jack.[42]

Therapeutic implications. These results have several implications for treatment of acute myocardial infarction with fibrinolytic agents. First, the occurrence of ICH following thrombolytic therapy for acute myocardial infarction may be difficult to predict. Second, the occurrence of a decreased level of alertness or appearance of a neurologic deficit, particularly in the 24 hours after initiation of thrombolytic therapy, must be suspected to reflect ICH until proven otherwise. Third, it may be informative to evaluate cognitive/neurologic function in older patients before giving thrombolytic therapy. Fourth, blood pressure should be carefully controlled before, during, and after infusion of the fibrinolytic agent. Finally, more data are needed to delineate the microvascular/microscopic pathology associated with ICH after thrombolytic therapy for acute myocardial infarction.

Acknowledgments

The authors express gratitude to the clinicians and pathologists who made data available for this study, and thank Myra Franklin and Patricia Haworth for preparation of the manuscript.

References

1. Gruppo Italiano per lo Studio della Streptochinasi nell'Infarto Miocardico (GISSI). Effectiveness of intravenous thrombolytic treatment in acute myocardial infarction. Lancet 1986;1:397-402.
2. Maggioni AP, Franzosi MG, Farina ML, et al. Cerebrovascular events after myocardial infarction. BMJ 1991;302:1428-1431.
3. ISAM Study Group. A prospective trial of intravenous streptokinase in acute myocardial infarction (ISAM). N Engl J Med 1986;314:1465-1471.
4. Schroder R, Neuhaus K-L, Leizorovicz A, Linderer T, Tebbe U, for the ISAM Study Group. A prospective placebo-controlled double-blind multicenter trial of intravenous streptokinase (ISAM): long-term mortality and morbidity in acute myocardial infarction. J Am Coll Cardiol 1987;9:197-203.
5. ISIS-2 (Second International Study of Infarct Survival). Randomized trial of intravenous streptokinase, oral aspirin, both or neither among 17,187 cases of suspected acute myocardial infarction: ISIS-2. Lancet 1988;2:349-360.
6. Gruppo Italiano per lo Studio della Sopravvivenza nell'Infarto Miocardico. GISSI-2. A factorial randomized trial of alteplase versus streptokinase and heparin versus no heparin among 12,490 patients with acute myocardial infarction. Lancet 1990;336:65-71.
7. International Study Group. In-hospital mortality and clinical course of 20,891 patients with suspected acute myocardial infarction randomized between alteplase and streptokinase with or without heparin. Lancet 1990;336:71-75.
8. Maggione AP, Franzosi MG, Santoro E, White H, Van de Werf F, Tognini G, Gruppo Italiano per lo Studio della Sopravvivenza nell'Infarto Miocardico II (GISSI II), and the International Study Group. The risk of stroke in patients with acute myocardial infarction after thrombolytic and antithrombotic treatment. N Engl J Med 1992;327:1-6.
9. ISIS-3. A randomized comparison of streptokinase versus tissue plasminogen activator versus anistreplase and of aspirin plus heparin versus aspirin alone among 41,299 cases of suspected acute myocardial infarctions. ISIS-3 (Third International Study of Infarct Survival) Collaborative Group. Lancet 1992;339:753-770.
10. de Jaegere PP, Arnold AP, Balk AH, Simoons ML. Intracranial hemorrhage in association with thrombolytic therapy: incidence and clinical predictive factors. J Am Coll Cardiol 1992;20:289-294.
11. Longstreth WT, Litwin PE, Weaver WD, for the MITI Project Group. Myocardial infarction, thrombolytic therapy, and stroke: a community-based study. Stroke 1993;24:587-590.
12. GUSTO Investigators. An international randomized trial comparing four thrombolytic strategies for acute myocardial infarction. N Engl J Med 1993;329:673-682.
13. Uglietta JP, O'Connor CM, Boyko CB, Aldrich H, Massey EW, Heinz ER. CT patterns of intracranial hemorrhage complicating thrombolytic therapy for acute myocardial infarction. Radiology 1991;181:555-559.
14. Anderson JL, Karagounis L, Allen A, Bradford MJ, Menlove RL, Pryor AT. Older age and elevated blood pressure are risk factors for intracerebral hemorrhage after thrombolysis. Am J Cardiol 1991;68:166-170.
15. Kase CS, Pessin MS, Zivin JA, et al. Intracranial hemorrhage following thrombolysis with tissue plasminogen activator. Am J Med 1992;92:384-390.
16. Gore JM, Sloan M, Price TR, et al, and the TIMI Investigators. Intracerebral hemorrhage, cerebral infarction, and subdural hematoma after acute myocardial infarction and thrombolytic therapy in the thrombolysis in myocardial infarction study. Thrombolysis in Myocardial Infarction, Phase II, Pilot and Clinical Trial. Circulation 1991;83:448-459.
17. De Bono DP, Simoons ML, Tijssen J, et al, for the European Cooperative Study. Effect of early intravenous heparin on coronary patency, infarct size, and bleeding complications after alteplase thrombolysis: results of a randomized double-blind European Cooperative Study Group trial. Br Heart J 1992;67:122-128.
18. LATE Study Group. Late assessment of thrombolytic efficacy (LATE) study with alteplase 6-24 hours after onset of acute myocardial infarction. Lancet 1993;342:759-766.
19. Passamani E, Hodges M, Herman M, et al, for the TIMI Investigators. The Thrombolysis in Myocardial Infarction (TIMI) Phase II Pilot Study: tissue plasminogen activator followed by percutaneous transluminal coronary angioplasty. J Am Coll Cardiol 1987;10(suppl):51B-64B.
20. TIMI Research Group. Immediate versus delayed catheterization and angioplasty following thrombolytic therapy for acute myocardial infarction: TIMI IIA results. JAMA 1988;260:2849-2858.
21. TIMI Study Group. Comparison of invasive and conservative strategies after treatment with intravenous tissue plasminogen activator in acute myocardial infarction: results of the Thrombolysis in Myocardial Infarction (TIMI) Phase II Trial. N Engl J Med 1989;320:618-627.
22. Braunwald E, Knatterud G, Passamani ER, Robertson TL. Announcement of protocol change in Thrombolysis in Myocardial Infarction Trial [letter]. J Am Coll Cardiol 1987;9:467.
23. Grossbard EB. Genentech experience with rt-PA (Activase®) [letter]. J Am Coll Cardiol 1987;9:467.
24. Braunwald E, Knatterud G, Passamani ER, Robertson TL, Solomon R. Update from the Thrombolysis in Myocardial Infarction trial [letter]. J Am Coll Cardiol 1987;10:970.
25. Hier DB, Davis KR, Richardson EP, Mohr JP. Hypertensive putaminal hemorrhage. Ann Neurol 1977;1:152-159.
26. Kase CS, Williams JP, Wyatt DA, Mohr JP. Lobar intracerebral hematomas: clinical and CT analysis of 22 cases. Neurology 1982;32:1146-1150.
27. Kitamoto T, Ogomori K, Tateishi J, Prusiner SB. Methods in laboratory investigation: formic acid pretreatment enhances immunostaining of cerebral and systemic amyloids. Lab Invest 1987;57:230-236.
28. Hsu S, Raine L, Fanger H. Use of avidin-biotin-peroxidase complex (ABC) in immunoperoxidase techniques. A comparison between ABC and unlabelled antibody (PAP) procedures. J Histochem Cytochem 1981;29:577-580.
29. Khachaturian ZS. The diagnosis of Alzheimer's disease. Arch Neurol 1985;42:1097-1105.
30. Mirra SS, Hart MN, Terry RD. Making the diagnosis of Alzheimer's disease. Arch Pathol Lab Med 1993;117:132-144.
31. Rutsch W, Schartl M, Mathey D, et al. Percutaneous transluminal coronary recanalization: procedure, results, and acute complications. Am Heart J 1981;102:1178-1181.
32. Ganz W, Geft I, Shah PK, et al. Intravenous streptokinase in evolving acute myocardial infarction. Am J Cardiol 1984;53:1209-1216.
33. PRIMI Trial Study Group. Randomized double-blind trial of recombinant prourokinase against streptokinase in acute myocardial infarction. Lancet 1989;1:863-868.
34. National Heart Foundation of Australia Coronary Thrombolysis Group. Coronary thrombolysis and myocardial salvage by tissue plasminogen activator given up to four hours after onset of a myocardial infarction. Lancet 1988;1:203-208.
35. Neuhaus K-L, Tebbe U, Gottwik M, et al. Intravenous recombinant tissue plasminogen activator (rt-PA) and urokinase in acute myocardial infarction: results of the German Activator Urokinase Study (GAUS). J Am Coll Cardiol 1988;12:581-587.
36. Califf RM, Topol EJ, George BS, et al, and the Thrombolysis and Angioplasty in Myocardial Infarction Study Group. Hemorrhagic complications associated with the use of intravenous tissue plasminogen activator in treatment of acute myocardial infarction. Am J Med 1988;85:353-359.

37. AIMS Trial Study Group. Effect of intravenous APSAC on mortality after acute myocardial infarction: preliminary report of a placebo-controlled clinical trial. Lancet 1988;1:545-549.

38. AIMS Trial Study Group. Long-term effects of intravenous anistreplase in acute myocardial infarction: final report of the AIMS study. Lancet 1990;335:427-431.

39. Proner J, Rosenblum BR, Rothman A. Ruptured arteriovenous malformation complicating thrombolytic therapy with tissue plasminogen activator. Arch Neurol 1990;47:105-106.

40. Pendlebury WW, Iole ED, Tracy RP, Dill BA. Intracerebral hemorrhage related to cerebral amyloid angiopathy and t-PA treatment. Ann Neurol 1991;29:210-213.

41. Ramsay DA, Penswick JL, Robertson DM. Fatal streptokinase-induced intracerebral hemorrhage in cerebral amyloid angiopathy. Can J Neurol Sci 1990;17:336-341.

42. Wijdicks CFM, Jack CR. Intracerebral hemorrhage after fibrinolytic therapy for acute myocardial infarction. Stroke 1993;24:554-557.

43. Eisenberg PR, Sherman LA, Tiefenbrunn AJ, Ludbrook PA, Sobel BE, Jaffe AS. Sustained fibrinolysis after administration of t-PA despite its short half life in the circulation. Thromb Haemost 1987;57:35-40.

44. Gorelick PB, Parikh M, McDonald L. Intracoronary streptokinase and fatal cerebellar hemorrhage. IMJ 1987;171:28-32.

45. Ropper AH, Davis KR. Lobar cerebral hemorrhages: acute clinical syndromes in 26 cases. Ann Neurol 1980;8:141-147.

46. Brott T, Thalinger K, Hertzberg V. Hypertension as a risk factor for spontaneous intracerebral hemorrhage. Stroke 1986;17:1078-1083.

47. Bahemuka M. Primary intracerebral hemorrhage and heart weight: a clinicopathologic case-control review of 218 patients. Stroke 1987;18:531-536.

48. Kase CS, Robinson RK, Stein RW, et al. Anticoagulant-related intracerebral hemorrhage. Neurology 1985;35:943-948.

49. Snyder M, Renaudin J. Intracerebral hemorrhage associated with anticoagulation therapy. Surg Neurol 1977;7:31-34.

50. Coon WW, Willis PW. Hemorrhagic complications of anticoagulant therapy. Arch Intern Med 1974;133:386-392.

51. Caplan L. Intracerebral hemorrhage revisited. Neurology 1988;38:624-627.

52. Miller DRW, Topol EJ. Selection of patients with acute myocardial infarction for thrombolytic therapy. Ann Intern Med 1990;113:949-960.

53. Kennedy JW. Expanding the use of thrombolytic therapy for acute myocardial infarction. Ann Intern Med 1990;113:907-909.

54. McCormick WF, Rosenfield DB. Massive brain hemorrhage: a review of 144 cases and an examination of their causes. Stroke 1973;4:946-954.

55. Weisberg L. Multiple spontaneous intracerebral hematomas: clinical and computed tomographic correlations. Neurology 1981;31:897-900.

56. Hickey WF, King RB, Wang AM, Samuels MA. Multiple simultaneous intracerebral hematomas: clinical, radiologic, and pathologic findings in two patients. Arch Neurol 1983;40:519-522.

57. Vonsattel JPG, Myers RH, Hedley-Whyte ET, Ropper AH, Bird ED, Richardson EP. Cerebral amyloid angiopathy without and with cerebral hemorrhages: a comparative histologic study. Ann Neurol 1991;30:637-649.

58. Kalyan-Raman UP, Kalyan-Raman K. Cerebral amyloid angiopathy causing intracranial hemorrhage. Ann Neurol 1984;16:321-329.

59. Vinters HV. Cerebral amyloid angiopathy: a critical review. Stroke 1987;18:311-323.

60. Itoh Y, Yamada M, Hayakawa M, Otomo E, Miyatake T. Cerebral amyloid angiopathy: a significant cause of cerebellar as well as lobar cerebral hemorrhages in the elderly. J Neurol Sci 1993;116:135-141.

61. Leblanc R, Haddad G, Robitaille Y. Cerebral hemorrhage from amyloid angiopathy after coronary thrombolysis. Neurosurgery 1992;31:586-590.

62. Sloan MA, Price TR. Intracranial hemorrhage following thrombolytic therapy for acute myocardial infarction. Semin Neurol 1991;11:385-399.

63. Sloan MA, Gore JM. Ischemic stroke and intracranial hemorrhage following thrombolytic therapy for acute myocardial infarction: a risk-benefit analysis. In: Gore JM, Becker RC, eds. A symposium: safety of thrombolytic agents. Am J Cardiol 1992;69:21A-38A.

64. Sloan MA, Price TR, Terrin ML, Forman S, for the TIMI Investigators. Ischemic cerebral infarction after rt-PA and heparin therapy for acute myocardial infarction. The TIMI II pilot and randomized trial combined experience [abstract]. Ann Neurol 1992;32:238.

65. Mutlu N, Berry RG, Alpers BJ. Massive cerebral hemorrhage: clinical and pathological correlations. Arch Neurol 1963;8:644-661.

66. Bogousslavsky J, Regli F, Uské A, Maeder P. Early spontaneous hematoma in cerebral infarct: is primary cerebral hemorrhage overdiagnosed? Neurology 1991;41:837-840.

67. Laureno R, Shields PW, Narayan T. The diagnosis and management of cerebral embolism and haemorrhagic infarction with sequential computerized cranial tomography. Brain 1987;110:93-105.

68. Lodder J, Krijne-Kubat B, van der Lugt PJM. Timing of autopsy-confirmed hemorrhagic infarction with reference to cardioembolic source. Stroke 1988;19:1482-1484.

69. Van de Werf F, Arnold AER, for the European Cooperative Study Group. Intravenous tissue plasminogen activator and size of infarct, left ventricular function, and survival in acute myocardial infarction. BMJ 1988;297:1371-1379.

70. Carlson S, Aldrich MS, Greenberg HS, Topol EJ. Intracerebral hemorrhage complicating intravenous tissue plasminogen activator treatment. Arch Neurol 1988;45:1070-1073.

71. Da Silva VF, Bormanis J. Intracerebral hemorrhage after combined anticoagulant-thrombolytic therapy for myocardial infarction: two case reports and a short review. Neurosurgery 1992;30:943-945.

72. Kase CS, O'Neal AN, Fisher M, Girgis GN, Ordia JI. Intracranial hemorrhage after use of tissue plasminogen activator for coronary thrombolysis. Ann Intern Med 1990;112:17-21.

73. Bovill EG, Terrin ML, Stump DC, et al, for the TIMI Investigators. Hemorrhagic events during therapy with recombinant tissue-type plasminogen activator, heparin, and aspirin for acute myocardial infarction. Ann Intern Med 1991;115:256-265.

74. Simoons ML, Maggioni AP, Knatterud G, et al. Individual risk assessment for intracranial hemorrhage during thrombolytic therapy. Lancet 1993;342:1523-1528.

75. Kase CS, Mohr JP. General features of intracerebral hemorrhage. In: Barnett HJH, Mohr JP, Stein BM, Yatsu FM, eds. Stroke, pathophysiology, diagnosis, and management. New York: Churchill Livingstone, 1986:497-523.

76. Portenoy RK, Lipton RB, Berger AR, Lesser ML, Lantos G. Intracerebral hemorrhage: a model for the prediction of outcome. J Neurol Neurosurg Psychiatry 1987;50:976-979.

77. Tuhrim S, Dambrosia JM, Price TR, et al. Prediction of intracerebral hemorrhage outcome. Ann Neurol 1988;24:258-263.

78. Tuhrim S, Dambrosia JM, Price TR, et al. Intracerebral hemorrhage: external validation and extension of a model for prediction of 30 day survival. Ann Neurol 1991;29:658-663.

Sudden Death in Young Competitive Athletes

Clinical, Demographic, and Pathological Profiles

Barry J. Maron, MD; Jamshid Shirani, MD; Liviu C. Poliac, MD; Robert Mathenge, MD; William C. Roberts, MD; Frederick O. Mueller, PhD

Objective.—To develop clinical, demographic, and pathological profiles of young competitive athletes who died suddenly.

Design.—Systematic evaluation of clinical information and circumstances associated with sudden deaths; interviews with family members, witnesses, and coaches; and analyses of postmortem anatomic, microscopic, and toxicologic data.

Participants and Setting.—A total of 158 sudden deaths that occurred in trained athletes throughout the United States from 1985 through 1995 were analyzed.

Main Outcome Measures.—Characteristics and probable cause of death.

Results.—Of 158 sudden deaths among athletes, 24 (15%) were explained by noncardiovascular causes. Among the 134 athletes who had cardiovascular causes of sudden death, the median age was 17 years (range, 12-40 years), 120 (90%) were male, 70 (52%) were white, and 59 (44%) were black. The most common competitive sports involved were basketball (47 cases) and football (45 cases), together accounting for 68% of sudden deaths. A total of 121 athletes (90%) collapsed during or immediately after a training session (78 cases) or a formal athletic contest (43 cases), with 80 deaths (63%) occurring between 3 PM and 9 PM. The most common structural cardiovascular diseases identified at autopsy as the primary cause of death were hypertrophic cardiomyopathy (48 athletes [36%]), which was disproportionately prevalent in black athletes compared with white athletes (48% vs 26% of deaths; P=.01), and malformations involving anomalous coronary artery origin (17 athletes [13%]). Of 115 athletes who had a standard preparticipation medical evaluation, only 4 (3%) were suspected of having cardiovascular disease, and the cardiovascular abnormality responsible for sudden death was correctly identified in only 1 athlete (0.9%).

Conclusions.—Sudden death in young competitive athletes usually is precipitated by physical activity and may be due to a heterogeneous spectrum of cardiovascular disease, most commonly hypertrophic cardiomyopathy. Preparticipation screening appeared to be of limited value in identification of underlying cardiovascular abnormalities.

JAMA. 1996;276:199-204

SUDDEN DEATH of a young competitive athlete is an unexpected and tragic event that continues to have great impact on both the community and the medical establishment.[1] Many such athletes are capable of exceptionally high levels of performance for long periods of time, even while harboring occult and potentially lethal cardiovascular malformations.[2,3] Some prior investigations of sudden death on the athletic field have been performed in highly selected and relatively small study populations, with few studies limited to highly trained athletes.[2,4-12] On occasion, these reports have provided conflicting characterization of the cardiac diseases responsible for such catastrophes.[2,3,8] Furthermore, the efficacy of preparticipation screening in identification of these cardiovascular abnormalities in athletes is unknown.[13,14] The objective of the present study was to develop a clinical and pathological profile for a broad-based and substantial group of young competitive athletes who had died suddenly.

METHODS

Since 1985, one of us (B.J.M.) has systematically assembled cases of competitive athletes who died suddenly. Athletes were identified from news media accounts, the National Center for Catastrophic Sports Injury Research registry, the cardiovascular pathology registry of Baylor University Medical Center, and informal communications and reports from high schools and colleges.

A subject was considered for inclusion if he or she (1) was a competitive athlete, ie, a participant in an organized sports program requiring regular training and competition with a premium placed on achievement[15]; (2) was younger than 35 years while an active athlete; (3) had no evidence of drug use on postmortem toxicologic examination of blood and urine; and (4) had accessible autopsy information from a complete or adequate postmortem examination. Data from our prior series of athletes[2,6] were not part of the present analysis.

A systematic process was used to assemble information for each case, including the autopsy report (with complete gross anatomic, microscopic, and toxicologic data), as well as pertinent clinical information, including the precise circumstances of collapse. Clinical data were derived from written accounts and from telephone interviews with family members, witnesses, or coaches. In selected instances, primary pathological materials were analyzed, and findings were verified by direct communication with medical examiners. Because few athletes had diagnostic cardiovascular evaluations during life, the diagnoses presented herein were necessarily based almost entirely on the necropsy findings.

Data analysis consisted of comparisons of proportions, using the χ^2 test where appropriate.

RESULTS

A total of 158 sudden deaths that occurred in young competitive athletes from 1985 through 1995 were analyzed. Of the

From the Division of Cardiovascular Research, Minneapolis Heart Institute Foundation, Minneapolis, Minn (Drs Maron, Poliac, and Mathenge); Albert Einstein College of Medicine, Bronx, NY (Dr Shirani); the National Center for Catastrophic Sports Injury Research and the University of North Carolina, Chapel Hill (Dr Mueller); and Baylor University Medical Center, Dallas, Tex (Dr Roberts).

Reprints: Barry J. Maron, MD, Minneapolis Heart Institute Foundation, 920 E 28th St, Suite 40, Minneapolis, MN 55407.

Primary Cardiovascular Lesion	No. (%) of Athletes	Median Age (Range), y
Hypertrophic cardiomyopathy	48 (36.0)	17.0 (13-28)
Unexplained increase in cardiac mass† ("possible hypertrophic cardiomyopathy")	14 (10.0)	17.0 (14-24)
Aberrant coronary arteries‡	17 (13.0)	15.0 (12-23)
Other coronary anomalies	8 (6.0)	17.5 (14-40)
Ruptured aortic aneurysm§	6 (5.0)	17.0 (16-31)
Tunneled LAD coronary artery	6 (5.0)	17.5 (14-20)
Aortic valve stenosis	5 (4.0)	14.0 (14-17)
Lesion consistent with myocarditis	4 (3.0)	15.5 (13-16)
Idiopathic dilated cardiomyopathy	4 (3.0)	18.0 (18-21)
ARVD	4 (3.0)	16.0 (15-17)
Idiopathic myocardial scarring	4 (3.0)	20.0 (14-27)
Mitral valve prolapse§	3 (2.0)	16.0 (15-23)
Atherosclerotic coronary artery disease	3 (2.0)	19.0 (14-28)
Other congenital heart diseases‖	2 (1.5)	13.5 (12-15)
Long QT syndrome¶	1 (0.5)	. . .
Sarcoidosis	1 (0.5)	. . .
Sickle cell trait#	1 (0.5)	. . .
"Normal" heart**	3 (2.0)	18.0 (16-21)

*LAD indicates left anterior descending; and ARVD, arrhythmogenic right ventricular dysplasia.

†Includes 1 athlete with grossly normal heart but distinctly abnormal histologic architecture with marked disorganization of cardiac muscle cells and bundles[26]; also, 2 of the 13 athletes with mildly increased mass had associated tunneled LAD coronary artery.

‡Anomalous origin of the left main coronary artery from the right sinus of Valsalva in 13 (1 of these also showed acute-angled takeoff of the right coronary artery and 1 had a tunneled segment of LAD), anomalous origin of the right coronary artery from the left sinus of Valsalva in 2, anomalous origin of the left main coronary artery (from between the left and posterior cusps) with acute-angled takeoff in 1, and origin of the LAD coronary artery from the pulmonary trunk in 1.

§Marfan syndrome was also present in 3 athletes with ruptured aortic aneurysm and in 1 with mitral valve prolapse.

‖One athlete with secundum atrial septal defect and 1 with coarctation of the aorta.

¶Also had anomalous origin of the right coronary artery from the left sinus of Valsalva.

#Judged to be the probable cause of death in the absence of any identifiable structural cardiovascular abnormality.[19]

**Absence of structural heart disease on standard autopsy examination.

158 athletes, 24 (15%) died of a variety of noncardiovascular causes; these included cardiac arrest due to blunt chest impact (7 cases),[16] but also drug abuse (2 cases),[17,18] pulmonary complications including bronchospasm (3 cases), heat stroke (1 case), peripheral embolization (1 case), and drowning (1 case). The remaining 134 athletes constitute the principal study group. For most of these athletes, several structural (and largely congenital) cardiovascular diseases were judged to be the probable cause of sudden death (Table; Figure 1).

Demographics

Of the 134 athletes, the median age was 17 years (range, 12-40 years); and 120 (90%) were male. The racial distribution included 70 whites (52%), 59 African Americans (44%), 3 Asians (2%), 1 Hispanic (0.5%), and 1 Native American (0.5%). The largest proportion of athletes were competing in high school (83 athletes [62%]), 30 (22%) were in college, and 9 (7%) were professional athletes; the remaining 12 athletes (9%) were aged 14 years or younger and in organized youth or junior high school sports. Sixteen elite athletes had achieved national or international levels of competition. A variety of 13 competitive sports were represented, with basketball and football the most common

(92 athletes [68%]) (Figure 2). Sudden deaths occurred in 35 states, with most cases in California (13 cases), Illinois (9 cases), and Georgia (8 cases).

Of the 134 athletes, 121 (90%) collapsed during or immediately after a training session (78 cases) or formal athletic contest (43 cases). The other 13 (10%) died while sedentary or during mild physical activity unrelated to sports, including 2 who died during sleep. Death was virtually instantaneous, although 4 athletes were conscious briefly after collapse and before cardiac arrest. In 12 athletes, prodromal complaints (eg, chest pain, dyspnea, dizziness, weakness) were described immediately before collapse.

The time of sudden death (ie, time of cardiovascular collapse) was determined for 127 athletes (95%). Sixty-three percent (80/127) of sudden deaths were clustered between 3 PM and 9 PM vs 37% (47/127) during the remainder of the day ($P<.003$), corresponding to the peak time for participation in most competitive team sports (Figure 3). This pattern was similar for athletes with hypertrophic cardiomyopathy (HCM) (64% [29/45] vs 36% [16/45]; $P<.01$) (Figure 3). Deaths were most common from August through January (62% [84/134]), corresponding to the competitive seasons for basketball and football.

Impact of Race and Sex

Hypertrophic cardiomyopathy occurred more commonly in black athletes (all male) than in white athletes (48% [28/59] vs 26% [18/70]; $P=.01$) (Figure 4). Aortic valve stenosis occurred only in white athletes (7% [5/70] vs 0/59 among blacks; $P=.02$), as did arrhythmogenic right ventricular dysplasia (ARVD) (6% [4/70] vs 0/59 among blacks; $P=.06$). The 14 female athletes were 15 to 31 years old and participated most commonly in basketball (5 cases) and track (5 cases); 6 had coronary anomalies, but only 2 had HCM.

Cardiac Symptoms

Only 24 athletes (18%) were known to have had symptoms judged to be cardiovascular in origin (eg, chest pain, exertional dyspnea, syncope, or dizziness) during the 36 months preceding death. These athletes had a variety of diseases, but most commonly had evidence of coronary anomalies (5 cases) and HCM (4 cases). Twelve athletes had 1 to 10 syncopal or near-syncopal episodes, including 3 with anomalous left main coronary artery, 2 with myocarditis, and 1 with HCM.

Specific Cardiac Diseases

Hypertrophic Cardiomyopathy.—Forty-eight athletes (36%) had probable or definite evidence of HCM. Each met our diagnostic criteria, with a hypertrophied, nondilated left ventricle (LV) in the absence of another cardiac or systemic disease capable of producing the degree of hypertrophy present[20] (Figure 1, A). With a heart weight of 500 g or more (to 675 g), at least 1 of the following supporting clinical or morphologic features was also required[21-27]: (1) a family history of HCM or premature sudden cardiac death; (2) gross anatomic abnormalities, including the description of an asymmetric pattern of LV hypertrophy, particularly marked ventricular septal thickening of 30 mm or greater, prominent bulging of the septum into the LV outflow tract, an enlarged left atrium with small ventricular cavities, and/ or greatly elongated mitral valve leaflets; (3) histologic abnormalities of the LV myocardium, including marked disorganization of cardiac muscle cells, abnormal intramural coronary arteries, and replacement fibrosis or scarring. With a heart weight of less than 500 g, a reported maximal LV wall thickness of 20 mm or greater and at least 1 of the aforementioned clinical or pathological features[21-27] were required for diagnosis of HCM. Six of 48 athletes with HCM had associated abnormalities that may have contributed to death, including hypoplastic coronary artery in 2, tunneled left anterior descending coronary artery in 2, and myocarditis or sickle cell trait in 1 each.

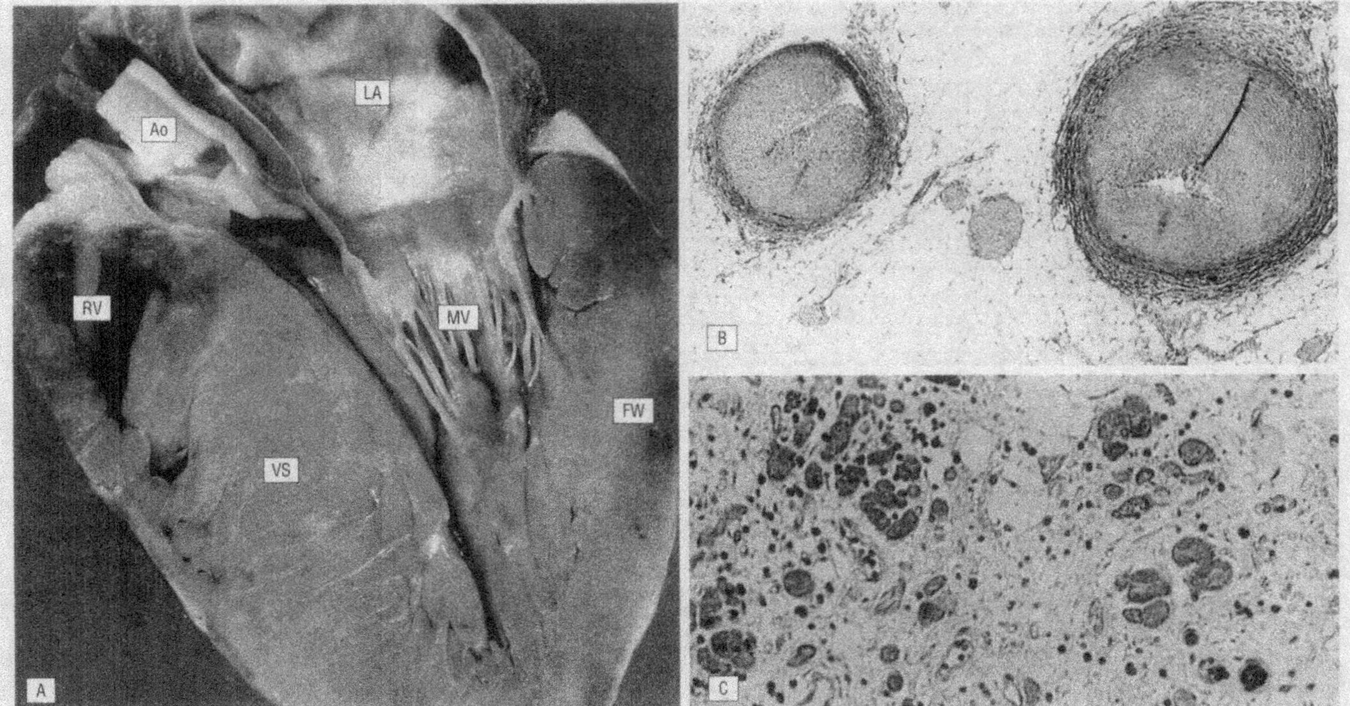

Figure 1.—Cardiac morphologic findings at autopsy in competitive athletes who died suddenly. A, Hypertrophic cardiomyopathy showing asymmetric hypertrophy of the ventricular septum (VS) with respect to the left ventricular free wall (FW) in the presence of a small cavity. Ao indicates aorta; LA, left atrium; RV, right ventricle; and MV, mitral valve. B, Histologic section of the left anterior descending coronary artery (right) and a branch (left) showing severe (>95%) cross-sectional luminal narrowing by atherosclerotic plaque (Movat stain, ×31). C, Histologic section of right ventricular wall showing islands of myocytes within a matrix of fatty and fibrous replacement, characteristic of arrhythmogenic right ventricular dysplasia; mononuclear cells are also evident (hematoxylin-eosin, ×63).

The hearts of 14 other athletes (11%) with a nondilated LV cavity were considered consistent with, but not diagnostic of, HCM ("possible HCM"). Thirteen showed a modest and unexplained increase in cardiac mass with heart weights of 400 to 499 g (≥350 g in females) and mild LV wall thickening (15-19 mm), but without any supporting clinical or pathological features of HCM.[21-27] The remaining heart was grossly normal (weight, 350 g) but showed markedly disorganized myocardial architecture and abnormal intramural coronary arteries typical of HCM.[24,26]

Coronary Artery Abnormalities.—A variety of congenital or acquired coronary artery abnormalities were judged to be the probable cause of death in 34 athletes (Table). Malformations involving anomalous coronary artery origin were most common (17 athletes [13%]), particularly anomalous origin of the left main coronary artery from the right sinus of Valsalva (13 cases) in which the left main coronary artery emanated from a slitlike ostium and made an acute-angled bend to course between the ascending aorta and pulmonary trunk.

Other coronary artery malformations judged to be of functional significance occurred in 8 other athletes (5%), including hypoplasia (ie, small size or shortened course),[28,29] or aneurysm, acute-angled takeoff of the left main coronary artery,[30] and intussusception (of ramus intermedius)[31] associated with hypoplastic left cir-

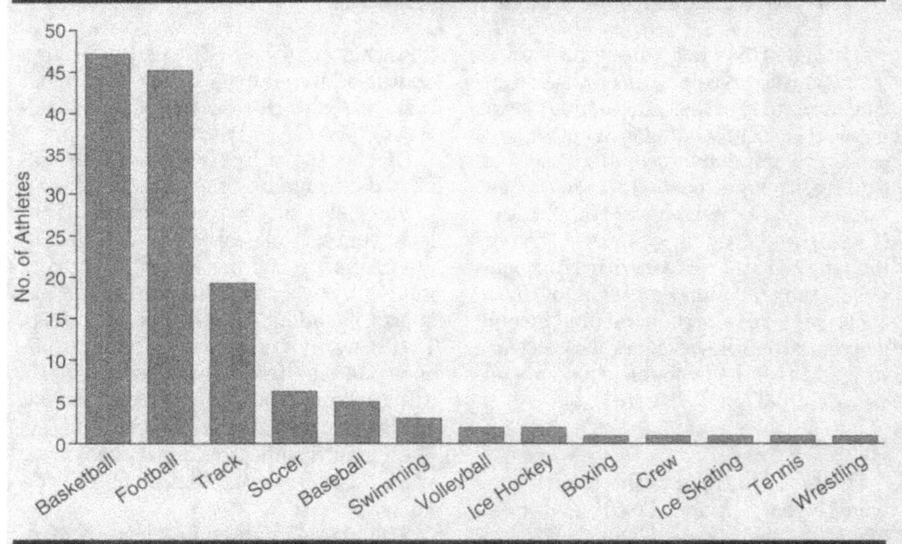

Figure 2.—Sports engaged in at the time of sudden death in 134 young competitive athletes. Those competing in track events were either distance runners or sprinters.

cumflex. In 4 of the 25 athletes with congenital coronary anomalies, small foci of myocardial necrosis or fibrosis were present in the LV myocardium.

In 3 other athletes, all male (2%), premature atherosclerotic coronary artery disease was the cause of sudden death at ages 14, 19, and 28 years, respectively. Epicardial coronary arterial narrowing of the cross-sectional luminal area by at least 75% was present in 1, 2, or 3 vessels, respectively (Figure 1, B); 1 athlete also had a healed anterior/apical myocardial infarction. In 6 other athletes, all male, the sole structural alteration was a relatively short tunneled segment (1-3 cm) of the left anterior descending coronary artery completely surrounded by myocardium and free of atherosclerotic plaques.

Myocarditis.—In 4 athletes without coronary atherosclerosis, areas of the LV myocardium showed histologic findings consistent with myocarditis of unknown cause, principally inflammatory mono-

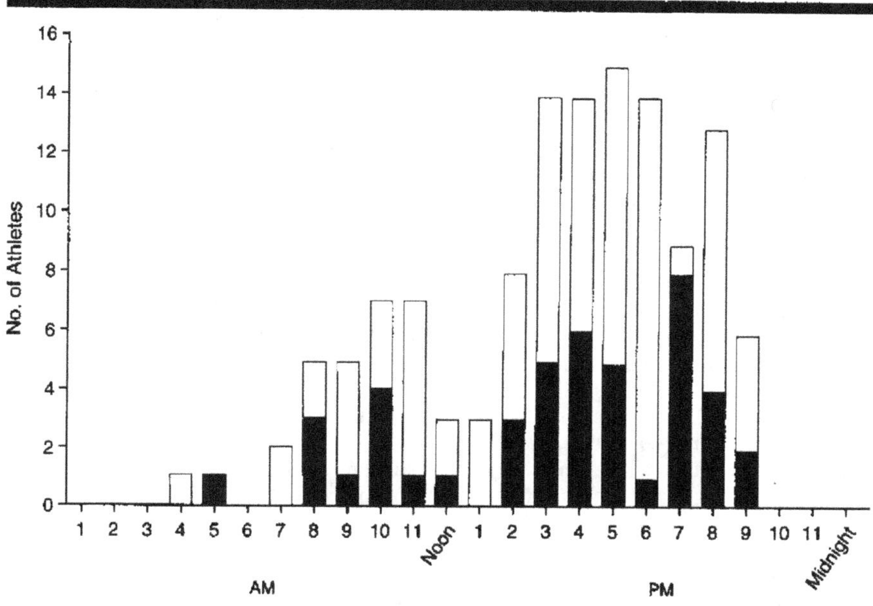

Figure 3.—Hourly distribution of sudden death in the 127 competitive athletes for whom these data were available. Shaded portions of the bars represent the hour of death for 45 athletes with probable or definite evidence of hypertrophic cardiomyopathy.

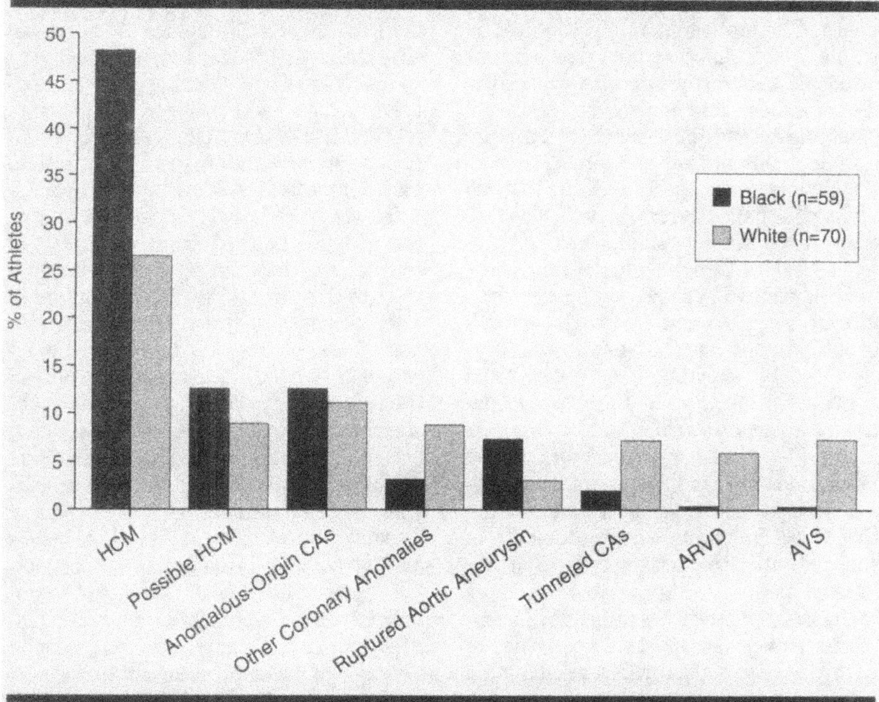

Figure 4.—Effect of race on cardiovascular causes of sudden death in competitive athletes, shown for those diseases with 5 or more deaths. The 5 Asian, Hispanic, or Native American athletes were not included in this analysis. Possible hypertrophic cardiomyopathy (HCM), as defined in the text, denotes those hearts with some morphologic features consistent with, but not diagnostic of, HCM. CAs indicates coronary arteries; ARVD, arrhythmogenic right ventricular dysplasia; and AVS, aortic valve stenosis.

nuclear cell infiltration associated with myocyte necrosis.[32] Four other athletes showed only isolated areas of idiopathic myocardial scarring, which could conceivably have represented the healing phase of myocarditis[33] (Figure 1, C).

Other Cardiomyopathies.—Four athletes had idiopathic dilated cardiomyopathy with substantial ventricular cavity dilatation in the absence of LV wall thickening[34]; 2 had cardiac symptoms, which in 1 were associated with atrial fibrillation. Three athletes had findings diagnostic of ARVD[35-37] with extensive fibrofatty replacement of myocytes in the right ventricular wall, including 1 each with LV free wall involvement and myocarditis; familial occurrence was documented in 1.

Valvular and Aortic Root Disease.—Three male athletes had myxomatous ("floppy") mitral valves[38,39]; however, each had other abnormalities that could have contributed to death: coronary artery hypoplasia in 2 and increased cardiac mass (475 g) in the other. Four male athletes had bicuspid aortic valves and anatomic evidence of aortic stenosis with leaflet thickening and fusion. Each had a systolic murmur due to outflow obstruction, including 1 with a peak transvalvular gradient of 50 mm Hg documented with cardiac catheterization. In 6 athletes, rupture of dissecting aneurysm of the ascending aorta with cardiac tamponade, which in 4 cases occurred during sedentary activities or light exercise, was the cause of death. Three of the 6 had physical signs consistent with Marfan syndrome.

Absence of Structural Cardiac Disease.—In 3 athletes, autopsy examination did not identify a cause of death; the hearts showed no morphologic abnormalities, and the toxicology results were negative. Only 1 of these was evaluated during life, an 18-year-old elite distance runner with recurrent exertional syncope, in whom clinical investigation (including electrophysiologic testing) showed no abnormalities.

Preparticipation Medical Evaluations

Standard medical history and physical examination, as part of the high school or college medical clearance process, had constituted the principal preparticipation evaluation for 115 athletes (Figure 5). In only 4 (3%) of these athletes had some aspect of the examination aroused suspicion of cardiac disease (ie, cardiac murmur, symptoms, other physical findings), and in just 1 athlete (0.9%) was the correct diagnosis ultimately made; this athlete with Marfan syndrome and a dilated aorta did not withdraw completely from collegiate sports and died 6 months later.

In another 15 athletes, signs or symptoms suggestive of cardiovascular disease had initiated an individualized medical evaluation with diagnostic testing, usually an electrocardiogram and echocardiogram. These evaluations led directly to the correct diagnosis in 7 athletes (most commonly, aortic valve stenosis in 3; HCM in 1), of whom 2 were disqualified from competitive sports. Of the 130 athletes with some form of preparticipation medical evaluation, an appropriate cardiovascular diagnosis was ultimately achieved during life in only 8 (6%).

Cardiovascular disease was suspected during medical evaluations in each of the 5 athletes with aortic stenosis, primarily by detection of a heart murmur. In contrast, overt evidence of other lesions was less common: eg, only 4 (31%) of 13 ath-

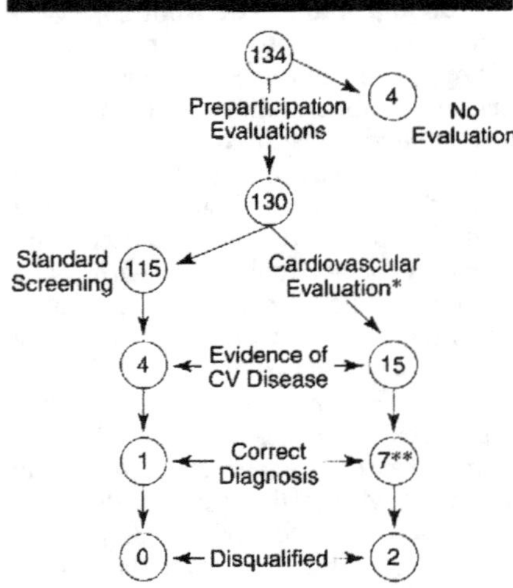

Figure 5.—Outcome of preparticipation medical examinations for the detection of structural cardiovascular (CV) disease and causes of sudden death, as well as subsequent disqualification from competitive athletics. Asterisk indicates CV evaluation with testing independent of standard school or institutional preparticipation screening, prompted in 15 athletes by symptoms, family history, cardiac murmur, or physical findings suggestive of heart disease. The 7 athletes designated with the double asterisk included 3 with aortic valve stenosis, 1 with dilated cardiomyopathy, 1 with hypertrophic cardiomyopathy, 1 with sarcoidosis, and 1 with a structurally normal heart.

letes with anomalous left main coronary arteries had symptoms (usually syncope or dizziness), and just 10 (21%) of 48 athletes with HCM had signs or symptoms of cardiac disease.

COMMENT

This study develops a clinical, demographic, and pathological profile for the phenomenon of sudden death in young, trained, competitive athletes. Over more than a decade we have assembled this large series of US athletes who died unexpectedly due to a variety of causes. In 80% of these athletes, a spectrum of more than 20 structural cardiovascular abnormalities were identified as definite or likely causes of death.

The most common single disease entity was HCM,[20-25] a disease known to be associated with a risk for sudden death during exercise,[40] which occurred in about one third of our cases. The second most frequent cause of death, encountered in about 15%, was a group of related malformations in which the origin of an epicardial coronary artery was anomalous[41-43]; the most common of these was anomalous origin of the left main coronary artery from the right sinus of Valsalva.[41] Several other diseases occurred less frequently, including myocarditis, ruptured aortic aneurysm, idiopathic dilated cardiomyopathy, aortic valve stenosis, and ARVD. The rare occurrence of ARVD in our series, while consistent with previous

observations in the United States,[44] contrasts sharply with the experience of investigators in northeastern Italy,[8,35] who reported ARVD to be the most common cause of sudden death in the competitive athletes they studied (in approximately 25% [6/22 deaths], predominantly among soccer players); HCM was particularly uncommon, occurring in only 2%. The explanation for discrepancies between the Italian data and those in our study is uncertain, although it is possible that the frequent occurrence of ARVD in a particular geographic region could reflect a unique genetic substrate.[45]

We found HCM to be a significantly more common cause of sudden death in black athletes than in white athletes. This preponderance of black athletes dying of HCM suggests its importance in the African-American population, a point not appreciated from previous analyses in hospital-based and selected referral populations with HCM. Also, only 15% of the athletes in our study were female. This may be explained on the basis of lower participation rates or less intensive training demands, but also because HCM appears to be less commonly recognized in women.[24,25] Finally, sudden death in our athletes occurred predominantly in the late afternoon and early evening, corresponding to the most common time period for competition and practice, particularly in team sports such as football and basketball. Therefore, while the diseases responsible for sudden death in athletes were heterogeneous, cardiovascular collapse was clearly associated with intense physical activity in the overall group, suggesting that death was precipitated by exercise. This observation supports prior consensus recommendations that many cardiovascular diseases in athletes represent risk factors during intense competitive sports, and also constitute a justification for recommending that these individuals not participate in such activities to diminish risk.[46] This relationship was also apparent in athletes in the present study having HCM, in contrast to our prior report that nonathletes with this disease showed a predilection for sudden death in the morning.[47]

Three subgroups of athletes identified in this study are of particular note. First, about 10% had morphologic findings at autopsy that could only be considered suggestive, but not diagnostic, of HCM (ie, idiopathic LV hypertrophy or possible HCM). It is uncertain whether some of these cases represent mild morphologic forms of HCM with little LV hypertrophy,[48-51] possibly at a point of incomplete structural evolution during adolescence,[52] or conceivably could represent unusual examples of athlete's heart[53-55] with nonbenign consequences. Second, 2% of our

athletes had no cause of death documented at autopsy. It is possible that these deaths were due to conditions such as long QT syndrome, which is not associated with gross morphologic abnormalities[56,57]; Wolff-Parkinson-White syndrome[58]; unrecognized drug use[17,18]; occult morphologic abnormalities of the cardiac conducting system and vasculature,[2,6,9,59,60] which require an analysis that is not a part of the standard medical examiners' protocol; or possibly undetected ARVD with segmental fibrofatty replacement.[35,36] Third, an intramural tunneled coronary artery was the sole morphologic alteration detected at autopsy in 5% of our athletes. This finding raises the possibility that myocardial bridging of coronary arteries, although a common anatomic variant and controversial risk factor for sudden death,[61] could have important clinical implications in a subset of individuals exposed to intense athletic activity.[62]

Assembly of a large series of athletic field deaths requires substantial reliance on news media accounts for identification of cases. This process may create certain selection biases, because media notifications are more likely to identify deaths in elite athletes, those participating in highly visible team sports during their competitive season, and athletes from urban population centers. Also, certain confidentiality issues (including pending litigation) may limit access to some information. Finally, we were largely dependent on primary data obtained from a variety of sources and medical examiners, in contrast to our prior investigations of highly selected cases in which the heart specimens could be examined directly.[2,6] Nevertheless, we believe that the large size of the present study population offers a substantial measure of compensation for these potential limitations in data acquisition.

This study does not address the prevalence of sudden death in young athletes. Because of unavoidable selection biases and lack of a systematic national reporting registry for these events, we do not believe that all relevant deaths were identified. Rather, our data, which suggest an average of 11 confirmed cardiovascular deaths per year from 1985 through 1995, almost certainly significantly underestimate the frequency of these events.

Based on the series of athletes analyzed herein, the standard preparticipation screening process appears to be limited in its power to identify those cardiovascular lesions ultimately responsible for death. For example, of the 115 athletes exposed to a standard screening examination, fewer than 5% were suspected of having cardiovascular disease, and the conditions of fewer than 1% were diagnosed accurately. Furthermore, of the 130 total athletes with either standard preparticipation screening or an individualized cardiovascular evaluation with testing, the abnormalities of only 6% were ultimately diagnosed correctly and just 2 of these athletes were denied sports eligibility.[46] Indeed, these medical evaluations failed to identify 47 of the 48 cases of HCM. This is perhaps understandable, given that most patients with HCM have the nonobstructive form in which no murmur or only a soft heart murmur would be apparent on routine examination under resting conditions. Furthermore, as demonstrated in the present series, few athletes with HCM have symptoms prior to collapse or report a definitive family history of the disease.

References

1. Maron BJ. Sudden death in young athletes: lessons from the Hank Gathers affair. *N Engl J Med.* 1993;329:55-57.

2. Maron BJ, Roberts WC, McAllister HA, Rosing DR, Epstein SE. Sudden death in young athletes. *Circulation.* 1980;62:218-229.

3. van Camp SP, Bloor CM, Mueller FO, Cantu RC, Olson HG. Nontraumatic sports death in high school and college athletes. *Med Sci Sports Exerc.* 1995;27:641-647.

4. Burke AP, Farb V, Virmani R, Goodin J, Smialek JE. Sports-related and non-sports-related sudden cardiac death in young adults. *Am Heart J.* 1991;121:568-575.

5. Thiene G, Pennelli N, Rossi L. Cardiac conduction system abnormalities as a possible cause of sudden death in young athletes. *Hum Pathol.* 1983;14:704-709.

6. Maron BJ, Epstein SE, Roberts WC. Causes of sudden death in competitive athletes. *J Am Coll Cardiol.* 1986;7:204-214.

7. Tsung SH, Huang TY, Chang HH. Sudden death in young athletes. *Arch Pathol Lab Med.* 1982;106:168-170.

8. Corrado D, Thiene G, Nava A, Rossi L, Pennelli N. Sudden death in young competitive athletes: clinicopathologic correlations in 22 cases. *Am J Med.* 1990;89:588-596.

9. James TN, Froggatt P, Marshall TK. Sudden death in young athletes. *Ann Intern Med.* 1967;67:1013-1021.

10. Furlanello F, Bettini R, Cozzi F, et al. Ventricular arrhythmias and sudden death in athletes. *Ann N Y Acad Sci.* 1984;427:253-279.

11. Drory Y, Turetz Y, Hiss Y, et al. Sudden unexpected death in persons <40 years of age. *Am J Cardiol.* 1991;68:1388-1392.

12. Topaz O, Edwards JE. Pathologic features of sudden death in children, adolescents and young adults. *Chest.* 1985;87:476-482.

13. Maron BJ, Bodison S, Wesley Y, Tucker E, Green KJ. Results of screening a large group of intercollegiate competitive athletes for cardiovascular disease. *J Am Coll Cardiol.* 1987;10:1214-1222.

14. Lewis JF, Maron BJ, Diggs JA, Spencer JE, Mehrotra PP, Curry CL. Preparticipation echocardiographic screening for cardiovascular disease in a large predominantly black population of collegiate athletes. *Am J Cardiol.* 1989;64:1029-1033.

15. Maron BJ, Mitchell JH. Revised eligibility recommendations for competitive athletes with cardiovascular abnormalities: introduction. In: Maron BJ, Mitchell JH, eds. 26th Bethesda Conference: Recommendations for Determining Eligibility for Competition in Athletes With Cardiovascular Abnormalities. *J Am Coll Cardiol.* 1994;24:848-850.

16. Maron BJ, Poliac LC, Kaplan JA, Mueller FO. Blunt impact to the chest leading to sudden death from cardiac arrest during sports activities. *N Engl J Med.* 1995;333:337-342.

17. Isner JM, Estes NAM III, Thompson PD, et al. Acute cardiac events temporally related to cocaine abuse. *N Engl J Med.* 1986;315:1438-1443.

18. Virmani R, Robinowitz M, Smialek JE, Smyth DF. Cardiovascular effects of cocaine: an autopsy study of 40 patients. *Am Heart J.* 1988;115:1068-1076.

19. Kark JA, Posey DM, Schumacher HR, Ruehle CJ. Sickle-cell trait as a risk factor for sudden death in physical training. *N Engl J Med.* 1987;317:781-787.

20. Maron BJ, Epstein SE. Hypertrophic cardiomyopathy: a discussion of nomenclature. *Am J Cardiol.* 1979;43:1242-1244.

21. Roberts CS, Roberts WC. Morphologic features. In: Zipes DP, Rowlands DJ, eds. *Progress in Cardiology 2/2.* Philadelphia, Pa: Lea & Febiger; 1989:3-32.

22. Olson EG. Anatomic and light microscopic characterization of hypertrophic obstructive and non-obstructive cardiomyopathy. *Eur Heart J.* 1983;4(suppl F):1-8.

23. Wigle ED, Sasson Z, Henderson MA, et al. Hypertrophic cardiomyopathy: the importance of the site and extent of hypertrophy—a review. *Prog Cardiovasc Dis.* 1985;28:1-83.

24. Maron BJ, Bonow RO, Cannon RO III, Leon MB, Epstein SE. Hypertrophic cardiomyopathy: interrelations of clinical manifestations, pathophysiology, and therapy. *N Engl J Med.* 1987;316:780-789, 844-852.

25. Klues HG, Schiffers A, Maron BJ. Phenotypic spectrum and patterns of left ventricular hypertrophy in hypertrophic cardiomyopathy. *J Am Coll Cardiol.* 1995;26:1699-1708.

26. Maron BJ, Anan TJ, Roberts WC. Quantitative analysis of the distribution of cardiac muscle cell disorganization in the left ventricular wall of patients with hypertrophic cardiomyopathy. *Circulation.* 1981;63:882-894.

27. Klues HG, Maron BJ, Dollar AL, Roberts WC. Diversity of structural mitral valve alterations in hypertrophic cardiomyopathy. *Circulation.* 1992;85:1651-1660.

28. Roberts WC, Glick BN. Congenital hypoplasia of both right and left circumflex coronary arteries. *Am J Cardiol.* 1992;70:121-123.

29. Menke DM, Waller BF, Pless JC. Hypoplastic coronary arteries and high take-off position of the right coronary ostium. *Chest.* 1985;88:299-301.

30. Virmani R, Chun PKC, Goldstein RE, et al. Acute takeoffs of the coronary arteries along the aortic wall and congenital coronary ostial valve–like ridges. *J Am Coll Cardiol.* 1984;3:766-771.

31. Roberts WC, Silver MA, Sapala JC. Intussusception of a coronary artery associated with sudden death in a college football player. *Am J Cardiol.* 1986;57:179-180.

32. Aretz HT, Billingham ME, Edwards WD, et al. Myocarditis: a histopathologic definition and classification. *Am J Cardiovasc Pathol.* 1986;1:3-14.

33. Lecomte D, Fornes P, Fouret P, Nicholas G. Isolated myocardial fibrosis as a cause of sudden cardiac death and its possible relation to myocarditis. *J Forensic Sci.* 1993;38:617-621.

34. Tamburro P, Wilber D. Sudden death in idiopathic dilated cardiomyopathy. *Am Heart J.* 1992;124:1035-1045.

35. Thiene G, Nava A, Corrado D, Rossi L, Penelli N. Right ventricular cardiomyopathy and sudden death in young people. *N Engl J Med.* 1988;318:129-133.

36. Daliento L, Turrini P, Nava A, et al. Arrhythmogenic right ventricular cardiomyopathy in young versus adult patients: similarities and differences. *J Am Coll Cardiol.* 1995;25:655-664.

37. McKenna WJ, Thiene G, Nava A, et al. Diagnosis of arrhythmogenic right ventricular dysplasia/cardiomyopathy. *Br Heart J.* 1994;71:215-218.

38. Chesler E, King RA, Edwards JE. The myxomatous mitral valve and sudden death. *Circulation.* 1983;67:632-639.

39. Dollar AL, Roberts WC. Morphologic comparison of patients with mitral valve prolapse who died suddenly with patients who died from severe valvular dysfunction or other conditions. *J Am Coll Cardiol.* 1991;17:921-931.

40. Maron BJ, Roberts WC, Epstein SE. Sudden death in hypertrophic cardiomyopathy: profile of 78 patients. *Circulation.* 1982;65:1388-1394.

41. Cheitlin MD, De Castro CM, McAllister HA. Sudden death as a complication of anomalous left coronary origin from the anterior sinus of Valsalva. *Circulation.* 1974;50:780-787.

42. Barth WC III, Roberts WC. Left main coronary artery originating from the right sinus of Valsalva and coursing between the aorta and pulmonary trunk. *J Am Coll Cardiol.* 1986;7:366-373.

43. Roberts WC, Siegel RJ, Zipes DP. Origin of the right coronary artery from the left sinus of Valsalva and its functional consequences: analysis of 10 necropsy patients. *Am J Cardiol.* 1982;49:863-868.

44. Goodin JC, Farb A, Smialek JE, Field F, Virmani R. Right ventricular dysplasia associated with sudden death in young adults. *Mod Pathol.* 1991;4:702-706.

45. Rampazzo A, Nava A, Danieli GA, et al. The gene for arrhythmogenic right ventricular cardiomyopathy maps to chromosome 14q 23-q24. *Hum Mol Genet.* 1994;3:959-962.

46. Maron BJ, Mitchell JH, eds. 26th Bethesda Conference: Recommendations for Determining Eligibility for Competition in Athletes With Cardiovascular Abnormalities. *J Am Coll Cardiol.* 1994;24:845-899.

47. Maron BJ, Kogan J, Proschan MA, Hecht GM, Roberts WC. Circadian variability in the occurrence of sudden cardiac death in patients with hypertrophic cardiomyopathy. *J Am Coll Cardiol.* 1994;23:1405-1409.

48. Rosenzweig A, Watkins H, Hwang D-S, McKenna WJ, Seidman JG, Seidman CE. Preclinical diagnosis of familial hypertrophic cardiomyopathy by genetic analysis of blood lymphocytes. *N Engl J Med.* 1991;325:1753-1760.

49. McKenna WJ, Stewart JT, Nihoyannopoulos P, McCinty F, Davies MJ. Hypertrophic cardiomyopathy without hypertrophy. *Br Heart J.* 1990;63:287-290.

50. Maron BJ, Kragel AH, Roberts WC. Sudden death in hypertrophic cardiomyopathy with normal left ventricular mass. *Br Heart J.* 1990;63:308-310.

51. Spirito P, Maron BJ. Relation between extent of left ventricular hypertrophy and occurrence of sudden cardiac death in hypertrophic cardiomyopathy. *J Am Coll Cardiol.* 1990;15:1521-1526.

52. Maron BJ, Spirito P, Wesley YE, Arce J. Development and progression of left ventricular hypertrophy in children with hypertrophic cardiomyopathy. *N Engl J Med.* 1986;315:610-614.

53. Pelliccia A, Maron BJ, Spataro A, Proschan MA, Spirito P. The upper limit of physiologic cardiac hypertrophy in highly trained elite athletes. *N Engl J Med.* 1991;324:295-301.

54. Maron BJ, Pelliccia A, Spirito P. Cardiac disease in young trained athletes. *Circulation.* 1995;92:1596-1601.

55. Huston TP, Puffer JC, Rodney WM. The athletic heart syndrome. *N Engl J Med.* 1985;313:24-32.

56. Moss AJ, Schwartz PJ, Crampton RS, et al. The long QT syndrome: prospective longitudinal study of 328 families. *Circulation.* 1991;84:1136-1144.

57. Vincent GM, Timothy KW, Leppert M, Keating M. The spectrum of symptoms and QT intervals in carriers of the gene for the long-QT syndrome. *N Engl J Med.* 1992;327:846-852.

58. Zipes DP, Garson A Jr. Arrhythmias: task force 6. In: Maron BJ, Mitchell JH, eds. 26th Bethesda Conference: Recommendations for Determining Eligibility for Competition in Athletes With Cardiovascular Abnormalities. *J Am Coll Cardiol.* 1994;24:892-899.

59. Burke AP, Subramanian R, Smialek J, Virmani R. Nonatherosclerotic narrowing of the atrioventricular node artery and sudden death. *J Am Coll Cardiol.* 1993;21:117-122.

60. Corrado D, Thiene G, Cocco P, Frescura C. Nonatherosclerotic coronary artery disease and sudden death in the young. *Br Heart J.* 1992;68:601-607.

61. Roberts WC, Dicicco BS, Waller BF, et al. Origin of the left main from the right coronary artery or from the right aortic sinus with intramyocardial tunnelling to the left side of the heart via the ventricular septum. *Am Heart J.* 1982;104:303-305.

62. Morales AR, Romanelli R, Boucek RJ. The mural left anterior descending coronary artery, strenuous exercise and sudden death. *Circulation.* 1980;62:230-237.

Frequency and Characteristics of Coronary Thrombosis in the Epicardial Coronary Arteries After Cardiac Transplantation

Eloisa Arbustini, MD, Barbara Dal Bello, MD, Patrizia Morbini, MD,
Maurizia Grasso, PhD, Marta Diegoli, ScD, Roberta Fasani, ScD, Andrea Pilotto, ScD,
Ornella Bellini, ScD, Carlo Pellegrini, MD, Luigi Martinelli, MD, Carlo Campana, MD,
Antonello Gavazzi, MD, Giuseppe Specchia, MD, Mario Viganò, MD,
and William C. Roberts, MD

We investigated at autopsy or at retransplantation the frequency and characteristics of coronary thrombosis in 76 cardiac allografts: 37 in place for ≤2 months (early) and 39 in place >2 to 99 months (late). The 76 allografts were inserted in 69 patients: a single 1 in 56 patients and 2 allografts in 13 patients, 7 of whom subsequently died and had an autopsy. An average of 140 sections from 70 5-mm-long segments of 8 epicardial coronary arteries were examined from each of the 76 allografts with both hematoxylin-eosin and Movat pentachrome stains. Thrombus was found in only 1 coronary artery (3%) (the right one) of the 37 early allografts, and in 24 of 39 late allografts (61%). Of the latter 39 grafts, 29 (79%) had allograft vascular disease (AVD) and 24 (83%) of them had coronary thrombosis. Of the 312 epicardial coronary arteries (4 major and 4 minor) examined in the 39 late cases, 66 arteries (21%) contained thrombus. Of the 24 late cases with thrombus in at least 1 artery, thrombus was present in 66 (34%) of the 192 epicardial coronary arteries examined: in 6 of the 8 arteries in 3 patients; in 5 arteries in 2 patients; in 4 arteries in 1 patient; in 3 arteries in 5 patients; in 2 arteries in 6 patients, and in a single artery in 7 patients. In all 66 arteries with thrombus (24 patients) the thrombus was longer than 5 mm. The thrombus in the late cases was entirely nonocclusive (mural) in 51 (77%) of the 66 epicardial coronary arteries containing thrombus and entirely occlusive in 10 arteries (15%). It consisted exclusively of multiluminal channels in 6 arteries (9%) and combinations in 1 artery (2%). Acute myocardial infarcts were present in 3 patients, all of whom had occlusive thrombi. In all 10 arteries with occlusive thrombi, the thrombus was larger than the underlying plaque and no occlusive thrombi were located over ulcerated plaques. These observations demonstrate that thrombus is common in epicardial coronary arteries >2 months after cardiac transplantation.

(Am J Cardiol 1996;78:795–800)

Allograft vascular disease (AVD) is a major cause of late failure of transplanted hearts.[1] The hallmarks of AVD include smooth muscle cell neointimal proliferation, extracellular matrix deposition, and mononuclear cells infiltration.[2–9] Coronary thrombus was not described in any of the 106 cases reported by Billingham[3] in 1987, or by Foerster[10] in 1992, or by several other authors.[2,4–10] In 1993, Rose et al[11] described 13 recent and 3 revascularized thrombi in the epicardial coronary arteries of 43 transplanted hearts. In an angiographic and morphologic study, Johnson et al[12] described fresh or organized thrombi in 21 of 67 type A lesions (31%) and in 1 of 14 type B lesions (7%) according to Gao et al.[13] Recently, however, Billingham observed that "it is not unusual to see mural thrombi in these hearts."[14] Most reported morphologic studies, however, have been based on examining only random sections of the coronary arteries from each case. Since our first cardiac transplantation in Pavia, Italy, in 1985, we have examined histologically at least 1 section from each 5-mm-long segment of each of the 4 major (right, left main, left anterior, left circumflex) epicardial coronary arteries, and from 4 minor (posterolateral, posterior descending, first diagonal, obtuse marginal) epicardial coronary arteries in patients dying after cardiac transplantation or having a second transplantation, irrespective of the cause of death or of graft failure. In the present study, we report the frequency and characteristics of coronary thrombi in 76 consecutive cardiac allografts in 69 patients.

METHODS

The 69 patients included 65 men and 4 women aged 9 to 65 years (mean 50 ± 10) who underwent cardiac transplantation and then died or underwent repeat transplantation at the Cardiac Surgery Department of Policlinico San Matteo–Pavia from No-

From the Pathologic Anatomy Institute, Cardiac Surgery Department, Cardiology Department, IRCCS-Policlinico San Matteo, University of Pavia, Pavia, Italy, and Baylor Cardiovascular Institute, Baylor University Medical Center, Dallas, Texas. This study was supported by grants "Trapianto Cardiaco," "Trapianto Cuore-Polmoni," and "Rigetto cronico nel cuore trapiantato" from Health Ministry to IRCCS Policlinico San Matteo, Pavia, Italy—Ricerche Finalizzate 1989 to 1990, 1991 to 1993, and 1993 to 1995. Manuscript received March 15, 1996; revised manuscript received and accepted June 14, 1996.

Address for reprints: Eloisa Arbustini, MD, Istituto di Anatomia Patologica, Viale Forlanini 16, 27100 Pavia, Italy.

TABLE I Clinical and Morphologic Data on 39 Patients Who Underwent Cardiac Transplantation and Survived >2 Months

| | Recipient | | Donor | | | | Thrombus in | Thrombus in Coronary Artery | | | | | | | | |
Patient	Age (yr) & Sex	Diagnosis	Age (yr) & Sex	Duration (mo) Allograft in Place	Cause of Allograft Failure	AVD Severity (0–4+)	any Coronary Artery	LM	LAD	LC	Right	FD	LOM	PD	PL	Myocardial Infarct
1	43 M	IC	17 M	3	AR	0	0	0	0	0	0	0	0	0	0	0
2*	52 M	IC	28 F	3	Graft failure	0	0	0	0	0	0	0	0	0	0	0
3	56 M	IC	36 M	3	M-O F	+	+ (3)	0	+‡	+	+	0	0	0	0	0
4	64 M	IC	14 M	3	Infection	0	0	0	0	0	0	0	0	0	0	0
5	39 F	IDC	45 F	4	PE	++	+ (2)	0	+	+	0	0	0	0	0	0
6	60 M	IDC	46 F	5	Infection	++	+ (1)	0	0	0	+	0	0	0	0	0
7	57 M	IC	39 F	6	Infection	0	0	0	0	0	0	0	0	0	0	0
8	60 M	IC	24 F	6	M-O F	0	0	0	0	0	0	0	0	0	0	0
9	44 M	IDC	18 M	7	Mediastinitis	0	0	0	0	0	0	0	0	0	0	0
10	47 M	IC	22 M	7	AVD	+++	+ (1)	0	0	0	+	0	0	0	0	0
11	23 M	IDC	19 M	8	Poisoning	0	0	0	0	0	0	0	0	0	0	0
12	47 M	IDC	36 M	8	AVD	+++	+ (1)	0	0	0	+	0	0	0	0	0
13*	48 M	IDC	44 M	11	AVD	+++	+ (6)	0	+	+	+	+ (Oc)	+	+	0	0
14	53 M	IC	25 M	11	Aortic rupture	0	0	0	0	0	0	0	0	0	0	0
15	54 M	IC	25 M	12	Neoplasm	++	+ (1)	0	+	0	0	0	0	0	0	0
16	58 M	IDC	26 M	12	AVD	+++	+ (2)	0	+ (Oc)	0	0	+ (Oc)	0	0	0	+ (Acute)
17	45 M	IDC	33 M	13	AVD	+++	+ (1)	0	0	0	+	0	0	0	0	0
18	60 M	VHD	56 M	14	Neoplasm	+++	+ (2)	0	+ (MLC)	0	+ (MLC)	0	0	0	0	0
19	46 M	IDC	34 M	15	Neoplasm	++	0	0	0	0	0	0	0	0	0	0
20	49 M	IDC	18 M	15	Infection	0	0	0	0	0	0	0	0	0	0	0
21	43 M	IC	43 F	16	AVD	+++	+ (3)	0	+ (Oc§)	0	+ (Oc)	0	0	+	0	+ (Acute)
22	61 M	IC	19 M	16	Neoplasm	++	0	0	0	0	0	0	0	0	0	0
23	50 M	VHD	14 M	21	AVD	+++	+ (3)	0	+ (Oc)	0	0	+ (Oc)	+ (Oc)	0	0	+ (Acute)
24	54 M	IC	19 M	22	Neoplasm	0	0	0	0	0	0	0	0	0	0	0
25	53 M	Amyloid	44 M	25	AVD	+++	0	0	0	0	0	0	0	0	0	0
26	35 M	IDC	17 M	33	PE	+++	+ (5)	+	+	+	+	0	0	0	+	0
27	47 M	IDC	20 F	34	Neoplasm	++	+ (2)	0	+	+	0	0	0	0	0	0
28*	28 M	IDC	34 M	40	AVD	+++	+ (5)	0	+	+	+	0	0	+	+	0
29*	45 M	IC	22 M	48	AVD	+++	+ (6)	+	+	+ (MLC§)	+ (MLC)	+	0	+ (Oc)	0	0
30	39 M	IC	32 M	55	AVD	+++	+ (2)	0	+	0	+	0	0	0	0	+ (Healed)
31	56 M	IDC	53 M	58	Infection	++	0	0	0	0	0	0	0	0	0	0
32	39 M	IC	14 F	60	Cirrhosis	+++	+ (3)	0	0	+	+	0	0	+ (Oc)	0	+ (Healed)
33	41 M	IC	15 F	70	AVD	+++	+ (2)	0	+	0	+ (MLC)	0	0	0	0	+ (Healed)
34	44 M	VHD	35 M	70	PE	++	+ (4)	+	+	+	+	0	0	0	0	0
35*	49 M	IC	46 M	72	AVD	+++	+ (6)	+	+ (MLC)	+	0	+ (MLC)	+	0	+	0
36†	44 M	IDC	18 F	83	M-O F	+++	+ (1)	0	+	0	0	0	0	0	0	0
37	46 M	IDC	8 M	91	Aortic rupture	+++	+ (3)	0	+	0	+	+	0	0	0	0
38*	53 M	IC	35 M	93	AVD	+++	+ (1)	0	0	0	+	0	0	0	0	0
39	42 M	HC	26 F	99	Neoplasm	++	0	0	0	0	0	0	0	0	0	0
TOTALS	38 M / 1 F	IC = 18; IDC = 16; VHD = 3; HC = 1; Amyloid = 1	28 M / 11 F		AVD = 14; Infection = 5; Neoplasm = 7; Misc. = 12; AR = 1	29	24 (66)	4	18	10	17	6	3	5	3	3 Acute / 3 Healed

*Heart obtained at retransplantation; † Heart obtained at necropsy from patients previously retransplanted; ‡ The + sign indicates mural thrombus only unless otherwise stated; § Also mural thrombus.

AVD = allograft vascular disease; AR = acute rejection; F = female; FD = first diagonal; HC = hypertrophic cardiomyopathy; IC = ischemic cardiomyopathy; IDC = idiopathic dilated cardiomyopathy; LAD = left anterior descending; LC = left circumflex; LM = left main; LOM = left obtuse marginal; M = male; MLC = multiluminal channels; MOF = multiorgan failure; Oc = occlusive; PD = posterior descending; PE = pulmonary embolism; PL = posterolateral; VHD = valvular heart disease.

vember 1985 to November 1995. Of the 69 patients, 56 had a single transplant and each died at varying intervals thereafter. The other 13 patients had 2 cardiac transplants: 6 of these patients are still alive and thus 6 allografts were available to be studied; the other 7 patients died from 3 days to 83 months after the second transplant, and therefore, 14 allografts were available to be studied in them. Of the 76 hearts studied, 63 were obtained at autopsy and 13 at retransplantation. The interval from first transplantation to death or to the second transplantation ranged from 4 hours to 99 months (mean 16 ± 26 months). The indications for heart transplantation were: idiopathic dilated cardiomyopathy in 30 patients, ischemic cardiomyopathy in 32, valvular heart disease in 4, hypertrophic cardiomyopathy in 1, cardiac amyloidosis in 1, and granulomatous myocarditis in 1. The indications for heart retransplantation were: graft failure in 4 cases, myocarditis in 1, persistent acute rejection in 1, hyperacute rejections in 2, and AVD in 5. One of the retransplanted patients had coronary artery bypass grafting for AVD of the first graft; analysis of the 2 aortocoronary bypass conduits in this patient is not included in this report. Twenty-five heart donors were women and 51 were men; their ages ranged from 6 to 61 years (mean 33 $\pm$ 15).

The major epicardial coronary arteries were dissected from either formalin-fixed or unfixed allograft hearts, according to previously described methods.[15,16] The left main, left anterior descending, left circumflex, and right coronary arteries were excised intact with attached closely adherent tissues and the latter 3 arteries were divided into proximal, middle, and distal portions. In all cases, the first diagonal, obtuse marginals, posterolateral, and posterior descending branches also were excised and also divided into 5-mm segments. Usually the tissues surrounding the coronary arteries were included in the tissues to be processed for histologic study. These techniques provided approximately 70 five-mm-long segments of the epicardial coronary arteries and 140 sections from each heart. Coronary artery samples were fixed in 10% buffered formalin solution, dehydrated, and then embedded in paraffin. Each paraffin block was sectioned at 5-μm intervals and the resulting 5-μm thick section was stained with hematoxylin-eosin and another with Masson's trichrome (3 cases) or Movat pentachrome (73 cases). Except for a few early cases with donor atherosclerosis, decalcification procedures were unnecessary in early and in all late cases. Three full thickness samples extending from endocardium to epicardium of the walls of both right and left ventricles were prepared for histologic study from each heart.

RESULTS

Early cases: Of all 76 allografts, 37 had been in place for $\leq$2 months (early) and 39 for >2 months (late) (Table I). The 37 early allografts had a mean follow-up of 17 ± 21 days. The causes of failure were: hyperacute rejection in 2 cases; acute rejec-

tions in 2 cases; graft failure in 13 cases; sepsis in 10 cases; multiorgan failure in 5; cerebrovascular events in 4; and eosinophilic myocarditis in 1 case. Seven hearts had been obtained during retransplantation for acute graft failure; 5 patients then died: 1 of graft failure, 1 of multiorgan failure, 1 of sepsis, 1 of acute rejection, and 1 of multiorgan failure with AVD. One heart had been obtained at autopsy from a patient who died 2 months after retransplantation for AVD (his first graft had a follow-up of 8 years); the cause of death had been graft failure. Twenty-three heart donors were men and 14 were women, aged 9 to 64 years (mean 37 ± 16).

In 11 of the 37 early allografts (30%) atherosclerosis of the native coronary arteries was found: in 3 the atherosclerosis caused critical stenosis ($\geq$75% cross-sectional area narrowing) of 1 major epicardial coronary artery (donor ages were 47, 48, 56 years, respectively, and donor cause of death was trauma in 1 and cerebral hemorrhage in 2).

In only 1 of the 37 patients (3%) surviving <2 months was thrombus found in a coronary artery. The thrombus was located at 2 sites in the right coronary artery, it was nonocclusive (i.e., mural) and the patient lived only 3 days after transplantation.

Late cases: Of the 39 late allografts, 6 were obtained at retransplantation (the indication was AVD in 5 cases and graft failure in 1) and 33 at autopsy. Findings in these 39 cases are tabulated in Table I. These 39 late grafts had been in place a mean of 32 $\pm$ 30 months. Four of the 5 patients retransplanted for AVD are alive; 1 died of acute graft failure 2 months later. The coronary bypass allograft patient survived 24 months after revascularization; then the patient underwent retransplantation and is alive 14 months after retransplantation. Of the 39 late grafts, 29 (74%) had AVD and 24 (83%) of them had coronary thrombus.

Of the 39 late allografts, thrombus was found in 1 or more epicardial coronary arteries in 24 (62%). Of the 312 epicardial coronary arteries (4 major, 4 minor) examined in the 39 late cases, 66 arteries (21%) contained thrombus. Of the 24 late cases with thrombus in at least 1 artery, thrombus was present in 66 (34%) of the 192 epicardial coronary arteries examined: in 6 of 8 arteries in 3 patients; in 5 arteries in 2 patients; in 4 arteries in 1 patient; in 3 arteries in 5 patients; in 2 arteries in 6 patients, and in a single artery in 7 patients. All thrombi in the 66 epicardial coronary arteries involved more than one 5-mm-long segment.

The thrombi in the right, left anterior descending, and left circumflex coronary arteries involved the proximal, middle, and distal portions of these 3 arteries or only 1 or 2 portions of these arteries. Thrombi were present in 18 left anterior descending arteries, involving the artery's proximal third in 16 allografts, the middle third in 9, and the distal third in 6. Thrombus was present in the left circumflex artery in 10 allografts: proximal portion in 6, middle portion in 6, and distal portion in 1. Thrombi involved the right coronary artery in 17 allografts:

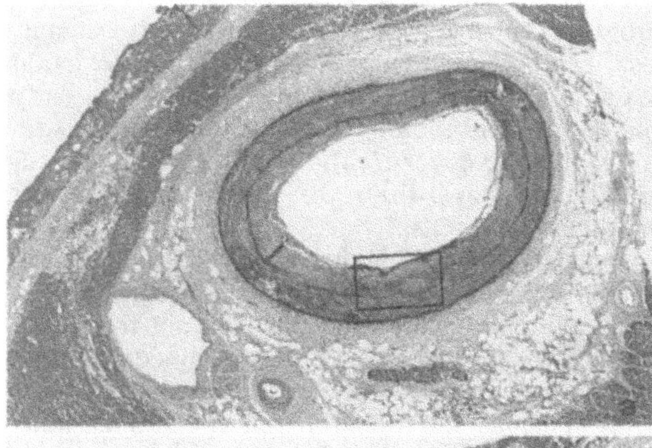

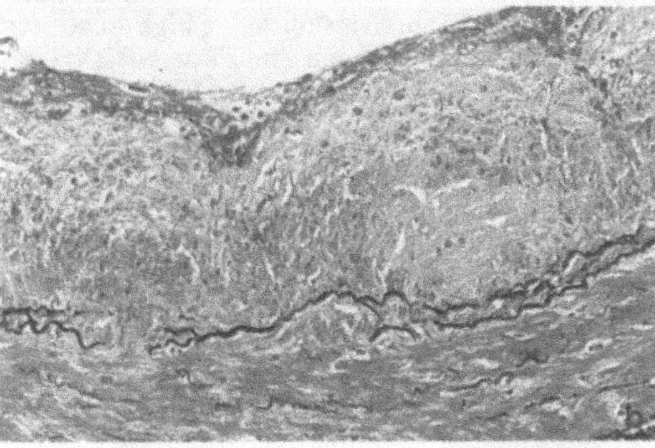

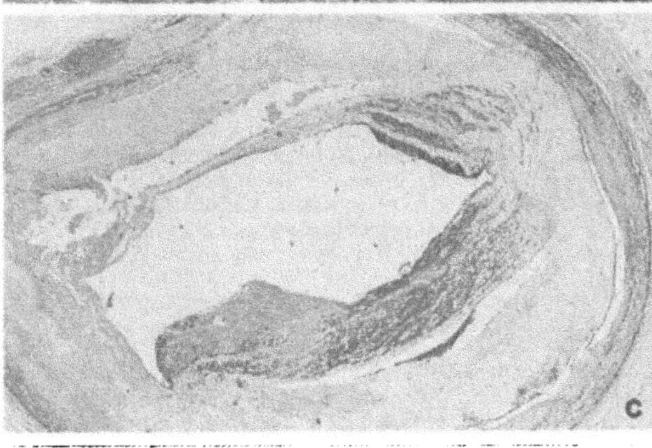

FIGURE 1. *A* and *B,* mural thrombus in the proximal tract of the first obtuse marginal branch from the allograft of a 44-year-old man who died 70 months after transplantation for postembolic lung infarctions. *C,* luminal nonocclusive thrombus partly incorporated into the plaque in the proximal portions of the right coronary artery from the same patient of *A* and *B.* (Movat pentachrome stain: *A,* ×102; *B,* ×280; *C,* ×102 [reduced by 55%].)

proximal portion in 12, middle portion in 8, and distal portion in 6.

The thrombi were entirely nonocclusive (mural) in 51 (77%) of the 66 epicardial coronary arteries containing thrombus (Figure 1); entirely occlusive in 10 arteries (15%) (Figure 2); it consisted exclusively of multiluminal channels in 6 arteries (9%) (Figure 3); and combinations in 1 artery (2%). Of the 6 patients with 1 or more occlusive thrombi, 3 had acute myocardial infarcts, and 1 had a healed myocardial infarct.

In addition to the luminal thrombi, fibrin deposits occurred within fibrous plaques in 15 patients. These fibrin deposits occurred only in the superficial layers of the fibrous plaques (Figure 4). The superficial intramural thrombi were of 2 patterns: (1) focal, so that only a portion of the arterial circumferential surface was covered by thrombotic material; and (2) diffuse along the entire internal lumen circumference. Multiple and large foci of endothelial cell denudation were commonly seen in the affected vessels.

DISCUSSION

These results indicate that coronary thrombosis is a frequent finding in the coronary arteries of transplanted hearts surviving >2 months after transplantation. Thrombus was found in 83% of late explanted hearts with AVD and in none of the late hearts without AVD. The frequency of coronary thrombus in our patients was much higher than reported previously.[2–12,14] Every 5-mm segment of 8 epicardial cor-

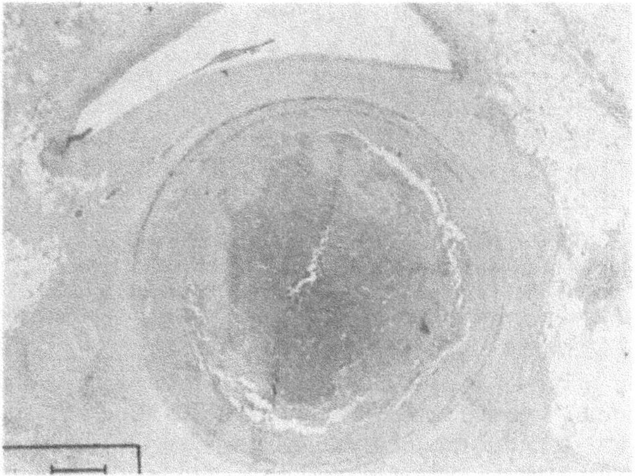

FIGURE 2. Endoluminal occlusive thrombus in the proximal portions of the left anterior descending coronary artery of a 50-year-old man who died from allograft vascular disease 21 months after transplantation. (Movat pentachrome stain, ×102 [reduced by 59%].)

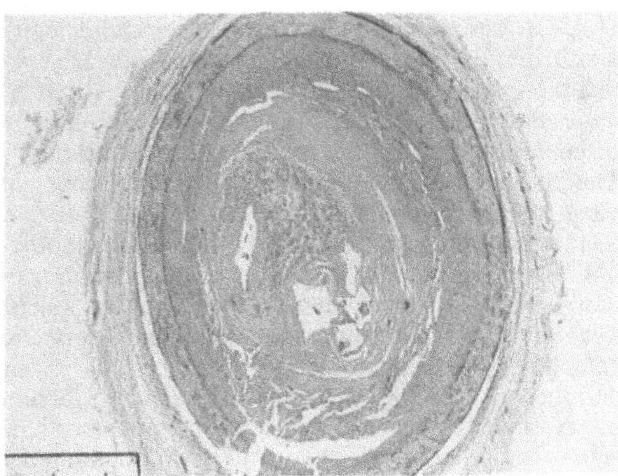

FIGURE 3. Multichannel pattern in the mid-left anterior descending coronary artery of an explanted graft that survived 72 months after transplantation. The patient, a 49-year-old man, is doing well 14 months after second transplantation. (Movat pentachrome stain, ×102 [reduced by 59%].)

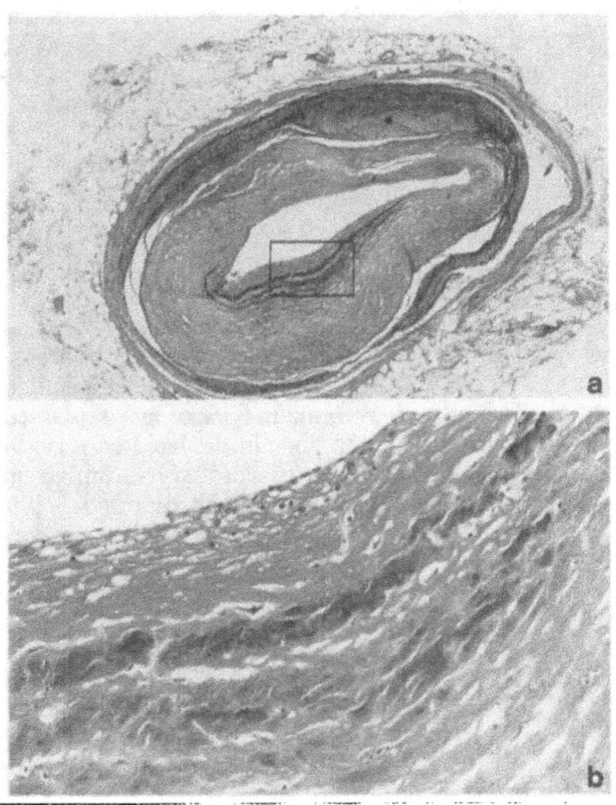

FIGURE 4. Fibrin deposits embedded within the superficial plaque layers in the posterolateral branch of a graft explanted 72 months after first transplantation (same patient as Figure 3). (Movat pentachrome stain: (a) ×102 and (b) high magnification view of the squared area ×340.)

onary arteries was examined in our 76 allografts, and this type of detailed examination has not been reported previously. Only random sections of coronary arteries have been studied histologically in nearly all previously reported studies.[5,9–11]

The occurrence of coronary thrombosis in a large percent (83%) of the late grafts with AVD and their absence in the late grafts without AVD suggest that coronary thrombosis plays a role in the progression of AVD. The neointimal hyperplasia, which usually dominates the morphologic picture of AVD[14] may result in part from the organization of these thrombi, given that platelets contain growth factors that may promote or favor smooth muscle cell proliferation.[17] The absence of continuous endothelial cell layer in most affected coronary arteries is a prothrombotic condition because of the exposure of the subendothelial collagen to blood flow. Intimal denudation provides an ideal substrate for adhesion of platelets. Several factors may cause endothelial cell injury and detachment: immunologic[18–22] or infectious[23,24] or common risk factors for atherosclerosis.[25,26] Recent intravascular ultrasound studies have emphasized the role of endothelial cell dysfunction in the pathogenesis of the AVD.[27]

Although thrombus has not specifically been dealt with in previous reports dealing with AVD in cardiac allografts, several observations support the concept that thrombosis may play a role in the progression of AVD: (1) the perturbed hemostasis with prothrombotic changes of heart transplanted patients, described by Hunt et al[28] in 1993; (2) the depletion of tissue plasminogen activator[29]; and 3) the early loss of the antithrombin component (of the heparin sulphate proteoglycan antithombin natural anticoagulant pathway) from the intima and vascular smooth muscle cells.[30]

Occlusive thrombi in our patients (also described by Johnson et al[12]) occurred over noncritically narrowed chronic lesions, and they did not form over ulcerated plaques. The AVD lesions underlying occlusive thrombosis clearly are different from those of spontaneous atherosclerotic plaques.[14] This study shows that in AVD patients there is a high frequency of coronary thrombosis, and that thrombosis probably accelerates the progression of AVD.

1. Hosenpud JD, Novick RJ, Breen TJ, Keck B, Daily P. The Registry of the International Society for Heart and Lung Transplantation: Twelfth Official Report. *J Heart Lung Transplant* 1995;14:805–815.
2. Kosek JC, Bibier CP, Lower RR. Heart graft arteriosclerosis. *Transplant Proc* 1974;3:512–514.
3. Billingham ME. Cardiac transplantation atherosclerosis. *Transplant Proc* 1987;19:19–25.
4. Billingham ME. Graft coronary disease: the lesions and the patients. *Transplant Proc* 1989;21:3665–3666.
5. Johnson DE, Gao SZ, Schroeder JS, DeCampli WM, Billingham ME. The spectrum of coronary artery pathology in human cardiac allografts. *J Heart Transplant* 1989;8:349–359.
6. Billingham ME. Histopathology of graft coronary disease. *J Heart Transplant* 1992;11:S38–S44.
7. Gravanis MB. Allograft heart accelerated atherosclerosis: evidence for cell-mediated immunity in pathogenesis. *Modern Pathol* 1989;2:495–505.
8. Pucci AM, Forbes RDC, Billingham ME. Pathologic features in long-term cardiac allografts. *J Heart Transplant* 1990;9:339–345.
9. Symmans WF, Nielsen H, Dell R, Rose E, Marboe CC. Cardiac allograft pathology: a clinicopathologic correlation. *Cardiovasc Pathol* 1994;3:249–256.
10. Foerster A. Vascular rejection in cardiac transplantation. A morphological study of 25 human cardiac allografts. *APMIS* 1992;100:367–376.
11. Rose AG, Viviers L, Odell JA. Pathology of chronic cardiac rejection: an analysis of the epicardial and intramyocardial coronary arteries and myocardial alterations in 43 human allografts. *Cardiovasc Pathol* 1993;2:7–19.
12. Johnson DE, Alderman EL, Schroeder JS, Gao SZ, Hunt S, DeCampli WM, Stinson E, Billingham ME. Transplant coronary artery disease: histopathologic correlations with angiographic morphology. *J Am Coll Cardiol* 1991;17:449–457.
13. Gao SZ, Alderman EL, Schroeder JS, Silverman JF, Hunt SA. Accelerated coronary vascular disease in the heart transplant patient: coronary arteriographic findings. *J Am Coll Cardiol* 1988;12:334–340.
14. Billingham ME. Pathology of graft vascular disease after heart and heart-lung transplantation and its relationship to obliterative bronchiolitis. *Transplant Proc* 1995;27:2013–2016.
15. Arbustini E, Grasso M, Diegoli M, Morbini P, Aguzzi A, Fasani R, Specchia G. Coronary thrombosis in non-cardiac death. *Coronary Artery Disease* 1993;4:751–759.
16. Arbustini E, Grasso M, Diegoli M, Pucci A, Bramerio M, Ardissino D, Angoli L, DeServi S, Bramucci E, Mussini A, Minzioni G, Viganò M, Specchia G. Coronary atherosclerotic plaques with and without thrombus in ischemic heart syndromes: A morphologic, immunohistochemical, and biochemical study. *Am J Cardiol* 1991;68:36B–50B.
17. Hayry P, Yilmaz S. Role of growth factors in graft vessel disease. *Transplant Proc* 1995;27:2066–2067.
18. Costanzo-Nordin MR. Cardiac allograft vasculopathy: relationship with acute cellular rejection and histocompatibility. *J Heart Lung Transplant* 1992;11:S90–103.
19. Paavonen T, Mennander A, Lautenschlager I, Mattile S, Hayry P. Endothelialitis and accelerated arteriosclerosis in human heart transplant coronaries. *J Heart Lung Transplant* 1993;12:117–122.
20. Hammond EH, Yowell RL, Price GD, Menlove RL, Olsen SL, O'Connell JB, Bristow MR, Doty DB, Millar RC, Karwande SV, Jones KW, Gay WA, Renlund DG. Vascular rejection and its relationship to allograft coronary artery disease. *J Heart Lung Transplant* 1992;11:S111–119.
21. Lowry RP, Takeuchi T, Cremesi H, Conieczny B, Someren A. Chronic rejection of organ allografts may arise from injuries sustained in recurring foci of acute rejection that resolve spontaneously. *Transplant Proc* 1993;25:2103–2105.
22. Hengstenberg C, Rose ML, Page C, Taylor PM, Yacoub MH. Immunocy-

tochemical changes suggestive of damage to endothelial cells during rejection of human cardiac allografts. *Transplantation* 1990;49:895–899.

23. Grattan MT, Moreno-Cabral CE, Starnes VA, Oyer PE, Stinson EB, Shumway NE. Cytomegalovirus infection is associated with cardiac rejection and atherosclerosis. *JAMA* 1989;261:3561–3566.

24. Loebe M, Schuler S, Zais O, Warnecke H, Fleck E, Hetzer R. Role of cytomegalovirus infection in the development of coronary artery disease in the transplanted heart. *J Heart Transplant* 1990;9:707–711.

25. Johnson MR. Transplant coronary disease: nonimmunologic risk factor. *J Heart Lung Transplant* 1992;11:S124–132.

26. Hess ML, Hastillo A, Thompson JA, Sansonetti DJ, Szentpetery S, Barnhart G, Lower RR. Lipid mediators in organ transplantation: does cyclosporine accelerate coronary atherosclerosis? *Transplant Proc* 1987;19:71–73.

27. Davis SF, Yeung AC, Meredith IT, Charbonneau F, Ganz P, Selwyn AP, Anderson TJ. Early endothelial dysfunction predicts the development of transplant coronary artery disease at 1 year posttransplantation. *Circulation* 1996;93:457–462.

28. Hunt BJ, Segal H, Yacoub M. Hemostatic changes in heart transplant recipients and their relationship to accelerated coronary sclerosis. *Transplantation* 1993;55:309–315.

29. Labarrere CA, Pitts D, Nelson DR, Faulk WP. Coronary artery disease in cardiac allografts: association with depleted arteriolar tissue plasminogen activator. *Transplant Proc* 1995;27:1941–1943.

30. Faulk WP, Labarrere CA, Nelson DR, Pitts D. Coronary artery disease in cardiac allografts: association with arterial antithrombin. *Transplant Proc* 1995;27:1944–1946.

Liver Transplantation After Coronary Artery Bypass Grafting

Frank Pelosi, Jr., MD, Goran B.G. Klintmalm, MD, PhD, Walter B. Simon, MD, and William C. Roberts, MD

ew patients have both coronary artery bypass grafting (CABG) and liver transplantation (LT). Indeed, only 7 patients have been reported to have had both procedures.[1–3] This article reviews findings in 12 patients who had CABG and then later had LT.

• • •

From December 1985 to July 1996, >1,150 patients have had LT at Baylor University Medical Center (BUMC) and since 1985 >8,000 patients have had CABG. The database of Baylor's LT unit was reviewed searching for patients who had had both LT and CABG. A total of 15 patients were retrieved and their clinical records were reviewed. Three patients had LT followed in 6, 36, and 72 months, respectively, by CABG. The 12 patients included in the present study had CABG followed by LT 1 to 228 months later. Pertinent data for each of these 12 patients are summarized in Table I.

Three patients (numbers 1, 2, and 3, Table I) were found to have evidence of myocardial ischemia and angiographic evidence of severe narrowing (>50% diameter reduction) of ≥ 3 major (right, left anterior descending, and left circumflex) epicardial coronary arteries when they were being evaluated for LT. In other words, when first seen at BUMC, each had evidence of both hepatic and cardiac dysfunction. Two of these patients underwent CABG followed within 1 month by LT; the third had LT 7 months after CABG. The cause of the hepatic dysfunction in these patients was methotrexate toxicity (treatment for psoriasis), biliary cirrhosis, and alcoholism, re-

spectively. Patients 1 and 3 have been reported previously.[3]

In the remaining 9 patients, CABG was performed before the development of serious hepatic disease. The cause of the hepatic dysfunction in these 9 patients was hepatitis C virus in 7, and habitual alcoholism in 2. These 9 patients had LT from 60 to 228 months (mean 129) after CABG. For those who had LT secondary to hepatitis C, the interval between CABG and LT ranged from 60 to 228 months (mean 134); for alcoholism, the interval was 72 and 156 months, respectively. Ten of the 12 patients had a single CABG operation, and only 2 of the 10 procedures (numbers 2 and 3, Table I) were performed at BUMC. Each of the remaining 2 patients (numbers 6 and 12, Table I) had 2 CABG procedures (1 before and 1 after LT), and none of these 4 CABG operations was performed at BUMC.

Of the 12 patients having LT after CABG, 6 are alive as of September 1996, a period ranging from 5 to 87 months (mean 59) after LT. Of the other 6, three died within 2 months of LT, and the other 3 at 42, 99, and 108 months, respectively, after LT. Patients 4 and 6 had fatal acute myocardial infarctions. The early deaths were attributed to renal failure (patient 9), gram negative sepsis (patient 8), and acute liver failure (patient 10).

• • •

This report describes 12 patients who had LT at varying intervals after CABG. Three patients were found to have coronary artery disease when they were being evaluated for LT, and in them it was elected to perform the CABG before the LT. The other 9 patients had no evidence of hepatic dysfunction at the time of CABG. In 7 of these 9 patients, hepatitis C virus was introduced via blood transfusions given at the time of CABG. The interval from CABG to LT in them is consistent with the natural course of hepatitis C infection.[4] Five of these 7 pa-

From the Baylor Cardiovascular Institute; the Baylor Institute for Transplantation Sciences; and the Departments of Internal Medicine (Division of Cardiology), Pathology and Surgery, Baylor University Medical Center, Dallas, Texas. Dr. Roberts' address is: Baylor Cardiovascular Institute, 3500 Gaston Avenue, Dallas, Texas 75246. Manuscript received October 3, 1996; revised manuscript received and accepted December 24, 1996.

TABLE I Certain Findings in 12 Patients Having Liver Transplantation After Coronary Artery Bypass Grafting

Case	Age (yr) at CABG	Age (yr) at LT	Date of CABG	Date of LT	Interval CABG to LT (mo)	Etiology of Liver Disease	Liver Weight (g)	CAs Narrowed ≥50% in Diameter				TC (mg/dl)		TG (mg/dl)		Alive (interval [mo] from LT to death or last follow-up)
								LM	LAD	LC	R	Pre LT	Post LT	Pre LT	Post LT	
1*	46	46	1988 (Dec 11)	1989 (Jan 13)	1	Methotrexate	1,570	0	+	+	+	—	—	—	—	0 (0.5)
2	50	50	1995 (Apr 24)	1995 (May 30)	1	Biliary cirrhosis	2,070	0	+	+	+	85	180	72	193	+ (12)
3*	63	63	1992 (Dec 11)	1993 (Mar 3)	7	Alcoholism	1,080	0	+	+†	+†	103	154	172	273	+ (37)
4	52	57	1981	1986 (May 12)	60	Hepatitis C	—	0	+†	+†	+†	300	120	28	286	0 (99)
5	55	61	1983	1989 (Mar 28)	72	Alcoholism	1,230	0	0	+†	+†	—	237	—	213	+ (87)
6**	40, 55	50	1975, 1990	1985 (Dec 19)	120	Hepatitis C	—	0	+†	+†	+†	—	197	—	314	0 (108)
7	46	56	1979	1989 (July 8)	120	Hepatitis C	2,200	+	+†	+†	+†	—	212	—	286	+ (84)
8	49	59	1975	1985 (Aug 4)	120	Hepatitis C	900	—	—	—	—	—	—	—	—	0 (2)
9	53	63	1977	1987 (Apr 22)	120	Hepatitis C	1,050	—	+†	+	+	—	—	—	—	0 (42)
10	47	60	1983	1996 (Mar 25)	156	Alcoholism	1,475	0	+†	+†	0	129	159	115	246	0 (0.5)
11	40	54	1982	1996 (Mar 29)	168	Hepatitis C	1,090	0	+†	0	+†	163	203	214	242	+ (5)
12**	40, 62	50	1972, 1994	1991 (May 29)	228	Hepatitis C	2,250	0	+†	+†	+†	107	173	59	324	+ (63)

*Previously reported by Morris JJ et al (Reference 3).

**CABG was performed both before and after LT.

†Patent bypass conduit at the time of LT.

CAs = coronary arteries; CABG = coronary artery bypass grafting; LAD = left anterior descending; LC = left circumflex; LM = left main; LT = liver transplantation; mo = months; R = right; TC = serum total cholesterol; TG = serum triglycerides; + = positive or present; 0 = negative or absent; — = not available.

tients had undergone CABG in the 1970s and 2 in 1982. During those decades, of course, blood for transfusion was not tested for hepatitis C virus antibody, and, furthermore, far more blood transfusions were given at the time of CABG than are given today.

The estimated frequencies of hepatitis C virus infection and its consequences among the approximately 500,000 patients undergoing CABG annually in the USA before and after the introduction of hepatitis C antibody serology are summarized in Figure 1. The frequencies for blood for transfusion among the 500,000 CABG patients in the USA before and after the introduction of hepatitis C antibody serology are summarized in Figure 2.

There has been an approximate 7-fold decrease in the frequency of development of end-stage liver disease after CABG since the development of hepatitis C antibody serology.[5] Likewise, there has been an approximate 17-fold decrease in the percentage of hepatitis C virus infected blood units used in transfusions during CABG since the introduction of the hepatitis C antibody serology.[5] The risk of acquiring hepatitis C virus after CABG will, of course, diminish further as fewer units of blood are used during CABG. For example, at BUMC in 1995, an average of 2.3 units of blood were used per CABG operation, and 47% of the patients undergoing CABG at BUMC in 1995 received no transfusion at all. Therefore, the patients who did receive a blood transfusion at the time of CABG averaged 4.4 units.

Only 3 previous reports including a total of 7 patients have been published of patients having both CABG and LT.[1-3] Four of the 7 patients had LT before the CABG and 1 patient had CABG and LT at the same operation. The remaining 2 patients had LT 33 and 210 days, respectively, after CABG. Each of these 2 patients have been reported previously.[3] Each of these 2 patients are like our patients numbers 1 and 2 (Table I) in that both were found to have coronary artery disease during their work-up for hepatic dysfunction and it was elected to do the CABG before the LT. None of the previously reported patients had LT late after CABG and normal hepatic function at the time of CABG, the situation in 9 of our 12 patients.

In summary, 12 patients are described who had LT after CABG. Nine of them had normal hepatic function at the time of LT and cirrhosis was precipitated by hepatitis C virus in 7 of the 9 patients. Because of the present policy of testing blood for hepatitis C before transfusion and because of the small numbers of blood transfusions now given at the time of CABG, it is predicted that LT after CABG will be much less of a problem in the future. Liver transplantation can be a life-saving procedure for serious hepatic dysfunction developing late after CABG.

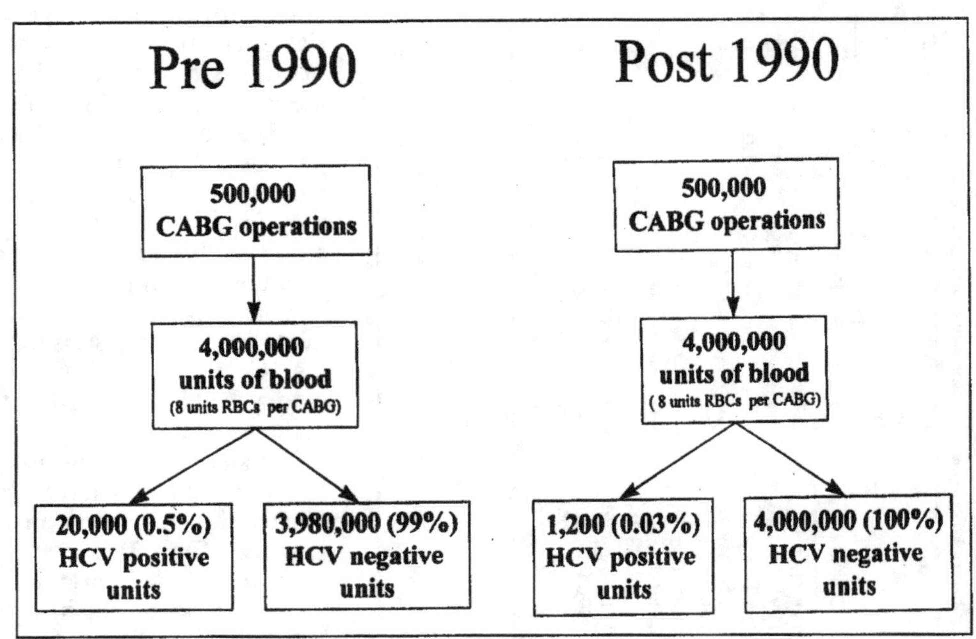

FIGURE 1. Estimated annual frequencies of sequelae of hepatitis C virus (HCV) infection from transfused blood products at the time of coronary artery bypass grafting (CABG) before and after the availability of hepatitis C antibody for donor screening.

FIGURE 2. Estimated annual frequency of hepatitis C virus (HCV) seropositivity in transfused units of red blood cells (RBCs) at the time of coronary artery bypass grafting (CABG) before and after the availability of hepatitis C antibody for donor screening.

1. Dillow JR, Larrieu AJ, Fine RH. Emergency coronary revascularization in liver transplant recipient. *Chest* 1995;108:1763–1764.

2. Dunton RF, Karlson KJ, Leonardi HK, Jenkins RL, Berger RL. Coronary artery bypass grafting in patients with transplanted livers. *Ann Thorac Surg* 1994;58:1054–1058.

3. Morris JJ, Hellman CL, Gawey BJ, Ramsey MAE, Valek TR, Gunning TC, Swygert TH, Shore-Lesserson L, Lalehzarian F, Brayman KL, Brennan TA. Three patients requiring both coronary artery bypass grafting and orthotopic liver transplantation. *J Cardiothorac Vasc Anesth* 1995;9:322–332.

4. Alter HJ. The hepatitis C virus and its relationship to the clinical spectrum of NANB hepatitis. *J Gastroenterol Hepatol* 1990;5(suppl 1):78–94.

5. Donahue JG, Munoz A, Ness PM, Brown DE, Yawn DH, McAllister HA, Reitz BA, Nelson KE. The declining risk of post-transfusion hepatitis C virus infection. *N Engl J Med* 1992;327:369–373.

Severe Mitral Regurgitation Late After Healing of Myocardial Infarction from Calcification of the Posteromedial Left Ventricular Papillary Muscle

Small calcific deposits occur commonly in the left ventricular papillary muscles of elderly persons, presumably a part of the aging process, and these small deposits do not appear to be related to coronary arterial disease. These small deposits are limited to the apices of the papillary muscles, and they are usually not discernible by currently available noninvasive techniques. Much larger calcific deposits occur on rare occasion in the left ventricular free wall and/or ventricular septum at sites of healed myocardial infarction.[1] These larger calcific deposits in these locations may be detected by radiographic means during life.[2] We studied a 72-year-old man who had had a transmural acute myocardial infarction 9 years earlier and now presented with severe mitral regurgitation. The echocardiogram (Figure 1) disclosed an echodense structure caudal to the mitral valve. The operatively excised mitral valve (Figure 2) disclosed the calcium to be located in the posteromedial papillary muscle.

John S. Gottdiener, MD

Washington, DC

William C. Roberts, MD

Dallas, Texas
11 January 1998

1. Roberts WC, Kaufman RJ. Calcification of healed myocardial infarcts. *Am J Cardiol* 1987;60:28–32.
2. Come PC, Riley MF. M-mode and cross-sectional echocardiographic recognition of fibrosis and calcification of the mitral valve chordae and left ventricular papillary muscles. *Am J Cardiol* 1982;49:461–466.

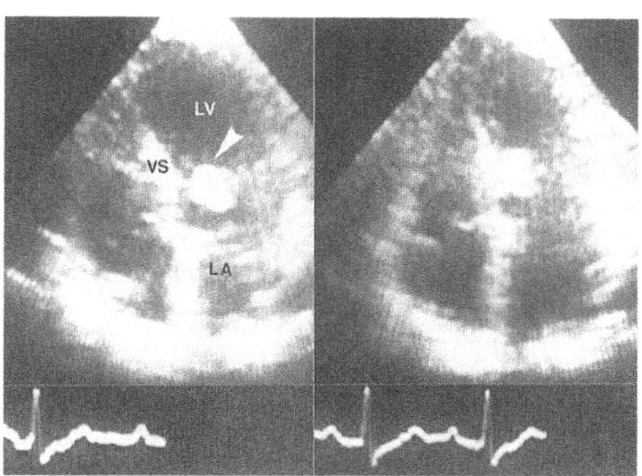

FIGURE 1. Diastolic (*left*) and systolic (*right*) frames of apical 4-chamber view showing echo dense structures (*arrowhead*) distal to the mitral valve, but which showed substantial motion within the left ventricular cavity (LV). LA = left atrial cavity; VS = ventricular septum.

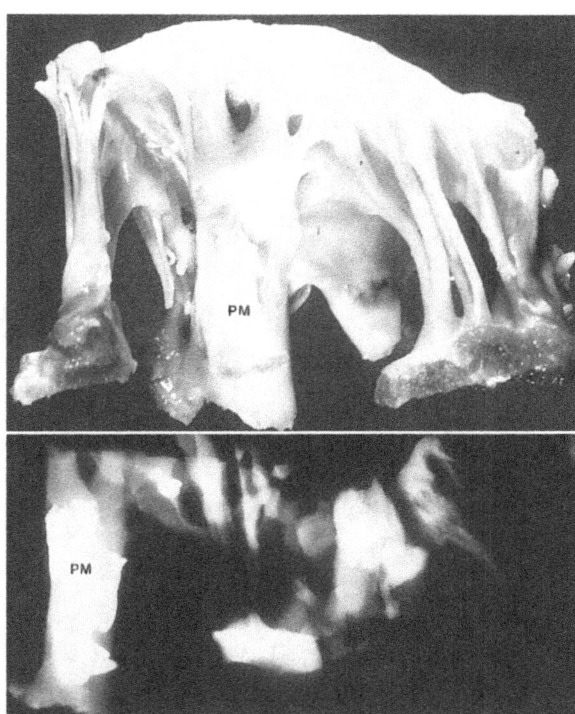

FIGURE 2. Operatively excised mitral valve (*upper*) with large calcified deposit replacing a large portion of the posteromedial papillary muscle (PM). Radiograph (*lower*) confirming calcium in the operatively excised valve.

Comparison of Cardiac Findings at Necropsy in Octogenarians, Nonagenarians, and Centenarians

William Clifford Roberts, MD, and Jamshid Shirani, MD

Certain clinical and necropsy cardiac findings are described and compared in 391 octogenarians (80%), 93 nonagenarians (19%), and in 6 centenarians (1%). The number of men and women was similar (248 [51%] and 242 [49%]). The cause of death was cardiac in 228 patients (47%), vascular but noncardiac in 71 (14%), and noncardiac and nonvascular in 191 (39%). The frequency of a cardiac condition causing death decreased with increasing age groups (51% vs 32% vs 0), and the frequency of a noncardiac, nonvascular condition causing death increased with increasing age groups (36% vs 47% vs 100%). Among the cardiac conditions causing death, coronary artery disease was found in 62% of cases (141 of 228), aortic valve stenosis in 16% (36 of 228), and cardiac amyloidosis in 10% of cases (22 of 228). Calcific deposits were found at necropsy in the coronary arteries in 81% of the patients (398 of 490), in the aortic valve in 47% (228 of 490), in the mitral annular area in 39% of the patients (190 of 490), and in 1 or both left ventricular papillary muscles in 25% of the patients (122 of 490). The calcific deposits tended to be less frequent in the octogenarians. Three hundred (61%) of the 490 patients had ≥1 major coronary arteries narrowed >75% in cross-sectional area by plaque and the percent of patients in each of the 3 age groups and the percent of coronary arteries significantly narrowed in each of the 3 age groups were similar. ©1998 by Excerpta Medica, Inc.

(Am J Cardiol 1998;82:627–631)

The amount of information at necropsy in very elderly persons is relatively sparse. In 1983, Waller and Roberts[1] described some clinical and necropsy findings in 40 American patients aged ≥90 years. In 1988, Lie and Hammond[2] reported findings at necropsy in 237 patients aged ≥90 years. In 1991, Gertz and associates[3] described composition of coronary atherosclerotic plaques in 18 persons ≥90 years of age. In 1993, Roberts[4] described cardiac necropsy findings in an additional 53 patients ≥90 years of age. In 1995, Shirani and colleagues[5] described cardiac findings at necropsy in 366 Americans aged 80 to 89 years, and in 1998 Roberts[6] described cardiac findings at necropsy in 6 centenarians. This study summarizes observations on the heart in these 459 patients,[1,4–6] aged 80 to 103 years, incorporates findings in 31 additional patients studied at necropsy since the previous publications, and compares findings in the octogenarians, nonagenarians, and centenarians.

METHODS

Patients: The files of the Pathology Branch, National Heart, Lung, and Blood Institutes, National Institutes of Health, Bethesda, Maryland, from 1959 to 1993, and those of the Baylor University Medical Center, Dallas, Texas, beginning January 1993, were searched for all accessioned cases of patients aged ≥80 years of age. Of 511 such cases found, adequate clinical information was available in 490 necropsy patients. These cases are the subject of this study. The clinical cardiac and morphologic records, photographs, and postmortem x-rays of the heart, histologic slides of the heart, and the initial gross description of the hearts were reviewed. All 490 hearts were originally examined by WCR, who recorded gross morphologic abnormalities in each case. The hearts in the octogenarians also were examined by JS.

Sources of patients: Of the 490 cases, the hearts in 412 were obtained from 12 hospitals in the Washington, DC, area, and the hearts in the other 78 cases from hospitals outside that area, including 25 from Baylor University Medical Center. Of the 490 hearts, 37 (8%) were examined in 1970 or before; 153 (31%) from 1971 to 1980; 244 (50%) from 1981 to 1990; and 56 (11%) were examined from 1991 to 1997.

Definitions: *Sudden coronary death* was defined as death within 6 hours from the onset of new symptoms of myocardial ischemia in the presence of morphologic evidence of significant atherosclerotic coronary artery disease (≥1 major epicardial coronary artery narrowed >75% in cross-sectional area by atherosclerotic plaque). Most patients who died suddenly did so outside a hospital; a few, however, died shortly after admission to an emergency room. Sudden, out-of-hospital death also occurred in some patients with cardiac diseases other than atherosclerotic coronary artery disease. In each case, an underlying cardiac disease generally believed to cause sudden death was present at necropsy. *Acute myocardial infarction* was defined as a grossly visible left ventricular wall lesion confirmed histologically to represent coagulation-type myocardial necrosis. *Ischemic cardiomyopathy* was defined as chronic congestive heart failure associated

From the Baylor Cardiovascular Institute, and the Departments of Medicine (Cardiology) and Pathology, Baylor University Medical Center, Dallas, Texas; and the Division of Cardiology, Department of Medicine, Albert Einstein College of Medicine, Bronx, New York. Manuscript received February 11, 1998; revised manuscript received and accepted April 15, 1998.

Address for reprints: William C. Roberts, MD, Baylor Cardiovascular Institute, Baylor University Medical Center, 3600 Gaston Avenue, Dallas, Texas 75246.

with a transmural healed myocardial infarct and a dilated left ventricular cavity.

CARDIAC MORPHOLOGIC DATA: Hearts were kept in 10% phosphate-buffered formalin for 3 to 15 days before examination. They were then "cleaned" of parietal pericardium and postmortem intracavity clot, and the pulmonary trunk and ascending aorta were incised approximately 2 cm cephalad to the sinotubular junction. *Heart weight* was then measured on accurate scales by WCR (Lipsaw scale before 1971, accurate to 10 g, and Mettler P1210 scale after 1971, accurate to 0.1 g). Heart weight was considered increased if it was ≥350 g in women and >400 g in men. Most hearts were studied by cutting the ventricles transversely at approximately 1-cm thick intervals from apex to base parallel to the atrioventricular groove posteriorly. In each heart, the visually estimated sizes of cardiac ventricular cavities, presence of left ventricular necrosis (acute myocardial infarct), fibrosis (healed myocardial infarct), status of the 4 cardiac valves, and the maximum degree of cross-sectional luminal narrowing in each of 3 major (left anterior descending, left circumflex, and right) epicardial coronary arteries were recorded.

RESULTS

Numbers of patients in each of the 3 groups: Certain clinical and necropsy cardiac findings in the 490 cases are summarized in Table I and their causes of death are listed in Table II. The 490 patients were divided into 3 groups: the octogenarians (80 to 89 years) (n = 391 [80%]); the nonagenarians (90 to 99 years) (n = 93 [19%]); and the centenarians (≥100 years) (n = 6 [1%]); 248 (51%) were women and 242 (49%) were men.

Clinical findings: The clinical manifestations of the various cardiac disorders probably represent minimal numbers: many patients apparently were unable to provide much clinical information, many came to the hospital from nursing homes, and many had varying degrees of dementia. Nevertheless, angina pectoris was noted in the records of 137 of the 391 octogenarians (35%), in 5 of the 93 nonagenarians (5%), and in none of the 6 centenarians. A history of a hospitalization for an illness compatible with acute myocardial infarction was present in 78 of the 391 octogenarians (20%), in 18 of the 93 nonagenarians (19%), and in none of the 6 octogenarians. Chronic congestive heart failure was present in 36% of the octogenarians (140 of 391), in 25% of the nonagenarians (23 of 93), and in none of the 6 centenarians. A history of systemic hypertension was present in 44% of the octogenarians (174 of 391), in 54% of the nonagenarians (50 of 93), and in none of the centenarians. Diabetes mellitus was present in 14% of the octogenarians (56 of 391), in 9% of the nonagenarians (8 of 93), and in none of the 6 centenarians.

Causes of death: The causes of death in the 490 patients are summarized in Table II. A cardiac condition was the cause of death in 51% of the octogenarians (198 of 391), in 32% of the nonagenarians (30 of 99), and in none of the centenarians. A noncardiac but vascular condition was responsible for death in 13% of the octogenarians (52 of 391) and in 20% of the nonagenarians (19 of 93). A noncardiac and a nonvascular condition was responsible for death in 36% of the octogenarians (141 of 391), in 47% of the nonagenarians (44 of 93), and in all 6 of the centenarians.

Cardiac necropsy findings: Cardiac findings at necropsy are shown in Table I.

HEART WEIGHT: The mean heart weights were largest in the octogenarians and smallest in the centenarians (449 g vs 420 g vs 328 g). Heart weight was increased (>400 g in men; >350 g in women) in 131 of 205 men (64%) and in 157 of 211 women (74%), and the percent was highest in the octogenarians.

CALCIFIC DEPOSITS IN THE HEART: Calcific deposits were present in the heart at necropsy in 444 of the 490 patients (91%) and were most common in the *coronary arteries*—in all cases being located in atherosclerotic plaques and not in the media—81% (398 of 490); in the *aortic valve cusps* in 47% (228 of 490)—heavy enough to result in aortic stenosis in 10% (51 of 490); *mitral valve annulus* in 39% (190 of 490)—very heavy deposits in 13% (63 of 490), and in the apices of 1 or both left ventricular *papillary muscles* in 17% (85 of 490). The cardiac calcific deposits were more frequent and heavier in the nonagenarians than in the octogenarians.

NUMBERS OF PATIENTS WITH NARROWING OF ≥1 MAJOR EPICARDIAL CORONARY ARTERIES: Among the 490 patients, 194 (40%) had none of the 3 major (right, left anterior descending, and left circumflex) epicardial coronary arteries narrowed by plaque >75% in cross-sectional area; 89 (18%) had 1 artery so narrowed; 105 (21%) had 2 arteries so narrowed, and 94 (19%) had all 3 arteries so narrowed. The percent of patients in each of the 3 groups with no arteries and 1, 2, and 3 arteries narrowed >75% was similar.

NUMBERS OF MAJOR CORONARY ARTERIES (3/PATIENT) NARROWED >75% IN CROSS-SECTIONAL AREA BY PLAQUE: Among the 490 patients, a total of 1,470 major epicardial coronary arteries were examined: 865 arteries (59%) had insignificant (<75% in cross-sectional area) narrowing and 605 (41%) had narrowing by plaque >75% in cross-sectional area. The percent of arteries significantly narrowed was similar in each of the 3 groups (42% vs 39% vs 33%).

ACUTE AND HEALED MYOCARDIAL INFARCTS: Grossly visible foci of left ventricular wall (includes ventricular septum) necrosis (acute infarcts) without associated left ventricular scars (healed infarcts) were found in 64 patients (13%); foci of left ventricular fibrosis without associated necrosis were observed in 123 patients (25%), and foci of both necrosis and fibrosis were found in 42 patients (9%). Thus, a total of 229 of the 490 patients (47%) had grossly visible evidence of acute or healed myocardial infarcts, or both. The percent of patients with myocardial lesions of ischemia was similar among the octogenarians and nonagenarians.

VENTRICULAR CAVITY DILATION: One or both ventricular cavities were dilated (by gross inspection) in

TABLE I Certain Clinical and Necropsy Findings in 490 Patients Aged 80 to 103 Years

Variable	Age Group (yrs)		
	80–89 (n = 391)	90–99 (n = 93)	≥100 (n = 6)
1. Mean age (yrs)	84 ± 4	93 ± 4	102
2. Men:women	194 (50%):197 (50%)	52 (56%):41 (44%)	2/4
3. Angina pectoris	137 (35%)	5 (5%)	0
4. Acute myocardial infarction	78 (20%)	18 (18%)	0
5. Chronic congestive heart failure	140 (36%)	23 (25%)	0
6. Systemic hypertension (history)	174 (44%)	50 (54%)	0
7. Diabetes mellitus	56 (14%)	8 (9%)	0
8. Atrial fibrillation	57 (15%)	35 (38%)	0
9. Heart weight (g):range (mean)	185–900 (449)	220–660 (420)	240–410 (328)
Men	230–830 (493)	285–660 (436)	335–410 (372)
Women	185–900 (409)	220–630 (406)	240–385 (306)
10. Cardiomegaly			
Men >400 g	103/154 (67%)	27/49 (55%)	1/2
Women >350 g	133/165 (81%)	23/42 (55%)	1/4
11. Cardiac calcific deposits			
None	43 (11%)	3 (3%)	0
Present	348 (89%)	90 (97%)	6 (100%)
Coronary arteries	304 (78%)	89 (96%)	5
Aortic valve cusps	164 (42%)	59 (63%)	5
Heavy (stenosis)	43 (11%)	8 (9%)	0
Mitral annulus	146 (37%)	42 (45%)	2
Heavy	52 (13%)	11 (12%)	0
Papillary muscle	37 (9%)	42 (45%)	6
12. No. of patients with 0,1,2, or 3 major (right, left anterior descending, left circumflex) coronary arteries ↓ >75% in cross-sectional area			
0	159 (41%)	33 (35%)	2
1	67 ⎱	20 ⎱	2 ⎱
2	71 ⎰ 232 (59%)	32 ⎰ 60 (65%)	2 ⎰ 4
3	94	8	0
Mean	1.7	1.5	1.5
13. Number of major coronary arteries (3/patient) ↓ >75% in cross-sectional area by plaque			
0	0/477	0/99	0/6
1	67/201	20/60	2/6
2	142/213	64/96	4/6
3	282/282	24/24	0
Totals	491/1,173 (42%)	108/279 (39%)	6/18 (33%)
14. Left ventricular necrosis/fibrosis			
Necrosis only	54 (14%)	10 (11%)	0
Fibrosis only	101 (26%)	20 (21%)	2
Both	37 (9%)	5 (5%)	0
15. Ventricular cavity dilation			
Neither	222 (57%)	58 (62%)	4
One	84 (21%)	4 (4%)	2
Right ventricle	42	2	2
Left ventricle	42	2	2
Both	85 (22%)	31 (34%)	0
16. Cardiac amyloidosis (massive)	14 (4%)	8 (9%)	0

218 of the 490 patients (44%) and no significant differences were observed in the 3 groups.

CARDIAC AMYLOIDOSIS: Grossly visible amyloid (confirmed histologically) in ventricular and atrial myocardium as well as in atrial mural endocardium was present in 22 patients (4%). In these 22 patients the amyloidosis was symptomatic and fatal. A number of other patients who had no gross evidence of cardiac amyloidosis had small foci in the heart on histologic study. These minute deposits did not cause symptoms of cardiac dysfunction. In the 22 patients with fatal cardiac amyloidosis, deposits of amyloid were also present in several other body organs at necropsy.

COMMENTS

This study describes findings in a large group (n = 490) of patients ≥80 years of age studied at necropsy, and it compares for the first time certain clinical and necropsy findings in octogenarians, nonagenarians, and centenarians. Despite this study of nearly 500 patients, only 6 patients lived ≥100 years (1%), and only 93 (19%) lived into the tenth decade of life. Nevertheless, the ratio of 1 centenarian for every 65 octogenarian is much higher than might be expected. In general, it takes 10,000 persons to reach age 85 before 1 reaches age 100.[7]

Another finding was the high frequency of men;

TABLE II Causes of Death in the 490 Necropsy Patients Aged 80 to 103 Years			
	Age Group (Years)		
	80–89 (n = 391)	90–99 (n = 93)	≥100 (n = 6)
I. Cardiac	198 (51%)	30 (32%)	0
A. Coronary artery disease	129/198 (65%)	12/30 (40%)	0
1. Acute myocardial infarction	90	12	0
2. Chronic congestive heart failure	15	3	0
3. Sudden	19	3	0
4. Coronary bypass	7	0	0
B. Valvular heart disease	41/198 (21%)	3/30 (10%)	0
1. Aortic stenosis	33	3	0
2. Aortic regurgitation	2	0	0
3. Mitral regurgitation	5	0	0
4. Mitral stenosis	1	0	0
C. Primary cardiomyopathy	7/198 (4%)	1/30 (3%)	0
1. Hypertrophic	4	0	0
2. Idiopathic dilated	3	1	0
D. Secondary cardiomyopathy	16/198 (8%)	8/30 (27%)	0
1. Amyloidosis	14	8	0
2. Hemosiderosis	1	0	0
3. Myocarditis	1	0	0
E. Pericardial heart disease	3/198 (2%)	0	0
II. Vascular, noncardiac	52 (13%)	19 (20%)	0
A. Stroke	17/52 (33%)	6/19 (32%)	0
B. Abdominal aortic aneurysm	14/52 (33%)	5/19 (26%)	0
C. Peripheral arterial disease	11/52 (21%)	5/19 (26%)	0
D. Aortic dissection	4/52 (8%)	0/19 (0)	0
E. Pulmonary embolism	6*/52 (11%)	3/19* (16%)	0
III. Noncardiac and Nonvascular	141 (36%)	44 (47%)	6 (100%)
A. Cancer	52/141 (37%)	13/44 (29%)	0/6
B. Infection	37/141 (26%)	17/44 (39%)	0/6
C. Fall complication	10/141 (7%)	3/44 (7%)	3/6
D. Other	42/141 (30%)	11/44 (25%)	3/6

*All had underlying chronic obstructive pulmonary disease.

there were 248 men (51%) and 242 (49%) women. A higher than expected percentage of men may have resulted in part from receiving a number of these cases from a Veterans Administration Hospital and from a retirement home filled almost entirely by men.

The causes of death were divided into 3 major types: cardiac = 228 of 490 (47%); vascular but noncardiac = 71 of 490 (14%), and noncardiac and nonvascular = 191 of 490 (39%). The frequency of a cardiac condition causing death decreased with increasing age groups (51% vs 32% vs 0), and the frequency of a noncardiac and nonvascular condition causing death increased with increasing age groups (36% vs 47% vs 100%). Among the cardiac conditions, coronary artery disease was found in 62% (141 of 228), and the other cardiac conditions, mainly aortic valve stenosis (36 of 228 [16%]) and cardiac amyloidosis (22 of 228 [10%]), in the other 38%. Stroke, rupture of an abdominal aortic aneurysm, and complications of peripheral arterial atherosclerosis were the major vascular (noncardiac) conditions causing death. Of the noncardiac and nonvascular causes of death, cancer and infection (mainly pneumonia) were the major conditions, 35% (65 of 185) and 29% (54 of 185), respectively, among the octogenarians and nonagenarians.

The cardiac necropsy findings focused primarily on calcific deposits in the coronary arteries, aortic valve cusps, and mitral valve annulus and their consequences, and to a lesser extent, on heavy amyloid deposits in the heart. Calcific deposits were present in the atherosclerotic plaques of ≥1 epicardial coronary arteries in 81% of the patients (398 of 490), on the aortic aspects of the aortic valve cusps in 47% (228 of 490), in the mitral annular regional in 39% (190 of 490), and in 1 or both left ventricular papillary muscles in 25% (122 of 490). The calcific deposits tended to be less frequent in the octogenarians. The frequent presence of calcific deposits in the coronary arteries, aortic valve cusps, and mitral annular region in the same patient suggests that the cause of the calcific deposits in each of these 3 locations is the same. The calcific deposits in the coronary arteries indicate the presence of atherosclerosis because calcium occurs in the coronary arteries, with 1 exception,[8] only in the plaques and not in the media. It is reasonable to believe that the calcific deposits in and on the aortic cusps, at least when this valve is 3 cuspid, are another manifestation of "atherosclerosis." Because mitral annular calcium in this older population is nearly always associated with calcium in the coronary arteries, it is also reasonable to believe that mitral annular calcium in persons ≥80 years of age also is a manifestation of "atherosclerosis."

When the deposits of calcium on the aortic aspects of the aortic valve cusps are extensive, the cusps may become relatively or absolutely immobile, resulting in aortic valve stenosis. These valves usually lack commissural fusion (i.e., adherence of 2 cusps together near the lateral attachments), and therefore, aortic regurgitation is usually absent. Although it most often is associated with some degree of mitral regurgitation, if the mitral annular calcium is "massive," and if the left ventricular cavity is also small and the wall quite thickened, this may result in mitral stenosis.[9]

Calcium in a papillary muscle appears to be a consequence of "aging" and not a direct manifestation of atherosclerosis.

The percent of patients with narrowing >75% in cross-sectional area by plaque of ≥1 major epicardial coronary artery was similar in all 3 age groups, as was the percent of major coronary arteries narrowed significantly.

1. Waller BF, Roberts WC. Cardiovascular disease in the very elderly. Analysis of 40 necropsy patients aged 90 years or over. *Am J Cardiol* 1983;51:403–421.
2. Lie JT, Hammond PI. Pathology of the senescent heart: anatomic observations on 237 autopsy studies of patients 90 to 105 years old. *Mayo Clinic Proc* 1988;63:552–564.
3. Gertz SD, Malekzadeh S, Dollar AL, Kragel AH, Roberts WC. Composition of atherosclerotic plaques in the four major epicardial coronary arteries in patients ≥90 years of age. *Am J Cardiol* 1991;67:1228–1233.
4. Roberts WC. Ninety-three hearts ≥90 years of age. *Am J Cardiol* 1993;71:599–602.
5. Shirani J, Yousefi J, Roberts WC. Major cardiac findings at necropsy in 366 American octogenarians. *Am J Cardiol* 1995;75:151–156.
6. Roberts WC. The heart at necropsy in centenarians. *Am J Cardiol* 1998;81:1224–1225.
7. Fries JF. Aging, natural death, and the compression of morbidity. *N Engl J Med* 1980;303:130–135.
8. Lachman AS, Spray TL, Kerwin DM, Shugoll GI, Roberts WC. Medial calcinosis of Monckeberg. A review of the problem and a description of a patient with involvement of peripheral, visceral and coronary arteries. *Am J Cardiol* 1977;63:615–622.
9. Hammer WJ, Roberts WC, deLeon AC Jr. "Mitral stenosis" secondary to combined "massive" mitral annular calcific deposits and small, hypertrophied left ventricles. *Am J Med* 1978;64:371–376.

Operative Therapy of Coronary Arterial Aneurysm

Safoora Harandi, MD, Stephen B. Johnston, MD, Richard E. Wood, MD, and William C. Roberts, MD

Although their involvement of the aorta and common iliac arteries is common, aneurysmal involvement of a coronary artery is uncommon. Most coronary aneurysms are surprise findings at coronary angiography or at necropsy. Relatively few reports are available describing operative therapy of coronary aneurysm. The present report describes operative therapy in a patient with large coronary aneurysms, and reviews previous reports[1–16] of patients having operative therapy for coronary aneurysm.

• • •

D.R.G., a 65-year-old obese white man was well, except for systemic hypertension, until January 1, 1997, when he developed nonexertional dyspnea associated with diaphoresis, and both recurred during the next 3 days when he was seen by a cardiologist. Blood pressure was 170/105 mm Hg. Electrocardiogram disclosed complete right bundle branch block. Cardiac catheterization on January 10, 1997, disclosed a huge aneurysm involving the proximal portion of the left anterior descending and first diagonal coronary arteries, and an even larger one involving the right coronary artery (Figure 1). The left main artery was normal and the left circumflex artery contained only luminal irregularities. Left ventriculography disclosed anteroapical wall hypokinesia without mitral regurgitation. Ejection fraction was about 35%. Magnetic resonance imaging disclosed thrombus within the aneurysm in

From the Departments of Internal Medicine (Division of Cardiology) and Thoracic & Cardiovascular Surgery, Baylor University Medical Center, Dallas, Texas. Dr. Roberts' address is: Baylor Cardiovascular Institute, Baylor University Medical Center, Dallas, Texas. Manuscript received November 4, 1998; revised manuscript received December 16, 1998, and accepted December 17.

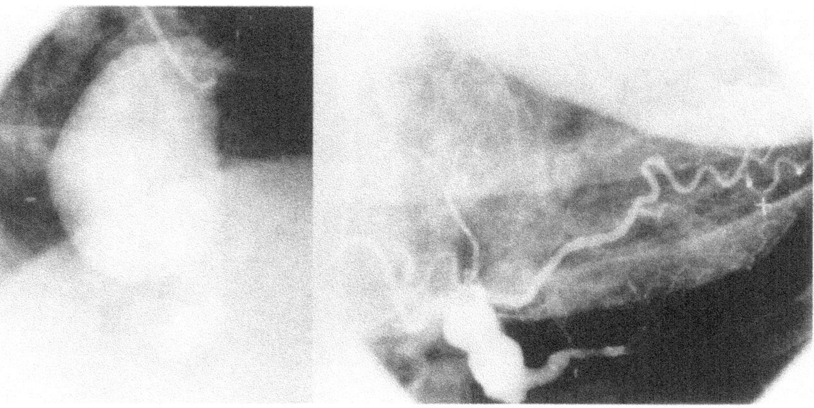

FIGURE 1. Coronary angiograms in the patient described. *Left,* aneurysm involving the right coronary artery: *right,* angiogram demonstrating an aneurysm in the left anterior descending coronary artery.

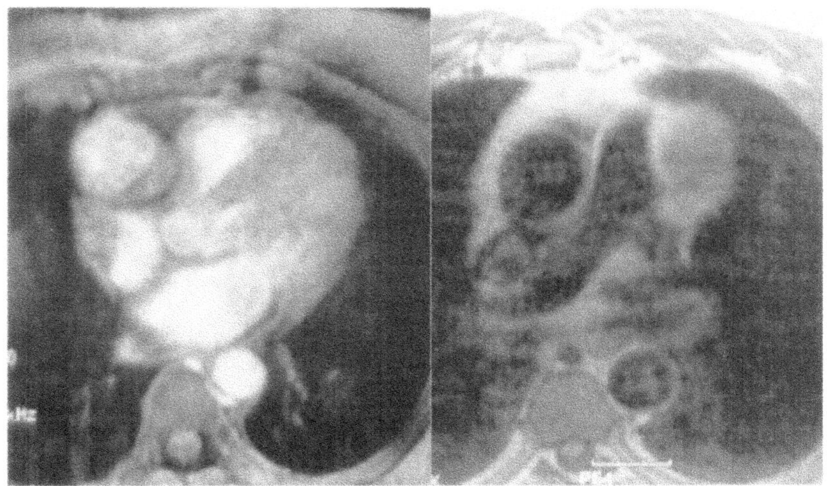

FIGURE 2. Magnetic resonance imaging of the heart in the patient described. *Left,* the aneurysm in the right coronary artery is shown. A thrombus is with the aneurysm. *Right,* the aneurysm involving the left anterior descending coronary artery is shown.

the right coronary artery; its dimensions were 5 × 8 cm (Figure 2). The aneurysm in the left anterior descending artery had a maximal dimension of 3 × 5 cm and it too contained thrombus (Figure 2). At operation, on January 14, 1997, the aneurysm of the left anterior descending coronary artery was ligated distally and a saphenous vein was inserted from aorta to this artery distally. The right coronary artery was ligated both proximal and distal to the aneurysm and a saphe-

nous vein conduit was inserted from aorta to the largest posterior descending branch. A conduit also was placed from aorta to first diagonal coronary artery. The early postoperative period was complicated by the appearance of a posterior wall acute myocardial infarction; creatine kinase rose to a peak of 2,739 U/L. Electrocardiogram postoperatively showed no bundle branch block, but Q waves and elevated ST segments were seen in leads III and aVF. In October 1998

TABLE I Previously Reported Patients With Operative Therapy of Coronary Artery Aneurysm and the Type of Operation Performed

| Case | First Author | CA Containing Aneurysm | Lumen of CA With Aneurysm Narrowed | Operative Procedure | | | | | |
				CABG	Aneurysm Resection	Proximal Ligation	Distal Ligation	T	Aneurysmorrhectomy (marsupilization)
1.	Anabtaui	LAD	+	+	0	0	0	+	+
2.	Oliver	LAD	0	+	0	0	0	0	0
3.	Wilson	LAD	+	+	0	0	0	0	0
		Right	+	0	0	0	0	0	0
4.	Glickel	Right	0	+	+	+	+	0	0
5.	Emmenrich (case 1)	Right	0	+	0	+	0	0	0
		LM	0	0	0	+*	0	0	0
		LAD	0	+	0	0	0	0	0
		LC	0	0	0	0	0	0	0
		FSP	0	0	0	0	0	0	0
6.	Selke	Right	0	+	0	0	0	0	+
7.	Chen	LAD	0	0	0	0	0	0	+
8.	Hawkins	Right	+	+	0	0	0	0	0
		LM	0	+	0	+	+	0	0
9.	Koike	Right	+	+	0	0	0	0	0
10.	Lenihan	LM	0	+	0	+	+	0	0
11.	Lazerus	LM	0	+	+†	0	0	0	+
12.	Eng	Right	0	+	0	+	+	0	0
13.	Lentini	LM	0	0	0	+	0	0	0
		LAD	0	+	0	0	0	0	0
14.	Vijayaragar	Right	+	+	0	+	0	0	+
		LC	+	+	0	0	0	0	0
		LAD	+	+	0	0	+	0	0
15.	Vijayaragar	LM	0	0	0	0	0	+	+
		LAD	—	+	0	0	+	+	+
16.	Wan	Right	0	0	0	+	+	0	0
17.	Sato	Right	+	+	0	0	0	0	0
		LAD	+	+	0	0	0	0	0

*Ostium of left main closed by a patch.

†Saccular aneurysm of left main resected but left main flow retained.

CA = coronary artery; CABG = coronary artery bypass grafting; FD = first diagonal; FSP = first septal perforator; LAD = left anterior descending; LC = left circumflex; LM = left main; T = thrombectomy; − = not applicable; + = present; 0 = absent.

(22 months after operation), he was asymptomatic, hunting nearly daily, and he slept flat in bed.

• • •

The heretofore described patient with preexisting systemic hypertension had an acute myocardial infarction without chest pain. Coronary angiography disclosed an aneurysm in the right and left anterior descending coronary arteries and magnetic resonance imaging disclosed their sizes to be 5 and 3.5 cm in maximal diameter, respectively. At operation, the coronary artery containing one aneurysm was ligated both proximally and distally, another aneurysm was ligated distally only, and aortocoronary conduits were inserted distally in each of the 2 arteries with aneurysms. Postoperatively, an acute myocardial infarct (posterior wall) was apparent by electrocardiographic changes and by elevation of the creatine kinase levels.

At least 17 patients >20 years of age having operative therapy for coronary arterial aneurysm unassociated with a coronary fistula or with Kawasaki disease have been reported (Tables I and II). The 17 patients at operation ranged in age from 28 to 68 years (mean 47); 13 (76%) were men and 4 (24%) were women. The event that brought the patients to medical attention was acute myocardial infarction in 6 patients (35%), angina pectoris in 12 patients (70%), and hemopericardium from coronary aneurysmal rupture in 2 (12%). In 10 patients (59%) only 1 coronary artery contained an aneurysm, and in 7 patients (41%) an aneurysm involved >1 coronary artery. Of the 28 aneurysms in the 17 patients (average 1.9/patient), 10 (36%) involved the right, 6 (21%) the left main, 9 (32%) the left anterior descending, 2 (7%) the left circumflex, and 1 (3%) another coronary artery. The largest diameter of the coronary aneurysm ranged from >1 to 8 cm. The country of origin of the 17 patients was USA in 9 (53%), Japan in 2 (12%), and 1 each from Belgium, Canada, China, France, India, and United Kingdom.

The variety of operative procedures performed in the 17 patients are summarized in Table II: coronary artery bypass grafting in 15 (88%) (alone in 4 and in association with another procedure in 11). The other procedures included total aneurysmal resection in 2 patients, proximal ligation in 9 and distal ligation in 7 (both in 5), aneurysmal thrombectomy in 3, and aneurysmorrhectomy in 7.

Despite the variety of operative procedures performed in the previously reported patients, the outcome in virtually all of them was uniformly good. From a follow-up period ranging from 42 to 1,440 days (mean 409) in 13 patients, 12

								Location of Aneurysm						Graft to							
Patient	Year of Report	Last Name of 1st Author	Age at Operation (yr)	Gender	AMI (location)	AP	Other	R	LM	LAD	LC	Other	CABG	R	LAD	LC	Other	Largest Dimension (cm) of CA Aneurysm	Interval (wk) Op to Latest Follow-Up	Number of CAs >50% ↓ in Diameter	Country of Patient
1	1974	Anabtaui	40	M	−	+	0	0	0	+	0	0	+	0	+	0	0	−	−	1 (LAD)	USA
2	1974	Olivers	62	F	0	+	0	0	0	+	0	0	+	0	0	0	+	>1	450	3 (LM,R)	USA
3	1975	Wilson	48	M	+ (I)	0	0	+	0	+	0	0	+	+	+	0	0	4	150	2 (LC,LAD,R)	USA
4	1978	Glickel	28	F	0	+	0	+	0	0	0	0	+	+	0	0	0	2	360	0	USA
5	1989	Emmerich	30	M	+ (A)	0	0	+	+	+	+	+	+	+	+	−	+	1.2	1440	0	India
6	1991	Selke	30	F	0	+	0	+	0	0	0	0	+	+	0	0	0	8	360	0	USA
7	1993	Chen	52	F	0	+	0	0	0	+	0	0	0	0	0	0	0	Large	−	0	China
8	1990	Hawkins	66	M	+ (NQ)	+	0	+	+	0	0	0	+	0	+	0	+	3	−	3 (LAD,LC,R)	USA
9	1990	Koike	46	M	+ (I)	0	0	+	0	0	0	0	+	+	0	0	0	2	42	1 (R)	Japan
10	1991	Lenihan	39	M	0	+	0	0	+	0	0	0	+	+	+	+	+	1.5	360	3 (LAD,RI,R)	USA
11	1992	Lazarus	49	M	0	+	0	0	+	0	0	0	+	+	+	0	+	−	180	2 (LAD,R)	France
12	1993	Eng	55	M	0	+	0	+	0	0	0	+	+	+	+	0	0	Large	60	1 (LAD)	UK
13	1994	Lentini	56	M	0	+	0	0	+	+	0	0	+	+	+	0	+	5	180	3 (LC,FD,R)	Canada
14	1994	Vijayanagar	68	M	0	0	+	+	0	+	+	0	+	+	+	LC	0	8	540	3 (LAD,LC,R)	USA
15	1994	Vijayanagar	32	M	+ (I)	+	0	0	+	+	0	0	+	−	+	−	+	3	540	Several	USA
16	1996	Wan	49	M	0	+	+	+	0	0	0	0	0	0	0	0	0	Small	150	0	Belgium
17	1997	Sato	44	M	+ (L)	0	0	+	+	+	0	+	+	+	+	0	+	2	−	3 (LM,LAD,LOM)	Japan

A = anterior; AMI = acute myocardial infarction; AP = angina pectoris; D = diameter; F = female; I = inferior; L = lateral; LOM = left obtuse marginal; M = male; NQ = non–Q-wave; OP = operation; R = right; RI = ramus intermedius; − = no information available or not applicable; + = positive or present; 0 = negative or absent; other abbreviations as in Table I.

(92%) were asymptomatic and 1 (case 3) had a single episode of chest pain (while casting for fish) during his 150-day postoperative period. Their outcomes were good despite the fact that our patient and also patient 4 (Table II) had a new acute myocardial infarction, and another patient (no. 13, Table II) had new complete heart block shortly after cardiac operation. It seems clear that the proper type of operative therapy for coronary aneurysm is as yet unclear. Whether the reported patients with coronary aneurysm and our patient would have done well without operative intervention also is unclear because there are no randomized studies available to answer these questions, and almost certainly there never will be any because of the comparative rarity of coronary aneurysm.

In summary, a patient with multiple coronary aneurysms and operative therapy is described and 17 previously reported similar cases are reviewed. The proper type of operation for this condition is as yet unclear, but, nevertheless, the reported cases and our case with operative therapy have done well postoperatively despite a variety of procedures performed.

1. Anabtawi IN, de Leon JA. Arteriosclerotic aneurysms of the coronary arteries. *J Thorac Cardiovasc Surg* 1974;68:226–228.
2. Oliveros RA, Falsetti HL, Carroll RJ, Heinle RA, Ryan GF. Atherosclerotic coronary artery aneurysm. Report of five cases and review of literature. *Arch Intern Med* 1974;134:1072–1076.
3. Wilson CS, Weaver WF, Forker AD. Bilateral arteriosclerotic coronary arterial aneurysms successfully treated with saphenous vein bypass grafting. *Am J Cardiol* 1975;35:315–318.
4. Glickel SZ, Maggs PR, Ellis FH Jr. Coronary artery aneurysm. *Ann Thorac Surg* 1978;25:372–376.
5. Emmerich J, Thomas D, Drobinski G, Canny M, Gandjbakhch I, Grosgogeat Y. Diagnosis of coronary aneurysms in siblings: treatment with a new surgical procedure. *Eur Heart J* 1989;10:91–96.
6. Selke KG, Vemulapalli P, Brodarick SA, Coordes C, Gowda S, Salem B, Alpert MA. Giant coronary artery aneurysm: detection with echocardiography, computed tomography, and magnetic resonance imaging. *Am Heart J* 1991;121:1544–1547.
7. Chen Y-T, Hwang C-L, Kan M-N. Large, isolated, congenital aneurysm of the anterior descending coronary artery. *Br Heart J* 1993;70:274–275.

8. Hawkins JW, Vacek JL, Smith GS. Massive aneurysm of the left main coronary artery. *Am Heart J* 1990;119:1406–1408.

9. Koike R, Oku T, Satoh H, Sawada Y, Suma H, Takeuchi A, Kato Y, Kita Y, Hirota Y, Kawamura K. *Jpn J Surg* 1990;20:463–467.

10. Lenihan DJ, Zeman HS, Collins GJ. Left main coronary artery aneurysm in association with severe atherosclerosis: a case report and review of the literature. *Cathet Cardiovasc Diagn* 1991;23:28–31.

11. Lazarus A, Donzeau-Gouge P, Spaulding C, Weber S, Guérin F. Surgical treatment of an atherosclerotic aneurysm of the left main coronary artery. *Am Heart J* 1992;123:222–224.

12. Eng J, Nair KK. Coronary artery aneurysm. *J Cardiovasc Surg* 1993;34:339–340.

13. Lentini S, Raymond G, Cartier P, Desaulniers D, Doyle D, Lemieux M, Métras J. Surgical treatment of left main coronary aneurysm. *J Cardiovasc Surg* 1994;35:311–314.

14. Vijayanagar R, Shafii E, DeSantis M, Waters RS, Desai A. Surgical treatment of coronary aneurysms with and without rupture. *J Thorac Cardiovasc Surg* 1994;107:1532–1534.

15. Wan S, LcClerc J-L, Vachiery J-L, Vincent J-L. Cardiac tamponade due to spontaneous rupture of right coronary artery aneurysm. *Ann Thorac Surg* 1996;62:575–576.

16. Sato T, Isomura T, Hayashida N, Aoyagi S. Coronary artery revascularization in an adult with coronary aneurysms probably secondary to childhood Kawasaki disease. *Eur J Cardiothorac Surg* 1997;12:312–314.

Twenty questions on atherosclerosis

WILLIAM C. ROBERTS, MD

1. Is atherosclerosis a disease affecting all animals or only certain animals?

Atherosclerosis affects only herbivores. Dogs, cats, tigers, and lions can be saturated with fat and cholesterol, and atherosclerotic plaques do not develop (1, 2). The only way to produce atherosclerosis in a carnivore is to take out the thyroid gland; then, for some reason, saturated fat and cholesterol have the same effect as in herbivores.

2. Are human beings herbivores, carnivores, or omnivores?

Although most of us conduct our lives as omnivores, in that we eat flesh as well as vegetables and fruits, human beings have characteristics of herbivores, not carnivores (2). The appendages of carnivores are claws; those of herbivores are hands or hooves. The teeth of carnivores are sharp; those of herbivores are mainly flat (for grinding). The intestinal tract of carnivores is short (3 times body length); that of herbivores, long (12 times body length). Body cooling of carnivores is done by panting; herbivores, by sweating. Carnivores drink fluids by lapping; herbivores, by sipping. Carnivores produce their own vitamin C, whereas herbivores obtain it from their diet. Thus, humans have characteristics of herbivores, not carnivores.

3. Is atherosclerosis genetic in origin?

Infrequently. Although many physicians and the lay public believe that atherosclerosis is genetic, the evidence for that is slim. One way to define the genetic variety of atherosclerosis is by the presence or absence of low-density lipoprotein (LDL) receptors in the liver (3–5). Patients with homozygous familial hypercholesterolemia have no LDL receptors in the liver, and their total cholesterol levels from birth are usually >800 mg/dL. The frequency of this genetic defect is 1 in 1,000,000. Patients with heterozygous familial hypercholesterolemia have only 50% of the normal number of LDL receptors in the liver. These patients generally have total cholesterol levels about 300 mg/dL, and they generally die (without lipid-lowering therapy) in their 40s or early 50s. The incidence of this familial defect is 1 in 500. The rest of us apparently have normal numbers of LDL receptors in the liver. Of course, a few patients have genetic defects involving high-density lipoprotein (HDL) cholesterol and triglyceride production and uptake, but these individuals are relatively few in number (6). Thus, the genetic defect producing atherosclerosis occurs in no more than 1 in 200 and possibly as low as 1 in 400 or 500 persons. This means, of course, that most persons with atherosclerosis acquire it by the types of calories they consume.

4. Is atherosclerosis a consequence of aging and therefore a degenerative disease?

No. When I was in medical school, I was taught that atherosclerosis was a disease of aging and that it was to be expected as we got older. It is true that symptomatic and fatal atherosclerosis is usually a problem of older people. But, not too old. Patients with homozygous familial hypercholesterolemia, however, may have lipid plaques in their arteries at the time of birth.

It appears that atherosclerosis requires certain serum cholesterol levels over certain periods of time. Therefore, if one has a serum total cholesterol of 1000 mg/dL, death usually occurs by age 15 (without lipid-lowering therapy). Those with total cholesterol levels of approximately 300 mg/dL live into their 30s and 40s. The average age of death from coronary artery disease in the USA is 60 years in men and 68 years in women (7). Sudden death is primarily a problem of young men. Therefore, those who make it to the hospital are usually older than these ages. Nevertheless, atherosclerosis is a disease of relatively young people as well as a disease of older persons. The point here is that atherosclerosis does not have to occur just because of aging. The more years we live, the longer the time period we have to keep our cholesterol levels elevated and thus to develop plaques. Multiplying our serum cholesterol level by our age in years may provide a rough indication of when we have developed enough atherosclerotic plaque to have symptomatic or fatal atherosclerosis.

5. What risk factors predispose to atherosclerosis?

Risk factors include hypercholesterolemia, systemic hypertension, diabetes mellitus, obesity, low HDL cholesterol, cigarette smoking, and inactivity.

6. Of the various atherosclerotic risk factors, which one is an absolute prerequisite for development of atherosclerosis?

The answer is hypercholesterolemia. What level of total cholesterol and specifically LDL cholesterol is required for atherosclerotic plaques to develop? Symptomatic and fatal atherosclerosis is extremely uncommon in societies where serum total cholesterol levels are <150 mg/dL and serum LDL cholesterol levels are <100 mg/dL (8). If the LDL cholesterol level is <100— and possibly it needs to be <80 mg/dL—the other previously mentioned risk factors in and of themselves are not associated with atherosclerosis. In other words, if the serum total choles-

From Baylor Cardiovascular Institute, Baylor University Medical Center, Dallas, Texas.

Corresponding author: William C. Roberts, MD, Baylor Cardiovascular Institute, Baylor University Medical Center, 3500 Gaston Avenue, Dallas, Texas 75246.

terol is 90 to 140 mg/dL, there is no evidence that cigarette smoking, systemic hypertension, diabetes mellitus, inactivity, or obesity produces atherosclerotic plaques. Hypercholesterolemia is the only *direct* atherosclerotic risk factor; the others are indirect. If, however, the total cholesterol level is >150 mg/dL and the LDL cholesterol is >100 mg/dL, the other risk factors clearly accelerate atherosclerosis.

7. What evidence connects atherosclerosis to cholesterol?

The connection between cholesterol and atherosclerosis is strong (9, 10):

a) Atherosclerotic plaques similar to those in humans can be produced in nonhuman herbivores by feeding them large quantities of cholesterol and/or saturated fat. It is not possible to produce atherosclerotic plaques experimentally in carnivores.

b) Cholesterol is found within atherosclerotic plaques.

c) In societies where the serum total cholesterol is <150 mg/dL, the frequency of symptomatic and fatal atherosclerosis is exceedingly uncommon; in contrast, in societies where the total cholesterol level is >150 mg/dL, the frequency of symptomatic and fatal atherosclerosis increases as the level above 150 increases.

d) The higher the serum total cholesterol level, and specifically the higher the serum LDL cholesterol, the greater the frequency of symptomatic atherosclerosis, the greater the frequency of fatal atherosclerosis, and the greater the quantity of plaque at necropsy.

e) In placebo-controlled, double-blind, lipid-lowering studies of adults without symptomatic atherosclerosis, the group with lowered serum LDL cholesterol developed fewer symptomatic and fatal atherosclerotic events compared with controls.

f) In placebo-controlled, double-blind, lipid-lowering studies of adults with previous symptomatic atherosclerosis, the group with lowered LDL cholesterol levels after the event had fewer subsequent atherosclerotic events than did the group that did not lower their cholesterol levels (controls).

g) LDL receptors were discovered in the liver by Brown and Goldstein, and the absence or decreased numbers of LDL receptors in patients with quite elevated serum cholesterol levels indicates a genetic defect in an occasional patient (3–5).

8. What are the major sources of cholesterol in calories?

Cholesterol comes from animals and their products. Therefore, if we do not eat animals and their products, we do not take in cholesterol. Most Americans now take in only about 300 to 400 mg of cholesterol daily. This amount is hardly enough to obtain a calorie from it. A toothpick weighs 100 mg, so most in the USA take in the equivalency of 3 or 4 toothpicks of cholesterol every day. There are 2 major sources of cholesterol in our diet: 1) *cows*, including their muscle (beef), milk, butter, and cheese, and 2) *eggs*. About 45% of the cholesterol we obtain in our diet comes from the visible and nonvisible eggs we eat, and about 40% comes from bovine muscle and bovine milk and its products.

9. What are the major sources of fat in calories?

Fat comes from many sources. A major source in the USA is bovine muscle (beef). Cows naturally do not have so much fat, but in the USA most are fattened before slaughter. They are placed in feed lots their last 4 to 6 months of life and fed 20 to 25 pounds of various grains and soybeans every day, and the result is a huge increase in body fat. Cows slaughtered directly from pasture have far less fat between their muscle fibers and that overlying them. In the USA most adults now consume approximately 140 grams of fat daily. Our upper limit should be 75 grams. (A deck of cards weighs 75 grams.) If we were to limit our fat intake to 50 grams a day, the health of the US population would skyrocket.

10. Which of the 3 components of fatty acids raise the serum total and LDL cholesterol levels?

Each triglyceride particle contains a saturated, a monounsaturated, and a polyunsaturated fatty acid. There is no such thing as a pure saturated fatty acid or a pure monounsaturated or a pure polyunsaturated fatty acid. The question is which one is dominant in the triglyceride particles. The saturated portion, when dominant, clearly raises our total and LDL cholesterol levels; the mono- and polyunsaturated, when dominant, either lower them or have a neutral effect. Saturated fatty acids are solid at room temperature, and that fact is easy to remember by the "s" in saturated. The fatty acids with the highest saturated component are coconut oil, palm kernel oil, beef tallow, and butter. Olive oil has the highest monounsaturated percentage (approximately 75%); peanut oil has approximately 50% monounsaturated fatty acids. Grundy and colleagues (11) have demonstrated that monounsaturated fatty acids have healthier features than do polyunsaturated fatty acids.

11. What percentage of reduction in the serum total and LDL cholesterol levels can be expected by decreasing the percentage of calories from fat by 25%, 50%, and 75%?

Hunninghake and colleagues (12) demonstrated that reducing the percentage of calories from fat from 40% to 30%, a 25% reduction, reduces *on average* the serum total cholesterol level by 5% and the LDL cholesterol level by 5%. Getting 30% of calories from fat is the most commonly prescribed diet by physicians in the USA, and its effect on cholesterol levels is relatively small. There is great individual variability, so that it is not possible to predict what drop in cholesterol levels will occur in a single individual. The drop in a single individual may be as high as 20%, but in some individuals the total and LDL cholesterol levels increase by as much as 20% (12). A reduction in percentage of calories from fat from 40% to 20%, a 50% reduction, generally leads to approximately a 20% reduction in both serum total and LDL cholesterol levels (13). A drop in percentage of calories from fat from 40% to 10%, a 75% reduction, generally leads to reductions in total and LDL cholesterol levels of about 40% (14). The 10% of calories from fat is a vegetarian-fruit diet.

12. What are the equivalent efficacious doses of the 6 statin drugs, and what are the average reductions in serum total and LDL cholesterol and average increase in HDL cholesterol from the various doses?

These are illustrated in the *Table* (15). These reductions in cholesterol are baseline independent—i.e., the percentage of reduction does not depend on what the baseline total cholesterol or baseline LDL might be. Furthermore, at the lower doses of the statin drugs, the increase in HDL cholesterol, which is generally about 6% to 7%, is also not baseline dependent. At the higher doses, the HDL becomes more baseline dependent, i.e., the lower the HDL, particularly when it is <35 mg/dL, the greater the increase in HDL produced by some statins but not by others (16, 17). Reductions in serum triglyceride levels by the statin drugs are baseline dependent, i.e., the higher the serum triglyceride level, the greater the reduction in triglycerides by the statin drugs. If the triglyceride level is >350 mg/dL, the statin drugs have the capacity to lower the triglyceride level by up to 40%; if, however, the serum triglyceride level is 100 mg/dL, even the higher doses of the statin drugs have essentially no effect on the triglyceride level.

13. What is the LDL cholesterol goal of lipid lowering?

The goals proposed by the National Cholesterol Education Committee are variable, depending on the baseline LDL cholesterol and the presence or absence of other atherosclerotic factors (18). Persons without an atherosclerotic event have LDL cholesterol goals of <160 or <130 mg/dL. The goal in persons with previous atherosclerotic events is LDL cholesterol <100 mg/dL. If it is useful to lower the LDL to <100 mg/dL after a heart attack, surely it must be useful to lower the LDL cholesterol level to <100 before a heart attack! Therefore, in my view, the LDL cholesterol goal for all persons should be <100 mg/dL.

Atherosclerosis might best be viewed as the pediatricians view measles, mumps, and pertussis. They are not satisfied with decreasing the risk of these 3 contagious diseases; their goal is complete prevention of these infectious diseases. I think the same philosophy needs to be applied to atherosclerosis (19). Because it is infrequently a disease related to defective genetic makeup, we should all try to get our serum LDL cholesterol levels down to the point where atherosclerotic plaques do not form, and that level is clearly <100 mg/dL and maybe <70 or 80 mg/dL. My goal for both primary and secondary prevention is the same—namely, serum LDL cholesterol <100 mg/dL.

The minimal HDL goal of therapy in men is >35 mg/dL and for women >45 mg/dL. Raising the HDL cholesterol, however, is usually more difficult than lowering the LDL cholesterol. And, finally, the ideal fasting serum triglyceride goal for everybody is <150 mg/dL.

14. How safe are the statin drugs?

These are some of the safest drugs that have been produced (20–28)! They are considerably safer than aspirin or nonsteroidal anti-inflammatory drugs. They are safer than many drugs presently available over the counter. At the lower doses there is no evidence that statin drugs have detrimental effects on the liver. The frequency of liver enzyme elevation at the lower doses is the same as in placebo groups (20). Evidence is now accumulating that possibly even at the higher doses the statin drugs do

not in themselves affect the liver detrimentally. Individuals with elevated liver enzymes associated with the intake of statin drugs have never had permanent damage to the liver produced by the statin drug. The only serious side effect of the statin drugs is myopathy, and that occurs in 1 of 10,000 persons taking the drug. The toxicity is not the statin drug; the toxicity is atherosclerosis! The risk-benefit ratio of using statin drugs in patients with atherosclerosis, either to prevent further plaque formation or to prevent its formation in the first place, favors drug use.

15. Who should be treated with the statin drugs?

Everyone who has had an atherosclerotic event, be it from involvement of the coronary arteries, carotid arteries, aorta, or peripheral arteries. The goal in patients with symptomatic atherosclerosis is LDL cholesterol <100 mg/dL. The goal in persons without symptomatic atherosclerosis should be the same. There is simply more time to work on dietary change in persons who have not had atherosclerotic events compared with persons who have. If dietary interventions are unsuccessful in lowering cholesterol levels in persons without atherosclerotic events, these drugs can be useful and should be used more freely as long as the users are >15 years of age. They also have proven benefit in the elderly.

16. Is it important to lower elevated serum triglyceride levels?

Yes. The most important lipoprotein to lower is the LDL cholesterol. The most important lipoprotein to raise is the serum HDL cholesterol. The third most important lipoprotein to alter is the serum triglyceride level (29). Although the LDL particles are the most atherogenic, the very-low-density lipoprotein particles contain atherogenic components as well. In general, the higher the serum triglyceride level, the lower the HDL cholesterol level. Thus, by lowering the serum triglyceride level, the effect often is to raise the serum HDL cholesterol level, and the higher the HDL cholesterol, the lower the risk of atherosclerotic events. When the triglyceride level is elevated, the LDL cholesterol particles tend to be small and dense, and these are the most atherogenic ones. When the triglyceride level is lowered, the LDL particle size tends to increase, and the larger and more buoyant LDL particles are not as atherogenic as the small dense ones. A third reason to lower the triglyceride levels is that elevated ones are associated with coagulation factors that promote thrombosis or retard thrombolysis. Platelet aggregation and therefore thrombosis is accelerated in patients with elevated triglyceride levels. And finally, elevated triglyceride levels are commonly associated with the metabolic syndrome (insulin-resistance syndrome). The components of this syndrome include obesity, systemic hypertension, the lipid triad (increased triglyceride, decreased HDL cholesterol, and predominance of small, dense LDL particles), glucose intolerance, insulin resistance, increased serum insulin levels, and diabetes mellitus.

The fibrates (fenofibrate and gemfibrozil) and niacin are the best triglyceride-lowering drugs. In my view, however, neither a fibrate nor niacin should be used as monotherapy. I think these drugs should be added to a statin drug, which in and of itself can reduce the triglyceride levels up to 40%, depending on the baseline level.

17. Can niacin and fibrates be used effectively and safely in combination with the statin drugs?

Yes. Liver enzyme elevations occur more frequently when either niacin or a fibrate is combined with a statin drug, and these enzyme levels should be checked more frequently in patients on this combination. The combination, however, is quite effective.

18. How effective are statin drugs compared with aspirin, beta-blockers, angiotensin-converting enzyme inhibitors, and calcium antagonists in preventing repeat atherosclerotic events?

At least among patients who have had an acute myocardial infarction and survived, daily aspirin decreases the chance of recurrence of an atherosclerotic event within a 5-year period by 25% (30), beta-blockers by 25% (31), angiotensin-converting enzyme inhibitors (at least the tissue inhibitors) by 25% (32), calcium antagonists by probably 0%, and statin drugs by >40% (21). Thus, if a person could take only 1 drug after a heart attack, the most effective one would be a statin.

19. How effective are the statin drugs in preventing strokes?

Very effective. The statin drugs decrease the frequency of strokes in a 5-year period by approximately 30% (33). Until recently the statin drugs were the only drugs other than an antihypertensive drug demonstrated to decrease the frequency of stroke. Recently, the angiotensin-converting enzyme inhibitor ramapril has been shown to decrease the frequency of strokes also by approximately 30% (32).

20. Do statin drugs have to be taken every day for the remainder of life?

Yes. Some patients apparently believe that the statin drugs need to be taken for only a few months—until the cholesterol levels come down. I believe that it is important to tell patients when they are first placed on a statin drug that they will need to take the drug every day for the remainder of their lives. Of course, if a patient subsequently becomes a pure vegetarian-fruit eater it might be possible to discontinue the statin drug, but few Americans are willing to go the vegetarian route.

1. Collens WS. Atherosclerotic disease: an anthropologic theory. *Medical Counterpoint* 1969;1:53–57.
2. Roberts WC. We think we are one, we act as if we are one, but we are not one. *Am J Cardiol* 1990;66:896.
3. Brown MS, Goldstein JL. How LDL receptors influence cholesterol and atherosclerosis. *Sci Am* 1984;251(5):58–66.
4. Brown MS, Goldstein JL. A receptor-mediated pathway for cholesterol homeostasis. *Science* 1986;232(4746):34–47.
5. Goldstein JL, Brown MS. Regulation of low-density lipoprotein receptors: implications for pathogenesis and therapy of hypercholesterolemia and atherosclerosis. *Circulation* 1987;76:504–507.
6. Havel RJ, Kane JB. Structure and metabolism of plasma lipoproteins. In Scriver CR, Beaudet AL, Sly WS, Valle D, eds. *The Metabolic Basis of Inherited Disease*. New York: McGraw Hill, 1989:1129–1164.
7. Roberts WC, Kragel AH, Potkin BN. Ages at death and sex distribution in age decade in fatal coronary artery disease. *Am J Cardiol* 1990;66:1379–1381.
8. Keys AB. *Seven Countries: A Multivariate Analysis of Death and Coronary Heart Disease*. Cambridge, Mass: Harvard University Press, 1980:381.
9. Roberts WC. Factors linking cholesterol to atherosclerotic plaques. *Am J Cardiol* 1988;62:495–499.
10. LaRosa JC, Hunninghake D, Bush D, Criqui MH, Getz GS, Gotto AM Jr, Grundy SM, Rakita L, Robertson RM, Weisfeldt ML, et al. The cholesterol facts. A summary of the evidence relating dietary fats, serum cholesterol, and coronary heart disease. A joint statement by the American Heart Association and the National Heart, Lung, and Blood Institute. The Task Force on Cholesterol Issues, American Heart Association. *Circulation* 1990;81:1721–1733.
11. Grundy SM, Ahrens EH Jr. The effects of unsaturated dietary fats on absorption, excretion, synthesis, and distribution of cholesterol in man. *J Clin Invest* 1970;49:1135–1152.
12. Hunninghake DB, Stein EA, Dujovne CA, Harris WS, Feldman EB, Miller VT, Tobert JA, Laskarzewski PM, Quiter E, Held J, Taylor AM, Hopper S, Leonard SB, Brewer BK. The efficacy of intensive dietary therapy alone or combined with lovastatin in outpatients with hypercholesterolemia. *N Engl J Med* 1993;328:1213–1219.
13. Leaf A. Dietary prevention of coronary heart disease: the Lyon Diet Heart Study. *Circulation* 1999;99:733–735.
14. Ornish D. Can life-style changes reverse coronary atherosclerosis? *Hosp Pract* 1991;26:123–132.
15. Roberts WC. The rule of 5 and the rule of 7 in lipid-lowering by statin drugs. *Am J Cardiol* 1997;80:106–107.
16. Jones P, Kafonek S, Laurora I, Hunninghake D. Comparative dose efficacy study of atorvastatin versus simvastatin, pravastatin, lovastatin, and fluvastatin in patients with hypercholesterolemia. *Am J Cardiol* 1998;81:582–587.
17. Crouse JR III, Frohlich J, Ose L, Mercuri M, Tobert JA. Effects of high doses of simvastatin and atorvastatin on high-density lipoprotein cholesterol and apolipoprotein A-I. *Am J Cardiol* 1999;83:1476–1477.
18. Grundy SM, Billheimer D, Chait A, Clark LT, Denke M, Havel RJ, Hazzard WR, Hulely SB, Hunninghake DB, Kreisberg RA, Kris-Etherton P, McKenney JM, Newman MA, Schaefer EJ, Sobel BE, Somelofski C, Weinstein, Brewer HB, Cleeman JI, Donato KA, Ernst N, Hoeg JM, Rifkind BM, Rossouw J, Sempos CT, Gallivan JM, Harris MN, Quint-Adler L. Summary of the second report of the National Cholesterol Education Program (NCEP) Expert Panel on Detection, Evaluation, and Treatment on High Blood Cholesterol in Adults. *JAMA* 1993;269:3015–3023.
19. Brown MS, Goldstein JL. Heart attacks: gone with the century? *Science* 1996;272:629.
20. Bradford RH, Shear CL, Chremos AN, Dujovne C, Downton M, Franklin FA, Gould AL, Hesney M, Higgins J, Hurley DP, Langendorfer A, Nash DT, Pool JL, Schnaper H. Expanded Clinical Evaluation of Lovastatin (EXCEL) study results. I. Efficacy in modifying plasma lipoproteins and adverse event profile in 8245 patients with moderate hypercholesterolemia. *Arch Intern Med* 1991;151:43–49.
21. Pedersen TR, Kjekshus J, Berg K, Haghfelt T, Faergeman O, Thorgeirsson G, Pyorala K, Miettinen T, Wilhelmsen L, Olsson AG, Wedel H. Randomised trial of cholesterol lowering in 4444 patients with coronary heart disease: the Scandinavian Simvastatin Survival Study (4S). *Lancet* 1994;344:1383–1389.
22. Kjekshus J, Pedersen TR. Reducing the risk of coronary events: evidence from the Scandinavian Simvastatin Survival Study (4S). *Am J Cardiol* 1995;76:64C–68C.
23. Shepherd J, Cobbe SM, Ford I, Isles CG, Lorimer AR, MacFarlane PW, McKillop JH, Packard CJ. Prevention of coronary heart disease with pravastatin in men with hypercholesterolemia. West of Scotland Coronary Prevention Study Group. *N Engl J Med* 1995;333:1301–1307.
24. Pedersen TR, Berg K, Cook TJ, Faergeman O, Haghfelt T, Kjekshus J, Miettinen T, Musliner TA, Olsson AG, Pyorala K, Thorgeirsson G, Tobert JA, Wedel H, Wilhelmsen L. Safety and tolerability of cholesterol lower-

ing with simvastatin during 5 years in the Scandinavian Simvastatin Survival Study. *Arch Intern Med* 1996;156:2085–2092.

25. Sacks FM, Pfeffer MA, Moye LA, Rouleau JL, Rutherford JD, Cole TG, Brown L, Warnica JW, Arnold JM, Wun CC, Davis BR, Braunwald E. The effect of pravastatin on coronary events after myocardial infarction in patients with average cholesterol levels. Cholesterol and Recurrent Events Trial Investigators. *N Engl J Med* 1996;335:1001–1009.

26. Pyorala K, Pedersen TR, Kjekshus J, Faergeman O, Olsson AG, Thorgeirsson G. Cholesterol lowering with simvastatin improves prognosis of diabetic patients with coronary heart disease. A subgroup analysis of the Scandinavian Simvastatin Survival Study (4S). *Diabetes Care* 1997;20:614–620.

27. Avorn J, Monette J, Lacour A, Bohn RL, Monane M, Mogun H, LeLorier J. Persistence of use of lipid-lowering medications: a cross-national study. JAMA 1998;279:1458–1462.

28. Pitt B, Waters D, Brown WV, van Boven AJ, Schwartz L, Title LM, Eisenberg D, Shurzinske L, McCormick LS. Aggressive lipid-lowering therapy compared with angioplasty in stable coronary artery disease. Atorvastatin versus Revascularization Treatment Investigators. *N Engl J Med* 1999;341:70–76.

29. Grundy SM, ed. A symposium: The role of statins in patients with hypertriglyceridemia. *Am J Cardiol* 1998;81(4A):1B–73B.

30. Manson JE, Tosteson H, Ridker PM, Satterfield S, Hebert P, O'Connor GT, Buring JE, Hennekens CH. The primary prevention of myocardial infarction. *N Engl J Med* 1992;326:1406–1416.

31. Braunwald E, Muller JE, Kloner RA, Maroko PR. Role of beta-adrenergic blockade in the therapy of patients with myocardial infarction. *Am J Med* 1983;74:113–123.

32. Yusuf S, Sleight P, Pogue J, Bosch J, Davies R, Dagenais G. Effects of an angiotensin-converting-enzyme inhibitor, ramipril, on cardiovascular events in high-risk patients. The Heart Outcomes Prevention Evaluation Study Investigators. *N Engl J Med* 2000;342:145–153.

33. Crouse JR III, Byington RP, Hoen HM, Furberg CD. Reductase inhibitor monotherapy and stroke prevention. *Arch Intern Med* 1997;157:1305–1310.

Wide Open Coronary Arteries at 103 Years of Age

When I was in medical school I was taught that atherosclerosis was a degenerative disease, and that if we lived long enough we could expect a good deal of it. I have examined the hearts of six people who lived 100 years or longer.[1] Although four had one or more major epicardial coronary arteries narrowed >75% in cross-sectional area by plaque, none had had apparent clinical evidence of myocardial ischemia or congestive heart failure during life. Two of the six patients had insignificant coronary narrowing. In one of the two, the four major (right, left main, left anterior descending, and left circumflex) epicardial coronary arteries were divided into 5 mm segments and a histologic section was prepared from each segment. All the resulting 45, 5 mm segments, were narrowed <25% in cross-sectional area (Figure). Thus, coronary narrowing does not have to be a consequence of living 100 years.

Editor's Note: This column appears three times annually.

REFERENCE

1 Roberts WC. The heart at necropsy in centenarians. *Am J Cardiol* 1998;81:1224–1225.

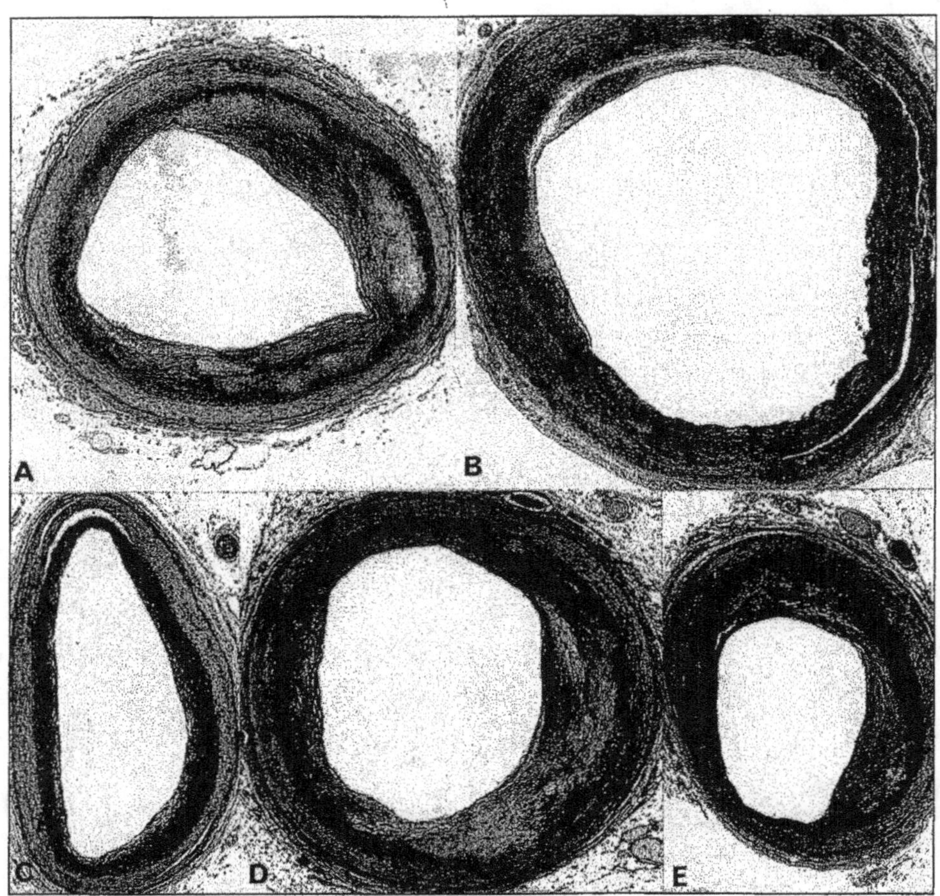

Figure. Coronary arterial narrowing of <25% as seen in 5 mm cross-sectional segments. A=right; B=left main; C=left anterior descending; D=left circumflex; E=left obtuse marginal.

Comparison of Modes of Death and Cardiac Necropsy Findings in Fatal Acute Myocardial Infarction in Men and Women >75 Years of Age

Jamshid Shirani, MD, Jamshid Alaeddini, MD, and William C. Roberts, MD

Age is an important risk factor for mortality after acute myocardial infarction (AMI).[1] The increased mortality in those >75 years old is only partially explainable by an increased incidence of multivessel coronary artery disease, prior myocardial infarction, and other comorbid conditions.[1,2] Recent studies have also indicated a difference in presentation and outcome of AMI in men and women.[3,4] Some studies have shown higher in-hospital mortality from AMI in women than in men.[4,5] The latter has been largely attributed to a combination of older age at the time of presentation,[5,6,7–10] higher prevalence of risk factors,[5–8] and lower likelihood of receiving aggressive therapy[7,8] including thrombolysis,[7] β-adrenergic blocking agents,[9,11,12] and coronary revascularization.[7,13] A recent study has noted a trend toward a difference in mode of death and frequency of mechanical complications after AMI in elderly men and women.[14] The present study compares modes of death and necropsy cardiac findings in men and women >75 years of age with fatal AMI.

• • •

The study patients consisted of 100 patients (60 women and 40 men, aged 76 to 95 years [mean 83 ± 3]) who died either suddenly outside or in a hospital within 25 days (mean 6) of onset of AMI. Among the 100 hearts examined, 68 were referred to the Pathology Branch of the National Heart, Lung, and Blood Institute, National Institutes of Health between 1980 and 1992, 12 were studied at the Medical College of Virginia Hospital in Richmond, Virginia, from 1992 to 1993, and the remaining 20 were examined at the Montefiore Medical Center in Bronx, New York, from 1993 to 1997. In all patients, records of clinical and pathologic findings, photographs of the heart, histologic slides, and descriptions of the cardiac morphologic abnormalities were reviewed. All hearts were examined either by WCR or by JS. All clinical information, including demographic and risk factor profile, was obtained from patients' medical records. Sudden death was defined as death within 6 hours from the onset of new symptoms of myocardial ischemia.

Hearts were fixed in 10% buffered formaldehyde before examination. Heart weight was obtained after removing the pericardium and all extraneous material

TABLE 1 Certain Clinical and Cardiac Morphologic Findings in 60 Women and 40 Men >75 Years of Age Who Died of Acute Myocardial Infarction

	Women (n = 60)	Men (n = 40)
Age (yrs) (mean ±)	76–89 (83 ± 3)	77–95 (83 ± 3)
White	48 (80%)	28 (70%)
Angina pectoris	36 (60%)	28 (70%)
Congestive heart failure	20 (33%)	18 (45%)
Systemic hypertension	31 (52%)	26 (65%)
Diabetes mellitus	10 (17%)	9 (23%)
Cerebrovascular accident	6 (11%)	8 (20%)
Sudden death	8 (13%)	1 (3%)
Thrombolytic therapy	2 (3%)	1 (3%)
Cardiac catheterization	6 (10%)	8 (20%)
Heart weight (g) (mean)	280–750 (421)	330–750 (527)*
Increased heart weight	43 (73%)	36 (90%)*
Location of acute infarct[†]		
Anterior wall, left ventricle	34 (57%)	15 (38%)*
Posterior wall, left ventricle	22 (37%)	20 (50%)
Lateral wall, left ventricle	8 (13%)	10 (25%)
Ventricular septum	19 (32%)	10 (25%)
Posterior wall, right ventricle	6 (10%)	1 (3%)
Papillary muscle, left ventricle	6 (10%)	5 (13%)
Location of healed infarct[†]		
Any location	9 (15%)	26 (65%)*
Anterior wall, left ventricle	3 (5%)	9 (23%)*
Posterior wall, left ventricle	5 (8%)	13 (33%)*
Lateral wall, left ventricle	1 (2%)	6 (15%)*
Ventricular septum	1 (2%)	5 (13%)*
Papillary muscle, left ventricle	4 (7%)	0
Dilated left ventricle	26 (43%)	28 (70%)*
Dilated right ventricle	18 (30%)	18 (45%)
Left ventricular thrombus	8 (13%)	9 (23%)
Rupture	25 (42%)	3 (8%)*
Left ventricular free wall	20 (33%)	2 (5%)*
Ventricular septum	4 (7%)	2 (5%)
Papillary muscle	2 (3%)	0

*p <0.05 versus women.

[†]More than 1 location may have been involved in the same patient.

and after cutting the large arteries at approximately 2 cm cephalad to the semilunar valve. Coronary artery disease was defined as the presence of >75% cross-sectional luminal narrowing by athersclerotic plaque in the 4 major (left main, left anterior descending, left circumflex, and right) coronary arteries. AMI was defined as a grossly visible myocardial lesion confirmed histologically to represent coagulation-type myocardial necrosis. Each heart was examined for weight, left ventricular size, location and extent of AMI, presence of mechanical complications (free wall, septal, or papillary muscle rupture), presence of valvular abnormalities, and number of major epicardial coronary arteries narrowed >75% in cross-sectional area by atherosclerotic plaque. Cardiac adipos-

From the Departments of Medicine (Division of Cardiology) and Pathology, Albert Einstein College of Medicine, Bronx, New York; and Cardiovascular Institute, Baylor University Medical Center, Dallas, Texas. Dr. Shirani's address is: Division of Cardiology, The Jack D. Weiler of the Albert Einstein College of Medicine, 1825 Eastchester Road, Room W1–70K, Bronx, New York 10461. E-mail: jshirani@montefiore.org. Manuscript received March 31, 2000; revised manuscript received and accepted May 5, 2000.

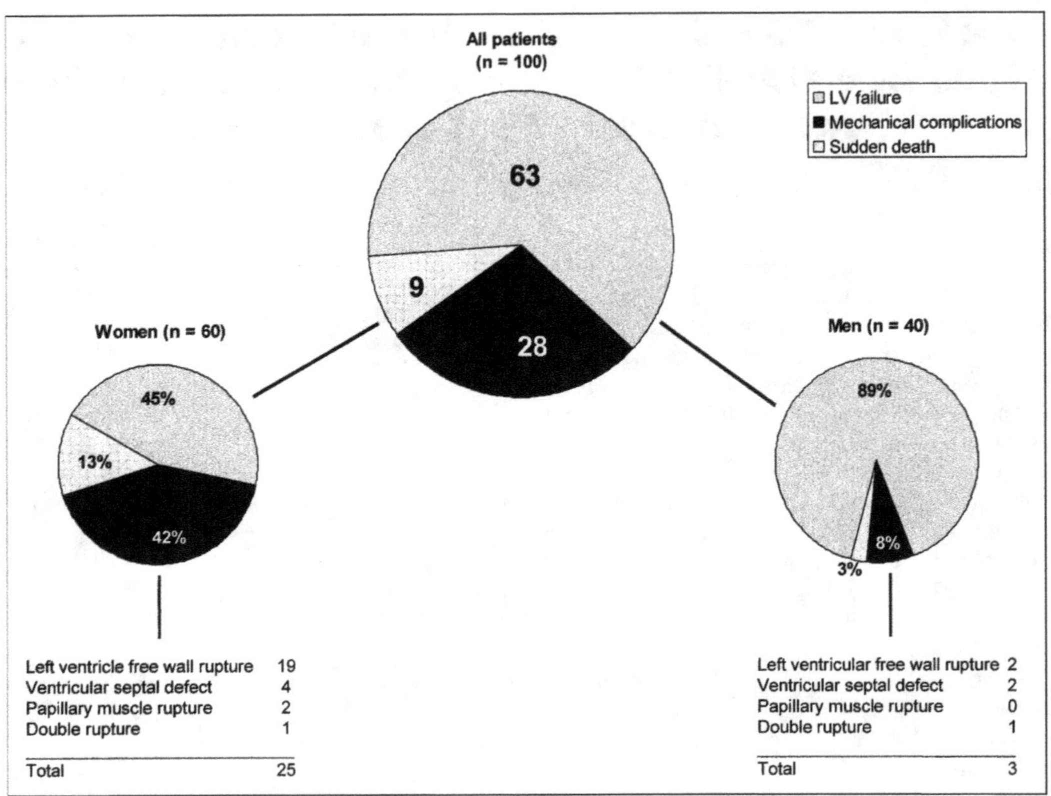

FIGURE 1. Diagram summarizing causes of death among 60 women and 40 men >75 years of age with fatal acute myocardial infarction.

TABLE 2 Coronary Artery Disease and Other Cardiac Morphologic Findings Among 60 Women and 40 Men >75 Years of Age Who Died of Acute Myocardial Infarction

	Women (n = 60)	Men (n = 40)
Coronary artery >75% ↓ in cross-sectional area by plaque		
Left main	8 (13%)	9 (23%)
Left anterior descending	50 (83%)	31 (78%)
Left circumflex	32 (53%)	29 (73%)
Right	39 (65)	31 (78)
No. of major coronary arteries >75% ↓ in cross-sectional area by plaque (mean)	2.2	2.5
1	13 (22%)	6 (15%)
2	23 (38%)	12 (30%)
3	23 (38%)	18 (45%)
4	1 (2%)	4 (10%)
Aortic stenosis	6 (10%)	6 (15%)
Calcific deposits in		
Aortic valve	25 (42%)	15 (38%)
Mitral annulus	22 (37%)	11 (28%)
Coronary arteries	57 (95%)	32 (80%)*
Papillary muscles	2 (3%)	3 (8%)
Cardiac amyloidosis	1 (2%)	3 (8%)
Cardiac adiposity	43 (74%)	18 (45%)*

*p <0.05 versus women.

ity was defined as an increased amounts of subepicardial fat as previously shown.[15]

Results are reported as range and mean ± 1 SD or as percentage of the population size. Differences between various subsets of patients were assessed with unpaired Student's *t* test for continuous variables and with chi-square analysis for noncontinuous variables. A p value <0.05 was considered statistically significant.

The predominant presenting symptom of AMI was chest pain that occurred in 21 of 60 women (35%) and in 30 of 40 men (75%; p <0.01). Proportionally, more women had an atypical presentation than with men: dyspnea (14 [23%] vs 4 [9%], p = 0.07), syncope (8 [13%] vs 1 [3%], p = 0.06), and weakness (4 [7%] vs 2 [5%], p = NS). One woman each presented with severe headache, epigastric discomfort, back pain, or feverish sensation. In 9 women and 1 man, the AMI was silent; 2 patients were postoperative (hip and abdominal surgery) and another 3 died suddenly outside the hospital without having had any manifest symptom of myocardial ischemia or cardiac dysfunction before death. A history of myocardial ischemia was elicited less often in women than in men (70% vs 93%, p <0.01).

Certain clinical and cardiac morphologic findings in the 60 women and 40 men are summarized in Table 1 and Figure 1. There were no significant differences between women and men with regard to symptoms of myocardial ischemia or cardiac dysfunction before AMI. In addition, a similar proportion of women and men received thrombolysis (both 3%) or underwent catheterization (10% vs 20%, p = NS). Women had significantly lower heart weights (421 ± 89 vs 527 ± 113 g, p <0.01), lower frequencies of cardiomegaly

(73% vs 90%, p = 0.04), and a higher frequency of anterior wall AMI (57% vs 38%, p <0.05). In addition, fewer women had healed infarcts (15% vs 65%, p <0.01) or dilated left ventricular cavities (43% vs 70%, p = 0.02). Left ventricular apical thrombi were present in 13% of women and in 23% of men (p = NS). More women had a mechanical complication of AMI (25 [42%] vs 3 [8%], p <0.01). Overall, mechanical complications involved the left ventricular free wall in 21 (75%), ventricular septum in 6 (21%), and papillary muscles in 2 (7%). Two patients (7%) had ruptures involving both free wall and ventricular septum.

There were no significant differences between women and men with regard to distribution or severity of epicardial coronary artery disease (Table 2). Compared with the 40 men, the 60 women had a higher frequency of calcific deposits in the coronary arteries (95% vs 80%, p = 0.02) and more cardiac adiposity (74% vs 45%, p <0.01).

To our knowledge, the present study is the only report comparing cardiac morphologic findings at necropsy in women and men >75 years of age with fatal AMI. Compared with men, women with AMI are reported to have a higher prevalence of risk factors.[5,7,8] These include diabetes mellitus,[4,5,16] systemic hypertension,[4,7,8,16] and cerebrovascular accident.[17] Women are also less likely to have had a previous AMI.[4,8] Some studies have suggested that in-hospital mortality from AMI in women may be higher than that in men.[5,8,11,16] This observation is supposedly related to a higher age at time of AMI and to the presence of more comorbid conditions in women.[18,19] Such differences between women and men are found in studies that have included patients from a wide age range and in which women are generally significantly older than men.[18]

We did not find any difference in women and men in the frequency of congestive heart failure, diabetes mellitus, systemic hypertension, cerebrovascular accident, or angina pectoris. Fewer women had evidence of a healed myocardial infarct. Typical chest pain was also less often the presenting symptom of AMI in women in this study.

Studies of mechanical complications of AMI have frequently found old age and female sex prominent risk factors.[20] We observed a higher frequency of mechanical complications among women with fatal AMI. Thus, 25 of the 60 women (42%) in this study died of left ventricular free wall rupture (33%), ventricular septal defect (7%), or papillary muscle rupture (3%). Mechanical complications of AMI occurred 5 times more frequently in women than in men. In a recent clinical study of 204 persons >75 years of age admitted with AMI, Bueno et al[14] noted a trend toward a higher incidence of mechanical complications

among the 105 women (14 [13%] vs 6 [6%], p = 0.08).

In conclusion, after AMI, women >75 years of age die more frequently from mechanical complications than age-matched men.

1. Devlin W, Cragg D, Jacks M, Freidman H, O'Neill W, Grines C. Comparison of outcome in patients with acute myocardial infarction aged >75 years with that in younger patients. *Am J Cardiol* 1995;75:537–576.
2. Suarez G, Herrera M, Vera A, Torrado E, Ferriz J, Arboleda A. Prediction on admission of in-hospital mortality in patients older than 70 years with acute myocardial infarction. *Chest* 1995;108:83–88.
3. Goldberg RJ, O'Donnell C, Yarzebski J, Bigelow C, Savageau J, Gore JM. Sex differences in symptom presentation associated with acute myocardial infarction: A population-based perspective. *Am Heart J* 1998;136:189–195.
4. Maynard C, Every NR, Martin JS, Kudenchuk PJ, Weaver WD. Association of gender and survival in patients with acute myocardial infarction. *Arch Intern Med* 1997;157:1379–1384.
5. Marrugat J, Sala J, Masià R, Pavesi M, Sanz G, Valle V, Molina L, Serés L, Elosua R. Mortality differences between men and women following first myocardial infarction. *JAMA* 1998;280:1405–1409.
6. Becker RC, Terrin M, Ross R, Knatterud GL, Desvigne-Nickens P, Gore JM, Braunwald E, and the Thrombolysis in Myocardial Infarction Investigators. Comparison of clinical outcome for women and men after myocardial infarction. *Ann Intern Med* 1994;120:638–645.
7. Maynard C, Litwin PE, Martin JS, Weaver WD. Gender differences in the treatment and outcome of acute myocardial infarction: result from the Myocardial Infarction Triage and Intervention (MITI) Registry. *Arch Intern Med* 1992;152:972–976.
8. Kudenchuk PJ, Maynard C, Martin JS, Wirkus M, Weaver WD. Comparison of presentation, treatment, and outcome of acute myocardial infarction in men versus women (the Myocardial Infarction Triage and Intervention registry). *Am J Cardiol* 1996;78:9–14.
9. Chandra NC, Zeigelstein RC, Roger WJ, Tiefenbrunn AJ, Gore JM, French WJ, Rubison M. Observation of the treatment of women in the United States with myocardial infarction. A report from the National Registry of Myocardial Infarction-I. *Arch Intern Med* 1998;158:981–988.
10. Malacrida R, Genoni M, Maggioni AP, Spatero V, Parish S, Palmer A, Collins R, Moccetti T. A comparison of the early outcome of acute myocardial infarction in women and men. *N Engl J Med* 1998;338:8–14.
11. Krumholz HM, Radford MJ, Wang Y, Chen J, Heiat A, Marciniak TA. National use and effectiveness of β-blockers for treatment of elderly patients after acute myocardial infarction: National Cooperative Cardiovascular Project. *JAMA* 1998;280:623–629.
12. Krumholz HM, Radford MJ, Wang Y, Chen J, Marciniak TA. Early β-blockers therapy for acute myocardial infarction in elderly patients. *Ann Intern Med* 1999;131:648–654.
13. Funk M, Griffey KA. Relation of gender to the use of cardiac procedures in acute myocardial infarction. *Am J Cardiol* 1994;74:1170–1173.
14. Bueno H, Vidán M, Almazán A, López-Sendón JL, Delcán JL. Influence of sex on the short-term outcome of elderly patients with a first acute myocardial infarction. *Circulation* 1995;92:1133–1140.
15. Shirani J, Berezowski K, Roberts WC. Quantitative management of normal and excessive (cor adiposum) subepicardial adipose tissue, its clinical significance and its effect on electrocardiographic QRS voltage. *Am J Cardiol* 1995;76:414–418.
16. Weaver WD, White HD, Wilcox RG, Aylward PE, Morris D, Guerci A, Ohman EM, Barbash GI, Bertiu A, Sadowski Z, Topol EJ, Califf RM. Comparison of characteristics and outcomes among women and men with acute myocardial infarction treated with thrombolytic therapy. *JAMA* 1996;275:777–782.
17. Lincoff AM, Califf RM, Ellis SG, Sigmon K, Lee KL, Leimbergr JD, Topol EJ. Thrombolytic therapy for women with myocardial infarction: is there a gender gap? Thrombolysis and Angioplasty in Myocardial Infarction (TAMI) Study Group. *J Am Coll Cardiol* 1993;22:1780–1787.
18. Vaccarino V, Krumholz HM, Berkman LF, Horwitz RI. Sex differences in mortality after myocardial infarction. Is there evidence for an increased risk for women? *Circulation* 1995;91:1861–1871.
19. Vaccarino V, Krumholz HM, Mendes de Leon CF, Holford TR, Seeman TE, Horwitz RI, Berkman LF. Sex differences in survival after myocardial infarction in older adults: A community-based approach. *J Am Geriatr Soci* 1996;44:1174–1182.
20. Rasmussen S, Leth A, Kjoller E, Pedersen A. Cardiac rupture in acute myocardial infarction: a review of 72 consecutive cases. *Acta Med Scan* 1979;205:11–16.

Thrombotic occlusion of the aortic ostia of saphenous venous grafts early after coronary artery bypass grafting by using the Symmetry aortic connector system

Alan S. Donsky, MD,[a,d] Jeffrey M. Schussler, MD,[a,d] Michael S. Donsky, MD,[a,d] William C. Roberts, MD,[b,d] and Baron L. Hamman, MD,[c,d] Dallas, Tex

St Jude Medical (St Paul, Minn) received Food and Drug Administration approval in May 2001 for a device to aid in the anastomosis of vein grafts to the aorta during coronary artery bypass grafting. This device, known as the Symmetry aortic connector system, allows the surgeon to connect a vein graft to the aorta without the use of sutures or an aortic clamp. To our knowledge, no reports have appeared describing complications from the use of this device. In this report we describe 2 patients who had complete thrombotic occlusions of the aortic ostia of saphenous venous grafts early postoperatively after the use of this device.

Clinical Summaries

PATIENT 1. A 66-year-old obese (body mass index, 45 kg/m^2) woman with type 2 diabetes mellitus, systemic hypertension, abdominal aortic aneurysm resection 4 years earlier, and heparin-induced thrombocytopenia was admitted for unstable angina pectoris. Coronary angiography disclosed that the left circumflex artery arose from the right sinus of Valsava and coursed in a retroaortic position to the left atrioventricular sulcus and distally

From the Departments of Internal Medicine (Division of Cardiology),[a] Pathology,[b] and Cardiothoracic Surgery[c] and the Heart and Vascular Institute,[d] Baylor University Medical Center, Dallas, Tex.

Received for publication Jan 22, 2002; accepted for publication Feb 16, 2002.

Address for reprints: Baron L. Hamman, MD, Baylor University Medical Center, Division of Cardiothoracic Surgery, 3500 Gaston Ave, Dallas, TX 75246 (E-mail: Bhamman@CDM.net).

J Thorac Cardiovasc Surg 2002;124:397-9

0022-5223/2002 $35.00+0   **12/54/124236**

doi:10.1067/mtc.2002.124236

was small and diffusely narrowed. The left anterior descending coronary artery was totally occluded in its midportion, and the right coronary artery was narrowed up to 75% in diameter. Left ventricular angiography disclosed normal systolic function with an estimated ejection fraction of 70%.

Off-pump coronary artery bypass grafting was performed through a left thoracotomy. Two saphenous venous grafts were attached to the ascending aorta by using the Symmetry system. One graft was anastomosed to the posterior descending branch of the right coronary artery, and the other graft was anastomosed to an obtuse marginal branch of the left circumflex coronary artery. The left internal thoracic artery (LITA) was anastomosed to the left anterior descending artery, but poor blood flow was noted through it, and a proximal obstruction of the LITA was assumed to be present. As a consequence, the LITA was severed, and the remaining 3-cm end was anastomosed to the vein graft supplying the obtuse marginal coronary artery, creating a Y-type composite graft. Lepirudin, instead of heparin, was used during the procedure because circulating heparin-associated antibodies were present.

The patient was extubated on the first postoperative day and transferred to the telemetry floor on aspirin and furosemide. Her recovery was complicated by persistent hypoxemia and increasing oxygen requirements despite rigorous diuresis. On postoperative day 7, severe hypoxemia and bradycardia occurred, followed by asystole; appropriate resuscitation efforts were unsuccessful.

Necropsy disclosed thrombi completely filling the ostia of both vein grafts at their anastomosis with the ascending aorta (Figure 1). The lumen of the vein graft to the posterior descending artery was otherwise widely patent. The LITA and the vein graft to the obtuse marginal artery were completely filled with thrombus. The left ventricular cavity was of normal size, and the heart weighed 515 g. A small area of necrosis (acute myocardial infarction) was seen in the myocardium adjacent to the anastomotic site of the vein graft to the obtuse marginal coronary artery.

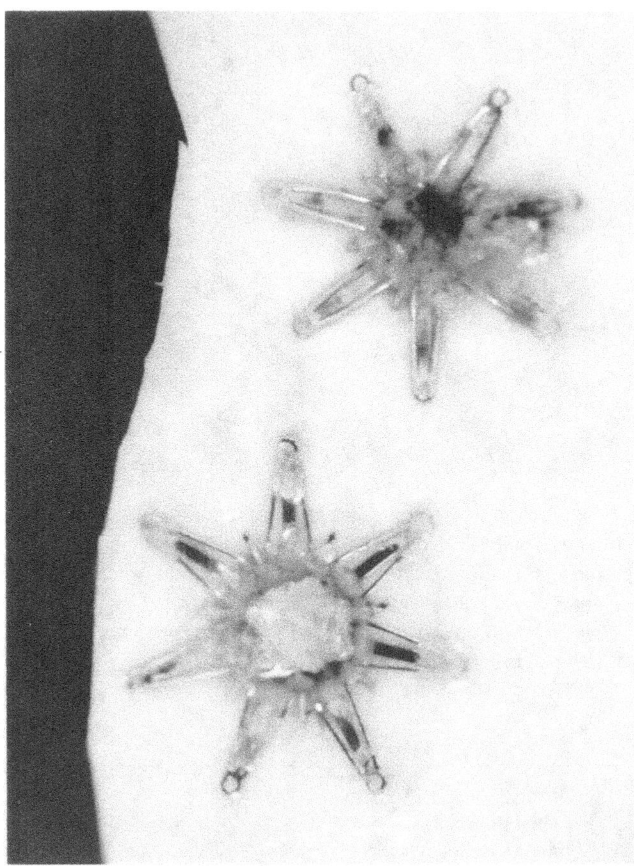

Figure 1. Patient 1: This photograph shows thrombus in the ostium of each of the 2 Symmetry aortic connector devices.

PATIENT 2. A 52-year-old obese (body mass index, 44 kg/m^2) white man with type 2 diabetes mellitus and systemic hypertension was admitted to an outside hospital for unstable angina pectoris. He had undergone coronary artery bypass surgery at age 39 years. At that operation, a LITA was attached to the left anterior descending coronary artery, and 2 saphenous venous grafts were attached to the obtuse marginal and right coronary arteries, respectively. He was transferred to Baylor University Medical Center on clopidogrel and enoxaparin. Coronary angiography showed complete occlusion of the vein graft to the obtuse marginal. The other 2 conduits were widely patent. The left main coronary artery was narrowed to 70% in diameter, and the proximal portion of the left circumflex was narrowed up to 95% in diameter. The ejection fraction by left ventricular angiography was estimated to be 30%.

Off-pump coronary artery bypass surgery through a left thoracotomy was performed. The Symmetry system was used in the anastomosis of a saphenous venous graft to the descending aorta, and it was then anastomosed to the obtuse marginal coronary artery. He was transferred to the telemetry floor on aspirin, metoprolol, and furosemide. On postoperative day 4, he had recurrent chest pain that was unresponsive to nitrates. An electrocardiogram now showed new T-wave inversions in the lateral precordial leads, and the troponin level was increased (1.9 ng/mL). Coronary angiography showed that contrast material injected into the left main coronary artery filled the distal end of the vein graft through the obtuse marginal coronary artery. However, contrast material injected into the descending aorta demonstrated total occlusion of the new vein graft at its ostium (Figure 2). Balloon angioplasty and stent placement was performed to the left main artery and the proximal portion of the circumflex artery with excellent angiographic results. The patient had no recurrence of chest pain and was discharged 2 days later.

Discussion

The Symmetry aortic connector system is a nitinol metallic device that functions somewhat like a grommet to attach a saphenous vein to a punched out portion of the aorta. This anastomosis is performed without sutures or an aortic clamp. This system has several potential advantages over the traditional suturing method. First, the time required to perform the anastomosis is reduced, and that might shorten recovery time. Second, minimizing aortic manipulation might reduce the risk of embolic events and thus reduce the incidence of neurologic complications. Finally, the size of the incision might be reduced because only limited exposure is needed to safely and consistently deploy the connector. Eckstein and associates[1] reported on their initial experience with this device in 20 patients undergoing off-pump coronary artery bypass surgery. They had excellent results, with no patient having any cardiac-related event within 3 months.

Each of the 2 patients described herein had thrombotic occlusion of the aortic ostia of saphenous venous grafts early after bypass surgery with the Symmetry aortic connector system. Such an occurrence in the early postoperative period with standard suture techniques is exceedingly uncommon. One of us (B.L.H.) has used this device in many patients, and the 2 described herein were the first encountered with known thrombotic complications at the aortic anastomotic sites.

Before concluding that the thrombotic complications were the direct result of one or more defects in the Symmetry system, several factors must be considered. Patient 1 had a history of heparin-induced thrombocytopenia with circulating antibodies, a circumstance recognized to be associated with a prothrombotic state. The saphenous venous graft attached to the left obtuse marginal coronary artery in the patient was totally occluded by thrombus, as was the LITA attached to it. The saphenous venous graft to the posterior descending artery, in contrast, was widely patent, except at its ostium. Patient 2 had the aortic anastomosis performed in the descending thoracic aorta. Both patients were extremely obese (grade 3/3) and had diabetes mellitus and systemic hypertension, features characteristic of the metabolic syndrome (insulin resistance syndrome), a condition recognized to be a prothrombotic state.[2,3] Whether these complicating factors played a role in the thrombotic occlusions of the aortic ostia in these 2 patients is, of course, unclear.

It is possible that the acute thrombosis seen in these 2 patients is similar in pathophysiology to that seen in acute stent thrombosis. The early experience with coronary artery stenting showed that acute thrombosis was a significant limiting factor. Improvements in stent design, deployment techniques, and the use of antiplatelet agents (ticlopidine and clopidogrel) dramatically reduced the incidence of acute stent thrombosis to less than 1%.[4] Although the use of clopidogrel is standard therapy after coronary artery stent-

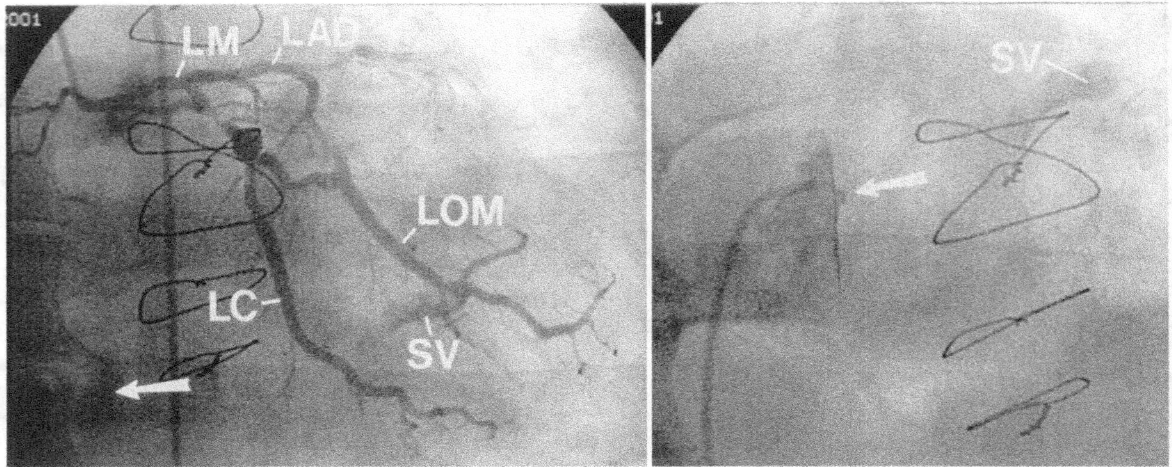

Figure 2. Patient 2: Coronary angiogram. *Left,* This photograph was taken after injection of contrast material into the left main *(LM)* coronary artery. The distal end of the saphenous venous graft *(SV)* fills through the left obtuse marginal *(LOM). LAD,* Left anterior descending artery; *LC,* left circumflex. *Right,* This photograph was taken after injection of contrast material into the descending aorta at the sight of the saphenous venous conduit *(arrow).* The ostium of the conduit is occluded. The upper right portion shows residual contrast material in the saphenous venous graft, which remained after the injection into the left main coronary artery.

ing, its use after placement of the Symmetry device has not been carefully studied.

In summary, 2 patients are described who underwent off-pump coronary artery bypass grafting with the Symmetry aortic connector system for the aortic anastomosis. Necropsy in one patient showed that the ostia of both aortic anastomotic sites were occluded by thrombus. In the second patient the aortic anastomotic site (in descending thoracic aorta) was demonstrated by angiography to be occluded. Although both patients had conditions predisposing to thrombus, such thrombotic occlusion of the aortic anastomotic sites are exceedingly rare in patients with an aortic anastomosis inserted by means of suture.

References

1. Eckstein FS, Bonilla LF, Strauffer E, Berg TA, Schmidli J, Carrel TP. Minimizing aortic manipulation during OPCAB using the Symmetry aortic connector system for proximal vein graft anastomosis. *Ann Thorac Surg.* 2001;72:S995-8.
2. Grundy SM. Hypertriglyceridemia, atherogenic dyslipidemia, and the metabolic syndrome. *Am J Cardiol.* 1998;81:18B-25B.
3. Juhan-Vague I, Alessi MC, Vague P. Increased plasma plasminogen activator inhibitor 1 levels: a possible link between insulin resistance and atherothrombosis. *Diabetologia.* 1991;34:457-62.
4. Schog A, Neumann FJ, Kastrati A, Schuhlen H, Blasini R, Hadamitzky M, et al. A randomized comparison of antiplatelet and anticoagulant therapy after the placement of coronary-artery stents. *N Engl J Med.* 1996;334:1084-9.

Syndrome of Protein C Deficiency and Anterior Wall Acute Myocardial Infarction at a Young Age From a Single Coronary Occlusion With Otherwise Normal Coronary Arteries

Mark A. Peterman, MD, and William C. Roberts, MD

Findings in a 19-year-old man with anterior wall acute myocardial infarction and total occlusion of the left anterior descending coronary artery associated with protein C deficiency are described. In addition, 5 previously reported patients with similar findings are summarized. ©2003 by Excerpta Medica, Inc.

(Am J Cardiol 2003;92:768–770)

Protein C deficiency in the heterozygous form occurs in approximately 1 in 500 persons[1] and is recognized to be associated with a relatively high frequency of venous thrombosis. Its association with arterial thrombosis is less appreciated. Herein, we describe a young man with protein C deficiency and anterior wall acute myocardial infarction associated with total occlusion of the distal left anterior descending coronary artery in the presence of an otherwise normal coronary arterial tree. Additionally, we review reported cases of protein C deficiency associated with acute myocardial infarction and coronary angiography.

• • •

A 19-year-old athletic African-American man, an inmate in a Texas prison, presented to an outlying hospital with sudden onset of severe, unremitting chest pain for the first time while doing push ups. Electrocardiography revealed ST elevation in leads I, AVL, and V_2 through V_6 (Figure 1). His troponin I level was 2.5 ng/ml. He was

From the Department of Internal Medicine and the Baylor Heart & Vascular Institute, Baylor University Medical Center, Dallas, Texas. Dr. Peterman's address is: Baylor University Medical Center, 3500 Gaston Avenue, Dallas, Texas 75246. E-mail: markpe@baylorhealth.edu. Manuscript received March 7, 2003; revised manuscript received and accepted May 28, 2003.

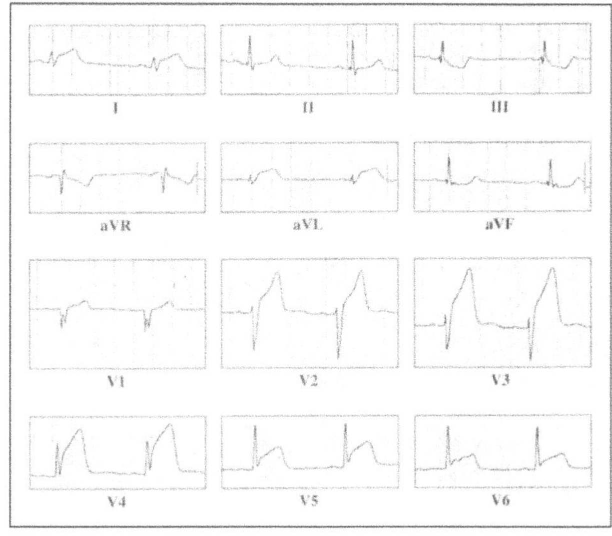

FIGURE 1. Electrocardiogram recorded immediately on presentation at the outlying hospital's emergency department.

treated with heparin, nitroglycerin, and tissue plasminogen activator without relief of chest pain or improvement in the electrocardiographic changes; the patient was transferred to Baylor University Medical Center. He denied illicit drug use since his incarceration 18 months earlier. He had had asthma during childhood. Six months earlier, his serum total cholesterol was 280 mg/dl and low-density lipoprotein cholesterol was 233 mg/dl. Two of his grandparents had coronary events. He had never smoked tobacco, but he had smoked cocaine and drank alcohol excessively before imprisonment. The patient was taking no medications.

On arrival, the patient's blood pressure was 105/60 mm Hg and heart rate was 59 beats/min. No precordial murmurs or abnormal sounds were heard, and his lungs were clear. He had normal electrolytes and renal function. The patient's hematocrit was 36 g/dl and his platelet count was 162,000/μl. The serum creatine kinase was 803

U/L with an MB fraction of 58 ng/ml; his troponin was 113 ng/ml. The electrocardiogram showed persistent anterolateral ST elevation.

Cardiac catheterization disclosed normal right, left main, and left circumflex coronary arteries and total occlusion of the distal left anterior descending coronary artery without collaterals (Figure 2). Balloon angioplasty did not relieve the obstruction. Left ventricular angiography disclosed apical akinesia. The creatine kinase level peaked at 1,865 U/L. The following day, chest pain recurred with additional ST elevations on electrocardiogram. Repeat coronary angiogram was unchanged. The ST segments were now elevated in multiple leads suggesting pericarditis, and a friction rub was heard. The pain lessened with rofecoxib therapy. In-hospital echocardiography on day 4 revealed a left ventricular ejection fraction of 30% with apical akinesia and anteroseptal hypokinesia. Due to a concern for paradoxical embolism via a

First Author	Year of Publication	Age (yrs)	Race	Sex	Interval: Chest pain to coronary angiogram (hours)	Coronary Artery Occluded	Peak CK (U/L)	Thrombolytic Therapy	Protein C Activity (% of normal)*	Protein C Deficiency in Family
Coller[10]	1987	28	W	M	—	+(LAD)	—	0	33	+(mother)
Hacker[11]	1991	28	W	M	<24	+(LM)	4200	+	51	+(father, uncle)
Kario[12]	1992	29	A	M	48	0	580	+	38	+(brother, mother)
Bux-Gewehr[13]	1996	35	W	F	"Days"	+(LAD)	—	+	57	—
Sadiq[14]	2001	22	—	F	<24	+(LAD,D)	—	0	33	—

*Normal was considered 70% to 130%.
A = Asian; CK = creatine kinase; D = diagonal; LAD = left anterior descending; LM = left main; W = white; — = no information available or not done.

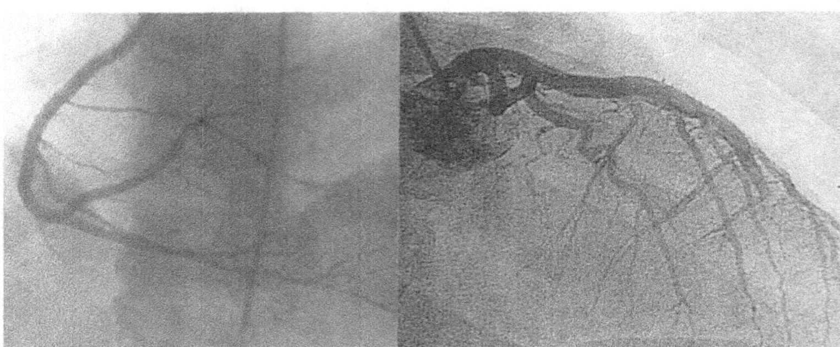

FIGURE 2. Coronary angiogram performed about 15 hours after onset of chest pain. *(Left panel)* Normal right coronary artery is shown. *(Right panel)* Injection of contrast material into the left main coronary artery is shown. The left anterior descending coronary artery is totally occluded distally.

patent foramen ovale, contrast echocardiography was also performed; it revealed no evidence of a right-to-left shunt.

A hypercoagulable workup was negative for homocystienemia (3 μmol/L), activated protein C resistance, and anticardiolipin antibodies. His functional protein C assay was low (45%), but the antigenic level was normal (116 U/dl). He was treated with heparin intravenously followed by warfarin and sent back to the prison infirmary to continue warfarin initiation and subcutaneous enoxaparin. A year later, the patient was well and active.

• • •

Although at least 22 patients with myocardial infarction and protein C deficiency have been reported, 17 did not have coronary angiography at the time of the infarct.[2–9] The remaining 5 previously reported patients[10–14] and the patient described herein had acute myocardial infarcts at a young age (19 to 35 years) and documented protein C deficiency of the heterozygous type (<60% of normal plasma levels of protein C).

The reason why protein C deficiency is not reported more often in patients, particularly young ones, with acute myocardial infarction is unclear but may simply result from the fact that the test is not commonly performed. Protein C deficiency occurs in approximately the same percentage of the population as the heterozygous form of familial hypercholesterolemia does (about 1 in 500 persons).

The patient described had a markedly elevated serum low-density lipoprotein cholesterol (233 mg/dl). In only 2 of the other previously reported 22 cases of protein C deficiency and acute myocardial infarction was this value mentioned: in 1 case, it was 102 mg/dl and in the other "normal."[11,14] Consequently, the relation of low-density lipoprotein cholesterol to protein C deficiency is unknown.

Thrombolytic therapy was administered in 3 of the 5 previously reported patients with this syndrome (Table 1) and to the presently reported patient. In 3 of these 4 cases, the major epicardial coronary artery remained totally oc-

cluded during angiography, a finding that suggests thrombolytic therapy in this group of patients may be of limited benefit.

The circumstances during which the acute myocardial infarction occurred in the present patient, namely while doing push-ups, is suggestive of paradoxical embolism. Paradoxical embolism most often occurs during a Valsalva maneuver in patients with a patent foramen ovale.[15] Contrast echocardiography, as was performed in our patient, excluded the presence of a right-to-left shunt.

1. Tait RC, Walker ID, Reitsma PH, Islam SIAM, McCall F, Poort SR, Conkie JA, Bertina RM. Prevalence of protein C deficiency in the healthy population. *Thromb Hemost* 1995;73:87–93.
2. Griffin JH, Evatt B, Zimmerman TS, Kleiss AJ, Wideman C. Deficiency of protein C in congenital thrombotic disease. *J Clin Invest* 1981;68:1370–1373.
3. Barbui T, Finazzi G, Mussoni L, Riganti M, Donati MB, Colucci M, Collen D. Hereditary dysfuncional protein C (protein C Bergamo) and thrombosis. *Lancet* 1984;2:819.
4. De Stefano V, Leone G, Micalizzi P, Teofili L, Falappa PG, Pollari G, Bizzi B. Arterial thrombosis as clinical manifestation of congenital protein C deficiency. *Ann Hematol* 1991;62:180–183.
5. Valla D, Denninger MH, Delvinge JM, Rueff B, Benhamou JP. Portal vein thrombosis with ruptured esophageal varices as presenting manifestation of hereditary protein C deficiency. *Gut* 1988;29:856–859.
6. Simioni P, Zanardi S, Saracino A, Girolami A. Occurrence of arterial thrombosis in a cohort of patients with hereditary deficiency of clotting inhibitors. *J Med* 1992;23:61–74.
7. Nakagawa K, Tsuji H, Masuda H, Kitamura H, Nakahara Y, Ogasahara Y, Okajima Y, Sawada S, Nakagawa M. Protein C deficiency found in a patient with acute myocardial infarction: a single base mutation 157 Arg (CGA) to stop codon (TGA). *Internat J Hematol* 1994;60:273–280.
8. Sakata T, Kario K, Katayma Y, Matsuyama T, Kato H, Miyata T. Analysis of 45 episodes of arterial occlusive disease in Japanese patients with congenital protein C deficiency. *Thromb Research* 1999;94:69–78.
9. Ninomiya M, Makuuchi H, Ohtsuka T, Takamoto S. Ischemic heart disease associated with protein C deficiency. *Eur J Cardio-thoracic Surg* 2001;20:883–885.
10. Coller BS, Owen J, Jetsy J, Horowitz D, Reitman MJ, Spear J, Yeh T, Comp PC. Deficiency of plasma protein S, protein C, or antithrombin III and arterial thrombosis. *Arteriosclerosis* 1987;7:456–462.

11. Hacker SM, Williamson BD, Lisco S, Kure J, Shoa M, Pitt B. Protein C deficiency and acute myocardial infarction in the third decade. *Am J Cardiol* 1991;68:137–138.

12. Kario K, Matsuo T, Tai S, Sakamoto S, Yamada T, Miki T, Matsuo M. Congenital protein C deficiency and myocardial infarction. *Thromb Res* 1992;67:95–103.

13. Bux-Gewehr I, Nacke A, Feurle GE. Recurring myocardial infarction in a 35-year-old woman. *Heart* 1999;81:316–317.

14. Sadiq A, Ahmed S, Karim A, Spivak J, Mattana J. Acute myocardial infarction: a rare complication of protein C deficiency. *Am J Med* 2001;110:414–415.

15. Ward R, Jones D, Haponik EF. Paradoxical embolism: an underrecognized problem. *Chest* 1995;108:549–558.

Late (≥6 Years) Results of Combined Coronary Artery Bypass Grafting and Mitral Valve Replacement for Severe Mitral Regurgitation Secondary to Acute Myocardial Infarction

Kevin Paul Theleman, MD, Phillip James Stephan, MD, Michael G. Isaacs, MD, Robert F. Hebeler, Jr., MD, A. Carl Henry III, MD, and William Clifford Roberts, MD

Analysis of outcomes in 31 patients who had combined mitral valve replacement (MVR) and coronary artery bypass grafting (CABG) for ischemic mitral regurgitation (MR) disclosed that 12 patients had MR because of papillary muscle rupture and that 19 patients had MR because of papillary muscle necrosis or fibrosis without rupture. Of the 12 patients with rupture, 6 died within 2 months of operation and the other 6 lived ≥6 years postoperatively; of the 19 patients without rupture, none died within 2 months of operation and 11 (58%) lived at least 6 years.   ©2003 by Excerpta Medica, Inc.

(Am J Cardiol 2003;92:1086–1090)

From the Departments of Internal Medicine (Cardiology), Cardiothoracic Surgery, and Pathology, and the Baylor Heart and Vascular Institute, Baylor University Medical Center; and Department of Surgery, Parkland Hospital, Southwestern Medical School, Dallas, Texas. Dr. Roberts' address is: Baylor Heart & Vascular Institute, Baylor University Medical Center, 3500 Gaston Avenue, Dallas, Texas 75246. E-mail: wc.roberts@baylorhealth.edu. Manuscript received June 11, 2003; revised manuscript received and accepted July 29, 2003.

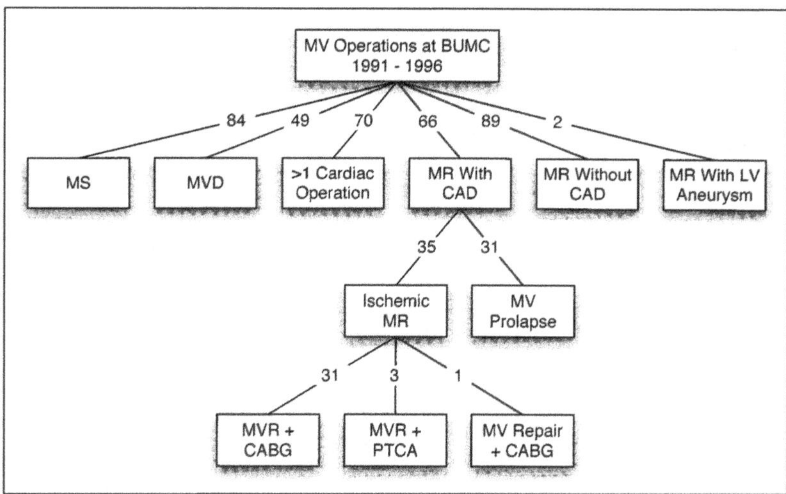

FIGURE 1. Diagram showing origin of the 31 patients with ischemic MR and combined MVR and CABG. BUMC = Baylor University Medical Center; CAD = coronary artery disease; LV = left ventricular; MS = mitral stenosis; MV = mitral valve; MVD = multivalvular disease; PTCA = percutaneous coronary angioplasty.

Mitral regurgitation (MR) is a major complication of acute myocardial infarction (AMI). When MR is severe, mitral valve replacement (MVR) or repair has proved beneficial, whether or not the mitral valve operation was performed during the period of AMI or after healing of the AMI. This report analyzes findings in 31 patients with MVR for severe MR that occurred during or after AMI with simultaneous coronary artery bypass grafting (CABG).

• • •

The names and numbers of patients who underwent mitral valve operations from January 1, 1991, to October 1, 1996, were obtained from a computer registry from the Department of Cardiovascular Surgery, Baylor University Medical Center. A total of 360 patients were found to have had mitral valve operations during this 69-month period, and the medical records of all 360 patients were reviewed to find those who had MVR because of ischemic MR and who underwent simultaneous CABG (Figure 1). Of the 360 patients, 329 were eliminated from further analysis for the following reasons: 84 had mitral stenosis; 89 had pure MR without angiographic evidence for coronary arterial narrowing; 70 had undergone a previous cardiac operation; 49 had ≥1 cardiac valves replaced in addition to the mitral valve; 2 had MVR associated with a left ventricular aneurysm; 31 had both MVR and CABG but the cause of MR was mitral valve prolapse; 3 had MVR and angioplasty rather than CABG; and 1 had mitral valve repair rather than MVR in addition to CABG. The remaining 31 patients had MVR and simultaneous CABG. This report focuses exclusively on these 31 patients.

The medical records, electrocardiographic, angiographic, operative, and morphologic (pathologic) reports were reviewed in detail in these 31 patients. The 31 patients included in this study were operated on by 12 different surgeons: 1 (ACH III) operated on 9 patients (29%); 1 (RFH) operated on 7 patients (23%);

5 different surgeons each operated on 2 patients; and 5 other surgeons each operated on 1 patient. Seventeen of the operatively excised valves were examined by WCR. In the remaining 14 valves, the status of the excised valves was determined from operative and pathologic reports. Of the 12 patients with ruptured papillary muscles, anterior and posterior leaflets were excised in 3 and only the anterior leaflet in the other 9; in the 19 patients without ruptured papillary muscles only the anterior leaflet was excised.

The Social Security Death Index (SSDI) was searched to learn how many of the 31 patients had died after hospital admission when the MVR and CABG had been performed. Each of the remaining patients whose names did not appear in the SSDI was contacted by telephone to determine their clinical status.

Pertinent findings in each of the 31 patients are provided in Table 1. The patients ranged in age at the time of MVR + CABG from 54 to 83 years (mean 69). AMI involved the anterior wall in 5 patients and the posterior (inferior) wall in 26 patients. All 31 patients were in New York Heart Association functional class III or IV just before MVR and CABG. The mean ejection fraction in the 31 patients was 49%. Ten patients (32%) were in shock preoperatively and 20 patients (64%) had intra-aortic balloon pumps inserted preoperatively. All 31 patients were followed at least 6 years, and 11 patients for at least 10 years. Twenty-six patients (83%) lived >30 days after combined MVR and CABG, 21 patients (65%) lived at least 1 year, and 18 patients (57%) lived at least 5 years. Of the 11 patients followed 10 years postoperatively, 4 (36%) are still alive. Survival in the 31 patients is graphically presented in Figure 2.

Twelve (39%) patients at operation had rupture of a portion of the left ventricular papillary muscle (Figure 3), and in each, the rupture was in the posteromedial papillary muscle (Table 1). In each, the electrocardiogram had indicated that the AMI involved the posterior wall. The interval from onset of AMI to MVR operation in 9 of these 12 patients ranged from 2 to 20 days (mean 7, median 4). The intervals from AMI to operation in the other 3 patients are unknown in 2 patients and was 6 months in the remaining patient. The left ventricular ejection fraction (from left ventriculography) was ≥45% in all 12 patients. Left ventricular cineangiography revealed 4+/4+ MR in 11 patients and 3+/4+ MR in the remaining patient. The left ventricular cavity in 6 patients was of normal size and was minimally dilated in another. Before operation, 9 of the 12 patients were in cardiogenic shock and each had an intra-aortic balloon pump inserted preoperatively. One additional patient also had an intra-aortic balloon pump inserted at operation.

TABLE 1 Observations in Each of the 31 Patients Who Underwent Coronary Artery Bypass Grafting (CABG) and Mitral Valve Replacement (MVR) for Pure Mitral Regurgitation (MR) Secondary to Myocardial Infarction

Case	Age (yr)/Sex	PMR	AMI Location	Interval (d) AMI to MVR	SH	DM	Pressures (mm Hg) LV (s/d)	SA (s/d)	PA (s/d)	PAW (mean)	EF (%)	MR by LV Cine (0 to 4+)	LV Dilated (0 to 4+)	Shock	IABP before MVR	No. CA >50%	No. CA A	Valve Inserted (size)	Interval (d) CC to MVR	Years Lived PO if Alive	Years Lived PO if Dead
1	59 M	+	Posterior	20	0	+	137/17	130/75	66/15	43	80	4+	0	0	0	2	1	SJM (29)	2	6	—
2	63 M	+	Posterior	4	0	+	73/0	77/55	37/24	19	46	4+	0	+	+	3	3	SJM (31)	1	—	7.4
3	63 M	+	Posterior	—	+	+		147/81	85/37	36	55	4+	3	0	+	3	4	SJM (27)	2	—	0.1
4	64 M	+	Posterior	4	0	0	100/21	93/68	33/18	15	64	4+	0	+	+	2	2	SJM (31)	2	9.6	—
5	64 F	+	Posterior	3	0	0	76/21	78/62	56/39	38	54	4+	0	+	+	1	1	SJM (27)	2	8.8	—
6	66 M	+	Posterior	8	+	0	78/28	77/62	60/34	42	64	4+	0	+	+	3	3	HPX (29)	7	—	0.2
7	66 F	+	Posterior	7	+	0	100/27	112/74	68/38	31	45	4+	4	+	+	1	1	SJM (25)	1	—	0.1
8	69 M	+	Posterior	11	0	0	76/17	83/47	44/21	22	49	4+	—	+	+	3	5	CE (27)	3	—	0.1
9	70 M	+	Posterior	—	+	0	115/17	97/63	47/22	25	50	3+	3	+	+	3	2	SJM (29)	3	—	0.1
10	71 F	+	Posterior	180	+	0	128/19	131/72	61/20	22	47	4+	4	0	0	3	4	CE (27)	1	—	11.3
11	79 M	+	Posterior	2	+	0	108/23	107/59	56/18	20	70	4+	0	+	+	3	5	HPX (29)	1	—	9.7
12	81 M	+	Posterior	2	0	0	62/9	62/45	50/16	20	50	4+	1	+	+	3	2	CE (31)	1	—	0.1
Subtotals	68 25%F	12	100% Posterior	24	6	3	96/18	100/64	55/25	28	56	3.9	1.4	9	10	2.5	2.8	7 mechanical	2.1	8.8 (3 alive)	3.2 (9 dead)
13	54 M	0	Posterior	720	0	0	—	128/80	21/10	—	55	4+	—	0	0	3	3	SJM (29)	—	9.3	—
14	54 F	0	Anterior	—	+	+	110/14	111/57	—	—	30	4+	1	0	+	3	3	SJM (27)	2	7.5	—
15	58 M	0	Posterior	60	+	0	101/12	101/58	49/17	22	49	3+	0	0	0	1	1	SJM (33)	30	10.3	—
16	63 F	0	Posterior	1710	0	+	132/28	131/71	63/7	37	41	4+	4	0	0	3	3	SJM (27)	11	—	10.8
17	64 M	0	Posterior	30	0	0	—	96/56	33/12	12	25	4+	1	0	+	3	3	CE (29)	1	10.4	—
18	64 M	0	Posterior	2	0	0	137/37	142/83	92/44	36	40	4+	2	0	+	3	3	SJM (31)	1	—	0.3
19	65 F	0	Posterior	—	+	0	101/20	99/49	40/19	26	50	4+	2	0	+	3	2	SJM (27)	1	—	7
20	66 M	0	Posterior	720	0	0	127/13	121/54	—	—	45	3+	0	0	0	3	5	HPX (29)	3	—	1.6
21	69 M	0	Posterior	360	0	0	142/19	143/83	37/16	18	45	4+	0	0	+	3	4	HPX (29)	1	9.6	—
22	70 M	0	Anterior	60	+	+	123/27	136/78	58/31	34	57	4+	2	0	+	3	4	SJM (29)	8	—	6.1
23	73 F	0	Anterior	1800	+	+	93/22	110/60	51/18	28	44	4+	1	0	+	3	3	CE (29)	5	—	0.7
24	73 F	0	Anterior	270	0	0	142/22	148/99	78/30	25	40	4+	4	0	+	2	1	SJM (29)	4	7.1	—
25	74 F	0	Anterior	1800	0	0	155/23	159/80	68/29	26	36	4+	3	0	0	3	3	CE (27)	3	9.7	—
26	76 F	0	Posterior	7	+	0	150/29	166/66	61/29	28	54	4+	0	0	+	3	3	HPX (25)	1	—	5.6
27	77 M	0	Posterior	12	+	+	197/24	198/98	—	—	51	4+	0	0	0	3	4	HPX (29)	11	—	4.6
28	77 F	0	Posterior	—	+	+	130/18	140/50	—	—	60	4+	—	0	+	3	3	SJM (27)	—	7.3	—
29	81 M	0	Posterior	13	+	+	113/19	114/55	40/16	25	55	4+	1	0	0	3	4	CE (29)	3	—	0.3
30	81 F	0	Posterior	720	0	0	152/15	147/69	—	—	44	3+	3	0	0	2	1	CE (25)	28	—	2.6
31	83 F	0	Posterior	15	0	+	86/14	82/35	33/17	18	49	4+	1	0	+	3	1	CE (27)	13	—	0.9
Subtotals	70 53% F	19	74% Posterior	519	9	8	129/21	130/67	51/21	26	46	3.9	1.4	1	10	2.8	2.8	9 Mechanical	7.4	8.9 (8 alive)	4 (11 dead)
Totals	69 42% F	39% Rupture	84% Posterior	328	15	11	116/20	118/66	53/23	27	50	3.9	1.4	10	20	2.7	2.8	16 Mechanical	5.2	9.7 (11 Alive)	3.5 (20 dead)

A = anastamoses; AMI = acute myocardial infarction; CC = cardiac catheterization; CA = coronary artery; CE = Carpentier-Edwards bioprosthesis; Cine = cineography; DM = diabetes mellitus; EF = ejection fraction; HPX = Hancock porcine xenograft; bioprothesis; IABP = intra-aortic balloon pump; LV = left ventricle; MR = mitral regurgitation; MVR = mitral valve replacement; PA = pulmonary artery; PAW = pulmonary artery wedge pressure; PMR = papillary muscle rupture; PO = postoperative; SA = systemic artery; SH = systemic hypertension; SJM = St. Jude Medical prothesis; s/d = peak systole/end diastole; + = present or positive; 0 = absent or negative; — = no information available or not applicable; ↓ = narrowed in luminal diameter.

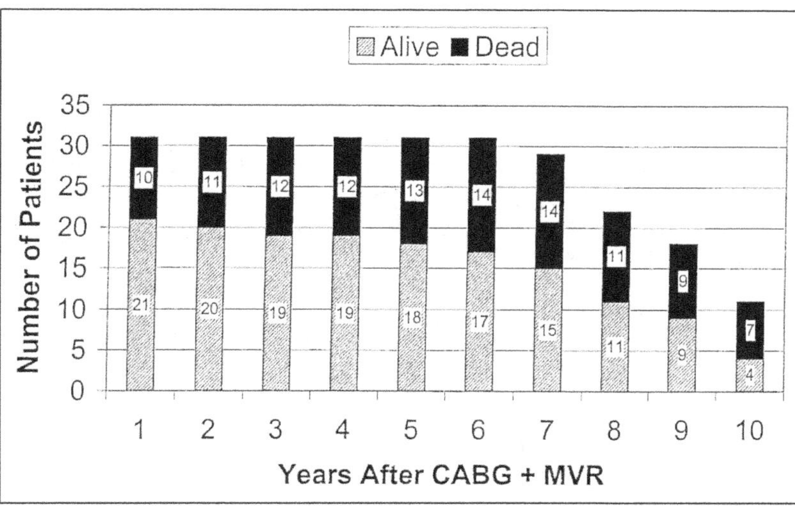

FIGURE 2. Survival in patients with combined CABG and MVR for severe MR secondary to myocardial infarction (n = 31). The column height represents the total number patients. The *striped portion* of the column represents the number of patients who are alive. The *black portion* of the column represents the number of patients who have died. All 31 patients were followed at least 6 years. Nineteen patients were followed at least 7 years, 22 were followed at least 8 years, 18 were followed at least 9 years, and 11 were followed at least 10 years.

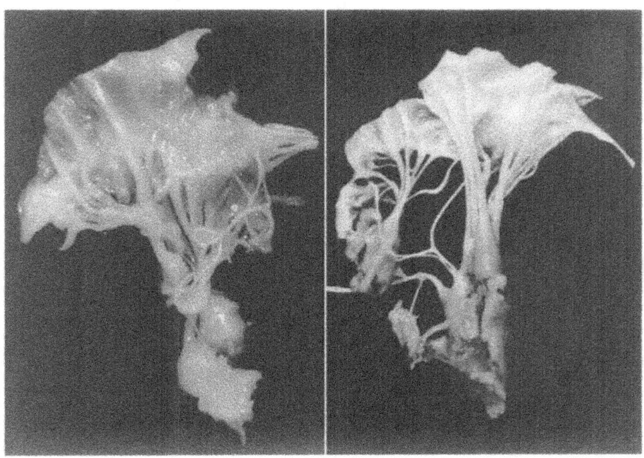

FIGURE 3. Photographs of the operatively-excised mitral valves in patient 1 *(left)* and in patient 8 *(right)*, respectively (Table 1). In both patients the posteromedial papillary muscle is ruptured. In patient 1, the chordae have twisted around the ruptured muscle.

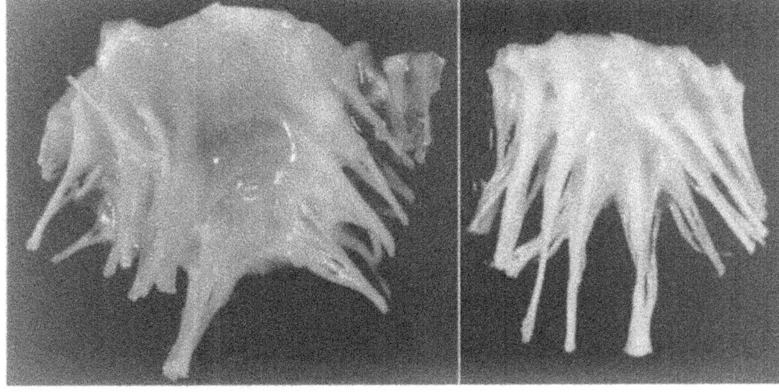

FIGURE 4. Photographs of anterior mitral leaflets excised in patients 14 *(left)* and 26 *(right)*, respectively (Table 1). Papillary muscle was not operatively excised in any of the 19 patients without papillary muscle rupture. Both leaflets have mildly thickened chordae, but otherwise are normal.

Mechanical mitral valve prostheses were placed in 7 patients and bioprostheses were placed in the other 5 patients. Of these 12 patients, 5 patients died within 30 days of operation and another died within 60 days of operation. The other 6 all lived at least 7 years postoperatively.

Nineteen of the 31 patients had severe MR due to papillary muscle necrosis or fibrosis rather than papillary muscle rupture (Figure 4 and Table 1). The location of the myocardial infarct by electrocardiogram was posterior in 14 patients (74%) and anterior in 5 patients (26%). The interval from the onset of AMI to operation in 16 of the 19 patients ranged from 2 days to 5 years (mean 1.6 years, median 270 days). The mean left ventricular ejection fraction was 46%. All but 3 patients had left ventricular ejection fractions $\geq$40%. Four of the 19 patients (21%) had 3 or 4+ left ventricular cavity dilatation, 7 (37%) had 1 or 2+ left ventricular cavity dilatation, and 8 (42%) had no left ventricular cavity dilatation. Left ventricular cineography revealed 4+ MR in 16 patients and 3+ in 3 patients. One patient was in cardiogenic shock before operation and 10 had an intra-aortic balloon pump inserted preoperatively. Of these 19 patients, none died within 60 days of MVR; 2 died within 6 months and another 2 died within 1 year. Mechanical mitral valve prostheses were placed in 9 patients and bioprostheses were placed in the other 10 patients. Eleven patients (57%) have died since operation with a mean survival of 4.0 years. Eight patients (43%) are still alive with a mean survival of 8.9 years.

• • •

This analysis of 31 patients who had combined CABG and MVR for ischemic MR disclosed that the long-term outcome was good. Of the 26 patients who survived the early operative period, 17 (65%) lived >6 years postoperatively, and of the total group of 31 patients, 55% lived >6 years. Of the 18 patients followed at least 8 years, 9 (50%) are still alive. The 12 patients who had ruptured papillary muscles as the cause of the MR did not have as favorable an outcome as the 19 patients who had necrosis or fibrosis of a papillary muscle as the cause of the MR. Of the 12 patients with a ruptured papillary muscle, 6 died within 60 days of the operation; the other 6 lived >7 years. Of the 19 patients with papillary muscle dysfunction without rupture, none died within 60 days of the operation; 10 lived >6 years, and all but 2 of them are alive >7 years after operation.

Previous reports of combined MVR and CABG for ischemic MR with follow-up of $\geq$5 years are summarized in Table 2. Of the 401 patients analyzed in these 5 reports, 336 patients (84%) survived the early oper-

TABLE 2 Previously Reported Studies of Coronary Artery Bypass Grafting and Mitral Valve Replacement for Pure Mitral Regurgitation Secondary to Myocardial Infarction

First Author	Year of Publication	No. of Cases	Mean Age (years)	Female	AMI Within 30 Days	MR 3+ or 4+	EF (%)	IABP before MVR	CABG @ MVR	Mean No. CA A	Papillary Muscle Rupture	Mechanical Valves	Mean Aortic Cross Clamp Time (min)	Survival After MVR		
														>30 Days	>1 Year	>5 Years
Connolly[1]	1986	16	64	31%	38%	100%	40	19%	100%	2.3	44%	13%	79	81%	81%	81%
Kay[2]	1986	40	—	—	—	—	—	—	100%	—	—	10%	—	65%	58%	27%
Colin[3]	1995	56	69	52%	48%	100%	—	—	89%	2	39%	29%	—	91%	91%	91%
Hausmann[4]	1999	197	64	—	—	100%	40	13%	88%	2	—	53%	—	86%	80%	73%
Bouchard[5]	2001	92	65	42%	16%	—	—	34%	77%	—	38%	87%	88	84%	82%	70%
Totals (sum or mean)		401	65	73 (45%)	48 (29%)	269 (100%)	40	60 (20%)	350 (87%)	2	64 (39%)	213 (53%)	87	336 (84%)	320 (80%)	283 (71%)

Abbreviations as in Table 1.

ative period and 283 patients (70%) survived >5 years. In the present study of 31 patients, 26 patients (84%) survived the early operative period and 18 patients (58%) survived >5 years. In the previously reported studies, it was not always clear how many patients had ruptured versus nonruptured left ventricular papillary muscles. Furthermore, whether the MR in some of the previously reported cases was due to mitral valve prolapse rather than papillary muscle ischemia (with or without rupture) was also not always clear.

The positive features of the present study include the relatively long follow-up, the division of the cases into those with and without papillary muscle rupture, and the careful study of the operatively-excised mitral valves to rule out mitral valve prolapse as the cause of MR. The present study is limited by the relatively small number of cases included.

1. Connolly MW, Gelbfish JS, Jacobwitz IJ, Rose DM, Mendelsohn A, Cappabianca PM, Acinapura AJ, Cunningham JN Jr. Surgical results for mitral regurgitation from coronary artery disease. *J Thorac Cardiovasc Surg* 1986;91:379–388.
2. Kay GL, Kay JH, Zubiate P, Yokoyama T, Mendez M. Mitral valve repair for mitral regurgitation secondary to coronary artery disease. *Circulation* 1986;74(suppl I):I88–I98.
3. Cohn LH, Rizzo RJ, Adams DH, Couper GS, Sullivan TE, Collins JJ Jr, Aranki SF. The effect of pathophysiology on the surgical treatment of ischemic mitral regurgitation: operative and late risks of repair versus replacement. *Eur J Cardiothorac Surg* 1995;9:568–574.
4. Hausmann H, Siniawski H, Hetzer R. Mitral valve reconstruction and replacement for ischemic mitral insufficiency: seven years' follow up. *J Heart Valve Dis* 1999;8:536–542.
5. Bouchard D, Pellerin M, Carrier M, Perrault LP, Pagé P, Hébert Y, Cartier R, Dyrda I, Pelletier LC. Results following valve replacement for ischemic mitral regurgitation. *Can J Cardiol* 2001;17:427–431.

Krakatoa—The Ultimate Heart Attack

Individuals when first developing chest pain that leads to cardiac arrest and/or acute myocardial infarction might describe the sudden initial cardiac event as *Krakatoa*, a name that has become a byword for cataclysmic disaster. In 1883, a volcano exploded on the island of Krakatoa, causing an immense tsunami that killed nearly 36,000 people! The waves were felt as far away as France. Barometers in Bogotá and Washington, DC, went haywire. The sound of the island's destruction was heard on islands thousands of miles away.

The author of *The Professor and the Madman* and *The Map that Changed the World* has now written *Krakatoa*. Most volcanoes, of course, continue to exist after erupting. Rarely is an eruption so great that it destroys an entire mountain. Such was the case with Krakatoa and a few others—Mount Mazana (leaving behind Crater Lake in Oregon), Santorini (which may have taken out the Minoan civilization and left a great hole in the Agean), and Yellowstone (in Montana).

Krakatoa was located in the Sundra Strait between the large islands of Sumatra and Java and was composed of 3 peaks: Rakata, at 2,600 ft; Danan, at nearly 1,500 ft; and Perboewatan, at 400 ft. The volcano began violent earthquakes in May 1883. After 3 months of earth tremors, the island blew up. (If Pike's Peak in Colorado had exploded with the same force, every person in the continental United States would have heard it!) There were 4 detonations over 5 hours. The last one occurred on Monday morning August 27, 1883; it was one of the largest explosions in recorded history.

At Krakatoa when cold sea water contacted the red-hot magma, the steam exploded with catastrophic violence, and 6 cubic miles of rock and ash were hurled >20 miles into the stratosphere. An hour after the explosion, as lightning lit up the blackening skies, a thick muddy rain fell on Batavia (now Jakarta). Boiling-hot debris from the blast, some chunks 3 feet around, fell over hundreds of square miles. Because the island was uninhabited at the time, nobody on Krakatoa was killed, but giant tsunamis rolled out in all directions, flooding the coast of Java and Sumatra, submerging nearly 300 towns and villages, and killing >36,000 people. It was as if a mountain-sized red-hot rock had been dropped into the ocean.

A 72-ft-high wave engulfed and totally destroyed the town of Telokbetong at the head of Sumatra's Lampong Bay, killing 2,200 people. Water cascaded into the town of Tangerang, and when it swept out again, it carried people, animals, houses, and trees. No one expected the waves to return after they had receded. It is likely that many people believed the worst was over and returned to their shore-side villages, only to experience another, more catastrophic inundation. The town of Merak, which had suffered little damage from the first wave, was destroyed by the second. The huge wave, after traveling at hundreds of miles per hour, entered the narrow bay, and as the shoaling beach slowed down the leading edge of the wave, millions of gallons of water began piling up behind until the wave reached the height of 135 ft, as tall as a 10-story building. This mountain of water rolled over Merak, obliterating everything in its path and drowning all but 2 of 2,700 inhabitants. Anjer was drowned by a 33-ft wave and Tyringin, 24 miles from the volcano, was smashed by 70-ft-high locomotive of rolling water. It was not the lava, noxious gases, flame, smoke, or volcanic bombs that destroyed those unfortunate thousands, it was the power of the water. In most instances death came at the hands of seismic sea waves.

Accompanied by thunderous explosions, the waves swept around St. Nicholas Point on Java and headed for Batavia, 94 miles from the epicenter. At approximately 12:15 P.M., 2 hours after the final explosion, the sea roared into the capital city. It receded and then came back. Thousands of ships, ranging in size from steamships to small proas, were destroyed in Batavia's harbor. Nine hours after the eruption, many riverboats were swamped and sunk in Calcutta, 2,000 miles away, and ships strained at their anchors in Port Elizabeth, South Africa, 5,000 miles from the blast.

What did not remain was the volcano that had caused it all. Krakatoa, after the final concatenation of seismic and tectonic climaxes that occurred just after 10:00 on that Monday morning, had simply and finally exploded itself out of existence. Where once there had been a tropical peak that was 2,600 ft tall, there was now a hole in the ocean floor that was 1,000 ft deep. Krakatoa's explosion generated a climate-altering ash cloud that produced lurid red, blue, green, and copper colored sunsets and lowered temperatures around the world.

Krakatoa (the volcano) was not the largest or deadliest of recent Indonesian volcanic eruptions. That dubious distinction goes to Tambora, which erupted with more than twice the power of Krakatoa, killed 10,000 people outright, and caused the deaths of another 82,000 by starvation and disease. *Krakatoa* (the book) must be one of the best books ever written about the history and significance of a natural disaster. And Simon Winchester, its author is a trained geologist.

William Clifford Roberts, MD
Editor in Chief
Baylor Heart & Vascular Institute
Baylor University Medical Center
Dallas, Texas

1. Winchester S. Krakatoa. The Day the World Exploded: August 27, 1883. New York: HarperCollins, 2003.

Acute myocardial infarction at 25 years of age

M. Wayne Falcone, MD, Paul A. Grayburn, MD, and William C. Roberts, MD

A 25-year-old black woman was found to have systemic hypertension when she was 18 years of age. She had 2 children in her early 20s; during both pregnancies, her blood pressure was extremely high, and both children were delivered early because of the hypertension. At age 24 she discontinued her antihypertensive medicines for unclear reasons. About 48 hours before hospital admission, she experienced various types of substernal chest pain, which occasionally radiated to her arms. In the emergency department, her blood pressure was 240/130 mm Hg and her serum troponin was 2.7 mg/mL. The electrocardiogram showed tall T waves anteriorly but no Q waves or S-T segment changes. The drug screen was positive for marijuana but negative for cocaine. She stated that she had never used cocaine but often used marijuana. She smoked about 20 cigarettes a day and was not aware of ever having her blood cholesterol tested. Her mother had diabetes mellitus and high blood pressure. Her father had died at age 51 of acute myocardial infarction.

When admitted to the ward, the patient's blood pressure was 140/90 mm Hg. She weighed 252 pounds and was 63 inches tall (body mass index 44 kg/m^2). Her lungs were clear. No precordial murmurs or abnormal sounds were heard.

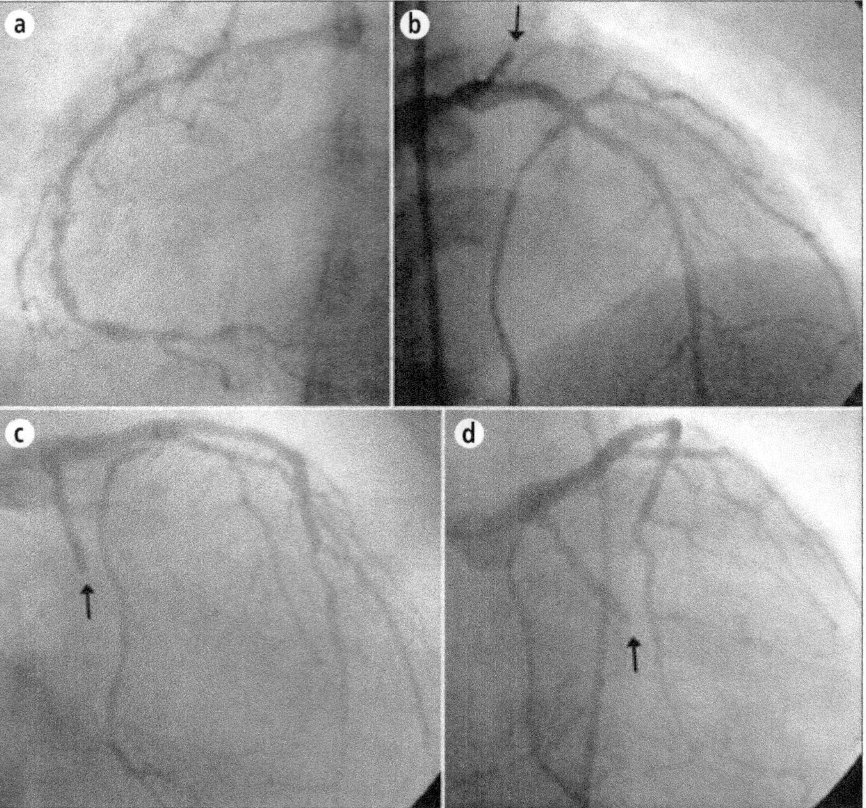

Figure. Coronary angiograms in the patient described. **(a)** Right coronary artery with numerous narrowings. **(b, c, d)** Injection of contrast material into the left main coronary artery showing total occlusion of the left circumflex (arrow) and multiple lesser narrowing in the left anterior descending artery.

The cardiac silhouette on chest radiograph was of normal size. The lung fields were clear. On chest computed tomography, the aorta appeared to be of normal size, and no dissection was present. The serum alanine aminotransferase was 33 U/L; aspartate aminotransferase, 61 U/L; and alkaline phosphatase, 73 U/L. The serum total protein was 7.8 g/dL; albumin, 3.1 g/dL; and globulin, 4.7 g/dL. The urine was negative for glucose, but a trace of protein was present. The serum total cholesterol was 375 mg/dL; the low-density lipoprotein cholesterol, 311 mg/dL; the high-density lipoprotein cholesterol, 47 mg/dL; the very-low-density lipoprotein cholesterol, 17 mg/dL; and the triglycerides, 83 mg/dL. The erythrocyte sedimentation rate was 89 mm/hour.

Cardiac catheterization during her first day in the hospital disclosed a large left main coronary artery, which contained a narrowing in its most distal portion, a relatively normal left anterior descending artery, and a totally occluded left circumflex coronary artery. The right coronary artery was the dominant one, and its interior lining was "ragged" with narrowing >90% in diameter. The distal left circumflex artery was filled by collaterals from the distal right coronary artery (*Figure*). A left ventricular angiogram showed the posterobasal portion of the left ventricular wall to be akinetic and the other portions of the left ventricular wall to contract well. The ejection fraction was estimated to be 50%.

During the cardiac catheterization, the totally obstructed obtuse marginal branch of the left circumflex coronary artery

From the Mid-Tex Cardiovascular Institute at Providence Health Center, Waco, Texas (Falcone); and the Baylor Heart and Vascular Institute (Grayburn and Roberts), Baylor University Medical Center, Dallas, Texas 75246.

Corresponding author: William C. Roberts, MD, Baylor Heart and Vascular Institute, 621 North Hall Street, Dallas, Texas 75226 (e-mail: wc.roberts@BaylorHealth.edu).

was opened and then 2 stents were placed in it. The patient was subsequently discharged, but about 1 month later, chest pain reccurred and she was rehospitalized. Cardiac catheterization again showed the left circumflex artery to be completely closed. It was not possible to open the total occlusion at the site of the stents. Additionally, a new narrowing was found in the left anterior descending coronary artery, and intravascular ultrasonic imaging showed it to be a 70% cross-sectional area narrowing. She also had evidence of severe narrowing by atherosclerotic disease of both the common and external iliac arteries and the femoral arteries bilaterally.

About a month later, she underwent an off-pump coronary bypass grafting procedure with a right internal mammary artery to the posterior descending branch of the right coronary artery and a left internal mammary artery to the left anterior descending coronary artery. Since the operation in March 2003, she has done remarkably well. Her chest discomfort has vanished, and she is now working full-time again.

• • •

The frequency of acute myocardial infarction in persons ≤45 years of age is relatively uncommon, particular in women. The *Table* lists publications describing patients ≤45 years of age with acute myocardial infarction (1–22). Excluding the 3 studies limited to women (2, 11, 16), acute myocardial infarction occurred in 303 woman (11%) and in 2488 men (89%) ≤45 years of age. Of the 303 women, only 5 (2%) were stated to be ≤25 years of age.

The hitherto described patient clearly had heterozygous familial hypercholesterolemia but also had systemic hypertension and diabetes mellitus and was a relatively heavy cigarette smoker. Additionally, she was obese. Nevertheless, acute myocardial infarction in the 20s is extremely rare. A number of studies have demonstrated that the number of atherosclerotic risk factors in young patients with acute myocardial infarction is considerably larger than in older patients with acute myocardial infarction (1–22). Additionally, coronary angiography in the younger patients compared with the older ones has shown less severe coronary narrowing, a lower frequency of death during the acute event, and a better prognosis with fewer long-term atherosclerotic events (3–16, 18, 21, 22). The present patient was unusual in this regard because of the extensive amount of coronary narrowing in all of her major coronary arteries.

Although a number of reports are available describing young patients with acute myocardial infarction, few focus exclusively on women. A most useful report was by Arnold and Moodie (11) in 1993. These authors described 32 women ≤30 years of age referred to the Cleveland Clinic for evaluation of coronary artery disease. Of the 32 patients, 22 had had an acute myocardial infarction. Although it was not possible to separate the findings in these 22 patients, serum cholesterol data (available in 28 of the 32 patients) disclosed mean fasting serum total cholesterol levels of 259 ± 78 mg/dL (range 155–500), mean low-density lipoprotein levels of 178 ± 64 mg/dL (range 120–305), triglyceride levels of 164 ± 86 mg/dL (range 44–465), and mean high-density lipoprotein levels of 49 ± 15 mg/dL (range 29–78). These mean values, of course, were similar to those in the patient described herein. Additionally, 9 of the 32 patients (28%) had juvenile diabetes mellitus, 12 (38%) had systemic hypertension, 23 (72%) smoked, and 9 (28%) used oral contraceptives. Fourteen patients (44%) had angiographic "single-vessel" coronary disease, 14 (44%) had multivessel involvement, and 4 (13%) had angiographically normal coronary arteries. Left ventricular dysfunction was documented in 27 (84%) of the 32 patients. Five patients (16%) died during the 3-month to 20-year follow-up (mean 10 years).

Table. Reported frequency of myocardial infarction in women ≤45 years of age

Reference	First author	Year of publication	Age (years) for inclusion	Number of patients	Number (%) of women	Number of women ≤25 years
1	Roth	1967	≤40	53	2 (4%)	1
2	Jick	1978	≤45	83	83 (100%)	0
3	Benacerraf	1978	≤35	20	4 (20%)	2
4	Glover	1982	≤35	120	10 (8%)	?
5	Uhl	1983	<40	165	10 (6%)	0
6	Puel	1983	<35	22	2 (9%)	?
7	Hoit	1986	<45	203	16 (8%)	?
8	Kaul	1986	<40	101	3 (3%)	?
9	Weinberger	1987	<30	30	4 (13%)	0
10	Klein	1987	<40	85*	13 (15%)	0
11	Arnold	1993	≤30	32	32 (100%)	2
12	Chouhan	1993	<35	62	1 (2%)	0
13	Badui	1993	≤40	142	18 (13%)	0
14	Negus	1994	≤40	129	11 (9%)	?
15	Teng	1994	<40	17	3 (18%)	0
16	Zimmerman	1995	≤35	210	210 (100%)	?
17	Barbash	1995	≤40	269	27 (10%)	?
18	Füllhaas	1997	≤40	75	11 (15%)	?
19	Doughty	2002	≤45	102	26 (25%)	?
20	Ranjith	2002	≤45	245	39 (16%)	0
21	Cole	2003	<40	843†	94 (11%)	?
22	Fournier	2004	≤40	108	9 (8%)	?

*Acute myocardial infarction in 59.
†Acute myocardial infarction in 451.

1. Roth O, Berki A, Wolff GD. Long range observations in fifty-three young patients with myocardial infarction. *Am J Cardiol* 1967;19:331–338.
2. Jick H, Dinan B, Herman R, Rothman KJ. Myocardial infarction and other vascular diseases in young women. *J Am Med Assoc* 1978;240:2548–2552.
3. Benacerraf A, Castillo-Fenoy A, Goffinet D, Krantz D. [Myocardial infarct before the age of 36: 20 cases]. *Arch Mal Coeur Vaiss* 1978;71:756–764.
4. Glover MU, Kuber MT, Warren SE, Vieweg WV. Myocardial infarction before age 36: risk factor and arteriographic analysis. *Am J Cardiol* 1982;49:1600–1603.
5. Uhl GS, Farrell PW. Myocardial infarction in young adults: risk factors and natural history. *Am Heart J* 1983;105:548–553.
6. Puel J, Robert J, Massabuau P, Cassagneau B, Miquel JP, Mimoun G, Fauvel

JM, Bounhoure JP. [Myocardial infarction before the age of 35. Clinical and coronarographic aspects]. *Presse Med* 1983;12:1911–1914.

7. Hoit BD, Gilpin EA, Henning H, Maisel AA, Dittrich H, Carlisle J, Ross J Jr. Myocardial infarction in young patients: an analysis by age subsets. *Circulation* 1986;74:712–721.

8. Kaul U, Dogra B, Manchanda SC, Wasir HS, Rajani M, Bhatia ML. Myocardial infarction in young Indian patients: risk factors and coronary arteriographic profile. *Am Heart J* 1986;112:71–75.

9. Weinberger I, Rotenberg Z, Fuchs J, Sagy A, Friedmann J, Agmon J. Myocardial infarction in young adults under 30 years: risk factors and clinical course. *Clin Cardiol* 1987;10:9–15.

10. Klein LW, Agarwal JB, Herlich MB, Leary TM, Helfant RH. Prognosis of symptomatic coronary artery disease in young adults aged 40 years or less. *Am J Cardiol* 1987;60:1269–1272.

11. Arnold AZ, Moodie DS. Coronary artery disease in young women: risk factor analysis and long-term follow-up. *Cleve Clin J Med* 1993;60:393–398.

12. Chouhan L, Hajar HA, Pomposiello JC. Comparison of thrombolytic therapy for acute myocardial infarction in patients aged <35 and >55 years. *Am J Cardiol* 1993;71:157–159.

13. Badui E, Rangel A, Valdespino A, Graef A, Plaza A, Chavez E, Ramos MA, Lepe L, Cruz H, Enciso R. [Acute myocardial infarct in young adults. A report of 142 cases]. *Arch Inst Cardiol Mex* 1993;63:529–537.

14. Negus BH, Willard JE, Glamann DB, Landau C, Snyder RW II, Hillis LD, Lange RA. Coronary anatomy and prognosis of young, asymptomatic survivors of myocardial infarction. *Am J Med* 1994;96:354–358.

15. Teng JK, Lin LJ, Tsai LM, Kwan CM, Chen JH. Acute myocardial infarction in young and very old Chinese adults: clinical characteristics and therapeutic implications. *Int J Cardiol* 1994;44:29–36.

16. Zimmerman FH, Cameron A, Fisher LD, Ng G. Myocardial infarction in young adults: angiographic characterization, risk factors and prognosis (Coronary Artery Surgery Study Registry). *J Am Coll Cardiol* 1995;26:654–661.

17. Barbash GI, White HD, Modan M, Diaz R, Hampton JR, Heikkila J, Kristinsson A, Moulopoulos S, Paolasso EA, Van der Werf T, Pehrsson K, Sandoe E, Simes J, Wilcox RG, Verstraete M, von der Lippe G, van de Werf F; the investigators of the International Tissue Plasminogen Activator/Streptokinase Mortality Trial. Acute myocardial infarction in the young—the role of smoking. *Eur Heart J* 1995;16:313–316.

18. Füllhaas JU, Rickenbacher P, Pfisterer M, Ritz R. Long-term prognosis of young patients after myocardial infarction in the thrombolytic era. *Clin Cardiol* 1997;20:993–998.

19. Doughty M, Mehta R, Bruckman D, Das S, Karavite D, Tsai T, Eagle K. Acute myocardial infarction in the young—the University of Michigan experience. *Am Heart J* 2002;143:56–62.

20. Ranjith N, Verho NK, Verho M, Winkelmann BR. Acute myocardial infarction in a young South African Indian-based population: patient characteristics on admission and gender-specific risk factor prevalence. *Curr Med Res Opin* 2002;18:242–248.

21. Cole JH, Miller JI III, Sperling LS, Weintraub WS. Long-term follow-up of coronary artery disease presenting in young adults. *J Am Coll Cardiol* 2003;41:521–528.

22. Fournier JA, Cabezón S, Cayuela A, Ballesteros SM, Cortacero JAP, de la Llera LSD. Longterm prognosis of patients having acute myocardial infarction when ≤40 years of age. *Am J Cardiol* 2004 (in press).

Clinical and necropsy findings in patients with calcified myocardial infarcts

CRAIG STEVEN CAMERON, MD, AND WILLIAM CLIFFORD ROBERTS, MD

Clinical and necropsy findings are described in 37 patients with grossly visible myocardial infarcts. At the time of the first infarct, the 31 men ranged in age from 25 to 72 years (mean, 47) and the 6 women, from 50 to 70 years (mean, 56). The interval from the first clinically apparent acute myocardial infarct to death varied from 2 to 28 years (mean, 13) and was ≥10 years in 24 of 32 patients (75%) for whom this information was available. The ages of death in the 31 men ranged from 39 to 75 years (mean, 61), and in the 6 women, from 62 to 75 years (mean, 69). The ages of death in the 9 patients having coronary bypass grafting was insignificantly different from that in the 28 patients not having this procedure. Most had chronic heart failure (73%), which was the most common mode of death. Nearly all had dilated left ventricular cavities, with left ventricular aneurysms in 43%. The hearts were increased in weight in 94%, and all had severe coronary arterial atherosclerosis. Thus, patients with calcified myocardial infarcts are usually men, the infarct that calcifies usually occurs at a relatively young age (mean, 50), the calcified wall is often aneurysmal, the left ventricular cavity is almost always dilated, the heart weight is increased, and heart failure is the predominant symptom and most common mode of death.

Calcific deposits often are observed in the hearts of older persons living in developed countries. These deposits are most commonly located in atherosclerotic plaques in the coronary arteries, in the mitral annulus, in the aortic valve cusps, and in the left ventricular papillary muscles (1). Stenotic mitral and aortic valves in adults are usually calcified (2, 3). Certain clinical and autopsy findings in 21 patients with grossly visible calcific deposits at sites of healed myocardial infarcts have been previously reported by one of us (WCR) (4). There have been no published reports on this topic since that publication in 1987. Since 1987, we have collected an additional 16 cases. This article summarizes clinical and necropsy findings in these 37 patients with calcified myocardial infarcts and compares findings in those having vs those not having coronary artery bypass grafting (CABG).

• • •

Certain clinical and necropsy findings in the 37 patients are summarized in *Tables 1–3*. All 37 hearts were examined by one of us (WCR). The cases were divided into 2 groups based upon whether or not the patient had CABG.

Non-CABG group: These 28 patients ranged in age from 39 to 78 years (mean, 62); 23 (82%) were men and 5 (18%) were women. Twenty-four had a history of ≥1 clinically apparent acute myocardial infarct, 17 (71%) with a single infarct and 7 (29%)

with ≥2 infarcts. The interval between the first clinically apparent infarct and death in these 24 patients ranged from 2 to 28 years (mean, 13). The ages at first acute myocardial infarct ranged from 25 to 72 years old (mean, 48). Two of the 4 patients with clinically silent infarcts (cases 13 and 22) had previous electrocardiograms consistent with healed myocardial infarction.

CABG group: These 9 patients at death ranged in age from 42 to 75 years (mean, 65); 8 (89%) were men and 1 (11%) was a woman. All 9 patients had a history of ≥1 clinically apparent acute myocardial infarcts, 2 patients with a single infarct and 7 patients with ≥2 infarcts. The interval between the first infarct and death ranged from 10 to >20 years (mean, 14). The ages at the first infarct spanned from 32 to 61 years (mean, 50) in the 8 patients whose ages at the first infarct are known. One of these 9 patients (case 9) had a history of 3 acute myocardial infarcts, including one at the time of his CABG 20 years before death.

In both groups, heart failure was the most common manifestation of cardiac disease: 20 of the 28 non-CABG cases (71%) had evidence of chronic heart failure, and 7 of the 8 remaining patients (cases 6, 7, 10, 13, 14, 18, and 24) had dilated left ventricular cavities at autopsy, including 2 with true left ventricular aneurysms (cases 13 and 24). Of the 9 CABG cases, 7 had evidence of heart failure, and the 2 remaining patients (cases 7 and 9) had dilated ventricles, including 1 with a true left ventricular aneurysm. Heart failure also was the most common mode of death in both groups (Table 3).

Of the 28 patients in the non-CABG group, 12 (43%) had true left ventricular aneurysms, and 5 had intraaneurysmal thrombus. Of the 16 patients in this group without aneurysms, 3 had thrombus in the left ventricular cavity at autopsy. In the CABG group, 4 patients (44%) had left ventricular aneurysms at autopsy, including 1 with intraaneurysmal thrombus.

All 37 patients had >75% reduction in cross-sectional area by atherosclerotic plaque in at least one major epicardial coronary artery and usually in ≥2 major arteries.

Photographs of several calcified myocardial infarcts are shown in *Figures 1–4*.

• • •

From the Division of Cardiology, Department of Internal Medicine, and Department of Pathology, Baylor Heart and Vascular Institute, Baylor University Medical Center, Dallas, Texas 75246.

Table 1. Calcified myocardial infarcts at autopsy among patients without coronary artery bypass grafting

Case	Age at death (yr)	Age at first AMI (yr)	Interval of first AMI to death (yr)	No. of AMIs	Gender	CHF	AP	VT	SH	DM	Stroke	Mode of death	HW (g)	Location of calcified infarct				LV aneurysm	LV T	Coronary artery decreased >75% in CSA by plaque			
														A	P	Apical	Basal			LM	LAD	LC	Right
1	39	30	9	2	M	+	+	+	0	0	0	AMI	615	+	0	+	+	+	+	0	+	+	+
2	43	37	6	1	M	+	0	0	0	0	0	CHF	610	+	0	+	+	+	0	--	+	+	+
3	49	42	7	1	M	0	0	0	+	+	+	--	480	0	+	+	0	0	0	--	--	--	--
4	50	36	14	1	M	+	+	+	0	0	0	AMI	480	+	0	+	+	+	0	--	+	0	0
5	52	25	27	1	M	+	0	0	0	0	0	Sudden	680	0	+	+	+	0	0	--	--	--	+
6	52	50	2	1	M	0	0	0	0	0	0	Suicide	475	+	0	+	+	0	0	--	+	0	+
7	52	46	6	1	M	0	0	0	+	0	0	Sudden	510	+	0	+	+	0	+	--	+	0	+
8	54	44	10	3	M	+	0	0	0	0	0	CVA	730	+	0	+	+	0	+	0	+	+	+
9	57	45	12	2	M	+	0	0	--	0	0	Sudden	540	+	0	+	+	0	0	--	+	0	+
10	57	43	14	1	M	0	0	+	+	0	0	HF	415	0	+	+	+	0	0	--	+	0	+
11	60	--	--	--	M	+	0	+	0	+	+	CHF	592	+	+	+	+	0	0	--	+	--	--
12	62	50	12	1	F	+	0	0	+	0	0	CHF	405	+	+	+	0	+	+	--	+	0	0
13	62	--*	--	--	M	0	0	0	0	0	0	Cancer	500	0	+	+	+	+	0	--	+	+	+
14	63	48	15	1	M	0	0	+	0	0	0	CVA	480	0	+	+	+	0	0	--	--	--	--
15	63	38	25	4	M	+	+	0	0	+	+	CHF	470	+	+	+	0	+	0	--	+	+	+
16	63	61	2	1	M	+	0	0	+	0	0	CHF	790	+	0	+	0	+	+	--	+	+	+
17	65	55	10	1	M	+	0	+	+	0	0	Sudden	570	+	0	+	0	+	+	0	+	+	0
18	66	--	--	--	M	0	0	0	+	0	0	Sudden	570	+	0	+	+	0	+	--	+	+	0
19	67	54	13	1	F	+	0	0	0	+	+	CVA	310	+	0	+	+	0	0	--	+	--	--
20	67	45	22	1	M	+	0	0	0	0	0	CHF	430	+	0	+	+	+	0	--	+	+	0
21	68	52	16	1	M	+	0	0	0	0	0	CHF	480	+	0	+	+	0	0	--	+	+	+
22	70	--†	--	--	M	+	+	0	0	0	0	Amyloidosis‡	430	0	+	0	+	0	0	0	+	0	+
23	74	62	12	1	F	+	+	+	+	0	0	AMI	--	+	0	+	0	0	0	--	+	+	+
24	75	47	28	2	F	0	+	0	+	0	0	Hip Fx	505	+	+	+	0	+	0	0	+	+	+
25	75	59	16	1	M	+	0	0	0	0	0	Infection	680	0	+	+	0	0	0	--	+	+	+
26	75	70	5	1	F	+	0	+	+	0	0	CHF	660	0	+	0	+	+	0	--	0	+	+
27	75	49	26	3	M	+	+	+	0	+	+	Hip Fx	700	0	+	+	+	0	0	--	+	+	+
28	78	72	6	2	M	+	0	0	0	0	0	CHF	680	+	+	+	0	+	+	--	+	0	0

*Electrocardiogram at age 43 was consistent with healed myocardial infarction.
†Electrocardiogram at age 67 was consistent with healed myocardial infarction.
‡No cardiac involvement.
A indicates anterior; AMI, acute myocardial infarction; AP, angina pectoris; CHF, chronic congestive heart failure; CSA, cross-sectional area; CVA, cardiovascular accident; DM, diabetes mellitus; Hip Fx, hip fracture; HW, heart weight; LAD, left anterior descending; LC, left circumflex; LM, left main; LV, left ventricular; P, posterior; SH, systemic hypertension; T, thrombus; VT, ventricular tachyarrhythmia; - -, no information available.

Table 2. Calcified myocardial infarcts at autopsy among patients having coronary artery bypass grafting

Case	Age at death (yr)	Age at first AMI (yr)	Interval of first AMI to death (yr)	Interval of CABG to death (yr)	No. of AMIs	Gender	CHF	AP	VT	SH	DM	Stroke	Mode of death	HW (g)	A	P	Apical	Basal	LV aneurysm	LV T	LM	LAD	LC	Right
															Location of calcified infarct				LV	LV	Coronary artery decreased >75% in CSA by plaque			
1	42	32	10	10	1	M	+	+	0	+	0	0	Sudden	735	+	+	+	+	0	0	+	+	+*	+
2	60	39	21	8	3	M	+	+	+	+	+	+	Stroke	695	+	+	+	0	+	+	+	+*	+*	+*
3	62	52	10	10	2	F	+	+	+	+	0	--	CHF	610	0	+	0	+	0	--	--	+*	+*	+
4	63	51	12	8	1	M	+	+	+	0	0	0	CHF	--	+	0	+	+	0	0	--	--	--	--
5	65	50	15	10	2	M	+	0	0	0	0	--	CHF	610	+	0	+	+	+†	0	--	+*	+	+
6	69	56	13	10	4	M	+	0	+	+	+	+	CHF	485	+	0	+	0	+†	0	0	+	+	+*
7	72	55	17	5	2	M	0	+	0	0	0	0	Cancer	390	0	+	0	+	+	0	0	+*	+*	+*
8	73	61	12	2 days	2	M	+	0	0	0	0	0	CHF	--	+	0	+	+	0	0	+	+*	0	+*
9	75	--	>20‡	20	3	M	--	--	--	--	0	0	Sudden	660	+	+	0	+	0	0	0	+*	--	+*

*Artery bypassed.

†Aneurysm excised at time of CABG.

‡Known myocardial infarction at time of CABG.

A indicates anterior; AMI, acute myocardial infarction; AP, angina pectoris; CABG, coronary artery bypass grafting; CHF, chronic congestive heart failure; CSA, cross-sectional area; DM, diabetes mellitus; HW, heart weight; LAD, left anterior descending; LC, left circumflex; LM, left main; LV, left ventricular; P, posterior; SH, systemic hypertension; T, thrombus; VT, ventricular tachyarrhythmia; - -, no information available.

Table 3. Comparison of findings in patients with and without coronary artery bypass grafting

	Coronary artery bypass grafting	
	No (n = 28)	Yes (n = 9)
Age (yr) at death: range (mean)	39–78 (62)	42–75 (65)
Women/men	5 (18%)/23 (82%)	1 (11%)/8 (89%)
Single myocardial infarct	17 (61%)	2 (22%)
Mean interval between first AMI and death (yr)	13	14
Age (yr) at first AMI: range (mean)	25–72 (48)	32–61 (50)
Chronic heart failure	20 (71%)	7 (78%)
Angina pectoris	7 (25%)	7 (78%)
Ventricular tachyarrhythmia	9 (32%)	4 (44%)
Systemic hypertension	10 (36%)	4 (44%)
Diabetes mellitus	5 (18%)	2 (22%)
Stroke	4 (14%)	2 (22%)
Mode of death		
Heart failure	9 (32%)	5 (56%)
Sudden	5 (18%)	2 (22%)
AMI	3 (11%)	0
Stroke	3 (11%)	1 (11%)
Noncardiovascular death	7 (25%)	1 (11%)
Heart weight (g)		
Women: range (mean)	310–660 (470)	610
Men: range (mean)	415–790 (562)	390–735 (596)
Location of calcified infarct		
Anterior only	14 (50%)	4 (44%)
Posterior only	9 (32%)	2 (22%)
Anterior + posterior	5 (18%)	3 (33%)
Apical only	9 (32%)	2 (22%)
Basal only	2 (7%)	3 (33%)
Apical + basal	17 (61%)	4 (44%)
Left ventricular aneurysm	12 (43%)	4 (44%)

AMI indicates acute myocardial infarction.

In 1908, Simmonds first described a patient with a calcified myocardial infarct grossly visible at autopsy (5). Over the next 96 years, 53 additional autopsy cases of calcified myocardial infarct were reported, including 21 cases previously reported by one of us (5) and included herein. Thus, grossly visible calcific myocardial infarcts are uncommonly seen at necropsy.

CABG probably did not alter the natural history of patients with calcified infarcts in the present study. The average age at death in the 9 patients in the CABG group was 65 years compared with 62 years in the 28 patients in the non-CABG group. Similarly, the interval between first infarct and death did not differ between the 2 groups (13 years in the non-CABG group vs 14 years in the CABG group).

Among the 37 patients with calcified myocardial infarcts included in the present study, most (84%) were men. Most had their first acute myocardial infarct at a relatively young age (range, 25–72 years; mean, 49; median, 50); only 5 (16%) of the 32 for which the information was known were >60 years of age at the time of their first acute myocardial infarct, presumably the one that later calcified. The 6 women ranged in age at the time of their first infarct from 50 to 70 years (mean, 56), and the 26 men,

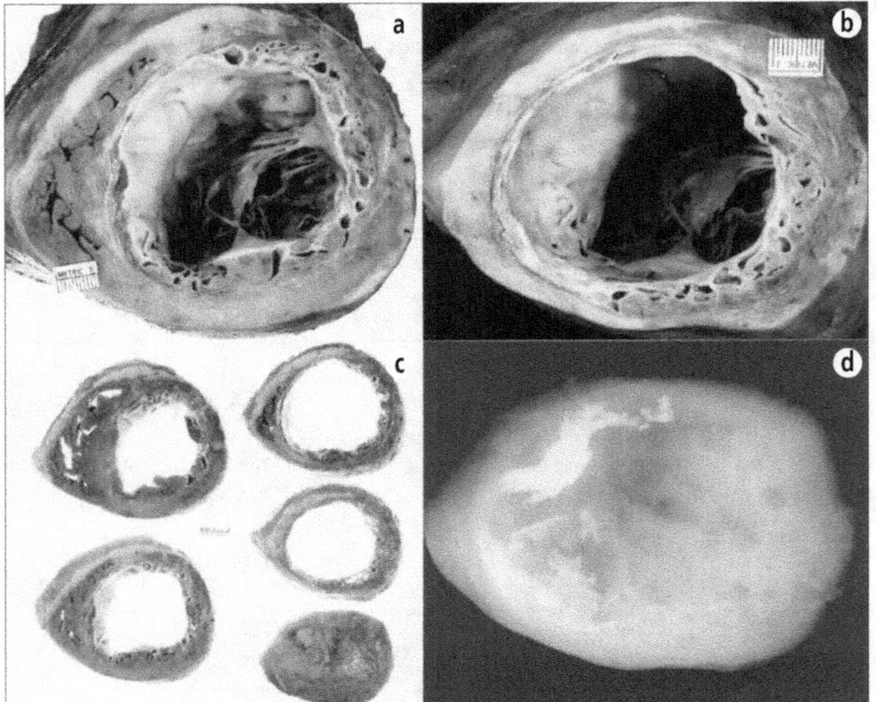

Figure 1. Case 1 in the coronary bypass group. Shown is the heart of a 42-year-old man who had had an acute myocardial infarct at age 32 and progressive heart failure thereafter. He died suddenly. **(a)** View of the left ventricular cavity from below showing marked dilatation and marked endocardial thickening and thinning of the ventricular septum. **(b)** A more apical view showing marked thinning of the left ventricular wall with heavy calcific deposits. **(c)** Views of slices of the ventricular walls showing marked left ventricular dilatation. **(d)** Radiograph of the heart specimen showing heavy calcific deposits primarily in the ventricular septum.

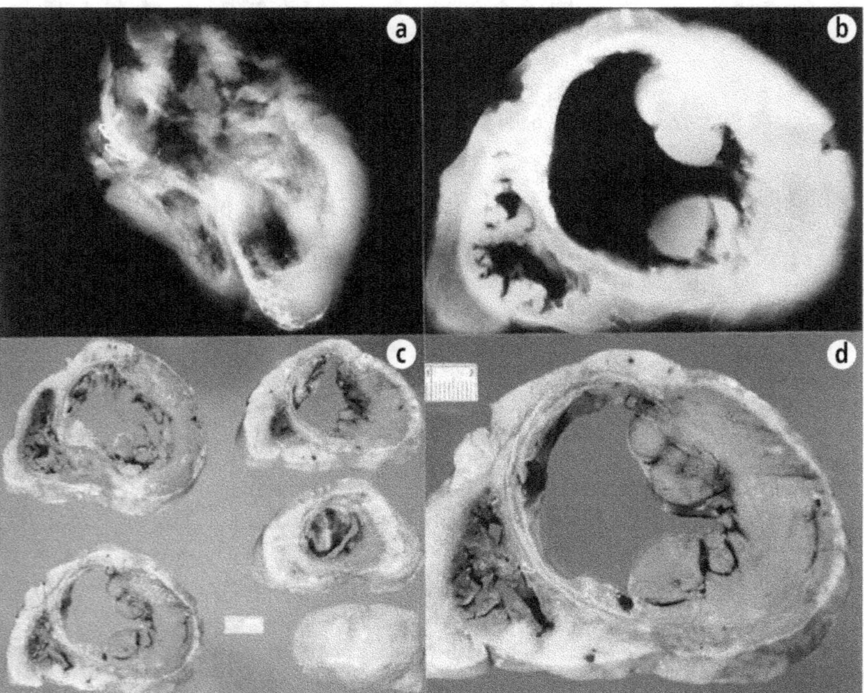

Figure 2. Case 2 in the coronary bypass group. This 60-year-old man had had an acute myocardial infarction at age 39 with chronic heart failure thereafter. He died of a stroke, presumably from embolic material originating in the left ventricular cavity overlying the calcified infarct. **(a)** Radiograph of the heart showing heavy calcific deposits in the anteroseptal wall. **(b)** Radiograph of one of the ventricular slices showing heavy calcific deposits in the anteroseptal wall. **(c)** Views of the ventricular walls showing marked thinning of the ventricular septum with heavy calcific deposits in that area with overlying thrombus in the more apical slices. **(d)** A close-up view showing the thinning of the anteroseptal wall with calcific deposits in the area of thinning.

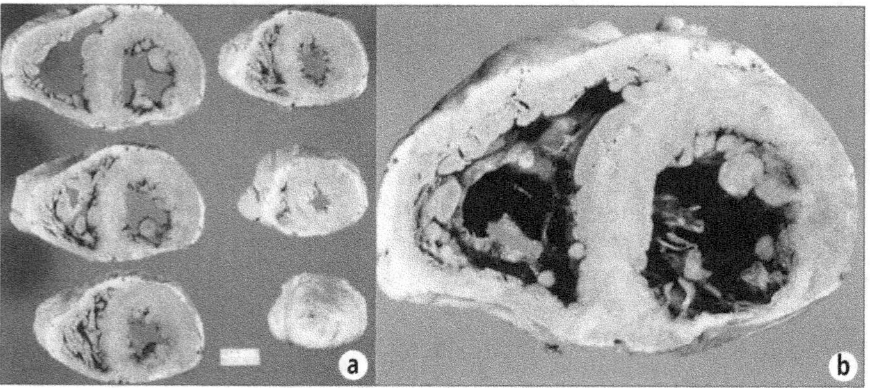

Figure 3. Case 22 in the noncoronary bypass group. This 70-year-old man had had an earlier infarct, but his age at the time was not known. He died of systemic amyloidosis rather than heart disease. There were no amyloid deposits in the myocardium. **(a)** Slices of the ventricular walls showing a healed infarct in the posterior portion of the left ventricular cavity. **(b)** A close-up view of the most basal portion of the ventricles. The posterior wall infarct is calcified. Both ventricular cavities are dilated.

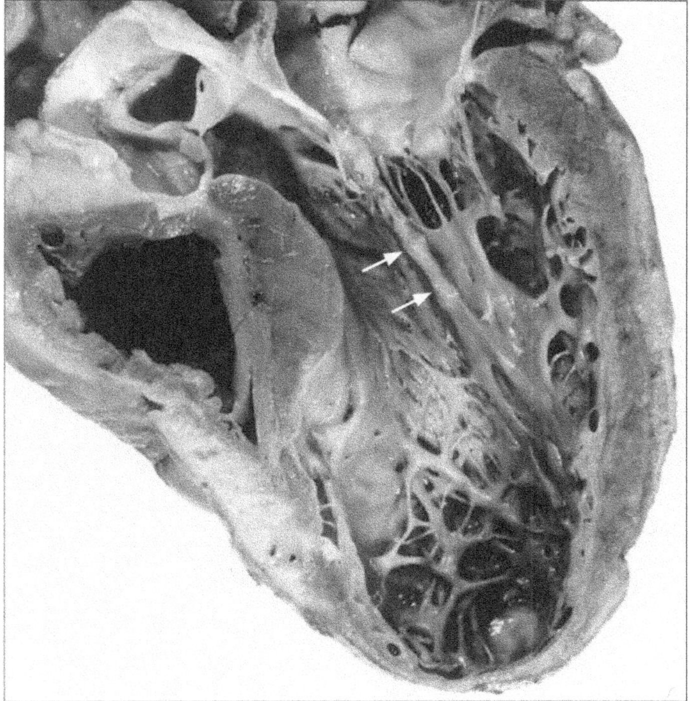

Figure 4. Case 24 in the noncoronary bypass group. The 75-year-old man whose heart is shown here had an acute myocardial infarction at age 47. The infarct involved the entire apical portion of the left ventricle, as well as the apical portion of the ventricular septum. A good bit of the infarcted wall is calcified. Calcium is also present in the posteromedial papillary muscle (arrows). The ventricular cavity is quite dilated. The patient died not from a cardiac condition but from consequences of a hip fracture.

from 25 to 72 years (mean, 47). Fifteen of the 26 men (58%) and only 1 of the 6 women were <50 years of age at the time of their first myocardial infarct.

The interval from the first acute myocardial infarction to death in the 32 patients for whom this information was available was much longer than in patients surviving acute myocardial infarction without calcification of the infarcted myocardium.

The intervals ranged from 2 to 28 years (mean, 13.5) and were similar in both men and women, 13.5 and 13.3 years, respectively. Thus, calcification of a myocardial infarct takes time and, from a prognostic standpoint, appears to be a favorable development despite the frequent association of ventricular arrhythmias, cardiomegaly, and left ventricular aneurysm.

Malignant ventricular arrhythmias were documented in 13 of the 37 patients (35%). These arrhythmias are recognized to be especially common in patients with dilated left ventricular cavities, particularly in the presence of left ventricular aneurysms, and the latter were present in 16 of the 37 patients (43%). Virtually all of the 21 patients without left ventricular aneurysms had dilated left ventricular cavities.

The hearts at necropsy were increased in weight (>350 g in women and >400 g in men) in 32 (94%) of the 34 patients for whom this information was available. The hearts in the 29 men ranged in weight from 390 to 790 g (mean, 568) and in the 5 women, from 310 to 660 g (mean, 498). At least 14 of the 37 patients (38%) had had a history of "elevated blood pressure" in the past, but none appeared to have had "hypertension" in their later months of life. Probably, most of the 37 patients had had hypertension at some time, but reliable information on this point was not available to us.

1. Roberts WC. The senile cardiac calcification syndrome. *Am J Cardiol* 1986;58: 572–574.
2. Lachman AS, Roberts WC. Calcific deposits in stenotic mitral valves. Extent and relation to age, sex, degree of stenosis, cardiac rhythm, previous commissurotomy and left atrial body thrombus from study of 164 operatively-excised valves. *Circulation* 1978;57:808–815.
3. Roberts WC, Ko JM. Weights of operatively-excised stenotic unicuspid, bicuspid, and tricuspid aortic valves and their relation to age, sex, body mass index, and presence or absence of concomitant coronary artery bypass grafting. *Am J Cardiol* 2003;92:1057–1065.
4. Roberts WC, Kaufman RJ. Calcification of healed myocardial infarcts. *Am J Cardiol* 1987;60:28–32.
5. Simmonds M. Uber der nachweis von verkalkungen am herzen durch das rontgenverfahren. *Fortschr Geb Rontgenstr* 1908;12:371–374.

Angina pectoris, dyspnea, fatigue, and edema after a non-ST-segment–elevation myocardial infarct

D. Luke Glancy, MD, and William C. Roberts, MD

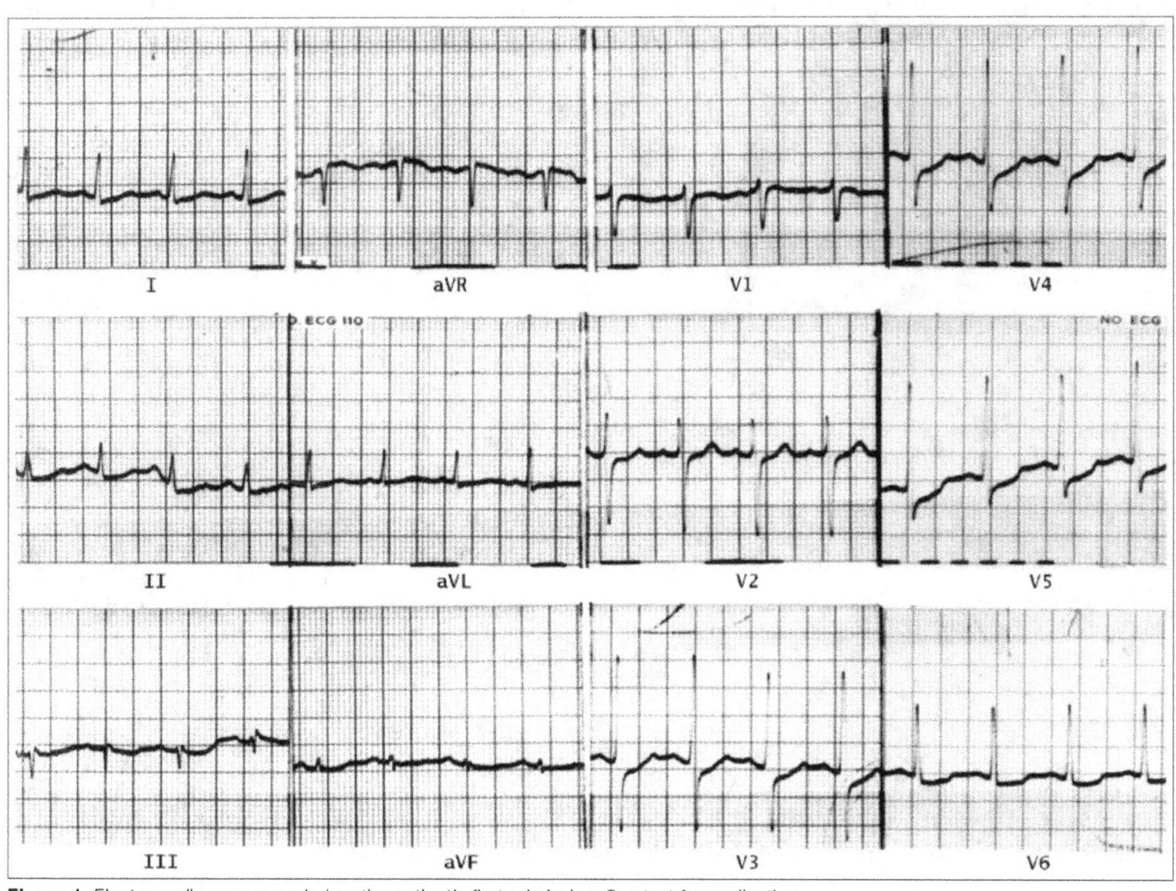

Figure 1. Electrocardiogram recorded on the patient's first admission. See text for explication.

A 65-year-old man came to the hospital because of retrosternal chest pain, and an electrocardiogram was recorded *(Figure 1)*. It showed sinus tachycardia and ST-segment depression in 8 leads (I, II, aVL, V_2–V_6) with slight reciprocal ST-segment elevation in lead aVR, findings of severe subendocardial ischemia and/or injury (1, 2). Serum markers confirmed non-ST-segment–elevation myocardial infarction. Despite the development of a systolic cardiac murmur, the patient had an uneventful recovery.

Over the ensuing 8 months, the patient had angina pectoris for the first time and gradually developed exertional dyspnea, fatigue, orthopnea, and marked peripheral edema. He returned to the hospital, and another electrocardiogram was recorded *(Figure 2)*. This one was quite different from the first electro-

cardiogram. Widespread ST-segment depression was no longer seen. The QRS axis in the frontal plane had shifted from approximately +10 degrees to about +75 degrees. The S wave in lead V_1 had shrunk, while the S waves in leads I, aVL, V_5, and

From the Section of Cardiology, Department of Medicine, Louisiana State University Health Sciences Center, New Orleans, Louisiana (Glancy) and the Baylor Heart and Vascular Institute, Baylor University Medical Center, Dallas, Texas (Roberts).

The patient described in this report is case 8 in the study cited in reference 3. The electrocardiograms and chest radiographs have not been published before.

Corresponding author: D. Luke Glancy, MD, Section of Cardiology, Department of Medicine, Louisiana State University Health Sciences Center, 1542 Tulane Avenue, Room 436, New Orleans, Louisiana 70112.

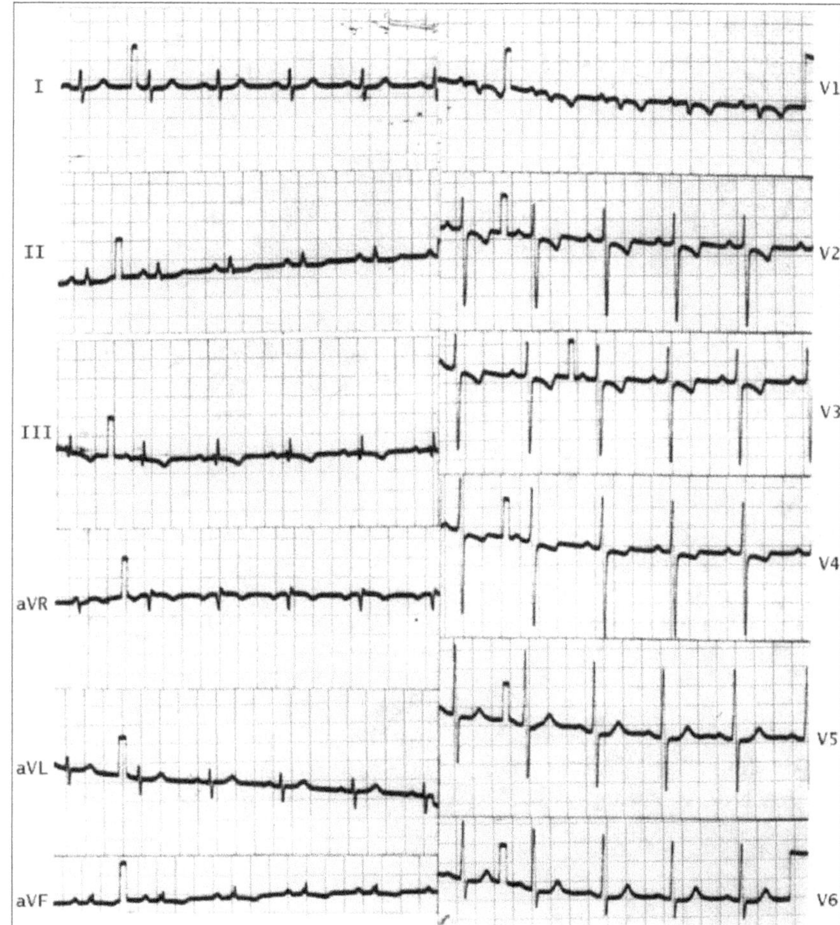

Figure 2. Electrocardiogram recorded on the patient's second admission. See text for explication.

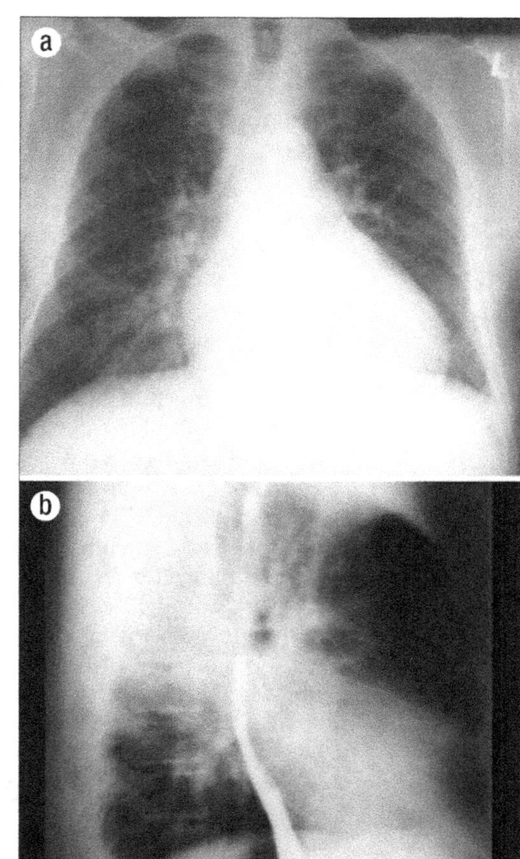

Figure 3. Chest radiographs taken during the patient's second admission. **(a)** The posteroanterior view shows plethoric lungs, prominent pulmonary arteries, and generalized cardiomegaly. **(b)** The lateral view shows indentation of the barium-filled esophagus by the enlarged left atrium.

V_6 had increased. T waves were now inverted in leads V_1 to V_4. These are signs of right ventricular enlargement.

What is the cause of the right ventricular enlargement? The most likely pulmonary cause of such a change in 8 months would be pulmonary embolic disease. The chest radiograph, however, showed pulmonary plethora rather than oligemia, and all of the cardiac chambers were large, including the left atrium *(Figure 3)*. Furthermore, a loud apical systolic murmur of mitral regurgitation had a definitely decrescendo quality, suggesting a large left atrial v wave with significant left atrial and, consequently, pulmonary arterial hypertension. This supposition was confirmed by pressures (in mm Hg) measured at cardiac catheterization: pulmonary arterial wedge mean of 35 with v waves of 60 and pulmonary arterial pressure of 95/40 with a mean of 60. A left ventriculogram showed severe mitral regurgitation and normal left ventricular systolic function (3).

At operation, a fibrotic posteromedial papillary muscle was found to be the cause of the severe mitral regurgitation. The valve was replaced, and the patient improved symptomatically

and hemodynamically (3). Thus, although the patient underwent operation 35 years ago without the benefit of myocardial revascularization, he was part of a study demonstrating that left ventricular function is the most important determinant of outcome in patients with ischemic mitral regurgitation.

1. Gorgels APM, Vos MA, Mulleneers R, de Zwaan C, Bar FWHM, Wellens HJJ. Value of the electrocardiogram in diagnosing the number of severely narrowed coronary arteries in rest angina pectoris. *Am J Cardiol* 1993;72: 999–1003.
2. Barrabes JA, Figueras J, Moure C, Cortedellas J, Soler-Soler J. Prognostic value of lead aVR in patients with a first non-ST-segment elevation acute myocardial infarction. *Circulation* 2003;108:814–819.
3. Glancy DL, Stinson EB, Shepherd RL, Itscoitz SB, Roberts WC, Epstein SE, Morrow AG. Results of valve replacement for severe mitral regurgitation due to papillary muscle rupture or fibrosis. *Am J Cardiol* 1973;32: 313–321.

Quantitative Comparison of Amounts of Cross-Sectional Area Narrowing in Coronary Endarterectomy Specimens in Patients Having Coronary Artery Bypass Grafting to Amounts of Narrowing in the Same Artery in Patients with Fatal Coronary Artery Disease Studied at Necropsy

William Clifford Roberts, MD[a,b,d,]*, Thomas Alpert Turnage II, BA[d], and
Lonnie Lee Whiddon, MD[c,†]

This study compares the amounts of cross-sectional area narrowing of the right coronary artery (RCA) in patients having endarterectomy of this artery at the time of coronary artery bypass grafting (CABG) to the amounts of narrowing in the same artery at necropsy in patients with fatal coronary artery disease (CAD). We examined histologically each 5-mm segment of endarterectomy specimens of the RCA in 39 patients having this procedure at the time of CABG and compared findings in them to the amounts of narrowing of 5-mm segments of the RCA in 141 patients with fatal CAD studied at necropsy. Of the 564 five-mm RCA segments in the endarterectomy patients, 371 (66%) were narrowed >75% in cross-sectional area by atherosclerotic plaque: another 112 (20%), 51% to 75%; 64 (11%), 26% to 50%, and 17 (3%), 1% to 25%. In contrast, of 2,699 five-mm segments of the RCA in 141 patients with fatal CAD, 1,217 (45%) were narrowed >75% in the cross-sectional area; another 966 (36%), 51% to 75%; 405 (15%), 26% to 50%, and 114 (4%), 1% to 25% by plaque. In conclusion, the amounts of severe narrowing found in coronary endarterectomy specimens excised at the time of CABG in live patients is at least as great as that found using the same technique in patients with fatal CAD studied at necropsy. This observation suggests that an even greater emphasis should be placed on primary prevention of atherosclerotic events and, indeed, of atherosclerotic plaques.   © 2007 Elsevier Inc. All rights reserved. (Am J Cardiol 2007;99:588–592)

Endarterectomy is a procedure to excise atherosclerotic plaque in an artery. It is performed most commonly in a carotid artery followed less commonly in other peripheral arteries. Coronary artery bypass grafting (CABG) is performed far more commonly than carotid endarterectomy, but coronary endarterectomy is infrequently performed. When endarterectomy is performed on a coronary artery, the artery is generally the *right* coronary artery (RCA). The purpose of this report is to describe quantitatively the amounts of cross-sectional area narrowing found in endarterectomy specimens of the RCA in patients who had this procedure at the time of CABG. Additionally, the amounts of narrowing are compared to the amounts of cross-sectional area narrowing of the RCA previously reported by 1 of us (WCR) in patients at autopsy with fatal coronary events. The hypothesis is that the amount of narrowing in the RCA in the living patients having coronary endarterectomy is similar to that in the same artery in patients with fatal coronary artery disease (CAD) studied at necropsy.

Methods

From January 1994 until May 2005, a total of 10,665 patients underwent CABG at Baylor University Medical Center (Dallas, Texas). Of this number, 167 (1.6%) patients underwent coronary endarterectomy of ≥1 epicardial coronary arteries at the time of CABG. Of these endarterectomy specimens, the RCA with or without portions of the posterior descending coronary artery were included in at least 92 (55%). Of the RCA endarterectomy specimens, 39 (42%) were divided into 5-mm long segments; each was processed in alchohols and xylene, embedded in paraffin blocks, and one 6-μm thick section was cut and stained by hematoxylin and eosin and another by the Movat method from each 5-mm long segment. Each prepared histologic section was examined by 1 of us (WCR), and the amounts of narrowing were determined from the Movat stained section because this section clearly outlines the internal elastic membrane. Each Movat stained cross section prepared from each 5-mm long coronary segment was mentally divided into 4 quadrants (0 to 25, 26 to 50, 51 to 75, and 76 to 100), and the amount of narrowing in each segment was recorded. The segments narrowed >75% in cross-sectional area were further subdivided into those narrowed 76% to 95% and into those narrowed >95% in cross-sectional area.

The original data tables were retrieved in published studies on quantitation of amounts of coronary narrowing in necropsy patients with fatal CAD performed in the Pathology Branch, National Heart, Lung, and Blood Institute, by 1

Departments of [a]Pathology, [b]Internal Medicine (Division of Cardiology) and [c]Cardiothoracic Surgery, and the [d]Baylor Heart & Vascular Institute, Baylor University Medical Center, Dallas, Texas. Manuscript accepted October 4, 2006.

*Corresponding author: Tel: 214-820-7911; fax: 214-820-7533.
E-mail address: wc.roberts@baylorhealth.edu (W.C. Roberts).

† Present address: Loyola University, New Orleans, Louisiana.

Table 1

Data in each of the 39 patients having coronary endarterectomy and 5-mm segments of right coronary artery studied histologically

Case	Age (Years) at CABG/Sex	Length (cm) Endarterectomy Specimen	No. of 5-mm Segments	No. of 5-mm Segments Narrowed to Various CSA categories					No. of 5-mm Segments With Calcium (1+–4+)	No. of 5-mm Segments With Media (circumferential media)
				0–25%	26–50%	51–75%	76–95%	>95%		
1	40M	9	20	0	0	1	17	2	2 (1+)	17 (9)
2	47M	10	23	0	0	2	20	1	3 (2+)	21 (8)
3	48M	8	16	0	0	9	7	0	0	12 (5)
4	49M	9	15	0	0	0	11	4	11 (4+)	11 (0)
5	53M	6	14	0	0	2	10	2	13	9 (1)
6	53M	10	20	0	2	4	7	7	2 (1+)	13 (3)
7	53F	3	4	0	0	0	1	3	4 (4+)	2 (0)
8	55M	4	7	1	0	0	3	3	0	3 (1)
9	55M	8	16	1	7	6	2	0	1 (1+)	16 (14)
10	56M	4	10	0	1	0	6	3	9 (4+)	9 (4)
11	59M	6	20	1	0	3	4	12	14 (4+)	6 (1)
12	61M	9	10	2	4	2	2	0	8	7 (5)
13	62M	10	8	0	0	4	4	0	1 (1+)	8 (6)
14	63M	6	11	0	1	0	10	0	8 (4+)	1 (0)
15	64M	2	6	0	0	0	3	3	2 (2+)	3 (1)
16	65M	4	5	0	1	1	3	0	0	3 (2)
17	65M	7	28	0	1	3	19	5	15 (4+)	22 (13)
18	65M	8	17	0	0	2	8	7	16 (4+)	17 (2)
19	66M	5	11	0	1	7	3	0	1 (4+)	11 (8)
20	67M	4	11	0	0	7	4	0	4 (3+)	6 (4)
21	68M	7	15	0	0	3	10	2	10 (4+)	6 (1)
22	68M	6	7	0	0	0	2	5	7 (4+)	5 (2)
23	68M	4	17	0	1	4	10	2	17 (4+)	15 (11)
24	68M	6	12	0	2	3	7	0	10 (4+)	13 (12)
25	69M	2	9	0	2	2	5	0	8 (4+)	5 (2)
26	70M	7	20	0	0	3	7	10	7 (2+)	18 (9)
27	71M	4	11	0	0	1	5	5	10 (4+)	4 (1)
28	73M	5	17	2	2	9	4	0	4 (2+)	10 (8)
29	73M	7	14	0	0	3	9	2	11 (4+)	9 (2)
30	73F	3	5	4	1	0	0	0	0	5 (5)
31	74M	7	16	0	0	1	13	2	8 (4+)	11 (1)
32	75F	8	22	0	0	3	11	8	9	22 (8)
33	76M	11	18	2	7	4	5	0	17 (4+)	13 (3)
34	77F	9	18	0	5	7	6	0	7 (3+)	15 (9)
35	78M	13	24	1	17	6	0	0	2 (1+)	24 (24)
36	79M	5	14	0	0	2	12	0	14 (4+)	12 (0)
37	80M	12	24	0	1	5	16	2	16 (4+)	18 (5)
38	82M	11	21	0	5	1	8	7	14 (4+)	11 (0)
39	83M	5	8	3	3	2	0	0	2 (3+)	5 (3)
	Mean 65	Mean 7	564	17	64	112	274	97	287	418 (193)
				3%	11%	20%	49%	17%	51%	74%

of us (WCR). These studies included histologic examination of each 5-mm coronary segment of the right, left main, left anterior descending, and left circumflex coronary arteries in patients with fatal acute myocardial infarction,[1] healed myocardial infarction,[2] sudden coronary death,[3] and unstable angina pectoris.[4] The data on the amounts of cross-sectional area narrowing of each 5-mm segment of the RCA only were retrieved.

The study protocol was approved by the Institutional Review Board of Baylor University Medical Center.

The authors had full access to the data and take responsibility for its integrity. All authors have read and agree to the manuscript as written.

Results

Findings in the 5-mm segments of the RCA in each of the 39 patients having coronary endarterectomy are shown in Table 1. The 39 patients ranged in age at the time of CABG from 40 to 83 years (mean 65); 35 were men and 4 were women. The endarterectomy specimens from the RCA with or without the posterior descending coronary artery measured from 2.0 to 13.0 cm (mean 7) in length (Figure 1). The number of 5-mm long segments from these specimens ranged from 5 to 28 (mean 14) per patient or per endarterectomy specimen. The cross-sectional area narrowing of each segment was determined

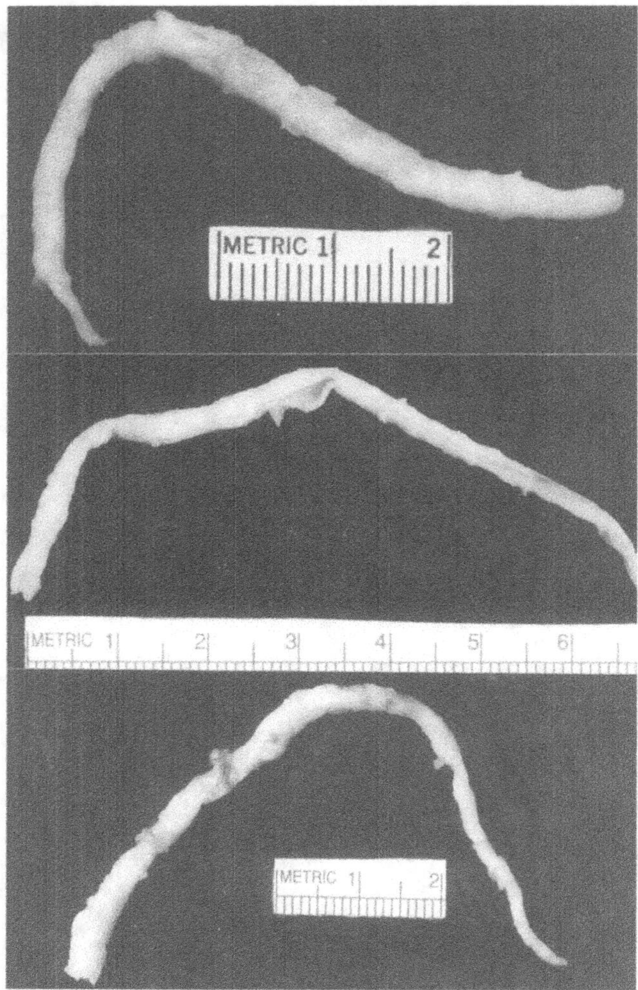

Figure 1. Right coronary arteries excised by endarterectomy procedure in 3 patients. *Top,* in a 48-year-old man; *Middle,* in a 73-year-old man; and *Bottom,* in a 53-year-old man.

from examination of the Movat-stained 6-μm thick section, 1 per 5-mm segment (Figure 2). Of the total of 564 segments, the amounts of cross-sectional area narrowing were as follows: 17 segments (3%) were narrowed 1% to 25%; 64 (11%) from 26% to 50%; 112 (20%), 51% to 75%; and 371 (66%), from 76% to 100%. Of the latter group, 274 segments (49%) were narrowed 76% to 95% and 97 (17%) were narrowed >95% in the cross-sectional area. Of the 564 five-mm segments, none was devoid of atherosclerotic plaque.

Calcium, confirmed by examination of the hemotoxylin-eosin sections, was present in 287 (51%) of the 564 segments and in 35 (90%) of the 39 patients. The calcific deposits were extensive (4+/4+) in at least 19 (54%) of the 35 patients with coronary calcium.

Of the 564 Movat-stained sections of the 564 five-mm long segments, 418 (74%) contained media, including 193 (46%) of the 418 sections in which the media was present over the entire circumference of the section. The dissection plane was the media in all 418 segments, and those without media at least contained the internal elastic membrane.

Thrombus was present in the residual lumen in 2 of the 39 patients, and these patients also were the only ones with plaque rupture with hemorrhage also into the plaque. The thrombus, plaque rupture, and plaque hemorrhage involved 4 five-mm segments. Thus, these acute lesions were present in 4 of the 564 five-mm segments or 560 of the 564 segments contained no acute lesions.

The findings in the 5-mm segments of RCA in the 141 previously reported patients with fatal coronary events are summarized in Table 2. In contrast to the 66% of the 5-mm segments of RCA narrowed >75% in the cross-sectional area by atherosclerotic plaque in the 39 coronary endarterectomy patients, the percent of 5-mm segments of the RCA narrowed >75% by plaque in the 141 patients with various fatal coronary events varied from 38% (acute myocardial infarction and sudden coronary death) to ≥50% (healed myocardial infarction and unstable angina pectoris). Additionally, none of the 2,699 five-mm RCA segments in the 141 patients with fatal coronary events was devoid of atherosclerotic plaque.

Discussion

This study describes, for the first time, the amounts of cross-sectional area narrowing by atherosclerotic plaque in endarterectomy specimens of the RCA in live patients having this procedure at the time of CABG, and it compares the amounts of cross-sectional area narrowing seen in them to that observed at necropsy in the same coronary artery among previously reported patients with fatal coronary events. The results of this study disclose that the percent of 5-mm segments of RCA narrowed >75% in the cross-sectional area by plaque in the endarterectomy specimens was at least as great as that observed in the same artery among patients with fatal coronary events (66% [371 of 564 segments] vs 45% [1,217 of 2,699 segments]).

It is important to realize that the "endarterectomy" specimens are not limited to intima, for if that were the case, it would not be possible to compare the amounts of cross-sectional area narrowing in them to that observed at necropsy. All of the 5-mm segments of the endarterectomy specimens contained internal elastic membrane with or without varying portions of media. In contrast to the necropsy specimens, however, the full thickness of the media was rarely present as evidenced by the absence of the external elastic membrane in all the endarterectomy specimens. The presence of the internal elastic membrane in the 5-mm segments of the endarterectomy specimens allows this coronary artery to be examined during life by the same technique, which was previously reserved only for necropsy examination. The present study indicates that the amounts of severe narrowing of the RCA in endarterectomy specimens excised at the time of CABG are similar to that observed in the same artery when studied at necropsy in patients with fatal CAD.

A possible conclusion from the present study is that the amounts of severe coronary narrowing in patients with coronary events leading to CABG is similar to that observed in patients with fatal coronary events. In other words, the amounts of severe coronary narrowing observed in patients with non-fatal coronary events may be similar to that ob-

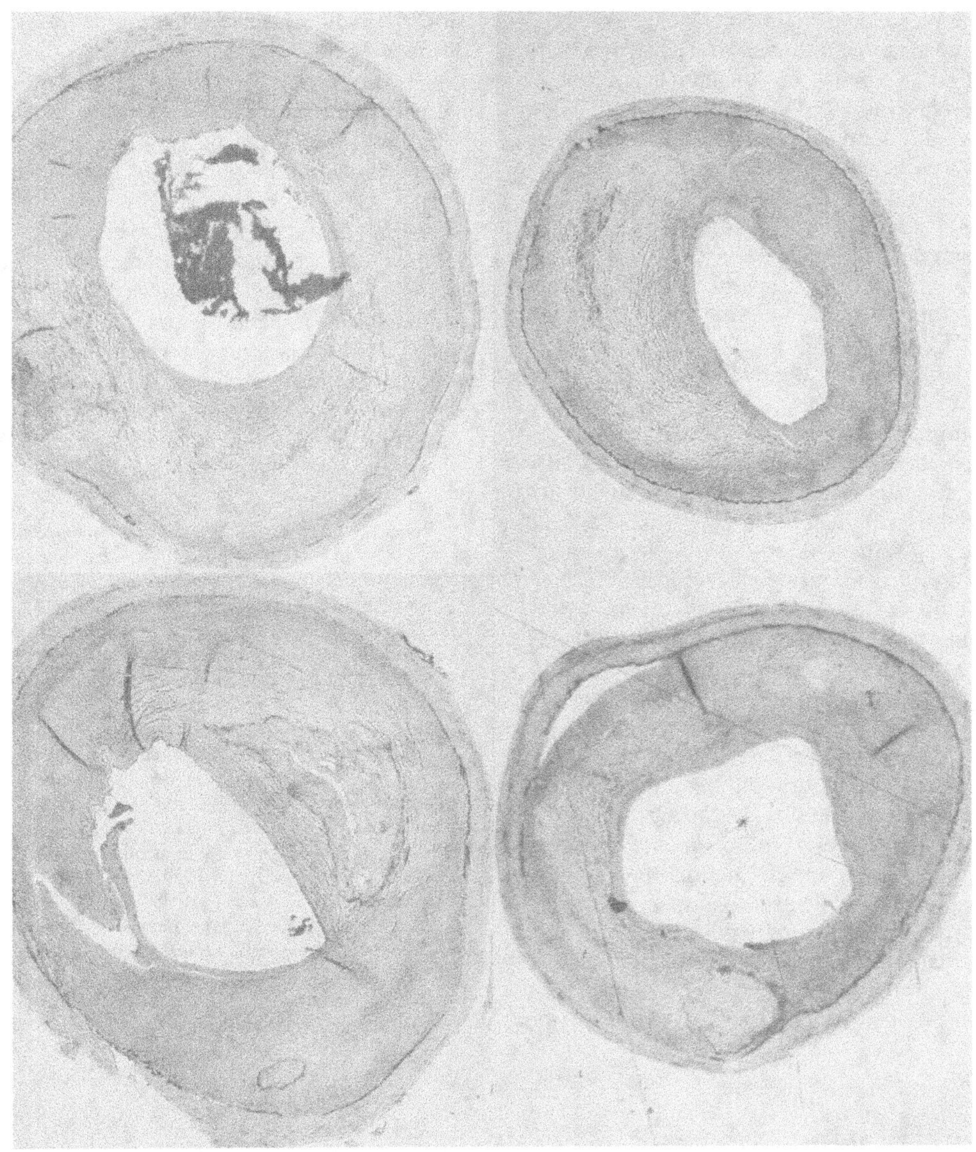

Figure 2. Four sections among 15 five-mm long cross sections of right coronary artery obtained by endarterectomy in patient #21 (Table 1), a 68-year-old man. The endarterectomy specimen was 4 cm in length. The lumen of each artery is narrowed by plaque that consists mainly of fibrous tissue. The black-staining internal elastic membrane is clearly visible in each, and the muscular media is present circumferentially in each. The external elastic membrane and adventitia is absent in each cross-section. Movat stains, each ×40.

Table 2

Quantitative comparison of the numbers and percentages of 5-mm long segments of the right coronary artery narrowed to four categories of cross-sectional area narrowing by atherosclerotic plaques in 39 live patients having coronary endarterectomy versus 141 patients having various fatal coronary events

Four Categories of Cross-Sectional Area Narrowing of the 5-mm Coronary Segments	Coronary Endarterectomy (n = 39)	Acute Myocardial Infarction (n = 27)	Healed Myocardial Infarction (n = 61)	Sudden Coronary Death (n = 31)	Unstable Angina Pectoris (n = 22)
76–100%	371 (66%)	210 (38%)	568 (50%)	232 (38%)	204 (52%)
51–75%	112 (20%)	230 (41%)	391 (34%)	238 (38%)	107 (28%)
26–50%	64 (11%)	100 (18%)	139 (12%)	124 (20%)	42 (11%)
0–25%	17 (3%)	14 (3%)	38 (3%)	25 (4%)	37 (9%)
5-mm segments	564	554	1,136	619	390

served in patients with fatal coronary events. Because the amounts of severe coronary narrowing differs little in patients with fatal and non-fatal coronary events (at least in those having CABG), an even greater emphasis on primary prevention, i.e., prevention of the first atherosclerotic event, appears warranted.

Some limitations need consideration. One could argue that the reason the coronary endarterectomy was performed was that the amount of narrowing encountered at the time of CABG was so severe that anastomosis of the bypass conduit to the distal RCA would not have been possible without the endarterectomy. We believe that to be an unlikely scenario. One of us (LLW) advocates coronary endarterectomy whenever feasible; in other words, the decision to do endarterectomy is simply an operative *preference*. Other cardiovascular surgeons with similarly good operative results do not advocate endarterectomy and rarely if ever do this procedure at the time of CABG.

Another limitation was that the endarterectomy series was not consecutive. We find this consideration, however, an unlikely limitation. In the early years, a number of endarterectomy specimens were simply laid aside after gross photography for later submission for histologic processing. In the several-year interval between excision and reexamination many specimens dried out (due to an unfortunate loss of air conditioning in the storage facility).

Another consideration is that the amounts of cross-sectional area narrowing by plaque were overestimated. If that were the case, one would have to conclude that the amounts of narrowing in the 5-mm segments of RCA in the 141 patients with fatal coronary events were also overestimated because all of the studies involved the same author (WCR) and the same laboratory. Estimating the amounts of cross-sectional area narrowing by microscopic examination has been found in a previous study to be almost as accurate as that determined by computer tracings.[5] Neither the coronary endarterectomy specimens nor the necropsy specimens were fixed in formaldehyde after pressure expansion. The 5-mm coronary segments that are the most narrowed, namely those >75% obliterated in cross-sectional area, are the least likely, however, to produce retraction of a portion of the artery's wall that may lead to an overestimation of the luminal stenosis.

The present study compares the quantity of plaque or the degree of cross-sectional luminal narrowing only in the RCA in the endarterectomy specimens in the live patients to that observed in the same artery at necropsy in patients with fatal CAD. The reason specimens of the left anterior descending or other left sided coronary arteries were not studied was because endarterectomy specimens from the non-RCA coronary arteries are usually very short (only about 1 cm in length) and the location of the excised specimen in this artery is rarely known. Furthermore, the external diameter of the RCA is about the same throughout its entire length, whereas the left anterior descending and other epicardial coronary arteries on the left side of the heart taper fairly rapidly.

1. Roberts WC, Jones AA. Quantification of coronary arterial narrowing at necropsy in acute transmural myocardial infarction: analysis and comparison of findings in 27 patients and 22 controls. *Circulation* 1980;61: 786–790.
2. Cabin HS, Roberts WC. Quantitative comparison of extent of coronary narrowing and size of healed myocardial infarct in 33 necropsy patients with clinically recognized and in 28 with clinically unrecognized ("silent") previous acute myocardial infarction. *Am J Cardiol* 1982;50:677–681.
3. Roberts WC, Jones AA. Quantitation of coronary arterial narrowing at necropsy in sudden coronary death. Analysis of 31 patients and comparison with 25 control subjects. *Am J Cardiol* 1979;44:39–45.
4. Roberts WC, Virmani R. Quantification of coronary arterial narrowing in clinically-isolated unstable angina pectoris. An analysis of 22 necropsy patients. *Am J Med* 1979;67:792–799.
5. Isner JM, Wu M, Virmani R, Jones AA, Roberts WC. Comparison of degrees of coronary arterial luminal narrowing determined by visual inspection of histologic sections under magnification among three independent observers and comparison to that obtained by video planimetry. An analysis of 559 five-millimeter segments of 61 coronary arteries from eleven patients. *Laboratory Invest* 1980;42:566–570.

Fatal Cardiac Arrest in the Hospital During Transfer from Gurney to Operating Table for Planned Coronary Artery Bypass Grafting and Mitral Valve Repair

William Clifford Roberts, MD;[1,2,3] Sharenda Lana Williams, MD;[2] Jong Mi Ko;[3] Johannes Jacob Kuiper, MD[1]

From the Department of Internal Medicine, the Division of Cardiology,[1] and the Department of Pathology;[2] and the Baylor Heart and Vascular Institute,[3] Baylor University Medical Center, Dallas, TX

Address for correspondence: William Clifford Roberts, MD, Baylor Heart and Vascular Institute, Baylor University Medical Center, 621 North Hall Street, Suite H-030, Dallas, TX 75226

E-mail: wc.roberts@baylorhealth.edu

A 76-year-old white man, who was born on March 3, 1930, and died on April 6, 2006, was apparently in his usual state of health until 1979, when at age 49 he had an acute myocardial infarction. In 1995, at age 65, chronic obstructive pulmonary disease was diagnosed and a left upper lobe noncancerous infiltrate was found and resected. He quit smoking at the time.

In March 2006 (age 76), the patient's chronic mild dyspnea worsened, a cough productive of green sputum developed, and he was hospitalized on March 21. A chest radiograph (Figure 1) disclosed near consolidation of the left lung with fluid-filled cavities (Figure 2) and he was intubated. His body mass index was 24 kg/m², and blood pressure was 85/65 mm Hg. A grade 2/6 holosystolic murmur was heard at the right sternal border. There was no subcutaneous edema. The leukocyte count was 23,000 m³, and the following levels were recorded: blood hematocrit, 43%; serum creatinine, 1.6 mg/dL; and troponin, 6.6 ng/mL, rising to 10 ng/mL. Electrocardiography showed sinus tachycardia; nonspecific T wave changes; small Q waves in leads 2, 3, and aVF; and no ST segment changes. Transthoracic echocardiography demonstrated normal left ventricular function despite posterior wall hypokinesis and mild to moderate mitral regurgitation and tricuspid regurgitation. Both right and left ventricular cavities were of normal size and both atria were

dilated. Cardiac catheterization (performed on March 31, 2006) disclosed the following pressures (in mm Hg): mean right atrial, 15; a wave, 14; v wave, 14; right ventricle, 43/16; pulmonary trunk, 43/31; mean pulmonary artery wedge, 22; a wave, 25; v wave, 24; aorta, 95/60. Left ventricular angiogram showed mild posterior wall hypokinesia, and severe (4+/4+) mitral regurgitation. Coronary angiography disclosed the following maximal diameter narrowings: left main, 95%; left anterior descending, >75%; left circumflex (proximal), 100%; and right, 100%. Both common iliac

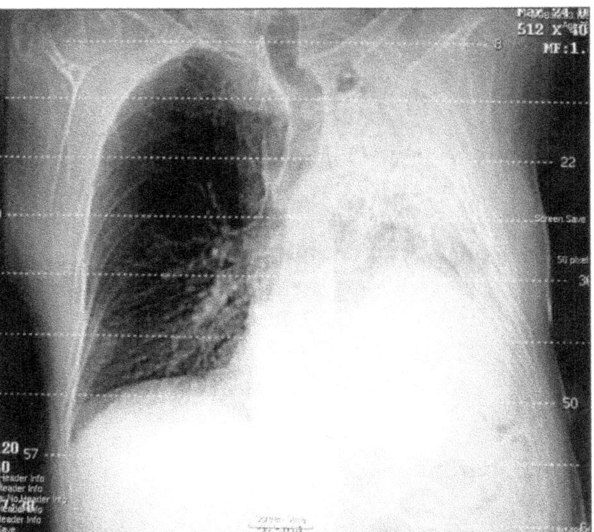

Figure 1. Chest radiograph performed 12 days before death, showing consolidation of most of the left lung.

www.lejacq.com   ID: 6222

arteries were narrowed (right, 80%; left, 60%). The former was dilated and an intra-aortic balloon pump inserted. Coronary bypass and mitral valve repair had been planned, but the patient arrested in the operating room before the operation was started.

At necropsy, both lungs contained bullae and focal organizing pneumonia (Figure 3). The coronary arteries (Figure 4) were removed from the 400-g heart, divided into 5-mm sections, and examined histologically (one section/5-mm segment) (Figure 5, Figure 6, Figure 7, Figure 8). Before the coronary arteries were removed, the cardiac ventricles were divided into 1-cm-thick cross-sections cut parallel to the posterior atrioventricular sulcus. The left ventricular cavity was of normal size and its wall was posteriorly thinned and focally scarred. The right ventricular cavity was mildly dilated (Figure 9). A radiograph of the base of the heart showed extensive calcific deposits in the 4 major epicardial coronary arteries, including the left main (Figure 10). Radiographs of the aorta and common iliac arteries showed focal but heavy calcific deposits (Figure 11, Figure 12).

COMMENTS

The hitherto described patient had severe coronary arterial disease and acute and chronic pulmonary disease. At age 49, an acute myocardial infarction was diagnosed and thereafter he was free of symptoms of myocardial ischemia for 27 years until his final illness prompted by pneumonia. Necropsy disclosed a small healed posterior wall infarct with some myofiber necrosis (acute myocardial infarction) at the borders of the healed infarct. To survive 27 years after an acute myocardial infarct is most unusual, assuming the accuracy of the history. McManus and Roberts[1] were able to document only 8 patients who survived 20 years or more after an acute myocardial infarct.

The degree of coronary narrowing in the patient described appeared out of proportion to the amount of myocardial damage, which was insufficient to result in dilation of the left ventricular cavity. The left main was severely narrowed (>95% in diameter), and that degree of narrowing is usually indicative of severe narrowing of the other 3 major coronary arteries (right, left anterior descending, and left circumflex), which certainly was the case in this patient.[2] The coronary atherosclerotic process was diffuse and extensive in the present case, as demonstrated by the finding that not a single 5-mm segment of any of the 4 major coronary arteries was devoid of plaque.[3] Plaque in

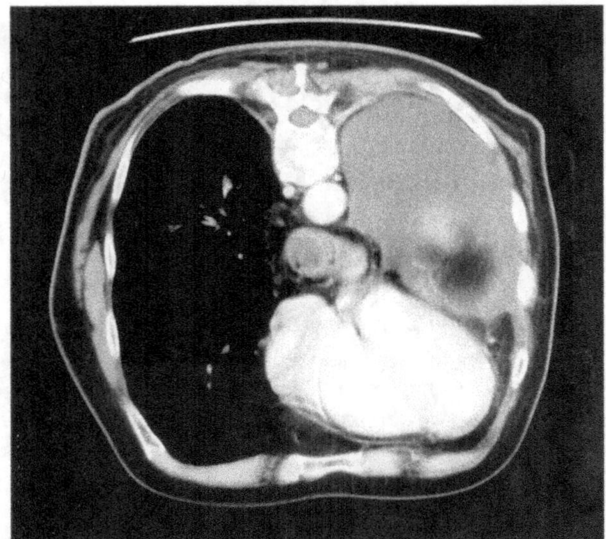

Figure 2. *Computed tomographic image showing consolidated left lung with abscess.*

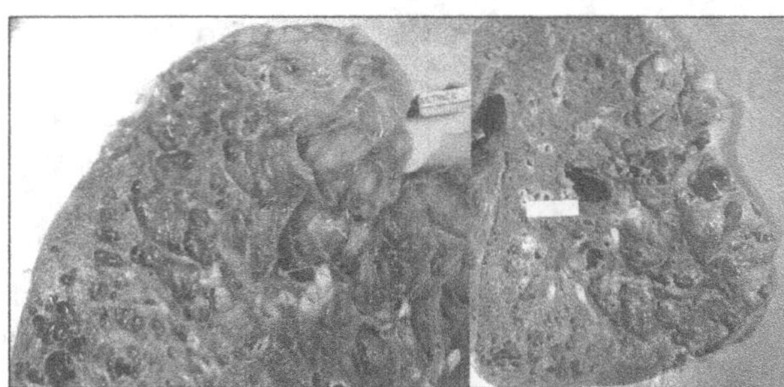

Figure 3. *Close-up view of the apex of the right lung (left) and of the base of the left lower lobe of the left lung (right) showing bullous emphysema.*

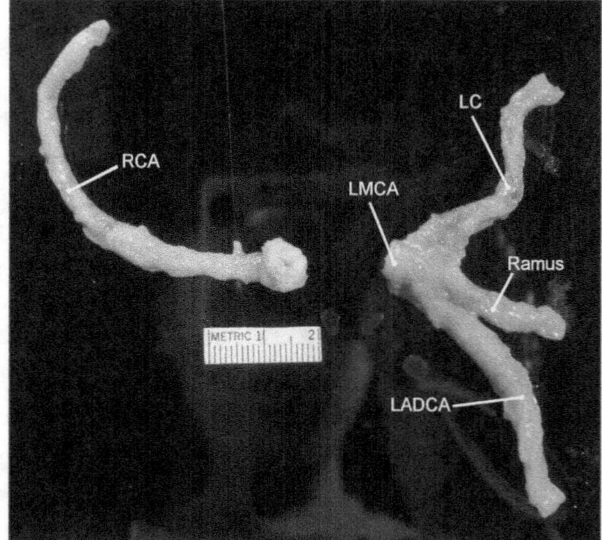

Figure 4. *Portions of the major epicardial coronary arteries after their removal from the heart. RCA indicates right coronary artery; LMCA, left main coronary artery; LC, left circumflex coronary artery; and LADCA, left anterior descending coronary artery.*

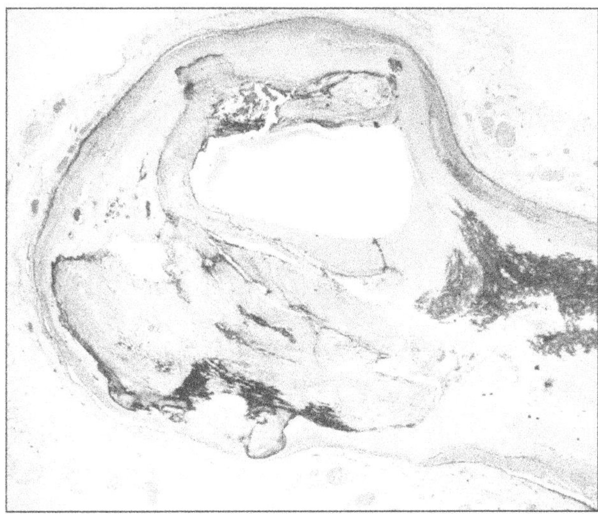

Figure 5. Photomicrograph of the left main coronary artery with the origin of the left anterior descending coronary artery. (Movat stain; original magnification ×20).

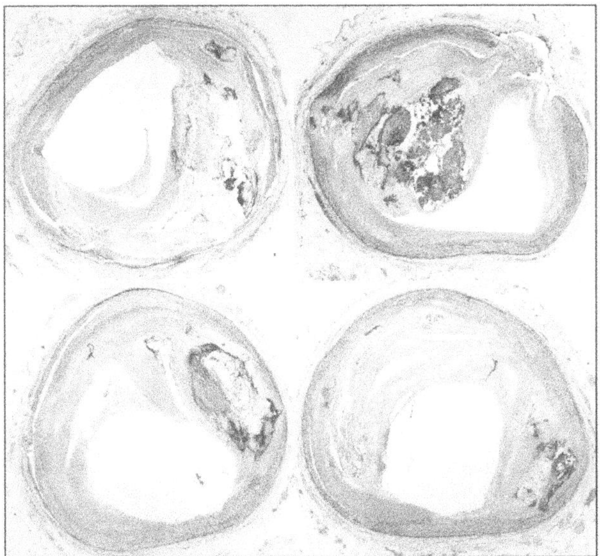

Figure 6. Photomicrographs of four 5-mm sections of the left anterior descending coronary artery proximally. (Movat stain; original magnification ×20).

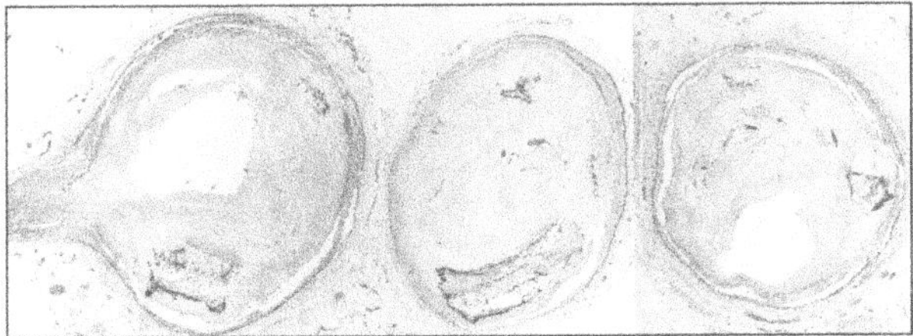

Figure 7. Photomicrographs of the left circumflex coronary artery proximally just after it arrives from the left main. (Movat stain; original magnification ×20).

one arterial system nearly always means plaque in another arterial system, as demonstrated by the large quantity of calcified plaques in the aorta and in its branches, including the noncoronary ones.[4,5]

The finding of severe mitral regurgitation on left ventricular cineangiography was a bit of a surprise. Transthoracic echocardiography disclosed only mild to moderate mitral regurgitation. The posteromedial papillary muscle was quite small in comparison to the anterolateral one and thus papillary muscle dysfunction is the presumed mechanism of the regurgitation.[6] The fact that the left ventricular cavity was not dilated and the systemic pressure was never elevated is surprising.

The extensive pulmonary disease with near obliteration of the left lung and severe emphysema of the upper lobe of the right lung certainly contributed considerably in making this patient a poor operative candidate, despite severe narrowing of the left main coronary artery.

REFERENCES

1 McManus BM, Roberts WC. Survival for 20 years or longer after transmural acute myocardial infarction: analysis of eight well-documented necropsy patients. *Am Heart J.* 1981;102:176–182.

2 Bulkley BH, Roberts WC. Atherosclerotic narrowing of the left main coronary artery: a necropsy analysis of 152 patients with fatal coronary heart disease and varying degrees of left main narrowing. *Circulation.* 1976;53:823–828.

3 Brosius FC 3rd, Roberts WC. Comparison of degree and extent of coronary narrowing by atherosclerotic plaque in anterior and posterior transmural acute myocardial infarction. *Circulation.* 1981;64:715–722.

4 Mautner GC, Mautner SL, Roberts WC. Amounts of coronary arterial narrowing by atherosclerotic plaque at necropsy in patients with lower extremity amputation. *Am J Cardiol.* 1992;70:1147–1151.

5 Mautner GC, Berezowski K, Mautner SL, et al. Degrees of coronary arterial narrowing at necropsy in men with large fusiform abdominal aortic aneurysm. *Am J Cardiol.* 1992;70:1143–1146.

6 Roberts WC, Cohen LS. Left ventricular papillary muscles: description of the normal and a survey of conditions causing them to be abnormal. *Circulation.* 1972;46:138–154.

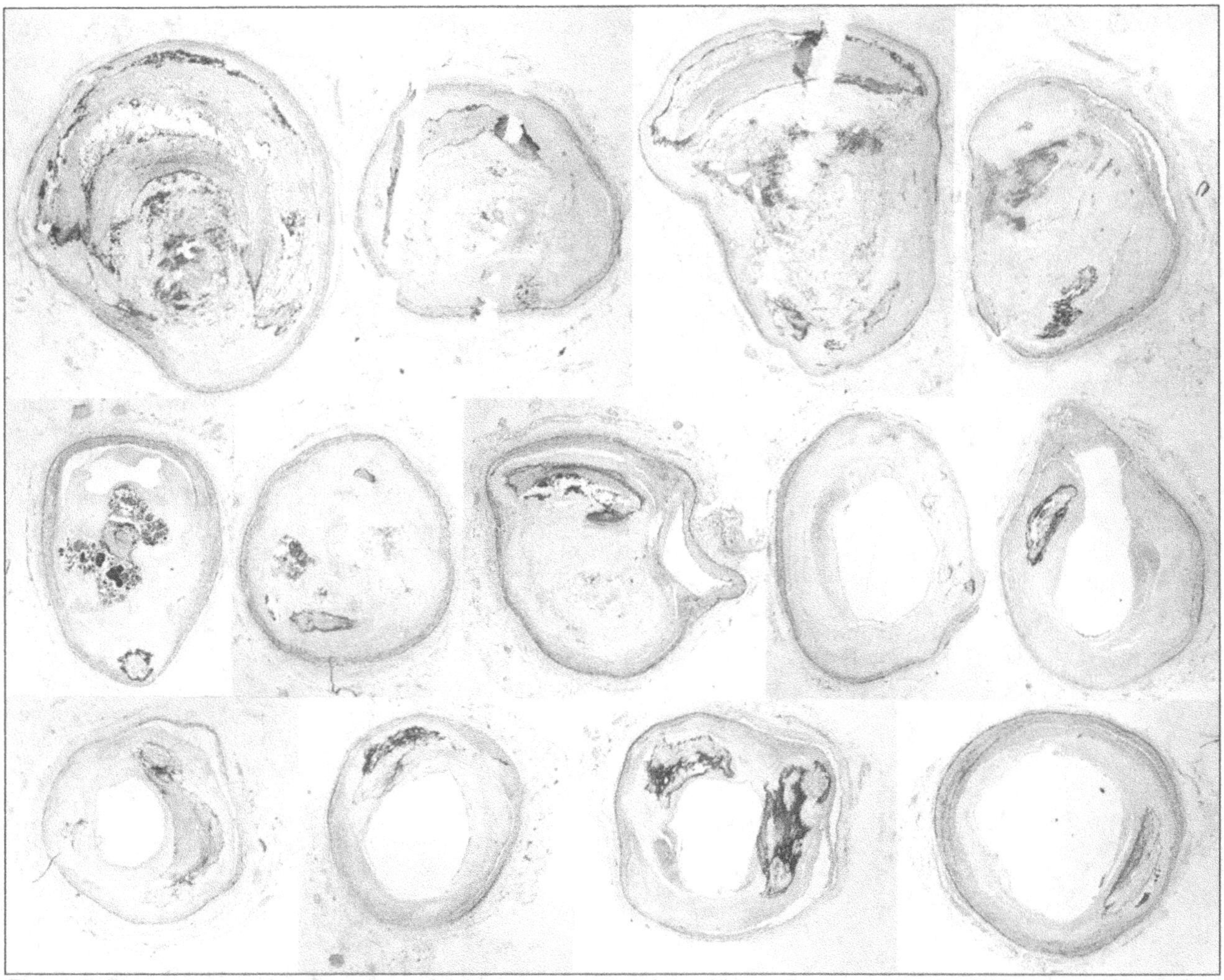

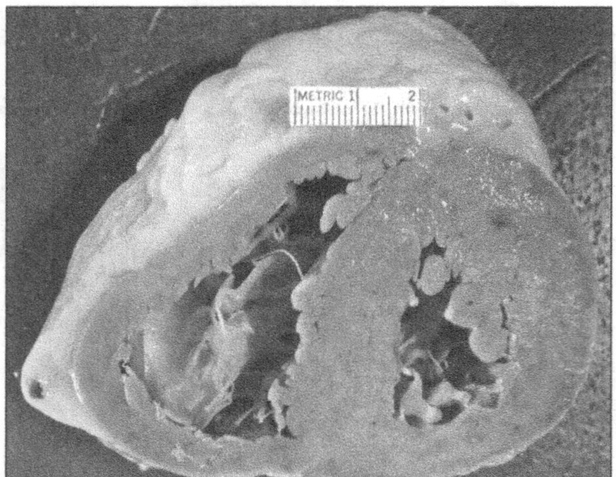

Figure 8. Photomicrographs of sections of right coronary artery from thirteen 5-mm segments of this artery. (Movat stain; original magnification ×20).

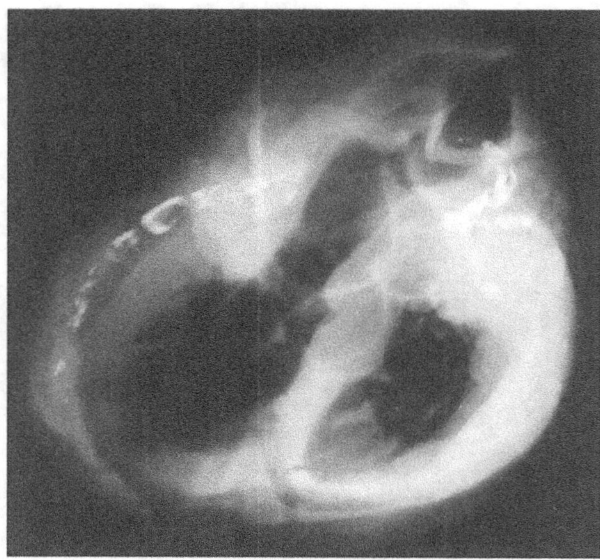

Figure 9. The heart. Base showing mild dilatation of the right ventricle and focal scarring and thinning of the posterior wall of left ventricle. The quantity of subepicardial adipose tissue is increased even though the patient's body weight was not increased.

Figure 10. Radiograph of the base of the heart showing the calcific deposits in major epicardial coronary arteries, including the left main.

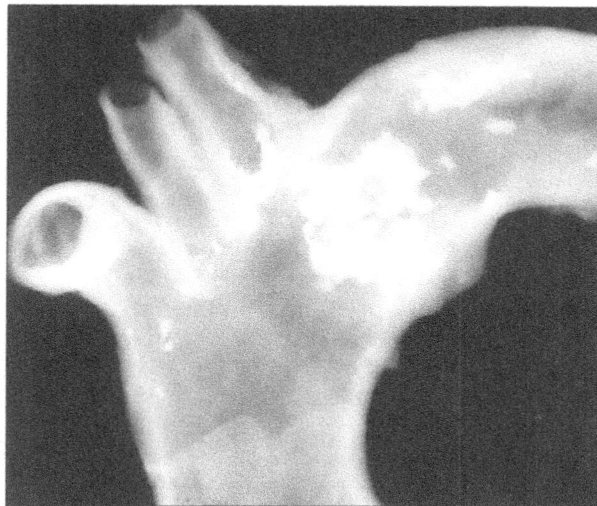

Figure 11. Radiograph of the aorta. At the arch, showing heavy calcific deposits in the aortic isthmic area, a common site of aortic calcific deposits.

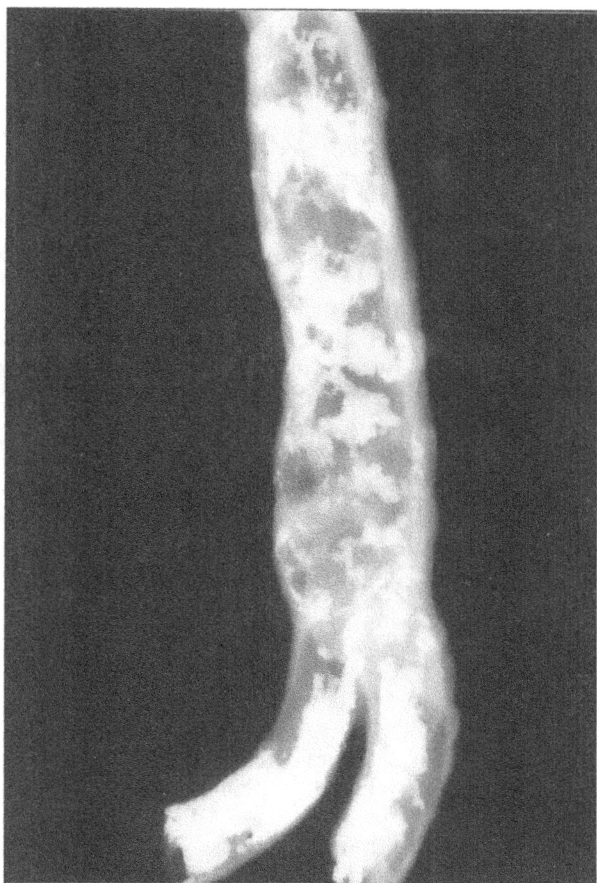

Figure 12. Radiograph of the aorta. Abdominal portion and proximal common iliac arteries showing heavy calcific deposits.

Comparison of Body Mass Index Among Patients With Versus Without Angiographic Coronary Artery Disease

Sabrina Deann Phillips, MD[†], and William Clifford Roberts, MD*

We examined body mass index (BMI) in kilograms divided by height in meters squared in 842 patients who underwent coronary angiography for suspected coronary artery disease (CAD) in a 2-month period in 2000 at Baylor University Medical Center. Comparison of the BMI in the 624 patients in whom ≥ 1 coronary artery was narrowed $>50\%$ in diameter to the BMI in the 218 patients with absent or lesser degrees of coronary narrowing disclosed the following: the BMI was >30 (obese) in 209 (33%) versus 92 (42%) patients (p 0.008): 26 to 30 (overweight but not obese) in 233 (37%) versus 80 patients (37%) (p = NS), and BMI ≤ 25 (ideal) in 182 (29%) versus 46 (21%) patients (p 0.01). Compared with the patients ≥ 65 years of age, the patients <65 years of age in both groups had a higher frequency of obesity and a lower frequency of ideal body weight. In conclusion, patients with coronary narrowing $>50\%$ in diameter were less likely to be obese and more likely to be at ideal body weight than the group of patients with absent or lesser degrees coronary narrowing by angiogram. © 2007 Elsevier Inc. All rights reserved. (Am J Cardiol 2007;100:18–22)

Although a number of previous articles have described body mass index (BMI) in patients with coronary artery disease (CAD), no study, to our knowledge, has compared BMI in both men and women with angiographic coronary narrowing ($>50\%$ in diameter) with similar age and sex and patients with absent or less degrees of angiographic coronary narrowing. We examined BMI in 842 patients who underwent coronary angiography at Baylor University Medical Center (BUMC) (Dallas, Texas) in a 2-month period in 2000 to determine if BMI differed among those with versus those without major coronary narrowing by angiography.

Methods

The Apollo Cardiovascular Data Base was searched for patients who had coronary angiography at BUMC in September and October 2000. A total of 889 patients underwent coronary angiography during the 2-month period. After excluding patients who underwent coronary angiography as part of post-cardiac transplant surveillance, prerenal transplant evaluation, and preoperative study before cardiac valve replacement or repair, 842 patients remained, and they are the subjects of this report. Indications for coronary angiography included suspected CAD, stable or unstable angina pectoris, positive stress test, or acute myocardial infarction (AMI). The degree of coronary arterial narrowing was determined by visual inspection of the angiogram and from the angiographic reports. The patients were divided into 2 groups: those with $>50\%$ diameter reduction of ≥ 1 coronary artery (hereafter considered to have CAD) and those with $<50\%$ diameter narrowing or no narrowing at all (hereafter considered not to have CAD). Body mass index was calculated as weight in kilograms divided by height in meters squared. *Obesity* was defined as BMI >30 kg/m^2; *overweight without obesity* as 26 to 30 kg/m^2, and *ideal weight* as BMI ≤ 25 kg/m^2.

Statistical analysis was performed on this data set using a z-test to determine the statistical significance (p <0.05).

Results

Of the 842 patients, 624 (74%) had ≥ 1 coronary artery narrowed $>50\%$ in diameter and 218 (26%) had no coronary artery narrowed to this degree (Table 1). A total of 474 patients (56%) were <65 years of age, and 330 (70%) had CAD; 368 patients were ≥ 65 years of age, and 294 (80%) had CAD (p <0.05). Of the 842 patients, 310 (37%) were women and 532 (63%) were men. Compared with the patients ≥ 65 years of age, the patients <65 years of age in both groups had a higher frequency of obesity and a lower frequency of ideal body weight.

Of the 301 obese patients, 209 (69%) had CAD; of the 313 patients overweight but not obese, 209 (67%) had CAD, and of the 228 lean or normal weight patients, 182 (80%) had CAD (p 0.0004). Of the 474 patients <65 years of age, 219 (46%) were obese, and 148 (68%) of them had CAD; 168 (35%) patients were overweight but not obese; and 117 (70%) of them had CAD, and 87 patients were of normal weight or lean, and 65 (75%) had CAD (p = NS). Of the 368 patients ≥ 65 years of age, 82 (22%) were obese, and 61 (74%) of them had CAD; 149 were overweight but not obese, and 116 (78%) had CAD; and 141 were lean or of normal weight, and 117 (83%) had CAD (p = NS).

Figure 1 is a scattergram comparing BMI to age in the 250 patients with ≥ 1 coronary artery narrowed $>50\%$ in diameter and either stable angina pectoris and/or positive exercise stress tests. Figure 2 is a similar scattergram com-

Baylor Heart & Vascular Institute and the Departments of Internal Medicine (Cardiology Division) and Pathology, Baylor University Medical Center, Dallas, Texas 75246. Manuscript received September 13, 2006; revised manuscript received and accepted February 5, 2007.

E-mail address: phillips.sabrina@mayo.edu or wcroberts@baylor.edu.

[†] Present address: Department of Internal Medicine, Division of Cardiovascular Diseases, Mayo Clinic, 200 First Street SW, Rochester, Minnesota 55905.

Table 1

Degree of coronary artery narrowing, gender, age group, and body mass index in 842 patients having coronary angiography for suspected coronary artery disease at Baylor University Medical Center in a 2-month period in 2000

Coronary Narrowing	Gender	Age (Years)	No. of Patients	Body Mass Index (kg/m^2)		
				≤25	26–30	>30
Stable Angina Pectoris and/or Positive Exercise Stress Test						
↑	Women	<65	26	6 (23%)	9 (35%)	11 (42%)
	Men	<65	95	23 (24%)	31 (33%)	41 (43%)
>50%	Women	≥65	53	25 (47%)	17 (32%)	11 (21%)
	Men	≥65	76	22 (29%)	40 (53%)	14 (18%)
↓	Subtotals		250	76 (30%)	97 (39%)	77 (31%)
Unstable Angina Pectoris and/or Acute Myocardial Infarction						
↑	Women	<65	47	7 (15%)	16 (34%)	24 (51%)
	Men	<65	162	29 (18%)	61 (38%)	72 (44%)
>50%	Women	≥65	68	32 (47%)	17 (25%)	19 (28%)
	Men	≥65	97	38 (39%)	42 (43%)	17 (17%)
↓	Subtotals		374	106 (28%)	136 (36%)	132 (35%)
Suspected Coronary Artery Disease						
↑	Women	<65	62	9 (15%)	17 (27%)	36 (58%)
	Men	<65	82	13 (16%)	34 (41%)	35 (43%)
<50%	Women	≥65	54	21 (39%)	19 (35%)	14 (26%)
	Men	≥65	20	3 (15%)	10 (50%)	7 (35%)
↓	Subtotals		218	46 (21%)	80 (37%)	92 (42%)

parison of the 374 patients with ≥1 coronary artery narrowed >50% in diameter and either unstable angina pectoris or AMI. Figure 3 is a scattergram showing the ages and BMI in the 218 patients who by angiography had coronary narrowing <50% in diameter. Figures 1 to 3 show that, among the 842 patients who underwent coronary angiography, the BMI correlated inversely with age: the older the patient the lower the BMI tended to be.

Table 1 compares the frequency of BMI ≤25, 26 to 30, and >30 kg/m^2 in the men versus women <65 and ≥65 years of age with versus without narrowing of ≥1 coronary artery >50% in diameter. The 2 groups in which ≥1 coronary artery was narrowed >50% in diameter had similar percentages of patients in each of the 3 groups of BMI. Compared with the younger (<65 years) patients within each of these 2 groups, the older (≥65 years) men and women had lower frequencies of obesity and higher frequencies of ideal body weight. The mean ages of the women and men with narrowing of ≥1 coronary artery >50% in diameter were 68 and 64 years, respectively, with BMI ≤25 kg/m^2; 62 and 62 years, respectively, with BMI 26 to 30 kg/m^2, and 60 and 57 years, respectively, in patients with BMI >30 kg/m^2. The group with clinically suspected CAD but no significant coronary artery narrowing on angiography had the highest frequencies of obesity and the lowest frequencies of ideal body weight. Both men and women in this group <65 years of age had much higher frequencies of obesity than both the men and women ≥65 years of age.

In an attempt to find a control population (of persons not undergoing coronary angiography), we reviewed data for the county of Dallas, Texas, collected from the Centers for Disease Control Behavioral Risk Surveillance System Questionnaire of 2002 to 2004. The average self-reported weight for the adult men was 187 pounds, and for the average adult women, 158 pounds. The average body weight of the 430 men with CAD in our study was 200 pounds and in the 102 men without CAD, 208 pounds. The average body weight of the 194 women in our study with CAD was 167 pounds, and in the 116 women without CAD, 178 pounds.

Discussion

The findings in the present study show that patients having had ≥1 coronary events (positive exercise stress test, stable and unstable angina pectoris, and/or AMI) are usually either overweight without obesity (BMI 26 to 30) or obese (BMI >30), but that similar aged men and women with suspected CAD but by angiography of <50% diameter narrowing of all coronary arteries have similar or even higher frequencies of obesity and lower frequencies of ideal body weight.

We found only 1 published report to which our data can be reasonably compared. Wessel et al[1] performed coronary angiography in 906 women (no men), who underwent coronary angiography because of "chest discomfort, suspected myocardial ischemia or both." Of the 906 women, 349 (39%) had narrowing of ≥1 coronary artery >50%: 81 (23%) had a BMI ≤25; 133 (38%), 26 to 30, and 135 (39%), a BMI >30. The other 557 (61%) had coronary narrowing <50%: 132 (24%) had a BMI ≤25; 186 (33%), 26 to 30, and 239 (43%) >30. Thus, those with and without angiographically demonstrated coronary narrowing had similar percentages in each of the 3 BMI categories. In contrast, of the 310 women in our study, 194 (62%) had narrowing >50% in ≥1 coronary artery: in 70 (36%), the BMI was ≤25; in 59 (30%), 26 to 30, and in 65 (34%), >30. The other 116 women had coronary narrowing <50%: in 30 (26%), the BMI was ≤25; in 36 (31%), 26 to 50, and in 50 (43%), >30. Thus, in our patients, the group without CAD had a higher frequency of obesity and a lower frequency of leanness than the group with CAD. We were unable to find similar data comparing BMI in men with and without angiographic CAD.

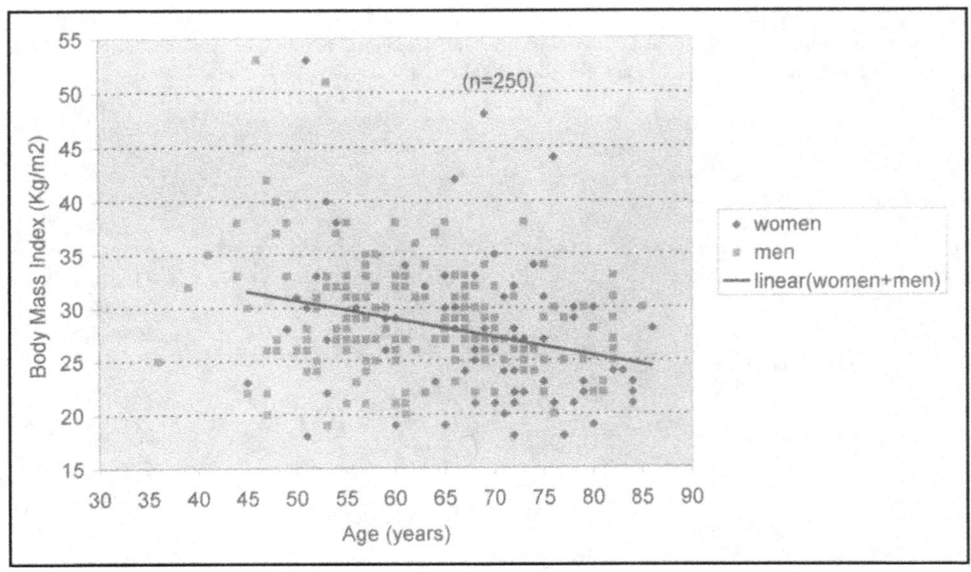

Figure 1. Scatterplot showing the relation of age to body mass index in patients with coronary narrowing >50% in diameter and stable angina pectoris and/or positive exercise stress test.

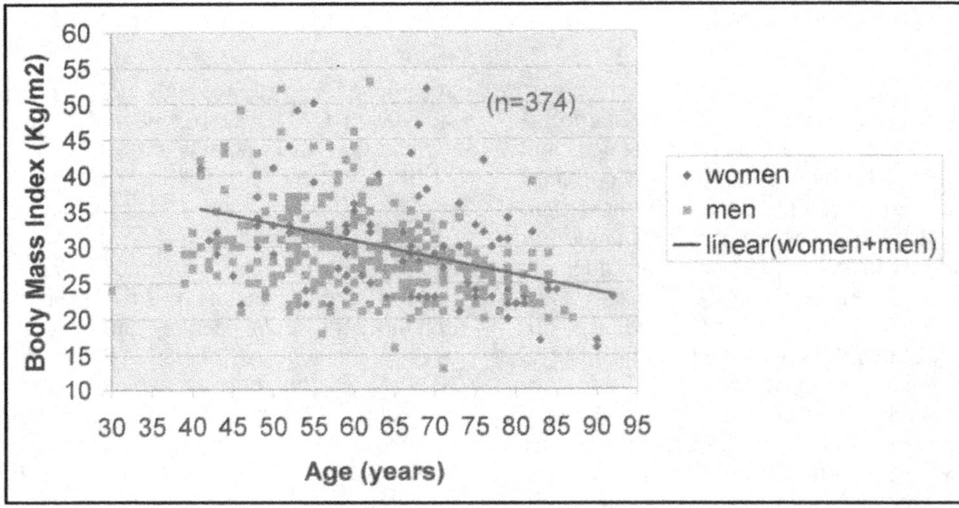

Figure 2. Scatterplot showing relation of age to body mass index in patients with coronary narrowing >50% with unstable angina pectoris or acute myocardial infarction.

The reported effect of obesity on total *mortality* and cardiovascular mortality has been variable. Hubert et al,[2] in 1983, found among their 5,209 men and women in Framingham that weight gain after the young adult years conveyed an increased risk of cardiovascular disease in the next 26 years in both sexes; they advised weight loss as a reasonable primary prevention of cardiovascular disease. Eckel and Krauss[3] in 1998 declared "obesity as a major risk factor for coronary heart disease . . . on a par with cigarette smoking, physical inactivity, and high blood cholesterol and emphasized that even a 5% to 10% reduction in body weight decreased blood pressure and total cholesterol, improved glucose tolerance, and reduced the severity of obstructive sleep apnea." Jonsson and colleagues[4] in 2002 followed 22,205 men for 23 years and found that the obese persons had a higher frequency of coronary events and death than the nonobese persons.

The findings of a high frequency of overweight in men with previous AMI was first reported by Garn and colleagues[5] in 1951 but they too found similar overweight in healthy men of similar age and sex. Lee and Thomas,[6] in 1956, compared body weights in both men and women at autopsy with fatal AMI with a group of patients who had died after a neurosurgical procedure. Of the 302 men with fatal AMI, 103 (34%) were >10% over ideal body weight (according to standard tables of the Metropolitan Life Insurance Company—1942 and 1943), and of the 60 men who died after a neurosurgical procedure (the control group), 19 (32%) were >10% over ideal body weight. Of the 148 women with fatal AMI, 69 (47%) were >10% over ideal body weight; of the 45 control women, 24 (41%) were similarly overweight. These authors also concluded that the weights of both men and women with fatal AMI were similar to those of patients "who had died of diseases that seem unlikely to be related to body weight (neurosurgical patients)." These 2 studies, of course, were performed before the presence or absence of coronary narrowing could be confirmed by angiogram.

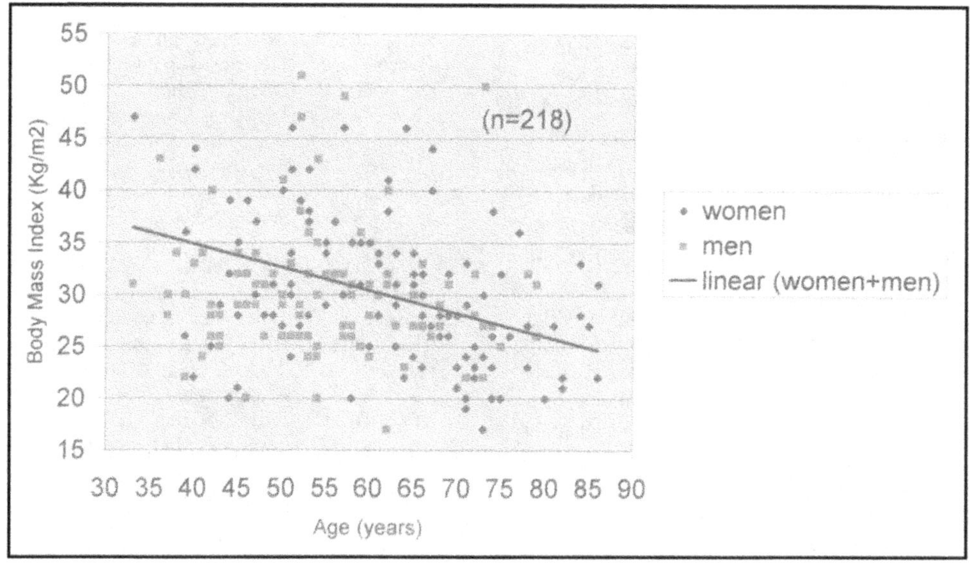

Figure 3. Scatterplot showing the relation of age to body mass index of patients with coronary narrowing <50% and clinically suspected coronary artery disease.

Tavani and colleagues,[7] in 1997, analyzed BMI in 432 women with non-fatal AMI and in 867 controls (hospitalized patients with "acute disease other than cardiovascular, neoplastic, digestive, and hormone-related conditions and any diseases associated with long-term modifications in diet"): 243 (65%) of the AMI women and 408 (47%) of the women controls had a BMI >25 kg/m². Nicoletti and colleagues,[8] in 2006, found BMI in survivors (n = 702) of AMI to be significantly higher than in nonsurvivors (n = 15) (26.1 ± 3.5 vs 23.3 ± 2.8 kg/m², respectively).

Kang and colleagues[9] determined BMI in 14,739 patients, 4,720 (32%) with "known coronary artery disease" (defined as history of myocardial infarction or coronary revascularization) and in 10,019 patients (68%) "without known coronary artery disease" as determined by resting and stress myocardial perfusion single-photon emission computed tomography. Of the 4,720 patients with clinical evidence of CAD, 1,865 (40%) had a BMI 18.5 to 24.9 (normal weight); 2,029 (43%), a BMI 25.0 to 29.9, and 826 patients (18%) had a BMI ≥30. Of the 10,019 patients with suspected CAD (but no clinical event of AMI or a coronary revascularization procedure), 3,850 (38%) had a normal BMI, 4,073 (41%) were overweight but not obese, and 2,096 (21%) were obese. Thus, the percent of overweight patients was similar in the patients with versus without clinical CAD (60% [2,855 of 4,720] vs 62% [6,169 of 10,019]). The obese and overweight groups and those with and without CAD were significantly younger than those at ideal body weight. In patients with but not those without known CAD, BMI was inversely related to cardiac death (mean follow-up approximately 3 years), i.e., an increased BMI was associated with a decreased risk of cardiac death.

Several investigators have observed that obese patients had lower mortality rates *after* AMI than nonobese patients. Hoit et al[10] followed 1,760 patients with AMI for 1 year. Although hospital mortality was higher in the obese (BMI >30) and overweight (BMI 25 to 30) patients compared with the normal weight (BMI <25) patients (13%, 14%,

9%), 1-year mortality was lower in the obese group compared with the other 2 groups (7%, 11%, 13%). Kennedy and colleagues[11] among 5,388 patients with AMI found that the overweight/obese patients had a lower risk of mortality and recurrent AMI than the normal weight patients. The underweight (BMI <22) group had the worst prognosis of all. Kragelund et al[12] studied 6,676 patients with AMI and also found BMI to be inversely related to mortality.

The relation of *heart failure* to body weight also has been variable. Kenchaiah et al[13] found among the 5,881 Framingham subjects that 496 developed heart failure in a mean of 14 years. Compared with the subjects with a BMI 18.5 to 24.9, those subjects with a BMI >30 had twice the risk of developing heart failure, and the higher the BMI the greater the risk. Curtis et al[14] studied 7,767 patients with "stable heart failure" and found that all-cause mortality rates decreased linearly from higher BMI (>25) groups (45%) to the underweight group (BMI <18.5) (25%). Gustafsson et al[15] also found among 4,700 hospitalized patients with heart failure that increasing BMI in heart failure was associated with a lower mortality.

The effect of body weight on outcomes of *percutaneous coronary intervention (PCI)* also appears to be variable. Ellis and colleagues[16] studied 3,571 PCI patients and found that in-hospital death after PCI correlated strongly with both low (BMI ≤25) and very high (BMI >35) body weight. Gruberg et al[17] found among 9,633 patients having PCI that the overweight and obese patients had a significantly lower frequency of major in-hospital complications, including death, and also lower 1-year mortality than the lean (BMI <18.5) and normal (BMI 18.5 to 24.9) weight patients. Gurm et al[18] studied 2,108 patients who had PCI and 1,526 patients who had coronary artery bypass grafting, and found among the PCI patients that each unit increase in BMI was associated with a 5.5% lower risk of a major in-hospital event (death, myocardial infarction, stroke, coma). No difference in in-hospital outcome was observed according to BMI in the coronary bypass group. Five-year mortality in the PCI group did not correlate with BMI; in the coronary bypass group, however, the higher the baseline BMI, the greater the 5-year mortality. Powell et al[19] reviewed data in 6,302 patients having PCI and followed a median of 2.1 years. The obese (BMI >30) patients had a similar to lower risk of late death after successful PCI compared with patients of normal weight (BMI 20 to 25), whereas underweight (BMI <20) patients had higher late mortality rates. Compared with the underweight and normal weight patients, the obese patients had lower rates of femoral arterial bleeding, hematoma, and blood loss that required transfusion after PCI.

The present report has limitations. There is probably more of a tendency to perform coronary angiography in overweight and obese patients than in those at ideal body weight. All patients in the present study had some symptoms or other manifestations clinically suggesting or at least arousing the suspicion of CAD. Coronary angiographic data are lacking in subjects without any suspicion of CAD. The degrees of narrowing by coronary angiography were determined by visual inspection, not by quantitative analysis, and by a number of different angiographers. Possibly there were more false positive noninvasive tests in the overweight and obese patients, prompting more coronary angiography in them than in patients at ideal body weight.

1. Wessel, TR, Arant CB, Olson MB, Johnson RD, Reis SE, Sharaf BL, Shaw LJ, Handberg E, Sopko G, Kelsey SF, Pepine CJ, Bairey Merz CN. Relationship of physical fitness vs body mass index with coronary artery disease and cardiovascular events in women. *JAMA* 2004;292:1179–1194.
2. Hubert HB, Feinleib M, McNamara PM, Castelli WP. Obesity as an independent risk factor for cardiovascular disease: a 26-year follow-up of participants in the Framingham Heart Study. *Circulation* 1983;67:968–977.
3. Eckel RH, Krauss RM, for the AHA Nutrition Committee. American Heart Association call to action: obesity as a major risk factor for coronary heart disease. *Circulation* 1998;97:2099–2100.
4. Jonsson S, Hedblad B, Engström, Nilsson P, Berglund G, Janzon L. Influence of obesity on cardiovascular risk. Twenty-three-year follow-up of 22,025 men from an urban Swedish population. *Int J Obesity* 2002;26:1046–1053.
5. Garn SM, Gertler MM, Levine SA, White PD. Body weight versus weight standards in coronary artery disease and a healthy group. *Ann Intern Med* 1951;34:1416–1420.
6. Lee KT, Thomas WA. Relationship of body weight to acute myocardial infarction. *Am Heart J* 1956;52:581–591.
7. Tavani A, Negri E, D'Avanzo B, La Vecchia C. Body weight and risk of nonfatal acute myocardial infarction among women: a case-control study from Northern Italy. *Prev Med* 1997;26:550–555.
8. Nicoletti I, Cicoira M, Morando G, Benazzi C, Prati D, Morani G, Rossi A, Zardini P, Vassanelli C. Impact of body mass index on short-term outcome after acute myocardial infarction: does excess body weight have a paradoxical protective role? *Int J Cardiol* 2006;107:395–399.
9. Kang X, Shaw LJ, Hayes SW, Hachamovitch R, Abidov A, Cohen I, Friedman JD, Thomas LEJ, Polk D, Germano G, Berman DS. Impact of body mass index on cardiac mortality in patients with known or suspected coronary artery disease undergoing myocardial perfusion single-photon emission computed tomography. *J Am Coll Cardiol* 2006;47:1418–1426.
10. Hoit BD, Gilpin EA, Maisel AA, Henning H, Carlisle J, Ross J Jr. Influence of obesity on morbidity and mortality after acute myocardial infarction. *Am Heart J* 1987;114:1334–1341.
11. Kennedy LMA, Dickstein K, Anker SD, Kristianson K, Willenheimer R, for the OPTIMAAL Study Group. The prognostic importance of body mass index after complicated myocardial infarction. *J Am Coll Cardiol* 2005;45:156–157.
12. Kragelund C, Hassager C, Hildrebrandt P, Torp-Pedersen C, Køber L, on behalf of the TRACE study group. Impact of obesity on long-term prognosis following acute myocardial infarction. *Int J Cardiol* 2005;98:123–131.
13. Kenchaiah S, Evans JC, Levy D, Wilson PWF, Benjamin EJ, Larson MG, Kannel WB, Vasan RS. Obesity and the risk of heart failure. *N Engl J Med* 2002;347:305–313.
14. Curtis JP, Selter JG, Wang Y, Rathore SS, Jovin IS, Jadbabaie F, Kosiborod M, Portnay EL, Sokol SI, Bader F, Krumholz HM. The obesity paradox. Body mass index and outcomes in patients with heart failure. *Arch Intern Med* 2005;165:55–61.
15. Gustafsson F, Kragelund CB, Torp-Pedersen C, Seibaek M, Burchardt H, Akkan D, Thune JJ, Køber L, for the DIAMOND study group. Effect of obesity and being overweight on long-term mortality in congestive heart failure: influence of left ventricular systolic function. *Eur Heart J* 2005;26:58–64.
16. Ellis SG, Elliott J, Horrigan M, Raymond RE, Howell G. Low-normal or excessive body mass index: newly identified and powerful risk factors for death and other complications with percutaneous coronary intervention. *Am J Cardiol* 1996;78:642–646.
17. Gruberg L, Weissman NJ, Waksman R, Fuchs S, Deible R, Pinnow EE, Ahmed LM, Kent KM, Pichard AD, Suddath WO, Satler LF, Lindsay J Jr. The impact of obesity on the short-term and long-term outcomes after percutaneous coronary intervention: the obesity paradox? *J Am Coll Cardiol* 2002;39:578–584.
18. Gurm HS, Whitlow PL, Kip KE, for the BARI Investigators. The impact of body mass index on short- and long-term outcomes in patients undergoing coronary revascularization. Insights from the Bypass Angioplasty Revascularization Investigation (BARI). *J Am Coll Cardiol* 2002;39:834–840.
19. Powell BD, Lennon RJ, Lerman A, Bell MR, Berger PB, Higano ST, Holmes DR Jr, Rihal CS. Association of body mass index with outcome after percutaneous coronary intervention. *Am J Cardiol* 2003;91:472–475.

Natural History, Clinical Consequences, and Morphologic Features of Coronary Arterial Aneurysms in Adults

William Clifford Roberts, MD[a,b,]*

Clinical and morphologic features are described in 20 adults (15 men) aged 17 to 85 years (mean 56) who at necropsy were found to have ≥1 aneurysm in ≥1 of their 3 major (right, left anterior descending, and left circumflex) epicardial coronary arteries. Of the 34 coronary aneurysms in the 20 patients (single in 10 patients, ≥2 in 10 patients), 27 (79%) contained intra-aneurysmal thrombi, and in each, the thrombus severely narrowed the lumen. Additionally, atherosclerotic plaque was present in the aneurysmal wall in all 27 aneurysms containing thrombi and also in the major coronary arteries uninvolved by aneurysm. The causes of the aneurysms in the 16 patients with intra-aneurysmal thrombi were therefore considered atherosclerotic. In the other 4 patients, with 7 aneurysms, none contained intra-aneurysmal thrombus or atherosclerotic plaque, and the aneurysms were considered congenital. Clinical diagnosis of coronary aneurysm was not made in any of the 20 patients, but none had proper imaging studies during life. Despite the coronary aneurysms and the associated luminal narrowing, only 8 patients (40%) had left ventricular wall scarring or necrosis or clinical evidence of myocardial ischemia. Proper therapy remains ill defined.   © 2011 Elsevier Inc. All rights reserved. (Am J Cardiol 2011;108:814–821)

Although atherosclerosis commonly involves the aorta, a common consequence of that involvement is aneurysmal dilatation, most commonly involving the abdominal portion, and significant narrowing or total occlusion of the aorta by this process is rare. In contrast, when atherosclerosis involves the coronary arteries, a common consequence is severe narrowing or total obstruction leading to myocardial ischemia and/or infarction, and aneurysmal dilatation involving these arteries is rare. Indeed, examination of several cardiac pathology books disclosed either no or minimal mention of coronary arterial aneurysm.[1–7] This report describes clinical and morphologic features in 20 adults with coronary arterial aneurysm observed personally during a 24-year period.

Methods

All hearts were initially examined by the author (W.C.R.), and most were reexamined all together at a later time. The hearts were submitted to W.C.R.'s cardiac pathology laboratory from 12 different medical institutions: 6 from 1 institution, 3 from another, 2 from another, and 1 each from 9 different institutions. The 20 cases were seen by W.C.R. during a 24-year period (1975 to 1999). The hearts were received after fixation in formaldehyde. After excising extraneous tissues, the hearts were weighted, described, and either photographed or illustrations prepared.

To be included in this study, ≥1 of the major epicardial coronary arteries (left anterior descending, left cir-

cumflex, and right) had to be focally dilated. The diameter of the aneurysm had to be ≥2 times the diameter of the right and left main coronary arteries in the first centimeter of their courses. Patients with previous cardiac surgery or percutaneous coronary intervention were excluded. Clinical records were obtained from the submitting institutions.

Results

Pertinent clinical and morphologic data for each of the 20 patients are listed in Table 1, and several hearts are illustrated in Figures 1 to 11.

The 20 patients ranged in age at death from 17 to 85 years: the 5 women from 17 to 85 years (mean 63) and the 15 men from 37 to 84 years (mean 56). Of the 20 patients, 10 (50%) had a single aneurysm in a single coronary artery; the other 10 (50%) had ≥1 aneurysm in ≥2 major coronary arteries. Of the latter 10 patients, 6 had aneurysms involving 2 major coronary arteries, and 4 patients had aneurysms in 3 major coronary arteries (right, left anterior descending, and left circumflex [excluding the left main]). Thus, the 20 patients had 34 coronary aneurysms: left anterior descending in 12, left circumflex in 9, and right in 13.

Intra-aneurysmal thrombi were present in 16 patients (80%), and 4 patients (20%) had no thrombi within coronary aneurysms. Of the total 34 coronary aneurysms in the 20 patients, 27 (79%) contained thrombi and 7 (21%) did not. Of the 34 aneurysms, 33 were fusiform (the entire wall was involved), and 1 (case 2) was saccular (only a portion of the wall was involved). In the latter patient, the aneurysm ruptured and led to fatal hemopericardium.

Maximal luminal narrowing at the coronary aneurysm, nearly entirely by thrombus, with some underlying atherosclerotic plaque was >75% in cross-sectional area in 28 aneurysms (82%) and zero or <25% in 6 aneurysms (18%).

[a]Baylor Heart and Vascular Institute of Baylor University Medical Center, Dallas, Texas; and [b]Pathology Branch, National Heart, Lung, and Blood Institute, National Institutes of Health, Bethesda, Maryland. Manuscript received April 14, 2011; revised manuscript received and accepted May 1, 2011.

*Corresponding author: Tel: 214-820-7911; fax: 214-820-7533.

E-mail address: wc.roberts@baylorhealth.edu (W.C. Roberts).

Table 1
Clinical and morphologic cardiac data in 20 necropsy patients with ≥1 aneurysm in ≥1 epicardial native coronary artery

Case	Age (Years)	Gender	CA With Aneurysm (n)	Coronary Aneurysm Diameter (cm)	Length (cm)	Maximal Diameter (cm) First 1 cm of RCA or LMCA	Intra-Aneurysmal Thrombus	Maximal Luminal Narrowing at Aneurysm (CSA)	Atherosclerosis in Aneurysmal Wall	Maximal Narrowing of Nonaneurysmal CAs
1	17	F	LAD (1)	1.5	1.8	0.4	0	0	0	0
2	37	M	LC (1)	3.0	Saccular	0.5	0	0	0	0
3	41	M	R (1)	1.0	1.0	0.4	+	>75%	+	>75%
4	41	M	LAD (1)	1.0	1.5	0.4	+	>95%	+	>75%
5	41	M	R (2)	2.0	4.0	0.5	+	>95%	+	>75%
			LAD (2)	1.5	4.0		0	0	+	26%–50%
			LC (1)	1.5	3.0		0	0	+	26%–50%
6	42	M	LAD (1)	2.0	4.0	0.5	+	>75%	+	51%–75%
7	50	M	R (1)	1.0	2.0	0.4	+	>95%	+	>75%
			LC (1)	0.9	1.5		+	>95%	+	
8	54	M	R (1)	1.5	8.0	0.5	+	>75%	+	>75%
			LAD (1)	1.5	4.0		+	>75%	+	
9	55	M	R (1)	1.5	3.0	0.4	+	>95%	+	>75%
10	56	M	R (1)	1.3	2.2	0.4	+	>95%	+	>75%
			LAD (1)	2.3	3.0		+	>95%	+	
11	61	M	R (1)	2.0	3.5	0.4	+	>95%	+	>75%
12	65	M	R (1)	1.1	7.0	0.5	0	51–75%	+	>75%
			LAD (1)	1.0	1.5		0	51–75%	+	
13	68	M	LAD (1)*	1.5	2.0	0.5	+	>75%	+	>75%
			LC (1)*	2.0	2.0		+	>75%	+	
14	68	F	R (1)	2.5	2.2	0.6	+	>95%	+	>75%
15	70	M	R (1)	5.0	7.0	0.5	+	>75%	+	>75%
			LAD (1)	2.0	3.0		+	>75%	+	>75%
			LC (1)	4.0	3.0		+	>75%	+	>75%
16	70	M	LC (1)†	2.5	9.0	0.5	0	0	0	<25%
17	72	F	R (2)	1.3	3.0	0.4	+	>75%	+	>75%
			LAD (1)	1.3	2.0		+	>75%	+	>75%
			LC (1)	1.4	2.0		+	>75%	+	>75%
18	74	F	R (1)	2.0	4.0	0.5	+	>75%	+	>75%
			LC (1)	2.0	2.5		+	>75%	+	
19	84	M	R (1)	8.0	10.0	0.7	+	>75%	+	>75%
			LAD (1)	5.0	3.5		+	>75%	+	>75%
			LC (1)	6.0	2.5		+	>75%	+	>75%
20	85	F	LAD (1)	1.5	2.0	0.4	+	>75%	+	>75%

*Also involved the distal LMCA.

†Dominate artery; went to the crux.

AAA = abdominal aortic aneurysm; AMI = acute myocardial infarction; AP = angina pectoris; C = cardiac; CA = coronary artery; CHF = chronic heart failure; CSA = cross-sectional area; DA = descending aorta; F = female; Fib = fibrosis; LAD = left anterior descending coronary artery; LC = left circumflex coronary artery; LMCA = left main coronary artery; LV = left ventricle; M = male; N = necrosis; R = right; RCA = right coronary artery; RV = right ventricle; SD = sudden death; SH = systemic hypertension; V = vascular; — = no information available.

Atherosclerotic plaques, usually calcified ones, were present in 31 (91%) of the 34 aneurysms in the 20 patients and were absent in 3 (9%) of the 34 aneurysms.

Of the 20 patients, 16 (80%) had ≥1 major epicardial coronary artery narrowed >75% in cross-sectional area by atherosclerotic plaque. Among these 16 patients with 48 major coronary arteries (left anterior descending, left circumflex, and right), 38 (79%) of the 48 arteries were narrowed >75% in cross-sectional area by atherosclerotic plaque alone. Of the 3 major coronary arteries in these 16 patients (excluding the left main), an average of 2.3 of the 3 arteries were narrowed >75% in cross-sectional area by plaque alone.

The heart weight in the 5 women ranged from 310 to 490 g (mean 400) and in the 14 men from 380 to 910 g (mean 503).

Grossly visible left ventricular scars were present in 8 patients (40%), and in 3 others (15%), grossly visible foci of necrosis (acute myocardial infarction) were present.

Clinically, 7 patients (35%) had clinical events in which acute myocardial infarction was diagnosed, 2 of whom also had angina pectoris. One other patient who did not have a myocardial infarct clinically had angina pectoris. Three patients (15%) had evidence of chronic heart failure. Eight patients (40%) died suddenly, and death in each was attributed to coronary heart disease.

Number of Major CAs ↓ >75% in CSA by Plaque	Heart Weight (g)	Left Ventricular Wall		Clinically							Cause of Death			Dilated	
		N	Fib	AP	AMI	CHF	SD	SH	DAA	AAA	C	Non-C, V	Non-C, Non-V	RV	LV
0	—	0	0	0	0	0	+	0	0	0	+	0	0	0	0
0	420	0	0	0	0	0	+	0	0	0	+	0	0	0	0
3	510	0	+	0	0	0	+	+	0	0	+	0	0	+	+
2	380	0	0	0	0	0	+	0	0	0	+	0	0	0	0
1	375	+	+	0	+	0	+	0	0	0	+	0	0	+	+
0	500	0	0	0	0	0	0	+	+	0	0	+	0	0	0
3	460	0	+	0	0	0	+	−	0	0	+	0	0	0	+
3	400	0	+	0	+	+	+	0	0	0	+	0	0	+	+
3	450	+	0	+	+	0	0	+	0	+	+	0	0	+	+
3	510	0	+	+	0	0	0	+	0	+	0	0	+	0	+
1	380	0	+	0	+	0	0	0	0	0	0	0	+	+	+
2	910	0	+	0	+	+	0	+	0	0	+	0	0	+	+
3	560	0	+	0	0	0	0	+	0	0	0	0	+	+	+
2	490	0	0	0	0	0	0	+	0	+	0	0	+	0	0
3	750	+	0	0	0	0	0	+	0	0	0	0	+	0	0
0	420	0	0	0	0	0	0	+	0	0	0	0	+	0	0
3	390	0	0	0	0	0	+	+	0	0	+	0	0	0	0
2	390	0	0	0	0	0	0	+	0	0	0	0	+	0	0
3	—	0	+	+	+	+	0	+	0	0	+	0	0	0	+
2	420	+	0	0	+	0	0	+	0	0	+	0	0	+	+

Of the 20 patients, 12 (60%) died from cardiac disease (including the 8 who died suddenly outside the hospital), 1 (5%) of noncoronary vascular disease, and 7 (35%), of noncardiac and nonvascular causes.

Discussion

The present study summarizes clinical and morphologic findings in 20 patients with ≥1 aneurysm in ≥1 of the major epicardial coronary arteries. Ten patients (50%) had a single aneurysm in a single coronary artery, and the other 10 had 2 or 3 major coronary arteries containing aneurysms. Of the 34 aneurysms in the 20 patients, 27 (79%) contained thrombus, which in most cases severely narrowed the lumens. The residual lumen in all 27 cases was eccentrically located and adjacent to the atherosclerotic, partially calcified, wall. Of the 16 patients with thrombus in ≥1 coronary aneurysm, all but 1 had severe luminal narrowing by atherosclerotic plaque in the coronary artery containing the aneurysm as well as in the major coronary arteries not

containing aneurysms. The largest coronary aneurysm in diameter was 8 cm, and this was also the longest (10 cm).

Of the 7 coronary aneurysms not containing intra-aneurysmal thrombus, 3 had none or insignificant quantities of atherosclerotic plaque within the aneurysms or in the nonaneurysmal portion of the artery containing the aneurysm or in the coronary arteries not containing an aneurysm. Thus, the cause of the coronary aneurysm in them was considered nonatherosclerotic, probably congenital in origin. Three other patients without thrombus in coronary aneurysm had insignificant atherosclerosis in the major coronary arteries; only 1 without intra-aneurysmal thrombus had severe coronary atherosclerosis. One patient without intra-aneurysmal thrombus had a large saccular aneurysm that ruptured, leading to fatal hemopericardium. The other 33 aneurysms were fusiform.

Despite the severe narrowing by intra-aneurysmal thrombus or by atherosclerotic plaque, only 8 patients (40%) had grossly visible left ventricular scars, and only 3 had grossly

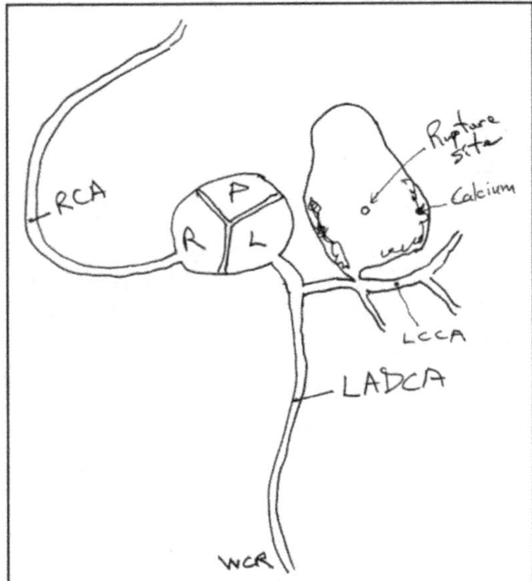

Figure 1. Case 2: diagram of the major coronary arteries in a 37-year-old man who collapsed at home. Necropsy disclosed hemopericardium and a large saccular aneurysm arising from the left circumflex coronary artery (LCCA). A perforation was present in the aneurysm. Calcific deposits were present in the basal portion of the wall of the aneurysm. The right coronary artery (RCA) and the left anterior descending coronary artery (LADCA) were free of atherosclerotic plaques. Cusps of the aortic valve: L = left; P = posterior; R = right.

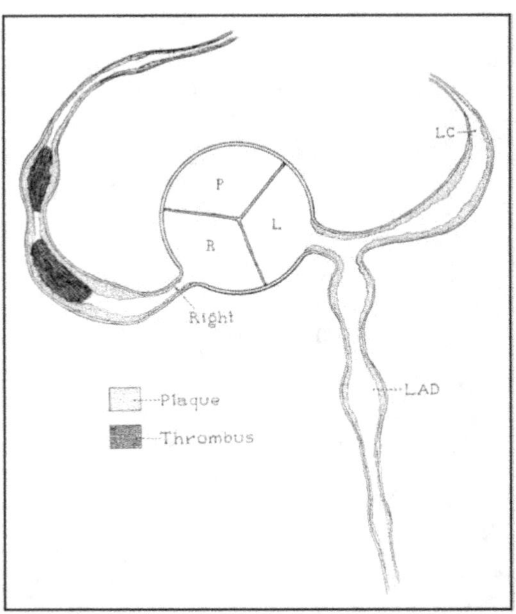

Figure 2. Case 5: diagram of the coronary arteries in a 41-year-old man with coronary aneurysms in the right, left anterior descending (LAD), and left circumflex (LC) coronary arteries. The 2 in the right contain large thrombi. He died from acute aortic dissection. Cusps of the aortic valve: L = left; P = posterior; R = right.

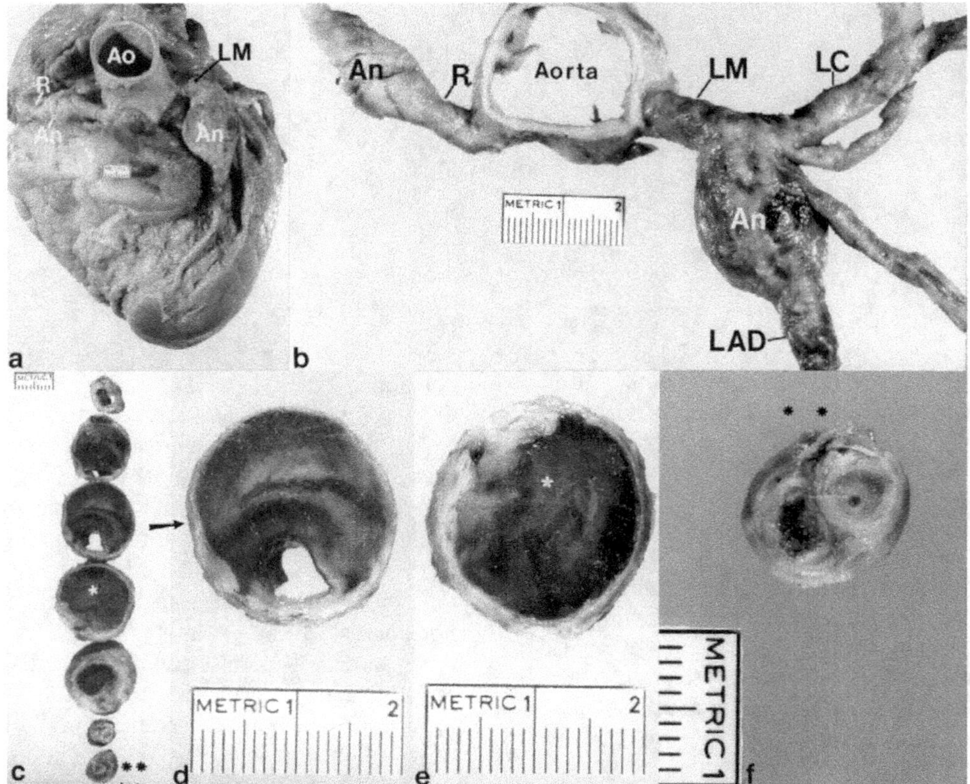

Figure 3. Case 10: the heart in a 56-year-old man with an aneurysm (An) in the right (R) and left anterior descending (LAD) coronary arteries. He died from cancer. (a) Anterior view of the heart showing the 2 aneurysms. (b) View of the R, left main (LM), and LAD coronary arteries showing the 2 aneurysms. The R and LM coronary arteries just after their origins from the aorta (Ao) are much smaller in diameter than either coronary aneurysm. (c) Cross sections of the LAD coronary artery with intra-aneurysmal thrombus. (d) Cross section of 1 section. The lumen is severely narrowed by intra-aneurysmal thrombus. (e) Another cross section of the same aneurysm. (f) Small coronary segment distal to the aneurysm. Its lumen is occluded by complicated plaque plus thrombus. LC = left circumflex.

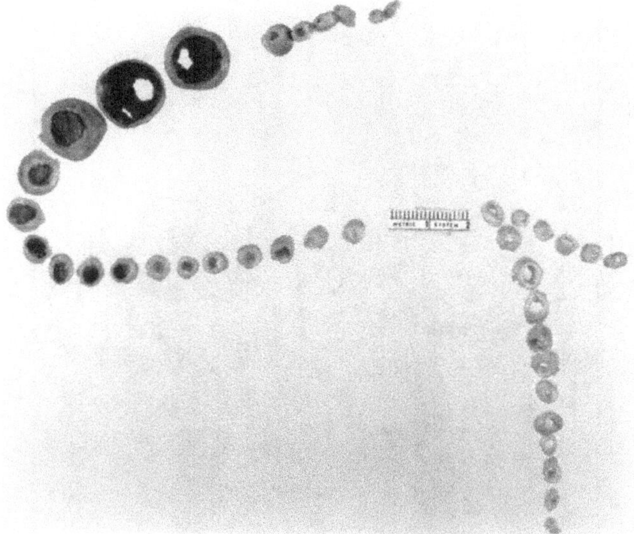

Figure 4. Case 11: coronary arteries in a 61-year-old man who died from complications of cancer. These cross sections of coronary arteries show a large aneurysm filled with thrombus in the distal right coronary artery.

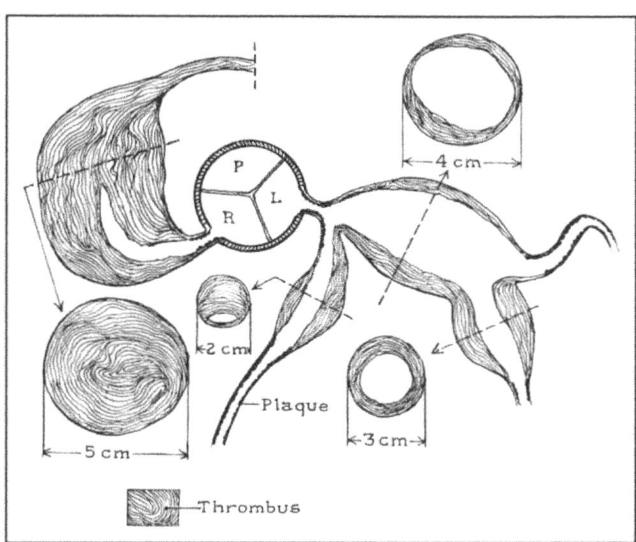

Figure 6. Case 15: diagram of coronary arterial aneurysms in a 70-year-old man who died from a gastrointestinal condition. Necropsy disclosed very large aneurysms in the right, left anterior descending, and left circumflex coronary arteries and in 1 of its obtuse marginal branches. Thrombus is present in each aneurysm and occludes the lumen of the right coronary artery. Cusps of the aortic valve: L = left; P = posterior; R = right.

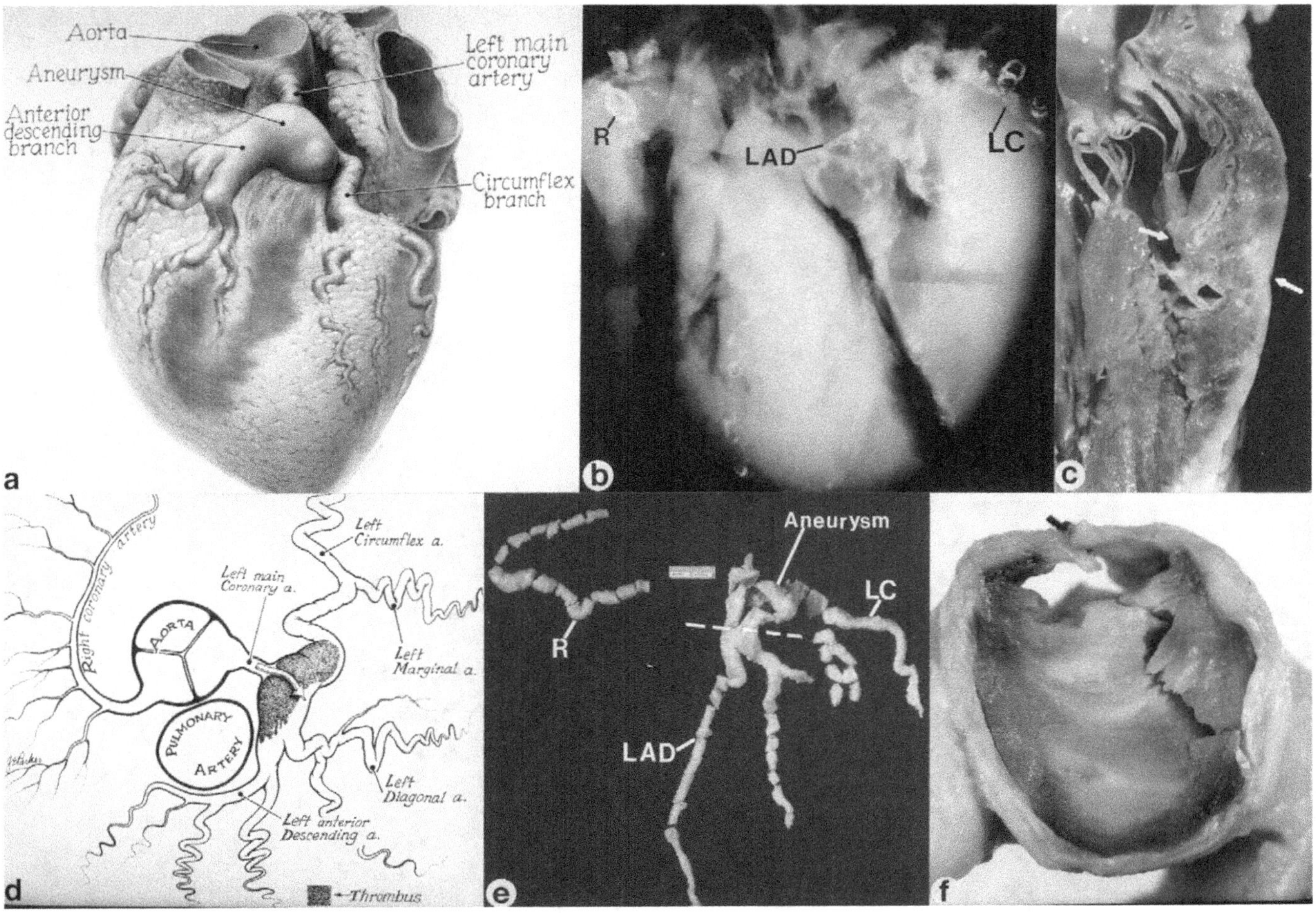

Figure 5. Case 13: heart in a 68-year-old man with a large aneurysm with intra-aneurysmal thrombus involving the proximal portion of the left anterior descending (LAD) and left circumflex (LC) coronary arteries (a,d). The walls of the coronary arteries are focally calcified (b). (c) A transmural scar (between the arrows) in the posterior wall of left ventricle. (e) View of the coronary arteries after their removal from the heart. (f) Cross section through the LAD aneurysm showing the large intra-aneurysmal thrombus.

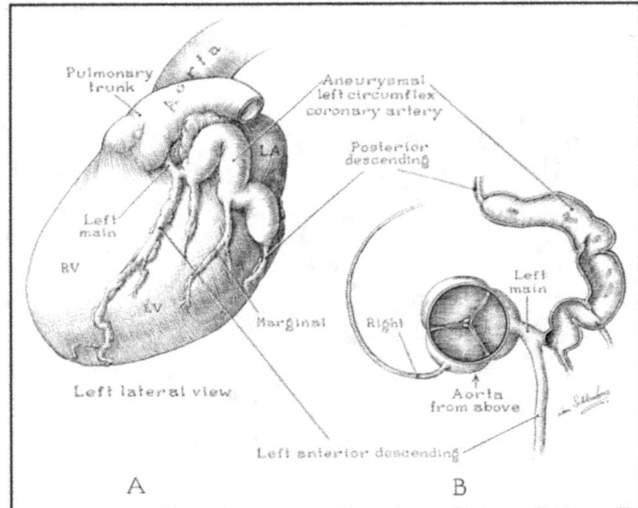

Figure 7. Case 16: diagram showing a large long aneurysm involving the left circumflex coronary artery in a 70-year-old man who died from a noncardiovascular condition (trauma). The coronary aneurysm is devoid of thrombus. LA = left atrium; LV = left ventricle; RV = right ventricle.

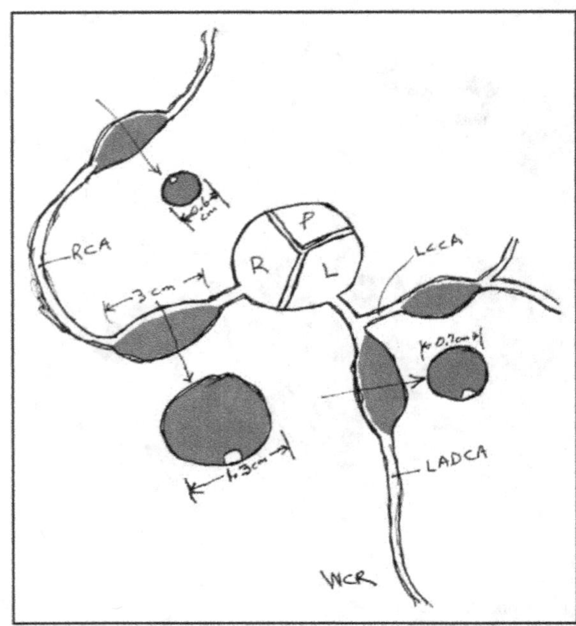

Figure 8. Case 17: diagram of coronary arteries in a 72-year-old woman who died suddenly and unexpectedly outside the hospital. She had never had clinical evidence of myocardial ischemia previously. Necropsy disclosed fusiform aneurysms filled with thrombi in each of the 3 major coronary arteries, including 2 aneurysms in the right coronary artery (RCA). At the sites of aneurysms, cross sections show thrombi filling most of the lumen, and the only residual opening is eccentric, adjacent to the artery's wall. LADCA = left anterior descending coronary artery; LCCA = left circumflex coronary artery. Cusps of the aortic valve: L = left; P = posterior; R = right.

visible foci of left ventricular necrosis, including 1 of the 8 with left ventricular scarring.

Only 3 patients had a diagnosis of angina pectoris, and 7 had a diagnosis of acute myocardial infarction during life. Three patients had evidence of chronic heart failure. Eight died suddenly outside the hospital. A diagnosis of coronary

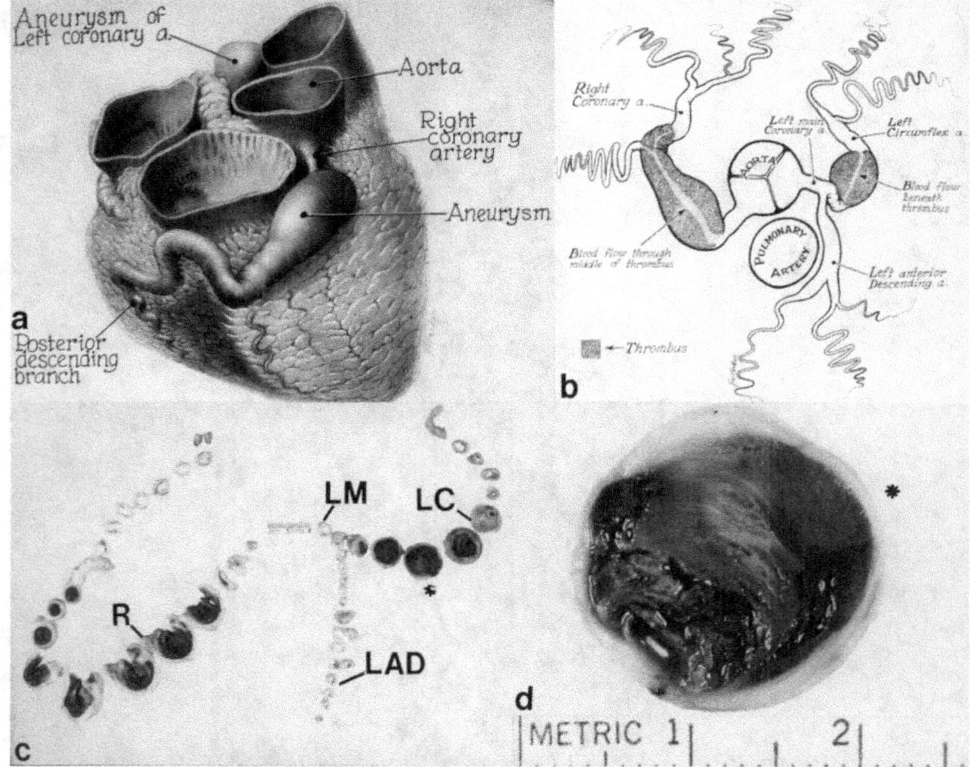

Figure 9. Case 18: coronary aneurysms of the left circumflex (LC) and right (R) coronary arteries in a 74-year-old woman who died from a noncardiovascular condition (chronic obstructive pulmonary disease). (a) Diagram of the heart. (b) Diagram of the coronary arteries showing that both coronary aneurysms contained thrombi. (c) Cross sections of the right R, left main (LM), left anterior descending (LAD), and LC coronary arteries. (d) Cross section of the LC coronary aneurysm showing its lumen to be virtually occluded by thrombus.

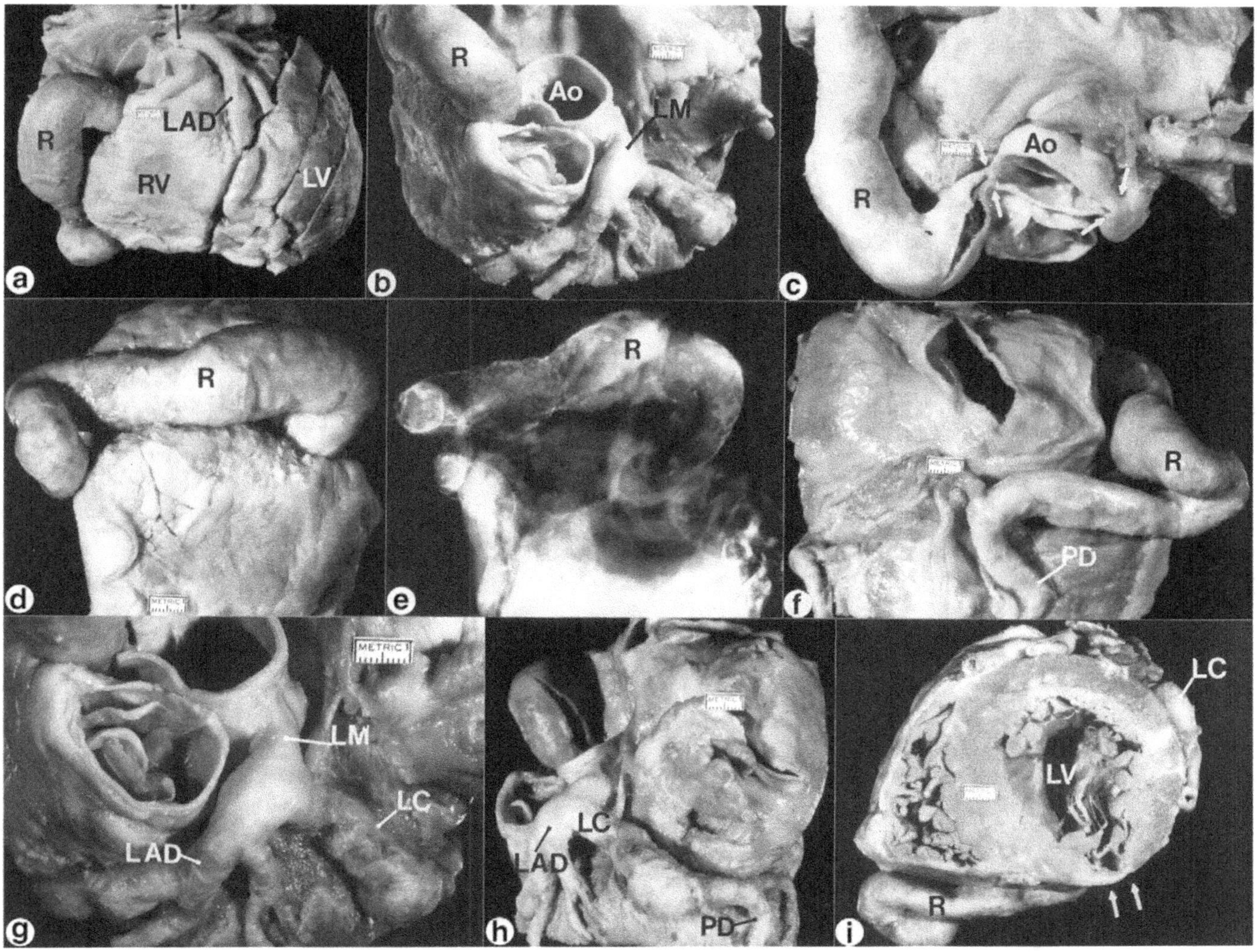

Figure 10. Case 19: heart in an 84-year-old man, who had a myocardial infarction at 80 years of age, showing a huge aneurysm involving nearly all the right (R) coronary artery, with smaller aneurysms involving the distal left main (LM) and proximal portions of the left anterior descending (LAD) and left circumflex (LC) coronary arteries. He died from pneumonia. (a) View of the anterior portion of the heart. Note the huge size of the R coronary artery. (b) View from above. (c) Another view of the aneurysm in the R coronary artery. (d) Still another view. (e) X-ray showing calcific deposits in the R coronary artery. (f) Distal portion of the right coronary artery and its posterior descending (PD) branch. i View of the left-sided coronary aneurysms. (h) Still another view. (i) Cross section of the cardiac ventricles showing transmural scars (arrows) in the left ventricular wall. Ao = aorta; LV = left ventricle; RV = right ventricle.

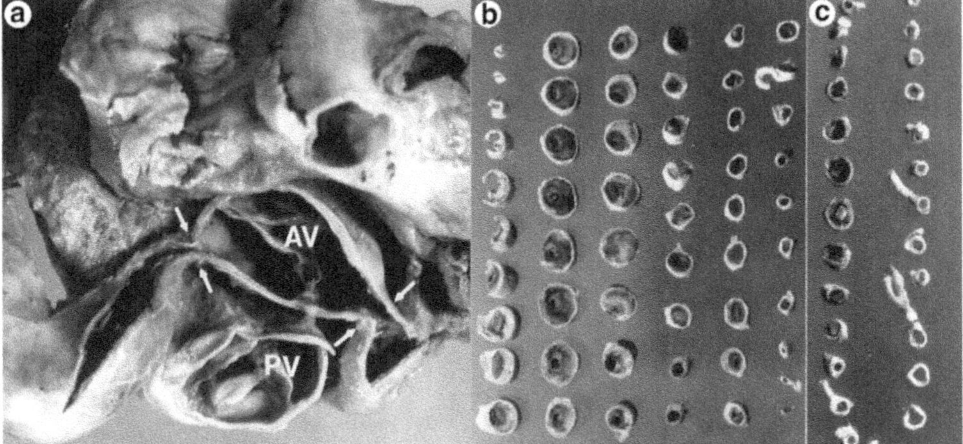

Figure 11. Case 19: (a) View of both coronary arteries from above showing that the most proximal portions of the right and left main coronary arteries (between the arrows) are of normal size. (b) Cross sections of the right coronary artery showing its lumen to be filled with thrombus. (c) Cross sections of the left anterior descending coronary artery. Again, the aneurysm is filled with thrombus. AV = aortic valve; PV = pulmonary valve.

aneurysm was not made in any patient during life. However, none had coronary angiographic or computed tomographic studies during life.

The cause of death was considered cardiac in 12 patients, 8 of whom died suddenly outside the hospital, and 4 others had fatal acute myocardial infarction within a hospital. Another patient died from noncoronary vascular causes, and 7 died from neither coronary nor noncoronary vascular causes. At necropsy, 3 patients were found to have abdominal aortic aneurysms, and 1 other patient had a saccular aneurysm of the descending thoracic aorta. At least 13 of the 20 patients had a history of systemic hypertension.

In the past 30 years, numerous reports on coronary artery aneurysm have been published. Most have been single case studies of "giant" coronary aneurysms diagnosed by computed tomography, magnetic resonance imaging, echocardiography, coronary angiography, and even routine chest radiography.[8–13] Many have been in patients with Kawasaki disease.[14] Most of the latter patients were aged <5 years, and they were excluded from the present study. (The youngest patient in the present study was 17 years of age.)

The largest reported necropsy study was that by Virmani et al[8] of 52 patients. Their patients ranged in age from 5 months to 80 years and included 14 patients in whom they attributed coronary aneurysms to inflammation (mean age 14 years) and 38 patients in whom the aneurysms were attributed to atherosclerosis (mean age 38 years). Of their 38 patients with atherosclerotic aneurysms, "20 (53%) had histories of ischemic heart disease." The coronary aneurysms involved a single coronary artery in 31 patients (82%) and >1 artery in 7 patients (18%). The data from their study were obtained from autopsy protocols and clinical records, not from examination of the hearts themselves.

When a coronary aneurysm is diagnosed during life, the best therapeutic course to follow has not been determined. In patients without evidence of myocardial ischemia the best course may be to do nothing unless the aneurysm is truly giant in size, such that rupture is a potential consequence. Because thrombi are present in most adults with coronary aneurysms, anticoagulation may be justified. In patients with symptomatic myocardial ischemia and ≥1 large coronary aneurysm, operative intervention has been the most common therapeutic option.[15] However, what is the proper operative procedure? Some surgeons have simply placed a bypass conduit distal to the coronary aneurysm with or without placing a ligature at both the proximal and distal ends of the

coronary aneurysm. Percutaneous coronary intervention in those circumstances appears less appealing (to me).

The positive feature of the present study was that all cases were studied by the same individual, namely the author, who has been studying hearts for 50 years. Most of the hearts were photographed and/or illustrated. The major deficiency of this study is that none of the coronary aneurysms were diagnosed clinically, and no echocardiographic, computed tomographic, magnetic resonance imaging, or coronary angiograms were available in any patient. The coronary aneurysms were surprise necropsy findings in all 20 patients. With autopsy rates in hospital deaths now about 5%, the "material" illustrated in the present study will be far less available in the future.

1. Hudson REB. Cardiovascular Pathology, Volume 1. Baltimore, Maryland: Williams & Wilkins, 1965:630–631.
2. Gould SE, Ioannides G. Diseases of the coronary vessels. In: Gould SE, ed. Pathology of the Heart and Blood Vessels. 3rd ed. Springfield, Illinois: Charles C. Thomas, 1968:557–558.
3. Davies MJ, Robertson WB. Diseases of the coronary arteries. In: Pomerance A, Davies MJ, eds. Pathology of the Heart. London, United Kingdom: Blackwell Scientific, 1975:114–115.
4. Olsen EGJ. The Pathology of the Heart. 2nd ed. Baltimore, Maryland: University Park Press, 1980:308.
5. Baroldi G. Diseases of the coronary arteries. In: Silver MD, ed. Cardiovascular Pathology, Volume I. New York, New York: Churchill Livingstone, 1983:362–364.
6. Virmani R, Robinowitz M, Darcy TP. Coronary vasculitis. In: Virmani R, Atkinson JB, Fenoglio JJ, eds. Cardiovascular Pathology. Philadelphia, Pennsylvania: W.B. Saunders, 1991:180–185.
7. Davies MJ, Mann JM. Part B: acquired diseases of the heart. In: Davies MJ, Mann JM. The Cardiovascular System. New York, New York: Churchill Livingstone, 1995:64–65.
8. Virmani R, Robinowitz M, Atkinson JB, Forman MB, Silver MD, McAllister HA. Acquired coronary arterial aneurysms: an autopsy study of 52 patients. Hum Pathol 1986;17:575–583.
9. Meinert D, Mohammed Z. MRI of congenital coronary artery aneurysm. Br J Radiol 2000;73:322–324.
10. Pahlavan PS, Niroomand F. Coronary artery aneurysm: a review. Clin Cardiol 2006;29:439–443.
11. Nichols L, Lagana S, Parwani A. Coronary artery aneurysm. A review and hypothesis regarding etiology. Arch Pathol Lab Med 2008;132:823–828.
12. Johnson PT, Fishman EK. CT angiography of coronary artery aneurysms: detection, definition, causes, and treatment. AJR Am J Roentgenol 2010;195:928–934.
13. Shambrook JS, Chowdhury R, Brown IW, Peebles CR, Harden SP. Cross-sectional imaging appearances of cardiac aneurysms. Clin Radiol 2010;65:349–357.
14. Sudo C, Monobe Y, Yashiro M, Sadakane A, Uehara R, Nakamura Y. Case-control study of giant coronary aneurysms due to Kawasaki disease: the 19th nationwide survey. Pediatr Int 2010;52:790–794.
15. Harandi S, Johnston SB, Wood RE, Roberts WC. Operative therapy of coronary arterial aneurysm. Am J Cardiol 1999;83:1290–1293.

Commonalities of Cardiac Rupture (Left Ventricular Free Wall or Ventricular Septum or Papillary Muscle) During Acute Myocardial Infarction Secondary to Atherosclerotic Coronary Artery Disease

William C. Roberts, MD[a,b,c,*], Kendall H. Burks[a,1], Jong Mi Ko, BA[a], Giovanni Filardo, PhD[d], and Joseph M. Guileyardo, MD[c]

Although mortality rates during acute myocardial infarction (AMI) continue to drop, cardiac rupture (left ventricular free wall [LVFW] or ventricular septum [VS] or papillary muscle [PM] or combination) remains relatively common. The aim was to identify commonalities among patients with AMI complicated by cardiac rupture. During a 22-year period (1993-2014) 64 patients hospitalized for AMI were studied and clinical and morphologic variables in those with (25 patients) — vs — those without (39 patients) cardiac rupture were compared, and previous reports on this topic were reviewed. Compared to the non-rupture cases, the rupture group was significantly older (71 years — vs — 60 years); had a much higher frequency of huge deposits of adipose tissue in the heart (floated in formaldehyde) (88% — vs — 20%) but a lower mean body mass index (28.2 Kg/m^2 — vs — 33.2 Kg/m^2); a much lower frequency of healed myocardial infarct (scar) (4% — vs — 28%); a lower frequency of diabetes mellitus (24% — vs — 47%), and a higher frequency of thrombolytic therapy during the fatal AMI (32% — vs — 10%). None of the rupture cases had evidence of dilated left ventricular cavities or evidence of heart failure before the AMI complicated by rupture. In conclusion, cardiac rupture appears to account for a high percent of deaths during a first AMI. It most commonly occurs in patients with extremely fatty hearts and in those without evidence of prior heart failure.   © 2015 Elsevier Inc. All rights reserved. (Am J Cardiol 2015;115:125—140)

During the last 80 years many publications on cardiac rupture complicating acute myocardial infarction (AMI) have appeared (Table 1).[1–29] Some have compared findings at necropsy in fatal AMI with — vs — without rupture of either the left ventricular free wall (LVFW) or ventricular septum (VS),[2,16,21,23,26–28] and others have described only the rupture cases.[8,13,19,26] Many previous publications provided no photographs of the ruptured hearts. One of us (WCR) has been involved since 1967 in a number of studies on cardiac rupture secondary to AMI,[25,30–42] including an examination at necropsy of 204 such patients with rupture of the LVFW or VS or papillary muscle (PM) studied from 1968 to 1989.[25] Despite these previous studies commonalities among these 3 types of cardiac rupture during AMI have not been clearly delineated. The present study attempts to fill that void by examining a new series of 25 patients with cardiac rupture studied at necropsy from 1993 to 2014, compares clinical and necropsy findings in them to 37 patients with fatal AMI without rupture, and focuses on commonalities observed in these patients and in previously reported ones.

Methods

The 64 patients with fatal AMI were seen at Baylor University Medical Center during a 22-year period (1993-2014). With 3 exceptions (gross photographs studied), all hearts were examined and described by WCR. At necropsy, the presence or absence of hemopericardium was determined by the prosector, most commonly under the supervision of JMG. At necropsy, the hearts were placed unopened in a container of formaldehyde, and after fixation for usually 3 to 5 days the hearts were opened and described by WCR, the specimens were photographed, (usually by JMK), and sections were cut by WCR for histologic study. After excising extraneous (non-cardiac) tissues, all hearts were placed in a container of 10% formaldehyde to see if they floated to the surface after removing any air inside of the cardiac chambers. Nearly all hearts were opened by cutting the ventricular walls parallel to the posterior atrioventricular sulcus at about 1 cm intervals, except for the most apical cut which was about 3 cm in thickness. All hearts were superficially dried with paper towels and weighed on an very accurate scale (to ± 1 g). The atria were incised by a cut about midway between the atrioventricular valve annulae and the most cephalad extension of the atrial walls. The pulmonary trunk was excised about 2 cm cephalad to its sinotubular junction and the ascending aorta about 3 cm cephalad to its sino-tubular junction. At least 4 histologic sections were

[a]Baylor Heart and Vascular Institute, Departments of [b]Internal Medicine (Division of Cardiology), and [c]Pathology, Baylor University Medical Center at Dallas, Texas; and [d]Department of Epidemiology, Office of Chief Quality Officer, Baylor Scott & White Health, Dallas, Texas. Manuscript received October 2, 2014; accepted October 4, 2014.

Funding: The study was funded by the Cardiovascular Research Review Committee of the Baylor Health Care System Foundation, Dallas, Texas.

See page 139 for disclosure information.

*Corresponding author: Tel: 214-820-7911; fax: 214-820-7533.

E-mail address: wc.roberts@baylorhealth.edu (W.C. Roberts).

———

[1] K.H.B is a sophomore, Rice University, Houston, TX 77005.

Table 1

Reported Frequency 1938-1968 of Rupture of the Left Ventricular Free Wall or Ventricular Septum in 12,984 Necropsy Patients with Fatal Acute Myocardial Infarction

Author (Year) [Reference]	No. Patients With Fatal AMI	Rupture Cases				
		Number Ruptured	Location		M/F	Ages (Years) Range (Mean)
			LV	VS		
BEFORE CORONARY CARE UNITS						
Bean (1938) [1]	300	17 (6%)	16	1	8/9	-
Edmonson and Hoxie (1942) [2]	865	72 (8%)	59	13	40/32	30-90 (-)
Friedman & White (1944) [3]	105	10 (10%)	10	0	7/3	51-80 (66)
Diaz-River & Miller (1948) [4]	53	5 (9%)	4	1	1/4	-
Wang et al (1948) [5]	267	23 (9%)	22	1	-	-
Selzer (1948) [6]	95	8 (8%)	7	1	-	-
Zinn & Cosby (1950) [7]	430	34 (8%)	34	0	12/22	54-82 (71)
Oblath et al (1952) [8]	1,026	80 (9%)	80	0	47/33	60-80 (-)
Wessler et al (1952) [9]	124	20 (16%)	15	5	-	-
Waldron et al (1954) [10]	545	40 (8%)	40	0	-	-
Goetz & Gropper (1954) [11]	145	14 (10%)	11	3	-	56-76 (-)
Maher et al (1956) [12]	183	21 (12%)	19	2	10/11	54-92 (69)
Griffith et al (1961) [13]	1,212	52 (4%)	44	8	-	-
Spiekerman et al (1962) [14]	87	21 (24%)	18	3	10/11	-
Ross & Young (1963) [15]	606	43 (7%)	43	0	27/16	35-90 (-)
London & London (1965) [16]	1,001	47 (5%)	42	5	27/20	- (69)
Sievers (1966) [17]	811	104 (13%)	104	0	52/52	- (69)
Sugiura et al (1968) [18]	50	8 (16%)	6	2	5/3	68-88 (77)
Lewis (1969) [19]	1,228	106 (9%)	106	0	52/54	42-92 (71)
Subtotal	9,133	725 (8%)	680 (94%)	45 (6%)	298/270 (52%)/(48%)	30-92 (-)
AFTER CORONARY CARE UNITS						
Hammer et al (1972) [20]	47	10 (21%)	7	3	6/4	55-80 (64)
Rasmussen et al (1979) [21]	401	64 (16%)	61	3	42/30	46-90 (-)
Dellborg et al (1985) [22]	329	56 (17%)	51	5	28/28	- (71)
Hiramori (1987) [23]	143	26 (18%)	20	6	-	23-92 (62)
Herlitz (1988) [24]	76	32 (42%)*	32	0	-	- (67)†
Reddy & Roberts (1989) [25]	648	204 (31%)‡	137	53	112/92	43-94 (68)
Batts et al (1990) [26]	1,251	100 (8%)	100	0	51/49	- (74)†
Pollak et al (1994) [27]	533	105 (20%)§	105	0	-	-
Hutchins et al (2002) [28]	153	47 (31%)‖	47	0	22/25	46-97 (70)
Markowicz-Pawlus et al (2012) [29]	270	49 (18%)	49	0	12/37	- (70)
Subtotal	3,851	693 (18%)	609 (90%)	70 (10%)	273/265 (51%)/(49%)	23-97 (-)

AMI = acute myocardial infarction; LV = left ventricular free wall; VS = ventricular septum; - = no information available.

* Study does not specify location of rupture.

† Mean age calculated as a weighted average of ages reported by the authors in separate patient groups.

‡ Five of these patients also had rupture of a left ventricular papillary muscle.

§ One case of rupture diagnosed intraoperatively.

‖ Includes one reported case of right ventricular free wall rupture.

prepared in each heart. Each was stained by hematoxylin-eosin and by the trichrome method and all sections were examined by WCR and frequently by JMG.

The medical records were obtained in all 64 patients and data in each of the variables listed in Tables 2 and 3 were sought.

Inclusion into this study required the presence at necropsy of AMI and the onset of the AMI *before* admission to BUMC. Patients who developed an AMI after admission to the hospital were not included. The later patients, for example, were those who developed an AMI after a percutaneous coronary intervention or after coronary bypass or cardiac valve replacement or ascending aorta resection or hepatic or renal or cardiac transplantation or during or shortly after hemodialysis (for chronic renal disease). Additionally, patients who developed a coronary embolus during active infective endocarditis were excluded. The attempt was to collect a non-rupture group of AMI patients as similar as possible to the rupture group of AMI patients.

Means, standard deviations (SDs) and percentages were calculated to describe the study cohort (n=64). Differences in demographic and clinical details were tested with a Wilcoxon (for continuous factors) or a chi-square (for categorical factors) test. Unadjusted p-values were also

Table 2

Clinical and Morphologic Findings in 25 Patients with Fatal Rupture of Left Ventricular Free Wall, Ventricular Septum, and/or Papillary Muscle Secondary to Acute Myocardial Infarction and Studied at Baylor University Medical Center from July 1993 through July 2014

Patient Number	Age	Race	Sex	BMI (kg/m^2)	DM	SH	BP	Rx	CABG	TT	PCI	LV Scar	Rupture Site	Location of AMI	Interval of Onset MI to Death (Days)	RV Infarct	HW (g)	Float	H	Figure Number
1	68	W	F	24.2	+	0	0		0	+	+	0	LVFW	A	2	0	375	+	+	-
2	70	B	F	-	+	+	-		0	0	0	0	LVFW	L	3	0	405	0	+	3
3	72	B	F	-	0	+	-		0	+	0	0	LVFW	Apical	1	0	415	-	+	-
4	72	W	F	28.2	0	+	0		0	+	+	0	LVFW	P	6	0	555	+	+	4
5*	78	W	F	23.9	0	+	0		+	+	+	0	LVFW	A	1	0	325	-	+	-
6	83	W	F	41.3	0	0	0		0	0	+	0	LVFW	P	4	+	415	+	+	5
7	47	W	M	28.3	0	0	0		0	0	+	0	LVFW	A	45	0	435	+	+	6
8	57	W	M	27.2	0	+	+		+	+	0	0	LVFW	A	15	0	640	+	+	-
9*	66	W	M	25.8	0	+	0		+	0	0	+	LVFW	A	2	0	430	+	+	-
10	67	W	M	28.4	0	+	0		0	0	+	0	LVFW	A	3	0	390	+	+	7
11	67	W	M	29.4	+	+	+		0	0	0	0	LVFW	P	3	0	660	+	+	8
12	70	W	M	24.3	+	+	+		0	0	+	0	LVFW	P	5	0	395	+	0	-
13	70	W	M	30.4	0	+	0		0	0	0	0	LVFW	P	4	0	530	+	+	-
14	75	W	M	30.1	0	+	0		0	0	+	0	LVFW	L	2	0	450	+	+	9
15	75	W	M	25.2	+	+	+		0	0	0	0	LVFW	P	3	+	575	+	+	-
16	78	W	M	26.8	0	+	+		0	+	0	0	LVFW	A	1	0	415	+	+	10
17	81	W	M	-	0	+	-		0	0	0	0	VS	A	1	0	500	+	0	-
18	80	W	F	27.4	0	-	-		0	0	+	0	PM[‡]	P	3	+	380	0	0	11
19	62	W	M	31.6	0	+	+		+[§]	0	0	0	PM[‡]	A	3	0	570	+	0	-
20*	63	W	M	27.1	0	+	+		0	0	0	0	PM[‡]	P	2	0	740	+	0	-
21	72	W	F	25.1	0	+	+		0	+	0	0	LVFW & VS	P	3	+	310	+	+	12
22	67	W	M	26.1	+	+	0		+	0	+	0	LVFW & VS	P	7	+	480	+	0	13
23	67	W	M	26.9	0	+	0		0	0	0	0	LVFW & VS	P	1	+	530	0	+	-
24	81	W	M	32.3	0	+	0		0	+	+	0	LVFW & VS	P	4	+	565	0	+	14
25	77	W	F	30.2	0	+	0		+	0	0	0	LVFW & PM	L	7	0	525	+	+	15

Abbreviations: A = anterior; AMI = acute myocardial infarct; B = black; BMI = body mass index; BP = blood pressure; C = circumferential; CABG = coronary artery bypass graft; DM = diabetes mellitus; F = female; HW = heart weight; H=hemopericardium; Hx = history; L = lateral; LV = left ventricular; LVFW = left ventricular free wall; M = male; P = posterior; PCI = percutaneous coronary intervention; PM = papillary muscle; RV = right ventricular; Rx = therapy; SH = systemic hypertension; TT=thrombolytic therapy; VS = ventricular septum; W = white; 0 = absent or negative; + = present or positive; - = no information available.

* Heart specimen was not examined by WCR, but photographs taken at autopsy were available.

[†] No hemopericardium due to earlier CABG causing absence of pericardial space (diffuse adherence of parietal and epicardial surface).

[‡] Partial rupture.

[§] Redo CABG performed.

estimated. A Bonferroni correction was employed to account for multiplicity.

The study protocol was approved by the Institutional Review Board of Baylor University Medical Center.

Results

Findings in each of the 25 patients with cardiac rupture secondary to AMI are detailed in Table 2 and the findings in them are compared to the 39 non-rupture patients in Table 3. The number of cases observed during each of the 22 years are shown in Figure 1. Of the 25 rupture cases, 16 (64%) had isolated rupture of the LVFW; 1 (4%), isolated rupture of the VS; 3 (12%), isolated rupture of a single PM, and 6 (24%) patients had combined rupture (both LVFW and VS in 4 and rupture of the LVFW plus PM [anterolateral] in 1.) (Figures 2-15).The interval from AMI to death varied from 1 to 45 days (median 3). Eight (32%) rupture patients received thrombolysis during the AMI, and 11 (44%) had percutaneous coronary intervention after admission for AMI. Five patients (20%) underwent coronary artery bypass grafting after onset of the AMI, all 5 within 5 days of death.

An additional patient had coronary artery bypass grafting 6 years before the fatal AMI.

In the 21 patients with LVFW rupture, the rupture site was at the junction of the LVFW and VS in 18 patients (82%): anterior in 7 and posterior in 10; in 3 others in the lateral wall, and in 1 at the apex (Figure 2). Of the 5 patients with rupture of the VS, 1 was anterior, and the other 4, all of whom also had LVFW rupture, was posterior. Of the latter 4 patients the rupture of the VS was partial, not complete. Of the 4 patients with PM rupture, all partial, the posteromedial muscle was involved in 2 and the anterolateral muscle in 2.

The unadjusted comparison of floating heart, left ventricular scar, diabetes mellitus, body mass index, age, and presence of hemopericardium between non-rupture and rupture patients were statistically significant (Table 3).

Discussion

The present study examines certain clinical and necropsy findings in 64 patients admitted to a single hospital during a 22-year period because of AMI, and compares the 25 (39%) with rupture of the LVFW or VS or PM or combinations to the

Table 3
Clinical and Necropsy Findings in 64 Patients with Fatal Acute Myocardial Infarction: 25 Patients with Cardiac Rupture and 39 without Rupture

Variable	Rupture		P Value[*]
	Yes (n=25)	No (n=39)	
Men : Women	16 (64%) : 9 (36%)	23 (59%) : 16 (41%)	0.690
Ages (years) range (mean)			0.001
Men	47-81 (68)	33-83 (56)	
Women	68-83 (75)	42-88 (65)	
Black : white	2 (8%) : 23 (92%)	10 (28%) : 26 (72%)[†]	0.060
Body mass index (kg/m^2)			0.048
Men	15/16	12/23	
Range (mean)	24.3-32.3 (28.0)	26.0-64.6 (35.3)	
Women	7/9	13/16	
Range (mean)	23.9-41.3 (28.6)	18.7-49.5 (31.2)	
Diabetes mellitus			0.034
Men	4 (25%)	6/19 (32%)	
Women	2 (22%)	12 (75%)	
Systemic hypertension (by history)			0.162
Men	15/16 (94%)	17/20 (85%)	
Women	6/8 (75%)	9 (56%)	
Coronary bypass	6 (24%)	11/35 (31%)	0.532
Thrombolytic therapy	8 (32%)	4 (10%)	0.031
Percutaneous coronary intervention	11 (44%)	17/38 (45%)	0.954
Left ventricular Scar	1 (4%)	11 (28%)	0.016
Location of AMI			0.470
Posterior	12 (48%)	22 (56%)	
Anterior	9 (36%)	10 (26%)	
Lateral	3 (12%)	5 (13%)	
Circumferential	0	2 (5%)	
Apical	1 (4%)	0	
Right ventricular Infarct	7 (28%)	5 (13%)	0.132
Heart weight (g) range (mean)			0.929
Men	390-740 (519)	375-1060 (565)	
Women	310-555 (412)	310-660 (402)	
Floating Heart	19/23 (83%)	6/30 (20%)	<0.001
Hemopericardium	19 (76%)	0	<0.0001

AMI=acute myocardial infarction.

[*] P-values account for multiple comparisons.

[†] Data missing in 3 patients.

39 patients (61%) studied in the same hospital and during the same time frame without cardiac rupture. Patients developing an AMI after admission to the hospital were excluded. Compared to the non-rupture cases, the rupture cases were significantly older (71 years — vs — 60 years); had a much higher frequency of huge deposits of adipose tissue in the heart (floated in formaldehyde) (88% — vs — 20%); a much lower frequency of having a healed myocardial infarct (scar) (4% — vs — 28%); a lower frequency of diabetes mellitus (24% — vs — 47%); a lower body mass index (28.2 kg/m^2— vs — 33.2 kg/m^2), and a higher frequency of thrombolytic therapy during the AMI (32% — vs — 10%).

Although the present report indicated a significant difference in age (mean 71 — vs — 60 years) between the rupture and none rupture groups, that has not been the case uniformly. Mann and Roberts (40), for example, found no significant difference in mean ages among men — vs — women in 138 necropsy patients with —vs — 50 without LVFW rupture (men: 63 years — vs — 63 years; women: 73 years — vs — 71 years) or a difference in 38 unoperated necropsy patients with — vs — without rupture of the VS (men: 65 years — vs — 63 years;

women: 74 years — vs — 71 years) (39). Of the 22 patients with rupture of the PM secondary to AMI reported by Barbour and Roberts,[36] the mean ages of the 15 men was 60 years (non-rupture mean age 63 years) and that in the 7 women, 75 years (non-rupture mean age 71 years). The mean ages of the women were significantly higher than that of the men in both the rupture and non-rupture groups in all these studies.

Because AMI is more common in men than women, the proportion of men in most published studies of rupture secondary to AMI is slightly higher in men but the percentage of men is less than in the AMI group without rupture. Of the 444 non-rupture cases of AMI studied at necropsy by Reddy and Roberts,[25] 70% were men and 30% were women; of the 204 rupture cases (LVFW or VS) studied by the same authors, 55% were men and 45% were women. Of the 22 cases of rupture of the PM reported by Barbour and Roberts,[36] 15 were men (68%) and 7 (32%) were women.

Although most patients with AMI have a body mass index $\geq$ 25 Kg/m^2, the mean BMI in the present study was significantly *lower* in the rupture group than in the non-rupture

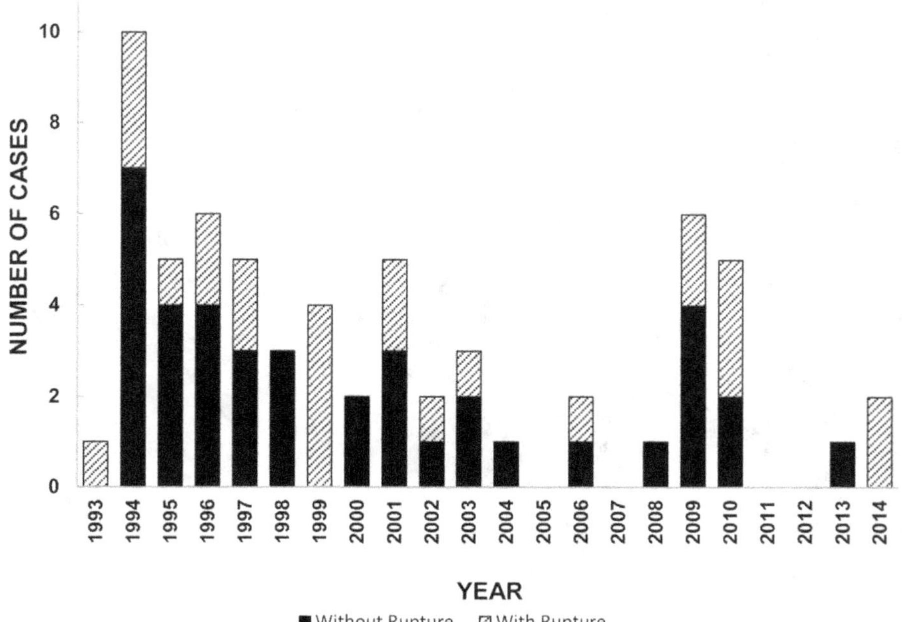

Figure 1. Bar graph Comparing the number of patients with fatal acute myocardial infarction at Baylor University Medical Center from 1993 through June 2014 showing the patients with acute myocardial infarction without rupture in black and those with rupture in gray. Of the total 64 patients studied both clinically and at necropsy, 25 had rupture of the left ventricular free wall or ventricular septum or left ventricular papillary muscle or combinations and 39 had fatal acute myocardial infarction without rupture.

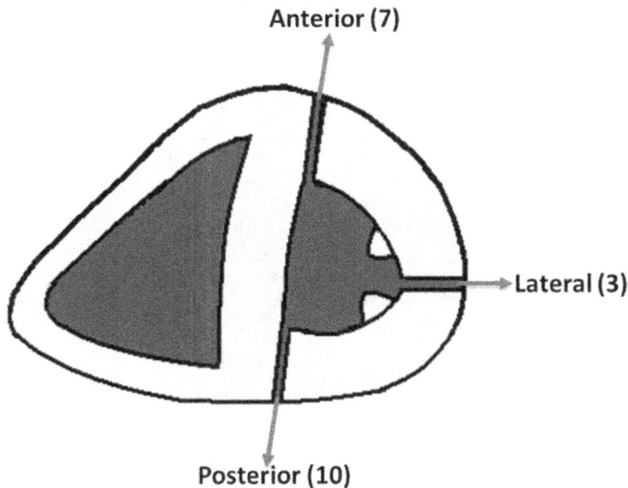

Figure 2. Diagram of cross-section of cardiac ventricles displaying the sites of the 21 left ventricular free wall ruptures. The left ventricular free wall ruptures were anterior in 7 patients, posterior in 10, and lateral (roughly between the 2 papillary muscles) in 3 patients. The left and right ventricular cavities are shown in red and the myocardium in yellow.

group. This finding is surprising because the quantity of adipose was significantly *greater* in the rupture — vs — the non-rupture groups. This finding was also observed in a previous LVFW rupture and VS rupture studies by Mann and Roberts.[37,38] The PM rupture study by Barbour and Roberts,[36] also disclosed a high frequency of cardiac adiposity, specifically a higher frequency of those with floating hearts among the PM rupture than the non-rupture cases. The greater the quantity of cardiac fat the greater the likelihood that the heart will float in a container of formaldehyde.[43] In the present study, 83% of the rupture hearts floated compared to only 20% of the non-rupture hearts. Because adipose tissue is lighter than formaldehyde (or water), hearts with enormous quantities of fat usually float except when the myocardial mass is particularly large. Shirani and colleagues[44] in a necropsy study of cardiac adiposity demonstrated that in the floating hearts the subepicardial adipose tissue constituted a mean of $32 \pm 9\%$ (range 21% to 52%) of the cardiac weight. Thus, irrespective of the rupture site, the quantity of cardiac adipose tissue in these patients is nearly always increased.

What does cardiac adipose tissue have to do with cardiac rupture? The cardiac adipose tissue is mainly in the subepicardial regions, particularly over the right ventricle, and around the epicardial coronary arteries particularly those in the atrioventricular sulci, and also in the atrial septa (lipomatous hypertrophy of the atrial septum), but not in the wall of the left ventricle or VS or in the left ventricular PM, the sites where rupture secondary to AMI occur. Although when excessive it usually penetrates the myocardial wall of the right ventricle, subepicardial adipose tissue does not infiltrate the left ventricular free wall, with the exception of sites of healed myocardial infarcts, an infrequent occurrence in patients with non-traumatic cardiac rupture. Cardiac adiposity can be viewed as a reflection of excessive adipose tissue in non-cardiac structures. One might assume from this observation that non-obese people infrequently have cardiac rupture as a consequence of AMI, but most individuals with AMI with or without subsequent rupture are overweight or obese.

Although a few patients with rupture during AMI have preexisting angina pectoris, the AMI complicated by rupture is nearly always the first AMI and virtually always the first clinically recognized AMI. This observation is confirmed by the infrequency of a grossly-visible scar in the left ventricular

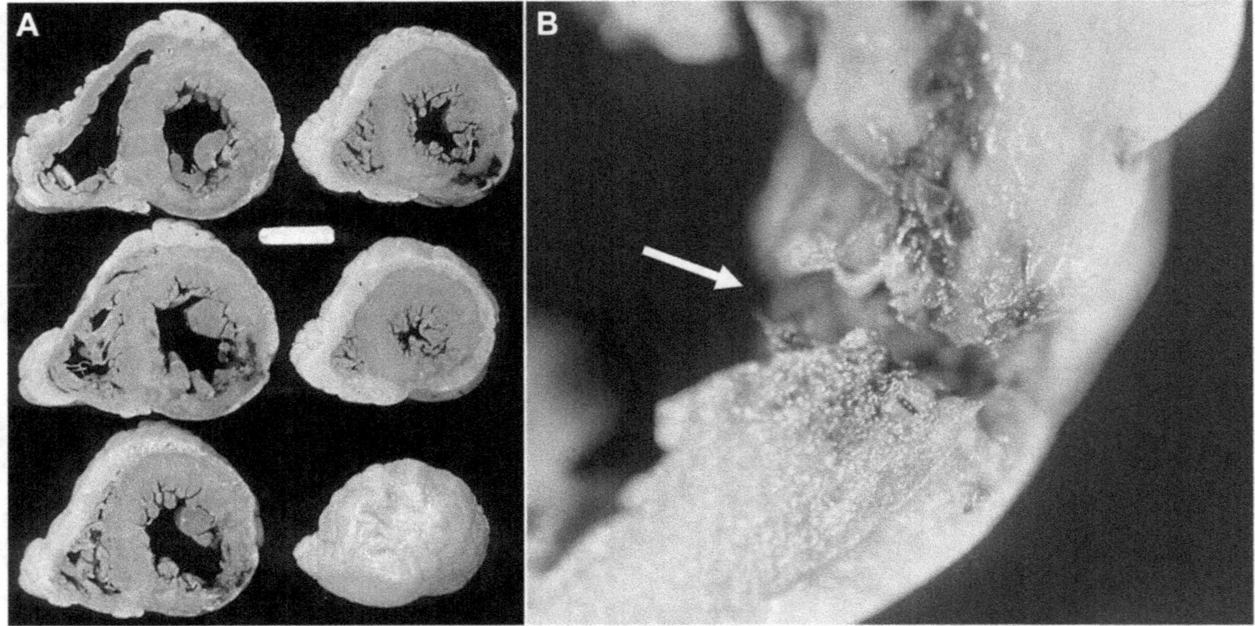

Figure 3. Case 2, Table 2. *(A)* Slices of the cardiac ventricles showing the infarct in the lateral wall and a great deal of subepicardial adipose tissue. *(B)* close-up of the lateral wall rupture showing the rupture site *(arrow)*.

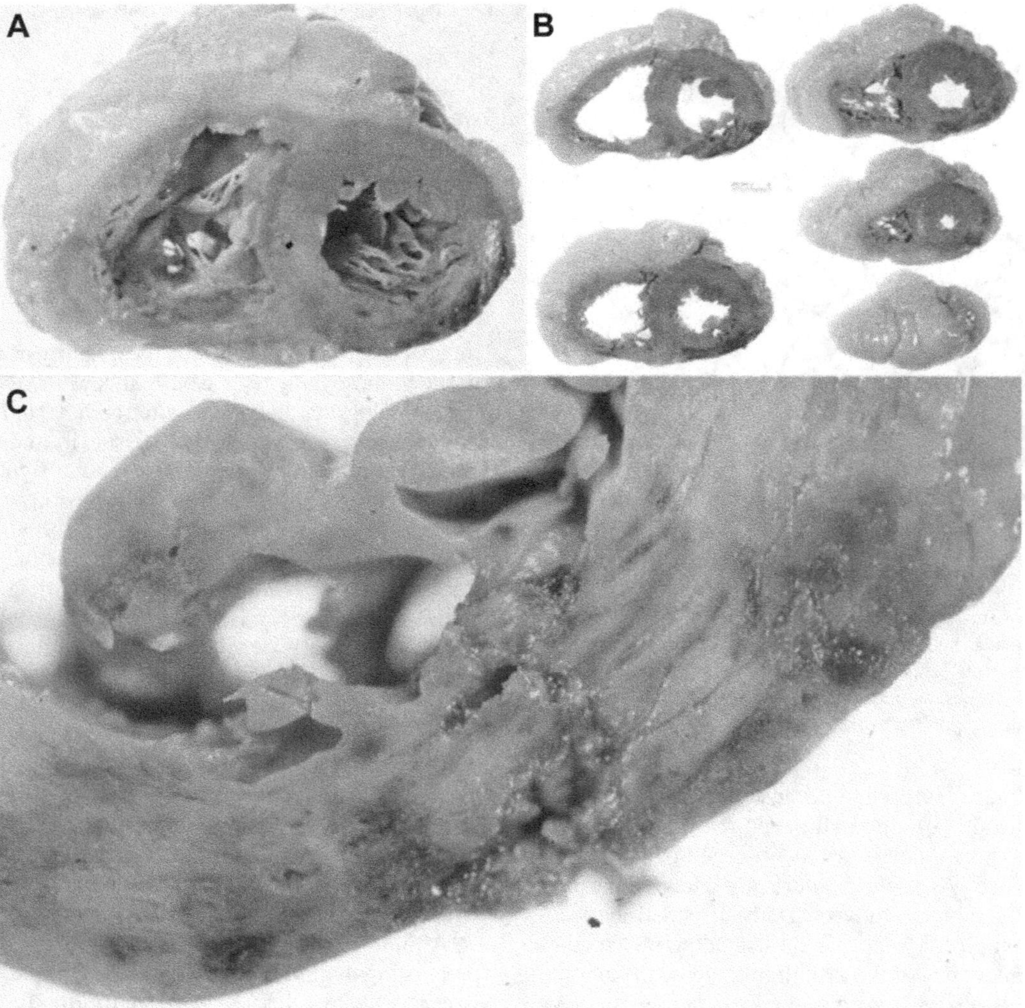

Figure 4. Case 4, Table 2. *(A)* View of both ventricles near the base of the heart. The infarct involves the left ventricular free wall just beneath the posteromedial papillary muscle. The quantity of subepicardial adipose tissue is huge. *(B)* Views of the ventricular cavities and walls caudal to the views shown in *(C)*. *Lower.* Close-up view of the ruptured site.

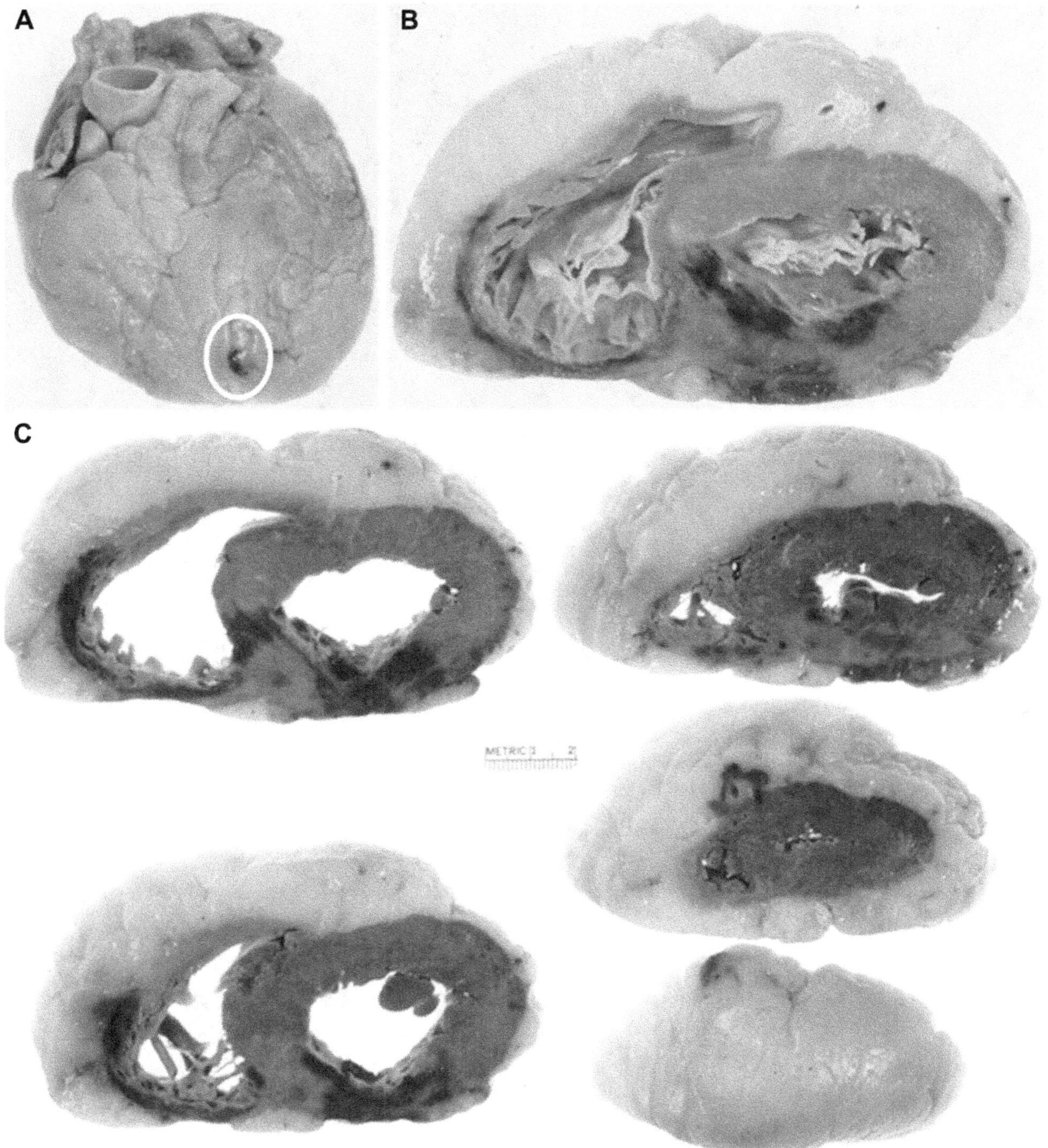

Figure 5. Case 6, Table 2. *(A)* View of the exterior of the heart anteriorly showing an enormous amount of subepicardial adipose tissue and the rupture site near the cardiac apex *(circle)*. *(B)* View of the more basal portion of the ventricles showing the tricuspid and mitral valves, an acute infarction involving the left ventricular free wall posteriorly, the ventricular septum, and a large portion of the right ventricular free wall. *(C)* Views of the ventricles caudal to the view shown in the *(B)*. The basal portions are quite dilated. The amount of infarction of the right ventricular free wall is enormous. The quantity of subepicardial adipose tissue is such that in some of these cross-sections no myocardium is visible exteriorly.

wall in the patients with rupture during AMI. In the present study, only 1 (4%) of the 25 rupture cases compared to 11 (28%) of the 39 non-rupture cases had a scar in the LVFW. In the necropsy study by Reddy and Roberts[25] of 648 cases of AMI, 29 (13%) of the 204 patients with rupture compared to 188 (42%) of 444 non-rupture cases had a preexisting left ventricular scar before the fatal AMI. The infrequency of

preexisting left ventricular scar strongly indicates that before the AMI which ruptured that systolic heart failure was absent. Indeed, examination of the hearts with LVFW rupture typically show a non-dilated left ventricular cavity; in contrast, those with rupture of the VS or a PM are usually dilated but the absence of left ventricular scar indicates that the dilatation occurred after the AMI which ruptured not before the event.

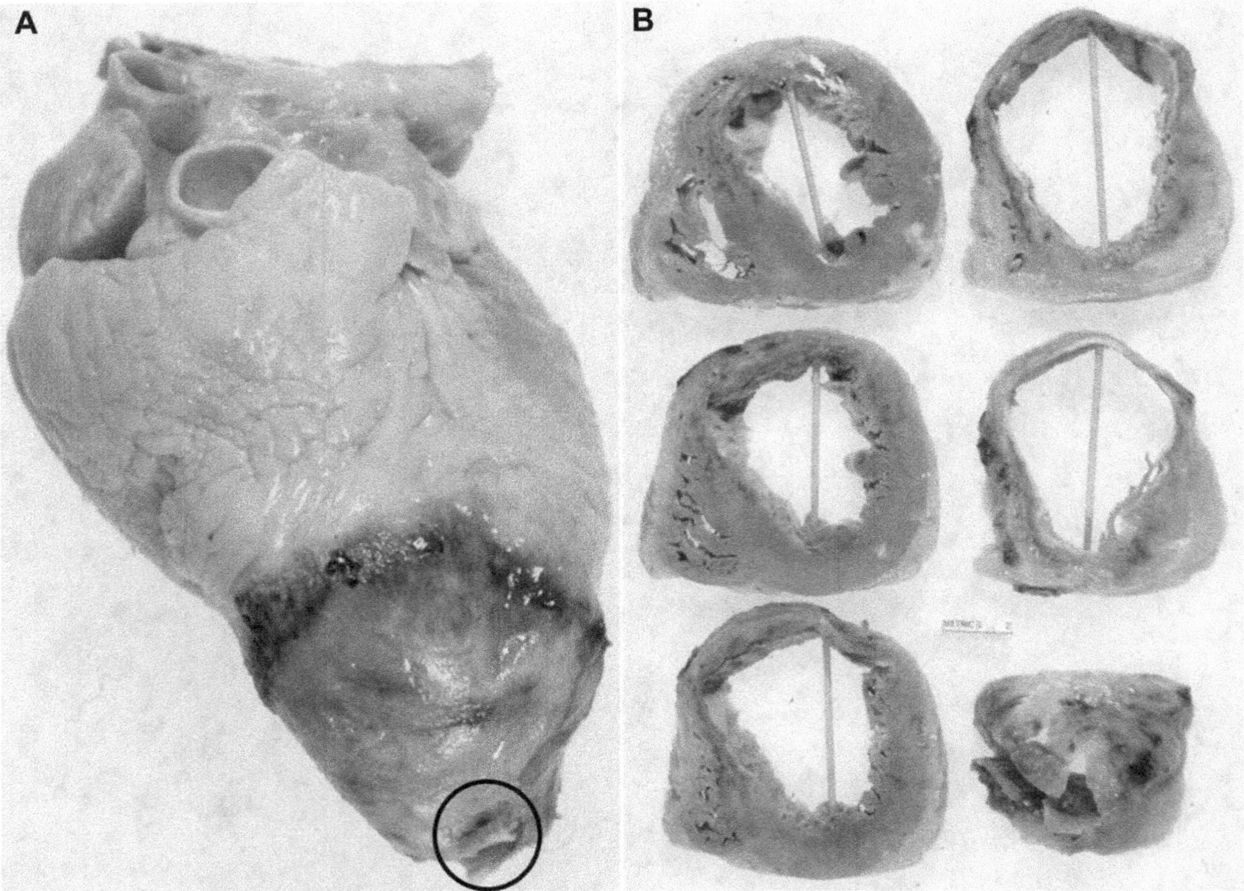

Figure 6. Case 7, Table 2. *(A)* Exterior of the heart, anterior view showing a large apical aneurysm which ruptured at the most apical portion *(circle)*. *(B)* Views of the ventricles showing severe dilatation of the left ventricular cavity, marked thinning of its wall, and, in some sections, nearly circumferential infarction). The rupture site is at the thinnest point shown best in *(B)*. The interval from onset of the acute myocardial infarction to rupture was 45 days, the longest of any of the 26 patients. This long interval allowed the free wall to thin considerably such that the rupture site was not between viable muscle and nonviable muscle but at the most central portion of the large myocardial infarct. Additionally, this was the largest infarct of any of the 25 patients with rupture.

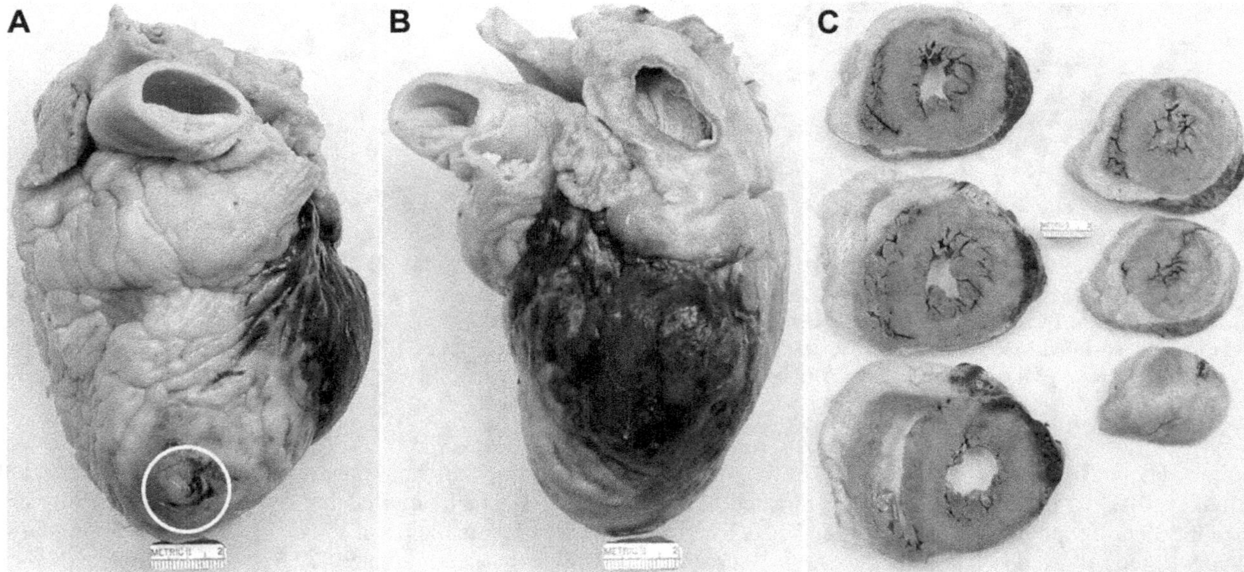

Figure 7. Case 10, Table 2. *(A)* View of the anterior wall of the heart showing hemorrhage into the subepicardial adipose tissue, which is excessive. The rupture site is circled. *(B)* View of the heart from the left lateral aspect showing the extent of the hemorrhage into the subepicardial adipose tissue. *(C)* Cross-sections of the cardiac ventricles showing the rupture site at the junction of the anterior freewall and ventricular septum.

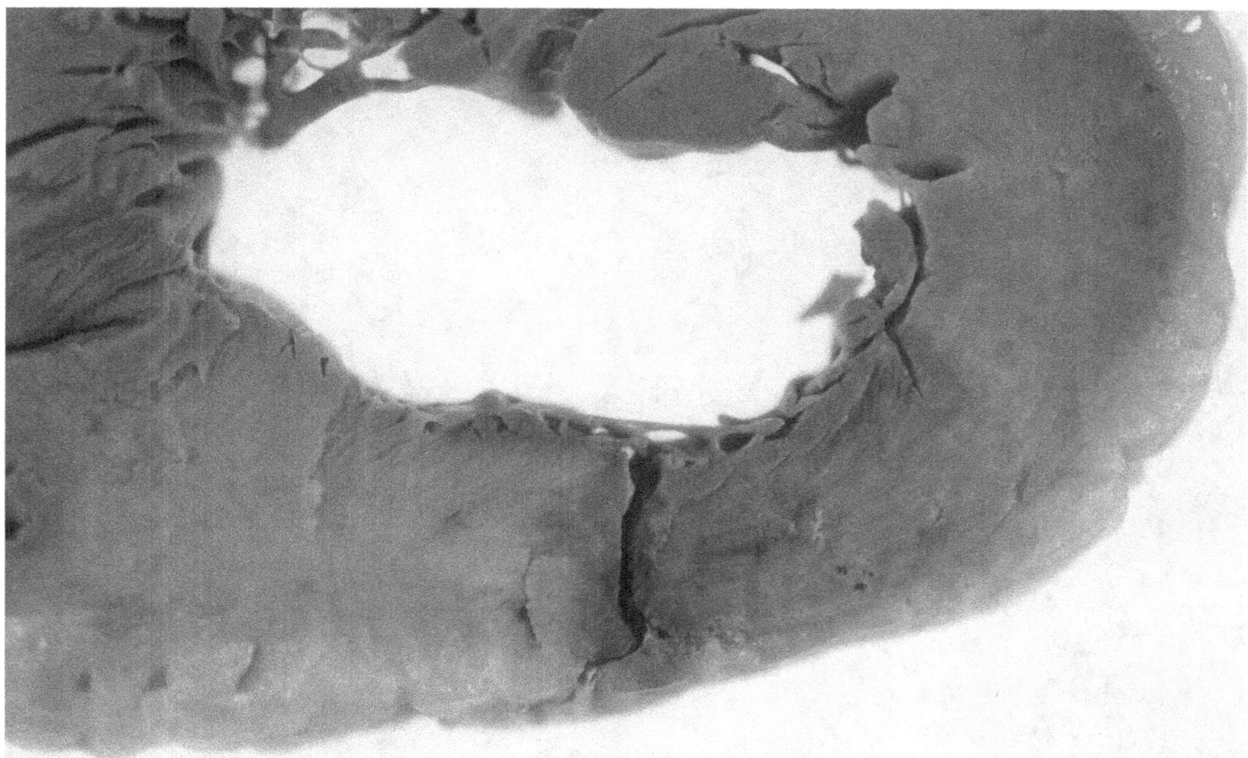

Figure 8. Case 11, Table 2. View of left ventricular freewall showing the rupture site. The size of the acute infarct was relatively small. The quantity of subepicardial adipose tissue is increased.

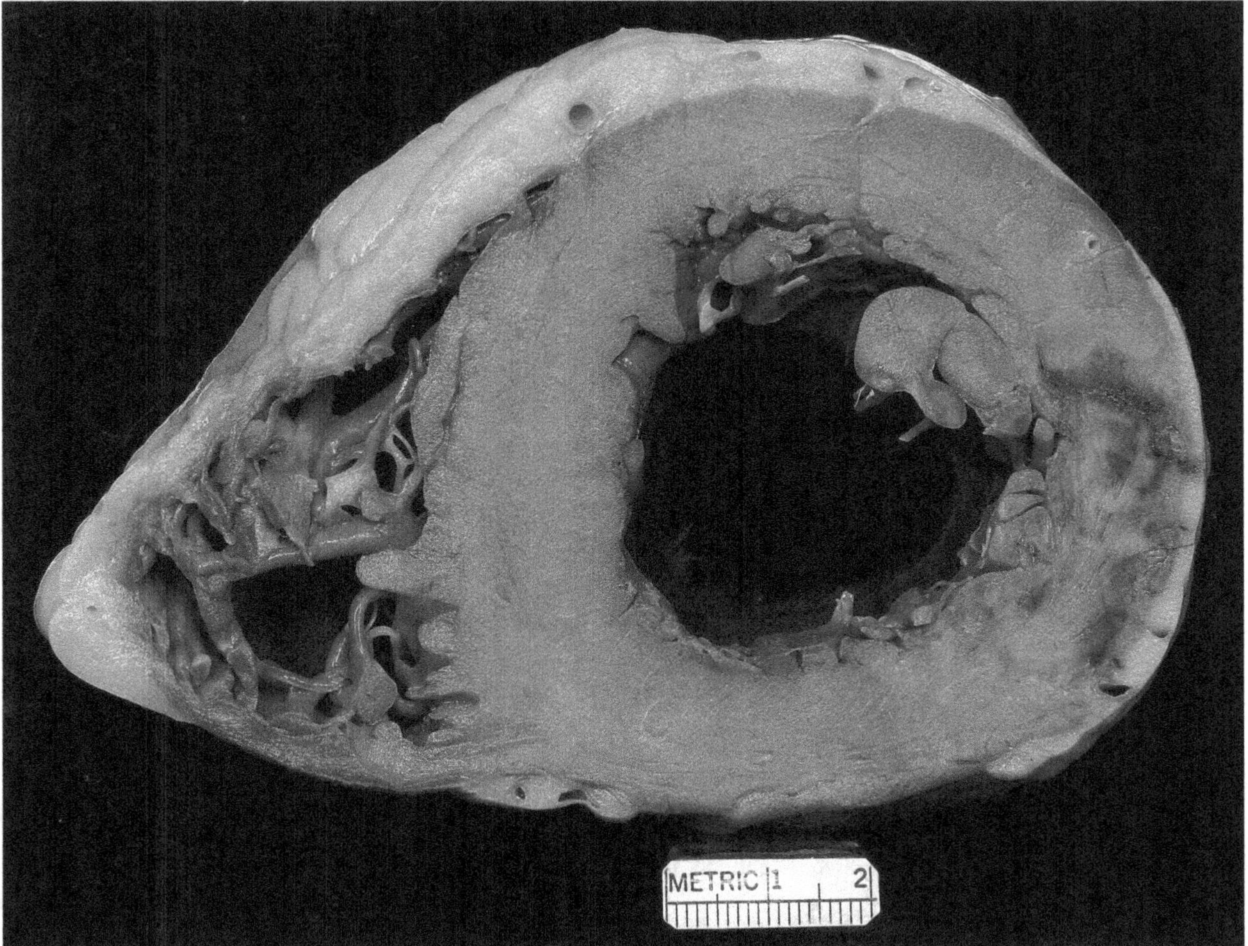

Figure 9. Case 14, Table 2. View of the ventricles showing rupture just beneath the posteromedial papillary muscle. The size of the infarct is relatively small.

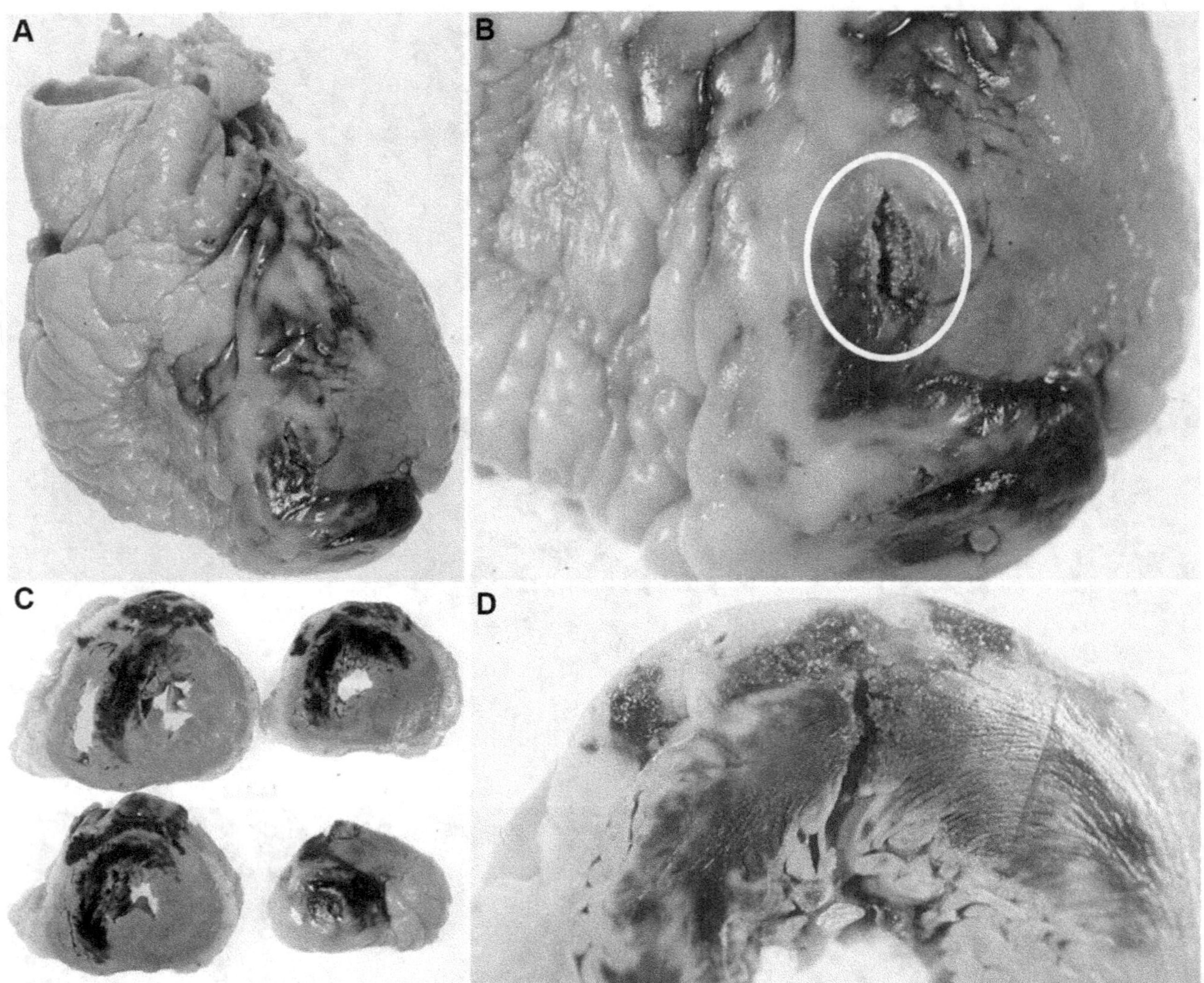

Figure 10. Case 16, Table 2. *(A)* View of the heart anteriorly showing patchy subepicardial hemorrhages. *(B)* View of the rupture site exteriorly *(circle)*. *(C)* Cross-section of the cardiac ventricles showing a large hemorrhagic infarct involving the anteroseptal walls. *(D)* Close up view of the rupture site. The patient received thrombolytic therapy.

Thus, the patient with preexisting heart failure from a previous AMI which healed is very unlikely to rupture with a subsequent AMI. Rupture during AMI generally indicates a good functioning left ventricle before the rupture event and usually up to the actual rupture event in the LVFW rupture cases. Furthermore and not surprisingly, the size of the acute infarct in the rupture cases is usually smaller than in the non-rupture cases. Saffitz and associates[45] compared at necropsy the size of the acute infarct in AMI patients in whom death was caused by cardiogenic shock, arrhythmia, or cardiac rupture, and found that the patients dying from cardiogenic shock had the largest acute infarcts ($37 \pm 11\%$ of the total left ventricular mass), and those who died of cardiac rupture had the smallest infarcts ($15 \pm 9\%$).

Much has been written on the relation of systemic hypertension *before* the AMI which ruptured but the results are conflicting. Although it appears logical that elevation of the peak left ventricular systolic pressure persisting *after* AMI would more likely lead to rupture compared to patients in whom the peak left ventricular systolic pressure fell to normal or lower levels, such evidence is speculative at best.

The frequency of systemic hypertension before the AMI was insignificantly different in the present study and in the previous Reddy and Roberts study between the rupture and non-rupture groups.[25] Additionally, heart weights were insignificantly different between the rupture and non-rupture cases in the present and in the previous Reddy and Roberts[25] study. Preexisting hypertension of course may cause thickening of the LVFW, VS, and PMs. One could reason that the thicker these structures the less likely they might rupture. In only 3 (12%) of the 25 rupture cases in the present study did the heart weigh > 600 g.

One might be surprised by the high frequency of rupture in the present study (39% of the total AMI cases). All of the patients included herein were studied in the last 2 decades, a period of improved medicines to manage patients with AMI and of course hospitalization in the coronary care units where now fatal arrhythmias are relatively infrequent. Reddy and Roberts[25] reviewed published reports of the frequency of rupture of the LVFW or VS among necropsy cases of AMI *before* and *after* the widespread use of coronary care units (Table 1): the frequency of rupture ranged

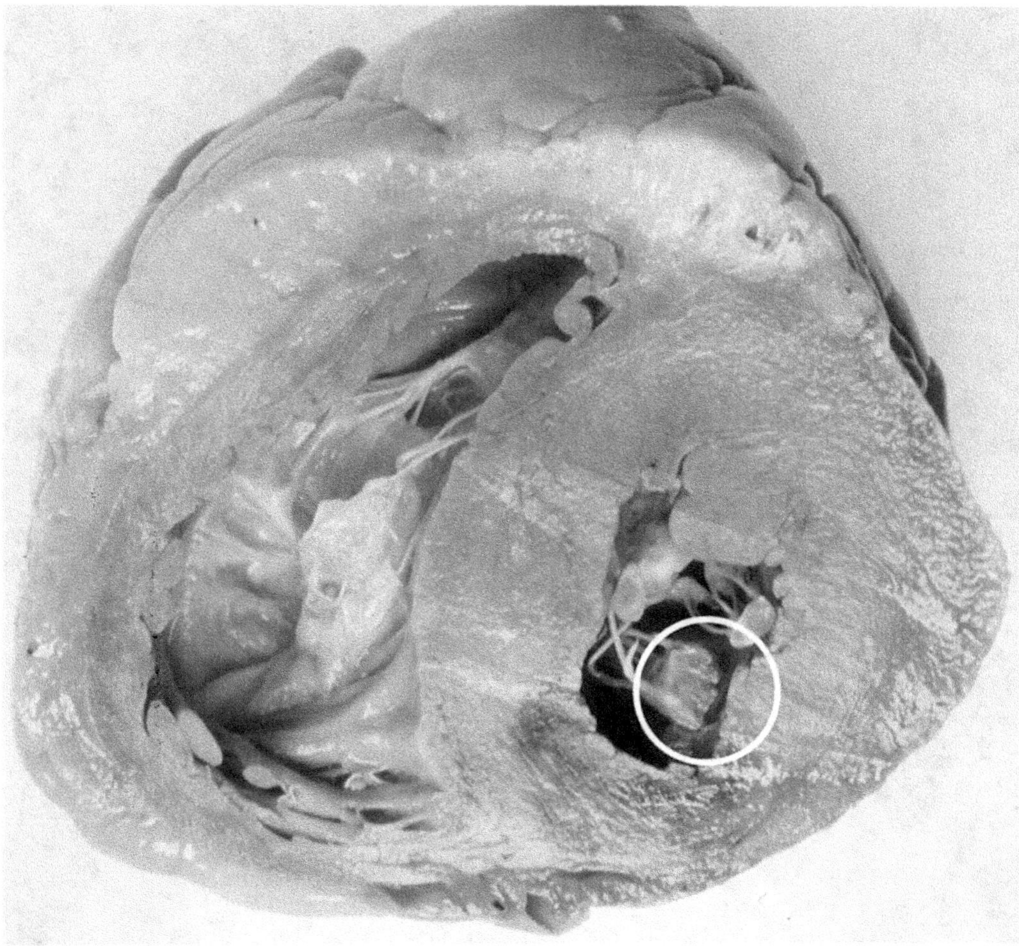

Figure 11. Case 18, Table 2. View of the base of the heart showing a ruptured posteromedial papillary muscle with an acute infarct involving the posterior wall and a portion of the ventricular septum. The ruptured muscle is circled.

from 4% to 24% (mean 8%) (680 of 9,133 cases); of the 3,851 necropsy patients reported by them *after* the common use of coronary care units, 693 (18%) ruptured the LVFW or VS (Table 1). Of the cases studied by Reddy and Roberts, however, 204 (31%) of the 648 necropsy patients with AMI ruptured.[25] Although the rupture cases are probably more likely to have an autopsy, the frequency of rupture of the LVFW or VS as a cause of death during AMI appears to have increased substantially since the widespread use of coronary care units, even though the total mortality from AMI has decreased dramatically (from roughly 35% to the present 5%).

The relation of thrombolysis therapy during AMI to the frequency of cardiac rupture remains unclear. Thrombolysis tends to convert an ischemic (pale) infarct into a hemorrhagic infarct. Roberts and colleagues[46] demonstrated experimentally in dogs that ischemic and hemorrhagic infarcts healed at the same rates. In the present study the frequency of thrombolysis therapy was significantly higher in the rupture cases compared to the non-rupture cases (32% − vs − 10%). Among the 648 AMI cases studied by Reddy and Roberts,[25] 56 (9%) had received streptokinase or recombinant tissue-type plasminogen activator during the first hours after onset of AMI: 18 (32%) had rupture of the LVFW or VS, a

percentage similar to that in the group who had not received thrombolytic therapy (186 of 592 [31%]). Pollak et al[27] found LVFW rupture during AMI in 3 (0.7%) of 447 patients treated with thrombolysis and in 102 (4%) of 2,403 patients not treated with thrombolysis (84% autopsy rate). Yusuf and colleagues[47] pooled the results of 33 randomized trials of thrombolytic agents for AMI, and found similar frequencies of cardiac rupture in patients and in control subjects. Honan et al[48] pooled the results of 4 randomized trials involving 1,638 patients, and observed that the risk of rupture (58 cases, autopsy rate $\geq$ 50%) was directly correlated with time to treatment.

Few studies have reported on the degrees of narrowing of the major epicardial coronary arteries in patients with cardiac rupture secondary to AMI. Mann and Roberts[39,40] compared the number of major (right, left anterior descending, and left circumflex) epicardial coronary arteries narrowed > 75% in cross-sectional area by atherosclerotic plaque alone and found that the rupture cases (LVFW or VS) had significantly less narrowing than did the non-rupture cases. As shown in Table 4, both the LVFW and the VS rupture cases had a lower percent of patients with all of these 3 major coronary arteries narrowed > 75% in cross-sectional area by plaque and also a lower percent of major

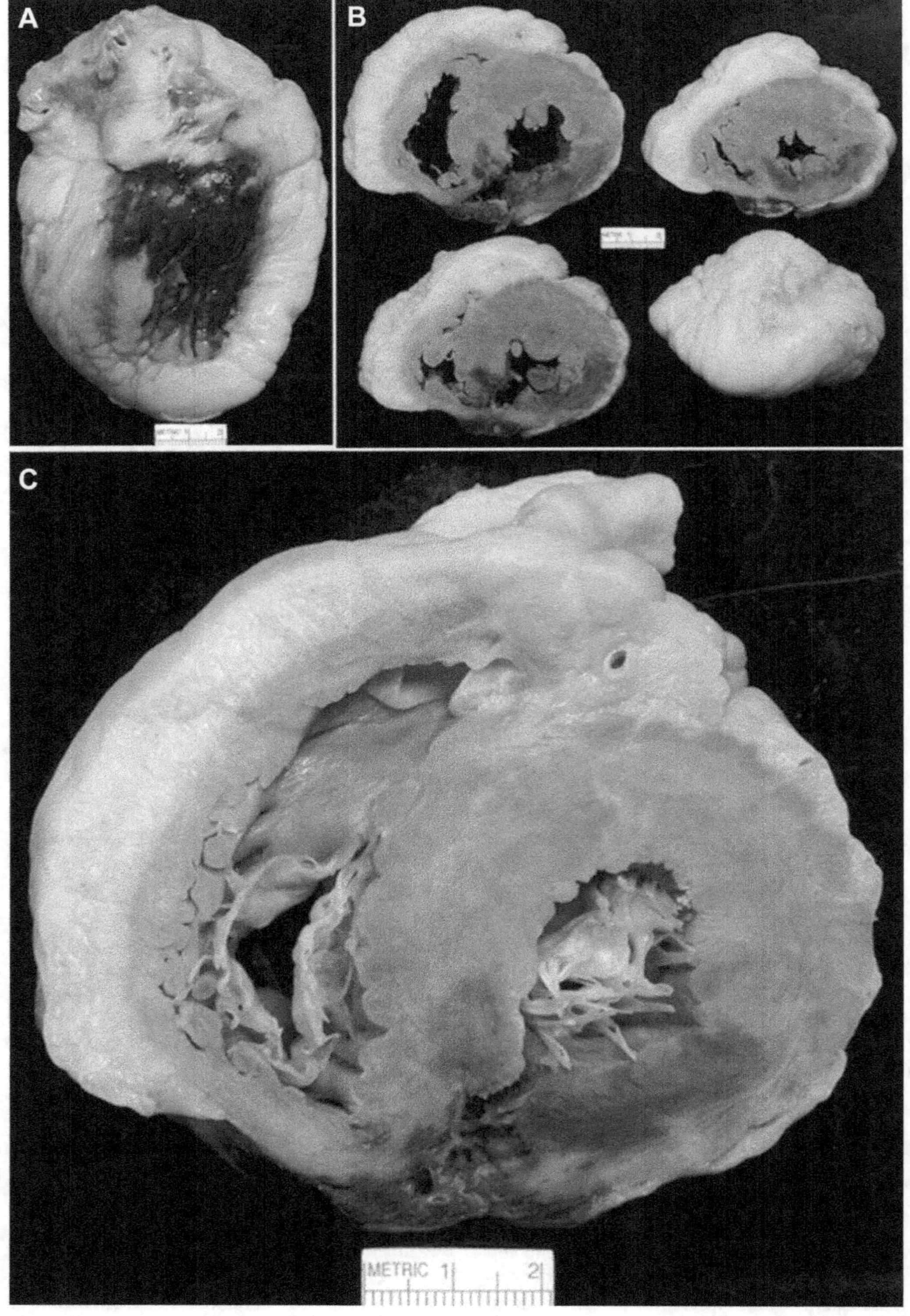

Figure 12. Case 21, Table 2. *(A)* View of the back of the heart showing a great deal of blood in the subepicardial adipose tissue. *(B)* View of the ventricles showing the rupture site involving both ventricular septum and left ventricular free wall. The quantity of subepicardial adipose tissue is enormous. *(C)* Close-up view of the rupture site. The infarct is hemorrhagic. The patient received thrombolytic therapy.

arteries narrowed insignificantly (≤25%) by plaque. Additionally, these authors[39,40] also studied the extent of the atherosclerotic process in these patients by examining each 5-mm long segment histologically of the 4 (includes left main) major epicardial coronary arteries. As shown in Table 5, the LVFW and VS rupture cases had 50% fewer

5-mm segments narrowed > 75% by atherosclerotic plaque and also about double the percent of segments narrowed ≤ 25% in cross-sectional area. The Mann and Roberts[39,40] studies were the first to examine carefully the status of the epicardial coronary arteries in rupture − vs − non-rupture cases. Barbour and Roberts[36] also studied the status of the

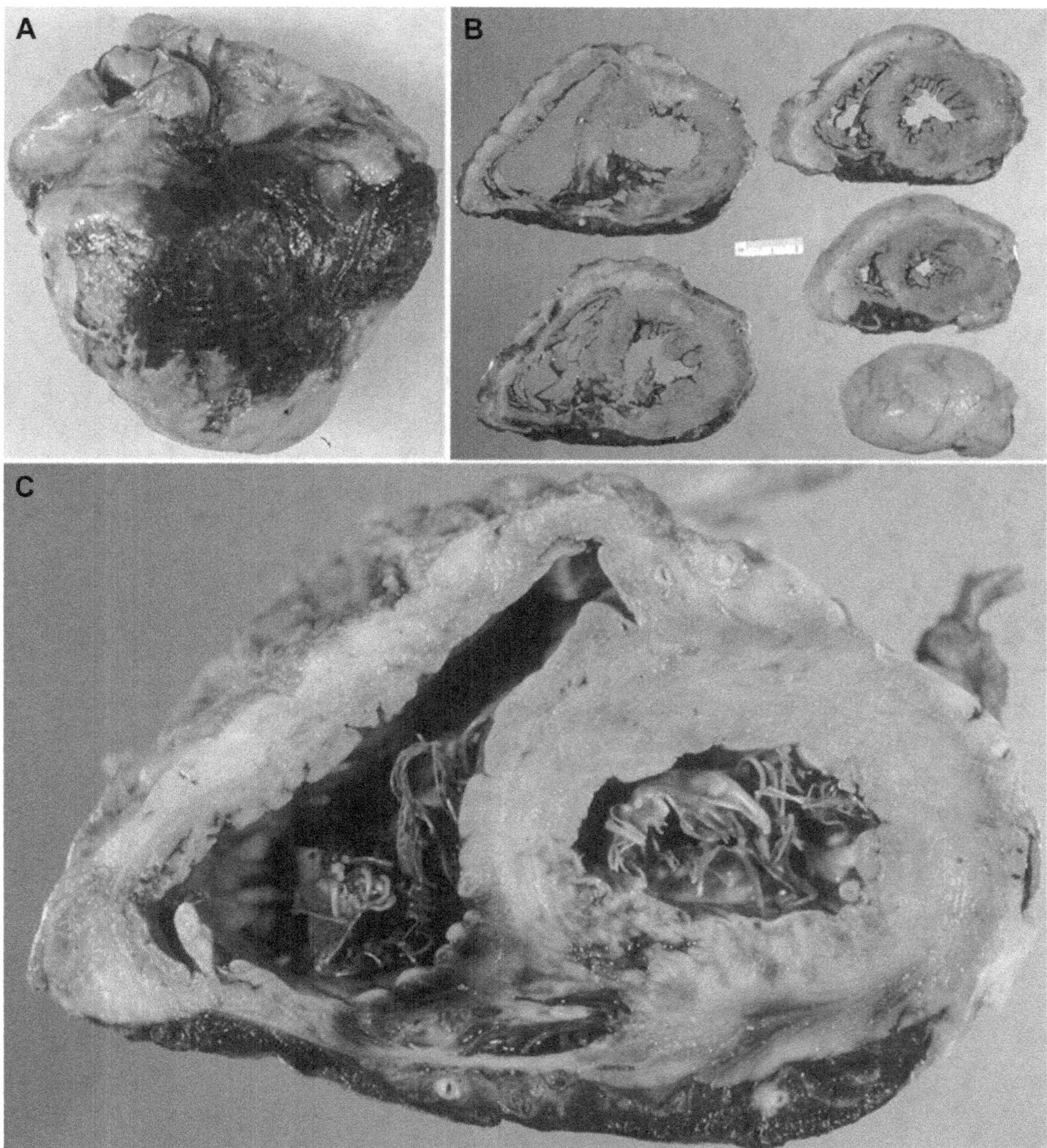

Figure 13. Case 22. Table 2. *(A)* Back of the heart showing a huge amount of hemorrhage into the subepicardial adipose tissue. *(B)* Cross-sections of the cardiac ventricles showing rupture of the ventricular septum and of the left ventricular free wall just posterior to the septum. *(C)* Close-up view of the ruptured site through the left ventricular free wall and ventricular septum show the ventricular septal rupture and also its exit from the right ventricular free wall.

epicardial coronary arteries in necropsy patients with PM rupture and also found significantly less coronary narrowing in the PM rupture group than in their non-rupture control group. A different control group was used than used in the LVFW and VS Mann and Roberts studies. In the LVFW and VS studies both patients and controls had no left ventricular scars (These cases were excluded.), whereas in the PM studies nearly half of the control group had left ventricular scars (a previously healed myocardial infarct).

Some features of the present study make it a bit different from previously reported ones on cardiac rupture. With the exception of 3 cases, all 64 hearts were studied at necropsy by the same individual (WCR) and described,

weighed, and sectioned by him. The information as a consequence would appear to be more reliable than that obtained simply by examining autopsy records produced by many different individuals with varying degrees of expertise in cardiovascular disease. A limitation of course of the present study is the number of cases studied in a 22-year-period at a very large tertiary hospital with an autopsy rate of approximately 4% among hospital deaths. As shown in Figure 1 the number of patients with onset of AMI before hospitalization with later autopsy ranged from none in 4 years to as high as 10 in one year; in 2 years all AMI cases coming to autopsy had rupture. There is likely a greater tendency among clinicians to get an autopsy if

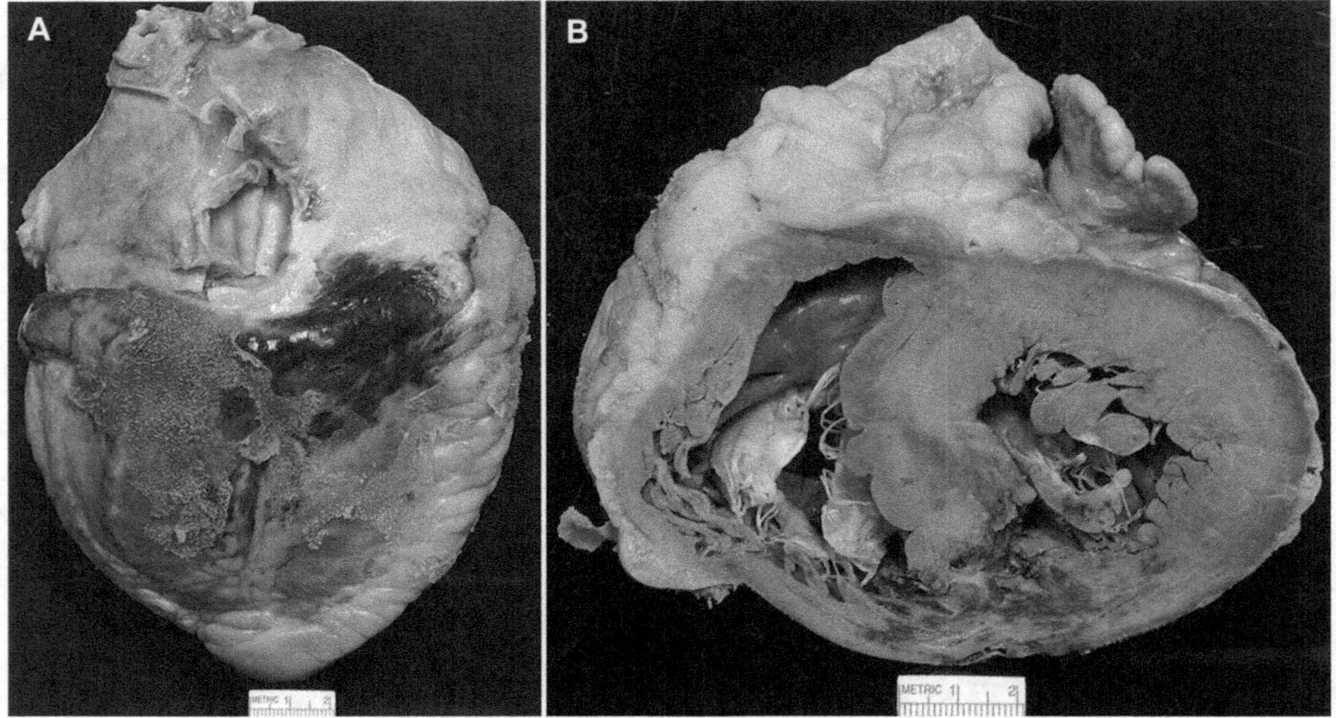

Figure 14. Case 24, Table 2. *(A)* View of the back of the heart showing extravasated blood in and around the right atrioventricular sulcus. *(B)* View of the base of the ventricles showing rupture of the ventricular septum and of the left ventricular free wall. The quantity of subepicardial adipose tissue is considerable.

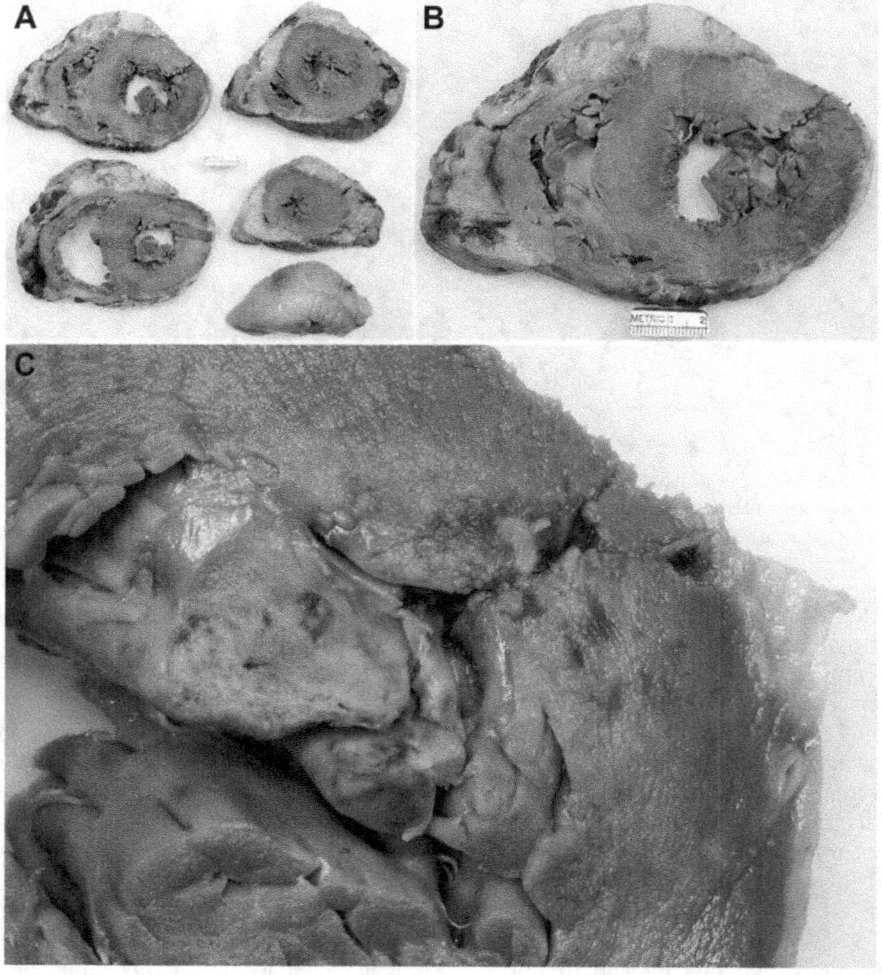

Figure 15. Case 25, Table 2. *(A)* View of the cardiac ventricles showing no dilatation of left ventricular cavity but a great deal of subepicardial adipose tissue. *(B)* View of the rupture site behind the anterolateral papillary muscle. *(C)* Close-up of the rupture site.

Table 4

Number of 3 Major Coronary Arteries (Right, Left Anterior Descending and Left Circumflex) Narrowed > 75% in Cross-Sectional Area by Atherosclerotic Plaque Alone in Patients with Rupture of the Left Ventricular Free Wall − vs − Rupture of the Ventricular Septum − vs − Non-Rupture Controls. All with Fatal First Acute Myocardial Infarction

Number of 3 major (R, LAD, LC) coronary arteries narrowed > 75% in CSA by plaque	Rupture		Non-rupture control (n=50)[*]
	LVFW (n=117)[*]	VS (n=33)[*]	
0	7 (8%)[†]	1 (3%)	11 (22%)
1	25 (28%)	8 (24%)	7 (15%)
2	24 (27%)	9 (27%)	12 (25%)
3	33 (37%)	15 (45%)	28 (58%)

CSA=cross-sectional area; LAD=left anterior descending; LC=left circumflex; LVFW=left ventricular free wall; R=right; VS=ventricular septum.

[*] Excludes patients with a left ventricular scar (healed myocardial infarct), in other words, all patients included in this table had only a first and only acute myocardial infarction.

[†] Of these 9 patients, 8 had total occlusion of the coronary artery by thrombus superimposed on atherosclerotic plaque.

Table 5

Analysis of the Extent of Atherosclerotic Plaque in the 4 Major (Right, Left Main, Left Anterior Descending and Left Circumflex) Epicardial Coronary Arteries in Patients with Rupture of the Left Ventricular Free Wall − vs − Rupture of the Ventricular Septum − vs − Non-Rupture Controls with Fatal First Acute Myocardial Infarction

Four categories of cross-sectional area narrowing (%)	Number of 5-mm long 5-mm segments of the 4 major coronary arteries		Non-rupture Group (Patients=50) (Five-mm segments=1848)
	Rupture		
	LVFW (Patients=66) (Five-mm segments=3287)	VS (Patients=18) (Five-mm segments=825)	
0-25	571 (17%)	118 (14%)	132 (7%)
26-50	1186 (31%)	287 (35%)	632 (34%)
51-75	1018 (14%)	319 (39%)	576 (31%)
76-100	513 (15%)	101 (13%)	508 (28%)

LVFW=left ventricular free wall; VS=ventricular septum.

the immediate cause of death is unclear or if rupture is suspected. This likely bias needs to be kept in mind when determining frequency of this particular event. In any study involving cardiac rupture, an autopsy is mandatory to achieve diagnostic accuracy.

Conclusion

Cardiac rupture is an increasingly more frequent cause of death during AMI. It complicates a first AMI, occurs in hearts which contain an enormous quantity of adipose tissue, the left ventricular cavity is usually of normal size until the rupture occurs, and the area of the infarct is usually relatively small.

Disclosures

There are no conflicts of interest and no author has any relation with industry.

1. Bean WB. Infarction of heart: III. Clinical course and morphological findings. Ann Intern Med 1938;12:71−94.
2. Edmondson HA, Hoxie HJ. Hypertension and cardiac rupture: A clinical and pathologic study of seventy-two cases, in thirteen of which rupture of the interventricular septum occurred. Am Heart J 1942;24:719−733.
3. Friedman S, White PD. Rupture of the heart in myocardial infarction. Ann Intern Med 1944;21:778−782.
4. Diaz-Rivera RS, Miller AJ. Rupture of heart following acute myocardial infarction: incidence in public hospital, with five illustrative cases including one of perforation of interventricular septum diagnosed ante mortem. Am Heart J 1948;35:126−133.
5. Wang CH, Bland EF, White PD. Note on coronary occlusion and myocardial infarction found post mortem at Massachusetts General Hospital during twenty year period from 1926 to 1945 inclusive. Ann Intern Med 1948;29:601−606.
6. Selzer A. Immediate sequelae of myocardial infarction: their relation to prognosis. Am J Med Sci 1948;216:172−178.
7. Zinn WJ, Cosby RS. Myocardial infarction: Statistical study of 679 autopsy-proven cases. Am J Med 1950;8:169−176.
8. Oblath RW, Levinson DC, Griffith GC. Factors influencing rupture of the heart after myocardial infarction. JAMA 1952;149:1276−1281.
9. Wessler S, Zoll PM, Schlesinger MI. The pathogenesis of spontaneous cardiac rupture. Circulation 1952;6:334−351.
10. Waldron BR, Fennell RH, Castleman B, Bland EF. Myocardial rupture and hemopericardium associated with anticoagulant therapy. N Engl J Med 1954;251:829−894.
11. Goetz AA, Gropper AN. Perforation of the interventricular septum. Report of three cases with ante-mortem diagnosis. Am Heart J 1954;48:103−140.
12. Maher JF, Mallory GK, Laurenz GA. Rupture of the heart after myocardial infarction. N Engl J Med 1956;255:1−10.
13. Griffith GC, Hedge B, Oblath RW. Factors in myocardial rupture: An analysis of 204 cases at Los Angeles County Hospital between 1924-1959. Am J Cardiol 1961;8:792−798.

14. Spiekerman RE, Brandeburg JT, Anchor RWP, Edwards JE. The spectrum of coronary heart disease in a community of 30,000. A clinicopathologic study. *Circulation* 1962;35:57—65.

15. Ross RM, Young JA. Clinical and necropsy findings in rupture of the myocardium. A review of 43 cases. *Scott Med J* 1963;8:222—226.

16. London RE, London SB. Rupture of the heart: A critical analysis of 47 consecutive autopsy cases. *Circulation* 1965;31:202—208.

17. Sievers J. Cardiac rupture in acute myocardial infarction. *Geriatrics* 1966;21:125—130.

18. Sugiura M, Okada R, Morii T, Hiraoka K, Shimada H, Nakanishi A. A clinicopathological study on the cardiac rupture following myocardial infarction in the aged. *Jpn Heart J* 1968;9:265—280.

19. Lewis AJ, Burchell HB, Titus JL. Clinical and pathologic features of postinfarction cardiac rupture. *Am J Cardiol* 1969;23:43—53.

20. Hammer J, Fabian J, Pavlovic J, Smid J. Myocardial rupture in acute myocardial infarction. *Cor Vasa* 1972;14:180—187.

21. Rasmussen S, Leth A, Kjoller E, Pedersen A. Cardiac rupture in acute myocardial infarction. *Acta Med Scand* 1979;205:11—16.

22. Dellborg M, Held P, Swedberg K, Vedin A. Rupture of the myocardium: Occurrence and risk factors. *Br Heart J* 1985;54:11—16.

23. Hiramori K. Major causes of death from acute myocardial infarction in a coronary care unit. *Jpn Circ J* 1987;51:1041—1047.

24. Herlitz J, Samuelsson SO, Richter A, Hjalmarson A. Prediction of rupture in acute myocardial infarction. *Clin Cardiol* 1988;11:63—69.

25. Reddy WG, Roberts WC. Frequency of rupture of the left ventricular free wall or ventricular septum among necropsy cases of fatal acute myocardial infarction since introduction of coronary care unit. *Am J Cardiol* 1989;63:906—911.

26. Batts KP, Ackermann DM, Edwards WD. Postinfarction rupture of the left ventricular free wall: Clinicopathologic correlates in 100 consecutive autopsy cases. *Hum Pathol* 1990;21:530—535.

27. Pollak H, Nobis H, Miczoch J. Frequency of left ventricular free wall rupture complicating acute myocardial infarction since the advent of thrombolysis. *Am J Cardiol* 1994;74:184—186.

28. Hutchins KD, Skurnick J, Lavenhar M, Natarajan GA. Cardiac rupture in acute myocardial infarction: A reassessment. *Am J Forensic Med Pathol* 2002;23:78—82.

29. Markowicz-Pawlus E, Nożyński J, Duszańska A, Hawranek M, Jarski P, Kalarus Z. The impact of a previous history of ischaemic episodes on the occurrence of left ventricular free wall rupture in the setting of myocardial infarction. *Kardiol Pol* 2012;70:713—717.

30. Roberts WC, Morrow AG. Pseudoaneurysm of the left ventricle: An unusual sequel of myocardial infarction and rupture of the heart. *Am J Med* 1967;43:639—644.

31. Morrow AG, Cohen LS, Roberts WC, Braundwald NS, Braunwald E. Severe mitral regurgitation following acute myocardial infarction and ruptured papillary muscle: Hemodynamic findings and results of operative treatment in 4 patients. *Circulation* 1968;37 (Suppl II):II-124—II-132.

32. Glancy DL, Stinson EB, Shepherd RL, Itscoitz SB, Roberts WC, Epstein SE, Morrow AG. Results of valve replacement for severe mitral regurgitation due to papillary muscle rupture or fibrosis. *Am J Cardiol* 1973;32:313—321.

33. Nagel MR, Ronan JA Jr, Roberts WC. Left-to-right shunt at atrial level after rupture of papillary muscle from acute myocardial infarction. *Am Heart J* 1973;86:112—116.

34. Hammer WJ, Ferrans VJ, Roberts WC. Myocardial embolus to coronary artery. *Chest* 1975;66:843—844.

35. Roberts WC. Cardiac rupture, abdominal aneurysmal rupture and dissecting aortic rupture. *Am J Cardiol* 1986;57:892—893.

36. Barbour DJ, Roberts WC. Rupture of a left ventricular papillary muscle during acute myocardial infarction: Analysis of 22 necropsy patients. *J Am Coll Cardiol* 1986;8:558—565.

37. Mann JM, Roberts WC. Fatal rupture of both left ventricular free wall and ventricular septum (double rupture) during acute myocardial infarction: analysis of seven patients studied at necropsy. *Am J Cardiol* 1987;60:722—724.

38. Mann JA, Kalan JM, Wallace RB, Roberts WC. Rupture of the ventricular septum or left ventricular free wall from acute myocardial infarction early after coronary artery bypass grafting. *Am J Cardiol* 1987;60:374—375.

39. Mann JM, Roberts WC. Acquired ventricular septal defect during acute myocardial infarction: Analysis of 38 unoperated necropsy patients and comparison with 50 unoperated necropsy patients without rupture. *Am J Cardiol* 1988;62:8—19.

40. Mann JM, Roberts WC. Rupture of the left ventricular free wall during acute myocardial infarction: Analysis of 138 necropsy patients and comparison with 50 necropsy patients with acute myocardial infarction without rupture. *Am J Cardiol* 1988;62:847—859.

41. Roberts WC. Rupture of the left ventricular free wall during acute myocardial infarction without hemopericardium. *Am J Cardiol* 1990;65:1033—1034.

42. Shirani J, Berezowski K, Roberts WC. Out-of-hospital sudden death from left ventricular free wall rupture during acute myocardial infarction as the first and only manifestation of atherosclerotic coronary artery disease. *Am J Cardiol* 1994;73:88—92.

43. Roberts WC, Roberts JD. The floating heart or the heart too fat to sink: Analysis of 55 necropsy patients. *Am J Cardiol* 1983;52:1286—1289.

44. Shirani J, Berezowski K, Roberts WC. Quantitative measurement of normal and excessive (cor adiposum) subepicardial adipose tissue, its clinical significance, and its effect on electrocardiographic QRS voltage. *Am J Cardiol* 1995;76:414—418.

45. Saffitz JE, Fredrickson RC, Roberts WC. Relation of size of transmural acute myocardial infarct to mode of death, interval between infarction and death and frequency of coronary arterial thrombus. *Am J Cardiol* 1986;57:1249—1254.

46. Roberts CS, Schoen FJ, Kloner RA. Effect of coronary reperfusion on myocardial hemorrhage and infarct healing. *Am J Cardiol* 1983;52:610—614.

47. Yusuf S, Collins R, Peto R, Furberg C, Stampfer MJ, Goldhaber SZ, Hennekens CH. Intravenous and intracoronary fibrinolytic therapy in acute myocardial infarction: overview of results on mortality, reinfarction and side-effects from 33 randomized controlled trials. *Eur Heart J* 1985;6:556—585.

48. Honan MB, Harrell FE, Reimer KA, Califf RM, Mark DB, Pryor DB, Hlatky MA. Cardiac rupture, mortality and the timing of thrombolytic therapy: a meta-analysis. *J Am Coll Cardiol* 1990;16:359—367.

Relation of left ventricular free wall rupture and/or aneurysm with acute myocardial infarction in patients with aortic stenosis

Irtiza N. Sheikh, BS, and William C. Roberts, MD

This minireview describes 6 previously reported patients with left ventricular free wall rupture and/or aneurysm complicating acute myocardial infarction (AMI) in patients with aortic stenosis. The findings suggest that left ventricular rupture and/or aneurysm is more frequent in patients with AMI associated with aortic stenosis than in patients with AMI unassociated with aortic stenosis, presumably because of retained elevation of the left ventricular peak systolic pressure after the appearance of the AMI.

In 1983, one of us (WCR) reported a patient with severe aortic stenosis (AS) and a healed left ventricular (LV) apical aneurysm (1). The authors speculated that LV aneurysm and LV free wall rupture would be more frequent in patients with acute myocardial infarction (AMI) associated with severe AS than in patients with AMI without AS. Herein, we summarize findings in 5 subsequently reported patients with LV rupture and/or aneurysm with AMI associated with severe AS.

METHODS

An initial PubMed search was conducted to locate publications of "cardiac rupture or aneurysm in patients with acute myocardial infarction complicated by aortic stenosis." A second search was made for publications of "myocardial infarction in patients with aortic stenosis."

RESULTS

Since the report by Roberts and colleagues (1) in 1983, we found 5 additional case reports of patients with AMI complicated by LV free wall rupture and/or aneurysm in patients with AS (2–6). The findings in them are summarized in the *Table 1*, which also includes the initial report by Roberts et al (1). No reported cases were found in the search for AMI associated with AS irrespective of whether an LV free wall rupture and/or aneurysm was present. At the time of AMI, the 6 patients ranged in age from 57 to 74 years (mean 64); 4 were women and 2 were men. The rupture site in all patients was the LV free wall, leading to hemopericardium. The interval from onset of AMI to rupture ranged from 1 to possibly 30 days. The AS appeared to be severe in all patients: the peak LV systolic gradients (reported in 4 patients) ranged from 50 to 177 mm Hg.

DISCUSSION

When AMI occurs in patients with systemic hypertension, the systemic arterial and LV pressures generally return to or toward normal if the AMI is fairly large. Several reports have demonstrated that systemic hypertension unassociated with

Table 1. Reported cases of acute myocardial infarction in patients with aortic valve stenosis with left ventricular free wall rupture or aneurysm

Variable	Reported cases: First author, year of publication					
	1 Roberts 1983	2 Duke 1984	3 Connary 1994	4 Kadri 1994	5 Ikeda 2002	6 Tanaka 2006
1. Age (years) at AMI	62	57	62	58	69	74
2. Sex	M	M	F	F	F	F
3. LV free wall rupture	0	+	+*	+	+	+
4. LV aneurysm	+	0	+	0	+	0
5. Days from AMI onset to rupture	–	6	?30	10	20	2
6. Previous hypertension (history)	+	0	–	+	–	+
7. ECG location of the infarct	–	Ant	Ant	Ant	–	Ant
8. Apical location of the infarct	+	+	0*	+	+	–
9. LV-SA psg (mm Hg)	–	–	50	105	70[†]	177[†]
10. Aortic valve area (cm^2)	–	–	0.4	–	0.7[†]	0.3[†]
11. Systemic artery (s/d) (mm Hg)	–	110/70	100/60	150/90	–	116/85
12. Heart weight (g)	630	610	–	–	–	–

*False left ventricular aneurysm.
[†]By echocardiogram.
AMI indicates acute myocardial infarction; Ant, anterior; ECG, electrocardiographic; LV, left ventricular; psg, peak systolic gradient; SA, systemic artery; s/d, peak systole/end diastole.

From the Baylor Heart and Vascular Institute and the Departments of Internal Medicine and Pathology, Baylor University Medical Center at Dallas (Roberts); and Texas College of Osteopathic Medicine, Fort Worth, Texas (Sheikh).

Corresponding author: William C. Roberts, MD, Baylor Heart and Vascular Institute, Baylor University Medical Center at Dallas, 3500 Gaston Avenue, Dallas, TX 75246 (e-mail: william.roberts1@bswhealth.org).

AS in patients with AMI is not a risk factor for LV free wall rupture and/or aneurysm formation (2, 3). When AMI occurs in patients with significant AS, however, the LV systolic pressure remains elevated and the continuation of this elevation appears to increase the likelihood of LV rupture and/or aneurysmal formation, particularly when the AMI involves the LV apical wall, which normally is several times thinner than the LV basal wall.

There is some data on the frequency of AS in older populations and on the frequency of AMI and sudden cardiac death among patients with AS. In an autopsy study, Roberts and Shirani (7) found severe AS to be present in 43 (11%) of 391 patients aged 80 to 89 years, in 8 (9%) of 93 patients aged 90 to 99 years, and in 0 of 6 patients aged ≥100 years, or in 51 (10%) of the total 490 patients aged 80 years or over. Of the 490 autopsied patients, 229 (47%) had acute and/or healed myocardial infarcts. Aronow and colleagues (8) studied by echocardiogram 1797 older patients (mean age 82 years) and found AS in 301 (17%)—severe in 40, moderate in 96, and mild in 165. Among their 301 patients with AS, 158 (52%) had had an earlier AMI that healed, and 217 (72%) had a new AMI or died suddenly. There was no mention of LV free wall rupture or LV aneurysm. There have been at least 2 case reports of AMI in patients with AS and normal epicardial coronary arteries (9, 10). Neither had LV free wall rupture or aneurysm.

The major limitation of this minireview is that the number of patients with AMI associated with AS without LV free wall rupture or LV aneurysm is entirely unknown. Conversely, the reported cases of LV free wall rupture and/or aneurysm complicating AMI in patients with AS may represent, of course, the tip of the iceberg.

1. Roberts WC, Arnett EN, Aisner SC, Techlenberg P. Aortic valve stenosis and left ventricular apical aneurysm and/or rupture: real or potential complications of persistent left ventricular systolic hypertension after acute myocardial infarction. *Am Heart J* 1983;105(3):513–514.

2. Duke M. Aortic stenosis, myocardial infarction and cardiac rupture: an unusual triad. *Tex Heart Inst J* 1984;11(1):96–97.

3. Connery CP, Dumont HJ, Dervan JP, Hartman AR, Anagnostopoulos CE. Transmural myocardial infarction with coexisting critical aortic stenosis as an etiology for early myocardial rupture. *J Cardiovasc Surg (Torino)* 1994;35(1):53–56.

4. Kadri MA, Kakadellis J, Campbell CS. Survival after postinfarction cardiac rupture in severe aortic valve stenosis. *Eur Heart J* 1994;15(1):140–142.

5. Ikeda M, Ohashi H, Tsutsumi Y, Kawai T, Ohnaka M. Endoventricular circular patch plasty with aortic valve replacement for post-infarction cardiac rupture complicated with aortic valve stenosis: case report. *Circ J* 2002;66(10):974–976.

6. Tanaka M, Goto Y, Suzuki S, Morii I, Otsuka Y, Miyazaki S, Nonogi H. Postinfarction cardiac rupture despite immediate reperfusion therapy in a patient with severe aortic valve stenosis. *Heart Vessels* 2006;21(1):59–62.

7. Roberts WC, Shirani J. Comparison of cardiac findings at necropsy in octogenarians, nonagenarians, and centenarians. *Am J Cardiol* 1998;82(5):627–631.

8. Aronow WS, Ahn C, Shirani J, Kronzon I. Comparison of frequency of new coronary events in older persons with mild, moderate, and severe valvular aortic stenosis with those without aortic stenosis. *Am J Cardiol* 1998;81(5):647–649.

9. Jondeau G, Dubourg O, Partovian C, Dib JC, Lacombe P, Chikli F, Bourdarias JP. Acute myocardial infarction in a patient with severe aortic stenosis and normal coronary arteries. *Eur Heart J* 1994;15(5):715–717.

10. Lin CF, Chu KC. Acute myocardial infarction in an elderly patient with severe aortic stenosis and angiographically normal coronary arteries. *Int J Gerontol* 2010;4(3):157–160.

Coronary arterial aneurysms in previously transplanted (donor) hearts

Nitin Kondapalli, MBBS, and William C. Roberts, MD

Described herein is a 57-year-old man who had had a cardiac transplant 5 years earlier (at age 52) and died of a ruptured abdominal aortic aneurysm. The donor heart was found to have a fusiform aneurysm, each filled with thrombus, in 2 major epicardial coronary arteries.

The occurrence of aneurysm involving the aorta is fairly common. In contrast, aneurysm involving one or more epicardial coronary arteries is extremely uncommon. In a 24-year period, Roberts (1) collected at necropsy the native hearts of 20 adults who had large aneurysms of one or more major epicardial coronary arteries. Those 20 cases were found from examining approximately 12,000 hearts during that time. Recently, we observed coronary aneurysms in a donor heart that had been transplanted 5 years earlier. A description of this unusual finding is the purpose of this report.

CASE STUDY

A 57-year-old white man who had had a heart transplant at age 52 died suddenly from a ruptured abdominal aortic aneurysm. The transplanted heart contained huge quantities of adipose tissue and floated in a container of formaldehyde. The left anterior descending and ramus intermedius coronary arteries each had a fusiform aneurysm filled with thrombus *(Figure)*. All of the major epicardial coronary arteries contained considerable quantities of atherosclerotic plaque that narrowed their lumens. Despite this narrowing, there were no grossly visible myocardial lesions, and neither ventricular cavity was dilated. The heart weighed 570 grams and the patient's body mass index was 36 kg/m^2.

DISCUSSION

The cause of aneurysmal formation in epicardial coronary arteries in native hearts is entirely unclear. The aneurysms in this location, with rare exception, are fusiform and contain thrombus superimposed on atherosclerotic plaque (1). Their rarity in coronary arteries in contrast to their relative frequency in the aorta may in part be related to their exposure to only a systemic diastolic pressure rather than to a peak systolic pressure, as occurs in the aorta. The aneurysms in native coronary arteries are not the consequence of an underlying arteritis.

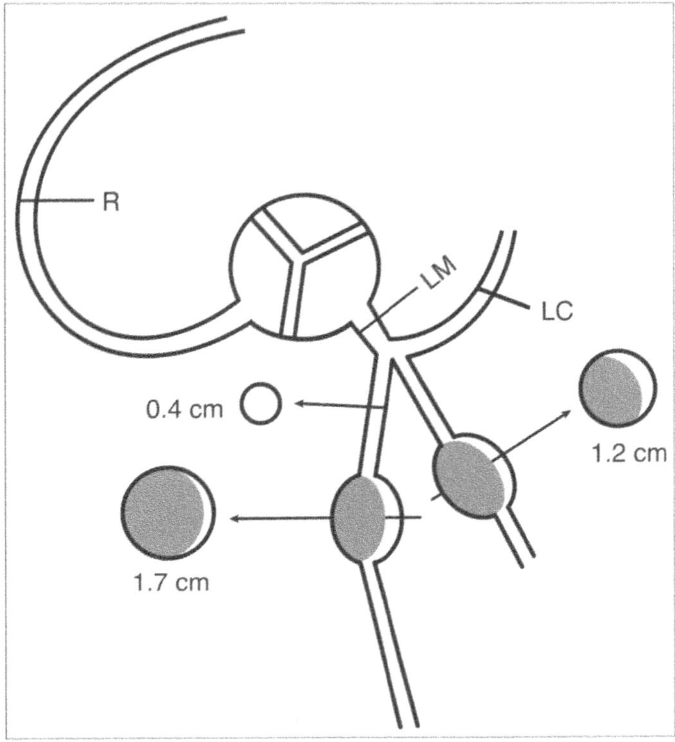

Figure. Diagram showing the aneurysms in the left anterior descending and ramus intermedius coronary arteries. Thrombus, shown in red, is present in each aneurysm. A cross-section is also shown of each aneurysm demonstrating that the thrombus does not involve all surfaces of the artery, thereby making the lumen at the site of the aneurysm eccentric. The largest diameter of each aneurysm was approximately 4 times that of the adjacent normal coronary artery. Heavy atherosclerotic plaque was present diffusely in all epicardial coronary arteries. LM indicates left main; R, right coronary artery.

The occurrence of aneurysm in one or more epicardial coronary arteries in donor hearts must be exceedingly uncommon. We have encountered coronary aneurysm in only one of 79 donor hearts studied at necropsy. (The longest interval from

From the Baylor Heart and Vascular Institute and the Departments of Internal Medicine (Cardiology) and Pathology, Baylor University Medical Center, Dallas, Texas.

Corresponding author: William C. Roberts, MD, Baylor Heart and Vascular Institute, 621 N. Hall Street, Suite H030, Dallas, TX 75226 (e-mail: william. roberts1@bswhealth.org).

heart transplant to death was 17 years.) Haddad and colleagues (2) described by computed tomography an aneurysm involving the left main and proximal left anterior descending artery in a 75-year-old woman who had had a heart transplant 18 years earlier; they also described a patient (age not given) who had a single aneurysm involving the right coronary artery also found by computed tomography 22 years after the heart transplant. These authors believed that the aneurysms in both patients contained thrombus. They speculated that the aneurysms in both patients were examples of "cardiac allograft vasculopathy." These 2 patients underwent heart transplantation nearly 2 decades earlier, and few patients have computed tomography that long after a heart transplant. In other words, the occurrence of coronary aneurysm after heart transplant may be much higher than presently recognized. Additionally, the autopsy rate in persons having earlier heart transplant is exceedingly low, a fact that might prevent recognition of coronary aneurysm if indeed it was present. Even if recognized, however, proper therapy is debated (3). Anticoagulation, because of the presence of intra-aneurysmal thrombus, certainly appears to be reasonable in patients with coronary arterial aneurysm.

1. Roberts WC. Natural history, clinical consequences, and morphologic features of coronary arterial aneurysms in adults. *Am J Cardiol* 2011; 108(6):814–821.
2. Haddad F, Perez M, Fleischmann D, Valantine H, Hunt SA. Giant coronary aneurysms in heart transplantation: an unusual presentation of cardiac allograft vasculopathy. *J Heart Lung Transplant* 2006;25(11):1367–1370.
3. Harandi S, Johnston SB, Wood RE, Roberts WC. Operative therapy of coronary arterial aneurysm. *Am J Cardiol* 1999;83(8):1290–1293.

Frequency of Coronary Endarterectomy in Patients Undergoing Coronary Artery Bypass Grafting at a Single Tertiary Texas Hospital 2010 to 2016 With Morphologic Studies of the Operatively Excised Specimens

William C. Roberts, MD*, and Anna E. Berry, BS

This study examines the frequency of coronary endarterectomy (CE) procedures during coronary artery bypass grafting (CABG), and determines the quantity of plaque in the specimens. Of the 2,268 CABG operations performed from January 2010 to June 2016, 35 patients had CE during CABG. The specimens were incised into 5-mm cross sections, stained by the Movat method, and examined. The number of CEs performed ranged from 0.21% to 4.01%. A total of 140 cm of specimens were examined, and all 140 cm contained considerable quantities of atherosclerotic plaque and narrowed lumens. The quantity of plaque present was similar to or greater than that observed in previously studied patients with fatal coronary artery disease. The frequency of CE during CABG varies greatly in surgeons. The quantity of plaque is enormous, and the lumens are severely narrowed.   © 2017 Elsevier Inc. All rights reserved. (Am J Cardiol 2017;120:2164–2169)

Coronary endarterectomy (CE) is occasionally performed in patients undergoing coronary artery bypass grafting (CABG). The frequency of performing CE at the time of CABG varies enormously in surgeons. Whether CE at the time of CABG improves outcomes is debatable.[1–12] In this study, we determined the frequency of CE at the time of CABG in 7 surgeons operating at Baylor University Medical Center (BUMC) at Dallas in the past 7 years, and we also describe results of histologic studies of the CE specimens, something rarely reported previously.[13–16]

Methods

Since March 1993, all cardiovascular surgical specimens submitted to the Surgical Pathology Division of the Department of Pathology at BUMC at Dallas have been described, and the final report was prepared by one of us (WCR). From January 2010 to June 2016, a total of 2,268 CABG operations were performed at BUMC at Dallas. Of that total, 35 patients (1.54%) had CE of 1 or more coronary arteries at the time of the CABG operation. The CE specimens were photographed, and then divided into 5-mm-long cross sections, processed in alcohols, and xylene, cut into 6 micro-thick sections, and 1 slide from each 5-mm segment was stained by hematoxylin-eosin and another by the Movat method. All slides

were then examined, and photomicrographs were obtained on many of the cross sections. The number of cross sections examined per patient ranged from 3 to 14 (mean 7). The clinical records were reviewed in all 35 patients having CE.

Results

Pertinent findings in the 35 patients are listed in Table 1. Of the 35 patients, 30 (86%) were men aged 39 to 88 years (mean 64), and 5 (14%) were women aged 49 to 64 (mean 56). The body mass index (kg/m^2) in the men ranged from 23.4 to 45.0 (mean 32.7), and in the women, from 19.7 to 31.9 (mean 28.1). A total of 37 CEs were performed in the 35 patients: in 33 patients, a CE was done in only 1 artery, and in 2 patients, 2 arteries. The arteries having CE were as follows: left anterior descending = 16; right = 10, obtuse marginal = 6; left circumflex = 1; intermedius = 1; and posterior descending = 3. The CE provided a single specimen in 24 patients (69%), 2 specimens in 8 (23%), and 3 specimens in 5 patients (14%). Small branches of the main artery were present in 4 patients, but their branches were not sectioned. The lengths of the major CE specimens ranged from 0.7 to 12.0 cm (mean 3.5).

The frequency of CE procedures performed by 7 different surgeons during 2.268 CABG procedures ranged from 0.21% (1 of 457) to 4.01% (14 of 349) (Figure 1). Two of the 35 patients died within 30 days of the combined CABG and CE procedures.

Photographs of 9 operatively excised endarterectomy specimens are shown in Figures 2 to 7, and photomicrographs of selected cross sections in Figures 3 to 7. Examination of the Movat-stained cross sections of the CE specimens disclosed at least 75% cross-sectional area narrowing in at least 1 section of coronary artery from each patient, and focal calcific plaques were present in 30 (86%) of the 35 patients. Every

Baylor Heart and Vascular Institute, The Departments of Internal Medicine (Division of Cardiology) and Pathology, Baylor University Medical Center, Dallas, Texas. Manuscript received August 31, 2017; revised manuscript received and accepted September 8, 2017.

Anna E. Berry is a Medical Student 1, Baylor College of Medicine, Houston, Texas 77030.

See page 2168 for disclosure information.

*Corresponding author: Tel: (214) 820-7911; fax: (214) 820-7533.

E-mail address: william.roberts1@bswhealth.org (W.C. Roberts).

Table 1

Pertinent data in each of the 35 patients having coronary endarterectomy at the time of coronary bypass

	Age (Years)	Gender	BMI (Kg/m^2)	Days in Hospital Postop	Interval CABG to Present (Years)	Number of Coronary Anastomoses	Coronary Artery Having Endarterectomy	Excised Pieces	Total Length (cm) of Endarterectomy	Calcium Present (+/0)
1	39	M	31	4	3.2	4	Right	2	5.3	+
2	41	M	28	6	6.3	3	Right	1	5	+
3	49	F	29	6	3.8	3	LAD	1	3	0
4	50	M	28	5	3.9	4	Right	1	5.8	+
5	51	M	31	45	4.3	3	Right	1	7.5	+
6	51	M	40	7	3.6	3	Right	1	6.8	+
7	51	F	29	7	3.1	4	Right	1	3	0
8	53	F	32	38	3.8	1	PD	2	1.3	+
9	53	M	32	4	0.2	4	LAD	2	3.7	+
10	54	M	27	5	2.7	3	LC	1	1.3	+
11	54	M	39	6	2.0	3	OM	1	0.7	+
12	55	M	34	7	5.1	4	I	3	1.8	+
13	57	M	33	20	4.9	6	LAD	3	4.5	+
14	57	M	37	8	4.7	5	LAD	1	2.5	+
15	58	M	39	8	1.1	3	Right	1	5	+
16	61	M	29	6	3.4	4	LAD + Right	4	12	+
17	63	F	20	7	3.5	3	OM	1	4.3	+
18	64	F	31	6	2.2	4	OM	2	0.3	+
19	66	M	27	7	4.8	4	OM	1	2.5	+
20	66	M	29	4	0.8	4	OM	1	1.8	+
21	67	M	28	6	5.8	5	PD	1	3	+
22	68	M	39	9	3.1	3	LAD	3	4.9	+
23	68	M	30	4	0.2	3	LAD	2	2	+
24	69	M	41	5	1.3	4	LAD	1	3	+
25	69	M	32	7 +	0.4	3	LAD + OM	3	7.7	+
26	70	M	31	5	6.3	4	Right	1	3.4	+
27	75	M	26	5	5.1	6	LAD	1	7	+
28	75	M	42	6	3.1	3	LAD	1	4.3	+
29	77	M	35	5	6.1	3	LAD	1	7.5	+
30	77	M	34	11	5.6	4	PD	1	1	+
31	78	M	27	18	5.9	1	LAD	1	3	0
32	78	M	45	1 +	5.7	4	LAD	1	2.5	0
33	78	M	33	5	1.0	2	LAD	2	5.3	+
34	80	M	31	7 +	0.4	5	Right	3	0	+
35	88	M	23	6	1.8	2	LAD	1	4.5	0

BMI = body mass index; CABG = coronary artery bypass grafting; F = female; I = intermedius; LAD = left anterior descending; LC = left circumflex; M = Male; OM = obtuse marginal; PD = posterior descending.

5-mm section in every patient contained large quantities of atherosclerotic plaque.

Discussion

This study shows that CE performed at the time of CABG at a single tertiary hospital in Texas from 2010 to 2016 is relatively infrequent, that its frequency varies considerably in surgeons performing CABG, and that the atherosclerotic process is diffuse in all endarterectomy specimens irrespective of the specific coronary artery having the CE. During the 7-year period, CE was performed by 7 different surgeons: the frequency of CE varied from as low as 0.22% (1 of 458 CABG procedures) to as high as 3.86% (14 of 363 total CABG procedures). In the 35 patients having CE, 33 (94%) had CE of a single coronary artery, and the other 2 (6%), of 2 coronary arteries. The total length of the CE specimens per patient ranged from 0.7 to 12.0 cm: 26 (74%) were >2.0 cm in length. A total of 140 cm of CE specimens were examined in the 35 patients, and all 140 cm contained considerable quantities of atherosclerotic plaque. The external elastic membrane and portions of media were present in all 140 cm.

The fact that the internal elastic membrane and portions of media were present on the histologic sections of all CE specimens allows comparisons of them with sections, at least of the right coronary artery, obtained from the same artery in patients with fatal coronary disease. Because the endarterectomy specimens of the left anterior descending and/or obtuse marginal coronary arteries are much shorter, the findings in them cannot readily be compared with those obtained in those arteries at necropsy.[16] A previous study by one of us (WCR) indicates that the degree of cross-sectional area narrowing in each 5-mm section of right coronary artery in the CE specimens is either more narrowed or similarly narrowed to the 5-mm cross sections of right coronary artery obtained in patients with fatal coronary disease.[16] This fact strongly suggests that lipid-lowering therapy must be started years before, probably decades before, the occurrence of a

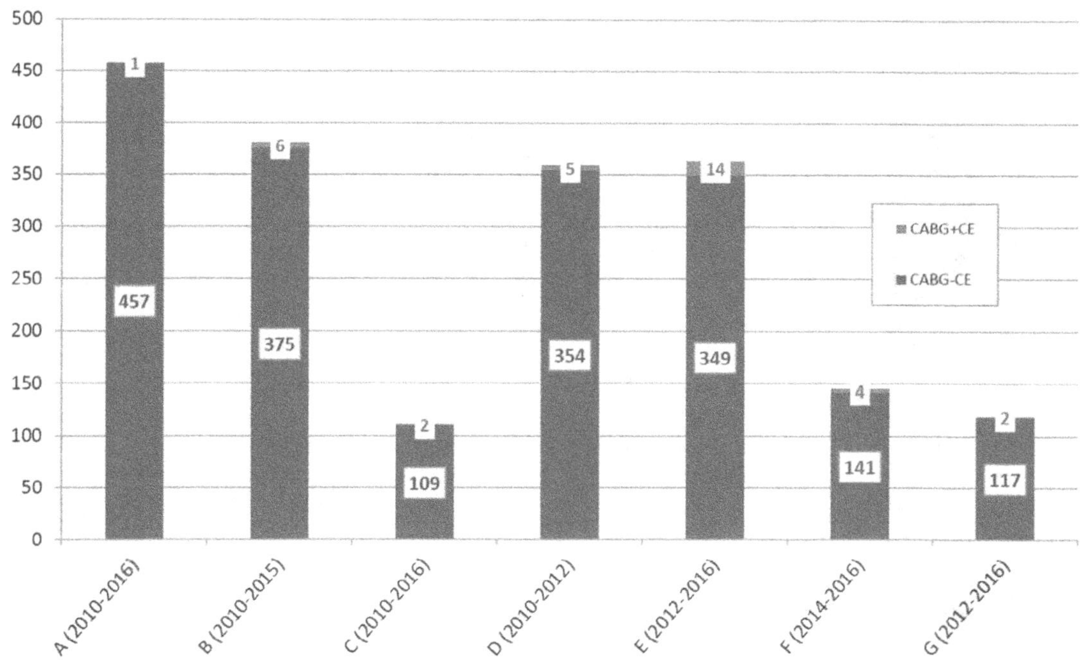

Figure 1. Bar graph showing the number of coronary endarterectomy procedures performed at the time of coronary bypass by each of 7 cardiac surgeons operating at Baylor University Medical Center at Dallas from January 2010 to June 2016.

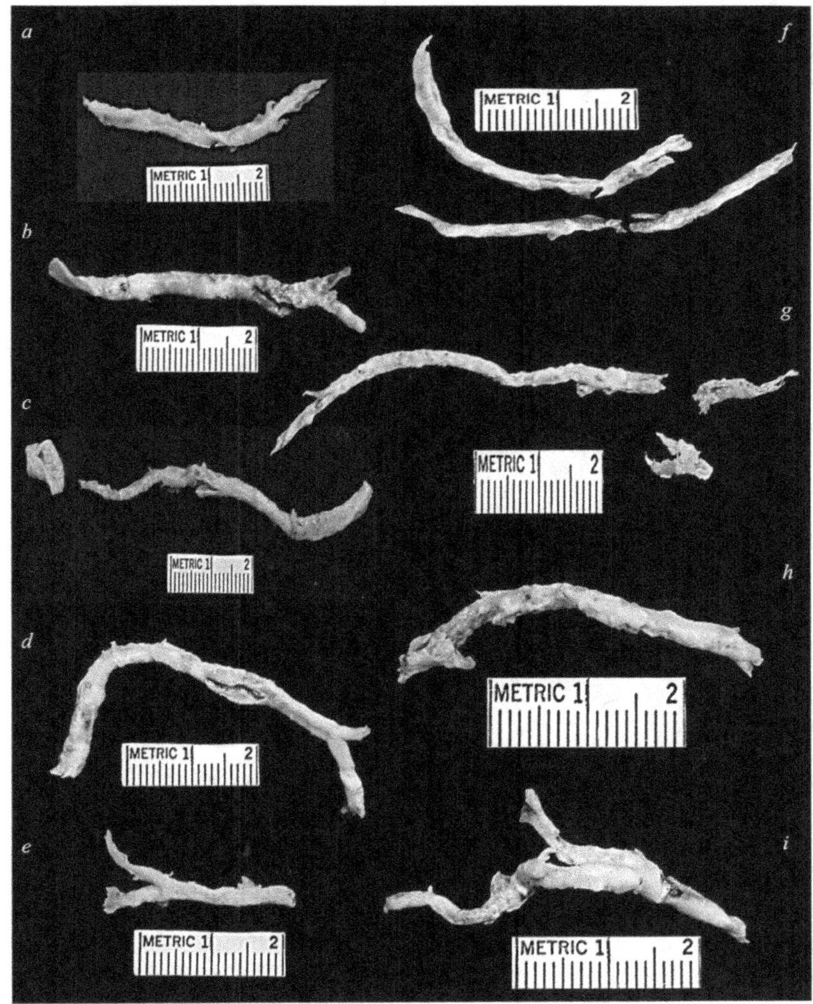

Figure 2. Photographs of the endarterectomy specimens in 9 patients: (A) case #2 (Table 1); (B) case #4; (C) case #5; (D) case #6; (E) case #26; (F) case #16; (G) case #25; (H) case #28; and (I) case #35.

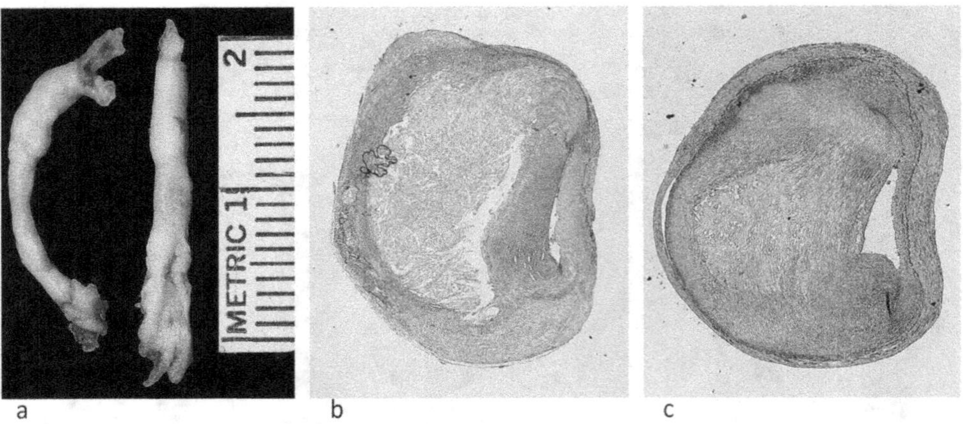

Figure 3. Case #1, Table 1. (*A*) Operatively excised endarterectomy specimen of the right coronary artery removed in 2 parts. (*B* and *C*) Photomicrographs of 2 cross sections of this coronary artery, with severe luminal narrowing of each. Portions of media are present in each cross section. Movat stains, ×40 (*B* and *C*).

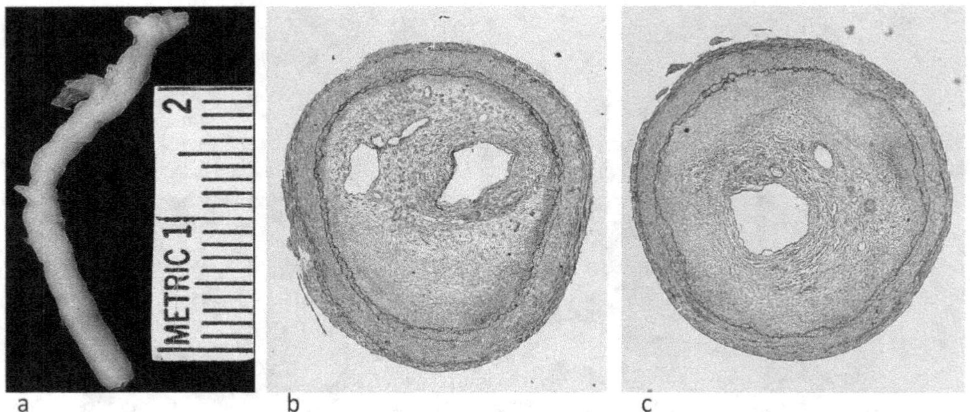

Figure 4. Case #7, Table 1. (*A*) Endarterectomy specimen from the right coronary artery. (*B* and *C*) Cross sections showing multi-luminal channels within the fibrous plaques. Most of the media is present in each. The multi-luminal channels suggest that the plaque was formed at least in part by organization of thrombus. Movat stains, ×40 (*B* and *C*).

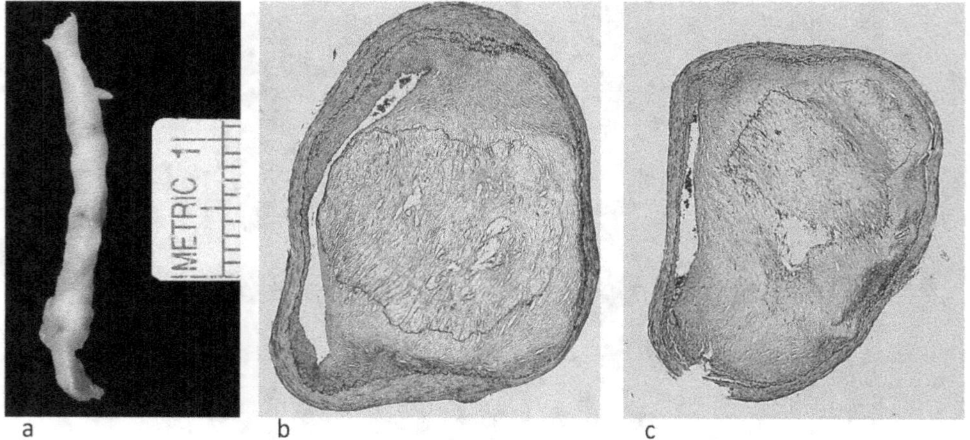

Figure 5. Case #9, Table 1. (*A*) Endarterectomy specimen from the left anterior descending coronary artery. (*B* and *C*) Cross sections at 2 sites, showing severe luminal narrowing mainly by calcified plaque. Movat stains, ×40 (*B* and *C*).

coronary event if the event is to be prevented or considerably delayed. That media is present in the entire specimen indicates that the split is in the media and not at the junction of intima and media. Additionally, the procedure might better be called "endomediaectomy" rather than endarterectomy. Additionally, the fact that plaque was present in every 5-mm cross section indicates that the atherosclerotic process was diffuse in all the patients.[17]

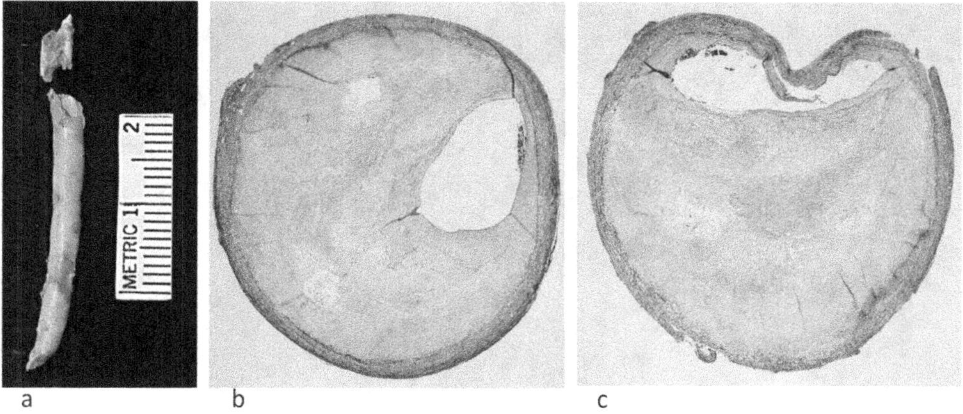

Figure 6. Case #24, Table 1. (*A*) Endarterectomy specimen from the left anterior descending coronary artery. (*B* and *C*) Cross sections at 2 sites. The luminal narrowing is by fibrous atherosclerotic plaque. Movat stains, ×40 (*B* and *C*).

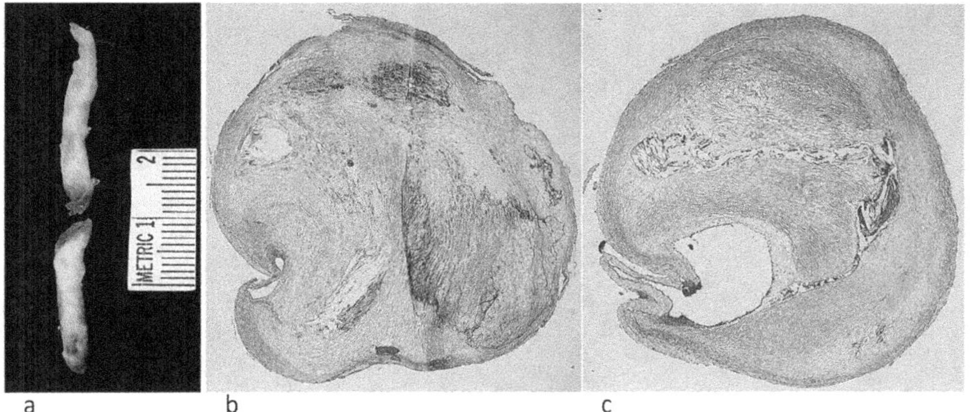

Figure 7. Case #29, Table 1. (*A*) Endarterectomy specimen from the left anterior descending coronary artery. (*B* and *C*) Cross sections at 2 sites, showing severe luminal narrowing mainly by calcified plaque. The media is circumferential in (*C*). Movat stains, ×40 (*B* and *C*).

Although the present study provides no useful information on whether CE added to CABG is better (fewer complications, longer survival) than CABG alone, some reports—all observational, none randomized—show more favorable and others less favorable results by the addition of CE.[1-12] Previous studies do demonstrate that the endarterectomized artery quickly develops fibrin deposits on its endarterectomized surfaces followed by conversion of these deposits to a rather uniform fibrous tissue, which too often is large enough to severely narrow or totally obstruct the lumen.[13,14]

Disclosures

The authors have no conflicts of interest to disclose.

1. Livesay JJ, Cooley DA, Hallman GL, Reul GJ, Ott DA, Duncan JM, Frazier OH. Early and late results of coronary endarterectomy. Analysis of 3,369 patients. *J Thorac Cardiovasc Surg* 1986;92:649–660.
2. Asimakopoulos G, Taylor KM, Ratnatunga CP. Outcome of coronary endarterectomy: a case-control study. *Ann Thorac Surg* 1999;67:989–993.
3. Ferraris VA, Harrah JD, Moritz DM, Striz M, Striz D, Ferraris SP. Long-term angiographic results of coronary endarterectomy. *Ann Thorac Surg* 2000;69:1737–1743.
4. Silberman S, Dzigivker I, Merin O, Shapira N, Deeb M, Bitran D. Does coronary endarterectomy increase the risk of coronary bypass? *J Card Surg* 2002;17:267–271.
5. Byrne JG, Karavas AN, Gudbjartson T, Leacche M, Rawn JD, Couper GS, Rizzo RJ, Cohn LH, Aranki SF. Left anterior descending coronary endarterectomy: early and late results in 196 consecutive patients. *Ann Thorac Surg* 2004;78:867–873.
6. Pardhy K, Narasimham SBR, Murthy GSRC, Chaganti VR, Kumar PVVNM, Rao MB, Kodem DR, Sinha GK, Saryanaryana PV. Coronary endarterectomy for diffuse extensive coronary artery disease. *Ind J Thorac Cardiovasc Surg* 2005;21:251–255.
7. Vohra HA, Kanwar R, Khan T, Dimitri WR. Early and late outcome after off-pump coronary artery bypass graft surgery with coronary endarterectomy: a single-center 10-year experience. *Ann Thorac Surg* 2006;81:1691–1696.
8. Marzban M, Karimi A, Ahmadi H, Davoodi S, Abbasi K, Movahedi N, Salehiomran A, Abbasi SH, Kawoosi Y, Yazdanifard P. Early outcomes of double-vessel coronary endarterectomy in comparison with single-vessel coronary endarterectomy. *Tex Heart Inst J* 2008;35:119–124.
9. Schmitto JD, Kolat P, Ortmann P, Popov AF, Coskun KO, Friedrich M, Sossalla S, Toischer K, Mokashi SA, Tirilomis T, Baryalei MM, Schoendube FA. Early results of coronary artery bypass grafting with coronary endarterectomy for severe coronary artery disease. *J Cardiothorac Surg* 2009;4:52.
10. LaPar DJI, Anvari F, Irvine JN Jr, Kern JA, Swenson BR, Kron IL, Ailawadi G. The impact of coronary artery endarterectomy on outcomes during coronary artery bypass grafting. *J Card Surg* 2011;26:247–253.

11. Wang J, Gu C, Yu W, Gao M, Yu Y. Short- and long-term patient outcomes from combined coronary endarterectomy and coronary artery bypass grafting: a meta-analysis of 63,730 patients (PRISMA). *Medicine (Baltimore)* 2015;94:1–16.

12. Stavrou A, Gkiousias V, Kyprianou K, Dimitrakaki IA, Challoumas D, Dimitrakakis G. Coronary endarterectomy: the current state of knowledge. *Atherosclerosis* 2016;249:88–98.

13. Kragel AH, McIntosh CM, Roberts WC. Morphologic changes in coronary artery seen late after endarterectomy. *Am J Cardiol* 1989;63:757–759.

14. Kragel AH, McIntosh CL, Roberts WC. Coronary arterial morphology 10 years after "endarterectomy." *Clin Cardiol* 1990;13:224–226.

15. Walley VM, Byard RW, Keon WJ. A study of the sequential morphologic changes after manual coronary endarterectomy. *J Thorac Cardiovasc Surg* 1991;102:890–894.

16. Roberts WC, Turnage TA 2nd, Whiddon LL. Quantitative comparison of amounts of cross-sectional area narrowing in coronary endarterectomy specimens in patients having coronary artery bypass grafting to amounts of narrowing in the same artery in patients with fatal coronary artery disease studied at necropsy. *Am J Cardiol* 2007;99:588–592.

17. Roberts WC. Coronary "lesion," coronary "disease," "single-vessel disease," "two-vessel disease": word and phrase misnomers providing false impressions of the extent of coronary atherosclerosis in symptomatic myocardial ischemia. *Am J Cardiol* 1990;66:121–123.